£ 100.00

5/12/2005

Geriatric Medicine

Fourth Edition

Springer
New York
Berlin
Heidelberg
Hong Kong
London
Milan
Paris
Tokyo

Geriatric Medicine
An Evidence-Based Approach
Fourth Edition

With 186 Illustrations in 217 Parts, 8 in Full Color

Editor

Christine K. Cassel, MD

Professor and Dean, Oregon Health & Science University, School of Medicine, Portland, Oregon

Deputy Editor

Rosanne M. Leipzig, MD, PhD

Vice-Chair for Education, Gerald and May Ellen Ritter Professor of Geriatrics, Brookdale Department of Geriatrics and Adult Development, Mount Sinai School of Medicine, New York, New York

Associate Editors

Harvey Jay Cohen, MD

Director, Center for the Study of Aging and Human Development, and Chief, Geriatrics Division, Duke University Medical Center; Director, Geriatric Research, Education, and Clinical Center, Veterans Affairs Medical Center, Durham, North Carolina

Eric B. Larson, MD, MPH

Director, Center for Health Studies, Group Health Cooperatives; Professor of Medicine, University of Washington Medical Center, Seattle, Washington

Diane E. Meier, MD

Director, Hertzberg Palliative Care Institute; Catherine Gaisman Professor of Medical Ethics; Professor, Brookdale Department of Geriatrics and Adult Development, Mount Sinai School of Medicine, New York, New York

Managing Editor

Carol F. Capello, PhD

Assistant Professor of Geriatric Education, Division of Geriatrics and Gerontology, Weill Medical College of Cornell University, New York, New York

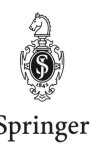

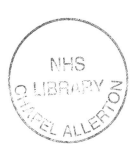

Springer

Christine K. Cassel, MD, Professor and Dean, Oregon Health & Science University, School of Medicine, Portland, OR, 97201-3098, USA

Rosanne M. Leipzig, MD, PhD, Vice-Chair for Education, Gerald and May Ellen Ritter Professor of Geriatrics, Brookdale Department of Geriatrics and Adult Development, Mount Sinai School of Medicine, New York, NY 10029, USA

Harvey Jay Cohen, Director, Center for the Study of Aging and Human Development, and Chief, Geriatrics Division, Duke University Medical Center; Director, Geriatric Research, Education, and Clinical Center, Veterans Affairs Medical Center, Durham, NC 27710, USA

Eric B. Larson, MD, MPH, Director, Center for Health Studies, Group Health Cooperatives; Professor of Medicine, University of Washington Medical Center, Seattle, WA 98195–6330, USA

Diane E. Meier, MD, Director, Hertzberg Palliative Care Institute; Catherine Gaisman Professor of Medical Ethics, Professor, Brookdale Department of Geriatrics and Adult Development, Mount Sinai School of Medicine, New York, NY 10029, USA

Carol F. Capello, PhD, Assistant Professor of Geriatric Education, Division of Geriatrics and Gerontology, Weill Medical College of Cornell University, New York, New York 10021, USA

Library of Congress Cataloging-in-Publication Data
Geriatric medicine: an evidence-based approach/editors, Christine K. Cassel . . . [et al.].—4th ed.
    p. ; cm.
  Includes bibliographical references and index.
  ISBN 0-387-95514-3 (h/c : alk. paper)
  1. Geriatrics. 2. Evidence-based medicine. I. Cassel, Christine K.
  [DNLM: 1. Geriatrics. 2. Evidence-Based Medicine. WT 100 G36635 2002]
  RC952 .G393 2002
  618.97—dc21   2002070548

ISBN 0-387-95514-3   Printed on acid-free paper.

Printed in the United States of America.

9 8 7 6 5 4 3 2 1   SPIN 10881173

www.springer-ny.com

Springer-Verlag New York Berlin Heidelberg
A member of BertelsmannSpringer Science+Business Media GmbH

*To the dedicated caregivers of older adults and
to the teachers and scientists devoted to
improving the care of the older population*

Preface

Since the publication of the third edition of *Geriatric Medicine*, extraordinary advances have occurred in the science of aging and the potential for biomedical research to give us answers to many, if not most, of the age-related disorders that threaten the quality of life in older years. At the most basic level, the successful mapping of the human genome was declared complete in the fall of 2000. Understanding the map of the human genome is as important as understanding the map of genomes of important laboratory species, ranging from the microscopic worms and fruitflies used in most classic genetic studies to rodents such as laboratory mice, and eventually to primates, on which much of the research on the aging human brain is done. The genetic maps of all of these species, including our own, does not answer clinical questions, but it does open the door to dramatic, rapid, and efficient answers to questions about the genetic polymorphisms related to diseases in humans.

The telomerase story also unfolded since the third edition. Telomerase is an enzyme responsible for maintaining the telomeres—the redundant DNA portions at the end of chromosomes—whose shortening seems to be linked directly to cell senescence, apoptosis, and the control over cell death, which, at the level of the individual cell, seems to be linked to the decline of organ function and eventually aging and death within the organism. The potential for genetic manipulations by which telomerase maintains and restores telomere length within individual tissue cultures gives great promise for potential approaches to restoring function lost through degenerative diseases, such as macular degeneration and other disorders related to epithelial aging. In addition, the maintenance of telomeres has been intriguingly associated with the malignant immortality of cancer cells, and yet it appears possible to prevent degeneration without creating uncontrolled growth or malignancy. Understanding this single genetic mechanism may give us clues not only to degenerative neurological and epithelial disease, but also perhaps to cancer, another age-related human disease. Scientists have also discovered that stem cells from embryonic and adult tissues can potentially create new tissues and new organs. Perhaps most excitingly, it appears that brain cells themselves can be replaced through this mechanism. Thus, stem cell research holds promise for treatment of Alzheimer's and Parkinson's disease, as well as for potentially growing new functioning organs that could be used for transplantation with much reduced risk of rejection because they are genetically fashioned to match the recipient's immune status.

Because of these and many more similar advances, it is more and more important for the practicing clinician to be conversant with the literature of basic science and to stay abreast of such developments. Our patients come to us having read about these developments or having seen television reports, and we should be able to answer their questions and share the excitement. We should also be educating them about the realistic limits, understanding that many of these developments will not provide immediate cures but are promising future developments.

Secondly, we owe it to ourselves to share the excitement of our colleagues in basic science, as well as the general public, in recognizing that aging research has come into real prominence in the last decade. We also need to be well informed about the rampant marketing of bogus dreams of anti-aging potions that the marketplace is all too ready to foist onto our patients. The aging of the baby boomers has created a huge and growing market for anti-aging therapies. Many are safe, effective, and worthwhile. However, in some instances, such as vitamin supplementation or hormone replacement, controversies exist and individual patient decision should be informed by knowledgeable and free discussions based on real science. This information can come from you, the clinician. It can also come from internet sources, but internet sources increasingly are also are full of inadequate and misleading information and, thus, it becomes even more important for us to be able to relay to our patients legitimate sources of information. Some of the most useful include the following:

- On terra firma, the *National Institutes of Health* is a complicated maze of 75 buildings. But on the Web (http://*www.nih.gov*), it is a snap to move from the National Cancer Institute to Mental Health to Alternative Medicine. Log on to www.clinicaltrials.gov to search for clinical trials by disease.
- The *National Institute on Aging*, one of 25 institutes and centers of the National Institutes of Health, leads a broad scientific effort to understand the nature of aging and to extend the healthy, active years of life. Visit *http://www.nia.nih.gov/* for a description of its mission, sponsored research programs, news and calendar of events, and health information, including NIA publications and videos, a resource directory for older adults, and various internet links of Federal websites of interest to the aging community.
- At their website, the *Centers for Disease Control and Prevention* (*www.cdc.gov*) provides a calendar of events, current topics, and recent reports and publications. Click on their "Data and Statistics" for CDC health data standards, scientific data, surveillance, health statistics reports, and laboratory information. The website also includes information about grant and cooperative agreement funding opportunities, as well as press releases and current health news. On their "Publications, Software, Products" link, one can order and download brochures, catalogs, publications, software, slides, and videos. Consumers can browse their "Health Topics" from A (Acanthamoeba infection) to Z (Zoster), get the latest on health "Hoaxes and Rumors" (i.e., deodorants cause breast cancer), or check out the travel section to find out if they will need vaccines for a trip abroad. Or stay close to home and find a link to your local state health department.
- The *Food and Drug Administration* is the primary resource for information about safety alerts/recalls and product approvals of drugs, cosmetics, foods, medical devices, biologics, animal feed and drugs, and radiation-emitting products. Ongoing clinical trials are also profiled. Go to http://*www.fda.gov*.
- *HealthWeb* (http://www.healthweb.org/) is a collaborative project of the health sciences libraries of the Greater Midwest Region of the National Network of Libraries of Medicine and those of the Committee for Institutional Cooperation. Currently, there are over 20 actively participating member libraries. The goals of the HealthWeb project include the development of an interface that provides organized access to evaluated noncommercial, health-related, internet-accessible resources, including those currently available, as well as new resources developed in collaboration with other organizations. The interface integrates educational information so the users has a one-stop entry point to learn skills and use material relevant to their discipline, including geriatrics and gerontology.
- The *National Aging Information Center* (*http://www.aoa.gov/NAIC/*) serves as a central source for a wide variety of information on aging for older people, their families, and those who work for or on behalf of older persons. NAIC resources include program and policy-related materials for consumers and practitioners and

demographic and other statistical data on the health, economic, and social conditions of older Americans. The NAIC bibliographic database contains references to program- and policy-related materials on aging not referenced in any other computer system or print resource.

- The *GeroWeb*, sponsored by the Geroinformatics Workgroup at the Wayne State University Institute of Gerontology, is designed as an online resource for researchers, educators, practitioners, and others interested in aging and older individuals. (*http://geroserver.iog.wayne.edu/GeroWebd/GeroWeb.html*)

- The *Alzheimer Research Forum*'s intended audience is Alzheimer researchers and other researchers whose work may bring understanding to Alzheimer's. The site has news, holds online forums, conducts online polls ("What are your 10 most wanted research tools?"), provides information on conferences, research funding, and includes a reagent company directory. Visit them at *http://www.alzforum.org/home.asp*.

- The Federal Interagency Forum on Aging-Related Statistics was initially established in 1986, with the goal of bringing together Federal agencies that share a common interest in improving aging-related data. The Forum has played a key role by criticially evaluating existing data resources and limitations, stimulating new database development, encouraging cooperation and data sharing among Federal agencies, and preparing collaborative statistical reports. Their website (*http://www.agingstats.gov/*) provides information from their latest report. Older *Americans 2000: Key Indicators of Well-Being*, as well as links to aging-related statistical information on Forum Member websites, ongoing Federal data resources relevant to the study of aging, past products of forum activities, and agency contacts.

- *AgeLine* is a free searchable electronic database of 60,000 summaries of publications about older adults and aging, including books, journal and magazine articles, and research reports. Coverage is sporadic between 1966–1977, but more comprehensive coverage exists from 1978–present. *http://research.aarp.org/ageline/home.html*)

- The Centers for Medicare and Medicaid (CMS), formerly the Health Care Financing Administration (HCFA), is a federal agency within the U.S. Department of Health and Human Services. CMS runs the Medicare and Medicaid programs and the State Children's Health Insurance Program (SCHIP), and also regulates all laboratory testing (except research) performed on humans in the U.S. By visiting the CMS website at *http://cms.hhs.gov* physicians and other health care professionals can gain quick access to professional publications and program forms and learn about the Medicare program and CMS contracts with Medicare health plans, as well as statistics, data, and the latest CMS research and program analysis. Consumers can find information on what Medicare covers, who is eligible, and how to enroll. They can also get a personalized report on Medicare health plans, nursing homes, dialysis facilities, participating physicians, and prescription drug programs in their area.

While we have a glut of information, we also have real ethical challenges facing us. The advances in genetic knowledge and potential alterations of genes through gene therapy have led to real caution because of highly visible adverse consequences to subjects of human studies. People are very concerned about the degree to which genetic information can be kept private and justifiably concerned that such information not fall into the hands of employers or insurers. The country will continue to be embroiled in deep disagreements about the use of human stem cells for research. The dramatic promise that they hold has come up against deep-seated religious beliefs of those who feel that embryos that are surplus and intended for discarding are indeed human life and ought not to be used for experimentation. These and other ethical issues will continue to be important as science progresses.

In their chapter, Greg Sachs and Harvey Cohen discuss the ethical issues in clinical research, including the ethics of research with Alzheimer's disease, a paradigmatic disorder where patients cannot fully make their own decisions and yet where research is very high stakes and needs to be offered to those suffering from the ravages of this disease. Ethical issues also continue to surround treatment decisions and, in particular, those around expensive potential life-prolonging and intrusive measures for older individuals. The challenge—especially in the United States—is how to balance the promise of these disorders with the increasing inequities in our health care system, in particular in a situation where more and more people under the age of 65 have no health insurance at all.

All of these issues will continue to intensely involve the public, and thus clinicians will need every possible resource to stay informed as citizens and to provide important answers for their communities and their patients. Along these lines, we have expanded this edition by 18 chapters, devoting an entire section to the emerging field of palliative medicine and increasing our coverage on surgical issues, care management, and pharmacology.

Health care providers will increasingly be called upon to practice what has come to be known as "evidence-based medicine." So much of health care—particularly the prescribing of medications—is extremely costly and, as we know well in geriatrics, carries risks of its own. For this reason, it is more and more important that clinicians understand the evidence behind the use of any interventions, both diagnostic and therapeutic. The science of evaluating evidence is a statistical one, and the standards for doing so have been articulated by leaders in the field. One of those leaders, Rosanne Leipzig, is deputy editor of this edition of *Geriatric Medicine*. She has looked at every single chapter through an evidence-based lens and, whenever possible, provided up-to-date information about the quality and strength of the evidence for the diagnostic and treatment recommendations included in each chapter. We are very fortunate that Dr. Leipzig has joined the *Geriatric Medicine*, 4/e, team and can give us this added dimension of balance and rigor to the expertise of our world-class roster of authors.

I also want to thank Harvey Cohen, Eric Larsen, and Diane Meier, Associate Editors, who have contributed enormously to the production of this book. We have worked hard together and learned a great deal from each other. Thanks also to Carol Capello in her role as Managing Editor. Carol has now taken us through two editions of *Geriatric Medicine*, and we hope we can persuade her to work with us on the fifth edition of *Geriatric Medicine*.

Christine K. Cassel

Contents

Part I   Basics of Gerontology

Part II   Changing Contexts of Care in Geriatric Medicine

Part III   Clinical Approaches to the Geriatric Patient

Part IV   Palliative Care

Part V Medical Care
Section A: Cancer in the Elderly

Section B: Organ System Diseases and Disorders

Section C: Common Problems in Older Adults

Part VI   Neurologic and Psychiatric Disorders

Part VII Ethics and Health Policy Issues for Older Adults

Contributors

Marilyn S. Albert, PhD, Professor of Psychiatry & Neurology, Harvard Medical School, Massachusetts General Hospital, Boston, MA 02114, USA

Angeles A. Alvarez, MD, Assistant Professor of Gynecology and Oncology, Division of Gynecology/Oncology, Duke University Medical Center, Durham, NC 27710, USA

Sonia Ancoli-Israel, PhD, Professor, Department of Psychiatry, University of California, San Diego, San Diego, CA 92161, USA

Sharon Anderson, MD, Professor of Medicine, Division of Nephrology and Hypertension, Oregon Health & Science University, Portland, OR 97201-2940, USA

Jerry Avorn, MD, Associate Professor of Medicine, Harvard Medical School; Chief, Division of Pharmacoepidemiology and Pharmacoeconomics, Brigham and Women's Hospital, Boston, MA 02115, USA

Patricia P. Barry, MD, Executive Director, Merck Institute of Aging and Health, Washington, DC 20005, USA

Judith L. Beizer, PharmD, Associate Clinical Professor, College of Pharmacy and Allied Health Professions, St. John's University, Jamaica, NY 11439, USA

Elizabeth M. Bengtson, MD, Assistant Professor, Department of Medicine, Dartmouth Hitchcock Medical Center, Lebanon, NH 03756, USA

Richard W. Besdine, MD, FACP, Greer Professor of Geriatric Medicine; Director, Center for Gerontology and Health Care Research, Brown University School of Medicine, Providence, RI 02912, USA

Susan A. Blackwell, PA-C, Senior Physician Assistant, Duke Comprehensive Cancer Center, Duke University Medical Center, Durham, NC 27710, USA

Dan G. Blazer, II, MD, PhD, J.P. Gibbons Professor of Psychiatry, Duke University Medical Center, Durham, NC 27710, USA

Harrison G. Bloom, MD, Clinical Associate Professor of Geriatrics and Medicine, Mount Sinai School of Medicine, New York, NY 10029, USA

Melissa A. Bottrell, MPH, PhD, Project Director, National Center for Ethics in Health Care, VA Puget Sound Health Care System, Seattle, WA 98108, USA

Daniel J. Brauner, MD, Associate Professor, Department of Medicine, University of Chicago, Chicago, IL 60637, USA

Robert A. Bruce, MD, Professor Emeritus of Medicine, University of Washington, Seattle, WA 98133-8065, USA

Kenneth Brummel-Smith, MD, Chair, Brain Center on Aging, Providence Health System, Portland, OR 97230, USA

Edith A. Burns, MD, Associate Professor of Medicine, Medical College of Wisconsin, Milwaukee, WI 53295, USA

Thierry Bussière, PhD, Elan Pharmaceuticals Inc., South San Francisco, CA 94080, USA

Joseph D. Buxbaum, PhD, Associate Professor, Department of Psychiatry, Mount Sinai School of Medicine, New York, NY 10029, USA

Daniel Callahan, PhD, Director of International Programs, The Hastings Center, Garrison, NY, 10524, USA

Maria Torroella Carney, MD, Assistant Professor of Clinical Medicine, State University of New York at Stony Brook School of Medicine; Mineola, NY 11501, USA

Christine K. Cassel, MD, Professor and Dean, Oregon Health & Science University, School of Medicine, Portland, OR 97201-3098, USA

Daniel L. Clarke-Pearson, MD, James M. Ingram Professor of Gynecologic Oncology, Duke University Medical Center, Durham, NC 27710, USA

Elizabeth C. Clipp, RN, PhD, Associate Director for Research, Geriatric Research, Education and Clinical Center (GRECC), Durham VA Medical Center; Professor, School of Nursing and Professor, Department of Medicine, Division of Geriatrics; Senior Fellow in the Center for the Study of Aging and Human Development, Duke University Medical Center, Durham, NC 27710, USA

Harvey Jay Cohen, MD, Director, Center for the Study of Aging and Human Development, and Chief, Geriatrics Division, Duke University Medical Center; Director, Geriatric Research, Education, and Clinical Center, Veterans Affairs Medical Center, Durham, NC 27710, USA

David S. Cooper, MD, Professor of Medicine, The Johns Hopkins University School of Medicine; Director, Division of Endocrinology, Sinai Hospital of Baltimore, Baltimore, MD 21215, USA

Jeffrey Crawford, MD, Professor of Medicine, Director, Clinical Research, Duke Comprehensive Cancer Center, Duke University Medical Center, Durham, NC 27710, USA

Jonathan Darer, MD, MPH, General Medicine Fellow, The Johns Hopkins Medical Institutions, Baltimore, MD 21205, USA

Catherine E. DuBeau, MD, Assistant Professor of Medicine, Harvard Medical School, Urban Medical Group; Research Physician, Hebrew Rehabilitation Center for Aged, Jamaica Plain, MA 02130, USA

Helen K. Edelberg, MD, Assistant Professor, Brookdale Department of Geriatrics and Adult Development, Mount Sinai School of Medicine, New York, NY 10029, USA

Michael H. Ellman, MD, Professor of Medicine, Rheumatology Section, Division of Medicine, University of Chicago, Chicago, IL 60637, USA

Peter C. Enzinger, MD, Department of Adult Oncology, Dana-Farber Cancer Institute, Boston, MA 02115-5013, USA

Emily R. Felzenberg, MPH, JD, Medical Student, New York College of Osteopathic Medicine, Old Westbury, NY 11568 USA

Bruce A. Ferrell, MD, Associate Professor, Department of Medicine, Division of Geriatrics, UCLA School of Medicine, Los Angeles, CA 90095-1687, USA

John R. Feussner, MD, MPH, Chief Research and Development Officer, Department of Veterans Affairs, Washington, DC 20420, USA

Linda P. Fried, MD, MPH, Director, Center on Aging and Health, The Johns Hopkins Medical Institutions, Baltimore, MD 21205, USA

Terry Fulmer, RN, PhD, FANN, Professor and Director for the Center of Nursing Research, and Head, Division of Nursing, New York University, New York, NY 10013, USA

George A. Gates, MD, Professor, Otolaryngology-Head and Neck Surgery; Director, Virginia Merrill Bloedel Hearing Research Center, University of Washington School of Medicine, Seattle, WA 98195, USA

Marc Gautier, MD, Associate Professor of Medicine, Section of Hematology and Oncology, Dartmouth Hitchcock Medical Center, Lebanon, NH 03756, USA

Gretchen Gibson, DDS, Director, Special Care Dental Programs, VA North Texas Health Care System, Clinical Associate Professor, Baylor College of Dentistry, Dallas, TX 75216, USA

Sarah Goodlin, MD, Assistant Professor of Medicine, Geriatrics Division, University of Utah School of Medicine; Director of Supportive Care and Palliative Medicine, LDS Hospital, Salt Lake City, UT 84143, USA

James S. Goodwin, MD, Professor of Medicine, Director, Geriatric Services, University of Texas Medical Branch, Galveston, TX 77555-0460, USA

Marsha Gordon, MD, Professor and Vice Chairman, Department of Dermatology, Mount Sinai School of Medicine, New York, NY 10029, USA

Jerry H. Gurwitz, MD, Professor of Medicine, University of Massachusetts Medical School; Executive Director, Meyers Primary Care Institute, Fallon Healthcare System, Worcester, MA 01605, USA

Tamara B. Harris, MD, MS, Chief, Laboratory of Epidemiology, Demography, and Biometry, National Institute on Aging, Bethesda, MD 20892, USA

Eric B. Haura, MD, Interdisciplinary Oncology Program, Thoracic Oncology Program, H. Lee Moffitt Cancer Center and Research Institute, Tampa, FL 33612, USA

Mitchell T. Heflin, MD, Assistant Professor, Department of Medicine, Division of Geriatrics, Duke University Medical Center, Durham, NC 27710, USA

Maria Hernandez, MD, Chief Medical Officer's Assistant, Hospital de Clinicas Caracas, San Bernardino, Caracas, Venezuela

William R. Hiatt, MD, Novartis Professor of Cardiovascular Research, Section of Vascular Medicine, Unversity of Colorado Health Sciences Center, Denver, CO 80203, USA

Patrick R. Hof, MD, Associate Regenstreif Professor of Neuroscience, Kastor Neurobiology of Aging Laboratories, Mount Sinai School of Medicine, New York, NY 10029, USA

Sharon K. Inouye, MD, MPH, Professor of Medicine, Department of Internal Medicine, Yale University School of Medicine, Yale-New Haven Hospital, New Haven, CT 06504, USA

Angela Inzerillo, MD, Assistant Professor of Medicine and Geriatrics, Mount Sinai School of Medicine, New York, NY 10029, USA

Jameel Iqbal, BS, Research Associate, Mount Sinai School of Medicine, New York, NY 10029, USA

Nancy S. Jecker, PhD, Professor, Department of Medical History and Ethics, University of Washington School of Medicine, Seattle, WA 98195, USA

Fran E. Kaiser, MD, Adjunct Professor of Medicine, St. Louis University School of Medicine, St. Louis, MO 63104, USA

Robert L. Kane, MD, Professor, Minnesota Chair in Long Term Care and Aging, University of Minnesota School of Public Health, Minneapolis, MN 55455, USA

Wishwa N. Kapoor, MD, MPH, Falk Professor of Medicine, Department of Medicine, University of Pittsburgh School of Medicine, Pittsburgh, PA 15213, USA

Marshall B. Kapp, JD, MPH, Professor, Departments of Community Health and Psychiatry; Director of Geriatric Medicine and Gerontology, Wright State University School of Medicine, Dayton, OH 45435-0001, USA

Jason H.T. Karlawish, MD, University of Pennsylvania, Institute on Aging, Philadelphia, PA 19104, USA

Gary J. Kennedy, MD, Professor of Psychiatry and Behavioral Science, Albert Einsteing College of Medicine; Director, Division of Geriatric Psychiatry and Fellowship Training Program, Montefiore Medical Center, Bronx Psychiatric Center, Bronx, NY 10024-2490, USA

Gerard J. Kerins, MD, FACP, Assistant Professor of Medicine, Division of Geriatrics, University of Connecticut Health Center, Farmington, CT 06030-3956, USA

Harold G. Koenig, MD, MHSc, Associate Professor of Psychiatry and Medicine, Department of Psychiatry and Behavioral Science, Duke University Medical Center, Durham, NC 27710, USA

Brandon Koretz, MD, Assistant Clinical Professor of Medicine, Division of Geriatrics, UCLA School of Medicine, Los Angeles, CA 90024, USA

Amy Krupnick Freeman, MD, Dermatology Resident, Department of Dermatology, Mount Sinai School of Medcine, New York, NY 10029, USA

Eric B. Larson, MD, MPH, Director, Center for Health Studies, Group Health Cooperatives; Professor of Medicine, University of Washington Medical Center, Seattle, WA 98195, USA

Rosanne M. Leipzig, MD, PhD, Vice-Chair for Education, Gerald and May Ellen Ritter Professor of Geriatrics, Brookdale Department of Geriatrics and Adult Development, Mount Sinai School of Medicine, New York, NY 10029, USA

Sharon A. Levine, MD, Associate Professor of Medicine, Director of Medical Education and the Geriatric Medicine, Dentistry, and Psychiatry Fellowship Program, Geriatrics Section, Boston University Medical Center, Boston, MA 02218, USA

Edward M. Liebers, MD, Clinical Fellow, Department of Medicine, Section of Hematology and Oncology, Dartmouth Hitchcock Medical Center, Lebanon, NH 03756, USA

David A. Lipschitz, MD, PhD, Chairman, Donald W. Reynolds Department of Geriatrics; Director, Center on Aging, Donald W. Reynolds Center on Aging, Little Rock, AK, 72205, USA

Deborah B. Marin, MD, Professor of Psychiatry, Vice Chair, Department of Psychiatry, Mount Sinai School of Medicine, New York, NY 10029, USA

Robert E. Martell, MD, PhD, Assistant Professor of Medicine, Divisions of Geriatrics and Medical Oncology, Duke University Medical Center, Durham, NC 27710, USA

José C. Masdeu, MD, PhD, Professor and Director of Neurology and the Neuroscience Center, Department of Neurology, University of Navarre Medical School, Pamplona, Spain

Khalid Matin, MD, Fellow, Division of Hematology-Oncology, Department of Medicine, University of Pittsburgh, Pittsburgh, PA 15213, USA

Robert J. Mayer, MD, Director, Center for Gastrointestinal Oncology; Professor of Medicine, Department of Adult Oncology, Harvard Medical School, Dana-Farber Cancer Institute, Boston, MA 02115-5013, USA

Wayne C. McCormick, MD, MPH, Associate Professor, Department of Medicine, Division of Gerontology and Geriatric Medicine, University of Washington Medical Center; Program Director, Long Term Care Services, Harborview Medical Center, Seattle, WA 98104, USA

Diane E. Meier, MD, Director, Hertzberg Palliative Care Institute; Catherine Gaisman Professor of Medical Ethics; Professor, Brookdale Department of Geriatrics and Adult Development, Mount Sinai School of Medicine, New York, NY 10029, USA

Kenneth L. Minaker, MD, Associate Professor of Medicine, Harvard Medical School; Chief, Geriatric Medicine Unit, Massachusetts General Hospital, Boston, MA 02114, USA

Charles Mobbs, PhD, Associate Professor, Neurobiology of Aging Laboratories, Brookdale Department of Geriatrics and Adult Development, Mount Sinai School of Medicine, New York, NY 10029, USA

Anna Monias, MD, Victory Springs, Inc., Premier Senior Health Care, Reisterstown, MD, 21136, USA

John H. Morrison, PhD, Professor and Director, Kastor Neurobiology of Aging Laboratories, Mount Sinai School of Medicine, New York, NY 10029, USA

R. Sean Morrison, MD, Associate Professor, Brookdale Department of Geriatrics, and Adult Development; Research Director, Hertzberg Palliative Care Institute, Mount Sinai School of Medicine, New York, NY 10029, USA

Thomas Mulligan, MD, AGSF, Chair, Consortium on Successful Aging, McGuire VAMC, Virginia Commonwealth University, Richmond, VA 23249, USA

Aman Nanda, MD, Assistant Professor of Medicine, Division of Geriatrics, Brown Medical School, Rhode Island Hospital, Providence, RI, 02903, USA

Mark R. Nehler, MD, Assistant Professor of Surgery, Section of Vascular Surgery, University of Colorado Health Sciences Center, Denver, CO 80203, USA

Linda C. Niessen, DM, MPH, MPP, Vice President, Clinical Education, DENTSPLY International, York, PA 17405, USA

Eugene Z. Oddone, MD, MHSc, Director, Center for Health Services Research in Primary Care, VA Medical Center; Chief, Divison of General Internal Medicine, Duke University Medical Center, Durham, NC 27710, USA

S. Jay Olshansky, PhD, Associate Professor, Department of Medicine, Harris Graduate School of Public Policy Studies, University of Chicago, Chicago, IL 60089, USA

Robert M. Palmer, MD, MPH, Department of General Internal Medicine, The Cleveland Clinic Foundation, Cleveland, OH 44195, USA

Cynthia X. Pan, MD, Assistant Professor and Director of Education, Palliative Care Program, Brookdale Department of Geriatrics and Adult Development, Mount Sinai School of Medicine, New York, NY 10029, USA

Ann Partridge, MD, Breast Oncology Center, Dana Farber Cancer Institute, Brigham and Women's Hospital, Boston, MA 02115, USA

Robert H. Pearlman, MD, MPH, Professor, Department of Medicine, University of Washington, VA Puget Sound Health Care System, Seattle, WA 98108, USA

Peter Pompei, MD, Associate Professor of Medicine, Stanford University School of Medicine, Veterans Affairs Palo Alto Health Care System, Stanford, CA 94305-5475, USA

Lawrence A. Pottenger, MD, PhD, Associate Professor, Orthopaedic Surgery; Director, Surgical Arthritis Clinic, University of Chicago Medical Center Chicago IL 60637, USA

Thomas S. Rees, PhD, Associate Professor of Otolaryngology-Head and Neck Surgery, University of Washington, Harborview Medical Center, Seattle, WA 98104, USA

Neil M. Resnick, MD, Professor of Medicine; Chief, Geriatric Medicine, University of Pittsburgh, Pittsburgh, PA 15213, USA

David B. Reuben, MD, Chief, Division of Geriatrics; Director, Multicampus Program in Geriatric Medicine and Gerontology; Professor of Medicine, UCLA School of Medicine, Los Angeles, CA 90095-1687, USA

Paula Rochon, MD, MPH, Assistant Professor of Medicine, University of Toronto; Scientist, Kunin Lunenfeld Applied Research Unit, Baycrest Center for Geriatric Care; Scientist, Institute for Clinical Evaluative Sciences, Toronto, Canada

María Cruz Rodriguez-Oroz, MD, Assistant Professor of Neurology, University of Navarre Medical School, Pamplona, Spain

Bruce P. Rosenthal, OD, FAAO, Chief, Low Vision Programs, Lighthouse International, New York, NY 10022, USA

Ronnie Ann Rosenthal, MD, Associate Professor of Surgery, Yale University School of Medicine; Chief, Surgical Service, VA Connecticut Healthcare System, West Haven, CT 06516, USA

Gerald Rothstein, MD, Chief of Geriatrics, University of Utah School of Medicine, Salt Lake City, UT 84132, USA

Laurence Z. Rubenstein, MD, MPH, Professor, Department of Medicine, Division of Geriatrics, UCLA School of Medicine; Director, Geriatric Research, Education, and Clinical Center, Sepulveda VA Medical Center, Sepulveda, CA 91343, USA

Greg A. Sachs, MD, Chief, Section of Geriatrics; Co-Director, Center for Comprehensive Care and Research on Memory Disorders, Department of Medicine, University of Chicago Medical Center, Chicago, IL 60637, USA

Steven C. Samuels, MD, Assistant Professor, Department of Psychiatry, Mount Sinai School of Medicine; Training Director, Geriatric Psychiatry Fellowship, Bronx Veterans Affairs Medical Center, Bronx Veterans Hospital, Bronx, NY 10468, USA

Kenneth Schmader, MD, Associate Professor of Medicine, Division of Geriatrics, Center for the Study of Aging, Duke University and Durham Veterans Affairs Medical Centers, Durham, NC 27710, USA

Tamar Shochat, PhD, Department of Psychiatry, University of California, San Diego, San Diego, CA 92161, USA

Waleed Siddiqi, MD, Staff Physician, Community Health Clinic of Clinch Valley Medical Center, Richlands, VA 24641, USA

Jeffrey H. Silverstein, MD, Associate Professor, Department of Anesthesiology/Surgery, Mount Sinai School of Medicine, New York, NY 10029, USA

Albert L. Siu, MD, MSPH, Chief, Division of General Internal Medicine, Mount Sinai School of Medicine, New York, NY 10029, USA

Leif B. Sorenson, MD, Professor of Medicine, Section of Rheumatology, University of Chicago Medical Center, Chicago, IL 60637, USA

Karen E. Steinhauser, PhD, Health Scientist, Program on the Medical Encounter and Palliative Care and Center for Health Services Research in Primary Care, Durham VA Medical Center; Research Assistant Professor, Department of Medicine, Division of General Internal Medicine, Duke University Medical Center, Durham, NC 27705, USA

Mark A. Supiano, MD, Associate Professor of Internal Medicine; Director, GRECC, VA Ann Arbor Health Care System, Ann Arbor, MI 48105, USA

Glendo L. Tangarorang, MD, Geriatrics Fellow, University of Connecticut Center on Aging, Farmington, CT 06030-5215, USA

George E. Taffet, MD, Associate Professor, Department of Medicine, Division of Geriatrics, Baylor College of Medicine, Houston, TX 77030, USA

David C. Thomas, MD, Assistant Professor, Departments of Internal Medicine and Rehab Medicine, Mount Sinai School of Medicine, New York, NY 10029, USA

David R. Thomas, MD, Professor of Medicine, Division of Geriatric Medicine, St. Louis University Health Sciences Center, St. Louis, MO 63104, USA

M. Chrystie Timmons, MD, FACOG, Director, Gerigyn, P.A., Chapel Hill, NC 27514, USA

Mary E. Tinetti, MD, Professor, Department of Medicine and Epidemiology and Public Health, Yale University; Chief, Section in Geriatrics, New Haven, CT 06520-8025, USA

Bruce Troen, MD, Associate Professor of Medicine, University of Miami School of Medicine, Miami Veterans Affairs Medical Center, Miami, FL 33125, USA

Donald L. Trump, MD, FACP, Chairman, Department of Medicine; Senior Vice President for Clinical Research, Roswell Park Cancer Institute, Buffalo, NY 14263, USA

Stanley Tuhrim, MD, Estelle and Daniel Maggin Department of Neurology, Brookdale Department of Geriatrics and Adult Development, Mount Sinai School of Medicine, New York, NY 10029, USA

James A. Tulsky, MD, Program on the Medical Encounter and Palliative Care, Durham VA Medical Center; Associate Professor of Medicine, Associate Director, Institute on Care at the End of Life, Duke University, Durham, NC 27705, USA

Bruce C. Vladeck, PhD, Professor of Health Policy and Geriatrics; Director, Institute for Medical Practice, Mount Sinai School of Medicine; Senior Vice President for Policy, Mount Sinai School of Medicine, New York, NY 10029, USA

Jeremy Walston, MD, Assistant Professor of Medicine; Medical Director, Terrrace Rehabilitation Unit, The Johns Hopkins Medical Institutions, Johns Hopkins Geriatric Center, Baltimore, MD 21224, USA

James R. Webster, Jr., MS, MD, Gertz Professor of Medicine, Northwestern University Medical School; Director Emeritus, Buehler Center on Aging, Chicago, IL 60611, USA

Nanette Kass Wenger, MD, Professor of Medicine, Division of Cardiology, Department of Medicine, Emory University School of Medicine; Chief of Cardiology, Grady Memorial Hospital; Consultant, Emory Heart and Vascular Center, Atlanta, GA 30303, USA

Joanne A. P. Wilson, MD, FACP, Professor of Medicine, Division of Gastroenterology, Department of Medicine, Duke University Medical Center, Durham, NC 27710, USA

Eric Winer, MD, Director of Breast Oncology Center, Dana Farber Cancer Institute, Boston, MA 02115, USA

Thomas T. Yoshikawa, MD, Chairman and Professor, Department of Internal Medicine, Charles R. Drew University of Medicine Science, Los Angeles, CA 90059, USA

Part I
Basics of Gerontology

1
Evidence-Based Medicine and Geriatrics

Rosanne M. Leipzig

The goal of evidence-based medicine is provision of care guided by the most up-to-date, scientifically sound evidence after careful investigation of the patient's history, physical condition, and expectations. Evidence-based medicine (EBM) is a term coined in 1992 by a group of clinical epidemiologists based at McMaster University in Hamilton, Ontario, to describe their transition from teaching clinicians how to read the medical literature[1] to teaching us how to use the literature in the care of an individual patient (Fig. 1.1).[2] This change emphasized three basic concepts.

Hierarchy of Evidence

The first concept is that "all evidence is not created equal." Depending on the type of clinical question—that is, therapeutic, diagnostic, prognostic, etc.—there is a hierarchy among study designs in terms of their ability to provide an accurate, less biased answer. For example, the Hormone and Estrogen Replacement Study (HERS) trial demonstrated in a randomized controlled trial (RCT) that hormone replacement therapy (HRT) given as 0.625 mg conjugated equine estrogens and 2.5 mg medroxyprogesterone acetate did not improve survival or decrease coronary events in women with existing coronary artery disease, even though several prospective cohort trials suggested that it would.[3] Results from two other RCTs to support this finding.[4] In the HRT observational trials, women who were offered and chose to take HRT differed systematically at baseline from those who did not; for example, they were more likely to be upper middle class, to be well educated, and to participate in more health promotion and disease prevention activities, and were therefore less at risk for death and coronary disease. These factors may account for their better outcomes after taking HRT.[5,6] Randomized controlled trials are superior to prospective cohort studies of the same population because the groups being compared are at equal risk of the outcome being studied, except for exposure to the intervention being tested. Risk factors associated with an outcome, whether they are known or not yet identified, are randomly distributed in RCTs. An observational trial can only identify known risk factors and then attempt to statistically adjust for discrepancies between them in the study groups.

Most clinical questions fall into one of seven categories: clinical findings, differential diagnosis, etiology, diagnostic tests, prognosis, therapy, or prevention.[62] Table 1.1 provides examples of important criteria that should be met to maximize the ability of clinical research to answer each type of clinical question. Some of these criteria have been used to create the "clinical query" search strategies on PubMed at the NLM's website ⟨http://www.ncbi.nlm.nih.gov/entrez/query/static/clinical.html⟩ and provide a filter for obtaining high-quality studies relating to therapy/prevention, diagnosis, etiology, and prognosis. Similar criteria have been developed for several other types of clinical questions.[7] For the past 10 years, studies that meet these validity criteria have been identified and published within the American College of Physicians (ACP) Journal Club, and are available online as well as in the print journal published by the ACP.[8] Clinical Evidence and the Cochrane Library are two other sources of systematic reviews of high-quality studies designed to answer specific medical questions.[9,10]

Clinically Meaningful Results

The second concept is that clinical, not statistical, significance is what matters in medicine. Many outcomes that are statistically significant are not clinically important. Some "clinical" outcomes are really intermediate, or surrogate, endpoints, not outcomes that make a difference to the patient. When these intermediate or

1. Convert daily clinical need for information into answerable questions.
2. Find best available evidence with which to answer each question.
3. Appraise the evidence critically and systematically with particular attention to its internal and external validity.
4. Integrate the evidence with the patient's unique biopsychosocial situation and the clinician's own expertise.
5. Evaluate clinical performance as well as the process of acquiring, integrating, and applying the new evidence.

FIGURE 1.1. Five tenets of evidence-based medicine. (From Ref. 62, with permission.)

surrogate outcomes are accepted, the treatment may result in an outcome that harms the patient. For example, before definitive studies using patient-oriented outcomes, suppression of ventricular premature contractions (VPB) was considered beneficial, as was increasing bone mineral density with fluoride. Yet when the studies were done, it was found that suppressing VPBs with certain agents increases patient mortality and increasing bone mineral density with fluoride increases fractures.[11,12]

Clinical significance also means that the magnitude of the effect is worth the costs of the intervention, including the inconvenience, adverse events, and psychologic or emotional as well as financial costs. The usual way of indicating a benefit, the relative risk reduction (RRR), may be quite large when the absolute risk reduction (ARR), or absolute benefit, is small (Table 1.2), as would be the case when, for example, a treatment reduces the risk of an outcome by 50% for an outcome that only occurs once in every million patients treated. In EBM, a term often used to define the size of the treatment benefit is the number needed to treat (NNT), which is the number of people who would need to be treated with the active intervention, rather than the control, over a specific time period to prevent one additional patient from having the bad outcome the treatment was given to prevent. These terms are illustrated in Figure 1.2, where stroke, the primary outcome of the Systolic Hypertension in the Elderly Program trial, is shown to occur in approximately 8% of control patients and 5% of treated patients.[13] Here the ARR is 3%, the RRR 36%, and the NNT is 33 over 4.5 years. In other words, treating 33 patients with isolated systolic hypertension (ISH) over 4.5 years will result in one fewer stroke than would have occurred if the ISH had not been treated. Similar terms describe the results of diagnostic tests, including the likelihood ratio, which compares the probability that people with an abnormal test actually have the disease in question to the probability that they have an abnormal test result but not the disease.

Applicability

The third concept is that studies are done on populations but clinicians need to apply them to an individual patient. This approach is relatively easy when the patient sitting in front of you meets the study inclusion and exclusion criteria, but it is far more difficult when the patient resembles those seen in most geriatric practices—old, somewhat frail, with multiple medical conditions and taking multiple medications, possibly with some cognitive, functional, or mood impairment.

In geriatrics, the primary challenge to practicing evidence-based medicine is the lack of high-quality studies that include older adults. There is a paucity of evidence on treating or diagnosing common conditions in relatively healthy elderly, let alone in patients like those just described. For example, how should patients with congestive heart failure (CHF) be treated? The range of mean ages of patients in the systolic CHF clinical trial literature is 58 to 65 years, with the median range being 61,[14] yet one recent population-based study found that almost 50% of new-onset CHF occurred in people age 80 or older and that approximately 50% of these had systolic CHF.[15] Will 80-year-olds be able to tolerate the recent standards for systolic CHF therapy, which include the addition of three to five new medications [i.e., aspirin, beta-blocker, HMG (3-hydroxy-3-methylgluaryl)-CoA reductase inhibitor, angiotensin-community enzyme (ACE) inhibitor, diuretic, digoxin]? How should the 40% to 50% of patients over 70 whose CHF is diastolic (an ejection fraction ≥45%)[16] be treated? The answer is unknown, as no large randomized trials have been published to date.

Treatment Studies: Applying Results to Older Adults

Figure 1.3 depicts several of the areas where differences in older adults might impact the benefit/risk ratio of a treatment. Several of these are key principles in geriatric medicine and overlap the specific biologic, social and economic, and epidemiologic issues discussed in the *User's Guide: How to Decide on the Applicability of Clinical Trial Results to Your Patient*.[17] In this chapter, disease, patient, and treatment differences that can influence the application of study results to older adults, as well as the intersections of each of these, are discussed.

Patient–Disease Interactions

Despite the concerns about reduced therapeutic efficacy that follow, it is important to recognize that older adults are often the group most likely to benefit from treatment

TABLE 1.1. Evidence-based medicine (EBM) criteria for evaluating studies.

Criteria	Therapy/prevention	Differential diagnosis	Diagnostic tests	Harm/etiology	Prognosis
Primary validity requirements	• Was the assignment of patients to treatments randomized? • Were all patients who entered the trial properly accounted for and attributed at its conclusion? • Was follow-up complete? • Were patients analyzed in the groups to which they were randomized?	• Did the study patients represent the full spectrum of those who present with this clinical problem? • Were the criteria for each final diagnosis explicit and credible?	• Was there an independent, blind comparison with a reference standard? • Did the patient sample include an appropriate spectrum of patients to whom the diagnostic test will be applied in clinical practice?	• Were there clearly identified comparison groups that were similar with respect to important determinants of outcome, other than the one of interest? • Were the outcomes and exposures measured in the same way in the groups being compared? • Was follow-up sufficiently long and complete?	• Was there a representative and well-defined sample of patients at a similar point in the course of the disease? • Was follow-up sufficiently long and complete?
Secondary Validity Requirements	• Were patients, health workers, and study personnel "blind" to treatment? • Were the groups similar at the start of the trial? • Aside from the experimental intervention, were the groups treated equally?	• Was the diagnostic workup comprehensive and consistently applied? • For initially undiagnosed patients, was follow-up sufficiently long and complete?	• Did the results of the test being evaluated influence the decision to perform the reference standard? • Were the methods for performing the test described in sufficient detail to permit replication?	• Is the temporal relationship correct? • Is there a dose–response gradient?	• Were objective and unbiased outcome criteria used? • Was there adjustment for important prognostic factors?
Results	• How large was the treatment effect? • How precise was the estimate of the treatment effect?	• What were the diagnoses and their probabilities? • How precise are these estimates of disease probability?	• Are likelihood ratios for the test results presented of data necessary for their calculation included?	• How strong is the association between exposure and outcome? • How precise is the estimate of the risk?	• How large is the likelihood of the outcome event(s) in a specified period of time? • How precise are the estimates of likelihood?
Applicability	• Can the results be applied to my patient care? • Were all clinically important outcomes considered? • Are the likely treatment benefits worth the potential harms and costs?	• Are the study patients similar to those in my own practice? • Is it unlikely that the disease possibilities or probabilities have changed since this evidence was gathered?	• Will the reproducibility of the test result and its interpretation be satisfactory in my clinical setting? • Are the results applicable to the patient in my practice? • Will the results change my management strategy? • Will patients be better off as a result of this test?	• Are the study results applicable to my practice? • What is the magnitude of the risk? • Should I attempt to stop the exposure?	• Were the study patients similar to my own? • Will the results lead directly to selecting or avoiding therapy? • Are the results useful for reassuring or counseling patients?

Source: From Refs. 52–54, with permission.

TABLE 1.2. Glossary of evidence-based vocabulary included in the fourth edition of *Geriatric Medicine*.

Terms relevant to study design

Case-control study	Case-control studies examine outcomes that are rare or take a long time to develop. Cases are identified in which the outcome occurred; controls are then selected with similar age, sex, and medical conditions excepting the target outcome. Investigators assess the relative frequency of exposure to the alleged harmful agent, controlling for differences in the variables.
Case series	Descriptions of a series of patients; case series lack a control group.
Cohort study	Involves identification of two or more groups (cohorts) of patients, one which did receive the exposure of interest, and one which did not, and following these cohorts forward for the outcome of interest.
Double-blind (DB)	A trial in which neither the patient nor the physician knows whether drug or placebo is being taken, or at what dosage.[58]
External validity	How well results fit populations other than the one in which the model was generated.
Heterogeneity	In a meta-analysis, results of individual studies suggest that they were performed in different populations. Can compromise the validity of a meta-analysis; significant heterogeneity indicates decreased likelihood that chance alone is responsible for any observed differences in treatment effects between studies.
Internal validity	How well results fit the population in which the model was generated.
Meta-analysis	Quantitative review of systematically chosen literature, the hallmark of which is statistical synthesis of the numerical outcomes of several trials that all asked the same question.
Multicenter	A clinical trial conducted at more than one site, but following the same protocol at all locations.
Placebo-controlled (PC)	A trial in which the effectiveness of the drug is compared to that of a placebo.
Prospective cohort study	An observational study that follows a large group (a cohort) of people forward in time
Randomized controlled trial (RCT)	Experiment in which individual are randomly allocated to receive or not receive an experimental preventative, therapeutic, or diagnostic procedure and then followed to determine the effect of the intervention.
Systematic review	Explicit, structured presentation of results of an unbiased literature review, using predetermined search and appraisal definitions. Based on deductive, rather than inductive, reasoning.

Terms relevant to study results

Absolute risk reduction (ARR)	The difference between the control event rate (CER) and the experimental treatment event rate (EER). Use restricted to a beneficial intervention. $$ARR = CER - EER$$
95% confidence interval (CI)	An estimate of the precision of a measurement by determining, with 95% accuracy, that the measurement includes the "true" value for the population. The broader the CI range, the more uncertain is the true value of the measurement; CIs that cross zero do not reach clinical significance.
Control event rate (CER)	Rate of the outcome in the control group.
Experimental event rate (EER)	Rate of the outcome in the experimental treatment group.
Intention-to-treat (ITT)	Results that include every individual originally randomized, regardless of whether or not they completed the trial.
Likelihood ratio (LR)	Positive LR = probability of an abnormal diagnostic or screening test result (including clinical signs or symptoms) in patients with the disorder of interest compared to the probability of the abnormal result in patients without the disorder (Sn/1 − Sp). Negative LR = probability of a normal diagnostic or screening test result (including clinical signs or symptoms) in patients without the disorder of interest compared to the probability of a normal result in patients with the disorder (Sp/1 − Sn).
Negative predictive value	The proportion of patients testing negative for the disorder who are actually disease free, of all the patients testing negative.
Number needed to treat (NNT)	The number of patients who must be treated with this intervention (rather than the control) over a specified time period to prevent one additional bad outcome. $$NNT = 1/ARR \text{ (as a decimal)}$$
Number needed to harm (NNH)	The number of patients who would need to be treated over a specific time period before one adverse side effect of the treatment will occur.
Odds ratio (OR)	The odds of an experimental patient suffering an adverse event relative to a control patient.
Per protocol analysis	Results that do not take into account all persons originally randomized, only those participants who followed the study protocol.
Positive predictive value	The proportion of patients testing positive for the disorder who actually have the disease, of all the patients testing positive.
Relative risk reduction (RRR)	Percent reduction in "bad" outcome events in the experimentally treated groups relative to the control groups. $$RRR = (CER - EER) / CER * 100$$
Sensitivity (Sn)	The proportion of diseased patients actually testing positive for the disorder, of all the diseased patients. SnNout: When a test has a high Sensitivity, a Negative test rules OUT the diagnosis.
Specificity (Sp)	The proportion of disease-free patients actually testing negative for the disorder, of all the disease-free patients. SpPin: When a test has a high Specificity, a Positive result rules IN the diagnosis.

Source: From Refs. 52, 55–60, with permission.

% Stroke/4.5 yrs

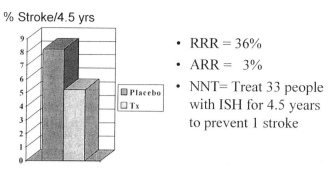

- RRR = 36%
- ARR = 3%
- NNT= Treat 33 people with ISH for 4.5 years to prevent 1 stroke

FIGURE 1.2. Stroke incidence in patients with isolated systolic hypertension. (From Ref. 13, with permission.)

of a given disorder. Benefits are almost always greatest in the population most likely to experience the bad outcome that the treatment is intended to avoid or improve. Treatment of hypertension can be used as an example. In Table 1.3, the NNTs over 5 years to prevent one additional death or cardiovascular or cerebrovascu-lar event are depicted for hypertensive patients. With increasing age, fewer patients need to be treated to obtain benefit, which is not surprising because the prevalence of death and cardiovascular events resulting from hyper-tension increases with age. In general, older adults have a similar decrease in relative risk and the same or a smaller NNT than middle-aged or younger adults, partic-ularly when risks of treatment are small. Table 1.4 illustrates this concept by summarizing the results of sub-group analyses by age from four RCTs of lipid-lowering agents in patients with known coronary disease.[18]

Disease Differences

Age-related differences in disease pathophysiology or in the multifactorial nature of a condition can decrease treatment efficacy. For example, agents effective at treat-ing pneumonia in community-dwelling adults may be less effective when treating nursing home-aquired pneumo-nia due to differences in the causative organisms and

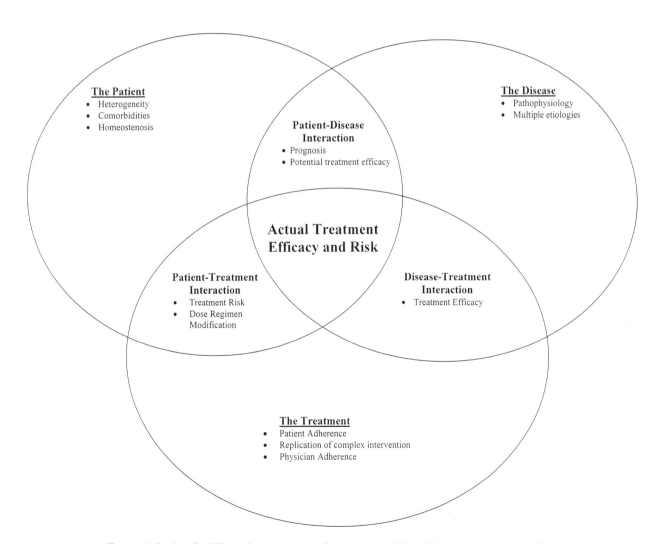

FIGURE 1.3. Applicability of treatment study results to older adults: domains to consider.

TABLE 1.3. Antihypertensive treatment NNT for 5 years to prevent one event.

	Older (>60 years old)	Younger
Mortality		
Total	72	167
Cardiovascular	58	205
Cerebrovascular	193	365
Coronary heart disease	88	NS
Morbidity and Mortality		
Cerebrovascular	46	168
Coronary heart disease	68	184
Cardiovascular	21	—

NNT, number needed to treat; NS, not statistically significant.
Source: From Ref. 61, with permission.

resistance patterns.[19,20] Sulfonylureas are effective in treating type II diabetes, but the lack of endogenous insulin makes them of little use in treating type I. The symptom complex of nocturia and leg edema may suggest CHF, yet diuretics will not improve nocturia caused by age-related temporal shifts in fluid elimination that are a result of loss of the circadian rhythm of antidiure-

tic hormone secretion, decreased renin-angiotensin-aldosterone, increased secretion of atrial naturetic hormone, and diminished renal concentrating and sodium-conserving ability,[21] or leg edema that is secondary to venous insufficiency.

Classic differential diagnosis teaches us to use Occam's razor; that is, scientists should assume no more causes than are absolutely necessary to explain their observations. A single diagnosis should be sought to account for all the patient's signs and symptoms. Many geriatric disorders, however, are multifactorial in that several different conditions contribute to the symptom complex. With multifactorial disorders, identifying and treating a single condition may result in some but not complete improvement. Intermediate outcomes may be improved, yet patients may not be aware of any improvement. For example, the single diagnoses most responsible for dyspnea on exertion (DOE) are pneumonia, asthma or chronic obstructive pulmonary disease (COPD), angina, or CHF. Specific treatment for the correct diagnosis results in resolution of the symptom. In older patients, a number of chronic conditions may contribute to the complaint of DOE. In addition to the disorders already noted, kyphosis, intrinsic lung disease, deconditioning,

TABLE 1.4. Secondary prevention: effects of age on lipid lowering in patients with congestive heart disease (CHD).

Reference	Agent/no. patients	Mean age, years (range)	Control event rate	Experimental event rate	Relative risk reduction (range)	Absolute risk reduction (range)	NNT/years (range)
4S (Lancet 1994)	Simvastatin/ 4444	58 (35–70)	28%	19%	32% (23%–41%)	9% (6.5%–11.5%)	11/5.4 (9–15)
Subgroup analyses	1021	67 (≥65)	33.4%	24%	28% (12%–45%)	9.4% (3.9%–14.9%)	11 (7–26)
	3423	56 (<65)	26.4%	18.1%	32% (21%–42%)	8.4% (5.6%–11.2%)	12 (9–18)
LIPID (Engl J Med 1998)	Pravastatin/ 9014	62 (31–75)	15.9%	12.3%	23% (14%–30%)	3.6% (2.2%–5.0%)	28/6.1 (20–46)
Subgroup analyses	3514	≥65	19.7%	16%	19% (6%–32%)	3.7% (1.2%–6.2%)	27 (16–85)
	5500	<65	13.4%	10%	25% (13%–38%)	3.4% (1.7%–5.1%)	29 (20–59)
CARE (Sacks et al., N Engl J Med 1996)	Pravastatin/ 4159	59 (21–75)	26.4%	21%	20% (11%–30%)	5.4% (2.8%–8.0%)	19/5 (13–35)
Subgroup analyses	2129	≥60	27%	20%	27% (12%–38%)	7.1% (3.5%–10.7%)	14 (9–28)
	2030	<60	26%	21%	20% (4%–33%)	4.7% (1%–8.4%)	21 (12–98)
VA-HIT (Rubins et al., N Engl J Med 1999)	Gemfibrozil/ 2531	64	26%	20%	23% (10%–36%)	6% (2.7%–9.3%)	17/5.1 (11–37)
Subgroup analysis	1266	≥66	29%	22%	26% (7%–40%)	6.7% (1.9%–11.5%)	15 (9–52)
	1265	<66	24%	19%	21% (2%–40%)	5.0% (0.5%–9.5%)	20 (11–207)

4S, Scandinavian Simvastatin Survival Study; LIPID, Long-Term Intervention with Pravastatin in Ischaemic Disease Study Group; CARE, Control and Recurrent Events trial; VA-HIT, Veterans Affairs Cooperative Studies Program High-Density Lipoprotein Cholesterol Intervention Trial.
    All studies were MC, PC, DB, RCTs, and examined CHD death and nonfatal myocardial infarction (MI) as outcomes in the treatment of hypercholesterolemia. Range in parentheses, 95% confidence intervals.
Source: From Ref. 18, with permission.

valvular heart disease, left ventricular dysfunction, tachyarrhythmias, and mild anemia may all exacerbate the patient's symptoms. Only some of these can be reversed, and treatment of any one ameliorates only some of the dyspnea, even if the laboratory or radiology results for that condition normalize.

Patient Differences

Older adults are more pathophysiologically heterogeneous than people at other stages of life as a result of the effects of aging itself, disease, lifestyle, and genetics. The concept of applying study results to "older adults" is actually misleading, as there appear to be multiple subsets with significantly different prognostic trajectories: successful agers, usual agers, chronically ill, dementing, or terminally ill agers. Even within each of these groups, the life expectancy trajectory has been shown to differ.[22–28] Prognostic indexes are better for some conditions than others, but generally even these only provide data on time to death or, occasionally, the need for institutional-type care.

Comorbid and age-related conditions can significantly alter the potential benefits and risks of treatment. The impact of comorbid illness on life expectancy can negate the benefit of treating certain conditions including early prostate cancer, where no outcome difference is seen between treatment and watchful waiting over 10 years,[29] and high cholesterol, where benefits are initially seen after 2 full years and reach a maximum at 5 years.[30] Other comorbidities allow parsimonious treatment to occur, resulting in an intervention having even greater benefit than usual: examples include anticoagulation in a person with both a deep venous thrombosis (DVT) and atrial fibrillation, or colchicine in someone with gout and significant obstipation. Comorbidities can also reduce the effect of treatment by producing a bad outcome through mechanisms not affected by the treatment. For example, cataract removal in older adults may not improve vision substantially if the patient has underlying macular degeneration or diabetic retinopathy, which is less likely to occur in middle-aged or younger adults.

Homeostenosis is a term that reflects the age-related decline in ability to maintain homeostasis and attenuate the impact of stressors. With aging, thermoregulation becomes more difficult, the immune system is not as responsive, and the maximal heart rate is not as high (see Chapter 3). This loss of physiologic flexibility and plasticity means that any intervention might have a more deranging influence than expected. For example, people with structurally abnormal brains due to either dementia or stroke are more likely to develop delirium from a small dose of an anticholinergic drug than age-matched people without these conditions.[31,32]

Treatment Differences

Patient adherence, and consequently therapeutic effect, can be markedly affected by the social and economic differences discussed in Chapters 6 and 82. In general, people who adhere to placebo in a study do better than study patients who do not adhere,[5] and many interventions have been found to have less benefit in practice than in an RCT. The ability of older adults to adhere to therapeutic regimens, including preparations for procedures, can be compromised by motivation, finances, social isolation, impaired ADLs (activities of daily living), IADLs (instrumental activities of daily living), and cognition, all of which usually are more common in study nonparticipants than participants. For other types of interventions, including test interpretation, provider and site experience and expertise are key to obtaining results comparable to those obtained in a clinical trial.[33–35]

Study interventions may be simple, such as a trial of a medication for a specific condition, or complex, for example, the effect of an Acute Care for Elders unit or a Delirium Prevention consultation team on functional change from preadmission to discharge. Complex interventions usually have several components including content variables, such as protocols for preventing and managing urinary incontinence or delirium, and process variables, such as the personnel, administrative structure, and methods for changing staff behavior. When a complex intervention is effective, it is often difficult to replicate and often unclear which components are critical to success and therefore required for replication.[36,37] Key components might be staff with specific personality traits or a culture that is supportive of change, both of which are more difficult to replicate than the administration of a medication.

Patient–Treatment Interactions

Older adults experience a variety of age-related changes in pharmacokinetics and pharmacodynamics (see Chapter 7), resulting in a need to modify drug dosing regimens from those used in a study. Comorbid conditions and their treatments result in novel drug–drug and drug–disease interactions that are not detected during phase III trials because of the stringent inclusion and exclusion criteria and the relatively small numbers of subjects tested. For example, treatment of atrial fibrillation with rate control agents such as beta-blockers is more likely to result in symptomatic bradycardia requiring a pacemaker in older adults[38] because it is more often a manifestation of sick sinus syndrome in this population. Treatment responsiveness may also vary with age, as demonstrated by the decreased immune response and efficacy of the influenza vaccine in nursing home patients.[39] The target range for therapeutic or

TABLE 1.5. Guide for using new therapy in an older adult.

Question	Supporting evidence and data sources
1. Could the disorder be secondary to a medication that could be tapered or stopped?	Leipzig RM. *Drug Prescribing for Older Adults: An Evidence-based Approach*. Philadelphia: American College of Physicians; 2003. Dukes MNG, ed. *Meyler's Side Effects of Drugs*, 13th Ed. New York: American Elsevier; 1996.

2. Has the treatment been shown to be superior to other accepted treatments in its effect on outcomes that matter to patients?	• Head-to-head trial against current standard treatment showing
	    Better efficacy
	    Fewer adverse events
	• More likely to be taken as directed (e.g., qd vs. qid)
	• Costs less
	In general, do not accept the following:
	    Improves disease-oriented outcomes
	    "Me-too" drug that differs chemically or pharmacokinetically but not in any of the above ways
	    Different mechanism of action without head-to-head trials

3. What is the patient's likelihood of a bad outcome if not treated?	• Estimation of the patient's life expectancy[22,25–28]
	• Studies that:
	    Identify prognostic factors and subgroups
	    Provide control group event rates

4. What is the effectiveness of the treatment for older adults?	Hierarchy of evidence
	• Systematic review of RCTs that include subjects similar to the patient
	• Single RCT that includes subjects similar to the patient
	• Analyses of the older adults within RCTs
	    Individual patient meta-analyses
	    Intentional subgroup analyses (appropriate power to show a difference)
	    Posthoc subgroup analyses
	• Prospective cohort studies
	• Retrospective cohort studies
	• Case-control studies

5. What are the risks of treatment? Is there any type of monitoring that will decrease this risk?	• Those identified in the studies (how large were the studies, who was excluded?)
	• What are the patient's "vulnerable" areas (balance, nutrition, hepatic and renal function, unable to comprehend instructions or report symptoms, etc)?
	Adverse event literature:
	    Goodman LS, Hardman JG, Limbird LE, Gilman AG, eds. *Goodman & Gilman's The Pharmacological Basis of Therapeutics*, 10th Ed. New York: McGraw-Hill; 2001.
	    Bennett WM. *Drug Prescribing in Renal Failure: Dosing Guidelines for Adults*, 3rd Ed. Philadelphia: American College of Physicians; 1994.
	    Semla TP, Beizer JL, Higbee MD. *Geriatric Dosage Handbook: Including Monitoring, Clinical Recommendations, and OBRA Guidelines 2002–2003*, 6th ed.: Lexi-Comp; 2002.
	    Hansten PD, Horn JR. *Hansten and Horn's Drug Interactions Analysis and Management*. (Updated quarterly.) Vancouver, WA: Applied Therapeutics; 1997–.

6. How important does the patient view avoiding the disorder's bad outcome compared to the risk of treatment?	Patient discussion; family and/or caregivers if patient unable to discuss

toxic drug levels may need to be adjusted due to differences in protein binding[25] or in recognition of the types of adverse events, such as delirium or falls, which commonly occur in older but not younger adults. This concern is particularly true for chronically ill or frail older adults, who may have compromised end organs that respond differently or in an exaggerated way to "usual" drug levels.[40]

In summary, it is often possible to identify factors that might change the benefit/risk ratio of an intervention in older adults from that estimated in an RCT performed mainly in younger or middle-aged persons. There are times, especially when the condition or the treatment are "high risk," when it is important to evaluate data obtained directly from the treatment's use in older adults themselves. An example of this is thrombolysis for acute myocardial infarction (MI), where RCTs suggest equal benefit up to the age of 75 but provide no data on persons 75 or older. Observational studies concur that 30-day or hospital survival improves up to age 75; however, these studies found that acute MI patients over this age treated with thrombolysis were more likely to die than sicker patients who did not receive thrombolysis.[41,42] Neither gastrointestinal nor brain hemorrhage in older adults, the major adverse effects of thrombolysis that lead to death, appear to be responsible for this increase. Table 1.5 suggests a series of questions to ask before applying the results of a therapeutic trial to older adults.

Diagnosis Studies—Diagnostic Tests, Differential Diagnosis, Screening, and Clinical Prediction Rules: Applying Results to Older Adults

Prevalence and competing diagnostic possibilities may differ between geriatric patients and the original study population. In a younger population in which a disease has low prevalence, a test may have a low positive predictive value and not be useful for screening; the positive predictive value, however, can increase in an older population where the disease has greater prevalence, making the same test appropriate as a screening test for older adults.

Differences in the differential diagnosis can affect diagnostic and screening test characteristics such as sensitivity, likelihood ratio, the accuracy of a clinical prediction rule, or the pretest probability of a diagnosis. For example, a clinical prediction rule derived and validated in middle-aged populations (with 20%–30% ≥60 years old), found that rales, fever, tachycardia, decreased breath sounds, and the absence of asthma were independent predictors of pulmonary infiltrates;[43] confusion and level of consciousness were not. In a similar derivation study conducted in nursing home residents, however,

TABLE 1.6. Select EBM resources.

Web sites	
Cochrane Collaboration	Online: www.cochrane.org
Clinical Evidence	Online: *www.clinicalevidence.org*
Centre for Evidence-Based Medicine	Online: http://cebm.jr2.ox.ac.uk/
Complementary and Alternative Medicine from Bandolier	Online: *http://www.jr2.ox.ac.uk/bandolier/booth/booths/altmed.html*
EBM Tutorial; University of North Carolina at Chapel Hill	http://www.hsl.unc.edu/lm/ebm/welcome.htm
Journal of Family Practice POEMS (Patient Oriented Evidence that Matters)	http://www.jfampract.com/display_archives.asp?YEA R=POEMs
MIAH (Merck Institute on Aging and Health)	*http://www.miahonline.org/resources/bibliographies/index.html*
	http://www.miahonline.org/resources/journalClub/index.html
Netting the Evidence	http://www.shef.ac.uk/~scharr/ir/netting/
Books	
Diagnostic Strategies for Common Medical Problems	Black ER. 2nd Ed. Philadelphia: American College of Physicians; 1999.
Evidence-Based Medicine: How to Practice and Teach EBM	Sackett DL. Edinburgh: Churchill Livingstone; 2000.
How to Read a Paper: The Basics of Evidence-Based Medicine	Greenhalgh T. BMJ Publishing; 1997.
PDQ: Evidence-Based Principles and Practice	McKibbon A, Eady A, Marks S. Hamilton, Ontario: Decker; 1999.
Users' Guides to the Medical Literature: A Manual for Evidence-Based Clinical Practice	Guyatt G, Rennie D, Evidence-Based Medicine Working Group, American Medical Association. Chicago: AMA Press; 2002.
Journals	
ACP Journal Club	Online: http://www.acponline.org/
Bandolier	Online: http://www.jr2.ox.ac.uk/bandolier/
Evidence-Based Cardiovascular Medicine	Journal
Evidence-Based Dentistry	Journal
Evidence-Based Nursing	Journal
Evidence-Based Occupational Therapy	Journal
Evidence-Based Healthcare	Journal
Evidence-Based Mental Health	Journal
Evidence-Based Oncology	Journal
Journal of Evidence-Based Health Care	Journal
Journal articles/series	
Basic Statistics for Clinicians Series	Guyatt G, Jaeschke R, Heddle N, Cook D, Shannon H, Walter S. Hypothesis testing. *Can Med Assoc J*. 1995;152(1):27–32. (First article in the series.)
Evaluation of diagnostic procedures (first in a series of five articles on the evidence base of clinical diagnosis)	Knottnerus JA, van Weel C, Muris JW. *Br Med J*. 2002;324(7335):477–480.
User's guide to the medical literature. I. How to get started	*JAMA*. 1993;270:2093–2095 (first in a series)
Databases/Tools	
CATmaker	http://cebm.jr2.ox.ac.uk/docs/catmaker.html
PubMed: clinical queries	Online: *http://www.ncbi.nlm.nih.gov/entrez/query/static/clinical.html*
TRIP (Turning Research Into Practice) Database	http://www.tripdatabase.com/

both acute confusion and somnolence and decreased alertness were independent predictors, along with all the other conditions except decreased breath sounds.[44] Similarly, a clinical prediction rule for hyperthyroidism or acute myocardial infarction may differ for middle-aged compared to older adults because of the difference in disease presentation in these two groups.[45–49]

For diagnostic tests, the competing diagnostic possibilities need to be those which are prevalent in the differential for people of that age presenting with a given symptom complex. In older adults, a diagnostic test for dementia due to Alzheimer's disease needs to differentiate this condition not simply from normal cognition or human immunodeficiency virus (HIV) dementia but from dementias due to Parkinson's disease or vascular causes. Younger patients presenting with fever and acute confusion undergo an urgent lumbar puncture and are immediately started on antibiotics because of the concern that they have bacterial meningitis, whereas this is rarely the cause of a febrile delirium in an older adult and a lumbar puncture is not often needed.[50] If the illness differs pathophysiologically in older and younger adults, diagnostic tests may be far less accurate. Pulse increase is a sensitive sign of orthostatic hypotension in younger adults, but not in older adults, probably because the hearts of older adults are relatively insensitive to the inotropic effects of beta-adrenergic agonists.[51]

Conclusion

Time pressures on the clinician make careful critique of individual trials difficult. Evidence-based resources such as those noted in Table 1.6 provide prescrutinized summaries for clinicians and allow one to be more informed of the results of high-quality studies that evaluate outcomes of concern to patients, not just to the disease. Table 1.2 defines some of the terms commonly used both in this chapter and in this edition of *Geriatric Medicine*.

The goal of this fourth edition is to provide, based on currently available sound data, an evidence-based approach to the older patient. We try to provide not only the best evidence available now, but also to set the stage for clinicians to rationally approach evidence that excludes the "real" geriatric patient. Finally, we hope to encourage research in those areas lacking evidence in older adults, with the full understanding that constantly updated editions will be required as new research is conducted.

References

1. How to read clinical journals: I. Why to read them and how to start reading them critically. *Can Med Assoc J.* 1981; 124(5):555–558.

2. Oxman A, Sackett D, Guyatt G. Users' guides to the medical literature. I. How to get started. The Evidence-Based Medicine Working Group. *JAMA.* 1993;270(17):2093–2095.

3. Hulley S, Grady D, Bush T, et al. Randomized trial of estrogen plus progestin for secondary prevention of coronary heart disease in postmenopausal women. Heart and Estrogen/progestin Replacement Study (HERS) Research Group. *JAMA.* 1998;280(7):605–613.

4. Writing Group for the Women's Health Initiative Investigators. Risks and benefits of estrogen plus progestin in healthy postmenopausal women: principal results from the Women's Health Initiative randomized controlled trial. *JAMA.* 2002;288:321–333.

5. Grady D, Hulley SB. Hormones to prevent coronary disease in women: when are observational studies adequate evidence? *Ann Intern Med.* 2000;133(12):999–1001.

6. Barrett-Connor E. Postmenopausal estrogen and prevention bias. *Ann Intern Med.* 1991;115(6):455–456.

7. Evidence-Based Medicine Working Group. *User's guides to the medical literature: a manual for evidence-based clinical practice.* Chicago: AMA Press; 2002.

8. ACP Journal Club. Vol. 2002. Philadelphia: American College of Physicians—American Society of Internal Medicine; 2002. http://www.acpjc.otg/.

9. Cochrane Library. Vol. 2002. Oxford: Cochrane Collaboration; 2002. Oxford, UK: Database, Published by Update Software.

10. American College of Physicians—American Society of Internal Medicine. *Clinical evidence*, 6th edn. London: BMJ Publishing ACP-ASIM; 2001.

11. Epstein AE, Hallstrom AP, Rogers WJ, et al. Mortality following ventricular arrhythmia suppression by encainide, flecainide, and moricizine after myocardial infarction. The original design concept of the Cardiac Arrhythmia Suppression Trial (CAST). *JAMA.* 1993;270(20):2451–2455.

12. Riggs BL, Hodgson SF, O'Fallon WM, et al. Effect of fluoride treatment on the fracture rate in postmenopausal women with osteoporosis. *N Engl J Med.* 1990;322(12):802–809.

13. SHEP Cooperative Research Group. Prevention of stroke by antihypertensive drug treatment in older persons with isolated systolic hypertension. Final results of the Systolic Hypertension in the Elderly Program (SHEP). *JAMA.* 1991;265(24):3255–3264.

14. Nguyen VH, McLaughlin MA. Congestive heart failure (CHF). In: Leipzig RM, ed. *Drug Prescribing for Older Adults: An Evidence-Based Approach.* Philadelphia: American College of Physicians; 2003. In press.

15. Senni M, Tribouilloy CM, Rodeheffer RJ, et al. Congestive heart failure in the community: a study of all incident cases in Olmsted County, Minnesota, in 1991. *Circulation.* 1998; 98(21):2282–2289.

16. Wong WF, Gold S, Fukuyama O, Blanchette PL. Diastolic dysfunction in elderly patients with congestive heart failure. *Am J Cardiol.* 1989;63(20):1526–1528.

17. Dans AL, Dans LF, Guyatt GH, Richardson S. Users' guides to the medical literature. XIV. How to decide on the applicability of clinical trial results to your patient. Evidence-

Based Medicine Working Group. *JAMA*. 1998;279(7):545–549.

18. Smith D. Hyperlipidemia. In: Leipzig RM, ed. *Drug Prescribing for Older Adults: An Evidence-Based Approach.* Philadelphia: ACP; 2003.

19. Yoshikawa TT, Norman DC. *Infectious Disease in the Aging: A Clinical Handbook.* Totowa, NJ: Humana Press; 2001.

20. Naughton BJ, Mylotte JM. Treatment guideline for nursing home-acquired pneumonia based on community practice. *J Am Geriatr Soc.* 2000;48(1):82–88.

21. Miller M. Nocturnal polyuria in older people: pathophysiology and clinical implications. *J Am Geriatr Soc.* 2000;48(10):1321–1329.

22. Knaus WA, Harrell FE, Jr, Lynn J, et al. The SUPPORT prognostic model. Objective estimates of survival for seriously ill hospitalized adults. Study to understand prognoses and preferences for outcomes and risks of treatments. *Ann Intern Med.* 1995;122(3):191–203.

23. Rowe JW, Kahn RL. Human aging: usual and successful. *Science.* 1987;237(4811):143–149.

24. Federal Interagency Forum on Aging-Related Statistics. Older Americans 2000: Key Indicators of Well-Being. Updated Detailed Tables, vol 2002. Hyattsville, MD: Federal Interagency Forum on Aging-Related Statistics.; April 10, 2002. http://www.agingstats.gov/chartbook2000/tables.html.

25. Anderson GD, Pak C, Doane KW, et al. Revised Winter-Tozer equation for normalized phenytoin concentrations in trauma and elderly patients with hypoalbuminemia. *Ann Pharmacother.* 1997;31(3):279–284.

26. Stern Y, Tang MX, Albert MS, et al. Predicting time to nursing home care and death in individuals with Alzheimer disease. *JAMA.* 1997;277(10):806–812.

27. Aguero-Torres H, Fratiglioni L, Guo Z, Viitanen M, Winblad B. Mortality from dementia in advanced age: a 5-year follow-up study of incident dementia cases. *J Clin Epidemiol.* 1999;52(8):737–743.

28. Heyman A, Peterson B, Fillenbaum G, Pieper C. Predictors of time to institutionalization of patients with Alzheimer's disease: the CERAD experience, part XVII. *Neurology.* 1997;48(5):1304–1309.

29. Lu-Yao GL, Yao SL. Population-based study of long-term survival in patients with clinically localised prostate cancer. *Lancet.* 1997;349(9056):906–910.

30. Law MR, Wald NJ, Thompson SG. By how much and how quickly does reduction in serum cholesterol concentration lower risk of ischaemic heart disease? *Br Med J.* 1994; 308(6925):367–372.

31. Sunderland T, Tariot PN, Cohen RM, Weingartner H, Mueller EA III, Murphy DL. Anticholinergic sensitivity in patients with dementia of the Alzheimer type and age-matched controls. A dose-response study. *Arch Gen Psychiatry.* 1987;44(5):418–426.

32. Dubois B, Danze F, Pillon B, Cusimano G, Lhermitte F, Agid Y. Cholinergic-dependent cognitive deficits in Parkinson's disease. *Ann Neurol.* 1987;22(1):26–30.

33. Criswell BK, Langsfeld M, Tullis MJ, Marek J. Evaluating institutional variability of duplex scanning in the detection of carotid artery stenosis. *Am J Surg.* 1998;176(6):591–597.

34. Hannan EL, Popp AJ, Feustel P, et al. Association of surgical specialty and processes of care with patient outcomes for carotid endarterectomy. *Stroke.* 2001;32(12):2890–2897.

35. Hannan EL, Siu AL, Kumar D, Kilburn H Jr, Chassin MR. The decline in coronary artery bypass graft surgery mortality in New York State. The role of surgeon volume. *JAMA.* 1995;273(3):209–213.

36. Wieland D, Stuck AE, Siu AL, Adams J, Rubenstein LZ. Meta-analytic methods for health services research—an example from geriatrics. *Eval Health Prof.* 1995;18(3): 252–282.

37. Applegate W, Deyo R, Kramer A, Meehan S. Geriatric evaluation and management: current status and future research directions. *J Am Geriatr Soc.* 1991;39(9 pt 2):2S–7S.

38. Rodriguez RD, Schocken DD. Update on sick sinus syndrome, a cardiac disorder of aging. *Geriatrics.* 1990;45(1): 26–30, 33–36.

39. Drinka PJ, Gravenstein S, Krause P, Schilling M, Miller BA, Shult P. Outbreaks of influenza A and B in a highly immunized nursing home population. *J Fam Pract.* 1997;45(6): 509–514.

40. Shannon M. Predictors of major toxicity after theophylline overdose. *Ann Intern Med.* 1993;119(12):1161–1167.

41. Thiemann DR, Coresh J, Schulman SP, Gerstenblith G, Oetgen WJ, Powe NR. Lack of benefit for intravenous thrombolysis in patients with myocardial infarction who are older than 75 years. *Circulation.* 2000;101(19):2239–2246.

42. Soumerai SB, McLaughlin TJ, Ross-Degnan D, Christiansen CL, Gurwitz JH. Effectiveness of thrombolytic therapy for acute myocardial infarction in the elderly: cause for concern in the old-old. *Arch Intern Med.* 2002;162(5):561–568.

43. Heckerling PS, Tape TG, Wigton RS, et al. Clinical prediction rule for pulmonary infiltrates. *Ann Intern Med.* 1990;113(9):664–670.

44. Mehr DR, Binder EF, Kruse RL, Zweig SC, Madsen RW, D'Agostino RB. Clinical findings associated with radiographic pneumonia in nursing home residents. *J Fam Pract.* 2001;50(11):931–937.

45. Samuels MH. Subclinical thyroid disease in the elderly. *Thyroid.* 1998;8(9):803–813.

46. Wallace K, Hofmann MT. Thyroid dysfunction: how to manage overt and subclinical disease in older patients. *Geriatrics.* 1998;53(4):32–38, 41.

47. Mokshagundam S, Barzel US. Thyroid disease in the elderly. *J Am Geriatr Soc.* 1993;41(12):1361–1369.

48. Solomon CG, Lee TH, Cook EF, et al. Comparison of clinical presentation of acute myocardial infarction in patients older than 65 years of age to younger patients: the Multicenter Chest Pain Study experience. *Am J Cardiol.* 1989;63(12):772–776.

49. Bayer AJ, Chadha JS, Farag RR, Pathy MS. Changing presentation of myocardial infarction with increasing old age. *J Am Geriatr Soc.* 1986;34(4):263–266.

50. Warshaw G, Tanzer F. The effectiveness of lumbar puncture in the evaluation of delirium and fever in the hospitalized elderly. *Arch Fam Med.* 1993;2(3):293–297.

51. Vestal RE, Wood AJ, Shand DG. Reduced beta-adrenoceptor sensitivity in the elderly. *Clin Pharmacol Ther.* 1979;26(2):181–186.

52. Guyatt G, Rennie D, Evidence-Based Medicine Working Group, American Medical Association. *Users' Guides to the Medical Literature: A Manual for Evidence-Based Clinical Practice.* Chicago: AMA Press; 2002.

53. Richardson WS, Wilson MC, Guyatt GH, Cook DJ, Nishikawa J. Users' guides to the medical literature. XV. How to use an article about disease probability for differential diagnosis. Evidence-Based Medicine Working Group. *JAMA.* 1999;281(13):1214–1219.

54. Centres for Health Evidence. Vol. 2002. May 10, 2002. Edmonton: 2002. http://www.cche.net/che/home.asp.

55. Evidence Based Medicine Glossary, vol. 2002. Oxford: Centre for Evidence Based Medicine; May, 31, 2002. http://163.1.96.10/docs/glossary.html.

56. Bigby M. Evidence-based medicine in a nutshell. A guide to finding and using the best evidence in caring for patients. *Arch Dermatol.* 1998;134(12):1609–1618.

57. ABC Data Companion, vol. 2002. New York: Susan G. Komen Breast Cancer Foundation; August 2001. http://www.komen.org/abc/dcldc_glossary.asp.

58. IBD Clinical Trials Registry, vol 2002. New York: Crohn's and Colitis Foundation of America; 2002. http://www.ccfa.org/clinical/trialp2.htm.

59. Greenhalgh T. *How to Read a Paper: The Basics of Evidence-Based Medicine,* 2nd ed. London: BMJ; 2000.

60. California Healthcare Institute Glossary Index, vol. 2002. LaJolla: California Healthcare Institute; 2002. http://www.chi.org/glossary.php.

61. Mulrow CD, Cornell JA, Herrera CR, Kadri A, Farnett L, Aguilar C. Hypertension in the elderly. Implications and generalizability of randomized trials. *JAMA.* 1994;272(24): 1932–1938.

62. Sackett DL. *Evidence-Based Medicine: How to Practice and Teach EBM,* 2nd Ed. Edinburgh: Churchill Livingstone; 2000.

2
Molecular and Biologic Factors in Aging

Charles Mobbs

Is "the biology of aging" a misnomer? Are there general principles that may usefully apply generally to senescence, or is senescence simply a collection of degenerative entropic processes that have in common only that they occur over time? Both views are supportable; indeed, the latter is perhaps the more common view among gerontologists and is the most supportable by evolutionary theory.[1]

However, gerontology, like geriatrics, has evolved into a discipline in part because senescence entails several general characteristics and because impairments associated with senescence are largely predictable within a species. For example, mortality (and other senescent changes) conform (within limits) to a precise mathematical description, the Gompertz curve, whose parameters are characteristic of each species.[2] Similarly, dietary restriction dramatically reduces many age-related impairments and increases maximum life span across a wide range of phyla.[3]

These general characteristics and the specificity of senescence require explanation, and seeking these explanations is the business of gerontology. Furthermore, recent studies have suggested that senescence may entail simpler and more orderly molecular processes than previously assumed. These general molecular processes may have profound consequences for geriatric practice, because far from ascribing age-related impairment merely to "old age," it may soon be as possible to treat some of these age-related impairments as any other disease.

Thus, some chronic age-related diseases may come to be viewed as symptoms of a more inclusive syndrome of senescence. This integration of geriatrics into the traditional medical model is an outcome of recent progress in gerontology.

Nomenclature

Aging: showing the effects of time; a process of change, usually gradual and spontaneous
Senescence: the loss of the power of cell division and growth (and function with time, leading to death) (*The New Shorter Oxford Dictionary*)

Gerontologists consider the term *aging* insufficiently precise because any process that occurs over time, for example, rusting or development, may be reasonably referred to as aging. Furthermore, although there are reasons to imagine that "aging" is a continuum beginning with development, these two terms are usually used to refer to distinct processes. Specifically, *development* (as in an embryo) refers to a *generative* process over time necessary for (and primarily evident at the beginning of) life, whereas *senescence* refers to a *degenerative* process ultimately incompatible with (and primarily evident at the end of) life. Whether development and aging form, in any informative way, a mechanistic continuum is a hypothesis that is far from proven. (Indeed, bibliographic database searches have been greatly complicated by the assignment of the term *aging* to the process of development, without a concomitant general use of the term *senescence*.) The distinction between aging and senescence is of more than academic interest because many changes that occur during aging may not be deleterious and may indeed be desirable. Thus, for example, the wisdom (or, at any rate, experience that ought to lead to wisdom) that increases with age is not usefully considered senescence, although it may be referred to as part of the aging process. Conversely, impairments in memory that occur during aging are usefully considered a manifestation of senescence. Thus, geriatrics is essentially concerned with senescence, not aging per se, except to promote aging with as little senescence as possible.

Theories of Aging

Is Senescence an Entropic Process?

The essential feature of degeneration as a concomitant to senescence immediately raises one of the most important questions in gerontology: is senescence merely a biologic manifestation of the second law of thermodynamics? An essential feature of life is the low level of internal entropy that characterizes biologic entities compared to the environment. Organisms maintain that low entropy state by conversion of external energy (with the result of a net increase in entropy, of course, when the organism and its environment are considered as a system). Mechanical objects such as automobiles or test tubes are also in a state of low entropy, but without the capacity to reduce internal entropy by converting external energy. Thus it is that mechanical objects accrue increased entropy over time "merely" as a mechanical manifestation of the second law and in that sense can plausibly be said to undergo senescence. Therefore the question arises: is senescence merely the accumulation of random events leading to a level of entropy that is incompatible with life? The key word in this formulation is *merely*. Ultimately, death is always a manifestation of entropy, but the pertinent question is, what is the proximal process that leaves the organism vulnerable to entropy? In short, do organisms senesce in a way fundamentally different from mechanical objects? By the view that senescence is merely a collection of degenerative processes that happen to occur over time, the second law would seem to be the only generally relevant principle operative. On the other hand, by the view that some general principles exist that subserve senescence, organisms would presumably differ fundamentally from mechanical objects.

The role of entropy may seem an abstraction, but an example will demonstrate its pertinence. A famous form of senescence is the death of the Pacific salmon.[4] After spawning, a predictable pattern of degenerative changes occurs, leading almost always to death. The question is, is this death "merely" the result of entropy? It would be as accurate to posit that death caused by smallpox (or starvation or myocardial infarction) is due to entropy. Such a formulation might be formally true, but it is more informative to ascribe the mechanism of senescence to its proximal biologic substrate—in the case of Pacific salmon, to the hyperactivity of the adrenal gland that accompanies the spawning process.[4]

In most forms of senescence, it has been much more difficult to determine the biologic substrate of the degenerative changes. This difficulty has given rise to the sense that degenerative changes with age are essentially random, for example, a manifestation of entropy. This view has been reinforced by the argument, developed convincingly by evolutionary biologists, that senescence did not evolve because it bestowed advantage on the species, but rather senescence is essentially an evolutionary by-product and, as such, is probably determined by the complex interaction of many genes with the environment.[1]

Evolutionary Theories of Aging

The fact that each species is characterized by a characteristic maximum life span whose value is essentially independent of environment indicates that, among species, senescence is determined genetically. The genetic constraint on maximum life span and rate of senescence has given rise to much speculation concerning the evolution of senescence. Early speculation around the turn of the nineteenth century was that senescence as a trait evolved, similar to most traits, because species that exhibited senescence would be more likely to survive than species which did not senesce. The general tone of such arguments was that species not exhibiting senescence would accumulate ill-adapted older members of the species that would compete with potentially better-adapted younger members of the species, effectively reducing the rate at which potentially adaptive mutations could be introduced into the species, thus slowing the rate of evolutionary adaptation. The lack of rigor of such arguments has long been recognized, and, particularly since Peter Medawar's landmark monograph in 1952,[5] there has been a consensus that senescence is not a trait that has been positively selected for but rather is a trait which has not been selected against. In particular, it has been assumed that the force of selection diminishes after reproduction, so that traits that facilitate successful reproduction will be selected for, even if such traits lead to death later in life. This general concept has been formulated mathematically by Charlesworth,[6] who concluded that even if an immortal species had ever existed, it would have eventually evolved to exhibit senescence.[7]

Although the mathematical formulation of Charlesworth is rigorous, there are challenges to the conclusions that may be drawn from this formulation because of the assumptions on which the analysis is based. For example, several species appear to exhibit extremely low, indeed virtually undetectable, rates of senescence.[8] Conversely, in some cases such as the Pacific salmon, there would indeed appear to be simple mechanisms that actively initiate and maintain senescent processes. Finally, as discussed below, several individual genes have been found whose continuing activity is by itself limiting to life span; furthermore, across phyla, these genes appear to be impinging on similar physiologic processes. If such a simple set of genes operated similarly in humans, it would be the object of great interest and perhaps a potential target for drug intervention. The existence of such genes poses a stark challenge to evolutionary analyses that imply that senescence could not be determined by the activity of a few genes or a developmental program.

Entropic Theories of Aging

The bewildering diversity of age-related impairments has led many gerontologists to conclude that no general mechanism is likely to underlie these changes. Furthermore, although there is a general sense that senescence might reflect an orderly unfolding of a genetic program as occurs during development, this view (which never had any real data to support it) has fallen out of favor with the rise of more sophisticated analyses of the evolution of senescence (see following). Nevertheless, gerontology has been a field characterized by a plethora of mechanistic theories. The most influential of these theories generally fall into two categories, which can broadly be referred to "loose cannon" theories and "weak link" theories.

The "loose cannon" theories posit that some entropy-producing agent is slowly wearing away at cellular macromolecular constituents. The most popular candidates have been free radicals[9,10] and glucose.[11–13] Free radicals are generated during oxidative phosphorylation and can, in theory, produce a variety of macromolecular modifications, primarily through oxidation. Considerable evidence suggests that oxidative damage increases with age.[14] This evidence includes the oxidation of specific amino acid residues in specific proteins that increases with age (having the effect of decreasing the specific activity of these proteins, a common observation during senescence),[15] and an increase in specific oxidized derivatives of nucleotides derived from DNA.[16–19] Furthermore, simultaneous overexpression of two different enzymes that attenuate free radical damage, superoxide dismutase and catalase, significantly increases the life span of fruit flies;[20] no effect was seen when only one enzyme was expressed. Similarly, exposure of nematodes to small molecules that mimic effects of superoxidase dismutase and catalse also increased life span.[21] These results are promising, but as yet the contribution of free radicals to senescence remains to be fully clarified.

The other popular candidate for a loose cannon is glucose. The major means by which glucose has been proposed to promote senescence is through nonenzymatic attachment to proteins and nucleic acids through Schiff base formation, followed by an irreversible formation of Amadori products, the same process that produces glycated hemoglobin.[11] As with oxidation, glycated proteins increase with age, and chemical blockade of the process of glycation delays at least some age-related

pathologies.[22] Furthermore, the fact that dietary restriction increases maximum life span and also reduces blood glucose and rate of glycation has continued to stimulate interest in the possible role glycation may play in the process of senescence.[12] It should also be noted that free radical mechanisms and glycation mechanisms are not mutually exclusive, because glycation can cause free radical production.[23] However, a major difficulty with the free radical and glycation theories, and indeed with all such theories, is that they are of little value in predicting the specific physiologic impairments that characterize the senescence of each species.

The "weak link" theories posit that a specific physiologic system is particularly vulnerable (presumably to entropic processes) during senescence, and when this system fails, it produces cascading effects that accelerate dysfunction of the whole organism. The two most popular candidates for the weak link theories are the neuroendocrine system and the immune system. Both the neuroendocrine system and the immune system exhibit profound and specific functional impairments during aging. Failure of the neuroendocrine system would be expected to produce profound impairments in homeostatic systems, including the loss of reproduction and metabolic regulation that is observed during aging. For example, secretion of growth hormone decreases robustly with age in humans and other species, and replacement of growth hormone has been reported to restore a variety of physiologic functions in aging rats and elderly men.[24] Similarly, failure of the immune system would be expected to produce increased susceptibility to infection and decreased ability to reject tumor cells, also observed during aging.

However, in general there is little evidence that failure of either system directly contributes to age-related diseases or mortality. For example, it now appears in fact that, far from the expected relationship between declining growth hormone and age-related mortality, mice with growth hormone deficiency exhibit increased life span compared to wild-type mice, whereas mice with elevated growth hormone exhibit reduced life span.[25] Similarly, although autoimmune processes cause type I (juvenile) diabetes, this form of diabetes occurs mainly in young individuals, whereas the form of diabetes that occurs during aging does not appear to involve immune impairments. Furthermore, even though neuroendocrine and immune systems do exhibit impairments with age, little is known about the more primary mechanisms that drive these changes. Therefore, in their current incarnations, none of the entropic theories of aging are complete, and it cannot be said that considerable evidence supports the idea that any of these mechanisms underlie the impairments and death that are associated with aging.

Physiology of Aging

As organisms age, they accrue functional impairments in virtually every physiologic system. In humans, Nathan Shock and his coworkers developed a general rule of thumb that many physiologic systems accrue impairments at a rate of about 5% to 10% per decade after the age of 30 or so.[26] A well-known example of this principle is the decrease in maximum tolerable heart rate.[27] In aerobic training, the maximum heart rate (Rh) recommended during training is given by the equation Rh = (244 − age) ∗ 0.8.

This equation is based on the general rule of thumb that a heart rate more than 80% of maximum attainable during a stress test is dangerous, and that the maximum heart rate attainable during a stress test reliably decreases by about 1 beat per minute each year during aging. The rate of this decline is reduced by about half in highly trained athletes, but even in such athletes, maximum heart rate and maximum oxygen consumption rate nevertheless decline with age.[27] Many other functions change gradually during aging (blood glucose, grip strength, fertility), and with time the death rate from many different causes increases.

The Gompertz Curve

The essential feature of senescence, at least when applied to mortality, is that the rate at which death occurs increases with time. If the rate at which death occurred were constant (e.g., age independent), then the term senescence would not be applicable. In most species, senescence, manifest as an increase in the rate of mortality with age, can be described by a remarkably simple mathematical function. The rate of mortality of most species that have been studied, including flies, nematodes, and rodents, increases exponentially with time, first observed in humans by Benjamin Gompertz after observing actuarial statistics and reported in 1825. The Gompertz equation can be stated succinctly as $Rm(t) = -(1/n)$ ∗ $dn/dt = R_0 e^{(at)}$, where $Rm(t)$ is the mortality rate at time or age t, $n =$ the number of survivors at time t, R_0 is the mortality rate at time $t = 0$, interpreted as a vulnerability factor depending on the hostility of the environment, and a is a rate constant dependent on the species. This equation can be linearized by log transform into $lnRm(t) = ln(R_0) + at$.

The intercept of this line is generally dependent on the hostility of the environment, whereas the slope is dependent on the genetic background of the population, for example, the species or strain. A goal of gerontology is to be able to derive the constants of the Gompertz curve, especially the slope of the linearized form, from the analysis of the biologic characteristics of the species.

Although this derivation is far from accomplished, simply being able to formulate such a precisely quantitative question is evidence of the state of gerontology as a scientific discipline. Analysis suggests that at least the form of the Gompertz curve may arise from evolutionary effects, involving a decline in the force of natural selection acting on age-specific mortality.[28] The extent to which this insight may contribute to a more mechanistic understanding of the process of senescence remains to be determined.

The relationship between the survival curves, rate of mortality, and the Gompertz transform is illustrated in by the idealized depictions of Figure 2.1. In the top panel (A), the survival curve (fraction of initial population left alive as age increases) of a typical ("normal") population is compared with the survival curve of a genetically similar population placed into an optimum environment ("enhanced environment") or a population modified genetically or subject to dietary restriction. Note that an enhanced environment can increase average life span by "rectangularization" of the survival curve, but the maximum life span (indicated by the age at which the fraction of the population left alive drops below an arbitrarily small number) is not influenced by environment. In contrast, genetic variance and dietary restriction can increase not only average life span but maximum life span as well. When these same data are plotted in terms of rate of mortality (the number of individuals that have died over an arbitrarily small unit of time), the mortality rate of all groups increases exponentially with age and reaches the same high rate toward the end of life; the groups differ in that environment can delay the exponential increase (although then the rate increases even faster toward the end of life), whereas genotype and dietary restriction can actually change the rate at which mortality rate increases. Because mortality rate increases exponentially with age, these effects are more easily understood by subjecting the rate data to a logarithmic transform. After such a transform, log (mortality rate) increases linearly with time. Normal and enhanced environment groups have similar slopes. If anything, the enhanced environment group may exhibit a slightly higher slope because the intercept is lower, whereas genotype and dietary restriction can actually decrease the slope of this transform.

When the rate of mortality becomes high enough, an arbitrarily small number of individuals will be left alive at time t_m, the maximum life span. In practice, maximum life span is determined empirically, and in humans is generally assumed to be around 125 years (for women; somewhat lower for men). Although the idealization of Figure 2.1 illustrates the case in which the Gompertz relation holds across the entire life span, in actual populations the Gompertz curve actually only applies to the rate of mortality between sometime after puberty and sometime well

FIGURE 2.1. Three views of mortality. (A) Fraction of population left alive as a function of age. *Normal*, standard population dynamics; *enhanced environment*, dynamic pattern as might be observed by idealized optimization of environment, leading to "rectangularization" of the survival curve; *enhanced genotype or dietary restriction*, dynamic pattern observed by single gene mutations that extend maximum life span (such as AGE-1) or by dietary restriction regimens that extend maximum life span. (B) View of the same data as in A, but plotted as rate of mortality. Depicted in this way, rate of mortality increases exponentially with age (Gompertz function). (C) Logarithmic transformation of the data in B. Note that rectangularization of the mortality curve may decrease initial rate of mortality but does not necessarily increase maximum life span and may indeed lead to increased mortality rate during the late period of life, whereas genetic or dietary enhancement of maximal life span is expected to entail decreased rate of mortality but not necessarily a decreased initial mortality rate.

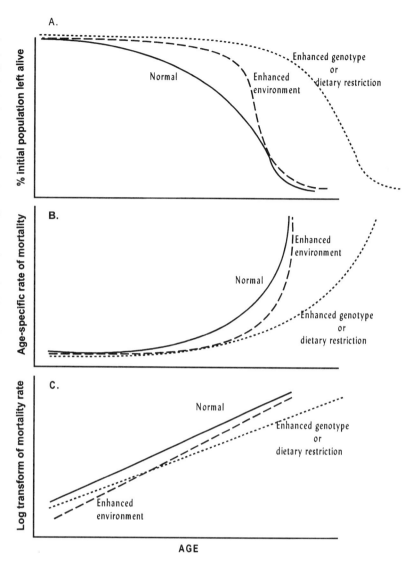

short of maximum life span. In humans, the generally accepted range of applicability is between ages 20 and 80 or so. A particularly interesting recent development is evidence in both humans and other species[29,30] that the slope of the linearized Gompertz equation (that is, the increase in the rate of mortality, or the second derivative of survival) begins to decrease at very old ages, and possibly the rate of mortality becomes constant (e.g., independent of age) in populations composed of very old individuals. These remarkable results have profound implications for our view of the process of senescence, because senescence necessarily entails an increased rate of mortality with age. Thus under some circumstances (in very old individuals), there is evidence that senescence itself may slow dramatically, possibly even to zero (keeping in mind, however, that even if the rate of mortality does not increase, the high rate of mortality already characteristic of old individuals ensures a fast depletion of the population). The role of selection from within a

population of heterologous individuals in this phenomenon has yet to be determined.

Pathology Versus Senescence

The Gompertz equation applies not only to mortality but also to diseases and may be used to resolve a major and controversial conceptual issue facing gerontologists and geriatricians: is there a valid distinction between pathology, or disease, and what is commonly (although, as we have seen, unrigorously) called normal aging? This distinction is not merely semantic but addresses fundamental questions of mechanism.

As with mortality, the rate of onset of many diseases increases exponentially with age. (In the following analysis, it is essential to keep in mind the difference between incidence, that is, the rate of new cases that occur at a given age, and prevalence, which is the total number of cases in a population of that age; rate equations such as the Gompertz curve only describe incidence, and thus incidence is the most informative from a mechanistic point of view. With regard to mortality, one generally is inherently referring to incidence, for example, the rate at which death occurs, because the equivalent of prevalence with respect to mortality, such as survival curves, would include the cumulative number of individuals who have died, not a particularly useful statistic with respect to mechanism. However, there is an extremely important difference in the application of rate equations to disease and mortality. As already described, the applicability of the Gompertz equation to mortality begins to break down at about age 85 or so, and the slope of the line (the second derivative of survival) begins to decrease. Nevertheless, the rate of mortality (the first derivative of survival) does not appear to decrease with time; that is, the rate of mortality continues to increase with age, or at least is constant at a very high level in very old individuals.

The incidence rate of diseases increases exponentially up to the age of maximum incidence, the age depending on the disease, but then the incidence of disease begins to decrease. Not only does the rate of increase of incidence begin to fall, but the absolute incidence of new cases declines after some age. For example, the incidence of new cases of type I diabetes increases from around 9 months of age and peaks around 14 years of age (depending on the population);[31,32] after this age, the incidence of type I diabetes declines[31] to a lower constant rate. Thus, after the age of peak incidence, the incidence rate decreases to a low rate that is independent of age, a common pattern for age-related diseases. Of course, the prevalence of the disease, representing the total accumulation of patients with the disease, increases over time. Type II diabetes follows a similar pattern, although shifted to much later ages, such that the peak incidence of type II diabetes occurs around 70 years to age, after which the age-specific incidence rate begins to decrease;[33] because the incidence rate falls or becomes constant after the peak age of incidence, it may be said that senescence is no longer operating on this disease after the age of peak incidence. Similarly, the age-specific incidence of Huntington's disease peaks around 40 years of age,[34] the age-specific incidence of Parkinson's disease peaks at about 75 years of age,[35] and the age-specific incidence rate of Alzheimer's disease appears to peak at about 90 years of age.[36]

These examples also indicate the important mechanistic implications of incidence rate data. Typically, the incidence rate of familial forms of age-related diseases peaks at earlier ages than the nonfamilial or sporadic forms. Thus, mutations in the *parkin* gene lead to juvenile-onset Parkinson's disease, whose incidence peaks around 20 years of age, and the incidence of Parkinson's disease from mutations in alpha-synuclein peaks around age 50.[37] In contrast, the incidence rate of Parkinson's disease in the population as a whole peaks around age 70.[35] Because twin studies have indicated that genotype makes little contribution to the late-onset (and most common) form of the disease, taken together these data imply that the contribution of genotype to Parkinson's phenotype increases with age up until about age 50, then begins to decline, such that by age 70 there is little contribution of genotype to phenotype.[37]

Gompertz analysis may also clarify the distinction between disease and nonpathologic processes of senescence, because processes whose incidence increases monotonically with age (including mortality) may be usefully considered a senescent process, whereas conditions whose incidences reach maxima before maximum life span are more usefully considered age-related pathology or disease. The mechanistic implications of the distinction between disease and senescence may be clarified by an example. As described, the incidence of Alzheimer's disease continues to increase until late in life. In addition, gradual impairments in memory functions also increase monotonically with age. A major question therefore has been: Is Alzheimer's disease an accentuated form of the more universal impairments in memory function? Were this hypothesis correct, one implication is that if we live long enough, everyone would contract Alzheimer's disease. However, careful analysis of the incidence of Alzheimer's disease has demonstrated that, as in all diseases, the incidence of Alzheimer's disease reaches a peak well before maximum life span. Thus, for example, centenarians exhibit a lower incidence of Alzheimer's disease than individuals between 70 and 80.[36] This finding indicates that Alzheimer's disease is not merely an accentuated form of "normal" age-related changes but is a distinct pathologic process (an conclusion supported by detailed analysis of brain tissue); conversely, the more universal (but milder) cognitive impairments observed during aging are not likely to be caused by the same mechanism as that which causes Alzheimer's disease. This conclusion is corroborated by rigorous clinical and pathologic analysis that demonstrates that neither the clinical nor the pathologic profile of Alzheimer's disease is in detail similar to the profile of normal aging.[38]

Nevertheless, one caveat must be made regarding the distinction between senescence and disease. Age-related diseases do, by definition, exhibit an age dependency, raising the question whether the development of these diseases is, in some fundamental sense, related to the underlying process of senescence, even if diseases can be dissociated from senescence. One reason for suspecting a mechanistic link between many diseases and senescence is that, in animal models, dietary restriction not only increases maximum life span but also dramatically decreases many age-related diseases such as cancer.[39–45] Naturally, much of the interest of gerontology is the possibility of some general principle subserving both senescence and the diseases associated with senescence. The fact that dietary restriction appears to concomitantly delay both senescence and disease suggests that such principles may exist.

Individual Variability

The Gompertz curve for both disease and senescence is essentially a mathematical statement of individual variability. Thus, a few individuals in the population die early, and increasingly more individuals die as the population ages. Similarly, a few individuals contract a disease (type II diabetes) at young ages, and increasingly more contract the disease as the population ages (until rate of incidence begins to decrease again, as discussed previously). Furthermore, a perhaps underappreciated fact is that senescence (in the United States, at least) is not usually accompanied by debilitating illness. For example, only 5.2% of the elderly is in nursing homes (a percentage that has been decreasing in recent years, despite the increase in the average age of the population over 65).[46–49] Similarly, recent studies indicate that more than 70% of persons between ages 75 and 84 report no disability, again a number that has decreased in recent years.[46–49]

These and other studies indicate that despite the fact that the population is growing older, the amount of debilitating illness is actually decreasing. Until recently, it had been assumed that reducing illness would increase average life span but not maximum life span. Thus it was assumed that eliminating disease would in effect increase average life span but increase the rate at which individuals die once advanced old age was attained (the so-called rectilinearization of the survival curve). However, recent evidence suggests that, remarkably, even though individuals are staying healthier longer, the rate of death is not increasing.[29] As already discussed, this remarkable and surprising phenomenon may be a reflection of the fact that the Gompertz slope begins to flatten after age 85 or so. If this analysis continues to pertain (and there is evidence from studies in flies that this flattening of the Gompertz curve is a general aspect of senescence), the implication is that very likely the apparent maximum life span of humans will continue to increase (although slowly).

These observations lead to two questions. First, what determines if an individual will contract an age-related disease? Second, what is the basis of the unexpected phenomenon that the incidence of age-related diseases is decreasing while average age (and possibly average life span) is increasing? Better medical technology is probably an important factor in facilitating survival after diseases are contracted, and if the diseases are entirely cured, as occurs with infectious diseases and sometimes cancer, although rarely with chronic diseases such as diabetes and cardiovascular disease, there is a higher probability that the individual will live beyond the age of high incidence of diseases. Nevertheless, the more important determinant of longevity is whether the individual contracts a major disease to begin with. The most general determinants of disease risk are hereditary and environment. At least with regard to longevity and average functionality, recent evidence suggests that in humans there is relatively little heritablity of longevity.[50] Therefore, at the moment, it appears that outcome during aging depends largely on what is generally referred to as lifestyle, such as decreased smoking, increased exercise, and better diet. In addition, the apparent increase in healthy (and perhaps maximum) life span is due to the logic of senescence versus pathology: once one has gotten past the age of maximum incidence of most diseases, one can live a relatively healthy life until true senescence becomes the limiting factor in the maintenance of function (which occurs in most humans only at very advanced age).

Aging: Usual Versus Successful

Consideration of individual differences in susceptibility to pathology and the trajectory of senescence has informed a very useful construct, developed by Rowe and Kahn,[51] between "usual aging" and "successful aging" (in this accessible formulation, aging is used as a synonym for senescence). Usual aging refers to the common complex of diseases and impairments that characterizes some of the aging population. However, as just discussed, individuals vary greatly in their manifestation of the diseases and impairments of aging, and some individuals seem to escape these diseases altogether, eventually dying, as former medical practice described it, of "old age," there not being any particularly more compelling pathology to which to ascribe the death. These individuals would certainly seem to exhibit the trajectory of senescence to which we would all aspire—an active healthy life until the very end. Indeed the very end of such individuals is usually rather late in life, because once one has aged past the time at which the incidence of most diseases is maximum, the probability of life-threatening disease, by definition, decreases.

The concept of successful aging has important implications for the practice of geriatrics. Thus, in the Neolithic period (and in some societies even now) near total tooth loss during aging was not only usual but almost universal; toothlessness was "usual," but not "successful." Nevertheless, it is now understood that toothlessness can be largely avoided, and clinicians encourage their patients to make the appropriate changes in personal habits to ensure successful (dental) aging. Although many, or perhaps most, aging individuals have in the past exhibited a range of debilitating diseases, a major and achievable goal is to decrease the incidence (and prevalence) of these diseases and risk factors in the elderly, rather than simply chalking them up to "old age." This approach implies that, from a clinical point of view, the temptation to "define deviancy down" during aging should be resisted, and the elderly should be held to the same criteria of health (glycemia, adiposity, etc.) as younger individuals are held. Such a position runs counter to the current practice of following age-adjusted charts for targeting physiologic parameters (such as blood pressure). Although maintaining a youthful profile (for example, with adiposity) becomes more difficult during aging, it is still an appropriate goal for physicians and their patients.

Molecular and Cellular Basis of Senescence

Limits to Cell Division: Role of Telomerase

The great diversity of age-related impairments, combined with the evolutionary arguments already described, have discouraged the idea that senescence could be an outcome of relatively simple and regulated molecular processes analogous with development. However, recent studies have suggested that reductionism is as powerful a strategy in gerontology as in other biologic disciplines.

One of the most important phenomena studied by gerontologists is the process by which cells lose their ability to divide over time unless the cells convert to an abnormal cancerous phenotype.[52,53] This limit to cellular replicative capacity can even be demonstrated in cell culture after removing the cells from the body. For example, when fibroblasts are removed from the umbilical cord of newborn humans and cultured in vitro, they will divide until they are dense enough to contact each other, then stop dividing, due to a phenomenon called contact inhibition. However, if the cells are diluted, they will divide again until a maximum density again occurs. This process can be repeated for about 50 times; each repeated division is called a passage. However, after about 50 passages, the cells cease to divide, regardless of the density. This limit to cellular replicative capacity is called the Hayflick phenomenon or Hayflick limit, in honor of its discoverer Leonard Hayflick. The Hayflick limit demonstrated in vitro has been thought to reflect actual processes that occur in vivo because fibroblasts removed from older individuals tend to exhibit a decreased number of maximum passages. The loss of replicative capacity is dependent not on the total amount of time that the cells are cultured (chronological age) but rather on the number of divisions (biologic age).[54]

For decades, the Hayflick phenomenon has been considered to be an excellent and experimentally accessible model of organismic senescence. When cells reach their final stages of division, they do not immediately die, but enlarge and may exist for some time before gradually dying. Cells in these final stages exhibit many differences from either "younger" dividing cells at earlier passages of division or younger cells whose division has been arrested by experimental manipulation. Thus, these "senescent" cells are like senescent organisms by virtue of these numerous differences. Over the years, many mechanisms have been suggested to mediate the Hayflick phenomenon, including free radicals, accumulated mutations, and overexpression of "gerontogenes" secondary to random epigenetic changes in DNA, such as loss of cytosine methylation, or, most likely, a combination of many different processes.

Nevertheless, it has now become clear that replicative senescence may, in fact, be regulated by a relatively small number of genes.[55] Among these, the gene coding for the enzyme telomerase may be particularly important.[56] Telomeres are stretches of DNA at the end of chromosome that serve essentially as handles by which the chromosomes are moved during the telophase of meiosis. In transformed cells and during meiosis, the enzyme telomerase is present, which lengthens the telomere after telophase. However, in normal cells after cessation of development, this enzyme is expressed at very low levels, so after each cell division the telomere becomes shorter and shorter.[56] After about 50 divisions (for human fibroblasts, at least), the telomeres are lost and mitosis is no longer possible. Although this observation by itself does not prove that the loss of the telomeres is the proximal cause of the cessation of mitosis, restoration of telomerase activity by genetic engineering dramatically increases the number of cell divisions of otherwise normal cells well past the Hayflick limit.[57]

This extension of in vitro life span by overexpression of telomerase, although dramatic, does not prove that telomerase shortening is the only mechanism by which cells senesce in vitro. For example, prior studies demonstrated that mRNA transferred from senescent cells into early passage cells would stop cell division in the young cells.[52] The normal function of such "gerontogenes" may be similar to that of anti-oncogenes, such as p53.[58] Mutations in p53 lead to uncontrolled cell division, cancer, and often death of the organism. There appear to be at least two classes of these gerontogenes, both of which must be inactivated to produce cellular immortalization.[59] It has now been shown that mutations in these classes of gerontogenes extend the number of cells past which cells may divide.[58,59]

Thus, as for many diseases, it may be said that in vitro senescence may be caused by a variety of factors, but on the other hand these factors are enumerable and specific. For example, diabetes may be caused by an autoimmune attack or a mutation in several different genes. However, the number of gene mutations that cause diabetes are probably small, and the genes whose mutations do cause diabetes are probably involved in a small number of specific metabolic pathways. Similarly, the molecular causes of in vitro senescence, although not confined to a single gene, are probably simpler than was once thought to be plausible.

Senescence in *Caenorhabditis elegans*: Role of Genes in an Insulin-Like Signaling Pathway Acting on Neurons

The relevance of the Hayflick phenomenon to senescence in the whole organism is not entirely clear. Certainly there are some cells that divide more or less continuously throughout life (intestinal epithelia, skin fibroblast), but it is unlikely that such cells approach the limit of 50 cell divisions. Even if they did, most gerontologists agree that the cells most likely to cause functional failure during senescence are cells that either divide very little (immune and endocrine cells) or not at all (neurons and muscle cells). Furthermore, many metazoans are composed entirely of postmitotic cells, yet exhibit senescence that is just as predictable and robust as the senescence of animals which contain mitotic cells.

The nematode *Caenorhabditis elegans* is precisely such an animal, consisting entirely of postmitotic cells that exhibit a reliable trajectory of senescence, including adherence to the Gompertz equation. *C. elegans* has become a useful model for genetic analysis because, owing to its optional hermaphroditic reproductive mode, genetic manipulation is relatively simple. In addition, all its postmitotic cells have been mapped. These properties have made *C. elegans* a dominant model in developmental biology and, beginning about 20 years ago,[60] *C. elegans* began to be studied as a potential model for aging research as well. One of the early dividends of this work was the establishment of a group of genetic mutations that lead to an extension of maximum life span, for example, genes that when active decrease maximum life span.[61–63] Particularly striking was the discovery that mutation in a single gene, termed *age-1*, reduces the Gompertz rate of mortality in *C. elegans*.[62] The existence of such a gene was largely unexpected, given evolutionary arguments implying that senescence is unlikely to be controlled by even a small number of genes.[1] When this gene was cloned, it was discovered to code for a homologue of mammalian phosphatidylinositol-3-OH kinase.[64] Although this clearly suggested a neuroendocrine mechanism, the ligand pathway mediated by this kinase was initially unclear. Subsequent to the discovery of *age-1*, however, other single genes were discovered that also extended life span in *C. elegans*; among these genes, DAF-2 was subsequently cloned and discovered to code for a homologue of the mammalian insulin receptor.[65]

Further genetic analysis has now conclusively demonstrated that single gene defects extending life span act through an insulin signaling pathway remarkably similar to the mammalian insulin signaling pathway.[66]

In essence, therefore, these studies indicate that senescence (or at least a major component of senescence, as defects in this pathway reduce the Gompertz slope) arises from the activity of an insulin-like pathway. As described below, considerable evidence has suggested that senescence may arise from metabolic activity. Therefore, a logical hypothesis is that an insulin-like pathway drives senescence in *C. elegans* by enhancing metabolic activity. On the other hand, transgenic manipulation has now demonstrated that it is activity of the insulin-like pathway specifically in neurons, not muscle or other highly metabolically active tissue, that regulates life span in *C. elegans*.[67] Furthermore, the life-extending effects of the insulin-like pathway appear to require activity of an unusual cytoplasmic catalase.[68] Taken together, these data suggest that reduction of senescence by attenuating the insulin-like pathway entails protection of neurons from free radical damage and that, conversely, integrity of neurons sensitive to this insulin-like pathway constitutes a limiting factor in the life span of *C. elegans*.[67] The specific nature of these neurons remains to be established, but in mammals the neurons most sensitive to insulin are probably the hypothalamic neurons that regulate metabolism and body weight, destruction of which leads to profound metabolic impairments.[69] Whether destruction of these neurons by free radical damage is a limiting factor in life span remains to be determined.

Other Single Genes Regulating Maximum Life Span

Single gene defects have now also been shown to increase maximum life span in fruit flies,[70,71] yeast,[72,73] and mice.[74–76] The function of all these "gerontogenes" is not yet completely determined, but it is plausible that, as in *C. elegans*, they all act through pathways that either mediate or are regulated by insulin-like signals. The clearest example would be in mice, in which genetic ablation of growth hormone or the growth hormone receptor extends maximum life span.[74,75] It is thought that most if not all major effects of growth hormone are mediated through the insulin-like growth factor pathway, whose molecular mechanisms are highly homologous to pathways mediating insulin signaling.[77] Ablation of p66Shc, which appears to mediate some effects of growth factors including insulin[78] and may also enhance oxidative damage,[76] also extends maximum life span in mice.[76] This latter observation was particularly striking because, unlike the gerontogenes studied in *C. elegans* or mutations in the growth hormone pathway in mice, ablation of p66Shc had no apparent effect on fertility or other functions,[76] suggesting that increased life span need not entail reduced functionality in adulthood. Thus, as in *C. elegans*, it appears that in mammals as well activity of an insulin-like pathway (possibly by enhancing oxidative damage) limits life span, and ablation of single genes that mediate this pathway extends life span. In *Drosophila*, ablation of two genes is also known to enhance life span. The first, termed *methuselah*, appears to code for a G-coupled protein receptor,[70] implying that this gene mediates an endocrine pathway, but the ligand for this receptor has not yet been identified. The second, termed *indy*, appears to code for a dicarboxylate cotransporter.[71] Thus, whereas interference with insulin-like pathways may extend life span by indirectly reducing metabolic function, a similar increase in life span may be obtained with direct interference with metabolism. As with ablation of p66Shc, partial ablation of *indy* increased life span in flies without producing any apparent deficit in fertility or other functions,[71] again indicating that increased life span need not entail impairments in functionality.

Possibly analogous with the effects of *indy*, a single gene, *SIR-2*, has been shown to regulate life span in yeast.[72,73] In this case, however, enhanced expression of *SIR-2* leads to increased life span, at least as measured in yeast.[72,73] *SIR-2* has been shown to regulate chromatin state through a histone acetylase activity, leading to a reduction in chromatin fragmentation that constitutes a concomitant of yeast senescence.[72,73] Although it is questionable if this property of *SIR-2* is relevant to aging in metazoans, a perhaps more pertinent property of *SIR-2* is that its activity is enhanced by the allosteric binding of NAD^+.[72] Thus, as glucose is metabolized to produce NADH from NAD^+, *SIR-2* would become less active, leading to a state more likely to senesce. Indeed, the investigators went on to demonstrate that, by analogy with dietary restriction, reduction in glucose concentration extends life span in yeast, and this effect requires the presence of *SIR-2* and also requires the synthesis of NAD^+.[73] These data suggest, consistent with results from other organisms, that metabolic activity does indeed drive the process of senescence. However, at least in yeast, it is not entropic effects of free radical damage, but the regulation of cellular processes by glucose metabolites (in particular AND^+), that drives the process of senescence.

Conclusion

Although senescence is undoubtedly a complex phenomenon, and there are sound reasons grounded in evolutionary theory to believe that the process cannot be simply explained in terms of a small number of genes, nevertheless much progress has been made using the same reductionist approach that has been successful in studying other aspects of biology. The specific examples presented in this brief review are by no means exhaustive. For example, a gene for Werner's syndrome, a progerioid syndrome in humans, has recently been cloned, and has proved to be a gene involved in DNA replication.[79] Thus, although the complexities of senescence continue to command considerable respect, there is also reason to be optimistic that more powerful simple mechanisms may be elucidated in the near future.

References

1. Rose MR. Can human aging be postponed? *Sci Am.* 1999; 281:106–111.
2. Riggs JE. The Gompertz function: distinguishing mathematical from biological limitations. *Mech Ageing Dev.* 1993; 69:33–36.
3. Masoro EJ. Caloric restriction and aging: an update. *Exp Gerontol.* 2000;35:299–305.
4. Robertson OH. Prolongation of the lifespan of kokanee salmon (*O. nerka kennerlyi*) by castration before beginning development. *Proc Natl Acad Sci USA.* 1961;47:609–621.
5. Medawar PB. *An Unsolved Problem in Biology.* London: Lewis, 1952.
6. Charlesworth B. Evolutionary mechanisms of senescence. *Genetica.* 1993;91:11–19.
7. Charlesworth B. *Evolution in Age-Structured Populations.* Cambridge Studies in Mathematical Biology, vol 13. Cambridge: Cambridge University Press; 1994:306.
8. Finch CE. Longevity, senescence, and the genome. The John D. and Catherine T. MacArthur Foundation Series on Mental Health and Development. Chicago: Chicago University Press; 1996.
9. Sohal RS, Weindruch R. Oxidative stress, caloric restriction, and aging, *Science.* 1996;273:59–63.
10. Beckman KB, Ames BN. The free radical theory of aging matures. *Physiol Rev.* 1998;78:547–581.
11. Cerami A. Hypothesis. Glucose as a mediator of aging. *J Am Geriatr Soc.* 1985;33:626–634.
12. Masoro EJ, Katz MS, McMahan CA. Evidence for the glycation hypothesis of aging from the food-restricted rodent model. *J Gerontol.* 1989;44:B20–B22.
13. Mobbs CV. Neurotoxic effects of estrogen, glucose, and glucocorticoids: neurohumoral hysteresis and its pathological consequences during aging. *Rev Biol Res Aging.* 1990;4:201–228.
14. Dubey A, Forster MJ, Lal H, Sohal RS. Effect of age and caloric intake on protein oxidation in different brain regions and on behavioral functions of the mouse. *Arch Biochem Biophys.* 1996;333:189–197.
15. Dulic V, Gafni A. Mechanism of aging of rat muscle glyceraldehyde-3-phosphate dehydrogenase studied byselective enzyme-oxidation. *Mech Ageing Dev.* 1987;40:289–306.
16. Shigenaga MK, Hagen TM, Ames BN. Oxidative damage and mitochondrial decay in aging. *Proc Natl Acad Sci USA.* 1994;91:10771–10778.

17. Ames BN. Measuring oxidative damage in humans: relation to cancer and ageing. *IARC Sci Publ.* 1988;89:407–416.

18. Wagner JR, Hu CC, Ames BN. Endogenous oxidative damage of deoxycytidine in DNA. *Proc Natl Acad Sci USA.* 1992;89:3380–3384.

19. Helbock HJ, Beckman KB, Shigenaga MK, et al. DNA oxidation matters: the HPLC-electrochemical detection assay of 8-oxo-deoxyguanosine and 8-oxo-guanine. *Proc Natl Acad Sci USA.* 1998;95:288–293.

20. Orr WC, Sohal RS. Extension of life-span by overexpression of superoxide dismutase and catalase in *Drosophila melanogaster. Science.* 1994;263:1128–1130.

21. Melov S, Ravenscroft J, Malik S, et al. Extension of life-span with superoxide dismutase/catalase mimetics. *Science.* 2000; 289:1567–1569.

22. Li YM, Steffes M, Donnelly T, et al. Prevention of cardiovascular and renal pathology of aging by the advanced glycation inhibitor aminoguanidine. *Proc Natl Acad Sci USA.* 1996;93:3902–3907.

23. Munch G, Schinzel R, Loske C, et al. Alzheimer's disease—synergistic effects of glucose deficit, oxidative stress and advanced glycation endproducts. *J Neural Transm.* 1998; 105:439–461.

24. Xu X, Sonntag WE. Growth hormone and the biology of aging. In: Mobbs CV, Hof P, eds. *Functional Endocrinology of Aging.* Basel: Karger; 1998:67–88.

25. Bartke A. Growth hormone and aging. *Endocrine.* 1998; 8:103–108.

26. Shock NW. Systems physiology and aging: introduction. *Fed Proc.* 1979;38:161–162.

27. Rogers MA, Hagberg JM, Martin WHd, Ehsani AA, Holloszy JO. Decline in VO$_2$max with aging in master athletes and sedentary men. *J Appl Physiol.* 1990;68: 2195–2199.

28. Mueller LD, Rose MR. Evolutionary theory predicts late-life mortality plateaus. *Proc Natl Acad Sci USA.* 1996;93:15249–15253.

29. Vaupel JW, Carey JR, Christensen K, et al. Biodemographic trajectories of longevity. *Science.* 1998;280:855–860.

30. Curtsinger JW, Fukui HH, Townsend DR, Vaupel JW. Demography of genotypes: failure of the limited life-span paradigm in *Drosophila melanogaster. Science.* 1992; 258:461–463.

31. Christau B, Kromann H, Christy M, Andersen OO, Nerup J. Incidence of insulin-dependent diabetes mellitus (0–29 years at onset) in Denmark. *Acta Med Scand Suppl.* 1979; 624:54–60.

32. Vandewalle CL, Coeckelberghs MI, De Leeuw IH, et al. Epidemiology, clinical aspects, and biology of IDDM patients under age 40 years. Comparison of data from Antwerp with complete ascertainment with data from Belgium with 40% ascertainment. The Belgian diabetes Registry. *Diabetes Care.* 1997; 20:1556–1561.

33. Rockwood K, Awalt E, MacKnight C, McDowell I. Incidence and outcomes of diabetes mellitus in elderly people: report from the Canadian Study of Health and Aging. *Can Med Assoc J.* 2000;162:769–772.

34. Greenamyre JT, Shoulson I. Huntington's disease. In: Calne DB, ed. *Neurodegenerative Diseases.* Philadelphia: Saunders; 1994:685–704.

35. Martilla RJ. Epidemiology. In: Koller W, ed. *Handbook of Parkinson's Disease.* New York: Dekker; 1987:55–50.

36. Lautenschlager NT, Cupples LA, Rao VS, et al. Risk of dementia among relatives of Alzheimer's disease patients in the MIRAGE study: what is in store for the oldest old? *Neurology.* 1996;46:641–650.

37. Langston JW. Epidemiology versus gentics in Parkinson's disease: progress in resolving an age-old debate. *Ann Neurol.* 1998;44:S45–S52.

38. Morrison JH, Hof PR. Life and death of neurons in the aging brain. *Science.* 1997;278:412–419.

39. Turturro A, Hart R. Dietary alteration in the rates of cancer and aging. *Exp Gerontol.* 1992;27:583–592.

40. Turturro A, Blank K, Murasko D, Hart R. Mechanisms of caloric restriction affecting aging and disease. *Ann NY Acad Sci.* 1994;719:159–170.

41. Sheldon WG, Bucci TJ, Hart RW, Turturro A. Age-related neoplasia in a lifetime study of ad libitum-fed and food-restricted B6C3F1 mice. *Toxicol Pathol.* 1995;23:458–476.

42. Sheldon WG, Warbritton AR, Bucci TJ, Turturro A. Glaucoma in food-restricted and ad libitum-fed DBA/2NNia mice. *Lab Anim Sci.* 1995;45:508–518.

43. Hart RW, Turturro A. Dietary restrictions and cancer. *Environ Health Perspect.* 1997;105(suppl 4):989–992.

44. Duffy PH, Leakey JE, Pipkin JL, Turturro A, Hart RW. The physiologic, neurologic, and behavioral effects of caloric restriction related to aging, disease, and environmental factors. *Environ Res.* 1997;73:242–248.

45. Wolf NS, Li Y, Pendergrass W, Schmeider C, Turturro A. Normal mouse and rat strains as models for age-related cataract and the effect of caloric restriction on its development. *Exp Eye Res.* 2000;70:683–692.

46. Manton KG, Corder L, Stallard E. Chronic disability trends in elderly United States populations: 1982–1994. *Proc Natl Acad Sci USA.* 1997;94:2593–2598.

47. Manton KG, Stallard E, Corder L. Changes in the age dependence of mortality and disability: cohort and other determinants. *Demography.* 1997;34:135–157.

48. Manton KG, Stallard E. Changes in health, mortality, and disability and their impact on long-term care needs. *J Aging Soc Policy.* 1996;7:25–52.

49. Manton KG, Stallard E, Corder L. Changes in morbidity and chronic disability in the U.S. elderly population: evidence from the 1982, 1984, and 1989 National Long Term Care Surveys. *J Gerontol B Psychol Sci Soc Sci.* 1995;50: S194–S204.

50. McGue M, Vaupel JW, Holm N, Harvald B. Longevity is moderately heritable in a sample of Danish twins born 1870–1880. *J Gerontol.* 1993;48:B237–B244.

51. Rowe JW, Kahn RL. Successful aging. *Gerontologist.* 1997; 37:433–440.

52. Campisi J, Dimri G, Hara E. Control of replicative senescence. In: Scheider EL, Rowe JW, eds. *Handbook of the Biology of Aging.* San Diego: Academic Press; 1996:121–149.

53. Hayflick L. The cell biology of aging. *Clin Geriatr Med.* 1985;1:15–27.

54. Hay RJ, Menzies RA, Morgan HP, Strehler BL. The division potential of cells in continuous growth as compared to cells subcultivated after maintenance in stationary phase. *Exp Gerontol.* 1968;3:35–44.

55. Ran Q, Pereira-Smith OM. Genetic approaches to the study of replicative senescence. *Exp Gerontol*. 2000;35:7–13.

56. Shay JW, Wright WE. Telomeres and telomerase: implications for cancer and aging. *Radiat Res*. 2001;155:188–193.

57. Bodnar AG, Ouellette M, Frolkis M, et al. Extension of lifespan by introduction of telomerase into normal human cells. *Science*. 1998;279:349–352.

58. Campisi J. Cancer, aging and cellular senescence. *In Vivo*. 2000;14:183–188.

59. Shay JW, Wright WE, Werbin H. Defining the molecular mechanisms of human cell immortalization. *Biochim Biophys Acta*. 1991;1072:1–7.

60. Johnson TE, Wood WB. Genetic analysis of life-span in *Caenorhabditis elegans*. *Proc Natl Acad Sci USA*. 1982;79:6603–6607.

61. Friedman DB, Johnson TE. A mutation in the age-1 gene in *Caenorhabditis elegans* lengthens life and reduces hermaphrodite fertility. *Genetics*. 1988;118:75–86.

62. Johnson TE. Increased life-span of *age-1* mutants in *Caenorhabditis elegans* and lower Gompertz rate of aging. *Science*. 1990;249:908–912.

63. Johnson TE, Lithgow GJ. The search for the genetic basis of aging: the identification of gerontogenes in the nematode *Caenorhabditis elegans*. *J Am Geriatr Soc*. 1992;40:936–945.

64. Morris JZ, Tissenbaum HA, Ruvkun G. A phosphatidylinositol-3-OH kinase family member regulating longevity and diapause in *Caenorhabditis elegans*. *Nature*. 1996;382:536–539.

65. Kimura KD, Tissenbaum HA, Liu Y, Ruvkun G. daf-2, an insulin receptor-like gene that regulates longevity and diapause in *Caenorhabditis elegans* [see comments]. *Science*. 1997;277:942–946.

66. Guarente L, Ruvkun G, Amasino R. Aging, life span, and senescence. *Proc Natl Acad Sci U S A*. 1998;95:11034–11036.

67. Wolkow CA, Kimura KD, Lee MS, Ruvkun G. Regulation of *C. elegans* life span by insulin-like signaling in the nervous system. *Science*. 2000;290:147–150.

68. Taub J, Lau JF, Ma C, et al. A cytosolic catalase is needed to extend adult lifespan in *C. elegans* daf-C and clk-1 mutants. *Nature*. 1999;399:162–166.

69. Woods SC, Seeley RJ, Porte D Jr, Schwartz MW. Signals that regulate food intake and energy homeostasis. *Science*. 1998;280:1378–1383.

70. Lin YJ, Seroude L, Benzer S. Extended life-span and stress resistance in the *Drosophila* mutant methuselah. *Science*. 1998;282:943–946.

71. Rogian B, Reenan RA, Nilsen SP, Helfand SL. Extended life span conferred by cotransporter gene mutations in *Drosophila*. *Science*. 2000;290:2137–2140.

72. Imai S, Armstrong CM, Kaeberlein M, Guarente L. Transcriptional silencing and longevity protein Sir2 is an NAD-dependent histone deacetylase. *Nature*. 2000;403:795–800.

73. Lin SJ, Defossez PA, Guarente L. Requirement of NAD and SIR2 for life-span extension by calorie restriction in *Saccharomyces cerevisiae*. *Science*. 2000;289:2126–2128.

74. Brown-Borg HM, Borg KE, Meliska CJ, Bartke A. Dwarf mice and the ageing process. *Nature*. 1996;384:33.

75. Coschigano KT, Clemmons D, Bellush LL, Kopchick JJ. Assessment of growth parameters and life span of GHR/BP gene-disrupted mice. *Endocrinology*. 2000;141:2608–2613.

76. Migliaccio E, Giorgio M, Mele S, et al. The p66shc adaptor protein controls oxidative stress response and life span in mammals [see comments]. *Nature*. 1999;402:309–313.

77. Myers MG Jr, Sun XJ, Cheatham B, et al. IRS-1 is a common element in insulin and insulin-like growth factor-1 signaling to the phosphatidylinositol 3′-kinase. *Endocrinology*. 1993;132:1421–1430.

78. Laurino C, Cordera R. Role of IRS-1 and SHC activation in 3T3-L1 fibroblasts differentiation. *Growth Horm IGF Res*. 1998;8:363–367.

79. Oshima J. The Werner syndrome protein: an update. *Bioessays*. 2000;22:894–901.

3
Physiology of Aging

George E. Taffett

Aging, from maturity to senescence, results in an apparent depletion of physiologic reserves that has been termed homeostenosis. This term suggests a narrowing of homeostatic reserve mechanisms. Homeostenosis leads to the increased vulnerability to disease that occurs with aging. Primary aging changes, upon which we focus here, are those that occur as a result of the passage of time and are independent of disease state, although there may be overlap between disease and these changes. The age changes may be accelerated or slowed by lifestyle but are usually evident by the fourth or fifth decade and are gradual and inexorable. Overall, primary aging changes result in little change in function when the older individual (or animal) is assessed in the unstressed state, but these age changes become readily evident when the older individual is stressed or moved away from homeostasis. Because disease produces such stresses, the impact, presentation, and natural history of diseases are modified with age because the substrate, perhaps more than the disease pathophysiology, has been modified.

The concept of homeostenosis—the characteristic, progressive constriction of homeostatic reserves that occurs with aging in every organ system—was recognized by the famous physiologist Walter Cannon in the 1940s.[1] Figure 3.1 graphically displays the traditional thinking about homeostenosis. With aging, the capacity of older persons to bring themselves back to homeostasis after a challenge becomes smaller. All challenges to homeostasis are movements off the baseline, and larger challenges require greater physiologic reserves to return to homeostasis. Aging itself brings the individual closer to the precipice or threshold by the loss of physiologic reserves. The "precipice" may be defined, for example, as death or ill enough to have a cardiac arrest or for hospital admission. The precipice may also be the appearance of common and protean symptoms, such as confusion, weight loss, sleep disorder, or weakness.

Although empirically this paradigm is true, direct evidence for this model may be derived from studying the physiologic deviation from normal using the APACHE severity of illness scales.[2] Acute physiologic assessment points are generated by increased deviation from homeostatic values for 12 variables, including vital signs, oxygenation, pH, electrolytes, hematocrit, white count, and creatinine. A normal person at homeostasis will have a zero score. A greater departure from homeostasis is measured by a greater point total.

Figure 3.2 shows young and old patients who experienced a cardiac arrest. The younger group (mean age, 59 years) had significantly higher (by 20%) acute physiologic assessment scores than the older group (mean age, 75).[3] The data represent the worst values available in the 24 h prearrest. These data support the concept that the threshold, in this case being "sick" enough to have a cardiac arrest, is closer to homeostasis for the older than for the younger group. In practice, the creators of the APACHE II or III scales recognized that advanced age adds to risk of physiologic impairment with intercurrent illness. Another way to say this is that age reduces reserve capacity and makes us less resilient. APACHE scales give "bonus points" for age so that the total scores are not different between the younger and older groups.[3]

Despite the summative evidence, there is high variability in these processes. Variation in the age effects on any parameter is large, and the variability appears to increase with age. These variations are present from individual to individual at the same age, within a given individual from organ system to system, and even from cell to cell isolated from the same person. For example, investigators of the Baltimore Longitudinal Study of Aging performed serial measurements of glomerular filtration rate (GFR) measured as creatinine clearance in healthy people. Overall, the mean GFR decreased 1 ml/year; however, almost 30% of patients showed no decrement in function in repeated studies over as long as 30 years. Others showed decreases in GFR of 2 ml/year or more.[4] Similarly, when lymphocytes are isolated from an older person and then studied in vitro, some of the cells func-

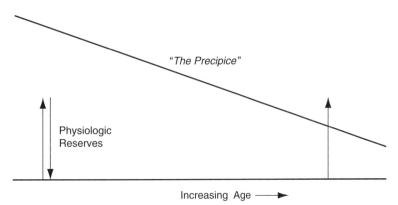

FIGURE 3.1. Standard schematic of homeostenosis. As the individual ages, there is no change in homeostasis, but the amount of physiologic reserves available to counter any challenge to homeostasis decreases with aging. Challenges to homeostasis are depicted as *arrows* moving away from the baseline. The "precipice" may be any clinically evident marker such as death, confusion, or cardiac arrest.

tion as well as those from a younger person[5]; of course, others function poorly, and it is the relative ratio of the two groups that impacts overall function. Therefore, as opposed to the pediatrician who can within a few weeks anticipate when a baby will start to walk, the geriatrician has a much harder time predicting when senescent changes will become clinically evident.

Another reason for the variability in the physiologic changes associated with aging is the contribution of behavioral factors such as exercise and diet, both of which are strong influences on healthy aging. Epidemiologists describe the growing rate of obesity, especially among older men, as an increasingly sedentary existence of most people beyond 30 years of age. For many of the variables listed in Table 3.1, exercise or other choices are known to attenuate but not totally abrogate aging effects. Some, such as the decrease in maximum heart rate attained with exercise, appear to be more predictable.

Table 3.1 summarizes many of the major changes in systems receiving further elucidation in respective sections of this volume. Data from the cardiovascular system are expanded here because the data in this area provide ample rationale to justify the necessity to reinterpret the traditional approach to homeostenosis. This reinterpretation helps one understand the phenomenon of frailty, a central concern of geriatrics. Frailty is the state when physiologic reserves are reduced to the point at which susceptibility to disability is increased. Frailty is, therefore, the clinical manifestation of the later stages of homeostenosis, an intolerance of homeostatic challenges. Additionally, the reinterpretation of homeostenosis makes those caring for the elderly appreciate and understand the complexities they face.

In the elderly, as in youth, maintaining homeostasis is a dynamic, active process. The reinterpretation of Figure 3.1 shown in Figure 3.3 is based on the concept that older persons are actively employing some of their physiologic reserves just to maintain homeostasis. Their available reserves appear depleted because they in are already in use by the old heart (or other organ or system) to compensate for primary age-related or other changes. The

physiologic reserves have not "disappeared," as suggested in Figure 3.1, but they remain unavailable to counter additional challenges. I focus on examples from the cardiovascular system, such as heart rate, cardiac hypertrophy, and diastolic function, because the data in this area provide an ample molecular, biochemical, and physiologic foundation to reinterpret the traditional approach to homeostenosis.

Although resting heart rate in unchanged with age, maximum heart rate attained with exercise or pharmacologic manipulation decreases with age. Baltimore Longitudinal Study data, obtained from healthy, highly screened individuals, give a regression equation of

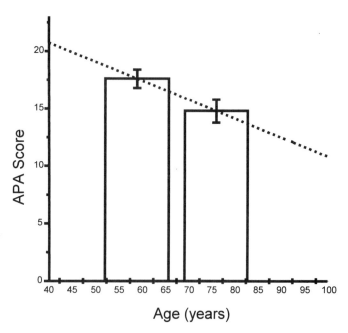

FIGURE 3.2. Age decreases the level of physiologic derangement associated with cardiac arrest. Acute physiologic assessment (*APA*) scores (from the APACHE II severity of illness scale) are shown from patients who subsequently experienced cardiac arrest and a resuscitation attempt. The data show the APA scores were significantly higher in the younger patients who arrested than the older ones ($p < 0.05$; Beer et al. 1994[3]).

TABLE 3.1. Major changes in system.

Endocrine system
  Impaired glucose tolerance (fasting glucose increased 1 mg/dl/decade; postprandial increased 10 mg/dl/decade)
  Increased serum insulin and increased HgbA1C nocturnal growth hormone peaks lost, decreased 1GF-1
  Marked decrease in dehydroepiandrosterone (DHEA)
  Decreased free and bioavailable testosterone
  Decreased T3
  Increased parathyroid hormone (PTH)
  Decreased production of vitamin D by skin
  Ovarian failure, decreased ovarian hormones
  Increased serum homocysteine levels

Cardiovascular
  Unchanged resting heart rate (HR), decreased maximum HR
  Impaired left ventricular filling
  Marked dropout of pacemaker cells in SA node
  Increased contribution of atrial systole to ventricular filling
  Left atrial hypertrophy
  Prolonged contraction and relaxation of left ventricle
  Decreased inotropic, chronotropic, lusitropic response to beta-adrenergic stimulation
  Decreased maximum cardiac output
  Decreased hypertrophy in response to volume or pressure overload
  Increased serum atrial natriuretic peptide (ANP)
  Large arteries increase in wall thickness, lumen, and length, become less distensible, and compliance decreases
  Subendothelial layer thickened with connective tissue
  Irregularities in size and shape of endothelial cells
  Fragmentation of elastin in media of arterial wall
  Peripheral vascular resistance increases

Blood pressure
  Increased systolic blood pressure (BP), unchanged diastolic BP
  Beta-adrenergic-mediated vasodilatation decreased
  Alpha-adrenergic-mediated vasoconstriction unchanged
  Brain autoregulation of perfusion impaired

Pulmonary
  Decreased FEV_1 and FVC
  Increased residual volume
  Cough less effective
  Ciliary action less effective
  Ventilation–perfusion mismatching causes PaO_2 to decrease with age: $100 - (0.32 * age)$
  Trachea and central airways increase in diameter
  Enlarged alveolar ducts due to lost elastic lung parenchyma structural support result in decreased surface area
  Decreased lung mass
  Expansion of thorax
  Maximum inspiratory and expiratory pressures decrease
  Decreased respiratory muscle strength
  Chest wall stiffens
  Diffusion of CO decreased
  Decreased ventilatory response to hypercapnia

Hematologic
  Bone marrow reserves decreased in response to high demand
  Attenuated reticulocytosis to erythropoeitin administration

Renal
  Decreased creatinine clearance and GFR 10 ml/decade
  Decrease of 25% in renal mass, mostly from cortex with a relative increased perfusion of juxtamedullary nephrons
  Decreased sodium excretion and conservation
  Decreased potassium excretion and conservation
  Decreased concentrating and diluting capacity
  Impaired secretion of acid load
  Decreased serum renin and aldosterone
  Accentuated ADH release in response to dehydration
  Decreased nitric oxide production
  Increased dependence of renal prostaglandins to maintain perfusion
  Decreased vitamin D activation

(Continued)

TABLE 3.1. *Continued*

Genitourinary (GU)
    Prolonged refractory period for erections for men
    Reduced intensity of orgasm for men and women
    Incomplete bladder emptying and increased postvoid residuals
    Decreased prostatic secretions in urine
    Decreased concentrations of antiadherence factor Tamm–Horsfall protein

Temperature
    Impaired shivering

Regulation
    Decreased cutaneous vasoconstriction and vasodilation
    Decreased sweat production
    Increased core temperature to start sweating

Muscle
    Marked decrease in muscle mass (sarcopenia) due to loss of muscle fibers
    Aging effects smallest in diaphragm (role of activity), more in legs than arms
    Decreased myosin heavy chain synthesis
    Small if any decrease in specific force
    Decreased innervation, increased number of myofibrils per motor unit
    Infiltration of fat into muscle bundles
    Increased fatigability
    Decrease in basal metabolic rate (decrease 4%/decade after age 50) parallels loss of muscle

Bone
    Slower healing of fractures
    Decreasing bone mass in men and women, both trabecular and cortical bone
    Decreased osteoclast bone formation

Joints
    Disordered cartilage matrix
    Modified proteoglycans and glycosaminoglycans

Peripheral nervous system
    Loss of spinal motor neurons
    Decreased vibratory sensation, especially in feet
    Decreased thermal sensitivity (warm–cool)
    Decreased sensory nerve action potential amplitude
    Decreased size of large myelinated fibers
    Increased heterogeneity of axon myelin sheaths

Central nervous system
    Small decrease in brain mass
    Decreased brain blood flow and impaired autoregulation of perfusion
    Nonrandom loss of neurons to modest extents
    Proliferation of astrocytes
    Decreased density of dendritic connections
    Increased numbers of scattered neurofibrillary tangles
    Increased numbers of scattered senile plaques
    Decreased myelin and total brain lipid
    Altered neurotransmitters, including dopamine and serotonin
    Increased monoamine oxidase activity
    Decrease in hippocampal glucocorticoid receptors
    Decline in fluid intelligence
    Slowed central processing and reaction time

Gastrointestinal (GI)
    Decreased liver size and blood flow
    Impaired clearance by liver of drugs that require extensive phase I metabolism
    Reduced inducibility of liver mixed-function oxidase enzymes Mild decrease in bilirubin
    Hepatocytes accumulate secondary lysosomes, residual bodies, and lipofuscin
    Mild decrease in stomach acid production, probably due to nonautoimmune loss of parietal cells
    Impaired response to gastric mucosal injury
    Decreased pancreatic mass and enzymatic reserves
    Decrease in effective colonic contractions
    Decreased calcium absorption
    Decrease in gut-associated lymphoid tissue

TABLE 3.1. *Continued*

Vision
  Impaired dark adaptation
  Yellowing of lens
  Inability to focus on near items (presbyopia)
  Minimal decrease in static acuity, profound decrease in dynamic acuity (moving target)
  Decreased contrast sensitivity
  Decreased lacrimation

Smell
  Detection decreased by 50%

Thirst
  Decreased thirst drive
  Impaired control of thirst by endorphins

Balance
  Increased threshold vestibular responses
  Reduced number of organ of Corti hair cells

Audition
  Bilateral loss of high-frequency tones
  Central processing deficit
  Difficulty discriminating source of sound
  Impaired discrimination of target from noise

Adipose
  Increased aromatase activity
  Increased tendency to lipolysis

Immune system
  Decreased cell-mediated immunity
  Lower affinity antibody production
  Increased autoantibodies
  Facilitated production of anti-idiotype antibodies
  Increased occurrence of MGUS (monoclonal gammopathy of unknown significance)
  More nonresponders to vaccines
  Decreased delayed-type hypersensitivity
  Impaired macrophage function (Interferon-gamma, TGF-beta, TNF, IL-6, IL-1 release increased with age)
  Decreased cell proliferative response to mitogens
  Atrophy of thymus and loss of thymic hormones
  Accumulation of memory T cells (CD-45+)
  Increased circulating IL-6
  Decreased IL-2 release and IL-2 responsiveness
  Decreased production of B cells by bone marrow

$208 - (0.95 \times \text{age})$ for maximum heart rate attained with exercise. It is likely that women have lower maximum heart rates at age 30 and a more gentle fall with aging than this equation predicts. This decrease in maximum heart rate responsiveness results from a combination of factors. First, primary aging decreases the intrinsic heart rate (the heart rate in the absence of sympathetic and parasympathetic stimulation), as well as invokes reserves just to maintain resting heart rate. Data from Jose,[6] although regretfully including only a modest number of elders, show a decrease in intrinsic heart rate from 120–130/min to less than 80. There is no difference

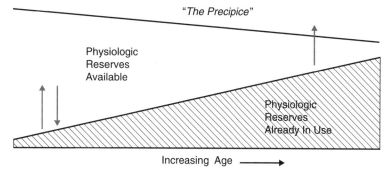

FIGURE 3.3. Revised schematic of homeostenosis. In comparison to Figure 3.1, this diagram shows that maintaining homeostasis is a dynamic process. The older person employs or consumes physiologic reserves just to maintain homeostasis, and therefore there are fewer reserves available for meeting new challenges.

in resting heart rate with age, so the extent of parasympathetic tone, slowing heart rate at rest, is decreased. Removal of parasympathetic tone, the first mechanism invoked to increase heart rate with exercise, is then less effective for the elderly because vagal tone is already diminished at rest; this is consistent with the attenuated heart rate response of healthy elders to administration of atropine. The decreased yield from lysis of parasympathetic tone is added to decreased beta-adrenergic chronotropic responsiveness to contribute to the overall decreased maximal heart rate in response to exercise (Fig. 3.4).

Importantly, the same limitation in maximum heart rate with exercise applies to that in response to other stimuli, such as infection or anemia. Therefore, an 80-year-old man with a sinus tachycardia of 120, mounting close to a maximum heart rate response, could be considered as a young man who had a heart rate of 170. In the setting of an infection, although a 120 heart rate would hardly raise eyebrows, a 170 would surely provoke serious concern. For their respective age groups, both values roughly represent an equivalent of 75% of maximum response.

A similar set of observations, that reserves are invoked to maintain homeostasis in the old, are seen following the response to another challenge, pressure overload induced by banding the aorta (Fig. 3.5).[7] In older male rats (18 months of age), there is only trivial increase in left ventricular mass in response to pressure overload. This same manipulation results in a 40% hypertrophy of the left ventricle in adult (9-month) animals. The molecular response to the pressure overload was markedly attenu-

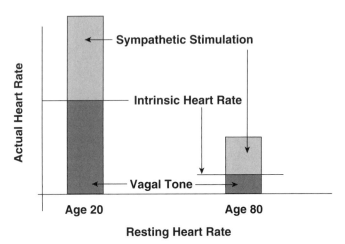

FIGURE 3.4. Resting and exercise heart rates. There are no differences in resting heart rate between the older and young person, but the extent of the resting vagal tone, slowing heart rate (*dark gray bar*), is decreased in the older person. With exertion, the removal of the vagal tone results in smaller increment in heart rate and the beta-adrenergic chronotropic responsiveness is also decreased (*light gray bar*), all contributing to the decreased maximum heart rate in the old. The straight line represents the intrinsic heart rate (absence of any sympathetic or vagal tone).

ated in the old heart, with little induction of the immediate early response genes c-*jun* and c-*fos*. Skeletal actin, which precedes cardiac actin when new contractile elements are laid down in the heart, was not increased in the older, banded heart. All these molecular markers confirmed the absence of hypertrophic response to banding in the old heart.

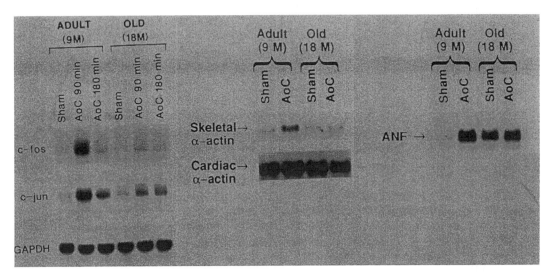

FIGURE 3.5. Decreased response to pressure stimulus in the old heart. After aortic banding in the young and old rat, there is a decreased elaboration of RNA for "early immediate response genes" (*fos* and *jun*) in the old heart, followed by decreased contractile protein response (skeletal actin). Ventricular atrial natriuretic peptide (ANP), a marker for myocyte hypertrophy, is increased in the control and old hearts, suggesting prior invocation of the hypertrophic response (Takahashi et al. 1992[7] with permission.)

In contrast, atrial natriuretic peptide (ANP), a marker for myocyte hypertrophy when it is expressed by the ventricular myocyte, is increased significantly after banding in the young heart. The ventricular ANP is not detectable in the control young heart. ANP is significantly elevated in the ventricle from both the banded and control older hearts, providing evidence that the old heart has already invoked the hypertrophic response even before the banding is applied.

Morphologic evidence of myocyte hypertrophy in aging is provided by examining myocyte size. Myocytes from the ventricles of older persons and animals are larger than those from young adults, consistent with ongoing myocyte hypertrophy in response to uncertain stresses. Various investigators report 25% increase in myocyte length and 50% or more increases in myocyte width.[8] There is likely a maximum size for the myocyte; therefore, myocytes in the old heart may be unable to hypertrophy further because they have already responded to prior or ongoing challenges.

With aging in animals and man, there are impairments in early cardiac relaxation, largely caused by alterations in cellular calcium flux. The increased dependence on transsarcolemmal calcium flux (in and out of the cell) seen in the old rat heart maintains adequate calcium availability for contraction. This adaptation appears to be a compensation for decreased transsarcoplasmic reticulum calcium flux. Therefore, the compensation comes at a cost, the lengthening of contraction by both slowing the development of force and slowing cardiac relaxation. Using gene therapy, a key sarcoplasmic reticulum calcium pump can be restored in old rats to levels found in the young heart, and cardiac relaxation improves significantly.[9] One manifestation of the impaired relaxation is the decreased effectiveness of early diastolic filling of the left ventricle. As a compensation to maintain ventricular filling, contribution of atrial systole to diastolic filling increases from 10% to 15% at age 20 to almost 50% at age 80.[10] In addition to explaining why atrial fibrillation (and the loss of atrial systole) becomes so devastating in the elderly, the ability to augment the atrial contribution to further increase cardiac output is limited. Therefore, the Frank–Starling mechanism is invoked; filling pressures increase to augment cardiac output.

There are numerous other changes in the cardiovascular system (CVS) that follow the paradigm just described, and the pattern is not at all limited to the CVS, such as the limited heat shock protein elaboration in response to certain stimuli. These changes support rethinking the concept of frailty. Frailty is not a static state of increased vulnerability to stressors; rather, it is a dynamic state in which the older person tolerates additional challenges poorly because reserves are already engaged in battles, seen or unseen. From a therapeutic standpoint, this suggests that efforts to disengage reserves may result

in decreasing vulnerability. To date, evidence for this opportunity to increase reserves remains unproven. Older persons are frailer, more likely to cross a given "precipice" after a stress, not only because they have lost some reserves because of aging, but because they are already utilizing other reserves to compensate for those lost just to maintain homeostasis. Older people are more likely to drown when thrown a brick, not because they cannot swim but because they are already treading water.

It is well known that the mortality associated with myocardial infarction (MI) increases dramatically with age. Although absolute death rates have improved with treatment for all ages, the 10-fold increase in mortality after MI from ages 40 to 80 has not been modified. This age-related increase in mortality has been variously attributed to increased infarct size in the old, comorbid conditions, less aggressive therapy for the old, noncompliance with medical regimens, or increased existence of multivessel coronary artery disease. Some of the points may be true, but in studies where all these factors are controlled, the mortality is still much higher in the older groups. Age is the key component, and I hypothesize that it is the age-related inability to respond to challenge, homeostenosis in the cardiovascular system, that results in the increased mortality.

A similar set of implications can be made relevant to the increased frequency of falls in response to challenge in the elderly. Decreases in baroreceptor sensitivity, arterial compliance, cardiac compliance (and greater dependence on cardiac filling to maintain cardiac output), renal sodium conservation, plasma volume, vasopressin response to standing, and renin, angiotensin, and aldosterone levels all contribute to the propensity to fall with postural change. Many of the problems with medications in the elderly, once attributed to altered pharmacodynamics, may be explained by this apparent depletion of physiologic reserves.

Data from the MacArthur Study of Aging support the concept that healthy elders are actively compensating just to maintain homeostasis and that the presence of invoked compensation is associated with poor outcomes.[11] Only 7% of those aged 70 to 79 had no evidence of such compensation, and the lack of compensation was associated with highest level of function. Seeman refers to this activation as "allostatic load," and while some of the markers, such as elevated cholesterol and systolic blood pressure, are known risk factors for CV events and death, others reflect the activity of sympathetic nervous system or the hypothalamic–pituitary–adrenal axis. Those patients with high allostatic load had decreased physical and cognitive function at 2-year follow-up.

There is some evidence that the inverse may also be true. Masoro believes that one mechanism by which the beneficial, life-prolonging effects of caloric restriction occur is precisely that the decreased availability of calo-

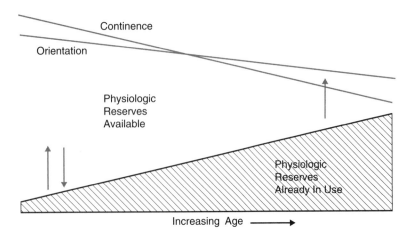

FIGURE 3.6. Altered presentation of illness may be another manifestation of homeostenosis. With age, the precipices may approach homeostasis at differing rates so that modest challenges produce clinically evident events, in this case, new onset of incontinence, and in others, disorientation or confusion.

ries is a low-intensity stress.[12] The beneficial effects of low-dose radiation may also be via this mechanism. Persistent, harmless stresses, such as caloric restriction or radiation, may be good for us; larger stresses may be harmful.

Invoking compensatory mechanisms has the additional effect of constraining the complexity of many variables. Heart rate variability decreases with aging, and this constriction of heart rate may be due to decreased parasympathetic tone and possible activation of the sympathetic nervous system while at rest.[13] A similar constriction is seen in blood pressure variability. The decrease in variability may correspond with the ongoing activation of compensatory reserves.

The concept of threshold is also useful in understanding the altered presentations of disease in the elderly. The extent that any threshold from Figure 3.1 or Figure 3.3 approaches homeostasis may determine whether that threshold is crossed by a given challenge. For example, delirium is a very common atypical presentation of a wide variety of illness in the elderly, a marker of the uneasy truce that the old brain maintains with its environment. The precarious balance is clearly evident but is not limited to the cholinergic pathways. While it seems strange that a given older person may have the same presentation (confusion) for a urinary tract infection, gastrointestinal bleeding, and a myocardial infarction, this phenomena may be relatively common because the systemic responses to these differing illnesses may be similar, involving cytokines, catecholamines, etc. In these patients, at homeostasis their "anticonfusion reserves" may be exhausted so the distance from homeostasis to the "precipice" becomes minimal and is easily crossed (Fig. 3.6).

Finally, the lines on these schematics (Figs. 3.1, 3.3, 3.6) are straight for convenience's sake, not because any of the processes described in Table 3.1 are necessarily linear. For example, the loss in muscle mass approaches 40% as one ages from 30 to 80, yet most of that loss happens after

age 60, indicating the rate of loss increases with increasing age. Strength follows mass in this pattern. It is likely that most age-related physiologic changes are not linear functions of age.

In summary, there is an apparent loss of physiologic reserves that leads to an intolerance of challenges to the homeostasis of older persons. One should appreciate that this frailty is, in part, present because the older person is continually expending reserves to compensate for primary age changes and other unseen processes absent or trivial in the younger individual.

Bibliography

Knaus WA, Wagner DP, Draper EA, et al. The APACHE III prognostic system. Risk prediction of hospital mortality for critically ill hospitalized adults. *Chest.* 1991;100:1619–1636.

Masoro EJ, ed. *Handbook of Physiology*, Section 11, Aging. American Physiological Society. New York: Oxford Press; 1995.

References

1. Cowdry EV, ed. *Problems of Ageing: Biological and Medical Aspects*, 2nd Ed. Baltimore: Williams & Wilkins; 1942.
2. Knaus WA, Draper EA, Wagner DP, Zimmerman JE. APACHE II: a severity of disease classification system. Crit Care Med. 1985;13:818–829.
3. Beer RJ, Teasdale TA, Ghusn HF, Taffet GE. Estimation of severity of illness with APACHE II: age-related implications in cardiac arrest outcomes. *Resuscitation.* 1994;27:189–195.
4. Lindeman RD, Tobin J, Shock NW. Longitudinal studies on the rate of decline in renal function with age. *J Am Geriatr Soc.* 1985;33:278–285.
5. Ghia P, Melchers F, Rolink AG. Age-dependent changes in B lymphocyte development in man and mouse. *Exp Gerontol.* 2000;35:159–165.

6. Jose AD. Effect of combined sympathetic and para-sympathetic blockade on heart rate and cardiac function in man. *Am J Cardiol.* 1966;18:476–483.

7. Takahashi T, Schunkert H, Isoyama S, et al. Age-related differences in the expression of proto-oncogene and contractile protein genes in response to pressure overload in the rat myocardium. *J Clin Investig.* 1992;88:939–946.

8. Lakatta EG. Cardiovascular regulatory mechanisms in advanced age. *Physiol Rev.* 1993;73:413–467.

9. Schmidt U, del Monte F, Miyamoto MI, et al. Restoration of diastolic function in senescent rat hearts through adenoviral gene transfer of sarcoplasmic reticulum Ca($^{2+}$)-ATPase. *Circulation.* 2000;101:790–796.

10. Swinne CJ, Shapiro EP, Lima SD, Fleg JL. Age-asociated changes in left ventricular diastolic performance during isometric exercise in normal subjects. *Am J Cardiol.* 1992;69: 823–826.

11. Seeman TE, Singer BH, Rowe JW, Horwitz RI, McEwen BS. Price of adaptation—allostatic load and its health consequences. MacArthur studies of successful aging. *Arch Intern Med.* 1997;157:2259–2268.

12. Masoro EJ. Commentary. *Hum Exp Toxicol.* 2000;19:340–341.

13. Lipsitz LA, Goldberger AL. Loss of "complexity" and aging. Potential applications of fractals and chaos theory to senescence. *JAMA.* 1992;267:1806–1809.

4
The Demography of Aging

S. Jay Olshansky

The demography of aging involves the investigation of trends in, and characteristics of, fertility, mortality, and migration and how these components of population change influence, and are influenced by, the physical and social environments in which people live. It is a relatively new area of scientific inquiry, principally because aging is a demographic phenomenon experienced within the past 200 years for the first time on a population scale by humans and only a few other species. Research on the demography of aging is conducted not only by demographers and actuaries but also by scientists representing a range of disciplines spanning the social and biological sciences from social psychology to evolutionary biology. It is an area of scientific inquiry that has important implications for public policy.

A central distinction exists between *population aging* and *individual aging*. *Population aging* refers to changes in the age structure of a population or, more specifically, an increase in the relative proportion of older persons to the total population alive at a single moment in time. Several measures are used to measure population aging, detect changes across time, and make comparisons between population subgroups. The most common measures include the median age, aged dependency ratio (ratio of the population aged 65+ to those aged 0–64), and the percentage of the total population aged 65 and older.

Individual aging refers to the length of life for individuals or an average length of life for population subgroups or species. Individual aging is measured in chronological time such as days, months, or years. A summary measure of individual aging for a population is most often represented by its expectation of life or life expectancy. Life expectancy is calculated from death probabilities observed throughout the age range over a selected time period, usually one calendar year, and may be estimated for a given birth cohort or for a population reaching any age or age range. The study of secular trends in life expectancy and changes in the underlying causes of death that comprise total death rates is one of many basic areas

of scientific inquiry in the demographic and actuarial sciences. Of particular interest at this time is how high life expectancy at birth and at older ages can increase, and how changes in individual aging influence, and are influenced by, the distribution of diseases and the health status of the population.

It is also important to distinguish between the terms *life expectancy, life span, average life span*, and *maximum life span potential* because they are often used interchangeably. As previously noted, life expectancy is a summary measure of the expected duration of life calculated from observed death rates for a population. Life span may be defined as the observed length of life for an individual. Average life span may be defined as the average of individual life spans in a population. Maximum life span potential (MLSP) has been used in the biologic literature to define the age of the longest-lived member of a species. The underlying premise behind the concept of average life span is the presumption that there are biologically based limits on the duration of life for individuals, and as the age-specific risk of death declines, the observed life expectancy approaches the average life span. However, because it is not possible to know the maximum duration of life for any individual, by extension it is not possible to know with certainty the maximum average life span for a population.

As individuals in a cohort pass through life from childhood to older ages, the observed probabilities of death take on a characteristic "bathtub" shape (Fig. 4.1). There is high mortality at birth, a rapid decline in the risk of death to its lowest point at sexual maturity, and an exponential rise in the death rate until very old ages (85+), after which the rate of increase in the death rate decelerates. This mortality curve has also been observed for other sexually reproducing species.[1–3] Although recent studies have documented decelerating increases in death rates at extreme old ages,[4] this phenomenon has been observed for humans and other species for more than 175 years.[5] Changes in individuals at the molecular and

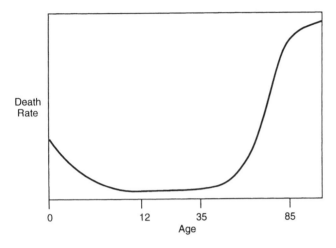

FIGURE 4.1. Characteristic "bathtub" shape of mortality.

cellular level that are observed across time and which are believed to bring forth these characteristic mortality patterns among populations are referred to collectively as *senescence*. Senescence may be thought of most appropriately as the passage of biologic time whereas *aging* is colloquially defined as the passage of chronologic time.[6] Thus, although individuals in a cohort age at exactly the same rate, the random or stochastic nature of damage that accumulates in the DNA, cells, and tissues of living organisms, when combined with genetic variability in inherited mortality risk, leads to different rates of senescence and thus varying mortality risks among individuals in a population across time.

Causes and Consequences of Population Aging

For most of recorded history, and probably dating back to the origin of anatomically modern humans approximately 100,000 years age, there has been a consistent (stable) pattern of birth rates and death rates (Fig. 4.2, phase 1). Under these "usual" demographic conditions, death rates fluctuated between peaks and troughs largely in response to the episodic influence of infectious and parasitic diseases. Birth rates remained extremely high during most of human history, barely exceeding death rates over the long term, but enough so to produce slow population growth. Death rates at middle and younger ages were so high that survival into what was then thought of as old age (65 years) was a rare event by comparison to today. Survival into extreme old age (85 years and older) was an even less frequent occurrence.

The age distribution of the population during most of human history (i.e., under phase I demographic conditions) resembles the shape of a pyramid (Fig. 4.3). The age pyramid of a population is a snapshot picture of the

number of people alive at all ages during a single moment in time, usually the middle of a calendar year (July 1). In a closed population with no migration, the horizontal bars reflect the number of people surviving to each age range from an original birth cohort based on prevailing death rates. However, with the more conventional interpretation of an open population with internal and external migration and changing vital rates, the age pyramid is a reflection of historical patterns of fertility, mortality, and migration.

During the nineteenth century, a combination of events led to dramatic changes in the stable patterns of birth rates and death rates that had existed for thousands of years. The development of consistent and clean sources of fresh water and refrigeration, the disposal of sewage, temperature-controlled indoor living and working environments, and developments in public health and medicine all contributed significantly to reductions in the transmission of air- and water-borne infectious and parasitic diseases.[7,8] The pervasive environmental conditions that permitted the easy transmission of infectious diseases which killed early in life had been profoundly altered within an extremely short time period. From a biologic perspective, modifications of this magnitude and importance lead to fundamental changes in the forces of natural selection operating on the human species.[9]

As a result of these advances in public health and medicine, the risk of death at younger ages, particularly among infants, children, and women of childbearing ages, declined rapidly; this eventually led to declines in total fertility rates as the need to replace children lost to early mortality waned. However, the decline in birth rates lagged behind the decline in death rates (Fig. 4.2, phase 2). The result was extremely high rates of population growth, with growth rates reaching as high as 3% to 4% among some population subgroups. A growth rate of 1% leads to the doubling of a population in about 70 years. Every time the growth rate doubles, the time it takes for a population to double in size is reduced by half. Thus, a growth rate of 4% leads to a population doubling time of about 18 years. The transformation of birth rates and death rates to a lower level of equilibrium at approxi-

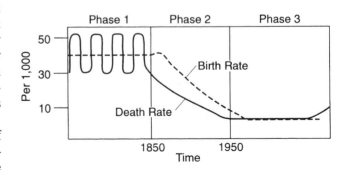

FIGURE 4.2. Demographic transition.

FIGURE 4.3. Age pyramid for humans before 1900.

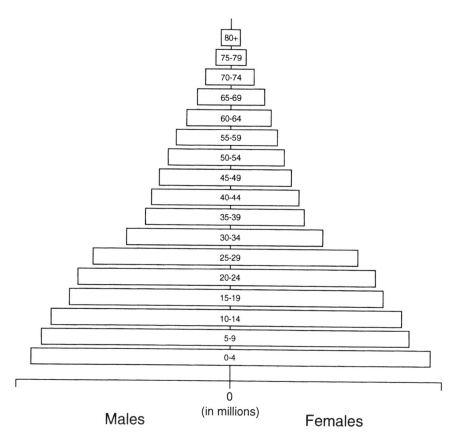

mately 10 per 1000 in most of today's developed nations (Fig. 4.2, phase 3) is what set the stage for population aging.

As the human population experienced declines in death rates at younger ages during the past 200 years, the base of the age pyramid expanded and its apex became smaller by comparison to the rest of the population. When the apex of an age pyramid decreases relative to its base, it may be said that a population is becoming younger. Thus, the first demographic consequence of declining early age mortality, at least with regard to a changing age composition, was a younger population.

Within one average human life span (about 85 years), those saved from dying at younger ages reach middle and older ages, thereby altering the population's age composition, with the middle and apex of the pyramid expanding relative to its base. Under conditions where death rates at younger ages have been reduced to extremely low levels (e.g., in populations with high life expectancies), the base of the age pyramid becomes stable, influenced almost entirely by changes in birth rates. With a stable base and a growing middle and apex, the stage is set for a permanent shift in the age structure from its historical pyramidal shape to that of a square or rectilinear form (Fig. 4.4). Although increasing birth rates (such as those that occurred during the post-World War II era) can slow population aging and even temporarily reverse

it, the new rectilinear age structure will eventually reassert itself as the children from the larger birth cohorts survive to older ages. Thus, the transformation from stable high birth and death rates to stable low birth and death rates, experienced only within the last 200 years, has produced fundamental and in all likelihood permanent changes in the age structure of the human species.[9]

The social, economic, health, and political implications associated with rapid changes in a population's age structure are profound.[10] Consider the example of what have become known as the compression and expansion of morbidity hypotheses. As the risk of death at younger ages declines, the proportion of each birth cohort surviving past ages 65 and 85 increases rapidly. For example, in the United States the proportion of the female birth cohort of 1900 that survived to ages 65 and 85 during the twentieth century was 57.8% and 25.5% respectively.[11] By comparison, the female birth cohort of 1996 is expected to have 85.7% and 41.6% survival past ages 65 and 85, respectively. These unprecedented patterns of survival into older ages have led scientists to identify the new patterns of mortality that lead to such improved survival chances and to evaluate how the health of cohorts surviving to older ages has already been influenced by these changing mortality patterns and how prospective mortality transitions might influence the future health of the older population.

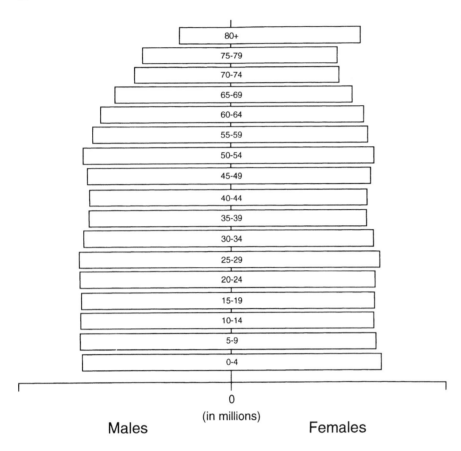

FIGURE 4.4. Age pyramid of the future.

One school of thought is based on a concept known as the compression of morbidity hypothesis. According to this hypothesis, lifestyle changes and advances in medicine will continue to reduce the risk of death from fatal diseases and simultaneously lead to a postponement in the onset and age progression of the nonfatal disabling diseases.[12] The underlying premise of this theory is that there is a fixed biologic limit to life of approximately 85 years toward which populations are headed. As improved lifestyles simultaneously postpone the onset and expression of fatal diseases and nonfatal but highly disabling diseases and disorders, more people will be pushed toward their biologic limit to life, and morbidity and disability will be compressed into a shorter duration of time before death.

A second school of thought is based on a concept known as the expansion of morbidity hypothesis. According to this hypothesis, the behavioral and biologic forces that are influencing the onset and age progression of the nonfatal diseases associated with senescence are believed to be largely independent of the forces influencing the risk of death from fatal diseases.[13–15] Thus, further reductions in death rates from fatal diseases are hypothesized to expose the saved population to a longer duration of time during which the nonfatal but highly disabling diseases and disorders of senescence have the opportunity to be expressed. Implicit in this theory is the etiologic

independence of fatal and nonfatal diseases and the premise that there are no active genetic programs for death (i.e., death genes) that evolved under the direct force of natural selection. The rationale supporting the latter premise is that it is not possible for the forces of natural selection to have favored the evolution of death (or longevity) genes that are expressed at older ages because selection does not operate in age ranges where few individuals normally live. That is, selection cannot effectively remove genes carried by those who have already made their genetic contribution to the next generation. The evolutionary explanation for why senescence arose is that it is a by-product of an evolved reproductive pattern and unprecedented survival into an older age range that permits its expression.[16–19]

A considerable debate has taken place in the literature regarding these two important hypotheses.[20–25] It is too early to determine which hypothesis will best characterize the future course of mortality and morbidity because recent studies have provided support for both trends.[25,26] However, research in this area should be interpreted with great caution because empirical studies addressed to this debate have focused on health transitions observed only during the past 20 years, with an emphasis placed on the decade of the 1980s. It is possible that healthy life expectancy (the proportion of total life expectancy free from disability) could improve at a faster pace in the short term, only to give way to a more rapid increase in disabled life expectancy at a later date when survival into older, more disabling age ranges becomes common.

Population aging not only has provided an opportunity for most people to survive into older ages, it has also fundamentally altered the age distribution of death, shifted the primary causes of death to chronic lethal conditions associated with senescence, and increased genetic heterogeneity at older ages. In addition to its impact on patterns of health and mortality, population aging has also had profound effects on the funding of age-entitlement programs such as Social Security and Medicare,[27,28] and in the coming decades it will likely have a profound influence on social institutions such as marriage, age at retirement, and even voting behavior. The social, economic, and health consequences associated with population aging are rapidly emerging as fertile areas of scientific inquiry.[10]

Individual Aging

The transformation of birth rates and death rates to their currently stable low levels not only brought forth rapid population growth and aging, it also led to unprecedented increases in life expectancy. It is estimated that during the Roman Empire life expectancy at birth was about 28 years.[29] By 1900, life expectancy at birth increased to 45 years in the nations with the lowest death rates of that time.[11] In low-mortality populations of the early twenty-first century, life expectancy at birth has now risen to between 75 and 80 years.

Most of the gains in life expectancy during the mortality revolution of the past two centuries are a result of dramatic reductions in death rates at younger ages. In fact, in today's high life expectancy populations of North America, Western Europe, Australia, Scandinavia, and Japan, death rates at younger ages have declined to such low levels that 98 of every 100 babies born will survive past 30 years of age. Deaths that occur among those younger than age 30 result mostly from accidents, homicide, suicide, congenital anomalies, and inherited lethal diseases.

What is perhaps most remarkable about the recent mortality transition is that, during the last third of the twentieth century, the majority of the gain in life expectancy at birth has been attributable to declines in death rates among those aged 50 and older. This latest trend in old-age mortality is so unique that it has been referred to as the fourth stage of the epidemiologic transition.[30–32] The first three stages are represented by the transition from high unstable mortality to low stable mortality as depicted in Figure 4.2.

Because declining death rates have been observed throughout the age structure, this raises questions about how much further death rates can decline and how high life expectancy can increase. Interestingly, the belief in a biologically based limit to life has its nonscientific origins in biblical references to a human life span of 120 years (Genesis 6 : 6). Early scientific studies addressed to a biologically based limit to life were often presented within the context of a fundamental "law of mortality" that would explain why different species have different life spans, and why the risk of death increases in a predictable fashion with the passage of time.[33–37]

The first scientists to speculate on a biologic limit to life looked to the world of chemistry for answers to why death rates increased predictably with time.[33] These researchers believed that chemical reactions took place within living organisms that resulted in the breakdown of cells and tissues, reactions that in the world of chemistry operated in a time-dependent fashion consistent with the age trajectory of death observed among living organisms. Although these early visions of a law of mortality have remarkable similarities to theories about the mechanisms of senescence that prevail today, scientists early in the twentieth century were unable to measure the chemical reactions that they believed led to increasing mortality with age. Subsequent studies addressed to the question of a law of mortality were focused on interspecies comparisons of mortality,[38] and these later gave way to more mathematically oriented models designed to characterize the pattern to the dying-out process of populations.[3]

The principal scientific basis for a biologic limit to life dates back to the pioneering work of Hayflick and Moorhead,[39] where it was shown that normal human fibroblasts have a limited number of doubling times, about 50, after which they die. This limited replicative capacity of fibroblasts has been interpreted as a form of programmed death, as if a death gene evolved that is triggered after a certain amount of elapsed time. In subsequent articles, Hayflick[40,41] made it clear that his findings should not have been interpreted as a biologic clock designed by evolution for the purpose of causing death. In spite of this clarification, the concept of a biologic limit to life based on these studies remains part of the scientific literature.[42]

Demographic estimates of how high life expectancy can rise has taken on various forms, from extrapolation and curve-fitting models[43–46] to reverse engineering approaches.[47] Extrapolating past mortality trends into the future has led some researchers to conclude that period life expectancy at birth in the United States will reach 100 years by the middle to latter part of the twenty-first century[43,48] and that cohort life expectancy at birth for females born since the early 1980s is already at 100. Other extrapolation models employed by the U.S. Census Bureau,[44] Social Security Administration (SSA),[11] and other researchers[45] project that life expectancy at birth will rise to between 81 and 87 years by the middle of the next century (based on middle-range assumptions).

The underlying premise behind demographic extrapolation models is that patterns of mortality decline from all causes of death combined that have occurred throughout the twentieth century have remained fairly stable.[28,45] More recent patterns of mortality decline indicate that, for some older age groups for some nations, mortality declines have even accelerated relative to earlier time periods.[49] This realization has led some demographers to conclude that extrapolating these mortality trends into the future is warranted and that there is reason to be optimistic that much higher life expectancies can still be achieved.[28,48–50] In addition, it has been argued that because declines in death rates have been documented reliably for the extreme elderly, if there is a biologically based limit to life it must be beyond the observed longevity horizon.[49,51–53] Additional support for this line of reasoning comes from research on the hypothetical relationship between risk factor modification and senescent mortality and the changes in behavior required to achieve high life expectancies.[50]

The reverse engineering approach developed by Olshansky et al.[47] demonstrated that to achieve a life expectancy at birth as high as 100 years for males and females combined, death rates from all causes of death combined would have to decline at every age by approximately 85%. Because mortality reductions of this magnitude require the near elimination of all senescent mortality throughout the age structure, it is difficult to justify assumptions that lead to such high life expectancies.[54,55] In addition, Olshansky and Carnes[55] demonstrated that the most optimistic demographic extrapolation models[48] rely on the underlying premise that dramatic reductions in cancer mortality are forthcoming, a condition that is inconsistent with the historical trend toward increasing death rates from this important cause of death. Furthermore, as death rates from other major killer diseases decline, the population saved from dying of these diseases remains exposed to the risk of developing cancer, a phenomenon known as competing risks (for more details on this concept, see Chapter 5). From the reverse engineering perspective, life expectancy at birth could rise beyond about 85 years only if advances are made in the biomedical sciences that somehow influence the basic rate of senescence itself.[47]

Conclusion

In the past 200 years, the demographic components of population change, principally birth rates and death rates, have been shifted from their "usual" historically high levels to more stable lower levels. This transformation has led to two unprecedented changes in the demography of humans—population aging and increased longevity. The social, economic, health, and political implications associated with both of these demographic phenomenon are profound.

With regard to population aging, rapid declines in death rates in the twentieth century have occurred throughout the age structure, leading to considerable increases in the proportion of each birth cohort surviving beyond age 65. Changes of this magnitude have undoubtedly led to increased heterogeneity at older ages, the health impacts of which have yet to be fully understood. Scientists involved in the debate on temporal trends in health expectancy are attempting to determine whether recent declines in old-age mortality have had a positive or negative impact on the health status of the older population, an issue directly related to increased heterogeneity. Because there is theoretical and empirical support for both the expansion and compression of morbidity hypotheses, it is premature to draw definitive conclusions abut the future course of health and longevity. Many other societal changes are expected to accompany rapid population aging, from changes in patterns of energy usage to the possible emergence of new senescent and infectious diseases at older ages.

Increased longevity among subgroups of the population is the other important demographic consequence of the transformation in death rates from high unstable levels to low stable levels. Although it is recognized that the majority of the rise in life expectancy at birth in the twentieth century is attributable to reductions in death rates at younger ages, reliable evidence has emerged to indicate that death rates are now declining, even among the extreme elderly (over age 85).[49] Demographic forecasts of human longevity have varied considerably, from optimistic estimates of about 85 years for men and women combined to extremely optimistic estimates of 100 years or higher.

Extrapolating past trends in mortality into the future is the conventional approach, and this appears quite reliable if the forecasts do not extend out too far into the future. Yet, during time periods when mortality rates either remain stable or decline rapidly, even short-term forecasts based on the extrapolation method will lead to substantial underestimates[56] or overestimates[55] of longevity. This difference has important policy implications for such agencies as the Social Security Administration or Census Bureau, which rely heavily on population forecasts to formulate public policy. Recently, scientists have questioned the use of statistical methods for speculating on trends in vital statistics that are ultimately determined by biologic phenomenon.[57] For example, one argument against a purely statistical approach to estimating the upper limit to life expectancy is that a linear extrapolation of past trends in mortality into the future would eventually lead to low death rates that are biologically implausible, which means that either a nonlinear assumption about the future course of mortality will eventually become necessary or justification for assuming zero death rates at any age must be provided. Because statistical approaches to extrapolating trends in death rates do not have either an implicit or explicit basis in biology, the only theoretical foundation for such assumptions is that the future will be some variation of the past. Determining the extent to which the past can be extrapolated into the future is critical in assessing the plausibility of such an assumption.

The future course of human longevity will be influenced by temporal trends in health practices, changes in the physical environments in which people live, advances in medical technology, and the degree to which humans lean how to modify the time-dependent expression of senescent mortality. The extent to which the expression of senescent mortality for humans can be modified remains uncertain, although there is theoretical and empirical evidence to indicate that low-mortality populations have already reached a point of diminishing returns with regard to future gains in life expectancy, although this is not to say that large declines in mortality at middle and older ages are impossible to achieve. To the contrary, such declines in death rates are anticipated. However, the measure of life expectancy is sufficiently insensitive to declining mortality in developed nations that it would take extremely large reductions in mortality to yield even small increases in life expectancy. Scientific advances that permit further modifications to the expression of senescent mortality may eventually lead to life expectancies for some population subgroups that exceed 85 years. There is reason to be optimistic that advances of this sort are forthcoming—although the social, economic, and health consequences of succeeding in altering the fundamental process of senescence are currently unknown.

References

1. Finch CE, Pike MC, Witten M. Slow mortality rate accelerations during aging in some animals approximate that of humans. *Science.* 1990;24:902–905.
2. Olshansky SJ, Carnes BA, Grahn D. Confronting the boundaries of human longevity. *Am Sci.* 1998;86(1):52–61.
3. Deevey ES Jr. Life tables for natural populations of animals. *Q Rev Biol.* 1947;22:283–314.
4. Thatcher AR. The long-term pattern of adult mortality and the highest attained age. *J R Stat Soc.* 1999;162(1):5–43.
5. Olshansky SJ, Carnes BA. Ever since Gompertz. *Demography.* 1997;34(1):1–15.
6. Carnes BA, Olshansky SJ. Evolutionary perspectives on human senescence. *Popul Dev Rev.* 1993;19:793–806.
7. McKinlay JB, McKinlay SM. The questionable contribution of medical measures to the decline of mortality in the United States in the twentieth century. *Milbank Q.* 1977; 55:405–428.
8. Olshansky SJ, Carnes BA, Rogers RG, Smith L. Infectious diseases—new and ancient threats to world health. *Popul Bull.* 1997;52(2):1–52.
9. Olshansky SJ, Carnes B, Cassel C. The aging of the human species. *Sci Am.* 1993;268(4):46–52.
10. National Research Council; Martin LA, Preston SH, eds. *Demography of Aging.* Washington, DC: National Academy Press; 1994.
11. Bell F, Wade AH, Goss SC. *Life Tables for the United States Security Area 1900–2080. Actuarial Study No. 107.* Washington, DC: Social Security Administration Publication 11-11536.
12. Fries JF. The compression of morbidity: near or far? *Milbank Q.* 1989;67:208–323.
13. Olshansky SJ, Rudberg MA, Carnes BA, et al. Trading off longer life for worsening health: the expansion of morbidity hypothesis. *J Aging Health.* 1991;3(2):194–216.
14. Rudberg M, Cassel C. Are death and disability in old age preventable? *Facts Res Gerontol.* 1993;7:191–202.
15. Verbrugge LM. Longer life but worsening health? Trends in health and mortality of middle-aged and older persons. *Milbank Q.* 1984;62:475–519.
16. Olshansky SJ, Carnes BA. *The Quest for Immortality.* New York: Norton Press; 2000.
17. Medawar PB. Old age and natural death. *Mod Q.* 1946; 2:30–49.
18. Williams GC. Pleiotropy, natural selection and the evolution of senescence. *Evolution.* 1957;11:398–411.
19. Kirkwood TBL. Comparative life spans of species: why do species have the life spans they do? *Am J Clin Nutr.* 1992; 55:1191S–1195S.
20. Crimmins E, Saito Y, Ingegneri D. Changes in life expectancy and disability-free life expectancy in the United States. *Popul Dev Rev.* 1989;15:235–267.
21. Mathers C. *Health Expectancies in Australia, 1981 and 1988.* Canberra, Australia: Australian Institute of Health Publications; 1999.
22. Robine JM, Ritchie K. Health life expectancy: evaluation of a new global indicator of change in population health. *Br Med J.* 1991;302:457–460.
23. Rogers R, Rogers A, Belanger A. Active life among the elderly in the United States: multi-state life-table estimates and population projection. *Milbank Q.* 1989;67:370–411.
24. Wilkins R, Adams OB. Health expectancy in Canada, late 1970s: demographic, regional and social dimensions. *Am J Public Health.* 1983;73:1073–1080.
25. Olshansky SJ, Wilkins R, eds. Special issue: policy implications of the measures and trends in health expectancy. *J Aging Health.* 1998;10(2).
26. Manton KG, Corder LS, Stallard E. Estimates of change in chronic disability and institutional incidents and prevalence rates in the United States elderly population from the 1992, 1984, and 1989 National Long-Term Care Survey. *J Gerontol.* 1993;48:S153–S168.
27. Bennett NG, Olshansky SJ. Forecasting U.S. age structure and the future of Social Security: the impact of adjustments to official mortality schedules. *Popul Dev Rev.* 1996;22(4): 703–727.

28. The 1999 Technical Panel on Assumptions and Methods. Report to the Social Security Advisory Board. Washington, DC: Social Security Administration; 1999.

29. Dublin LI, Lotka AJ, Spiegelman M. *Length of Life: Study of the Life Table.* New York: Ronald Press; 1949.

30. Olshansky SJ, Ault B. The fourth stage of the epidemiologic transition: the age of delayed degenerative diseases. *Milbank Q.* 1986;64:355–391.

31. Rogers R, Hackenberg R. Extending epidemiologic transition theory: a new stage. *Soc Biol.* 1989;34(3–4):234–243.

32. Olshansky SJ, Rogers R, Carnes BA, Smith L. Emerging infectious diseases: the fifth stage of the epidemiologic transition? *World Health Stat Q.* 51(2,3,4):207–217.

33. Loeb J, Northrop JH. Is there a temperature coefficient for the duration of life? *Proc Natl Acad Sci* USA. 1916;2:456.

34. Brownlee J. Notes on the biology of a life-table. *J R Stat Soc.* 1919;82:34.

35. Brody S. The kinetics of senescence. *J Gen Physiol.* 1924; 6:245–257.

36. Greenwood M. Laws of mortality from the biological point of view. *Q Rev Biol.* 1928;28:267–294.

37. Pearl R, Miner JR. Experimental studies on the duration of life. XIV. The comparative mortality of certain lower organisms. *Q Rev Biol.* 1935;10:60–79.

38. Pearl R. A comparison of the laws of *Drosophila* and in man. *Am Nat.* 1922;56:39.

39. Hayflick L, Moorhead PA. The serial cultivation of human diploid cell strains. *Exp Cell Res.* 1961;25:585–621.

40. Hayflick L. Theories of biological aging. *Exp Gerontol.* 1985;20:145–159.

41. Hayflick L. Why do we live so long? *Geriatrics.* 1988; 43(10):77–87.

42. Fries JF. Aging, natural death, and the compression of morbidity. *N Engl J Med.* 1980;303(3):130–135.

43. Vaupel JW, Gowan AE. Passage to Methuselah: some demographic consequences of continued progress against mortality. *Am J Public Health.* 1986;76:430–433.

44. Day JC. Population projections of the United States, by age, sex, race, and Hispanic origin. *Current Population Reports*, Series P-25, No. 1092. U.S. Census Bureau, Washington, DC, 1992.

45. Lee RD, Carter LR. Modeling and forecasting United States mortality. *J Am Stat Assoc.* 1992;87(419):659–671.

46. Stoto M, Durch JS. Forecasting survival, health, and disability: report on a workshop. *Popul Dev Rev.* 1993; 19(3):557–582.

47. Olshansky SJ, Carnes BA, Cassel C. In search of Methuselah: estimating the upper limits to human longevity. *Science.* 1990;250:634–640.

48. Ahlburg DA, Vaupel JW. Alternative projections of the US population. *Demography.* 1990;27:639–652.

49. Kannisto V, Lauritsen J, Thatcher AR, et al. Reductions in mortality at advanced ages: several decades of evidence from 27 countries. *Popul Dev Rev.* 1994;20:793–810.

50. Manton KG, Stallard E, Tolley HD. Limits to human life expectancy. *Popul Dev Rev.* 1991;17:603–637.

51. Carey JR, Liedo P, Orozco D, et al. Slowing of mortality rates at older ages in large medfly cohorts. *Science.* 1992; 258:457–461.

52. Curtsinger JW, Fukui, HH, Townsend JW, et al. Demography of genotypes: failure of the limited life-span paradigm in *Drosophila melanogaster. Science.* 1992;258: 461–463.

53. Fukui HH, Xiu L, Curtsinger JW. Slowing of age-specific mortality rates in *Drosophila melangaster. Exp Gerontol.* 1993;28:585–588.

54. Carnes BA, Olshansky SJ. Evolutionary perspectives on human senescence. *Popul Dev Rev.* 1993;19:793–806.

55. Olshansky SJ, Carnes BA. Demographic perspectives on human senescence. *Popul Dev Rev.* 1994;20:57–80.

56. Olshansky SJ. On forecasting mortality. *Milbank Q.* 1988; 66:482–530.

57. Olshansky SJ, Carnes BA, Cassel C. The future of long life [letter]. *Science.* 1998;281:1611–1612.

5
Epidemiology and Aging

Tamara B. Harris

The growing numbers of older people and the implications for the health care system, including higher costs of inpatient and outpatient treatments, drugs, and physician care, are inescapable in geriatric medicine. What is the relevance of epidemiology to these issues?

Generally defined, epidemiology is the "science which investigates the causes and control of ... disease in a community."[1] However, epidemiology, more specifically, is a methodology by which patterns of risk factors, health behaviors, and environmental and genetic factors are systematically studied for their impact on health outcomes. Application of this methodology to problems of aging has proven useful not only in understanding the relationship of factors contributing to disease but also in gaining insights into the potential age-related biologic processes that underlie these relationships and in defining how these processes are modifiable. This chapter presents an overview of some of the lessons learned from application of epidemiologic methods to problems of old age, highlighting illustrative advances in recognition and treatment of hypertension and new strategies to prevent hip fractures.

The Aging Population

In 2000, there were an estimated 35 million people aged 65 years or older, and this number will increase to 70 million by 2030. The proportion of persons older than age 85 will grow and, if current projections hold, this population will also be increasingly female, with relatively greater numbers of Hispanics and African-Americans. Life expectancy in old age continues to increase, and death rates for heart disease and stroke continue to decline while deaths from cancer are slightly increasing.[2] Older Americans continue to be more affluent than previous generations and less dependent on Social Security for exclusive income support. This situation will continue to be true in the future, reflecting the demo-

graphic trend for greater current workforce participation by women.[3]

One of the first lessons from epidemiology, however, is that not all older persons are alike. Chronic health conditions are a major source of heterogeneity in the older population, with hypertension and osteoarthritis among the most common chronic conditions, affecting upwards of 40% of men and almost 50% of women. Other specific diagnoses, such as cancer or heart disease, affect about 20% of the population, with diagnosed diabetes and stroke around 10%. The proportion with cognitive impairment or Alzheimer's disease is more difficult to estimate, owing to the greater difficulty with disease ascertainment, but estimates by age range from about 4% in those age 65 to 69 to as high as 20% or more in those age 80 and older.[4] What can be forgotten is that a substantial proportion of the older population remains free of disease and does not even use prescription medication. It is not surprising then that this heterogeneity in health status, coupled with heterogeneity of socioeconomic status and social factors, translates into heterogeneity in functional status.

Functional Status: More Differences Than Expected

The frailest older persons have been the major focus of epidemiologic studies of aging. This group is both the most vulnerable and also the most costly in terms of expenses related to long-term care, medical illness, and medication expenditures. However, it has become clear the frail elderly represent a relatively small proportion of those age 65 and older. A major contribution of epidemiology of aging has been the characterization of the heterogeneity of function in the older population, including the course of disability trajectories and a nascent understanding of factors contributing to these trajectories. In addition, recent studies have emphasized understanding how even the most disabled preserve social integrity and provide context in their lives.

In terms of the range of disability in the older population, data suggest that, even accounting for those who are institutionalized or have severe enough disability problems to have difficulty with an activity essential for daily living, only approximately 17% of the population over age 65 have some disability. Furthermore, data from repeated waves of national surveys suggest that this proportion is declining over time.[5] Even more important, among those age 80 and older, there is a substantial proportion, upwards of a fifth of both men and women, who not only report no difficulty with activities of daily living, but also report that they are fully independent, including meeting criteria established by Nagi for being able to work full-time.[6] Thus, although the very disabled elderly are most visible in institutions and health care facilities and as users of health care resources, the range of capacities across the spectrum of aging is very large.

These differences have been highlighted by a number of studies targeted to identification of this heterogeneity and to examination of some of the earliest factors contributing to functional decline. These studies have identified new ways to measure disability, including using a wider range of reported items to cover the entire spectrum of function, especially among those with no limitations in activities of daily life; these include drawing on Nagi items to examine mobility-related problems and questions regarding ease of performance or change in performance.[7] Objective measures involving timed tasks mirroring clinical assessments of daily life tasks have been used to augment the self-report and to provide measures that facilitate comparisons of populations.[8] These measures, analogous to mental status testing, draw on simple tasks basic to a standard neurologic examination but refined and standardized to be administered and scored by nonmedical personnel. Both sets of measures augment approaches specifically targeted to establishing need for supportive services by self-report of simple, necessary activities of daily living.

Epidemiologic and clinical studies have shown that much of disability reflects a failure of compensatory mechanisms either on an organ-specific physiologic basis, as in the case of congestive failure, pulmonary disease, or renal disease, or on a societal level, where the capacity of the person to be maintained in independent living may be compromised by a lack of ability to obtain the basic necessities of life. Disability trajectories also may reflect the underlying severity of factors contributing to functional decline. Catastrophic disability is associated with irreparable organ failure that cannot be compensated, for instance, from a stroke, whereas progressive disability tends to occur with small decrements which, cumulatively over time, result in failure of compensation, although each insult alone might not result in disability.[9] Further-

more, in the case of progressive disability, deficits that are quite profound may not be recognizable for some time because individuals may successfully adjust to their deficits either by altering what they do or by altering the manner in which they perform necessary life tasks so that they can continue to function, albeit in a different manner.[10] Last, we have also begun to recognize that disability in one area of function, such as physical function, may not be accompanied by disability in another area of function, such as cognitive or social. For instance, epidemiologists have recently described the phenomenon of emotional vitality, identifying the preserved quality of life experienced by severely disabled older women who continue to maintain an active and supportive social network.[11] Religion and religiosity may play a role in this area as well,[12] although social vitality may exist quite apart from the religious community.

Thus, a major contribution of population epidemiology has been to identify the heterogeneity within the older population—developing methods to allow evaluation of the prevalence and causes of disability and to address the question of how people age differently, how aging reflects both biology and life events, and how older people maintain and consolidate their level of independence in the face of major challenges to mind, body, and spirit. These efforts continue to help in identification of new risk factors for disease that will help to further limit loss of independence in old age and in the formulation of preventive interventions appropriate for each level of functioning in old age.

How Heterogeneity Affects Our View of Age-Related Changes and Risk

Epidemiologic tools have been also useful in development of a fundamental principle of gerontologic research: that longitudinal age-related changes are exaggerated by using cross-sectional populations.[13] Because of the difficulty of performing longitudinal studies across the entire life span, a number of different approaches have been used in studies of age-related changes. The easiest type of study to perform to assess age-related trends involved identification of groups of individuals of different ages, measuring the trait of interest in each of these groups. The results, comparing the older age groups with the youngest group participating, were considered in indicative of "normal" trends with age. A number of problems were identified with this approach. There were secular factors that could distort "age" trends, that is, a decrease in cholesterol following major health education campaigns regarding the risks associated with cholesterol.[14] Cohort factors that might change from one generation to another could confound observed patterns. For instance, although height does decrease with age, this effect is exaggerated if one looks across successive generations because more recent generations enjoy better nutrition and health, which translates into taller maximal heights.[15] Younger individuals have at least two reasons for taller heights. Their generation grew to taller maximal heights because of better nutrition, and they have not yet suffered age-associated height loss, effects that may be difficult to separate. Similar issues are seen for cognitive function, where declines with age are exaggerated by better educational status associated with better test performance in more recent generations.[16] Other investigators identified preagonal patterns affecting the data. For instance, in the years before death, even in seemingly healthier older people, cognitive performance was lower or slower than in those who were likely to survive the same period of time.[17]

Even among well-screened volunteers, groups of subjects of different ages were likely to vary by health status, and the trajectories of longitudinal trends might differ reflecting patterns of lifelong contributing factors. For instance, mean creatinine clearance declines with age when comparing subjects of different ages who have been similarly screened. However, at least part of this effect is secondary to the fact that renal function reflects lifelong health factors such as ambient blood pressure. Data from the Baltimore Longitudinal Study of Aging demonstrated that there is little change in renal function among those who have been stable normotensives, whereas among those with poorly controlled hypertension, the trajectory of decline in renal function was very steep.[18] Among people in each age group, the proportion with underlying factors that would contribute to decline in kidney function increases with age, and therefore the mean creatinine clearance appears to markedly decline with "normal" aging. As with renal function, once all these issues were taken into account, many changes in function with age were noted to be much smaller than suggested by either the cross-sectional data or by methodologically poor longitudinal studies.

A second major issue with regard to risk assessment follows from these studies. As the population ages, the proportion of individuals with subclinical illness that could affect the status of other health markers increases. This factor has led to a series of paradoxical findings in elderly populations that have confused efforts to counsel older individuals regarding weight, cholesterol, and other health behaviors and risk factors important in younger populations. For instance, studies of weight and mortality in old age have shown no risk, an increased risk with thinness, an increased risk with heavier weight, and a protective effect of heavier weight, especially in the oldest-old.[19–21] Although it is biologically plausible that the relationship of weight to mortality could change with age, these disparate findings may also reflects shifts in weight that occur with age. People in the developed world tend to gain weight over their lifetime, so that by late middle age there are few individuals who have been thin throughout most of life. In old age, many people lose weight, either directly because of illness or to ameliorate weight-related risk, and therefore their thinness reflects risk secondary to poor health.[22] Thus, most thin older people have not been thin throughout life but rather have become thin in old age. It is hardly surprising then that this group has an increased risk of mortality that approaches and may even surpass that of the heavier population. Among heavy older persons, most have also not been heavy all throughout their lives but have gained weight in late middle age. This group may have lower risk of mortality secondary reflecting their midlife weight. Consideration of lifelong patterns of risk factors may help to clarify the results of relationships based on a one-point-in-time measurement. This life-course approach, another contribution of epidemiology to aging research, may identify whether the pathophysiology of disease really does differ in old age or whether age-related changes merely obscure a consistent biologic pattern.

Contributions of Epidemiology to Clinical Practice: Hypertension Control in Old Age

Epidemiology has also been important in the "medicalization" of processes previously thought to be a part of normal aging, with conditions once accepted as normal now being identified as associated with risk or as disease states. This reclassification from "normal" to "disease" has allowed formulation of methods of prevention or treatment. Among these conditions is cognitive impairment. Over time, the definition of acceptable cognitive loss with age has become substantially narrower as researchers investigate patterns of cognitive function and risk factors for change. As more "normal aging" becomes understood to represent pathology secondary to disease, health-related behaviors, or environmental factors that change with age, efforts to delineate causal factors increase in parallel with efforts to remediate the condition.

One important example, one of the major successes of aging research, is the recognition and treatment of hypertension, particularly isolated systolic hypertension. As recently as 30 years ago, it was still believed that development of systolic hypertension in old age was "natural" process stemming from atherosclerosis.[23] Autoregulation of cerebral blood flow that reflected hypertension suggested that older people required a "higher head of steam" to perfuse the brain.[24] Efforts to treat hypertension, particularly isolated systolic hypertension, were postulated as not only unlikely to benefit the patient but potentially contributing to risk. These theories did not yield easily to data. Studies began to demonstrate that systolic blood pressure tended to increase later in life and that this increase might represent a distinct physiologic process from diastolic hypertension.[25] Although cross-sectional and longitudinal studies showed that blood pressure tended to increase with age in most populations, studies from isolated populations such as lifetime residents of mental hospitals showed that blood pressure did not increase very much at all over the life span.[26] These studies called into question whether blood pressure rise with age should be considered as an inevitable consequence of aging. Studies of the outcomes of systolic hypertension demonstrated that this was not a benign condition, but rather, whether in combination with diastolic hypertension or when isolated, resulted in increased risk of stroke and coronary heart disease.[27,28] Thus, studies of blood pressure change with age showed that these changes were not "normal" with age and that hypertension carried an increased risk of poor health outcomes.

However, demonstration of the poor health risks associated with systolic hypertension was not enough. Clinical trials were needed to demonstrate that there was a benefit to treatment in terms of reduction of risk of cardiovascular complications. The first clinical trials for hypertension did not really address the issue of treatment of systolic hypertension; in fact, the clinical trials focused primarily on diastolic blood pressure, the most common type of elevated blood pressure in middle-aged individuals.[29] Even the gradual recognition that treatment of diastolic blood pressure often resulted in lowering of systolic blood pressure was not believed to clearly address the question of whether older persons with isolated systolic hypertension should be treated aggressively to lower blood pressure.

Several major clinical trials were undertaken to address the issue of hypertension in old age. The first was the European Isolated Systolic Hypertension Study, which enrolled 840 older persons in 11 countries throughout Europe.[30] In the United States, the Systolic Hypertension in the Elderly Program (SHEP) was established, enrolling 4736 persons in a complicated protocol that involved screening thousands of participants.[31] Both studies demonstrated conclusively that treatment of systolic hypertension resulted in lower mortality and cardiovascular morbidity in the elderly, and these results were supported by additional studies.[32,33] Even with a much more limited group of medications than is available today, blood pressure could be treated safely, effectively, and cheaply using a stepped protocol in older persons.

These studies established important principles for research in aging. First, age-related changes that were so common as to seem "normal" can carry risk. Second, medical conditions in the elderly could be successfully treated to alter the course of health outcomes associated with these conditions. Thus, even in older persons, prevention is important. Third, older persons could be recruited successfully to participate in clinical trials; they would comply with the treatments and provide analyzable data that could help to guide clinical reommendations for other older persons. This realization established the viability of clinical trials in old age; however, even today there remain major barriers to the participation of older persons in clinical trials, primarily based on misconceptions about the compliance of older persons in the trials. Last, results from trials of conditions common in old age could provide important information about the biology of disease in old age and the causes of these conditions and, if not the reversibility of biologic effects, at least the prevention of secondary outcomes.

Population epidemiology continues to provide new information on hypertension risk and the benefits of treatment that could be very important in old age. Although the role of hypertension in cardiovascular disease has been appreciated for some time, the potential contribution of hypertension to other conditions is only beginning to be understood. For instance, recent data on population-based magnetic resonance imaging studies of the brain have suggested that hypertension may make a major contribution to risk of small silent brain infarctions that may contribute to cognitive decline[34] and that treatment of hypertension can lower risk of congestive heart failure.[35] Other data suggest that even apart from risk of stroke, hypertension in midlife may contribute to cognitive decline in old age.[36] This area continues to be one of active research.

Epidemiology and the Geriatric Perspective on Hip Fracture

Epidemiology of aging has contributed a novel perspective on how to attack the problem of fracture risk in osteoporosis. Osteoporosis and associated risk of fracture is a major health problem for both elderly men and women.[37] There have been major improvements in understanding of the best techniques and timing for surgery, but outcomes associated with hip fracture are still poor. Risk of mortality in the 6 months postfracture remain high, and odds of full recovery of function are low.

The medical community has gained remarkably in terms of understanding osteoporsis and risk of fracture from clinical research, population studies, and clinical trials targeting osteoporosis and fracture-associated risk. In the course of these studies, a perspective on fracture has emerged that gives weight to both the classical endocrinologic perspective of hormones determining osteoporotic risk and the geriatric perspective, which suggests that factors associated with frailty and increased risk of falling contribute to fracture risk as well. The benefit has been a comprehensive and integrated approach to fracture prevention.

By the mid-1980s, the role of estrogen decline in women contributing to bone loss was well established. Patterns of change in bone mineral relating to periods of hormonal change over the lifetime had been identified and a threshold for risk of osteoporotic fracture established.[38] The primary goal of therapy was to boost women over the fracture threshold so long as possible, with manipulations targeted to increasing peak bone mass and reducing bone loss at critical periods, such as during the perimenopausal period.[39]

During this same period, a group of geriatricians and general internists began to question whether bone mass alone was the key to the entire risk of fracture. Equally, if not more important, were risk factors that contributed to the fall leading to fracture. Early studies identified those at risk of falling and demonstrated some overlap with known risk factors for fracture.[40] These studies also established methodologies that could be used to track the frequency and severity of falls in population studies to better prospectively establish the role of falling in relation to risk of fracture.

At the same time, techniques were developed that allowed the measurement of bone mineral density in populations, and several studies were initiated that incorporated a holistic overview of putative risk factors for fracture. The largest of these, the Study of Osteoporotic Fractures, established that bone mineral density and falls were both risk factors for fracture. Furthermore, risk factors contributing to both lower bone mineral density, such as smoking, and risk factors contributing to risk of falling, such as reduced vision and strength, also contributed to risk of fracture.[41] Thus, new avenues for intervention to reduce risk of fracture were identified.

Subsequent clinical trials have addressed the potential modifiability of each of these factors. Tinetti and colleagues identified that risk of falling was modifiable by testing an algorithmic approach to diagnosis and intervention of risk factors for falling.[42] In addition, Tinetti contributed seminal work defining that the risk factors for falling could be used to identify those most at risk and therefore most likely to benefit from intervention and that the interventions might differ depending on the functional status of the older person.[43,44] Interventions needed to prevent fracture needed to account for the heterogeneity in the at-risk population, as the goal was to prevent fractures without increasing fear of falling, which could itself lead to decline in functional independence.

Clinical trials have also provided a number of interventions to modify bone mineral. The Fracture Intervention Trial established the efficacy of alendronate first in prevention of vertebral fractures and later for hip frac-

ture.[45] Other more specific estrogen agonists, such as raloxifene, have also been identified as useful to prevent osteoporotic bone loss.[46] Most surprising, however, have been the clinical trials of estrogen. Although a staple of therapy for osteoporosis for years, estrogen had not been tested in a randomized clinical trial. Potential biases related to the characteristics of women given estrogen therapy in clinical practice, including the fact that these women were often thinner and healthier than other women, raised questions about whether this therapy would prove as efficacious when tested in a randomly assigned population. The Women's Health Initiative, a multioutcome trial of estrogen use as protective for hip fracture and heart disease and enhancing the risk of breast cancer, is now underway.[47] Surprisingly, the only finding thus far is a modest increase in risk of cardiovascular deaths in the first several years of the study. This finding, plus options now available with other medications, have opened the questin of whether estrogen is the first-line treatment for osteoporosis.

A third potential avenue for prevention of fractures is dietary supplementation with calcium, also part of the Women's Health Initiative. In addition, following the observation that older men are experiencing a major increase in the numbers of fractures, a large population-based study has been initiated to further understand risk factors for fracture in older men, which is likely to add to the already large list of factors that contribute to fracture.

Summing Up

Thus, epidemiologic methods have contributed to a complex and dynamic understanding of risk of disease in old age, identifying factors that are related to "classical" medical disciplines, such as endocrinology, but also a host of new risk factors that could be regarded as "geriatric." These latter risk factors tend to be more holistic in that they relate not to one organ system specifically, but identify how even small deficits in multiple organ systems can contribute to risk of poor health outcomes in old age.

The tools and principles of epidemiology have had an important impact on our view of the capabilities and heterogeneity of the older population, on the differentiation of disease from normal aging, on a life-course perspective for risk, and on the types of interventions available to contend with the problems of old age. Many of these contributions have been incorporated in a variety of evidence-based practice guidelines, and the possibilities for the future are bright. Epidemiology can be an important tool to help researchers who study the problems of old age to learn more about the range of health, social, and psychologic problems of the elderly, to identify new avenues for intervention and to test these interventions, and to adapt the interventions to the practical realities of growing old. In this way, epidemiologic method can function as an important adjunct in the mission of promoting independence and providing evidence-based health care for older people.

References

1. *Webster's New Twentieth Century Dictionary*, 2nd Ed. New York: Simon Schuster; 1979.
2. Federal Interagency Forum on Aging-Related Statistics. *Older American 2000: Key Indicators of Well-Being*. Washington, DC: Sauls Lithograph; 2000.
3. Federal Interagency Forum on Aging-Related Statistics. *Older American 2000: Key Indicators of Well-Being*. Washington, DC: Sauls Lithograph; 2000. p 19.
4. Federal Interagency Forum on Aging-Related Statistics. *Older American 2000: Key Indicators of Well-Being*. Washington, DC: Sauls Lithograph; 2000. pp 24, 25.
5. Manton KG, Stallard E, Corder LS. The dynamics of dimensions of age-related disability 1982 to 1994 in the U.S. elderly population. *J Gerontol A Biol Sci Med Sci*. 1998;53: B59–B70.
6. Harris T, Kovar MG, Suzman R, et al. Longitudinal study of physical ability in the oldest-old. *Am J Pubic Health*. 1989;79:698–702.
7. Simonsick EM, Newman AB, Nevitt MC, et al. Measuring higher level physical function in well-functioning older adults: Expanding familiar approaches in the Health ABC study. *J Gerontol Series A-Biol Sci Med Sci*. 2001;56: M644–M649.
8. Guralnik JM, Ferrucci L, Simonsick EM, et al. Lower-extremity function in persons over the age of 70 years as a predictor of subsequent disability. *N Engl J Med*. 1995; 332:556–561.
9. Ferrucci L, Guralnik JM, Simonsick EM, et al. Progressive versus catastrophic disability: a longitudinal view of the disablement process. *J Gerontol A Biol Sci Med Sci*. 1996;51: M123–M130.
10. Fried LP, Herdman SJ, Juhn K, et al. Preclinical disability: Hypotheses about the bottom of the iceberg. *J Aging Health*. 1991;3:285–300.
11. Penninx BW, Guralnik JM, Bandeen-Roche K, et al. The protective effect of emotional vitality on adverse health outcomes in disabled older women. *J Am Geriatr Soc*. 2000; 48:1359–1366.
12. Koenig HG, Hays JC, George LK, et al. Modeling the cross-sectional relationships between religion, physical health, social support, and depressive symptoms. *Am J Geriatr Psychiatry*. 1997;5:131–144.
13. Bleich HL, Boro ES, Rowe JW. Clinical research on aging: strategies and directions. *N Engl J Med*. 1977;297:1332–1336.
14. Herschcopf RJ, Elahi D, Andres R, et al. Longitudinal changes in serum cholesterol in man: An epidemiologic search for an etiology. *J Chronic Dis*. 1982;35:101–114.
15. Cline MG, Meredith KE, Boyer JT, et al. Decline of height with age in adults in a general population sample: estimat-

16. ing maximum height and distinguishing birth cohort effects from actural loss of stature with aged. *Hum Biol*. 1989; 61:415–425.
16. Schaie KW, Parham IA. Cohort-sequential analyses of adult intellectual development. *Dev Psychol*. 1977;13:649–653.
17. White N, Cunningham WR. Is terminal drop pervasive or specific? *J Gerontol*. 1988;43:P141–P144.
18. Lindeman RD, Tobin J, Shock NW. Longitudinal studies on the rate of decline in renal function with age. *J Am Geriatr Soc*. 1985;33:278–285.
19. Stevens J, Cai J, Pamuk ER, et al. The effect of age on the association between body-mass index and mortality. *N Engl J Med*. 1998;338:1–7.
20. Diehr P, Bild DE, Harris TB, et al. Body mass index and mortality in nonsmoking older adults: the Cardiovascular Health Study. *Am J Public Health*. 1998;88:623–629.
21. Rajala SA, Kanto AJ, Haavisto MV. Body weight and the three-year prognosis in very old people. *Int J Obes*. 1990; 14:997–1003.
22. Harris TB, Launer LJ, Madans J, et al. Cohort study of effect of being overweight and change in weight on risk of coronary heart disease in old age. *Br Med J*. 1997;314:1791–1794.
23. Busse EW. Biologic and sociologic changes affecting adaptation in mid and late life. *Ann Intern Med*. 1971;75: 115–120.
24. Standgaard S, Olesen J, Skinhoj E, et al. Autoregulation of brain circulation in severe arterial hypertension. *Br Med J*. 1973;1:507–510.
25. Koch-Weser J. The therapeutic challenge of systolic hypertension. *N Engl J Med*. 1973;289:481–484.
26. Main CJ, Masterton G. The influence of hospital environment on blood pressure in psychiatric in-patients. *J Psychosom Res*. 1981;25:157–163.
27. Lew EA. High blood pressure, other risk factors and longevity: the insurance viewpoint. *Am J Med*. 1973;55: 281–287.
28. Shekelle RB, Ostfield AM, Klawans HL Jr. Hypertension and risk of stroke in an elderly population. *Stroke*. 1974;5: 71–75.
29. Hypertension Detection and Follow-Up Program Cooperative Group. Five-year findings of the hypertension deterction and follow-up program. II. Mortality by race, sex, and age. *JAMA*. 1979;242:2572–2577.
30. Amery A, Birkenhager W, Brixho P, et al. Mortality and morbiditiy results from the European working party on high blood pressure in the elderly trial. *Lancet*. 1985;i: 1349–1354.
31. SHEP Cooperative Research Group. Prevention of stroke by antihypertensive drug treatment in older persons with isolated systolic hypertension. Final results of the Systolic Hypertension in the Elderly Program (SHEP). *JAMA*. 1991;265:3255–3264.
32. Australian Therapeutic Trial Management Committee. Treatment of mild hypertension in the elderly: a study initiated and administered by the National Heart Foundation of Australia. *Med J Aust*. 1981;ii:398–402.
33. Dahlof B, Lindholm LH, Hansson L, et al. Morbidity and mortality in the Swedish trial in old patients with hypertension (STOP-Hypertension). *Lancet*. 1991;338:1281–1285.

34. Price TR, Manolio TA, Kronmal RA, et al. Silent brain infarction on magnetic resonance imaging and neurological abnormalities in community-dwelling older adults. The cardiovascular Health Study. *Stroke.* 1997;28:1158–1164.

35. Kostis JB, Davis BR, Cutler J, et al. Prevention of heart failure by antihypertensive drug treatment in older persons with isolated systolic hypertension. SHEP Cooperative Research Group. *JAMA.* 1997;278:212–216.

36. Launer LJ, Masaki K, Petrovitch H, et al. The association between midlife blood pressure levels and late-life cognitive function. The Honolulu-Asia Aging Study. *JAMA.* 1995;274:1846–1851.

37. Kanis JA, Johnell O, Oden A, et al. Risk of hip fracture derived from relative risks: an analysis applied to the population of Sweden. *Osteoporosis Int.* 2000;11:120–127.

38. Riggs BL, Melton LJ III. Involutional osteoporosis. *N Engl J Med.* 1986;314:1676–1686.

39. Richelson LS, Wahner HW, Melton LJ III, Riggs BL. Relative contributions of aging and estrogen deficiency to postmenopausal bone loss. *N Engl J Med.* 1984;311:1273–1275.

40. Cummings SR, Nevitt MC. A hypothesis: the causes of hip fractures. *J Gerontol.* 1989;44:M107–M111.

41. Nevitt MC, Cummings SR. Type of fall and risk of hip and wrist fractures: the Study of Osteoporotic Fractures. *J Am Geriatr Soc.* 1993;41:1226–1234.

42. Tinetti ME, Speechley M, Ginter ST. Risk factors for falls among elderly persons living in the community. *N Engl J Med.* 1988;319:1701–1707.

43. Tinetti ME, Baker DI, McAvay G, et al. A multifactorial intervention to reduce the risk of falling among elderly people living in the community. *N Engl J Med.* 1994;331:821–827.

44. Speechley M, Tinnetti M. Falls and injuries in frail and vigorous community elderly persons. *J Am Geriatr Soc.* 1991;39:46–52.

45. Cummings SR, Black DM, Thompson DE, et al. Effect of alendronate on risk of fracture in women with low bone denisty but without vertebral fractures: results from the Fracture Intervention Trial. *JAMA.* 1998;280:2077–2082.

46. Prestwood KM, Gunness M, Muchmore DB, et al. A comparison of the effects of raloxifene and estrogen on bone in postmenopausal women. *J Clin Endocrinol Metab.* 2000;85:2197–2202.

47. The Women's Health Initiative Study Group. Design of the Women's Health Initiative clinical trial and observational study. *Control Clin Trials.* 1998;19:61–109.

6
Psychosocial Influences on Health in Later Life

Elizabeth C. Clipp and Karen E. Steinhauser

Geriatricians face an enormous intellectual and personal challenge in understanding the interactive complexities—physical, psychosocial, functional, and spiritual—of caring for elderly patients. Successful geriatric assessment and treatment depend not only on recognition of pathology but, perhaps more importantly, on understanding how such pathology relates to the "whole person."

The interactive complexities of geriatric medicine have led geriatricians to consider relatively unique care approaches, most notably the multidisciplinary approach, which utilizes expertise from a number of disciplines in the care of older adults. It is the geriatrician's challenge to move beyond medical opinion and integrate the observations of multidisciplinary team members before implementing an overall plan of care. Equally important to the recognition of pathologic processes in geriatrics is the impact of disease on function. As such, the practice of multidimensional geriatric assessment focuses heavily on the social, psychologic, and environmental factors that influence function, such as the elderly patient's social milieu.

Several key observations in geriatrics highlight the links between psychosocial factors and patient functioning. First, psychosocial and cultural factors influence differences in illness behavior between older and younger patients. Second, these differences in illness behavior interact with age-related physiologic organ change leading to delayed or altered disease presentation and multiple concurrent pathology. Third, variation in disease presentation and comorbidity profiles gives rise to different trajectories of recovery and clinical outcomes. These observations anticipated the introduction of "nonmedical supports" as important to geriatricians' goals of maintaining and improving patient outcomes. Geriatric assessment often includes patients' emotional tone and lifelong habits. In some settings, teams expand the social history component in geriatric assessment to include social interaction, support systems, and community resources, factors likely to influence the future functioning and disability management of the patient in the community.

Now considered the optimal standard of care, a systematic approach to comprehensive geriatric assessment attends to multiple personal domains, including but not limited to physical health, mental health, function, and social situation. This scope of inquiry is significantly broader than other medical specialities and makes performing comprehensive assessment a formidable task within the shorter encounter time frames of most managed care environments. Although early, single-site studies of this approach showed impact on survival and improved functional outcomes, more recent randomized controlled trials have shown little impact on survival but do show benefits in functional outcomes.[1,2] Tension between managed care time constraints, the geriatrician's need to integrate multiple data sources, and the potential benefits of applying comprehensive assessment to functionally compromised patients gives rise to two questions. First, what psychosocial aspects of aging are most likely to affect clinical outcomes? And second, how can geriatricians efficiently capture these data in standard clinical encounters?

The clinical focus of this chapter necessitates the omission of many of the more traditional topics usually associated with the psychological aspects of aging (e.g., personality, behavioral processes, memory, learning, perception) and social aspects of aging (e.g., demographic patterns, social structure, housing and living arrangements, work and retirement, economic status). Readers interested in comprehensive reviews on such topics are referred to the recently released fifth editions of the *Handbook of the Psychology of Aging* and the *Handbook of Aging and the Social Sciences*, 2001.[3,4]

This chapter identifies seven key psychosocial domains that should be part of the geriatrician's perspective: gender, ethnicity and class; historical influences (i.e., military experience); social relationships; spirituality;

caregiving; elder mistreatment; and successful aging. This list is by no means exhaustive, but rather offers an initial framework for assessment. We present the proposed mechanisms linking these domains to health in later life and conclude with a set of probes that may be used by practicing geriatricians to capture these key psychosocial domains in everyday practice.

The Role of Gender, Ethnicity, and Class

It has long been known that one's position in society —being female or male, richer or poorer, African-American, Caucasian, or Latino—is strongly associated with different levels of health and illness. Beyond differences in physiology, individuals live in psychosocial environments in which health is either enhanced or put at risk. Gender, ethnicity, and socioeconomic status or class are three predominant features of these contexts.

What accounts for these predictable differences in health outcomes? A variety of explanations have been proposed.[5,6] Demographic categories may function as proxies for inherent physiologic disparities between various population subgroups. Alternatively, demographics may be proxies for other social factors. First, each social location category offers different access to health care. Second, differential socialization affects health behaviors. For example, poorer individuals may be more likely to smoke; men are less likely to formally report health problems; women have higher rates of health care utilization; and persons experiencing discrimination may be less likely to trust physicians of other ethnicities, which may reduce both utilization and compliance. Third, social location may produce varying levels of stress that increase susceptibility to disease. For example, poorer individuals may live in more toxic, crowded, or hazardous environments. Finally, physicians may treat individuals differently on the basis of gender, ethnicity, or class. There are well-documented examples of minorities receiving different cardiac care when presenting the same symptoms as Caucasian patients.[7] No one explanation is sufficient. Rather, clinicians should be aware of the variety of causal processes—physiologic, psychosocial, environmental— that impact health or contribute to illness.

We offer here a brief general overview of some evidence-based differences in health associated with gender, ethnicity, and socioeconomic status that may be useful in the clinical encounter, highlighting differences in general patterns of chronic disease, functional impairment, self-rated health, depressive symptoms, psychologic distress, and mortality. At the end of each subsection, we direct the reader to full reviews, but offer summaries of those reviews.

Gender

For most health indicators, except mortality, women have poorer health than men. Older women report more chronic disease; however, as compared to men, those illnesses generally are less serious or catastrophic.[8] Women show higher prevalence of functional impairment than men, but there are no gender differences in incidence. This discrepancy is most likely caused by earlier onset and increased longevity for women. Perception of one's own health, or self-reported health, is lower for women than men. However, one study shows a gender and age interaction, whereby gender differences in self-rated health are greatest among young adults and least during old age. Studies show that the onset of depression is more common in younger women than among younger men but equally common in men and women at older ages.[9]

Race and Ethnicity

Chronic diseases are more prevalent among older African-Americans. Functional decline, according to most studies, is also greater among African-Americans; Latino functional status falls between that of African-Americans and Caucasian older adults. However, research has shown a crossover among the oldest-old, where African-Americans over 85 function at higher levels than whites. It has been hypothesized that this crossover represents a "hardiness factor," whereby because African-Americans are at higher risk for mortality and morbidity for the majority of the life course, those who survive to 85 represent a select group in terms of function. African-Americans over 75 have lower mortality than Caucasian older adults. As such, these results represent not an elevated functional status enjoyed by older African-Americans, but rather a remarkable selection effect from a lifetime of poorer health risk.[10] Research shows no differences in self-rated health or depressive symptoms among older African-American and Caucasian adults.[9,10]

Some have proposed a double-jeopardy hypothesis in that being African-American and older gives double risk for adverse health consequences. Evidence does not support this. However, leading health and ethnicity researchers suggest this hypothesis remains an important part of the theoretical landscape by emphasizing the racial disparity in health outcomes throughout most of the life course.[10]

Social Class or Socioeconomic Status

Research shows that, in general, lower socioeconomic status (SES) is related to increased mortality and disproportionate impairment from major diseases, such as cardiovascular disease, diabetes, and cancer.[10] Socioeconomic status is measured in several ways, including education, occupation, and income; conclusions about the effects of SES on health are often dependent on the particular indicator used. Higher levels of education are significantly related to lower prevalence of chronic illness, lower functional impairment, and higher self-rated health. Lower income has been found to predict functional decline among men but not women. Both income and education are inversely related to depressive symptoms. However, SES interacts with ethnicity for this health outcome, such that among highly educated individuals, African-Americans report fewer depressive symptoms and, among lower-education adults, African-Americans report more depressive symptoms. Evidence is not convincing regarding the relationship between SES and depressive disorders.[9]

Socioeconomic status also can mediate the relationship between social factors and health. Education and income have been shown to partially explain functional status differences among blacks and whites and fully explain the relationship between gender and functional decline. These findings suggest that if women had equal socioeconomic resources, they would attain higher functional levels than men. Similarly, data show that SES explains gender differences in self-rated health. Finally, the influence of socioeconomic status on health varies across the life course with differences small in childhood, increasing in middle age, and decreasing again in later life. The lessening effects of SES in late adulthood are hypothesized to be related to policies, such as Medicare, that are aimed at increasing population-wide access to health care resources.[9,10]

Physician–Patient Relationship and Health

Some discrepancies in health outcomes are associated with ethnic and gender differences between patients and physicians. For example, evidence suggests that gender and ethnicity do influence patient–physician communication and patient decision making.[11] In particular, minority patients and those with lower education report less participation with their physicians; women report more participation, receive more information, and ask more questions. Female physicians have been rated as having a higher participatory style and empathy, which is associated with higher patient satisfaction and lower rates of malpractice. These differences may be due to perceived stereotypes, a lack of understanding of cultural differences in disease models, and lack of awareness regarding difference expectation among those with lower education, health literacy, or health care autonomy.[11] Some clinician-researchers recommend that physicians may

work to develop their own communication skills, as well as empower patients to increase participation. Furthermore, acquiring "cultural competence" may improve interaction. That competence is developed with three components: knowledge of variation in health-related beliefs and values, disease incidence and prevalence, and differential treatment efficacy.[11]

Time

It is important to emphasize the role of time in predicting health. Much of gerontologic research focuses on documenting age differences in health. However, we are less clear about the underlying causal processes and whether measurable health differences are age related, age dependent, or time dependent. For example, are the differences we see in older adults the result of an age-dependent process, whereby after 80 years of life, organisms generally function in a relatively predictable way? Or are the observed health differences the result of historical effects, such as the long-term effects of military experience? An entire group or cohort not permitted to attend public school may express the effects of lower education across a lifetime. In fact, no reductionist explanation is sufficient. Individuals, with their unique physiology, move across the life course and through historical time being shaped by and, in turn, shaping their world. Identification of the source of idiosyncrasy apparent in old age is multifaceted and presents researchers with a conundrum, frequently referenced as the age–period–cohort issue in gerontology. Its resolution will appear only as we accrue longitudinal health outcome data on multiple generations across long periods of time that permit us to test the effects of age, controlling for time and generational influences. Until such data are available, clinicians may be reminded of the fluidity of aging processes; aging today will be different from aging tomorrow. A clear example of a cohort or historical effect present in many geriatric patients today is that of military experience.

Historical Influences: The Example of Military Experience

It is well recognized that the entire American population is aging but infrequently acknowledged that the increase of elderly U.S. veterans is even more rapid. Specifically, the number of veterans over age 65 peaked in 2000 at 9 million, making them a majority proportion (63%) of all elderly males in the United States. It is therefore highly likely that currently practicing geriatricians will encounter substantial numbers of older male veterans in their practices. How does former military experience influence health in later life? Why is knowledge of veteran status important in geriatric assessment?

The majority of studies linking military experience, especially combat exposure, to war and postwar health have concentrated on emotional manifestations, such as psychiatric syndromes and posttraumatic stress disorder (PTSD). Research also has explored veteran postwar and longer-term health trajectories and somatic indicators of war stress, but postwar and long-term pathogenesis (e.g., cardiovascular disease, cancer) has been neglected. Little attention has been given to military experience in the development of health risk factors, and virtually nothing is known about the military precursors of postwar mortality. One model emerging in the behavioral medicine literature that explores potential relationships among war stress, disease risk, and mortality focuses on mechanisms linked to coronary artery disease (CAD), the impairment of immunocompetence, and health risk behaviors. Unfortunately, little work has applied these models to long periods of the life span, as between military service in the twenties and later-life health.

An extensive recent literature now links psychosocial factors (e.g., acute and chronic stress), social isolation, and character traits (e.g., hopelessness) to the pathogenesis of CAD.[12] For each of these factors, behavioral and physiologic mechanisms are implicated in the disease process. Behavioral mechanisms suggest that certain factors (e.g., social isolation) influence the extent to which individuals engage in high-risk behaviors (e.g., consuming high-fat foods, problem drinking, and smoking) that promote CAD. Physiologic mechanisms operate between acute psychologic stress and sympathetic nervous system hyperresponsivity. In the example of social isolation, studies suggest a relationship between lower levels of social support and higher resting heart rates, which suggest altered autonomic arousal.[13] Blood pressure and cardiovascular responses to stress also may be attenuated by the presence of social support.[14,15] Our earlier work on the social dislocation hypothesis suggested that men who served overseas, leaving behind families and careers, experienced adverse health effects.[16]

War experiences also may engender persistent feelings of hopelessness among aging veterans. In observational studies, hopelessness has been linked to sudden death in humans and prospectively to the development of carotid atherosclerosis and CAD.[14,17,18] Recent studies using a multi-item measure of fatigue, irritability, and demoralized feelings, termed "vital exhaustion," show that this symptom triad significantly predicts future CAD or cardiac events in both healthy and CAD populations.[19–21] Early observations of combat exhaustion, indicated by persistent fatigue, irritability, and feelings of inadequacy led to decades of military studies and clinical case reports of "vital exhaustion" that marked many veterans' lives initially and in the longer term (e.g., shell shock, combat neurosis, battle fatigue, Vietnam syndrome, and, more recently, PTSD). In addition, hostility, an individual attribute and major element of the type A behavior pattern, also has been implicated in the development of CAD.[12]

A CAD model thus links the heightened arousal of war stress to cardiovascular reactivity and an array of other CAD symptoms, including an elevated resting heart rate and hypertension, as well as damaged arteries.[22] Excessive cardiovascular arousals can, over time, promote damaged arteries through mechanical injury of the arterial endothelium.[23] Cardiovascular reactivity refers to the duration and magnitude of cardiovascular response to acute stress or change. The greater such reactivity, the greater the CAD risk, as in the prediction of problematic blood pressure.

More specifically, war experiences constitute acute and sometimes chronic levels of stress that stimulate the sympathetic nervous system, leading to a variety of physiologic effects (e.g., heart rate and blood pressure stimulation, direct effects on coronary vascular endothelium). Known clinical consequences of these effects include myocardial ischemia, arrhythmias, more vulnerable vessel plaques, and hemostatic changes. According to Rozanski and colleagues, these changes position the individual for the development of acute myocardial infarction and sudden cardiac death.[12] Combat veterans may thus become increasingly more vulnerable and reactive in cardiovascular symptoms to change and stress as they age.

Finally, war stress has probable consequences for immune system impairments through a complex set of hormonal and neural pathways.[24] The biobehavioral pathways described in the CAD model also could act on the cellular and molecular biology of the monocyte–macrophage system to promote arterial lesions that compromise the immune system's ability to disable malignant cells.[25] Although the immune system is clearly responsive to changing behaviors and moods, and trauma studies postulate a weakening of previously adequate defenses with age, it is unclear at this time whether altered immune function influences aging changes that can be linked to disease vulnerability.

Given the substantial proportion of veterans in the elderly population and the potential links between war stress and health, veteran status should be ascertained on all geriatric patients. If indicated, patients should be referred for assessment and treatment of posttraumatic stress disorder (PTSD). Even in the absence of formally diagnosed PTSD, current research suggests that military experience can constitute a form of chronic stress that may be associated with deleterious physiologic processes, including hyperarousal or compromised immune function continuing into old age.

Social Relationships

Military experience illustrates the powerful influence of earlier stress and social dislocation on lifelong risk of illness. The corollary also has received considerable attention, in that health has been shown to be related to one's degree of connectedness or one's social relationships. Research has shown that multiple roles are related to better health, lower functional impairment, and multiple indicators of physical illness and symptoms. For example, unmarried and socially isolated individuals are at risk for higher mortality and morbidity, including tuberculosis, accidents, and psychiatric disorders.[5,9]

For decades, much of the research on social relationships documented patterns of greater and lesser health and illness associated with social relationships. More recently, researchers are exploring the underlying mechanisms linking social ties and health. Do social relationships prevent people from becoming ill? Do they help in recovery from illness? Do social relationships foster health by improving a sense of meaning or coherence in an individual's life, by promoting healthy behaviors, or perhaps by neuroendocrine response?

Evidence began to accumulate in the 1970s, when researchers such as Cassel and Cobb and Berkman and Syme pioneered the notion that social relationships were protective.[5,26] Experimental and quasi-experimental research showed that the presence of a familiar member of the species could buffer the impact of experimentally produced stress on ulcers, hypertension, and neurosis in rats, mice, and others. In addition, it was shown to reduce anxiety and physical arousal (via secretion of fatty acids) in humans. Physical contact and the presence of others were shown to modulate cardiovascular activity and reactivity in general and stressful contexts. Handling reduced the arteriosclerotic impact of high-fat diets in rats. Bovard proposed a psychophysiologic theory suggesting social relationships, mediated through the amygdala, activated the anterior hypothalmic zone and, hence, secretion of adrenocorticotropic hormone, cortisol, catecholamines, and associated sympathetic autonomic activity.[27]

Similar to socioeconomic status, links between social relationships and health outcomes vary depending on the measurement of this social indicator. Researchers in this tradition have focused particularly on the effects of two types of connectedness: social integration (i.e., the degree to which individuals have formed attachments to social structure) and social support (i.e., the degree to which

individuals have formed attachments to other individuals). Examples of the former include role types, church attendance, and participation in voluntary organizations. The latter contains at least five dimensions: (1) the size of an individual's social network; (2) the type of support they receive (e.g., emotional or tangible assistance); (3) the source (friends or family); (4) the frequency of that support; and (5) the perceived quality referred to as subjective social support.[28]

Social integration, in the form of church attendance, has been shown to be related to lower functional impairment, better immune function, and reduced depressive symptoms. Among older African-American men, it also has been shown to decrease subsequent mortality. Participation in voluntary organizations also is related to lower mortality. Social support in the form of marriage has been empirically linked to fewer depressive symptoms, decreased psychiatric disorders, and less functional impairment. Some data suggest marriage is more protective against mental illness for Caucasians than for African-Americans. Higher levels of subjective social support have been related to lower functional impairment, better self-rated health, fewer depressive symptoms, and more rapid recovery from depressive disorders. There is no evidence, however, relating this support to mortality.[9]

In general, the data on the influence of social support on health have been mixed. However, based on the evidence to date, leading researchers in the field offer three conclusions. First, social support shows robust direct effects on health outcomes. Second, the most powerful component is subjective social support; "feeling" supported is more important for health than objective levels of support received. Third, support from friends is more strongly related to health outcomes than family support.[9] It is hypothesized that the voluntary nature of friend support may increase quality. Or friends, as peers, are more likely to offer mutually appealing support.[9]

As researchers continue to identify the mechanisms that link social relationships to health, clinicians should proceed by recognizing the importance of their patients' social integration and support and assess it as part of a normal social history. One may ask what kinds of organizations and activities are important to the patient. A comprehensive assessment of a patient's level of social support should include questions regarding amount, frequency, and kind of support. Gathering such information does not require the physician to resolve support issues. It does, however, offer a window into the social context in which medications or other health regimens are prescribed. If recommending dietary adjustments, increased physical activity, or drug regimens, geriatricians should consider the odds that such recommendations will be taken based on the nature of elderly patients' social relationships and support. Similarly, when patients are recovering from illness or medical intervention, providers should assess the nature of support that is in place. Perhaps most importantly, physicians should ascertain the extent to which their patients "feel" supported.

Spirituality and Health

One important form of social integration involves the spiritual involvement and religious participation of older patients. In recent years, the medical community has become increasingly interested in the role that religion or spirituality plays in the lives of patients. When patients refer to their faith or spirituality, there are at least three possible aspects of this experience: religion, religious participation, and religiosity. Religion refers to attachment to a formal organization, denomination, or set of formal beliefs. Religious participation involves attendance, particularly its frequency, and is associated with the concept of social integration. Religiosity refers to the personal or intrinsic meaning associated with specific religious or spiritual practices; it can be associated with coping. Patients' lives may include all, some, or none of these components. Each is hypothesized to have a different relationship to health and illness. In the next section, we provide an overview of the most recent evidence linking religion and spirituality with health.[29]

Onset of Illness

Research has shown significant relationships between religion and a reduction in the onset of a variety of physical illnesses, including coronary disease and myocardial infarction, emphysema, cirrhosis and other liver disease, hypertension, and disability. Of the multiple dimensions of religion, religious participation is the strongest predictor of prevention practices, longevity, and reduced mortality.[29]

Recovery from Illness

Research suggests religion can influence the trajectory of illness. It is associated with better recovery patterns among heart transplant patients, reduced risk of heart attacks, reduced mortality among breast cancer patients, increased tolerance of pain, and higher quality of life. Religious coping is the dimension most strongly related to recovery.[29]

Mental Health and Substance Abuse

Religious involvement has been shown to be associated with reduced likelihood of anxiety disorders, depression,

and alcohol and drug abuse and dependence. It also is associated with increased likelihood of recovery from mental illness and substance abuse or dependence. Religious participation is the dimension most strongly associated with better mental health.[29]

Evidence linking religion to health and illness proposes three possible mechanisms. First, many religions encourage healthy behaviors. These differences also can be seen between religious denominations. For example, Mormons, Seventh Day Adventists, and members of other religions with strict behavioral prohibitions around health, on average, are healthier and live longer. Second, religious participation may offer a form of social support and thereby be associated with improved health outcomes. Finally, although the studies exploring the mechanisms of religious coping and health are limited, research suggests religion may buffer the effects of stress via an increased sense of coherence or meaning.[29]

Although it is important to know the evidence regarding religion and spirituality and health outcomes, a more essential clinical question may be what patients want from physicians in relation to their religion or spirituality. A number of recent studies document the overwhelming importance of religion for patients, and most suggest patients would like their physicians to acknowledge its importance in their lives. Specifically, one investigation found that 77% of patients said physicians should consider patient spiritual needs, 37% wanted their physician to discuss religious beliefs with them more frequently, and 48% wanted their physician to pray with them. Interestingly, 68% said their physician had never discussed religious beliefs with them.[30] In another study, 70% of patients said they would welcome the question, "Do you have spiritual or religious beliefs that would influence your medical decisions if you became gravely ill?" The large majority of patients (84%) answered affirmatively. However, only 15% recalled ever being asked this.[31]

In one study, an overwhelming majority (more than 85%) of patients rated prayer and coming to peace with God as an important component of end-of-life care; in fact, patients ranked coming to peace with God as equal in importance to freedom from pain.[32] There was less consensus, however, about the role of the physician regarding patient spirituality issues: 50% agreed that they wanted to discuss spiritual beliefs with their doctor, and 50% felt otherwise. These results reinforce the notion that spirituality is a highly individual value; cues about its expression must come from the patient. Furthermore, these results imply that resolving the spiritual needs of patients may not be the physician's responsibility, but that acknowledging the existence of such needs and making appropriate referrals is a way of affirming the whole person.

Caregiver Issues

Many elderly patients presenting to geriatricians for evaluation or follow-up are accompanied by their informal caregivers. These providers are most often related to the older patient, such as a spouse or adult child, but also may be a close personal friend. Geriatricians know that it would be impossible for many of their elderly patients to function in noninstitutional settings, were it not for this occasional or routine assistance. Caregivers provide the critical support that compensates for the older person's limitations caused by chronic illness, disability, or physical or mental frailty. Their dedication stems from deep commitments to their elderly loved ones and because the need for long-term care exceeds formal services and public policy support. Many elderly caregiving spouses take seriously their marital vows, "til death do us part," and adult child providers tend to assume the caregiving role because of desires to reciprocate help that their parents once gave to them. In this section we describe the informal caregivers that geriatricians should expect to meet in their practices, what challenges they face as caregivers, the consequences of meeting those challenges, and why geriatricians should be aware of these informal providers functioning.

Who are the caregivers? The National Academy on an Aging Society recently profiled elderly care recipients and their informal caregivers using Wave 1 data from the NIA-funded study of Assets and Health Dynamics Among the Oldest Old (AHEAD).[33] From this, we learn that some 8.5 million individuals over age 70 are impaired in activities of daily living (ADLs; e.g., using the toilet, eating) or instrumental activities of daily living (IADLs; e.g., taking medications, making phone calls), such that some level of assistance is necessary for them to function in the community. By 2030, this number may be as high as 21 million. For the practicing geriatrician, this translates to approximately two of five older patients in their practices who need assistance with one or more of these routine activities.

AHEAD data suggest that most caregivers are family members (72%), the majority of which are adult children (42%) and spouses (25%), and identifies significant ethnic variation in typical caregiving arrangements. For example, white elderly patients tend to receive help from spouses, Hispanics from adult children, and blacks from informal providers outside the family. Most of the caregivers surveyed provide daily care; about 21% assist several times a week. The large majority (80%) allocates up to 5 h of assistance per day, and a small group, approximately 7%, provides care 24 h a day.

Clearly caregiving can be and usually is time consuming, labor intensive, and stressful. In shouldering this burden, caregivers often experience substantial levels of emotional distress and physical exhaustion. Caring for an elderly individual with physical impairment involves organizing ADLs and orchestrating medical and home care arrangements. Caring for an elderly person with cognitive impairment requires this same organization of ADLs and health services, plus additional burdens associated with progressive memory loss, complex decisions about health care, legal arrangements and finances, personal control and autonomy issues, challenging behavior problems and communication deficits, and anticipatory grief.

Overall, about 15% of caregivers in the AHEAD study reported experiencing a physical or mental health problem because of their caregiving responsibilities. Among dementia caregivers, links have been found between caregiving and anxiety and depression symptomatology, psychotropic drug use, lower ratings of self-rated health, less optimum health-related behaviors such as getting enough exercise or sleep, and changes in immune function.[34] Perhaps the most provocative research to date, from a population-based cohort, suggests that being an elderly spousal caregiver under mental or emotional strain is an independent risk factor for mortality.[35]

Clearly all caregivers, but especially those coping with progressive dementia disorders in their care recipients, constitute a vulnerable population at high risk for adverse health consequences, including death. Geriatricians attempting to identify caregivers in their practices that may be at risk for adverse health outcomes are aided by two sets of caregiver characteristics identified by Schulz.[34] The first set includes characteristics associated with adverse health outcomes in any population, such as being female, low means, high stress, and lower feelings of mastery. Two aspects of caregiving, severity of patient problem behaviors and extent of patient cognitive impairment, complete the risk factor profile.

The wealth of data identifying health risks associated with informal care provision underscores the importance of family assessment in geriatric patient evaluations. Clinicians should inquire about the level (unskilled versus skilled) and intensity (occasional, daily, round-the-clock) of care and the caregiver's needs for additional assistance or services. By identifying at-risk caregivers and referring them to appropriate community resources or to other health care professionals before irreversible health problems arise, geriatricians increase the likelihood that dedicated caregivers continue to provide care and that elderly impaired patients are able to age in place. As most clinicians are acutely aware, however, not all presumably supportive relationships are, in fact, supportive. Some compromise or seriously threaten an elderly patient's health and well-being.

Elder Mistreatment

Caregiving relationships sometimes exacerbate physical violence or other forms of elder mistreatment including verbal, financial, sexual, or emotional abuse, abandonment, or intentional neglect. An in-depth analysis of elder abuse can be found in Chapter 72; the discussion here focuses specifically on elder mistreatment within the informal dementia caregiving relationship. Geriatricians hold key positions to detect such abuse because of the frequency with which they interface with older patients and their family members and are required by statutes in the majority of U.S. states to report suspected abuse to adult protective services. For an in-depth discussion of the physical, emotional, and behavioral indicators of possible elder mistreatment, see Gall and Szwabo in the fourth edition of the *Geriatric Review Syllabus*.[36]

Among caregivers of elderly persons with dementing disorders, abuse by spouses is more common than abuse by children.[37,38] Pillemer and Suitor suggest that elder mistreatment is more likely to occur when a potential perpetrator has problems, such as mental illness or substance abuse, when the recipient of the abuse is financially or otherwise dependent on the abuser, in socially isolated environments, and in the presence of external stress.[38]

Research suggests that characteristics of the dementia caregiver, such as older age, being the patient's spouse, and experiencing some form of violence from the cognitively impaired patient, increase the likelihood that caregivers act violently. Geriatricians should be knowledgeable of assessment components of quality care: *physical abuse* (e.g., excessive sedation, restraining to bed or chair, hitting/pinching), *psychologic abuse* (e.g., threats or physical force or to institutionalize, locking in room), *physical neglect* (e.g., failure to provide food, medical care, safe environment), *psychologic neglect* (e.g., failure to provide affection or to include in family celebrations), and *exploitation* (e.g., theft or misuse of resources).[39] Asking about the nature of informal care may identify the need to refer caregivers for support services to prevent elder mistreatment from occurring or escalating.

In assessing elder mistreatment, it is important to ask, in separate sessions, the caregiver and the patient about their relationships with each other; this provides an opportunity for each to speak privately and frankly. Geriatricians suspecting mistreatment problems need to consider the safety of sending the older patient back home, the services that may be available to reduce caregiver stress, and the need for closer than usual follow-up. Fortunately, most home care situations involving caregivers and elderly care recipients do not involve abuse. Most informal caregivers are deeply committed to the health and well-being of their care recipients and work to help them age as successfully as possible.

Successful Aging

Since the publication in 1976 of *The Quality of American Life* by Campbell, Converse, and Rogers, social scientists have understood that definitions of successful aging include multiple domains, including education, income, health, marriage, children, and neighborhood and community life. Gerontologic studies subsequently demonstrated the obvious, that most older adults do not expect to age well at all times across all these domains. Campbell and associates also contributed an important distinction between "satisfaction" with life or the perception that goals have been achieved, and "happiness," a positive affective state. Specifically, they observed that younger persons are more likely than older persons to be happy and that older people are more likely than younger individuals to be satisfied. Over the next several decades, social scientists repeatedly observed that older persons typically want to live well, to age "successfully," adaptively, or in some other way that signifies that living is more than surviving.

Geriatricians have been understandingly hesitant in addressing such concepts as aging well or successful aging, primarily because they observe firsthand the heterogeneity of the older population and know that there cannot be any single pattern of successful aging. In addition, their clinical assessment processes rely largely on objective indicators of health, illness, and function; concepts such as successful aging appear value laden and proscriptive rather than objective and descriptive. From a practical standpoint, the notion of successful aging presents a complexity requiring data about a wide range of parameters that attempt to capture the essence of an elderly person's life. Such breadth is increasingly difficult or impossible to cover in busy practice settings. Yet despite these reasons for not thinking in terms of aging successfully, all geriatricians devote their energies to facilitate aging well.

The most significant articulation of the successful aging concept occurred with the publication of results from the MacArthur Foundation successful aging studies in a recent volume by Rowe and Kahn, entitled *Successful Aging*.[40] The authors merged their perspectives from geriatrics and social science, rejected the established approach of studying aging in terms of decline, and used data to show that lifestyle choices rather than genetic inheritance are key factors that determine how successfully people age. Basically, Rowe and Kahn point to three tightly interrelated critical components of successful aging: avoidance of disease, lifestyle choices, and engagement with life. Obviously, the avoidance of acute and chronic disease is critical. However, equally important are certain lifestyle choices that maintain or improve physical and mental function and social engagement with life.

More specifically, the MacArthur studies showed that one of the most statistically significant predictors of maintaining cognitive functioning with age was the older patient's sense of self-efficacy, or the belief in one's own ability to handle various situations. Rowe and Kahn call self-efficacy the "can-do factor."[40] Other predictors were physical exercise, education, and lung function. People demonstrating this "can do" attitude also demonstrated higher levels of productivity (e.g., gardening, homemaking, volunteering). Physical functioning was more dependent on an elderly person's level of social support, specifically emotional support as opposed to instrumental support or tangible assistance. Elderly with higher levels of emotional support (i.e., expressions of affection, respect, love, encouragement) were more likely to engage in physical activity, such as brisk walking and substantial housework, whereas instrumental support (direct, hands-on assistance, provision of resources) was associated with lower physical performance. These data suggest the importance of providing adequate emotional support to older persons, but at the same time not limiting their autonomy by doing things that they are able to do themselves.

Perhaps the most exciting conclusion of these studies is that lifestyle factors and choices, such as adopting a positive attitude about meeting challenges (i.e., self-efficacy), engaging in routine exercise, and seeking opportunities to engage others are modifiable. With this knowledge, more geriatricians currently are shifting their goals from identifying and managing disease to preventing or delaying disease and promoting health. Because many older individuals have multiple comorbid illnesses, delaying the onset of one condition through lifestyle changes may also reduce risks associated with the development of other medical problems as well. More aggressive attempts to modify risk in elderly patients through exercise, diet, and efforts to detect and prevent disease are important. However, recent data on successful aging suggest that to reduce the total period of disability for any one patient, efforts should be made to enhance patient self-efficacy by promoting their beliefs that challenges can be met and by encouraging close relationships with others. Geriatricians should make their older patients aware that they are more responsible than anyone else for their own health in later life.

Summary

We began this chapter by acknowledging the geriatric perspective as broadly comprehensive with a focus on the "whole person"—biological, philosophical, and psychosocial. Regarding the psychosocial component, we posed two questions. The first sought to identify the psychosocial aspects of aging likely to affect clinical outcomes, and the second challenged us to make recommendations to geriatricians on how best to assess these aspects of their patients during standard clinical encounters. To address the first, we examined the evidence linking seven psychosocial factors to later life health: social characteristics of the older patient (i.e., gender, race, and socioeconomic status); historical influences (i.e., military experience); social relationships; spirituality; caregiving; elder mistreatment; and behaviors linked to successful aging. The potential for each of these domains to affect older patient health and well-being suggests their importance in geriatric assessment practices. The second question asked how best to assess elderly patients along these dimensions. The following questions may assist clinicians in probing these domains with the goal of identifying modifiable areas.

Gender, Ethnicity, and Socioeconomic Status

- Observe gender and inquire about education or years of formal schooling. Assess level of knowledge; do not assume. For example, older patients with lower levels of education have been shown to confuse the concept of a living will with a legal or financial document.
- In the absence of financial information (e.g., income, assets), geriatricians can probe their patients' *perceived* adequacy of financial resources, often a more powerful predictor of well-being than objective income. "Are your bills difficult to meet? Does your money take care of your needs? Can you afford to buy those little extras, that is, those small luxuries?" Such questions may open doors for discussion of unmet needs.

Historical Influences (Military Experience)

- Are you a veteran? Which war? Did you experience combat? If yes, probe into the meaning of that experience in day-to-day life. Consider potential links between chronic stress and CAD. If patient mentions PTSD symptoms (e.g., nightmares, flashbacks, or re-experiencing), make appropriate referral.
- Were you born in the United States? If not, were the circumstances of immigration likely to be traumatic (e.g., Holocaust, revolution)?

Social Relationships

- The structure of a patient's social networks can be appreciated by asking about the people with whom the patient interacts and the assistance, if any, provided by those persons. For example, with whom do you live? One of the strongest predictors of noninstitutionalization is presence of a spouse. How many people are in your support network? What kinds of things do they do for you? How often?
- The adequacy of emotional support can be probed by such questions as the following: "Do you feel supported by and close to those around you?" "Do you feel the need for more assistance than you are currently receiving?" "Is there someone in your life with whom you can discuss your deepest concerns and feelings?"
- Whom would you contact if you needed help?

Spirituality

- What role does faith or spirituality play in your life? This brief question may help the clinician understand for whom spiritual activity (including formal religious participation and private practices) is a critical component in coping with illness, decision making, and general well-being.

Caregiving

- Determine caregiver status by asking patient or family member if they are "providing care for anyone on a routine basis." If yes:
- Ask about the intensity of care provision (primary versus secondary provider, daily basis or less often) and type of care (personal management, household, physical care).
- Identify potential stressors (use of alcohol or drugs to cope) and feelings of helpless and hopelessness that could lead the caregiver to mistreat the patient.
- Ask about the caregiver's needs for assistance—what would help caregiver most (e.g., support group, respite, in-home care, sitter service, chore worker).

Elder Mistreatment

- Ask the patient if problem behavior exists in the family, such as acts of violence or excessive force. "Has anyone tried to hurt or hit you?" "Has anyone made you do things that you did not want to do?" "Has anyone taken your things?"

- The next steps may involve notifying Adult Protective Services or other state-specific agencies and creating a safety plan for the patient.

Successful Aging

- Are measures being taken to avoid disease and maintain optimal cognitive and physical function (e.g., scheduling regular checkups, eating a nutritious diet, engaging in regular, moderate physical activity, and avoiding high-risk behaviors such as smoking)?
- Does the patient cope well with setbacks?
- In general, does the patient have a positive attitude?
- Is the patient socially connected and engaged with life?

References

1. Schmitt MH, Heinemann GD, Farrell MP, Feussner JR, Cohen HJ. Evaluation of the process of care in the VA cooperative study of the outcomes of geriatric evaluation and management inpatient and outpatient care. *Gerontologist.* 2000;40. (Special Issue) p. 343.
2. Wieland D, Rubenstein LZ. What do we know about patient targeting in geriatric evaluation and management (GEM) programs? [Review]. *Aging* (Milano). 1996;8:297–310.
3. Birren J, Schaie K. *Handbook of Psychology and Aging.* San Diego: Academic Press; 2001.
4. Binstock R, George L. *Handbook of Aging and the social Sciences.* San Diego: Academic Press, 2001.
5. House J, Landis K, Umberson D. Social relationships and health. In: Conrad P, Kern R, eds. *The Sociology of Health and Illness.* New York: St. Martin's Press, 1990.
6. House JS, Kessler RC, Herzog AR. Age, socioeconomic status, and health. *Milbank Mem Q.* 1990;68:383–412.
7. Wenneker J, Epstein A. Racial inequalities in the use of procedures for patients with ischemic heart disease in Massachusetts. *JAMA.* 1989;261:253–257.
8. Verbrugge LM. The twain meet: empirical explanations of sex differences on health and mortality. *J Health Soc Behav.* 1989;30:282–304.
9. George L. Social factors and illness. In: Binstock R, George L, eds. *Handbook of Aging and the Social Sciences.* San Diego: Academic Press, 1996; pp. 229–252.
10. Markides K, Black S. Race, ethnicity, and aging: the impact of inequality. In: Binstock R, George L, eds. *Handbook of Aging and the Social Sciences.* San Diego: Academic Press; 1996. pp. 153–170.
11. Cooper-Patrick L, Gallo J, Gonzales J, et al. Race, gender, and partnership in the patient-physician relationship. *JAMA.* 1999;282:583–589.
12. Rozanski A, Blumenthal JA, Kaplan J. Impact of psychological factors on the pathogenesis of cardiovascular disease and implications for therapy [Review]. *Circulation.* 1999; 99:2192–2217.
13. Unden AL, Orth-Gomer K, Elofsson S. Cardiovascular effects of social support in the work place: twenty-four-hour

ECG monitoring of men and women. *Psychosom Med.* 1991;53:50–60.

14. Kamarck TW, Manuck SB, Jennings JR. Social support reduces cardiovascular reactivity to psychological challenge: a laboratory model. *Psychosom Med.* 1990;52:42–58.

15. Gerin W, Pieper C, Levy R, Pickering TG. Social support in social interaction: a moderator of cardiovascular reactivity. *Psychosom Med.* 1992;54:324–336.

16. Elder GH Jr, Shanahan MJ, Clipp EC. Linking combat and physical health: the legacy of World War II in men's lives. *Am J Psychiatry.* 1997;154:330–336.

17. Everson SA, Kaplan GA, Goldberg DE, Salonen R, Salonen JT. Hopelessness and 4-year progression of carotid atherosclerosis. The Kuopio Ischemic Heart Disease Risk Factor Study. *Arterioscler Thromb Vasc Biol.* 1997;17: 1490–1495.

18. Everson SA, Kauhanen J, Kaplan GA, et al. Hostility and increased risk of mortality and acute myocardial infarction: the mediating role of behavioral risk factors. *Am J Epidemiol.* 1997;146:142–152.

19. Appels A, Falger PR, Schouten EG. Vital exhaustion as risk indicator for myocardial infarction in women. *J Psychosom Res.* 1993;37:881–890.

20. Appels A, Mulder P. Excess fatigue as a precursor of myocardial infarction. *Eur Heart J.* 1988;9:758–764.

21. Pignalberi C, Patti G, Chimenti C, Pasceri V, Maseri A. Role of different determinants of psychological distress in acute coronary syndromes. *J Am Coll Cardiol.* 1998;32:613–619.

22. Krantz DS, Manuck SB. Acute psychophysiologic reactivity and risk of cardiovascular disease: a review and methodologic critique [review]. *Psychol Bull.* 1984;96:435–464.

23. Kaplan JR, Pettersson K, Manuck SB, Olsson G. Role of sympathoadrenal medullary activation in the initiation and progression of atherosclerosis [review]. *Circulation.* 1991;84:VI23–VI32.

24. Maier SF, Watkins LR. Cytokines for psychologists: implications of bidirectional immune-to-brain communication for understanding behavior, mood, and cognition [review]. *Psychol Rev.* 1998;105:83–107.

25. Adams DO. Molecular biology of macrophage activation: a pathway whereby psychosocial factors can potentially affect health [review]. *Psychosom Med.* 1994;56:316–327.

26. Berkman L, Syme S. Social networks, host resistance, and mortality: a nine-year follow-up study of Alameda County residents. *Am J Epidemiol.* 1979;109:186–204.

27. Bovard E. Perspectives on behavioral medicine. In: Williams R, ed. *Perspectives on Behavioral Medicine,* vol 2. New York: Academic Press; 1985.

28. Broadhead W, Gehlback S, de Gruy F, et al. The Duke-UNC Functional Social Support Questionnairre: measurement of social support in family medicine patients. *Med Care.* 1988;26:709–723.

29. George L, Larson D, Koenig H, McCullough M. Spirituality and health: what we know, what we need to know. *J Soc Clin Psychol.* 2000;19:102–116.

30. King D, Bushwick B. Beliefs and attitudes of hospital inpatients about faith healing and prayer. *J Fam Pract.* 1994;39:349–352.

31. Ehman J, Ott B, Short T, Ciampa R, Hansen-Flaschen J. Do patients want physicians to inquire about their spiritual or religious beliefs if they become gravely ill? *Arch Intern Med.* 1999;159:1803–1806.

32. Steinhauser K, Christakis N, Clipp E, McNeilly M, McIntyre L, Tulsky J. Factors considered important at the end of life by patients, family, physicians and other care providers. *JAMA.* 2000;284:2476–2482.

33. Shirley L, Summer L. *Caregiving: Helping the Elderly with Activity Limitations.* National Academy on an Aging Society Series, vol 7. Washington, DC: The Gerontological Society of America; 2000.

34. Schulz R. *Handbook on Dementia Caregiving.* New York: Springer; 2000.

35. Schulz R, Beach S. Caregiving as a risk factor for mortality: the Caregiver Health Effects Study. *JAMA.* 1999;282: 2215–2219.

36. Gall JS, Szwabo PA. Psychosocial aspects of aging. In: Cobbs EL, Duthie EH, Murphy JB, eds. *Geriatric Review Syllabus: A Core Curriculum in Geriatric Medicine.* Dubuque: Kendall/Hunt; 1999.

37. Pillemer K, Suitor JJ. Sharing a residence with an adult child: a cause of psychological distress in the elderly? *Am J Orthopsychiatry.* 1991;61:144–148.

38. Pillemer K, Finkelhor D. Causes of elder abuse: caregiver stress versus problem relatives. *Am J Orthopsychiatry.* 1989; 59:179–187.

39. Schulz R, Williamson G. The measurement of caregiver outcomes in Alzheimer disease research. *Alzheimer Dis Assoc Disord.* 1997;11:117–124.

40. Rowe JW, Kahn RL. *Successful Aging.* New York: Pantheon; 1998.

7
Principles of Pharmacology

Jerry Avorn, Jerry H. Gurwitz, and Paula Rochon

It is much easier to write upon a disease than upon a remedy. The former is in the hands of nature and a faithful observer with an eye of tolerable judgement cannot fail to delineate a likeness. The latter will ever be subject to the whim, the inaccuracies, and the blunder of mankind.
　　　　　　　　　　　　William Withering, 1741–1799

The proper use of medications represents one of the most crucial ways in which the practice of geriatric medicine differs from conventional medical care. Pharmacotherapy is probably the singly most important medical intervention in the care of elderly patients, and its appropriate implementation requires a special understanding of the unique pharmacologic properties of drugs in this population, as well as a grasp of the clinical, epidemiologic, sociocultural, economic, and regulatory aspects of medication use in aging.

Pharmacokinetics

Of the four traditional components of pharmacokinetics—absorption, distribution, metabolism, and excretion—only the last three are meaningfully affected by age. In the absence of malabsorptive syndromes, traditional oral formulations of drugs are absorbed as well in old age as in youth. Of course, the same concerns apply in elderly patients as in those of any age concerning the possible adsorption of medications by antacids and the relation between the ingestion of meals and the taking of medications. However, the well-reported changes in gastric motility and blood flow to the gut with aging do not appear to alter meaningfully the efficiency with which medications move from the gastrointestinal tract into the systemic circulation.[1,2] Nonetheless, many slow-release drug preparations have undergone little or no study of potential age-related changes in their delivery rates. Similarly, data on the kinetics of transdermal, transbuccal, and transbronchial drug administration in the elderly are too limited to allow conclusions regarding age-related

changes in drug absorption via those routes,[3] even though the elderly are among the most prominent users of such drug delivery systems.

Another aspect of drug distribution that is likewise not affected by normal aging is the binding of drugs to carrier proteins such as serum albumin. In large populations, clinically meaningful decreases in serum albumin have not been found, although there is a very modest reduction with advancing age.[4,5] Previous studies that purported to show a large age-related decline in serum albumin levels were probably marred by the problem of confounding illness with aging. Despite these observations on serum proteins in healthy aging, it is crucial to consider that serum albumin levels may be markedly decreased in older patients suffering from malnutrition or severe chronic disease,[6,7] with important consequences for drug binding.

One of the more important risks of diminished binding proteins is an iatrogenic one, resulting from misinterpretation of serum drug levels. Many assays measure the total amount of drug that is present in serum, both protein-bound and unbound ("free"). The unbound concentration is more clinically relevant than the total concentration because only unbound drug is pharmacologically active. For a patient with hypoalbuminemia or another deficiency in binding protein, any given serum drug level reflects a greater concentration of unbound drug than the same level would signify in a patient with normal protein-binding capacity. A hypoalbuminemic patient with a "normal" total serum drug concentration may actually have an unbound drug concentration that is unacceptably high. By contrast, the same patient with a slightly lower than normal total serum concentration may have an unbound drug concentration that is in a reasonable range. For extensively protein-bound drugs whose binding is reduced as a result of hypoproteinemia, clinicians should expect both therapeutic and toxic events at lower total serum concentrations.[8] Phenytoin, which is highly bound to albumin, is one example of a drug for which the interpretation of serum levels reflecting total drug concentration (rather than the free drug concentration) can be difficult in malnourished or chronically ill elderly patients.

In evaluating serum drug levels in the older patient, it is also important to recall that the therapeutic range routinely reported on such assays may not be an accurate guide to either efficacy or toxicity in the geriatric patient. Such ranges have typically been defined in nonelderly subjects and cannot take into account pharmacodynamic differences (see following) or idiosyncratic aspects of specific patients.

One aspect of drug distribution that varies importantly with age is the volume of distribution, which is the theoretical space in a given patient which a particular drug occupies. The volume of distribution is heavily influenced by the relative proportions of lean body mass versus fat. Because the latter increases in the elderly at the expense of the former, lipid-soluble drugs (such as some benzodiazepines) will have a greater volume of distribution in an older patient and water-soluble drugs (such as lithium) will have a smaller volume of distribution.[9] Combined with changes in clearance (discussed below), these alterations in body composition can have important implications for both the half-life and the steady-state concentration of many medications. Women comprise an increasingly large majority of the aging population, making it important to also consider gender differences in drug distribution and effects. Women have a lower lean body mass compared with men at all ages, and there may be gender differences in other pharmacokinetic and pharmacodynamic functions as well.[10]

Drug Clearance and Aging

The liver represents the major site of metabolism for many medications. Hepatic biotransformations of drugs are categorized into phase I (preparative) and phase II (synthetic) reactions. Phase I reactions include oxidations (hydroxylation, N-dealkylation, and sulfoxidation), reductions, and hydrolyses. Phase II reactions involve conjugation of the drug molecule to glucuronides, sulfates, or acetates.

Earlier studies in animals had suggested that normal aging is accompanied by reduced activity of liver microsomal drug-metabolizing enzymes as well as diminished microsomal enzyme induction, but data on hepatic drug metabolism in aging human subjects are much more limited. However, it is clear that normal aging is associated with a reduction in the liver mass, as well as in hepatic blood flow. These changes are likely responsible for the reduction in hepatic metabolism of drugs, which can be as great as 25% over the life span.[11,12] Autopsy and ultrasound studies have found a progressive decrease in liver mass after age 50. Regional blood flow to the liver at age 65 is reduced by 40% to 45% relative to that in a 25-year-old; this observation may partially reflect a fall in cardiac output wiht advancing age. Such changes can also result in reduced clearance rates for drugs exhibiting flow-dependent clearance characteristics ("first-pass effects").[13]

Antipyrine is frequently used as a marker compound to evaluate hepatic metabolizing capacity. Although many studies have reported reduced metabolic clearance of antipyrine in older subjects, as with many age-related differences interindividual variation is substantial.[14] This finding suggests that genetic, environmental, and other patient-specific factors often have a greater important on hepatic drug metabolism than the aging process itself. Therapeutic considerations therefore should be based on individual patient characteristics as well as expected physiologic changes due to aging.

Renal Excretion

Several commonly used drugs are excreted primarily by the kidney, including digoxin, ranitidine, and the aminoglycoside antibiotics.[15] Early cross-sectional studies of renal function in aging suggested that there is a linear decrease in renal function between young adulthood and old age, amounting on average to a reduction in glomerular filtration rate by nearly a third.[16] Although this is true in the aggregate, longitudinal studies indicate that some subjects evidence no changes or only small changes in creatinine clearance with advancing age; another subgroup showed a linear decrease with age; still others appeared to show some improvement in renal function as they became older.[17] Thus, although the aggregate findings have been enshrined in conventional gerontologic wisdom and in nomograms used to calculate drug dosing with age, these longitudinal studies make it clear that the effect of age on renal function (and therefore on the excretion of many drugs) can be quite variable. Here, too, differences among patients often will be as important as the changes attributed to the aging process itself.

Although blood urea nitrogen (BUN) and serum creatinine levels may be useful (albeit crude) markers of renal function, it must be remembered that each is susceptible in its own way to perturbations that can occur with aging but have nothing to do with renal function itself. For example, the BUN reflects the concentration of urea in the blood. However, the origin of much of this urea is ingested protein, so that a malnourished older patient may not consume enough nitrogen to produce an appropriate rise in BUN, even in the face of renal impairment. Similarly, serum creatinine is produced by muscle, and if a patient has a markedly diminished muscle mass, whether because of chronic illness or any other cause, he or she may not produce enough creatinine to reflect a change in the ability of the kidney to excrete this substance. Thus, overreliance on "normal-appearing" BUN and creatinine in older patients can severely underestimate the degree of renal impairment.

The Cockcroft–Gault formula[18] is sometimes used to estimate renal function in older patients who are to receive potentially nephrotoxic drugs (e.g., aminoglycosides) or drugs that are primarily excreted by the kidneys (e.g., digoxin):

$$\text{Estimated creatinine crearance} = \frac{(140 - \text{age}) \times (\text{body weight in kg})}{\text{serum creatinine} \times 72}$$

(for women, multiply $\times 0.85$).

It should be emphasized that these estimates are valid only in patients whose renal function is in steady state and who are not taking medications that directly alter renal function or affect creatinine excretion. This formula has some utility in assessing renal function in healthy ambulatory individuals, but it has limited utility and can be misleading in severely ill, clinically unstable, elderly patients.[19]

Drug Elimination Half-Life and Steady-State Concentration

The elimination half-life of a medication ($t_{1/2}$) is determined by the volume of distribution (V_d) for that medication in a given individual, divided by its clearance (Cl) in that subject (generally through metabolism in the liver and/or renal excretion); this can be expressed as follows:

$$t_{1/2} = 0.693 \times V_d / Cl$$

Thus, the half-life of a medication will increase as the clearance (Cl) decreases if the volume of distribution (V_d) remains constant. If the volume of distribution is also increased (as with a lipophilic drug in an older patient), the half-life will be prolonged still further.[20]

The clinical implications of these pharmacokinetic relationships are illustrated by the benzodiazepine hypnotic flurazepam. In a study comparing the kinetics of flurazepam in young and elderly subjects, the drug was found to have an elimination half-life of 160 h in elderly men, compared with 74 h in young men.[21] This difference probably is accounted for by an age-related reduction in the clearance of flurazepam by the oxidative pathways in the liver and an increase in the volume of distribution for this highly lipid-soluble drug. The clinical impact of such massive prolongation of flurazepam half-life is fur-

ther magnified by its biotransformation into the active metabolite desalkylflurazepam, which also has benzodiazepine effects on the central nervous system.

It is frequently assumed that the duration of clinical action of a drug is related to its half-life. Under this assumption, long elimination half-life implies a long duration of action and short elimination half-life implies a short duration of action. Although this presumption is sometimes incorrect,[22] some epidemiologic data support an association between use of agents with long elimination half-lives and the occurrence of drug side effects in the elderly.[23–25] However, other observational studies suggest that dose is a more important determinant of risk than half-life.

Steady-State Drug Concentration

A common goal of long-term pharmacotherapy is to achieve and maintain a therapeutic steady-state serum concentration. The steady-state drug concentration is proportional to the medication dosing rate (dose/dosing interval) and is inversely proportional to drug clearance. Assuming complete bioavailability, the equation for steady-state concentration (Css) can be expressed as follows:

$$Css = (\text{dose} / \text{dosing interval}) / \text{clearance}$$

This equality has a number of important ramifications for the prescriber. Although drug clearance is a biologically determined characteristic of each patient over which the prescriber has no control, dose and dosing interval are variables that can be modified. To prevent the excessive accumulation of a drug when its clearance is reduced (as is often the case in an elderly patient), one can reduce the dose, increase the interval between doses, or both, depending on the situation.[26]

Pharmacodynamics

Pharmacodynamic changes with aging (i.e., end-organ effects) have been more difficult to define than pharmacokinetic changes. The study of this phenomenon is complicated by the fact that the effect of many drugs is magnified in the elderly because of reduced drug clearance, resulting in higher serum levels.[27] Therefore, in studying the effects of aging on pharmacodynamics, one must control for the age-related changes in pharmacokinetics already discussed. A small but growing number of ingeniously conducted studies are helping to clarify the unique contribution of age-related pharmacodynamic changes to the overall picture of drug response in aging.

One of the first studies describing changes in drug sensitivity with aging involved patients between the ages of 30 and 90 years who underwent elective cardioversion.[28] The clinical endpoint used was the patient's inability to respond to voice, with preservation of response to a painful stimulus. The serum level of diazepam at which this effect occurred was significantly lower in elderly patients than in younger ones, suggesting that the older brain was sensitive to smaller concentrations of circulating drug. Analogous findings emerged from a study of the performance of patients given a single dose of another benzodiazepine, nitrazepam.[29] Serum levels of the drug were similar in both young and old, but elderly subjects showed a deterioration in performance on psychomotor testing after administration of a single dose of the drug, while comparable deterioration was not seen in younger patients. Similarly, in another study of i.v. midazolam, a lower dose was administered to older patients compared with younger ones, overcoming the expected pharmacokinetic differences between the two age groups. However, elderly subjects still demonstrated greater sedation than younger subjects, probably because of greater central nervous system sensitivity.[30] Details of the neuroreceptor explanation for such changes in intrinsic sensitivity to these agents are still obscure. In vitro assessment of benzodiazepine receptor binding and function in brain tissue from young and aged rodents has not revealed clear age-related differences in benzodiazepine receptor number or affinity.[31] Age-related changes in pharmacodynamics can result in greater therapeutic effect as well as an increased potential for toxicity. Increases in medication sensitivity with age have also been suggested for a number of other medications, including warfarin[32–34] and the opioids.

Special care must be taken in drawing conclusions from the results of studies examining age-related changes in pharmacodynamics.[35] The interpretation of results of some pharmacodynamic investigations may be complicated by baseline differences between young and elderly study populations, which in turn may confound assessment of drug-associated changes.[36] For example, in a study examining the effects of diphenhydramine on psychomotor performance, impairment was reported to be unaffected by the age of subjects when differences were expressed as the percentage change from baseline.[37] However, in absolute terms, the elderly demonstrated a greater impairment (expressed as time required to react to a stimulus) than did younger subjects; this yielded a similar percentage change because at baseline younger subjects performed better than older subjects. Thus, the presentation of research data in terms of percentage change from baseline (rather than absolute change) can obscure clinically important differences in pharmacodynamic effects between young and old study groups.

Recognizing and Preventing Adverse Drug Events in Older Adults

Many hospital-based studies have suggested that risk for the occurrence of adverse drug reactions increases with advancing age.[38] Unfortunately, this finding is of limited usefulness in guiding medical practice because most investigations have assessed all adverse drug reactions from all medication exposures as a single outcome category. Most studies have not controlled for important variables including the clinical status of the patient, length of hospitalization, and number of medications taken concurrently.

Assessing risk for adverse drug reactions in the individual elderly patient remains a difficult clinical challenge. Patient-specific physiologic and functional characteristics are probably far more important than chronologic age in predicting either the adverse or beneficial effects of specific therapies.[39] Nonetheless, from a population standpoint, older patients consume far more medications than younger patients. Taken together with the age-related pharmacologic changes described here, the physiologic declines associated with aging, and the increasing burden of chronic illness in the older population, assessing and reducing the risks for adverse drug effects becomes critically important in the practice of geriatric medicine.

Adverse drug effects can mimic almost any clinical syndrome in geriatrics. Clinicians are most familiar with mental status changes as adverse effects of psychoactive drugs in the elderly;[40] indeed, one study of reversible dementia found that drug-induced cognitive impairment was among the most common and treatable causes of syndromes that could be mistaken for dementia in the elderly.[41] It is less commonly recognized that some "nonpsychoactive" medications (e.g., anticholinergics) also have the potential to cause central nervous system toxicity in elderly patients.[42,43]

Equally important are the somatic side effects that can be caused by any drug, including psychoactive medications. Falls can be precipitated by a wide variety of drugs.[44] Drugs with strong anticholinergic properties run the gamut from antiarrhythmics to antipsychotics, and anticholinergic toxicity can be responsible for numerous symptoms apparently unrelated to the indication for which the drug was prescribed. Because acetylcholine serves as a neurotransmitter in numerous key roles in both the parasympathetic and central nervous systems, its blockade by medications with strong anticholinergic properties can yield a host of problems including dry mouth, constipation, urinary retention, blurred vision, and confusion. Conversely, cholinesterase inhibitors used in Alzheimer's disease, such as donepezil, can have the opposite effect: hypersalivation, diarrhea, nausea.

Another example of drug-induced illness is provided by the neuroleptic drugs often used for the management of behavioral disorders associated with dementia. These drugs can produce extrapyramidal effects including rigidity, bradykinesia, tremor, difficulty swallowing and walking, and loss of facial expression. When they occur, such side effects can be clinically indistinguishable from idiopathic Parkinson's disease. The most common offenders are the high-potency neuroleptic medications (e.g., haloperidol).

If the prescriber does not consider the possibility that neuroleptic therapy could be responsible for the patient's symptoms, additional drug therapy may be started inappropriately. Preferably, the neuroleptic therapy could be discontinued on a trial basis and nonpharmacologic approaches tried. If a neuroleptic therapy is required, it would be critical to choose the drug with the fewest adverse events.[45,46] Because adverse effects are generally dose related, it is important to choose the lowest dose required for clinical benefit.[47] Prescribing an additional drug therapy to treat an adverse drug effect should be considered a last resort in the care of older patients.

Adverse Drug Effects Associated with Commonly Used Drug Therapies

A group of drug-related medical problems has been called the "prescribing cascade".[48] The prescribing cascade develops when a drug complication is mistaken as a new medical problem. Instead, a new drug is prescribed with the patient now placed at the additional risk of developing yet another drug-related problem as a result of the new drug therapy. There are numerous examples of prescribing cascades: the use of nonsteroidal anti-inflammatory drugs and the initiation of antihypertensive therapy,[49] the use of thiazide diuretic therapy and the initiation of treatment for gout,[50] and the use of metoclopramide followed by treatment with levodopa therapy.[51] Finally, a patient who develops constipation while taking a strongly anticholinergic antidepressant such as amitriptyline has a resulting dependency on laxatives.[52,53]

The diagnosis of drug-induced illness in elderly patients is further complicated by lack of awareness of the physiology of normal aging and the tendency by patients, families, and even physicians to mislabel many symptoms as signs of "just growing old." As a result, drug-induced incontinence, confusion, fatigue, depression, and many other problems may be attributed to the human condition, when they may well be amenable to appropriate diagnosis and therapeutic action. A useful antidote to these problems is a very high index of suspicion for drug-induced illness in elderly patients. An overstatement that is of great clinical use and forms a good starting point for clinical evaluation can be stated as follows: "Any symptom in an elderly patient may be a drug side effect until proved otherwise."

Side Effects of Psychoactive Drugs

Psychotropic drugs have been associated with the occurrence of hip fracture in a number of epidemiologic studies. One study examining risk for hip fracture in older patients exposed to psychotropic medications indicated that a significantly increased risk was associated with use of hypnotic-anxiolytics with long (>24-h) elimination half-lives (odds ratio, 1.8; 95% confidence interval, 1.3–2.4), tricyclic antidepressants (odds ratio, 1.9; 95% confidence interval, 1.3–2.8), and neuroleptics (odds ratio, 2.0; 95% confidence interval, 1.6–2.6).[54] The long elimination half-life hypnotics-anxiolytics included flurazepam, diazepam, and chlordiazepoxide. More recent studies have suggested that it is the dose of benzodiazepine rather than the drug half-life that is the most important risk factor for drug-induced accidents.[55,56] Until this issue is resolved, it is prudent to avoid both long-acting drugs and high doses of any benzodiazepine in older patients unless there is a compelling reason to do otherwise.

The tricyclic antidepressants most often implicated in drug-induced injury in the elderly include the older tertiary amines amitriptyline, doxepin, and imipramine. However, more recent findings[57,58] suggest that risk of falls and fractures is seen as well with selective serotonin reuptake inhibitors (SSRIs) as well as with the older heterocyclic antidepressants. Indeed, one of these studies[59] found that depressed older patients appeared to be at increased risk of falls even before antidepressant therapy had been started.

Anticoagulants

Ample data exist regarding the benefits of anticoagulation in patients with atrial fibrillation.[60] Both a substantial increase in the incidence of nonrheumatic atrial fibrillation (AF) with age and an increased association between AF and stroke in the elderly have been found.[61-63] The proportion of strokes that can be attributed to AF increases consistently with age, after adjusting for the effects of systolic blood pressure.

Long-term oral anticoagulant therapy with warfarin is essential for the management or prevention of many thromboembolic and vascular disorders whose prevalence is increased in elderly patients. In fact, anticoagulation in patients with chronic nonrheumatic AF can reduce the risk of stroke by more than two-thirds. However, willingness to initiate anticoagulant therapy in an older patient is often tempered by concerns about the risk of bleeding, despite the fact that these patients may have the most to gain from anticoagulant therapy. The extent of anticoagulation, as reflected by the international normalized ratio (INR), is the dominant risk factor for hemorrhagic complications.[64] Several studies have presented conflicting findings on whether there is a greater risk of anticoagulant-induced hemorrhage in elderly patients, which may be explained to a large extent by differences in treatment setting and in the attention given to monitoring.[65,66] Specialized anticoagulation consultation services and clinics can assess risks for bleeding, monitor closely for potential warfarin–drug interactions, and pay close attention to target therapeutic ranges. Risk of anticoagulant-related bleeding appears to be reduced when expert consultation is provided at the start of anticoagulant therapy and when patients are monitored in specialized anticoagulation clinics.[67,68] Careful assessment of the appropriate indications for anticoagulant therapy, the optimal target INR, and the use of potentially interacting medications are the most important strategies for reducing the risk of bleeding complications in older patients.

Nonsteroidal Anti-Inflammatory Drugs

Nonsteroidal anti-inflammatory drugs (NSAIDs) are very widely used in the management of arthritis; because the prevalence of degenerative joint disease increases substantially with advancing age, the elderly are among the most frequent users of these medications. The NSAIDs encompass several different chemical entities, each with the common ability to inhibit cyclooxygenase, a major enzyme in the synthesis of prostaglandins. It is important to consider, however, that prostaglandins also mediate a variety of important protective physiologic effects in a number of organ systems. For example, prostaglandins maintain renal blood flow and glomerular filtration in the face of a reduction in the effective or actual circulatory volume (e.g., congestive heart failure, cirrhosis with ascites, volume depletion due to diuretic therapy, and hemorrhage with hypotension). Under such conditions, vasodilatory renal prostaglandins mitigate vasoconstrictive effects on renal blood flow. In this way, renal perfusion is maintained, preventing prerenal azotemia and eventual ischemic damage to the kidney. When this prostaglandin-mediated compensatory mechanism is suppressed by NSAID therapy, impairment in renal function can result. A prospective study of elderly residents of a large long-term care facility who were newly treated with NSAID therapy demonstrated that 13% developed azotemia over a short course of therapy.[69] Risk factors associated with this adverse effect included higher NSAID dosage and concomitant loop diuretic therapy.

Prostaglandins also mediate a range of effects that protect the mucosa of the stomach and duodenum from injury; these include the inhibition of acid secretion, an increase in mucous secretion and bicarbonate, and enhancement of mucosal blood flow. When the biosynthesis of prostaglandins is impaired by NSAIDs, this can lead to impaired mucosal defense; acid and peptic activity can then produce ulcers. A meta-analysis of epidemiologic studies investigating the association between NSAIDs and severe upper gastrointestinal tract disease indicated that older patient age was associated with a higher risk of gastrointestinal toxicity.[70]

The risks associated with NSAID use in the elderly emphasize the need for careful monitoring of patients with risk factors for NSAID-associated nephrotoxicity and gastropathy. To limit the occurrence of side effects, NSAID therapy should be limited to those clinical situations where it is absolutely required. The lowest feasible dose should be prescribed for the shortest time necessary to achieve the desired therapeutic effect. Because of the iatrogenic nature of these disorders, the best treatment for NSAID-associated nephrotoxicity or gastropathy is discontinuation of the NSAID. Alternative analgesic therapies are available and effective for many patients. For example, nonacetylated salicylates may be a safer alternative to NSAIDs. Another effective analgesic choice is acetaminophen. One study comparing the analgesic effects of acetaminophen (4 g/day) to ibuprofen (1.2 g/day and 2.4 g/day) in patients with osteoarthritis found no difference in pain relief in patients treated with acetaminophen compared to those given NSAID therapy.[71] Although acetaminophen is free of NSAID-related side effects, its use should not exceed 4 g/day in most patients; its toxicity is increased in the presence of hepatic insufficiency, heavy alcohol intake, or fasting.[72]

Recently, two cyclooxygenase-2 receptors (Cox-2 inhibitors) were approved for use in North America for arthritis treatment: celecoxib and rofecoxib.[73] Cox-2 inhibitors are similar to nonselective NSAIDs in terms of efficacy but have a more favorable side effect profile. However, adverse events, including gastrointestinal hemorrhage and reduced renal function, have been associated with use of Cox-2 inhibitors. Relative to nonselective NSAIDs, Cox-2 inhibitors are less likely to produce gastrointestinal ulcers, although ulcers do occur and this complication can be serious and even fatal.[74] The Cox-2 inhibitors have an effect on renal function similar to that of NSAIDs. A randomized controlled trial compared the effect of rofecoxib relative to indomethacin on glomerular filtration rates in 75 patients between the ages of 60 and 80.[75] The investigators found that the effect of the Cox-2 inhibitors was similar to that of nonselective NSAIDs in decreasing glomerular filtration rate. These findings indicate the need for caution when prescribing Cox-2 inhibitors for older adults.

The Context of Adverse Drug Effects in Frail Elderly

As the setting of care for more than 1.5 million Americans, the number of beds committed to nursing home care in the United States exceeds the number of acute care beds.[76] Of all types of therapeutic interventions, medications are the most commonly utilized in the nursing home setting. The average U.S. nursing home resident takes 6 different medications; more than one-fifth use 10 or more different drugs.[77]

The occurrence of adverse drug events that may be preventable is among the most serious concerns regarding medication use in the nursing home setting. Few studies have systematically examined the incidence of adverse drug events in the nursing home population.[78] A retrospective review of incident reports relating to adverse and unexpected events in one academically affiliated, 700-bed long-term care facility identified 50 reports of adverse drug reactions over a 1-year period.[79] Skin rashes were the most frequently reported events, and antibiotics were the most commonly implicated medication category. The limited number of periodically documented reports of drug-related events in that study suggested that voluntary reporting systems in the nursing home setting lead to very low reporting rates of only a very narrow spectrum of events. In a recent study of all long-term care residents of 18 community-based nursing homes in Massachusetts over a 12-month observation period, drug-related incidents were detected by stimulated self-report by nursing home staff and by periodic review of all nursing home resident records by trained nurse and pharmacist investigators.[80] Incidents were subsequently classified by physician reviewers as to whether they represented adverse drug events, their severity (significant, serious, life-threatening, and fatal), and preventability.

During 28,839 nursing home resident-months of observation in the 18 participating nursing homes, 546 adverse drug events were identified (1.89 adverse drug events per 100 resident-months). Of all adverse drug events, 1 was fatal, 31 (6%) were life threatening, 206 (38%) were serious, and 308 (56%) were significant. Overall, 50.5% of adverse drug events were judged preventable. Of the 238 fatal, life-threatening, or serious adverse drug events, 72% were considered preventable, compared with 34% of the 308 significant adverse drug events. Errors resulting in preventable adverse drug events occurred most often at the stages of ordering and monitoring; transcription, dispensing, and administration errors were less commonly identified. Psychoactive drugs (antipsychotics, antidepressants, and sedatives/hypnotics) and anticoagulants were the most commonly implicated drug categories associated with the occurrence of preventable adverse drug events (Table 7.1). Neuropsychiatric events (confusion, oversedation, delirium), falls, and hemorrhagic events were the most commonly identified preventable adverse drug events (Table 7.2).

Suboptimal prescribing of psychoactive medications in the nursing home setting has long been an issue of substantial concern,[81] leading to federal regulations to control their use in this setting.[82] Various interventions have been developed and tested to reduce the risks of psychoactive drug use in the nursing home setting.[83] "Academic detailing" to educate physicians and nursing home staff about the principles of geriatric psychoactive medication use has been utilized with success to improve the quality of drug prescribing, specifically in regard to antipsychotic medications and long elimination half-life benzodiazepine therapy.[84,85]

Next to psychoactive drugs, anticoagulants have been found to be the next leading cause of adverse drug events in long-term care facilities. Concerns have been raised regarding the quality of anticoagulant use in the nursing home setting,[86] with evidence for both undertreatment and poor control of INR. A more systematic approach to decision making regarding the use of warfarin for stroke prevention in the frail elderly is required, as well as a more consistent approach to the management of therapy. More widespread use of specialized anticoagulation clinics to provide coordinated anticoagulation care may offer an option to improve the effectiveness and safety of warfarin therapy in this particularly high-risk group of patients.

If the findings of the study just described are generalizable to all U.S. nursing homes, then one would predict that at least 24 adverse drug events and 8 potential adverse drug events would be identifiable over a 1-year period in the average facility, with half of these adverse drug events being preventable. Thus, in the 1.5 million residents of U.S. nursing homes, as many as 350,000 adverse drug events are likely to occur annually, with more than half preventable. Similarly, almost 20,000 fatal or life-threatening adverse drug events would be expected per year in nursing homes, of which 80% are likely to be preventable.

One flawed approach to preventing medication errors emphasizes seeking out and punishing health care providers who make errors that lead to adverse drug events. However, this ignores the fact that failures in the design of systems of care often contribute to the occurrence of medical errors, as well as the injuries that result from some of those errors.[87–90] Instead, enhanced surveillance and reporting systems for adverse drug events occurring in the nursing home setting are required, along with continued educational efforts relating to the optimal use of drug therapies in the frail elderly patient population. However, preventive efforts that focus solely on the individual provider or which rely on inspection alone

TABLE 7.1. Frequency of adverse drug events and potential adverse drug events by drug class.[a]

Drug class	Adverse drug events, no. (%) ($n = 546$)	Preventable adverse drug events, no. (%) ($n = 276$)	Nonpreventable adverse drug events, no. (%) ($n = 270$)
Antipsychotics	125 (23)	72 (26)	53 (20)
Antibiotics/antiinfectives	109 (20)	13 (5)	96 (36)
Antidepressants	68 (13)	50 (18)	18 (7)
Sedatives/hypnotics	68 (13)	49 (18)	19 (7)
Anticoagulants	51 (9)	37 (10)	14 (5)
Antiseizure	47 (9)	27 (10)	20 (7)
Cardiovascular	35 (6)	25 (9)	10 (4)
Hypoglycemics	27 (5)	14 (5)	13 (5)
Nonopioid analgesics	22 (4)	13 (5)	9 (3)
Opioids	15 (3)	7 (3)	8 (3)
Antiparkinsonians	12 (2)	7 (3)	5 (2)
Gastrointestinal	11 (2)	6 (2)	5 (2)
Diuretics	10 (2)	9 (3)	1 (0.4)
Antigout	6 (1)	4 (1)	2 (0.7)
Muscle relaxants	6 (1)	4 (1)	2 (0.7)
Alzheimer's disease	4 (0.7)	3 (1)	1 (0.4)
Nutrients/supplements	3 (0.5)	1 (0.4)	2 (0.7)
Ophthalmics	3 (0.5)	1 (0.4)	2 (1.0)
Antineoplastics	2 (0.4)	2 (0.7)	0 (0.0)
Respiratory	2 (0.4)	1 (0.4)	1 (0.4)
Osteoporosis	2 (0.4)	0 (0.0)	2 (0.7)
Steroids	1 (0.2)	1 (0.4)	0 (0.0)
Nonophthalmic topicals	1 (0.2)	0 (0.0)	1 (0.4)
Antihistamines	0 (0.0)	0 (0.0)	0 (0.0)
Antihyperlipidemics	0 (0.0)	0 (0.0)	0 (0.0)
Miscellaneous	2 (0.4)	0 (0.0)	2 (0.7)

[a] Drugs in more than one category were asociated with some events. Frequencies in each column sum to greater than the total number of events.

have limited impact. As Leape has noted, "Analysis and the correction of underlying systems faults is much more likely to result in enduring changes and significant error reduction."[89]

A systems-based approach to addressing the problem of medication errors emphasizes that the most important cause of error is faulty systems or design. Such approaches include improving information access for health care providers at the time drugs are prescribed,[91] reducing reliance on memory by standardizing approaches to clinical management (e.g., use of protocols when appropriate), and enhancing the education and training of health care professionals around the principles of geriatric pharmacotherapy.[92] As stated in the recent Institute of Medicine report entitled *To Err Is Human: Building a Safer Health System*, "Errors can be prevented by designing systems that make it hard for people to do the wrong thing and easy for people to do the right thing."[93]

Ordering and monitoring errors in the nursing home may be particularly amenable to prevention strategies utilizing systems-based approaches. The benefits of such an approach to error reduction in the hospital setting utilizing computerized order entry have recently been reported; such a system could be designed to focus on ordering and monitoring issues in the nursing home.[94]

Successes in the hospital setting pave the way for similar efforts in the nursing home setting aimed at reducing drug-related injuries and disability and improving the quality of care provided to the frail elderly patient population.[93]

Clinician Initiatives in Preventing Adverse Drug Events

Explicit criteria have been published for determining potentially inappropriate medication use by the elderly,[95,96] but most drug-related problems for the elderly are caused by medications that are not on any "bad drug" list. Nonetheless, such criteria are increasingly utilized in quality improvement efforts by health care systems and managed care plans. However, it should be recognized that these criteria generally cover a relatively small number of agents, some of which are rarely used in current practice.[97] Most suboptimal prescribing relates to drugs that are not included on these lists. Common examples include the excessive use of antibiotics for nonbacterial infections,[98] overuse or misuse of "acceptable" psychoactive drugs in all categories, and suboptimal management

TABLE 7.2. Frequency of adverse drug events by type.[a]

Type	Adverse drug events, total (n = 546) n (%)	Preventable events (n = 276) n (%)
Neuropsychiatric	150 (27)	83 (30)
Falls	67 (12)	55 (20)
Gastrointestinal	65 (12)	30 (11)
Dermatologic/allergic	59 (11)	7 (3)
Hemorrhage	57 (10)	40 (14)
Extrapyramidal symptoms/tardive dyskinesia	52 (6)	19 (7)
Infection	34 (6)	1 (0.4)
Metabolic/endocrine	27 (5)	14 (5)
Anorexia/weight loss	20 (4)	14 (5)
Ataxia/difficulty with gait	18 (3)	9 (3)
Cardiovascular	15 (3)	10 (4)
Electrolyte/fluid balance abnormality	9 (2)	5 (2)
Syncope/dizziness	8 (1)	5 (2)
Functional decline[b]	7 (1)	6 (2)
Respiratory	3 (0.5)	3 (1)
Anticholinergic[c]	3 (0.5)	2 (0.7)
Renal	3 (0.5)	1 (0.4)
Hematologic	2 (0.4)	2 (0.7)
Hepatic	1 (0.2)	1 (0.4)

[a] Adverse drug events could manifest as more than one type.
[b] Adverse drug event manifested only as decline in activities of daily living without any other more specific type of event. Other types of events may have been associated with functional decline.
[c] Anticholinergic effects include dry mouth, dry eyes, urinary retention, and constipation.

of warfarin therapy in patients with appropriate indications for treatment (e.g., chronic atrial fibrillation).[99]

There are a number of steps that prescribers can take to minimize the risk of adverse drug events in the elderly outside or within long-term care facilities. First, the physician must be aware of precisely what medications the patient is taking, which is best accomplished by a rigorous periodic review (at least every 6 months in a stable patient) of *all* medications taken by each elderly patient. Careful drug regimen review has been said to be one of the most useful interventions available to modern geriatric medicine, yet it fails to receive the attention it merits. Particular attention should be paid to eliciting information about medications that are (1) prescribed by another physician, (2) used only sporadically, (3) obtained over the counter, or (4) taken by some route other than by mouth and hence often not thought of by patients as "drugs" (e.g., eyedrops for glaucoma, estrogen or steroid cream, medications applied via transdermal patch). Periodic drug regimen review makes it possible to identify those medications that are truly enhancing a patient's clinical status and those which have become accidents of history and pose nothing but an ongoing risk.

Second, consider a "therapeutic un-trial" of a medication of dubious value that is currently in a patient's regimen. Older patients are at risk of accumulating layers and layers of drug therapy as they move through time, and often from physician to physician, forming the pharmacologic equivalent of a reef with accumulating layers of coral. Medications used for symptomatic relief are fairly easy to "prune," as their removal is less likely to put the patient at risk. However, even this must be done carefully, as chronic benzodiazepine users who have become habituated to their hypnotic may be at high risk of the serious withdrawal symptoms that can occur after discontinuation of the drug.[100,101]

More challenging is the reassessment of medications that could be vital to the patient's regimen or may be presenting the risk of toxicity with no therapeutic benefit; common examples include digoxin, quinidine, thiazides, antihypertensives, and anticonvulsants. Very often, these agents have been prescribed many years previously, for reasons that were either poorly documented or transitory (e.g., digoxin for mild transient congestive heart failure following a myocardial infarction, or phenytoin for a poorly described seizure occurring immediately after a stroke or in the setting of alcohol withdrawal). Some clinicians argue that if a patient is stable and in no overt distress, it is too risky to change the regimen by removing drugs that may not be needed. However, any medication that has the potential for toxicity with no continuing indication can also represent a "time bomb" for the patient. Progressive diminution of renal or hepatic clearance, an acute hypovolemic state accompanying a transient respiratory or gastrointestinal illness, confusion on the part of the patient or caregiver regarding dosing—each of these situations can result in unexpected toxicity from a medication that is not currently producing symptoms.

Another form of risk is the unrecognized diminution in function that may result from the unwise use of a medication. Examples include slight postural instability from excessive diuretic therapy, blunting of affect or cognitive function with psychoactive drug use, and so forth. Often, the presence of these symptoms is clear only in retrospect, when they have disappeared after withdrawal of the offending drug.

A number of investigators have engaged in careful withdrawal of several medications from patients in whom no clear ongoing indication was apparent. In a study of the feasibility of discontinuing potentially unnecessary antihypertensive medications in elderly persons, 105 patients who were normotensive on therapy were withdrawn from their medication. Eleven months later, 41% of them remained normotensive without treatment.[102] However, in a more recent study of withdrawal of diuretic therapy in the elderly, a substantial number of patients randomized to thiazide withdrawal had to have their regimen restored because of exacerbation of congestive heart failure or uncontrolled hypertension.[103] A number of studies have suggested that many patients with compensated heart failure in sinus rhythm can be withdrawn from digoxin with no adverse clinical or hemodynamic effects; this may be particularly true of patients receiving concurrent diuretic and vasodilator therapy.[104–106] In a study of nursing home residents (mean age, 87 years) receiving long-term digoxin therapy; three-quarters had normal ejection fractions (50% or greater); and, of these, two-thirds were in normal sinus rhythm. None of the patients in whom digoxin was discontinued had ejection fractions fall below 50%, and none showed signs of clinical deterioration over a 2-month follow-up period.[107] Although these were the first such data from a long-term care setting, they replicated findings from earlier studies conducted in community settings. By contrast, other investigators have reported that withdrawal of digoxin in patients with *impaired* systolic function can be detrimental.[108]

When a drug therapy is required, it is vital to use the minimum effective dose. Most adverse drug reactions are dose related. Accordingly, it makes sense to "start low and go slow." Following this strategy of using titrated dosing may be difficult. For many drug therapies, the low-dose therapy commonly used in clinical practice is not manufactured. For example, thiazide diuretic therapy is widely used in low doses (i.e., 12.5 mg) for the management of hypertension. However, the lowest manufactured dose in Canada is a 25-mg tablet, twice the dose recommended in guidelines for the initiation of this therapy in older patients. In one study of older adults in Ontario, Canada's largest province, almost 27% were dispensed a low dose of the thiazide diuretic therapy, with low-dose therapy being more common with increasing age. To achieve this low-dose therapy, older adults were required to split their pills.[109]

An additional issue is that for many drug therapies the minimum effective dose is not known for older people, particularly those of advanced age. Among commonly used drug therapies, many older people are prescribed doses much lower than were evaluated in clinical trials. For example, beta-blocker therapy is widely recommended for patients for secondary prevention of post-myocardial infarction. However, the minimum effective dose has not been fully determined for older people. Among more than 13,000 myocardial infarction survivors, use of beta-blocker therapy was associated with improved survival and decreased heart failure admissions relative to patients not prescribed beta-blocker therapy. However, among the 4681 older adults prescribed beta-blocker therapy, the risk of rehospitalization with heart failure was greater in the high-dose relative to the low-dose group. This finding suggests that although beta-blocker therapy is beneficial, it may be prudent to start

with low-dose therapy and to slowly titrate upward as tolerated.[110]

A similar issue of dose, risk, and benefit has recently been identified in relation to thrombolytic therapy in older patients with acute myocardial infarction. Older patients were either excluded from or underrepresented in the initial trials of these agents, even though they are the age group with the highest incidence of heart attack. Years after thrombolysis became the treatment of choice for this condition on the basis of those trials, evidence has emerged that the risk of thrombolytic-induced stroke is greater than expected in older patients being treated for myocardial infarction,[111] raising the question of whether the benefit–risk relationship for these drugs might be quite different for older patients.

Although almost 50% of older adults report some form of arthritis, randomized control trials of NSAIDs include few older people and hardly any over the age of 85 years.[112] Selecting the right dose may therefore be difficult because so little research evidence is available to guide choices. There are, however, a series of studies that suggest that adverse effects, including peptic ulcer disease, renal impairment, and hypertension, associated with the use of NSAID therapy are all dose related. Griffin et al.[113] evaluated older Medicaid enrollees to explore the relation between NSAID use and the development of peptic ulcer disease. Among NSAID users, the relative risk for the development of peptic ulcer disease increased from 2.8 for the lowest to 8.0 for the highest dose group. In a systematic review of epidemiologic studies, Henry et al.[114] found that the lower risk of serious gastrointestinal complications associated with the use of certain NSAIDs was attributable mainly to the low doses of those drugs generally used in clinical practice. Gurwitz et al.[115] conducted a study of 114 long-term care patients and documented the nephrotoxic effects of short-term NSAID therapy. They found that use of a high NSAID dose was a significant predictor of a greater than 50% increase in serum urea nitrogen level. In a further study, the same investigators studied 9411 patients newly started on an antihypertensive therapy.[116] NSAID users were significantly more likely than nonusers to be initiated on an antihypertensive, with the risk of starting up antihypertensive therapy increasing with increasing NSAID dose. These examples illustrate the dose-related development of a range of adverse effects associated with the use of NSAID therapy.

Concerns about preventable drug-induced illness have been amplified in recent years by the increasingly widespread use by older patients of vitamin supplements[117] and unproven over-the-counter (OTC) remedies to treat a wide variety of conditions ranging from memory loss[118] and depression to erectile dysfunction and arthritis. Following Congressional legislation in 1994 ending the supervisory role of the FDA (U.S. Food and Drug Administration) over claims made for OTC products, a menagerie of supplements and herbal remedies has sprung up, often marketed directly at the geriatric population, making claims that are completely unsubstantiated. Several related problems have resulted from this proliferation of untested therapies. Their use increases patient health care expenses at a time when it is difficult for many older Americans to afford effective drugs. Further, a growing body of evidence indicates that although most of the newer herbal remedies may lack efficacy, they have a genuine potential for toxicity, with numerous interactions between herbal medicines and conventional drug therapies documented as leading to adverse events.[119,120] Their presence in the marketplace further increases the need for the physician to take a detailed history of *all* substances the patient ingests in pursuit of health.

Although there is a tendency to focus on the excessive use of medications in the elderly patient population, the underuse of potentially beneficial medications is also a problem. An increasing number of examples suggest that adverse clinical consequences are associated with underprescribing of potentially beneficial drug therapies, including beta-blocker therapy after acute myocardial infarction, drugs for osteoporosis prevention, and the pharmacologic treatment of hypertension.[121]

Quality improvement efforts must also focus on underuse of specific classes of drugs and undertreatment of specific medical conditions. Efforts that seek only to reduce the total numbers of drugs prescribed to elderly patients to below an arbitrary threshold have a lower likelihood of providing real health benefits, as compared with carefully considered evidence-based efforts that focus on reducing the use of specific categories of medications that pose a high risk of adverse effects (e.g., long elimination half-life benzodiazepines or highly anticholinergic tricyclic antidepressants).

Clinical Decision Making in the Institutional Setting

Beyond the general aspects of geriatric pathophysiology and pharmacology, the unique situation of the long-term care facility adds another set of influences to prescribing for elderly patients. Drug use in the nursing home occurs in some of the most frail patients in the population, in institutions with the potential for supervised, round-the-clock observation. However, the nursing home environment is also one in which there is sometimes little physician input, particularly in light of the clinical complexity of the patients receiving care.[122] Nursing homes are complicated social institutions in which physicians, nurses, consultant pharmacists, other health professionals, aides, and administrators interact to make drug prescribing and drug administration decisions. Although the physician writes a prescription, this decision is often spurred by a nurse (or an aide) in much closer contact with the resident, who often guides the physician's prescribing decisions by telephone or in brief visits. When a drug is written for prn use (e.g., psychoactive medications, analgesics, and laxatives), it is the nursing staff or their assistants who frequently make the crucial decision as to whether an as-needed drug is actually administered, at what frequency, and often in what dose and by what route.[123]

For decades, the Health Care Financing Administration has required that a consultant pharmacist periodically review the drug regimens of all residents of skilled nursing facilities.[124] Thus, the nursing home is the only component of the health care system with required, regular pharmacist involvement in monitoring the appropriateness of specific prescribing decisions. While often dramatic in individual instances, the overall impact of this mandated review has been more modest than originally anticipated and was not successful in controlling the very high levels of psychoactive drug use often reported in such settings.

Adding still another dimension to the influences on drug use in the nursing home is the fiscal situation of such facilities. Although most U.S. hospitals are nonprofit institutions, the majority of long-term care facilities in the United States are for-profit entities. Even those that are not face reimbursement constraints that influence many aspects of care; because Medicaid programs are the main payors for about half the nation's nursing home residents, nonprofit facilities must also confront the limited per diem reimbursement rate provided by these state programs. Although drugs are generally covered separately and in full, limited reimbursement to the institution can constrain the level of staffing in both nonprofit and for-profit homes. Insufficient staffing in turn can influence the incentive for use of psychoactive medications, as well as the capacity to monitor the consequences of drug use, both therapeutic and adverse.

Regulatory changes may have brought about some change, but numerous studies during the 1990s indicated that about half of all nursing home residents were regularly administered one or more psychoactive drugs. Until recently, antipsychotic drugs were taken by a quarter or more of all nursing home residents.[125–128] Although a few studies suggest some efficacy of antipsychotics in the treatment of agitation in geriatric patients with dementia,[129] the literature is both limited and ambiguous in this area. However, there is clear evidence linking the use of such drugs with extrapyramidal symptoms, gait instability, falls, and hip fractures. Benzodiazepines, frequently used for dementia-associated agitation, can also be troublesome; long elimination half-life benzodiazepines pose their own risks of falls and fractures and other side effects including daytime somnolence, confusion, and ataxia, although not parkinsonian symptoms. Cross-national studies indicate that apparently comparable patients with dementia are managed in long-term care facilities in western Europe and Japan with much less reliance on sedating medications, and apparently with good control of agitated behavior.

In a randomized trial of a comprehensive educational outreach program to reduce the use of psychoactive drugs in nursing homes, the use of antipsychotic drugs was discontinued in significantly more residents in nursing homes receiving the intervention than in control homes (32% versus 14%); these reductions occurred without adversely affecting the overall behavior and level of functioning of the residents[130] or level of distress among staff.[131] In a similar study, Ray et al. also reported large reductions in antipsychotic drug use.[132]

Considerably more needs to be learned about the relative clinical efficacy of interpersonal interventions, benzodiazepines, and antipsychotic agents in calming agitated demented nursing home residents. Some studies have found that reliance on sedative drugs was more common in larger nursing homes, facilities with lower staff-to-patient ratios, or by physicians with larger nursing home practices[133]; however, these findings have not been consistently replicated. The interplay among economic constraints, staffing patterns, and sedative use is a crucial topic for further investigation.

In considering whether pharmacologic intervention is required to manage agitated behavior in an elderly nursing home resident, two basic facts should be considered. The first is that unusual behavior in the elderly is not necessarily an indication for drug intervention. Incoherent babbling or constant repetition of inappropriate requests may merely require a greater level of tolerance on the part of staff members, rather than sedation. Other problems, such as wandering, might be approached by environmental solutions, such as facility designs that enable disoriented patients to move about freely while preventing their escape from the range of staff supervision. If intervention is warranted, the safest therapeutic approach (and one which can be highly effective) is interpersonal attention, which is often preferable to sedation. Whether in the institutional or the ambulatory setting, programs to improve prescribing quality may lead to increased costs in the short term but can lead to long-term improvements in outcome. Such interventions to improve the quality of health care provided to the elderly have been shown to prevent readmission of elderly patients with congestive heart failure,[134] reduce the risk of falls,[135] and improve the quality of care in patients requiring chronic warfarin therapy.[136]

Development and Testing of New Therapeutic Agents

Even though many drugs are likely to be used heavily by the geriatric population, progress has been slow toward systematic inclusion of older patients in the drug evaluation and approval process. In the past, it has been advantageous for pharmaceutical manufacturers and clinical researchers to test new drugs before marketing primarily in healthy younger patients, because they are likeliest to yield "clean" results uncomplicated by concomitant therapy with other drugs, comorbidity, or pharmacokinetic abnormalities. However, this leaves open the possibility that one of these "complicating factors" will have a clinically meaningful effect on the new drug once it is marketed and taken by large numbers of elderly persons.

Unfortunately, much time can pass before studies are mounted to address important therapeutic issues in the elderly (e.g., the Systolic Hypertension in the Elderly Program[137]), and clinicians and patients are forced to make pressing clinical decisions in the absence of an adequate knowledge base. Perceptions about the difficulty of involving elderly subjects in research protocols can lead to study designs that prevent a study from yielding the very information necessary to clarify or refute such preconceptions about the drug's effects in elderly patients. This a priori exclusion of elderly has been particularly problematic in clinical trials in the prevention and treatment of heart disease.[138] For example, age restrictions excluded older patients from most of the pivotal studies of lipid-lowering drugs in both primary and secondary prevention. Some clinicians and payors then responded to this lack of information with the conclusion that "there is no evidence to justify the use of lipid-lowering drugs in the elderly," and advocated withholding such therapy from older patients. However, when age-stratified analyses have been performed to determine whether the benefits of cholesterol reduction are attenuated with age (most notably in the CARE trial, which included patients up to age 75),[139] it was found that the risk reduction afforded by pravastatin remained constant throughout the age range studied.[140] Cost-effectiveness modeling suggested that the intervention remained a "good buy" for older patients as well.[141] Definitive results are expected from an ongoing randomized trial of pravastatin in elderly patients, PROSPER.[142]

Over a decade ago, the Food and Drug Administration issued a guideline on the testing of drugs in the elderly.[143] The guideline was intended to encourage routine and thorough evaluation in elderly populations of the effects of new medications proposed for FDA approval, so that physicians would have sufficient information to use drugs properly in their older patients. The recommendations state that "there is no good basis for the exclusion of patients on the basis of advanced age alone, or because of the presence of any concomitant illness or medication, unless there is reason to believe that the concomitant illness or medication will endanger the patient or lead to confusion in interpreting the results of the study. Attempts should therefore be made to include patients over 75 years of age and those with concomitant illness and treatments, if they are stable and willing to participate." The FDA guideline presented a reasonable and practical approach to the study of drugs in the elderly, with implications for the design of future clinical trials of both new and existing drug therapies. However, few data are available to document its effect on the demographics of premarketing trials.

Conclusion

As the most prominent consumers of prescription medications, elderly patients stand to benefit the most and are also at greatest risk of toxicity from our increasingly complex, effective, and costly pharmacopoeia. When pharmacotherapy is indicated, choosing the right drug in the right dose for an elderly patient represents one of the most difficult challenges in all of medicine, but also can yield the most gratifying outcomes. Likewise, few interventions in geriatric practice are as elegant in process, and as "heroic" in outcome, as identifying and treating adverse drug effects. Thorough knowledge of some of the principles outlined here will enable the clinician to wield this powerful double-edged sword with the least possible risk and with the maximum benefit for patients.

References

1. Schmucker DL. Aging and drug disposition: an update. *Pharmacol Rev.* 1985;37:133–148.
2. Castleden CM, Volans CN, Raymond K, et al. The effect of ageing on drug absorption from the gut. *Age Ageing.* 1977;6:138–143.
3. Schwartz JB. Clinical pharmacology. In: Hazzard WR, Bierman EL, Blass JP, Ettinger WH Jr, Halter JB, eds. *Principles of Geriatric Medicine and Gerontology*, 3rd Ed. New York: McGraw-Hill; 1994.
4. Campion EW, deLabry LO, Glynn RJ. The effect of age on serum albumin in healthy males: report from the Normative Aging Study. *J Gerontol.* 1988;43:M18–M20.
5. Grandiston MK, Boudinot FD. Age-related changes in protein binding of drugs: implications for therapy. *Clin Pharmacokinet.* 2000;38:271–290.
6. MacLennan WJ, Martin P, Mason BJ. Protein intake and serum albumin levels in the elderly. *Gerontology.* 1977; 23:360–367.
7. Conti MC, Goralnik JH, Salive ME, Sarkin JD. Serum albumin level and physical disability as predictors of mortality in older persons. *JAMA.* 1994;272:1036–1042.
8. Greenblatt DJ, Sellers EM, Koch-Weser J. Importance of protein binding for the interpretation of serum or plasma drug concentrations. *J Clin Pharmacol.* 1982;22:259–263.
9. Frontera WR, Hughes VA, Lutz KJ, Evans WJ. A cross-sectional study of muscle strength and mass in 45- to 78-yr-old men and women. *J Appl Physiol.* 1991;71:644–650.
10. Thurmann PA, Hompesch BC. Influence of gender on the pharmacokinetics and pharmacodynamics of drugs. *Int J Clin Pharmacol Ther.* 1998;36:586–590.
11. Vestal RE. Aging and pharmacology. *Cancer.* 1997;80: 1302–1310.
12. Kinirons MT, Crome P. Clinical pharmacokinetic considerations in the elderly. *Clin Pharmacokinet.* 1997;33: 302–312.
13. Mooney H, Roberts R, Cooksley WGE, et al. Alterations in the liver with aging. *Clin Gastroenterol.* 1985;14:757–771.
14. Vestal RE, Norris AH, Tobin JD, et al. Antipyrine metabolism in man: influence of age, alcohol, caffeine, and smoking. *Clin Pharmacol Ther.* 1975;18:425–432.
15. Muhlberg W, Platt D. Age-dependent changes of the kidneys: pharmacological implications. *Gerontology.* 1999; 45:243–253.
16. Rowe JW, Andres R, Tobin JD, et al. The effect of age on creatinine clearance in man. *J Gerontol.* 1976;31:155–163.
17. Lindeman RD, Tobin JD, Shock NW. Longitudinal studies on the rate of decline in renal function with age. *J Am Geriatr Soc.* 1985;33:278–285.
18. Cockcroft DW, Gault MH. Prediction of creatinine clearance from serum creatinine. *Nephron.* 1976;16:31–41.
19. Friedman JR, Norman DC, Yoshikawa TT. Correlation of estimated renal function parameters versus 24-hour creatinine clearance in ambulatory elderly. *J Am Geriatr Soc.* 1989;37:145–149.
20. Abernethy DR. Aging effects on drug disposition and effect. *Geriatr Nephrol Urol.* 1999;9:15–19.
21. Greenblatt DJ, Divoll M, Harmatz JS, et al. Kinetics and clinical effects of flurazepam in young and elderly insomniacs. *Clin Pharmacol Ther.* 1981;30:475–486.
22. Greenblatt DJ. Benzodiazepine hypnotics: sorting the pharmacokinetic facts. *J Clin Psychiatry.* 1991;52(suppl 9): 4–10.
23. Ray WA, Griffin MR, Downey W. Benzodiazepines of long and short elimination half-life and the risk of hip fracture. *JAMA.* 1989;262:3303–3307.
24. Greenblatt DJ, Allen MD, Shader RI. Toxicity of high-dose flurazepam in the elderly. *Clin Pharmacol Ther.* 1977;21: 355–361.
25. Greenblatt DJ, Harmatz JS, Shader RI. Clinical pharmacokinetics of anxiolytics and hypnotics in the elderly: therapeutic considerations (part I). *Clin Pharmacokinet.* 1991; 21:165–177.
26. Turnheim K. Drug dosage in the elderly. Is it rational? *Drugs Aging.* 1998;13:357–379.

27. Greenblatt DJ, Harmatz JS, Shapiro L, Engelhardt N, Gouthro TA, Shader RI. Sensitivity to triazolam in the elderly. *N Engl J Med.* 1991;324:1691–1698.

28. Reidenberg MM, Levy M, Warner H, et al. Relationship between diazepam dose, plasma level, age, and central nervous system depression. *Clin Pharmacol Ther.* 1978; 23:371–374.

29. Castleden CM, George CF, Marcer D, et al. Increased sensitivity to nitrazepam in old age. *Br Med J.* 1977;1:10–12.

30. Fischer M. Effect of age on pharmacokinetics and pharmacodynamics in man. *Int J Clin Pharmacol Ther.* 1998; 36:581–585.

31. Greenblatt DJ, Harmatz JS, Shader RI. Clinical pharmacokinetics of anxiolytics and hypnotics in the elderly: therapeutic considerations (part II). *Clin Pharmacokinet.* 1991;21:262–273.

32. O'Malley K, Stevenson IH, Ward CA, et al. Determinants of anticoagulant control in patients receiving warfarin. *Br J Clin Pharmacol.* 1977;4:309–314.

33. Shephard AMM, Hewick DS, Moreland TA. Age as a determinant of sensitivity to warfarin. *Br J Clin Pharmacol.* 1977;4:315–320.

34. Gurwitz JH, Avorn J, Ross-Degnan D, Choodnovskiy I, Ansell J. Aging and the anticoagulant response to warfarin. *Ann Intern Med.* 1992;116:901–904.

35. Hammerlein A, Derendorf H, Lowenthal DT. Pharmacokinetic and pharmacodynamic changes in the elderly. Clinical implications. *Clin Pharmacokinet.* 1998; 35:49–64.

36. Greenblatt DJ, Shader RI, Harmatz JS. Implications of altered drug disposition in the elderly: studies of benzodiazepines. *J Clin Pharmacol.* 1989;29:866–872.

37. Berlinger WG, Goldberg MJ, Spector R, Chiang CK, Ghoneim M. Diphenhydramine: kinetics and psychomotor effects in elderly women. *Clin Pharmacol Ther.* 1982;32:387–391.

38. Nolan L, O'Malley K. Prescribing for the elderly. Part I: Sensitivity of the elderly to adverse drug reactions. *J Am Geriatr Soc.* 1988;36:142–149.

39. Gurwitz JH, Avorn J. The ambiguous relation between aging and adverse drug reactions. *Ann Intern Med.* 1991;114:956–966.

40. Flaherty JH. Psychotherapeutic agents in older adults. Commonly prescribed and over-the-counter remedies: causes of confusion. *Clin Geriatr Med.* 1998;14:101–127.

41. Larson EB, Kukull WA, Buchner D, et al. Adverse drug reactions associated with global cognitive impairment in elderly persons. *Ann Intern Med.* 1987;107:169–173.

42. Cantu TG, Korek JS. Central nervous system reactions to histamine-2 receptor blockers. *Ann Intern Med.* 1991;114:1027–1034.

43. Gray SL, Lai KV, Larson EB. Drug-induced cognition disorders in the elderly: incidence, prevention, and management. *Drug Saf.* 1999;21:101–122.

44. Verhaeverbeke I, Mets T. Drug-induced orthostatic hypotension in the elderly: avoiding its onset. *Drug Saf.* 1997;17:105–118.

45. Sweet RA, Pollock BG. New atypical antipsychotics. Experience and utility in the elderly. *Drugs Aging.* 1998;12:115–127.

46. Chan YC, Pariser SF, Neufeld G. Atypical antipsychotics in older adults. *Pharmacotherapy.* 1999;19:811–822.

47. Cohen JS. Avoiding adverse reactions. Effective lower-dose drug therapies for older patients. *Geriatrics.* 2000;55: 54–56, 59–60, 63–64.

48. Rochon PA, Gurwitz JH. Optimising drug treatment for elderly people: the prescribing cascade. *Br Med J.* 1997;315:1096–1099.

49. Gurwitz JH, Avorn J, Bohn RL, Glynn RJ, Monane M, Mogun H. Initiation of thiazide diuretic therapy during nonsteroidal anti-inflammatory drug therapy. *JAMA.* 1994;272:781–786.

50. Gurwitz JH, Kalish SC, Bohn RL, et al. Thiazide diuretics and the initiation of anti-gout therapy. *J Clin Epidemiol.* 1997;50:953–959.

51. Avorn J, Gurwitz JH, Bohn RL, et al. Increased incidence of levodopa therapy following metoclopramide use. *JAMA.* 1995;274:1780–1782.

52. Monane M, Avorn J, Beers MH, Everitt DE. Anticholinergic drug use and bowel function in nursing home patients. *Arch Intern Med.* 1993;153:633–638.

53. Rochon PA, Gurwitz JH. Drug therapy. *Lancet.* 1995;346: 32–36.

54. Ray WA, Griffin MR, Schaffner W, et al. Psychotropic drug use and the risk of hip fracture. *N Engl J Med.* 1987; 316:363–369.

55. Wang PS, Bohn RL, Glynn RJ, Mogun H, Avorn J. Zolpiderm use and hip fractures in older people. *J Am Geriatr Soc.* 2001;49:1685–1690.

56. Herings RMC, Stricker BHC, de Boer A, Bakker A, Sturmans A. Benzodiazepines and the risk of falling leading to femur fractures. *Arch Intern Med.* 1995;155:1801–1807.

57. Liu B, Anderson G, Mittmann N, To T, Axcell T, Shear N. Use of selective serotonin-reputake inhibitors of tricyclic antidepressants and risk of hip fractures in elderly people. *Lancet.* 1998;351:1303–1307.

58. Thapa PB, Gideon P, Cost TW, Milam AB, Ray WA. Antidepressants and the risk of falls among nursing home residents. *N Engl J Med.* 1998;339:875–882.

59. Thapa PB, Gideon P, Cost TW, Milam AB, Ray WA. Antidepressants and the risk of falls among nursing home residents. *N Engl J Med.* 1998;339:875–882.

60. Fifth ACCP Consensus Conference on Antithrombotic Therapy (1998): summary and recommendations. *Chest* 1998;114(suppl):439S–769S.

61. Wolf PA, Abbott RD, Kannel WB. Atrial fibrillation: a major contributor to stroke in the elderly. The Framingham Study. *Arch Intern Med.* 1987;147:1561–1564.

62. Feinberg WM, Blackshear J, Laupacis A, Kronmal R, Hart RG. Prevelance, age distribution, and gender of patients with atrial fibrillation: analysis and implications. *Arch Intern Med.* 1995;155:469–473.

63. Atrial Fibrillation Investigators. Risk factors for stroke and efficacy of antithrombotic therapy in atrial fibrillation: analysis of pooled data from five randomized controlled trials. *Arch Intern Med.* 1994;154:1449–1457.

64. Hylek EM, Singer DE. Risk factors for intracranial hemorrhage in outpatients taking warfarin. *Ann Intern Med.* 1994;120:897–902.

65. Fihn SD, McDonell M, Martin D, et al. Risk factors for complications of chronic anticoagulation: a multicenter study. Warfarin Optimized Outpatient Follow-up Study Group. *Ann Intern Med.* 1993;118:511–520.

66. Kalish S, Gurwitz JH, Avorn J. Anticoagulant therapy in the elderly. *Prim Cardiol.* 1993;7:34–42.

67. Landefeld CS, Anderson PA. Guideline-based consultation to prevent anticoagulant-related bleeding. A randomized, controlled trial in a teaching hospital. *Ann Intern Med.* 1992;116:829–837.

68. Poller L, Shiach CR, MacCallum PK, et al. Multicentre randomised study of computerised anticoagulant dosage. European Concerted Action on Anticoagulation. *Lancet.* 1998;352:1505–1509.

69. Gurwitz JH, Avorn J, Ross-Degnan D, Lipsitz LA. Non-steroidal anti-inflammatory drug-associated azotemia in the very old. *JAMA.* 1990;264:471–475.

70. Bollini P, Garcia Rodriguez LA, Perez Gutthann S, Walker AM. The impact of research quality and study design on epidemiologic estimates of the effect of non-steroidal anti-inflammatory drugs on upper gastrointestinal tract disease. *Arch Intern Med.* 1992;152:1289–1295.

71. Bradley JD, Brandt KD, Katz BP, Kalasinski LA, Ryan SI. Comparison of an antiinflammatory dose of ibuprofen, an analgesic dose of ibuprofen, and acetaminophen in the treatment of patients with osteoarthritis of the knee. *N Engl J Med.* 1991;325:87–91.

72. Whitcomb DC, Block GD. Association of acetaminophen hepatotoxicity with fasting and ethanol use. *JAMA.* 1994;272:1845–1850.

73. Feldman M, McMahon AT. Do cyclooxygenase-2 inhibitors provide benefits similar to those of traditional nonsteroidal anti-inflammatory drugs, with less gastrointestinal toxicity? *Ann Intern Med.* 2000;132:134–143.

74. Feldman M, McMahon AT. Do cyclooxygenase-2 inhibitors provide benefits similar to those of traditional nonsteroidal anti-inflammatory drugs, with less gastrointestinal toxicity? *Ann Intern Med.* 2000;132:134–143.

75. Swan SK, Rudy DW, Lasseter KC, et al. Effect of cyclooxygenase-2 inhibition on renal function in elderly persons receiving a low-salt diet. *Ann Intern Med.* 2000;133:1–9.

76. Strahan GW. An overview of nursing homes and their current residents: data from the 1995 national nursing homes survey. *Advance Data from Vital and Health Statistics*, no. 280. Hyattsville, MD: National Center for Health Statistics; 1997.

77. Bernabei R, Gambassi G, Lapane K, et al. Characteristics of the SAGE database: a new resource for research on outcomes in long-term care. SAGE (Systematic Assessment of Geriatric drug use via Epidemiology) Study Group. *J Gerontol Ser A Biol Sci Med Sci.* 1999;54:M25–M33.

78. Gerety MB, Cornell JE, Plichta DT, Eimer M. Adverse events related to drugs and drug withdrawal in nursing home residents. *J Am Geriatr Soc.* 1993;41:1326–1332.

79. Gurwitz JH, Sanchez-Cross MT, Eckler MA, Matulis J. The epidemiology of adverse and unexpected events in long-term care setting. *J Am Geriatr Soc.* 1994;42:33–38.

80. Gurwitz JH, Field TS, Avorn J, et al. Incidence and preventability of adverse drug events in nursing homes. *Am J Med.* 2000;109:87–94.

81. Rango N. Nursing home care in the United States. *N Engl J Med.* 1982;307:883–889.

82. Elon R, Paulson LG. The impact of OBRA on medical practice within nursing facilities. *J Am Geriatr Soc.* 1992; 40:958–963.

83. Ray WA, Taylor JA, Meador KG, et al. A randomized trial of a consultation service to reduce falls in nursing homes. *JAMA.* 1997;278:557–562.

84. Avorn J, Soumerai SB, Everitt DE, et al. A randomized trial of a program to reduce the use of psychoactive drugs in nursing homes. *N Engl J Med.* 1992;327:168–173.

85. Ray WA, Taylor JA, Meador KG, et al. Reducing antipsychotic drug use in nursing homes. A controlled trial of provider education. *Arch Intern Med.* 1993;153:713–721.

86. Gurwitz JH, Monette J, Rochon PA, Eckler MA, Avorn J. Atrial fibrillation and stroke prevention with warfarin in the long-term care setting. *Arch Intern Med.* 1997;157: 978–984.

87. Berwick DM. Continuous improvement as an ideal in health care. *N Engl J Med.* 1989;320:53–56.

88. Leape LL. Error in medicine. *JAMA.* 1994;272:1851–1857.

89. Leape LL, Bates DW, Cullen DJ, et al. Systems analysis of adverse drug events. *JAMA.* 1995;274:35–43.

90. Horton R. The uses of error. *Lancet.* 1999;353:422–423.

91. Teich JM, Merchia PR, Schmiz JL, Kuperman GJ, Spurr CD, Bates DW. Effects of computerized physician order enty on prescribing practices. *Arch Intern Med.* 2000;160:2741–2747.

92. Rothschild JM, Bates DW, Leape L. Preventable medical injuries in older patients. *Arch Intern Med.* 2000;160: 2717–2728.

93. Kohn LT, Corrigan JM, Donaldson MS, eds. *To Err Is Human: Building a Safer Health System.* Washington, DC: National Academy Press; 1999.

94. Bates DW, Leape LL, Cullen DJ, et al. Effect of computerized physician order entry and a team intervention on prevention of serious medication errors. *JAMA.* 1998; 280:1311–1316.

95. Beers MH, Ouslander JG, Rollingher I, Reuben DB, Brooks J, Beck JC. Expliit criteria for determining inappropriate medication use in nursing home residents. *Arch Intern Med.* 1991;151:1825–1832.

96. Beers MH. Explicit criteria for determining potentially inappropriate medication use by the elderly: an update. *Arch Intern Med.* 1997;157:1531–1536.

97. Gurwitz JH. Suboptimal medication use in the elderly. The tip of the iceberg. *JAMA.* 1994;272:292–296.

98. Gonzales R, Steiner JF, Lum A, Barrett PH Jr. Decreasing antibiotic use in ambulatory practice: impact of a multidimensional intervention on the treatment of uncomplicated acute bronchitis in adults. *JAMA.* 1999;281: 1512–1519.

99. Gurwitz JH, Monette J, Rochon PA, Eckler MA, Avorn A. Atrial fibrillation and stroke prevention with warfarin in the long-term care setting. *Arch Intern Med.* 1997;157: 978–984.

100. Greenblatt DJ, Harmatz JS, Zinny MA, et al. Effect of gradual withdrawal on the rebound sleep disorder after discontinuation of triazolam. *N Engl J Med.* 1987;317:722–728.

101. Busto U, Sellers EM, Naranjo CA, et al. Withdrawal reaction after long-term therapeutic use of benzodiazepines. *N Engl J Med.* 1986;315:854–859.

102. Danielson M, Lundback M. Withdrawal of antihypertensive drugs in mild hypertension. *Acta Med Scand.* 1981; 646(suppl 1):127–131.

103. Walma EP, Hoes AW, van Dooren C, Prins A, van der Does E. Withdrawal of long-term diuretic medication in elderly patients: a double blind randomised trial. *Br Med J.* 1997; 315:464–468.

104. Fleg JL, Gottlieb SH, Lakatta EG. Is digoxin really important in treatment of compensated heart failure? A placebo-controlled crossover study in patients with sinus rhythm. *Am J Med.* 1982;73:244–250.

105. Gheorghiade M, Beller GA. Effect of discontinuing maintenance digoxin therapy in patients with ischemic heart disease and congestive heart failure in sinus rhythm. *Am J Cardiol.* 1983;51:1243–1250.

106. Yusuf S, Garg R, Held P, Gorlin R. Need for a large randomized trial to evaluate the effects of digitalis on morbidity and mortality in congestive heart failure. *Am J Cardiol.* 1992;69:64G–70G.

107. Forman DE, Coletta D, Kenny D, et al. Clinical issues related to discontinuing digoxin therapy in elderly nursing home patients. *Arch Intern Med.* 1991;151:2194–2198.

108. Packer M, Gheorghiade M, Young JB, et al. Withdrawal of digoxin from patients with chronic heart failure treated with angiotensin-converting-enzyme inhibitors. *N Engl J Med.* 1993;329:1–7.

109. Rochon PA, Anderson GM, Tu JV, et al. Age and gender-related use of low-dose drug therapy: the need to manufacture low-dose therapy and evaluate the minimum effective dose. *J Am Geriatr Soc.* 1999;47:954–959.

110. Rochon PA, Tu JV, Anderson GM, et al. Rate of heart failure and 1-year survival for older people receiving low-dose beta-blocker therapy after myocardial infarction. *Lancet.* 2000;356:639–644.

111. Gurwitz JH, Gore JM, Goldberg RJ, et al., for the participants in the National Registry of Myocardial Infarction. *Ann Intern Med.* 1998;129:597–604.

112. Rochon PA, Fortin PR, Dear KBG, Minaker KL, Chalmers TC. Reporting of age data in clinical trials of arthritis: deficiencies and solutions. *Arch Intern Med.* 1993;153:243–248.

113. Griffin MR, Piper JM, Daugherty JR, Snowden M, Ray WA. Nonsteroidal antiinflammatory drug use and increased risk for peptic ulcer disease in elderly persons. *Ann Intern Med.* 1991;114:257–263.

114. Henry D, Lim LL, Garcia Rodriguez LA, et al. Variability in risk of gastrointestinal complications with individual non-steroidal anti-inflammatory drugs: results of a collaborative meta-analysis. *Br Med J.* 1996;312:1563–1566.

115. Gurwitz JH, Avorn J, Ross-Degnan D, Lipsitz LA. Nonsteroidal anti-inflammatory drug-associated azotemia in the very old. *JAMA.* 1990;264:471–475.

116. Gurwitz JH, Avorn J, Bohn RL, Glynn RJ, Monane M, Mogun H. Initiation of antihypertensive treatment during nonsteroidal anti-inflammatory drug therapy. *JAMA.* 1994;272:781–786.

117. Schumann K. Interactions between drugs and vitamins at advanced age. *Int J Vitam Nutr Res.* 1999;69:173–178.

118. Coleman LM, Fowler LL, Williams ME. Use of unproven therapies by people with Alzheimer's disease. *J Am Geriatr Soc.* 1995;43(7):747–750.

119. Fugh-Berman A. Herb–drug interactions. *Lancet.* 2000; 355:134–138.

120. Gold JL, Laxer DA, Dergal JM, Lanctot KL, Rochon PA. Herb–drug therapy interactions: A focus on dementia. *Curr Opin Clin Nutr Metab Care.* 2001;4(1):29–34.

121. Rochon PA, Gurwitz JG. Prescribing for seniors: neither too much nor too little. *JAMA.* 1999;282:113–115.

122. Mitchell JB. Physician visits to nursing homes. *Gerontologist.* 1982;22:45–48.

123. Gurwitz JH, Soumerai SB, Avorn J. Improving medication prescribing and utilization in the nursing home. *J Am Geriatr Soc.* 1990;38:542–552.

124. Anonymous. Conditions of participation-pharmaceutical services. *Fed Reg.* 1974;39:12–17.

125. Ray WA, Federspiel CF, Schaffner W. A study of antipsychotic drug use in nursing homes: epidemiologic evidence suggesting misuse. *Am J Public Health.* 1980;70: 485–491.

126. Ingman SR, Lawron IR, Pierpaoli PG, et al. A survey of the prescribing and administration of drugs in a long-term care institution for the elderly. *J Am Geriatr Soc.* 1975;23: 309–316.

127. Beers M, Avorn J, Soumerai SB, et al. Psychoactive medication use in intermediate-care facilities. *JAMA.* 1988;260:3016–3020.

128. Buck JA. Psychotropic drug practice in nursing homes. *J Am Geriatr Soc.* 1988;36:409–418.

129. Schneider LS, Pollock VE, Lyness SA. A metaanalysis of controlled trials of neuroleptic treatment in dementia. *J Am Geriatr Soc.* 1990;38:553–563.

130. Avorn J, Soumerai SB, Everitt DE, et al. A randomized trial of a program to reduce the use of psychoactive drugs in nursing homes. *N Engl J Med.* 1992;327:168–173.

131. Everitt DE, Fields DR, Soumerai SS, Avorn J. Resident behavior and staff distress in the nursing home. *J Am Geriatr Soc.* 1991;39:792–798.

132. Ray WA, Taylor JA, Meador KH, et al. Reducing antipsychotic drug use in nursing homes: a controlled trial of provider education. *Arch Intern Med.* 1993;153:713–721.

133. Svarstad BL, Mount JK. Nursing home resources and tranquilizer use among the institutionalized elderly. *J Am Geriatr Soc.* 1991;39:869–875.

134. Rich MW, Beckham V, Wittenberg C, Leven CL, Greedland KE, Carney RM. A multidisciplinary intervention to prevent the readmission of elderly patients with congestive heart failure. *N Engl J Med.* 1995;333:1213–1214.

135. Tinetti ME, Baker DI, McAvay G, et al. A multifactorial intervention to reduce the risk of falling among elderly people living in the community. *N Engl J Med.* 1994;331: 872—873.

136. Elston Lafata J, Martin SA, Kaatz S, Ward RE. The cost-effectiveness of different management strategies for patients on chronic warfarin therapy. *J Gen Intern Med.* 2000;15:31–37.

137. SHEP Cooperative Research Group. Prevention of stroke by antihypertensive drug treatment in older persons with isolated systolic hypertension: final results of the Systolic Hypertension in the Elderly Program (SHEP). *JAMA.* 1991;265:3255–3264.

138. Gurwitz JH, Col NF, Avorn J. The exclusion of the elderly and women from clinical trials in acute myocardial infarction. *JAMA.* 1991;268:1417–1422.

139. Sacks FM, Pfeffer MA, Moye LA, et al. The effect of pravastatin on coronary events after myocardial infraction in patients with average cholesterol levels. *N Engl J Med.* 1996;335:1001–1009.

140. Lewis SJ, et al. Effect on pravastatin on cardiovascular events in older patients with myocardial infraction and cholesterol levels in the average range. *Ann Intern Med.* 1998;129:681–689.

141. Ganz DA, Kuntz KM, Jacobson GA, Avorn J. Cost-effectiveness of 3-hydroxy-3-methylglutaryl coenzyme A reducatase inhibitor therapy in older patients with myocardial infraction. *Ann Intern Med.* 2000;132:780–787.

142. Shepherd J, et al. The design of a prospective study of *pravastatin* in the elderly at risk (PROSPER). *Am J Cardiol.* 1999;84:1192–1197.

143. *Guideline for the Study of Drugs Likely to Be Used in the Elderly.* Rockville, MD: Center for Drug Evaluation and Research, Food and Drug Administration; 1989.

8
Clinical Strategies of Prescribing for Older Adults

Judith L. Beizer

Appropriate prescribing of medication for elderly patients involves more than knowledge of the pharmacology of the medications. Clinical issues, as well as practical and regulatory issues surrounding medication use in the older population, must also be taken into consideration.

Medication History

Before even considering any of the issues involving drug therapy in a given patient, it is essential that the prescriber know exactly what medications the patient is taking, achieved by taking a thorough and accurate medication history. When asking the patient about their medications, it is important to be specific. The interviewer should specifically ask about prescription medications, over-the-counter (OTC) products, as needed (prn) medications, vitamins and minerals, herbal products, and home remedies. The questions can be asked by category of product or as a review of systems. For example, "Do you take anything for your eyes, ears, etc.?" The interview should end with the question, "Do you do anything else for your health?" With the widespread interest in complementary and alternative medicine, this last question may provide some interesting and unusual responses. Another useful technique is to have patients bring in all their medications and medicinal products for review by the physician, nurse, or pharmacist. Ideally the medication history and inventory should be updated at each office visit, and a complete history should be obtained at least every 6 months. Asking what health care providers the patient has seen since their last visit with you often serves as a prompt to remember other medications.

Minimizing Medication

One of the most crucial elements of geriatric pharmacotherapy is not to overmedicate the patient. Polypharmacy, the use of many medications, is a major cause of noncompliance, adverse effects, and drug interactions. Before adding a new medication to a patient's regimen, current therapy should be assessed. Questions that should be addressed include: Is the new symptom a side effect of an existing medication, or can the problem be handled by adjusting the dose of current medications or discontinuing a medication? An important point to remember is that it is usually easier to not start a medication that may not be necessary than it is to stop a current medication.

When withdrawing medications thought to be unnecessary, it is crucial to monitor the patient for recurrence of symptoms. Walma et al. conducted a double-blind randomized controlled trial of diuretic withdrawal in elderly patients with no symptoms of heart failure or hypertension.[1] Of the 102 patients in the withdrawal group, 50 patients needed to be restarted on diuretics, 25 of them because of heart failure. Other studies have examined the effect of drug withdrawal in elderly populations. Gerety et al. studied adverse drug events (ADEs) and adverse drug withdrawal events (ADWEs) in a Veteran Affairs (VA) nursing home;[2] 190 medications were withdrawn and 62 patients experienced 94 ADWEs, 72% of which were minor. The most common risk factors for ADEs and ADWEs were the number of diagnoses, number of medications, and hospitalization during the nursing home stay. The most common medications associated with ADWEs were cardiovascular, central nervous system (CNS), and gastrointestinal (GI) drugs. Of note, 60% of the medications did not need to be reinstituted. A similar study was conducted in a VA outpatient setting:[3] 238 medications were discontinued in 124 patients, resulting in 62 ADWEs; 74% of the medications were not restarted, and the most common medications involved were cardiovascular and CNS medications.

When choosing the dose of a medication for an older patient, the motto has always been "start low, go slow." The other half of that statement should be "but don't stop too soon." Although doses of medications used in the elderly should be held to a minimum, the "right" dose in an elderly patient is the dose that is both effective and well tolerated.[4] Initially, doses should be modified based on pharmacokinetic predictions, but actual pharmacodynamic responses to the medication should then be used to adjust the dose. When pharmacokinetic data are not available, whenever practical, doses can be initiated at one-half the usual adult dose; this can be achieved by splitting tablets or by extending the dosing interval. Some manufacturers, realizing the need for smaller doses in the elderly, have marketed smaller dosage forms or liquid formulations to facilitate dosing.

The scheduling of medications is another important factor to consider when prescribing for the older patient. Minimizing the number of doses per day is easier for the patient and can improve compliance. The use of sustained-release dosage forms or taking advantage of prolonged elimination half-lives in the elderly can decrease the number of doses per day. For example, ciprofloxacin can often be dosed once a day in elderly patients.[5] Scheduling is also important as to the time of day. Medications that can cause drowsiness should be dosed at bedtime.

Economics

At the time of this writing, Medicare still does not include a prescription drug benefit, and many elderly patients do not have prescription coverage. As the cost of medication soars, elderly patients on fixed incomes may have difficulty affording their drug therapy. Prescribers need to learn the costs of medications, specifically the cost of 30 days at a geriatric dose. It is also useful to be familiar with therapeutic alternatives, and which one is most cost-effective. For example, one angiotensin-converting enzyme (ACE) inhibitor may be less expensive than another.

It is also important to be aware which medications are available generically. There are few data on the use of generic medications in the elderly and whether any significant pharmacokinetic or pharmacodynamic changes are evident. A study of generic verapamil products found that there was a significant amount of variability in the maximum serum concentration and the area under the curve in older adults.[6] A follow-up study in elderly hypertensive patients found that, despite pharmacokinetic differences, no significant clinical differences were seen when comparing a generic verapamil to the brand product.[7] It is important to consider that even though the FDA (U.S. Food and Drug Administration) may find that the generic products are bioequivalent, most of these studies are done in younger adults and therefore these products may not actually be bioequivalent in the elderly. Even if elderly subjects are included in the studies, their

data may not be separated from the rest of the study population.

A study comparing generic Warfarin and the brand Coumadin found no significant difference between the two products in respect to average international normalized ratio (INR) values.[8] The median age of the study population was 79 years (range, 42–96), so it can be inferred that there was no difference between the products in the older patients in the study, but no specific geriatric data were reported.

Patient attitudes about generic medications may influence a physician's prescribing habits. A survey was conducted to assess patient perceptions of the risk of generic medications versus brand products.[9] The more serious the condition (e.g., heart disease), the more patients perceived generics as risky compared to the brand. For less severe conditions (e.g., cough), more respondents were willing to accept generic products and perceived them to be the same as the brand product. Patient education about the safety and appropriateness of generics may help improve their acceptance.

Compliance

There is no strict definition of noncompliance, but it can be defined as a patient's intentional or unintentional deviation from the medication regimen prescribed or recommended by the health care professional. Noncompliance includes omitting doses, adding doses, taking doses at the wrong time, or incorrectly administering the medication, to name only a few noncompliant behaviors.

Studies reporting compliance rates in elderly patients have found that the adherence rate ranges from 26% to 59%.[10] In the elderly, there are numerous causes of noncompliance or barriers to good compliance with medication regimens. Changes in functional and cognitive status are some of the key causes, and creative solutions are sometimes needed to overcome these barriers (Table 8.1).

Specific dosage forms may be particularly difficult for the older patient to manage. For example, in a study by Brown et al., 70% of patients could not adequately instill an ophthalmic preparation into their eyes.[11] In another study on eye medications, 21% of patients reported difficulty administering the medication due to the force

TABLE 8.1. Changes in functional status affecting compliance.

Decreased vision
Decreased hearing
Decreased manual dexterity
Dysphagia
Impaired mobility

required to squeeze the bottle, unsteadiness of their hand, difficulty raising their arm, difficulty tilting their head, or difficulty opening the tamper-proof seal on the new bottle.[12] Eyedrop guides, which fit onto the eyedrop bottle, can help steady the hand and direct the drop into the eye. When using the guide, the percent of people who could instill a drop on the first try increased from 20% to 87%.[12]

In all patients, difficulties in properly using a metered-dose inhaler (MDI) can impair the effectiveness of the medication.[13,14] Assessment of technique and education are essential for compliance and efficacy. Newer versions of MDIs are breath activated, making it easier for the older patient who may not be able to coordinate their breathing with pressing down on the canister. Additionally, there are a variety of devices that can adapt MDIs for patients with arthritis, making it easier to press down on the canister. There are various inhalation aids and spacer devices, such as the InspirEase and Aerochamber, which can improve the delivery of the medication to the airways.

Even child-resistant caps, which have been required on prescription medications in the United States since 1970, can be barriers to compliance in the older patient. In one study, one-third of patients over 60 years of age could not remove tablets from a vial with a child-resistant cap.[15] Of these patients, 91% either left the cap off the vial, changed containers, or did something else to be able to get to their medications; 9% of the patients simply discontinued the medication. Obviously, none of these options is optimal. It is the responsibility of the prescriber and the pharmacist to ask the elderly patient if they need a non–child-resistant cap. The prescriber can note it on the prescription or the patient can tell the pharmacist directly. The pharmacist should document this information on the individual's patient profile for further prescriptions.

Visual problems can affect the patient's ability to read the medication label or patient education material and may even impair their ability to discriminate between colors of tablets. Decreased hearing can make patient counseling challenging for the health professional. When interacting with sensory-impaired patients, it is important to ensure that they are accurately receiving the information.

Besides alterations in functional status, there are other reasons for noncompliance in the elderly patient. Economic issues, as mentioned earlier, can force a patient to compromise their compliance. Attitudes about illness, aging, and even the medications themselves can impair compliance. Medications may be a reminder of illness and growing older, and the patient may resist or ignore the medications. Living alone, with no support system to remind them to take their medication, may also lead to noncompliance.

Cognitive status can also be an impediment to compliance. Simply remembering to take the medication can be difficult for the cognitively impaired patient. Actions requiring judgment, such as recognizing adverse events or self-monitoring their therapy, may be impossible. Simplifying the regimen, reminder aids, and family or caregiver involvement are the best methods to improve compliance in these patients.

It would seem logical that the most significant risk factors for noncompliance are simply the number of medications and the number or severity of illnesses. However, a review of compliance studies found conflicting results.[10] Noncompliance and its reasons are still not well understood. Studies have also examined the relationship between knowledge about the medications or illnesses and compliance.[16] Unfortunately, they do not always correlate, in that educating the patient does not always result in good compliance.

Methods to Improve Compliance

The first step to improve compliance should be to simplify the regimen. The minimum number of medications and doses per day should be the goal. It is advisable to avoid medications that must be given more than twice a day.

Patient Education

Even though knowledge does not always equal compliance, patient education is still important. The National Council on Patient Information and Education (NCPIE) recommends that patients know, at a minimum, the following information about their medications:

1. Name of the medication and its indication
2. Dose and schedule of the medication and how long to take it
3. What to avoid while on the medication
4. Major adverse effects and what to do if they occur
5. Any written information about the medication

With elderly patients, it is advisable to include a family member or caregiver in the education process. Supplementing verbal information with written information is also important. When developing patient education materials, it is important to utilize a large font size and aim for a reading level not greater than sixth grade. Black print on nonglare white or yellow paper can ease the readability.

The effect of an education program on compliance and control of illness was assessed in an elderly population with osteoarthritis.[17] Patients in the intervention group were educated about their disease and their medications via a computer program. The control group was only exposed to information about osteoarthritis. The intervention group had a significantly higher rate of appropriate use of medication. However, the only difference seen between the groups in regard to the severity of illness measures was in the extent of stiffness. The intervention group also had a greater sense of confidence in their ability to be compliant with the drug regimen.

Another difficulty with compliance lies in the ability of the patient to read and understand the label. Directions should be simple and easy to understand. Ideally the prescription directions for all patients should state exactly how, when, and why to take the medication, for example: "Take one tablet every morning for high blood pressure." Large type should be used when possible, or the patient should be encouraged to use a magnifier.

Medication Administration Skills

One of the simplest ways to assess compliance is to watch the patient take the medication. The patient should be able to open the vial, count out the correct number of tablets or capsules, and swallow them. Assessment of the elderly patient's functional ability to take medication has been reported in several studies.[18–21] It is important to check their technique for using inhalers, instilling ophthalmic preparations, injecting insulin, and even applying a transdermal patch or creams and ointments. Before prescribing a liquid form of a medication, it should be ensured that the patient can accurately measure liquids. Patients with difficulties with these special dosage forms should be referred to their pharmacist, who can recommend compliance aids. For example, for diabetics, there are magnifiers that fit onto the insulin syringes. For liquid medications, there are a variety of dosing spoons, cups, and oral syringes. Even transdermal patches can present a problem, as an elderly patient with visual problems or arthritis may have difficulty peeling off the protective backing on the patch. For vials, easy-to-open caps are available. It is also important to check the size of the vial. A very small vial may be difficult to manage for a patient with severely arthritic hands or who has hemiplegia. In these cases, a larger vial may be easier to grasp.

Tablet splitters and crushers can be used for those patients who have difficulty swallowing tablets. Before splitting or crushing a tablet, the patient or prescriber should check with the pharmacist or the manufacturer's information to make sure that the medication will not be affected by breaking the tablet. Sustained-release formulations and enteric-coated medications should not be split or crushed.

If despite compliance aids the patient is still having difficulty administering the medication, alternative dosage forms may be necessary. For example, a patient having difficulty with a transdermal nitroglycerin patch may be better managed on isosorbide mononitrate once a day. In other cases, a family member or caregiver may need to be trained to help with the medications.

One of the medication compliance problems that is often overlooked is the problem of the family caregiver and medication administration difficulties. Travis et al. assessed the difficulties that family caregivers had when giving medications.[22] The difficulties were described as scheduling logistics (29.5%), administration procedures (32%), and safety issues (38.5%). The three most common difficulties were (1) giving medications to a confused or uncooperative person; (2) working the medication schedule into the care routines; and (3) recognizing adverse or toxic effects. This study demonstrates that family caregivers must be given proper instructions on how to administer medications and be educated about the medications themselves.

Reminder Aids

A variety of reminder aids can be used to help patients remember to take their medications. The simplest method is to design a calendar that lists the medications and the time of day to take them. The calendar can be posted on the refrigerator or other prominent place in the home. Weekly or monthly calendar cards with boxes to check off each dose can be used and correlated with tablet counts to assess level of compliance.

Commercially available medication boxes can aid in compliance. These boxes hold 1 day or 1 week or medication, and some have compartments for up to four dosing times per day. Electronic aids also have been developed. These devices can be set to beep at the correct times, and some even provide a warning if a dose has been missed. Some systems are locked and tamperproof and actually dispense the medication only at the correct time.

Studies on compliance measures have shown that no one intervention is universally better than another.[16] Rather, a compliance plan should be individualized to the needs of the patient and should include a combination of interventions focusing on behavioral as well as educational interventions.

Utilizing the Pharmacist

Assessing and improving compliance requires a multidisciplinary effort. Prescribers should utilize the patient's pharmacist and keep the lines of communication open. The pharmacist can provide advice on compliance and reminder aids and also can suggest alternative dosage forms, such as sustained-release formulations or smaller tablet sizes. The pharmacist can also track compliance via refill records and note what OTC products the patient is using. The pharmacist is a ready source of drug information for both the patient and the prescriber. By federal law, the pharmacist must offer to counsel all Medicaid patients on prescription medications.[23] Many states have expanded this regulation to include all patients. All patients, particularly the elderly, should be encouraged to consult their pharmacist when purchasing OTC medications and other health-related products. Most important, it should be stressed to the patient that it is safer to use only one pharmacy so that all their prescription and OTC medications are entered into one computer profile. This method allows the pharmacist to monitor for drug interactions, duplications, and potential adverse effects.

For the prescriber, the pharmacist can provide information about the availability of new medications, dosage forms, or newly approved indications, as well as drug interactions, adverse effects, and special concerns in the elderly. Since 1997, pharmacists who specialize in geriatrics have had the opportunity to become certified in the area of geriatric pharmacy. The Commission for Certification in Geriatric Pharmacy offers an examination covering various areas of geriatric pharmacy practice. These pharmacists carry the title of Certified Geriatric Pharmacist (CGP), demonstrating their expertise in the area.

Nursing Home Issues

Residents of nursing homes are generally among the frailest of the elderly and are often on many chronic medications. The decision to institute a new medication may be the result of the input of a variety of disciplines. Because the physician may only be making monthly visits to the facility, the nursing staff is the "front line." The nurses or nursing aides often are the ones to suggest that an intervention is necessary. The consultant pharmacist is another active voice in the drug use process. Since 1974, the Federal government has required that a pharmacist review the drug regimen of all residents in long-term care facilities (LTCF) on a monthly basis.[24] This drug regimen review is based on a set of guidelines or "indicators" that are used by the state surveyors when they review medication use in a facility.[25] The pharmacist must provide comments about the drug regimen to the physician of record, who must respond to these comments. A recent study assessing the impact of drug regimen review in nursing homes estimated that the pharmacists' reviews saved $3.6 billion annually in drug-related costs.[26] Despite these savings, it is estimated that for every dollar spent on medications in LTCFs, $1.33 is spent on drug-related problems.[26]

Since the implementation of drug regimen review, the nursing home regulations affecting medications have been modified several times. One of the most significant changes was in 1987 with the passage of the Nursing Home Reform Amendments of the Omnibus Budget

TABLE 8.2. Definition of "unnecessary drugs" according to OBRA 1987 guidelines.

An unnecessary drug is any drug when used:

1. In excessive dose (including duplicate drug therapy); or
2. For excessive duration; or
3. Without adequate monitoring; or
4. Without adequate indications for its use; or
5. In the presence of adverse consequences that indicate the dose should be reduced or discontinued; or
6. Any combination of the reasons above.

Source: Omnibus Budget Reconciliation Act of 1987.[27]

Reconciliation Act (OBRA '87).[27] This regulation requires that "each resident's drug regimen must be free from unnecessary drugs"[27] (Table 8.2). The Interpretive Guidelines accompanying this regulation, which were implemented in 1990, focused on the appropriate use of psychotropic medications, most specifically antipsychotics, anxiolytics, and hypnotics.[28] OBRA '87 also states that "the resident has the right to be free from any physical restraints imposed or psychoactive drug administered for purposes of discipline or convenience and not required to treat the resident's medical symptoms."[27] The Interpretive Guidelines include a list of appropriate indications for the use of antipsychotics, anxiolytics, and hypnotics and explain under what circumstances these medications should be used. Nonpharmacologic interventions are considered first-line therapy, and medications should only be used if the interventions fail. Justification for use of psychoactive medication is based on improving or maintaining the resident's functional status. Emphasis is placed on length of therapy and maximum recommended dosages. For anxiolytics and hypnotics, the guidelines discourage the use of long-acting benzodiazepines and older agents such as meprobamate. They also discourage the use of the antihistamines, diphenhydramine and hydroxyzine, as hypnotics or anxiolytics.

Later modifications to the guidelines focused on antidepressants and their underutilization in nursing facilities. It has been shown that depression is often unrecognized and therefore left untreated in elderly nursing home residents.[29] The appropriate diagnosis and treatment of depression are stressed.

In all the psychotropic drug guidelines, the use of the lowest effective dose is emphasized. It must be noted that as new psychoactive medications are marketed, the impact of the guidelines on their use in LTCFs must be established.

Studies assessing the impact of the psychotropic guidelines on prescribing patterns in nursing homes have found significant decreases in the use of antipsychotics.[30–32] In some cases, reductions in antipsychotics resulted in adjustment in the use of other psychoactive

TABLE 8.3. Nursing facility quality indicators directly involving medications.

Prevalence of:

- Symptoms of depression without antidepressant therapy
- Residents who take nine or more different medications
- Antipsychotic use, in the absence of psychotic or related conditions
- Antianxiety/hypnotic use
- Hypnotic use more than two times in the last week

---

medications, such as an increase in the use of antidepressants.[33] Multidisciplinary and educational interventions were most effective in ensuring appropriate use of psychoactive medications.[34–36]

Additions to the Interpretive Guidelines in 1999 focused on the choice of medications for elderly nursing home residents.[37] The "Beers criteria," a set of guidelines concerning "potentially inappropriate" medications for the elderly, were incorporated into the nursing home regulations.[38] Medications with a high-severity risk were placed under the definition of "unnecessary medications," and those with a low-severity risk were placed under the drug regimen review regulations. In either case, use of these medications must be justified in the patient's chart. Department of Health surveyors will scrutinize residents on one of these "potentially inappropriate" medications to make sure that they are not suffering adverse outcomes. Also, 1999 saw the implementation of Quality Indicators for assessing the quality of care in nursing facilities; 5 of these 24 indicators specifically refer to medications (Table 8.3).

A major change in nursing homes that affected medication is the change in reimbursement for Medicare patients. The Prospective Payment System (PPS) provides a per diem rate based on level of care. The payment segment that includes medication is relatively stable across the levels of care. This plan encourages the use of the least expensive medication, which may not necessarily be the best for the elderly patient and, in the end, may not be the most cost-effective. For example, the older tricyclic antidepressants (TCAs) are less expensive than the newer selective serotonin reuptake inhibitors (SSRIs), but the TCAs have more side effects and the outcomes of these side effects may be costly. The effect of the PPS on medication usage and clinical outcomes in LTCFs remains to be seen.

Assisted Living Facilities

At the time of this writing, there are no national guidelines concerning medication use in assisted living facilities. Some states are requiring or suggesting pharmacist drug regimen reviews, and the impact of these interventions is still unknown. Depending on the level of care of the individual facility, some provide medication administration, some only supervision (reminding the resident to take the medication), and some require that the resident be able to self-medicate. Medication use in assisted living is still an uncharted area in geriatrics.

Conclusion

Appropriate drug therapy in the older patient is the result of assessing all the complexities of the geriatric patient. Factors to be considered are pharmacologic, physiologic, sociologic, practical, and, in the case of nursing homes, regulatory. Once the decision is made to prescribe a medication, the right agent and patient-specific dose must be chosen. Care then must be taken to ensure that the patient will be able to comply with the regimen. Consideration of the patient's functional and cognitive status and their living environment may influence the choice of medication. By balancing all these factors and being sensitive to the special needs of the elderly, safe and effective medication regimens can be achieved.

References

1. Walma EP, Hoes AW, van Dooren C, et al. Withdrawal of long term diuretic medication in elderly patients: a double blind randomized trial. *Br Med J.* 1997:315:464–468.
2. Gerety MB, Cornell JE, Plichta DT, et al. Adverse events related to drugs and drug withdrawal in nursing home residents. *J Am Geriatr Soc.* 1993:41:1326–1332.
3. Graves T, Hanlon JT, Schmader KE, et al. Adverse events after discontinuing medications in elderly outpatients. *Arch Intern Med.* 1997:157:2205–2210.
4. Cohen JS. Avoiding adverse reactions. Effective lower-dose drug therapies for older patients. *Geriatrics.* 2000;55(2): 54–64.
5. Semla TP, Beizer JL, Higbee MD. *Geriatric Dosage Handbook,* 5th Ed. Hudson, OH: Lexi-Comp; 2000:216–217.
6. Carter BL, Noyes MA, Demmler RW. Differences in serum concentrations of and responses to generic verapamil in the elderly. *Pharmacotherapy.* 1993:13:359–368.
7. Saseen JJ, Porter JA, Barrette DJ, et al. Postabsorption concentration peaks with brand-name and generic verapamil: a double-blind, crossover study in elderly hypertensive patients. *J Clin Pharmacol.* 1997:37:526–534.
8. Swenson CN, Fundak G. Observational cohort study of switching wafarin sodium products in a managed care organization. Am J Health Syst Pharm. 2000:57:452–455.
9. Ganther JM, Kreling DH. Consumer perceptions of risk and required cost savings for generic prescription drugs. *J Am Pharm Assoc.* 2000:40:378–383.
10. Balkrishnan R. Predictors of medication adherence in the elderly. *Clin Ther.* 1998:20:764–771.

11. Brown MM, Brown GC, Spaeth GL. Improper self-administration of ocular medication among patients with glaucoma. *Can J Ophthalmol.* 1984:19:2–5.
12. Winfield AJ, Jessiman D, Williams A, et al. A study of causes of non-compliance by patients prescribed eye-drops. *Br J Ophthalmol.* 1990:74:477–480.
13. Armitage JM, Williams SJ. Inhaler technique in the elderly. *Age Ageing.* 1988:17:275–278.
14. Daniels S, Meuleman J. Importance of assessment of metered-dose inhaler technique in the elderly. *J Am Geriatr Soc.* 1994:42:82–84.
15. McIntire MS, Angle CR, Sathees K, et al. Safety packaging: what does the public think? *Am J Public Health.* 1977: 67:169–171.
16. Roter DL, Hall JA, Merissa R, et al. Effectiveness of interventions to improve patient compliance: a meta-analysis. *Med Care.* 1998:36:1138–1161.
17. Edworthy SM, Devins GM. Improving medication adherence through patient education distinguishing between appropriate and inappropriate utilization. *J Rheumatol.* 1999:26:1793–1801.
18. Hurd PD, Butkovich SL. Compliance problems and the older patient: assessing functional limitations. *Drug Intell Clin Pharm.* 1986:20:228–231.
19. Meyer ME, Schuna AA. Assessment of geriatric patients' functional ability to take medication. *Drug Intell Clin Pharm.* 1989:23:171–174.
20. Atkin PA, Finnegan TP, Ogle SJ, et al. Functional ability of patients to manage medication packaging: a survey of geriatric inpatients. *Age Ageing.* 1994:23:113–116.
21. Fitten LJ, Coleman L, Siembeda DW, et al. Assessment of capacity to comply with medication regimens in older patients. *J Am Geriatr Soc.* 1995:43:361–367.
22. Travis SS, Bethea LS, Winn P. Medication administration hassles reported by family caregivers of dependent elderly persons. *J Gerontol Med Sci.* 2000:55A:M412–M417.
23. Anonymous. Omnibus Budget Reconciliation Act of 1990. (PL101-508) 01, *Health Care Financing Review.* 1991; 13(2):115–134.
24. Anonymous. Conditions of participation—pharmaceutical services. *Fed Reg.* 1974:39:12–17.
25. State Operations Manual Provider Certification. Transmittal 174. Washington, DC: Health Care Financing Administration, Department of Health and Human Services; 1985.
26. Bootman JL, Harrison DL, Cox E. The health care cost of drug-related morbidity and mortality in nursing facilities. *Arch Intern Med.* 1997:157:2089–2096.
27. Omnibus Budget Reconciliation Act of 1987. (PL100-203). See Anonymous. Quarterly listing of program issuances–HCFA. General notice. *Fed Reg.* 1988, June 9; 53(111): 21730–21737.
28. State Operations Manual: Provider Certification. Transmittal 232. Washington, DC: Health Care Financing Administration, Department of Health and Human Services; 1989.
29. Rovner BW, German PS, Brant LJ, et al. Depression and mortality in nursing homes. *JAMA.* 1991:265:993–996.
30. Rovner BW, Edelman BA, Cox MP, et al. The impact of antipsychotic drug regulations on psychotropic prescribing practices in nursing homes. *Am J Psychiatry.* 1992:149: 1390–1392.
31. Neel AB, Pittman JC, Marasco RA, et al. Psychoactive drug use in Georgia nursing homes: effects of aggressive intervention. *Consult Pharm.* 1993:8:245–248.
32. Semla TS, Palla K, Poddig B, et al. Effect of the Omnibus Reconciliation Act 1987 on antipsychotic prescribing in nursing home residents. *J Am Geriatr Soc.* 1994:42:648–652.
33. Somani SK, Cooper SL. Outcomes of antipsychotic drug withdrawal in elderly nursing home residents. *Consult Pharm.* 1994:9:789–802.
34. Avorn J, Soumerai SB, Everitt DE, et al. A randomized trial of a program to reduce the use of psychoactive drugs in nursing homes. *N Engl J Med.* 1992:327:168–173.
35. Hirshfield JS. Positive patient outcomes from interdisciplinary assessments of psychoactive drug use. *Consult Pharm.* 1993:8:532–534.
36. Lattari LP, Chesley LD. Reducing use of psychoactive medications through quality assurance. *Consult Pharm.* 1993:8:523–526.
37. State Operations Manual Provider Certification. Washington, DC: Department of Health and Human Services, Health Care Financing Administration; 1999.
38. Beers MH. Explicit criteria for determining potentially inappropriate medication use by the elderly: an update. *Arch Intern Med.* 1997:157:1531–1536.

Part II
Changing Contexts of Care in Geriatric Medicine

9
Contexts of Care

Laurence Z. Rubenstein

Geriatric medicine is characterized by multiple levels or contexts of care. The geriatrician and their team typically care for elderly patients along a continuum of these contexts, stretching from hospitalization for an acute problem, such as a stroke, to rehabilitation on a subacute ward, to convalescence in a nursing home, to continued care at home via a home care program, and finally to a return to primary care in the office. (Conversely, one can view this continuum from the opposite direction, beginning in primary and preventive care and spanning to institutional care.) Each of these contexts of care has its own scope of purpose, its own rationale, its own teams of care professionals, and its own financial considerations and incentives, all of which are actively evolving along with changes in the overall health care system and larger society. Proper geriatric care requires familiarity with all these contexts and an understanding of how best to manage patients within them.

In several countries with well-organized health care systems (e.g., Great Britain), the geriatrician serves as the manager/gatekeeper of a variety of geriatric care services, such as hospital geriatric assessment and management units, rehabilitation wards, day hospitals, nursing homes, and home care service. In all these contexts, the geriatrician can function as the primary care provider or as a consultant physician. In other countries with less-developed geriatric care systems, these services, when available, tend to be autonomous, and geriatricians play more consultative roles.

Some common threads shared by most of these programs include their focus on functionally impaired elderly persons, their focus on optimizing functional status and quality of life, and their employment of interdisciplinary teams, comprehensive geriatric assessment techniques, and principles of case management. This chapter provides an overview of these contexts of geriatric care and how they can and should be coordinated, serving as an introduction to the more detailed program-specific chapters that follow.

Use of Services by Older Persons

The population aged 65 and older uses a greatly disproportionate amount of most health services. In developed countries, older persons typically use most services at a rate three to four times higher than their proportion in the general population, which primarily reflects the increased prevalence of most diseases and physical disabilities among older persons.[1] This trend, together with the continual expansion of the older population segment worldwide, has been one of the major factors leading to dramatic cost inflation of health services globally. With medical care responsible for 8% to 14% of the gross national product in most developed countries, public resources have increasing difficulty sustaining these services. Health care cost containment is now an international watchword. The difficulty in attaining this objective without sacrificing the older person's need for adequate care has become a universal and growing challenge. Understanding health services utilization, its determinates, and ways to effectively manage it are major priorities for health services research and policy analysis worldwide.

In 1998, 13.5% of the United States gross domestic product was spent on health care, or $3632 per capita.[2] Of this, 33.3% went for hospital services 20.0% for physician services, 10.6% for drugs and other medical nondurales, 7.6% for nursing home care, 4.7% for dental services, 5.8% for other professional services, 3.2% for government public health activities, 1.3% for vision products, 2.5% for home health care, 5.0% for insurance administrative expenses, 3.1% for research and construction, and 2.8% for miscellaneous services. Figure 9.1 shows health care expenditures by older persons in the United States for major service categories by age subgroup and highlights the progressive increase and changing patterns after age 65.[3]

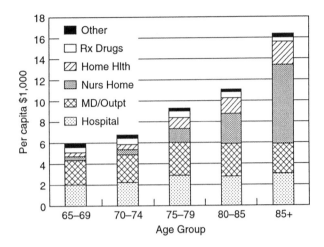

FIGURE 9.1. United States per capita health care expenditures by older persons, by service type and age group. (Data from 1996 Medicare Current Beneficiary Survey, Older American 2000.)

Hospital Use

Hospital use is by far the largest single health expense category, and it dramatically increases with age, as indicated clearly in Figure 9.2, which shows data on annual per capita hospital discharges in the United States by age group. This age trend is true whether considering discharges, total hospital days per year, or per capita expenditures. Persons age 75 years and over use five times as many annual per capita hospital days as persons 45 to 64 years of age (30.3 versus 6.0 day per year, in 1998 in the United States).[2]

A number of studies have identified predictors of hospital use that largely explain this disproportionately heavy use of hospital services by older persons. In one study, the most important predictors were hospital use in the previous year, poor perceived health status, more than six physician visits in the past year, and lack of an

informal caregiver.[4] In a more detailed study using the behavioral model, which subdivided potential predictors of hospital use into the three traditional categories of predisposing, enabling, and need characteristics, significant predictors of hospital use included lower functional status, poorer perceived health, lack of social supports, and health concerns.[5] In all studies, age has been one of the major predictors of hospitalization.

The most common diagnoses responsible for hospitalization among older persons in the United States in 1996 were, in decreasing order, heart disease, cancer, cerebrovascular disease, injuries, pneumonia, and eye diseases.[2] Hospitalization rates for all these disorders continue to increase with increasing age, except for neoplastic disease, which tends to decline after age 75. Mean hospital length of stay in 1998 for persons age 65 and older was 6.2 days, down from 10.7 days in 1980. Among the most common diagnoses, mean hospital length of stay was longest for hip fractures (8.2 days), followed by pneumonia (7.1 days), heart disease (5.6 days), and cerebrovascular disease (5.4 days). Over the past two decades, diagnosis-specific length of stay has been dramatically falling, largely in response to economic incentives from the payors. For example, length of stay for hip fracture patients over age 74 has declined from 19.2 days in 1985 to 8.2 days in 1998, and for cerebrovascular disease from 10.0 days to 5.4 days. This shortening of length of stay has been the major factor behind the declining proportion of the health care dollar spent on hospital care—from 42% in 1980 to 33% in 1998—and has been a major factor in the slowing of health care inflation.

A number of studies have looked at factors predictive of hospital outcomes. In an article that reviewed 15 studies, the most commonly found predictors of adverse hospital outcomes (i.e., mortality, nursing home placement, or long length of stay) were advancing age (9 of 11 studies), impaired functional status (8 of 11), impaired

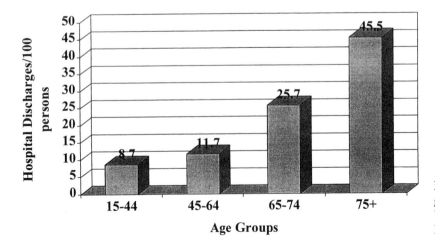

FIGURE 9.2. U.S. hospital discharges by age group, per 100 persons/year. (Data from 1996 U.S. National Hospital Discharge Survey, Health United States 2000.)

FIGURE 9.3. U.S. hospital discharge locations for older adults (1987 data, vs DHHS, 1993).

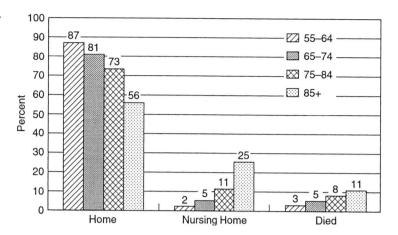

mental function (7 of 11), and problematic living location (6 of 11).[6] In a more recent study that was able to include illness severity in the model, severity was an important predictor of adverse outcome, along with impaired functional status.[7] Figure 9.3 shows the changing patterns of hospital discharge location after age 65, indicating the progressive increase in mortality and nursing home placement and decreasing likelihood of returning home.

Nursing Home Use

Although nursing homes account for only 7.6% of all health care expenditures for the entire U.S. population, the older population expends more than 20% of its health care dollar on nursing home care, and this proportion approaches 46% for the population age 85 and over (see Fig. 9.1).[2] Between 1974 and 1997, the U.S. nursing home population grew by more than 52%. Currently, about 4.3% of persons age 65 and over reside in nursing homes; however, more than 22% of women age 85 and over live in nursing homes. As discussed in Chapter 11, the nursing home clientele is highly diverse. This diversity presents itself in several areas, including the degree of physical or mental impairment, the type of care required, and the duration of stay. The important distinction has been made between short stayers (less than 6 months) and long stayers (more than 6 months). Short stayers include patients needing rehabilitation or convalescent care after an acute illness and who are expected to go back home, as well as patients who are terminally ill from endstage cancer or dementia and who are expected to die in the nursing home. Long stayers include three large subgroups: those with cognitive impairment; those with physical impairment (largely musculoskeletal, neurologic, cardiac, or pulmonary disease); and those with both cognitive and physical impairments. The proportion of short stayers has increased in the past two decades in response to fiscal pressures to shorten hospital length of stay.

Several studies have examined predictors of nursing home use. The most common factors that correlate with use include age, diagnostic condition, living alone, functional impairment, being unmarried, white race, weak social support, poverty, hospital admission, bed disability, female sex, and use of an ambulation aid.[8] Most studies have found that women have a much higher probability of nursing home use. For instance, the lifetime probability of nursing home use in the United States is about 45% for women versus 28% for men.[9] This gender gap can be partially explained by the greater longevity of women with decreased likelihood of spousal support, their higher prevalence of disabilities, their lower functional status score, and their lower incomes. It has been argued that when the effects of such variables are controlled for, older women may actually have a lower risk of nursing home use than men. Be that as it may, the current prototype of the nursing home dweller is still that of an older woman with multiple pathologies, taking several medications, most likely widowed and incontinent.

Use of Physician Services

A physician contact can take place in the office setting or clinic, in the hospital, in the nursing home, in the patient's home, or by telephone. In 1996, the U.S. population age 65 and over had a mean of 11.7 physician contacts per year[2]; this included 10.2 annual contacts for persons age 65 to 74 years and 13.7 contacts for persons age 75 years and over. Of these contacts, about 49% took place in the office, 10% in the hospital, 19% in the home or nursing home, 9% on the phone, and 12% in other places such as clinics. Factors shown to correlate with physician utilization include perceived health status, having an active health problem, having a functional impairment, and having a regular primary care physician.[10]

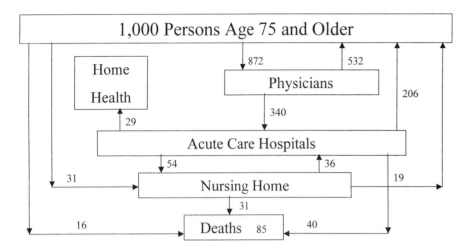

FIGURE 9.4. Movement of the elderly population through the U.S. health care system (US DHHS, 1993).

Use of Community Health Care Services

This category covers auxiliary and support health services and is usually subdivided into the two subcategories of home care services (which include visiting nurses, hot meals, home health aides, or other special care delivered at home) and ambulatory care services (which include rehabilitation, counseling, and speech therapy). Also sometimes considered are services offered by community centers, such as day hospitals and senior citizen centers. Utilization of these services has been traditionally low. In the 1980 National Health Interview Survey, only 4% of respondents had reported using any of these services. However, in more recent years, use of these services has grown faster than for any other type of service. The proportion of the health care dollar paying for home care alone has increased from 0.5% to 3.0% between 1975 and 1997.[2]

The most important predictor of community services use is a recent discharge from an acute hospital.[11,12] Age is also a major predictor, largely related to increased needs.[13] Although community care services are often advocated as "alternatives" to more costly institutional services, most studies have been unable to show a substantial substitution effect. Many people will use community services when offered, as add-ons to their current care rather than as substitutes for more intensive levels of care. In fact, several studies suggest that use of community services may actually lead to increased use of other health care services, albeit often appropriately so. Thus, issues of unproven cost-effectiveness have often been cited as reasons why community care services are not more widely available. However, efforts to contain costs are often influential and may be more important than true effectiveness in determining availability of some of these services.

Interrelationships of Service Use

Utilization of each service in the health care system is inexorably linked to that of other services. These linkages are difficult to analyze because of the complexity of the relationships as well as the lack of accurate information. In a 1991 study of the U.S. Agency for Health Policy Research, Denson attempted to construct a diagrammatic movement pathway for the U.S. population through the health care system,[14] which is shown in simplified fashion in Figure 9.4. One can see that, in a given year, about 87% of the U.S. population age 75 and over will see a physician, 34% will be hospitalized, 8.5% will enter a nursing home, 2.9% will receive home health care, and 8.5% will die. Also shown is the complexity of movement between many of the services. This pattern of movement with its specific rates should be viewed as a snapshot in time because changes in availability in certain types of services and changes in reimbursement systems have dramatic effects on service utilization and on the rates of transition. For example, the prospective payment system of hospital care introduced by Medicare in 1984 led to dramatically shortened hospital lengths of stay and increasing proportions of hospital patients discharged to nursing homes and using home health service.

References

1. Ebrahim S, Kalache A, eds. *Epidemiology of Old Age.* London: British Medical Journal Publications; 1995.
2. *Health United States, 2000.* Hyattsville, MD: National Center for Health Statistics; 2000.
3. *Key Indicators of Well-Being.* Hyattsville, MD: Federal Interagency Forum on Aging-Related Statistics Older Americans 2000; 2000.

4. Boult C, Dowd B, McCaffrey D, et al. Screening elders for risk of hospital admission. *J Am Geriat Soc.* 1993;41:811–817.

5. Wolinsky FD, Johnson RJ. The use of health services by older adults. *J Gerontol Soc Sci.* 1991;46(6):S345–S357.

6. Narain P, Rubenstein LZ, Wieland D, et al. Predictors of immediate and 6-month outcomes in hospitalized elderly patients: the importance of functional status. *J Am Geriatr Soc.* 1988;36:775–783.

7. Pompei P, Charlson ME, Ales K, et al. Relating patient characteristics at the time of admission to outcomes of hospitalization. *J Clin Epidemiol.* 1991;44:1063–1069.

8. Kane RL. The risk of placement in a nursing home after acute hospitalization. *Med Care.* 1983;21:1055–1061.

9. Kemper P, Murtaugh CM. Lifetime use of nursing home care. *N Engl J Med.* 1991;324:595–600.

10. Branch L, Jette A, Polansky M, et al. Toward understanding elders' health services utilization. *J Community Health.* 1981;7(2):80–92.

11. Evashwick C, Rowe G, Diehr P, et al. Factors explaining use of health care services by the elderly. *Health Serv Res.* 1984;19(3):357–382.

12. Hawe P, Gebski V, Andrews G. Elderly patients after they leave hospital. *Med J Aust.* 1986;145(6):251–254.

13. Daatland SO. Use of public services for the aged and role of the family. *Gerontologist.* 1983;23:650–656.

14. Denson PM. *Tracing the Elderly Through the Health Care System.* AHCPR-91-11. Washington, DC: Agency for Health Research and Quality; 1991.

10
The Long and the Short of Long-Term Care

Robert L. Kane

Long-term care (LTC) is an amorphous concept. It is more readily defined by what it is not than by what it is. Clinicians tend to view it as what is left over after acute care has been addressed, but in an era of chronic disease, even the concept of acute care is blurred. For many, LTC is synonymous with nonmedical care; but in fact most LTC recipients need active medical care, and close coordination of both types of care is important to obtaining maximum benefit.

It may come as no surprise then that there is no common definition of LTC. One that seems to serve well is the following: Long-term care is assistance given over a sustained period of time to people who are experiencing long-term disabilities of difficulties in functioning because of a disability.

Several implications flow from this definition.

1. Functioning is a central theme of LTC. It serves as the lingua franca (common tongue) that facilitates communication among those involved in planning and delivering care. It is an important basis for assessing the outcomes of such care. For reasons that are not altogether clear, the age-specific prevalence of disability has actually been decreasing slightly.[1] However, the growth in the aging population will far outweigh this modest decrease.

2. LTC is not limited to one age group. Although our attention here is directed at LTC for older persons, people of all ages may need such care. Indeed, especially if one includes chronic mental illness as a cause, those under age 65 far outnumber those above it. Each age group has a different set of goals for the care they receive. Younger persons are more interested in living a normal life, or mainstreaming. For them, the best care is that which supports them in performing their age-appropriate social roles, be it education, employment, or social activities. Many older persons have more modest goals. They seek assistance to help them cope with the disabilities they face. They accept the idea of restricted social roles.

Not surprisingly, leaders of the young disabled movement suggest that older persons are settling too cheap and need to be reeducated to seek more.

3. Even within older clientele, the goals for LTC may vary widely. Some seek active rehabilitation with the expectation of substantial functional improvement. Others seek assistance in coping with their functional deficits, relying on human or mechanical assistance to compensate for losses they have sustained. Still others share the desire of their younger colleagues to maintain an active participation in social affairs.

4. These different goals for LTC can be linked to two fundamentally different conceptual models of this care. One approach can be thought of as "compensatory." Under this model, activity is focused on assessing functional dependencies and prescribing services to compensate for these deficiencies. Good care is defined as that which matches the needs with appropriate services without creating untoward effects. This approach is often associated with the term social model. The other approach can be thought of as "therapeutic." Under this model, care should be expected to make a difference. Because the natural clinical trajectory of many people needing LTC is decline, good care may yield simply a slowing of that path. Unfortunately, it may be difficult to detect a positive effect in the absence of good data as to what would have occurred without such care. The ultimate comparison will be actual versus expected course. The therapeutic model is often referred to as the medical model. These two approaches are frequently presented as being in opposition, but it is possible to find common ground by viewing each as necessary but not sufficient. Good care should respond to assessed needs, but it should also make a positive difference. This difference need not be restricted to medically germane concepts; it can include quality of life issues as well.

5. LTC is often linked closely to chronic disease. Much of the disability that underlies it is a result of such disease, often more than one acting simultaneously. Hence,

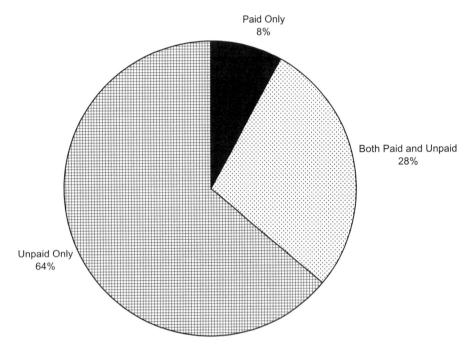

Paid Only
8%

Both Paid and Unpaid
28%

Unpaid Only
64%

FIGURE 10.1. Sources of long-term care. Most long-term care is provided by informal caregivers, either alone or in combination with formal care. (From Georgetown University Institute for Health Care Research and Policy. Based on Liu K, Manton K, Aragon C. Changes in home care use by disabled elderly persons: 1982–1994. Washington, DC: The Urban Institute, September 1998, with permission.)

persons needing LTC are also very likely to need aggressive primary care to manage their chronic disease. Attitudes that attempt to categorize people as needing either medical or social care are thus dysfunctional.

6. Nothing about the definition of LTC implies care given at a particular site. Practice has historically confused the site of care with the nature of the services rendered. That artifact has hindered developing more creative and efficient approaches to such care. Indeed, if one looks back on what has happened in delivering acute medical care, there has been a dramatic revolution in how such care is provided. Care that used to be considered as needing a hospital is now provided in an ambulatory setting or even at home. Likewise, LTC can likely be offered in a wider variety of settings than is currently the case.

7. The backbone of LTC is informal care provided by family (and to a lesser extent by others). As shown in Figure 10.1, only about 8% of care provided to persons living in the community comes exclusively from formal (i.e., paid) sources; another 28% is provided by a combination of formal and informal care, and almost two-thirds comes solely from informal sources. This pattern appears to be amazingly stable. It is encountered in countries that have gone through the demographic revolution, including places where universal paid LTC is available. This stability is especially comforting in the face of predictions about the death of the American family. Because informal care has traditionally been a euphemism for care provided by women, the observation that larger numbers of women are entering the labor market, combined with

high divorce rates and smaller family sizes, raises serious concerns about whether this cadre of informal care providers will be available in the years to come. Losing this informal care would place enormous strains on the formal care system. It is, therefore, not surprising to find many policy analysts urging ways to support the informal care system.

Figure 10.2 shows the extent of informal care services provided to frail older people. The proportion of persons receiving assistance increases with their age. Women receive more help than men. The more care given, the more caregivers are involved.

Even with the substantial amount of informal care being provided, many older people still do not receive needed help. Figure 10.3 shows the proportion of persons aged 70 and older who have unmet needs with regard to activities of daily living (ADL) and instrumental ADL (IADL) dependencies. The rates of unmet IADL needs decrease with age among women, while the rates for unmet ADL assistance remain constant.

Figure 10.4 describes the sources of payment for long-term care in general and nursing homes in particular, which are presented together to highlight the differences in funding patterns. Medicare and Medicaid together account for about 60% of LTC expenditures and about the same proportion of nursing home expenditures. However, Medicaid plays a much larger role in the latter, whereas Medicare is major funder of home care (and hence LTC in general). Because a substantial portion of LTC comes from public funds, there is inevitably some

FIGURE 10.2. Proportion of persons 70 years and older with one or more ADL or IADL dependencies receiving informal assistance. The rate of receiving assistance increases with age. The rates for women are consistently higher than those for men. Many older people receive care from more than one person. (From Centers for Disease Control and Prevention, National Center for Health Statistics. 1994 National Health Interview Survey. Second Supplement on Aging.)

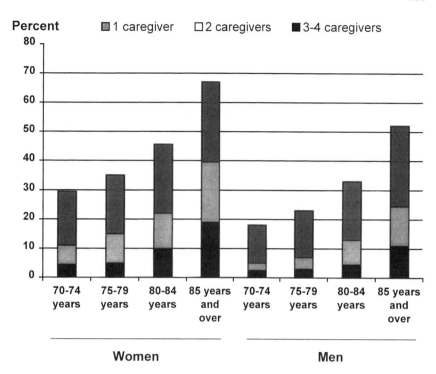

degree of age competition, especially with regard to Medicaid. This welfare-based program was designed to provide medical insurance for poor persons, especially mothers and children. An unanticipatedly large proportion of Medicaid funds, however, went to cover the costs of older persons who were in nursing homes. Indeed, a disproportionately large share of Medicaid payments go to older persons. Although the amount spent per recipient is much greater for developmentally disabled children, there are far fewer of them.

Medicare, which is basically a universal health insurance program for persons age 65 and older, was not intended to cover LTC, but it has been used for this purpose by means of two developments. The first was the imposition of prospective payment for hospitals, whereby they were paid a fixed amount based on each Medicare patient's Diagnosis-Related Group. When hospitals were paid for all their costs, there was no incentive to make care more efficient. The Medicare provisions that allowed payment for posthospital care at home or in a nursing

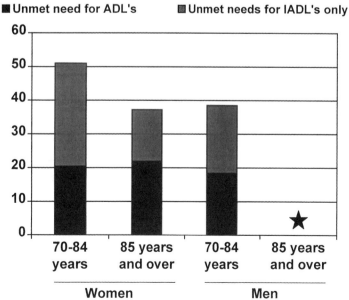

FIGURE 10.3. Percent of persons 70 years of age and over who need help with one or more activities of daily living or instrumental activities of daily living by age and sex, 1995. The overall rate of disability among older women is higher for those 70–84 than for those 85+, but the proportion of those with ADL dependencies increases. Older women are more disabled than older men. (From Health, United States, 1999.)

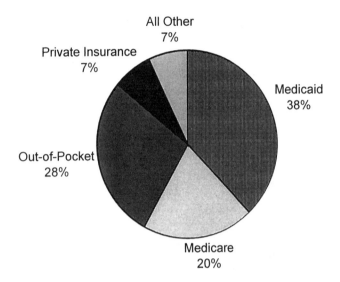

Long-Tem Care Expenditures: $115 Billion

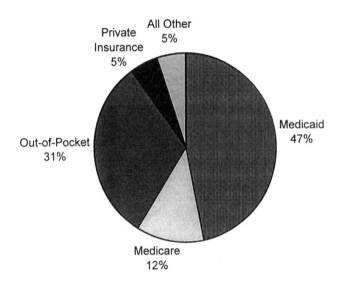

Nursing Home Expenditures: $83 Billion

FIGURE 10.4. Sources of long-term care expenditures, 1997. Payments for LTC in general come more equally from Medicare and Medicaid, whereas those nursing homes come more heavily from Medicaid. (From Georgetown University Institute for Health Care Research and Policy, with permission.)

home lay dormant. However, once hospitals were paid a fixed amount, the incentives changed drastically. Patients were discharged "quicker and sicker," creating a new demand for what came to be called postacute care (PAC).

As the use of Medicare to pay for nursing homes increased, Congress applied prospective payment to them as well. The system used differs from that used in hospitals. Instead of calculating the expected costs of an episode of care, Medicare payments to nursing homes are based on the costs of each day of care. These costs are calculated by estimating the personnel needed to provide various levels of care, called Resource Utilization Groups (RUGs). Linking greater disability to higher RUG payments inadvertently created an incentive to preserve disability.

This care-mix approach is mandated only for Medicare payments to nursing homes. Medicaid payment approaches are left at the discretion of the states. Of the fewer than half the states that use some variant of case-mix-based payments, most have opted to make these payments compatible with the RUGs approach for the sake of simplicity.

The enthusiasm for prospective payment has extended to all forms of PAC. However, each modality is paid separately. Whereas nursing homes are paid on a daily basis, home health care is paid for a 60-day episode and rehabilitation for 30-day episode.

As shown in Table 10.1, 38% of all Medicare-covered hospital discharges in 1995 received one or more forms of PAC. The dominant model was home health care, accounting for more than half of all PAC usage. About 20% of those using PAC used more than one type of service.[2] The use of PAC, like many other forms of care, varies considerably from one part of the country to another. Table 10.2 shows the extent of the variation across the major census regions for each of four diagnoses associated with substantial PAC use. Several lessons emerge. The likelihood of using PAC varies with both diagnosis and location. Hip fracture patients are more likely to get some type of PAC than are stroke patients, and both use PAC more than congestive heart failure patients. Within a given diagnosis, for example, stroke, the likelihood of getting some PAC varies from

TABLE 10.1. Proportion of hospital discharges using postacute care (PAC), 1995.

Type of PAC service	Use of PAC (%)
None	62.0
Rehabilitation	0.9
Skilled nursing facility	9.3
Home health	19.5
2+ PAC services	8.3

Source: Gage. Health Care Financing Review, 1999.

TABLE 10.2. Percent of Medicare recipients discharged from hospital using no postacute care, 1998.

Census Region	Stroke		Hip fracture		Hip Procedure		Congestive heart failure	
	Rank	%	Rank	%	Rank	%	Rank	%
East North Central	6	30.4	4	12.5	4	19.5	3	55.1
East South Central	1.5	37.4	7	10.3	1	21.9	2	56.9
Mid-Atlantic	7	29.0	8	8.9	9	13.4	8	49.1
Mountain	3	35.8	3	12.7	5	18.8	7	52.7
New England	9	25.5	5	11.0	6	17.7	9	39.6
Pacific	8	28.4	9	7.4	7	15.1	6	53.5
South Atlantic	4	35.0	6	10.8	8	13.6	1	58.1
West North Central	5	32.2	2	14.9	2	21.6	4	54.9
West South Central	1.5	37.4	1	15.6	3	21.1	5	54.1

63% to 75%. For hip fracture patients, the variation is from 85% to 93%.

One reflection of the impact of the hospital DRG payment system can be seen in Figure 10.5, which compares the payment sources for nursing home care in 1985 and 1995. Over that decade, the proportion of funds covered by private payment decreased, while the contributions of Medicare, and to a lesser degree Medicaid, increased.

The Nursing Home

The nursing home has served as the touchstone for LTC. For better or worse, other forms of LTC are usually considered in relationship to the nursing home. This institution can be said to have a mixed heritage, descended from the almshouse on one side and the hospital on the other. Skeptics would say it has inherited the worst traits from each parent. Because nursing home care has been closely associated with Medicaid, a welfare program, it carries the welfare stigmata. At the same time, early federal regulations used small hospitals as the template for nursing home standards. What might be tolerable for a brief spell in an acute hospital where one expects to derive substantial benefit becomes unbearable in a longer stay in a nursing home where the expectation of benefit is far less.

Institutional practices that rob patients of their identity and their dignity, which impose rules developed to make care more efficient but less personalized, are never welcome, but they are even less so when the quality of one's environment dramatically affects the quality of one's life. The standard hospital model of multiple persons in a room, fixed hours for eating and being awake, limited choice of food, and a general sense of being driven by a therapeutic philosophy does not jibe well with a sense of creating a more normal living environment. The de facto linking of services and hotel func-

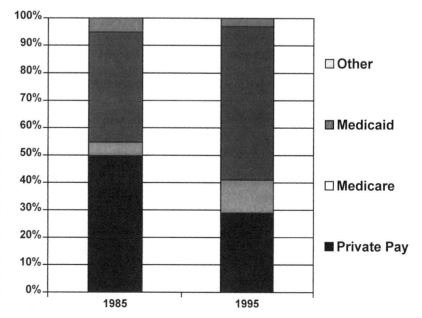

FIGURE 10.5. Changes in the sources of payment for nursing home residents age 65 and older from 1985 to 1995. The proportion of coverage from Medicare and Medicaid increased while that from private pay declined. (From Hing E. (1985). Use of Nursing Home by the Elderly: Preliminary Data from the 1985 National Nursing Home Survey. Advance Data from Vital and Health Statistics no. 135. DHHS Pub. No. (PHS)87-1250. Hyattsville, MD: Public Health Service; 1987, Table 9; and Georgetown University Institute for Health Care Research and Policy, 1995.)

TABLE 10.3. Nursing home constituencies.

Population	Other sources of care for this group
Physically frail	Home care
	Assisted living
	Day care
Cognitively impaired	Home care
	Assisted living
	Day care
Postacute care	Inpatient rehabilitation units
	Outpatient rehabilitation units
	Home health care
Terminally ill	Hospice
	Home care
Total vegetative state	

tions, inherent in the notion of a nursing home, may impose a high price on one's lifestyle. In fact, one might argue that the very term "nursing home" is a misnomer, because it provides neither much nursing (on average, about 90 min/day, primarily from nursing aides) nor a very homelike atmosphere.

The plight of the nursing home has been made more serious by asking it to play multiple roles in the lives of very different types of clients. In many instances the nursing home is not the only institution serving this group. Table 10.3 shows the various populations served and some of the alternative sources of care for each group. Trying to fill so many roles makes it difficult to achieve good results.

The use of nursing homes is linked to age. Summary numbers about the average use of nursing home are misleading. As shown in Figure 10.6, the use of nursing homes is much higher among those aged 85 and above. Indeed, it makes much more sense to report nursing

home use rates as a function of the population in this range rather than 65 and above.

For a long time, even though the supply of nursing homes varied greatly across the country, the demand for nursing home care was perceived to be so strong that utilization would rise to meet the supply. However, that situation seems to be changing. As shown in Figure 10.7, the use of nursing homes per capita fell from 1985 to 1995. For the first time, nursing homes are now facing the potential of empty beds. Several factors likely contribute to this shift.

1. Nursing home, are increasingly being used for post-acute care, where the expectation is for a finite stay and discharge to the community. Shorter lengths of stay are inevitably associated with lower occupancy.
2. Nursing homes are facing new competition from assisted living. Private-paying clients especially are attracted to the idea of being able to live in more commodious settings, often at lower costs.
3. People are entering nursing homes later in their medical careers and thus dying sooner, lowering the average length of stay.

Nursing homes entering the postacute care market may find themselves disadvantaged and unable to provide the services they wish. In general nursing homes do not have the nursing staff, especially professional nurses, to meet the needs of patients just discharged from the hospital. Medical attention is often less than that which is needed. Doctors who make hospital rounds are less inclined to make comparable nursing home rounds, certainly not as frequently, nor is Medicare as likely to pay for such care. Ironically, a patient may be covered in a hospital one day and a day later be a nursing home patient, virtually identical clinically, but with much lower

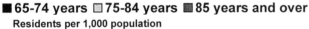

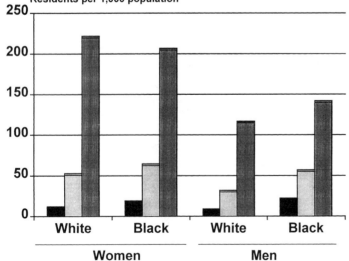

FIGURE 10.6. Nursing home residents among persons 65 years of age and over by age, sex, and race, 1997. The proportion of older persons in nursing home homes increases dramatically with older ages. Women use more nursing home care than men. Black persons now use as much or more nursing home care as do whites. (From Health, United States, 1999.)

FIGURE 10.7. Nursing home residents 65+ per 1000 elderly, 1985 and 1995. The use of nursing home declined from 1985 to 1995. The reasons for this drop are being debated. (From Georgetown University Institute for Health Care Research and Policy, with permission.)

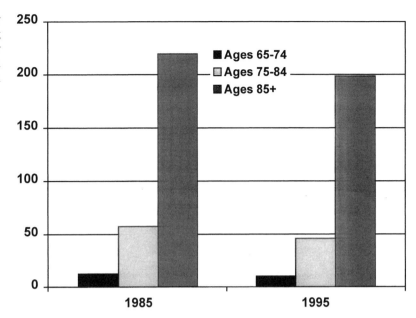

expectations for medical care. Concerned doctors may have to spend considerable effort arguing why they should be paid for their work. Likewise, nursing homes may not be able to provide the rehabilitation needed. Some homes have physical therapists on staff, and others contract for such care, but few have the full gamut of a rehabilitation team.

The nature of medical care in nursing homes has changed. Although nurse practitioners have been shown to improve primary care in nursing homes for some time,[3,4] they have not been widely utilized. With the emergence of managed care, dedicated teams of physicians and nurse practitioners have been effectively used to follow nursing home residents.[5,6] Special managed care programs directed specifically at nursing home residents have been created under the belief that aggressive primary care will prove cost-effective by reducing hospitalizations.[7]

Home and Community-Based Care

The nursing home finds itself squeezed at both ends. On the one hand, it must compete with rehabilitation units and hospitals that are turning their new excess capacity into long-stay or subacute care units. At the other end, it must compete for chronic care business with assisted living and home care, both of which may offer more attractive settings in which to live.

This situation is a new one for nursing homes, which have for years served as the touchstone of long-term care. All other modalities were considered in terms of alternatives to the nursing home. This "alternatives paradigm" has persisted for some time. The search for suitable alter-

natives that were both more effective and less costly has proven frustrating, in part because long-term care is, at its base, a social construction. The solution to the problem ultimately was to redefine the needs.

The search for alternatives faced many obstacles.

1. It was hard to target services accurately. Many people who seemed to be eligible for or at risk for nursing home services never used them. Hence, an intervention designed to decrease nursing home use could not show an impressive difference against a low rate in the control group.

2. Calculating comparable costs was a challenge. In one sense, the nursing home is a good buy, as it includes room and board as well as services. Purchasing room and board in the community is an added expense, but one may get much more than in a nursing home, where rooms are not private and little choice of food is offered. Simply adding the costs of room and board to services in the community seems to artificially raise community-based costs, especially if one is, in fact, buying more than would be available in the nursing home. On the other hand, much of the care in the community relies on informal care, which is not charged. Shadow pricing this care implies (1) that the care would be given in the same amount if it were paid for and (2) that the costs would be equivalent to the going wage for an appropriate level of caregiver.

3. The effects of community care may be delayed. The window for detecting a benefit may be too narrow to reflect the effect of delaying institutionalization.

4. The evidence of benefit may extend beyond reduced hospitalizations or nursing home admissions. Getting care in one's own home might be what most people want; there may be intangible benefits.

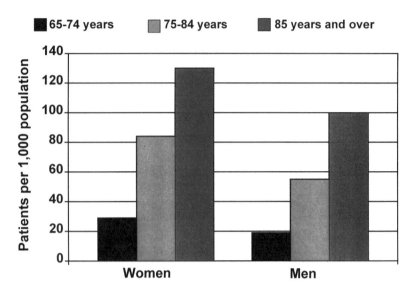

FIGURE 10.8. Home health care patients among persons 65 years of age and over by age and sex, 1996. The use of home health care increases with age. Women use home health more than men. (From Centers for Disease Control and Prevention, National Center for Health Statistics. National Home and Hospice Care Survey.)

The most prevalent type of home- and community-based care is home care. Care at home comes in two forms that are often difficult to distinguish. Home health care is usually covered by Medicare and is built around a nursing model, although most of this care is given by home health aids. Homemaking services, usually provided by persons termed personal care attendants, are more likely to be covered from other sources, such as Medicaid. As Figure 10.8 indicates, the pattern of home health care closely resembles that for nursing home care, with a rapid increase in use with age. Home health care has experienced a dramatic growth, spurred by the shortening of hospital stays and the removal of coverage constraints. As a result, home health care, which is presumably treated as a postacute care service under Medicare, was often providing care to persons more than 120 days after discharge from a hospital. Changes in the 1997 Balanced Budget Act and the subsequent revisions in the 1999 Act were introduced to constrain this rapidly growing area. The prospective payment system uses data from the mandated Outcome and Assessment Information Set (OASIS), which is used to track the outcomes of home health care. Table 10.4 shows the effectiveness of the short-term changes in Medicare payment in reducing the numbers of visits per episode. The median number of visits fell from 26 to 28 in 1994 and 1997 to 21 in 1998.

The concept of home- and community-based care conjures up images of care at home, but in some instances housing may be required as well, either because the person's original home has been lost during a period of institutionalization or because the nature of the care required implies a need for frequent brief visits, where the costs of travel time may exceed those of the care itself. Such a situation is best addressed by some form of congregate housing whereby services can be affordably provided to many people living close together.

An emerging form of LTC is assisted living. Although there is no consistent definition of this style of care, most people agree that it includes an opportunity to live alone with quarters that provide their own toilet and bathing facilities and some means to preserve and prepare food. At the heart of this concept is the idea that people are first seen as inhabitants of their space with control over their lives. Services are provided as conditions dictate. Some may be offered as a part of an overall package (e.g., congregate dining, a minimum number of service hours per week); others can be purchased as needed.

Questions have been raised about how well this modality can handle very frail individuals. Although the case mix of assisted living is usually less complex than that of nursing homes, the clinical trajectories seem to be fairly equivalent.[8] No one has yet probed the limits of such care.

Anecdotal reports feature care of very frail persons, but the wholesale expansion of assisted living has resulted in a proliferation of forms and shapes. The term no longer conveys a clear message. Persons interested in such services must examine carefully just what is promised and for how long. Cost pressures have encouraged many ALs to seek ways to discourage clients once their care needs become heavy or to demand that families hire personal care attendants. States are currently struggling

TABLE 10.4. Use of home health, FY1994–1998.

	1994	1997	1998
Home health users (million)	3.1	3.5	3.0
Users per 1000 fee-for-service beneficiaries	87	103	90
Average visits per user	63	73	51
Median visits per user	26	28	21

Source: Medicare Payment Advisory Commission. Report to the Congress: Medicare payment policy. Washington, DC, March 2000.

TABLE 10.5. States most committed to home and community-based care (HCBS).

Commitment based on HCBS utilization		Commitment based on HCBS expenditure	
Strong demographic pressure for LTC	Milder demographic pressure for LTC	Strong demographic pressure for LTC	Milder demographic pressure for LTC
Kentucky	Alaska	Texas	California
New Mexico	California	West Virginia	Idaho
New York	Idaho	New York	Illinois
Texas	Maine	North Carolina	Michigan
Arkansas	Michigan		Nevada
Louisiana	Nevada		Oregon
North Dakota	Oregon		Virginia
	Washington		Alaska
	Delaware		Maine
	Illinois		
	Montana		

LTC, long-term care.
Source: State LTC Profiles Report, 1996.[24]

with how to accommodate AL within their LTC Medicaid programs. The results to date are very varied.

Although the initial efforts to establish the benefits of home- and community-based care were frustrating and the research results proved unconvincing;[9,10] the press for such care continued. Policies influencing the amount of such care given in proportion to the amount spent on institutional care showed great variation from state to state. Even when demographic and other factors are considered, there continues to be a big national discrepancy.[11] Table 10.5 shows the states in 1996 that had the most and the least commitment to home- and community-based care, arrayed by the amount of demographic pressure on them to generate long-term care. Although most of the states with heavy commitments to home- and community-based care have less demographic pressure to develop LTC programs, a few states with high demand have responded creatively.

Until now, LTC has been largely a state responsibility because of the heavy role Medicaid has played. The result has been the wide variety of programs and level of effort reflected here. Some observers view this variation as a positive phenomenon. They see the states as the national laboratory, experimenting to find better programs. Others view this variation as an indication that more federal attention is needed to provide a more equal basis for care. For them, geography should not determine one's destiny.

LTC Policy Dilemmas

Quality

As the population ages and as older people become more affluent, our society faces several conflicting demands. Consumers have long held a preference for receiving care

in the community, preferably in their own homes. Those needing housing, either because they had no shelter or because logistics required some sort of congregate living arrangement to make home care affordable, prefer a livable environment where they have maximal control and autonomy. At the same time, our society continues to view older people as vulnerable and in need of protection.

Heavy regulations dominate the nursing home scene and indeed have shaped the nature of that care. The impetus for active regulation goes back to a series of scandals in the nursing home industry in the 1960s and 1970s that featured both inflated prices and neglectful care.[12,13] A turning point was the report of the Institute of Medicine,[14] which led to the Nursing Home Reform Act of 1987. In addition to requiring more training and better staffing, the Act mandated a uniform data system. The Resident Assessment Inventory (RAI) is composed of the Minimum Data Set (MDS) and the Resident Assessment Protocols (RAPs), which provides suggestions for further evaluations that should form the basis of care planning. The underlying idea held that collecting more systematic data would improve care planning and could provide the basis for better oversight of the care provided.

The RAI represents an important step forward, although the MDS approach has serious limitations, largely attributable to the plan to collect data from the observations of those who provide the care rather than talking directly to residents, and hence the requirement that many salient domains be inferred or ignored.[15] Although some states had already created strong assessment tools, many states had not. A national standard not only raises the mean performance, it allows comparisons. Whether causal or coincidental, the introduction of the MDS has been associated with improvement in several aspects of nursing home care, including improvements in function,[16] hospitalization,[17] and health conditions.[18]

At the same time, the MDS approach has an important limitation. Because its data come exclusively from staff observations, they cannot address the equally important issues around quality of life. Such critical information is highly subjective and cannot be inferred.

Assessing problems is not the same as fixing them. Nursing home regulations have been much better at detecting care deficiencies than correcting them. Such corrective actions involve sanctions and often result in litigation. The threat of litigation and the demand for objective documentation of poor care has led regulators to emphasize those aspects of care that best lend themselves to quantification. Unfortunately, these may not be the ones most closely related to a decent quality of life or even to good care.

Some have argued for a shift in emphasis away from the process and structure of care to a focus on the outcomes of care. In a situation such as LTC, outcomes can be easily misunderstood. Because the normal course favors decline in function, it may be hard to demonstrate a positive outcome. Thus, even good care can appear to create a poor result. The key to understanding LTC outcomes is the recognized need to demonstrate the difference between observed and expected results. Good care may be best portrayed as slowing the rate of decline. Unfortunately, in many instances this favorable result is hard to demonstrate in the absence of any data to show the expected course with such care. Thus, benefits must be expressed as the difference between observed and expected outcomes. Achieving this end requires having access to data that can describe the clinical course associated with typical care and with the care actually being rendered.

This approach is useful beyond regulatory purposes. LTC workers may readily become discouraged and dissatisfied from seeing decline in so many of their clients. Without some means of appreciating the differences their care is making on the lives of those they care for, they may assume a reaction of learned helplessness, feeling that their efforts cannot change the course of their charges. At least some of the high turnover and low prestige of nursing home work may be traceable to this problem.

An outcomes focus also allows comparisons across modalities of care. As new forms of care emerge, such as assisted living, those in the nursing home arena cry foul, claiming that assisted living is allowed to live under a different (i.e., lower) standard. On the other hand, if assisted living is required to meet all the mandates of nursing home care, it will inevitably become nursing home care and any possible benefits will be lost. By shifting the emphasis away from mandating components and methods of care to accountability for case-mix-adjusted outcomes, it is possible to preserve flexibility and still assure accountability.

One issue that runs through all the discussions about quality is the extent to which frail older people should be placed at risk, or even allowed to take risks. One faction holds that all frail older persons are vulnerable elders and hence must be treated as wards of the state, protected from all potential sources of harm. An alternative formulation suggests that older people should be allowed the right to take risks so long as they do so knowledgeably. This construct, called managed risk, emphasizes the need for responsible decision making and the obligation to provide older persons and their families with better information about the risks and benefits (and costs) of alternative modes of care.

Financing

A continuing issue is how to finance LTC. As noted earlier, a considerable amount of the money is public dollars and many of the costs are hidden as informal care. Despite efforts to push the idea, private long-term care insurance has not really caught on. People seem reluctant to commit their disposable income early in their lives when the risk of LTC seems very remote. As people age and the chances of LTC increase, so do the costs of the policies. Another related problem is that inflation plays a big role in determining the value of such a policy purchased well in advance of needing it. Adding an inflation adjuster raises the cost considerably. From the states' perspective, buying private long-term care can reduce the likelihood of needing Medicaid coverage. Hence many states have tried to create inducements for older people to buy such coverage, usually offering to exclude more assets in determining eligibility for Medicaid. For many people, private LTC insurance is really asset insurance. It offers a means to assure that assets will not be depleted and can be left as a legacy.

The better the LTC coverage offered under Medicaid, the fewer the incentives to purchase LTC insurance. It would be perverse public policy, however, to make Medicaid-covered care so unattractive to induce more people to buy LTC insurance.

One possible way out of this policy dilemma would be to redefine the state's responsibility for providing LTC coverage. So much of these considerations is driven by the nursing home model, which combines room and board with services. An alternative formulation would have public funds cover only the services component of LTC, leaving the responsibility for the housing aspect to the individual. This formulation has several potential advantages. It could lay the groundwork for a universal LTC benefit restricted to services only. It could allow a more even footing for comparing the costs and value of different modalities of LTC. It could emphasize the need to offer a reasonable living situation as well as the requisite care. In effect, it would end the distinction between institutional and community-based care. All care would offer the same range of services to people living in a variety of settings with varying levels of amenities. The latter would reflect their affluence but would not affect the receipt of care.

Another direction being explored is to translate public obligations for financing LTC into strict accounts. Those eligible for such payments would be given the option of in effect cashing out their benefits by receiving a cash payment in lieu of services. This arrangement has been used in several European countries, most notably Germany, which has a universal long-term care insurance program.[19] A crucial question is, of course, how the conversion rate should be established. Traditionally, it has been quite deeply discounted (paying only about 65% of estimated costs). People's willingness to accept such a deep discount raises interesting questions. Either the cost of LTC is overpriced or many people expect that they can obtain these services less expensively from informal sources, including family members.

These cash and counseling programs raise a number of questions. Historically, public agencies have had a much harder time relinquishing responsibility compared to the relationship between private agencies and clients. Given this vulnerability, public agencies are reluctant to simply cash out benefits. Instead, they prefer to provide some sort of vouchers that would limit the range of services that could be bought or to insist on some sort of counseling to enhance the likelihood of wise decisions. The other large concern is the so-called woodwork effect. Offering home and community care has always raised fears that the availability of such services would induce demand. In the main, these fears have never materialized. However, the offer of cash should prompt more people to demand care (or its cash equivalent) and hence raise the overall costs.

Balancing Long-Term Care

If long-term care is acknowledged as a social construct, then the goal should be to improve the lives of the people served. From this starting point, planning the future would better start from the vantage point of the type of care we want rather than how to revise what we have. We need a wider array of choices that can provide care at varying levels of intensity, combined with housing and supportive services. The housing can be the client's or congregate housing may be needed, either to meet a person's needs for housing or because colocation is necessary to achieve efficiency.

Long-term care is primarily a state-level issue because of the central role played by the Medicaid program. As a result, there is wide geographic variation in the nature

TABLE 10.6. Proportion of total and of Medicaid LTC expenditures going to HCBS, 1996.

	LTC expenditures to HCBS (%)	
	Total	Medicaid
Alaska	47	14
Oregon	46	44
Idaho	37	28
New York	34	34
California	33	21
West Virginia	28	28
North Carolina	28	27
Texas	28	25
Arkansas	26	24
Maryland	9	6
New Hampshire	9	8
Alabama	9	8
Ohio	8	6
South Dakota	7	3
Rhode Island	7	6
Mississippi	7	5
Louisiana	7	6
North Dakota	7	3
Pennsylvania	7	0.6
Tennessee	2	0.6

Source: State LTC Profiles Report, 1996.[24]

and extent of care. The extent of balance in current long-term care programs varies widely across the states. A few vanguard states, such as Oregon and Washington, have made deliberate efforts to redirect Medicaid expenditures from nursing homes to community care, including institutional options like assisted living, but most states have been hesitant or unable to make such a shift. Table 10.6 illustrates the level of variation in the balance of nursing home and community expenditures for Medicaid and total LTC dollars. The range in expenditures on home- and community-based services (HCBS) as a percentage of total LTC expenditures runs from 47% (Alaska) to 2% (Tennessee). The proportion of expenditures is generally quite similar for Medicaid funds, but there are some exceptions (e.g., Alaska, Idaho, California, Pennsylvania, and Tennessee).

A commitment to a balanced LTC program requires both the creation of options for care and the flexibility to spend money on a variety of services. While one might expect the market to respond to more flexible payment policies, some proactive effort from the state seems to be required to provide assurance of demand as an inducement for innovation.

The debate goes on as to whether LTC should continue to be a state-level issue or should move toward a more national standard. The argument for the latter is one of equity. Geography should not determine services. On the other hand, reality suggests that conditions vary widely across the country, and states have been the primary innovators. No single model that could be adopted as the national prototype has yet emerged as clearly preferable, nor is there any reason to believe that there will ever be a single best way to deliver such care. At least some consistent set of expectations (beyond the general list of mandatory services that are now part of Medicaid) seems reasonable, leaving the specific modes of implementation to the discretion of states, given that these are publicly funded programs with major federal subsidies.

Integrating Medical and Social Services

Long-term care may be primarily a social service, but many of the people receiving it suffer from serious chronic diseases. At a minimum, these people need close medical attention. Some would advocate merging both long-term and acute care elements into a single program. Others fear that this merger would create an overly medical model that might compromise the quality of life of participants.

One way to provide integrated care is to capitate the total care under a single managed care aegis. The experience with this approach is still preliminary. The best known model of this approach to care is PACE (Program for All-inclusive Care for Elders). This approach places great emphasis on active primary care, provided by a comprehensive care team, with a strong commitment to keeping clients out of institutions, both hospitals and nursing homes.[20] Preliminary data suggest that the PACE programs have succeeded in reducing utilization of both types of institutions; however, the overall impacts of the program on health status show little benefits over conventional care.[21] These results have not impeded PACE in becoming an official option under Medicare + Choice.

It is not yet clear how widely programs like PACE can be replicated, nor whether they really operate within the prescribed budgets they receive.[22] Presently, the PACE model has several limitations, which have affected marketing. (1) It serves a select dually eligible (for Medicare and Medicaid) population who are eligible for nursing home care but still in the community. (2) It requires clients to change their doctors to use a PACE physician who is comfortable with the PACE team approach. (3) It requires clients to use adult day health care. Newer forms have been developed that try to adapt the overall PACE philosophy to more flexible models that permit maintaining existing doctor–patient relationships.[23]

Quality Concerns

One potential for addressing the quality conundrum posed by the diversity of LTC programs may lie in moving toward establishing accountability on the basis of outcomes in lieu of process and structure. It seems more sensible to hold all providers equally accountable for outcomes adjusted for case mix. However, many advocates are reluctant to give up the hard-won regulations that have historically emphasized process and structure; they acknowledge the desirability of looking more at outcomes, but they are not yet convinced that outcomes can be used exclusively, or even primarily, as an enforceable tool in regulation.[24]

Another quality issue addresses the relationship between medical care and other care on behalf of nursing homes. At present, most of the attention is directed at nursing-related items; exceptions include the use of psychoactive medications. It seems likely that future regulation will raise expectations about medical care for nursing home residents, including the failure to track problems with sufficient vigilance to prevent unnecessary hospitalizations. The shared responsibility (leading to an implicit partnership relationship) of hospitals and attending physicians will likely be repeated in the context of the nursing home.

Summary

LTC is changing. Its final form is hard to foresee, but it will inevitably require a close linkage between those providing the supportive services needed to compensate for functional losses and those providing the active medical care needed to manage the underlying chronic conditions. Ironically, although such care is often held in low esteem, it represents an area where a modest input can reap large dividends in terms of both avoiding catastrophes and improving patient quality of life.

References

1. Cutler DM. Declining disability among the elderly. *Health Affairs*. 2001;20(6):11–27.
2. Gage M. The patient-driven interdisciplinary care plan. *J Nurs Admin*. 1994;24:26–35.
3. Kane RL, Jorgensen LA, Teteberg B, Kawahara J. Is good nursing-home care feasible? *JAMA*. 1976;235:516–519.
4. Kane RL, Garrard J, Buchanan JL, Rosenfeld A, Skay C, McDermott S. Improving primary care in nursing homes. *J Am Geriatr Soc*. 1991;39:359–367.
5. Reuben DB, Schnelle JF, Buchanan JL, et al. Primary care of long-stay nursing home residents: approaches of three health maintenance organizations. *J Am Geriatr Soc*. 1999; 47:131–138.
6. Farley DO, Zellman G, Ouslander JG, Reuben DB. Use of primary care teams of HMOs for care of long-stay nursing home residents. *J Am Geriatr Soc*. 1999;47:139–144.
7. Kane RL, Huck S. The implementation of the EverCare demonstration project. *J Am Geriatr Soc*. 2000;44:218–228.
8. Frytak J, Kane R, Finch M, Kane R, Maude-Griffin R. Outcome trajectories for assisted living and nursing facility residents in Oregon. *Health Serv Res*. 2001;36:91–111.

9. Kemper P. Evaluation of the National Channeling Demonstration: overview of the findings. *Health Serv Res.* 1988;23:161–174.

10. Carcagno GJ, Kemper P. The evaluation of the national long term care demonstration: an overview of the channeling demonstration and its evaluation. *Health Serv Res.* 1988; 23:1–22.

11. Kane RL, Kane RA, Ladd RC, Nielsen W. Variation in state spending for long-term care: factors associated with more balanced systems. *J Health Polit Policy Law.* 1998;23: 363–390.

12. Mendelson MA. *Tender Loving Greed.* New York: Knopf; 1974.

13. Moss FE, Halamandaris VJ. *Too Old, Too Sick, Too Bad: Nursing Homes in America.* Germantown, MD: Aspen Systems; 1977.

14. Institute of Medicine. *Improving the Quality of Care in Nursing Homes.* Washington, DC: National Academy Press; 1986.

15. Kane RL. Assuring quality in nursing home care. *J Am Geriatr Soc.* 1998;46:232–237.

16. Phillips CD, Morris JN, Hawes C, et al. Association of the Resident Assessment Instrument (RAI) with changes in function, cognition, and psychosocial status. *J Am Geriatr Soc.* 1997;45:986–993.

17. Mor V, Intrator O, Fries BE, et al. Changes in hospitalization associated with introducing the Resident Assessment Instrument. *J Am Geriatr Soc.* 1997;45:1002–1010.

18. Fries BE, Hawes C, Morris JN, Phillips C, Mor V, Park PS. Effect of the National Resident Assessment Instrument on selected health conditions and problems. *J Am Geriatr Soc.* 1997;45:994–1001.

19. Cameron KA, Firman JP. *International and Domestic Programs Using "Cash and Counseling" Strategies to Pay for Long-Term Care* (draft report). Washington, DC: National Council on the Aging; 1995.

20. Eng C, Pedulla J, Eleazer GP, McCann R, Fox N. Program of All-inclusive Care for the Elderly (PACE): an innovative model of integrated geriatric care and financing. *J Am Geriatr Soc.* 1997;45:223-232.

21. Abt Associates Inc. *Evaluation of the Long Term Care Survey Process.* Cambridge: Abt Associates; 1996.

22. Branch LG, Coulam RF, Zimmerman YA. The PACE evaluation: initial findings. *Gerontologist.* 1995;35:349–359.

23. Kane RL, Homyak P, Bershadsky B, Lum Y-S. Consumer responses to the Wisconsin Partnership Program for elderly persons: A variation on the PACE.

24. Ladd RC, Kane RL, Kane RA. *State LTC Profiles Report, 1996.* Minneapolis: Division of Health Services Research and Policy, School of Public Health, University of Minnesota; 1999.

11
The Geriatrician in the Nursing Home

Wayne C. McCormick

Imagine this practice. You arrive to see your patients when it is convenient for you (morning, afternoon, or evening; it does not matter)—sometimes scheduled, sometimes unannounced. The staff is glad to see you, bringing you current information on your patients, as well as documents for your signature, as necessary. Your patients are all present—100% show rate, every time! They are also delighted to see you and will see you when convenient; they are in no hurry—they literally have all day. They are extremely needy of your services; many are quite debilitated, and quite a few have very interesting and challenging medical problems. A substantial diagnostic armamentarium is available to you: standard clinical laboratory tests, radiology, and electrocardiograms; even ultrasound abdominal and vascular studies can be obtained. Reimbursement has steadily improved for your services, as has the knowledge base and quality of care in your practice environment, thanks to a number of national provider organizations and other advocacy groups.[1] And the overhead expenses and hassle factor of your practice are quite low relative to those of other office-based physicians you know.

Welcome to practice in the modern skilled nursing facility (SNF), or nursing home. Many health care providers have poorly conceived prejudices about nursing homes, viewing them as many lay people do—as warehouses for the ill elderly, where care is poor and staff is made up of persons who cannot get a job anywhere else. These prejudices are pervasive because many physicians, like many lay people, have never set foot in a nursing home and are averse to debility and chronic disease. In fact, no two nursing homes are alike. Many are quite fancy; some are highly specialized (catering to patients with head injury, or those with AIDS), whereas others may be more humble physical plants; they are often replete with dedicated and skilled staff with substantial altruism and medical knowledge.

What nursing homes do have in common nationwide is a dedication to care of persons with chronic disease, an emphasis on patient autonomy, and a daunting regulatory structure that (since an Institute of Medicine report and resultant enactment of federal legislation more than a decade ago[2]) has standardized patient assessment and quality of care to a large degree. In fact, most nursing homes today deliver good-quality care, and many deliver care that can only be described as outstanding. Certainly, a substantial number need to make quality improvements, which is probably true in any category of medical care. At least assessment of quality of care is more elaborate, codified, and complete, thanks to legislation and a regulatory structure that encourages comprehensive assessment in a uniform manner for all patients.[3]

In modern times, most nursing homes function in a multidisciplinary manner similar to geriatric evaluation teams or units in other settings. By regulation, most members of a typical geriatric evaluation team are available in the nursing home, including physical therapists, occupational therapists, speech pathologists, social workers, recreational therapists, and, of course, nurses and nurses' aides. It is quite typical for skilled nursing facility nurses to specialize in some aspect of chronic care, such as wound care, dementia, AIDS, or spinal cord injury. This approach is facilitated by the existence of specialized units within many nursing homes, such as high-intensity subacute rehabilitation or ventilator units, or low-intensity dementia or head injury units. It is also common to have team meetings, as is done in geriatric evaluation units, and the family of the patient is often included to help in sharing perspectives and care planning.

Hierarchy of Influence in the Nursing Home

Nursing homes are well named; they are run by nurses. The most powerful and influential administrator in the modern nursing home is not necessarily the executive director, and certainly not the Medical Director or the

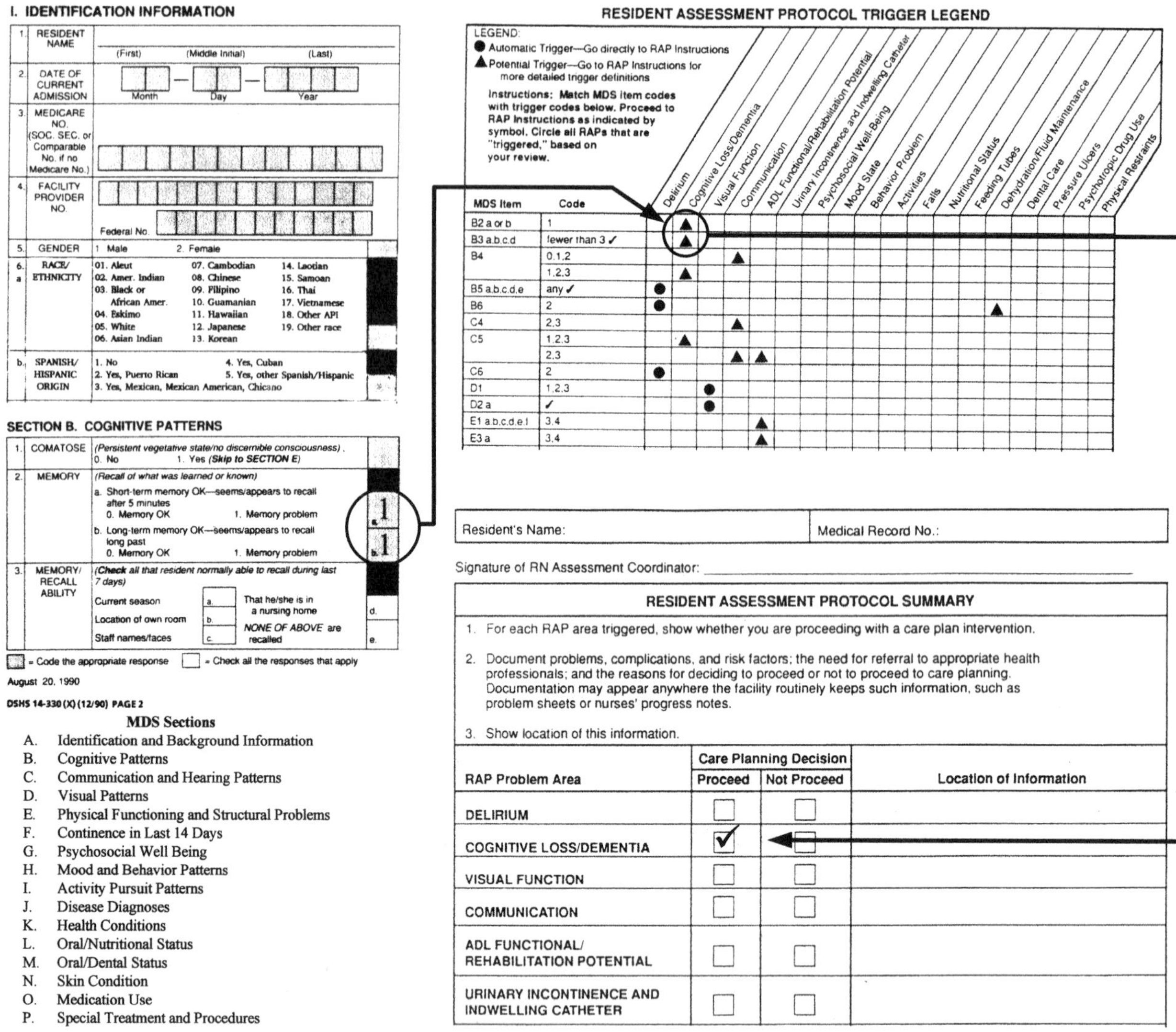

I. IDENTIFICATION INFORMATION

1.	RESIDENT NAME	(First) (Middle Initial) (Last)
2.	DATE OF CURRENT ADMISSION	Month — Day — Year
3.	MEDICARE NO. (SOC. SEC. or Comparable No. if no Medicare No.)	
4.	FACILITY PROVIDER NO.	Federal No.
5.	GENDER	1. Male 2. Female
6. a	RACE/ ETHNICITY	01. Aleut 02. Amer. Indian 03. Black or African Amer. 04. Eskimo 05. White 06. Asian Indian 07. Cambodian 08. Chinese 09. Filipino 10. Guamanian 11. Hawaiian 12. Japanese 13. Korean 14. Laotian 15. Samoan 16. Thai 17. Vietnamese 18. Other API 19. Other race
b.	SPANISH/ HISPANIC ORIGIN	1. No 2. Yes, Puerto Rican 3. Yes, Mexican, Mexican American, Chicano 4. Yes, Cuban 5. Yes, other Spanish/Hispanic

SECTION B. COGNITIVE PATTERNS

1.	COMATOSE	*(Persistent vegetative state/no discernible consciousness).* 0. No 1. Yes *(**Skip to SECTION E**)*	
2.	MEMORY	*(Recall of what was learned or known)* a. Short-term memory OK—seems/appears to recall after 5 minutes 0. Memory OK 1. Memory problem	a. 1
		b. Long-term memory OK—seems/appears to recall long past 0. Memory OK 1. Memory problem	b. 1
3.	MEMORY/ RECALL ABILITY	*(**Check** all that resident normally able to recall during last 7 days)* Current season a. Location of own room b. Staff names/faces c. That he/she is in a nursing home d. *NONE OF ABOVE* are recalled e.	

▒ = Code the appropriate response ☐ = Check all the responses that apply

August 20. 1990

DSHS 14-330 (X) (12/90) PAGE 2

MDS Sections

A. Identification and Background Information
B. Cognitive Patterns
C. Communication and Hearing Patterns
D. Visual Patterns
E. Physical Functioning and Structural Problems
F. Continence in Last 14 Days
G. Psychosocial Well Being
H. Mood and Behavior Patterns
I. Activity Pursuit Patterns
J. Disease Diagnoses
K. Health Conditions
L. Oral/Nutritional Status
M. Oral/Dental Status
N. Skin Condition
O. Medication Use
P. Special Treatment and Procedures

RESIDENT ASSESSMENT PROTOCOL TRIGGER LEGEND

LEGEND:
● Automatic Trigger—Go directly to RAP Instructions
▲ Potential Trigger—Go to RAP Instructions for more detailed trigger definitions

Instructions: Match MDS item codes with trigger codes below. Proceed to RAP Instructions as indicated by symbol. Circle all RAPs that are "triggered," based on your review.

MDS Item	Code	Delirium	Cognitive Loss/Dementia	Visual Function	Communication	ADL Functional/Rehabilitation Potential	Urinary Incontinence and Indwelling Catheter	Psychosocial Well-Being	Mood State	Behavior Problem	Activities	Falls	Nutritional Status	Feeding Tubes	Dehydration/Fluid Maintenance	Dental Care	Pressure Ulcers	Psychotropic Drug Use	Physical Restraints
B2 a or b	1		▲																
B3 a.b.c.d	fewer than 3 ✓		▲																
B4	0.1.2				▲														
	1.2.3		▲																
B5 a.b.c.d.e	any ✓	●																	
B6	2	●													▲				
C4	2.3				▲														
C5	1.2.3		▲																
	2.3				▲	▲													
C6	2	●																	
D1	1.2.3			●															
D2 a	✓			●															
E1 a.b.c.d.e.f	3.4					▲													
E3 a	3.4					▲													

Resident's Name:	Medical Record No.:

Signature of RN Assessment Coordinator: ____________

RESIDENT ASSESSMENT PROTOCOL SUMMARY

1. For each RAP area triggered, show whether you are proceeding with a care plan intervention.
2. Document problems, complications, and risk factors; the need for referral to appropriate health professionals; and the reasons for deciding to proceed or not to proceed to care planning. Documentation may appear anywhere the facility routinely keeps such information, such as problem sheets or nurses' progress notes.
3. Show location of this information.

RAP Problem Area	Care Planning Decision: Proceed	Care Planning Decision: Not Proceed	Location of Information
DELIRIUM	☐	☐	
COGNITIVE LOSS/DEMENTIA	☑	☐	
VISUAL FUNCTION	☐	☐	
COMMUNICATION	☐	☐	
ADL FUNCTIONAL/ REHABILITATION POTENTIAL	☐	☐	
URINARY INCONTINENCE AND INDWELLING CATHETER	☐	☐	

FIGURE 11.1. Minimum data set for nursing home resident assessment and care screening (MDS): Background information/intake at admission.

attending physicians—it is the Director of Nursing. The language of the clinical staff of nursing homes is the language of nursing, built on the basic needs of persons with chronic diseases. For example, common nursing diagnoses include "alteration in bowel function," "alteration in nutrition," or "alteration in cognition." The underlying medical diagnoses are only of passing interest, whether Alzheimer's disease, multiple sclerosis, or AIDS: the drivers of care day in and day out are the nursing diagnoses.

Little wonder, then, that all basic assessments are headlined by nursing diagnoses, including the national, mandatory assessment completed on admission and serially (at least quarterly) on all patients admitted to skilled nursing facilities—the Minimum Data Set (MDS).[4] This arcane five-page document is becoming more familiar to physicians practicing in nursing homes, who may over time be called upon to verify the data contained in the MDS. The MDS drives nursing home care and reimbursement in an absolute and powerful way nationwide, through severity of illness indices derived directly from the data elements in the MDS.

Figure 11.1 shows a typical portion of a page and section list of the MDS. Debility identified on the MDS "triggers" a Resident Assessment Protocol, or RAP, which is essentially a codified care plan for each triggered problem. The more RAPs that are triggered, the more care plans that are applicable and the more complex the care of the patient. Progressive debility in basic activities of dally living (ADLs), cognition, behavior, and other realms that translate into higher skilled care needs also translates into higher reimbursement categories, known as Resource Utilization Groups (RUGS),[5] a classification system analogous to the Diagnosis-Related Group (DRG) system in hospitals and similar in that it dictates prospective payment. The reader will note, however, that the prospective payment in the nursing home is not built on medical diagnoses, but rather on the level of debility implicit in the nursing diagnoses. This fundamental principle highlights the importance of nursing function and lingo in the SNF, and many physicians practicing in the SNF are slow to understand the pervasiveness of this principle; it is much like learning a foreign language while living abroad.

The Nursing Home Medical Record

Physicians are often struck by the volume of the typical nursing home medical record; it is huge. The first reaction of doctors when confronted with the patient record is, "What are all these sections for?" The typical record has two dozen sections. Table 11.1 lists the usual makeup of the record in order; advance directives invariably follow demographic face sheets as the first section. It is nearly impossible to be admitted to the modern nursing home without declaring one's code status. Admitting history and physical examination, orders, and progress notes usually follow. The progress note section often demon-

TABLE 11.1. Sections of the nursing home medical record.

Demographic Face Sheet
Advance Directive/Code Status
Orders
History and Physical
Admission Records (from previous care, e.g., hospital)
Minimum Data Set (MDS)
Total Parenteral Nutrition
Active Care Plans
Progree Notes
Resolved Care Plans
Care Conference Records
Vital Signs
Lab and Special Reports
Medication Administration Record (MAR)
Treatments
Dietary
Occupational Therapy
Physical Therapy
Speech Therapy
Quality of Life/Activities
Social Work
Miscellaneous

strates a frank economy of space, with all disciplines represented in close succession; typically, 6 to 10 notes can fit on the face of one page. This economy is to account for long stays so the chart can contain a lengthy record without thinning. Most of the sections that follow are nursing driven, with care plans, the MDS, and each discipline (physical therapy, occupational therapy, recreational therapy, social services, medication delivery records, treatment records, etc). Although it is not necessary for the physician to read completely the entire chart of every patient, it pays to do so for a substantial minority to get an impression of the total care rendered. In aggregate, the total nursing home record of patient care captures the comprehensiveness of the experience better than a typical hospital chart, certainly with regard to care rendered.

Patient Autonomy

The second fundamental principle that pervades nursing home practice is that of patient autonomy. The volumes of regulations pertinent to nursing home care (second only to the regulatory burden of the airline and nuclear power industries) has at its core patient autonomy. Every conceivable effort is expended to ensure this principle in the SNF. For example, patients are not to be restrained in any way, whether chemically (via sedatives or neuroleptics) or physically, without extensive documentation and monitoring (Fig. 11.2). Most nursing homes find it far easier to find creative ways to avoid restraint through behavior management than to use restraints. Regarding physical restraints, the rules go beyond what many might consider restraints, not just wrist restraints or waist restraints. For instance, lap trays on wheelchairs and bed rails are considered restraints. Not only are residents not to be restrained; they are also encouraged to participate in as many activities as possible to replicate the day-to-day rights and activities of nondebilitated citizens. By regulation, this autonomy and independence is to be fostered, which implies that it must be assessed in the first place. Residents are strongly encouraged to take meals in groups, to see movies or watch television together, to attend musical events, and to vote. These activities are either brought to them in the facility or arranged in "field-trip" fashion. Again, physicians may be slow to comprehend this fundamental atmosphere of patient autonomy. Physicians are used to meting out admonitions and directives to patients in the office, clinic, or hospital. Patients are referred to as "residents" in the SNF—this is their home, where they are boss. The admonitions and directives are supposed to come from them to the staff and physicians, not the other way around.

Resident Behavior and Facility Practices (483.13)

A. Level B requirement: Restraints
1. The resident has the right to be free from any physical restraints imposed or psychoactive drug administered for purposes of discipline or convenience and not required to treat the resident's medical symptoms.
2. Physical restraints are any manual method of physical or mechanical device, material, or equipment attached or adjacent to the resident's body that the individual cannot remove easily which restricts freedom of movement or access to one's body (includes leg and arm restraints, hand mitts, soft ties or vest, wheelchair safety bars, and gerichairs).
3. Psychoactive drugs are covered below, under "Quality of Care."
4. There must be a trial of less restrictive measures unless the physical restraint is necessary to provide lifesaving treatment.
5. The resident or his/her legal representative must consent to the use of restraints.
6. Residents who are restrained should be released, exercised, toileted, and checked for skin redness every 2 h.
7. The need for restraints should be reevaluated periodically.

Drug therapy

a. Each resident's drug regimen must be free from unnecessary drugs
   (1) "Unnecessary drugs" are drugs that are given in excessive doses, for excessive periods of time, without adequate monitoring, or in the absence of a diagnosis or reason for the drug. An unnecessary drug is a drug for which monitoring data, or undue adverse consequences indicates that the drug should be reduced or discontinued entirely. An unnecessary drug is also one which is prescribed only in anticipation of an adverse consequence of another prescribed drug.
   (2) In deciding whether an unnecessary drug is being used, surveyors are instructed to be very sure that reputable literature and thorough understanding of the resident's clinical condition justifies this judgment. (HCFA is developing additional guidelines for surveyors for determining unnecessary drugs which will include specific drugs and dosages.)

b. Antipsychotic drugs
   (1) Residents who have not used antipsychotic drugs are not given these drugs unless antipsychotic drug therapy is necessary to treat a specific condition.
      (a) Antipsychotic drugs should not be used unless the clinical record documents that the resident has one or more of the following "specific conditions":

1. Schizophrenia
2. Schizoaffective disorder
3. Delusional disorder
4. Psychotic mood disorders (including mania and depression with psychotic features)
5. Acute psychotic episodes
6. Brief reactive psychosis
7. Schizophreniform disorder
8. Atypical psychosis
9. Tourette's disorder
10. Huntington's disease
11. Organic mental syndromes (including dementia) with associated psychotic and/or agitated features as defined by
   • Specific behaviors as quantitatively (number of episodes) and objectively (e.g., biting, kicking, and scratching) documented by the facility which causes residents to
      —Present a danger to themselves
      —Present a danger to others (including staff)
      —Actually interfere with staff's ability to provide care
   • Psychotic symptoms (hallucinations, paranoia, delusions) not exhibited as specific behaviors listed above but *which cause the resident frightful distress*
12. Short-term (7 days) symptomatic treatment of hiccups, nausea, vomiting, or pruritus
      (b) Antipsychotics should not be used if one or more of the following is/are the *only* indication
1. Simple pacing
2. Wandering
3. Poor self-care
4. Restlessness
5. Crying out, yelling, or screaming
6. Impaired memory
7. Anxiety
8. Depression
9. Insomnia
10. Unsociability
11. Indifference to surroundings
12. Fidgeting
13. Nervousness
14. Uncooperativeness
15. Any indication for which the order is on an "as needed" basis
   (2) Residents who use antipsychotic drugs must receive gradual dose reductions, drug holidays, or behavioral programming (unless clinically contraindicated) in an effort to discontinue these drugs.

FIGURE 11.2. Summary of new federal regulations relevant to primary physicians and medical directors in nursing homes: 1987 Omnibus Budget Reconciliation Act (OBRA).

Code Status

When physicians enter the nursing home, it is well to remember these two fundamental principles: one, the nursing home is run by nurses and patients, and, two, patients' rights and autonomy rule the day—after all, the nursing home is their home. The lion's share of physician discomfort with nursing home practice might be traced to misunderstanding, and not embracing, these two principles. A sentinel example of this is the typical decision making and ordering regarding cardiopulmonary resuscitation (CPR), or its avoidance [do not resuscitate (DNR)];

this is a "patient order," not necessarily a physician order, in the nursing home. Generally, the patient or surrogate decision maker signs the CPR/DNR order. If the physician is called upon to sign the form as well, it is often merely an acknowledgment, almost an afterthought. Many nursing homes simply dispense with the physician signature. The MD signature merely confuses the issue as they are not the decider; the patient is. On the other hand, if a code status decision is reached that the physician feels is not appropriate, the onus is on the doctor to work with the family and staff to establish goals appropriate to severity of illness and prognosis—an "incorrect" code status is often a good stimulus for such a heart-to-heart discussion. The physician can and should discuss code status issues with patients; in the nursing home this is primarily to inform, which may or may not influence their decisions.

Physician Visits

Physician participation in the care of nursing home patients is also regulated. By federal law (and as amended in some states), minimum visitation by the physician to nursing home patients includes the initial order and approval for admission in the form of an admitting history, physical, and orders. An annual review similar to the admission work is also prudent. After admission, monthly visits (every 30 ± 10 days) should ensue for at least one quarter, then every other month thereafter. In many states, subsequent visits may be alternated with a physician assistant or nurse practitioner. Some states continue to require monthly visits indefinitely. Again, this is the minimum. So long as medical necessity can be documented, the physician or nurse practitioner can round on the patients (and bill for these services) as often as medically necessary, daily, if need be, as occurs in some high-intensity nursing home wings variously known as rehabilitation or subacute units. Nurse practitioners are highly effective partners in the nursing home because they speak the language of nursing and also have prescriptive authority and diagnostic decision-making skills. Their autonomy and ability to bill effectively for their services have recently been enhanced by federal legislation.

During the physician visit, the doctor must sign all orders (including therapy or telephone orders that have accumulated between visits) and approve the plan of care, usually by signing monthly orders after review, a review that should include review of the MDS. Physicians may also include multidisciplinary care conferences in rounds and, at a minimum, should touch base with nurses and therapists involved in the care of patients, either face to face or by phone. The physician who does not actively interact with nurses and therapists runs the risk of being left out of the picture entirely. Remember, the physician is not running the show, is not present day to day, and needs this interaction to be at all effective in patient care. Communication with staff should take advantage of every available device, including communication logs or books on nursing home units, voice mail, and e-mail, reserving paging for emergencies. Paradoxically, the more available and responsive the physician team is to communications, the fewer calls generated, as the nursing staff feels the confidence of support. Concentrated physician/nurse practitioner presence in the nursing home with good communication can reduce unnecessary readmissions to hospitals by employing the full diagnostic and therapeutic means available in the nursing home (with

attention to patient wishes and directives).[6] It is not unusual for patients to request "DNH" (do not hospitalize) when they are confident of physician care in the nursing home.

Patient Population Dynamics in the Modern Nursing Home

Most patients admitted to nursing homes in this day and age are rehabilitated over a period of a month or two and discharged alive.[7] That said, the majority of bed-days are accounted for by long-stayers, patients with slow trajectories of improvement or decline, with chronic illnesses such as Alzheimer's disease or other debilitating neurologic diseases. These persons can be expected to succumb to their illness in the nursing home setting. A substantial minority of residents, perhaps a quarter to a third, are admitted with a clearly terminal illness, such as advanced carcinoma, amyotrophic lateral sclerosis, or AIDS, and stay only a few weeks for end-of-life care. Small wonder that the staffs of most nursing homes are quite proficient in end-of-life care, with attention to patient and family goals of care first and foremost, with penultimate importance placed on symptom relief, pain management, and smoothness of comfort measure decisions and resuscitation avoidance. This focus of care is considerably easier to arrange (and to attain unanimity of thinking among staff and family) in the nursing home than in the hospital.

Importantly, most nursing homes cannot necessarily provide the full panoply of hospice care, with expert nursing, social services, clergy, and volunteer support all directed toward typical hospice goals. This distinction is highlighted by two phenomena: (1) the common practice of patients receiving care in the nursing home, with the addition of the full hospice team from a home health agency; and (2) the relative lack of family support and bereavement services in nursing home settings. Generally, the nursing staffing ratio in nursing homes may vary from 20:1 to 40:1 (patients: RN or LPN), with nurses' aide staffing of about 10:1 to 15:1, for an average patient to staff ratio of about 10:1. Nurses are generally occupied with medication passes and wound care; and aides with the physical movement, hygiene, and feeding of patients. This staffing ratio allows enough staff to fulfill the physical, medication, and treatment needs of patients, but not necessarily the time to spend supporting a grieving family. Hence, what appears to be "too many cooks" for a terminally ill patient (i.e., both hospice and nursing home staff) can actually be an excellent team approach in practice. The nursing home staff is free to concentrate on the patient's comfort, and the hospice team can concentrate on counseling and bereavement, in collaboration with each other. When done well, this nursing home/hospice team collaboration is synergistic; when done poorly, it is indeed "too many cooks," and the physician is often in the best position to emphasize synergy and discourage the opposite. This attitude implies enough physician input and involvement in the case to manage both the nursing home staff and hospice team effectively.

In fact, this example highlights the certain value of the physician in the nursing home: not as boss, but as manager, consultant, and team player. The physician brings a crucial medical perspective of disease process and medical diagnosis, of medication use and interactions, of prognosis, and of counseling techniques in dealing with patients and families, often at truly the most dire turning point in many patients' and families' lives. One cannot imagine a better-trained specialist than the geriatrician to perform this task—a specialist trained and skilled in management of multidisciplinary teams, in rehabilitation and end-of-life care, and in counseling those with chronic illnesses.

Medical Directorship of the Skilled Nursing Facility

Most nursing homes seek out geriatricians to be medical directors of their facilities for these same reasons. Medical directorship enhances the professional experience of physicians in nursing home practice in several ways, not the least of which is the influence, over time, in the overall quality of care of all patients in the facility, not just those being directly managed by that physician. Table 11.2 lists common types of activities of medical directors in skilled nursing home facilities. Excellent courses are now available with certification in medical directorship through national physician organizations.[1] For physicians attracted to a modest administrative role, medical directorship of the nursing home provides a stimulating forum and reasonable reimbursement to enhance the physician's role in the nursing home. And, the physician's perspective is truly valued in this role. No one else in the nursing home can provide it. The administration of the nursing home basically wants the medical perspective

TABLE 11.2. Potential roles of the medical director in the nursing home.

Participate in medical decision making
Organize and coordinate physician services
Help ensure appropriate high-quality care
Develop and conduct educational programs
Participate in employee health, safety, and welfare
Articulate mission to the physician and wider community
Interact with regulators, government officials, and payors
Assure rights of residents, staff, and volunteers

from the physician medical director and someone to interact with the physician's peers, other attending physicians. Geriatricians should not be daunted by this role; it is truly enjoyable and not taxing by any means.

Understanding the Patient Experience of Nursing Home Care

Understanding the experience of the nursing home from the patient's perspective is perhaps the most challenging exercise in empathy a physician can undergo, at once heartwarming and heartrending. It is hard to imagine a more depressing event than entering a nursing home; a concrete marker of likely permanent debility and disease, joining with many others of the same (or worse) fate, in turn a forced admission of frailty and mortality.

The admission process to the nursing home is also highly regulated. It is a prolonged process involving the signing of stacks of papers and discussions of illness, code status, funeral home choice, relinquishment of belongings, and embracing the frightening and the unfamiliar. Given the multiplicity of legal forms and the lengthy discussions during the admission process, which usually exceeds 2 h, the pervasive feeling is akin to buying a house—a house you do not want. The physical and emotional tolls are sometimes eclipsed by the financial toll. Nearly half of nursing home care is paid for by private funds; that is, the patient or family writes a check every month for several thousand dollars to cover the nursing home daily rate, not to mention medications and doctor visit co-pays. Typical daily cost for nursing home care is of the order of $100 to $150, for a monthly cost of about $4000. The other half of nursing home payment is largely through Medicaid for persons impoverished by fate or illness or by previous medical and nursing home bills (so-called spend down). A small proportion of payment is from Medicare, and an even smaller part from long-term care insurance, the latter still being rare at this point in the evolution of payment for medical services in the United States. The Medicare category of payment is almost entirely for relatively short rehabilitation stays. Medicare was never intended to cover typical long-term care, and legislators have systematically maintained this short-term, rehabilitation focus of the Medicare benefit. Given the daunting costs of typical long-term care for chronic illness, this attitude is unlikely to change in the foreseeable future. The Medicare benefit will cover 100 days per year for a rehabilitation stay after hospitalization, and only fully covers the first 20 days with a substantial co-pay (20%) after that; small wonder that many Medicare stays are less than 20 days. It can only be invoked for skilled services: parenteral therapy (not including insulin), complex wound care, or daily physical, occupational, or speech therapy. Daily compliance and consistent improvement are necessary to retain the benefit. If patients cannot meet these requirements, the Medicare benefit is terminated, and the remainder of the nursing home stay cost is covered by private pay or Medicaid. This change is a source of consternation for patients and families, and that consternation is often conveyed to the nursing home staff and to physicians. This eventuality cannot be prepared for enough—indeed, much of the staff and physician effort for nursing home patients is in the setting of realistic goals—physical, cognitive, prognostic, and financial. The physician cannot escape participation in all four areas.

Conclusion

For a growing number of physicians, nursing home practice is the most rewarding part of geriatric medicine. Some of the most wonderful and fulfilling experiences of doctoring can be shared with patients and families in nursing homes. Of course, some of the more depressing and occasionally awful experiences also occur, just as they do in hospitals or other clinical settings. In the nursing home, it is often possible to coordinate a compassionate approach to care of persons with chronic or terminal illnesses if the geriatrician knows how to effectively lead the multidisciplinary team and work with nurses. The nursing home is a nursing engine, for nursing-intensive, hands-on care, as opposed to the hospital, which serves more as a diagnostic machine for doctor-intensive workup and intervention. For patients who no longer need the latter, the hospital can be a dangerous place, filled with iatrogenic pitfalls. The hospital is usually the wrong modality for care of persons with debilitating chronic disease or terminal illness. Often, the nursing home can meet the needs of these patients far better than the hospital. Skilled geriatricians know which type of facility their patients need and can enjoy caring for them in any setting, including the nursing home, to fulfill the primary care bond engendered by the care of older persons with chronic disease.

References

1. The American Medical Directors Association, *www.amda.com*.
2. Institute of Medicine. *Improving the Quality of Care in Nursing Homes*. Washington, DC: National Academy Press; 1986.
3. Morris JN, Hawes C, Fries BE, et al. Designing the National Resident Assessment Instrument for nursing facilities. *Gerontologist*. 1990;30:293–307.
4. Hawes C, Morris JN, Phillips CD, et al. Reliability estimates for the Minimum Data Set for nursing home resident assessment and care screening. *Gerontologist*. 1995;35:172–178.
5. Fries BE, Schneider D, Foley WJ, et al. Refining a case-mix measure for nursing homes: resource utilization groups (RUG-III). *Med Care*. 1994;32:668–680.
6. Reuben DB, Schnelle JF, Buchanan JL, et al. Primary care of long-stay nursing home residents: approaches of three health maintenance organizations. *J Am Geriatrics Assoc*. 1999;47: 131–138.
7. Characteristics of elderly nursing home current residents and discharges: data from the 1997 National Nursing Home Survey. DHHS (PHS) 2000-1250. Washington, DC: National Center for Health Statistics, 2000.

12
Home Care

Sharon A. Levine and Patricia P. Barry

Until the 1940s, primary care was often delivered in the home. As medical technology grew more complex and patients became more mobile, care switched to hospitals, clinics, and offices; the prevalence of house calls gradually diminished to less than 1% of practice activity.[1,2] But while physicians were deemphasizing house calls, home care—providing health and social services in the home—was becoming the fastest growing service industry in the United States. The reasons include the growth of the elderly population, an increase in the number of functionally impaired elders residing in the community, a decline in the number of nursing home beds, and the preference of many elders to receive care at home.[3,4] There are economic factors, too; prospective payment systems and managed care programs encourage early discharge of patients from hospitals, and Medicare allows home care services without prior hospitalization. From 1990 to 1997, Medicare home care expenditures increased from $3.9 billion to an estimated $17.2 billion. However, since then, Congressional initiatives have slowed the growth of the industry. Early in 2000, data from the Congressional Budget Office showed that Medicare spending on home health care dropped to $9.7 billion in 1999. This sharp decline in spending stems from changes imposed by the Balanced Budget Act of 1997.[5–7]

There is little formal home care training in most medical schools and residency programs, but many physicians need to understand the basics of health care delivery in the home, including the range of services available and the sources of funding. Most primary care physicians will be responsible for authorizing and supervising complex care plans for homebound patients. They will need to coordinate care among an interdisciplinary variety of service providers. In addition, they must be able to answer patients' and caregivers' questions about home care.

Definitions

The term *home care* includes all health and social services that may be provided in the home, ranging from homemaker, chore, and meal services to nursing and physician care. (The American Medical Association defines home care as "the provision of a wide range of services and equipment to the patient in the home for the purpose of restoring and maintaining the maximal level of comfort, function, and health").[8] *Home health care* is the term used for health services provided by health aides, nurses, physical and occupational therapists, and physicians. *Home medical care*, or the *house call*, usually involves a physician or other primary care provider, such as a physician assistant or nurse practitioner.

In 1990, the American Medical Association suggested that medical care at home be categorized as follows:

1. Preventive, including home safety evaluation, patient education, provision of assistive equipment, or monitoring
2. Diagnostic, including home assessment, comprehensive geriatric assessment, or evaluation of functional capacity and the environment
3. Therapeutic, from "high tech" to hospice
4. Rehabilitative, especially with family involvement
5. Long-term maintenance for chronically ill and disabled patients, with supportive care by formal and informal caregivers[8]

Effectiveness of Home Care

Evidence is accumulating that some targeted, home-based interventions are effective in changing clinical outcomes or affecting costs of care. Tinetti and colleagues demonstrated that an in-home fall-reduction program was successful.[9] A 1995 randomized controlled trial evaluated the usefulness of annual in-home comprehensive geriatric assessment by a gerontologic nurse practitioner that focused on evaluating problems and risk factors for disability and providing specific recommendations and health education for the intervention group.[10] Three-year results found less disability, fewer nursing home admissions, and more physician visits for the intervention group. A 1998 randomized controlled trial evaluated the utility of a single home visit after discharge from acute hospital care by a nurse and a pharmacist to patients at high risk of readmission to optimize compliance and identify clinical deterioration.[11] Six-month results in the intervention group found fewer unplanned hospital readmissions, fewer out-of-hospital deaths, fewer total deaths, and fewer emergency department visits. Another randomized controlled trial has also demonstrated the effectiveness of home interventions in reducing unplanned admissions, out-of-hospital deaths, adverse events, days in the hospital, and overall deaths in patients discharged after hospital admissions for congestive heart failure.[12] An earlier prospective randomized study of patients aged 70 and older who were hospitalized for congestive heart failure used a nurse-directed multidisciplinary intervention that followed Agency for Health Care Policy and Research (AHCPR) guidelines in an effort to reduce readmissions. The trial showed fewer readmissions, better quality of life scores, and lower costs in the intervention group.[13]

These recent trials stand in contrast to older studies that failed to demonstrate the benefits of multiple interventions provided to unselected populations of community-residing elderly. A 1986 critical review of 12 experimental or quasi-experimental studies of home care concluded that there was no evidence of a consistent effect on mortality, hospitalization, physical/functional status, or nursing home placement.[14] Similarly, a 1987 review of 16 waiver-financed demonstration projects, including the well-described Channeling Project, which substituted community care for nursing home care by comprehensive case management, concluded that overall costs were increased by additional case management and community services.[15] Most subjects, apparently, were not actually at high risk of nursing home care. Subsequently, Weissert and Hedrick suggested that targeting might improve outcomes, and that costs must be aggressively controlled and services limited for these programs to be cost-effective.[16]

Physicians in Home Care

The role of physicians in home care may include authorization of services, communication with providers, patients, and families, or even actual home visits. However, few physicians provide home visits. In an

TABLE 12.1. The physician's role in home care.

Management of medical problems
Identification of home care needs of the patient
Establishment/approval of a plan of treatment with identification of both short- and long-term goals
Evaluation of new, acute, or emergent medical problems based on information supplied by other team memebers
Provision for continuity of care to and from all settings (institutions, home, and community)
Communication with the patient and other team members and with physician consultants
Support for other team members
Participation, as needed, in home care/family conferences
Reassessments of care plan, outcomes of care
Evaluation of quality of care
Documentation in appropriate medical records
Provision for 24-h on-call coverage by a physician

Source: Adapted from the Amerian Medical Association, with permission.[33]

analysis of 1993 Part B Medicare claims, Meyer and Gibbons focused on a 5% random sample of more than 1.3 million beneficiaries aged 65 or more who were not in health maintenance organizations.[1] They determined that 36,350 house calls were made to 11,917 patients. Extrapolation from this sample to all Medicare beneficiaries over age 65 suggested that 727,000 house calls were provided to 238,340 patients, which in turn implied that only 0.88% of all Medicare beneficiaries received house calls from physicians, at a cost of $63 million. Patients who received house calls were noted to be very sick and near the end of life.

In an accompanying editorial, Campion reviewed the disadvantages of house calls: they are time consuming, inefficient, and poorly reimbursed, and there are concerns about safety and lack of equipment.[17] The advantages include patient convenience, support, and reassurance, and the availability of assessment information. He also reported that an elderly patient is significantly more likely to receive a CT scan or a cardiac catheterization than a home visit.

A survey of 389 Virginia primary care physicians found that family physicians and general practitioners were significantly more likely to do home visits than were internists[18]; a subsequent national survey of 1161 internists and family physicians found similar results, with physicians noting that, although house calls were important, reimbursement was poor.[19]

The American Medical Association has outlined the responsibilities of the physician as a member of an interdisciplinary home care team (Table 12.1).

Home Care Recipients

Homebound patients are community-dwelling individuals who depend on the assistance of others to perform some activities of daily living (ADLs) because of acute or chronic medical conditions or disabilities. In the absence of this help, they would be at high risk of institutionalization. Nationwide, some 9.5 million people older than 50 receive help with at least one of the ADLS—bathing, dressing, eating, toileting, continence, transferring, and ambulating—or instrumental activities of daily living (IADLs)—management of finances, use of the telephone, organizing transportation, meal planning and cooking, shopping, and taking medications).[4] The Medical Expenditure Panel Survey findings indicated that 7.2 million individuals received formal home care services in 1996.[7] Of people receiving home health services in 1996, 72% were aged 65 or older, 67% were female, 65% were white, 29% were married, and 35% were widowed, according to the National Center for Health Statistics.[20] These data also showed that 22% of patients discharged from home health agencies in 1995–1996 had as their primary admission diagnoses diseases of the circulatory system, including heart disease and hypertension. Other common admission diagnoses were cancer and diabetes. Medicare data regarding principal diagnoses of home care recipients show a similar profile.[21]

Patients receiving medical care, as opposed to other services, at home have been described in at least two studies. Fried and colleagues described 71 patients cared for in an academic medical house calls program.[22] Eligibility included being homebound and residing within a 15-min drive of the academic medical center. Visits were scheduled every 3 months; unscheduled visits were provided on weekdays as needed. Eighty-one percent of patients were female; 52% were age 85 or older; only 23% had independent mobility at home; and 16% had cognitive impairment. Services included an average of five visits per year, 52% of which were for treatment of acute illness; 25% of patients refused hospital care. Social support was provided by children (32%), spouses (21%), or other family members (24%); 14% of patients received no such support. Referral sources included visiting nurses (25%), previous physicians (23%), and the patients themselves or the patient's families (20%).

Barry and colleagues studied the records of 480 patients enrolled in the Home Medical Service of Boston University Medical Center Hospital (now Boston University Geriatrics Services at Boston Medical Center) between January 1, 1992, and October 18, 1994, to better characterize the frail, elderly residents of urban Boston.[23,24] The study used baseline data from a comprehensive initial assessment that consisted of demographic, social, financial, medical, and functional information. Follow-up data on service utilization and outcome were obtained from Home Medical Service and hospital records. Most patients were female (72%) and elderly (mean age, 80.0 ± 9.1 years); 61% were white; 47% lived alone; and 28% had no informal caregivers. Forty-one

percent had Mini Mental State Examination (MMSE) scores suggestive of cognitive impairment (23%, under 20; 19%, 20–24). One-third reported visual (36%) and hearing (33%) deficits. Many could not independently bathe (53%), ambulate in their own homes (55%), use the toilet (25%), or eat (20%). Only 31% were free of functional impairments; 50% had two or more functional deficiencies. Other characteristics included:

- Women were older than men (59% vs. 46% over 80; $p = 0.03$) and were more likely to have an MMSE score of less than 25 ($p = 0.01$). Women were not significantly more likely to be depressed, live alone, or have two or more ADL deficiencies.
- Age alone was not associated with number of ADL deficiencies or living alone, but age was a risk factor for death or nursing home placement for those over 70 years of age.
- Impaired functional status was associated with several findings, including lower MMSE scores ($p < 0.02$), being unable to live alone ($p < 0.01$), requiring more home visits and more hospital admissions ($p < 0.001$), and increased likelihood of death ($p < 0.01$).
- Subjects who lived alone demonstrated significantly higher MMSE scores and better functional status, and required fewer admissions but did not differ by age or prevalence of depression from those who did not live alone.

Over an average follow-up period of 13 months, patients received an average of 9.6 home visits annually and were hospitalized 0.96 times per year. Increased numbers of home visits were associated with depression ($p = 0.04$) and impaired ambulation ($p = 0.005$) but not with increasing age ($p = 0.48$). Increased frequency of hospitalization was associated with depression ($p = 0.03$) and impaired ambulation ($p = 0.02$) but not with increasing age ($p = 0.70$). Patients who lived alone were less likely to be hospitalized ($p = 0.03$). At the end of the follow-up period, 61% were still being seen in the home, 16% had died, 11% were in a nursing home, and 12% had otherwise been discharged. Dying was associated with being older ($p < 0.01$) and impaired ambulation ($p = 0.01$). Similarly, significant relationships were seen between dying and other impairments in activities of daily living ($p < 0.01$). Living alone was not associated with differences in placement outcomes.

Caregivers

The vast majority of care provided in the home is unpaid, nonmedical, informal care. Data from the Informal Caregivers Survey, which was part of the 1982 National Long Term Care Survey, show that 72% of caregivers are female, mostly wives and daughters, and more than one-third of all caregivers are 65 or older. One-third of care-givers themselves are in fair or poor health and most are poor or near poor (31%) or low- to middle-income (57%). Because of the competing demands of elder care-giving with child care or employment, 9% have left work and 20% have reduced work hours. These informal care-givers spend approximately 4 h extra on an average day on caregiver tasks; 80% provide this care 7 days a week.[25] For people over age 65 who require help with at least one ADL, professional caregivers constitute the largest cate-gory of caregivers at 30%.[4]

Services Available at Home

An impressive array of professional, ancillary, diagnostic, and therapeutic services can be provided in the home, including technologically advanced services and tele-medicine (Table 12.2). In the United States, the service used most frequently by home care patients 65 and older

TABLE 12.2. Services available in the home.

Professional
  Physician
  Nurse
  Dentist
  Podiatrist
  Optometrist
  Rehabilitation therapists:
    Occupational
    Physical
    Speech
    Respiratory
  Psychologist
  Dietitian
  Pharmacist
  Social worker
Diagnostics
  Phlebotomy
  X-rays
  Electrocardiograms
  Holter monitoring
  Oximetry
  Blood cultures
Ancillary/supportive
  Home health aides
  Personal care assistants
  Homemakers
  Chore aides
  Volunteers
  Home-delivered meals
Medical equipment
  Intravenous infusion for hydration, chemotherapy, blood
    transfusion, antibiotics, total parenteral nutrition, pain
    management and other medications
  Mechanical ventilators
  Dialysis
  Medical alert devices
  Glucometers

is skilled nursing, used by 81% of patients; this is followed by personal care (57%) and homemaker services (23%).[26]

Funding for Home Care

Funding for home care services comes from a variety of public and private sources (Fig. 12.1). According to the Health Care Financing Administration, Medicare is the largest single payor of home care services, accounting for 39.6% of total estimated home care expenditures in 1997, followed by private out-of-pocket spending (21.7%) and Medicaid (14.9%).[27] Other public funding sources in-clude Title XX of the Social Security Act, the Older Americans Act, the Veterans Administration, and the Civilian Health and Medical Program of the Uniformed Services (CHAMPUS). Private sources include research and demonstration grants, charities, and commercial insurers, including managed care plans.

The interim payment system of the Balanced Budget Act of 1997 introduced a new per beneficiary limit designed to slow the growth of Medicare home health expenditures. The results were dramatic. In 1997, home health spending was 9% of total Medicare benefit pay-ments; in fiscal year 2000, home health benefits accounted for only 4% of total Medicare spending. A further 15% reduction in home health payments was scheduled to take effect in October 2001. About 3.5 million Medicare enrollees received fee-for-service home health services in 1997, a twofold increase from 1990. After the enactment of the Balanced Budget Act in 1997, however, utilization of the home care benefit markedly decreased; approxi-mately 500,000 fewer beneficiaries used the benefit in 1998 than in 1997.[7] Some beneficiaries may have difficulty

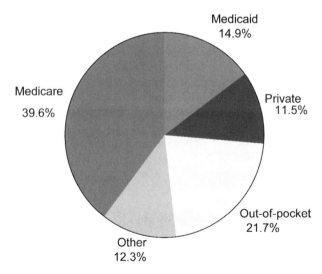

FIGURE 12.1. Sources of payment for home care (1997).

gaining access to home care services.[28] In a report to Congress, the General Accounting Office states that in response to the changes imposed by the interim payment system, home health agencies may be less likely to care for patients who require costly intensive services.[29]

Medicaid spending for home health services has also grown enormously in the past two decades, from $70 million in 1975 to $12 billion in 1997. Home care services made up 9.8% of Medicaid payments in 1997; payments to hospitals and institutions, by contrast, accounted for nearly half of Medicaid spending.[7]

Medicare

Medicare covers services deemed to be "reasonable and necessary for the treatment of an illness or injury." To qualify for home care benefits under Medicare, the patient must be *homebound* by Medicare's definition (Table 12.3), services must be *provided under a plan of care established and approved by a physician*, and the patient must be *in need of reasonable and necessary skilled nursing services* on an *intermittent* or *part-time* basis. In other words, Medicare is not intended to cover long-term care by an individual or a nursing home, nor is it designed to pay for services for patients who leave home regularly for work, recreation, or even social programs such as senior centers. In addition to a home care benefit, Medicare has a home hospice benefit that is reimbursed separately.

Services that are 100% covered under Medicare Part A include skilled nursing, skilled therapy, home health aide services, and social services (Table 12.4). However, the beneficiary must be in need of nursing, physical therapy, or speech therapy to be reimbursed for other services such as occupational therapy, personal care, or social work.[30] *Skilled nursing* includes evaluation of the patient's condition; services and procedures that can only be performed by a skilled professional; assessment or management of the patient's plan of care; and patient education. *Skilled therapy* includes restorative therapy, which is based on the expectation that the patient will improve in a reasonable amount of time, and maintenance therapy, which consists of activities that the bene-

TABLE 12.3. Medicare definition of homebound.

To qualify for Medicare Home Care benefits, a patient must meet the following criteria:
  A normal inability to leave home
  Medically contraindicated to leave home
  Leaving home requires a considerable and taxing effort
  Inability to leave home except with the aid of supportive devices, special transportation, or the assistance of another person
  Leaves home only infrequently or for short duration of time, or for the purpose of receiving medical treatment

Source: From the Health Care Financing Administration.[30]

TABLE 12.4. Services covered by Medicare.

Part A (100%)	Part B (20% co-payment)
Home health aide	Physician visit
Visiting nurse: RN	Certain durable medical equipment
Observation/assessment, management and evaluation of care plan	Some diagnostic labs, electrocardiography, and X-rays
Social service	
Physical therapy, occupational Therapy, speech therapy	

ficiary or caregivers will be taught and supervised in carrying out. *Home health aide services* include personal care, dressing changes that do not require the skills of a licensed nurse, assistance with self-administered medication, assistance with exercises not requiring a therapist, and routine care of prosthetic or orthotic devices. *Medical social services* include psychosocial and economic assessment, counseling services for the patient and caregivers, and aid in referring the patient to services in the community.

Medicare services covered under Part B (see Table 12.4), which requires a monthly premium and 20% co-payment, include physician home visits; certain medical equipment ordered by a physician, including hospital beds, wheelchairs, commodes, pumps, tube feeds, and other assistive devices; and diagnostic laboratory studies, electrocardiograms, and portable radiography.

It is important to be aware of exclusions in Medicare coverage, including homemaker services, long-term care nursing, home-delivered meals, transportation that is nonemergent, all bathroom equipment, and patient care for those who do not require skilled nursing services.

Since 1998, physicians providing home health and hospice care have been able to bill Medicare for Care Plan Oversight (Table 12.5). To bill for services, a physician must do at least 30 min or more of documented work per patient within a calendar month. The work can include development or revision of care plans, review of care plans, review of studies and test results, communication with home health agency personnel, coordinating care with consultants, and arranging other services (including by telephone).

Medicaid

Medicaid funding for home care services is provided jointly by the federal and state governments. The regulations are federal, but eligibility is determined on a state-by-state basis. Coverage is designed for those who not only meet state income eligibility guidelines but also are blind or disabled. The majority of states cover nursing and home health aide services, durable medical equip-

TABLE 12.5. Massachusetts Medicare fee schedule for home care, fiscal year 2000.

Visit type charges	Level	CPT Code	Fee in 2000	M.D. receives 80% of allowed
New patient	1	99341	$63.55	$50.84
	2	99342	$90.92	$72.74
	3	99343	$135.55	$108.44
	4	99344	$170.42	$136.34
	5	99345	$205.55	$164.44
Established patient	1	99347	$50.28	$40.22
	2	99348	$76.56	$61.25
	3	99349	$115.02	$92.02
	4	99350	$165.61	$132.49
Care plan oversight	(30 min or more)	99375	$100.00	
	(Hospice)	99378	$92.00	

Source: Data from the Health Care Financing Administration.[36]

ment, and medical supplies. Coverage for diagnostics, medication, transportation, adult day care, social work, personal care, and physical, speech, or occupational therapy varies from state to state. Medicaid payments for home health services fall into three main categories: the traditional home health benefit, which is a mandatory benefit provided by all states, and two optional programs—the personal care option and home- and community-based waivers. Hospice is an optional Medicaid service that is presently offered by 42 states.

Private Insurance and Managed Care

Private insurers and managed care organizations generally follow Medicare guidelines, although benefits and eligibility may vary. There may be caps on the number of visits. Long-term care insurance policies may be purchased privately; eligibility is usually based on functional or cognitive limitations.

Practical Aspects of Home Care

Indications for a Home Care Referral

Indications for a home care referral include advanced age and frailty, multiple comorbidities, recurrent and frequent admissions, homeboundedness, impaired psychosocial or functional status, and terminal care. Often the first sign of decline in status is the inability to keep scheduled office or clinic appointments. A single house call, as part of comprehensive geriatric assessment, helps to identify medical, psychosocial, and environmental factors that affect functional ability (Tables 12.6, 12.7). Problems identifiable by house calls include alcoholism (finding bottles or cans), incontinence (by odor), sensory impairment, pain, medical noncompliance, falls (with special attention to environmental factors), elder abuse, and depression.

In a randomized controlled trial with 1-year follow-up, veterans 70 or older were screened by a physician assistant or registered nurse for medical, functional, and social problems. The results included the discovery of four new or suboptimally treated problems in each patient, on average, and an improvement in immunization rate and IADL scores.[31] In another study of 154 patients, home visits revealed an average of two new problems per patient and from one to eight new recommendations for the treatment plan, when compared with office-based assessment. About 23% of the newly diagnosed problems indicated extreme morbidity and were potentially life threatening.[32]

The house call can also be used to find the causes of known problems (e.g., falls or medical noncompliance), to determine whether there is a need for nursing home placement, to make emergency evaluations that otherwise would require a trip to the emergency department, to conduct posthospitalization follow-up, to provide ter-

TABLE 12.6. Medical problems frequently identified by house calls.

Alcoholism
Incontinence
Sensory impairment
Pain
Compliance and medication errors
Falls
Depression

TABLE 12.7. Other problems identified by house calls.

Safety/environmental
Psychobehavioral
Caregiver stress
Elder abuse and neglect
Nutrition
Finances
Limitations in ADLs/IADLs

minal care, or to deliver primary care to the truly home-bound population.

Perceived Barriers to Home Care

Reasons given for the low frequency of home visits by doctors include time constraints, inefficiency, concerns about safety, low reimbursement, concerns about liability, lack of physician training, and institutional barriers. To relieve time constraints and improve efficiency, visits can be carefully planned and clustered geographically. In the Boston University practice, patients or their families are phoned 1 day in advance, and a time for the visit is planned so that family members can be present, which is especially useful in the case of non-English-speaking patients. Practices that employ physician assistants or nurse practitioners can integrate them into the home care team as another way to improve efficiency. Physicians can enhance their safety by traveling with students or other members of the team, scheduling visits early in the day, and carrying cellular telephones.

Current Medicare reimbursement for home visits is higher, in some cases, than outpatient visit reimbursement. For instance, Medicare reimbursement in Massachusetts for the lowest level of care for an established home care patient was $50.28 in 2000, compared with $10.67 for a similar ambulatory patient. The highest level of care for a new home care patient was reimbursed at $205 per visit versus $135.10 for a new ambulatory clinic patient at the same level of care (see Table 12.5). Physician documentation should be complete, for several reasons: it ensures that physicians will receive compensation; it substantiates the physician oversight that is necessary for other home care providers to receive payment; and it provides important evidence in case of a malpractice suit, although such lawsuits are rare.

What Is in the Doctor's Bag

The old-time doctor's "black bag" is probably not large enough to accommodate the items that most home care physicians might need on a routine or emergent home visit. In the Boston University practice, we use a light-weight diaper bag with multiple pockets. Others use medium-sized overnight bags. A bag on wheels might also be appropriate in the case of a long walk from the car to the patient's home. Table 12.8 shows items that can be included in the doctor's bag.

Interdisciplinary Teams

The home is the ideal location to identify the elder's strengths, abilities, and supports, both formal and informal. These factors are important in developing a care plan that can be put into operation realistically and that

TABLE 12.8. Supplies in the home care doctor's bag.

Blood pressure cuff (including large and thigh-sized cuffs) with handheld gauge
Stethoscope
Oto-ophthalmoscope
Thermometer with disposable covers
Gloves
Phlebotomy supplies including vacutainers, syringes, needles, tourniquets, alcohol swabs, specimen tubes, labels
Containers for transporting lab specimens
Basic wound care supplies: 2×2 gauze, 4×4 gauze, tape, iodine, Kerlix, gloves
Wound debridement supplies: disposable scalpel, debridement kits
Suture removal kit
Measuring tape
Shears
Stool guaiac materials and lubricant
Sharps container
Urinary catheter supplies including catheterization kit, catheters, specimen containers
Prescription pad
Tongue depressor
Culture swab
Medications: steroid for joint injections, local anesthetic, intravenous furosemide
Optional: glucometer, nail clippers, scale, nasogastric tubes

Note: In the summer, it is wise to have a cooler for laboratory specimens.

Source: Adapted from Boling, with permission.[37]

complies with the patient's and family's wishes. An interdisciplinary team approach and the use of a home care coordinator for case management are essential in implementing complex plans that may include numerous referrals and services as well as education for the patient and family (Table 12.9). This approach also allows continuous assessment of outcomes over time so that the plan can be revised as the patient's needs and health status change. The collaborative nature of this practice requires communication among the varied disciplines that provide services in the home. In addition, there may be overlap of shared tasks. In the case of a patient undergoing poststroke rehabilitation, for example, a speech-and-swallowing specialist might work closely with a nutritionist and visiting nurse in providing a patient with a safe plan for eating. A physical therapist must work with the family, patient, home health aide, and visiting nurse on a plan for safe transfers.

Leadership for a given service may be transferred from one discipline to another, depending on the goal being addressed. If communication is adequate, the entire team should be apprised of current and future plans. In small practices where the physician does not have the luxury of an interdisciplinary team, the physician must act as the case manager in concert with a visiting nurse. Although most patients receiving home care services do not receive house calls from physicians, the physician

TABLE 12.9. Possible members of a home care interdisciplinary team.

Physician
Licensed nurse
Physical therapist
Nurse practitioner
Occupational therapist
Speech therapist
Home health aide
Homemaker
Physician assistant
Social worker
Pharmacist
Dentist
Podiatrist
Audiologist
Chore aide
Optometrist
Nutritionist
Dietician
Friendly visitor
Volunteer
Psychologist
Personal care assistant
Laboratory assistant
Home repairman
Rehabilitation personnel

Source: Adapted from the American Medical Association, with permission.[33]

remains an important member of the team and must remain in close communication with those who provide services. Situations in which a visit by the physician may be required include discrepancies in reports of the patient's status, acute declines in health or function in frail patients, unexplained failure to thrive, unexplained failure of the care plan, request for physician evaluation in the home by another team member, need for a patient/family meeting to make an important decision, and routine medical care for the patient who cannot leave home.[33]

Conducting the Home Visit

Before the home visit, the physician or team should gather important data, including the patient's medical diagnoses, current community-based services, formal and informal supports, insurance information, and medications. The doctor's bag should be stocked as already described. Patients should be clustered geographically and the most efficient route planned. The family should be contacted to ensure that key members or significant others are present so that communication can be enhanced. If the patient is non-English-speaking, it is especially helpful to have English-speaking caregivers present to ensure that problems are identified and the plan of care can be carried out. Interpreter services should be employed if available.

The initial home visit to a medically and socially complicated patient who will receive ongoing primary care in the home may pose formidable challenges. It may take several home visits for the physician or team to gather all the information in a comprehensive geriatric assessment. A checklist can be helpful.

Basic elements of the house call should include the history and physical exam, social interaction that solidifies the doctor–patient relationship, assessment of caregivers and their burden, environmental safety assessment, psychosocial assessment, nutritional assessment, financial assessment, cognitive assessment, a medication review (including prescribed and over-the-counter medications), functional assessment, an introduction to a discussion of advance directives and personal preferences, an exploration of spiritual needs, and a discussion of the care management plan.

The physician may have to take into account various environmental barriers when taking the history in the home setting. Families may need to be asked to leave the room for private conversations, and the television or radio may need to be turned off. The physical examination poses its own problems. If lighting is poor, the physician should have a light source available; to avoid self-injury, the physician should use caution when examining patients who are immobile or who are in low, wide beds or chairs. The physician may need to bring disposal containers for needles, syringes, and other instruments. Although the first physical exam must be comprehensive, subsequent exams can be focused on the patient's particular needs. For instance, a look at the feet of a diabetic patient with neuropathy may be more important than weighing the patient.

Social interaction is essential in the development of the doctor–patient relationship. The home environment alters the traditional doctor–patient relationship in that the patient is on his or her own "turf" and therefore has increased autonomy. Some providers may feel uncomfortable about having less control, but the situation sets the stage for more realistic establishment of goals and involvement of the family. As a guest in someone's home, a physician should ask permission to walk through the house, turn off the television, wash hands, use the telephone, or even simply sit at the bedside. Because caregivers provide the bulk of home care, assessment of their level of stress is important. It is also important to identify and enlist the support of potential informal caregivers.

A thorough environmental safety assessment cannot be performed anywhere but in the home. In Ramsdell's study, home safety problems posed great risks to patients.[32] The safety of the neighborhood and the patient's access to shopping and other services can be ascertained on the visit. A walk through the home can reveal potential hazards for falls or injury such as loose wires and tile, poor lighting, and clutter (Table 12.10). The odors of garbage, urine, animal waste, and vermin can point to an unhealthy environment. When alcohol or drug abuse on the part of the patient or caregivers is suspected, bottles or other containers can provide evidence. Faulty wiring, lack of smoke detectors, evidence of burned pots, and lack of heat and hot water are clues to the patient's safety, functional status, or possible impaired cognition or judgment.

The psychosocial assessment can reveal important family ties, depression, or social isolation. A walk through the kitchen will reveal the nutritional status and food preferences of the patient. An empty refrigerator and kitchen cupboards may point to previously undiagnosed functional impairment, such as dementia or decreased mobility, and may show the need for interventions, such as home health aides, transportation, and shopping services. Problems such as malnutrition, vitamin B_{12} deficiency, and dietary indiscretion in patients on special diets can be addressed and a plan formulated that includes the services of a dietician or nutritionist for patient and family education.

A review of the patient's finances is helpful in determining which services the patient may be eligible for. For instance, in Massachusetts, patients who are Medicaid eligible will qualify for adult day care, which may mean the difference between independent community living and nursing home placement.

The home visit may enhance the physician's ability to conduct cognitive assessment because it may provide evidence of self-neglect, memory impairment, or medication noncompliance. Also, research suggests that in some cases, cognitive assessment in the clinic setting may produce misleading results. In one study, the scores of one-quarter of patients were significantly different when the Mini Mental State Examination was performed at home versus the clinic; of that group, 76% scored higher in the home setting.[34] Sometimes the condition of a patient's home environment raises questions about his or her capacity to make decisions, such as whether to remain at home at all. In such situations, the physician can refer to guidelines regarding the complex and nuanced issue of decision-making capacity, an issue discussed in Chapter 85.

A medication review at home can provide more information on medication noncompliance than a drug history in an outpatient clinic. It can reveal that patients are not taking medications they have listed in drug histories at clinics, or, conversely, that they are taking medications they have not listed.[35] Dosages, frequency, and modes of medication delivery can be examined more thoroughly in the home. A review of over-the-counter medications, such as analgesics or nonsteroidal anti-inflammatory agents for pain, may point to undiagnosed medical problems. Additionally, such a review may reveal that certain medical problems are caused by adverse drug reactions, drug–drug reactions, or drug–food reactions involving nonprescription drugs. A visit to the home is also the best way to determine which dispensing device—Mediplanner, bottle, or blister pack, for example—would meet the patient's needs.

TABLE 12.10. Elements of home safety assessment.

Areas to be assessed	Questions to consider
Kitchen safety (especially use of gas stove)	Is it easy to tell when a burner or oven gas is turned on or off?
	Does the patient wear loose garments when cooking?
Bathroom safety	Are handholds in appropriate places?
	Can the toilet seat be raised, if needed?
	Does the shower or bathtub have a nonslip surface?
	Is the floor of the bathroom slick?
Stairs	Are the stairs well lit?
	If carpeting is present, is it secure?
Gas or electric utilities	Which systems does the home have?
	Are systems checked and properly maintained?
Heating and air-conditioning	Are the controls accessible and easy to read?
Hot water heater	Is the temperature below 49°C (120°F)?
Water source	Is water from a public service or a well?
Emergency actions and evacuation route	Are emergency numbers on or near the telephone?
	Is there a means of exit in case of emergency?
Electrical cords	Are cords frayed or lying across walking paths?
Lighting and night lights	Is the wattage sufficient?
Fire and smoke detectors and fire extinguishers	Are fire extinguishers persent and accessible?
	Are fire and smoke detectors present?
	Are batteries charged or changed regularly?
Loose carpets and throw rugs	Can loose carpets and throw rugs be secured or removed?
Tables, chairs, and other furniture	Is furniture sturdy and well-balanced?
Pets	Are the animals easy to care for and to feed?

Source: Adapted from Unwin and Jerant, with permission.[38]

Assessment of ADLs and IADLs is readily accomplished in the home setting. The physician can observe bathing, dressing, ambulation, transfers, continence, the distance to the bathroom, and the patient's ability to prepare meals, use a phone, take medications, and manage finances. Further, discussions regarding spiritual needs, the patient's advance directives, surrogate decision making, and personal preferences are accomplished comfortably in the privacy of the patient's home.

On occasion, the physician finds that a patient's needs are inadequately met in the home or discovers a home environment that is unsafe. Often, the physician's first instinct is to recommend placement in a more supervised setting. But we believe that if the patient and the caregivers want the patient to remain at home, all efforts should be made to honor that wish—assuming the patient has the capacity to make such a decision. Physicians should investigate whether maximizing services can help such individuals maintain their autonomy.

Conclusion

Demographics, patient and family preference, insurance reimbursement, and the availability of sophisticated technology in the home guarantee that home health care will continue to grow as an element of community-based long-term care. Care in the home will therefore remain an important aspect of health care policy. Additionally, physicians will continue to be responsible for providing supervision of home care and, when appropriate, making home visits to enhance the well-being of patients. Home care will therefore remain a vital part of the education of physicians. This truly holistic approach to patient care can be among the most rewarding aspects of the doctor–patient relationship for both the physician and the patient.

References

1. Meyer GS, Gibbons RV. House calls to the elderly—a vanishing practice among physicians. *N Engl J Med*. 1997;337:1815–1820.
2. Keenan JM, Bland CJ, Webster L, et al. The home care practice and attitudes of Minnesota family physicians. *J Am Geriatr Soc*. 1991;39:1100–1104.
3. Bayer A, Harper L. *Fixing to Stay: A National Survey on Housing and Home Modification Issues. Executive Summary*. Washington, DC: Matthew Greenwald and Associates for the American Association of Retired Persons; 2000.
4. Kassner E, Bectel RW. *Midlife and Older Americans with Disabilities: Who Gets Help? A Chartbook*. Washington, DC: Public Policy Institute, American Association of Retired Persons; 1998.
5. Pear R. Medicare spending for care plunges by 45%. *New York Times*. April 21, 2000.
6. *Medicare Projections and the President's Medicare Proposals. An Analysis of the President's Budgetary Proposals for the Fiscal Year 2000*. Washington, DC: Congressional Budget Office; 2000.
7. *Basic Statistics About Home Care*. Washington, DC: National Association for Home Care; March 2000.
8. American Medical Association Council on Scientific Affairs. Home care in the 1990's. *JAMA*. 1990;263:1241–1244.
9. Tinetti ME, Baker DI, McAvay G, et al. A multifactorial intervention to reduce the risk of falling among elderly people living in the community. *N Engl J Med*. 1994;331:821–827.
10. Stuck AE, Aronow HV, Steiner A, et al. A trial of annual in-home comprehensive geriatric assessments for elderly people living in the community. *N Engl J Med*. 1995;333:1184–1189.
11. Stewart S, Pearson S, Luke CG, et al. Effects of home-based intervention on unplanned readmissions and out-of-hospital deaths. *J Am Geriatr Soc*. 1998;46:174–180.
12. Stewart S, Pearson S, Horowitz JD. Effects of a home-based intervention among patients with congestive heart failure discharged from acute hospital care. *Arch Intern Med*. 1998;158:1067–1072.
13. Rich MW, Beckham V, Wittenberg C, et al. A multidisciplinary intervention to prevent the readmission of elderly patients with congestive heart failure. *N Engl J Med*. 1995;333:1190–1195.
14. Hedrick S, Inui T. The effectiveness and cost of home care: an information synthesis. *Health Serv Res*. 1986;20:851–880.
15. Kemper P, Applebaum R, Harrigan M. *A Systematic Comparison of Community Care Demonstrations*. Washington, DC: National Center for Health Services Research; 1987.
16. Weissert WG, Hedrick SC. Lessons learned from research on effects of community-based long term care. *J Am Geriatr Soc*. 1994;42:348–353.
17. Campion EW. Can house calls survive? *N Engl J Med*. 1997;337:1840–1841.
18. Boling PA, Retchin SM, Ellis J, et al. The influence of physician specialty on house calls. *Arch Intern Med*. 1990;150:2333–2337.
19. Keenan JM, Boling PA, Schwartzberg JG, et al. A national survey of the home visiting practice and attitudes of family physicians and internists. *Arch Intern Med*. 1992;152:2025–2032.
20. Haupt BJ. *An Overview of Home Health and Hospice Care Patients: 1996 National Home and Hospice Care Survey*. Advance Data, No. 297. Hyattsville, MD: National Center for Health Statistics; 1998.
21. Health Care Financing Review Annual Statistical Supplement, table 52. Washington, DC: Health Care Financing Administration; 1999.
22. Fried T, Tinetti ME. When the patient cannot come to the doctor: a medical house calls program. *J Am Geriatr Soc*. 1998;46:226–231.
23. Barry P, Markson L, Atkinson L. Physician home care: patient characteristics and outcomes. *J Am Geriatr Soc*. 1995;43:SA40.

24. Barry PP, Levine SA. Home care and medical education: the Boston University experience. In: Michel JPRL, Vellas BJ, Albarede JL, eds. *Facts, Research, and Intervention in Geriatrics: Geriatric Programs and Departments Around the World.* New York: Springer; 1998.

25. Stone R, Cafferata GL, Sangl J. Caregivers of the frail elderly: a national profile. *Gerontologist.* 1987;27:616–626.

26. Dey Achintya N. *Characteristics of Elderly Home Health Care Users: Data from the 1994 National Home and Hospice Care Survey.* Advance Data No. 279. Hyattsville, MD: National Center for Health Statistics; 1996.

27. *National Health Expenditures Projections: 1998–2008.* Washington, DC: Health Care Finance Administration, Office of the Actuary; 1997.

28. Smith BMMK, Hawkins DJ. *An Examination of Medicare Home Health Services: A Descriptive Study of the Effects of the Balanced Budget Act Interim Payment System on Access to and Quality of Care.* Washington, DC: George Washington University Center for Health Services Research and Policy; 2000.

29. *Medicare Home Health Agencies: Closures Continue with Little Evidence Beneficiary Access Is Impaired.* No. HEHS-99-120. Washington, DC: General Accounting Office; 1999.

30. *Home Health Agency Manual Section 205–206; Section 204.1.* Washington, DC: Health Care Financing Administration; 2000.

31. Fabacher D, Josephson K, Pietruszka F, et al. An in-home preventive assessment program for independent older adults: a randomized controlled trial. *J Am Geriatr Soc.* 1994;42:630–638.

32. Ramsdell JW, Swart J, Jackson JE, et al. The yield of a home visit in the assessment of geriatric patients. *J Am Geriatr Soc.* 1989;37:17–24.

33. *Medical Management of the Home Care Patient: Guidelines for Physicians.* Chicago: American Medical Association; 1998.

34. Ward HW, Ramsdell JW, Jackson JE, et al. Cognitive function testing in comprehensive geriatric assessment: a comparison of repeated test performance in residential and clinic settings. *J Am Geriatr Soc.* 1990;38:1088–1092.

35. Jackson JE, Ramsdell JW, Fenvall M, et al. Reliability of drug histories in a specialized geriatric outpatient clinic. *J Gen Intern Med.* 1989;4:39–43.

36. *Medicare B 2000 Fee Schedule.* Washington, DC: U.S. Department of Health and Human Services, Health Care Financing Administration; 2000.

37. Boling PA. *The Physician's Role in Home Health Care.* New York: Springer; 1997.

38. Unwin BK, Jerant AF. The home visit. *Am Fam Physician.* 1999;60:1481–1488.

39. *Home Health Care Expenditures and Average Annual Percentage Change, by Source of Funds: Selected Calendar Years 1970–2009.* Washington, DC: Health Care Financing Administration; 1997.

13
Acute Hospital Care

Robert M. Palmer

For older patients, hospitalization is a two-edged sword. Hospitalization for acute illness offers older patients the hope of relief of symptoms and cure of disease, but it also exposes them to the adverse risks of hospitalization—functional decline (a loss of independence in activities of daily living), iatrogenic illness, and possible institutionalization. Recent studies have identified risk factors for functional decline in hospitalized elderly patients and opportunities for improving the process of care to improve functional and psychosocial outcomes of hospitalization.

Epidemiology of Hospitalization

Although rates of hospitalization have declined in the past two decades for all age groups, since the introduction of the prospective payment system and Medicare/managed care programs, the proportion of hospitalized patients who are age 65 years and older is increasing. In nonfederal acute hospitals, elderly patients account for 37% of all discharges and 47% of inpatient days of care.[1] Hospitalization rates are more than twice as great for patients 85 years and older compared with patients aged 65 to 74 years. The oldest patients have longer hospitalizations, higher mortality rates, and higher rates of nursing home placement.[1] Among noninstitutionalized adults, patients age 75 years and over have the greatest number of hospitalizations, with nearly 15% being hospitalized yearly and 5.3% hospitalized two or more times per year.[2] A small portion of older patients consistently make extensive use of hospital services. In the Longitudinal Study of Aging, which followed nearly 7500 patients age 70 years and older for 7 years, 43% had no hospital admissions and another 25% had infrequent hospitalizations.[3] Fewer than 5% had consistently higher rates of hospitalization, averaging one or more admissions annually. A prospective cohort study identified eight independent variables that are risk factors for repeated hospital admission among people age 70 years

or older: older age, male sex, poor self-rated general health, availability of an informal caregiver, having ever had coronary artery disease, having had a hospital admission during the previous year, more than six doctor visits, or diabetes mellitus.[4] The presence of these risk factors more than doubled the risk of hospital admission compared to low-risk patients and was associated with a higher cumulative rate of mortality, hospital days per person-year survived, and higher hospital charges.[4] The cost of acute hospitalization peaks in the 70- to 79-year-old age group and declines with age, reflecting lower ancillary costs in the oldest patients.[5]

In-hospital mortality rates are age related and increase from 5% among those 65 to 74 years of age to 10% in those 85 years of age and older. In the hospitalized elderly longitudinal project (HELP), a prospective cohort study of seriously ill patients age 80 years and older, major variables predictive of 2-year mortality included weight loss, cognitive dysfunction, impaired functional status, chronic disease class, and adult physiology score (from the Acute Physiology and Chronic Health Evaluation [APACHE]).[6] Most elderly patients—one-third of patients aged 65 to 74 years and 46% of those 75 years and older—are admitted to the hospital from the emergency department.[7] Among nursing home residents referred to the emergency department, more than 40% are admitted to the hospital.[8]

Taken together, these data suggest that rates of hospitalization, total cost of hospital care, mortality rates, and nursing home discharges will continue to be greater in the elderly population compared to younger patients.

Risks of Hospitalization

Functional Decline

Hospitalization for an acute illness often results in an older patient's loss of independent self-care (functional decline). A study of functional morbidity in hospitalized older patients with a mean age of 84 years found that 65% of patients experienced a decline in mobility scores between baseline and day 2 of hospitalization.[9] By hospital discharge, 67% showed no improvement and another 10% deteriorated further. Recent prospective cohort studies found that 20% to 32% of patients admitted to general medical units lose independence in their ability to perform one or more basic activities of daily living (ADL) at discharge.[10–12]

Risk factors for functional decline, its natural history, and sequelae have been identified. In a study of more than 1200 community-dwelling patients aged 70 years and older hospitalized with acute medical illnesses, 31% lost independence in one or more of five basic ADLs when compared to their baseline status 2 weeks before admission.[13] A loss of independence in one or more instrumental ADL occurred in 40% of survivors 3 months after hospital discharge. Functional decline occurred more frequently in patients who were over 75 years of age, had some disability in the performance of an instrumental ADL before admission, and had lower mental status scores on admission.[12] Other studies have identified pressure sore, low social activity level, delirium, and depressive symptoms as risk factors for functional decline in hospital.[10,14] In hospitalized patients aged 80 years and older, independent predictors of functional decline after hospitalization included poorer baseline quality of life, lower serum albumin level, being bedridden, and documented need for nursing home admission.[15]

Cognitive impairment and depressed psychosocial functioning are important predictors of posthospital outcomes.[16] Depressive symptoms at hospital admission independently predict mortality in the ensuing 3 years, even when controlling for disease severity and baseline functional status.[17] The loss of independent functioning during hospitalization is associated with serious sequelae, including prolonged hospital stay, nursing home placement, and mortality. Functional measures are strong predictors of mortality and contribute prognostic ability beyond that obtained with combined measures of disease comorbidity, severity, disease staging, and diagnosis-related groups.[18] Three independent risk factors—impairment in the patient's performance of instrumental activities of daily living (IADL), cognitive impairment, and depressive symptoms—predict subsequent mortality in elderly patients adjusted for disease burden and severity.[18]

The conceptual basis for functional decline is shown in Figure 13.1.[19] The cause of functional decline is complex and involves the interaction of aging, hospitalization, and comorbid illness. Physiologic impairments, multiple comorbid conditions, impaired homeostatic reserves, and elements of hospitalization interact to predispose the

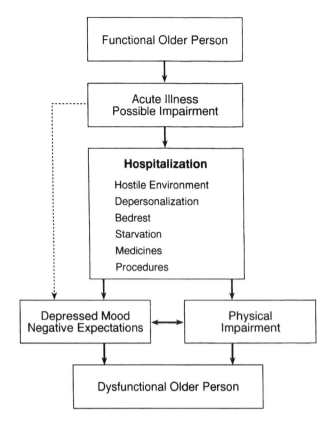

FIGURE 13.1. Conceptual basis for functional decline. (From Palmer RM, Counsell S, Landefeld CS,[19] by permission of W.B. Saunders Company.)

patient to functional decline. The physical features of the hospital may render it a "hostile environment," structured to meet the needs of professional caregivers rather than patients.[19] Hospitalization is often perceived as depersonalizing, and patients may be subjected to bed rest, undernutrition or starvation, and adverse events resulting from medications and diagnostic or therapeutic procedures. These elements can interact with depressed mood, negative expectations, and physical impairments to result in a dysfunctional older person. Identification of patients at risk for functional decline begins with the recognition of predisposing factors, as accomplished by a comprehensive geriatric assessment conducted by nurses, physicians, or other health professionals.

Iatrogenic Illness

Iatrogenic illness is any illness that results from a diagnostic procedure or therapeutic intervention and is not a natural consequence of the patient's disease.[20] Iatrogenesis is often categorized as illness that results from medications, diagnostic and therapeutic procedures, nosocomial infections, or environmental hazards.[21] Adverse drug events are the most commonly cited iatrogenic illness in hospitalized patients and are associated with significantly prolonged length of stay, higher costs of care, and increased risk of death. Virtually any class of medication can cause an adverse event, but antibiotics and cardiovascular drugs have been most commonly implicated in studies of hospitalized patients. The increased risk for adverse drug events is also attributable to alterations in drug disposition and tissue sensitivity associated with usual aging and to drug–drug interactions (see Chapter 7). Nosocomial (hospital-acquired) infections are common complications of hospitalization. Common nosocomial infections are those of the urinary tract, pneumonia, and blood (due to intravascular catheters). Colonization or infection with resistant or opportunistic infections may complicate hospitalization.[21]

Guidelines for the potential prevention of iatrogenic illnesses are shown in Table 13.1.

Medical Errors

Medical errors, which have recently received widespread attention, also appear to be more common in elderly hospitalized patients. For example, in one study, patients over age 65 had twice the chance of sustaining injury during hospitalization as younger patients, with most events being judged as potentially preventable.[22] Concerns over the reported incidence of medical error led the Institute of Medicine to release a report advocating dramatic systemwide changes in hospitals to reduce these rates.[23] Medical errors can contribute to death or injury of hospitalized patients.

TABLE 13.1. Keys to prevention of iatrogenic illness.

Iatrogenic problem	Common reasons	Keys to prevention
Adverse drug effects	Polypharmacy; drug–drug interactions; altered drug disposition and tissue sensitivity with aging	Rational drug prescribing: review all medications taken before admission; use lower-than-usual maintenance doses when geriatric dose is unknown; limit the addition of psychoactive drugs; avoid whenever possible multiple drugs that inhibit or induce cytochrome P-450 hepatic metabolism or are highly albumin bound
Falls/immobility	Weakness of leg muscles; postural hypotension; deconditioning due to prolonged bed rest; cognitive impairment; sensory impairment	Assess falls risk at admission (multiple chronic diseases, cognitive dysfunction, neuromuscular dysfunction, multiple sensory impairments); avoid physical restraints; order physical therapy for transfer-dependent and gait-impaired patients; prescribe assistive devices (e.g., canes,. walkers); modify environment (e.g., add handrails, grab bars to rooms; prophylactic anticoagulation with unfractionated heparin is warranted in immobile patients to prevent deep venous thrombosis
Pressure ulcers	Immobility; sustained point pressure over bones; excess moisture, friction and shearing forces	Pressure ulcer risk assessment: paresis, cognitive dysfunction, incontinence, malnutrition; turn immobile patients at least every 2 h; lubricate skin with cream; correct nutritional deficiencies; order pressurized bed mattresses; use patient lifts
Dehydration/ undernutrition	Chronic disease predisposing to protein-calorie malnutrition; poor oral intake due to acute illness; anorexia; preparation for diagnostic studies	Assess nutritional status at admission: low body weight; muscle wasting; low levels of serum albumin, cholesterol, hemoglobin; prescribe and monitor daily calorie and fluid intake; obtain dietitian consult; give intravenous fluids when oral intake is inadequate or prohibited; consider enteral alimentation or peripheral hyperalimentation when oral intake is inadequate or contraindicated
Nosocomial infection	Transmission of resistant/opportunistic microorganisms by caregivers or hardware; use of broad-spectrum antibiotics that eliminate normal flora; instrumentation (e.g., urethral catheters); pulmonary aspiration	Hygienic hand-washing techniques; sterilization of medical equipment; narrowing the spectrum of antibiotics when feasible; aspiration precautions in high-risk patients; disinfection of patient's skin before insertion of intravenous or intra-arterial line; urethral catheterization intermittently rather than continuously when indicated
Contrast-associated nephropathy	Hypertonic contrast agents given intravenously for diagnostic studies; dehydration; renal disease; myeloma	Avoid contrast whenever possible; maintain adequate hydration before and after study; avoid giving contrast to patients with underlying renal diseases, dehydration, multiple myeloma; use noncontrast studies (e.g., renal ultrasound rather than intravenous pyelography); consider N-acetylcysteine prophylaxis

Errors leading to adverse drug events are the most commonly recognized medical error in hospitalized patients. The use of computerized and other support systems is advocated to reduce the rate of errors.[23] Computerized medical information systems can improve the quality of patient care. A computerized decision support program linked to computer-based patient records has been shown to assist physicians in the use of antimicrobial agents and to improve patient care.[24] Computer-assisted decision support programs, using practice guidelines, can improve antibiotic use, reduce associated costs, and appear to limit the emergence of antibiotic-resistant pathogens.[25] Hospital information systems can be programmed to generate alerts in clinical situations associated with an increased risk for injury resulting from adverse drug events.[26] A physician computer order entry system combined with a pharmacist intervention decreases the rate of nonintercepted serious medication errors, thereby providing evidence that information systems can be effective in reducing medical error.[27] In addition, computerized databases enable health professionals to access relevant laboratory results, diagnostic studies, and consultation notes, even when they are outside the hospital.

Geriatric Comorbid Problems

Common geriatric problems often complicate the medical management of acute illness during hospitalization.

Immobility

Immobility is associated with functional decline, increased risk of nursing home placement after discharge, medical complications (including deep venous thrombosis, urinary incontinence, pressure sores, joint contractures, cardiac deconditioning, and muscle weakness), and fall.[28] Cardiac and muscular deconditioning occur within days of sustained bed rest. Loss of muscle strength is proportionally greater in the lower extremities than the upper extremities. Enforced bed rest and immobility are abetted by high beds, intravenous lines and catheters, and both physical and chemical restraints. Physical restraints include vest, belt, mitten, jacket, wrist, and ankle restraints. Bed rails, geriatric chairs and wheelchairs, and full rails are also often classified as mechanical restraints.[29] Restraints are most often used to control problematic behaviors, prevent disruption of treatment, and prevent falls, although their effectiveness is not established.[29] Both the Joint Commission on Accreditation of Healthcare Organizations and the Health Care Financing Administration (HCFA) require hospitals to have policies and procedures related to physical restraint of hospitalized patients. Mechanical restraints and drugs used as restraints should be avoided unless they are medically necessary and less restrictive measures have been deemed ineffective.

To enhance patient mobility, physical therapy or graded exercises should be prescribed on the first hospital day, particularly for bedbound and severely deconditioned patients.[28] Exercises should also be prescribed for patients admitted for acute or elective surgery to speed the process of recovery and rehabilitation from the operation. For patients with impaired independence in gait or bed transfers, physical therapy consultation and bedside therapy should be considered. Exercises should include passive and active range of motion exercises to enhance flexibility, low-intensity resistive exercises of the lower extremities, and assisted ambulation. Ideally, patients should be allowed free movement to reduce the risk of physical deconditioning, postural hypotension, venous thrombosis, and joint contractures. Patients often need encouragement to sit up or to get out of bed even when they prefer bed rest.[28]

Undernutrition

Undernutrition and frank protein-energy malnutrition are common in hospitalized older patients. The importance of undernutrition is underscored by prospective studies that link protein-energy malnutrition evident at admission to increased hospital and posthospital mortality. In one study, the prevalence of malnutrition at admission was 30% in male and 41% in female patients 70 years of age or older.[30] In-hospital mortality was associated with low serum albumin and prealbumin levels and decreased midarm circumference and triceps skin fold thickness.[30] A prospective cohort study found that 20% of elderly patients consumed an average daily in-hospital nutrient intake of less than 50% of their calculated maintenance energy requirements.[31] These patients had lower discharge levels of total cholesterol and albumin and prealbumin concentrations and a higher rate of in-hospital mortality.[31] Patients often had orders for nothing by mouth, and canned supplements often were not consumed.

Malnutrition is suspected in patients with a history of weight loss of 5% to 10% of their body weight over a 6-month period and physical signs of malnutrition such as muscle wasting. The laboratory evaluation of malnutrition is confounded by the effects of inflammation and chronic diseases, associated with the elaboration of cytokines and interleukins, that reduce the serum levels of nutritional markers.[32]

The subjective global assessment (SGA), a validated measure of nutritional status based on medical history and physical examination findings, accurately classifies patients as severely, moderately, or well nourished.[33] The SGA combines elements of the patient's nutrition history (weight loss in previous 6 months) and physical examination (e.g., muscle wasting) to generate a subjective impression of nutritional status.[33] In a study controlling for acute illness severity, comorbidity, and functional status, severely malnourished patients as determined by the SGI had poorer outcomes of hospitalization. They were more likely than well-nourished patients to die within 1 year of discharge; to be dependent in activities of daily living 3 months after discharge; and to spend time in a nursing home during the year after discharge.[33]

Acutely ill patients have greater nutritional requirements than well elderly patients. Nutritional consultation is warranted for patients at risk for malnutrition. Oral and enteral alimentation, with a high-protein and calorie-dense diet, are the preferred routes of nutrition. Nutritional supplements have benefits based on studies of elderly patients with femoral neck fractures or chest infections.[34,35] Food and fluids should be prescribed and monitored daily. Patients at risk for aspiration should be formally evaluated by speech therapist or by a modified barium swallow.[36] For patients with dysphagia for liquids, a pureed diet or thickened liquids may restore their ability to safely swallow and to obtain sufficient calories and hydration. Patients with severe oropharyngeal dysphagia or significant risk of aspiration may require enteral or parenteral alimentation. The placement of a nasoenteric tube should be consider for a brief duration, with the consent of patient and family for patients with malnutrition and dysphagia. Parenteral alimentation is indicated when there is a contraindication to enteral alimentation. If the patient's dysphagia is severe and unlikely to resolve in the near future, a percutaneous endoscopic gastrostomy tube may be warranted. Active patient and family participation, however, is needed in making the decision to use a feeding tube, with consideration given to the balance between potential benefits, burdens, and limitations in patients with severe irreversible illnesses.[37]

Delirium

Delirium, an acute disorder of attention and cognition, occurs in 20% to 30% of elderly patients admitted with an acute medical diagnosis. Risk factors for incident delirium in hospitalized elderly patients include baseline dementia, severe underlying illness, sensory impairment, and dehydration.[38] Delirium may be precipitated by processes of hospital care, including immobilization of the patient, use of an indwelling bladder catheter, use of physical restraints, dehydration, malnutrition, iatrogenic complications, and psychosocial factors.[39] Delirium prolongs hospital length of stay, increases costs of care, and increases the risk of nursing home placement or death.[40] Delirium can be detected through repeated observations of patients at the bedside and through application of screening instruments and scales. The

prevention and treatment of delirium are discussed in Chapter 77.

Depression

Depressive symptoms are present in 20% to 25% of medically ill elderly patients in hospital.[14] Depression may be difficult to diagnose in patients with critical illnesses or cognitive impairment. Depression may be suspected in patients who appear withdrawn, uncooperative, and intermittently agitated or have a history of functional decline, social withdrawal, and weight loss. Detection for depression is easily performed and aided by screening instruments. Therapy of patients with depression includes environmental, psychosocial, and pharmacologic interventions (see Chapter 80). Environmental changes (for example, a brighter room), physical and occupational therapy, increased frequency of family visits, and psychological counseling may be of immediate benefit to the depressed patient.

Comprehensive Discharge Planning

Comprehensive discharge planning begins on the day of hospitalization. The process of discharge planning often requires an interdisciplinary team, case manager, or advanced practice nurse.[41,42] The objectives of comprehensive discharge planning are to identify patients at risk of nursing home placement related to nonmedical issues including inadequate social support network or cognitive impairment; to estimate the patient's hospital length of stay; and to identify the need for functional assistance or formal supports at home. Patients and their families may be educated about diagnosis, prognosis, and the need for medications, home safety following discharge, and plans to coordinate posthospital care with physicians and other health professionals.

A "functional trajectory" projects the patient's discharge functional status and disposition from hospital[43] (Fig. 13.2). The functional trajectory assesses the patient's current ability to perform activities of daily living, mobility, cognition, affect, and nutritional status. This information is contrasted to the patient's baseline functional status before the acute illness and hospitalization. This review includes the patient's performance of both basic and instrumental ADL, living situation, and the patient's informal and formal support network.[43] The functional trajectory predicts nursing home placement in patients with a decline from baseline to admission in their activities of daily living.[44] Patient-centered interventions, commonly physical therapy, occupational therapy, medication review, and nutritional support, are implemented as required to achieve the anticipated discharge status and disposition.[11,43,45]

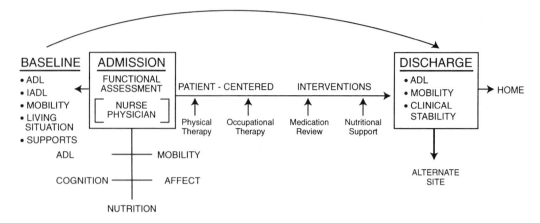

FIGURE 13.2. The functional trajectory. (From Palmer RM,[43] by permission of Marcel Dekker, Inc.)

Most medically ill older patients return home after hospitalization, but some patients will require rehabilitation, short-term nursing home care or care at other alternate sites, or home care skilled nursing services (Table 13.2). Patients with a self-limited illness who are able to perform daily activities independently may return to home without the need for formal services. Some patients will benefit from short-term skilled nursing care or other restorative services to assess, treat, or monitor new medical problems. Subacute care units or inpatient rehabilitation hospitals are appropriate options for patients with categorical illnesses, such as hip fracture or stroke, and for patients who require extensive physical therapy and skilled nursing services before their return home.[46] Home health care is warranted when patients or their families prefer to receive restorative services in the home rather than the subacute care or skilled nursing unit. However, for patients who are dependent in basic ADL, have limited rehabilitative potential, or lack adequate informal supports at home, placement in a long-term care facility may be warranted. Alternatives to hospitalization may include home care for patients with acute but nonlife-threatening illnesses, hospice or palliative care for patients with terminal illness, or direct admissions to a skilled nursing facility for patients who have managed care insurance. Discharge planning that is conducted by Advance Practice Nurses reduces the risk of hospital readmission of patients who are discharged to home.[41,42]

Patients should not be discharged from the hospital if there is evidence of clinical instability. Signs of instability on the day preceding the planned discharge include (1) a new finding of incontinence, chest pain, dyspnea, delirium, tachycardia, or hypotension; (2) temperature above 38.3°C; or (3) diastolic blood pressure of 105 mmHg or more.[47] Elderly patients who are sent home in an unstable condition have twice the risk of mortality 30 days after hospitalization compared with those whose condition is stable.

Patient Values and Comfort

The personal values and priorities of patients and the wishes of their families should be addressed early in the course of hospitalization. Hospitals are required to ascertain whether patients have Advance Directives. The patient's Advance Directive should be reviewed with the appropriate family member or power of attorney for health care throughout the hospitalization. A review of the objectives of hospitalization, the diagnostic evaluation, and probable outcome should be discussed early in hospitalization. Periodic conferences with the patient and family will serve to update them about the patient's diagnosis, prognosis, length of stay, and probable disposition.

The value of knowing the patient's values becomes most evident when considering the use of potentially futile but life-extending interventions. One study of health values in very old hospitalized patients revealed that most patients were unwilling to trade much time to live for excellent health.[48] Discussions with the patient may revolve around end-of-life care, including cardiopulmonary resuscitation, intensive care, or nutritional support in the event of acute or end-stage illness.

Although palliative care is often the most appropriate approach for patients with incurable illness, very few elderly patients with incurable illness receive palliative interventions at the end of life.[49] In a prospective study, most elderly and seriously ill patients died in acute hospitals and had pain or other troubling symptoms.[50] Spirituality may be an important predictor of hospital prognosis. In one prospective study of patients aged 60 years and older admitted with depressive symptoms to a medical unit, greater intrinsic religiosity independently predicted shorter time to remission; depressed patients with higher intrinsic religiosity scores had more rapid remissions than patients with lower scores.[51]

TABLE 13.2. Discharge disposition of hospitalized patients.

Disposition site	Patient characteristics	Usual source of payment	Example	Comments
Home without formal (paid) support services	Independent in ADL, self-limited acute illness; stable chronic disease; adequate informal (family) supports	Self	Cellulitis; acute gastroenteritis; atrial arrhythmia	Most older patients admitted to hospital from home return to independent living; greater family support often needed for a short time
Home with formal support services	Recovering independence in ADL, or return to stable baseline; good informal supports; skilled nursing care or physical therapy needed	Medicare, third party	New medications (e.g., insulin instructions); pressure ulcer; intravenous antibiotics; gastrostomy tube	Home care needs identified early in hospitalization through process of comprehensive discharge planning; skilled services covered by Medicare for finite time; "custodial" services not included; need to monitor for family caregiver strain or elder mistreatment
Subacute care/ skilled nursing unit	Dependence in ADL or ambulation preventing discharge to home; home supports adequate for chronic care, but not subacute; skilled nursing care or physical therapy needed; patient too impaired for rehabilitation hospital	Medicare, third party	Postoperative patients; intravenous antibiotics; heart failure and deconditioning	Often a fine line between patients going to rehabilitation hospital, subacute care unit, or home with formal support services; growth of subacute care is related to the greater severity of illness of hospitalized patients and increasing tendency to discharge patients "quicker and sicker"; short-term (<2 months) placement is typical
Long-term care (intermediate care) facility	Dependent in ADL; unable to return to independent living; ineligible for subacute or rehabilitative services; inadequate informal home supports (e.g., lives alone)	Self, Medicaid	Dementia; end-stage lung or heart disease	Most often needed when informal (family) supports are inadequate or the costs of home care are prohibitive
Hospice (palliative care)	Patients with terminal illness (prognosis ≤6 months)	Medicare, third party	Metastatic cancer; terminal heart failure	Provides comfort measures in home (or inpatient unit); palliative, not "curative" interventions covered; provided in hospital, home, or long-term care facility
Rehabilitation hospital	Categorical illness; likely improvement in ADL or ambulation; good home (informal) supports	Medicare, third party	Hip fracture; stroke	Eligible patients must be able to participate in physical therapy ≥3 h/day and demonstrate potential for improvement in ADL/ambulation

Personal comfort should be addressed throughout hospitalization. Privacy and quiet at night are important. Family members should be encouraged to visit patients. A normal bowel and bladder regimen is maintained with a toileting schedule, a bedside commode, or urinal for men. Fiber supplements or hyperosmolar laxatives are helpful to prevent fecal impaction in immobilized patients or those taking opiates or anticholinergic agents.

Controlled Clinical Trials Designed to Improve Outcomes of Hospitalization

Models of care designed to enhance patient functioning during hospitalization or immediately postdischarge have emerged in the past decade (Table 13.3). Early studies of hospitalized patients supported the value of comprehensive geriatric assessment when linked to direct care of selected patients.[52–54] They demonstrated that geriatric assessment units might be effective for carefully targeted patients. Subsequent clinical trials have been nurse directed or employed the interventions of geriatric consultation and acute care units. The usual objectives of the studies are to improve functional outcomes of hospitalization, reduce hospital lengths of stay, prevent nursing home admissions, or prevent rehospitalization.

The Acute Care of Elders (ACE) Unit intervention includes four main components: a prepared environment to foster patient self-care; patient-centered care, including guidelines for maintaining or restoring patient functioning; interdisciplinary team rounds; and discharge planning and medical care review.[11,43,45] ACE Units have

TABLE 13.3. Controlled clinical trials to improve outcomes of hospitalization.

Study	Design	Patients	Setting	Intervention	Primary outcome measures	Results	NNT
Inouye et al. 1993[56]	Stratified and matched cohort analysis	$N = 216$; age ≥70 years, targeted conditions	General medicine wards: two intervention, three control; university teaching hospital	Geriatric care program: Geriatric CNS Geriatric resource nurse Geriatricians on one ward Daily surveillance of Frail patients Weekly rounds	Incidence of functional decline (net loss of 1 or more basic ADL) from baseline to discharge	No benefit by stratified analysis: RR = 0.64 (95% CI, 0.43–0.96) by matched analysis (targeted conditions)	4 by matched analysis
Thomas et al. 1993[63]	Randomized clinical trial	$N = 132$ (analysis on $N = 120$) age ≥70 years	General medical and surgical wards at nonacademic community hospital	Comprehensive geriatric assessment by interdisciplinary team consultation	Mortality at 6 months	6-month mortality significantly decreased ($p = 0.01$); hospital readmissions decreased ($p = 0.02$); no significant differences in functional status	7 to prevent one death
Winograd et al. 1993[60]	Randomized clinical trial	$N = 197$; age ≥65 years; targeted conditions (frailty)	Medical and surgical services at a Veterans Affairs teaching hospital	Comprehensive geriatric assessment by interdisciplinary team consultation; limited direct patient care; limited in-service education	Differences in basic and instrumental ADL, morale, and cognition at discharge and 1 year	No differences in ADL, or morale, at discharge or follow-up for 1 year; cognition better at 1 year follow-up	N/A
Landefeld et al. 1995[11]	Randomized clinical trial	$N = 651$; age ≥70 years	General medicine wards: one intervention; university teaching hospital	Acute care of elders (ACE): Prepared environment Patient-centered care Planning for discharge Medical care review	Change in 1 or more of 5 ADL between admission and discharge	ACE improved performance of ADL ($p = 0.009$); nursing home discharges decreased ($p = -0.01$)	6 to prevent loss of 1 or more ADL; 15 to prevent first-time nursing home discharge
Reuben et al. 1995[59]	Randomized clinical trial	$N = 2553$; age ≥65 years; targeted conditions	General medicine wards, four staff-model HMO hospitals	Comprehensive geriatric assessment by an interdisciplinary team (social worker, nurse practitioner, geriatrician) after hospital admission; daily team conferences; minor changes in therapy made by geriatrician	One-year mortality	No differences in 1-year survival; no differences in functional status at 3 and 12 months	N/A

Study	Design	Population	Intervention	Outcome measures	Results	NNT
Rich et al. 1995[64]	Randomized clinical trial	N = 282; age ≥70 years; congestive heart failure, risk factors for readmission	Intensive education about CHF by cardiovascular research nurse; dietary instruction by dietitian; social service consultation; geriatric cardiologist recommendations; home care visits; telephone calls	Survival without readmission for 90 days	No differences in 90-day survival ($p = 0.09$); decrease in hospital readmissions ($p = 0.02$) and CHF readmissions ($p = 0.04$); higher quality of life; lower costs	10 to prevent survival without readmission; 8 to prevent ≥1 readmission; 5 to prevent readmission for CHF
SUPPORT Principal Investigators 1995[65]	Phase II: randomized clinical trial	Age ≥18 years (median age = 65); advanced states of ≥1 defined illnesses	Physicians given estimates of 6-month survival, outcomes of CPR and 2-month functional disability; elicit/document patient/family preferences and understanding of disease prognosis and treatment	The timing of written DNR orders; patient–physician agreement on DNR preferences; days spent in ICU comatose or on mechanical ventilation before death; pain frequency and severity; hospital resources used	No significant differences in median time to DNR order, DNR agreement, undesirable state, or resource use. No improvement in level of reported pain	N/A
Siu et al. 1996[61]	Randomized clinical trial	N = 354; age ≥65 years; unstable medical problems, recent functional decline or geriatric problems	Geriatric assessment and limited examination before discharge by nurse practitioner; home visits 1–3 days after discharge by NP; home evaluations by health professionals; interdisciplinary team meetings; recommendations to primary physicians	Nursing home admission, hospital readmission, mortality at 30 and 60 days after discharge	No differences in survival, hospital readmission or nursing home placement by 60 days; no benefits on functional status	N/A
Ronning et al. 1998[58]	Quasi-randomized clinical trial	N = 570 (analysis on 550); age ≥60 years; acute stroke	Stroke Unit: Standardized neurologic and laboratory examination aspirin multidisciplinary stroke team	Death, long-term care placement, ADL, after 7 months	No significant differences in death (OR = 0.87, 95% CI, 0.59–1.28); or long-term care	N/A

(Continued)

TABLE 13.3. *Continued*

Study	Design	Patients	Setting	Intervention	Primary outcome measures	Results	NNT
Inouye et al. 1999[57]	Controlled trial, individual matching strategy	$N = 852$; age ≥70 years; risk factors for delirium	General medical wards; one intervention, two control; university teaching hospital	Elder Life Program, targeted at six risk factors for delirium: Cognitive impairment Sleep deprivation Immobility Visual impairment Hearing impairment Dehydration Interdisciplinary team	Delirium incidence	First episode (incident) of delirium reduced (OR = 0.60, 95% CI, 0.39–0.92); total days of delirium decreased ($p = 0.02$); no difference in delirium severity	20 to prevent a first case of delirium
Naylor et al. 1999[42]	Randomized clinical trial	N-363; age ≥65 years; selected common diagnoses, risk factors for poor postdischarge outcomes	Medical and surgical services; one university and one community teaching hospital	Comprehensive discharge planning and home follow-up for 4 weeks by advanced practice nurse	Time to first hospital readmission, 24 weeks after discharge	Time to first readmission was significantly increased ($p ≤ 0.001$); readmissions decreased ($p ≤ 0.001$); fewer hospital days per patient ($p < 0.001$)	6 to prevent 1 readmission in 24 weeks
Counsell et al. 2000[55]	Randomized clinical trial	$N = 1531$; age ≥70 years	General medicine wards; one intervention; community teaching hospital	ACE Unit: Prepared environment Patient-centered care Planning for discharge Medical care review	Change in one or more of 5 ADL from 2 weeks preadmission to discharge	No significant difference in ADL ($p = 0.33$ by intent to treat, 0.07 per protocol); decreased composite outcome of ADL decline or NH placement ($p = 0.027$)	18 to prevent either ADL decline or NH placement

NH, nursing home; NP, nurse practioner; ADL, activities of daily living; NNT, number needed to treat.

shown the potential to reduce the incidence of functional decline in older patients, the length of hospital stay, and the risk of nursing home admission from hospital.[11,43,55]

In the Geriatric Care Program, a gerontologic clinical nurse specialist working with trained resource nurses focuses nursing care on patients at high risk for functional decline.[56] The intervention includes identification and monitoring of frail older patients, twice-weekly rounds of a multidisciplinary "Geriatic Care Team," and a nursing-centered educational program. In a clinical trial, when patients were matched on number of target conditions and risks for functional decline at baseline, the intervention resulted in a significant beneficial effect with a reduction in functional decline.[56]

In the Elder Life Program, patients at risk for incident delirium are identified shortly after hospital admission, using the Confusion Assessment Method.[57] An array of protocols targeted at specific risk factors serve to optimize cognitive function (reorientation, therapeutic activities), prevent sleep deprivation (relaxation, noise reduction), avoid immobility (ambulation, exercises), improve vision (visual aids, illumination), improve hearing (hearing devices), and treat dehydration (volume repletion). A clinical trial of intervention protocols targeted at risk factors for delirium resulted in a 40% reduction in the incidence of delirium but had no significant effect on the severity of delirium or on recurrence rates.[57]

Several studies demonstrate the effectiveness of specially trained nurses to coordinate discharge planning and reduce the rate of hospital readmissions of at-risk elderly patients. In one clinical trial, an advanced practice nurse-centered discharge planning and home care intervention for at-risk hospitalized elders reduced readmissions, lengthened the time between discharge and readmission, and decreased the costs of providing health care.[42]

Stroke units appear to reduce rates of patient mortality, institutionalization, and functional dependency in comparison to general medical wards, although long-term benefits are less evident.[58] The stroke unit interdisciplinary team, including the patient's physician, social worker, physical and occupational therapist, speech therapist, and neurologist, uses a systematic approach to enhance patient recovery after admission and to begin diagnostic and rehabilitative services.

In general, comprehensive geriatric assessment performed by consultation teams fails to improve functional outcomes of hospitalization.[54,59–61] However, a recent clinical trial found that comprehensive assessment on a geriatric unit reduced hospital length of stay for patents with acute and subacute illnesses.[62]

These studies in perspective offer hope that the adverse consequences of hospitalization can be attenuated through comprehensive assessment, special units, and comprehensive discharge planning.

References

1. Graves EJ, Gillum BS. National Hospital Discharge Survey: Annual Summary, 1994. National Center for Health Statistics. *Vital Health Stat.* 1997;13:128.
2. Benson V, Marano MA. Current estimates from the National Health Interview Survey, 1995. National Center for Health Statistics. *Vital Health Stat.* 1998;10:199.
3. Wolinsky FD, Stump TE, Johnson RJ. Hospital utilization profiles among older adults over time: consistency and volume among survivors and decedents. *J Gerontol (Soc Sci).* 1995;50B:S88–S100.
4. Boult C, Dowd B, McCaffrey D, et al. Screening elders for risk of hospital admission. *J Am Geriatr Soc.* 1993;41: 811–817.
5. Perls TT, Wood ER. Acute care costs of the oldest old: they cost less, their care intensity is less, and they go to non-teaching hospitals. *Arch Intern Med.* 1996;156:754– 760.
6. Teno JM, Harrell FE, Knaus W, et al. Prediction of survival for older hospitalized patients: the HELP survival model. *J Am Geriatr Soc.* 2000;48:S16–S24.
7. Schappert SM. National Hospital Ambulatory Medical Care survey: 1992 emergency department summary. National Center for Health Statistics. *Vital Health Stat.* 1997;13:125.
8. Ackermann RJ, Kemle KA, Vogel RL, et al. Emergency department use by nursing home residents. *Ann Emerg Med.* 1998;31:749–757.
9. Hirsch C, Sommers L, Olsen A, et al. The natural history of functional morbidity in hospitalized older patients. *J Am Geriatr Soc.* 1990;38:1296–1303.
10. Inouye SK, Wagner DR, Acampora D, et al. A predictive index for functional decline in hospitalized elderly medical patients. *J Gen Intern Med.* 1993;8:645–652.
11. Landefeld CS, Palmer, RM, Kresevic D, et al. A randomized trial of care in a hospital medical unit especially designed to improve the functional outcomes of acutely ill older patients. *N Engl J Med.* 1995;332:1338–1344.
12. Sager MA, Rudberg MA. Functional decline associated with hospitalization for acute illness. *Clin Geriatr Med.* 1998;14:669–679.
13. Sager MA, Franke T, Inouye SK, et al. Functional outcomes of acute medical illness and hospitalization in older persons. *Arch Intern Med.* 1996;156:645–652.
14. Covinsky KE, Fortinsky RH, Palmer RM, et al. The relationship of depressive symptoms to health outcomes in acutely ill hospitalized elders. *Ann Intern Med.* 1997;126: 417–425.
15. Wu AW, Yasui Y, Alzola C, et al. Predicting functional status outcomes in hospitalized patients aged 80 years and older. *J Am Geriatr Soc.* 2000;48:S6–S15.
16. Magaziner J, Simonsick EM, Kashner TM, et al. Predictors of functional recovery one year following hospital discharge for hip fracture: a prospective study. *J Gerontol (Med Sci).* 1990;45:M101–M107.
17. Covinsky KE, Kahana E, Chin MH, et al. Depressive symptoms and three year mortality in older hospitalized medical patients. *Ann Intern Med.* 1999;130:563–569.

18. Inouye SK, Peduzzi PN, Robinson JT, et al. Importance of functional measures in predicting mortality among older hospitalized patients. *JAMA*. 1998;279:1187–1193.

19. Palmer RM, Counsell S, Landefeld CS. Clinical intervention trials: the ACE Unit. *Clin Geriatr Med*. 1998;14:831–849.

20. Steele K, Gertman PM, Crescenzi C, et al. Iatrogenic illness on a general medical service at a university hospital. *N Engl J Med*. 1981;304:638–642.

21. Riedinger JL, Robbins LJ. Prevention of iatrogenic illness: adverse drug reactions and nosocomial infections in hospitalized older adults. *Clin Geriatr Med*. 1998;14:681–698.

22. Brennan TA, Leape LL, Laird NM, et al. Incidence of adverse events and negligence in hospitalized patients. *N Engl J Med*. 1991;324:370–376.

23. Kohn L, Corrigan J, Donaldson M, eds. *To Err Is Human: Building a Safer Health System*. Committee on Quality of Health Care In America, Institute of Medicine. Washington, DC: National Academy Press; 1999.

24. Evans RS, Pestotnik SL, Classen DC, et al. A computer-assisted management program for antibiotics and other anti-infective agents. *N Engl J Med*. 1998;338:232–238.

25. Pestotnik SL, Classen DC, Evans RS, et al. Implementing antibiotic practice guidelines through computer-assisted decision support: clinical and financial outcomes. *Ann Intern Med*. 1996;124:884–889.

26. Raschke RA, Gollihare B, Wunderlich TA, et al. A computer alert system to prevent injury from adverse drug events. Development and evaluation in a community teaching hospital. *JAMA*. 1998;280:1317–1320.

27. Bates DW, Leape LL, Cullen DJ, et al. Effect of computerized physician order entry and a team intervention on prevention of serious medication errors. *JAMA*. 1998;280:1311–1316.

28. Mahoney JE. Immobility and falls. *Clin Geriatr Med*. 1998;14:699–726.

29. Mion LC, Minnick A, Palmer R, et al. Physical restraint use in the hospital setting: unresolved issues and directions for research. *Millbank Q*. 1996;74:411–433.

30. Constans T, Bacq Y, Brechet JF, et al. Protein-energy malnutrition in elderly medical patients. *J Am Geriatr Soc*. 1992;40:263–268.

31. Sullivan DH, Sun S, Walls RC. Protein-energy undernutrition among elderly hospitalized patients. A prospective study. *JAMA*. 1999;281:2013–2019.

32. Rosenthal AJ, Sanders KM, McMurtry CT, et al. Is malnutrition overdiagnosed in older hospitalized patients? Association between the soluble interleukin-2 receptor and serum markers of malnutrition. *J Gerontol (Med Sci)*. 1998;53:M81–M86.

33. Covinsky KE, Martin GE, Beyth RJ, et al. The relationship between clinical assessment of nutritional status and adverse outcomes in older hospitalized medical patients. *J Am Geriatr Soc*. 1999;47:532–538.

34. Delmi M, Rapin CH, Bengoa JM, et al. Dietary supplementation in elderly patients with fractured neck of the femur. *Lancet*. 1990;335:1013–1016.

35. Woo J, Ho SC, Mak YT, et al. Nutritional status of elderly patients during recovery from chest infection and the possible role of nutritional supplementation assessed by a prospective, randomized, single-blind trial. *Age Ageing*. 1994;23:40–48.

36. Drickamer MA, Cooney LM. Geriatrician's guide to enteral feeding. *J Am Geriatr Soc*. 1993;41:672–679.

37. Quill TE. Utilization of nasogastric feeding tubes in a group of chronically ill, elderly patients in a community hospital. *Arch Intern Med*. 1989;149:1937–1941.

38. Inouye SK, Viscoli CM, Horwitz RI, et al. A predictive model for delirium in hospitalized elderly medical patients based on admission characteristics. *Ann Intern Med*. 1993;119:474–481.

39. Inouye SK, Charpentier PA. Precipitating factors for delirium in hospitalized elderly persons. Predictive model and interrelationship with baseline vulnerability. *JAMA*. 1996;275:852–857.

40. Inouye SK, Rushing JT, Foreman MD, et al. Does delirium contribute to poor hospital outcomes? A three-site epidemiologic study. *J Gen Intern Med*. 1998;13:234–242.

41. Naylor M, Brooten D, Jones R, et al. Comprehensive discharge planning for the hospitalized elderly. A randomized clinical trial. *Ann Intern Med*. 1994;120:999–1006.

42. Naylor MD, Brooten D, Campbell R, et al. Comprehensive discharge planning and home follow-up of hospitalized elders. A randomized clinical trial. *JAMA*. 1999;281:613–620.

43. Palmer RM. Acute hospital care: future directions. In: Yoshikawa TT, Norman DC, eds. *Acute Emergencies and Critical Care of the Geriatric Patient*. New York: Dekker; 2000;461–486.

44. Fortinsky RH, Covinsky KE, Palmer RM, et al. Effects of functional status changes before and during hospitalization on nursing home admission of older adults. *J Gerontol Med Sci*. 1999;54:M521–M526.

45. Palmer RM, Landefeld CS, Kresevic D, et al. A medical unit for the acute care of the elderly. *J Am Geriatr Soc*. 1994;42:545–552.

46. Mistry PR, Sandhu S, Hopkins M. Subacute care: which patients benefit? *Clevel Clin J Med*. 1999;66:443–446.

47. Brook RH, Kahn KL, Kosecoff J. Assessing clinical instability at discharge. The clinician's responsibility. *JAMA*. 1992;268:1321–1322.

48. Tsevat J, Dawson NV, Wu AW, et al. Health values of hospitalized patients 80 years or older. *JAMA*. 1998;279:371–375.

49. Ahronheim JC, Morrison RS, Baskin SA, et al. Treatment of the dying in the cute care hospital: advanced dementia and metastatic cancer. *Arch Intern Med*. 1996;156:2094–2100.

50. Lynn J, Teno JM, Phillips RS, et al. Perceptions by family members of the dying experience of older and seriously ill patients. *Ann Intern Med*. 1997;126:97–106.

51. Koenig HG, George LK, Peterson BL. Religiosity and remission of depression in medically ill older patients. *Am J Psychiatry*. 1998;155:536–542.

52. Rubenstein LZ, Josephson KR, Wieland GD, et al. Effectiveness of a geriatric evaluation unit. A randomized clinical trial. *N Engl J Med*. 1984;311:1664–1670.

53. Applegate WB, Miller ST, Graney MJ, et al. A randomized controlled trial of a geriatric assessment unit in a community rehabilitation hospital. *N Engl J Med*. 1990;22:1572–1578.

54. Stuck AE, Siu Al, Wieland GD, et al. Comprehensive geriatric assessment: a meta-analysis of controlled trials. *Lancet.* 1993;342:1032–1036.
55. Counsell SR, Holder CM, Liebenauer LL, et al. Effects of a multicomponent intervention on functional outcomes and process of care in hospitalized older patients: A randomized controlled trial of acute care of elders (ACE) in a community hospital. *J Am Geriatr Soc.* 2000.
56. Inouye SK, Wagner DR, Acampora D, et al. A controlled trial of a nursing-centered intervention in hospitalized elderly medical patients: the Yale geriatric program. *J Am Geriatr Soc.* 1993;41:1353–1360.
57. Inouye SK, Bogardus ST, Carpentier PA, et al. A multicomponent intervention to prevent delirium in hospitalized older patients. *N Engl J Med.* 1999;340:669–676.
58. Ronning OM, Guldvog B. Stroke units versus general medical wards. I: 12- and 18-month survival. A randomized, controlled trial. *Stroke.* 1998;29:58–62.
59. Reuben DB, Borok GM, Wolde-Tsadik G, et al. A randomized trial of comprehensive geriatric assessment in the care of hospitalized patients. *N Engl J Med.* 1995;332:345–1350.
60. Winograd CH, Gerety MV, Lai NA. A negative trial of inpatient geriatric consultation. Lessons learned and recommendations for future research. *Arch Intern Med.* 1993;153:2017–2023.
61. Sui AL, Kravitz RL, Keeler E, et al. Post-discharge geriatric assessment of hospitalized frail elderly patients. *Arch Intern Med.* 1996;156:76–81.
62. Nikolaus T, Specht-Leible N, Bach M, et al. A randomized trail of comprehensive geriatric assessment and home intervention in the care of hospitalized patients. *Age Ageing.* 1999;28:543–550.
63. Thomas DR, Brahan R, Haywood BP. In-patient community-based geriatric assessment reduces subsequent mortality. *J Am Geriatr Soc.* 1993;41:101–104.
64. Rich MW, Beckham V, Wittenberg C, et al. A multidisciplinary intervention to prevent the readmission of elderly patients with congestive heart failure. *N Engl J Med.* 1995;333:1190–1195.
65. The SUPPORT principal investigators. A controlled trial to improve care for seriously ill hospitalized patients. The study to understand prognoses and preferences for outcomes and risks of treatments (SUPPORT). *JAMA.* 1995;274:1591–1598.

Part III
Clinical Approaches to the Geriatric Patient

14
Clinical Approach to the Older Patient: An Overview

Glendo L. Tangarorang, Gerard J. Kerins, and Richard W. Besdine

Impact of Aging on Disease

Health and Disease Behavior in Older Adults

Health and disease behavior in older adults refers both to differences in the way diseases behave when occurring in older persons and to differences in the way older persons behave when afflicted with disease.[1] Behavior is the summation of social, cultural, psychologic, and clinical influences. Perceived severity of illness, the impact of disease on everyday function, denial, and local resources for help all play into behavior.[2,3]

Although *self-perception of health* is heavily influenced by an individual's disease burden and its current activity, norms and expectations concerning health in the group against which one measures health and dependence also can be powerful determinants of perceived health.[4] A robust 80-year-old widow, independent in a community of active and energetic retired persons, self-sufficient in ADL (activities of daily living), IADL (instrumental ADLs), and executive functions, is likely to perceive difficulty walking or remembering which of the 20 identical entrance doors on the street is hers far more seriously than is her cousin living in a nursing home.

Aging is associated with a decline in expectation of healthiness. Those over age 65 generally give more positive evaluations of their healthiness in the face of increasing burden of disease and disability.[5,6] The older the person, the more likely they are to report very good health status.[7] However, overestimating healthiness (also called normalization) often results in explaining away symptoms or problems as caused by minor illnesses or even by external events. In either case, late recognition and delayed intervention are the usual outcome. Previous neglect of symptoms by health care professionals is also likely to teach older patients that frailty and loss of independence are normal and to be expected with aging; again, late detection and intervention are likely, resulting in high cost and discouraging outcomes. Perhaps these attitudes explain the finding of greater pessimism in older persons compared with those middle-aged, even when health status was factored in.[4]

Underreporting of symptoms is a common theme in discussions of illness behavior of older persons. First reported in the 1950s by Scottish geriatricians who screened older individuals and discovered surprising numbers of unrecognized disorders,[8,9] underreporting has been documented repeatedly. Major burdens of unreported and thus undiagnosed and untreated medical conditions were detected in these investigations. The British studies are doubly noteworthy. First, all patients were served by the National Health Service, which appeared to have requisite features for satisfactory geriatric care. All enrollees had a designated primary care community physician, who received an annual sum to provide care at no cost to the patient. Second, the problems identified were common and usually treatable diseases[9]; congestive heart failure, correctable hearing and vision deficits, tuberculosis, incontinence, anemia, bronchitis, claudication, cancers, malnutrition, diabetes, immobility, oral disease preventing eating, dementia, and depression were frequent.

Shanas reported that 90% of community-dwelling persons had symptoms in the previous 30 days, but only 30% had consulted their physicians about them.[10] When relatives were questioned about their older family members, one-third responded that medical care was insufficient; they further thought that their elderly relatives attributed most of their symptoms to aging, not disease. Brody also demonstrated minimizing of problems[11]; of 20 potentially serious symptoms (e.g., chest pain, bleeding, shortness of breath, ankle swelling, unsteady on feet), only a slight majority were reported at all, and most of the reports were to a family member rather than a health professional. Explanations were "no big deal; nobody cares; nothing can be done about it" or "don't want to bother people."

Considerable underreporting was also seen among people with chronic diseases. More than half of chronically ill individuals who were surveyed in one study failed to report at least one disease. "Number of diseases" and age were notable factors that independently accounted for this problem.[12] In another survey of community-dwelling elderly people, the independent influence of age on reporting chronic diseases was again demonstrated. Older people tend to inaccurately report cardiac disease, arthritis, and stroke.[13]

Among patients seen in the emergency room for chest pain due to cardiac ischemia, elderly patients were more likely to wait more than 6 h before going to the emergency room, even though more than half of them had documented coronary artery disease. Among elderly (70–80 years old) and very elderly patients (>80 years old) whose chest pain represented acute myocardial infarction, hospital mortality was double and triple, respectively, when compared to that in younger patients (<70 years old).[14]

Morgan et al.[15] emphasized the need for increased health education in older people. Morgan reported that many symptoms classically associated with common diseases were often considered by community-dwelling elderly *to be normal for old people.* Some important symptoms, such as blackouts or paralysis of a limb, were understandably not considered to be normal. However, although nonspecific symptoms of psychiatric disturbances were also frequently considered not normal, they were not considered to represent disease. Whether a doctor would be consulted was often, but not always, related to whether a symptom was thought to represent a disease.[15]

In addition to provider-related reasons, failure by older persons to recognize symptoms as abnormal may help explain why depression is frequently underreported and undertreated.[16] Undetected depression in older persons assumes more importance, because it has been shown that, compared with younger suicide cases, older suicides planned more carefully the fatal suicide attempt, *and* they were more secretive about their intent.[17] Even among patients meeting full criteria for major depression, aging is associated with a sharp decrease in self-reported depressive symptoms, as measured by the Beck Depression Inventory.[18] In fact, among older adults, depression is commonly underdiagnosed and undertreated.[19] As a result, clinicians should be cautious in using screening instruments (e.g., Geriatric Depression Scale) or accepting self-report data when trying to exclude depression.

Although the oldest subjects had the highest levels of health-promoting behavior, they were also least likely to take action in response to symptoms of serious illness.[20] In one study, older patients with community-acquired pneumonia reported respiratory and nonrespiratory symptoms less commonly than younger patients, even after controlling for increased comorbidity and severity of illness.[21] Older persons most often attributed symptoms to aging and reacted to those symptoms by (1) waiting and watching, (2) accepting symptoms, (3) denying danger, or (4) delaying or rejecting medical care. Although underreporting of symptoms by older persons has been identified as a common illness behavior with dangerous consequences, many clinicians have an image of older patients with infinite complaints whose investigation lead nowhere. As with many "old saws" about older persons, the stereotypical image of hypochondriacal older patients could not be documented.[22] Instead, it appears that hypochondriasis is less common among older people than among the middle-aged. In addition, among nonhypochondriacal patients, complaints in older adults are more often "validated" by the identification of disease than in younger persons.[23]

The riskiness of underreporting of symptoms by older patients is obvious; late identification of disease leads to late initiation of treatment, usually after substantial morbidity associated with advanced pathology has already occurred and caused major functional losses. Rehabilitation to independence from these losses is difficult; permanent dependence in spite of "successful" treatment may occur. The message to clinicians is clear: aggressive case-finding and surveillance of at-risk older persons is necessary to prevent perpetuation of the discouraging and expensive pattern of late discovery of disease resulting from insufficient symptom reporting by older patients.[24] This aggressive approach must include the patient, and family when appropriate, in the decision process when surveillance uncovers the need for more intensive investigation and intervention. It may be that underreporting is a cohort phenomenon, likely to abate as contemporary generations of Americans age, aware of the benefits of medical intervention and having heightened consciousness of wellness. For the present, clinicians should expect symptom underreporting by their older patients.

The Role of Cultural Diversity

Cultural beliefs and factors exert important influences on provision of medical care to older adults. Social supports, perceptions of wellness or illness, and health expectations are all influenced by one's cultural beliefs. Use of alternative and nontraditional therapies may also be culturally based and must be considered when providing medical care. Recent data suggest that African-American and Hispanic women use complementary and alternative medicine for a wide range of health conditions.[25] Social supports that may affect health care utilization and use of long-term care can be influenced by culture and tradition, which vary greatly among different ethnic and socioeconomic groups. Accordingly, appreciating the influence of cultural diversity and beliefs on health and health care demands that physicians and other providers understand diversity and its relationship to care.[26]

Goldstein and Griswold[27] point out that the challenge to acquire competence and sensitivity in dealing with patients of diverse cultures is especially important for health professionals in gateway cities, in urban communities along the U.S. border, and in rural areas with migrant workers or Native Americans. The broad categories commonly used to define ethnic minorities—African-Americans, American and Alaskan Natives, Asian-Americans, and Hispanics—do not capture the wide array of cultural differences that can affect definition of illness and selection of treatment. It is important to view elders with multicultural sensitivity and to understand that there may be great heterogeneity within cultural or ethnic groups.[27] Clinicians should always consider the epidemiology of diseases in various cultures, the acculturation process, and the potential for misdiagnosis resulting from cultural differences. Another unique challenge is presented by the care of persons who have come to the United States in late life, often to join sons and daughters who previously emigrated.[27] Continuing research is addressing these issues.

Multiple Pathology

Multiple pathology, or concurrence of diseases, is common among older persons. An early Scottish study of community-dwelling persons over age 65 reported 3.5 major problems per person[9]; for those being admitted to hospitals, 6 disorders were documented per patient.[28]

Multiple pathology poses multiple risks to older patients and their physicians.[29] The first hazard is that active medical problems frequently interact with one another to the detriment of the patient—*disease–disease interactions*. The more frail and delicately compensated the patient, the more quickly unattended disease produces major functional losses; these can be permanent in spite of subsequent detection and treatment.

Illustrative is the story of a 70-year-old community-dwelling widow who walks slowly and limps because of left knee pain, who chews incompletely because of gum pain, who sees poorly, and who has urinary urgency and "a touch of diabetes." She develops lethargy and fever over several days, and oral intake declines; one night, on her way to the bathroom to urinate, she is incontinent of a large volume of urine. Stepping into the puddle, she slips, falls backward onto her right greater trochanter, and sustains a hip fracture. In the hospital, preoperative evaluation identifies hyperosmolar dehydration resulting from out-of-control diabetes and right intertrochanteric hip fracture. Bacteremia is discovered; it and fever are attributed to periodontal abscess. Treatment is initiated for all these conditions and, on the 5th day, the hip fracture is successfully repaired with a compression screw.

That night, she develops atrial fibrillation; evaluation reveals transmural myocardial infarction. Over the next 5 days, although hemodynamically stable, she is in and out of atrial fibrillation; she is found hemiplegic and aphasic on the 6th postoperative day. Evaluation reveals mural thrombus and left ventricular clot. After a 2-week hospitalization, she is discharged to a nursing home, doubly incontinent, confused, aphasic, and requiring total nursing care.

Her prefracture problem list of (1) degenerative osteoarthritis of the knee causing slow gait, (2) atrophic vaginitis causing urinary urgency, (3) osteoporosis, (4) cataracts, (5) periodontal disease, (6) type II diabetes mellitus, and (6) coronary insufficiency had never been assembled or considered by her physician, who thought of her as a "delightful old dear." Her root caries and gingivitis had never been treated, nor had her difficulty with chewing been considered as a risk factor for dehydration. Her gait had not been evaluated, either for primary treatment of the underlying arthritis nor for support with a walking aid. Her cataracts had not been considered, nor had her vaginitis been identified or treated with estrogens for comfort or reduction of urinary urgency; her osteoporosis had not been addressed. Late detection of treatable problems whose neglect and interaction have led to functional decline is common in older patients and can be one of the few discouraging features of geriatric care. Preventive dental and medical care could have avoided the sepsis, worsening of diabetes, fall, hip fracture, postoperative heart attack, stroke, and loss of independent living.

A second risk is that unidentified multiple pathologies can interact with diagnostic studies or treatment undertaken to manage a diagnosed problem and produce iatrogenic harm, or *disease–treatment interaction*. An 82-year-old man with coronary heart disease and impaired systolic function presents to an urgi-center for shortness of breath; treatment is begun with furosemide and digoxin, resulting in reduced symptoms and improved physical findings. Diabetes mellitus (type II, diet-controlled), prostatism, and early Parkinsonian gait are not considered. Dehydration is precipitated by furosemide and exacerbated by poor oral intake resulting when his already loose upper denture falls out and breaks. The intense diuresis also results in urinary retention with overflow incontinence. Blood sugar rises and further exacerbates dehydration. Now confused, dribbling urine, and unsteady, he falls, hits his head on the toilet, and sustains a subdural hematoma. The clinical outcome is dismal; no longer able to walk, confused, and afflicted with three pressure sores and a urethral catheter, he requires permanent nursing home residence. Ignoring his (1) poorly fitting dentures, (2) diabetes, (3) prostatism, and (4) gait difficulty has transformed a well-intentioned intervention into an iatrogenic catastrophe.

Functional Loss

Functional loss is a final common pathway for most clinical problems in older persons, especially in persons over age 75.[30] Additionally, it may be the only sign or symptom of important underlying disease when more specific and typical symptoms of a particular disease are absent. Functional impairment means decreased ability to meet one's own needs and is easily measured by assessing activities of daily living (ADL) and instrumental activities of daily living (IADL). In addition, objective assessments of cognition and behavior and of social, economic, and emotional state are required to document health-related function of older persons[31–35] (see Chapter 17). A systematic literature review[36] identified risk factors highly correlate with functional decline, including cognitive impairment, depression, comorbidity/disease burden, increased and decreased body mass index, lower extremity functional limitation, low frequency of social contacts, low level of physical activity, no alcohol use compared to moderate use, poor self-perceived health, smoking, and vision impairment. Among the very old (85 years and older), impaired functioning and cognition predict institutionalization.[6]

Presentation of illness in older persons less often is a single, specific symptom or sign, which in younger patients, announces the organ with pathology. Older persons often present with nonspecific problems that are in fact functional deficits.[29,37] Stopping eating and drinking, or the new onset of falls, confusion, lethargy, dizziness, or incontinence in older patients may be the primary or sole manifestation of diseases with classic signs and symptoms in the young (e.g., pneumonia, myocardial infarction, pulmonary embolus, alcoholism or myxedema). These deficits have been named *geriatric syndromes*; they devastate independence without producing obvious or typical indications of disease. Geriatric syndromes may be defined as a set of lost specific functional capacities potentially caused by a multiplicity of pathologies in multiple organ systems. For example, dizziness among community-dwelling elderly people was shown to be associated with seven characteristics: anxiety; depressive symptoms; impaired hearing; use of five or more medications; postural hypotension; impaired balance, and past myocardial infarction.[38] Comprehensive evaluation is usually required to identify and treat underlying causes. Although in many instances a geriatric syndrome has several contributing causes, remedying even one or a few may result in major functional improvement.

Nonspecific Presentation of Disease

The most likely explanation for nonspecific presentation is that the additive effects of aging restrict capacity to maintain homeostasis. Perturbation of homeostasis by disease, trauma, or drug toxicity will be manifest in the most vulnerable organ, or weakest link, resulting from interactions of biologic aging and chronic disease. The locus of deficit, which reliably identifies the root of pathology in younger patients (immobility originates in musculoskeletal or neurologic disorders, confusion arises from brain disease, incontinence stems from urinary tract problems, and undernutrition is gastrointestinal), is a less reliable guide in older patients. Instead, especially vulnerable systems are likely to decompensate from systemic impact of disease anywhere in the body. The lesson for physicians and for older persons and their families is that functional loss, especially if abrupt, is a reliable sign of disease; rapid and comprehensive evaluation is the only appropriate clinical response.

Altered Presentation of Disease

In addition to nonspecific presentation, disease in older patients can present in other atypical ways. Blunting or absence of typical or classic symptoms and signs is well described in many conditions.[39–44] In a study of 55 elderly patients presenting to the emergency room with suspected hypovolemia, seven signs correlated best with dehydration: confusion; extremity weakness; nonfluent speech; dry mucous membranes; dry tongue; furrowed tongue; and sunken eyes. None of these findings is particularly helpful when present in isolation.[39] Painless myocardial infarction[41,42] is well documented as more common in older patients. Hypothyroidism has been shown in a prospective study to occur with fewer symptoms and to be more difficult to diagnose in older patients.[43] Likewise, among patients 70 years and older, hyperthyroidism *infrequently* presented with tremor, hyperactive reflexes, increased sweating, heat intolerance, nervousness, polydipsia, and increased appetite. More commonly found in the older hyperthyroid patients than in younger patients were anorexia and atrial fibrillation. Only three signs occurred in more than half the older patients: tachycardia, fatigue, and weight loss. Goiter, seen in 94% of younger patients, presented in only 50% of the older subjects.[44] Osler first drew attention to the muted picture of lobar pneumococcal pneumonia: "Pneumonia in the aged may be latent and set in without a chill; the cough and expectoration are slight, the physical signs ill-defined and changeable, and the constitutional symptoms out of all proportion to the extent of the local lesion."[45] Finally, a few diseases have specific presentations usually found only in older patients; diabetes out of control presents as hyperosmolar state,[46,47] hyperthyroidism presents as apathetic thyrotoxicosis,[48] and depression presents as blunted cognition.[49–51]

Evaluating the Patient

Much of what has been written on evaluation of the older patient is simply attention to the details of careful clinical assessment. Contemporary emphasis on efficiency and effectiveness of clinical care requires thoughtfulness about any extension of the already lengthy evaluation of complex chronic medical problems that commonly cluster in older persons. Brief screening questions rather than elaborate instruments are appropriate for first encounters[52]; more detailed assessment should be reserved for patients with demonstrated deficits.[35] Even at its most parsimonious, the initial evaluation of older patients with multiple disorders and treatments will generally be prolonged, as compared with time needed for younger persons. Dividing the new patient assessment into two sessions can spare both patient and physician an exhausting and inefficient 2-h encounter. Other office personnel can collect much information by questionnaire before the visit, from previous records, and from patient and family before the physician's contact. It is essential that good care, fully informed by current geriatrics knowledge, be delivered within a reasonable time allocation consistent with contemporary patterns of primary care. One hour for a new visit and 30 min for a follow-up are an absolute maximum in most environments.

Completing a home visit may also provide valuable insight into a patient's environment and daily functional status. How mobility may affect function in a particular environment, real insight into nutrition, medication use and compliance, and social interactions and support can all be assessed quickly by a home visit. In one well-designed trial, in-home comprehensive geriatric assessment delayed onset of disability and reduced future need for skilled placement.[53] Medicare now provides appropriate reimbursement for a home visit with the proper code (CPT code 99341–99350, depending on the various conditions). Comprehensive geriatric evaluation and management by an interdisciplinary team in selected populations may improve overall health outcomes, maintain function, and possibly reduce health care utilization[54,55] (see Chapter 18).

The Setting

Ambulatory Office Care

The common occurrence of physical frailty among older persons demands particular attention to providing both a comfortable and safe environment for evaluation. Autonomic dysfunction, reflected by the occurrence of accidental hypothermia and hyperthermia, is commonly encountered in older persons and increases vulnerability to excessively cool or warm settings, especially when the patient is dressed appropriately to the outside temperature. Accordingly, examining rooms should be kept between 70°F and 80°F. Brighter lighting is required for adequate perception of the physician's facial expression and gestures by the older patient, whose lenses admit less than half the light they did in youth, due to cross-linking of lens proteins.

Presbycusis (present in >50% of older persons) makes background noise more distracting and interferes with the patient's hearing. Even in a quiet setting, the high-tone loss of presbycusis makes consonants most difficult to discriminate; speaking in a lower-than-usual pitch will help the patient hear, and facing the patient directly will improve communication by allowing lip reading. The patient's eyeglasses, dentures (to enhance the patient's speech), and hearing aid (with a functional battery) should always be brought to and used at the physician visit. Chairs with a higher-than-standard seat or a mechanical lift to assist in arising are useful for frail older persons with quadriceps weakness, and a broad-based step stool with handrail can make mounting and dismounting the examining table safe. Drapes for the patient should not exceed ankle length so as not to be a risk for tripping and falling.

The Acute Hospital or Nursing Home

The patient room is commonly the site of evaluation for the nursing home resident or hospitalized older adult. Little is different in evaluating older persons in the hospital; the patient is usually confined to bed, so that safety and comfort are dictated by the hospital amenities. All other considerations relevant in the ambulatory setting apply. Respect demands either drawing the privacy curtain or, in the nursing home, asking a roommate to leave if possible. In the nursing home, a good strategy, if space allows, is to do everything except emergency evaluation and treatment in set-aside office space rather than in the resident's room. The room is home for the resident; using that space for clinical purposes risks implying that the resident has no personal space and that the room and bed are part of the medical care environment. Privacy and identification of the nursing home room as living space, rather than medical care space, are important issues for the nursing home resident and staff.

The History

Although it is important to discover the patient's "reliability" as soon as possible, one should not simply dismiss patients with dementia as unreliable and confine data collection to other informants or previous records.[52] Dementia produces a spectrum of cognitive function loss, ranging from detectable only on exhaustive neuropsychologic testing to mutism or gibberish. Beginning history taking with questions whose answers will illuminate mental status (e.g., time and place orientation, reasons for the visit, previous health care contacts, biographic data, problem solving) can quickly establish credibility of responses.[56] Even in cases of severe impairment, questions concerning current symptoms may still give useful information,[57] and interaction at any level is an essential part of conveying a caring and respectful attitude.

Regardless of mental status, it is common for older patients to be accompanied by family members. Always give the patient the option of being interviewed and examined alone; including family members or companions during the visit should only occur at the patient's request. Certain older adults may be more comfortable meeting the physician with others present, but this decision should be left to the patient.

Generally, it is best to ask if the patient wants a relative or other concerned person present for history or physical examination; getting *some* time alone with the patient is essential for the patient to communicate any information he or she regards as confidential for the physician.[58] If the relative is present during the history, it is critical to make clear that *the patient* is to answer all questions; the relative should answer only if the physician asks for clarification. In cases of cognitive impairment or simply a long and complex history, family members, previous medical records, and other providers can provide supplementary data.

Structuring the History

A single or chief complaint is less common among older patients; more often, multiple diseases and problems have multiple symptoms and complaints associated with them. Accordingly, trying to structure the history in the standard format of "chief complaint," "history of present illness," and "past medical history" usually results in frustration for the clinician. More useful is the enumeration of a comprehensive problem list, followed by complaints, recent and interval history, and remote information for each of the active problems being considered at a visit. The first evaluation, regardless of setting, requires creating a complete database; its future utility justifies the initial time allocation. It may be easiest to commence the history with an open-ended question, such as "What do you feel interferes most with your day-to-day activities?" Such a question is usually very helpful in focusing the clinical evaluation.

Another common finding in older patients is that the law of parsimony, or Occam's razor, is not valid—multiple complaints and abnormal findings arise from multiple diseases; discovering a diagnosis that unifies multiple signs, symptoms, and laboratory data is uncommon and, although welcome in patients of any age, should not be expected in older persons. The classic paradigm in which clinical findings lead directly to a unifying diagnosis has been found to operate in fewer than half of older patients studied; other models, which included major roles for comorbidities, for functional status, and for psychosocial factors, were found to operate in 60% of patients evaluated.[59]

Medications

The importance of collecting and inquiring about each and every medication taken by or in the possession of the older patient cannot be overemphasized.[60] Older adults often take duplicate, overlapping, and conflicting drugs,[61] usually acquired from multiple prescribing physicians and over-the-counter sources. All drugs owned by the patient, including supplements, herbals, vitamins, laxatives, sleeping pills, and cold preparations, should be gathered from bathroom cabinet, bedside table, purse, kitchen drawer, and relatives and brought to the office visit. Ask patients specifically about food and vitamin supplements and the use of any other alternative medications or remedies they may take. A national survey of alternative medicine use in the United States documented that 42% of 2055 adults used alternative therapies during the previous year, mostly for chronic conditions such as back pain, anxiety, depression, and headache. In addition, a sizable number of people who are taking alternative medicines fail to inform the clinician, emphasizing the need for the clinician to specifically inquire about nonprescription drug use.[62] All containers should be placed on a table and the patient asked how often each drug is taken and for what, if any, symptomatic indication.[60] Consider review of all types of medications every 3 months. Ascertaining pneumococcal, influenza, and tetanus vaccination status can be conveniently done as part of the medication history.

In the hospital, caution should be exercised in ordering all drugs that have been prescribed; toxic accumulation of one or several agents is common, usually because the patient has not been taking prescribed medications as instructed. "Self-protective nonadherence" to the regimen, often in response to adverse reactions when drugs were taken as ordered, has led to reduction in dosage or frequency by the patient. Return to originally prescribed schedules produces toxicity.

In the nursing home, the major additional caution concerns the continued administration of unnecessary drugs that were initiated for transient problems arising during hospitalization. Sedative, antipsychotic, diuretic, antiarrhythmic, and anti-infective drugs are often continued indefinitely at the nursing home on the incorrect assumption that they are needed.[63] Careful winnowing of the medication list is indicated at least every 3 months and following any hospitalization.

Social History

Crucial information for developing a coherent and feasible care plan at home includes detailed knowledge of any change in living arrangements, who is available at home or in the local community, and what plans if any exist for coverage in times of illness or functional decline. Although a home visit is the best way to evaluate risks or limitations, inquiring about stairs, rugs, thresholds, bathing facilities, heating, and crime can increase the care plan's utility. Stable and durable plans for care at home both fulfill the patient's goal to remain at home and the system's goal to control costs of institutional care. Extent of social relationships is a powerful predictor of functional status and mortality for older adults[64]; accordingly, determining the patient's friendship network and recommending ideas for increased socialization can be an appropriate clinical role. Even social and productive activities that involve little or no physical exertion may lower the risk of all cause mortality as much as fitness activities do.[65] Encouraging older persons to become involved with local senior center activities may be one mechanism to enhance social relationships, reduce isolation, and improve daily functioning.

Nutrition History

Although independent elders in the community are generally adequately nourished, the prevalence of under- and overnutrition increases in older persons. Undernutrition is most often unrecognized.[66] Most of the undernutrition occurs in those with chronic diseases that directly or indirectly interfere with nutrition. Oral or gastrointestinal disorders, drug effects on appetite, systemic illness, and psychiatric disease increase the risk of undernutrition. Screening questions include a diet history (within the past few days), pattern of weight during recent years, and shopping and food preparation habits.[67] Other questions should include any recent intentional efforts to gain or lose weight or any history of eating disorders. Sites of eating, companionship, and skipped meals are also relevant. Serum albumin is a good marker of nutritional status over the preceding 3 months and is correlated with mortality rates.[68] The prealbumin reflects nutrition during the past 20 days.

Although it is not strictly part of the nutritional history, this is a convenient time to inquire about alcohol and tobacco use. Alcohol misuse by older persons is often overlooked in all but florid situations, in part because symptoms and signs are often attributed to other problems common in older persons.[69] However, alcohol-related hospitalizations are more common than expected, as frequent as for myocardial infarction.[70] Alcohol can dramatically affect health status and function. Furthermore, alcoholism increases the older patient's risk of

dying within 2 years.[71] Accordingly, it is important to include routine questions in the history[72]; the CAGE (*Cut down, Annoyed, Guilty feelings, Eye-opener*) questionnaire has been validated in older persons.[73] In a study of 120 elderly male veterans, the MAST-G (Michigan Alcoholism Screening Test—Geriatric Version) and the CAGE had comparable sensitivity and specificity (70% and 81%, respectively, for MAST-G score ≥5, and 63% and 82% for CAGE score ≥2). The CAGE is more useful, as it requires only four easily memorized questions.[74] A positive response to two of four questions has traditionally been considered a positive screen. However, in a patient population with high prevalence of drinking problems, even a score of one should trigger appropriate investigation.[75] In elderly medical outpatients, the CAGE may miss half the cases of alcohol abuse or dependence.[76] Occult alcohol ingestion contributing to cognitive deficits, falls, depression, and exacerbation of diabetes or heart disease is common; specific questions are required for detection. Smoking cessation at any age, even beyond 80, rapidly improves health[77,78]; a minority of physicians counsel older persons to quit.

Family History

Although causes of mortality among relatives are usually irrelevant, history of Alzheimer's disease or nonspecified dementia appears to be important. Likewise, certain psychiatric disorders, such as depression and dysthymia, appear to cluster within families. From a mental health perspective, the medical family history also can identify caregiving *by* the older person. Caregiving of a disabled spouse and its attendant stress confer substantial mortality risk for the caregiver. Persons who were providing care and who were experiencing strain have a 50% greater risk of dying within 4 years, compared to noncaregiving controls.[79]

Sexual History

Older persons continue to be sexually active unless inhibited by the absence of a partner or the occurrence of a disease that reduces libido, makes intercourse painful, or prevents it mechanically.[80] Discomfort or awkwardness may result from physician rather than patient attitudes; a simple open-ended question, such as "Tell me about your sex life" or "Are you satisfied with sex?" may encourage the older person to give information not spontaneously reported.

Miscellaneous History

Routine questions should be asked regarding driving habits, seatbelt use, recreational activities, and gambling history. The Lie/Bet questionnaire[81] may be a useful screening tool. A positive response to either of two ques-

TABLE 14.1. Brief screening instrument for common problems in older persons.

Problem	Screening measure	Positive screen
Vision	Two parts: Ask: "Do you have difficulty driving or watching television, or reading, or doing any of your daily activities because of your eyesight? If yes, then: Test each eye with Snellen chart while patient wears corrective lenses (if applicable)	Yes to question and inability to read greater than 20/40 on Snellen chart
Hearing or	Use audioscope set at 40 dB	Inability to hear 1000 or 2000 Hz in both ears
	Test hearing using 1000 and 2000 Hz	either of these frequencies in one ear
Leg mobility	Time the patient after asking: "Rise from the chair; walk 20 feet briskly, turn, walk back to the chair, and sit down"	Unable to complete task in 15 s
Urinary incontinence	Two parts: Ask: "In the last year, have you ever lost your urine and gotten wet?" If yes, then ask: "Have you lost urine on at least 6 separate days?"	Yes to both questions
Nutrition/weight loss	Two parts: Ask: "Have you lost 10 lb over the past 6 months without trying to do so?" Weigh the patient	Yes to the question or weight <100 lb
Memory	Three-item recall	Unable to remember all three items in 1 min
Depression	Ask: "Do you often feel sad or depressed?"	Yes to the question
Physical disability	Six questions: Are you able to: "Do strenuous activities like fast walking or bicycling?" "Do heavy work around the house like washing windows, walls, or floors?" "Go shopping for groceries or clothes?" "Get to places out of walking distance?" "Bathe, either a sponge bath or shower?" "Dress, like putting on a shirt, buttoning and zipping, or putting on shoes?"	No to any of the questions

Source: Modified with permission from Moore AA, Siu AL.[85]

tions: (1) "Have you ever felt the need to bet more and more money?" and (2) "Have you ever had to lie to people important to you about how much you gambled?" is highly sensitive and specific for a gambling problem.

Functional Status

Data support the validity of self-reported physical functional status. The patient should be asked screening questions about independence and self-care—ability to get out of bed, dress, shop, and cook.[82,83] Any reported or observed difficulty should provoke more elaborate questions concerning dependence in activities of daily living (ADLs: mobility, bathing, transferring, toileting, continence, dressing, hygiene, and feeding[84]) and in instrumental activities of daily living (IADLs: shopping, cooking, cleaning, managing money, telephoning, laundry, and travel out of house[28]). Questions should also be asked about vision, hearing, continence, and depression; deficits should be followed up. A brief screening instrument for common impairments,[85] administered by trained nonmedical personnel, was found to be inexpensive and clinically useful (i.e., good validity and reliability). Appropriate use of such an instrument may help identify

specific problems and issues that can then be addressed in a more detailed manner by the clinician (Table 14.1).

Preferences for Care

Although not classically part of the history, before discussing end-of-life decision making and advance directives, it is wise to take a values history: the patient's beliefs about technologic interventions to prolong life, what defines life quality for the patient as an individual, and with what decrements the patient would still think life were worth living. Documenting discussions, executing a living will, and designating a proxy decision maker and durable power of attorney for health care are part of this process of helping the patient have a voice in decisions that may need to be made when the patient, by reason of illness, cannot participate.[86]

Physical Examination

General appearance of the older patient should include any noteworthy features; vitality, markedly youthful or aged appearance, and any indicators of frailty or clinical problems (e.g., odor of urine or stool; signs of abuse, neglect, or poverty; hygiene and grooming) deserve mention. Merely observing how long it takes for the patient to get ready for examination and the extent and nature of help that may be required remains a useful and reliable tool to measure functional capacity.

Vital signs do not change with age. Hypothermia is more common, and reliable low-reading thermometers are essential, especially for emergency room and wintertime use. Blood pressure should be taken in the supine position after at least 10 min rest, and immediately and 3 min after standing. Orthostatic hypotension, defined as either 20 mmHg drop in systolic pressure or any drop accompanied by typical symptoms, occurs in 11% to 28% of individuals older than 65 years.[87,88] In acute moderate blood loss, postural hypotension is a fairly specific but poorly sensitive sign of hypovolemia.[89] Blunting of the baroreflex mechanism with age makes cardioacceleration with the upright position a late and unreliable sign of volume depletion in older persons.

Although pseudohypertension is often mentioned as a consideration when blood pressure is refractory to treatment, the condition is extremely rare. Osler's maneuver, widely recommended in the past, is not reliable in older people.[90] Tachypnea at a rate of more than 25 per minute is a reliable sign of lower respiratory infection, even in very elderly patients.[91] Weight is the most reliable measure of undernutrition in older outpatients and should be carefully recorded under comparable conditions at each visit. Specific assessment of general or localized pain should be considered as the fifth vital sign and should be recorded using a uniform scale (e.g., 0–10).[92]

Skin undergoes many changes with age, including dehydration, thinning, and loss of elastic tissue. Wrinkling is more powerfully predicted by sun exposure and cigarette smoking than by age. Most proliferative lesions, benign and malignant, are related to sun exposure; accordingly, basal and squamous cell cancers and melanomas should be most aggressively hunted on exposed skin. Because of skin aging, turgor is not a reliable sign of hydration status. All skin should be examined, exposed to sun or not, for evidence of established or incipient (nonblanching redness) pressure sores. Ecchymoses should also be noted, whether due to purpura of thin old skin or trauma; the possibility of abuse should be considered.

Head and neck examination begins with careful observation of sun-exposed areas for premalignant and malignant lesions (as above). Palpation of temporal arteries for pain, nodularity, and pulse is recommended, but asymptomatic temporal or giant cell arteritis or polymyalgia rheumatica is not common,[93] and palpation is an insensitive test. Arcus ocularis, or cornealis, a white-to-yellow deposit at the outer edge of the iris, along with xanthelasma, predicts premature coronary disease in young

adults. Beyond age 60, these signs do not identify increased risk.

Visual acuity and hearing screening are necessary, given the high prevalence of impaired vision and auditory acuity among older persons. Impairment in either sense predicts subsequent functional loss. Measured visual impairment was found predictive of mortality in 10 years, whereas combined impairment confers the highest risk of 10-year functional dependence.[94] For most clinical situations, a pocket Snellen chart, held 14 in. from the eye, is more practical than a wall-mounted chart. The whispered voice is as sensitive as an audioscope for detection of hearing loss,[95,96] but the latter is, to date, the best objective measurement of hearing and more accurate at following changes over time. Inspecting the ear canals and drums using an otoscope is especially necessary if hearing loss is detected; removing impacted cerumen is a common quick-fix intervention for many older patients.

Oral examination for denture sores, tooth and gum health, and oral cancers is essential and should include inspection and palpation with dentures out.[97] The earliest detectable malignant oral lesion is red and painless; if persistent beyond 2 weeks, biopsy is mandatory. Although on the decline, oral cancers are most common in older persons with long-standing alcohol or tobacco use or poor hygiene.

Vascular sounds in the neck usually arise from vessels other than the carotid artery;[98] true carotid bruits confer more risk for coronary events and contralateral stroke than for ipsilateral stroke, and may cease unpredictably.[99]

Breast examination is generally simpler in older women. Fat diminished, making breast tissue and the tumors that arise from it more easily palpable. Routine screening mammograms annually or every other year should be continued lifelong or until a decision is reached that a discovered cancer would not be treated[100]; age-specific breast cancer incidence increases at least until age 85, and no evidence indicates that treatment is not effective in older women.[101,102] Current recommendations for breast cancer screening suggest yearly mammography until age 69, but there has been much discussion about revising the age to 74, 79, or removing an upper age limit entirely. Routine screening mammography annually is part of the Medicare benefit, and age cutoffs or stopping screening on the basis of age alone is controversial (see Prevention, Chapter 17). Routine screening mammograms should be continued with the understanding that the patient and/or family are aware that an abnormal result will provoke more aggressive evaluation. Many elderly women experienced considerable anxiety concerning more testing when their mammographies appeared suspicious, even though the vast majority did not have breast cancer.[103] Accordingly, discussions as to how the information will be utilized should take place before testing is initiated.

Lung examination is little different in the older patient. Rales are abnormal at any age; evanescent crackles of atelectasis are the most common cause of rales in the absence of pathology.

Cardiac examination has several special features in aged patients. Both atrial and ventricular ectopy are common at baseline without symptoms or ominous prognosis.[104,105] Although S_4 is common among older persons free of cardiac disease, S_3 is associated with congestive heart failure. The ubiquitous systolic ejection murmur is less reliable as a sign of hemodynamically significant aortic stenosis in older individuals. A loud murmur (>2/6), diminution of the aortic component of S_2, narrowed pulse pressure, and dampening of the carotid upstroke suggest aortic stenosis, but each may be absent and be falsely reassuring.[106] Although not specific to older patients, true aortic stenosis may be detected by the simple bedside maneuver of simultaneous palpation of brachial and radial arteries and noting a delay between their pulsations.[107] Absence of a murmur over the right clavicle rules out moderate or severe aortic stenosis, whereas the presence of three of the following four associated findings makes moderate to severe aortic stenosis likely: slow carotid artery upstroke, reduced carotid artery volume, maximal murmur intensity at the second right intercostal space, and reduced intensity of the second heart sound.[108] In the absence of typical symptoms, a systolic ejection murmur lacking any of the features of stenosis may be followed without cardiac imaging. Although for decades aortic sclerosis was considered benign, it has recently been associated with increased risk for myocardial infarction, congestive heart failure, stroke, and death from cardiovascular causes, even without evidence of significant outflow tract obstruction.[109]

Abdominal and rectal examination have few additional or special components for the older patient. Unsuspected fecal impaction is common and, despite no complaint of constipation, should be treated with a bowel regimen that includes fiber and scheduled toileting. Evidence of fecal or urinary incontinence is usually obvious to the alert examiner. A chronically overfilled and distended bladder should be suspected in men who are incontinent. Although part of the screen for prostate cancer, prostatic masses detected on digital rectal examination may also reflect granuloma, calcification, or hyperplasia, and benign causes outnumber malignant ones; differentiation by imaging is thought not to be reliable unless calcification is present. Prostatic enlargement of benign hyperplasia (because cell proliferation occurs, hypertrophy is an incorrect term) correlates poorly with both urethral obstruction and symptoms of prostatism; anterior periurethral encroachment causes symptoms, but it is the posterolateral portions of the gland that are accessible on digital examination. The need for and utility of screening for fecal occult blood in the early detection and reduction of mortality and morbidity of colon cancer is established in patients of all ages.[110,111]

Musculoskeletal examination, often a source of abundant complaints and pathology in older adults, begins with simple screening. In the absence of complaints or loss of function, brief tests of function are adequate to reveal unsuspected limitations. For upper extremity, "Touch the back of your head with your hands" and "Pick up the spoon" are sensitive and specific.[52] Gait and mobility can be assessed by the timed "up and go" test[112] (arise from a chair, walk 3 m, turn, walk back, and sit down); requiring that each foot be off the floor in the "up and go" yields a test that is a better predictor of functional deficits than standard detailed neuromuscular examination.[113] Neuromuscular abnormalities may not identify persons with mobility deficits and demonstrable difficulties in the "up and go." Simple physical-diagnostic tests, such as stance and balance assessments, timed walking of 8 feet at a normal pace, and timed rising from a chair and sitting back down five times in succession identified patients with increased risk of disability in 4 years.[114] When deficits are detected in any screening test, more detailed evaluation, including neuromuscular exam and longer standard objective tests,[35,115] and likely inclusion of a physical therapist in evaluation and treatment, are indicated.

Pelvic examination in older women often is neglected. Atrophic vaginitis, with associated urinary incontinence, or itching or dyspareunia, is remarkably easy and gratifying to treat. Topical (often difficult for the elderly woman with arthritis to manage) or oral conjugated estrogen may often be discontinued after a few weeks without return of symptoms. Ovaries or uterus palpable more than 10 years beyond the menopause usually indicate pathology, often tumor. Any adnexal mass in a woman over 50 years is considered malignant until proven otherwise.[116] If arthritis or frailty makes stirrups uncomfortable for the patient, examination in bed or on a table with the patient positioned on her side with knees drawn up will allow speculum exam and Papanicolau smear. The bimanual exam can be done with the patient supine, again avoiding use of stirrups. Signs of abuse may only be apparent on pelvic examination.

Neurologic examination of older patients is confusing for many physicians. Abnormalities are thought to be common and their clinical importance is sometimes uncertain, because of either lack of data or existence of conflicting data. Odenheimer[117] has approached the problem rationally; in an age-stratified (65–74, 75–84, >85) random sample of nearly 500 community-dwelling older persons, comprehensive physical, psychiatric, neuropsychologic, and neurologic examinations were performed. In addition, medical histories, functional status, and medication use were inventoried. Data were used to determine whether neurologic abnormalities could be attributed to identifiable disease or existed in the absence of detectable medical or neurologic conditions.

The most important principle found in this study is that although abnormalities are common in the neurologic examination of the older patient, one-third to one-half the abnormal findings have no identifiable disease causing them. Abnormalities were classified as (a) attributable to a disease or an isolated abnormality; and (b) more common with increasing age or not. Abnormalities occurring in the absence of detectable disease and more common with increasing age are the best current definition of "changes of aging" in the nervous system. Abnormalities attributable to disease and more common with increasing age simply reflect diseases that are more common in older persons and have nervous system findings. Abnormalities occurring in the absence of dectectable disease but not more common with increasing age are most likely individual variations not attributable to aging; the unlikely possibility also exists that lack of progression occurs following changes that developed before age 65.

Analysis of previous reports of abnormal neurologic signs in older persons helps explain sources of confusion. Most studies include subjects screened inadequately or not at all for diseases that can be expected to produce the abnormal findings. Accordingly, caution must be used in interpreting reports of very high prevalence of abnormalities in older persons. On the other hand, the considerable prevalence of neurologic abnormalities in older persons carefully evaluated and found to have no disease explaining the finding demands even greater caution in attributing predictive significance to the abnormality. For example, frontal release signs (also called "primitive" reflexes)—snout, palmomental, root, suck, grasp, glabellar tap—have been reported to identify patients with dementia[118–120] or with Parkinson's disease. Because these signs appear in 10% to 35% of older adults screened to exclude disease,[117,121,122] it is difficult to accept reports of these signs as identifiers of disease, at least in older persons. Ankle jerks, reported to be absent among many otherwise healthy older persons, turn out to be just a bit more difficult to elicit. Using a high-quality, round neurologic hammer rather than a lightweight, red triangulated hammer and striking briskly will improve accuracy. It appears that reports of loss of ankle jerk with age may be a result of the care and expertise with which the reflex is elicited, rather than an aging effect.[117,123]

Peripheral neuropathy, which is common in older adults, increases risk for falls by causing impairments of proprioception and strength that hinder balance. Suggestive of functionally significant neuropathy are absent heel reflexes, reduced vibratory sense, impaired position sense at the great toe, and inability to maintain unipedal stance for 10 s in three attempts.[124,125] Unipedal stance time is particularly helpful in assessing the severity and functional importance of peripheral neuropathy. Persons with healthy peripheral nerves are generally able to stand for more than 10 s, while patients with significant peripheral neuropathy rarely keep the stance for more than 5 s. The precise prevalence of peripheral neuropathy in elderly persons is yet unknown (estimates vary from 10% in the nondiabetic population to around 50% among diabetic patients older than 60 years), but the presence of disease, particularly diabetes, accounts for the majority of cases.

References

1. Levkoff SE, Cleary PD, Wetle T, et al. Illness behavior in the aged, implications for clinicians. *J Am Geriatr Soc.* 1988;36:622–629.
2. Mechanic D. *Medical Sociology*, 2nd Ed. New York: Free Press; 1978.
3. Besdine RW, Levkoff SE, Wetle T. Health and illness behaviors in elder veterans. In: Wetle T, Rowe JW, eds. *Older Veterans: Linking VA and Community Resources.* Cambridge: Harvard University Press; 1984.
4. Levkoff SE, Cleary PD, Wetle T. Differences in the appraisal of health between aged and middle-aged adults. *J Gerontol.* 1987;42:114.
5. Ferraro K. Self-ratings of health among the old and the old-old. *J Health Soc Behav.* 1980;21:377.
6. Hogan DB, Fung TS, Ebly EM. Health, function and survival of a cohort of very old Canadians: results from the second wave of the Canadian Study of Health and Aging. *Can J Public Health* 1999;90:338–342.
7. Ebly EM, Hogan DB, Fung B. Correlates of self-rated health in persons aged 85 and over: results from the Canadian Study of Health and Aging. *Can J Public Health* 1996;87(1):28–31.
8. Anderson WF. *The Prevention of Illness in the Elderly: The Rutherglen Experiment in Medicine in Old Age.* Proceedings of a conference held at the Royal College of Physicians of London. London: Pitman; 1966.
9. Williamson J, Stokoe IH, Gray S, et al. Old people at home: their unreported needs. *Lancet.* 1964;1:1117–1120.
10. Shanas E. *The Health of Older People.* Cambridge: Harvard University Press; 1961.
11. Brody EM. Tomorrow and tomorrow and tomorrow: toward squaring the suffering curve. In: Gaitz CM, Wilson NL, Niederene G. *Aging 2000: Our Health Care Destiny, II.* New York: Springer-Verlag; 1985.
12. Gross R, Bentur N, Einayany A, et al. The validity of self-reports on chronic disease: characteristics of underreporters and implications for the planning of services. *Public Health Rev.* 1996;24(2):167–182.
13. Kriegsman DM, Penninx BW, van Eijk JT, et al. Self-reports and general practitioner information on the presence of chronic diseases in community-dwelling elderly. A study on the accuracy of patients' self-reports and on determinants of inaccuracy. *J Clin Epidemiol.* 1996;49(12):1407–1417.

14. Tresch DD, Brady WJ, Aufderheide TP, et al. Comparison of elderly and younger patients with out-of-hospital chest pain. *Arch Intern Med.* 1996;156:1089–1093.

15. Morgan R, Pendleton N, Clague JE, et al. Older people's perceptions about symptoms. *Br J Gen Pract.* 1997; 47(420):427–430.

16. Lecrubier Y. Is depression under-recognised and under-treated? *Int Clin Psychopharmacol.* 1998;13(suppl 5): S3–S6.

17. Duberstein PR, Conwell Y, Seidlitz L, et al. Age and suicidal ideation in older depressed inpatients. *Am J Geriatr Psychiatry.* 1999;7(4):289–296.

18. Lyness JM, Cox C, Curry J, et al. Older age and the under-reporting of depressive symptoms. *J Am Geriatr Soc.* 1995; 43:216–221.

19. NIH Consensus Development Panel on Depression in Late Life. Diagnosis and treatment of depression in late life. *JAMA.* 1992;268:1018–1024.

20. Leventhal EA, Prohaska TR. Age, symptom interpretation and health behavior. *J Am Geriatr Soc.* 1986;34:185.

21. Metlay JP, Schulz R, Li YH, et al. Influence of age on symptoms at presentation in patients with community-acquired pneumonia. *Arch Intern Med.* 1997;157(13):1453–1459.

22. Costa PT Jr, McCrae RR. Somatic complaints in males as a function of age and neuroticism: a longitudinal analysis. *J Behav Med.* 1980;3:245.

23. Stenback A, Kumpulainen M, Vauhkonen ML. Illness and health behavior in septuagenarians. *Gerontologist.* 1978; 33:57.

24. Besdine RW. Clinical approach to the elderly patient. In: Rowe JW, Besdine RW, eds. *Geriatric Medicine,* 2nd Ed. Boston: Little, Brown; 1988:23–36.

25. Cushman LF, Wade C, Factor-Litvak P, et al. Use of complementary and alternative medicine among African-American and Hispanic women in New York City: a pilot study. *J Am Med Women's Assoc.* 1999;54(4):193–195.

26. Stolley JM, Koenig H. Religion/spirituality and health among elderly African-Americans and Hispanics. *J Psychosoc Nurs.* 1997;35:32–38.

27. Goldstein MZ, Griswold K. Cultural sensitivity and aging. *Psychiatr Serv.* 1998;49(6):769–771.

28. Wilson LA, Lawson IR, Brass W. Multiple disorders in the elderly. *Lancet.* 1962;2:841–843.

29. Besdine RW. Geriatric medicine: an overview. *Annu Rev Gerontol Geriatr.* 1980;1:135.

30. Besdine RW. The educational utility of comprehensive functional assessment in the elderly. *J Am Geriatr Soc.* 1983;31:651.

31. Kane RA, Kane RL. *Assessing the Elderly: A Practical Guide to Measurement.* Lexington, MA: Lexington; 1981.

32. National Institutes of Health. Consensus Development Conference Statement: geriatric assessment methods for clinical decision-making. *J Am Geriatr Soc.* 1988;36:342–347.

33. Besdine RW, Wakefield KM, Williams TF. Assessing function in the elderly. *Patient Care.* 1988;22:69–79.

34. American College of Physicians, Health and Public Policy Committee. Comprehensive Functional Assessment for Elderly Patients. *Ann Intern Med.* 1988;109:70–72.

35. Applegate WB, Blass JP, Williams TF. Instruments for the functional assessment of older patients. *N Engl J Med.* 1990;322:1207–1214.

36. Stuck AE, Walthert JM, Nikolaus T, et al. Risk factors for functional status decline in community-living elderly people: a systematic literature review. *Soc Sci Med.* 1999; 48:445–469.

37. Hodkinson HM. Non-specific presentation of illness. *Br Med J.* 1973;4:94.

38. Tinetti ME, Williams CS, Gill TM. Dizziness among older adults: a possible geriatric syndrome. *Ann Intern Med.* 2000;132:337–344.

39. Cross CR, Lindquist RD, Woolley AC, et al. Clinical indicators of dehydration severity in elderly patients. *J Emerg Med.* 1992;10:267–274.

40. Perez-Guzman C, Vargas MH, Torres-Cruz A, et al. Does aging modify pulmonary tuberculosis? a mentaanalytical review. *Chest.* 1999;116(4):961–967.

41. Bayer AJ, Chadha JS, Farag RR, et al. Changing presentation of myocardial infarction with increasing old age. *J Am Geriatr Soc.* 1986;34:263.

42. Kannel WB, Abbott RD. Incidence and prognosis of unrecognized myocardial infarction. *N Engl J Med.* 1984; 311:1144.

43. Doucet J, Trivalle CH, Chassagne PH, et al. Does age lay a role in clinical presentation of hypothyroidism? *J Am Geriatr Soc.* 1994;42:984–986.

44. Trivalle C, Doucet J, Chassagne P, et al. Differences in the signs and symptoms of hyperthyroidism in older and younger patients. *J Am Geriatr Soc.* 1996;44:50–53.

45. Osler W. *Principle and Practice of Medicine.* New York: Appleton;1982:95.

46. Podolsky S. Hyperosmolar nonketotic coma in the elderly diabetic. *Med Clin North Am.* 1978;62:815.

47. Wachtel TJ, Silliman RA, Lamberton P. Prognostic factors in the diabetic hyperosmolar state. *J Am Geriatr Soc.* 1987;35:737–741.

48. Thomas FB, Mazzaferri EL, Skillman TG. Apathetic thyrotoxicosis: a distinctive clinical and laboratory entity. *Ann Intern Med.* 1970;72:679.

49. Arie T. Pseudodementia [Editorial]. *Br Med J.* 1983;286: 1301.

50. Kiloh LG. Pseudo-dementia. *Acta Psychiatr Neurol.* 1961; 37:336.

51. Reding M, Haycox J, Blass J. Depression in patients referred to a dementia clinic. A three-year prospective study. *Arch Neurol.* 1985;42:894.

52. Lachs M, Feinstein A, Cooney L, et al. A simple procedure for general screening of functional disability in elderly patients. *Ann Intern Med.* 1990;112:699–706.

53. Stuck AE. A trial of annual in-home comprehensive geriatric assessments for elderly people living in the community. *N Engl J Med.* 1995;333:1184–1189.

54. Burns R, Nichols LO, Martindale-Adams J, et al. Interdisciplinary geriatric primary care evaluation and management: two year outcomes. *J Am Geriatr Soc.* 2000;48(1): 8–13.

55. Stuck AE, Siu AL, Wieland GD, et al. Comprehensive geriatric assessment: a meta-analysis of controlled trials. *Lancet.* 1993;342:1032–1036.

56. Lagaay AM, van der Meij JC, Hijmans W. Validation of medical history taking as part of a population based survey in subjects aged 85 and over. *Br Med J.* 1992;304:1091–1092.

57. Davis PB, Robins LN. History-taking in the elderly with and without cognitive impairment. *J Am Geriatr Soc.* 1989; 37:249–255.

58. Greene MG, Majerovitz SD, Adelman RD, Rizzo C. The effects of the presence of a third person on the physician-older patient medical interview. *J Am Geriatr Soc.* 1994; 42:413–419.

59. Fried LP, Storer DJ, King DE, et al. Diagnosis of illness presentation in the elderly. *J Am Geriatr Soc.* 1991;39: 117–123.

60. Nolan L, O'Malley K. Prescribing of the elderly. Pat I: Sensitivity of the elderly to adverse drug reactions. *J Am Geriatr Soc.* 1988;36:142–149.

61. Montamat SC, Cusack BJ, Vestal RE. Management of drug therapy in the elderly. *N Engl J Med.* 1989;321:303–309.

62. Eisenberg DM, Davis RB, Ettner SL, et al. Trends in alternative medicine use in the United States, 1990: results of a follow-up national survey. *JAMA.* 1998;280(18):1569–1575.

63. Beers MH, Ouslander JG, Fingold SF, et al. Inappropriate medication prescribing in skilled-nursing facilities. *Ann Intern Med.* 1992;117:684–689.

64. Berkman LF. Social networks, support, and health: taking the next step forward. *Am J Epidemiol.* 1986;123:559.

65. Glass TA, de Leon C, Marottoli RA, et al. Population-based study of social and productive activities as predictors of survival among elderly Americans. *Br Med J.* 1999;319:478–483.

66. Morley JE. Why do physicians fail to recognize and treat malnutrition in older persons? *J Am Geriatr Soc.* 1991;39: 1139–1140.

67. Detsky AS, Smalley PS, Chang J. Is this patient malnourished? *JAMA.* 1994;271:54–58.

68. Corti M-C, Guralnik JM, Salive ME, et al. Serum albumin level and physical disability as predictors of mortality in older persons. *JAMA.* 1994;272:1036–1042.

69. Graham K. Identifying and measuring alcohol abuse among the elderly: serious problems with existing instrumentation. *J Stud Alcohol.* 1986;47:322–325.

70. Adams WL, Yuan Z, Barboriak JJ, et al. Alcohol-related hospitalizations of elderly people. *JAMA.* 1993;270:1222-1225.

71. Callahan CM, Tierney WM. Health services use and mortality among older primary care patients with alcoholism. *J Am Geriatr Soc.* 1995;43(12):1378–1383.

72. Naik PC, Jones RG. Alcohol histories taken from elderly people on admission. *Br Med J.* 1994;308:248.

73. Buchsbaum DG, Buchanan RG, Welsh J, et al. Screening for drinking disorders in the elderly using the CAGE questionnaire. *J Am Geriatr Soc.* 1992;40:662–665.

74. Morton JL, Jones TV, Manganaro MA. Performance of alcoholism screening questionnaires in elderly veterans. *Am J Med.* 1996;101(2):153–159.

75. Buchsbaum DG, Buchanan RG, Welsh J, et al. Screening for drinking disorders in the elderly using the CAGE questionnaire. *J Am Geriatr Soc.* 1992;40:662–665.

76. Jones TV, Lindsey BA, Yount P, et al. Alcoholism screening questionnaires: are they valid in elderly medical outpatients? *J Gen Intern Med.* 1993;8(12):674–678.

77. LaCroix AZ, Lang J, Scherr P, et al. Smoking and mortality among older men and women in three communities. *N Engl J Med.* 1991;324:1619–1625.

78. Kawachi I, Colditz GA, Stampfer MJ, et al. Smoking cessation and decreased risk of stroke in women. *JAMA.* 1993;269:232–236.

79. Schulz R, Beach SR. Caregiving as a risk factor for mortality: the caregiver health effects study. *JAMA.* 1999; 282:2215–2219.

80. Bretschneider JG, McCoy NL. Sexual interest and behavior in healthy 80 to 102 year olds. *Arch Sex Behav.* 1988;17:109–129.

81. Johnson EE, Hamer R, Nora RM, et al. The Lie/Bet questionnaire for screening pathological gambler. *Psychol Rep.* 1997;80(1):83–88.

82. Guralnik JM, Simonsick EM, Ferrucci L, et al. A short physical performance battery assessing lower extremity function: association with self-reported disability and prediction of mortality and nursing home admission. *J Gerontol.* 1994;49:M85–M94.

83. Reuben DB, Siu AL, Kimpau S. The predictive validity of self-report and performance-based measures of function and health. *J Gerontol.* 1992;47:M106–M110.

84. Katz S, Ford AB, Moskowitz RW, et al. Studies of illness in the aged: the index of ADL, a standardized measure of biological and psychosocial function. *JAMA.* 1963;185: 914–919.

85. Moore AA, Siu AL. Screening for common problems in ambulatory elderly: clinical confirmation of a screening instrument. *Am J Med.* 1996; 100:438–440.

86. Cassell EJ. Art of medicine. In: Reich Warret T, ed. *Encyclopedia of Bioethics, vol III.* New York: Simon & Schuster Macmillan; 1995:1674–1679.

87. Oowi WL, Barrett S, Hossain M, et al. Patterns of orthostatic blood pressure change and their clinical correlates in a frail elderly population. *JAMA.* 1997;277:1299-1304.

88. Raiha I, Luntonen S, Piha J, et al. Prevalence, predisposing factors and prognostic importance of postural hypotension. *Arch Intern Med.* 1995;155:930–935.

89. Witting MD, Wears RL, Li S. Defining the positive tilt test: a study of healthy adults with moderate acute blood loss. *Ann Emerg Med.* 1994;23(6):1320–1323.

90. Prochazka AV, deRois S, Holdcrost C, et al. Observer variation in Osler's maneuver, abstracted. *Clin Reg.* 1987;35: 756.

91. McFadden JP, Price RC, Eastwood HD, et al. Raised respiratory rate in elderly patients: a valuable physical sign. *Br Med J.* 1982;284:626–627.

92. AGS Panel on Chronic Pain in Older Persons, American Geriatrics Society. The management of chronic pain in older persons. *J Am Geriatr Soc.* 1998;46(5):635–651.

93. Hunder G, Bloch DA, Michel BA, et al. The American College of Rheumatology 1990 criteria for the classification of giant cell arteritis. *Arthritis Rheum.* 1990;33:1122–1128.

94. Reuben DB, Mui S, Damesyn M, et al. The prognostic value of sensory impairment in older persons. *J Am Geriatr Soc.* 1999;47(8):930–935.

95. Swan IRC, Browning GG. The whispered voice as a screening test for hearing impairment. *J R Coll Gen Pract.* 1985;35:197.

96. Lichtenstein MJ, Bess FH, Logan SA. Validation of screening tools for identifying hearing-impaired elderly in primary care. *JAMA.* 1988;259:2875–2878.

97. Gordon SR, Jahnigen DW. Oral assessment of the dentulous elderly patient. *J Am Geriatr Soc.* 1986;34:276–281.

98. Ruiswyk JV, Noble H, Sigmann P. The natural history of carotid bruits in elderly persons. *Ann Intern Med.* 1990; 112:340–343.

99. Heyman A, Wilkinson WE, Heyden S, et al. Risk of stroke in symptomatic persons with cervical arterial bruits. *N Engl J Med.* 1980;302:838.

100. Mandelblatt JS, Wheat ME, Monane M, et al. Breast cancer screening for elderly women with and without comorbid conditions. *Ann Intern Med.* 1992;116:722–730.

101. Horm JW, Asire AJ, Young JL, et al. *SEER Program: Cancer Incidence and Mortality in the US, 1973–1981.* NIH Pub 85–1837. Bethesda, MD: Dept. of Health and Human Services; 1985.

102. Yancik R, Ries LG, Yates JW. Breast cancer in aging women. *Cancer.* 1989;63:976–981.

103. Welch HG, Fisher ES. Diagnostic testing following screening mammography in the elderly. *J Natl Cancer Inst.* 1998; 90(18):1389–1392.

104. Fleg JL, Kennedy HL. Long-term prognostic significance of ambulatory electrocardiographic findings in apparently healthy subjects ≥60 years of age. *Am J Cardiol.* 1992;70: 748–751.

105. Aronow WS, Mercando AD, Epstein S. Prevalence of arrhythmias detected by 24-hour ambulatory electrocardiography and value of antiarrhythmic therapy in elderly patients with unexplained syncope. *Am J Cardiol.* 1992;70: 408–410.

106. Lembo NJ, Dell'Italia LJ, Crawford MH, et al. Bedside diagnosis of systolic murmurs. *N Engl J Med.* 1988;318: 1572–1578.

107. Leach RM, McBrien DJ. Brachioradial delay: a new clinical indicator of the severity of aortic stenosis. *Lancet.* 1990; 335:119–201.

108. Etchells E, Glenns V, Shadowitz S, et al. A bedside clinical prediction rule for detecting moderate or severe aoric stenosis. *J Gen Intern Med.* 1998;13:699–704.

109. Otto CM, Lind BK, Kitzman DW, et al. Association of aortic valve sclerosis with cardiovascular mortality and morbidity in the elderly. *N Engl J Med.* 1999;341:142–147.

110. Mandel JS, Bond JH, Church TR, et al. Reducing mortality from colorectal cancer by screening for fecal occult blood. *N Engl J Med.* 1993;328:1365–1371. [Editorial: Winawer SJ. Colorectal cancer screening comes of age. 1993;328:1416–1417.]

111. Winawer SJ, Zauber AG, Ho MN, et al. Prevention of colorectal cancer by colonoscopic polypectomy. *N Engl J Med.* 1993;329:1977–1981.

112. Podsiadlo D, Richardson S. The timed "up and go": a test of basic functional mobility for frail elderly persons. *J Am Geriatr.* 1991;39:142–148.

113. Tinetti ME, Ginter SF. Identifying mobility dysfunctions in elderly patients: standard neuromuscular examination or direct assessment? *JAMA.* 1988;259:1190–1193.

114. Guralnik JM, Ferrucci L, Simonsick EM, et al. Lower-extremity function in persons over the age of 70 years as a predictor of subsequent disability. *N Engl J Med.* 1995;332:556–561.

115. Reuben DB, Siu AL. An objective measure of physical function of elderly outpatients, the physical performance test. *J Am Geriatr Soc.* 1990;38:1105–1112.

116. Dumesic DA. Pelvic examination: what to focus on in menopausal women. *Consultant.* 1996;36:39–46.

117. Odenheimer G, Funkenstein H, Beckett L, et al. Comparison of neurologic changes in "successfully aging" persons vs the total aging population. *Arch Neurol.* 1994; 51:573–580.

118. Thomas RJ. Blinking and the release reflexes: are they clinically useful? *J Am Geriatr Soc.* 1994;42:609–613.

119. Forstl H, Burns A, Levy R, et al. Neurologic signs in Alzheimer's disease. Results of a prospective clinical and neuropathological study. *Arch Neurol* 1992;49:1038–1042.

120. Backine S, Lacomblez L, Palisson E, et al. Relationship between primitive refelxes, extra-pyramidal signs, reflective apraxia and severity of cognitive impairment in dementia of the Alzheimer's type. *Acta Neurol Scand.* 1989;79:38–46.

121. Jenkyn LR, Reeves AG, Warren T, et al. Neurologic signs in senescence. *Arch Neurol.* 1985;42:1154–1157.

122. Forgotten symptoms and primitive signs [Editorial]. *Lancet* 1987;1(8537):841–842.

123. Impallomeni M, Kenny RA, Flynn MD, et al. The elderly and their ankle jerks. *Lancet.* 1984;670–672.

124. Richardson JK, Ashton-Miller JA. Peripheral neuropathy: an often overlooked cause of falls in the elderly. *Postgrad Med.* 1996;99(6):161–172.

125. Richardson JK, Hurvitz EA. Peripheral neuropathy: a true risk factor for falls. *J Gerontol A Biol Sci Med Sci.* 1995;50(4):M211–M215.

15
Chronic Disease Management

Harrison G. Bloom

The term *disease management* has evolved within the past decade to become defined as a systematic, population-based approach to identify persons with a given disease or persons at risk for that disease, followed by implementation of therapeutic or preventive interventions, finally followed by measurement of clinical and other (e.g., utilization of services, costs) outcomes.[1,2] Chronic disease management places an emphasis upon coordination and comprehensiveness of care along the continuum of disease, not just the acute episode or exacerbation, and across health care delivery systems.[3] Promotion of high-quality, better coordinated, and appropriately utilized care, coupled with control of costs, are its major goals. Components of disease management programs include the following[3]: presence of an integrated health delivery system that has the capability to coordinate care along the continuum; a thorough understanding of the disease in question, including approaches to prevention, diagnosis, treatment, and palliation; information systems for clinical and administrative data that allow for continuing analysis of practice patterns and outcomes; and a philosophy and active program for continuous quality improvement. Developing an evidence-based disease management program requires a series of steps as outlined in Table 15.1.[3] Schematically, the disease management process would encompass a process illustrated in Figure 15.1.[4]

Overall objectives of disease management programs include the following[5]:

- Encourage disease prevention
- Promote correct diagnosis and treatment planning
- Maximize clinical effectiveness of interventions
- Eliminate duplication of effort and activity
- Utilize only cost-effective diagnostic and therapeutic strategies
- Maximize the efficiency of health care delivery while maintaining appropriate standards of quality
- Continually improve the outcomes of the process, and the process itself

The proliferation of managed care has given great impetus to the establishment of disease management programs with considerable help from pharmaceutical companies. A push by insurers and employers to measure clinical and other outcomes has also contributed to its growth. Indeed, some would argue that such programs are simply marketing and packaging devices, yet there is a small but growing literature indicating significant value for properly designed and implemented programs.[6]

A significant majority of individuals over 75 years of age suffer from chronic medical conditions. The prevalence of congestive heart failure, hypertension, diabetes mellitus, depression, osteoarthritis, Alzheimer's, and other dementias are high among the older population. There are, therefore, unique aspects of chronic disease management that apply to programs aimed at older individuals. These aspects include attention to syndromes, not just diseases; the frequent presence of accompanying comorbidities; cognitive impairment as a frequent complicating factor; the high prevalence of functional dependencies; the involvement of family caregivers; and the realization that self-care may or may not play a significant role.

Although emphasis may vary among programs, most comprehensive chronic disease management programs include care in the patient's home, office-based care, and care in the acute hospital setting. Additionally, careful attention to the transition between these settings (e.g., hospital to home in the community) can be a key component as well. Interventions can range from very "low-tech" patient-focused steps (e.g., providing educational materials about a disease) to specialized units with sophisticated monitoring (e.g., inpatient stroke units).[7]

A variety of examples of chronic disease management programs that have had some degree of success follow.

For patients requiring lifelong oral anticoagulation therapy, a program utilizing a structured educational approach to patient self-management of anticoagulation resulted in improved accuracy of anticoagulation control

TABLE 15.1. Steps for developing an evidence-based disease management program.

Formulate a clear definition of the disease, its scope, and its impact over time using a multidisciplinary team
Develop comprehensive baseline information to understand current health care delivery and resource utilization
Generate specific clinical and economic questions and search the literature
Critically appraise and synthesize the evidence
Evaluate the benefits, harms, and costs
Develop evidence-based practice guidelines, clinical pathways, and algorithms
Create a system for process and outcome measurement and reporting
Implement the evidence-based guidelines, pathways, and algorithms
Complete the quality improvement cycle

Source: From Ref. 3, with permission.

and improved treatment-related quality of life.[8] Other programs targeting older patients with chronic non-valvular atrial fibrillation have utilized expert nurses as teachers and managers to assist physicians by helping educate patients about the condition, its potential complications, and the rationale and method of medication management with attention to dietary interactions with anticoagulants.[9]

A number of programs and studies have targeted congestive heart failure.[10–13] Most were multidisciplinary approaches implemented in the patient's home immediately after a hospitalization for congestive heart failure (CHF). The major goals of the programs were to improve patient adherence with therapeutic recommendations, increase patients' understanding of their disease, allow for and provide easy access for communication during careful follow-up surveillance, decrease unplanned hospital readmission, improve functional status, and reduce overall medical costs. Most studies were at least 3 months in duration, with 6- to 18-month follow-up periods. One randomized controlled trial enrolled patients (mean age, 79) at a large urban teaching hospital in the Midwest.[10,11] Protocols emphasizing education about CHF and careful clinical follow-up were carried out by a nurse manager-led multidisciplinary team including a geriatric cardiologist, dieticians, social workers, and home health professionals. The control group received usual care and follow-up. Positive outcomes included improved quality of life measures, a 56% reduction in hospital admission

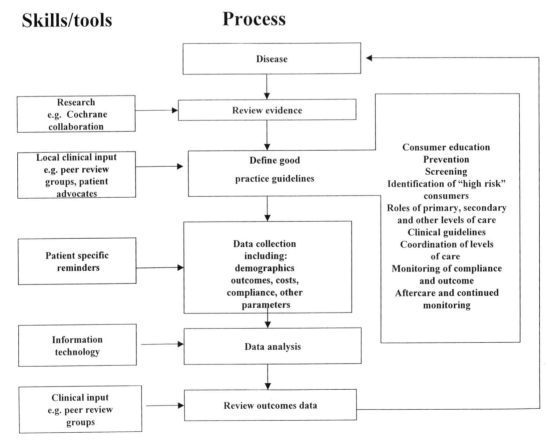

FIGURE 15.1. Disease management process.

rate, and a savings of $1,058 per patient in health care costs. Another study with 97 individuals whose intervention was a single home visit by a nurse and a pharmacist 1 week after hospital discharge for acute heart failure resulted in a significant reduction in unplanned hospital readmissions, hospital-based costs, total hospital stay, and mortality.[13]

With Alzheimer's disease, any chronic disease management program must involve caregivers because patient self-directed care and self-help are, at best, limited. Because the prevalence of Alzheimer's disease is increasing dramatically as the population ages and because the natural course of the disease often can be over 10 years, programs attempting to work with patients and caregivers are potentially important and helpful. One randomized controlled intervention study carried out in a large urban area with 206 spouse-caregivers of Alzheimer's disease patients utilized counselors (clinicians with master's degrees or doctorates in social work, gerontology, or psychiatry) whose primary goal was to help caregivers better cope with caring for their Alzheimer's spouse.[14] A series of individual and family counseling sessions, support groups, and additional counseling availability were provided to the intervention group. The control group received usual care. The major positive outcome was a significant increase in time that Alzheimer's patients, especially those with mild to moderate disease, were able to continue living at home rather than being placed in a long-term care facility.

Accidental falling is not a disease, nor are those at risk for injurious falls a homogeneous group. The morbid sequelae of injurious falls in older people are well known, hip fracture being one of the most common. Prevention of falls, however, is a good example of a variation of chronic disease management applicable to the older population. By identifying individuals at risk, a falls prevention program can theoretically thwart the acute and chronic complications of falls by preventing them from occurring. One study of 301 community-dwelling individuals utilized a multifactorial intervention for the study group and usual care plus social visits for the control group.[15] To be enrolled, individuals had to be at least 70 years old and have at least one risk factor for falling. The risk factors identified were postural hypotension; use of sedatives; use of four or more prescription drugs; impairment in arm or leg strength or range of motion; problem with balance or gait; and difficulty with transfer skills (e.g., bed to chair). The study group received some or all of the following in their homes from a nurse practitioner and a physical therapist: medication adjustments, behavioral instructions, and exercise programs, all aimed at modifying their risk factors. Outcomes resulted in a significant reduction in the risk of falling, as well as reduction in the number of actual risk factors for falling. Another study of 530 older individuals (mean age, 77

years) demonstrated that home visits by occupational therapists making environmental modifications could prevent falls among those at risk of falling by both home environmental modifications and subsequent behavioral changes in those at risk.[16]

Some chronic illness management programs are less disease specific. A randomized controlled study examining a heterogenous group of patients (mean age, 65 years) demonstrated that a community-based self-education course could result in positive outcomes for those participating in this chronic disease self-management program.[17] Participants included 952 patients with a diagnosis of heart disease, lung disease, arthritis, or stroke, most also having comorbidities. The self-education course addressed the following issues: use of cognitive symptom management techniques; nutrition; fatigue and sleep management; use of community resources; medication use; dealing with fear, anger, and depression; communicating with health care professionals; problem solving; and decision making. The intervention group demonstrated improved health behaviors, improved health status, fewer hospitalizations, and fewer days of hospitalization. This study showed that, for individuals able to learn and self-manage, a multifaceted educational program could be effectively utilized for those with a variety of chronic conditions and comorbidities.

A somewhat similar randomized controlled study of 201 chronically ill adults (mean age, 77 years) paired community primary care providers with managed care organization nurse practitioner-led interventions.[18] The multicomponent disability prevention and disease self-management program addressed risk factors for disability such as inactivity, smoking, misuse of alcohol, use of psychoactive drugs, depression, and poor nutrition. The program also taught self-management of chronic illness. The geriatric nurse practitioner met individually with each participant from one to eight times (median, three) during the 1-year study period. Participant chronic conditions included heart disease, hypertension, arthritis, cancer, stroke, and diabetes. Significant outcomes in the study versus control group were as follows: less functional decline, less hospitalization and fewer total inpatient days, greater levels of physical activity, and less use of psychoactive medications. Another 1-year randomized study of 200 older individuals utilizing an approach integrating social and medical care along with case management also demonstrated less functional decline, less hospitalization, and less nursing home placement, as well as considerable cost savings in the intervention group.[19]

An additional variation of chronic disease management is sometimes called high-risk case management. High risk could refer to susceptibility to or a specific disease syndrome, or it could refer to an individual's overall health status. For example, hazards of hospitalization for older adults have been well documented.[20]

Also, the hospital readmission rate for a subset of older patients is high, especially during the first month after hospital discharge. A study to examine the effectiveness of intensive pre- and posthospital care, the transitional care period, by interventions by experienced advanced practice nurses with at-risk older patients, demonstrated significant reductions in unplanned hospital readmissions and overall health care costs.[21] The advance practice nurses coordinated and actively participated in hospital discharge planning, made regular posthospital discharge home visits, which included thorough clinical assessments, and were available 24 h per day, 7 days per week, by telephone.

Chronic disease management programs have been implemented and utilized far more often in the Medicare managed care sector than in the regular Medicare fee-for-service arena. Managed care organizations view such programs as an opportunity to significantly decrease health care costs while maintaining or even improving quality of care. Also, because managed care companies deal with large populations and often have the capability of collecting and tracking large volumes of data, they are much better positioned than individual physicians or small physician groups to implement and evaluate disease management programs. Additionally, they can distribute educational materials and flexibly fund, as well as quickly modify or cancel programs, if necessary. Until the Center for Medicare and Medicaid Services (CMS) endorses and funds chronic disease management programs in the traditional system, this discrepancy will persist.

Nevertheless, in spite of the advantages managed care organizations have in creating, implementing, and evaluating chronic disease management programs, significant barriers to success exist even within managed care. Such barriers include the cost of program development and implementations, limited data systems, resistance by physicians to participate in or support programs, and the difficulty in measuring any dollar savings. Additionally, overlapping programs can interfere with the coordination of care. If, for example, a managed care organization has programs in both diabetes and congestive heart failure, which program will be primarily responsible for a member with both conditions?[22]

Chronic disease management programs implemented in the older adult population hold promise for better quality care and decreased costs. The systematic and evidence-based approach to specific at-risk populations, not just individual patients, has the possibility to improve overall health care status. It is, however, still a relatively new and very heterogeneous field that will require many additional methodologically sound studies, especially in the nonmanaged care arena where most Medicare beneficiaries are still insured, before it can be accepted as a standard of treatment for chronic diseases.

References

1. Bodenheimer T. Disease management—promises and pitfalls. *N Engl J Med*. 1999;340:1202–1205.
2. Epstein RS, Sherwood LM. From outcomes research to disease management: a guide for the perplexed. *Ann Intern Med*. 1996;124:832–837.
3. Ellrodt G, Cook DJ, Lee J, Cho M, Hunt D, Weingarten S. Evidence-based disease management. *JAMA*. 1997;278:1687–1692.
4. Mallarkey G, Sutherland J. *Disease Management Handbook*. Hong Kong: Adis; 1999:5.
5. Mallarkey G, Sutherland J. *Disease Management Handbook*. Hong Kong: Adis; 1999;8.
6. Hunter DJ, Fairfield G. Disease management. *Br Med J*. 1997;315:50–53.
7. Harris JM. Disease management: new wine in new bottles? *Ann Intern Med*. 1996;124:838–842.
8. Sawicki PT. A structured teaching and self-management program for patients receiving oral anticoagulation: a randomized controlled trial. Working Group for the Study of Patient Self-Management of Oral Anticoagulation. *JAMA* 1999;281:145–150.
9. Matchar DB, Samsa GP, Cohen SJ, Oddone EZ. Community impact of anticoagulation services: rationale and design of the Managing Anticoagulation Services Trial (MAST). *J Thromb Thrombolysis*. 2000;9(suppl 1):S7–S11.
10. Philbin EF. Comprehensive multidisciplinary programs for the management of patients with congestive heart failure. *J Gen Intern Med*. 1999;14:130–135.
11. Rich MW, Beckham V, Wittenberg C, Leven CL, Freedland KE, Carney RM. A multidisciplinary intervention to prevent the readmission of elderly patients with congestive heart failure. *N Engl J Med*. 1995;333:1190–1195.
12. Cline CM, Israelsson BY, Willenheimer RB, Broms K, Erhardt LR. Cost effective management programme for heart failure reduces hospitalisation. *Heart*. 1998;80:442–446.
13. Stewart S, Vandenbroek AJ, Pearson S, Horowitz JD. Prolonged beneficial effects of a home-based intervention on unplanned readmissions and mortality among patients with congestive heart failure. *Arch Intern Med*. 1999;159:257–261.
14. Mittelman MS, Ferris SH, Shulman E, Steinberg G, Levin B. A family intervention to delay nursing home placement of patients with Alzheimer disease. A randomized controlled trial. *JAMA* 1996;276:1725–1731.
15. Tinetti ME, Baker DI, McAvay G, et al. A multifactorial intervention to reduce the risk of falling among elderly people living in the community. *N Engl J Med*. 1994;331:821–827.
16. Cumming RG, Thomas M, Szonyi G, et al. Home visits by an occupational therapist for assessment and modification of environmental hazards: a randomized trial of falls prevention. *J Am Geriatr Soc*. 1999;47:1397–1402.
17. Lorig KR, Sobel DS, Stewart AL, et al. Evidence suggesting that a chronic disease self-management program can improve health status while reducing hospitalization: a randomized trial. *Med Care*. 1999;37:5–14.

18. Leveille SG, Wagner EH, Davis C, et al. Preventing disability and managing chronic illness in frail older adults: a randomized trial of a community-based partnership with primary care. *J Am Geriatr Soc.* 1998;46:1191–1198.

19. Bernabei R, Landi F, Gambassi G, et al. Randomised trial of impact of model of integrated care and case management for older people living in the community. *Br Med J.* 1998; 316:1348–1351.

20. Creditor MC. Hazards of hospitalization of the elderly. *Ann Intern Med.* 1993;118:219–223.

21. Naylor MD, Brooten D, Campbell R, et al. Comprehensive discharge planning and home follow-up of hospitalized elders: a randomized clinical trial. *JAMA.* 1999;281:613–620.

22. Coucheditor J. *The Health Care Professional's Guide to Disease Management.* Gaithersburg, MD: Aspen; 1998:211.

16
Prevention

Harrison G. Bloom

Disease prevention and health promotion are important aspects of health for older individuals. Between 40% and 70% of all diseases are partially or totally preventable through lifestyle modification, risk factor management, and primary or secondary preventive practices.[1–3] Despite a lack of definitive data regarding preventive interventions for a number of diseases and occasional disagreements among organizations publishing preventive guidelines, there is consensus on the value of many preventive measures. However, the underutilization of recommended preventive services remains a major challenge in medicine, including geriatric medicine.

Because significant barriers preventing the implementation of recommendations exist for both clinicians and individuals, creative ways to deliver preventive services have become increasingly important. Offering and incorporating such services at worksites, schools, senior centers, and churches could significantly help improve the numbers of older people receiving preventive care. Using nonphysician assistants, nurses, technicians, and others can also greatly facilitate the delivery of preventive services.

Primary, secondary, and tertiary prevention are all important. Primary prevention is the avoidance of a disease before it can begin. Secondary prevention, or screening for occult disease, is looking for early markers of a disease before it becomes symptomatic and then intervening early enough to positively affect outcomes. Tertiary prevention emphasizes rigorously treating established disease to prevent adverse outcomes and complications from the natural course of that disease.

Important criteria for deciding upon which diseases to apply primary or secondary preventive interventions are addressed here and apply to all age groups, including individuals 65 and over. Differentiating recommendations for the general population of older adults as opposed to a high-risk group within that population is also important. For example, yearly influenza vaccination is recommended for all adults age 65 and older. Regular

Papanicolaou smears to detect early cervical cancer, on the other hand, are recommended after age 65 mainly for women with high-risk sexual behavior or those without a previous Pap smear. Additionally, life expectancy and quality of life are especially important considerations for older individuals when deciding upon preventive interventions. Table 16.1 outlines typical life expectancies.

Criteria for screening tests include the following:

1. *The disease must have a significant effect on the quality and quantity of a patient's life.* Screening for common warts, for example, may be simple and inexpensive, but there are no adverse health effects from their presence and hence no reason to screen.

2. *Acceptable methods of treatment must be available.* Discovering a potentially serious condition at an early stage via screening is only useful if there is a treatment available to cure or significantly decrease morbidity from that condition. If effective treatment does not exist or if any individual is unable to access treatment after screening, screening is not indicated.

3. *Early treatment should yield a therapeutic result superior to that obtained by delaying treatment.* If early treatment does not lead to a better outcome, detecting a condition earlier by screening is not warranted.

4. *The disease must have an asymptomatic period during which detection and treatment significantly reduce morbidity or mortality.* By definition, screening is performed on individuals asymptomatic for the condition. If symptoms are present, any testing is diagnostic. Not only must an asymptomatic period exist, but finding and treating the condition at that earlier time must significantly reduce morbidity or mortality.

5. *Tests must be available at a reasonable cost to detect the condition in the asymptomatic period.* This criterion is more of an administrative or policy consideration. Individuals may be willing to pay for a screening test that their insurance company will not cover. Before Medicare covered screening mammography, women had to pay for

TABLE 16.1. Life expectancy, United States, 1997: additional years of life.

Age (years)	All races (years)
65	17.7
70	14.3
75	11.2
80	8.5
85	6.3
90	4.5
95	3.3
100	2.5

Source: Adapted from Anderson RN. United States Life Tables, 1997. National Vital Statistics Reports; Vol 47(28). Hyattsville, Maryland: National Center for Health Statistic; 1999.

the test. More recently, some groups have advocated utilizing helical computerized tomography to screen for lung cancer in smokers. The test is costly, and to date there is only limited evidence of its efficacy as a screening tool.

6. *The incidence of the condition must be sufficient to justify the cost of screening.* This point is also an administrative consideration. A physician may decide that if a patient can afford it, screening for a condition with an extremely low incidence is worthwhile. Conversely, the medical director of a health center, managing a limited budget, would likely not want to spend scant resources screening for a condition that would very likely never occur in that health center's population.

Influenza Prevention

Yearly vaccination against influenza is one of the most important primary preventive practices readily available for older individuals. Influenza and pneumonia together rank as the sixth leading cause of death in persons aged 65 to 74, the fifth leading cause between the ages of 75 and 84, and the fourth leading cause in persons 85 years of age or older.[4]

Inactivated influenza virus vaccine is strongly recommended for all persons 65 and older.[5] Vaccination is safe and cost-effective, particularly for individuals at high risk for influenza infection.[6,7] Medicare covers the cost of the vaccine and its administration. The vaccine needs to be given annually because of antigenic drift (variation in infectious strains) and antibody levels that wane with time.[8] October to mid-November are usually the best times to administer influenza vaccine, but any time from September to the end of flu season is appropriate.

Among community-dwelling older adults, one randomized controlled trial (RCT) found a 58% reduction in relative risk of clinically and serologically confirmed influenza infection for those who received an annual influenza vaccination compared to those receiving a placebo.[9] An intranasal live attenuated influenza vaccine has recently undergone several clinical trials and is nearing approval.[10] Like the inactivated vaccine, it will be useful preventively for influenzas A and B.

In nursing homes, vaccination of both patients and staff reduces patient morbidity and mortality. A large meta-analysis of cohort studies in nursing homes demonstrated the effectiveness of annual influenza vaccination in reducing relative risk of respiratory illness, pneumococcal pneumonia, hospitalization, and death compared to unvaccinated controls.[11] A resident vaccination rate of at least 80% should be met to establish herd immunity in institutionalized populations during active influenza outbreaks.[12] Staff vaccination in long-term care facilities provides additional protection to older institutionalized patients and in two RCTs was associated with a 40% reduction in relative risk for patient mortality.[13,14]

During institutional influenza outbreaks, chemoprophylaxis in combination with timely annual influenza vaccination has been shown to be highly effective in preventing influenza complications in small cohort studies.[15,16] M2 channel inhibitors (amantadine or rimantadine) and the neuraminidase inhibitor oseltamivir are approved for chemoprophylaxis in older adults with known or anticipated influenza A exposure. For influenza B prophylaxis, only neuraminidase inhibitors are effective. Unfortunately, there are very few randomized trials assessing efficacy of these agents in older adults, and the data are hampered by limited population size and low influenza incidence in control groups. Zanamivir, an inhaled neuraminidase inhibitor recently approved by the U.S. Food and Drug Administration (FDA) for influenza prevention, has demonstrated a nonsignificant trend toward efficacy against clinical and laboratory-confirmed influenza in a nonblinded randomized nursing home trial.[17] Persons with underlying airway diseases should not be given zanamivir.

Chronically ill or immunodeficient older persons, those who have not received the yearly influenza vaccination or received it too late to be of use in an active outbreak, and those who received a vaccine poorly matched to the outbreak antigen are particularly likely to benefit from chemoprophylaxis during influenza outbreaks. In institutional outbreaks, 14-day chemoprophylaxis for residents and staff, (with dosage adjusted for renal function) is warranted, continuing at least 7 days past the onset of the last case.[18] For community-dwelling older patients and their close personal contacts, 10-day prophylaxis is usually sufficient. Drug resistance is a concern with the M2 channel inhibitors, and the side effect profile of these agents appears slightly worse than the neuraminidase inhibitors. Both drug classes can also be used for treatment of acute influenza infection if begun within 48 h of symptom onset.

Handwashing, isolating infected persons, and restricting ill visitors and staff also reduce infection transmission in nursing homes.[19–21] Because of the very significant morbidity and mortality associated with outbreaks of influenza, both community surveillance and rapid diagnosis are important. Community surveillance can alert health care workers as to whether an outbreak is influenza A, B or both, as well as when influenza entered and exited the area.

Other Immunizations

Vaccines recommended for older individuals include influenza, pneumococcal, and tetanus. Influenza A and B and pneumococcal disease are common diseases frequently associated with significant morbidity and mortality. Tetanus, although rare, is a serious disease often resulting in death.

The 23-valent pneumococcal vaccine is between 50% and 80% effective in preventing invasive pneumococcal disease, but not pneumococcal pneumonia, in older adults who are immunocompetent.[22–25] The vaccine is safe, has only rare serious adverse effects, is inexpensive, and is covered by Medicare. There are no definite data on whether the vaccine should be given only once in a lifetime or repeated every 5 to 6 years. Although its efficacy in high-risk groups, particularly immunocompromised patients,[26,27] is questionable, the U.S. Preventive Service Task Force and the CDC's Advisory Committee on Immunization Practices recommend its use in this population because of the low risk of harm. The vaccine can be administered at any time during the year, including the same time influenza vaccine is given (in a different extremity).

Although tetanus is rare in the United States, it is a serious disease and more than 60% of tetanus infections occur in older individuals.[28,29] Current recommendations call for booster vaccinations every 10 years, although 15 to 30-year intervals are probably adequate in the United States for those properly vaccinated in childhood. If never previously vaccinated, older adults can be given a primary series that includes doses at 0, 2, and 8 to 14 months.[30] The vaccine is safe, effective, and covered by Medicare.

Colorectal Cancer Screening and Prevention (See Chapters 32 and 34)

More than 55,000 deaths yearly with 140,000 new cases per year place colorectal cancer as the second most common form of cancer, as well as the cancer with the second highest mortality rate, in the United States. The incidence of both invasive colorectal cancer and mortal-

ity increase sharply with advancing age (see Chapter 32).

Early detection in the asymptomatic period is associated with better prognosis. For patients at average risk of colon cancer, the American Cancer Society (ACS) recommends screening with fecal occult blood tests (FOBT) annually in combination with flexible sigmoidoscopy (FSIG) every 5 years (either test alone is sufficient, but the ACS prefers the combination), or a total colon exam with either a double-contrast barium enema every 5 years or colonoscopy every 10 years. As with other cancers, older adults at higher risk for colorectal cancer (e.g., those with inflammatory bowel disease or a strong family history of colorectal cancer, adenomatous polyposis, and nonpolyposis colorectal cancer) should be screened more frequently than the general older population.[31] The ACS does not impose an upper age limit at which to discontinue screening, suggesting instead that continued screening is of benefit to older patients with continued good health. The most frequently studied form of screening, fecal occult blood testing, has been shown to significantly reduce the rate of death from colorectal cancer.[32–34] There is also evidence that fecal occult blood testing done annually reduces the actual incidence of colorectal cancer by detecting premalignant adenomatous polyps.[35] Adding fecal occult blood testing to sigmoidoscopy improves the sensitivity of sigmoidoscopy, although recent studies suggest that the combination may miss as many as 50% to 60% of advanced proximal lesions.[36,37] Double-contrast barium enemas are less useful in older adults, as uninterpretable results occur because many patients cannot move as required while on the radiography table[38,39] and biopsy cannot be done at the time of the exam, making a second bowel prep necessary. Colonoscopy is the most accurate of the available tests and is becoming the modality of choice for many physicians.[40–42] "Virtual colonoscopy," three-dimensional computed tomographic colography, is a new technique promising fewer complications than endoscopic colonoscopy, does not require sedation, and requires less time. However, a number of improvements and more controlled studies are necessary before it can be recommended for population-based routine screening.[43] Although very uncommon, serious complications do occur with screening sigmoidoscopy and colonoscopy, making the choice of screening tests, especially for older persons, an individual choice as much as a clinician preference.[44]

Primary prevention of colorectal cancer with diet remains controversial. Observational data have yielded conflicting results,[45,46] and there are no randomized controlled trials (RCTs) on the efficacy of fiber in primary prevention of colon cancer. In an RCT, neither a wheat bran-supplemented diet nor a low-fat, high-fruit and -vegetable diet were found to affect the incidence of new colorectal adenomas (which can then progress to cancers).[47–49] It is important, however, to encourage measures to reduce known risk factors for colorectal cancer through weigh control, smoking cessation, regular exercise, and less red meat intake.[50]

These has been increasing interest in chemoprevention of colorectal cancer utilizing one or a combination of substances. Although future research may prove utility, there is currently no evidence from double-blind, placebo-controlled, randomized studies that aspirin, other NSAIDs, supplemental folate and calcium, or postmenopausal hormone replacement therapy are efficacious in the primary prevention of colorectal cancer.[50] Cohort and other studies of observational design do suggest a beneficial association, and the reader is referred to Chapter 34 for a summary of these studies.

Screening for Breast Cancer (See Chapters 32 and 33)

Approximately one in eight women will develop breast cancer during her lifetime. There are more than 176,000 new cases of breast cancer yearly, making it the most common cancer in women and the second leading cause of cancer death in women.[51] Advanced age is an important risk factor both for developing breast cancer and for death from breast cancer.[52]

The use of screening mammography has been highly recommended for women aged 50 to 69, with a decrease in the rate of late-stage disease detection correlating well with an increase in the use of mammography.[53–55] Recently a Cochrane Review of the randomized controlled trials upon which these recommendations are based strongly questioned the validity of five of the seven trials, only "accepting" two which together suggested that mammography does not save lives.[56] The National Cancer Institute's independent panel of experts, the PDQ, reviewed this evidence and concurred.

Most completed clinical trials have not included women over age 70 and therefore the effectiveness of screening mammography is not known in women 70 and older. Additionally, mortality is not the only endpoint of interest to women who may develop breast cancer; the effect of breast cancer diagnosis at a later stage on function and quality of life is not known. There is some evidence from a retrospective cohort study that screening mammography is effective in women at least up to age 79.[57] In fact, if women 70 and older are cognitively and functionally intact with a life expectancy of 5 or more years, there is little reason to exclude routine mammography at any age in spite of there being no definitive evidence yet that this decreases breast cancer mortality. The American Geriatrics Society recommends annual or biennial screening mammography until age 75, and every 1 to 3 years after that with no upper age limit for nondemented women with life expectancies of at least 4 years.[58] For women with family history of breast cancer or ongoing or previous long-term exposure to hormone replacement therapy, screening should be more frequent.

Fewer than half of all women over age 65 undergo regular screening mammography. Primary care physicians are encouraged help older patients overcome physical, economic, or other barriers to receiving screening. Medicare covers annual mammography screening for all female beneficiaries 40 and older, with patients paying 20% of approved charges but no deductible.[59]

Other modalities used to screen for breast cancer include clinician breast exam and teaching breast self-examination. There is not sufficient evidence at this time to recommend in favor of or against including these in periodic screening exams.[60] Nevertheless, long-standing clinical practice habits usually include periodic breast exams, and there is little reason to exclude performing these exams.

Regarding primary prevention of breast cancer, raloxifene and the antiestrogen tamoxifen have been recommended for women at increased risk of developing breast cancer, but not for the general risk population.[61] In a large RCT in which 30% of the participants were over age 65, tamoxifen was associated with as much as a 50% reduction in invasive breast cancer incidence, particularly estrogen receptor-positive cancers, compared to placebo. Use of the drug in older women, however, was associated with a 4-fold increased risk of endometrial cancer, however (RR 4.01).[62] In an RCT in which breast cancer development was a secondary outcome, raloxifene use over 3 years effectively reduced incidence of invasive breast cancer compared to placebo by as much as 40% and was not associated with elevated risk of endometrial cancer. Again, protective effects were mainly observed against the development of estrogen receptor-positive cancers.[63]

Physical activity may also reduce the risk of cancer. A review of 13 mostly observational studies found lower incidence of breast cancer among physically active adults than in sedentary adults.[64]

Screening for Prostate Cancer (See Chapters 32 and 36)

Routine screening for prostate cancer using prostate-specific antigen (PSA) remains very controversial in older men. Although prostate cancer is common in older men and it can be aggressive and lethal, there are currently no reliable ways to distinguish small early cancers that will become aggressive from those that are slow growing and non–life-threatening even if left untreated. Additionally, false-positive PSA tests are frequent, and treatment is associated with the potential for significant complications.[65,66] For these reasons, a number of organizations advise that an individual patient be educated about the potential benefits and risks of routine screening PSA testing followed by diagnostic confirmation and treatment and decide for himself whether or not to pursue testing.

Digital rectal exam by itself is not effective as a screening test for prostate cancer.[67] In one study, the most valid screening results were obtained when suspicious digital rectal exam was combined with PSA values greater than 4 ng/ml (sensitivity, 95%; positive predictive value, 62%).[68] Medicare covers annual digital rectal exams as well as annual PSA screening test without deductibles or coinsurance payments or male beneficiaries aged 50 and over.[69]

Screening for Cervical Cancer (See Chapters 32 and 37)

Positive Pap smears are more often associated with invasive disease in older women.[70,71] A significant percentage of women over age 65 have never had a Pap smear. There is some debate as to what age to discontinue Pap screening. For women who have a cervix, the U.S. Preventive Service finds no solid evidence to impose an upper age limit, but suggests testing be discontinued after age 65 for those who have up until that time had regular and normal screenings.[72] For women at higher risk of cervical cancer (including older patients with a personal or family history of cervical cancer, previous abnormal smears, or high-risk sexual behavior), testing should continue annually.[73] Medicare covers annual cervical cancer screening for women at higher risk for cervical cancer; screening for all other female beneficiaries is covered every 3 years.

The validity of the Pap test as a screening instrument varies with the technique of the individual physician, sample method used, and laboratory interpretation; sensitivity ranges from 30% to 87% while specificities range from 86% to 100%.[74] Obtaining a proper specimen can sometimes be difficult in older women for a number of reasons, including vaginal atrophy and narrow cervical os. Musculoskeletal disorders can make lying in the usual supine position with legs in stirrups quite difficult. Using the left lateral position may be preferable. For these reasons, if a primary care clinician is not experienced in performing Pap smears in older women, referral to a gynecologist is appropriate.

Screening: Other Cancers (See Chapter 32)

There are currently no reliable screening modalities for cancers of the lung, ovary, thyroid, kidneys, brain, skin, pancreas, or hematologic system.

Screening for High Blood Pressure (See Chapter 40)

Hypertension is a chronic, highly prevalent, generally asymptomatic condition that is safely and effectively treatable in older adults. Treatment of hypertension in older persons has played a key role in leading to a significant reduction in morbidity and mortality from congestive heart failure, myocardial infarction, and stroke.[75–77] Controlling hypertension can also decrease risks for renal disease, retinopathy, and ruptured aortic aneurysm.[78]

All forms of hypertension, including isolated systolic, isolated diastolic, and mixed systolic/diastolic, should be screened for at least every 2 years and treated.[33,79] Annual screening is appropriate for patients whose most recent diastolic blood pressure was between 85 and 89 mmHg and/or systolic blood pressure was 130 to 139; higher measurements should provoke more immediate evaluation.[80] Proper cuff size and technique are especially important in older individuals, and, as with younger adults, hypertension should only be diagnosed if present at more than one reading on three separate visits.[81,82]

Screening for Lipid Disorders (See Chapter 39)

Whether to routinely screen older individuals for high cholesterol and other lipid abnormalities remains controversial. The American College of Physicians guidelines neither recommend nor discourage cholesterol screening in patients 65 to 75 years of age and find it unnecessary in patients older than 75 years with no evidence of coronary disease. However, the evidence upon which these recommendations were based, that is, studies showing no association between coronary heart disease (CHD) mortality and high cholesterol in old age, may have been confounded by inclusion of frail elderly persons with low cholesterol. A study of 4066 older persons, after adjustment for frailty, found an association between total cholesterol and increased risk for CHD mortality.[83] Older age (>45 years for men, >55 years for women) is itself an accepted risk factor for coronary artery disease.

After reviewing evidence on whether identification and treatment of asymptomatic people with abnormal lipid levels can substantially reduce the risk of coronary heart disease, the U.S. Preventive Services Task Force recently extended its recommendations to include routine lipid screening for older and middle-aged persons. Neither an optimal screening interval for older adults nor an upper age limit at which to discontinue screening has been set, but the Task Force has suggested that repeated screening may be less important in older people because lipid levels are less likely to increase after age 65 years. Five-year intervals have been suggested as a benchmark for the general U.S. population, with longer or shorter intervals dictated by patient risk; intervals longer than 5 years may be sufficient for older persons who have had low-risk results on previous lipid tests whereas elderly patients showing higher-risk lipid levels should be screened more frequently. Older individuals who have never been screened should be.[84]

The U.S. Preventive Services Task Force strongly recommends measurement of total cholesterol (TC) and high-density lipoprotein cholesterol (HDL-C), but finds insufficient evidence to recommend for or against triglyceride measurement. The American College of Physicians has set ranges for total cholesterol (>240 mg/dL), LDL-C (≥160 mg/dL), and triglycerides (>400 mg/dL) that it considers associated with high risk for coronary heart disease. The National Cholesterol Education Program sets a high-risk range for HDL-C (<40 mg/dL) levels.[85–89] The Canadian Task Force on the Periodic Health Exam is in the process of revising its earlier screening recommendations.

Diabetes (See Chapter 46)

Noninsulin-dependent diabetes mellitus (NIDDM) is an increasingly common disease in older adults. Weight loss and increased physical activity are simple lifestyle changes that significantly reduce the risk of diabetes. At least three studies have found marked benefits from lifestyle modifications in preventing the development of diabetes in middle-aged adults with impaired glucose tolerance,[90–92] and the latter of these studies showed benefit for older patients as well. Even relatively modest weight loss (mean, 7.7 lb) over 2 years is associated with significant reductions in risk in persons already at high risk for diabetes. These studies are summarized in Chapter 46.

For screening purposes, the American Diabetes Association lowered its normal fasting glucose level for adults over age 45 to less than 126 and suggested screening occur every 3 years.[93,94] Although the value of rigorous

glucose control in older diabetics to prevent end-organ damage (tertiary prevention) has not been definitively demonstrated, consensus expert opinion believes it will be equally beneficial in older as well as younger (insulin-dependent) individuals.[95–97] Medicare covers home glucose monitoring kits for its beneficiaries.

Prevention and Screening for Osteoporosis (See Chapter 43)

Even in asymptomatic older women, the prevalence of low bone mineral density (BMD) is widespread. The National Osteoporosis Risk Assessment study, a longitudinal observation of 200,160 postmenopausal women, offered bone mineral density screening at primary care sites and revealed previously undiagnosed osteoporosis in 7.2% of those screened and a further 36.9% with undiagnosed osteopenia. The consequences of undiagnosed low bone mineral density (BMD) in the year following testing, compared to those with normal BMDs, were a 4-fold-greater incidence of fracture with osteoporosis and a 1.8-fold-greater rate of fracture with osteopenia.[98] History of smoking or cortisone use was associated with significantly elevated risk of fracture.

As a primary preventive measure, discussing and offering hormone prophylaxis to perimenopausal and postmenopausal women is recommended. Fracture and bone mass decline is most effectively prevented when hormone replacement therapy begins close to menopause and is continued for longer than 5 years. Benefits are observed only while estrogen use is continued, and a history of past estrogen use provides little or no current bone mass protection for women over age 75. No upper age limit to stopping prophylaxis has yet been established.[99]

Hormone prophylaxis carries its own set of risks, including risk of cardiovascular events during the initial period of treatment and of breast or endometrial cancer with long-term use. Lifestyle changes are viable alternatives to HRT in the prevention of bone loss for most older women, and include adequate calcium intake, routine exercise, and cessation of smoking.[100,101] Adequate intake of Vitamin D is also prudent.

Bone densitometry to screen for osteopenia in asymptomatic women at risk for osteoporosis is recommended, and if osteopenia is present, prophylactic treatment to avert frank osteoporosis should be recommended utilizing estrogen, raloxifene, or alendronate.[102] National Osteoporosis Foundation (NOF) guidelines, issued in 1998, recommend testing for women over age 65 regardless of risk factors. (NOF recommendations are summarized in Chapter 43, Table 43.4.) Although the efficacy of osteoporosis screening in men is unproven, longevity is a risk factor in itself, and a one-time screening can establish which men need preventive treatment.

Malnutrition (See Chapter 68)

Obesity, malnourishment, and failure to maintain adequate fluid intake are all common, significant problems in older adults, associated with increased mortality and morbidity, including cognitive dysfunction, depression, and delayed wound healing. Up to 15% of community-living elders may be considered malnourished if the term is defined as a decrease in nutrient reserves.[103] Among hospitalized or institutionalized patients the prevalence is much higher. Chronically ill persons, cognitively impaired elderly, and those with excessive alcohol intake are particularly prone to malnourishment;[104] malnourishment can in turn exacerbate these same problems. Vitamin D deficiency is common in elderly populations with limited exposure to sunlight. Protein-energy malnourishment is common among older persons following elective surgical procedures or minor infections. Physicians should maintain a high index of suspicion for nutritional deficiencies in these patients, as well as in patients with low incomes, social isolation, multiple medication use, malabsorption syndromes, or chronic myocardial, renal, or pulmonary illnesses.

The U.S. Preventive Services Task Force recommends that all patients, regardless of age, be administered periodic height and weight measurements. Body mass index (BMI) is the recommended gauge, although obtaining accurate height measurements may be difficult in bed-bound elders. BMI below 22 or above 29 should raise red flags. Use of the single question: "Have you lost 10 pounds over the last 6 months without trying to do so?" in combination with measurement of BMI or use of height/weight charts is an effective and simple screen for malnourishment. Persons weighing less than 100 lb (45.5 kg) are more likely to be malnourished, and involuntary weight loss may indicate elevated risk of death. Older patients of normal weight or who are overweight can also be malnourished. The Nutrition Screening Initiative Checklist, with 10 yes/no questions, can also help physicians identify older persons at risk for malnourishment. Scores of 6 points or higher warrant concern. Nearly one-quarter of a noninstitutionalized Medicare population surveyed with this tool was found to be at risk.[105] Other nutritional screening tools validated among older adults in various settings are reviewed by Reuben et al.[103]

A thorough physician assessment of patient access to nutritious foods with counseling on daily multivitamin use and adequate water intake can prevent or alleviate many problems. Chapter 68 details management of nutritional deficiencies common in older adults.

Screening for Depression and Dementia (See Chapters 74 and 79)

Depression is a common and treatable condition in older individuals. Early diagnosis (case finding) and appropriate treatment with medication or psychotherapy are critical to management; unfortunately, however, it is both underdiagnosed and undertreated once diagnosed in the elderly population. The U.S. Preventive Services Task Forces recommends that physicians maintain a high index of suspicion for elderly patients, especially those with a family or personal history of depression, chronically ill or homebound elders, and those with recent personal loss, sleep disorders, and memory impairment.

A "yes" response to the question "Do you often feel sad or depressed?" has a sensitivity of 83% and specificity of 79%,[106] and should provoke a more thorough assessment. The Geriatric Depression Scale (GDS 15 or 30) is even more sensitive. In a random sample of community-living persons over the age of 75 in the United Kingdom, a GDS 15 cutoff score of 3 had 100% sensitivity and 72% specificity in detecting cases of depression, more than three-quarters of which had been undiscovered by the primary care physicians at least as long as the year before the clinical interview.[107] The GDS, however, is a screening instrument and does not make the diagnosis. Fewer than one in five of those testing positive with the GDS 15 in this study reached the diagnostic threshold for depression upon further testing by researchers blinded to GDS score.

Dementia, particularly Alzheimer's disease, increases in prevalence as the population ages. It is a chronic, progressive disease whose etiology is not yet known and for which there is currently no effective curative treatment. A systematic review of studies by the American Academy of Neurology indicates that individuals classified as having mild cognitive impairment (but not meeting clinical criteria for dementia) have a high risk of progressing to dementia or Alzheimer's disease (estimated rate, 6%–25% per year, compared to incident dementia in the overall population of older persons of 0.2% in the 65–69 age range to 3.9% in the 85–89 age range).[108] For the purposes of the systematic review, criteria for mild cognitive impairment included objective memory impairment as well as patient memory complaint, preferably corroborated by an informant, but normal general cognitive function and activities of daily living.

Early diagnosis (case-finding) is increasingly important as potentially helpful palliative treatments are available, but as yet there is insufficient evidence to screen elderly adults in whom there is no suspicion of cognitive impairment. When patients or family informants reporting memory difficulties, the U.S. Preventive Task Force advises screening; recommended instruments include the

Mini-Mental Status Exam (MMSE), the Short Portable Mental Status Questionnaire, and the Clock-Drawing Test. A very simple three-item recall test has a sensitivity of 90% for patients unable to remember all three items after 1 min.[109] In general, mild to moderate cognitive impairment is indicated by scores between 18 and 24 on the Mini-Mental Status Exam. The MMSE must be adjusted for high education or intelligence levels. The Clock-Drawing Test, despite multiple scoring systems, has a mean sensitivity and specificity of 85% and a likelihood ratio greater than 10.[110] Abnormal entries in the fourth quadrant of the clock alone are almost diagnostic of dementia.[111] For an excellent review of studies on the sensitivity and specificity of the various instruments, the reader is referred to Petersen et al.[108] It is important to note that depression, language differences, hearing impairment, and aphasia can affect the accuracy of cognitive screening tests. In addition, because dementia cannot reliably be screened in the presence of delirium, differentiating between the two must be a priority. The Confusion Assessment Method has a high specificity for delirium.[112,113]

Screening for Visual Acuity and Glaucoma (See Chapter 59)

Routine vision screening utilizing Snellen acuity testing to detect diminished visual acuity is recommended for older individuals although there have not been any trials in older individuals that primarily assessed vision per se.[114,115] Analysis of multiphasic assessment trials where visual acuity testing was included has not revealed a benefit.[116] Despite a lack of evidence supporting routine screening for glaucoma, screening older persons can be justified but is best done by eye specialists, not primary care physicians.[117]

Screening for Hearing Impairment (See Chapter 60)

A very common problem in older adults, hearing impairment is most easily and reliably screened for by periodically asking individuals whether they are experiencing any problems with their hearing.[118] If yes, referral for formal hearing evaluation is indicated. Even those already wearing hearing aids can benefit from routine screening: in one study, 10 of 11 older hearing aid users were discovered upon testing in a screening clinic to require major readjustment or complete replacement of the device.[119] Hearing aids are often helpful in appropriate persons and are smaller and consmetically more appealing than in the past.

The audioscope and the self-administered Hearing Handicap Inventory for the Elderly—Screening Version (HHIE-S) are both valid screening tools with similar specificities and likelihood ratios, but audioscope testing is the more sensitive test in both older[120–122] and younger[123] adults and is considered to be the gold standard. The majority of older adults receiving both these screening tests in one primary care setting preferred audioscope testing (60%) to the HHIE-S (13%) because they believed it to be more "reliable," an important consideration as many older adults are reluctant to follow through on recommendations to get further testing and fitting for amplification devices. Depending on whether a cutoff score of 8 or 24 is used, the HHIE-S has a sensitivity ranging from 29% to 63%, specificity ranging from 75% to 93%, and positive likelihood ratio ranging from 2.42 to 4.27. The audioscope, depending on reference standard used, has a sensitivity range of 64% to 96%, specificity of 80% to 91%, and positive likelihood ratio of 4.86 to 7.52.[124] Another simple screening test, the whisper test, may be inadequate in the primary care setting due to broad variation in outcomes between examiners.[125] For more details on screening for hearing impediments, the reader is referred to Chapter 60.

Incontinence (See Chapters 50 and 63)

Patients are often reluctant to mention or seek help for urinary or fecal incontinence, yet both are common problems with aging, affecting independence and quality of life. In a cross-sectional survey conducted in Minnesota, the age-adjusted prevalence of any episode of fecal incontinence in 1540 community-living adults over the age of 50 was 11.1% for men and 15.2% for women; for urinary incontinence, 25.6% of men and 48.4% of women reported problems. Approximately 6% of men and 9.4% of women reported dual incontinence.[126]

In addition to the significant social and emotional toll, incontinence may be both a marker for and a contributing cause of frailty in elderly patients. Frequent urinary incontinence (weekly or more often) is associated with an increased risk of falls and nonspinal fractures in older women.[127] Onset of incontinence after age of 65 has also been associated with increased risk of functional impairment in one elderly Hispanic population.[128]

Screening is simple. All older patients should be asked, "Do you ever lose your urine and get wet?" Affirmative answers should be followed up with the question, "Have you lost urine on at least 6 separate days?" Chapter 63 provides follow-up questions regarding frequency, quantity, and situations under which incontinence occurs and management of the problem. Fecal incontinence can be screened for in a similar manner. Few trials have evaluated the outcomes of screening for either condition on function or quality of life, but incontinence is a common and potentially treatable cause for nursing home admissions.

Exercise (See Chapter 69)

Regular physical activity has been shown in numerous studies to be an extremely important preventive intervention for older adults. Exercise promotes health and stimulates a sense of well-being. Included among the many benefits of regular exercise for older people are the following: an increase in lean body mass and strength; a reduction in risk for coronary artery disease, hypertension, and diabetes; a diminished risk for falling; a delay in overall functional decline; a decrease in depression; a reduction in pain from arthritis; and improved longevity.[129,130] Of all the benefits, perhaps the most important are those gleaned from preventing age-associated functional decline and the reversal of effects of adverse health episodes.[131–140]

Exercise, if approached properly, is safe even into advanced age.[141] Jogging may be one exception: in a randomized trial of 70- to 79-year-old men and women, injury rates were 57% for those who jogged during weeks 14 to 26 and had walked during the first 14 weeks compared to 5% to 9% injury rates for walking and strength training groups in the first 14 weeks.[142] Both resistance training and aerobic exercise are important and efficacious. Resistance training is most helpful for improving balance and muscular strength. Aerobic exercise is most helpful for improvement in cardiopulmonary fitness and stamina.[143]

Giving permission to older patients and encouraging regular physical activity are more important than the exact exercise program undertaken. Regular activity along with the older individual's preference and adherence are key factors for success. Appropriate exercise can include regimens easily integrated into a routine day such as walking, climbing and descending stairs, swimming, gardening, and bicycling (mobile or stationary). For individuals unable to ambulate or transfer independently, exercises can be done in bed or in a chair. Regular exercise is therefore appropriate for people at any age and almost all stages of functional status.

Functional Decline and Frailty (See Chapters 17 and 73)

Frailty, loss of function, and disability are common among older individuals. Preservation of as much independence as possible is a major goal in caring for older individuals, especially the older old. Prevention of disability is a multifaceted task encompassing all the preventive measures reviewed in this chapter plus very careful and thorough generalized overall physical and cognitive assessment. Interventions must be individualized. Ultimately, geriatric medicine strives to limit functional loss and disability to the extent possible, thereby improving quality of life.

Table 16.2 provides likelihood ratios and sensitivities for several common in-office geriatric screening instruments. Tables 16.3 through 16.5 summarize evidence-based recommendations for inclusion or exclusion of preventive measures for the older adult population. How often to perform various preventive measures and at what age (chronologic or physiologic) to stop certain

TABLE 16.2. Sensitivity and specificity of common screening instruments by blinded assessment (±95% CI).

Condition	Description of screening test	Sensitivity	Specificity	Likelihood ratio
Nutrition	Ask: Have you lost 10 lb, over the past 6 months without trying to do so? Weigh the patient.	0.65 (0.56, 0.74)	0.87 (0.81, 0.93)	5.0
Vision	Ask: "Do you have difficulty driving, watching TV, or reading, or doing any of your daily activities because of your eyesight?" If yes, test each eye with Snellen chart while patient wears corrective lenses (if applicable).	0.67 (0.58, 0.76)	0.86 (0.79, 0.93)	4.8
Hearing	Set audioscope to 40 dB. Test hearing using 1000 and 2000 Hz.	0.93 (0.88, 0.98)	0.60 (0.51, 0.69)	2.3
Cognition/ memory	Three-item recall test.	0.90 (0.84, 0.96)	0.64 (0.55, 0.73)	2.5
Incontinence	Ask: "In the last year, have you ever lost your urine and gotten wet?" If yes, ask: "Have you lost your urine on at least 6 separate days?"	0.89 (0.83, 0.95)	0.95 (0.91, 0.99)	17.8
Depression	Ask: "Do you often feel sad or depressed?"	0.83 (0.76, 0.90)	0.79 (0.71, 0.87)	4.0
Physical disability	Ask six questions: Are you able to: Do strenuous activities like fast walking or bicycling? Do heavy work around the house like washing windows, walls, or floors? Go shopping for groceries or clothes? Get to places out of walking distance? Bathe, either a sponge bath, tub bath, or shower? Dress, like putting on a shirt, buttoning and zipping, or putting on shoes?	0.91 (0.86, 0.96)	0.50 (0.41, 0.59)	1.8

Source: Adapted from Moore AA, Siu AL. Screening for common problems in ambulatory elderly: clinical confirmation of a screening instrument. *Am J Med*. 1996;100(4):438–443, with permission.

TABLE 16.3. Common screening measures recommended on good evidence for the geriatric patient.

Screening or counseling	USPSTF	CTF	AAFP	ACP	AMA	Specialist organizations	High-risk elderly patients
Screening for hearing impairment	Y	Y	Y				
Screening for visual impairment	Y	Y	Y			American Academy of Opthamologists, American Optometric Association	African-Americans and Caucasians; diabetics; family history of ocular disease
Counseling on well-balanced diet/ use of BMI tables	Y	Y	Y			Institute of Medicine, American Academy of Clinical Endocrinologists	
Counseling on physical activity	Y	Y					
Counseling on falls/injury prevention	Y	I					
Screening for elder abuse	Y*	I					Injured older patients
Screening for IADL/ADL limitations						Lachs; Moore and Siu (see references)	
Screening for substance abuse	Y	Y				Substance Abuse and Mental Health Administration	Personal history of substance abuse; patients with major life changes
Screening for hypertension (BP)	Y	Y	Y	Y		American Heart Association	
Screening for lipid disorders	Y		Y	I		National Cholesterol Education Program Adult Treatment Panel II, National Institutes of Health, American Heart Association	
Screening for oral health	Y	I				National Cancer Institute, American Cancer Society	Tobacco or alcohol users; patients with suspicious lesions
Annual influenza vaccination	Y	Y	Y		Y	American College of Preventive Medicine, CDC Advisory Committee on Immunization Practices	Patients with chronic pulmonary, cardiovascular, or metabolic disorders; institutionalized patients
Pneumococcal vaccination	Y	I*	Y		Y	American College of Preventive Medicine, CDC Advisory Committee on Immunization Practices	Patients with chronic pulmonary, cardiovascular, or metabolic disorders; institutionalized immunocompetent elderly patients
Tetanus-diptheria vaccination	Y	Y	Y	Y		CDC Advisory Committee on Immunization Practices	
Screening for breast cancer, ages 50–69 (mammography)	Y	Y	Y	Y	Y	American College of Preventive Medicine; NIH consensus conference, National Cancer Institute, American Cancer Society, American College of Radiologists, American College of Obstetricians & Gynecologists, American Geriatric Society	
Screening for breast cancer, ages 50–69 (clinical breast exam)	Y	Y	Y	Y		National Cancer Institute; American College of Obstetricians & Gynecologists; American Cancer Society; American College of Radiology; American Society of Clinical Oncology	
Screening for breast cancer (breast self-exam)	I					American College of Radiology, American Society of Clinical Oncology	
Screening for cervical cancer (PAP smear, up to age 69)	Y*	Y	Y	Y		American College of Preventive Medicine; National Cancer Institute	Previous irregular tests; immigrants from developing nations who have never been screened
Screening for colorectal cancer (annual FOBT)	Y	I	Y	Y		American Cancer Society, American Gastroenterology Association	Familial polyposis; family history of colorectal cancer in a first-degree relative; inflammatory bowel disease
Screening for colorectal cancer (sigmoidoscopy)	Y	I	Y	Y		American Cancer Society	Same as above
Screening for colorectal cancer (colonoscopy)	I	I*	Y	Y*		American Cancer Society	Same as above

USPSTF, The U.S. Preventive Services Task Force; CTF, Canadian Task Force on the Periodic Health Examination (1997); AAFP, The American Academy of Family Physicians (2002); ACP, American College of Physicians; AMA, American Medical Association; Y, yes; N, no; I, insufficient evidence; *, screen high-risk patients.

TABLE 16.4. Common screening measures to consider recommending, despite lack of conclusive evidence.

Screening measure	USPSTF	CTF	AAFP	ACP	AMA	Amer Coll Preventive Medicine	Specialty organizations recommending	High-risk patients
Screening for cognitive impairment (MMSE, SPMSQ, or clock-drawing test)	I*	I*						Difficulties in daily activities, self-reported (or reported by reliable informant)
Screening for depression (GHQ or Zung self-rating scale)	I*	N						Family/personal history of depression; patients with chronic illness, pain, sleep disorders, or multiple unexplained somatic complaints
Screening for gait/mobility problems		Y						Over age 75; using ≥4 prescription medications, especially psychoactive or antihypertensive drugs
Screening for diabetes mellitus (plasma glucose measurement)	I*	N*	N*	N*			American Diabetes Association	Obese patients; family history of disease; Native Americans, Hispanics, African Americans
Screening for thyroid disease (thyroid function tests)	I	I	Y	Y*			American Thyroid Association, American Academy of Clinical Endocrinologists	Postmenopausal women with vague complaints; patients with possible symptoms
Screening for thyroid disease (neck palpation)	N*	N	N*				American Cancer Society	Patients with history of head/neck irradiation
Screening for prostate cancer (DRE)	N	I		N		N	American Cancer Society, American Urologic Society, American College of Radiology	
Screening for prostate cancer (PSA)	N	N		N		N	American Cancer Society, American Urologic Society, American College of Radiology	
Screening for prostate cancer (TRUS)	N	N						
Screening for skin cancer (clinical skin exam)	I*	N*	N*		N	N	American Cancer Society, National Institutes of Health, National Cancer Institute, American Academy of Dermatologists, American College of Preventive Medicine*	Fair-skinned men and women aged >65, patients with atypical moles, and those with >50 moles
Screening for ovarian cancer	N	N	Y	N*	Y		National Institutes of Health, American Cancer Society, National Cancer Institute, American Medical Women's Association	Family history of ovarian cancer

USPSTF, The U.S. Preventive Services Task Force (1996); CTF, Canadian Task Force on the Periodic Health Examination (1997); AAFP, The American Academy of Family Physicians (2002); ACP, American College of Physicians; AMA, American Medical Association; CDC, Center for Disease Prevention and Control; Y, yes; N, no; I, insufficient evidence; *, screen high-risk patients.

TABLE 16.5. Screening measures for which evidence does not support recommendation.

Screening measure	Does not recommend				Recommends	Screen high-risk individuals
	USPSTF	CTF	AAFP	ACP		
Annual electrocardiogram	I	N		N	American College of Cardiologists/ American Heart Association, American College of Sports Medicine	
Screening for osteoporosis (bone densitometry)	I*	N*			National Osteoporosis Foundation, American Academy of Clinical Endocrinologists*	Women with history of fractures; loss of height with back pain; advanced age; Caucasian race; low body weight; bilateral oophorectomy before menopause; women considering estrogen prophylaxis
Screening for lung cancer	N		N	N		
Screening for pancreatic cancer	N	N	N			
Screening for bladder cancer	N*	N				Smokers; patients who worked in rubber or dye professions
Screening for asymptomatic carotid disease	I	N	N*	N		Patients with risk factors for cardio- or cerebrovascular disease
Screening for peripheral artery disease	N*		N		American Heart Association*	Diabetics
Screening for abdominal aortic aneurysm	I*	I*				Men over 60 who are smokers, hypertensives, claudicants, or have family history of AAA
Screening for asymptomatic bacteriuria	I	I				
Screening for iron-deficiency anemia	N	N	N*			Recent immigrants from developing nations
Screening for tuberculosis	N*	N*	N*	N*		Recent immigrants from developing nations; patients from underserved, low-income populations, patients with diabetes, renal failure, HIV; substance abusers; nursing home residents

USPSTF, The U.S. Preventive Services Task Force (1996); CTF, Canadian Task Force on the Periodic Health Examination (1997); AAFP, The American Academy of Family Physicians (2002); ACP, American College of Physicians; AMA, American Medical Association; Y, yes; N, no; I, insufficient evidence; *, screen high-risk patients.

interventions, with few exceptions (e.g., influenza vaccine yearly), has not been well studied. Until better evidence is available, common sense should prevail.

Conclusion

As the quantity of prevention-related information increases and dissemination becomes quicker and more widespread, shared decision making between clinician and patient will become increasingly important. Availability of sites beyond the physician's office—the Internet, the workplace, senior centers, and schools, for example—will facilitate broader access to disease prevention and health promotion measures. As more individuals live longer and more active lives, attention to lifestyle habits, quality of life issues, risk factors for diseases, and genuine health promotion activities will demand more attention in the disease prevention/health promotion arena. The medical community, however, will need to be vigilant in its surveillance of "new breakthrough prevention measures" to guard the general older public from the unscientific claims of those purporting to practice "anti-aging" medicine (see Chapter 62).

References

1. U.S. Department of Health and Human Services. *Healthy People 2000: National Health Promotion and Disease Prevention Objectives.* DHHS pub PHS 91-50213. Washington, DC: Government Printing Office; 1991.
2. Fries JF, Koop CE, Beadle CE, et al. Reducing health care costs by reducing the need and demand for medical services. *N Engl J Med.* 1993;329:321–325.
3. Patterson C, Chambers LW. Preventive health care. *Lancet.* 1995;345:1611–1615.
4. Centers for Disease Control and Prevention. CDC surveillance summaries, Dec. 17, 1999. *MMWR.* 1999;48(no SS-8).
5. Centers for Disease Control and Prevention. Prevention and control of influenza: recommendations of the Advisory Committee on Immunization Practices (ACIP). *MMMW.* 2000;49:1–38.
6. Patriarca PA, Weber JA, Parker RA, et al. Efficacy of influenza vaccine in nursing homes. Reduction in illness and complications during an influenza A (H3N2) epidemic. *JAMA.* 1985;253:1136–1139.
7. Gross PA, Hermogenes AW, Sacks HS, Lau J, Levandowski RA. The efficacy of influenza vaccine in elderly persons. A meta-analysis and review of the literature. *Ann Intern Med.* 1995;123:518–527.
8. Couch RB. Drug therapy: prevention and treatment of influenza. *N Engl J Med.* 2000;343:1778–1787.
9. Govaert TM, Thijs CT, Masurel N, et al. The efficacy of influenza vaccination in elderly individuals. A randomized double-blind placebo-controlled trial. *JAMA.* 1994; 272(21):1661–1665.
10. Couch RB. Drug therapy: prevention and treatment of influenza. *N Engl J Med.* 2000;343:1778–1787.
11. Gross PA, Hermogenes AW, Sacks HS, Lau J, Levandowski RA. The efficacy of influenza vaccine in elderly persons. A meta-analysis and review of the literature. *Ann Intern Med.* 1995;123:518–527.
12. Arden NH, Kendal AP, Patriarca PA. Influenza prevention and treatment. In: *Managing an Influenza Vaccination Program in the Nursing Home.* U.S. DHHS Public Health Services. Atlanta: Centers for Disease Control; 1987:3–7.
13. Carman WF, Elder AG, Wallace LA, et al. Effects of influenza vaccination of health-care workers on mortality of elderly people in long-term care: a randomised controlled trial. *Lancet.* 2000;355(9198):93–97.
14. Potter J, Stott DJ, Roberts MA, et al. Influenza vaccination of health care workers in long-term-care hospitals reduces the mortality of elderly patients. *J Infect Dis.* 1997; 175(1):1–6.
15. Mast EE, Harmon MW, Gravenstein S, et al. Emergence and possible transmission of amantadine-resistant viruses during nursing home outbreaks of influenza A (H3N2). *Am J Epidemiol.* 1991;134(9):988–997.
16. Libow LS, Neufeld RR, Olson E, Breuer B, Starer P. Sequential outbreak of influenza A and B in a nursing home: efficacy of vaccine and amantadine. *J Am Geriatr Soc.* 1996;44(10):1153–1157.
17. Schilling M, Povinelli L, Krause P, et al. Efficacy of zanamivir for chemoprophylaxis of nursing home influenza outbreaks. *Vaccine.* 1998;16(18):1771–1774.
18. Drinka PJ, Gravenstein S, Schilling M, Krause P, Miller BA, Shult P. Duration of antiviral prophylaxis during nursing home outbreaks of influenza A: a comparison of 2 protocols. *Arch Intern Med.* 1998;158(19):2155–2159.
19. Degelau J, Somani SK, Cooper SL, Guay DR, Crossley KB. Amantadine-resistant influenza A in a nursing facility. *Arch Intern Med.* 1992;152(2):390–392.
20. Drinka PJ, Gravenstein S, Krause P, et al. Outbreaks of influenza A and B in a highly immunized nursing home population. *J Fam Pract.* 1997;45(6):509–514.
21. Bradley SF. Prevention of influenza in long-term-care facilities. Long-Term-Care Committee of the Society for Healthcare Epidemiology of America. *Infect Control Hosp Epidemiol.* 1999;20(9):629–637.
22. Sims RV, Steinmann WC, McConville JH, King LR, Zwick WC, Schwartz JS. The clinical effectiveness of pneumococcal vaccine in the elderly. *Ann Intern Med.* 1988;108: 653–657. (Published erratum appears in *Ann Intern Med.* 1988;109(9):762–763).
23. Shapiro ED, Berg AT, Austrian R, et al. The protective efficacy of polyvalent pneumococcal polysaccharide vaccine. *N Engl J Med.* 1991;325:1453–1460.
24. Butler JC, Breimen RF, Compbell JF, Lipman HB, Broome CV, Facklam R. Pneumococcal polysaccharide vaccine efficacy. An evaluation of current recommendations. *JAMA.* 1993;270:1826–1831.
25. Farr BM, Johnston BL, Cobb DK, et al. Preventing pneumococcal bacteremia in patients at risk. Results of a matched case-control study. *Arch Intern Med.* 1995;155: 2336–2340.

26. Shapiro ED, Berg AT, Austrian R, et al. The protective efficacy of polyvalent pneumococcal polysaccharide vaccine. *N Engl J Med.* 1991;325(21):1453–1460.

27. Butler JC, Breiman RF, Campbell JF, Lipman HB, Broome CV, Facklam R. Pneumococcal polysaccharide vaccine efficacy. An evaluation of current recommendations. *JAMA.* 1993;270:1826–1831.

28. Prevots R, Sutter RW, Strebel PM, et al. Tetanus surveillance—United States 1989–1990. *MMWR.* 1992:41–49.

29. Sutter RW, Cochi SL, Brink EW, Sirotkin BI. Assessment of vital statistics and surveillance data for monitoring tetanus mortality, United States, 1979–1984. *Am J Epidemiol.* 1990;131:132–142.

30. U.S. Preventive Services Task Force. *Adult Immunizations. Guide to Clinical Preventive Services.* Baltimore: Williams & Wilkins; 1996:791–814.

31. Smith RA, von Eschenbach AC, Wender R, et al. American Cancer Society guidelines on screening and surveillance for the early detection of adenomatous polyps and cancer: update 2001. In: American Cancer Society Guidelines for the Early Detection of Cancer. Update of Early Detection Guidelines for Prostate, Colorectal, and Endometrial Cancers. Also Update 2001: Testing for Early Lung Cancer Detection. *CA Cancer J Clin.* 2001;51(1):38–75.

32. Mandel JS, Church TR, Ederer F. Colorectal cancer mortality: effectiveness of biennial screening for fecal occult blood. *J Natl Cancer Inst.* 1999;91:434–437.

33. Hardcastle JD, Chamberlain JO, Robinson MH, et al. Randomised controlled trial of faecal-occult-blood screening for colorectal cancer. *Lancet.* 1996;348:1472–1477.

34. Kronborg O, Fenger C, Olsen J, Jorgensen OD, Sondergaard O. Randomised Study of screening for colorectal cancer with faecal-occult-blood test [see comments]. *Lancet* 1996;348:1467–1471.

35. Mandel JS, Church TR, Bond JH, et al. The effect of fecal occult-blood screening on the incidence of colorectal cancer. *N Engl J Med.* 2000;343:1603–1607.

36. Imperiale TF, Wagner DR, Lin CY, Larkin GN, Rogge JD, Ransohoff DF. Risk of advanced proximal neoplasms in asymptomatic adults according to the distal colorectal findings. *N Engl J Med.* 2000;343(3):169–174.

37. Lieberman DA, Weiss DG, Bond JH, Ahnen DJ, Garewal H, Chejfec G. Use of colonoscopy to screen asymptomatic adults for colorectal cancer. Veterans Affairs Cooperative Study Group 380. *N Engl J Med.* 2000;343(3):162–168.

38. Tinetti ME, Stone L, Cooney L, Kapp MC. Inadequate barium enemas in hospitalized elderly patients. Incidence and risk factors. *Arch Intern Med.* 1989;149(9):2014–2016.

39. Gurwitz JH, Noonan JP, Sanchez M, Prather W. Barium enemas in the frail elderly. *Am J Med.* 1992;92(1):41–44.

40. Woolf SH. The best screening test for colorectal cancer. *N Engl J Med.* 2000;343:1641–1643.

41. Winawer SJ, Zauber AG, Ho MN, et al. Prevention of colorectal cancer by colonoscopic polypectomy. The National Polyp Study Workgroup. *N Engl J Med.* 1993;329:1977–1981.

42. Rex DK, Johnson DA, Burt R. Colorectal cancer prevention 2000: screening recommendations of the American College of Gastroenterology. American College of Gastroenterology. *Am J Gastroenterol.* 2000;95:868–877.

43. Bond JH. Virtual colonoscopy—promising, but not ready for widespread use. *N Engl J Med.* 1999;341:1540–1542.

44. Woolf SH. The best screening test for colorectal cancer. *N Engl J Med.* 2000;343:1641–1643.

45. Jansen MC, Bueno-de-Mesquita HB, Buzina R, et al. Dietary fiber and plant foods in relation to colorectal cancer mortality: the Seven Countries Study. *Int J Cancer.* 1999;81(2):174–179.

46. Fuchs C, Giovannucci E, Colditz G, et al. Dietary fiber and the risk of colorectal cancer and adenoma in women. *N Engl J Med.* 1999;340:169–176.

47. Byers T. Diet, colorectal adenomas, and colorectal cancer. *N Engl J Med.* 2000;342:1206–1207.

48. Schatzkin A, Lanza E, Corle D, et al. Lack of effect of a low-fat, high-fiber diet on the recurrence of colorectal adenomas. Polyp Prevention Trial Study Group. *N Engl J Med.* 2000;342(16):1149–1155.

49. Alberts DS, Martinez ME, Roe DJ, et al. Lack of effect of a high-fiber cereal supplement on the recurrence of colorectal adenomas. Phoenix Colon Cancer Prevention Physicians' Network. *N Engl J Med.* 2000;342(16):1156–1162.

50. Janne PA, Mayer RJ. Chemoprevention of colorectal cancer. *N Engl J Med.* 2000;342(26):1960–1968.

51. Minton SE. Chemoprevention of breast cancer in the older patient. *Hematol Oncol Clin N Am.* 2000;14:113–130.

52. Smith-Bindman R, Kerlikowske K, Gebretsadik T, Newman J. Is screening mammography effective in elderly women? *Am J Med.* 2000;108:112–119.

53. Smith-Bindman R, Kerlikowske K, Gebretsadik T, Newman J. Is screening mammography effective in elderly women? *Am J Med.* 2000;108:112–119.

54. Chu KC, Tarone RE, Kessler LG, et al. Recent trends in U.S. breast cancer incidence, survival, and mortality rates. *J Natl Cancer Inst.* 1996;88:1571–1579.

55. Kerlikowske K, Barclay J. Outcomes of modern screening mammography. *J Natl Cancer Inst Monogr.* 1997;63:105–111.

56. Olsen O, Gotzsche PC. Screening for breast cancer with mammography (Cochrane Review). *Cochrane Database Syst Rev.* 2110;4:CD001877.

57. Smith-Bindman R, Kerlikowske K, Gebretsadik T, Newman J. Is screening mammography effective in elderly women? *Am J Med.* 2000;108:112–119.

58. Breast cancer screening in older women. AGS Clinical Practice Committee. *J Am Geriatr Soc.* 2000;48:842–844.

59. De Parle N. From the Health Care Financing Administration. *JAMA.* 2000;283(12):1558.

60. U.S. Preventive Services Task Force. Screening for breast cancer. In: DiGuiseppi C, ed. *Guide to Clinical Preventive Services.* Baltimore: Williams & Wilkins; 1996:73–87.

61. Minton SE. Chemoprevention of breast cancer in the older patient. *Hematol Oncol Clin N Am.* 2000;14:113–130.

62. Gail MH, Brinton LA, Byar DP, et al. Projecting individualized probabilities of developing breast cancer for white females who are being examined annually. *J Natl Cancer Inst.* 1989;81(24):1879–1886.

63. Cummings SR, Eckert S, Krueger KA, et al. The effect of raloxifene on risk of breast cancer in postmenopausal women: results from the MORE randomized trial. Multiple Outcomes of Raloxifene Evaluation. *JAMA*. 1999;281(23):2189–2197.

64. Kiningham RB. Physical activity and the primary prevention of cancer. *Prim Care*. 1998;25(2):515–536.

65. Flood AB, Wennberg JE, Nease RF, Fowler FJ, Ding J, Hynes LM. The importance of patient preference in the decision to screen for prostate cancer. Prostate Patient Outcomes Research Team. *J Gen Intern Med*. 1996;11: 342–349.

66. Friedrich MJ, Issues in prostate cancer screening. *JAMA*. 1999;281:1573–1575.

67. U.S. Preventive Services Task Force. *Guide to Clinical Preventive Services*. Baltimore: Williams & Wilkins; 1996.

68. Martinez de Hurtado J, Chechile Toniolo G, Villavicencio Mavrich H. The digital rectal exam, prostate-specific antigen and transrectal echography in the diagnosis of prostatic cancer. *Arch Esp Urol*. 1995;48(3):247–259.

69. De Parle N. From the Health Care Financing Administration. *JAMA*. 2000;283(12):1558.

70. Siegler EE. Cervical carcinoma in the aged. *Am J Obstet Gynecol*. 1969;103:1093–1097.

71. Mandelblatt JS, Hammond DB. Primary care of elderly women: is Pap smear screening necessary? *Mt Sinai J Med*. 1985;52:284–290.

72. U.S. Preventive Services Task Force. *Guidelines from Guide to Clinical Preventive Services*, 2nd Ed. Baltimore: Williams & Wilkins; 1996.

73. Cervical cancer. NIH Consens Statement. 1996; 14(1):1–38.

74. Nanda K, McCrory DC, Myers ER, et al. Accuracy of the Papanicolaou test in screening for and follow-up of cervical cytologic abnormalities: a systematic review. *Ann Intern Med*. 2000;132:810–819.

75. U.S. Preventive Services Task Force. Screening for hypertension. In: *Guide to Clinical Preventive Services*. Baltimore: Williams & Wilkins; 1996:39–51.

76. Gorelick PB, Sacco RL, Smith DB, et al. Prevention of a first stroke: a review of guidelines and a multidisciplinary consensus statement from the National Stroke Association. *JAMA*. 1999;281:1112–1120.

77. Mulrow CD, Cornell JA, Herrera CR, Kadri A, Farnett L, Aguilar C. Hypertension in the elderly. Implications and generalizability of randomized trials. *JAMA*. 1994;272: 1932–1938.

78. U.S. Preventive Services Task Force. Screening for hypertension. In: *Guide to Clinical Preventive Services*. Baltimore: Williams & Wilkins; 1996:39–51.

79. SHEP Cooperative Research Group. Prevention of stroke by antihypertensive drug treatment in older persons with isolated systolic hypertension. Final results of the Systolic Hypertension in the Elderly Program. *JAMA*. 1991;245: 3255–3264.

80. *The Sixth Report of the Joint National Committee on Prevention, Detection, Evaluation, and Treatment of High Blood Pressure*. The National Heart, Lung, and Blood Institute (NHLBI). Bethesda: National Institutes of Health; 1997.

81. SHEP Cooperative Research Group. Prevention of stroke by antihypertensive drug treatment in older persons with isolated systolic hypertension. Final results of the Systolic Hypertension in the Elderly Program. *JAMA*. 1991;245:3255–3264.

82. Joint National Committee on Detection, Evaluation, and Treatment of High Blood Pressure. The fifth report of the Joint National Committee on Dection, Evaluation, and Treatment of High Blood Pressure. NIH Pub: 93–1088. Bethesda: National Institutes of Health, 1993.

83. Corti MC, Guralnik JM, Salive ME, et al. Clarifying the direct relation between total cholesterol levels and death from coronary heart disease in older persons. *Ann Intern Med*. 1997;126:753–760.

84. U.S. Preventive Services Task Force. Screening for Lipid Disorders: Recommendations and Rationale. *Am J Prev Med*. 2001;20(3S):73–76 (*http://www.elsevier.com/locate/ajpmonline*).

85. Guidelines for using serum cholesterol, high-density lipoprotein cholesterol, and triglyceride levels as screening tests for preventing coronary heart disease in adults. American College of Physicians. Part 1. *Ann Intern Med*. 1996;124(5):515–517.

86. Garber AM, Browner WS, Hulley SB. Cholesterol screening in asymptomatic adults, revisited. Part 2. *Ann Intern Med*. 1996;124(5):518–531.

87. Leaf DA. Lipid disorders: applying new guidelines to your older patients. *Geriatrics*. 1994;49(5):35–41.

88. Ginsberg HN, Goldberg IJ. Disorders of lipoprotein metabolism. In: Harrison's *Principles of Internal Medicine*. McGraw-Hill, New York, 2001.

89. Executive Summary of the Third Report of the National Cholesterol Education Program (NCEP) Expert Panel on Detection, Evaluation, and Treatment of High Blood Cholesterol in Adults (Adult Treatment Panel III). *JAMA*. 2001;285(19):2486–2497.

90. Pan XR, Li GW, Hu YH, et al. Effects of diet and exercise in preventing NIDDM in people with impaired glucose tolerance. The Da Qing IGT and Diabetes Study. *Diabetes Care*. 1997;20(4):537–544.

91. Tuomilehto J, Lindstrom J, Eriksson JG, et al. Prevention of type 2 diabetes mellitus by changes in lifestyle among subjects with impaired glucose tolerance. *N Engl J Med*. 2001;344(18):1343–1350.

92. U.S. Department of Health and Human Services, Diabetes Prevention Program. Information available online: *http://www.hhs.gov/news/press/2001pres/20010808a.html*.

93. Goldberg TH, Chavin SI, Preventive medicine and screening in older adults. *J Am Geriatr Soc*. 1997;45:344–354.

94. Butler RN, Rubenstein AH, Gracia AM, Zweig SC. Type 2 diabetes: causes, complications, and new screening recommendations. I. *Geriatrics*. 1998;53(3):47–50, 53–54.

95. Goldberg TH, Chavin SI. Preventive medicine and screening in older adults. *J Am Geriatr Soc*. 1997;45:344–354.

96. Goldberg TH. Update: Preventive medicine and screening in older adults. *J Am Geriatr Soc*. 1999;47:122–123.

97. Association AD. Report of expert committee on the diagnosis and classification of diabetes mellitus. *Diabetes Care*. 1997;20:1183–1197.

98. Siris ES, Miller PD, Barrett-Connor E, et al. Identification and fracture outcomes of undiagnosed low bone mineral density in postmenopausal women: results from the National Osteoporosis Risk Assessment. *JAMA*. 2001; 286(22):2815–2822.

99. U.S. Preventive Services Task Force. Guidelines *Guide to Clinical Preventive Services*, 2nd Ed. Section I. Screening Part H. Musculoskeletal Disorders; Section III, Immunizations and Chemoprophylaxis. Baltimore: Williams & Wilkins; 1996.

99. Panel NCD. Osteoporosis prevention, diagnosis, and therapy. *JAMA*. 2001;285:785–795.

100. Hough S. Osteoporosis clinical guideline. South African Medical Association—Osteoporosis Working Group. *S Afr Med J.* 2000;90(9 pt 2):907–944.

101. Goldberg TH. Update: Preventive medicine and screening in older adults. *J Am Geriatr Soc.* 1999;47:122–123.

102. Writing Group for the Women's Health Initiative Investigators. Risks and benefits of estrogen plus progestin in healthy postmenopausal women: principal results from the Women's Health Initiative randomized controlled trial. *JAMA* 2002;288:321–333.

103. Hulley S, Grady D, Bush T, et al. Randomized trial of estrogen plus progestin for secondary prevention of coronary heart disease in postmenopausal women. Heart and Estrogen/progestin Replacement Study (HERS) Research Group. *JAMA*. 1998;280:605–613.

104. Grady D, Herrington D, Bittner V. Cardiovascular disease outcomes during 6.8 years of hormone therapy. Heart and Estrogen/Progestin Replacement Study Follow-up (HERS II). *JAMA*. 2002;288:49–57.

105. Hulley S, Furberg C, Barrett-Connor E. Non-cardiovascular disease outcomes during 6.8 years of hormone therapy. Heart and Estrogen/Progenstin Replacement Study Follow-up (HERS II). *JAMA*. 2002;288:58–66.

106. Reuben DB, Greendale GA, Harrison GG. Nutrition screening in older persons. *J Am Geriatr Soc.* 1995;43(4): 415–425.

17
Instruments to Assess Functional Status

Brandon Koretz and David B. Reuben

Geriatric assessment refers to an overall evaluation of the health status of the elderly patient. The well-being of any person is the result of the interactions among a number of factors, only some of which are medical. In the geriatric population, these various factors may have become impaired at different rates. Thus, an overall functional assessment is more holistic than the traditional medical evaluation. The ultimate goal of these evaluations is to improve or maintain function.

Frequently, assessment instruments are used to evaluate the various components of patients' lives that contribute to their overall well-being. These components, or domains, include cognitive function, affective disorders, sensory impairment, functional status, nutrition, mobility, social support, physical environment, caregiver burden, health-related quality of life, and spirituality. The instrument itself can take many forms: it can be a structured interview, a self-reported questionnaire, a physical or mental task, or a blood test. Assessment instruments usually produce scores that can be compared to established normal ranges. The results from an individual patient assessment can be used to establish a baseline for future comparisons, form diagnoses, monitor the course of treatment, provide prognostic information, and screen for occult conditions. This last application is the most common use for instruments that are employed in the outpatient setting.

This chapter provides an overview of geriatric assessment instruments. We begin by briefly describing some of the basic psychometric attributes that should guide the use of any instrument. Next, we discuss the strengths and weaknesses of different types of instruments. Finally, we end with a review, arranged by functional domain, of some useful instruments. The emphasis is on those instruments that are easy for a single healthcare provider to apply in the outpatient setting. A list of some suggested instruments appears in Table 17.1.

Psychometric Attributes of Instruments

As there are a wide variety of assessment instruments, it is important for practitioners to chose those that have been appropriately evaluated for validity, reliability, and, if possible, responsiveness.

Validity

Validity is the extent to which an assessment instrument accurately measures the quality it is intended to measure. Usually, validity is the relationship between an instrument's performance and a "gold standard," another instrument, or a future event.

Sensitivity and specificity are both components of validity. Sensitivity is the extent to which a test is able to detect persons with a disorder.[1] Specificity is the extent to which those with a negative test result do not have a disorder.[1] Both these characteristics refer to the intrinsic qualities of the instrument itself and are not dependent upon disease prevalence in the population being examined. However, they are frequently combined with prevalence rates to estimate positive and negative predictive values. For screening purposes, it is appropriate to maximize sensitivity at the expense of specificity to capture as many patients with the condition as possible.

Reliability

Reliability is the ability of a test to arrive at the same result with repeated measurements. The two most important types are interrater and test–retest. Interrater reliability refers to the degree of similarity between two scores obtained by two simultaneous observers. Test–retest reliability refers to the similarity between two scores obtained serially by the same observer over a time period when change is not expected.

TABLE 17.1. Suggested brief geriatric assessment instruments.

Domain	Instrument	Sensitivity	Specificity	Time (min)	Cutpoint	Comments
Cognition						
Dementia	MMSE[7]	79%–100%[a]	46%–100%	9	<24[b]	Widely studied and accepted
	Timed time and change test[20]	94%–100%	37%–46%	<2	<3 s for time and <10 s for change	Sensitive and quick
Delirium	CAM[23]	94%–100%	90%–95%	<5		Sensitive and easy to apply
Affective disorders	GDS 5 question form[33]	97%	85%	1	2	Rapid screen
Visual impairment	Snellen chart[4]	Gold standard	Gold standard	2	Inability to read at 20/40 line	Universally used
Hearing impairment	Whispered voice[4,40]	80%–90%	70%–89%	0.5	50% correct	No special equipment needed
	Pure tone audiometry[40,41]	94%–100%	70%–94%	<5	Inability to hear ≥2 of 4 40-db tones (0.5, 1, 2, and 3 kHz)	Can be performed by trained office staff
Dental health	DENTAL[46]	82%	90%	<2 (estimated)	Score ≥2	
Nutritional status	Weight loss of >10 pounds in 6 months or weight <100 lb[3]	65%–70%	87%–88%		Yes to either	
Gait and balance	Timed Get Up and Go[3,70]	88%	94%	<1	>20 s	Requires no special equipment

[a] Some studies have found lower sensitivites, but most studies of dementia subjects fall in this range.[7]

[b] Cutoff is dependent on a number of variables including age, education, and racial or ethnic background.[7]

Responsiveness

Responsiveness refers to an instrument's ability to detect clinically significant changes over time, even if these changes are small.[2] Tests demonstrating a high sensitivity to small changes may have an increased rate of false positives. Although in general reliable measurements are likely to be responsive, the two terms are not interchangeable.

Strengths and Weaknesses of Instruments

Assessment instruments are simply tools to begin an evaluation process. It is easy to overestimate their value and make their application an end unto itself. The crucial step in the use of assessment instruments is the interpretation of their findings. Knowing how to proceed based on positive or negative results is one of the most important duties of the clinician.

The choice of which assessment instrument to use is based on a careful consideration of its relative strengths and weaknesses as they apply to a given clinical situation. For instance, comprehensive but lengthy interview-based questionnaires may be appropriate for research settings but not in clinical practice. Patients are usually unwilling to submit to prolonged interviews, and practitioners are unlikely to have enough time to conduct them. Thus, clinically useful assessment instruments must be concise. This criterion does not mean, however, that they must be administered by the primary clinicians. The costs and utilities of administering various instruments in clinical settings by nonphysician office staff are reasonably inexpensive and effective.[3,4] Furthermore, patients can complete self-administered surveys at home.

The mode of administration (i.e., who performs the rating) can affect a test's results. The rater can be the patient, a proxy, or an interviewer. Self-administered questionnaires, although efficient and inexpensive, may introduce elements of underreporting or overreporting because of lack of motivation or denial of dysfunction. Furthermore, elderly patients may require or request assistance from family members when completing the questionnaire, thus introducing the biases of a second reporter; this may be especially true for those with cognitive impairments. However, even trained interviewers can introduce their own biases during the information-gathering process.[5]

Another element to consider is the contrast between measures of capacity and those of performance. There are advantages and disadvantages to each approach. Capacity refers to what patients report they are able to do. As the task or skill at issue is not actually performed in an observed setting, the rating process can be completed quickly. Similarly, there is no need for any special equipment. The chief disadvantage of capacity assessment is the reliance on patients' subjective estimates of their abilities. Thus, clinicians frequently ask what patients actually do instead of what they can do. Because some patients function substantially below their capacity, this approach may underestimate their functional ability. Performance-based measures are direct observations of particular actions. Advantages include an increase in objectivity as patients' biases and those of their proxies are minimized. Disadvantages include the need to train the observer and the costs for specialized equipment to create the task being observed: an audiometer to create a tone, stairs to climb, etc. Some tasks (e.g., role functions), however, cannot be measured in clinical settings.

Patient factors may also affect the performance of the instrument in clinical settings; these include educational level, social background, gender, and ethnicity.[6–8] An additional element—patient fatigue—can affect scores on cognitive or performance-based measures.

Finally, each test has a limited range in which it is sensitive, commonly referred to as ceiling and floor effects. A ceiling effect describes limited usefulness of an instrument because virtually everyone scores at the top. Conversely, a floor effect is when everyone scores at the bottom of the scales. For example, in a population of healthy community-dwelling older persons, the ceiling effect would apply if one measured basic activities of daily living (BADL, discussed below); almost all the patients are able to complete all the relevant tasks. Similarly, in a nursing home population, almost all patients will be dependent in all items of the instrumental activities of daily living scale (IADL; discussed below); thus, the instrument does not capture a range of function—a floor effect. Practitioners must be aware of the range of sensitivity of the tools they employ and select tests that are appropriate for the population.

Screening

Many assessment instruments applied in the outpatient setting are used to detect asymptomatic conditions. The principles of screening derive from preventive services research. Screening has been defined as using "a test or other standardized examination procedure ... to identify patients requiring special intervention."[9] There are at least five requirements for screening: (1) a screening test must have acceptable sensitivity and specificity; (2) the test must detect a condition in a presymptomatic stage; (3) there must be a proven treatment for this condition; (4) there must be additional benefit derived from receiving the treatment in the presymptomatic stage; and (5) the condition that the screening is targeting must be common and be associated with a significant burden.[10] Although geriatric assessment instruments usually do not

fulfill all these requirements, these principles should be considered when deciding whether it is worth assessing a particular dimension.

Dimensions of Geriatric Assessment

Cognitive Function

Assessment of the cognition of elderly patients generally focuses on detection of dementia and delirium. Although these two conditions can be distinguished by time course, pathophysiology, and clinical features, they may coexist. In fact, the presence of dementia is a risk factor for the development of delirium in elderly hospitalized patients.[11]

Cognitive Impairment

The prevalence of dementia, an acquired, progressive impairment of multiple cognitive domains, is age dependent. Therefore, the yield of screening for cognitive impairment increases as the population ages. Because the initial phases of impairment can be quite subtle, it can be difficult for a clinician to make the incidental discovery of cognitive impairment. Structured examination techniques may be helpful in detecting early dementia. Such detection has become increasingly important because a number of pharmacologic and behavioral interventions have been shown to slow the progression of symptoms and delay nursing home placement for patients with moderate Alzheimer's disease.[12,13] Additionally, early detection of cognitive impairment allows family members and caregivers to plan for the future.

The most widely used assessment tool for cognitive status is the Mini-Mental State Exam (MMSE).[14] Originally developed to detect delirium, dementia, and affective disorders in inpatient settings, it has since been validated in a number of other settings.[15] In a 5- to 10-min period, the MMSE tests a number of cognitive domains: orientation, registration, attention and calculation, language, recall, and visual-spatial orientation. It is easy to apply and interpret. In fact, the instrument can be given by office staff after minimal training. The Short Portable Mental Status Questionnaire[16] is similar in design but has a more narrow focus. It requires that the patient answer many of the same orientation questions as the MMSE but also asks for the name of the current and past president, the patient's mother's maiden name, and his or her birthday, address, and phone number. As the questionnaire is shorter, it takes less time to administer. A disadvantage to both these performance tests is that they measure functions that are not particularly relevant in everyday life, such as drawing intersecting pentagons and performing serial subtraction.

Other useful and rapidly administered tests are the Clock Drawing task and the Time and Change test. Both are performance-based tests. The former assesses executive function and visuospatial skills by having the patient draw a clock face and place the hands at 10 min after 11 o'clock. There are standardized scoring methods[17] for the drawing, and the test has been shown to have a high negative predictive value for Alzheimer's disease.[18] The latter is a brief performance based test in which a patient must read a clock face set at 11:10 and separate $1.00 in change from a collection of coins totaling $1.80.[19,20] It has been shown to be accurate in both inpatient and outpatient populations.[19,20] To improve sensitivity, time thresholds may be applied—taking longer than 3 s to correctly tell the time and longer than 10 s to correctly make change indicate the need for further evaluation.

A very different type of cognitive assessment is the Set Test.[21] As originally described, the patients are given four categories (colors, fruit, towns, and animals) and an unlimited amount of time to list as many members of that category as possible. The maximum score in each category is 10. A score under 15 is considered abnormal,[22] although there are concerns about its sensitivity even at higher cutpoints. In one trial, 17% of demented patients demonstrated a perfect score.[23] Patients are not exposed to any lists of relevant words before the test begins and are expected to create their list de novo. This test examines a number of cognitive domains including language, executive function, and memory. Unimpaired older persons should be able to generate a list of 10 items within 1 min.

Delirium

Delirium is an acute, fluctuating alteration in level of consciousness and attention. It is a common occurrence, particularly in hospitalized elderly patients. Because its manifestations can be variable, it is often overlooked. Delirium is associated with increased morbidity and cost of care.

Several assessment instruments can facilitate the detection of delirium.[24] The most commonly used is the Confusion Assessment Method.[25] When using it, the examiner diagnoses delirium based on the demonstration of (1) an altered mental status with an acute onset and fluctuating course, (2) impaired attention, and (3) either disorganized thinking or a change in level of consciousness. Its high sensitivity and brevity make the Confusion Assessment Method a clinically useful instrument. Other cognitive tests that have been used to detect delirium are the MMSE, the Dementia Rating Scale,[26] and the Mental Status Questionnaire.[27] All have adequate reliability.[28] Disadvantages of these latter instruments include their substantial false-negative rates and their inability to distinguish delirium from dementia. Clinical tests of

attention, such as digit span or stating the months of the year backward, may also help detect delirium at an early stage. Because of the temporal variability that is the hallmark of delirium, a patient may seem entirely lucid at the time of evaluation. For this reason, it is important to seek out reports from collateral informants, family or nurses.

Affective Disorders

Depression is one of the most common psychiatric disorders affecting older persons. It is associated with significant morbidity and mortality.[29] The earliest depression scales relied heavily on the presence of somatic symptoms.[30,31] Hence, the scales may be less useful in geriatric populations with a high prevalence of such symptoms caused by other comorbid medical illness.[32] The Geriatric Depression Scale (GDS) was specifically designed for elderly patients.[33] Initially validated in a 30-question format, 15- and 5-question versions have been described.[34,35] The threshold scores for a positive depression screen are 11, 7, and 2, respectively.[33,34,35] An even more concise approach, a single question screen, "Do you often feel sad or depressed?" has been suggested.[36] If answered affirmatively, it should be followed by the 30-question form of the GDS. The single question may be as accurate in identifying depression as the long version of the GDS,[37] although this technique identifies too many false positives to be useful as a screening instrument.[38]

Visual Impairment

Although the treatment of visual impairment is beyond the scope of the primary practitioner, the leading causes of visual loss in older adults—cataract, glaucoma, age-related macular degeneration, and diabetic retinopathy—are prevalent and treatable. One accepted method of screening is having patients read the letters from the handheld Jaeger card at a distance of 14 in. from their eyes. Decreased visual acuity is defined as the patient begin unable to read the 20/40 line. The wall-mounted Snellen chart, generally considered to be the gold standard, can be similarly employed. Visual acuity tests do not assess the functional impact of visual impairment, but three self-report instruments have been developed. The Activities of Daily Vision Scale,[39] the VF-14,[40] and the National Eye Institute Visual Function Questionnaire,[41] although not typically used in the primary practice setting, each assess the patient's perceptions of impairments of their visual function.

Hearing Impairment

Hearing impairment can result in social isolation, depression, and decreased functional status. Treatment by amplification with a hearing aid has been demonstrated to improve quality of life. Analogous to the visual impairment screens, both performance-based and self-reported measuring tools are used to determine hearing loss.

Performance tests include the whispered voice, finger rub, and tuning forks. Of these, the whispered voice test has been shown to have acceptable sensitivity and specificity to be useful as a screen.[42] The examiner performs it by initially asking the patient to repeat a series of words. Then the examiner stands out of sight of the patient, occludes one of the patient's ears, and whispers one of the previously spoken words at a minimum of 6 cm from the patient's ear. A passing score is the ability to correctly repeat at least 50% of the whispered words. Screening can also be accomplished with the Welch–Allyn audioscope, a handheld otoscope with a built-in audiometer capable of delivering a 40-dB tone at frequencies of 500, 1000, 2000, and 4000 Hz. Patients fail the screen if they are unable to hear at least two of the four tones. Compared to pure tone audiometry, the audioscope has a sensitivity of 94% and a specificity of 72% for detecting hearing impairment. Its positive predictive value in the elderly is 60%.[43]

The Hearing Handicap Inventory for the Elderly—Screening version is a self-reported questionnaire designed to evaluate the effects of hearing loss on the social and emotional well-being of elderly patients.[44] A newer scale, developed from an analysis of data from the National Health and Nutrition Examination Survey, also accurately predicts hearing loss.[45] It incorporates age, gender, and education, in addition to specific questions about decreased hearing. However, because it was developed using data from a relatively young population, aged 50 to 74, its value in those who are older remains uncertain. Neither questionnaire is commonly used in primary care settings.

Dental Health

Dental disease, similar to visual or hearing impairment, requires a specialist for management. Nevertheless primary care providers should recognize dental problems and the resulting functional impact so that they can make appropriate referrals. Two of the assessment instruments available are the Geriatric Oral Health Assessment Index (GOHAI) and the DENTAL instrument. The GOHAI[46] is a 12-item self-report measure that assesses the impact of oral disease in three domains—physical function, psychosocial function, and discomfort. It is sensitive to the change of function and symptoms that occur after the subject receives dental care.[47] The DENTAL instrument, on the other hand, is used for screening purposes and to provide dental referrals from primary care practices.[48] It is composed of a list of six conditions: dry mouth, oral pain, oral lesions, difficulty eating, altered food selection,

and no recent dental care. The presence of one of the first three or two of the latter three conditions should trigger a dental referral.

Functional Status

Functional status has been defined as "a person's ability to perform tasks and fulfill social roles associated with daily living cross a broad range of complexity."[49] Measures of functional status are used for a wide variety of purposes. Clinicians apply them to establish baselines, to monitor the course of treatment, or for prognostic purposes. These assessments can also be used for screening. For instance, health maintenance organizations may use them to identify frail elderly who can be targeted for case management efforts.

Examinations of function may be divided into three levels: basic activities of daily living (BADL),[50] instrumental activities of daily living (IADL),[51] and advanced activities of daily living (AADL).[52] BADL refer to those functions that are necessary, but not sufficient, for maintaining an independent living status. Katz described basic functional tasks: feeding, maintaining continence, transferring, toileting, dressing, and bathing. Individuals with multiple dysfunctions at this level will require significant in-home support, such as 24-h care, or nursing home admission.

IADL are more complicated levels of activity that are necessary to maintain an independent household; these include tasks such as paying bills, taking medications, shopping, and preparing food. People with several deficiencies in these areas usually require an assisted living situation, extensive community services, or some in-home support. At this level, opportunity and motivation are important contributors to maintaining function.[53]

The highest level of activity is represented by the AADL. These are tasks such as working, attending religious services, volunteering, and maintaining hobbies. These pursuits, because they are the most complex and require the highest levels of multiple abilities to complete, are likely to be the most sensitive to changes in health status.

Self-reported measures of functional status can be administered by questionnaire or by interview. As the scales tend to follow a hierarchical ordering,[54] the clinician can efficiently assess a patient's level of function by asking about more advanced items first. Performance-based measures of functional status provide useful prognostic information. Several instruments have been developed including those that focus on lower extremity function (e.g., standing balance, gait speed, and rising from a chair[55]) and those that include upper extremity function.[56] These instruments predict functional decline, institutionalization, and mortality.

Nutritional Status

Malnutrition occurs frequently among elderly patients, particularly those residing in nursing facilities. It has been associated with increased mortality, morbidity, and admission to nursing homes.[57] Nutritional status can be evaluated by self-report screens, biochemical markers, and anthropometric measures. The most widely used self-report screen is the 10-question, self-administered checklist portion of the Nutrition Screening Initiative.[58,59] A score of six or more indicates that a patient is at risk for malnutrition. If patients score at this level, they are prompted to see health care providers for more in-depth evaluations. Checklist scores can predict future disability and persons at high risk for hospitalization.[60] The checklist has been criticized for being no more accurate as a multi-item instrument than some of the individual component items and for having poor predictive value in general.[61,62]

Biochemical markers, although not specific for malnutrition, can be used as prognostic indicators. The most studied serum marker is the serum albumin, which predicts morbidity and mortality in community-dwelling, hospitalized, and institutionalized patients.[63] Hypocholesterolemia is also associated with increased mortality.[64] The combination of hypoalbuminemia and hypocholesterolemia can be used to predict long-term mortality and functional decline.[65]

Anthropometric tools have been used to assess nutrition. The easiest one for the primary practitioner to employ is the body mass index (BMI), which is calculated by dividing the body weight in kilograms by the square of the height in meters. BMI less than 22 indicates undernutrition and predicts future mortality.[66] Measurements of skin folds assess nutritional status. However, these measurements require specialized equipment and training and may not be reliable in elderly patients.[67]

Assessment methods employing combinations of these approaches can be used to determine nutritional status. The Mini Nutritional Assessment (MNA)[68] creates a composite score from the results of anthropometric measurements, general assessment, dietary factors, and patient self-report. Subjects are then classified as either well nourished, at risk of malnutrition, or malnourished. The Subjective Global Assessment also uses information from the history and physical examination to categorize patients into one of three groups—the same three as the MNA—which can be used to predict major postoperative complications.[69]

Gait and Balance Impairment

Falls are a major cause of morbidity and mortality in geriatric patients. Assessments of gait and balance impairment should begin with the clinician asking patients about their histories of falls, including frequency, resulting injury, and circumstances surrounding each incident. However, because many patients do not recall previous falls,[70] self-report measures alone may not be sufficient. Performance-based assessment instruments can be more useful. For example, the Performance-Oriented Assessment of Mobility[71] employs a series of simple tasks: sitting and standing balance, turning, standing without the use of upper extremities for a push-off, and gait. Five other common maneuvers—head turning, reaching, bending over, back extension, and standing on one leg—can be added for a further assessment of balance. All these simulate real-life situations in which the patient may be at increased risk for falls. Although an impairment in these activities is not diagnostic of a particular pathologic process, clinicians can use this information to identify those in need of further diagnostic evaluation.

Other screening instruments include the Timed Get Up and Go Test[72] and the Functional Reach.[73] In the Timed Get Up and Go Test, patients arise from a seated position, walk 3 m, turn around, return to the chair, and sit down. A healthy, elderly individual should be able to complete this task in less than 10 s; any score greater than 20 s should prompt a more in-depth evaluation. This test may also be useful to follow patients over time for functional decline. The Functional Reach is a measure of patient ability to stretch forward without moving their feet. Limited ability to reach forward predicts the occurrence of future falls.

Although falls themselves create disability, even the fear of falling can produce functional limitation. The Survey of Activities and Fear of Falling in the Elderly is an instrument designed to evaluate how this fear contributes to the restriction of physical activity.[74]

Social Support

There is a strong association between patients' social functioning and health status. Clinicians should be familiar with their patients' levels of social interaction. During times of physical or emotional stress, these social networks may mean the difference between remaining independent in the community or requiring nursing home care. Although there are a number of scales to assess social well-being and interaction, they are too detailed to be useful when applied by a primary care practitioner in interview form.[75] As part of the social history, the health care provider should ask about who lives with the patient, who provides meals and transportation if the patient is unable to do so, and if the patient provides care for anyone else. These questions are particularly important because any subsequent absence of a caregiver, if present, would have major implications for the patient's well-being. For example, if the caregiver becomes ill, the patient may need to find an alternative source of food and transportation. Simple ways to assess a patient's social supports are to ask if there is someone whom the patient could call for help or if there are friends or relatives with whom the patient has contact more than once a month.[76]

Environment

Physicians rarely perform home safety evaluations themselves, but many home health providers are trained to do so. These evaluations are covered by Medicare for those who are eligible for home health services. Environmental hazards that may lead to falls are common in community-based housing and in retirement communities.[77] The most common hazards are poor lighting, pathways that are not clear, and loose rugs or other "slip and trip" threats.

Caregiver Burden

Because dementia and other chronic illnesses affecting the elderly are prevalent, older persons are frequently caregivers for their spouses or other relatives. The psychologic, physical, and economic burden associated with caregiving can be substantial. Moreover, such stress also has effects on patients who are recipients of care. Increased caregiver burden independently predicts use of medical services and nursing home placement.[78] Interventions to decrease the stress of caregivers may delay nursing home placement.[79]

Scales to assess caregiver burden are primarily used for research,[80] but some may have clinical applications. The Screen for Caregiver Burden,[81] which evaluates spouse caregivers of patients with Alzheimer's disease, is a 25-item self-administered questionnaire that is sensitive to changes over time. The Caregiving Hassles Scale also evaluates the stress experienced by the caregivers of family members with Alzheimer's disease.[82] This 42-item self-administered instrument focuses on the minor irritations associated with providing care on a daily basis.

Quality of Life

Many elderly patients have chronic diseases that result in discomfort and disability. As it is impossible to cure these problems, the goal is to ameliorate suffering and improve patients' perceptions of their lives. Measurements of health-related quality of life provide feedback to researchers and clinicians so they can better target their efforts. Unfortunately, there is not yet any brief, widely accepted quality of life scale specifically targeting the geriatric population. The Geriatric Quality of Life Questionnaire (GQLQ) was designed to measure the health-related quality of life of community-dwelling elderly. However, in spite of being specifically designed for a frail elderly population, the GQLQ is neither more responsive nor more valid than other generic scales with regard to measurement of ADL function and emotional function.[83] The Medical Outcomes Short Study Form-36, a brief questionnaire, has been extensively studied and is widely used.[84] It is more appropriate for healthier community-dwelling older persons rather than the frail or institutionalized population.

Spirituality

For many older patients, spiritual beliefs are very important components of quality of life. Furthermore, attendance at religious services has been associated with decreased mortality.[85] The SPIRIT mnemonic provides a structure for taking a patient's spiritual history.[86] The interview covers personal spirituality and beliefs, involvement in a spiritual community and rituals, as well as the implications of these beliefs and practices on medical care and advanced directives. These issues may be particularly important for patients who are approaching death. As with problems in other domains, clinicians should not hesitate to involve specialists. Clergy members can be helpful, especially during times of health crisis.

Incorporating Assessment Instruments

The biggest challenge for clinicians with regard to assessment instruments is incorporating them into a busy practice. The particular combination of self-reported and performance instruments that will result in the best yield, highest accuracy, and most efficient use of time will vary from practice to practice. Similarly, how to best utilize trained ancillary staff to maximize the amount of useful information obtained during each office visit will depend on the patient populations and resources of each practitioner. Finally, assessment instruments are valuable only if the practitioner can respond to abnormal findings. Hence, clinicians should be knowledgeable and skilled in the management of the conditions detected, including having available referral resources (e.g., rehabilitation therapy).

References

1. Applegate WB. Use of assessment instruments in clinical settings. *J Am Geriatr Soc.* 1987;35:45–50.
2. Guyatt GH, Deyo RA, Charlson M, et al. Responsiveness and validity in health status measurement: a clarification. *J Clin Epidemiol.* 1989;42:403–408.
3. Moore A, Siu A. Screening for common problems in ambulatory elderly: clinical confirmation of a screening instrument. *Am J Med.* 1996;100:438–443.

4. Miller DK, Brunworth D, Brunworth DS, et al. Efficiency of geriatric case-finding in a private practitioner's office. *J Am Geriatr Soc.* 1995;43:533–537.

5. Rubenstein L, Schairer C, Wieland GD, et al. Systemic biases in functional status assessment of elderly adults: effects of different data sources. *J Geriatr.* 1984;39:686–691.

6. O'Connor DW, et al. The influence of education, social class and sex on mini-mental state scores. *Psychol Med.* 1989;19: 771–776.

7. Tombaugh T, McIntyre N. The mini-mental state examination: a comprehensive review. *J Am Geriatr Soc.* 1992;40: 922–935.

8. Weiss B, Reed R, Kligman E, et al. Literacy and performance on the mini-mental state examination. *J Am Geriatr Soc.* 1995;43:807–810.

9. Report of the U.S. Preventive Services Task Force. *Guide to Clinical Preventive Services*, 2nd Ed. Alexandria, VA: International Medical, 1996;XLI.

10. Rush D. Evaluating the nutritional screening initiative. *Am J Public Health.* 1993;83:944–945.

11. Elie M, Cole MG, Pimeau FJ, et al. Delirium risk factors in elderly hospitalized patients. *J Gen Intern Med.* 1998;13: 204–212.

12. Rogers SL, Farlow MR, Doody RS, et al. A 24-week, double-blind, placebo controlled trial of denepezil in patients with Alzheimer's disease. *Neurology.* 1998;50:136–145.

13. Mittleman MS, Ferris SH, Shulman E, et al. A family intervention to delay nursing home placement of patients with Alzheimer's disease: a randomized controlled trial. *JAMA.* 1996;276:1725–1731.

14. Folstein MF, Folstein SE, McHugh PR. Mini-mental state: a practical method for grading the cognitive state of patients for the clinician. *J Psychiatr Res.* 1975;12:189–198.

15. Tombaugh TN, McIntyre NJ. The mini-mental state examination: a comprehensive review. *J Am Geriatr Soc.* 1992;40: 922–935.

16. Smyer MA, Hofland BF, Jonas EA. Validity study of the short portable mental status questionnaire for the elderly. *J Am Geriatr Soc.* 1979;27:263–269.

17. Sunderland T, Hill JL, Mellow AM, et al. Clock drawing in Alzheimer's disease: a novel measure of dementia severity. *J Am Geriatr Soc.* 1989;37:725–729.

18. Esteban-Santillan C, Praditsuwan R, Ueda H, et al. Clock drawing test in very mild Alzheimer's disease. *J Am Geriatr Soc.* 1998;46:1266–1269.

19. Inouye SK, Robinson JR, Froehlich TE, et al. The time and change test: a simple screening test for dementia. *J Gerontol.* 1998;53A:M281–M286.

20. Froehlich TE, Robinson J, Inouye S. Screening for dementia in the outpatient setting: the time and change test. *J Am Geriatr Soc.* 1998;46:1506–1511.

21. Isaacs B, Akhtar AJ. The set tes: a rapid test of mental function in old people. *Age Ageing.* 1972;1:222–226.

22. Isaacs B, Kennie AT. The set test as an aid to the detection of dementia in old people. *Br J Psychiatry.* 1973;123:460–470.

23. Oeksengaard AR, Braekhus A, Laake K, et al. The set test as a diagnostic tool in elderly outpatients with suspected dementia. *Aging Clin Exp Res.* 1995;7:398–401.

24. Trzepacz P. A review of delirium assessment instruments. *Gen Hosp Psychiatry.* 1994;16:397–405.

25. Inouye SK, van Dyck CH, Alessi C, et al. Clarifying confusion: the confusion assessment method. *Ann Intern Med.* 1990;113:941–948.

26. Mattis S. Mental status examination for organic mental syndromes in the elderly patient. In: Bellak L, Karasu TE, eds. *Geriatric Psychiatry.* New York: Grune & Stratton; 1976.

27. Kahn RL, Goldfarb AI, Polack M, et al. Brief objective measures for the determination of mentals status in the aged. *Am J Psychiatry.* 1960;117:326–328.

28. Nelson A, Fogel B, Faust P. Bedside cognitive screening instruments a critical assessment. *J Nerv Ment Dis.* 1986; 174:73–83.

29. NIH consensus conference. Diagnosis and treatment of depression in late life. *JAMA.* 1992;268:1018–1024.

30. Beck AT, Ward CH, Mendelson M, et al. An inventory for measuring depression. *Arch Gen Psychiatry.* 1961;4:561–571.

31. Zung WWK. A self-rating depression scale. *Arch Gen Psychiatry.* 1965;12:63–70.

32. Van Gorp WG, Cummings JL (as cited by Applegate W, Blass JP, Williams TF). Instruments for the functional assessment of older patients. *N Engl J Med.* 1990;322:1207–1213.

33. Yesavage JA, Brink TL. Development and validation of a geriatric depression screening scale: a preliminary report. *J Psychiatr Res.* 1983;17:37–49.

34. Sheikh JI, Yesavage JA. Geriatric depression scale (gds): recent evidence and development of a shorter version. In: Brink TL, ed. *Clinical Gerontology: A Guide to Assessment and Intervention.* New York: Haworth, 1986.

35. Hoyl MT, Alessi CA, Harker JO, et al. Development and testing of a five-item version of the GDS. *J Am Geriatr Soc.* 1999;47:873–878.

36. Lachs M, Feinstein AR, Conney LM, et al. A simple procedure for general screening for functional disability in elderly patients. *Ann Intern Med.* 1990;112:699–706.

37. Mahoney J, Drinka TJK, Abler R, et al. Screening for depression: single question versus GDS. *J Am Geriatr Soc.* 1994;42:1006–1008.

38. Maly RC, Hirsch SH, Reuben DB. The performance of simple instruments in detecting geriatric conditions and selecting community-dwelling older people for geriatric assessment. *Age Ageing.* 1997;26:223–231.

39. Mangione CM, Phillips RS, Seddon JM, et al. Development of the activities of daily vision scale. *Med Care.* 1992;30: 1111–1126.

40. Steinberg EP, Tielsch JM, Schein OD, et al. The vf-14: an index of functional impairment of patients with cataracts. *Arch Ophthalmol.* 1994;112:630–638.

41. Managione CM, Lee PP, Pitts J, et al. Psychometric properties of the National Eye Institute visual function questionnaire. *Arch Ophthalmol.* 1998;116:1496–1504.

42. Uhlmann RF, Rees TS, Psaty BM, et al. Validity and reliability of auditory screening tests in demented and non-demented older adults. *J Gen Intern Med.* 1989;4:90–96.

43. Lichtenstein MJ, Bess FH, Logan S. Validation of screening tools for identifying hearing impaired elderly in primary care. *JAMA.* 1988;259:2875–2878.

44. Ventry IM, Weinstein BE. The hearing handicap inventory for the elderly: a new tool. *Ear Hearing.* 1982;3:128–134.

45. Reuben DB, Walsh K, Moore AM, et al. Hearing loss in community-dwelling older persons: national prevalence data and identification using simple questions. *J Am Geriatr Soc.* 1998;46:1008–1011.

46. Atchinson KA, Dolan TA. Development of the geriatric oral health assessment index. *J Dent Educ.* 1990;11:680–687.

47. Dolan TA. The sensitivity of the geriatric oral health assessment index to dental care. *J Dent Educ.* 1997;61:37–46.

48. Bush LA, Horenkamp N, Morley JE, et al. D-e-n-t-a-l: a rapid self-administered screening instrument to promote referrals for further evaluation in older adults. *J Am Geriatr Soc.* 1996;44:979–981.

49. Reuben DB, Wieland DL, Rubensein LZ. Functional status assessment of older persons: concepts and implications. *Facts Res Gerontol.* 1993;7:232.

50. Katz S, Downs TD, Crash H, et al. Progress in development of the index of ADL. *Gerontologist.* 1970;10:20–30.

51. Lawton MP, Brody EM. Assessment of older people: self-maintaining and instrumental activities of daily living. *Gerontologist.* 1969;9:179–186.

52. Reuben DB, Solomon DH. Assessment in geriatrics of caveats and names. *J Am Geriatr Soc.* 1989;37:570–572.

53. Feinstein AR, Josephy BR, Wells CK. Scientific and clinical problems in indexes of functional disability. *Ann Intern Med.* 1986;105:413–420.

54. Siu AL, Reuben DB, Hays RD. Hierarchical measures of physical function in ambulatory geriatrics. *J Am Geriatr Soc.* 1990;38:1113–1119.

55. Guralnik JM, Simonsick EM, Ferrucci L, et al. A short physical performance battery assessing lower extremity function: association with self-reported disability and prediction of mortality and nursing home admission. *J Gerontol Med Sci.* 1994;49:M85–M94.

56. Reuben DB, Siu AL. An objective measure of physical function of elderly patients: the physical performance test. *J Am Geriatr Soc.* 1990;38:1105–1112.

57. Covinsky KE, Martin GE, Beyth RJ, et al. The relationship between clinical assessments of nutritional status and adverse outcomes in older hospitalized medical patients. *J Am Geriatr Soc.* 1999;47:532–538.

58. White JV, Dwyer JT, Posner BM, et al. The validity of nutritional status as a marker for future disability and depressive symptoms among high-risk older adults. *J Am Geriatr Soc.* 1999;47:995–999.

59. Lipshitz DA, Ham RJ, White JV. An approach to nutritional screening for older americans. *Am Fam Physician.* 1992;45:601–608.

60. Boult C, Krinke UB, Urdangarin CF, et al. The validity of nutritional status as a marker for future disability and depressive symptoms among high-risk older adults. *J Am Geriatr Soc.* 1999;47:995–999.

61. Reuben DB, Greendale G, Harrison GG. Nutritional screening in older persons. *J Am Geriatr Soc.* 1995;43:415–425.

62. Rush D. Evaluating the nutrition screening initiative. *Am J Public Health.* 1993;83:944–945.

63. Committee of Nutrition Services for Medicare Beneficiaries. Undernutrition. In: *The Role of Nutrition in Maintaining Health in the Nation's Elderly. Evaluating Coverage of Nutrition Services for Medicare Beneficiaries.* National Washington, DC: Academy Press; 2000.

64. Harris T, Feldman JJ, Kleinman JC, et al. The low cholesterol-mortality association in a national cohort. *J Clin Epidemiol.* 1992;45:595–601.

65. Reuben DB, Ix JH, Greendale GA, et al. The predictive value of combined hypoaluminemia and hypocholesterolemia in high functioning community-dwelling older persons: Macarthur studies of successful aging. *J Am Geriatr Soc.* 1999;47:402–406.

66. Landi F, Zuccali G, Gambassi G, et al. Body mass index nd mortality among people living in the community. *J Am Geriatr Soc.* 1995;47:1072–1076.

67. Sullivan DH, Patch GA, Baden AL, et al. An approach to assessing the reliability of anthropometrics in elderly patients. *J Am Geriatr Soc.* 1989;37:607–613.

68. Guigoz Y, Vellas B, Garry PJ. Assessing the nutritional status of the elderly; the mini nutritional assessment as part of the geriatric evaluation. *Nutr Rev.* 1996;54:S59–S65.

69. Detsky AS, Smalley PS, Chang J. Is this patient malnourished? *JAMA.* 1994;271:54–58.

70. Cummings SR, Nevitt ML, Kidd S. Forgetting falls: the limited accuracy of recall of falls in the elderly. *J Am Geriatr Soc.* 1988;36:613–616.

71. Tinetti, ME. Performance-oriented assessment of mobility problems in elderly patients. *J Am Geriatr Soc.* 1986;34:119–126.

72. Podsiadlo D, Richardson J. The timed "up and go": a test of basic functional mobility for frail elderly persons. *J Am Geriatr Soc.* 1996;39:142–148.

73. Duncan PW, Weiner DK, Chandler J, et al. Functional Reach: a new clinical measure of balance. *J Gerontol Med Sci.* 1990;45:M192–M197.

74. Lachman ME, Howland J, Tennstedt S, et al. Fear of falling and activity restriction: the survey of activities and fear of falling in the elderly (safe). *J Gerontol Psychol Sci.* 1998;53:P43–P50.

75. Kane RA, Kane RL. *Assessing the Elderly: A Practical Guide to Measurement.* Lexington, MA: Health; 1981.

76. Kane RA. Instruments to assess functional status. In: Cassel C, ed. *Geriatric Medicine*, 3rd ed. New York: Springer; 1996.

77. Gill TM, Willimas CS, Robinson JT, et al. A population-based study of environmental hazards in the homes of older persons. *Am J Public Health.* 1999;89:553–556.

78. Brown LJ, Potter JF, Foster BG. Caregiver burden should be evaluated during geriatric assessment. *J Am Geriatr Soc.* 1990;38:455–460.

79. Mittelman MS, Ferris SH, Shulman E, et al. A family intervention to delay nursing home placement of patients with Alzheimer disease. *JAMA.* 1996;276:1725–1731.

80. Vitaliano PP, Young HM, Russo J. Burden: a review of measures used among caregivers of individuals with dementia. *Gerontologist.* 1991;31:67–75.

81. Vitaliano PP, Russo J, Young HM, et al. *Gerontologist.* 1991; 31:76–83.

82. Kinney JM, Stephens MAP. Caregiving hassles scale: assessing the daily hassles of caring for a family member with dementia. *Gerontologist.* 1989;29:328–332.

83. Guyatt GH, Eagle DJ, Sackett B, et al. Measuring quality of life in the frail elderly. *J Clin Epidemiol.* 1993;46:1433–1444.

84. Ware JE, Sherbourne CD. The MOS 36-item short-form health survey (sf-36). i. Conceptual framework and item selection. *Med Care.* 1992;30:473–483.

85. Oman D, Reed D. Religion and mortality among the community dwelling elderly. *Am J Public Health.* 1998;88:1 469–1475.

86. Maugans TA. The spiritual history. *Arch Fam Med.* 1996;5: 11–16.

18
Comprehensive Geriatric Assessment and Systems Approaches to Geriatric Care

David B. Reuben

During the past quarter century, the health care delivery of older persons has evolved from a traditional medical framework to a broader recognition of the relationship between an older person's health and their environment, beliefs, support system, and societal roles. Accordingly, new systems of care have been developed that recognize the complexity of this health-related ecosystem and attempt to organize and enhance it to improve the overall health and well-being of the individual. The initial attempts at organizing this care focused on the frail elderly population, based upon the belief that this population was most needy and most likely to benefit from a geriatric approach. Early descriptive studies indicated that among many institutionalized older persons, treatable problems could be uncovered by systematic evaluation of multiple dimensions of health. These dimensions and specific approaches to evaluation are covered in Chapter 17. Because of the frailty of the population initially considered and because physicians had little training or skill in many aspects of this broader evaluation, teams of health care professionals were assembled to provide comprehensive geriatric assessment (CGA). A 1987 National Institutes of Health Consensus Development Conference defined CGA as a "multidisciplinary evaluation in which the multiple problems of older persons are uncovered, described, and explained, if possible, and in which the resources and strengths of the person are catalogued, need for services assessed, and a coordinated care plan developed to focus interventions on the person's problems."[1]

Over the past two decades, research on the effectiveness of CGA has led to changes in both the target population for geriatric assessment and the approaches employed. Simultaneously, the overall health care system has evolved in response to financial, technologic, and cultural forces. This chapter first describes traditional comprehensive geriatric assessment and then traces the evolution of the next generation of health service delivery innovations that are derived from CGA. Finally, I speculate on the future of CGA-like interventions.

Comprehensive Geriatric Assessment

Overview

The premise behind comprehensive geriatric assessment is the belief that a systematic evaluation of frail older persons by a team of health professionals can uncover treatable health problems and lead to improved health outcomes. Early randomized clinical trials provided convincing evidence that such programs conducted in hospital-based and rehabilitation units, which typically required several weeks of treatment, could lead to better survival rates, improved functional status, and more desirable placement (e.g., home rather than nursing home) following discharge from the hospital. Since these first trials were published in the early 1980s, the health care delivery system in the United States has changed and there has been an increased focus on the costs of delivering care. Such emphasis on controlling costs has led to a shift from hospital to outpatient care, growth in managed care, and case management of frail older persons. In response to these changes, many programs have attempted to retain principles of CGA yet streamline the process of care, frequently relying on postdischarge and community-based assessment. Furthermore, most of the early programs focused on restorative or rehabilitative goals (tertiary prevention) whereas many newer programs are aimed at primary and secondary prevention. Finally, many of the principles of CGA are being incorporated into the practices of individual clinicians (both physicians and nurse practitioners), whereas in CGA the assessments are conducted by a team of health care professionals rather than by one solitary clinician. As a result, most of today's CGA programs bear little resemblance to the traditional models of the 1980s. Nevertheless, reviewing the basic principles of CGA provides an understanding of both the evolution of this method of health care delivery and the framework for CGA-like interventions that are currently available or are in development.

Process of Care

Conceptually, comprehensive geriatric assessment is a three-step process: (1) screening or targeting of appropriate patients; (2) assessment and development of recommendations; and (3) implementation of recommendations, including physician and patient adherence to recommendations. Each of these steps is essential if the process is to be successful at achieving health and functional benefits. Within this broad conceptualization, CGA has been implemented using many different models in various health care settings.

Screening and Selection of Appropriate Patients

Most CGA programs have used some type of identification (targeting) of high risk parents as a criterion for inclusion in the program. The purpose of such selection is to match health care resources to patient need. For example, it would be wasteful to have multiple health care professionals conduct assessments on older persons who are in good health and have only needs for preventive services. Rather, the intensive (and expensive) resources needed to conduct CGA should be reserved for those who are at high risk of incurring adverse outcomes. Such targeting criteria have included:

- Chronologic age
- Functional impairment
- Geriatric syndromes (e.g., falls, depressive symptoms, urinary incontinence, functional impairment)
- Specific medical conditions (e.g., congestive heart failure)
- Expected high health care utilization

Each of these criteria has been shown to be effective in identifying patients who may benefit from some type of geriatric assessment and management. However, none of these criteria are effective in identifying patients who would benefit from all geriatric assessment and management programs. Accordingly, the specific targeting criteria should be matched to the type of assessment and intervention that is being implemented. For example, a geriatric evaluation and case management program might focus on persons at high risk of health care utilization. Conversely, a preventive program might rely solely on age (e.g., >75 years) as the entry criterion.

Assessment and Development of Recommendations

Once patients have been identified as being appropriate for CGA, the traditional model of CGA invokes a team approach to assessment. Such teams are intended to improve quality and efficiency of care of needy older persons by delegating responsibility to the health professionals who are most appropriate to provide each aspect of care. Appropriateness in this case indicates both special expertise (e.g., social workers have unique knowledge about community resources) and costs of providing care (e.g., a nurse may be able to conduct some medical assessments as well as a physician). Such team care requires a set of operating principles and governance. Otherwise, it can result in uncoordinated, redundant, or dysfunctional care. First among these principles is an understanding of the roles of each member of the team and mutual respect among the different professions. The team must also establish rules for process of care including the conduct of team meetings, communication, and follow-up on each professional's assigned responsibilities and tasks. Although such teams have been embraced in principle by health care systems, in practice they often run counter to the training of health professionals. In particular, physicians have had little training in working with health care teams, and their basic training emphasizes a medical model.

The composition of the CGA team has traditionally included core and extended team members. Core members evaluate all patients; whereas extended team members are enlisted to evaluate patients on an "as-needed" basis. Most frequently, the core team consists of a physician (usually a geriatrician), a nurse (nurse practitioner or nurse clinical specialist), and a social worker.

The extended members of the team include a variety of rehabilitation therapists (e.g., physical, occupational, speech therapy), psychologists or psychiatrists, dietitians, pharmacists, and other health professionals (e.g., dentists, podiatrists). Frequently, the constituency of the team is determined more by the local availability of professionals with interest in CGA than by programmatic needs.

To increase efficiency, the concept of a core and extended team is gradually yielding to a strategy that relies on flexibility in team composition so that patients are assessed by only those providers who are likely to benefit the patient. In this model, the only consistent member of the team would be the primary care provider. Brief screens, as described in Chapter 17, might identify which providers need to conduct further assessment and therapy. Thus, team members would only assess the patient briefly to determine whether a more in-depth evaluation is necessary. The overriding approach of this strategy is that each patient receives the only the amount of assessment that is necessary.

Regardless of the composition of the team, a key element is the training of the team. Such training should serve several purposes: (1) to ensure that team members have an adequate understanding of the CGA process; (2) to raise the level of expertise of team members in their specific contribution to the team; (3) to develop standard approaches to problems that are commonly identified through CGA; (4) to define areas of responsibility of individual team members; and (5) to learn to work effectively as a team. Such training can begin as a retreat or through a series of in-service seminars and should be reinforced periodically. When new members of the team are added, they should receive the basic components of the initial team training.

If CGA is to be effective, the following six components of the process of care must be addressed:

1. Data gathering
2. Discussion among team members
3. Development of a treatment plan
4. Implementation of the treatment plan
5. Monitoring response to the treatment plan
6. Revising the treatment plan as necessary

The approach to gathering clinical data is changing. Traditionally, data gathering for outpatient-based comprehensive geriatric assessment has been conducted by all team members during the course of one long visit, often lasting 3 to 4 h. This scheduling has traditionally been to accommodate the health care providers schedules but must be balanced with considerations of potential patient fatigue. As a result, there has been increasing flexibility in scheduling outpatient CGA so that is more convenient for patients and their families. In inpatient and home settings, different providers usually conduct their assessments over the course of several days before convening as a team.

The content of clinical data that are collected is also evolving. Although health care professionals receive broad and patient-specific training in their discipline that is relevant to assessment of older persons, what actually happens in the clinical encounter is highly variable. Therefore, many CGA programs have turned toward structured professional evaluations so that each patient receives a similar evaluation. Of course, when appropriate, health professionals may depart from the standard evaluation to pursue problems in greater depth. These structured evaluations may take the form of assessments that the team has developed and believes to be clinically relevant for their population or may rely on validated instruments. The latter allows comparisons of assessments with those conducted in other programs but, because these instruments are usually developed for research purposes, they may be less useful for clinical decision making.

With increased flexibility in team structure and scheduling, team discussions in outpatient and home settings are increasingly changing from face-to-face meetings to conference calls or conferencing via Internet. In this manner, discussions can occur at convenient times, even though team members may be in geographically disparate locations. However, in inpatient settings, where discharge planning is an exceptionally important role for the team, most meetings still occur face to face.

The process of management of clinical disorders can also be structured (e.g., protocols for managing geriatric syndromes). However, as discussed next, the implementations of such protocols have frequently met with considerable resistance or have been ignored in clinical settings. Nevertheless, common approaches to these problems that span across providers participating in the CGA team are important to ensure that a similar intervention is being rendered to all patients.

Implementing Recommendations from CGA

In inpatient settings where the assessment team has primary care of the patient, generally implementation of recommendations is not a problem, provided that there are adequate resources (e.g., sufficient number of rehabilitation therapists available at the hospital). However, patients may refuse to participate in diagnostic or therapeutic plans. When the CGA team is providing consultative services, the link between recommendations and implementation is less certain. In outpatient settings, the implementation of CGA recommendations is particularly tenuous because the process can fail at several points, including lack of implementation of CGA recommendations by primary care physicians (in consultative CGA models) and poor adherence to CGA recommendations by patients. The later can range from patients choosing not to see recommended consultants or refusing to undergo recommended tests to choosing not to adhere to prescribed exercise, nutrition, or rehabilitation regimens.

Successful strategies to increase adherence to CGA recommendations have included geriatrician-to-referring-physician telephone calls with follow-up patient-specific recommendations by mail, and patient and family education including empowerment techniques. Newer technologies, including fax and e-mail, are increasingly being used to communicate recommendations. Even when primary care physicians and patients are in agreement with CGA recommendations, access barriers to receiving indicated services may limit the effectiveness of outpatient CGA. These access barriers include lack of transportation, fragmented services, and gaps in insurance coverage. For example, patients may not be able to get to needed physical therapy three times a week because they do not drive, have no nearby family, or are too disabled to use public transportation. In community-based settings, needed referral services may not be available or, more commonly, are not covered by Medicare. A potential solution to some of these obstacles is use of home health agencies, which can provide a wide range of services to those who are homebound. Similarly, establishing a network of health professionals in the community is essential in developing CGA programs in office-based practices.

Outcomes of Traditional CGA

In virtually all studies of CGA, the process itself has resulted in improved detection and documentation of geriatric problems. However, such identification of problems has not always led to improved outcomes. A 1993 meta-analysis of five models of CGA (geriatric evaluation and management units, inpatient geriatrics consultation services, home assessment services, home assessment services for patients who had recently been discharged, and outpatient assessment services) summarized the evidence to date on traditional models of CGA.[2] The principal findings of the meta-analysis indicated that the hospital or rehabilitation unit model of CGA had the strongest and most consistent benefits on mortality, living at home, and functional status. Home assessment programs, all of which were implemented and tested in Europe, demonstrated survival benefit at 36 months. None of the other models demonstrated consistent benefits across studies, outcomes, and time points.

Further studies of these traditional models have supported these findings including negative randomized clinical trials of inpatient geriatric assessment consulation,[3] in-home assessment by a geriatric nurse practitioner for patients who had recently been discharged from the hospital,[4] and outpatient geriatric consultation.[5] Even the most robust traditional CGA model, the geriatric evaluation and management unit, may no longer confer the same benefits in the current environment. A recently completed multisite randomized clinical trial within the Department of Veterans Affairs demonstrated little benefit of such units when compared to usual care, which may have improved considerably since the early 1980s.[6] Nevertheless, many CGA programs continue despite the lack of strong supporting evidence from clinical trials. Reasons include perceptions among teams and health systems that this is a better way to deliver care to frail older persons, regardless of whether clinical or cost benefits can be demonstrated, and a sense that traditional outcome measures employed in previous research do not adequately capture the benefits of CGA.

New Models of CGA

In light of the potential benefits that CGA can provide when physician implementation and patient adherence are high, new strategies have focused on geriatric management with continuity by the geriatrics team[7–9] and CGA consultation coupled to an adherence intervention that emphasizes patient empowerment.[10] Recently, some of these models have achieved health benefits in randomized clinical trials. Geriatric evaluation and continuity management has resulted in better perceived health, life satisfaction, affective health status, and quality of health and social care.[7,8,11,12] Another type of continuity

geriatric evaluation and management assumes primary care of older persons who are at high risk for high health care utilization for an average of 6 months and then returns patients to the care of their primary care physicians. When evaluated in a randomized clinical trial, this approach prevented functional decline and reduced the likelihood of depression at a modest cost.[13] A model of geriatric preventive services for unselected community-dwelling older persons utilized a geriatric nurse practitioner to provide periodic in-home assessments that were subsequently discussed with a multidisciplinary team.[14] This intervention delayed functional decline and reduced nursing home placement in a randomized clinical trial. In a replication study, however, the benefit was confined to persons who were at low risk for nursing home admission.[15] Finally, a model that combines CGA with an adherence intervention has been developed and tested. This program provided single outpatient comprehensive geriatric assessment for community-dwelling older persons with functional impairment, urinary incontinence, falls, or depressive symptoms. The team consisted of a geriatrician, nurse practitioner, social worker, and physical therapist (when needed). The assessment was then linked to an adherence intervention that was designed to empower the patient to take action and to educate the physician. In a randomized clinical trial, this strategy was associated with less functional decline, less fatigue, and better social functioning[16] and was cost-effective when compared with many commonly used treatments.[17]

New Models of Care That Have Roots in CGA

As traditional models have been tested and modified, several new models of care have been developed and tested that could be considered the progeny of CGA. These models differ from traditional and modified CGA in some important characteristics. First, they are increasingly being developed outside of academic settings. This shift is noteworthy because of the increased difficulty of conducting studies in such settings where change is so rapid. Nevertheless, these studies are exceptionally valuable because they frequently test effectiveness rather than efficacy (i.e., the ability to work under "real-world" circumstances as well as in the "idealized" research settings). As a result, when successful, these interventions are frequently retained. Second, there has been increasing emergence of nursing-based interventions, both in hospital and community-based settings. Third, many new interventions have focused on self-management and increased patient empowerment in caring for their diseases. Such approaches, including those using volunteer

FIGURE 18.1. Functional and clinical outcomes.

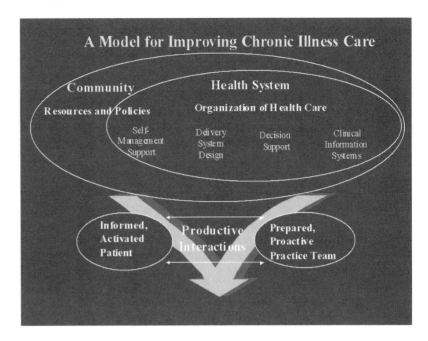

lay class leaders, have demonstrated improvement in health status among person with chronic diseases.[18] Fourth, there has been an emphasis, perhaps a predominance, of the importance of cost savings as an outcome. However, reliance on costs as a sole outcome may result in programs that improve health care delivery but do not benefit patients directly. Although the argument that a financially secure health care system will be able to afford to provide other benefits to its patients, improved patient health outcomes should not be forgotten as an important goal of these interventions. Finally, many programs have begun adopting more of a systems approach to providing care that also includes the community and patient as well as the health care system.

One example of such a model of health care for chronic diseases is provided in Figure 18.1.[19] Within the health care system, information support is used (e.g., to identify patients through a registry), the manner in which health care is provided is changed to meet the needs of both patients and providers (e.g., group visits or condition-specific visits), and decision support for providers is readily available (e.g., through telephone or on-line consultants or ready references). This model focuses on self-management as a major philosophic tenet and practical approach (e.g., through self-management classes or other methods of empowering patients to assume responsibility for their diseases). In the best cases, there is partnership with community agencies and resources to provide complementary education and services.

An important caveat in interpreting these new CGA-like interventions is that their effectiveness may be dependent upon the health care system where they are implemented. Variations in health care delivery and financing systems across nations and within the United States may override the effectiveness of these interventions. As a result, the same intervention may be effective in one setting yet ineffective in another. Even within the same health care system, effectiveness may vary between experimental and practice conditions and may diminish with changes in the environment (e.g., downsizing or merging). Finally, as health care evolves, the concept of a "shelf life" of clinical interventions must be recognized. In other words, health services delivery innovations may be effective for a time and then no longer retain the same value when the entire health care system and reimbursement system change. Examples include the inpatient geriatrics evaluation and management units and hospital-based postacute units; in these instances, economic forces have rendered effective interventions untenable.

Outpatient Models

Several new models of outpatient care for older persons modify the basic structure of care; these adopt various components of CGA including targeting, assessment, and interventions. One approach has been to utilize gerontologic nurse practitioners who are based at senior centers and develop a targeted health management plan that addresses risk factors for disability.[20] This health management plan emphasizes physical activity and chronic illness self-management, including attending a 7-week course. Although the intervention did not demonstrate functional or health status benefits, total hospital days were reduced.

Another approach that focuses on older persons who have high predicted health care utilization is the Chronic

Care Clinics developed at Group Health Cooperative of Puget Sound. These clinics are actually special sessions within the primary care physicians practices in which a team of health providers (including a nurse, social worker, and pharmacist) are convened to care for patients who have similar health problems. In one randomized clinical trial, significant benefits on health, functional status, or costs could not be demonstrated at 24 months.[21]

Another comprehensive care model that uses an interdisciplinary team of health professionals is the Cooperative Health Care Clinics developed at Kaiser-Permanente, Colorado, and widely replicated elsewhere. This model of care focuses on older persons who have at least one of four chronic conditions (heart, lung, or joint disease, or diabetes) and high outpatient utilization. However, the intervention is unique, consisting of monthly group visits led by a physician, a nurse, and a guest speaker. Typically, 20 to 25 members attend the group. At the end of these 90-min sessions, 30 min are set aside for brief one-on-one visits with the physician, if necessary. In a randomized clinical trial, such care was associated with increased visits and calls to nurses but fewer emergency room and subspecialist visits and fewer hospitalizations. Although there were no differences in health and functional status measures, participants were more satisfied with their care and the overall costs of care were less.[22]

In-Hospital Settings

Several interventions have incorporated CGA principles into hospital care of older persons. Acute care of the elderly (ACE) units have been developed and widely replicated. The care of elderly patients in these units focuses on environmental changes, patient-centered care, discharge planning, and intensive review of medications and procedures (including protocols) to minimize the adverse effects of medications and procedures. The initial randomized clinical trial of these units demonstrated their effectiveness in reducing functional decline and discharge to nursing homes among unselected older hospitalized persons.[23] In a subsequent replication study at a community hospital, the benefits were less dramatic.[24]

More recently, programs have been developed to identify hospitalized older persons who are at risk for functional and cognitive decline and intervene regardless of where the patient is located in the hospital.[25] Such an approach obviates the need for a dedicated unit. The intervention includes geriatric assessment and interdisciplinary involvement as needed, as well as specific interventions to address the multiple dimensions of geriatric syndromes. A prototype program has demonstrated

reduction in new cases of delirium and hospitalized costs.[26]

Disease Management

A major trend in the management of chronic illness has been disease management in which health care delivery has been focused around a single disease (target condition) with the goal of optimizing the care of this disease. These programs adopt the assessment and intervention approach of CGA, frequently using an interdisciplinary team. The prototype condition has been congestive heart failure. A multidisciplinary program (geriatrics cardiologist, nurse, dietitian, and social worker) for elderly patients with heart failure who were at risk for readmission has been demonstrated to reduce readmission rates and cost of care.[27]

More recently, this concept has been extended beyond a disease-specific model. A nursing-led program of comprehensive discharge planning and home follow-up has been developed and tested. It uses series of targeting criteria, a program of comprehensive discharge planning (including multidimensional assessment), and home follow-up with advanced practice nurses who visited the patients at least every other day during the hospitalization and at least twice during the 4 weeks following discharge; these visits were supplemented by telephone calls.[28] In a randomized clinical trial, this intervention was associated with reduced hospital readmissions and costs (both reduced by approximately 50%).

Case/Care Management

Case management has been defined as a process designed to allocate services appropriately and organize them efficiently.[29] This innovation was initially implemented in managed care settings, which were free to allocate funds to support such services, and is beginning to be integrated into fee-for service Medicare where it has traditionally been excluded as a benefit. However, the practice of case management varies considerably in terms of types of health care professionals and their responsibilities.[27] Some programs have relied on nurse case managers and others have used social workers; some have used both interchangeably. Similar to CGA, case management virtually always begins with some method of screening to identify high-risk older persons (case selection). Usually, these targeting criteria have been functional impairment or predicted high health care utilization. Following identification, the roles of case managers differ, though components frequently including problem identification, planning, coordinating or implementation, monitoring, and evaluation.[27,30] However, within this broad framework, there is considerable variation especially with respect to caseload, how services are provided (e.g., face to face versus on the telephone), assessment, and provision of specific services (e.g., home visits, education, counseling).[27]

Research support for health benefits or cost savings of case management has been limited by both the paucity of studies and methodologic issues in some studies. In randomized clinical trials and pre–post studies, case management has had variable success in providing health or functional status benefits or reducing costs. In an Italian study of persons who were already receiving conventional home health services, case management in conjunction with a geriatric evaluation unit resulted in improved physical function, less cognitive decline, and reduced health care costs.[31,32] A Kaiser-Permanente of Northeast Ohio study demonstrated attenuation of functional decline[33] but at higher cost than conventional care. Another trial of nurse case managers assigned to frail older persons discharged from a hospital emergency department failed to demonstrate health or economic benefits and resulted in higher readmission rates to emergency departments.[34] A social work model of case management for health maintenance organization enrollees at high risk of using health care services heavily in the future did not demonstrate cost savings in a randomized clinical trial.[35]

The Future

The place of traditional comprehensive geriatric assessment in future health care delivery is likely to be quite limited. Although some programs remain, usually at academic health centers, the expense and logistics of such programs preclude their widespread proliferation. Such programs may be largely confined to teaching settings where they provide excellent environments for teaching geriatrics and team care. Rather, new generations of programs will need to be created that draw upon the lessons learned from these well-studied programs. These programs will need to be efficient yet comprehensive. The best of these programs will adopt the chronic illness care model similar to that described in Figure 18.1 that relies on partnerships between health care systems and the community.

Under the current system of health care reimbursement, such major restructuring of health care for older persons is extremely difficult. Within fee-for-service health care delivery, there is no financial incentive to make health care more efficient. In fact, many of the innovations that have been most successful are not covered benefits under traditional Medicare. With managed care, such global changes are equally difficult to implement in independent provider models despite the incentive to reduce costs. Logistic and reimbursement difficulties usually preclude such innovation. Such change is easier within group or staff managed care models but still requires vision, leadership, and willingness to overcome inertia.

Nevertheless, future models of geriatric care are likely to be guided by the following principles:

- Comprehensive provision of preventive services (including lifestyle modification) and basic and episodic care for older persons who have few health care needs. These services will likely be provided as inexpensively as possible, using community educational and preventive care resources and trained health care providers who are mostly not physicians.
- Increased use of technology (e.g., Internet) for delivery of health care information to both professionals and patients.
- Systematic identification of older persons who have more extensive health care needs and design of systems to meet such needs on an ongoing basis. Such care is likely to be best provided by teams of health care providers, but such teams must reflect more efficient care rather than simply more care. Communication among teams will be increasingly electronic.
- Increased patient (and family) participation in management of diseases and health care decision making.
- The traditional distinction of roles among health care professionals will become increasingly obscured. Nurses will be increasingly responsible for care management and continuity for older persons who have chronic illnesses.

Such changes will not come easily; they reflect departures from the traditional health care delivery system, and resistance and inertia will be formidable barriers. As noted by the Institute for the Future, "There has been little real change in the way physicians practice medicine since the invention of the telephone."[36] Nevertheless, there is enormous incentive to make basic changes in health care delivery. Even in times of economic prosperity, health care in the United States and other countries has remained under continued pressure to reduce costs. Such pressures are unlikely to abate, and "smarter" systems of care that improve patient outcome within cost constraints will be the only systems that survive.

References

1. National Institute of Health Consensus Development Conference Statement. *Geriatric Assessment Methods for Clinical Decisionmaking.* Washington, DC: U.S. Department of Health and Human Services; 1987:6(13).

2. Stuck AE, Siu AL, Wieland GD, Adams J, Rubenstein LZ. Comprehensive Geriatric Assessment: a meta-analysis of controlled trial. *Lancet.* 1993;342:1032–1036.

3. Reuben DB, Borok GM, Wolde-Tsadik G, et al. A randomized trial of comprehensive geriatric assessment in the care of hospitalized patients. *N Engl J Med.* 1995;332:1345–1350.

4. Siu AL, Kravitz RL, Keeler E, et al. Postdischarge geriatric assessment of hospitalized frail elderly patients. *Arch Intern Med.* 1996;156:76–81.

5. Silverman M, Musa D, Martin DC, Rave JR, Adams J, Ricci EM. Evaluation of outpatient geriatric assessment: a randomized multi-site trial. *J Am Geriatr Soc.* 1995;43:733–740.

6. Cohen HJ, Feussner JR, Weinberger M, et al. A Controlled trial of inpatient and outpatient generic evaluation and mangement. *N Engl J Med.* 2002;346(12):905–912.

7. Engelhardt JB, Toseland RW, O'Donnell JC, Richie JT, Jue D, Banks S. The effectiveness and efficiency of outpatient geriatric evaluation and management. *J Am Geriatr Soc.* 1996;44:847–856.

8. Burns R, Nichols LO, Graney MJ, Cloar T. Impact of continued geriatric outpatient management on health outcomes of older veterans. *Arch Intern Med.* 1995;155:1313–1318.

9. Boult C, Boult, L, Morishita L, Smith SL, Kane RL. Outpatient geriatric evaluation and management (GEM). *J Am Geriatr Soc.* 1998;46(3):296–302.

10. Reuben DB, Maly RC, Hirsch SH, et al. Physician implementation of and patient adherence to recommendations from comprehensive geriatric assessment. *Am J Med.* 1996;100:444–451.

11. Toseland RW, O'Donnel JC, Engelhardt JB, Hendler SA, Richie JT, Jue D. Outpatient geriatric evaluation and management: results of a randomized trial. *Med Care.* 1996;34:624–640.

12. Burns R, Nichols LO, Martindale-Adams J, Graney MJ. Interdisciplinary geriatric primary care evaluation and management: two-year outcomes. *J Am Geriatr Soc.* 2000;48(1):8–13.

13. Boult C, Boult LB, Morishita L, Dowd B, Kane RL, Urdangarin CF. A randomized clinical trial of outpatient geriatric evaluation and management. *J Am Geriatr Soc.* 2001;49:351–359.

14. Stuck AE, Aronow HU, Steiner A, et al. A trial of annual in-home comprehensive geriatric assessments for elderly people living in the community. *N Engl J Med.* 1995;333:1184–1189.

15. Stuck AE, Minder CE, Peter-Wuest I, et al. A randomized trial of in-home visits for disability prevention in community-dwelling older people at low and high risk for nursing home admission. *Arch Intern Med.* 2000;160:977–986.

16. Reuben DB, Frank JC, Hirsch SH, McGuigan KA, Maly RC. A randomized clinical trial of outpatient comprehensive geriatric assessment coupled with a intervention to increase adherence to recommendations. *J Am Geriatr Soc.* 1999;47:269–276.

17. Keeler EB, Robalino DA, Frank JC, Hirsch SH, Maly RC, Reuben DB. Cost-effectiveness of outpatient geriatric assessment with an intervention to increase adherence. *Med Care.* 1999;37:1199–1206.

18. Lorig KR, Sobel DS, Stewart AL, et al. Evidence suggesting that a chronic disease self-management program can improve health status while reducing hospitalization: a randomized trial. *Med Care.* 1999;37:5–14.

19. Wagner EH. Chronic disease management: what will it take to improve care for chronic illness? *Effective Clin Pract.* 1998;1:2–4.

20. Leveille SG, Wagner EH, Davis C, et al. Prevention disability and managing chronic illness in frail older adults: a randomized trial of a community-based partnership with primary care. *J Am Geriatr Soc.* 1998;46:1191–1198.

21. Coleman EA, Grothaus LC, Sandhu N, Wagner EH. Chronic care clinics: a randomized controlled trial of a new model of primary care for frail older adults. *J Am Geriatr Soc.* 1999;47:775–783.

22. Beck A, Scott J, Williams P, et al. A randomized trial of group outpatient visits for chronically ill older HMO members: the Cooperative Health Care Clinic. *J Am Geriatr Soc.* 1997;45:543–549.

23. Landefeld CS, Palmer RM, Kresevic DM, Fortinsky RH, Kowal J. A randomized trial of care in a hospital medical unit especially designed to improve the functional outcomes of acutely ill older patients. *N Engl J Med.* 1995;332:1338–1344.

24. Counsell SR, Holder CM, Liebenauer LL, et al. Effects of a multicomponent intervention on functional outcomes and process of care in hospitalized older patients: a randomized controlled trial of acute care for the elders (ACE) in a community hospital. *J Am Geriatr Soc.* 2000;48:1572–1581.

25. Inouye SK, Bogardus ST Jr, Baker DI, Leo-Summers L, Cooney LM. The Hospital Elder Life Program: a model of care to prevent cognitive and functional decline in hospitalized older patients. *J Am Geriatr Soc.* 2000;48:1697–1706.

26. Inouye SK, Bogardus ST, Charpentier PA, et al. A multicomponent intervention to prevent delirium in hospitalized older patients. *N Engl J Med.* 1999;340:669–676.

27. Rick MW, Beckham V, Wittenberg C, et al. A multidisciplinary intervention to prevent the readmission of elderly patients with congestive heart failure. *N Engl J Med.* 1995;333:1190–1195.

28. Naylor MD, Brooten D, Campbell R, et al. Comprehensive discharge planning and home follow-up of hospitalized elders: a randomized clinical trial. *JAMA.* 1999;281(7):613–620.

29. Pacala JT, Boult C, Hepburn KW, Kane RA, Kane RL, Malone JK, et al. Case management of older adults in health maintenance organizations. *J Am Geriatr Soc.* 1995;43:538–542.

30. Case Management Society of America. *Standards of Practice for Case Management.* Little Rock, AR: Case Management Society of America; 1995.

31. Bernabei R, Landi F, Gambassi G, et al. Randomised trial of impact of model of integrated care and case management for older people living in the community. *Br Med J.* 1998;316:1348–1351.

32. Landi F, Gambassi G, Pola R, et al. Impact of integrated home care services on hospital use. *J Am Geriatr Soc.* 1999;47:1430–1434.

33. Marshall BS, Long MJ, Voss J, Demma K, Skerl KP. Case management of the elderly in a health maintenance organization: the implications for program administration under managed care. *J Healthcare Manage.* 1999;44(6): 477–491.

34. Gagnon AJ, Schein C, McVey L, Bergman H. Randomized controlled trial of nurse case management of frail older people [special series]. *J Am Geriatr Soc.* 1999;47:1118–1124.

35. Boult C, Rassen J, Rassen A, Moore R, Bouquillon S. Does case management save money in Medicare HOMs? Presented at the 2000 Annual Scientific Meeting of the American Geriatrics Society/American Federation for Aging Research, 17–21 May 2000, Nashville, TN.

36. The Institute for the Future. In: Grosel C, Hamilton M, Koyano J, Eastwood S, eds. *Health and Health Care 2010: The Forecast, the Challenge.* San Francisco: Jossey-Bass; 2000.

19
Neuropsychological Testing

Marilyn S. Albert

A variety of cognitive disorders occur with increasing frequency as people age; these include progressive dementing disorders, acute confusional states, and cognitive disorders secondary to psychiatric syndromes. Epidemiologic studies indicate that approximately 15% of the population over 65 years of age suffers from some form of dementia.[1] However, the probability of having a dementing disorder increases dramatically with age. Data concerning the prevalence of dementia in a community-dwelling population indicate that between the ages of 65 and 74 years the prevalence of dementia ranges from 2% to 3%; this increases to 22% to 23% among those persons 75 to 84 years and to 47% to 48% among those persons aged 85 years and older.[2] Similarly striking figures pertain to the incidence and prevalence of acute confusion in hospitalized elderly patients. Several studies have reported that 25% to 35% of hospitalized geriatric patients on a general medical service who are cognitively intact at admission develop acute confusion. The incidence of acute confusion in younger subjects is approximately 3%, whereas among individuals 70 and older the prevalence has been estimated to be at least 10 fold higher.[3,4] There are few systematic studies of the prevalence of cognitive disorders secondary to psychiatric syndromes, but numerous clinical reports state that their prevalence is greater among elderly patients than young patients.[5]

These cognitive disorders produce considerable morbidity and mortality, and although only some of them can be completely reversed with treatment, appropriate management can substantially improve the quality of life and reduce the development of secondary conditions. Thus, it is in the best interests of the patient if one can become increasingly attuned to the possible presence of cognitive dysfunction in older individuals and to be knowledgeable about procedures for workup and referral. This chapter focuses on the role of neuropsychologic testing in the assessment of cognitive dysfunction in elderly patients, particularly as it applies to the geriatrician, because there

is much that a geriatrician can do to identify the presence of cognitive dysfunction and see that it is properly assessed.

Interview with Patient

There are two sources of information concerning the cognitive status of patients: (1) patients themselves and (2) patients' families. Unless a family member has approached the physician with concerns about the patient's cognitive function, it is not likely a family member will be routinely involved in a geriatric assessment. Therefore, the physician is initially limited to information that is obtainable from the patient. This information can be most easily gathered in two ways: (1) from an interview of the patient in the course of conducting a medical evaluation and (2) from brief mental status testing.

Observation During the Medical Examination

In the course of a routine medical examination, there is ample opportunity to converse with patients and gather information about their cognitive status. Because the most common causes of cognitive decline in elderly patients produce a memory disorder (specifically a difficulty with learning and retaining new information), greatest emphasis should be placed on ascertaining information about the memory function of the patient. This may be accomplished by a discussion of current events. Appropriate subjects will differ according to the educational and socioeconomic background of the patient. For one patient; it may be politics, for another, sports, and for another, the stage of the planting season. If there is a particularly dramatic event in the news that most people are likely to have heard of (e.g., a presidential election, a plane crash), this may be useful for persons of diverse backgrounds. In any case, the task is to determine whether the person is familiar with the event in question and, if so, if it is familiarity that is more than general. Many patients in the early stages of dementing disorder can make general all-purpose remarks that appear to be appropriate while obscuring the fact that they do not have any substantive knowledge of the subject at hand.

In the course of conversing, one can also listen to the nature of the patient's linguistic output. Language problems are important to assess because they are common in both cerebrovascular disorders (e.g., stroke) and dementing disorders. The patient's comprehension ability can be evaluated during a medical examination with relative ease because the patient is generally asked to perform tasks (e.g., open your mouth; life up an arm), and the ability to comprehend these simple directions can be ascertained. Speech fluency also is relatively easy to observe. Patients who are nonfluent have an effortful and halting quality to their speech. Substantive words, such as nouns and verbs, are present, but small connective words (e.g., "if," "and", "but") are generally missing. Disturbances in speech fluency and problems with comprehension often are indicative of a stroke, unless the patient has a long-standing dementing disorder.[6]

Naming ability also can be assessed in the course of conversation. A person with naming problems frequently hesitates over names of objects or persons and may attempt to circumvent the difficulty in a variety of ways (e.g., giving a lengthy description of the object or person; substituting associated words). If naming problems are suspected, a further evaluation can be carried out by using common objects at hand. Very familiar objects, such as a watch or a door, are easy to name. Thus, only a person with a relatively severe naming problem will have difficulty with them. In general, however, parts of objects are harder to name (e.g., the stem of a watch; the knob on a door). The use of both common objects and parts of objects as stimuli will assess a range of naming ability.

Thus, with little additional expenditure of time, memory and language, that is, the two aspects of cognitive function most frequently affected by cerebrovascular disease and common dementing disorders, can be briefly assessed. The goal is not to undertake a detailed or thorough evaluation, but to determine whether any problems are present that suggest an underlying abnormality.

Mental Status Testing

It should, however, be pointed out that it takes a considerable amount of experience to become skilled in drawing sound clinical conclusions from a conversational approach to the assessment of cognitive function. Therefore, it is ideal if this can be supplemented by a brief test of mental status.

The most widely used tests are the Mini-Mental State Exam (MMSE),[7] the Blessed Dementia Scale (BDS),[8] and the Short Portable Mental Status Questionnaire (SPMSQ).[9] In addition, a test known as the 7-Minute Screen was recently developed for use by the practicing physician.[10] These tests all take approximately 10 min to administer and have high test–retest reliability.

Of these, the MMSE has most commonly been used in clinical settings. Its strength is that it assesses a broad range of cognitive abilities (i.e., memory, language, spatial ability, set shifting) in a simple and straightforward manner. In addition, the wide use of the MMSE in epidemiologic studies has yielded cutoff scores that facilitate the identification of patients with cognitive dysfunction. The other screening tests have been used in a variety of experimental settings, but epidemiologic data are limited. Finally, the extensive use of the MMSE has produced widespread familiarity with its scoring system, facilitating communication among clinicians. Until additional data are available on newer tests, such as the 7-Minute Screen, the MMSE still seems most appropriate for inclusion in the standard clinical evaluation of a patient.

Scores on the MMSE range from 0 to 30. In general, scores greater than 26 are considered to be excellent and reflective of normal cognitive function. Mildly impaired patients typically obtain scores of 18 to 26, moderate impairment is reflected by scores of 11 to 18, and severe impairment by scores of 10 or lower. A cutoff score of 23 is generally recommended as indicative of cognitive dysfunction; however, the application of this cutoff value must be modified by knowledge of the educational level of the patient. For example, patients with a substantial amount of education can experience a considerable amount of cognitive decline before a score of 23 is achieved. On the other hand, persons with little education may obtain a score of 23 at baseline. The rigid use of cutoff scores is difficult because some items on the MMSE, or other comparable screening tests, require minimal educational background. For example, serial sevens, which contribute heavily to the score on both the MMSE and SPMSQ, can be difficult for most elderly persons with limited education. This difficulty may lower the total score such that, with a few other minor errors, the result falls below the cutoff point on the test.

Several studies have examined subjects of varying educational levels, racial backgrounds, and age to identify some guidelines for adjusting MMSE cutoff scores according to the premorbid level of the patient.[11–13] Their findings suggest that a cutoff score of 17 is appropriate for persons with 8 or fewer years of education. The standard cutoff score of 23 was optimal for subjects with 8 to 15 years of education. For persons with higher educational levels (i.e., 16 or more years), a cutoff score of 27 appeared more appropriate. No consistently significant differences were found between black and white subjects with equal education, suggesting that education, not race, is the important factor that influences test performance. Moreover, persons with little or no formal education may vary in terms of literacy; those who report that they never learned to read and write will perform more poorly on cognitive tests than those who learned these skills outside the normal education channels.[14]

It is also important to note that screening tests, such as the MMSE, by their very nature were not designed to measure subtle aspects of behavior. In addition, because there is less redundancy in a brief screening test and it is brief, its measurement error may be close to the amount of decline one might expect with a dementing disease, such as Alzheimer's disease (AD). Thus, the scores may show little or no decline over time in patients whose conditions can be shown, by other measures, to have declined substantially.[15]

Despite these shortcomings, mental status screening tests are extremely useful tools. In a brief period of time, one can administer a standardized series of questions that have proved to be helpful in identifying persons with cognitive dysfunction. Most of the tests are effective in screening memory ability. Thus, they are useful in identifying persons with dementing disorders, such as Alzheimer's disease, or acute confusion, conditions that are particularly difficult to diagnose. If used repeatedly over time, they are helpful in establishing a numerical baseline against which future performance can be compared. And, if clinicians use the same test with frequency, they will begin to learn how to use test results to formulate referral questions. It is, for example, much more useful for a patient to be referred for further neuropsychologic testing with a statement such as "the patient has declined four points on the Mini-Mental State Exam over the last year and appears to have particular difficulty with memory testing" rather than "referral for question of dementia."

Obtaining a Cognitive History

If cognitive dysfunction is suspected, it is extremely important to obtain a good history of the cognitive changes that have occurred over time. As the patient's self-report may be unreliable, it is important to obtain a cognitive history from one or more family members (or equivalent caregivers).

When obtaining this information, it is often helpful to begin by asking about the nature of the patient's personality and cognitive skills many years before the onset of the symptoms (e.g., "Can you tell me whether, 15 years ago, the patient was outgoing or quiet, organized or dis-organized; did he/she have a good memory or a bad memory?"). This type of information helps to provide an anchor against which reports of the onset and progression of symptoms can be judged, because the issue at hand is whether there has been a true change and what the nature of the change has been.

Obtaining a good cognitive history is one of the most difficult and yet important aspects of an evaluation for cognitive dysfunction. A comprehensive history should include information concerning the onset, nature, and progression of behavioral change. Cognitive histories are difficult to obtain because most patients and family members are not attuned to subtle behavioral symptoms. They do not know how to isolate important aspects of the medical history or how to focus on individual cognitive functions in isolation from one another. For example, the family may state that the first symptom of disease was the patient's anxiety and depression about work and, only when asked, may remember several episodes that preceded the onset of work-related anxiety in which the patient could not remember how to handle a complex situation or how to use new equipment in the workplace.

Family members also may have difficulty in understanding why certain subtle distinctions are important for diagnosis. For example, a family member may say that the patient's first symptom was forgetfulness, but when asked to provide instances of forgetfulness, the family member may explain that the patient had trouble installing a new drawer pull in the kitchen or had trouble knowing how to find a familiar location, both of which would suggest spatial difficulty more than memory difficulty. In addition, an unwillingness to admit that certain impairments exist can prevent family members from providing accurate information.

Finally, family members can sometimes misinterpret even fairly direct questions. For example, a history of a gradually progressive disorder is essential to the diagnosis of Alzheimer's disease. Yet, frequently family members say that a disorder came on suddenly when it did not. The realization that the patient is having cognitive problems often coincides with an unusual external event, such as a trip to an unfamiliar place. An unfamiliar environment generally prevents persons from employing overlearned habits and routines and thus exposes their cognitive problems. As family members notice these difficulties suddenly, they may conclude that the disease onset is sudden. Likewise, an illness or hospitalization can exacerbate an underlying cognitive impairment that suddenly makes the family aware that a problem exists. If either of these situations appear to be the case, it is necessary to determine whether any symptoms of cognitive change preceded the external or precipitating event. Most commonly, family members then recall episodes of an earlier change in cognitive function.

Time Since Onset

As mentioned earlier, a good cognitive history must first establish the time at which cognitive changes became apparent. This background will provide important clues regarding the nature of the disorder because some diseases are well known for their particularly rapid rate of decline (e.g., Creutzfeldt–Jakob disease). It will also enable the clinician to give the family some tentative feedback regarding the course of the illness. If the point at which the disorder began is known, the rate of decline can be determined by seeing how long it has taken the patient to reach the present level of function. Although estimates of the rate of progression can be only roughly approximated, it is extremely helpful for the family to have an estimate in making plans for the future. Repeated cognitive testing can provide further help in establishing the course of disease.

Initial Symptoms

Second, it is important to determine the nature of the cognitive or behavioral changes that were evident when the disease began; this also will provide essential information regarding the diagnosis. For example, an early symptom of frontotemporal dementia or Pick's disease is often a change in personality (e.g., inappropriate behavior), whereas the most common early symptom of Alzheimer's disease is a gradually progressive decline in the ability to learn new information.[16] Several years after the disease has begun, which is when most patients' conditions are actually diagnosed, the cognitive symptoms of the two disorders may be very similar, so that information regarding the initial symptoms may be critical to accurate diagnosis.

Type of Onset

Third, it is important to determine whether the initial symptoms came on suddenly or gradually. If the onset of illness is gradual and insidious, as in Alzheimer's disease, it is often only in retrospect that the family realizes that a decline has occurred. In contrast, a series of small strokes, even if not evident on computed tomographic or magnetic resonance imaging scans, generally produce a history of sudden onset and stepwise progression. There may, for example, be an incident (e.g., a fall or a period of confusion) that marks the beginning of the disorder. Acute confusional states generally have an acute onset as well, although if they are the result of a condition such as drug toxicity, this may not be the case.

The manner in which the symptoms have progressed over time also provides important diagnostic information. A stepwise deterioration, characterized by sudden exacerbations of symptoms, is most typical of multi-infarct dementia. However, a physical illness in a patient with Alzheimer's disease (e.g., pneumonia, hip fracture) can cause a rapid decline in cognitive function. The sudden worsening of symptoms in a psychiatric patient (e.g., depression) also can produce an abrupt decrease in mental status. Careful questioning is therefore necessary to determine the underlying cause of a stepwise decline in function.

It is also important to determine the patient's current functional status. This information is most easily elicited by asking about what the patient does during the course of a usual day. A substantial discrepancy between the functional and cognitive status of the patient suggests the presence of a psychiatric illness. For example, a report that the patient tends to sit all day doing very little in an individual with an MMSE score of 20 suggests a level of functional impairment that is substantially beyond what would be expected. If physical limitations, such as difficulty in walking, are not present, then careful questioning for evidence of depression is warranted.

Detailed Neuropsychologic Testing

If one suspects the presence of cognitive deficits and is going to refer a patient for neuropsychologic testing, it is helpful to know that there are two basic approaches to the selection of a neuropsychologic test protocol. Some neuropsychologists use a predetermined battery, such as the Halstead Reitan Battery[17] or the Luria Nebraska Battery.[18] Other neuropsychologists select a set of tests from among a group that seems to be particularly relevant to the diagnostic question. Even in the latter case, however, there tends to be a core set of tests that are relied on more heavily than others. However, regardless of the approach of the neuropsychologist, it is reasonable to expect the neuropsychologist's report to be formed in terms of the following major areas of cognitive ability: attention, language, memory, spatial ability, executive function, and general information.

Attention is important to consider because simple attentional abilities must be preserved for any other task to be performed adequately. If the subject has difficulty in keeping his or her mind on a task for 1 to 3 min at a time, it will not be possible to assess other areas of function. Commonly used tests of simple attention are digit span,[19] reaction time,[20] and the continuous performance test.[21]

In the digit span test, the individual is asked to repeat a series of numbers of increasing length, first in order forward and then a similar series backward. Reaction time is generally tested on a computer, where the individual is asked to press a key in response to a specific stimulus (e.g., pattern, sound, etc). The continuous performance test generally asks the subject to identify a particular letter ("A") or series of letters ("I before X") in a continuous series of letters; the series can be written or spoken out loud.

If aphasia is not suspected, the language evaluation is likely to be limited to an assessment of confrontation naming because decreases in naming ability are a prominent symptom of a number of cognitive disorders common in the elderly (e.g., Alzheimer's disease). The most common method for assessing naming is to present drawings of common objects or the actual objects to be named. The Boston Naming Test[22] and the Alzheimer's Disease Assessment Scale[23] include such assessments of naming.

Verbal fluency is also commonly assessed, as it is a reflection of both linguistic and executive function skills. Both letter fluency and category fluency are generally evaluated. In both these tests, the individual is asked to generate within 1 min all the words they can think of within a particular category (e.g., the letters F, A, S; or animals; or vegetables).[24]

If a more extensive language evaluation seems desirable, then it will generally include an assessment of naming, fluency, grammar, comprehension, repetition, vocabulary, reading, and writing. This step can be done briefly with a short screen for each of these areas[25] or with a lengthy and more comprehensive assessment of language, with such batteries as the Boston Diagnostic Aphasia Exam[26] and the Western Aphasia Battery.[27]

A careful evaluation of memory is perhaps the most essential to the cognitive workup of an older person. Memory dysfunction occurs in almost all the cognitive disorders common in the elderly, and the nature and severity of the memory impairment can serve as one of the major guidelines in the diagnosis. The neuropsychologic assessment of memory should at least distinguish between the patient's immediate and delayed memory function, because the difference between immediate and delayed recall is strikingly impaired in early Alzheimer's disease and, if present, can be diagnostic. By contrast, normal aging individuals typically take longer to learn something new, but retain that information well over brief delays.[28] Moreover, patients with other dementing disorders, such as frontotemporal dementia and psychiatric disorders (e.g., major depressive disorder) can have difficulty with memory, but the loss of information over a brief delay is less severe than in AD.[29,30] Commonly used tests of memory include the California Verbal Learning Test,[31] Wechsler Memory Scale,[32] and Cued Selective Reminding Test.[33]

The assessment of visuospatial ability should, if at all possible, include figure copying. Such figures can be chosen to span a great range of difficulty and to include both two-dimensional and three-dimensional figures. If the patient has visuosensory deficits, the visual stimuli to be used for copying can be adapted (by using enlarge-ments of drawings or making figures with a felt-tipped pen). A number of shorter test batteries that have been developed for use with dementia patients contain an array of figures that are easy to use; these include the CERAD Battery[34] and the Alzheimer's Disease Assessment Scale.[23] Other tests of spatial ability can be used that employ blocks, sticks, or design recognition; these include the Benton Visual Retention Test[35] and the Block Design subtest of the Wechsler Adult Intelligence Scale—III (WAIS).[19]

Tasks that examine executive function ability evaluate a variety of functions, including set formation, set shifting, self-monitoring, and abstraction. These abilities are affected in most of the major dementing disorders (such as Alzheimer's disease and frontotemporal dementia), as well as in psychiatric disorders such as depression. Therefore, executive function should be carefully assessed. Examples of such tests that can be used include the Trail Making Test,[36] Stroop Test,[37] Self-Ordering Test,[38] Proverbs Test,[39] and the Similarities subtest of WAIS.[19]

Individuals who are having trouble performing tasks with multiple steps that must be integrated with one another, such as cooking or balancing a checkbook, will usually demonstrate impairments on tests that evaluate set shifting, such as the Trail Making Test. Individuals who have trouble understanding complex ideas or planning for the future, such as required for planning a trip or deciding how to handle one's finances, will often have problems on tests of abstraction, such as the Similarities subtest of the WAIS.

Tests of general intelligence are also useful to administer, if time permits; this will allow one to determine whether the individual has access to previously acquired knowledge. For example, early in the course of Alzheimer's disease, some patients have a normal IQ although they have a striking memory deficit and difficulty with executive function. A relatively preserved IQ in a patient with Alzheimer's disease often relates to higher levels of functioning at home and tends to be a good prognostic sign.

Full-scale IQ tests are, however, very lengthy. It is therefore likely that the neuropsychologist may administer a brief test that provides a good estimate of general intelligence. One such test is a reduced version of the WAIS.[40] Alternatively, one can use a brief test that estimates IQ, based on the ability to read irregular words.[41]

The referring physician should encourage the neuropsychologist to formulate their clinical report in terms of the six broad areas of cognitive function described here. A neuropsychologic report organized in this fashion will make it easier for an individual with less neuropsychologic expertise to interpret the results. It will also be easier to determine whether the patient has spared areas of cognitive function. This understanding is important, because knowing the patient's pattern of spared and

TABLE 19.1. Strengths and weaknesses in mildly and moderately impaired patients with Alzheimer's disease (AD).

Mild AD
    Memory: very defective new learning, relatively preserved recall of remote events
    Conceptualization: defective ability to plan and execute complex activity, problems switching from one task to another, impaired ability to form conceptual generalities, and preserved ability to understand concrete ideas
    Language: word-finding deficits, preserved conversational abilities
    Visuospatial skills: difficulty with complex spatial tasks, relatively preserved figure copying and spatial skills needed for activities of daily living (dressing, bathing, sports, etc.)
    Personality: less interest in usual activities, occasional irritability, paranoia in some patients, preserved general personality profile

Moderate AD
    Memory: severely defective new learning, moderately affected remote memory, preserved recall of most distant remote events
    Conceptualization: difficulty with anything requiring abstract thinking, can understand only simplest concrete ideas
    Language: increased word-finding deficits, difficulty with comprehension of complex language, relatively fluent speech
    Visuospatial skills: difficulty in copying simple drawings; problems with spatial skills needed for activities of daily living (dressing, bathing, sports, etc.); can engage in physical activity, such as walks and simple exercise
    Personality: increased likelihood of behavioral disturbances, such as hallucinations, delusions and agitation; can enjoy simplified and restructured activities

impaired abilities can provide an important guide to diagnosis. For example, patients with Alzheimer's disease have an approximately equal impairment in both verbal and nonverbal memory. Therefore, a patient whose verbal memory skills are disproportionately deficient relative to nonverbal testing is unlikely to have Alzheimer's disease.

The description of a patient's major cognitive impairments and major cognitive strengths also can be used to maximize function. For example, early in the course of Alzheimer's disease, most patients have striking difficulty in retaining new information during a brief delay and have problems with conceptualization that make it hard for them to integrate a number of individual tasks into a complex whole or to plan activities in the future. However, mildly impaired patients with Alzheimer's disease frequently have spared spatial abilities and a preservation of well-learned skills; therefore, they can be encouraged to carry out a wide variety of sports and leisure activities with the knowledge that they will be successful. Table 19.1 provides a summary of the major strengths and weaknesses in mild and moderately impaired patients who have typical symptoms of Alzheimer's disease.

The number and nature of the patient's impairments will also enable the skilled clinician to formulate a reasonable prognosis. For example, even though a patient with Pick's disease might have only a mild memory deficit, early evidence of severe conceptualization difficulties and inappropriate behavior suggests that the patient will need to be in a supervised environment relatively soon and the family needs to plan for that eventuality. On the other hand, a patient with Alzheimer's disease with a striking memory deficit who has some preservation of conceptualization skills and shows good judgment by, for example, not cooking when food has been repeatedly burned, or not going for a long walk if

this has previously led to being lost, is likely to be able to remain in a relatively unsupervised environment for a long period of time.

The assessment of cognitive function in an older person can thus serve many useful purposes if it is well focused and integrated into the general evaluation of the patient. A geriatrician who understands the potential utility of neuropsychologic testing can substantially contribute to its appropriate application.

Acknowledgments. This chapter represents a revision and expansion of the one that appeared in the 3rd edition of *Geriatric Medicine.* The preparation of this chapter was supported in part by funds from NIH grant P01-AG04953.

References

1. Katzman R, Kawas C. The epidemiology of dementia and Alzheimer disease. In: Terry RD, Katzman R, Bick KL, eds. *Alzheimer Disease.* New York: Raven Press; 1994:105–122.
2. Evans D, Funkenstein H, Albert M, et al. Prevalence of Alzheimer's disease in a community dwelling population of older persons: higher than previously reported. *JAMA.* 1989;262:2551–2556.
3. Schor J, Levkoff S, Lipsitz L, et al. Risk factors for delirium in hospitalized elderly. *JAMA.* 1992;267:827–831.
4. Inouye SK. Prevention of delirium inhospitalized older patients: risk factors and targeted intervention strategies. *Ann Med.* 2000;32:257–263.
5. Kramer S, Reifler B. Depression, dementia and reversible dementia. *J Clin Geriatr Med.* 1992;8:289–297.
6. Nadeau S, Gonzalezrothi L, Crosson B, Gonzalez-Rothi L. *Aphasia and Language: Theory and Practice.* New York: Guilford; 2000.

7. Folstein M, Folstein S, McHugh P. "Mini-Mental State". A practical method for grading the cognitive state of patients for the clinician. *J Psychiatr Res.* 1975;12:189–198.

8. Blessed G, Tomlinson BE, Roth M. The association between quantitative measures of dementia and of senile changes in the cerebral gray matter of elderly subjects. *Br J Psychiatry.* 1968;114:797–811.

9. Pfeiffer E. A short portable mental status questionnaire for the assessment of organic brain deficit in elderly patients. *J Am Geriatr Soc.* 1975;23:433–441.

10. Solomon P, Hirschoff A, Kelly B, et al. A 7-minute neurocognitive screening battery highly sensitive to Alzheimer's disease. *Arch Neurol.* 1998;55:349–355.

11. Murden R, McRae T, Kaner S, Buckram M. Mini-Mental State Exam scores vary with education in blacks and whites. *J Am Geriatr Soc.* 1991;39:149–155.

12. Hereen T, Lagaay A, Beek W, et al. Reference values for the Mini-Mental State Examination (MMSE) in octo- and nonagenarians. *J Am Geriatr Soc.* 1990;38:1093–1096.

13. Bleeker M, Colla-Wilson K, Kawas C, Agnew J. Age-specific norms for the Mini-Mental State Exam. *Neurology.* 1988;38:1565–1568.

14. Manly J, Jacobs D, Sano M, et al. Effect of literacy on neuropsychological test performance in nondemented, education-matched elders. *J Int Neuropsychol Soc.* 1999;5: 191–202.

15. Clark C, Sheppard L, Fillenbaum G, et al. Variability in annual Mini-Mental State Examination score in patients with probable Alzheimer's disease: a clinical perspective of data from the Consortium to Establish a Registry for Alzheimer's Disease. *Arch Neurol.* 1999;56:857–862.

16. Neary D, Snowden JS, Gustafson L, et al. Frontotemporal lobar degeneration: a consensus on clinical diagnostic criteria. *Neurology.* 1998;51:1546–1554.

17. Halstead WC. *Brain and Intelligence.* Chicago: University of Chicago Press; 1947.

18. Golden CJ, Hammeke TA, Purisch AD. *Manual for the Luria–Nebraska Neuropsychological Battery.* Los Angeles: Western Psychological Services; 1980.

19. Wechsler D. *Wechsler Adult Intelligence Scale—III.* New York: Psychological Corporation; 1997.

20. Baker EL, Letz R, Fidler AT. A computer administered neurobehavioral evaluation system for occupational and environmental epidemiology. *J Occup Med.* 1985;27:206–212.

21. Mirsky A. Attention: a neuropsychological perspective. In: Chall J, Mirsky A, eds. *Education and the Brain.* Chicago: University of Chicago Press; 1978.

22. Kaplan E, Goodglass H, Weintraub S. *Boston Naming Test.* Philadelphia: Lea & Febiger; 1982.

23. Stern R, Mohs R, Davidson M, et al. A longitudinal study of Alzheimer's disease: measurement, rate, and predictors of cognitive deterioration. *Am J Psychiatry.* 1994;151:390–396.

24. Benton AL, Hamsher K. *Multilingual Aphasia Examination.* Iowa City: University of Iowa Press; 1976.

25. Halstead WC, Wepman JM. The Halstead–Wepman aphasia screening test. *J Speech Hearing Disord.* 1979;14:9–15.

26. Goodglass H, Kaplan E. *The Assessment of Aphasia and Related Disorders.* Philadelphia: Lea & Febiger; 1972.

27. Kertesz A. *Western Aphasia Battery.* London, Ontario: University of Western Ontario; 1980.

28. Petersen R, Smith G, Kokmen E, Ivnik R, Tangalos E. Memory function in normal aging. *Neurology.* 1992;42:396–401.

29. Binetti G, Locascio J, Corkin S, Vonsattel J, Growdon J. Differences between Pick disease and Alzheimer disease in clinical appearance and rate of cognitive decline. *Arch Neurol.* 2000;57:225–232.

30. Nebes R, Butters M, Mulsant B, et al. Decreased working memory and processing speed mediate cognitive impairment in geriatric depression. *Psychol Med.* 2000;30:679–691.

31. Delis D, Kramer J, Kaplan E, Ober B. *The California Verbal Learning Test.* New York: Psychological Corp.; 1987.

32. Wechsler D. *Wechsler Memory Scale—III.* New York: Psychological Corporation; 1997.

33. Grober E, Buschke H. Genuine memory deficits in dementia. *Dev Neuropsychol.* 1987;3:13–36.

34. Welsh KA, Butters N, Mohs RC, et al. The Consortium to Establish a Registry for Alzheimer's Disease (CERAD). Part V. A normative study of the neuropsychological battery. *Neurology.* 1994;44:609–614.

35. Benton AL. *The Revised Visual Retention Test.* New York: Psychological Corp.; 1974.

36. Reitan RM. Validity of the Trail Making Test as an indicator of organic brain damage. *Percept Mot Skills.* 1958;8:271–276.

37. Stroop JR. Studies of interference in serial verbal reactions. *J Exp Psychol.* 1935;18:643–662.

38. Petrides M, Milner B. Deficits in subject-ordered tasks after frontal and temporal lobe lesions in man. *Neuropsychologia.* 1982;20:249–262.

39. Gorham DR. A proverbs test for clinical and experimental use. *Psychol Rep.* 1956;1:1–12.

40. Satz P, Mogel S. An abbreviation of the WAIS for clinical use. *J Clin Psychol.* 1962;18:77–79.

41. Nelson H, O'Connell A. Dementia: the estimation of premorbid intelligence levels using the new adult reading test. *Cortex.* 1978;14:234–244.

20
Preoperative Assessment and Perioperative Care

Peter Pompei

The increasing number of older persons undergoing surgery stems from both our aging population and important recent advances in surgical and anesthetic techniques. Currently, about one-third of all operations are performed on persons 65 years of age and older, compared to about 20% in 1980.[1] The types of surgical procedures commonly performed on older persons reflect the prevalence of chronic diseases: intraocular lenses for cataracts, resections of hypertrophied prostate glands, colorectal procedures for cancer, arthroplasties for osteoarthritis and fractures, and arterial reconstruction for vascular disease. The introduction of neuroleptic anesthesia, sophisticated perioperative monitoring technology, and effective prophylaxis against deep venous thrombosis have contributed to lower surgical mortality for older adults.[2] Endoscopic and other minimal access techniques have added to the ease and safety of operative therapy and have led to reduced mortality, increased ambulatory surgery, and shorter-stay hospitalizations.[3,4] Returning patients quickly to their usual environment and functional status can reduce complications so commonly related to medications and immobilization associated with hospitalization. The lowered risk of operative morbidity and mortality has encouraged physicians and patients to consider surgical therapy more readily.

With the increasing rate of operative therapy among older patients, there is an increasing demand by surgeons for medical consultation in the perioperative period. Although the request is often for "preoperative clearance," both the unstated expectations of the requesting physician and the responsibilities of the consultant are much more specific. The purpose of a preoperative assessment is to identify factors associated with increased risks of specific complications related to the anticipated procedure and to recommend a management plan that would minimize these risks. The consultant must give careful attention to the extent and severity of comorbid conditions, the current and anticipated pharmacologic therapy, and the functional and psychologic state of the patient. These patient-specific risk factors are only part of the required assessment; the type and technical difficulty of the procedure, the skill of the surgeon, and the anesthetic management all contribute to the risks of complications.[2] The most common postoperative medical complications include respiratory problems, congestive heart failure, delirium, and thromboembolism.[5] This chapter reviews the risk factors for and management of these and other common perioperative problems of older persons.

Perioperative Risk Stratification

Assessing a patient's risk for postoperative complications is an important aspect of preoperative evaluation. This process allows physicians to focus treatments on modifiable factors, anticipate specific problems, and provide patients and families with more precise, individual-specific, prognostic information.

Since 1941, anesthesiologists have stratified patients according to a physical status classification system that has been modified over the years and now consists of the five classes shown in Table 20.1.[6] Although developed to describe the preoperative condition of patients in a subjective but standardized way, several reports indicate an important relationship between the American Society of Anesthesiologists (ASA) score and operative mortality.[7,8] The ASA status has become a useful global index of operative risk despite institutional differences in death rates and the subjective nature of the ratings.

In a large study of complications associated with anesthesia done in France, the rate of complications, although rising with advancing age, was largely dependent on the number of associated diseases per person.[9] Among patients 75 years of age and older, those with three or more associated diseases had a complication rate 10 times greater than those with no associated diseases. This observation supports the hypothesis that physiologic

TABLE 20.1. The American Society of Anesthesiologists (ASA) physical status classification system.

Class I	A normal healthy patient for elective operation
Class II	A patient with mild systemic disease
Class III	A patient with severe systemic disease that limits activity but is not incapacitating
Class IV	A patient with incapacitating systemic disease that is a constant threat to life
Class V or	A moribund patient not expected to survive 24 h with without operation

Source: New Classification of Physical Status,[6] with permission.

TABLE 20.2. The Charlson weighted index of comorbidity.

Condition	Weight
Myocardial infarction	1
Congestive heart failure	1
Peripheral vascular disease	1
Cerebrovascular disease	1
Dementia	1
Chronic pulmonary disease	1
Connective tissue disease	1
Ulcer disease	1
Mild liver disease	1
Diabetes	1
Hemiplegia	2
Moderate or severe renal disease	2
Diabetes with end-organ damage	2
Any tumor	2
Leukemia	2
Lymphoma	2
Moderate or severe liver disease	3
Metastatic solid tumor	4
AIDS	4

Weights are assigned for each of the patient's conditions; the score is the sum of the weights.
Source: From Ref. 12, with permission.

reserve and ability to regain homeostasis is affected partly by changes associated with aging but, more importantly, by the deleterious consequence of accumulating disease among older persons. To determine predictors of 30-day mortality among 92 patients undergoing pneumonectomy, investigators examined the contribution of the following comorbid conditions: cardiac disease, diabetes, hypertension, respiratory disease, pulmonary cancer, peripheral vascular disease, liver disease, renal insufficiency, and inflammatory bowel disease.[10] The presence of one or more of these conditions was associated with an increased risk of 30-day mortality. Similarly, in a study of about 100 patients undergoing total knee arthroplasty, comorbidity was quantified by counting how many of the following conditions were present: hypertension, diabetes mellitus, coronary artery disease, atherosclerotic heart disease, peripheral vascular disease, chronic renal failure, and asthma.[11] Patients with four or more of these comorbid conditions were found to have longer hospital stays and a worse functional status at 3 months compared to those with fewer than four of the conditions. These results indicate that a simple count of selected diagnoses can help identify patients at risk for untoward outcomes such as decreased survival, functional recovery, and longer duration of hospitalization.

A tool commonly used to measure comorbidity is the Charlson index,[12] an empirically derived prognostic taxonomy of comorbid conditions relevant to short-term survival. It was derived from a cohort of about 600 patients admitted to the medical service of New York Hospital during a 1-month period in 1984. Comorbid conditions judged cogent to short-term prognosis were included in the index. Weights were assigned to each condition based on the association with 1-year mortality of the patients enrolled. The specific conditions considered and their associated weights are shown in Table 20.2. The index has proven useful in many clinical studies, including predicting 5-year mortality among older men undergoing prostatectomy for benign prostatic hypertrophy[13] and estimating the risk of 30- and 90-day mortality in more than 21,000 cases of open cholecystectomy among older persons.[14]

Two patient-specific factors other than comorbidity associated with poor surgical outcomes are hypoalbu-

minemia and severely limited physical activity level. Two reports from a study of more than 200,000 patients treated at Department of Veterans Affairs Medical Centers highlight the importance of a low serum albumin in predicting poor surgical outcomes. Among about 54,000 cases of major noncardiac surgery, a low serum albumin level was the strongest predictor of morbidity and 30-day mortality when compared to 61 other preoperative patient risk variables.[15] In the subset of patients undergoing proctectomy for rectal cancer, presurgical hypoalbuminemia was associated with an increased 30-day mortality rate.[16] It is not yet known whether preoperative correction of hypoalbuminemia will alter patient outcomes. Similarly, an impaired physical functional status has been associated with poor postoperative outcomes. In a study of 474 male veterans (mean age, 68 years) undergoing noncardiac surgery, the risk of death was significantly increased among those patients with severely limited preoperative activity level, defined as bedridden or bed-to-chair movement.[17] Awareness of patient-specific factors associated with a high risk of poor surgical outcomes is useful in providing realistic prognostic information to patients and their families.

Assessing the Risk of Cardiac Complications

Because cardiac complications are among the most common and most serious postoperative problems, significant attention has been focused on estimating the risk of cardiac complications, especially in noncardiac surgical procedures. Goldman and associates pioneered the association of preoperative factors with the development of cardiac complications among patients over 40 years of age.[18] In their initial work, nine independent predictors of cardiac complications after noncardiac surgery were identified, the most important of which included recent myocardial infarction, uncompensated congestive heart failure, electrocardiographic evidence of a rhythm other than sinus or premature atrial contractions, and more than five premature ventricular contractions per minute. The usefulness of the multifactorial index of cardiac risk that was developed has been repeatedly confirmed.[19–23] Most recently, Goldman and others have revised and validated a simple index for predicting cardiac risk of noncardiac surgery.[24] Stable patients undergoing nonurgent, major, noncardiac surgery were assessed for the presence or absence of the following six factors: high-risk type of surgery, history of ischemic heart disease, history of congestive heart failure, history of cerebrovascular disease, preoperative treatment with insulin, and preoperative

serum creatinine greater than 2.0 mg/dL. The rates of major cardiac complications among patients with zero, one, two, and three or more of these factors were 0.5%, 1.3%, 4%, and 9%, respectively. This index performed better than the original Goldman index and several other risk prediction indices.

Beyond the identification of groups of patients at increased risk for developing cardiac complications are management algorithms that can guide the physicians beyond the assessment phase.[25,26] The guideline for assessing and managing the risk of perioperative cardiac complications in noncardiac surgery from the American College of Physicians is shown in Figure 20.1. The algorithm begins with an assessment of the patient's risk for cardiac complications using the Modified Cardiac Risk Index. Patients in the low-risk category can proceed to surgery without additional evaluation or treatment. Patients in the intermediate-risk category not undergoing a vascular procedure can also proceed to surgery. Patients in the intermediate-risk category undergoing vascular surgery are advised to have a cardiac stress test.

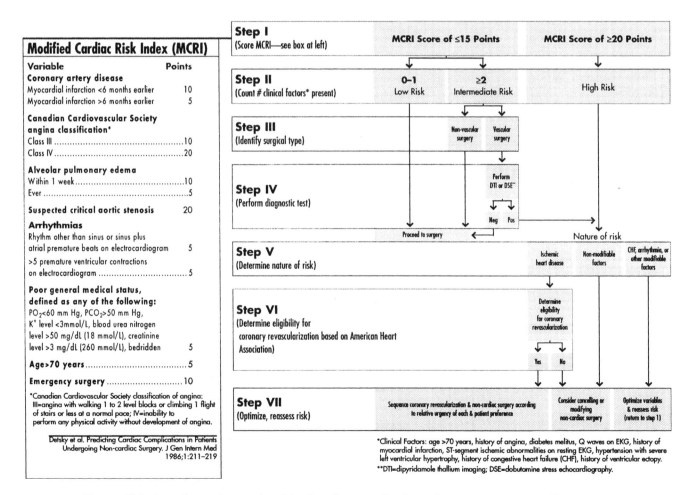

FIGURE 20.1 Assessing and managing risk of cardiac complications of nonemergent, noncardiac surgery.

If negative, they can proceed to surgery; if positive, they are treated like patients who fall into the high-risk category based on the Modified Cardiac Risk Index.

Patients in the high-risk category and those in the intermediate-risk category with an abnormal cardiac stress test should have a further evaluation of the nature of their risk. If the risk is due to ischemic heart disease, eligibility for coronary revascularization should be considered before proceeding with elective noncardiac surgery. If the risk is due to congestive heart failure, dysrhythmias, or other modifiable factors, these should be optimally managed before proceeding to surgery. If the risks are nonmodifiable, consideration should be given to canceling or altering the anticipated surgery. The stepwise approach of this guideline provides the clinician with an organized, systematic approach to assessment and management. The clinical outcomes to be expected by following this approach are still being studied. Results of some large studies support the recommendation that preoperative stress testing be done in selected patients undergoing vascular surgery.[27,28]

Management of Selected Problems

In addition to identifying and quantifying the risks older patients face when surgery is being planned, geriatricians are also called upon to assist in minimizing these risks by managing specific medical problems. A comprehensive review of the management of all possible medical problems in surgical patients and of the specific problems related to particular operations is beyond the scope of this chapter. The reader is referred to other publications that address many of these important issues.[29–33] The remainder of this chapter focuses on the management of selected perioperative medical problems commonly faced by medical consultants.

Hypertension

The prevalence of hypertension among Hispanic and non-Hispanic white Americans aged 60 years and older was found to be about 60%; in non-Hispanic African-Americans of the same age group, 70% had hypertension.[34] Uncontrolled hypertension is a well-established risk factor for stroke, myocardial infarction, and renal dysfunction. In the preoperative period, when the blood pressure is 180/110 mmHg or greater, elective operations should be postponed until better control of the hypertension is achieved.[25] An increased incidence of myocardial ischemia is seen not only among patients with preoperative hypertension, but also in those patients who have major fluctuations in blood pressure during a

surgical procedure.[35,36] This variability is more common in patients with established hypertension: significant elevations in blood pressure were observed in 25% of hypertensive patients during the perioperative period, irrespective of the control of their blood pressure preoperatively.[37]

The causes of variability in blood pressure among older persons perioperatively include anesthetic agents and other medications, age-related changes in the cardiovascular system, changes in intravascular volume, and pain or other stimuli to the nervous system. The work of Prys-Roberts[36] has demonstrated some of the expected changes in blood pressure during surgery. Induction of anesthesia usually results in a reduction in systemic vascular resistance. The normal compensatory responses of increased heart rate and increased stroke volume may be limited in older persons; this limitation may result in a reduced cardiac output and a fall in blood pressure. Endotracheal intubation generally causes significant stimulation of the sympathetic nervous system and a sharp rise in blood pressure. Changes in intravascular volume and depth of anesthesia contribute to fluctuations in blood pressure during the operation.

Although the anesthesiologist attends to the variability of blood pressure in the immediate perioperative period, the geriatric consultant is more likely to have a role in preoperative assessment and the management of the patients once they have left the recovery room. Patients with chronic hypertension undergoing elective operations are probably at no increased risk for cardiac complications so long as the preoperative diastolic pressure is stable and less than 110 mmHg and large fluctuations in the mean arterial pressure can be avoided intraoperatively.[37] For this reason, and because of the potential for untoward responses to newly introduced antihypertensive agents, it generally is not advisable to begin a new drug regimen for blood pressure control in the few days before surgery. When therapy needs to be initiated or adjusted, it is preferable to postpone the procedure until the patient's response to a new regimen can be observed and a steady state achieved. Oral medications used to control hypertension preoperatively should be given on the day of surgery with a sip of water and restarted as soon as possible postoperatively.[38] The risks of severe hypertension from withholding antihypertensive medications far outweigh the potential adverse effects of giving these medications preoperatively. Clinicians must be alert to the negative chronotropic and inotropic effects of some beta-adrenergic blockers and calcium channel antagonists that may exacerbate similar pharmacologic effects of inhalation anesthetics.

In the postoperative period, patients with significant elevations in blood pressure should be fully evaluated. Occasionally, uncontrolled pain or a distended bladder is the cause of the hypertension, and treatment is directed at these precipitating factors. If secondary causes of hypertension are excluded, antihypertensive drug treatment is indicated. Parenteral calcium channel antagonists, beta-blockers, and drugs that block both alpha- and beta-adrenergic receptors have been very useful in controlling postoperative hypertension in older patients. Intravenous angiotensin-converting enzyme inhibitors, such as enalaprilat, have been used for postoperative hypertension and hypertensive crises and may be appropriate for patients with congestive heart failure and hypertension. The ability to quickly titrate the dose of parenterally administered medications to blood pressure response is a significant advantage. Beta-blockers must be used cautiously in patients predisposed to congestive heart failure because of negative inotropic effects. The negative chronotropic effects of this class of drugs can blunt the normal compensatory response of increased heart rate to a sudden loss of intravascular volume, such as a major postoperative bleeding episode. Other relative contraindications to beta-blockers include a history of bronchospasm, claudication, and diabetes mellitus. Orally administered calcium channel antagonists have been successfully used to control postoperative hypertension in older patients undergoing cataract surgery.[39] Potent vasodilators, such as hydralazine, can be hazardous in the subset of patients with hypertensive, hypertrophic cardiomyopathy who have a small left ventricular chamber and good contractile function; these patients depend heavily on adequate diastolic filling that can be compromised by rapid vasodilation and reflex tachycardia. Nitroprusside can effectively control significant hypertension, but its use requires careful monitoring of the patient, usually in an intensive care unit with an intra-arterial catheter to continuously measure the blood pressure response.

Atherosclerotic Disease

Many older surgical patients can be expected to have atherosclerosis. The identification and management of occlusive coronary disease in the surgical patient is especially important because the mortality of perioperative myocardial infarction has been estimated to be about 40%.[40] Useful guidelines for the assessment and management of patients with coronary artery disease have been developed, and one has been outlined in the previous section on Assessing the Risk of Cardiac Complications.[25,26,41] Management of patients with known or suspected coronary artery disease should include the perioperative use of beta-blockers. The use of these medications has been shown to significantly reduce the risk of postoperative cardiac complications among patients undergoing noncardiac surgery, including vascular procedures.[42–44]

Carotid occlusions and peripheral vascular disease are prevalent among older persons and raise important management questions. The presence of a carotid bruit has been judged to be supportive evidence of atherosclerosis but has not been shown to increase the risk of postoperative stroke.[45] Clinical factors that have been shown to increase the incidence of perioperative stroke include cerebrovascular disease, chronic obstructive pulmonary disease, and peripheral vascular disease.[46] Patients experiencing transient ischemic attacks for whom carotid endarterectomy is recommended should have this procedure done before elective noncardiac surgery. Peripheral vascular disease very commonly coexists with significant atherosclerotic coronary artery disease. If the peripheral vascular disease is serious enough to limit the patient's activity, exertional angina may be masked. Symptoms or signs of arterial disease should prompt the consultant to evaluate the patient for the presence of ischemic heart disease.

Congestive Heart Failure

Congestive heart failure is an important complication of ischemic heart disease, but it can also result from other cardiomyopathies or valvular heart disease. In the original Goldman index of cardiac risk factors in noncardiac surgery, the preoperative conditions associated with the most points predictive of an adverse outcome are the presence of an S_3 gallop and jugular venous distension, two of the classic signs of uncompensated congestive heart failure. In the management of surgical patients with congestive heart failure, it is important to optimize their medication regimen and to monitor carefully their volume status and cardiac output. The standard treatment of systolic cardiac dysfunction includes the use of diuretics, positive inotropic agents, and medications to reduce afterload. Heart rate and rhythm contribute significantly to cardiac output and may require special interventions; this is especially true in patients with diastolic dysfunction, often caused by hypertensive cardiomyopathy, in which the left ventricular end-diastolic volume is so dependent on atrial contraction and adequate filling time. Swan–Ganz catheters have significantly improved our ability to monitor accurately the volume status of patients and optimize ventricular filling pressures. The intraoperative transesophageal echocardiogram has become popular in some centers, especially for cardiothoracic procedures.[47] The advantages of this device over the Swan-Ganz catheter are that continuous estimates of left ventricular end-diastolic volumes can be made, changes in regional wall motion can be monitored, and the observed ejection fraction area can be used to assess contractility. The disadvantage is that the device is only used intraoperatively, and unless a right heart catheter is also placed, management of postoperative volume status must rely on imprecise clinical measures.

Valvular Heart Disease

The primary perioperative risks associated with valvular heart disease are congestive heart failure and bacterial endocarditis. It has been estimated that 20% of surgical patients who have significant valvular heart disease will develop new or worsening congestive heart failure perioperatively.[48] Critical aortic stenosis has been identified as the valvular lesion most commonly associated with complications. Preoperative identification of this lesion by history and physical examination alone may be difficult. Clinical findings include a harsh systolic murmur radiating to the neck, occurring late in systole, that is prolonged and may obscure the second heart sound; diminished carotid pulses; and left ventricular hypertrophy on the electrocardiogram and radiographic evidence of aortic valvular calcification. A bedside clinical prediction rule has been proposed to detect moderate or severe aortic stenosis. The absence of a murmur over the right clavicle is a useful sign that significant aortic stenosis is unlikely. When such a murmur is heard, the presence of three of the following four associated findings is useful to confirm the presence of aortic stenosis: reduced carotid artery volume, slow carotid artery upstroke, maximum murmur intensity at the second right intercostal space, and reduced intensity of the second heart sound.[49] If significant aortic stenosis is suspected, an echocardiogram can confirm the diagnosis. It has been suggested that patients with angina, heart failure, or syncope who have significant aortic stenosis established by echocardiography should undergo cardiac catheterization to assess the need for valve replacement before elective operations.[50] Other types of valvular heart disease are not absolute contraindications to elective surgery. Nevertheless, patients with stenotic or incompetent valves require careful hemodynamic monitoring during perioperative fluid management.

Certain valvular and other cardiac conditions predispose the patient to endocarditis, and prophylactic antibiotics should be used in selected operative settings. Patients with a high risk of endocarditis are those with prosthetic cardiac valves, previous bacterial endocarditis, complex congenital heart disease, and surgically constructed systemic pulmonary shunts or conduits. Patients considered to be at moderate risk for endocarditis are those with most other congenital cardiac malformation, acquired valvular dysfunction, hypertrophic cardiomyopathy, and mitral valve prolapse with valvular regurgitation and/or thickened leaflets.[15] The procedures for which prophylactic antibiotics are indicated are listed in Table 20.3;[51] the recommended antibiotic regimens are summarized in Table 20.4.[51]

TABLE 20.3. Procedures for which endocarditis prophylaxis is recommended.

Dental procedures
  Dental extractions
  Periodontal procedures including surgery, scaling and root
    planning, probing, and recall maintenance
  Dental implant placement and reimplantation of avulsed teeth
  Endodonic (root canal) instrumentation or surgery only beyond
    the apex
  Subgingival placement of antibiotic fibers or strips
  Initial placement of orthodontic bands but not brackets
  Intraligamentary local anesthetic injections
  Prophylactic cleaning of teeth or implants where bleeding is
    anticipated

Respiratory, gastrointestinal, and genitourinary tract procedures
  Tonsillectomy and/or adenoidectomy
  Surgical procedures that involve respiratory mucosa
  Bronchoscopy with a rigid bronchoscope
  Sclerotherapy for esophageal varices
  Esophageal stricture dilation
  Endoscopic retrograde cholangiography with biliary obstruction
  Biliary tract surgery
  Surgical procedures that involve intestinal mucosa
  Prostatic surgery
  Cystoscopy
  Urethral dilation

Source: Dajani AS, Taubert KA, Wilson W, et al. Copyright 1997, American Medical Association,[51] with permission.

Rhythm Disturbances and Heart Block

A cardiac rhythm other than sinus rhythm is associated with an increased risk of cardiac complications, most commonly myocardial ischemia or congestive heart failure.[50] If a patient is on an antiarrhythmic medication, this should be given on the day of surgery and restarted as soon as possible postoperatively. Parenteral forms of many of these drugs are available and can be used until the patient can tolerate oral medications. Supraventricular tachycardia is commonly encountered in older persons undergoing noncardiac surgery. A recent study of more than 4000 patients undergoing major, nonemergency, noncardiac procedures who were in sinus rhythm at the preoperative evaluation identified 12 risk factors for developing perioperative supraventricular arrhythmia: male gender, age 70 years and older, significant valvular disease, history of a supraventricular arrhythmia, asthma, congestive heart failure, premature atrial complexes on preoperative electrocardiogram, ASA class III or IV, abdominal aortic aneurysm repair, and abdominal, vascular, or intrathoracic procedures.[52]

Efforts to restore sinus rhythm often begin with an infusion of adenosine; for patients who do not convert with this intervention, intravenous infusion of a betablocker or calcium channel blocker has been shown to accelerate the conversion to sinus rhythm.[53] Ventricular dysrhythmias during the perioperative period occur in

TABLE 20.4. Regimens of prophylactic antibiotics for patients at risk for bacterial endocarditis.

Drug	Dosing regimen
Dental, oral, respiratory tract, or esophageal procedures:	
Standard regimen	
Amoxicillin	2 g orally 1 h before procedure
Amoxicillin-/penicillin-allergic patients	
Clindamycin or	600 mg orally 1 h before procedure
Cephalexin or cefadroxil or	2 g orally 1 h before procedure
Azithromycin or clarithromycin	500 mg orally 1 h before procedure
Patients unable to take oral medications	
Ampicillin	2 g intravenously (i.v.) or intramuscularly (i.m.) within 30 min before procedure
Penicillin-allergic patients unable to take oral medications	
Clindamycin or	600 mg intravenously (i.v.) within 30 min before procedure
Cefazolin	1 g intravenously (i.v.) or intramuscularly (i.m.) within 30 min before procedure
Genitourinary and gastrointestinal (excluding esophageal) procedures:	
High-risk patients	
Ampicillin and gentamicin	Intravenous (i.v.) or intramuscular (i.m.) administration of ampicillin 2 g, plus gentamicin 1.5 mg/kg (not to exceed 120 mg), 30 min before the procedure; followed by ampicillin 1 g i.m./i.v. or amoxicillin 1 g, orally 6 h after initial dose
High-risk patients allergic to ampicillin/amoxicillin	
Vancomycin and gentamicin	Intravenous administration of vancomycin 1 g, over 1–2 h, plus gentamicin 1.5 mg/kg i.m./i.v. (not to exceed 120 mg); complete injection/infusion within 30 min of starting procedure
Moderate-risk patients[a]	
Amoxicillin or ampicillin	Amoxicillin 2 g orally 1 h before procedure, or ampicillin 3 gm i.m./i.v. within 30 min of starting procedure
Moderate-risk patients allergic to ampicillin/amoxicillin	
Vancomycin	1 g i.v. over 1–2 h; complete infusion within 30 min of starting procedure

[a] Patients with prosthetic heart valves and those with a previous history of endocarditis are considered to be in a high-risk category and should not be considered for this regimen.
Source: Dajani AS, Taubert KA, Wilson W, et al. Copyright 1997, American Medical Association, with permssion.

almost half of older men with known or suspected coronary artery disease undergoing noncardiac surgery, but unless they occur with other symptoms or signs of myocardial ischemia, they may not require monitoring or treatment.[54] The indications for a pacemaker are not influenced by an anticipated operative procedure. Patients with an asymptomatic chronic bifascicular block or left bundle branch block rarely progress to complete heart block in the perioperative period. Bradyarrhythmias can occur but are successfully managed with medications so that prophylactic insertion of a temporary pacemaker in such patients should be questioned.[55]

Pulmonary Disease

Pulmonary problems are among the most common postoperative complications.[56] Older persons may be particularly prone to pulmonary complications because of the age-related changes in the respiratory system. At the alveolar level, there is a decrease in elasticity due to alterations in collagen content and structure. Functionally, this leads to an increase in the closing volume, that lung volume at which airway closure is first detected. As the closing volume approaches the functional residual capacity, the risk for atelectasis increases. There is also increased chest wall stiffness due to calcification of cartilage, arthritic changes, and diminished intervertebral space combined with insufficient respiratory muscle strength to match the added work load of breathing imposed by the increased chest wall stiffness.[57] These structural changes can increase residual volume and reduce the expiratory flow rates in older persons.

There are also important changes in respiratory function resulting from anesthesia and surgery that are superimposed on the age-related changes. The combination of the supine position, general anesthesia, and abdominal incisions leads to a significant reduction in functional residual capacity and an associated increase in airway resistance.[58] The decline in functional residual capacity is most severe on about the fourth postoperative day but can persist for more than a week.[59] The combination of a reduced functional residual capacity and an age-associated increase in closing volume predisposes patients to atelectasis with the attendant risks of hypoxemia and infection. Vital capacity can be decreased as much as 25% to 50%, especially after upper abdominal incisions.[59] Postoperative pain and analgesics both contribute to a reduction in tidal volume and impaired clearing of secretions through normal cough mechanisms.

The geriatric consultant can be most helpful by anticipating patients at high risk for complications and then recommending strategies to reduce these risks. In addition to the well-recognized risk for pulmonary complications, such as significant lung disease and type and duration of operation, a patient's functional level should be taken into account. Patients with better exercise tolerance by self-report or by the measured distance during a timed walk have fewer pulmonary complications than those with poorer exercise tolerance.[60] Other patient characteristics used to identify those at increased risk for pulmonary complications include dementia, recent cigarette smoking, age of 60 years or more, a history of cancer or angina, location and length of the incision, and ASA class of 3 or greater.[61] Continued research is needed to establish a valid risk index for pulmonary complication for older persons undergoing noncardiac surgeries.

Considerable attention has been focused on pulmonary function tests to identify patients at high risk for respiratory complications.[59,62] Functional and anatomic tests have proven helpful to clinicians in managing patients facing pulmonary resections. In such patients, the quantitative ventilation–perfusion scan can accurately predict postoperative flow rates; when the predicted postoperative forced expiratory volume in 1 s is 0.8 L or greater, the operative risk is often considered acceptable.[63,64] In contrast, the predictive value of pulmonary function tests for patients undergoing abdominal procedures is unproven.[65,66] Additional studies are needed to address whether pulmonary function test results contribute significant additional information to what is known from the clinical examination and whether this information has a beneficial effect on patient outcomes.

Prospective studies in high-risk patients have identified specific interventions that reduce morbidity and mortality from respiratory problems. Stein and Cassara found that "poor-risk" patients treated with a regimen of preoperative smoking cessation, antibiotics "when indicated," perioperative bronchodilator therapy, inhalation of humidified gas, postural drainage, and chest physiotherapy had fewer pulmonary complications, lower mortality, and shorter hospital stays than nontreated patients.[67] Data on the impact of cigarette smoking suggest that as much as 6 weeks of abstinence may be required before there is improvement in small airways disease, hypersecretion of mucus, tracheobronchial clearance, and immune function, although cardiovascular function can be enhanced through the elimination of carbon monoxide and nicotine for even 12 to 24 h.[68] Benefits of antibiotics, chest physiotherapy, and incentive spirometry have been reported,[69–71] but more information is needed regarding these interventions, especially which patients to target and for which operative procedures.

There is little consensus about the benefit of other treatments, such as instruction in respiratory maneuvers, bronchodilators, minimization of postoperative narcotic analgesics, and early mobilization of the older patient.[72] In the absence of an evidence-based practice guideline for the perioperative management of an older person at increased risk of pulmonary complications, a pragmatic approach is required. Preoperatively, it is important to encourage abstinence from cigarettes, eradicate tracheobronchial infections, relieve airflow obstruction, and instruct the patient in lung expansion maneuvers. Intraoperative goals would include limiting the duration of the operation to less than 3 h using limited access surgical procedures when possible, and considering spinal or epidural anesthesia. Postoperatively, deep-breathing exercise and incentive spirometry should be encouraged, and consideration should be given to continuous positive airway pressure devices and regional analgesia via epidural or local nerve blocks.[73]

Thromboembolic Disease

Thromboembolic complications are prevalent in the perioperative period. It has been estimated that between 20% and 30% of patients undergoing general surgery develop deep venous thrombosis, and the incidence is as high as 40% in hip and knee surgery, gynecologic cancer operations, open prostatectomies, and major neurosurgical procedures.[74] Although fatal pulmonary embolism occurs in 1% to 5% of all surgical patients, it accounts for a larger proportion of operative deaths in middle-aged and older individuals.[75] Because venous thrombosis and pulmonary emboli can be difficult to diagnose and treat, considerable effort has been focused on prophylaxis. Various regimens to reduce deep venous thrombosis and pulmonary emboli, including heparin, warfarin, aspirin, dextran, and leg compressive devices, have been used. The recommendations for prevention of venous thromboembolism of the Sixth American College of Chest Physicians Consensus Conference on Antithrombotic Therapy related to older surgical patients are summarized in Table 20.5.[76] Clinical risk factors identified by this group include: increasing age; prolonged immobility, stroke or paralysis; previous venous thromboembolism; cancer and its treatment; obesity; varicose veins; cardiac dysfunction; indwelling central venous catheters; inflammatory bowel disease; nephrotic syndrome; and estrogen use.

Renal, Fluid, and Electrolyte Disorders

The kidneys play a critical role in drug metabolism and fluid and electrolyte balance during the perioperative period. The age-related changes in kidney structure and

TABLE 20.5. Prevention of venous thromboembolism.

Clinical setting	Recommended prophylaxis
General surgery	
>40 years old, nonmajor surgery, no other risk factors	LDUH, LMWH, ES or IPC
>40 years old, major surgery or >60 years old, nonmajor surgery, with other risk factors	LDUH, LMWH, or IPC
Higher risk patients with a greater than usual risk of bleeding	ES or IPC
Very high risk patients with multiple risk factors	LDUH or LMWH combined with ES or IPC
Orthopaedic surgery	
Hip replacement	LMWH or adjusted dose warfarin (INR 2-3)
Knee replacement	LMWH or adjusted dose warfarin (INR 2-3)
Hip fracture repair	LMWH or adjusted dose warfarin (INR 2-3)
Neurosurgery	
Intracranial operations	IPC with or without ES

LDUH, low dose unfractionated heparin; LMWH, low molecular weight heparin; ES, elastic stockings; IPC, intermittent pneumatic compression
Source: Geerts et al., Chest, 2001;119(1):132S–175S.

function, combined with the effects of anesthesia and surgery, can have important consequences in the management of the older surgical patient. With aging, there is a loss of renal mass, primarily in the cortex, that results in a 30% to 50% decrease in the number of glomeruli by the seventh decade.[77] This loss of filtering surface is associated with a fall in renal blood flow and reduction in glomerular filtration rate (GFR). The decrease in GFR is generally coincident with a decline in muscle mass so that the serum creatinine levels may remain normal. Accurate measurements of glomerular filtration rates can be very helpful to the clinician but may not be readily available. Estimates of GFR can be calculated using the following equation proposed by Cockcroft and Gault[78]:

$$C_{Cr}(ml/min) = [140 - age\ (yr)] \times [weight\ (kg)]/ [72 \times serum\ Cr\ (mg/dL)]$$

where C_{Cr} indicates creatinine clearance and Cr is the serum creatinine level. (This formula is for men; the estimate is adjusted for women by multiplying the result by 0.85.) The estimates obtained from this formula have been shown to correlate with measured creatinine clearance in older patients.[79,80] This measure, although not precise, is sufficiently accurate for appropriate medication dose adjustments when Cr < 5 mg/dl and relatively stable.

Diminished preoperative renal function increases the risk of postoperative acute renal failure. Renal blood flow can be compromised intraoperatively because of a decline in cardiac output secondary to the negative inotropic effects of inhalational anesthetic agents, the effects of positive pressure ventilation, and loss of intravascular volume. These factors and nephrotoxic medications can result in postoperative acute reversible intrinsic renal failure.[81] Oliguria, isosthenuria, and a rising serum creatinine are early clinical signs of this syndrome.

When acute renal failure is suspected, the urine sediment should be examined for epithelial cell casts, granular casts, and tubular epithelial cells. The urine sodium is generally greater than 40 mEq/L, and the urine to plasma creatinine ratio is generally less than 10:1. In contrast, prerenal azotemia is associated with a urine sodium of less than 40 mEq/L and a urine to plasma creatinine ratio of greater than 10:1. Management of acute intrinsic renal failure includes discontinuing potentially nephrotoxic drugs and carefully monitoring volume status. Dialysis is occasionally necessary to manage hypervolemia, hyperkalemia, metabolic acidosis, or uremic encephalopathy. Even with appropriate treatment, acute postoperative renal failure has a mortality rate between 40% and 80%.[82] Obstructive nephropathy is a concern in older patients because of sensitivity of the bladder to anticholinergic medications and the prevalence of associated problems such as prostatic hypertrophy and detrusor and urethral sphincter dysfunction from a variety of causes.

The ability of the kidneys to regulate body osmolality and fluid volume can be compromised by both aging and surgery. With aging, the loss of functioning nephrons increases the solute load per nephron, and renal blood flow patterns favor the medulla; these changes adversely affect the normal countercurrent concentrating mechanism[77]; this can lead to volume depletion through a reduction in renal concentrating capacity and excessive losses of free water. Older individuals also have a diminished thirst perception that compromises their ability to respond to significant free water loss and hyperosmolality.[83] This change is particularly important postoperatively, when third-space losses of fluid and bleeding may cause severe intravascular volume depletion. Conversely, volume overload sometimes results from the delayed response to sodium restriction and salt wasting observed in older individuals,[84] which can be exacerbated by the elevated levels of vasopressin seen in the postoperative state. Sodium and water retention after surgery may last for several days. These physiologic changes are compounded by the difficulties in the clinical assessment of volume status in older persons. Postural hypotension is an important sign of intravascular volume depletion but can be observed in euvolemic older patients and may be difficult to assess properly in the immediate postoperative period. When the assessment of volume status becomes critically important, it is often necessary to measure pulmonary capillary wedge pressure using a Swan–Ganz catheter.

Intravenous fluid administration must be adjusted for the older surgical patient because there is a decline in both total body water and intracellular water with advancing age. For men between 65 and 85 years of age and weighing between 40 and 80 kg, the intracellular volume represents 25% to 30% of body weight.[85] For women of the same age and weight ranges, the intracellular volume is approximately 20% to 25% of body weight. In the absence of acute stress and conditions known to affect salt and water balance, the daily metabolic requirements per liter of intracellular fluid are as follows:

Water, 100 mL
Energy, 100 kcal
Protein, 3 g
Sodium, 3 mmol
Potassium, 2 mmol

For example, an 80-year-old woman weighing 40 kg has an estimated intracellular volume of 10 L. Daily maintenance requirements would be 1 L water, 1000 kcal, 30 g protein, 30 mmol sodium, and 20 mmol potassium. Fluid and electrolyte status must be closely monitored and adjusted according to the response of the patient and the development of other pathophysiologic conditions.

Endocrine Disorders

Diabetes mellitus, usually type II, is common among older persons. It has been estimated that of diabetic patients undergoing surgery, more than 75% are over the age of 50.[86] Diabetes not only complicates the management of surgical patients but also predisposes the patient to an increased risk of morbidity and mortality from cardiovascular and infectious complications.[87,88] Several predictable perioperative metabolic changes can exacerbate hyperglycemia. With the stress and tissue injury of surgery, there is an increase in many of the counterregulatory hormones: cortisol, epinephrine, glucagon, and growth hormone. These changes stimulate gluconeogenesis, and the catecholamines can directly depress the release of insulin from the pancreas and blunt insulin activity at the cellular level.

In all diabetic patients undergoing surgery, it is important to monitor blood sugar frequently. Values should be obtained preoperatively, during the procedure, and in the recovery room. Afterward, the frequency of monitoring will be determined by the treatment regimen, the patient's condition, and glucose control. For patients whose blood sugar can be maintained in the normal range by diet and exercise therapy, no special preoperative preparation is required. Hyperglycemia can be effectively treated with supplemental short-acting insulin preparations given subcutaneously. The patients receiving oral hypoglycemic medications should have these held on the day of the operation. Hyperglycemia can be treated with short-acting insulin. For patients receiving insulin, several management regimens are possible. Constant insulin infusions can be used successfully but require careful monitoring because of the rapid changes in glucose and potassium levels. More commonly, for patients normally treated with a single dose of insulin each day, one-half to two-thirds of the usual dose of insulin is given on the morning of surgery, and a glucose-containing intravenous solution is administered at a rate of 5 to 10 g glucose per hour.

For patients who are normally managed with multiple does of insulin throughout the day, one-third the usual morning dose is administered on the morning of surgery, and a glucose-containing solution is infused intravenously.[89] Blood sugar control is easier if a constant rate of infusion of the glucose solution is maintained while nonglucose-containing intravenous fluids are used to adjust for changes in intravascular volume. Additional doses of regular insulin should be administered to control blood sugar levels; a 6-h interval between glucose measurements is commonly used. In addition to meticulous attention to blood sugar levels, it is important to monitor diabetic surgical patients for infections and impaired wound healing.[90] Cardiovascular complications are also common because diabetes is an important risk factor for atherosclerosis. Myocardial ischemia can be silent and may be detected unexpectedly on postoperative electrocardiograms.

Thyroid disease is not as prevalent as diabetes but, if undetected, can result in major complications perioperatively. The prevalence of hypothyroidism in hospitalized older patients has been reported to be 9.4% and the prevalence of hyperthyroidism 0.8%.[91] It is well known that older persons may have nonspecific or atypical manifestations of thyroid illness, so it is important to maintain a high index of suspicion for thyroid illness in this population. The consequences of operating upon a patient with unsuspected hypothyroidism can be significant. These patients metabolize medications more slowly, and their increased sensitivity to central nervous system depressants can result in respiratory insufficiency. In addition, cardiac reserve is diminished and the response to pressors may be blunted. While the potential for these complications should be suspected and preventive measures instituted, hypothyroidism should not be considered an absolute contraindication to necessary operative procedures.[92] Emergency surgery and trauma are indications for rapid replacement of thyroid hormone. When hypothyroidism is severe, an intravenous dose of 300 to 500 µg L-thyroxine will significantly improve basal metabolic rate within 6 h. Corticosteroids should also be given in the perioperative period because the acute rise in basal metabolic rate can exhaust adrenal reserves.

The increased perioperative risks associated with hyperthyroidism include hyperpyrexia, arrhythmias, and congestive heart failure. Older persons may be particularly prone to iodine-induced hyperthyroidism from non-ionic contrast radiography.[93] Elective operations should be delayed until treatment with thionamide medications render the patient euthyroid. When an emergency operation is necessary, the patient can be treated with 1000 mg propylthiouracil by mouth and a beta-blocker to control the increased catecholamine effects. Sodium iodide is often given to inhibit the release of thyroid hormone and transiently inhibit organification. Iodide can be given either by mouth or intravenously; administration should be delayed until at least 1 h after the propylthiouracil to allow time for the latter to block organification. Supplemental corticosteroids are also recommended for hyperthyroid patients undergoing emergency operations. These supplements are given to protect against the possibility of adrenal insufficiency related to the chronic hyper-metabolic state and because corticosteroids may lower serum thyroxine and thyroid-stimulating hormone levels.

Nutrition

Surgery and wound healing cause increased energy demands. Patients who are malnourished preoperatively are likely to quickly deplete their body's carbohydrate stores, which will lead to protein catabolism and a negative nitrogen balance. In some malnourished or high-risk patients, preoperative total parenteral nutrition has been shown to reduce morbidity and mortality rates.[94,95] Whenever possible, preoperative nutritional supplements should be delivered via the gastrointestinal system. Total parenteral nutrition should be reserved for those patients in whom the gastrointestinal tract cannot be used.

Especially for older patients, there is no consensus on the best method for assessing nutritional status.[95,96] In addition, it is not clearly established that improvements in commonly used nutritional indices are associated with reduced perioperative morbidity; hence, the optimal duration of nutritional support is unknown. Additional studies are needed in patients most likely to benefit from perioperative nutritional supplements: those who are severely malnourished before major surgery; and those who undergo operations resulting in prolonged periods of inadequate enteral intake. Until more is known, it is common to provide postoperative enteral tube feedings to patients with a functioning gastrointestinal tract who were malnourished preoperatively and who are unable to consume adequate calories orally. Total parenteral nutrition is indicated for malnourished patients who have a nonfunctioning gastrointestinal tract or for whom enteral feedings are contraindicated.[97] (See Chapter 68 for a more complete discussion of nutrition.)

Neuropsychiatric Disorders

Neuropsychiatric problems are common among older persons and can be associated with an increased risk of perioperative complications. The prevalence of dementia is about 5% among persons aged 65 years; it increases to about 25% in those 80 years of age and older. A study of older patients admitted for repair of hip fractures in Sweden reported a prevalence of dementia of 15%.[98] Depression also is prevalent among older persons and can be exacerbated by any acute illness or hospitalization. Anesthesia and surgery can have profound effects on mental functioning. The metabolic changes associated with surgery along with the previously discussed effects on all the vital organ system can compromise cerebral function and exacerbate or precipitate neuropsychiatric disorders. The physiologic and behavioral manifestations of neuropsychiatric disorders can significantly complicate perioperative care and often lead to prolonged hospital stays.

The most common psychiatric problem in the postoperative period is delirium. The major manifestation of this condition is an alteration in consciousness, and it is, by definition, a transient disorder.[99] One prospective study reported delirium in 44% of older patients undergoing repair of hip fractures.[100] The presence of depression, use of anticholinergic medications, and hypoxemia were associated with delirium. Neither the duration of the procedure nor the type of anesthetic used (halothane versus epidural) were predictors of an acute confusional state. In another study of older patients undergoing elective noncardiac surgery, 9% of patients developed delirium postoperatively. Risk factors included age 70 years and older; self-reported alcohol abuse; poor cognitive status; poor functional status; markedly abnormal preoperative serum sodium, potassium, or glucose level; noncardiac thoracic surgery; and aortic aneurysm surgery.[101]

The differential diagnosis of delirium is very broad. A careful clinical assessment of the patient should focus on the possibility of infection, metabolic derangements, central nervous system events, myocardial ischemia, sensory deprivation, or drug intoxication. Lidocaine, cimetidine, atropine, aminophylline preparations, antihypertensives, steroids, and digoxin are medications commonly associated with delirium, but all drugs should be considered as possible causes. The best management strategy is prevention; the incidence of delirium can be significantly reduced by meticulous attention to precipitating factors. A multicomponent intervention that addressed the six risk factors—cognitive impairment, sleep deprivation, immobility, visual impairment, hearing impairment, and dehydration—was successful in reducing the incidence of delirium from 15% to 9%.[102] When it cannot be prevented, it is important to recognize the syndrome early, then identify and treat the underlying cause. When medications are necessary to protect the patient and others from agitated behaviors, 0.5 mg haloperidol can be given parenterally and repeated every 30 min as necessary. The minimum dose sufficient to control symptoms is recommended, and doses exceeding 6 mg over a 24-h period are rarely indicated. Frequent assessment of patients suffering from delirium is mandatory to monitor both response to therapy and potential drug toxicity. It is important to ask patients about their hallucinations and illusions, to discuss and clarify these frightening experiences, and to reassure them if the underlying cause is reversible.

Alcoholism is another serious and common problem among older persons; it has been estimated that there are at least 1.5 million alcoholics in this country who are 65 years of age of older.[103] The geriatric consultant should carefully explore current ethanol use with all patients, and a screening tool such as the Michigan Alcoholism Screening Test may be useful in identifying alcohol abuse preoperatively.[104] When there is suspicion of alcoholism, the patient should be evaluated for symptoms or signs of physiologic dependence and organ damage.

Chronic alcohol use can cause important metabolic derangements, as well as cardiac, hepatic, hematologic, and neurologic dysfunction. Liver disease has a variable effect on drug metabolism. The rate of metabolism of many drugs is slowed, but microsomal enzyme induction may result in increased dose requirements of many anesthetic agents. The patients for whom a withdrawal syndrome seems likely should be treated with thiamine and short-acting benzodiazepines, and elective surgery should be delayed. The consultant is commonly called to assist in the management of delirium tremens or alcohol withdrawal seizures occurring postoperatively. Withdrawal seizures are effectively treated with benzodiazepines and often do not require long-term antiepileptics. Delirium tremens usually occurs 24 to 48 h after the last drink but can occur after 7 to 10 days of abstinence. The classic signs are fever, tachycardia, confusion, and visual hallucinations. Oxazepam or lorazepam are given in sufficient doses to sedate the patient. The other principles of treating patients with delirium also apply.

Summary

Operative therapy is an important option for many of the health conditions experienced by older persons. Although the risks of perioperative complications are increased in individuals with multiple chronic conditions and impaired functional status, with careful preoperative assessment and perioperative management, these risks can be minimized and successful outcomes can be achieved.

References

1. Lawrence L, Hall MJ. *1997 Summary: National Hospital Discharge Summary. Advance Data from Vital and Health Statistics, no. 308.* Hyattsville, MD: National Center for Health Statistics; 1999.
2. Thomas DR, Ritchie CS. Preoperative assessment of older adults. *J Am Geriatr Soc.* 1995;43:811–821.
3. Owings MF, Kozak LJ. Ambulatory and inpatient procedures in the United States, 1996. National Center for Health Statistics. *Vital Health Stat.* 1998;13(139):1–9.
4. Maxwell JG, Taylor BA, Rutledge R, Brinker CC, Maxwell BG, Covington DL. Cholecystectomy in patients aged 80 and older. *Am J Surg.* 1998;176(6):627–630.
5. Seymour DG, Pringle R. Post-operative complications in the elderly surgical patient. *Gerontology.* 1983;29:262–270.
6. New classification of physical status. *Anesthesiology.* 1963; 24:111.
7. Arvidsson S, Ouchterlony J, Sjostedt L, Svardsudd K. Predicting postoperative adverse events. Clinical efficiency of four general classification systems: the project perioperative risk. *Acta Anaesth Scand.* 1996;40(7):783–791.
8. Cook TM, Day CJE. Hospital mortality after urgent and emergency laparotomy in patients aged 65 years and over. *Br J Anaesth.* 1998;80(6):776–781.
9. Tiret L, Desmonts JM, Hatton F, Vourc'h G. Complications associated with anaesthesia—a prospective survey in France. *Can Anaesth Soc J.* 1986;33:336–344.
10. Swartz DE, Lachapelle K, Sampalis J, Mulder DS, Chiu R C-J, Wilson J. Perioperative mortality after pneumonectomy: analysis of risk factors and review of the literature. *Can J Surg.* 1997;40:437–444.
11. Wasielewski RC, Weed H, Prezioso C, Nicholson C, Puri RD. Patient comorbidity: relationship to outcomes of total knee arthroplasty. *Clin Orthop Relat Res.* 1998;356:85–92.
12. Charlson ME, Pompei P, Ales KL. MacKenzie CR. A new method of classifying prognostic comorbidity in longitudinal studies: development and validation. *J Chron Dis.* 1987;40:373–383.
13. Krousel-Wood MA, Abdah A, Re R. Comparing comorbid-illness indices assessing outcome variation: The case of prostatectomy. *J Gen Intern Med.* 1996;11:32–38.
14. Escarce JJ, Shea JA, Chen W, Qian Z, Schwartz JS. Outcomes of open cholecystectomy in the elderly: a longitudinal analysis of 21,000 cases in the prelaparoscopic era. *Surgery.* 1995;117:156–164.

15. Gibbs J, Cull W, Henderson WG, Daley J, Hur K, Khuri SF. Preoperative serum albumin level as a predictor of operative mortality and morbidity: Results from the National VA surgical risk study. *Arch Surg*. 1999;134:36–42.

16. Longo WE, Virgo KS, Johnson FE, et al. Outcome after proctectomy for rectal cancer in Department-of-Veterans-Affairs hospitals: a report from the national surgical quality improvement program. *Ann Surg*. 1998;228:64–70.

17. Browner WS, Li J, Mangano DT. In-hospital and long-term mortality in male veterans following noncardiac surgery. *JAMA*. 1992;268:228–232.

18. Goldman L, Caldera DL, Nussbaum SR, et al. Multifactorial index of cardiac risk in noncardiac surgical procedures. *N Engl J Med*. 1977;297:845–850.

19. Zeldin RA, Math B. Assessing cardiac risk in patients who undergo noncardiac surgical procedures. *Can J Surg*. 1984;27:402–404.

20. Jeffrey CC, Kunsman J, Cullen DJ, et al. A prospective validation of the cardiac risk index. *Anesthesiology*. 1983;58:462–464.

21. Gerson MC, Hurst JM, Hertzberg VS, et al. Cardiac prognosis in noncardiac geriatric surgery. *Ann Intern Med*. 1985;103:832–837.

22. Detsky AS, Abrams HB, McLaughlin JR, et al. Predicting cardiac complications in patients undergoing non-cardiac surgery. *J Gen Intern Med*. 1986;1:211–219.

23. Goldman L. Multifactorial index of cardiac risk in non-cardiac surgery: ten-year status report. *J Cardiothoracic Anesth*. 1987;1:237–244.

24. Lee TH, Marcantonio ER, Mangione CM, et al. Derivation and prospective validation of a simple index for prediction of cardiac risk of major noncardiac surgery. *Circulation*. 1999;11(10):1043–1049.

25. Eagle KA, Brundage BH, Chaitman BR, et al. Guidelines for perioperative cardiovascular evaluation for noncardiac surgery: a report of the American Heart Association/American College of Cardiology Taskforce on Assessment of Diagnostic and Therapeutic Cardiovascular Procedures. *J Am Coll Cardiol*. 1996;27:910–948.

26. American College of Physicians. Clinical Guideline, Part I: Guidelines for assessing and managing the perioperative risk from coronary artery disease associated with major noncardiac surgery. *Ann Intern Med*. 1997;127:309–312.

27. Fleisher LA, Eagle KA, Shaffer T, Anderson GF. Perioperative and long-term mortality rates after major vascular surgery: the relationship to preoperative testing in the Medicare population. *Anesth Analg*. 1999;89(4):849–855.

28. Sicari R, Ripoli A, Picano E, et al. Perioperative prognostic value of dipyridamole echocardiography in vascular surgery: a large-scale multicenter study of 509 patients. *Circulation*. 1999;100(19)(suppl):II-269–II-274.

29. Goldmann DR, Brown FH, Levy WK, Slap GB, Sussman EJ. *Medical Care of the Surgical Patient*. Philadelphia: Lippincott; 1982.

30. Litaker D. Preoperative screening. *Med Clin North Am*. 1999;83:1565–1581.

31. Brindley GV Jr. Common surgical problems. *Geriatr Clin North Am*. 1985;1:311–495.

32. Stone DJ. *Perioperative Care: Anesthesia, Medicine, Surgery*. St. Louis: Mosby-Year Book; 1998.

33. Caputo GM, Gross RJ. Medical consultation on surgical services: an annotated bibliography. *Ann Intern Med*. 1993;118:290–297.

34. Burt VL, Whalton P, Rocella EJ, et al. Prevalence of hypertension in the U.S. adult population: results from the third National Health and Nutrition Examination Survey, 1988–1991. *Hypertension*. 1995;25:305–313.

35. Prys-Roberts C, Meloche R, Foex P. Studies of anesthesia in relation to hypertension. I. Cardiovascular responses of treated and untreated patients. *Br J Anaesth*. 1971;43:122–137.

36. Prys-Roberts C, Greene LT, Meloche R, Foex P. Studies of anesthesia in relation to hypertension. II. Haemodynamic consequences of induction and endotracheal intubation. *Br J Anaesth*. 1971;43:531–546.

37. Goldman L, Caldera DL. Risks of general anesthesia and elective operation in the hypertensive patient. *Anesthesiology*. 1979;50:285–292.

38. National Heart, Lung, and Blood Institute. *The Sixth Report of the Joint National Committee on Prevention, Detection, Evaluation, and Treatment of High Blood Pressure*. NIH pub 98-4080. Bethesda, MD: U.S. Department of Health and Human Services, National Institutes of Health; 1997.

39. Adler AG, Leahy JJ, Cressman MD. Management of perioperative hypertension using sublingual nifedipine: experience in elderly patients undergoing eye surgery. *Arch Intern Med*. 1986;146:1927–1930.

40. Mangano DT. Perioperative cardiac morbidity. *Anesthesiology*. 1990;72:153–184.

41. Palda VA, Detsky AS. Perioperative assessment and management of risk from coronary artery disease. *Ann Intern Med*. 1997;127:313–328.

42. Mangano DT, Layug EL, Wallace A, Tateo I. Effect of atenolol on mortality and cardiovascular morbidity after noncardiac surgery. *N Engl J Med*. 1996;335:1713–1720.

43. Wallace A, Layug EL, Tateo I, et al. Prophylactic atenolol reduces postoperative myocardial ischemia. *Anesthesiology*. 1998;88:7–17.

44. Poldermans D, Boersma E, Bax JJ, et al. The effect of bisoprolol on perioperative mortality and myocardial infarction in high-risk patients undergoing vascular surgery. *N Engl J Med*. 1999;341:1789–1794.

45. Ropper AH, Wechsler LR, Wilson LS. Carotid bruit and the risk of stroke in elective surgery. *N Engl J Med*. 1982;307:1388–1390.

46. Limburg M, Wijdicks EFM, Li HZ. Ischemic stroke after surgical procedures: clinical features, neuroimaging, and risk factors. *Neurology*. 1998;50:895–901.

47. Cahalan MK, Litt L, Botvinick EH, Schiller NB. Advances in noninvasive cardiovascular imaging: implications for the anesthesiologist. *Anesthesiology*. 1987;66:356–372.

48. Goldman L, Caldera DL, Southwick FS, et al. Cardiac risk factors and complications in non-cardiac surgery. *Medicine*. 1978;47:357–370.

49. Etchells E, Glenns V, Shadowitz S, et al. A bedside clinical prediction rule for detecting moderate of severe aortic stenosis. *J Gen Intern Med*. 1998;13:699–704.

50. Goldman L. Cardiac risks and complications of noncardiac surgery. *Ann Intern Med.* 1983;98:504–513.

51. Dajani AS, Taubert KA, Wilson W, et al. Prevention of bacterial endocarditis: recommendations of the American Heart Association. *JAMA.* 1997;277:1794–1801.

52. Polanczyk CA, Goldman L, Marcantonio ER, Orav EJ, Lee TH. Supraventricular arrhythmia in patients having noncardiac surgery: clinical correlates and effect on length of stay. *Ann Intern Med.* 1998;129:279–285.

53. Balser JR, Martinez EA, Winters BD, et al. Beta-adrenergic blockade accelerates conversion of postoperative supraventricular tachyarrhythmias. *Anesthesiology.* 1998;89:1052–1059.

54. O'Kelly B, Browner WB, Massie B, et al. Ventricular arrhythmias in patients undergoing noncardiac surgery. *JAMA.* 1992;268:217–221.

55. Hubner GA, Radermacher P, Schutz GM. Perioperative risk of bradyarrhythmias in patients with asymptomatic chronic bifascicular or left bundle branch lock: does an additional first-degree atrioventricular block make any difference? *Anesthesiology.* 1998;88:679–687.

56. Lawrence VA, Hilsenbeck SG, Mulrow CD, Dhanda R, Sapp J, Page CP. Incidence and hospital stay for cardiac and pulmonary complications after abdominal surgery. *J Gen Intern Med.* 1995;10:671–678.

57. Mahler DA, Rosiello RA, Loke J. The aging lung. *Geriatr Clin North Am.* 1986;2:215–225.

58. Jackson CV. Preoperative pulmonary evaluation. *Arch Intern Med.* 1988;148:2120–2127.

59. Tisi GM. Preoperative evaluation of pulmonary function: validity, indications, and benefits. *Am Rev Respir Dis.* 1979; 119:293–310.

60. Williams-Russo P, Charlson ME, MacKenzie CR, Gold JP, Shires GT. Predicting postoperative pulmonary complications: is it a real problem? *Arch Intern Med.* 1992;152: 1209–1213.

61. Brooks-Brunn JA. Validation of a predictive model for postoperative pulmonary complications. *Heart Lung.* 1998; 27:151–158.

62. Gass GD, Olsen GN. Preoperative pulmonary function testing to predict postoperative morbidity and mortality. *Chest.* 1986;89:127–135.

63. Wernly JA, DeMEester TR, Kirchner PT, Myerowitz PD, Oxford DE, Golomb HM. Clinical value of quantitative ventilation-perfusion scans in the surgical management of bronchogenic carcinoma. *J Thorac Cardiovasc Surg.* 1980; 80:835–843.

64. Boysen PG, Block AJ, Olsen GN, et al. Prospective evaluation for pneumonectomy using the technitium lung scan. *Chest.* 1977;72:422–425.

65. Lawrence VA, Page CP, Harris GD. Preoperative spirometry before abdominal operations: a critical appraisal of its predictive value. *Arch Intern Med.* 1989;149:280–285.

66. Zibrak JD, O'Donnel CR, Marton K. Indications for pulmonary function testing. *Ann Intern Med.* 1990;112: 763–771.

67. Stein M, Cassara EL. Preoperative pulmonary evaluation and therapy for surgery patients. *JAMA.* 1970;211:787–790.

68. Jones RM. Smoking before surgery: the case for stopping. *Br Med J.* 1985;290:1763–1764.

69. Collins CD, Darke CS, Knowelden J. Chest complications after upper abdominal surgery: their anticipation and prevention. *Br Med J.* 1968;1:401–406.

70. Morran CG, Finlay IG, Mathieson M, McKay AJ, Wilson N, McArdle CS. Randomized controlled trial of physiotherapy for postoperative pulmonary complications. *Br J Anaesth.* 1983;55:1113–1117.

71. Olsen MF, Hahn I, Nordgren S, Lonroth H, Lundholm K. Randomized controlled trial of prophylactic chest physiotherapy in major abdominal surgery. *Br J Surg.* 1997;84: 1535–1538.

72. Mohr DN, Jett JR. Preoperative evaluation of pulmonary risk factors. *J Gen Intern Med.* 1988;2:277–287.

73. Smetana GW. Preoperative pulmonary evaluation. *N Engl J Med.* 1999;340:937–944.

74. National Institutes of Health Consensus Conference. Prevention of venous thrombosis and pulmonary embolism. *JAMA.* 1986;256:744–749.

75. Dalen JE, Paraskos JA, Ockene IS, Alpert JS, Hirsh V. Venous thromboembolism: scope of the problem. *Chest.* 1986;89(suppl):370S–373S.

76. Geerts WH, Heit JA, Clagett GP, et al. Prevention of venous thromboembolism. *Chest.* 2001;119(1):132S–175S.

77. Frocht A, Fillit H. Renal disease in the geriatric patient. *J Am Geriatr Soc.* 1984;32:28–39.

78. Cockroft DW, Gault MH. Prediction of creatinine clearance from serum creatinine. *Nephron.* 1976;16:31–41.

79. Gral T, Young M. Measured versus estimated creatinine clearance in the elderly as an index of renal function. *J Am Geriatr Soc.* 1980;28:492–496.

80. Goldberg TH, Finkelstein MS. Difficulties in estimating glomerular filtration rate in the elderly. *Arch Intern Med.* 1987;147:1430–1433.

81. Kellerman PS. Perioperative care of the renal patient. *Arch Intern Med.* 1994;154:1674–1688.

82. Beck LH. Postoperative acute renal failure. In: Goldmann DR, Brown FH, Levy WK, Slap GB, Sussman EJ, eds. *Medical Care of the Surgical Patient.* Philadelphia: Lippincott; 1982:201–217.

83. Phillips PA, Rolls BJ, Ledingham JGC, et al. Reduced thirst after water deprivation in healthy elderly men. *N Engl J Med.* 1984;311:753–759.

84. Epstein M, Hollenberg NK. Age as a determinant of renal sodium conservation in normal man. *J Lab Clin Med.* 1976;87:411–417.

85. Miller RD. Anesthesia for the elderly. In: Miller RD, ed. *Anesthesia.* New York: Churchill Livingstone; 1986:1801–1818.

86. Galloway JA, Shuman CR. Diabetes and surgery. A study of 667 cases. *Am J Med.* 1963;34:177–191.

87. Hirsch IB, McGill JB, Cryer PE, White PF. Perioperative management of surgical patients with diabetes mellitus. *Anesthesiology.* 1991;74:346–359.

88. Golden SH, Peart-Vigilance C, Kao WHL, Brancati FL. Perioperative glycemic control and the risk of infectious complications in a cohort of adults with diabetes. *Diabetes Care.* 1999;22:1408–1414.

89. Jacober SJ, Sowers JR. An update on perioperative management of diabetes. *Arch Intern Med.* 1999;159:2405–2411.

90. MacKenzie CR, Charlson ME. Assessment of perioperative risk in the patient with diabetes mellitus. *Surg Gynecol Obstet*. 1988;167:293–299.

91. Livingston EH, Hershman JM, Sawin CT, Yoshikawa TT. Prevalence of thyroid disease and abnormal thyroid tests in older hospitalized and ambulatory persons. *J Am Geriatr Soc*. 1987;35:109–114.

92. Ladenson PW, Levin AA, Ridgway EC, Daniels GH. Complications of surgery in hypothyroid patients. *Am J Med*. 1984;77:261–266.

93. Martin FIR, Tress BW, Colman PG, Deam DR. Iodine-induced hyperthyroidism due to nonionic contrast radiography in the elderly. *Am J Med*. 1993;95:78–82.

94. Bellatone R, Doglietto GB, Bossola M, et al. Preoperative parenteral nutrition in malnourished high-risk surgical patients. *Nutrition* 1990;6:168–170.

95. Detsky AS, Baker JP, O'Rourke K, Goel V. Perioperative parenteral nutrition: a meta-analysis. *Ann Intern Med*. 1987;107:195–203.

96. Baker JP, Detsky AS, Wesson DE, et al. Nutritional assessment. A comparison of clinical judgment and objective measurements. *N Engl J Med*. 1982;306:969–972.

97. Ellis LM, Copeland EM, Souba WW. Perioperative nutritional support. *Surg Clin North Am*. 1991;71:493–507.

98. Gustafson Y, Berggren D, Brannstrom B, et al. Acute confusional states in elderly patients treated for femoral neck fracture. *J Am Geriatr Soc*. 1988;36:525–530.

99. Tune L, Folstein F. Post-operative delirium. *Adv Psychosom Med*. 1986;15:51–68.

100. Berggren D, Gustafson Y, Eriksson B, et al. Postoperative confusion after anesthesia in elderly patients with femoral neck fractures. *Anesth Analg*. 1987;66:497–504.

101. Marcantonio ER, Goldman L, Mangione CM, et al. A clinical prediction rule for delirium after elective noncardiac surgery. *JAMA*. 1994;271:134–139.

102. Inouye SK, Bogardus ST, Charpentier PA, et al. A multicomponent intervention to prevent delirium in hospitalized older patients. *N Engl J Med*. 1999;340:669–676.

103. Solomon DH. Alcoholism and aging. *Ann Intern Med*. 1984;100:411–412.

104. Willenbring ML, Christensen KJ, Spring WD Jr, Rasmussen R. Alcoholism screening in the elderly. *J Am Geriatr Soc*. 1987;35:864–869.

21
Anesthesia for the Geriatric Patient

Jeffrey H. Silverstein

Anesthesia is a reversible state that permits procedures to be performed on the human body. Based principally on the early experience with ether, the anesthetic state was thought to be a single entity as described by the unitary theory of narcosis. In recent years, it has become clear that various physiologic phenomena that can be controlled independently combine to produce the anesthetic state. These phenomena are analgesia, hypnosis or amnesia, control of the physiologic responses to surgical stimuli, and maintenance of adequate operating conditions, primarily muscle relaxation.

In the first third of the twentieth century, surgery was considered a desperate measure for patients over 50 years of age, who were believed to be incapable of sustaining the rigors of even an inguinal hernia repair.[1] Advances in anesthesia have allowed surgeons to develop an extraordinary array of procedures with excellent outcomes in an increasingly aging population. The number of patients over age 65 who undergo noncardiac surgery are now projected to increase from 7 million to 14 million over the next three decades.[2] Geriatric patients are becoming an increasing part of the anesthesia workload.[3]

Because intraoperative mortality is now rare and intensive care can prolong short-term survival, the current standard for comparing rates of perioperative complications is 30 days from the time of surgery. Current estimates of 30-day perioperative mortality for properly prepared surgical patients over age 65 are 5% to 10%.[4–6] These figures are less than half the mortality recorded a few decades ago but are still higher than for younger patients. Denney and Denson reported on 272 nonagenarians undergoing 301 operations.[7] Their initial belief was that surgery was not justified in such old patients; however, they reported that in more than 70%, the benefit justified the risk they underwent. Only serious small bowel obstruction was associated with prohibitive perioperative mortality (63%). Studying 500 patients over age 80 who had undergone surgery in the Harvard

System, Djokovic and Hedley-Whyte found that the American Society of Anesthesiologists (ASA) physical status classification (see p. 213–214) predicted mortality.[5] This finding is consistent with an earlier large French study by Tiret et al., in which age is seen to be an important modifier of comorbid conditions[8] (Fig. 21.1).

Lawrence and colleagues studied 372 patients undergoing elective abdominal surgery in San Antonio, Texas.[9] Patients were evaluated preoperatively and postoperatively at 1, 3, and 6 weeks and at 3 and 6 months using a battery of instruments to capture multiple dimensions of functional health. Figure 21.2 shows the recovery status for activities of daily living (ADLs) across the follow-up assessments. Using ADL and instrumental activities of daily living (IADL) summary scores, patients were dichotomized as not recovered or recovered/improved at each assessment point. Mean change scores were significantly different from preoperative assessment at 1, 3, and 6 weeks. For IADLs (Fig. 21.3), mean scores were significantly below baseline at 1, 3, and 6 weeks and 3 months. At 3 months after surgery, 14% of patients had disability in ADLs; for IADLs, 20% had persistent disability at 6 months after surgery. Thus, although surgery is feasible for elderly patients, it remains an important and potentially debilitating experience.

General Anesthesia and Anesthetic Agents

Anesthesia generally consists of analgesia, control of the physiologic responses to surgical stimuli, hypnosis or amnesia, and maintenance of adequate operating conditions, primarily muscle relaxation. Analgesia, the absence of pain, is the cornerstone of the anesthetic state. Pain pathways have been described in great depth and can be altered by a variety of different methods.[10] Other integrated systems also respond to surgical stimuli. The most

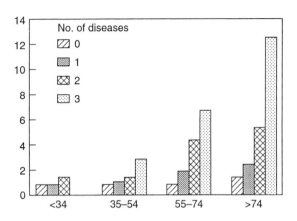

FIGURE 21.1. Major anesthesia complications per 1000 as a function of age and associated disease (Modified from Tiret et al. *Can Anaesth Soc J.* 1986;33:336,[8] with permission.

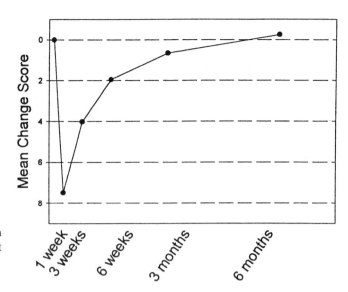

FIGURE 21.3. Patients aged 60 and greater ($n = 372$) on average return to baseline levels of independent activities of daily living by 3 months following elective abdominal surgery under general anesthesia. (From Ref. 9, with permission.)

important clinically is sympathetic nervous activity, which manifests principally as increased pulse and blood pressure. Blood pressure and pulse are the principal endpoints by which adequacy of anesthesia is gauged. Hypothalamic–pituitary–adrenal and acute-phase reactions also occur. Anesthesia does not completely block all these reactions, but they are reduced orders of magnitude from what would occur in the absence of anesthesia. Hypnosis or amnesia is a state in which conscious awareness is suppressed. Awareness under anesthesia is considered an adverse event. The amnesia produced by various hypnotic agents is not necessarily complete in that, even under deep general anesthesia, it is possible to demonstrate learning. Finally, it is important to maintain adequate operating conditions to facilitate surgery.

Aside from a lack of movement, muscle relaxation is frequently required to facilitate surgery, for example, on the abdominal cavity. In addition, the anesthesiologist is responsible for maintenance of the patient's homeostasis during and immediately following surgery.

The spectrum of activity of the drugs available to the anesthesiologist varies tremendously (Fig. 21.4). Agents are chosen to produce the desired effect and minimize side effects. In this chapter, I first describe the agents and techniques used to produce anesthesia. Selection of different anesthetic techniques for elderly surgical patients and their advantages and disadvantages follow.

Volatile Anesthetics

The commonly used volatile anesthetic agents are isoflurane, ethrane, halothane, sevoflurane, and desflurane. They are administered by inhalation as part of the gas mixture used to ventilate patients under general anesthesia. All agents are principally agonists of the $GABA_A$ chloride channel.[11] Volatile agents have a broad spectrum of action and are capable of producing a complete anesthetic state. Induction of anesthesia can be accomplished simply by breathing a mixture of a volatile agent in air or oxygen. Certain of the volatile agents (isoflurane, ethrane, and desflurane) are considered too pungent (produce gagging and coughing) to accomplish an inhalation induction; however, halothane and sevoflurane are commonly used for this purpose. This type of induction is reserved almost exclusively for young children who will not allow an intravenous catheter to be placed before anesthesia; it is essentially never done for an adult.

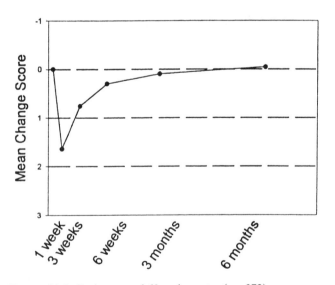

FIGURE 21.2. Patients aged 60 and greater ($n = 372$) on average return to baseline levels of activities of daily living by approximately 3 months following elective abdominal surgery under general anesthesia. (From Ref. 9, with permission.)

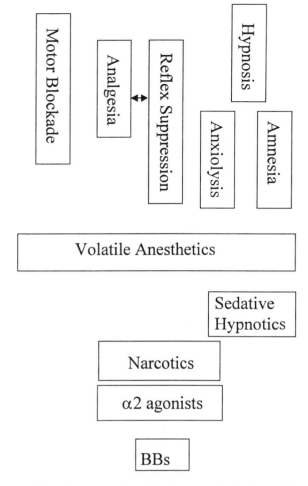

FIGURE 21.4. Spectrum of activity for anesthetic drugs. Physiologic aspects of the anesthetic state are displayed in the *vertical boxes*. The ability of various medications to provide all or parts of that state are displayed in *horizontal bars*. Volatile anesthetic agents can produce a complete anesthetic state, but their use alone is limited by side effects.

TABLE 21.1. Alteration in volatile anesthetic doses for the elderly.

Agent	Young adults	Elderly adults
Isoflurane	1.15	1.05[a]
Sevoflurane	2.6	1.4[b]
Desflurane	6	5.2[b]

[a] Age 64 years.
[b] Age 80 years.

principal advantage of a rapid induction of unconsciousness. The old adage to count backward from 99 is rarely employed because a patient almost never gets beyond 97. The principal agents are the barbiturates thiopental (Pentothal), thiamylal (Surital), and methohexital (Brevital), and an agent of a unique class called propofol (Diprivan). Ketamine, etomidate, and benzodiazepines may also be employed. Apart from ketamine, the sedative hypnotic agents do not provide analgesia. The barbiturates are antianalgesic; that is, on their own, they make pain worse.

Following the introduction of barbiturates, a lack of understanding of their pharmacokinetics led to their use for induction and maintenance of general anesthesia in the manner of diethyl ether and chloroform, with frequently disastrous results, including prolonged sleeping times and hypotension. Administration of thiopental to the causualties at Pearl Harbor resulted in large numbers of deaths and the statement that intravenous anesthesia was "an ideal method of euthanasia."[14] A subsequent understanding that the effects of small doses of barbiturates were terminated not by metabolism but rather by redistribution from their sites of actions to other body tissues set the groundwork for thiopental to become the standard drug for induction of anesthesia. This experience is an important example of the importance of an in-depth understanding of the pharmacology of anesthetic agents.

The most likely site of action for the barbiturates is the γ-aminobutyric acid (GABA) receptor complex. GABA is the principal inhibitory neurotransmitter found in mammalian central nervous systems. Barbiturates both enhance and mimic the action of GABA on the ion channels.[15] Studies on the effect of aging on the pharmacodynamics and pharmacokinetics of thiopental suggest that the principal effect is based on a reduction of volume of distribution in the elderly, resulting in a higher concentration of the drug at the effect site for any given dose. There is considerable interindividual variation in the dose of thiopental required to induce anesthesia. A healthy 80-year-old requires approximately 85% as much drug as a 20-year-old. It appears that the elderly brain is not more sensitive to the effects to thiopental. A more complete description of the pharmacology of barbiturates in the elderly is provided by Shafer.[16]

The pharmacologic equivalent of an ED$_{50}$ (median effective) dose for volatile anesthetics is defined as the minimum alveolar concentration (MAC),[12] the concentration of an agent at which 50% of subjects no longer produce purposeful movement in response to a skin incision. Anesthesia can be maintained with any of these agents at 1.25 to 1.3 times MAC. Relatively lower concentrations are usually employed in combination with other agents in a standard general anesthetic. Halothane has been associated with hepatitis and is rarely used in adult patients. Anesthetic requirements decrease progressively with advancing age, a phenomenon thought to be primarily a pharmacodynamic alteration[13] (Table 21.1).

Sedative Hypnotic Agents

Induction of anesthesia is most commonly undertaken with intravenous hypnotic agents, which have the

Propofol (diisopropylphenol) is the newest intravenous anesthetic, one that has become very popular for the induction and maintenance (by continuous infusion) of anesthesia and for sedation. The exact mechanism of action of propofol has not been completely elucidated. There is evidence that is acts through activation of the $GABA_A$ β_1-subunit, as well as by inhibition of the N-methyl-D-aspartate (NMDA) subtype of the glutamate receptor.

The induction dose varies from 1.0 to 2.5 mg/kg. Premedication with a benzodiazepine and or an opiate substantially reduces the induction dose of propofol. A dose of 1 mg/kg (with premedication) to 1.75 mg/kg (without premedication) appears to be appropriate for patients over age 60.[17] Side effects associated with the induction of anesthesia with propofol include a decrease in arterial blood pressure, pain on injection, myoclonus, apnea, and rarely thrombophlebitis of the vein where the propofol is injected. Apnea is very common, with an incidence similar to thiopental or methohexital; however, the apnea is likely to last longer.[18]

Propofol has been used for sedation during surgical procedures and in the ICU for sedation during mechanical ventilation. The level of sedation is readily titratable and recovery occurs rapidly on termination of the infusion, regardless of the duration of infusion.[19,20] Infusion rates must be markedly reduced in elderly and sicker patients.

Etomidate is an imidazole derivative that was introduced into practice in the United States in 1972. Its properties include minimal respiratory depression, cerebral protection, rapid recovery, and hemodynamic stability. Reports that the drug can temporarily inhibit steroid synthesis and hence decrease adrenal activity,[21,22] along with a side effect profile that includes myoclonus, pain on injection, and high incidence of nausea and vomiting, tremendously decreased the enthusiasm for this drug.[23] In recent years, the drug has regained some of its popularity, particularly for sick and elderly patients. Increasing age is associated with a smaller initial volume of distribution and decreased clearance of etomidate.[24]

Ketamine is the one phencyclidine currently available for clinical use. Although phencyclidine, the prototype of this class of drugs was a promising anesthetic agent, it was associated with an unacceptably high incidence of psychologic effects, including hallucinations and delirium. Phencyclidine is currently available only for illicit recreational use ("angel dust"). Ketamine (Ketalar) was released for clinical use in humans in 1970 and is still used for a variety of clinical circumstances. Ketamine is unique among the injectable hypnotic agents because it provides significant analgesia. In addition, it does not depress the cardiovascular system (i.e., does not produce hypotension) or the respiratory system.[25] Indeed, ketamine manifests both sympathomimetic and bronchodi-

lalting effects. Nonetheless, it does possess some potential to create the same adverse psychologic effects found with other phencyclidines. Poor-risk (ASA IV) patients with respiratory and cardiovascular disorders represent the majority of candidates for ketamine. The drug is used with some frequency for sedation of children outside the operating room and for dressing changes in settings such as burn units. When used in combination with a benzodiazepine, emergence delirium is considerable less frequent, and this combination has recently been advocated for routine use in the elderly (R. Roy, personal communication).

The principal benzodiazepines utilized for anesthetic care are midazolam, diazepam, and lorazepam. Midazoloam (Versed) is the only water-soluble benzodiaepine and thus causes considerably less irritation of the vein at the site of infusion and less thrombophlebitis. It has a faster onset of action. These properties have made midazolam the benzodiazepine of choice for most anesthetic use. Midazolam may be used for the induction of anesthesia. Awakening times following a benzodiazepine induction are much longer than for either thiopental or propofol, and thus benzodiazepines are rarely used for the induction of anesthesia. As an adjunct to general anesthesia, benzodiazepines provide better amnesia than thiopental. Elderly patients require lower doses of midazolam than younger patients.[26] This phenomenon was well illustrated in a series of 800 cases of sedation for upper gastrointestinal endoscopy in which the dose decreased from an average of 10 mg for a 20-year-old patient to 2.4 mg in 80-year-old patients[27] (Fig. 21.5).

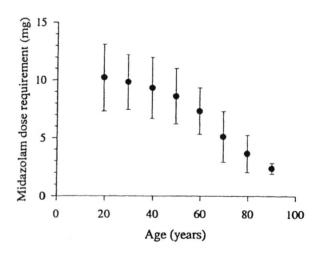

FIGURE 21.5. The influence of age on the intravenous dose of midazolam required to produce sedation in 800 patients undergoing endoscopic procedures. (Adapted from Bell GD, Spickett GP, Reeve PA, Morden A, Logan RF. Intravenous midazolam for upper gastrointestinal endoscopy: a study of 800 consecutive cases relating dose to age and sex of patient. *Br J Clin Pharmacol.* 1987;23:241–243.[27])

Anecdotal evidence suggests that some elderly patients manifest a paradoxic reaction to benzodiazepines, becoming agitated rather than sedated.

Flumazenil is the only available competitive antagonist for the benzodiazepine receptor. In the absence of a benzodiazepine, flumazenil has little discernable effect. When administered to patients who have benzodiazepine-induced CNS depression, flumazenil produces rapid and dependable reversal of unconsciousness, respiratory depression, sedation, amnesia, and psychomotor dysfunction.[28] There is little substantial information concerning alteration of flumazenil pharmacology for elderly patients. It should be emphasized that flumazenil is rarely used by experienced anesthesiologists, who greatly prefer to titrate the initial drug effect carefully rather than depend on functional antagonism. Repeated doses of flumazenil may be necessary because the effect of the initial benzodiazepine is likely to last longer than that of flumazenil and resedation may easily occur.

Opioids

The opioids are those endogenous and exogenous substances that bind to the opiate receptors. The principal use of opioids is to provide analgesia, and the primary downside is respiratory depression.

Pain perception is altered with aging, but this does not mean that pain is either less common or less important in the elderly. There is a dramatic decrease in myelinated and unmyelinated nerve fibers in older patients.[29,30] Elderly patients report pain primarily following activation of C fibers, whereas younger patients require A δ fiber activation before reporting pain.[31,32] These types of alterations in pain perception, with alterations in pharmacokinetics of analgesics, provide direction for both the anesthesiologist and physicians involved in postoperative pain management.

The most used opioid in modern anesthetic practice is fentanyl, a synthetic opioid with a short half-life. Using EEG, Scott and Stanski observed a 50% decrease in the concentration at which 50% inhibition occurs (IC_{50}) from age 20 to age 85.[33] However, unlike may drugs, the pharmacokinetics of fentanyl are not altered by age, except for a small change in rapid intercompartmental clearance. Thus, the dose of fentanyl is decreased for pharmacodynamic reasons.

Remifentanil was recently introduced to clinical practice under the new FDA guidelines that require pharmacodynamic and pharmacokinetic evaluation of special populations, including the elderly. Minto et al. reported on the age-adjusted pharmacology in two manuscripts that formed the basis for age-adjusted dosing in the remifentanil package insert.[34,35] In addition to a similar pharmacodynamic alteration, the volume of the central compartment decreases about 20% from age 20 to 80,

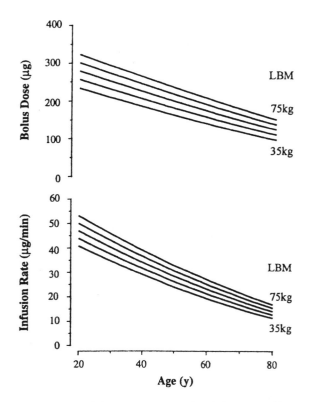

FIGURE 21.6. The influence of age and weight on remifentanil dose. The bolus dose should be reduced by 50% in elderly patients, and the infusion rate should be reduced by two-thirds. The dose adjustment for age is considerably larger than the dose adjustment for weight. (Adapted from Minto CF, Schnider TW, Shafer SL. The influence of age and gender on the pharmacokinetics and pharmacodynamics of remifentanil. II. Model application. *Anesthesiology.* 1997;86:24–33, with permission.[34])

and the clearance concurrently decreases about 30%. Figure 21.6 presents a series of nomograms that may be used to calculate remifentanil doses for elderly patients.

Muscle Relaxants

To facilitate endotracheal intubation and provide an optimal surgical field, an anesthesiologist must frequently control muscle tone, which may be accomplished with high concentrations of volatile anesthetic agents. The concentrations necessary to produce an adequate effect are frequently associated with hemodynamic instability. A regional anesthetic technique will provide muscle relaxation for operations amenable to this approach (see following). The third, and by far most common, approach is to utilize agents that disrupt neuromuscular transmission. The available agents are either depolarizing agents, such as succinylcholine, or competitive antagonists such as pancuronium, vecuronium, or atracurium. Depolarizing agents exert the same effect at the neuromuscular junction as acetylcholine, depolarizing the endplate and causing muscle contraction; this is seen clinically as fasciculation, an uncoordinated contraction of muscle. Because succinylcholine is not eliminated as rapidly as acetylcholine, depolarization of the endplate persists and the muscle remains flaccid for a relatively short period of time (about 2 min). This short-acting phenomenon is frequently used for facilitation of endotracheal intubation and for muscle relaxation during electroconvulsive therapy. Patients frequently complain of muscle soreness following succinylcholine, and it has been associated with rapid, sometimes fatal, increases in serum potassium levels, particularly in patients with recent trauma, extensive burns and possibly hemi or paraplegia.

The competitive antagonists combine with the acetylcholine receptor but do not activate them. Their presence on the receptor prevents access of the transmitter. At sufficient concentration, muscle relaxation occurs. Many different agents have become available in recent years. All manifest a minor increase in duration with age, but doses are not significantly altered. None of these agents should ever be used in the absence of both the equipment and expertise necessary to maintain adequate ventilation.

Regional Anesthesia

A different method of allowing a procedure to proceed without pain and its sequelae is to block the nerve fibers that subserve pain to the region of interest. Neural blockade is produced by local anesthetic agents. All currently available clinically useful agents are either aminoamides or aminoesters. When applied in sufficient concentration at a site of action, these drugs prevent conduction of electrical impulses by the nerve. When these drugs are administered systemically, the function of cardiac, skeletal, and smooth muscle, as well as peripheral and central nerves, is altered. Care must be taken to prevent toxicity that may occur either locally or systemically. The principal forms of acute toxicity affect the CNS (seizures) and cardiovascular system (arrhythmias and sudden death).

Local anesthetics are thought to act by blockade of neural sodium channels that block the conduction of signals along the nerve. The clinically observed rates of onset and recovery from local anesthetic blockade are governed by the relatively slow diffusion of local anesthetic molecules in and out of the nerve, rather than by their binding and dissociation from ion channels. For many years, the prevailing dogma was that minimal alterations in the pharmacokinetics or pharmacodynamics of local anesthetic occurred with aging.[36] In recent years, increasing knowledge has refined our understanding of the effects of age on local anesthetic agents; however, the effects are not as prominent as for many of the general anesthetic agents.[37]

Local anesthetic agents may be used for infiltration anesthesia where the agent is injected into the area required for a procedure; this is commonly done for small dermal surgeries but may be used for larger areas. Toxicity limits the total dose and therefore the area that may be anesthetized by this method. Intravenous regional anesthesia involves the intravenous infusion of local anesthetic into a tourniquet-occluded limb, almost always the arm; this procedure is called a Bier block. The anesthetic agent diffuses from the vascular space to the surrounding nerve endings. Peripheral nerve blockade techniques inject local anesthetic around specific nerves or nerve trunks that innervate particular areas of the body. Central neural blockade techniques encompass primarily epidural and spinal or subarachnoid anesthesia. Some local anesthetic preparations are available for topical administration. These techniques provide relatively short lived anesthesia for a very circumscribed area of limited depth. Finally, a relatively new technique, called tumescent anesthesia, applies a large volume of dilute local anesthetic into the subcutaneous tissue; this has been used by plastic surgeons for liposuction procedures.

Regional anesthesia is frequently advocated for the elderly patient because of the presumed advantage of reduced stress and less mental confusion in the perioperative period. Unfortunately, no large study has been able to confirm this perception.[38] A large international study examining neurocognitive function in patients randomized to regional versus general anesthesia is currently underway, and results should be available in 2003.

Neuraxial Anesthesia

Neuraxial anesthesia involves blockade of nerves within the spinal cord, which may be accomplished by injecting agents into the cerebrospinal fluid that surrounds the spinal nerves in the subarachnoid space. This technique is referred to as spinal or subarachnoid anesthesia. Epidural anesthesia involves the placement of drug in the epidural space, which is the area outside the dural sac but inside the vertebral canal (Fig. 21.7). Despite the apparent similarities, there are significant pharmacologic and physiologic differences between these two techniques. Spinal anesthesia utilizes a small volume of concentrated anesthetic that produces profound anesthesia and very low systemic levels of drug. Although continuous techniques exist, for the most part spinal anesthesia is a one-shot process. Epidural anesthesia requires a larger volume of anesthetic that produces pharmacologically significant blood levels of anesthetic. Epidural techniques are usually associated with the placement of an indwelling catheter, thus permitting long-term anesthesia and analgesia. A recent trend toward combined spinal epidural anesthesia tends to blur the difference.

Spinal anesthesia is the most easily mastered technique and is frequently selected for elderly patients. However,

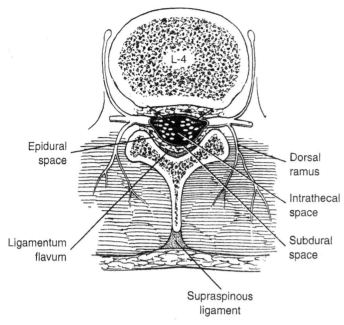

FIGURE 21.7. Cross-sectional anatomy of the lumbar spine. Needles for neuraxial anesthesia are usually inserted at the lumbar levels, seeking to place medication outside the dura mater, in the epidural space, or directly into the cerebrospinal fluid that is contained in the intrathecal space.

TABLE 21.2. Types of operations undertaken with nerve blocks.

Nerve or trunk	Area of operation
Cervical plexus	Carotid endarterectomy
Brachial plexus	Shoulder operations
Optic nerve	Eye surgery
Axillary nerve	Lower arm surgery
Femoral nerve[a]	Upper leg
Popiteal nerve	Below-knee surgery
Ankle block[b]	

[a] Sometimes combined with sciatic and obturator blocks for leg surgery.
[b] Ankle block invovles the deep and superficial peroneal, saphenous, sural, and posterior tibial nerves.

Nerve Blocks

Blockade of specific nerves or nerve trunks may be accomplished by injecting local anesthetic agents around the nerve. Examples of operations of the area subtended by specific nerves are listed in Table 21.2.

Sedation

"Sedation and analgesia describes a state that allows patients to tolerate unpleasant procedures while maintaining adequate cardiorespiratory function and the ability to respond purposefully to verbal command and tactile stimulation."[42] Sedation is a frequent accompaniment to regional anesthetic techniques or may be used to facilitate minor procedures that do not require full anesthesia, such as endoscopy. Sedation/analgesia is preferred to the more common term "conscious sedation," which is difficult to define. The American Society of Anesthesiologists supports a practice guideline development process based on evidence linkages from exhaustive literature reviews and expert opinion from 60 to 150 external consultants. The Task Force on Sedation and Analgesia published their work in 1996.[42]

Recommendations for sedation/analgesia include a patient evaluation and preprocedure preparation, including fasting. The patient should be monitored, and a record of the monitored parameters should be maintained. The patient's level of consciousness may be assessed using spoken responses. Patients whose only response is reflex withdrawal from painful stimuli may be approaching a state of general anesthesia. Sedation/analgesia is expertly performed by many medical practitioners; however, general anesthesia should be administered by trained anesthesia personnel. Respiratory activity can be monitored by observation of spontaneous respiration, auscultation of breath sounds, but other methods, such as detection of exhaled carbon dioxide, may be required if access to the patient is limited, such as in a CAT scan bay. Although there are insufficient data to support regular monitoring of blood pressure and heart rate or electro-

the high incidence of osteoarthritis in the spinal column frequently diminishes flexion and impairs positioning of the patient that is necessary to institute spinal anesthesia. Alterations of the technique are available to facilitate placement of the needle into the subarachnoid space.[39] Spinal anesthesia is frequently associated with profound decreases in cardiac output and blood pressure. Young patients may be relatively resistant to hypotension, but patients over 60 years of age frequently manifest 30 to 40 mmHg decrease in blood pressure with anesthetic levels up to the T5 dermatome.[40,41] Another important complication of spinal anesthesia is the development of a postspinal headache; this can be a severe and debilitating headache that requires that placement of an epidural blood patch, 10 to 20 ml of the patient's blood that must be acquired sterilely and injected into the epidural space near the site of the previous spinal puncture. Fortunately, spinal headache is principally a complication of younger patients and is relatively rare in the elderly.

Epidural techniques require similar modifications to cope with the anatomic alterations of age.[39] Dosage may be slightly decreased to compensate for increased permeability of the dura mater, and the onset of anesthesia may be somewhat more rapid.

In addition to local anesthetics, opioids are frequently administered into either the subarachnoid or epidural space as a means of pain control.

cardiogram (ECG), most experts suggest vital sign monitoring for patients undergoing sedation/analgesia. ECG is recommended only for patients with cardiovascular disease. Acknowledging that patients at the extremes of age or with severe cardiac, pulmonary, hepatic, or renal disease are at increased risk for developing complications related to sedation/analgesia, no specific recommendations were advanced by the expert panel to address sedation/analgesia in the elderly.

Choice of Anesthetic Technique

The choice of anesthetic techniques for any given patient is the province of the anesthesiologist. Notations in a medical chart indicating that a patient should undergo one or the other type of anesthesia are inappropriate and place the practitioner in the unfortunate position of conducting an argument in a medical record. An excellent review of the issues associated with choosing anesthetic techniques for elderly patients was recently compiled by Roy.[43] Although there are theoretical considerations and clinical perceptions that regional anesthetics should be safer for elderly patients than general anesthetics, most major studies fail to support this idea. A recent meta-analysis, not focused on elderly patients, concluded that, "Neuraxial blockade reduces postoperative mortality and other serious complications. The size of some of these benefits remains uncertain, and further research is required to determine whether these effects are due solely to benefits of neuraxial blockade or partly to avoidance of general anaesthesia."[44] There is a developing consensus that overall perioperative care, as opposed to the choice of anesthetic technique, is more likely to have a positive impact on the elderly surgical patient.[43]

Indications for Intraoperative Monitoring

Blood pressure, ECG, and oxygen saturation should be monitored in all elderly patients undergoing any procedure. Automated blood pressure cuffs are common and accurate. The measurement should be made at least every 5 min. Accurate reading may be difficult in patients with highly irregular cardiac rhythms. Application of the cuff should be done with care in frail individuals, who may require a thin layer of webril padding to protect the skin. The ECG should be configured to observe both p waves and the lateral wall of the left ventricle (i.e., II and V5, or MCV1). The pulse oximeter measures oxygen saturation of arterial blood using a probe that is typically placed on the finger. Frequently, signal quality is inadequate due to a decrease in pulsatile flow. The probe can be repositioned, or other forms of probes can be used on other anatomic sites, such as ear lobes. Anesthesia or sedative drugs should not be administered in the absence of a satisfactory pulse oximeter reading. For lengthy procedures, a urinary catheter is usually needed to monitor urine output. If the operative field involves the pelvis, draining the bladder often aids operative exposure.

Temperature should be measured and recorded during all major operations because significant hypothermia is a common sequela of a long procedure, particularly when the viscera are exposed. After a complicated operation, a core temperature of 32.2° to 35°C (90°–95°F) can occur. Many elderly patients begin with lower core temperatures. The importance of maintaining temperature is due to the metabolic cost of rewarming the body. Elderly patients do not maintain temperature as well as young patients, and the mechanisms used to increase body temperature, such as shivering, can require excessive portions of a patient's oxygen consumption. Severe hypothermia [<31.5°C (89°F)] is associated with cardiac dysrhythmias. Core temperature is commonly measured with either an esophageal or rectal temperature probe. During large operations, measures to maintain a reasonable body temperature are essential. Convection warming systems operate like a large hair dryer, inflating a blanket that directs warm air over the patient's body. Intravenous fluids can be warmed, the operating room can be maintained at a reasonable ambient temperature, the abdominal viscera can be maintained in the abdominal cavity as long as possible, and lavage fluids can be warmed. In spite of these attempts, patients may lose significant body heat. Elderly patients emerging from general anesthesia should not be extubated until body temperature is within 0.5°C of their baseline core body temperature. End-tidal carbon dioxide measurement is used to evaluate ventilation and should be used whenever intubation is required.

For larger or prolonged surgeries, invasive monitoring should be considered. Continuous peripheral arterial blood pressure measurement may be taken by placing an intra-arterial catheter in the radial artery and connecting it to a transducer. Other arterial sites include the axillary and femoral arteries. Both radial arteries should be palpated before selecting a cannulation site to be sure that they are equal. If blood flow to one limb is diminished, the arterial monitor should be placed elsewhere. The advantages of continuous monitoring include beat-to-beat blood pressure information and the ability to acquire multiple blood samples without further venipuncture.

Central venous pressures can be monitored with a catheter placed in an intrathoracic vein, such as the superior vena cava. With major limitations, these pressures reflect intravascular volume, which is very important when the cardiovascular system responds primarily to Starling forces, rather than altering heart rate and contractility (see Chapter 39). The normal pressure is 8 to 10 mmHg. Lower pressures generally indicate the need for blood or fluid replacement; elevated pressures may occur with right ventricular or biventricular heart failure. Pulmonary arterial hypertension secondary to pulmonary disease, high bronchial airway pressure, and right ventricular failure may elevate central venous pressure out of proportion to the left ventricular end-diastolic pressure and volume. Such an elevation suggests adequate blood volume when, in fact, blood volume is inadequate. If major blood loss or fluid shifts (e.g., major peritoneal dissections) occur, central venous pressure should be instituted from the outset of surgery. If a patient shows signs of hypovolemia, tachycardia (which may not occur), hypotension, or decreased urine output, isotonic fluid should be administered in bolus form (250–500 ml in ≤10 min, as tolerated). If signs fail to resolve with one or two bolus infusions, placement of a central venous catheter is indicated. In addition, a central catheter may be indicated for venous access if irritating medications need to be administered or if the patient has difficulty maintaining a peripheral intravenous line for multiple days.

The next level of monitoring is the use of balloon-tipped pulmonary artery catheter (PAC), which is passed through the right ventricle into the pulmonary artery. Occluding a small pulmonary artery with the flotation balloon allows measurement of the pulmonary capillary wedge pressure (PCWP). This measurement removes any right ventricular and most pulmonary artery contribution to the pressure measurement. Normal PCWP is 4 to 12 mmHg. PACs also allow measurement of cardiac output and mixed venous blood gas analysis, which can be useful in managing hemodynamics. Patients with severe cardiac dysfunction and patients in whom the CVP is high when other signs suggest hypovolemia should be considered for PAC monitoring. In left ventricular failure, wedge pressures may rise to 40 mmHg or more. These measurements are particularly valuable guides to intraoperative management of fluid replacement therapy and management of cardiac inotropic activity and peripheral vascular resistance when vasopressor support is used in patients with cardiac dysfunction. When available, this level of monitoring can be supplemented or replaced by the use of transesophageal echocardiography.

Intraoperative fluid replacement should be carefully considered, providing maintenance fluids and replacing lost blood and fluids. The elderly may have difficulty eliminating any excess fluid because of exaggerated or prolonged aldosterone and antidiuretic hormone (ADH) responses postoperatively.

Conclusion

Anesthesiology has followed the general specialty of geriatrics in developing a wealth of information that can be brought to bear on the care of elderly surgical patients. This chapter provides an overview of some of the issues

associated with anesthetic care of the elderly. Interested readers are referred to a number of recent publications that expand greatly on the knowledge presented here.[45–47]

References

1. Ochsner A. Is risk of operation too great in the elderly? *Geriatrics.* 1927;22:121.
2. Mangano DT. Preoperative risk assessment: many studies, few solutions. Is a cardiac risk assessment paradigm possible? *Anesthesiology.* 1995;83:897–901.
3. Klopfenstein CE, Herrmann FR, Michel JP, Clergue F, Forster A. The influence of an aging surgical population on the anesthesia workload: a ten-year survey. *Anesth Analg.* 1998;86:1165–1170.
4. Valentin N, Lomholt B, Jensen JS, Hejgaard N, Kreiner S. Spinal or general anaesthesia for surgery of the fractured hip? A prospective study of mortality in 578 patients. *Br J Anaesth.* 1986;58(3):284–291.
5. Djokovic JL, Hedley-Whyte J. Prediction of outcome of surgery and anesthesia in patients over 80. *JAMA.* 1979;242(21):2301–2306.
6. Davis FM, Woolner DF, Frampton C, et al. Prospective multicentre trial of mortality following general or spinal anaesthesia for hip fracture surgery in the elderly. *Br J Anaesth.* 1987;59(9):1080–1088.
7. Denney JL, Denson JS. Risk of surgery in patients over 90. *Geriatrics.* 1972;27(1):115–118.
8. Tiret L, Desmonts JM, Hatton F, Vourch G. Complications associated with anaesthesia—a prospective survey in France. *Can Anaesth Soc J.* 1986;33:336–344.
9. Lawrence VA. Postoperative functional outcomes in Elders. National Institute of Aging RO1 AG14304. 1999 (personal communication).
10. Yaksh TL. An introductory perspective on the study of nociception and its modulation. In: Yaksh TL, Lynch C III, Zapol WA, Maze M, Biebuyck JF, Saidman LJ, eds. *Anesthesia: Biologic Foundations.* Philadelphia: Lippincott-Raven; 1998:471–482.
11. Krasowski MD, Harrison NL. General anaesthetic actions on ligand-gated ion channels. *Cell Mol Life Sci.* 1999; 55(10):1278–1303.
12. Eger E III, Saidman LJ, Brandstater B. Minimum alveolar anesthetic concentration: a standard of anesthetic potency. *Anesthesiology.* 1965;26:756–763.
13. Gold MI, Abello D, Herrington C. Minimum alveolar concentration of desflurane in patients older than 65 yr. *Anesthesiology.* 1993;79:710–714.
14. Halfond FJ. A critique of intravenous anesthesia in war surgery. *Anesthesiology.* 1943;4:67.
15. Carlson BX, Hales TG, Olsen RW. GABAÂ receptors and anesthesia. In: Yaksh TL, Lynch C III, Zapol WA, Maze M, Biebuyck JF, Saidman LJ, eds. *Anesthesia: Biologic Foundations.* Philadelphia: Lippincott-Raven; 1998:259–275.
16. Shafer SL. Pharmacokinetics and pharmacodynamics of the elderly. In: McLeskey CH, ed. *Geriatric Anesthesiology.* Baltimore: Williams & Wilkins; 1997:123–142.
17. Steib A, Freys G, Beller JP, Curzola U, Otteni JC. Propofol in elderly high risk patients. A comparison of haemody-

namic effects with thiopentone during induction of anaesthesia. *Anaesthesia.* 1988;43(suppl):111–114.

18. Turtle MJ, Cullen P, Prys-Roberts C, Coates D, Monk CR, Faroqui MH. Dose requirements of propofol by infusion during nitrous oxide anaesthesia in man. II: Patients premedicated with lorazepam. *Br J Anaesth.* 1987;59(3):283–287.

19. Wilson E, MacKenzie N, Grant IS. A comparison of propofol and midazolam by infusion to provide sedation in patients who receive spinal anaesthesia. *Anaesthesia.* 1988; 43(suppl):91–94.

20. Grounds RM, Lalor JM, Lumley J, Royston D, Morgan M. Propofol infusion for sedation in the intensive care unit: preliminary report. *Br Med J (Clin Res Ed).* 1987; 294(6569):397–400.

21. Wagner RL, White PF. Etomidate inhibits adrenocortical function in surgical patients. *Anesthesiology.* 1984;61(6): 647–651.

22. Wagner RL, White PF, Kan PB, Rosenthal MH, Feldman D. Inhibition of adrenal steroidogenesis by the anesthetic etomidate. *N Engl J Med.* 1984;310(22):1415–1421.

23. Owen H, Spence AA. Etomidate. *Br J Anaesth.* 1984;56(6): 555–557.

24. Arden JR, Holley FO, Stanski DR. Increased sensitivity to etomidate in the elderly: intial distribution versus altered brain response. *Anesthesiology.* 1986;65:19–27.

25. White PF, Way WL, Trevor AJ. Ketamine—its pharmacology and therapeutic uses. *Anesthesiology.* 1982;56(2):119–136.

26. Jacobs JR, Reves JG, Marty J, White WD, Bai SA, Smith LR. Aging increases pharmacodynamic sensitivity to the hypnotic effects of midazolam. *Anesth Analg.* 1995;80(1): 143–148.

27. Bell GD, Spickett GP, Reeve PA, Morden A, Logan RF. Intravenous midazolam for upper gastrointestinal endoscopy: a study of 800 consecutive cases relating dose to age and sex of patient. *Br J Clin Pharmacol.* 1987;23(2): 241–243.

28. Amrein R, Hetzel W, Hartmann D, Lorscheid T. Clinical pharmacology of flumazenil. *Eur J Anaesthesiol Suppl.* 1988; 2:65–80.

29. Ochoa J, Mair WG. The normal sural nerve in man. II. Changes in the axons and Schwann cells due to ageing. *Acta Neuropathol* (Berl). 1969;13(3):217–239.

30. Ochoa J, Mair WG. The normal sural nerve in man. I. Ultra-structure and numbers of fibres and cells. *Acta Neuropathol* (Berl). 1969;13(3):197–216.

31. Harkins SW, Davis MD, Bush FM, Kasberger J. Suppression of first pain and slow temporal summation of second pain in relation to age. *J Gerontol A Biol Sci Med Sci.* 1996;51(5): M260–M265.

32. Chakour MC, Gibson SJ, Bradbeer M, Helme RD. The effect of age on A delta- and C-fibre thermal pain perception. *Pain.* 1996;64(1):143–152.

33. Scott JC, Stanski DR. Decreased fentanyl and alfentanil dose requirements with age. A simultaneous pharmacokinetic and pharmacodynamic evaluation. *J Pharmacol Exp Ther.* 1987;240:159–166.

34. Minto CF, Schnider TW, Shafter SL. Pharmacokinetics and pharmacodynamics of remifentanil. II. Model application. *Anesthesiology.* 1997;86(1):24–33.

35. Minto CF, Schnider TW, Egan TD, et al. Influence of age and gender on the pharmacokinetics and pharmacodynamics of remifentanil. I. Model development. *Anesthesiology.* 1997;86(1):10–23.

36. Nation RL, Triggs EJ, Selig M. Lignocaine kinetics in cardiac patients and aged subjects. *Br J Clin Pharmacol.* 1977;4(4):439–448.

37. Bowdle TA, Freund PR. Effects of age on local anesthetic agents. In: McLeskey CH, ed. *Geriatric Anesthesiology.* Baltimore: Williams & Wilkins; 1997:367–380.

38. Nielson WR, Gelb AW, Casey JE, Penny FJ, Merchant RN, Manninen PH. Long-term cognitive and social sequelae of general versus regional anesthesia during arthroplasty in the elderly. *Anesthesiology.* 1990;73(6): 1103–1109.

39. Mulroy ME. Modifications of regional anesthetic techniques. In: McLeskey CH, ed. *Geriatric Anesthesiology.* Baltimore: Williams & Wilkins; 1997:381–388.

40. Economacos G, Skountzos V. Clinical aspects of high spinal anesthesia in urological surgery on 3012 patients. *Acta Anaesthesiol Belg.* 1980;31(suppl):183–186.

41. Graves CL, Klein RL. Central venous pressure monitoring during routine spinal anesthesia. *Arch Surg.* 1968;97(5):843–847.

42. Practice guidelines for sedation and analgesia by non-anesthesiologists. A report by the American Society of Anesthesiologists Task Force on Sedation and Analgesia by Non-Anesthesiologists. *Anesthesiology.* 1996;84(2):459–471.

43. Roy RC. Choosing general versus regional anesthesia for the elderly. *Anesth Clin North Am.* 2000;18(1):91–104.

44. Rodgers A, Walker N, Schug S, et al. Reduction of postoperative mortality and morbidity with epidural or spinal anaesthesia: results from overview of randomised trials. *Br Med J.* 2000;321(7275):1493.

45. Silverstein JH (ed). Geriatric anesthesia. *Anesth Clin North Am.* 2000;18(1).

46. McLeskey CH. *Geriatric Anesthesiology.* Baltimore: Williams & Wilkins; 1997.

47. Muravchick S. *Geroanesthesia. Principles for Management of the Elderly Patient.* St. Louis: Mosby; 1997.

22
Surgical Approaches to the Geriatric Patient

Ronnie Ann Rosenthal

Operative Outcomes

Surgery, as a therapeutic alternative, has an essential role in the medical care of the geriatric patient. Certain types of cancer, coronary artery disease, and arthritis, common diseases that accompany aging, can be effectively treated and often cured by operation. Yet concern about the risk of surgery in patients with diminished reserves and multiple comorbid illnesses, although sometimes warranted, may prevent the appropriate referral of older patients for this care. With careful attention to detail and an understanding of how elderly patients differ from younger patients, many of these hazards can be at least partially avoided (see Chapter 13 and 20).

Changing Patterns of Surgical Care

It should be emphasized that reluctance to offer surgical treatment at a point in time when elective operation can be conducted with minimal risk leaves the patient vulnerable to progression of the disease. As a consequence, emergency surgery may become necessary at some point in the future when reserves are further compromised. Operative mortality and morbidity increase at least threefold when surgery is performed under emergent rather than elective conditions, almost regardless of the type of procedure. In a series of 42 operative procedures in 31 men and women over age 100 years, all the perioperative deaths occurred in patients requiring emergency operation.[1] However, the percent of operations done on an emergent basis in patients over age 85 is twice that of patients under age 65.

As the size and general health of the population over age 65 has increased, attitudes toward surgery in older patients have become more liberal. Discharge data from acute care hospitals in the United States[2] show that the portion of all operations performed in which the patient is over age 65 has increased from 19% in 1980 to 36% in 1998. When obstetric procedures are excluded, the percentage increases to 43%. The distribution of common operations performed on the elderly in 1998 is shown in Table 22.1: 38% of cholecystecomies, 56% of coronary artery bypass grafts, 60% of bowel resections, and 67% of total joint replacements. It is now estimated that at least 50% of patients in most general surgical practices are over age 65.

The pattern of surgical management of malignant disease in the elderly is an example of the changing views on surgery in this age group. Using data from the National Cancer Institute's Surveillance, Epidemiology, and End Results (SEER) Program, Farrow et al.[3] compared operative percentages for various cancers by age in three time periods: 1973–1978, 1979–1985, and 1986–1991. With increasing age, there was a persistent decline in the percentage of patients receiving surgical treatment for cancer. However, the gap between younger and older patients narrowed over the three time periods for certain cancers. The likelihood of receiving surgery when indicated for cancers of the breast, ovary, uterus, colon, and rectum increased more rapidly among patients over age 75 than in those younger than 55 (Fig. 22.1). For cancers that required extensive surgery and for those from which survival is poor even with surgery, there was less of a change, even for early-stage disease (Fig. 22.2). At present, it is still unclear whether this is the result of appropriate decision making based on the overall health of the patient and the patient's preference for treatment or a consequence of unfounded age bias.

The increased willingness to consider surgery in the elderly patient is also a reflection of the improvements in surgical and anesthetic techniques that presently allow us to operate safely on even the oldest patient. With the question of "can we operate?" less of an issue, the question "should we operate?" becomes the principal concern. To answer this question, we must understand the goals and expectations of treatment in the context of the individual patient.

TABLE 22.1. Common operations performed on elderly patients.

Operation	Total patients (×1000)	Patients of age >65	Percent (%)
Coronary bypass	553	304	55
Total joint replacement	426	286	67
Open reduction and Internal fixation	416	184	44
Cholecystectomy	438	165	38
Large bowel resection	242	146	60
Lysis of adhesions	310	87	27
Appendectomy	278	16	5

Source: From CDC Advanced Data No. 316,[2] with permission.

Mortality and Morbidity

For surgeons, the traditional measures of outcome have always been postoperative mortality and morbidity, with mortality used as the endpoint in the determination of "operative risk." For the elderly patient, however, restoration of functional capacity to at least the preoperative level and quality of life may be far more important considerations than survival alone. It is shown that when the perioperative course in an elderly patient is uncomplicated, results are nearly indistinguishable from those of younger patients. However, when a complication occurs, the elderly are far less able to muster the reserves to overcome the complication without significant overall decline. Strategies to improve surgical care for the elderly, therefore, should be designed to identify and address concomitant diseases that predispose to complications, thereby minimizing the influence of these factors on all outcome measures. Chapter 20 details the essential considerations in the preoperative assessment and perioperative care of the aged patient. With careful attention to the details described therein, surgical care can

be provided with excellent results in a cost-effective manner.

In the recent debates over containing rising health care costs, this latter consideration has gained attention. The efficacy and cost-efficiency of major surgery as a treatment modality for the elderly is demonstrated in a recent study of coronary artery bypass surgery versus medical management in octogenarians. Outcome was assessed in terms of cost and quality life-year survival.[4] The cost of surgical care per quality life-year saved was only $10,424, less than the cost for many common procedures such as screening mammography. The survival in the surgery group was 80% and 69% at 3 and 4 years, respectively, whereas in the medical group, comparable survival was 64% and 32%. Using a validated health status assessment tool, the EurQol Questionnaire,[5] the authors assessed the quality of life in five domains: pain, activity, mobility, self-care, and depression/anxiety. In all areas, quality of life was better in the surgically treated than in the medically treated groups. Quality of life in the group of 80-year-old patients who selected Coronary Artery Bypass Grafting (CABG) was found to be equal to that of an average 55-year-old in the general population.

Unfortunately, data on functional outcomes for surgical procedures that are not specifically designed to improve functional outcome, as are coronary revascularization and joint replacement, are not yet abundant. Where available, these data are included with the more traditional data on operative outcomes of mortality and morbidity.

Reviews of several series of operative procedures in elderly patients have reported a decline in overall operative mortality over the past several decades, from 10% to 25% in the 1960s to less than 5% in 1990s.[6] The reason for this is unclear. Series of this kind are primarily retrospective with a wide variety of procedures from a wide

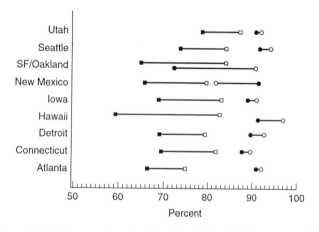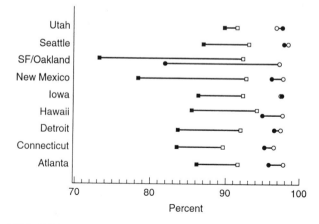

FIGURE 22.1. Temporal and regional variations in the percent of patients treated surgically for rectal cancer (*left*) and breast cancer (*right*). *Solid symbols*, 1973–1978; *open symbols*, 1986–1991; *squares*, patients over 75 years of age; *circles*, patients under 55 years of age. (From Farrow et al.,[3] with permission.)

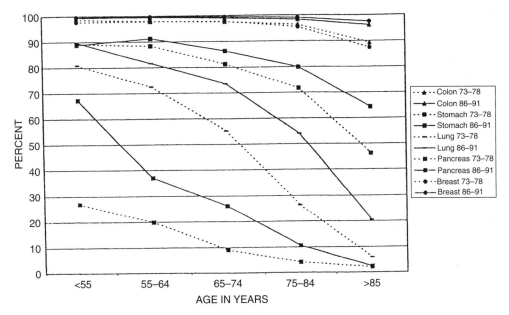

FIGURE 22.2. Temporal variation in the percent of patient treated surgically for local stage cancer, with age. *Broken lines*, 1973–1978; *solid lines*, 1986–1991. (From Farrow et al.,[3] with permission.)

variety of institutions and without standardized methodology to allow comparison among of the patient groups for comorbidity and severity of illness.

Prospective data on declining postoperative morbidity and mortality over the past decade, adjusted for the risk imposed by comorbidity and other pre- and intraoperative factors, can be found in the National VA Surgical Quality Improvement program (NSQIP).[7] Since 1991, this program has been prospectively collecting data on patient risk and surgical outcome from 44 Veterans Affairs Medical Centers across the country. The study was designed to provide risk-adjusted mortality and morbidity figures for the comparison of surgical care across institutions in the VA Hospital system. At present, there are more than 1 million cases enrolled in the database. Although this study was not designed to look at older patients specifically, nearly half the patients are over age 65 because of the nature of the VA population. Interrogations into the data to obtain age-specific data are presently underway.

From 1991 to 1999, overall postoperative mortality in the NSQIP population has fallen from 3.1% to 2.4%, and overall morbidity has decreased from 17.6% to 9.6%, while the mean age of the patients has increased slightly from 60.1 to 60.6 years.[8] Complication rates in this study appear to increase as a function of age, from 7.1% in patients less than 65 years of age to 17.6% for those over age 85. Risk-adjusted complications rates as a function of age are not yet available; however, it is likely that this increase in morbidity is in great part related to patient comorbidity rather than chronologic age alone.

Better data on the effect of age specifically on mortality can be found by looking at the results of a single type of operation. In one such study[9] examining the results of open cholecystectomy in the prelaparoscopic era in 21,000 elderly patients, mortality clearly increased with increasing age, from 0.7% in patients aged 65 to 69 years to 7.5% in those over age 85 (Table 22.2). However, increasing comorbidity with age, rather than chronologic age alone, was shown to be responsible for this effect. Similar results can be found in studies of other procedures.

Pathophysiologic Considerations

Aging influences surgical outcome in two major ways: first, because of the increased incidence of comorbid disease, and second, because of changes in the presenta-

TABLE 22.2. Effect of age and comorbidity on mortality from open cholecystectomy.

	Mortality (%)
Age (years)	
65–69	0.7
70–74	1.4
75–79	2.2
80–84	4.4
>85	7.5
Comorbid index	
0	1.5
1	2.3
2	3.7
>3	6.1

Source: From Escarce et al.,[9] with permission.

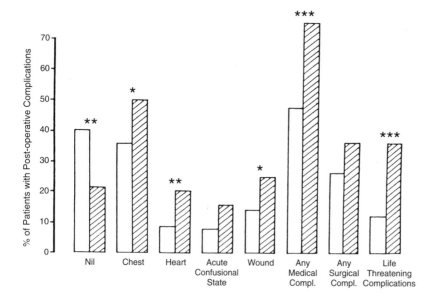

FIGURE 22.3. Incidence of postoperative complications in active and inactive patients. Inactivity was defined in this study as the inability to leave the home by one's own effort at least twice at week. Cross-hatched rectangle = inactive patients, * p < 0.05; ** p < 0.01, *** p < 0.001. (From Seymour and Pringle,[14] with permission.)

tion and natural history of the primary surgical disease. Although the latter is far less well characterized, each plays an extremely important role.

Effect of Aging on the Surgical Patient

A thorough review of the importance of comorbid conditions on surgical outcome can be found in Chapter 20. Here, however, we address four general factors that are of particular importance because they are either sensitive predictors of outcome (functional capacity and nutritional status) or are subtle and difficult to quantitate (cognitive status and wound-healing capacity).

Functional Status

For decades, the American Society of Anesthesiologists (ASA) Physical Status Classification has been one of the most reliable and accurate predictors of surgical mortality. This simple classification ranks patients according to the functional limitations imposed by coexisting disease (see Chapter 20). Curves for mortality versus ASA class in older patients are nearly superimposable on those of younger patients[10]; even in patients over age 80, ASA classification has been shown to accurately predict postoperative mortality.[11] Data from the NSQIP study indicate that ASA classification ranks as either the first or second most predictive factor for mortality and among the top three for morbidity for all types of surgical procedures combined.[12]

Other standard measures of functional status have also proven to be predictive of postoperative outcome. The ability to perform the activities of daily living (ADL) has been correlated with postoperative mortality and morbidity.[13] In one study, patients identified as inactive were

shown to have a higher incidence of all major surgical complications (Fig. 22.3).[14] Inactivity was defined as the inability to leave the home by one's own efforts at least twice a week. In another study of noncardiac surgical cases, mortality in patients with severely limited activity was 9.7 times higher than in active patients.[15] In this study, limited activity was defined as confined to bed or, at maximum, able to transfer from bed to chair. Of the risk factors studied, inactivity was found to be the strongest single predictor of death.

Preoperative functional deficits contribute to postoperative immobility, with associated complications such as atelectasis and pneumonia, venous stasis and pulmonary embolism, pressure ulcers, and multisystem deconditioning. Deconditioning is an important clinical entity characterized by depression and lethargy; anorexia and dehydration; neuromuscular instability, decreased bone density, muscular weakness, and incoordination; altered bladder and bowel function with retention and constipation; and urinary and fecal incontinence. Deconditioning leads to further functional decline despite improvement in the acute illness.[16] The recovery period from deconditioning after surgery can be three or more times longer than the period of immobilization that led to the decline (see Chapter 13).

Even for patients with less obvious limitations, functional capacity as demonstrated by exercise tolerance is the single most important predictor of cardiac and pulmonary complications following noncardiac surgery. In a study comparing ASA criteria, several other objective clinical risk measures, and exercise tolerance, Gerson et al. demonstrated that the inability to raise the heart rate to 99 beats/min while doing 2 min of supine bicycle exercise was the most sensitive predictor of both postoperative cardiac and pulmonary complications and death.[17,18]

TABLE 22.3. Estimated energy requirements for various activities.

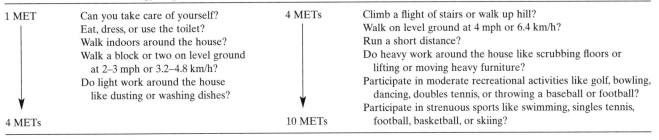

1 MET	Can you take care of yourself?	4 METs	Climb a flight of stairs or walk up hill?
	Eat, dress, or use the toilet?		Walk on level ground at 4 mph or 6.4 km/h?
	Walk indoors around the house?		Run a short distance?
	Walk a block or two on level ground at 2–3 mph or 3.2–4.8 km/h?		Do heavy work around the house like scrubbing floors or lifting or moving heavy furniture?
	Do light work around the house like dusting or washing dishes?		Participate in moderate recreational activities like golf, bowling, dancing, doubles tennis, or throwing a baseball or football?
4 METs		10 METs	Participate in strenuous sports like swimming, singles tennis, football, basketball, or skiing?

MET, metabolic equivalent (see text).
Source: Reprinted with permission from Eagle KA, et al. Guidelines for perioperative cardiovascular evaluation for noncardiac surgery. *Circulation* 1996;93:1279,[20] with permission.

A recent study in which oxygen consumption was quantitated during exercise demonstrated that subjects unable to increase oxygen delivery by threefold over basal levels during exercise were unable to meet the metabolic demands of surgical stress and therefore had much higher rates of postoperative cardiac ischemia and death.[19] Energy requirements for many types of activities have already been determined in terms of metabolic equivalents (METs), with one MET being equal to the basal oxygen consumption of a 40-year-old, 70-kg man at rest.[20] Using a simple questionnaire about activity level,[21] a quantitative estimate of the ability to meet the metabolic demands of surgery can be determined (Table 22.3).

Nutritional Status

Nutrition is an extremely important factor in surgical care, so much so that surgical nutrition is a topic in the curricula of all surgical residency training programs. In fact, the scientific basis and clinical development of total parenteral nutrition (TPN) was largely the work of one famous surgeon, Dr. Stanley Dudrick. Yet, the presence and importance of preoperative malnutrition in the elderly surgical patient is often not appreciated. Surgeons rarely perform more of a nutritional assessment than querying weight loss.

Physiologic dysfunctions, comorbid conditions, and a variety of psychosocial issues common to the elderly place this population at high risk for nutritional deficits. Malnutrition occurs in approximately 0% to 15% of community-dwelling elderly persons, 35% to 65% of older patients in acute care hospitals, and 25% to 60% of institutionalized elderly.[22] Factors that may lead to inadequate intake and utilization of nutrients include the ability to get food (e.g., financial constraints, availability of food, limited mobility), the desire to eat food (e.g., living situation, mental status, chronic illness), the ability to eat and absorb food (e.g., poor dentition, chronic gastrointestinal problems such as gastroesophageal reflux disease or diarrhea), and medications that interfere with appetite or nutrient metabolism (Table 22.4).[23]

Although complete assessment and specific markers are necessary to identify deficits and direct correction, simple measurement of the body mass index [BMI = weight in kilograms/(height in meters)^2] is a useful guide. It is generally accepted that a BMI between 24 and 29 is appropriate for persons over age 65. The Subjective Global Assessment (SGA) is one relatively simple, reproducible tool for assessing nutritional status from the history and physical exam.[24] SGA ratings are most strongly influenced by loss of subcutaneous tissue, muscle wasting, and weight loss. In a study of patients undergoing elective gastrointestinal surgery, both SGA and serum albumin were predictive of postoperative nutrition-related complications.[25]

In the face of stress from either illness, injury, infection, or even elective surgery, in nutritionally compromised elderly patient quickly develops protein-energy malnutrition. This metabolic response to the release of cytokines and hormones is characterized by increased requirements for energy and protein. The increased catabolism, however, is not matched by increased intake because of anorexia or other limitations to ingestion imposed by the disease process. When exogenous energy is not provided, endogenous protein stores are mobilized

TABLE 22.4. Historical findings associated with an increased risk of nutritional deficiency.

Recent weight loss
Restricted dietary intake
    Limited variety, food avoidances
Psychosocial situation
    Depression, cognitive impairment, isolation, economic difficulties
Problems with eating, chewing, swallowing
Previous surgery
Increased losses due to GI disorders such as malabsorption and diarrhea
Systemic disease interfering with appetite or eating (chronic lung, liver, heart and renal disease, abdominal angina, cancer)
Excessive alcohol use
Medications that interfere with appetite or nutrient metabolism

Source: From Rosenberg,[23] with permission.

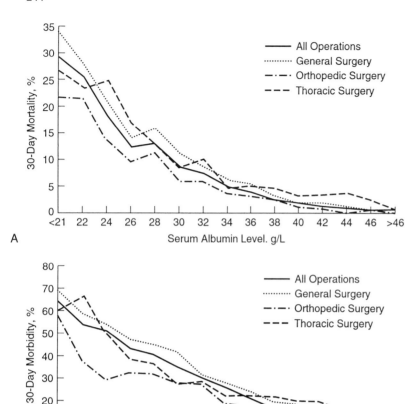

Figure 22.4. Thirty-day mortality rate (A) and morbidity rate (B) as a function of serum albumin for all operations combined and for three sub-specialties. (From Gibbs et al.,[28] with permission.)

and depleted to meet the metabolic demands. Serum albumin levels fall and hepatic function declines, further impairing endogenous protein synthesis. Dysfunction in those tissues with high cell turnover (the skin, the hematopoetic and immune system, and gastrointestinal organs) leads to breakdown in barrier function, increased susceptibility to infection, and further impairment of absorption of essential nutrients.[26] This cycle of worsening nutrition is compounded by dehydration, as the thirst drive declines with advancing age as well.

In the elderly surgical patient with protein-energy malnutrition, these changes are further aggravated by the increased energy requirements for wound healing. Additional deficits in vitamins, particularly A and C, and in trace minerals such as zinc can adversely effect enzymes systems necessary for wound repair. Further, major tissue injury and sepsis is associated with large fluid shifts and sequestration of extracellular water in the interstitial space. Compared to a younger patient, the mobilization of this fluid is delayed following large-volume resuscitation in the elderly. It is postulated that this prolonged sequestration is related to alterations in the structural elements of the interstitium with age and sepsis, which are exacerbated when endogenous

protein stores are depleted and protein synthesis is impaired.[27]

It should not be surprising that low serum albumin is a very sensitive predictor of complications and deaths for the hospitalized elderly whether hospitalization is the result of medical or surgical illness. In a subgroup of data from the NSQIP study mentioned earlier, both 30-day operative mortality and overall morbidity clearly rose as a function of declining serum albumin for a variety of different types of operations (Fig. 22.4A,B).[28] The incidence of several major infectious complications, including pneumonia and systemic sepsis, were approximately four times higher in patients with albumin levels below 3.5 g/dL when compared to those with higher albumin levels.

Cognitive Function

The importance of cognitive status as a determinant of surgical outcome is also underappreciated. Most surgeons do not perform tests of cognition before surgery, even when cognitive decline is a reported consequence of the procedure, as it is in cardiopulmonary bypass. Yet, a change in mental status postoperatively is frequently the first clinical sign of other serious complications, and

TABLE 22.5. Association of postoperative delirium with other surgical outcomes.

| Outcome | Delirium | | p |
	Yes (n = 117)	No (n = 1124)	
Major complication	18 (15%)	28 (2%)	<0.001
Death	5 (4%)	3 (0.2%)	<0.001
Mean length of stay (days)	15	7	<0.001
Discharge to long-term care or rehabilitation facility	43 (36%)	136 (11%)	<0.001

Source: From Marcantonio et al.,[29] with permission.

the occurrence of delirium in the postoperative period has a significant negative effect on all the markers of outcome. In one study,[29] mortality was increased 17 fold, major complications were increased 7 fold, length of stay was doubled, and patients returned to independence only one-third as often (Table 22.5). In another subgroup of patients from the NSQIP study undergoing operations for rectal cancer (mean age, 66 years), acute confusion was also associated with a number of other complications. Postoperative pneumonia, unplanned intubation, and failure to wean from the ventilator were 14.3, 15, and 5.7 times more likely to occur, respectively, in patients with cognitive changes than in those without. The chance of death within 30 days was 8.1 times higher in patients with delirium.

The impression that the cognitive consequences of surgery and anesthesia are transient recently has been disproven; deficits can persist for months, even years, after the operative event. One prospective study of noncardiac surgery patients over age 60 years demonstrated that cognitive deficits persisted in nearly 10% of patients for more than 3 months after hospital discharge.[30] In another study of coronary artery bypass patients of mean age 61 years, the incidence of cognitive decline was 53% at discharge, 36% at 6 weeks, 24% at 6 months, and 42% at 5 years.[31]

Postoperative delirium may be the manifestation of unrecognized preexisting disease or the result of intra- or postoperative events. Over the past several years, several studies have attempted to identify risk factors for delirium in hospitalized elderly surgical and medical patients. Although the results vary somewhat with the reasons for hospitalization, type of surgery, and the variables studied, age, polypharmacy, preoperative cognitive impairment, and poor functional status are among the most frequently associated factors.

A "predictive rule" for postoperative delirium has been developed from a large prospective study of major elective noncardiac surgery patients over age 50 years.[29] Independent correlates for postoperative delirium in this study included age over 70 years; self-reported alcohol abuse; poor cognitive function; poor functional status; markedly abnormal serum sodium, potassium, or glucose; aortic aneurysm surgery; and noncardiac thoracic surgery. A point system was devised to quantify these factors. Postoperative delirium developed in 2% of patients with 0 points; 8% with 1 point; 13% with 2 points; and 50% with more than 3 points.

Intraoperative and postoperative factors have also been studied. No association has been found with the route of anesthesia, epidural versus general,[32,33] or the occurrence of intraoperative hemodynamic complications. Intraoperative blood loss, the need for blood transfusion, and postoperative hematocrit below 30%, however, are associated with a significant increased risk of postoperative delirium.[33] Alteration in the sleep–wake cycle following surgery has also been associated with delirium.[34] In nonsurgical hospitalized elderly patients, independent precipitating factors for delirium include malnutrition, the use of physical restraints, the use of bladder catheters, the need for more than three medications, and any iatrogenic event during hospitalization.[35] These factors no doubt have similar influence on the incidence of delirium in elderly postoperative patients.

Specialized hospital programs designed to maintain functional status and minimize delirium in the elderly with medical illness have had a positive effect on outcome. In one such program entitled Hospital Elder Life Program, Inouye and colleagues[36] used a multicomponent strategy with standard protocols to manage six risk factors for delirium in hospitalized medical patients: cognitive impairment, sleep deprivation, immobility, visual impairment, hearing impairment, and dehydration. With this strategy, they were able to reduce the number of episodes of delirium and prevent cognitive and functional decline in at-risk older patients. This strategy, with minor modification, is presently under investigation as a method for reducing delirium and related complications among elderly postoperative patients.

Wound Healing

Wound healing is a complex constellation of coordinated events requiring adequate nutrition, adequate perfusion, and immunocompetence to support the cellular mechanism of tissue repair. Many of the processes involved in normal wound healing are susceptible to the changes of aging. Although it is generally thought that wounds in the elderly heal more slowly, this impression is largely unsubstantiated. Actual clinical differences in wound healing have been difficult to demonstrate because of myriad interacting and uncontrollable factors. Certain changes in the skin, subcutaneous tissue, muscle, and bones are documented,[37] but the effect of these changes, and others, on the orchestrated process of tissue repair is more elusive. Although tissue friability and easy inadvertent injury are observed in the elderly, as they are in infants and small children, the quantitation of these observations is lacking. A brief review of normal wound healing and the changes observed in the elderly is presented. It is more likely, however, that comorbidity with poor perfusion, poor nutrition, and immunosuppression rather than physiologic decline alone is responsible for most clinically relevant wound problems seen in elderly surgical patients.

Normal wound healing is described in three overlapping phases: inflammation/coagulation, proliferation, and remodeling. In large healing wounds, fibrinous exudate and eschar represent the inflammatory phase; granulation tissue, the proliferative phase; and contracting edges, the remodeling phase.[38]

The initial response to tissue injury is hemostasis and inflammation. When endothelial disruption occurs, platelets exposed to collagen adhere, aggregate, and release coagulation factors, vasoactive amines, and many of the cytokines essential for coordination of ensuing events. A fibrin mesh is formed that traps platelets, RBCs, and inflammatory cells and seals the wound. Increased capillary permeability from histamine, serotonin, and bradykinin release from platelets and mast cells facilitates diaphedisis of lymphocytes, macrophages, and neutrophils in response to chemotactic factors such as interleukin-1 (IL-1), transforming growth factor-beta (TGF-β), and platelet-derived growth factor (PDGF) produced by platelets and macrophages. By 24 h, activated neutrophils predominate; they scavenge debris and phagocytize and kill bacteria. In the process, however, oxidative bursts and release of proteases may further damage surrounding uninjured tissue. Removal of as much nonviable tissue as possible limits the extent of neutrophil migration and subsequent inflammation and scarring. When there is extensive bacterial contamination, macrophages process necrotic material and bacteria for presentation to lymphocytes. These, in turn, proliferate and release cytokines, including interferon-γ and IL-2, which stimulates the antimicrobial activities of monocytes and inhibits their migration out of the wound. Lymphocytes have a smaller role in less-contaminated wounds.[38]

By 48 h, macrophages progressively replace neutrophils. In response to debris, fibrin, low tissue oxygen tension, and high lactate levels, macrophages release the large array of cytokines and growth factors essential for repair; these include IL-1, IL-6, IL-8, tumor necrosis factor-alpha (TNF-α), TGF-β, insulin-like growth factor (IGF-1), fibroblast growth factor (FGF), and epidermal growth factor (EGF), which stimulate migration and proliferation of fibroblasts and endothelial cells.[39] As TGF-β increases, fibroblasts are stimulated to synthesize

collagen and proteoglycans, and the proliferative phase begins.

The proliferative phase is characterized by fibroplasia, angiogenesis, and epithelialization. By 72 h, fibroblasts have begun to proliferate and synthesize collagen and proteoglycan elements of the extracellular matrix. FGF stimulates the angiogenesis cascade and hypoxia, and TNF-α, among other growth factors, stimulates the migration and proliferation of endothelial cells. Extracellular matrix materials such as fibronectin, hylauronic acid, laminin, and fibrin form the framework on which new vessels can form. Epithelial cells migrate from the margin of the wound or from the bottom of epithelial-lined skin appendages as an intact sheet, facilitated by matrix material and endogenous proteases. Reepithelialization restores the barrier function.

Remodeling is the prolonged phase characterized by collagen synthesis, remodeling, and wound contraction. By 9 days, collagen synthesis declines as fibroblasts begin to disappear, neovascularity regresses, and mature scar is formed. Wound strength continues to increase from 1 to 6 weeks as collagen is cross-linked. Although this cross-linking increases strength and contraction, it renders the scar less elastic than unwounded skin.

Changes in wound healing with aging have been identified in each phase, but the translation of these changes into consistent clinical findings is not clear. Changes in coagulation and immune function with age might be expected to have a detrimental effect on the early events in wound healing. In a study of experimental human wounds, there was an exaggerated peak of neutrophils early in the inflammatory phase with a delay in the appearance of macrophages and lymphocytes.[40] In young mice, 7-day-old wounds showed mature granulation tissue and few inflammatory cells while those of older animals were still in the inflammatory phase.[41] Platelet and macrophage adherence to substrate seems to increase with age, whereas there is a decline in macrophage function in mice and humans.[42,43] In other experiments, the addition of macrophages from young animals to the wounds of old animals accelerated the healing rate.[44]

In addition, T-cell-mediated functions decline with age; there is a decreased proliferative capacity, decreased cytotoxic activity, and a decreased release of IL-2. This decreased release of IL-2 may further impair monocyte efficiency.[39]

In the proliferative phase, there is a deficit in the cellular responsiveness to certain cytokines, with decline in motility and proliferation of fibroblasts.[45,46] The rate of epithelialization of open wounds has been shown to be delayed in older patients compared to younger patients.[47,48] A few studies have demonstrated changes in angiogenesis, and there is a consensus that aged endothelium has a reduced proliferative capacity. The expression of endothelial adhesion molecules is also delayed with increasing age in human wounds.[40]

There are contradictory data on changes in collagen synthesis in the remodeling phase with age. In one study of experimental human wounds, the collagen content of wounds appeared equal regardless of age, but the accumulation of noncollagenous proteins was decreased in the older group.[47] Others report variations in collagen content, and there is no consensus. The breaking strength of some wounds may be lower in older animals,[49] but age alone does not suppress experimental anastamotic healing in the intestines.[50]

Improving wound healing in the elderly is not primarily directed at the cellular events identified above but at the comorbid conditions that cause hypoperfusion and subsequent tissue hypoxia, immunosuppression, and inadequate nutrition. Sufficient tissue perfusion to allow appropriate delivery of nutrients and oxygen to the wound is of paramount importance. In the elderly, conditions such as diabetes, congestive heart failure, arteriosclerosis, and venous insufficiency commonly compromise this perfusion.

Growing evidence supports the importance of adequate tissue oxygenation for the biochemical and cellular aspects of wound healing and infection control. Collagen synthesis requires oxygen as a cofactor, and the rate of collagen deposition is directly proportional to oxygen tension in the wound.[51] The enzymatic hydroxylation of proline and lysine residues on forming collagen chains also requires oxygen. Inadequate hydroxylation of proline results in instability of the collagen molecules and decreased strength of the resulting scar.[52] Collagen content in subcutaneous test wounds of general surgery patients has been shown to correlate with tissue oxygen tension during the first 48 h after surgery.[51] In animals, angiogenesis[53] and the rate of epithelialization[54] are accelerated in hyperoxic environments. In addition, the rate of healing of ischemic wounds in old animals is impaired by 40% to 65% compared to that of younger animals.[55]

Local wound infection is the most significant cause of impaired wound healing. The inflammatory response to infection further increases the inflammatory phase of wound healing and disrupts the balance toward collagen degradation rather than synthesis. Bacterial control in wounds is also an oxygen-dependent process. The ability of leukocytes to effectively kill bacteria requires local tissue oxygen tension of 30 mmHg or more.[56] In a study of general surgery patients, wound infections occurred in 43% of those with measured tissue oxygen tension of 40 to 50 mmHg compared to 0% in those with tissue oxygen tension over 90 mmHg.[57]

Systemic sepsis, in addition to local infection, can also interfere with proper wound healing. In one study, experimental systemic sepsis impaired collagen synthesis, resulting in defective healing of bowel anastamoses and reduced anastamotic bursting strength.[58] Transient bacteriemia from instrumentation of the oropharynx, trachea, and urinary tract in the perioperative period may seed newly created wounds. Eliminating possible sources of local wound contamination and eradicating all treatable infections before any elective disruption of tissue can decrease the incidence of wound complications. The high prevalence of bacteriuria in the elderly (approximately 20% in men and 20%–50% in women over age 80 years), most of which is asymptomatic, mandates preoperative microscopic exam of the urine followed by culture/sensitivity and treatment if positive.[59] The colonization of the oropharynx with gram-negative bacteria may predispose to gram-negative pneumonia postoperatively, although the clinical relevance to postoperative infection is not well established.

Adequate tissue perfusion and oxygenation require appropriate hydration. Increasing volume resuscitation as a therapy to improve wound healing has recently been studied in patients undergoing abdominal operations. Patients randomized to receive modest fluid supplements showed higher tissue oxygen tension on the 1st postoperative day and higher hydroxyproline content of test wounds on the 7th postoperative day.[60]

In the elderly, maintenance of adequate hydration may be difficult. Preoperative bowel preps and periods of forced abstinence from oral intake combined with age-related decline in thirst drive may quickly result in dehydration, which is often unrecognized. In elderly patients with compensated congestive heart failure, overzealous hydration will decrease tissue perfusion. However, in those with diastolic rather than systolic failure, the maintenance of adequate preload is essential for optimum cardiac output.[61] Finding the appropriate balance may be challenging for the anesthesiologist, particularly when the procedure is long and there are large volume losses.

Cold ambient temperatures may exacerbate the effects of underhydration on tissue perfusion by causing vasoconstriction. In the elderly, the declining metabolic rate and decreased function of the hypothalamic thermal regulatory centers lead to rapid decreases in core and peripheral temperature. Studies have shown that wound infection rates,[62] as well as cardiac-related complications,[63] go up if temperatures are allowed to fall intraoperatively. Higher room temperature, warmed infusions, and forced-air warming devices are useful in maintaining body temperature and limiting vasoconstriction. Radiant heat, which has been shown to increase blood flow to wounds, is being studied with regard to effects on actual wound healing.

Pain and stress with the release of catecholamines have also been shown to induce vasoconstriction and decrease tissue perfusion. Activation of the sympathetic nervous system during the stress response shunts blood away from the periphery to support the heart and brain. Sympathetic blockade with epidural anesthetic has been shown to improve wound healing in vascular surgical procedures.[64] Although epidural anesthesia is an excellent method for decreasing postoperative pain without the sedation of systemic agents (see pain, following), its utility in improving wound healing in other settings remains to be determined.

The benefit of supplemental oxygen in routine clinical practice to improve tissue oxygenation and thereby improve wound healing has not been well established. Tissue oxygen levels fall as a result of surgery alone,[65] but tissue perfusion depends on many factors in addition to the oxygen saturation of the blood. It makes sense, however, that in patients at risk for tissue hypoxia either because of preexisting diseases or the length, contamination level, and location of the operation, supplemental oxygen might be of benefit.[52]

The importance of adequate nutrition for wound healing was mentioned earlier. The incidence of major complications and death in a variety of settings increases as a function of falling serum albumin.[28] Experimental wounds in elderly surgical patients show delayed wound-healing response, even with a mild degree of protein-calorie malnutrition (mean weight loss, 9%; mean albumin, 3.9 g/dL).[66] Nutritional supplements given both pre- and postoperatively have been shown to improve wound healing. One study demonstrated that healing was better when both preoperative and postoperative nutritional supplementation were given.[67,68]

In patients with significant preoperative deficits, several weeks of supplementation to reverse these deficits before the operation would be ideal, but this is rarely feasible. In one study, wound healing as assessed by hydroxyproline accumulation increased in surgical patients receiving only 1 week of intravenous alimentation.[69] In another study, recent preoperative food intake was found to be more important than overall nutritional status.[70] A short course of enteral supplements is worthwhile in patients with moderate deficits who can tolerate the delay in operation. For those who cannot, enteral or parenteral nutrition should be started immediately postoperatively. A recent randomized trial of postoperative enteral supplementation showed a decrease in morbidity and an improvement in nutritional status and quality of life.[67]

Replacement of specific nutrients is also important. Vitamins A, B, C, and possibly E and trace elements such as zinc are essential for wound healing. Vitamin C is a cofactor for the enzymes involved in proline and lysine hydroxylation during collagen synthesis, and it is also important in leukocyte function and production of growth factors such as IGF-1. Vitamin A promotes the early inflammatory phases of wound healing and is particularly important in reversing the wound-healing deficits that accompany the use of steroids and chemotherapeutic agents. Zinc is involved in at least 300 enzyme reactions and is essential for DNA synthesis, cell division, protein synthesis, and lymphocyte proliferation. Although replacement of these nutrients is essential for wound healing, supplementation beyond replacement has not been shown to improve healing.[39]

Other specific nutrients including the amino acid arginine have recently generated significant interest as a stimulant of both wound healing and immune function. In animals, wound breaking strength and collagen synthesis have been shown to improve with arginine supplementation.[71] In healthy humans, oral arginine increased wound collagen deposition and lymphocyte response to mitogens.[72] Supplemental arginine has also been shown to increase IGF-1 and improve nitrogen balance.[73] The effects of arginine may be the result of stimulation of growth hormone secretion or increased T-cell recruitment and activation of fibroblasts.[74] Alternatively, arginine is converted to citruline and nitric oxide (NO) by nitric oxide synthase. NO in low concentration stimulates collagen synthesis. The impaired wound collagen synthesis seen in protein-energy malnutrition may reflect low NO synthesis in the wound. The deficit may be corrected by the addition of exogenous arginine.[75]

Growth hormone (GH) has also been studied as a stimulant to wound healing. In animal models, GH has been shown to increase collagen content in wounds and bowel anastamoses.[76,77] It has also been shown to accelerate the rate of donor site healing in pediatric burn patients.[78,79] GH effects are exerted through the induction of synthesis of endogenous growth factors such as IGF-1. IGF-1 is secreted early in the inflammatory phase and stimulates fibroblast and endothelial proliferation and collagen synthesis; there are no studies documenting its clinical utility specifically in wound healing in the elderly. Other growth factors, such as PDF and PDGF, have been shown in prospective randomized studies to accelerate the rate of closure of chronic wounds such as diabetic ulcers, venous status ulcers, and pressure sores. The cost of these therapies, however, is prohibitive.[38]

Effect of Age on the Presentation and Natural History of Disease

With age, there are changes in the pattern of presentation of certain diseases. Although these changes are not well characterized, they are real and frequently observed. For example, surgical disease in the elderly is often described as atypical and acute because the signs and symptoms tend to be less severe early in the course of the disease and a complication is often the presenting finding.[80] With gallbladder disease, for example, the classic pattern of worsening biliary colic leading to elective cholecystectomy is replaced by acute cholecystitis, cholangitis, or pancreatitis at presentation without antecedent symptoms.[81] Even when acute inflammatory changes are present, as many as one-half of elderly patients with acute cholecystitis fail to have signs of peritoneal inflammation in the right upper quadrant, one-third have normal white blood cell counts, and one-third are afebrile.[82] In the previously mentioned study of open cholecystectomy, more than 60% of operations on the elderly were performed as emergencies, as compared less than to 20% in the general population. With appendicitis, more than 50% of elderly patients are found to have perforation at the time of operation, compared to less than 25% in younger patients.[83]

This advanced progression of disease at the time of surgery occasionally makes the technical execution of the operation more difficult. With biliary tract disease, for example, older age is associated with a higher rate of conversion from laparoscopic to open technique because of the technical difficulties encountered due to the long-standing inflammation.[84] At operation for perforated appendicitis, inflammatory changes may be so severe that right hemicolectotomy rather than appendectomy is required to rule out the possibility of perforated cecal cancer.

Even when the presentation of disease is similar in the elderly, there may be a delay in diagnosis because the symptoms are attributed to other diseases found more commonly in old age. Such is the case with Crohn's disease, in which the basic symptoms of diarrhea, pain, and weight loss occur with about equal frequency in the elderly; the correct diagnosis, however, is initially made in only 64% of patients over age 65 years compared to 96% of younger patients.[85]

The natural history of surgical disease in the elderly is also not well defined in many cases. In both Crohn's disease and ulcerative colitis, for example, there are conflicting reports about the relative frequency of disease location, the need for surgery, the response to treatment, and the prognosis.[86] The characteristics of tumors may vary also with age. In elderly women, for example, breast cancers are found more often to be moderately to well differentiated, have estrogen receptors, and have a low thymidine labeling index.[87] The biologic behavior of tumors in the elderly may also be different. In a series of patients with gastric cancer, for example, 5-year survival was 23% for older patients compared to 11% for younger patients.[88] In those with stage IV disease, no younger patient survived 3 years, while several elderly patients were alive at 5 years.

Great care must be taken, however, to avoid inappropriately treating cancer in the elderly because of the impression that the disease may have a less virulent course. Although there have been improvements in the

SEER database about the approach to surgery for cancer treatment in the elderly over the past two decades, patients in this age group are still often excluded from many types of treatment trials. Data from the 1990 SEER database, for example, indicated that 47.7% of breast cancer occurred in patients over age 65, but only 17.3% of women treated in National Cancer Institute-sponsored trials were in this age group.[89] Until more elderly patients are included in treatment trials, conclusions about the safety and efficacy of these treatments in the elderly will continue to be made without firm evidential support.

Minimizing the Impact of Surgery

Many of the negative consequences of surgery in the elderly are the same as those of hospitalization for any reason in this age group (see Chapter 13), although the additional stress of tissue damage, blood loss, and anesthesia is not insignificant. Table 22.6 lists the most common and potentially preventable hazards of hospitalization for both medical and surgical patients.[90] The use of prophylactic measures, monitoring devices, and alternate approaches to operation can minimize the risk of many of these adverse outcomes.

Prophylactic Measures

Anticoagulation

The annual incidence of deep venous thrombosis (DVT) and pulmonary embolism (PE) at ages 65 to 69 is 1.3 and 1.8 per 1000, respectively. At ages 85 to 89, this incidence rises to 2.8 and 3.1 per 1000.[91] In the elderly surgical patient, the factors favoring the development of DVT and PE abound: included are surgery-induced hyper-

TABLE 22.6. Hazards of hospitalization and surgery.

Acute renal failure
Adverse drug event
Inappropriate bladder catheterization
Deconditioning and immobility
Delirium
Depression
Electrolyte disturbance
Falls
Functional decline
Incontinence
Infection
Malnutrition
Stress-induced GI ulceration
Thromboembolism
Untreated or undertreated pain

Source: From The Interdisciplinary Leadership Group of the American Geriatrics Society Project to Increase Geriatric Expertise in Surgical and Medical Specialties,[90] with permission.

coagulability; stasis from postoperative immobility and decreased lower extremity musculature; frequent operation for malignancy or injury; and age-associated coagulation changes, with hypercoagulable states particularly involving factor X_a, decreased vascular wall fibrinolysis, and decreased antithrombin levels.[92] In spite of these risks, the incidence of clinically significant postoperative DVT and PE is lower than that of many other operative complications overall. In the VA NSQIP study mentioned earlier, the overall incidence DVT is 0.3% and PE is 0.1%. The incidence of PE is twice as high in orthopedic procedures[8] and five times as high for patients over age 85. In certain operations such total hip replacement, the risk of thromboembolic complications has been reported to be as high as 20% to 50%.[93] The mortality for PE in the hospitalized elderly exceeds 20%.[94]

Prophylaxis for DVT and PE is now a standard part of perioperative care for a variety of moderate- and high-risk procedures. Regimens include adjusted-dose subcutaneous heparin, low molecular weight heparin, or warfarin, combined with sequential compression devices (see Chapter 20). DVT and PE still occur, however, even when prophylactic measures are properly employed. Newer regimens using synthetic oligosaccharides that are selective, antithrombin-dependent indirect inhibitors of factor Xa have recently been reported. These agents potentiate the neutralization of factor Xa, inhibiting the generation of thrombin from prothrombin and thus preventing clot formation. In a recent report comparing one of these agents, Org3150/SR90907A, with low molecular weight heparin in patients undergoing total hip replacement (median age, 66 years), the oligosaccharide was shown to increase the risk/benefit ratio for the prevention of DVT; at a dose that produced bleeding rates equivalent to the standard dose of low molecular weight heparin, there was an 82% reduction; the risk of thromboembolism was 82% less.[95]

Antibiotics

As already mentioned, a leading cause of wound-healing failure is infection. Older persons are potentially more susceptible to wound infection because of the changes in the nutrition, perfusion, and immunocompetence that accompany aging and the high prevalence of comorbid conditions, such as diabetes mellitus. Appropriate utilization of methodology to decrease wound infection is, therefore, particularly important when operating on elderly patients. The Centers for Disease Control and Prevention provide excellent guidelines for the prevention of surgical site infection.[96] While the recommendations for skin preparation and operating room environment are important, they are well accepted and uniformly employed. The importance and correct use of antibiotic prophylaxis, however, is less well understood and less uniformly applied.

According to the CDC guidelines, antibiotic prophylaxis is "a critically timed adjunct used to reduce the microbial burden of intra-operative contamination to a level that cannot overwhelm the host." Four basic principles guide the use of antibiotic prophylaxis[96]:

1. *Prophylaxis should be used for all operations in which it has been shown to reduce the incidence of surgical site infections, or where the risk of infection would be catastrophic.* This condition includes all operations in which there is controlled entry into a hollow viscus (clean-contaminated) and clean operations in which a prosthetic material, particularly an intravascular graft or prosthetic joint, is being implanted. Cardiac, neurosurgical, and certain operations on the eye also meet this criteria because of the catastrophic consequences of infection in these organs (Table 22.7).

2. *The agent used should be safe, inexpensive, and bactericidal with an in vitro spectrum that covers the organisms that are likely to be encountered with that specific procedure* (see Table 22.7).

3. *The agent should be given before the skin is incised so the tissue and serum levels of the agent are adequate at the time the potential contamination might occur.*

4. *Therapeutic levels should be maintained throughout the operation by redosing until a few hours after the procedure is over and the skin is closed.* The frequency of redosing depends on the tissue levels normally achieved, serum half-life of the drug, and the MIC_{50} of the agent for the organisms likely to be encountered.

TABLE 22.7. Guidelines for antibiotic prophylaxis.

Operation	Likely pathogen
Placement of prosthetic	*Staphylococcus aureus*, coagulase-negative staphylococci
Cardiac	*S. aureus*, coagulase-negative staphylococci
Neurosurgery	*S. aureus*, coagulase-negative staphylococci
Breast	*S. aureus*, coagulase-negative staphylococci
Ophthalmic[a]	*S. aureus*, coagulase-negative staphylococci Streptococci, Gram-negative bacilli
Orthopedic	*S. aureus*, gram-negative bacilli, coagulase-negative staphylococci
Noncardiac thoracic	*S. aureus*, coagulase-negative staphylococci *Streptococcus pneumoniae*, gram-negative bacilli
Vascular	*Staphylococcus aureus*, coagulase-negative staphylococci
Appendectomy	Gram-negative bacilli, anaerobes
Biliary tract	Gram-negative bacilli, anaerobes
Colorectal	Gram-negative bacilli, anaerobes
Gastroduodenal	Gram-negative bacilli, streptococci Oropharyngeal anaerobes (peptostreptococci)
Head and neck	*S. aureus*, streptococci Oropharyngeal anaerobes (peptostreptococci)
Urologic	Gram-negative bacilli

[a] Limited data but used for anterior segment resection, vitrectomy, scleral buckle.
Source: From Mangram et al.,[96] with permission.

Special note should be made about controlling infections during operations in which the colon may be resected. Oral nonabsorbable antibiotics are usually given as part of the mechanical bowel preparation before all such procedures, in addition to parenteral prophylactic antibiotics. Although there is some controversy about the need for both, most colorectal surgeons use oral and parenteral prophylaxis.[97]

In colon surgery, however, the most important part of the preparation is the mechanical cleaning of the bowel to decrease the enormous bacterial load, not the antibiotics alone. Mechanical preparation is accomplished with cathartics or gastrointestinal lavage solutions containing polyethylene glycol and electrolytes. Lavage solutions are commonly used in the elderly because they are isosmotic and the risk of dehydration is less than with the effective saline cathartics. Nausea and vomiting from lavage can still lead to dehydration. Monitoring of the preparation is extremely important because the large volume (4 L) required for lavage to be effective can lead to compliance problems in elderly patients, particularly those who have mobility constraints. In the past, bowel preparation was usually performed in the hospital where patients could be observed. With present health insurance mandates for same-day admission for surgery, preparation is now routinely done at home the night before operation. In the frail or compromised elderly, home nursing support should be used if preoperative hospitalization is not possible because of the high rate of infection if preparation is inadequate.

Swallowing Dysfunction: A Less Well Appreciated Risk

The most common and one of the most resource-intensive complications in the elderly in the postoperative period is pneumonia. In the NSQIP study for 1998, the incidence of postoperative pneumonia was nearly 5% in patients more than 85 years of age compared to 1% for those aged less than 65 years. Although the explanation for this increase is multifactorial, one factor that has only recently been studied is the effect of swallowing dysfunction on the incidence of postoperative aspiration.

The majority of community-acquired bacterial pneumonias in the elderly are the result of microaspiration of oral flora.[98] Alterations in deglutition secondary to stroke and other central nervous system disease, dementia, medications, and generalized decline predispose to the aspiration of oral contents. In the postoperative period, nausea and vomiting from anesthetic medications combined with the decline in level of consciousness and the further pharyngeal dyscoordination caused by endotracheal, nasogastric, and transesophageal echocardiogra-phy (TEE) probes exacerbates the risk for aspiration of gastric, as well as oral, contents.

Most surgeons are aware that the incidence of swallowing dysfunction following endotracheal extubation in postoperative and critically ill patients correlates with the length of intubation.[99] It is less well appreciated that other tubes that traverse the oropharynx can alter swallowing function in the elderly and also cause postoperative aspiration. TEE has gained great favor as a less-invasive method to monitor intravascular volume and cardiac performance during operation. The safety and efficacy of this form of monitoring is generally accepted. The utility of TEE in cardiac surgery has been particularly impressive. However, in a study of swallowing dysfunction after cardiac surgery,[100] the two independent predictors by multivariate logistical regression analysis were length of endotracheal intubation and the use of TEE. Swallowing dysfunction in this study was documented in 4% of patients, 90% of whom had documented aspiration. The incidence of pneumonia, need for tracheostomy, length of ICU stay, and length of hospital stay were all significantly increased in the TEE group. In another study of cardiac surgery patients,[101] the relative risk for dysphagia in the postoperative period was 7.8 times greater for TEE than for non-TEE patients.

Similar negative consequence of pharyngeal intubation occur with nasogastric (NG) tubes. In a meta-analysis[102] of all published trials comparing routine versus selective use of nasogastric tubes after elective laparotomy, fever, atelectasis, and pneumonia were significantly less common in patients managed without an NG tube. There was, however, significantly more abdominal distension and vomiting in the group managed without the NG tubes, but these episodes did not translate to a higher incidence of aspiration pneumonia. Caution should be exercised when reviewing these data because the study was for elective operation only and results are not reported as a function of age. However, there are putative advantages and disadvantages with either method of management in this age group. If gastric distension is unrecognized in the sedated elderly patient, vomiting and aspiration is a serious risk. If an NG tube is functioning properly, gastric decompression will prevent vomiting, but aspiration of oral secretions may still occur. If the NG tube is functioning improperly, the risk of aspiration is probably higher than without an NG tube because the normal protective mechanism of the lower esophageal sphincter is disturbed by the presence of the tube. The data seem to firmly support the use of NG tubes only when specifically indicated for control of distension and vomiting in selected cases. The NG tube is still an important adjunct to treatment for procedures on the esophagus or stomach, where they are placed for technical reasons, and in emergencies when the likelihood of prolonged distension is high.

Minimal Access Surgery

Over the past decade, the growing applications of minimal access techniques to a large number of disciplines has allowed surgeons to perform a wide variety of complex major operations through small incisions. Smaller incisions are associated with less postoperative pain, less atelectasis, less postoperative ileus, fewer wound complications, and quicker return to normal activities. It is logical that the elderly patient with marginal reserves would benefit most from this minimal invasive approach. However, the extent to which the traumatic response to surgery is moderated by minimal incisions in the elderly is a subject of active investigation. It is still unclear whether the hemodynamic and cardiorespiratory consequences of pneumoperitoneum are completely offset by the benefits of decreased inflammatory, hormonal, and metabolic stress.[103]

The cardiorespiratory consequences of pneumoperitoneum are attributable both to the use of CO_2 as the insufflating gas and to mechanical forces associated with increased intra-abdominal pressure. Although hypercarbia and respiratory acidosis from CO_2 absorption are common, pH can usually be well controlled with adequate mechanical ventilation. Hypercarbia becomes a serious problem only when there is preexisting pulmonary disease. The consequences of increased intra-abdominal pressure, although not insignificant, are usually easily controlled with adequate volume loading and mechanical ventilation as well. Although the overall consequences of laparoscopy and pneumoperitoneum are not inconsequential, with adequate preload and careful mechanical ventilation laparoscopic procedures can be safely performed in most elderly patients. In those with severe cardiac and or pulmonary compromise, invasive monitoring to maintain adequate volume loading and alternate gas sources or gasless techniques may eliminate most of the negative sequelae of CO_2 insufflation.[104]

The largest amount of data on the outcome of laparoscopic surgery in the elderly is found in the biliary literature, although a wide range of other major intra-abdominal and intrathoracic procedures are being reported.[105] Laparoscopic cholecystectomy is associated with fewer complications and shorter length of stay than open procedures. Results of one study comparing laparoscopic to open cholecystectomy in patients over 65 years of age is shown in Table 22.8.[106] However, when compared to younger patients, the elderly still experience more postoperative complications. In addition, operative times are longer in elderly patients with complicated cholelithiasis and in those classified ASA 3 or 4. Both age greater than 70 years and ASA 3 or 4 are also associated with higher rates of conversion from laparoscopic to open procedures.[107] In one study comparing patients with acute cholecystitis, the conversion rate to open operation

TABLE 22.8. Prospective randomized trial of laparoscopic versus open cholecystectomy in the elderly.

Factor	Open	Laparoscopic	p
Number of patients	131	133	ns
Age	72 (65–88)	71 (65–87)	ns
Acute cholecystitis (%)	29.7	32.3	ns
Operative minutes	70.9	75.0	ns
Hospital days	9.9	3.7	<0.05
Complications	31 (23.6%)	18 (13.5%)	<0.05

Source: From Brunt and Soper,[105] with permission.

was 23.3% in older patients compared to 2.5% in younger patients.[108]

As with open cholecystectomy, the mortality rate for laparoscopic cholecystectomy is largely a function of comorbidity and acuity of the disease. Mortality rates are reported from 0% to 2.0%. Two studies comparing mortality of laparoscopic versus open operation by logistical regression analysis indicated reduced odds of death from the laparoscopic approach.[105] Present comparisons are less meaningful because conversion to open procedure usually indicates complicated disease.

The presence of common bile duct (CBD) stones requires additional intervention by either minimal access or open procedure. Although laparoscopic CBD explorations are successful in more than 90% of reported cases,[105] the technical skills to do this procedure are greater than those required for routine cholecystectomy. Many surgeons, therefore, address CBD stones with endoscopic techniques either preoperatively or postoperatively.

The laparoscopic technique for colon resection has also been reported in the elderly, although fear of port site implantation of tumor during laparoscopy for malignant disease slowed the development of this technique for that indication. In a matched control study of laparoscopic versus open colectomy in patients over age 75, the morbidity rate in the open group was 33.3% compared to 14.3% for the laparoscopic group. There were no deaths in either group. Narcotic use, return to normal bowel function, and length of hospital stay were all also significantly shorter in the laparoscopic group. Of the 37 laparoscopic patients and 38 open patients documented as independent in ADLs on admission, 35 in the laparoscopic group and 29 open group ($p < 0.025$) were independent at discharge.[109] These data indicate that laparoscopic colectomy is not only safe but is associated with a better outcome in terms of morbidity and maintenance of function.

As mentioned earlier in the chapter, surgical options for malignant disease in the elderly are not offered when the surgery is high risk and the chance of survival even with surgery is low; this was the case with lung cancer in the past. With careful patient selection, mortality for thoracotomy in elderly patients over the past decade has ranged from 3% to 5%. Recent experience with video-assisted thoracic surgery (VATS) suggests that this technique may result in much lower morbidity and mortality and should be evaluated in more rigorous clinical trials. VATS procedures use small incisions and preserve respiratory muscle function by not spreading the ribs and by avoiding rib fractures. In a study from the Brigham and Women's Hospital,[110] there was no mortality when VATS was used to perform 32 lobectomies or segmentectomies in patients over age 65 and only one death when used in 156 other thoracic procedures. Length of stay was 4 days for patients aged 65 to 79 and 5 days for those aged 80 to 89. Of particular note is that the incidence of delirium in the postoperative VATS patients was 2.7% compared to 13% to 19% for elderly patients undergoing traditional thoracic procedures.

Similarly encouraging results have been reported for retroperitoneal laparoscopic radical nephrectomy and nephroureterectomy in patients over age 80.[111] In a small series, laparoscopically treated patients had quicker return to oral intake, lower narcotic requirements, and shorter hospital stay. In addition, total convalescence time was 14 days in the laparoscopic group compared to 42 days in the open group.

The laparoscopic approach has also been studied for splenectomy, antireflux procedures, staging of malignancy, and the diagnosis of acute abdominal pain. Although the series are few and the number of elderly patients studied is small, results in these areas also appear favorable when compared to open procedures.

Postoperative Pain Management

Untreated or undertreated postoperative pain can have significant negative impact on the recovery of the elderly patient following surgery. Pain causes tachycardia, increases myocardial oxygen consumption, and may lead to myocardial ischemia. The anticipation of pain after major abdominal and thoracic procedures leads to splinting and poor inspiratory effort with subsequent atelectasis and increased risk of pneumonia. Because pain is exacerbated by moving, untreated pain results in immobility with all the sequelae of prolonged bed rest including pressure ulcers, thromboembolic disorders, and the declines associated with deconditioning; depression and lethargy; anorexia and dehydration; neuromuscular instability, decreased bone density, muscular weakness, and incoordination; altered bladder and bowel function with retention and constipation; and urinary and fecal incontinence.

Several clinical observations suggest pain perception is altered with increasing age: the incidence of silent myocardial infarction rises from less than 20% in patients aged 45 to 54, to more than 40% in those aged 75 to 84[112];

more than 35% of elderly patients with duodenal ulcer disease report no epigastric pain compared to only 8% of younger patients.[113] However, experimental data do not support changes attributed to aging alone. Therefore, pain must be actively assessed and treated in the elderly as it would in any other postoperative patient.

Pain assessment should be based on the patient's perception of pain, not on the assumptions of the caregivers. Simple tools such as a numerical rating for severity of pain or a visual analogue scale are usually adequate to document the patient's perceived level of pain. In the cognitively impaired or acutely delirious patient, this assessment is much more difficult. Patients with chronic dementia can often respond to direct questioning about the presence and intensity of pain, although concern about inducing or exacerbating acute confusion with opioids may result in inadequate treatment of the pain. This undertreatment itself may be a cause of worsening agitation and confusion. When coherent verbal communications are not helpful, other verbal cues such as groaning and nonverbal signs such as facial expressions and body language can be used to guide treatment.

Opioids are the ideal agents for treating the acute postoperative pain because they have no ceiling to the analgesic effect.[114] However, the side effects of confusion and sedation are rate limiting in the elderly patient. Of the opioids used outside the operating room, morphine is the most commonly used and most predictable. The previous enthusiasm for meperidine is unfounded for the treatment of pain in the elderly: it is associated with CNS excitatory effects, particularly in patients with renal insufficiency, and its metabolites can cause grand mal seizures.

Parenteral nonsteroidal anti-inflammatory drugs (NSAIDS) when first introduced were widely accepted because of their excellent analgesic effects without the sedation associated with opioids. However, the incidence of gastrointestinal bleeding in the elderly with parenteral NSAIDs has greatly limited their usefulness.

The route of administration of the analgesic agent is extremely important. For elderly patients the epidural infusion of opioids combined with local anesthetic agents is an excellent intra- and postoperative method of pain control, providing excellent analgesia with less sedation.[115] The local anesthetic agents also provide sympathetic blockade, which ameliorates some of the negative sequelae of sympathetic activation associated with general anesthetics. Local anesthetics, however, can cause orthostatic hypotension, urinary retention, and muscle weakness, while the opioids cause urinary retention and itching.[114] Overall, however, the improved risk/benefit profile of the epidural route more than justifies the additional invasive procedure.

Patient-controlled analgesia (PCA) is also an important improvement in the way pain medications are now delivered. The patient is given a button to push to deliver a fixed dose of drug when needed. A lock-out interval between doses prevents overdose, which is also unlikely because the patient must be conscious enough to push the button. Low-dose continuous infusion can run simultaneously when the pain is most severe in the first few days after surgery. PCA allows for a much more constant level of analgesia without the peaks and troughs associated with conventional intramuscular (i.m.) injections. In a randomized study comparing PCA with conventional i.m. injections in elderly men, PCA gave better pain control with few complications, less sedation, and better patient satisfaction.[116] The only caveat for using the PCA is that the patient must be able to understand the instructions and must be encourage to use the button before the pain becomes intense to maintain the effective level of pain control.

References

1. Warner MA, Saletel RA, Schroeder DR, et al. Outcome of anesthesia and surgery in people 100 years of age and older. *J Am Geriatr Soc.* 1998;46:988–993.
2. Centers for Disease Control and Prevention. *Advanced Data* no. 316. Washington, DC: National Center for Health Statistics; June 30, 2000.
3. Farrow DC, Hunt WC, Samet JM. Temporal and regional variability in the surgical treatment of cancer among older people. *J Am Geriatr Soc.* 1996;44:559–564.
4. Sollano JA, Rose EA, Williams DL, et al. Cost-effectiveness of coronary artery bypass surgery in octogenarians. *Ann Surg.* 1998;228:297–306.
5. Kind P. Measuring valuations for health states. A survey of patients in general practice. Discussion paper 76. York: Center for Health Economics, University of York; 1990.
6. Thomas DR, Ritchie CS. Preoperative assessment of older adults. *J Am Geriatr Soc.* 1995;43:811–821.
7. Khuri SF, Daley J, Henderson W, et al. The National Veterans Administration Surgical Risk Study: risk adjustment for the comparative assessment of the quality of surgical care. *J Am Coll Surg.* 1995;180:519–531.
8. Khuri SF, Daley J, Henderson W. National Surgical Quality Improvement Program (NSQIP). *Annual Report*; Hines, IL: Department of Veteran Affairs, FY 1999;A-5.
9. Escarce JJ, Shea JA, Chen W, et al. Outcomes of open cholecystectomy in the elderly: a longitudinal analysis of 21,000 cases in the prelaparoscopic era. *Surgery.* 1995;117:156.
10. Buxbaum JL, Schwartz AJ. Perianesthetic considerations for the elderly patient. *Surg Clin North Am.* 1994;74:41–61.
11. Djokovic JL, Hedley-White J. Prediction of outcome of surgery and anesthesia in patients over 80. *JAMA.* 1979;242:2301–2304.
12. Khuri SF, Daley J, Henderson W, et al. Department of Veterans Affairs' NSQIP. The first national, validated, outcome-based, risk adjusted, and peer-controlled

program for the measurement and enhancement of the quality of surgical care. *Ann Surg.* 1998;228:491–507.
13, Narain P, Rubenstein LZ, Wieland GD, et al. Predictors of immediate and 6 month outcome in hospitalized elderly patients. The importance of functional status. *J Am Geriatr Soc.* 1988;36:775–783.
14. Seymour DG, Pringle R. Post-operative complications in the elderly surgical patient. *Gerontology.* 1983;29:262–270.
15. Browner WS, Manganese DT. In hospital and long-term mortality in male veterans following non-cardiac surgery: The study of perioperative ischemia research group. *JAMA.* 1992;268:228–232.
16. Shahar A, Powers KA, Black JS. The risk of postoperative deconditioning in older adults. *J Am Geriatr Soc.* 1996;44:471–474.
17. Gerson MC, Hurst JM, Hertzberg VS, et al. Cardiac prognosis in noncardiac geriatric surgery. *Ann Intern Med.* 1985;103:832–837.
18. Gerson MC, Hurst JM, Hertzberg VS, et al. Prediction of cardiac and pulmonary complications related to elective abdominal and noncardiac thoracic surgery in geriatric patients. *Am J Med.* 1990;88:101–107.
19. Older P, Smith R, Courtney P, et al. Preoperative evaluation of cardiac function and ischemia in elderly patients by cardiopulmonary exercise testing. *Chest.* 1993;103:701–705.
20. Eagle KA, Brundage BH, Chaitman BR, et al. ACC/AHA Task Force Report: guidelines for perioperative cardiovascular evaluation for noncardiac surgery. *Circulation.* 1996;93:1278–1317.
21. Hlatky MA, Boineau BE, Higginbotham MB, et al. A brief self-administered questionnaire to determine functional capacity (the Duke's Activity Status Index). *Am J Cardiol.* 1989;64:651–656.
22. Reuben DB, Greendale GA, Harrison GG. Nutrition screening in older persons. *J Am Geriatr Soc.* 1995;43:415–420.
23. Rosenberg IH. Nutrition and aging. In: Hazzard WR, Bierman EL, Blass JP, et al, eds. *Principles of Geriatric Medicine and Gerontology*, 3rd Ed. New York: McGraw-Hill; 1994:49–60.
24. Detsky AS, Mclaughlin JR, Baker JP, et al. What is subjective global assessment of nutritional status? *J Parenter Enteral Nutr.* 1987;11:8–13.
25. Detsky AS, et al. Predicting nutrition-associated complications for patients undergoing gastrointestinal surgery. *J Parenter Enteral Nutr.* 1987;11:440–446.
26. Lipschitz DA. Nutrition. In: Cassel CK, Cohen HJ, Larson EB, et al. eds. *Geriatric Medicine*, 3rd Ed. New York: Springer-Verlag; 1996:801–813.
27. Cheng ATH, Planck LD, Hill GL. Prolonged overexpansion of the extracellular water in elderly patients with sepsis. *Arch Surg.* 1998;133:745–751.
28. Gibbs J, Cull W, Henderson W, et al. Preoperative serum albumin level as a predictor of operative mortality and morbidity. *Arch Surg.* 1999;134:36–42.
29. Marcantonio ER, Goldman L, Mangione CM, et al. A clinical prediction rule for delirium after elective noncardiac surgery. *JAMA.* 1994;271(2):134–139.

30. Moller JT, Cluitmans P, Rasmussen LS, et al. Long-term postoperative cognitive dysfunction in the elderly: ISPOCD1 study. *Lancet.* 1998;351:857–861.

31. Newmann MF, Kirchner JL, Phillips-Bute B, et al. Longitudinal assessment of neurocognitive function after coronary-artery bypass surgery. *N Engl J Med.* 2001;344: 395–401.

32. Williams-Russo P, Urquhart BL, Sharrock NE, et al. Postoperative delirium: predictors and prognosis in elderly orthopedic patients. *J Am Geriatr Soc.* 1992;40:759–777.

33. Marcantonio ER, Goldman L, Orav JE, Cook FE, Lee TH. The association of intraoperative factors with the development of postoperative delirium. *Am J Med.* 1998;105(5): 380–387.

34. Kaneko T, Takahashi S, Naka T, et al. Postoperative delirium following gastrointestinal surgery in elderly patients. *Surg Today.* 1997;27(2):107–110.

35. Inouye SK, Charpentier PA. Precipitating factors for delirium in hospitalized elderly persons. Predictive model and inter-relationship with baseline vulnerability. *JAMA.* 1996;275:852–857.

36. Inouye SK, Bogardu ST, Baker DI, et al. The hospital elder life program: a model of care to prevent cognitive and functional decline in older hospitalized patients. *J Am Geriatr Soc.* 2000;48:1697–1706.

37. Fedarko NS, Shapiro JR. Physiologic changes in the soft tissue and bone as a function of age. In: Rosenthal RA, Zenilman ME, Katlic MR, eds. *Principles and Practice of Geriatric Surgery.* New York: Springer-Verlag; 2000:850–866.

38. Phillips LG. Wound healing. In: Townsend CM, et al, eds. *Sabiston Textbook of Surgery*, 16th Ed. Philadelphia: Saunders; 2000:131–144.

39. Jacobs DO, Lara TM. Nutrition, metabolism and wound healing in the elderly. In: Rosenthal RA, Zenilman ME, Katlic MR, eds. *Principles and Practice of Geriatric Surgery.* New York: Springer-Verlag; 2000:65–87.

40. Ashcroft GS, Horan MA, Ferguson MWJ. Aging alters the inflammatory and endothelial cell adhesion profiles during human cutaneous wound healing. *Lab Investig.* 1998;78: 47–58.

41. Ashcroft GS, Horan MA, Ferguson MWJ. Aging is associated with reduced deposition of specific extracellular matrix components, and upregulation of angiogenesis and an altered inflammatory response in murine incisional wound healing model. *J Investig Dermatol.* 1997;108:430–437.

42. Cohen BJ, Danon D, Roth GS. Wound repair in mice as influenced by age and anti-macrophage serum. *J Gerontol.* 1987;42:295–301.

43. Marcus JR, Tyrone JW, Bonomo S, et al. Cellular mechanisms for diminished scarring with aging. *Plast Reconstr Surg.* 2000;105:1591–1599.

44. Danon D, Kowatch MA, Roth GS. Promotion of wound repair in old mice by local injection of macrophages. *Proc Natl Acad Sci USA.* 1989;86:2018–2020.

45. Rattan SI, Derventzi A. Altered cellular responsiveness during ageing. *Bioessays.* 1991;13:601–606.

46. Phillips PD, Kaji K, Cristofalo VJ. Progressive loss of proliferative response of senescing WI-38 cells to platelet derived growth factors, epidermal growth factor, insulin, transferrin, and dexamethasone. *J Gerontol.* 1984;39:11–17.

47. Holt DR, Kirk SJ, Regan MC, et al. Effect of age on wound healing in healthy human beings. *Surgery.* 1992;112:293–298.

48. Grove GL, Kligman AM. Age-associated changes in human epidermal cell renewal. *J Gerontol.* 1983;38:137–142.

49. Holm-Pedersen P, Zederfeldt B. Strength development in skin incisions in young and old rats. *Scand J Plast Reconstr Surg.* 1971;5:7–12.

50. Stoop MJ, Dirksen R, Hendriks T. Advanced age alone does not suppress healing in the intestines. *Surgery.* 1996;119:15–19.

51. Jonsson K, Jensen JA, Goodson WH, et al. Tissue oxygenation, anemia, and perfusion in relation to wound healing in surgical patients. *Ann Surg.* 1991;214:605–613.

52. Whitney JA, Heitkemper MM. Modifying perfusion, nutrition and stress to promote wound healing in patients with acute wounds. *Heart Lung.* 1999;28:123–133.

53. Knighton DR, Sliver IA, Hunt TK. Regulation of wound healing angiogensis—effect of oxygen gradients and inspired oxygen concentration. *Surgery.* 1981;90:262–269.

54. Pai MP, Hunt TK. Effect of varying oxygen tensions on healing of open wounds. *Surg Gynecol Obstet.* 1972;135: 756–758.

55. Quirina A, Viidik A. The influence of age on the healing of normal and ischemic incisional skin wounds. *Mech Ageing Dev.* 1991;58:221–232.

56. Hohn DC, Mackay RD, Halliday BJ, Hunt TK. Effect of O$_2$ tension on microbial function of leukocytes and wounds and in vitro. *Surg Forum.* 1976;27:18–20.

57. Hopf HW, Hunt TK, West JA, et al. Wound tissue oxygen predicts the risk of wound infection in surgical patients. *Arch Surg.* 1997;132:997–1004.

58. Thornton FJ, Ahrendt GM, Schaffer MR, et al. Sepsis impairs anastamotic collagen gene expression and synthesis: a possible role for nitric oxide. *J Surg Res.* 1997;69: 81–86.

59. Bentzen A, Vejlagaard R. Asymptomatic bacteriuria in the elderly subject. *Dan Med Bull.* 1980;27:101–105.

60. Hartmann M, Jonsson K, Zederfeldt B. Effects of tissue perfusion and oxygenation on the accumulation of collagen in healing wounds. *Eur J Surg.* 1992;158:521–526.

61. Rosenthal RA, Zenilman ME. Surgery in the elderly. In: Townsend CM, et al, eds. *Sabiston Textbook of Surgery*, 16th ed. Philadelphia: Saunders; 2000:226–246.

62. Kurtz A, Sessler DI, Rainer L. Perioperative normothermia to reduce the incidence of surgical wound infection and shorten hospitalization. *N Engl J Med.* 1996;334: 1209–1215.

63. Frank SM, Fleisher LA, Breslow MJ, et al. Perioperative maintenance of normothermia reduces the incidence of morbid cardiac events: a randomized clinical trial. *JAMA.* 1997;277:1127–1134.

64. Perler BA, Christopherson R, Rosenfeld BA, et al. The influence of anethestic method on infringuinal graft patency: a closer look. *Amer Surg.* 1995;61:784–789.

65. Chang N, Goodson WH, Gottrup F, Hunt TK. Direct mea-

surement of wound and tissue oxygen tension in post-operative patients. *Ann Surg*. 1983;197:470–478.

66. Haydock DA, Hill GL. Impaired wound healing in surgical patients with varying degrees of malnutrition. *J Parenter Enteral Nutr*. 1986;10:150–154.

67. Beattie AH, Prach AT, Baxter JP, Pennington CR. A randomized controlled trial evaluating the use of enteral nutritional supplements postoperatively in malnourished surgical patients. *Gut*. 2000;46:813–818.

68. MacFie J, Woodcock NP, Palmer MD, et al. Oral dietary supplement in pre- and postoperative surgical patients: a prospective randomized clinical trial. *Nutrition*. 2000;16:723–728.

69. Haydock DA, Hill GL. Improved wound healing response in surgical patients receiving intravenous nutrition. *Br J Surg*. 1987;74:320–323.

70. Windsor JA, Knight GS, Hill GS. Wound healing response in surgical patients: recent food intake is more important than nutritional status. *Br J Surg*. 1988;75:135–137.

71. Barbul A, Rettura G, Leveson S, et al. Wound healing and thymotrophic effects of arginine; a pituitary mechanism of action. *Am J Clin Nutr*. 1983;37:786–794.

72. Barbul A, Lazarou SA, Efron DT, et al. Arginine enhances wound healing and lymphocyte immune responses in humans. *Surgery*. 1990;108:331–337.

73. Hurson M, Regan MC, Kirk SJ, et al. Metabolic effects of arginine in a healthy elderly population. *J Parenter Enteral Nutr*. 1995;19:227–230.

74. Barbul A. Role of the immune system. In: Cohen IK, Diegelmann RF, Lindblad WJ, eds. *Wound Healing: Biochemical and Clinical Aspects*. Philadelphia: Saunders; 1992:282–291.

75. Schaffer MR, Tantry U, Ahrendt GM, et al. Acute protein-calorie malnutrition impairs wound healing: a possible role of decreased wound nitric oxide synthesis. *J Am Coll Surg*. 1997;184:37–43.

76. Belcher HJRC, Ellis H. Somatropin and wound healing after injury. *J Clin Endocrinol Metab*. 1990;70:939–943.

77. Christensen H, Oxlund H. Growth hormone increases the collagen deposition rate and breaking strength of the left colonic anastamoses in rats. *Surgery*. 1994;116:550–556.

78. Herndon DN, Barrow RE, Kunkel KR, et al. Effects of recombinant human growth hormone on donor-site healing in severely burned children. *Ann Surg*. 1990;212:424–431.

79. Herndon DR, Pierre EJ, Stokes KN, et al. Growth hormone treatment for burned children. *Horm Res*. 1996;45(suppl 1):29–31.

80. Bell R, Rosenthal RA. Surgery in the elderly. In: Hazzard WR, Blass JP, Ettinger WH, et al, eds. *Principles of Geriatric Medicine and Gerontology*, 4th Ed. New York: Mc Graw-Hill; 1999:391–412.

81. Rosenthal RA, Andersen DK. Surgery in the elderly: observations on the pathophysiology and treatment of cholelithiasis. *Exp Gerontol*. 1993;28:459–464.

82. Morrow DJ, Thompson J, Wilson SE. Acute cholecystitis on the elderly. *Arch Surg*. 1978;113:1149–1153.

83. Thornton SC. Diverticulitis and appendicitis in the elderly. In: Rosenthal RA, Zenilman ME, Katlic MR, eds. *Princi-*

ples and Practice of Geriatric Surgery. New York: Springer-Verlag; 2000:620–634.

84. Fried GM, Clas D, Meakins JL. Minimally invasive surgery in the elderly. *Surg Clin North Am*. 1994;74:375–384.

85. Stalnikowicz R, Eliakim R, Diab R. Crohn's disease in the elderly. *J Clin Gastroenterol*. 1989;11:411–415.

86. Rosenthal RA. Small-bowel disorders and abdominal wall hernia in the elderly patient. *Surg Clin North Am*. 1994;74:261–291.

87. Hansen N, Morrow M. Breast cancer in elderly women. In: Rosenthal RA, Zenilman ME, Katlic MR, eds. *Principles and Practice of Geriatric Surgery*. New York: Springer-Verlag; 2000:331–342.

88. Coluccia C, Ricci EB, Marzola GG, et al. Gastric cancer in the elderly: results of surgical treatment. *Int Surg*. 1987;72:4–9.

89. Trimble EL, Carter CL, Cain D, et al. Representation of older patients in cancer treatment trials. *Cancer*. 1994;74:2208–2212.

90. The Interdisciplinary Leadership Group of the American Geriatric Society Project to Increase Geriatric Expertise in Surgical and Medical Specialties. A statement of principles: toward improving care of older patients in surgical and medical specialties. *Ann Long Term Care*. 2000;8:21–24.

91. Kniffin WD, Baron JA, Barrett J, et al. The epidemiology of diagnosed pulmonary embolism and deep venous thrombosis in the elderly. *Arch Intern Med*. 1994;154:861–866.

92. Ibbotson SH, Tate GH, Davies JA. Thrombin activity by intrinsic activation of plasma in vitro acceleration with increasing age of the donor. *Thromb Haemost*. 1992;67:377–380.

93. Clagett GP, Anderson FA, Geerts W, et al. Prevention of venous thromboembolism. *Chest*. 1998;114(suppl):531s–560s.

94. Chan ED, Welsh CH. Geriatric respiratory medicine. *Chest*. 1998;114:1704–1733.

95. Turpie AGG, Gallus AS, Hoek JA, for the pentasaccharide investigators. A synthetic pentasaccharide for the prevention of deep-vein thrombosis after total hip replacement. *N Engl J Med*. 2001;344:619–625.

96. Mangram AJ, Horan TC, Pearson ML, et al. Guidelines for the prevention of surgical site infection, 1999. *Infect Control Hosp Epidemiol*. 1999;20:247–278.

97. Nichols RL, Smith JW, Garcia RY, et al. Current practices of preoperative bowel preparation among North American colorectal surgeons. *Clin Infect Dis*. 1997;24:609–619.

98. Niederman M, Fein A. Community-acquired pneumonia in the elderly. In: Niederman M, ed. *Respiratory Infections in the Elderly*. New York: Raven Press; 1991:45–72.

99. DeVita MA, Spierer-Runback L. Swallowing disorders in patients with prolonged orotracheal intubation or tracheostomy tubes. *Crit Care Med*. 1990;14:1328–1330.

100. Hogue CW, Lappas GD, Creswell LL, et al. Swallowing dysfunction after cardiac operations. *J Thorac Cardiovasc Surg*. 1995;110:517–522.

101. Rousou JA, Tighe DA, Garb JL, et al. Risk of dysphagia after transesophageal echocardiography during cardiac operations. *Ann Thorac Surg*. 2000;69:486–490.

102. Cheatham ML, Chapman WC, Key SP, Sawyers JL. A meta-analysis of selective versus routine nasogastric decompression after elective laparotomy. *Ann Surg*. 1995; 221:476–478.

103. Peters JH, Katkhouda N. Physiology of laparoscopic surgery. In: Rosenthal RA, Zenilman ME, Katlic MR, eds. *Principles and Practice of Geriatric Surgery*. New York: Springer-Verlag; 2000;331–342:1021–1035.

104. Rosenthal RA. Laparoscopic surgery in the elderly. In: Merrell RC, ed. Laparoscopic surgery: a colloquium. New York: Springer-Verlag; 1998:186–196.

105. Brunt LM, Soper NJ. Outcomes of minimal access vs. open surgical procedures in the elderly. In: Rosenthal RA, Zenilman ME, Katlic MR, eds. *Principles and Practice of Geriatric Surgery*. New York: Springer-Verlag; 2000: 1036–1053.

106. Lujan JA, Sachez-Bueno F, Parrilla P, et al. Laparoscopic vs. open cholecystectomy in patients aged 65 and older. *Surg Laparosc Endosc*. 1998;8:208–210.

107. Jones DB, Soper NJ, Brunt M, et al. Effect of age and ASA status on the outcome of laparoscopic cholecystectomy. *Surg Endosc*. 1996;10:238 [abstract].

108. Lo C, Lai E, Fan S, et al. Laparoscopic cholecystectomy for acute cholecystitis in the elderly. *World J Surg*. 1996;20: 983–987.

109. Stocchi L, Nelson H, Young-Fadok, et al. Safety and advantages of laparoscopic vs. open colectomy in the elderly: matched-control study. *Dis Colon Rectum*. 2000;43:326–332.

110. Jaklitsch MT, Bueno R, Swanson SJ, et al. New surgical options for elderly lung cancer patients. *Chest*. 1999;116(suppl):480s–485s.

111. Hsu TH, Fazeli-Matin S, Soble JJ, et al. Radical nephrectomy and nephrouretectomy in the octogenarian and nonagenarian. Comparison of laparosocpic and open approaches. *Urology*. 1999;53:1121–1125.

112. Kannel WB, Dannenberg AV, Abbott RD. Unrecognized myocardial infarction and hypertension: Framingham study. *Am Heart J*. 1985;109:581–585.

113. Clinch D, Banerjee AK, Ostick G. Absence of abdominal pain in the elderly with peptic ulcer. *Age Ageing*. 1985;13: 120–123.

114. Morrison RS, Carney MT, Manfredi PL. Pain management. In: Rosenthal RA, Zenilman ME, Katlic MR, eds. *Principles and Practice of Geriatric Surgery*. New York: Springer-Verlag; 2000:160–173.

115. Yeager M, Glass D, Neff R, et al. Epidural anesthesia and analgesia in high risk surgical patients. *Anesthesiology*. 1987;66:729–736.

116. Egbert A, Parks L, Short L, et al. Randomized trial of postoperative patient-controlled analgesia vs. intramuscular narcotics in frail elderly men. *Arch Intern Med*. 1990; 150:1897–1903.

23
Rehabilitation

Kenneth Brummel-Smith

Rehabilitation is a process of care directed at restoring or maintaining a person's ability to live independently. Interventions are directed at helping the patient to recover from and adapt to the loss of physical, psychologic, or social skills lost as a result of illness or trauma. This chapter primarily considers rehabilitation from physical illnesses, but geriatrics always involves attention to the psychologic and social aspects of care.

Disability is a common problem among older Americans. Kunkel and Applebaum estimated that by the year 2020, between 9.7 and 13.6 million older people will have moderate to severe disability, an increase of 85% to 167% over current levels.[1] Clinical geriatrics emphasizes the "functional approach" in the care of the patient. By enhancing the person's functional abilities, the impact of a disability can be lessened. Rehabilitation is a basic foundation of geriatric care. All health care providers should promote a rehabilitation orientation when caring for older persons.[2]

Ultimately, those receiving rehabilitation hope to live in personally satisfying environments and maintain meaningful social relationships. In geriatrics, rehabilitation shifts from a goal of returning the patient to gainful employment to helping the older person live more independently. This type of care can be provided in any health care setting, including the home, office, acute or rehabilitation hospital, and long-term care facility. An interdisciplinary team approach is required because of the complex nature of the various interventions. Patients and their families must be involved in decisions regarding rehabilitation treatment.

Rehabilitation is a philosophic approach to the patient that recognizes that improvement in functional abilities is an important goal of medicine, that having a disability does not diminish one's social worth, and that the psychosocial aspects of care are at least as important as its medical aspects. Rehabilitation is an essential component of quality geriatric care that should be available to all those who might benefit. The American Geriatrics Society has recognized the importance of rehabilitation in a position statement.[3] The Society has also proposed training guidelines in rehabilitation for geriatric fellows.[4] All persons caring for older patients should have some knowledge of rehabilitation.[5]

Functional disability had been on the rise for a number of years but appears to be decreasing.[6] The 1994 National Long Term Care Survey showed the overall prevalence of disability (21.3%) to have fallen by 3.6% from 1982. However, the rate of disability in individuals increases markedly with age. In 1995, among noninstitutionalized persons over the age of 70, 32% had difficulty performing and 25% were unable to perform at least one of nine physical activities, such as dressing or bathing.[7] Activity limitations increase with age and are more prevalent in females and in African-Americans. Those persons over age 85 are 2.6 times as likely to be unable to perform physical activities.

Disability is costly, consuming more than $170 billion per year.[8] Rehabilitation services are but one part of that cost. Equipment use in disabling conditions is common and expensive. Most elderly patients with disability require assistance from family members or special community services. At higher levels of disability [>3 activities of daily living (ADLs) impaired], either personal assistance only or equipment use only appeared insufficient to support the patient remaining in the community.[9] Disability measures strongly predict cost of Medicare services.[10]

Definitions of Disability

The World Health Organization's classification system is useful when discussing geriatric rehabilitation[11] (Table 23.1). In this system, *disease* refers to intrinsic pathology that may or may not be evident clinically. *Impairment* refers to alterations of function at the organ level. Older persons may have many impairments. Some physiologic

TABLE 23.1. World Health Organization definitions of disability.

- Disease—an intrinsic pathology or disorder . . . [which] may or may not make [itself] evident clinically
- Impairment—a loss or abnormality of structure or function at the organ system level
- Disability—a restriction or lack of ability to perform an activity in a normal manner, a disturbance in the performance of daily tasks
- Handicap—a disadvantage resulting from impairment or disability that limits or prevents fulfillment of a role that is normal

decline in organ function is seen in almost all systems. These declinations, however, may not affect the person's ability to perform daily activities. An impairment severe enough to affect the person's daily functioning is a *disability*. When persons with disability have received appropriate rehabilitation training and have adapted to the change in functional status, they often can be fully independent. However, if subjected to policies that limit rehabilitation interventions or services because of age, these persons become *handicapped*. Therefore, by this definition, there are no handicapped persons; there are only handicapping societies. Unfortunately, there is evidence that such factors as race and hospital size can affect whether older people receive rehabilitation interventions.[12] Although this chapter is devoted to the problems of aged persons with a disability, the sociopolitical implications of rehabilitation must not be forgotten.

Demographics of Disability

A large percentage of persons with a disability are elderly. Conditions for which rehabilitation interventions are beneficial disproportionately affect the elderly population. Arthritis is the most common condition affecting older persons and the most common cause of disability.[13] The incidence of stroke peaks in the seventh and eighth decades.[14] The average 80-year-old white woman has a 1% to 2% risk of hip fracture per year.[15] Most amputations are performed in the geriatric age group.[16] Even without such catastrophic diagnoses, the prevalence of limited activities due to chronic conditions is very high, particularly in those over age 75.

The type of disability also is important in the way it affects the caregiving system. A decreased ability to walk, feed, or toilet indicates greater dependency and increases the burden on caregivers. The decision to institutionalize an older family member is very much related to the level of disability, in that a greater burden of illness creates greater needs for care. Interventions designed to enhance functional abilities and support caregivers have been shown to be cost-effective and lead to fewer hospitalizations, greater levels of independence, and lower mortal-

ity.[17] Access to rehabilitation for older persons, however, is sometimes restrictive. The prospective payment systems for reimbursement for acute care and short hospital stays provide disincentives for physicians and hospitals to offer rehabilitation interventions while the patient is in the hospital. A study of attitudes and knowledge of a large sample of policy makers in the federal and state governments indicated that comprehensive rehabilitation programs were widely unavailable because few of these officials considered it a priority need.[18]

Rehabilitation Principles

Components of Rehabilitation

Rehabilitation comprises a number of components of care, as summarized in Table 23.2. Each of these components requires special attention in geriatric patients. With older persons, it is not always possible to completely stabilize the primary problem. Furthermore, there often is more than one "primary problem." An 80-year-old man with a recent amputation may have underlying cardiac disease, diabetes, and mild renal failure, necessitating close supervision by the geriatric provider during an inpatient rehabilitation stay. He also may be more prone to secondary complications than a younger person. Preventing such complications is crucial in geriatric populations because of the remarkable ease with which such events develop and the great risks involved. Secondary complications are frequently seen in older patients, including such conditions as falls, pressure sores, deep venous thrombosis, contractures, deconditioning, malnutrition, incontinence, family discord, and depression.

These complications also disproportionately affect older patients. Decreased subcutaneous fat, poor capillary function, and low blood volumes increase the risk of developing pressure sores. Besides adding great costs to the care of the patient, a sacral pressure sore may delay wheelchair training after a stroke. The enforced lack of exercise may then increase the risk of other secondary complications, such as deconditioning or psychologic dependence. Contractures, that is, muscle shortening causing a decrease in the functional range of motion, begins to develop within 24 h of the cessation of activity. Some contractures may lead to permanent disability,

TABLE 23.2. Components of rehabilitation.

- Stabilize the primary disorder
- Prevent secondary complications
- Treat functional deficits
- Promote adaptation:
    - Adaptation of the person to their disability
    - Adaptation of the environment to the person
    - Adaptation of the family to the person

TABLE 23.3. Tools for activities of daily living.

- Bathing—handheld shower hoses, bath seats and benches, long-handled scrubbers, grab bars
- Ambulation—canes, walkers, special shoes, wheelchairs
- Toileting—raised toilet seats, arm attachments, grab bars
- Transfers—side rails, sliding boards, trapeze bars
- Eating—large-handle utensils, rocker knives, plate guards, plate holders, hand braces
- Dressing—button hooks, Velcro closures, sock-donners, clothes hooks

while others may require months of intense physical therapy and serial casting to recover the full range of motion. Muscle strength rapidly declines with acute immobilization or chronic decreased physical activity.[19] Recovery of lost strength occurs at a much slower rate. Last, the quality of "help" given may contribute to the development of secondary complications. Patients encouraged to maintain activities of daily living may lose abilities less rapidly than those who are helped with all such activities.[20] A conscious effort by all members of the team, including the patient, is required to prevent the development of secondary disabilities.

The foundation of rehabilitation is the restoration of lost functional abilities. By using directed exercises, with the assistance of physical, occupational, and often communication therapists, the patient can "relearn" how to carry out daily activities. Various adaptive equipment, such as rocker knives, sock-donners, and dressing sticks have been shown in randomized trials to enable a person to function independently and reduce health care costs[21] (Table 23.3).

Another key component in geriatric rehabilitation is adaptation of the environment to the disabled person. The older person may be less able than a younger person to maintain an activity that is extremely demanding physiologically. For instance, a 20-year-old paraplegic may be able to walk using canes and braces. An 80-year-old with spinal stenosis and diminished cardiac reserve most often needs to learn wheelchair mobility skills. Similarly, the evaluation of the home environment plays an important

role in geriatrics. Financial concerns and personal preferences may limit opportunities for obtaining new housing or for modifying the home.

Finally, the family must be assisted in the adaptation and support of the older person with a disability. The family provides 85% of all health care for dependent elders.[22] Often the caregivers themselves are elderly (spouses and older children). Families play a vital role in determining rehabilitation outcomes. Families may perceive the disability as a threat, or as a challenge, or be overwhelmed by it. They will cope using the preexisting rules and roles that existed before the disability.[23] In a study of outcomes in a geriatric rehabilitation unit, 78% of the patients who had family members that participated in the inpatient program returned home, whereas only 54% of those patients whose families did not participate returned to the home setting.[24] Rehabilitation in the home prevents hospitalizations and nursing home use.[25] The approach to the training of family caregivers is similar to that used with other students. Their knowledge regarding the disabilities and caregiving needs must be assessed and enhanced, their skills in providing care should be evaluated, and their attitudes toward the caregiving role should be elicited.

In summary, each component of rehabilitation must receive attention from a team of clinicians to ensure that the greatest level of functional independence is achieved.

Rehabilitation Teams

Both multidisciplinary and interdisciplinary teams are used in rehabilitation (Table 23.4). Geriatric providers and physiatrists (specialists in physical medicine and rehabilitation) are often involved in interdisciplinary teams, while most primary care physicians function in a multidisciplinary setting. A multidisciplinary team works in a consulting relationship, each person seeing the patient individually and communicating with other team members by written notes or telephone calls. The decision to involve other team members usually is made by the physician. An interdisciplinary team functions in a

TABLE 23.4. Roles of selected team members.

- Physiatrist—provides consultation regarding complex functional limitations and interventions to improve function; conducts diagnostic tests such as nerve conduction studies and may perform invasive interventions such as nerve blocks
- Physical therapist—deals with problems in mobility and transfers, gait training, use of braces for mobility; involved in training in the use of canes, walkers, and wheelchairs
- Occupational therapist—works with patient to improve skills in activities of daily living, uses a variety of interventions, and teaches the patient how to use assistive devices for ADL; may also produce or train in the use of splints
- Recreation therapist—helps the patient to recover or learn new skills in vocational activities (many older adults continue to have vocational activities, extending from volunteer work to income-generating activities)
- Speech and language pathologist—helps the patient to improve communication skills; trains patient to use alternative forms of communication if needed; may be involved in swallowing programs
- Orthotist—fashions braces and splints
- Rehabilitation nurse—in addition to providing nursing care, assists the patient in utilizing new techniques learned from the above-mentioned therapists; involved in family training

setting where all team members can meet periodically to discuss the patient's problems and progress. Although each team member has a specific area of expertise, often there is considerable overlap in roles. With more complex cases, such as those seen in inpatient or long-term care rehabilitation, an interdisciplinary team is usually required.

Different team members address specific areas of functioning. Speech and language pathologists or communication disorders specialists do much more than help people talk. In addition to training patients in a wide variety of communication techniques and helping the family adapt to the patient's communication needs, they assess cognitive skills. Occupational therapists are primarily concerned with assessment and treatment of the patient's deficits in basic and instrumental activities of daily living. Cognitive retraining programs, as well as perceptual and sensory evaluations, are also provided by occupational therapists. Some occupational therapists can assist the geriatric provider by providing driver training and by making recommendations for automobile modifications.[26]

Physical therapists assess strength, range of motion, coordination, balance, and gait, but these are only a few of the services they provide. Some also assess bulbar function and provide swallowing training programs. The use of electrical stimulation for functional activities and pain control often is managed by physical therapists. Retraining in ambulation, the use of walking aids (canes and walkers), general strengthening, and wheelchair mobility are within the province of physical therapists. As there are hundreds of types of wheelchairs, these are best prescribed by physical therapists. Many of these activities are also conducted by kinesiotherapists, particularly in Veterans Administration hospitals.

Recreation therapists serve an important role in geriatric rehabilitation. The ability to resume one's favorite leisure activity can be a powerful force encouraging participation in the rehabilitation program. The quality of life can be greatly enhanced by the resumption or learning anew of hobbies and enjoyable activities.

Each of these specialists has specific requirements for certification or registration. Most have certified aides, assistants, or technicians who provide some portion of the therapeutic program under the supervision of the registered therapist. In some states, physical and occupational therapists are in private practice and available for outpatient consultation and referral. When this is not the case, consultation can be obtained by referral to the appropriate hospital department.

Rehabilitation nurses play a crucial role in promoting the gains made by all the other therapists. Besides attending to the patient's nursing needs, they help the patient practice activities of daily living, make transfers in and out of bed or to the toilet, and learn new medication regimens. They also train family members in caregiving skills and encourage patients and their families to bring up questions, discuss concerns and fears, and learn to cope with disability.[27]

Ideally, team members should meet periodically to discuss their assessments, establish goals, provide updates on progress toward those goals, and estimate the length of the program needed to meet the goals. A written summary of the meeting is placed in the patient's record. Some teams also provide a copy to the patient and the family.

Every attempt should be made to incorporate the patient and family into the rehabilitation process. Patients often find attendance at team meetings to be stressful. Many teams regularly report the patient's and family members' views of the course of rehabilitation and facilitate a discussion after a team meeting.

The role of the physician on the team is to provide medical expertise and often to serve as facilitator of the team process. Physicians must be extremely careful in this dual role as both the "expert" and the "facilitator." Hierarchical relationships are common in medical settings, and the physician-expert may inhibit the functioning of other team members. If that happens, the flow of information necessary to make critical decisions may be impeded. Although the final responsibility of the clinical decision rests with physicians, they must always promote the reasoned deliberation of other team members. Group communication skills and knowledge of team dynamics, attributes often ignored in medical school training, are important for efficient and mutually satisfying teamwork.

Rehabilitation in Different Care Sites

Rehabilitation interventions can be provided in a variety of continuing care sites (Table 23.5). Medicare covers most of these services, but Medicaid's reimbursement policies vary from state to state. Medicare and most third-party reimbursement requires that there be documenta-

TABLE 23.5. Sites for rehabilitation.

- Home—requires a committed in-home caregiver, reasonably accessible (or modifiable) environment, and access to home health services
- Outpatient facility—requires a dependable means of transportation, enough medical stability to tolerate outings into the community, reasonable cognition to retain newly learned information between visits
- Nursing home—best if a rehabilitation-oriented facility, needs dependable access to therapists, burden of documentation by physicians and therapy staff is high
- Acute hospital—limited time available for providing rehabilitation; even small amounts of therapy may be beneficial; attention should be paid to limiting functional decline
- Rehabilitation hospital—intensive services (minimum 3 h/day) may limit ability of frail elders to participate; evidence that greatest gains in stroke rehabilitation happen in this setting

tion that the patient is progressing toward goals and that therapy must not be used for "maintenance" of function only. Algorithms have been developed for determining the proper site of rehabilitation for older persons with functional decline[5] and for stroke.[28]

An ideal site for providing rehabilitation is the patient's home.[29] The problem of transportation is relieved, and services can be rendered at lower costs than in hospitals. In a small, randomized trial in England, patients with stroke who received rehabilitation at home had similar outcomes, at lower costs, than those treated in the hospital.[30] The patient's ability to function in a familiar environment with available equipment can be assessed, the family is usually supportive, and carryover of techniques taught during therapy can be monitored. In one study, patients cared for at home obtained the greatest degree of functional improvement from home modifications, the next best improvement from instruction in the proper use of assistive aid devices, and the least from exercises.[31] For the patient thought to be able to benefit from rehabilitation in outpatient settings but unable to attend clinics because of transportation difficulties, limited endurance, psychologic reasons, or personal choice, home care is a valuable option.

Outpatient centers provide a large proportion of rehabilitation services. These centers may be found in physicians' offices, private physical (and occupational) therapy practices, Certified Outpatient Rehabilitation Facilities (CORF), day health centers, specialized senior clinics,[32] and hospital-affiliated facilities. Their advantages are (1) access to a wider variety of practitioners and technology, (2) the stimulation for patients of being around other people (a disadvantage to some patients with cognitive deficits), and (3) their ability to serve more patients with fewer practitioners. Transportation to the clinic often is a major problem with the very old.

Perhaps the greatest unmet need for rehabilitation is in the acute hospital. The potential negative effects of acute hospitalization have been well documented.[33–35] Many elderly patients have difficulties with activities of daily living, and the hospital environment itself may interfere with functional recovery. With the advent of prospective payment, patients are being discharged "quicker and sicker." It is essential to obtain early allied health consultation and discharge planning. When possible, patients should be kept out of their beds, walked to the bathroom or diagnostic studies, and encouraged to dress and feed themselves.

The classic site for providing rehabilitation is the specialized rehabilitation unit. Such facilities may be freestanding or affiliated with an acute hospital. A full complement of rehabilitation specialists is on site. Usually, a physiatrist (or, in the case of geriatric rehabilitation units, a geriatrician) coordinates the team. To receive Medicare reimbursement, patients must undergo 3 h per day of physical, occupational, or speech therapy and must make regular progress toward specific goals. Periodic team meetings are held at least biweekly, and progress must be documented in the chart. Because of these criteria, older persons may have restricted access to inpatient programs. In one study, only 21% of patients who met criteria for rehabilitation actually received rehabilitation services. At follow-up, those participants in rehabilitation had lower mortality, spent less time in skilled nursing care, and were less frequently hospitalized.[36] With the expansion of the use of health maintenance organizations (HMOs), there has been a decrease in the use of hospital-based rehabilitation units.[37,38] In part, this change is based upon there being little evidence from randomized controlled trials that specialized units provide added benefits. In fact, although the Agency for Health Care Policy and Research (AHCPR) algorithm for choice of a rehabilitation unit appears to function reasonably well,[39] the factors that guide choices were all based solely upon expert opinion.

Some hospitals have developed specialized geriatric rehabilitation units. Patients at moderate, rather than high, risk for nursing home placement appear to do the best in geriatric rehabilitation units. In a randomized trial, such patients had improved function, fewer nursing home placements, and a trend toward reduced mortality when compared to older patients cared for in traditional hospital units.[40] Geriatric-orthopedic units[41] have shown similar success, as have stroke rehabilitation units,[42] although there is controversy whether they offer benefits over traditional rehabilitation units. Geriatric rehabilitation has been shown to be effective,[43,44] and age need not be a deterrent to providing rehabilitation. In a prospective evaluation of factors that may predict rehabilitation outcomes, Rondinelli et al. were able to show that age was not a good predictor of outcomes (length of stay or functional improvement).[45] Preadmission functional status and social supports were strong predictors, as would be expected.

The nursing home is another important site for providing rehabilitation.[46] For patients in a skilled facility requiring physical, occupational, and speech therapy, Medicare reimbursement is available. With implementation of the Balanced Budget Act of 1997, changes in Medicare reimbursement have led to an increase in the number of nursing homes providing rehabilitation services.[47,48] In fact, the highest rate of Medicare reimbursement is provided for the most complex rehabilitation patient. Some community-dwelling elderly persons may be able to use the nursing home as a primary site of rehabilitation because of the slower pace allowed. However, in the fee-for-service setting, current Medicare regulations require a 3-day stay in an acute hospital before allowing reimbursement. This requirement is waived for HMOs, so direct admission to a nursing home can be arranged. Outcomes from nursing home rehabilitation are beginning to be demonstrated with various studies showing improvements in mobility and the use of assistive devices,[40] muscle strength and gait velocity,[50] and general activity levels.[51]

It is possible, however, that nursing home-based rehabilitation is less effective than hospital-based programs. A recent study compared patients admitted either to a skilled nursing facility or to a rehabilitation facility for treatment of stroke or hip fracture. Patients were matched according to seven groups of patient characteristics: basic demographics; social support measures; premorbid functional status, using the ADL index; acute medical or surgical characteristics; conditions at admission to rehabilitation, derived from nursing staff or patient record; functional status at rehabilitation admission, using the number of ADL dependencies and the Barthel index; and cognitive and psychologic status, assessed using Mini-Mental State Exam and Geriatric Depression Scale (GDS) scale scores. Enhanced outcomes were found for elderly patients with stroke who were treated in rehabilitation hospitals, but not for patients with hip fracture. Rehabilitation-oriented nursing homes were more effective than traditional nursing homes in returning patients with stroke to the community, despite comparable functional outcomes.[52]

Assessment for Rehabilitation Potential

The first step in the assessment for rehabilitation potential is awareness that rehabilitation interventions may be of benefit. Once that idea is entertained, a number of features must be considered. Factors associated with a better prognosis include recent (rather than long-term) health changes, less severe deficits, an assertive personality, a supportive family system, and adequate economic resources. A poorer prognosis exists for patients with low motivation, more severe health problems (especially if associated with cognitive impairments), and inadequate economic resources or support systems. However, because of the great variability seen in older persons, no single factor should automatically exclude a person from a trial of rehabilitation interventions.

When there is doubt, the patient should undergo a comprehensive assessment before a final determination is made. The assessment should identify what demands the patient will encounter in the expected living environment and whether he or she has the ability to meet those demands. A complete assessment includes evaluation of the patient's physical impairments, cognitive and psychologic functioning, the social environment, and economic resources.[53] The patient's prior levels of functioning and present capabilities should both be determined.

Two scales have been widely used to measure progress in rehabilitation. The oldest is the Barthel index[54] (Table 23.6). Using this 100-point scale, some investigators have

TABLE 23.6. Barthel index.

Activity	Score
Bowels	0 = incontinent (or needs to be given enemas) 5 = occasional accident 10 = continent
Bladder	0 = incontinent, or catheterized and unable to manage alone 5 = occasional accident 10 = continent
Grooming	0 = needs help with personal care 5 = independent face/hair/teeth/shaving (implements provided)
Toilet use	0 = dependent 5 = needs some help, but can do some things alone 10 = independent (on and off, dressing, wiping)
Feeding	0 = unable 5 = needs help cutting, etc., or requires modified diet 10 = independent
Transfers (bed to chair and back)	0 = unable, no sitting balance 5 = major help (one or two people, physical), can sit 10 = minor help (verbal or physical) 15 = independent
Mobility (on level surfaces)	0 = immobile or <50 yards 5 = wheelchair independent, including corners, >50 yards 10 = walks with help of one person (verbal or physical), >50 yards 15 = independent (but may use any aid; for example, stick), >50 yards
Dressing	0 = dependent 5 = needs help but can do about half unaided 10 = independent (including buttons, zips, laces)
Stairs	0 = unable 5 = needs help (verbal, physical, carrying aid) 10 = independent
Bathing	0 = dependent 5 = independent (or in shower)
Total (0–100)	

Source: Adapted from Mahoney and Barthil,[54] with permission.

shown that discharge to home is unlikely with scores below 29 and very likely with scores above 60. The most widely used scale in rehabilitation at this time is the Functional Independence Measure (FIM)[55] (Table 23.7).

Rehabilitation of Common Geriatric Conditions

Stroke

Stroke is one of the most common conditions for which older people receive rehabilitation. (Risks, prevention, and early treatment of stroke are covered in Chapter 78.) Rehabilitation interventions begin during the acute hos-

TABLE 23.7. The functional independence measure (FIM): areas of assessment (A–R).

FIM (motor):
  Self-care
    A.   Self-care
    B.   Grooming
    C.   Bathing
    D.   Dressing upper body
    E.   Dressing lower body
    F.   Toileting
  Sphincter control
    G.   Bladder management
    H.   Bowel management
  Mobility (transfer)
    I.   Bed, chair, wheelchair
    J.   Toilet
    K.   Tub, shower
  Locomotion
    L.   Walk/wheelchair
    M.   Stairs

FIM (cognitive):
  Communication
    N.   Comprehension
    O.   Expression
  Social cognition
    P.   Social integration
    Q.   Problem solving
    R.   Memory

Scoring:
  Independence: 7—complete independence (timely, safely)
                       6—modified independence (device used)
  Modified dependence: 5—supervision
                       4—minimal assistance (subject performs >75% of task)
                       3—moderate assistance (subject performs 50%–74% of task)
                       2—maximal assistance (subject performs 25%–49% of task)
  Complete dependence: 1—total assistance (subject performs <25% of task)

Source: Adapted from Granger et al.,[55] with permission.

pital phase, primarily directed at preventing secondary complications. The geriatric provider will need to be involved in many aspects of the patient's care, in reducing ongoing risk factors, minimizing medications, providing the family with information, and care planning.

Although impairment and disability depend on the size, location, and nature of the offending lesion(s), functional return is to some degree dependent on chance. However, even in the case when the patient is fortunate to have significant return of motor or sensory function, the occurrence of a secondary disability may limit the maximum independence the patient may achieve. Hence, rehabilitation should be considered in all patients as they progress.

Most of the return of function is seen in the first month. In some cases, however, motor function may return as late as 6 months after the stroke. Sensory deficits or swallowing problems may improve later. In spite of these endogenous improvements, rehabilitation efforts following stroke are cost-effective and lead to higher functional levels.[56] A meta-analysis of rehabilitation research determined that the average person in treatment functioned better than 66% of the participants in the control group. ADL performance and visual-perceptual function improved the most consistently. Younger patients fared better than older, but gains were seen among the older subjects.[57] Age, by itself, does not affect rehabilitation outcome.[58]

Patients and their families need accurate prognostic information soon after the stroke to make informed decisions about care. They should be told that most patients survive infarcts and that the highest mortality is in the first week. Many survivors will have residual deficits longer than 6 to 12 months after the acute event (Table 23.8). Rehabilitation interventions help survivors adjust to these disabilities even if they cannot be eliminated through therapy.

Acute Care Phase

Initially, rehabilitation efforts are geared toward preventing secondary disabilities and identifying patients who need more intensive rehabilitation. Prevention of secondary disabilities should begin soon after admission. The patient must be turned regularly to prevent the development of pressure sores. Sitting up, daily range of motion of the extremities, and exercise of the uninvolved limbs to prevent deconditioning should be provided. Constipation or dehydration must be avoided. Although most have some urinary incontinence initially, patients with persistent problems should receive appropriate investigation for treatable causes (see Chapter 63).

Immediately after the stroke, the patient's affected limbs are often flaccid. The arm needs to be properly positioned to prevent subluxation of the shoulder, so that

TABLE 23.8. Neurologic deficits following stroke.

Neurological deficit	Finland (% at 12 months)	Framingham (% at 6 months)
Motor coordination	61	NR
Hemiparesis	37	48
Visual-perceptual deficits	41	NR
Memory deficits	31	NR
Aphasia	30	18
Depression	29	NR
Sensory deficits	NR	24
Dysarthria	21	16
Hemianopsia	NR	13
Incontinence	9	NR

NR, not reported.
Source: Adapted from Table 2, Epidemiology and natural history of stroke, in Gresham GE, Duncan PW, Stason WB, et al. Post-stroke rehabilitation: assessment, referral, and patient management. Clinical Practice Guideline: Quick reference guide for clinicians, No. 16. Rockville, MD: U.S. Department of Health and Human Services, Public Health Service, Agency for Health Care Policy and Research. AHCPR publication No. 95-0663, May 1995, with permission.

when motor function returns the arm will be more functional. Shoulder-hand syndrome (a form of reflex-sympathetic dystrophy) may be prevented by regular range of motion exercises ("ranging"), close attention to proper bed positioning, and protecting the shoulder when moving the patient. Systemic corticosteriods may be helpful in its treatment.[59] Proper body positioning will usually prevent nerve palsies from developing. The use of a footboard to prevent plantar flexion contractures is controversial and should not take the place of active ranging of the patient's ankles.

Predictions of eventual recovery are difficult during the acute phase. Factors associated with a poor prognosis include flaccid hemiplegia of more than 2 months duration, dementia, persistent bowel or bladder incontinence, severe neglect or sensory deficits, and global aphasia.[60] Certain features, such as a depressed caregiver, those caregivers not married to the patient, and family dysfunction have been shown to predict which patients may not benefit from home rehabilitation.[61]

The choice of which site, whether inpatient unit, nursing home, or the patient's home, to provide rehabilitation is complex. Recently, the algorithm provided in the Post-Stroke Rehabilitation Guidelines[28] has been evaluated and revised slightly[62] (Fig. 23.1). Rehabilitation "services" refer to a single discipline or type of therapy, whereas a rehabilitation "program" refers to multidisciplinary, coordinated services. The algorithm was found to have good reliability for home and nursing facility placement with rehabilitation services but with no multidisciplinary rehabilitation program. In fact, more than one type of placement was appropriate for 65% of patients. Hence, the most appropriate choice must often be negotiated between the clinician and the patient based upon patient-specific desires and available resources.

Rehabilitation Phase

Once the patient's condition is reasonably stable, intensive rehabilitation can begin. Total stability is elusive in the older person, and risks of an intervention must be weighed against risks of continued bed rest and deconditioning. Motor return follows a fairly predictable pattern. Initially, the limbs are flaccid with hyperactive reflexes. The next stage is mass flexor synergism; that is, the limb will flex at multiple joints when movement is attempted. A mass extensor synergism usually occurs next. Once the patient has an extensor synergy pattern, even with poor control, ambulation may be possible with a brace and adequate physical training. If the motor return progresses, selective flexion of individual joints usually follows, and finally selective extension with decreased flexor tone returns. Unfortunately, the return of sensory function is much less predictable. Although the return of motor function most affects ambulation (a value held

highly by patients), sensory return often determines upper extremity function and ability to accomplish activities of daily living. There are many interventions that can be used to accommodate for weak muscles. However, patients who are oblivious of their deficit due to perceptual neglect will have a much more difficult time learning new techniques.

It is in this phase that rehabilitation therapists play crucial roles. Physical therapists work with patients to develop strength, augment balance (first while sitting, then when standing), enhance transfer ability, and increase endurance. When being tested for strength, patients should attempt to stand (with assistance if necessary), because supine testing may give falsely weak results. When the lower extremities have "good strength" (4/5) and the patient can balance on the uninvolved side, gait training can be initiated.

For those patients with difficulty advancing the limb or maintaining stability, the patient should be evaluated for a brace and walking aid. For instance, a platform cane or hemiwalker may be required (Fig. 23.2). Ankle-foot orthoses (AFO) are most commonly used in the elderly stroke patient (Fig. 23.3). Two types are commonly employed: the double adjustable upright metal ankle-foot orthosis, used to stabilize a spastic ankle and provide some proprioceptive feedback to the knee; and the posterior plastic AFO, which prevents footdrop but requires a more stable ankle. Seventy-eight percent to 85% of patients are able to walk after 6 months.[28]

The occupational therapist works with the patient to provide training in daily self-care activities. Occupational therapy has been shown to significantly reduce functional deficits in a randomized trial of stroke survivors.[63] Perceptual deficits are commonly seen, particularly in right hemispheric strokes. The patient's deficits may go undetected until the patient's ability to organize motor tasks in sequence is evaluated. Simple remedies may provide great self-care benefits. For instance, spasticity sometimes can be controlled with the use of weighted utensils. Other types of special utensils, such as rocker knives, plate guards, and reachers, enable persons with hemiplegia to function more independently. A cognitive retraining program also may be provided by occupational therapists or sometimes by speech therapists. Early assessment for aphasia is critical to providing other team members with recommendations regarding communication needs. Approximately 24% to 53% of stroke survivors are partially or totally dependent 6 months after their strokes.[64]

Special attention must be given to two common, and often related, problems. Poststroke depression is very common, affecting about 30% of survivors. It is especially likely with left hemisphere damage. Depression is often recognized 2 to 3 weeks after the stroke. Depression retards functional recovery and may be misinterpreted as "poor motivation."[65] Treatment of depression facilitates

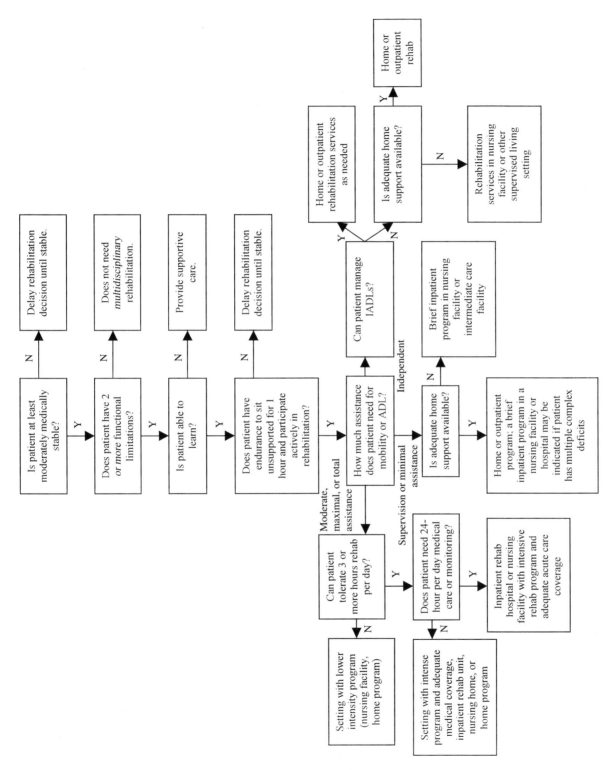

FIGURE 23.1. Algorithm for rehabilitation placement decisions for stroke patients. *Y*, yes; *N*, no; (Adapted from Johnston et al.,[62] with permission.)

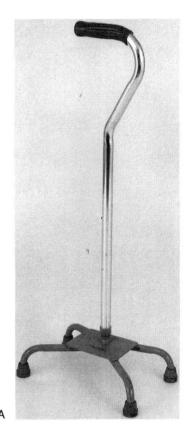

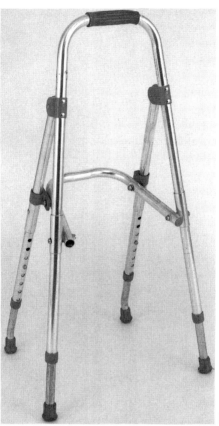

FIGURE 23.2. Walking aids used in stroke. (A) A platform cane offers moderate stability on smooth, flat surfaces but can be unsafe when negotiating uneven ground. (B) A hemiwalker offers much more stability for patients with more limited ambulation skills.

A

B

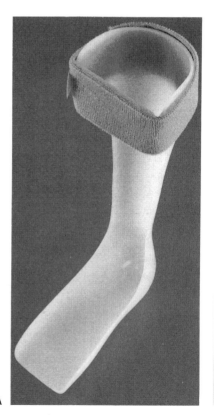

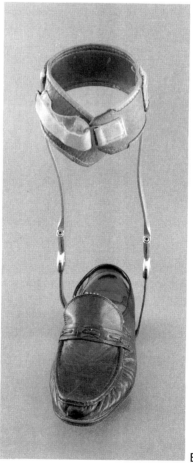

A

B

FIGURE 23.3. Lower extremity braces (ankle-foot orthoses, AFO). (A) plastic AFO provides some stability to a weak ankle but will usually not be appropriate when control of spasticity is required. (B) A metal AFO is useful to control the effects of spasticity but is more difficult to don and is physically unattractive.

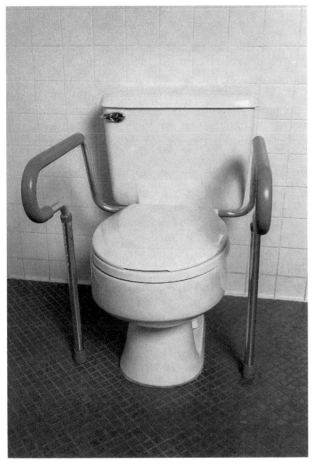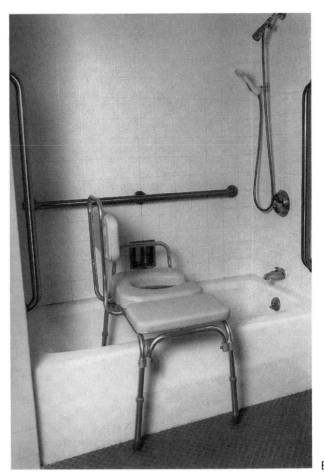

A   B

FIGURE 23.4. Bathroom modifications. (A) Toilet arm attachments facilitate standing with weak hip extensors. (B) A bath bench and handheld shower hose allow the patient to bathe independently.

the gains made in rehabilitation. Psychotherapy and the judicious use of antidepressant medication are usually needed. The choice of an antidepressant medication is usually made based on the side effect profile because all have more or less the same response rate. However, because most agents require at least 2 weeks to produce a response, some have advocated early use of methylphenidate to accelerate the response.[66] Depression must be distinguished from uncontrolled crying, which is also common after a stroke. This condition, thought to be caused by "disinhibition," responds to selective serotonin reuptake inhibitors.[67]

Malnutrition is another problem seen too often in rehabilitation. A bedside swallowing evaluation by a speech and language pathologist has been shown to be valuable,[68] and early dietary consultation should occur on all persons after stroke. In some cases, short-term use of enteral feedings may be required.

Attention to premorbid problems must be especially vigilant in geriatric patients. Having access to one's dentures, eyeglasses, and clothing promotes self-esteem and

may enhance the ability to participate in the rehabilitation program. The patient's family should be involved in the treatment program through training in caregiving skills. A bedside graph to document progress made by the patient and a chart that specifies goals to be achieved can also be helpful.

Chronic Phase

The chronic phase begins when the person who has suffered a stroke returns to society as a person with a disability. The home, especially the bathroom, will usually need modifications. Raised toilet seats with arm frames, grab bars, and a bathtub bench with a handheld shower hose will often be required (Fig. 23.4). Kitchen modification also may be necessary. Before discharge, the home should be assessed for door widths to assure passage of walkers or wheelchairs, the presence of steps and stairs, the need for ramps, the adequacy of lighting, and safety features that may need modifications.

Because the adjustment process to a major disability may take up to 2 years, ongoing psychologic support often is necessary. The patient may benefit from individual or group psychotherapy, a day health center, or a stroke recovery group. Frank information should be provided regarding the fact that sexual activities following a stroke are quite safe, although new techniques are often needed.

Social activities should be strongly encouraged. A vocational rehabilitation counselor can assess and help with the return to employment if appropriate. Arrangements for transportation are particularly important, as many geriatric patients stop driving after a stroke. For patients with right hemisphere lesions and neglect, driving is inadvisable unless the neglect resolves.

The question of whether patients should receive further evaluations by rehabilitation therapists 1 to 2 years after the stroke is controversial. In a randomized trial, physical therapy was offered to study patients with mobility problems seen more than 1 year after their stroke. Therapy was provided in the home, with most patients seen one to six times. Follow-up was for 6 months. The intervention group showed an improvement in their gait speed (while the controls declined). This benefit was lost, however, if patients stopped having therapy.[69] In another study, intensive rehabilitation was provided in a stroke clinic to 40 patients who were, on average, 3 years poststroke. Patients received 2 h of therapy, four times a week, for 4 weeks. Significant improvements in balance and ADL performance were achieved. Three months following the intervention, the patients' skills in balance and weight shifting, as well as their ADL scores, were maintained.[70]

Hip Fractures

Many patients with hip fractures can benefit from rehabilitation. Unfortunately, since the advent of prospective payment in hospitals, more patients with hip fracture are sent to nursing homes for longer periods of time.[71,72] Rehabilitation in the home and nursing home setting has been shown to be cost-effective,[73,74] but inpatient rehabilitation has not.[75] Early surgical repair and more than five physical therapy/occupational therapy (PT/OT) sessions per week postoperatively are associated with better health outcomes.[76] Unfortunately, in this age of short hospital stays, many patients may not be afforded adequate hospital-based physical therapy, in spite of evidence showing that such interventions decrease the number and the length of nursing home stays.[77] Certain features predict more successful outcomes with hip fracture, which include intact mental orientation, younger age, independence in bathing and transfers, family involvement, and the number of hours received in physical

therapy.[78] Other features, such as being over age 85 and poor prefracture functional status, predict poor outcomes.[79] Mild to moderate dementia should not preclude providing the patient with rehabilitation.[80]

Weightbearing after surgery is often a source of confusion. The ideal surgical result would promote maximum independence and allow early ambulation to prevent deconditioning and prevent venous thrombosis. Many orthopedists order weeks of nonweightbearing after the placement of pins or nails, the most common type of surgery used in elderly patients. It is very difficult for older persons to bear weight with only touching their foot on the ground ("toe-touch" weightbearing) during ambulation, owing to general deconditioning and weak upper extremities. There is no evidence that this practice is needed, and early weightbearing according to the patient's tolerance of pain is recommended.[81,82] It does not appear that hip replacement facilitates better functional outcomes over other surgical approaches.[83]

Two types of hip fractures, femoral neck and intertrochanteric, are most common. The distinguishing feature is the high rate of avascular necrosis of the femoral head seen in subcapital fractures. Impacted and nondisplaced fractures are often treated with internal fixation, using nails or pins. As already noted, weightbearing can begin usually by the 3rd day. In osteoporotic patients, subcapital fractures may be treated with installation of an Austin–Moore (or similar) prosthesis. Weightbearing to tolerance is allowed by the 2nd or 3rd day. Trochanteric fractures are treated using open reduction and internal fixation, often using a compression screw. With this procedure, the patient usually can bear weight as tolerated by the 2nd day. In the patient with a femoral neck fracture who has preexisting joint disease, a total hip prosthesis also may be indicated.[84]

Rehabilitation efforts should begin as soon as the patient is admitted to the hospital. Stabilization of life-threatening medical problems should occur before surgical repair. If the patient is alert, preoperative evaluation by physical and occupational therapy and training in the exercises to be performed in bed can begin immediately. The patient can begin quadriceps contractions and, on the 1st postoperative day, can sit up and perform isometric exercises as well as gentle flexion and extension at the hip. Adduction, excessive flexion, and abduction at the hip should be avoided if the joint has been replaced.

The patient can begin supervised ambulation with parallel bars by the 2nd or 3rd postoperative day, advancing to the use of a walker or cane. A properly fitted cane should have a 1-in. (or 2–3 cm) rubber tip and be long enough to allow 20° to 30° of flexion at the elbow when held at the side (Fig. 23.5). The patient should support no more than 20% to 25% of total body weight on a cane. The patient should hold the cane in the hand opposite the

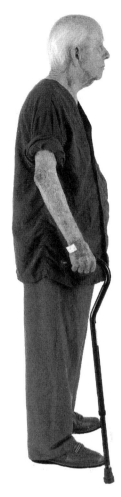

FIGURE 23.5. Proper cane length. The elbow is flexed 20° to 30° when holding the cane at the side.

injured hip. Stair training begins during the second week and consists of going up stairs with the uninvolved leg first and coming down with the involved leg first ("up with the good, down with the bad").

If the patient lacks upper body strength or is unstable with a cane, a pick-up walker should be prescribed (Fig. 23.6A). Patients need to practice advancing the walker about 20 to 30 cm, then advancing the weak leg, and then the good leg. Some older persons may find it easier to advance the good leg first, but this practice increases the risk of falls. Crutches are very difficult for most older persons to use. It must be remembered that special walkers are needed for going up stairs and that it is very difficult to carry objects while using a walker. New walkers with three or four wheels are available that are much easier to negotiate and have carrying baskets[85] (Fig. 23.6B). Patient acceptance of these walkers is better than for the standard issue models.

Depending on the preexisting health and social support status of the patient, the site for rehabilitation

after hip fracture will vary. Early discharge and home rehabilitation should be considered for those with (1) good health (the absence of significant medical problems), (2) strong social supports (someone who can provide assistance), and (3) adequate performance of ambulation and activities of daily living within 2 weeks of surgery. The remainder may require more intensive therapy that can be effectively provided in a rehabilitation nursing facility.

Lower Extremity Amputation

Although most patients who experience a lower extremity amputation (LEA) are between 51 and 69 years old, the age-related incidence of LEA in persons over age 80 has increased significantly.[86] More than 1.5 million people in the United States live with some form of major limb amputation.[87] Of the 127,000 limb amputation procedures done in acute care, nonfederal hospitals in 1993, 98,000 involved the lower extremity. The direct medical cost for a single LEA procedure is approximately $46,900.[88] Below-the-knee (BK) amputations are used in two-thirds of patients and above-knee (AK) in one-third.[89] The predominant cause is peripheral vascular disease. The older person's care is more complex after amputation because of upper extremity weakness, underlying cardiovascular problems, skin that is prone to breakdown, and poor balance mechanisms. Older persons are more likely to have subsequent amputations on the contralateral side.[86] The geriatric provider plays a crucial role in managing these problems and in helping to determine the most appropriate surgical intervention.

In frail older persons, the decision as to level of amputation is often difficult. An ankle-brachial Doppler index ratio of greater than 0.5 is associated with a greater than 90% success rate for healing a transtibial amputation.[90] Others believe that a transcutaneous oximetry measurement provides better determination of the appropriate level of surgery.[91] Sometimes the surgeon cannot determine the best level until the amount of blood flow to the tissues can be observed during surgery. Above all, attempts should be made to avoid serial amputations (e.g., partial foot, followed by transtibial, followed by transfemoral) because prolonged bed rest and its attendant complications are more likely.

There are three major types of lower extremity amputations: partial foot, transtibial (also called a below-the-knee or BK amputation), and transfemoral [above-the-knee (AK)]. Partial foot amputations generally do not require postoperative rehabilitation. The older person with a BK amputation has a much greater chance of achieving independent ambulation. With a BK procedure, there is a lower postoperative mortality rate, the energy costs of using a prosthesis are less, and the chance of walking without the use of canes or walkers is better.

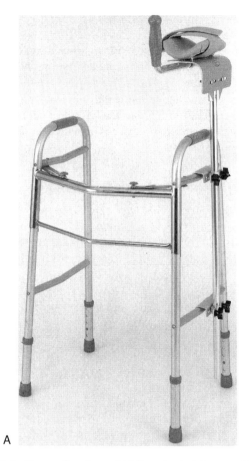

A

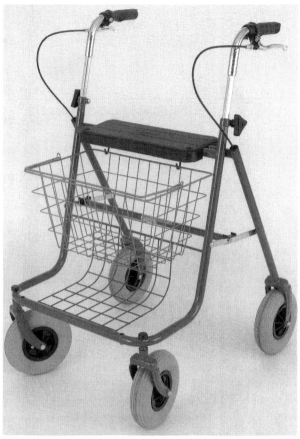

B

FIGURE 23.6. Types of walkers. (A) Standard pick-up walker is very stable. Patient is able to put full weight on handholds. Promotes a slow and abnormal gait. Useful in early rehabilitation of hip fractures. (B) Rolling four-wheeled walker is very mobile, easy to maneuver in tight spaces. Patient must have good balance and control to use safely.

Indeed, the energy cost of walking with bilateral BK amputations is lower than that of walking with a single AK amputation (Table 23.9). In a younger person such energy costs may be insignificant, but in the older patient they may precipitate angina when there is underlying coronary insufficiency.

Barriers to successful use of a prosthesis include hip or knee contractures, preexisting joint disease of the affected knee, contralateral sensory deficits (e.g., periph-eral neuropathy), and significant comorbid disease (congestive heart failure, angina, chronic lung disease).[92] Those patients with cognitive deficits that interfere with learning may have difficulties learning to use a BK pros-thesis.[93] If the patient has contralateral vascular disease, a prosthesis may be contraindicated. However, this is a very individual decision, and the motivated patient still may benefit from a prosthesis trial. It has been shown that measurements of transcutaneous oxygen tension on the

TABLE 23.9. Lower extremity amputation (LEA) in the elderly patient.

Type of LEA	Percent of total number of LEA	Percent recommended for prosthetic gait training	Percent using prosthesis after intensive physical therapy program	Percent additional energy required for normal bipedal ambulation
Transtibial	25	60–80	60–90	Unilateral TTA: 40–60 Bilateral TTA: 60–100
Transfemoral or higher	25	20–30	0–40	90–120

TTA, transtibial amputation.
Note: 50% of all LEA are partial foot amputations that generally do not require rehabilitation.
Source: Adapted from Coletta EM. Care of the elderly patient with lower extremity amputation. *J Am Board Fam Pract.* 2000;13:23–34,[87] with permission.

stump skin may be valuable in predicting success at prosthesis fitting. Levels above 40 mmHg are associated with successful fitting, while below 15 mmHg there are often complications.[94]

Even if a prothesis is not going to be used, patients can benefit from rehabilitation. Training in the use of a special amputation-style wheelchair should be provided. Bed, chair, and toilet transfers also must be learned. Home modifications will be needed. Because the energy costs of using a wheelchair are higher than those of walking, patients with chronic obstructive pulmonary disease and cardiovascular insufficiency must be stabilized.

All geriatric patients should be considered for the fitting of a prosthesis. Age should not be a determinative factor in this consideration. The decision should be based on the patient's medical state, motivation, and mobility needs. As in the case of hip fractures, rehabilitation should begin before the surgical procedure.[95] Exercise training, including strengthening of the upper body, quadriceps, and hip extensors and practice lying prone, should begin as soon as the amputation is considered. Upper extremity bicycle ergometry is particularly useful for this purpose.[96] Contractures of the hip and knee are the most common complications of amputations and must be prevented by active and passive ranging daily. The bed should be kept flat, and pillows should not be placed under the knees.

Following the operation, the patient must be trained in care of the stump. Massage techniques, wrapping with an elastic bandage or stump shrinker, inspection for skin integrity, and hygiene should receive attention. Semirigid dressings may also be used and appear to accelerate the time to prosthesis fitting.[97] The patient should begin transfers with and without the prosthesis immediately postoperatively. Many geriatric patients will use a wheelchair for longer distances, so they also must receive training in its use. Sitting and single-limb balance training also are important.

A permanent prosthesis is usually fitted 6 to 8 weeks postoperatively to allow for stump shrinkage and wound healing. A temporary pylon prosthesis is often employed in the meantime. Some surgeons have used casts placed at the time of the operation to promote early ambulation.[98] The experience of using casts or prostheses in older persons is limited. A physiatrist or orthotist usually prescribes and fits a prosthesis. A patella-tendon supracondylar socket with a solid-ankle, cushioned heel (SACH) foot is often used in elderly patients because it is lightweight and easy to use.

The outcome of prosthetic training in elderly persons is good, with between 60% and 80% of unilateral BK amputees achieving independent ambulation. Unfortunately, only 50% of bilateral BK amputees and less than 50% of unilateral AK amputees will walk with a prosthesis.[99] Most amputees will have some residual sensations long after surgery. In one study, 79% reported phantom limb sensations, 72% reported phantom limb pain, and 74% reported residual limb pain. However, most described their phantom limb and residual limb pain as episodic and not particularly bothersome.[100] Massage and physical therapy, along with small doses of antidepressant medication, usually suffice to treat such pain. The older person also may experience a change in the socket size with large weight changes (weight loss affects size more than weight gain), and neuroma formation and local skin problems can occur.

Parkinson's Disease

The peak incidence of Parkinson's disease is between the ages of 60 and 69 years, with as many as 40,000 to 50,000 new cases per year. Drug treatment has led to significant improvements in the care of patients with Parkinson's disease (see Chapter 78). Physical therapy, including passive and active mobilization exercises, walking, and range of motion exercises, when combined with medication treatment, may be superior to medication treatment alone.[101] Many rehabilitative therapies, such as speech therapy and music therapy, have been studied in Parkinson's patients.[102,103] All have shown improvements in functioning during treatment, but many report that the positive gains are not maintained once the treatment concludes. There have been no randomized, controlled trials showing long-term, sustained effects on function from rehabilitation alone. Hence, the physical treatment of Parkinson's disease can be considered an example of "preventive" geriatric rehabilitation.

The patient should be trained in techniques used to counter the effects of the disease. Strengthening and endurance training and proper use of assistive equipment also are important. Such training is best provided early in the course of the illness as an outpatient. Involvement in a support group may help to maintain newly learned skills.

Gait and balance training emphasizes a safe gait and improved balance. The patient should be taught to keep the head up, to counter the flexed posture consciously, and to lift the toes during the swing phase of the gait.[104] It also may help to take longer steps and widen the base. The therapist often prescribes a home program of regular exercises to maintain or improve strength, range of motion, and flexibility. Other patients find singing to be helpful. In a recent 3-month randomized, controlled, single-blinded study, researchers explored the efficacy of active music therapy (MT) on motor and emotional functions in Parkinson's patients. The MT group showed significant improvements in their bradykinesia, as measured by the Unified Parkinson's Disease Rating Scale.[103]

Canes should be avoided when walking aids become necessary. Due to the posture of Parkinson's disease, protraction and internal rotation of the shoulder may place the tip of the cane between the legs, causing a fall. When the walker is prescribed, it should be fitted with front wheels, as pick-up walkers may induce a backward fall. In the home, shag or throw rugs should be removed, rails should be installed on all steps, and bathroom equipment (including a raised toilet seat or arm frames and grab bars) should be prescribed.

Deconditioning and Immobility

Deconditioning, which usually can be traced to excessive bed rest in the home or institution, is a common geriatric phenomenon. With modern medical therapies, there are few diseases for which absolute bed rest is indicated. Conditioning reflexes can be maintained by simply sitting in a chair for 1 to 2 h. Following hospitalization, some patients may be unable to return home because of deconditioning, in spite of having had their admitting diagnoses "successfully" treated. Therefore, the mainstay of treatment is prevention. In the acute hospital, patients should have orders for regular out-of-bed activities, be encouraged to walk to diagnostic studies if possible, and be taught bed and chair exercises if activities are limited. In some cases, group exercise programs may be better tolerated and less costly.

If patients do not stress their cardiopulmonary or muscular systems, the presence of deconditioning may go unnoticed. This disorder can be recognized by a rise in the resting heart rate or an exaggerated blood pressure response to exercise, decreased muscle power, decreased endurance, and fatigue during simple activities of daily living. Measurements of a person's "capacity" for exercise should be based on the expected demand in the anticipated living environment. One does not need to achieve total cardiovascular fitness to improve skills in independent living. Gait velocity and safety, not cardiovascular fitness, determine how well the person functions in community settings.

Rehabilitation is directed at enhancing strength, gait stability, and velocity in building endurance.[105] In severely deconditioned patients, the time required to recover lost strength can be estimated to be three times as long as they were immobilized. Patients with premorbid cardiac or pulmonary disease may need inpatient rehabilitation to regain independence. Over the long run, low-intensity, low-frequency (two times per week) walking exercise is associated with improvements in cardiovascular fitness in older women. After 26 weeks of training in a supervised walking program, the experimental group had lower heart rates, both at rest and during exercise.[106] Regular exercise also improves gait stability in disabled elders.[107]

Arthritis

A wide variety of other problems are amenable to rehabilitation interventions. The most common chronic illness in the geriatric age group is arthritis. Rehabilitation techniques are used to maintain function of arthritic joints, enhance mobility, and prevent deterioration. In one study, an 8-week course of comfortable walking enabled walkers to improve 70 m over their maximum distance achieved, while controls decreased 17 m. Improvements in functional status (as measured by the Arthritis Impact Measurement Scale) were observed in the walking group but not in the control group ($p < 0.001$); patients assigned to the walking program improved 39%. Walkers used fewer medications and had a 27% decrease in arthritis pain.[108] A longer randomized trial in patients with osteoarthritis using either an aerobic or a resistance exercise program showed improvements in walking speed, pain, stair climbing, and lower rates of disability.[109] Regular exercise should be encouraged in all elders with osteoarthritis to prevent deconditioning and promote independence. The Arthritis Foundation has an extensive array of educational materials for patients.[110]

Joint replacement surgery is being used increasingly in older populations, and rehabilitation is very important following these procedures. The cornerstones of arthritis rehabilitation are the use of adaptive equipment and training in joint protection and energy conservation techniques.

Conclusion

Rehabilitation should be considered in all geriatric patients with functional losses. Every intervention provided to older persons has the potential for enhancing functional abilities or limiting disabilities. A rehabilitation approach can be adopted in any care setting, including the acute hospital. The patient's premorbid functional status, cognitive capabilities, and support system are strong predictors for success in rehabilitation interventions.

References

1. Kunkel SR, Applebaum RA. Estimating the prevalence of long-term disability for an aging society. *J Gerontol.* 1992; 47:S253–S260.
2. Frieden RA. Geriatrics and rehabilitation medicine: common interests, common goals. *Mt Sinai J Med.* 1999;66: 145–151.
3. *http://www.americangeriatrics.org/products/positionpapers/index.shtml.*

4. *http://www.americangeriatrics.org/products/ positionpapers/trainfel.shtml.*

5. Hoenig H, Mayer-Oakes A, Siebens H, et al. Geriatric rehabilitation: what do physicians know about it and how should they use it? *J Am Geriatr Soc.* 1994;42:341–347.

6. Manton KG, Corder L, Stallard E. Chronic disability trends in elderly United States populations: 1982–1994. *Proc Natl Acad Sci USA.* 1997;94:2593–2598.

7. Centers for Disease Control, National Center for Health Statistics. *Health and Aging Chartbook from Health, United States, 1999.* PHS 99-1232-1. *http://www.cdc.gov/nchs/data/hus99cht.pdf.*

8. Pope AM, Tarlov AR, eds. *Disability in America.* Washington, DC: National Academy Press; 1991:1–15.

9. Manton KG, Corder L, Stallard E. Changes in the use of personal assistance and special equipment from 1982 to 1989: results from the 1982 and 1989 National Long Term Care Surveys. *Gerontologist.* 1993;33:168–176.

10. Salas M, Bubolz T, Caro JJ. Impact of physical functioning of health status on hospitalizations, physician visits, and costs in diabetic patients. *Arch Med Res.* 2000;31:223–227.

11. World Health Organization. *International Classification of Impairments, Disabilities, and Handicaps: A Manual of Classifications Relating to the Consequences of Disease.* Geneva: World Health Organization; 1990.

12. Hoenig H, Rubenstein L, Kahn K. Rehabilitation after hip fracture—equal opportunity for all? *Arch Phys Med Rehabil.* 1996;77:58–63.

13. Boult C, Kane RL, Louis TA, et al. Chronic conditions that lead to functional limitation in the elderly. *J Gerontol.* 1994;49:M28–M36.

14. Lorish TR. Stroke rehabilitation. *Clin Geriatr Med.* 1993;4: 705–716.

15. Ackerman RJ. Medical consultation for the elderly patient with hip fracture. *J Am Board Fam Pract.* 1998;11:366–377.

16. Esquenazi A, Vachranukunkeit T, Torres M, et al. Characteristics of a current lower extremity amputee population: review of 918 cases. *Arch Phys Med Rehabil.* 1984;65:623.

17. Rubenstein LZ, Josephson KR, et al. Effectiveness of a geriatric evaluation unit: a randomized trial. *N Engl J Med.* 1984;31:1664–1670.

18. Wray LA, Torres-Gil FM. Availability of rehabilitation services for elders: a study of critical policy and financing issues. *Generations.* 1992;16:31–36.

19. Siebens H. Deconditioning. In: Kemp B, Brummel-Smith K, Ramsdell JW, eds. *Geriatric Rehabilitation.* Austin: Pro-Ed; 1990:183.

20. Avorn J. Induced disability in nursing home patients. *J Am Geriatr Soc.* 1980;30:397–400.

21. Mann WC, Ottenbacher KJ, Fraas L, Tomita M, Granger CV. Effectiveness of assistive technology and environmental interventions in maintaining independence and reducing home care costs for the frail elderly. A randomized controlled trial. *Arch Fam Med.* 1999;8:210–217.

22. Brody E. Informal support systems in the rehabilitation of the disabled elderly. In: Brody SJ, Ruff GE, eds. *Aging and Rehabilitation.* New York: Springer; 1986.

23. Youngblood NM, Hines J. The influence of the family's perception of disability on rehabilitation outcomes. *Rehabil Nurs.* 1992;17:323–326.

24. Gregor S, McCarthy K, Chwirchak D, et al. Characteristics and functional outcomes of elderly rehabilitation patients. *Rehabil Nurs.* 1986;11:10–14.

25. Intrator O, Berg K. Benefits of home health care after inpatient rehabilitation for hip fracture: health service use by Medicare beneficiaries, 1987–1992. *Arch Phys Med Rehabil.* 1998;79:1195–1199.

26. Retchen SH. Evaluation of the older driver. In: Yoshikawa TT, Cobbs EL, Brummel-Smith K, eds. *Practical Ambulatory Geriatrics.* St. Louis: Mosby; 1998:111.

27. Hamberger SG, Tanner RD. Nursing interventions with families of geriatric patients. *Top Geriatr Rehabil.* 1988;4: 32–39.

28. Gresham GE, Duncan PW, Stason WB, et al. Post-stroke rehabilitation: assessment, referral, and patient management. *Clinical Practice Guideline: Quick Reference Guide for Clinicians*, No. 16. Rockville, MD: U.S. Department of Health and Human Services, Public Health Service, Agency for Health Care Policy and Research; 1995.

29. Portnow J, Kline T, Daly MA, et al. Multidisciplinary home rehabilitation: a practical model. *Clin Geriatr Med.* 1991; 7:695–706.

30. Wolfe CD, Tilling K, Rudd AG. The effectiveness of community-based rehabilitation for stroke patients who remain at home: a pilot randomized trial. *Clin Rehabil.* 2000;14:563–569.

31. Liang MH, Partridge AJ, Larson MG, et al. Evaluation of comprehensive rehabilitation services for elderly homebound patients with arthritis and orthopedic disability. *Arthritis Rheum.* 1984;27:258–266.

32. Coleman EA, Grothaus LC, Sandhu N, Wagner EH. Chronic care clinics: a randomized controlled trial of a new model of primary care for frail older adults. *J Am Geriatr Soc.* 1999;47:775–783.

33. Counsell SR, Holder CM, Liebenauer LL. Effects of a multicomponent intervention on functional outcomes and process of care in hospitalized older patients: a randomized controlled trial of Acute Care for Elders (ACE) in a community hospital. *J Am Geriatr Soc.* 2000;48:1572–1581.

34. Gorbien MJ, Bishop J, Beers MH, et al. Iatrogenic illness in hospitalized elderly people. *J Am Geriatr Soc.* 1992;40: 1031–1042.

35. Sager MA, Franke T, Inouye SK, et al. Functional outcomes of acute medical illness and hospitalization in older persons. *Arch Intern Med.* 1996;156:645–652.

36. Evans RL, Haselkorn JK, Bishop DS, Hendricks RD. Characteristics of hospital patients receiving rehabilitation: an exploratory outcome comparison. *Arch Phys Med Rehabil.* 1991;72:685–689.

37. Hill JW, Brown RS, Chu D. The impact of the Medicare risk program on the use of services and expenditure to Medicare. Princeton: Mathematica Policy Research; 1992.

38. Von Sternberg T, Hepburn K, Cibuzar P, et al. Posthospital sub-acute care: an example of a managed care model. *J Am Geriatr Soc.* 1997;45:87–91.

39. Bates BE, Stineman MG. Outcome indicators for stroke: application of an algorithm treatment across the contin-

uum of postacute rehabilitation services. *Arch Phys Med Rehabil.* 2000;81:1468–1478.

40. Applegate WB, Miller ST, Graney MJ, et al. A randomized, controlled trial of a geriatric assessment unit in a community rehabilitation hospital. *N Engl J Med.* 1990;322: 1572–1578.

41. Cameron ID. Accelerated rehabilitation after hip fracture: a randomized controlled trial. *Disabil Rehabil.* 1993;15: 29–34.

42. Langhorne P, Williams BO, Gilchrist W, Howie K. Do stroke units reduce mortality? *Lancet.* 1993;342:395–398.

43. Liem PH, Chernoff R, Carter WJ. Geriatric rehabilitation unit: a 3-year outcome. *J Gerontol.* 1986;41:44–50.

44. Asplund K, Gustafson Y, Jacobsson C, et al. Geriatric-based versus general wards for older acute medical patients: a randomized comparison of outcomes and use of resources. *J Am Geriatr Soc.* 2000;48:1381–1388.

45. Rondinelli DRD, Murphy JR, Wilson DH, Miller CC. Predictors of functional outcome and resource utilization in inpatient rehabilitation. *Arch Phys Med Rehabil.* 1991;72: 447–453.

46. Joseph CL, Wanlass W. Rehabilitation in the nursing home. *Clin Geriatr Med.* 1993;4:859–871.

47. Chan L, Ciol M. Medicare's payment system: its effect on discharges to skilled nursing facilities from rehabilitation hospitals. *Arch Phys Med Rehabil.* 2000;81:715–719.

48. Murray PK, Singer ME, Fortinsky R, Russo, Cebul RD. Rapid growth of rehabilitation services in traditional community-based nursing homes. *Arch Phys Med Rehabil.* 1999;80:372–378.

49. Mulrow CD, Gerety MB, Kanten D, et al. A randomized trial of physical rehabilitation of very frail nursing home residents. *JAMA.* 1994;271:519–524.

50. Fiatarone MA, O'Neill EF, Ryan ND, et al. Exercise training and nutritional supplementation for physical frailty in very elderly people. *N Engl J Med.* 1994;330:1769–1775.

51. Gishert NM, Pendergast DR, Calkins E. Muscle rehabilitation in impaired elderly nursing home residents. *Arch Phys Med Rehabil.* 1991;72:181–185.

52. Kramer AM, Steiner JF, Schlenker RE, et al. Outcomes and costs after hip fracture and stroke. A comparison of rehabilitation settings. *JAMA.* 1997;277:396–404.

53. Mosqueda LA. Assessment of rehabilitation potential. *Clin Geriatr Med.* 1993;4:689–703.

54. Mahoney F, Barthel D. Functional evaluation: Barthel index. *Md State Med J.* 1965;14:61–65.

55. Granger C, Hamilton B, Keith R, et al. Advances in functional assessment for medical rehabilitation. *Top Geriatr Rehabil.* 1986;3:59–74.

56. Stroke Unit Trialists' Collaboration. Collaborative systematic review of the randomised trials of organised inpatient (stroke unit) care after stroke. *Br Med J.* 1997; 3154:1151–1159.

57. Ottenbacher KJ, Jannell S. The results of clinical trials in stroke rehabilitation research. *Arch Neurol.* 1993;50:37–44.

58. Falconer JA, Naughton BJ, Strasser DC, Sinacore JM.

Stroke inpatient rehabilitation: a comparison across age groups. *J Am Geriatr Soc.* 1994;42:39–44.

59. Braus DF, Krauss JK, Strobel J. The shoulder-hand syndrome after stroke: a prospective clinical trial. *Ann Neurol.* 1994;36:728–733.

60. Dombovy M, Sandok B, Basford J. Rehabilitation for stroke: a review. *Stroke.* 1986;8:651–656.

61. Evans RL, Bishop DS, Haselkorn JK. Factors predicting satisfactory home care after a stroke. *Arch Phys Med Rehabil.* 1991;72:144–147.

62. Johnston MV, Wood K, Statson WB, Beatty P. Rehabilitative placement of poststroke patients: reliability of the clinical practice guideline of the Agency for Health Care Policy and Research. *Arch Phys Med Rehabil.* 2000;81:539–548.

63. Walker MF, Gladman JR, Lincoln NB, Siemonsma P, Whiteley T. Occupational therapy for stroke patients not admitted to hospital: a randomised controlled trial. *Lancet.* 1999;354:278–280.

64. Kojima S, Omura T, Wakamatsu W, et al. Prognosis and disability of stroke patients after 5 years in Akita, Japan. *Stroke.* 1990;21:72–77.

65. van de Weg FB, Kuik DJ, Lankhorst GJ. Post-stroke depression and functional outcome: a cohort study investigating the influence of depression on functional recovery from stroke. *Clin Rehabil.* 1999;13:268–272.

66. Lazarus LW, Winemiller DR, Lingam VR, et al. Efficacy and side effects of methylphenidate for poststroke depression. *J Clin Psychiatry.* 1992;53:447–449.

67. Burns A, Russell E, Stratton-Powell H, Tyrell P, O'Neill P, Baldwin R. Sertraline in stroke-associated liability of mood. *Int J Geriatr Psychiatry.* 1999;14:681–685.

68. Mann G, Hankey GJ, Cameron D. Swallowing disorders following acute stroke: prevalence and diagnostic accuracy. *Cerebrovasc Dis.* 2000;10:380–386.

69. Wade DT, Collen FM, Robb GF, Warlow CP. Physiotherapy intervention after stroke and mobility. *Br Med J.* 1992;304:609–613.

70. Tangemen PT, Banaitis DA, Williams AK. Rehabilitation of chronic stroke patients: changes in functional performance. *Arch Phys Med Rehabil.* 1990;71:876–880.

71. Fitzgerald JF, Moore PS, Dittus RS. The care of elderly patients with hip fracture. Changes since implementation of the prospective payment system. *N Engl J Med.* 1988;319:1392–1397.

72. Zuckerman JD. Hip fracture. *N Engl J Med.* 1996;334: 1519–1525.

73. Kane RL, Chen Q, Finch M, Blewett L, Burns R, Moskowitz M. Functional outcomes of posthospital care for stroke and hip fracture patients under Medicare. *J Am Geriatr Soc.* 1998;46:1525–1533.

74. Hollingworth W, Todd C, Parker M, et al. Cost analysis of early discharge after hip fracture. *Br Med J.* 1993;307:903–906.

75. Kramer AM, Steiner JF, Schlenker RE, et al. Outcomes and costs after hip fracture and stroke. A comparison of rehabilitation settings. *JAMA.* 1997;277:396–404.

76. Hoenig H, Rubenstein LV, Sloane R, Horner R, Kahn K. What is the role of timing in the surgical and rehabilitative care of community-dwelling older persons with acute hip fracture? *Arch Intern Med.* 1997;157:513–520.

77. Harada ND, Cuh A, Chiu V, Pakalniskis A. Patterns of rehabilitation utilization after hip fracture in acute hospitals and skilled nursing facilities. *Med Care.* 2000;38: 1119–1130.

78. Bonar SK, Tinetti ME, Speechley M, Cooney LM. Factors associated with short- versus long-term skilled nursing facility placement among community-living hip fracture patients. *J Am Geriatr Soc.* 1990;38:1139–1144.

79. Koval KJ, Skovron ML, Aharonoff GB, Zuckerman JD. Predictors of functional recovery after hip fracture in the elderly. *Clin Orthop.* 1998;348:22–28.

80. Huusko TM, Karppi P, Avikainen V, Kautiainen H, Sulkava R. Randomised, clinically controlled trial of intensive geriatric rehabilitation in patients with hip fracture: subgroup analysis of patients with dementia. *Br Med J.* 2000;321: 1107–1111.

81. Hotz TK, Zellweger R, Kach KP. Minimal invasive treatment of proximal femur fractures with the long gamma nail: indication, technique, results. *J Trauma.* 1999;47:942–945.

82. Koval KJ, Sala DA, Kummer FJ, Zuckerman JD. Postoperative weight-bearing after a fracture of the femoral neck or an intertrochanteric fracture. *J Bone Joint Surg Am.* 1998;80:352–366.

83. Burns RB, Moskowitz MA, Ash A, Kane RL, Finch M, McCarthy EP. Do hip replacements improve outcomes or hip fracture patients? *Med Care.* 1999;37:285–294.

84. Zuckerman JD. Hip fracture. *N Engl J Med.* 1996;334: 1519–1525.

85. Mahoney J, Euhardy R, Carnes M. A comparison of a two-wheeled walker and a three-weeled walker in a geriatric population. *J Am Geriatr Soc.* 1992;40:208–212.

86. Pernot HF, de Witte LP, Lindeman E, Cluitmans J. Daily functioning of the lower extremity amputee: an overview of the literature. *Clin Rehabil.* 1997;11:93–106.

87. Coletta EM. Care of the elderly patient with lower extremity amputation. *J Am Board Fam Pract.* 2000;13: 23–34.

88. Rith-Najarian S, Branchaud C, Beaulieu O, Gohdes D, Simonson G, Mazze R. Reducing lower-extremity amputations due to diabetes. Application of the staged diabetes management approach in a primary care setting. *J Fam Pract.* 1998;47:127–132.

89. Campbell WB, St. Johnston JA, Kernick VF, Rutter EA. Lower limb amputation: striking the balance. *Ann R Coll Surg Engl.* 1994;76:205–209.

90. Sarin S, Shami S, Shields DA, Scurr JH, Smith PD. Selection of amputation level: a review. *Eur J Vasc Surg.* 1991;5:611-620.

91. Misuri A, Lucertini G, Nanni A, Viacava A, Belardi P. Predictive value of transcutaneous oximetry for selection of the amputation level. *J Cardiovasc Surg* (Torino). 2000; 41:83–87.

92. Cutson TM, Bongiorni DR. Rehabilitation of the older lower limb amputee: a brief review. *J Am Geriatr Soc.* 1996;44:1388–1393.

93. Leung EC-C, Rush PJ, Devlin M. Predicting prosthetic rehabilitation outcome in lower limb amputee patients with the functional independence measure. *Arch Phys Med Rehabil.* 1996;77:605–608.

94. Casillas JM, Michel C, Aurelle B, Becker F, et al. Transcutaneous oxygen pressure. An effective measure for prosthesis fitting on below-knee amputations. *Am J Phys Med Rehabil.* 1993;72:29–32.

95. Esquenazi A, Meier RH III. Rehabilitation in limb deficiency. 4. Limb amputation. *Arch Phys Med Rehabil.* 1996; 77(suppl 3):S18–S28.

96. Davidoff GN, Lampman RM, Westbury L, et al. Exercise testing and training of persons with dysvascular amputation: safety and efficacy of arm ergometry. *Arch Phys Med Rehabil.* 1992;73:334–338.

97. MacLean N, Fick GH. The effect of semirigid dressings on below-knee amputations. *Phys Ther.* 1994;74:668–673.

98. Folsom D, King T, Rubin JR. Lower-extremity amputation with immediate postoperative prosthetic placement. *Am J Surg.* 1992;164:320–322.

99. Brodzka WK, Thornhill HL, Zarapkar SE, et al. Long-term function of persons with atherosclerotic bilateral below-knee amputation living in the inner city. *Arch Phys Med Rehabil.* 1990;71:895–900.

100. Ehde DM, Czerniecki JM, Smith DG, et al. Chronic phantom sensations, phantom pain, residual limb pain, and other regional pain after lower limb amputation. *Arch Phys Med Rehabil.* 2000;81:1039–1044.

101. Formisano R, Pratesi L, Modarelli FT, et al. Rehabilitation and Parkinson's disease. *Scand J Rehabil Med.* 1992; 24:157–160.

102. Nagaya M, Kachi T, Yamada T. Effect of swallowing training on swallowing disorders in Parkinson's disease. *Scand J Rehabil Med.* 2000;32:11–15.

103. Pacchetti C, Mancini F, Aglieri R, Fundaro C, Martignoni E, Nappi G. Active music therapy in Parkinson's disease: an integrative method for motor and emotional rehabilitation. *Psychosom Med.* 2000;62:386–393.

104. Viliani T, Pasquetti P, Magnolfi S, et al. Effects of physical training on straightening-up processes in patients with Parkinson's disease. *Disabil Rehabil.* 1999;21:68–73.

105. Vorhies D, Riley BE. Deconditioning. *Clin Geriatr Med.* 1993;9:745–763

106. Hamdorf PA, Withers RT, Penhall RK, Haslam MV. Physical training effects on the fitness and habitual activity patterns of elderly women. *Arch Phys Med Rehabil.* 1992;73:603–608.

107. Krebs DE, Jette AM, Assmann SF. Moderate exercise improves gait stability in disabled elders. *Arch Phys Med Rehabil.* 1998;79:1489–1495.

108. Kovar PA, Allegrante JP, MacKenzie R, et al. Supervised fitness walking in patients with osteoarthritis of the knee. *Ann Intern Med.* 1992;116:529–534.

109. Ettinger WH Jr, Burns R, Messier SP, et al. A randomized trial comparing aerobic exercise and resistance exercise with a health education program in older adults with knee osteoarthritis. The Fitness Arthritis and Seniors Trial. *JAMA.* 1997;277:25–31.

110. *http://www.arthritis.org/answers/exercise_info.asp.*

Part IV
Palliative Care

24
Old Age and Care Near the End of Life

Diane E. Meier

Popular images of death and dying are a jumble of gun violence; young and middle-aged adults on television fighting for life; with the help of tubes, ICUs, and other modern machinery, and nineteenth-century images of feverish mothers or children attended at home by their grieving families and helpless physicians. In reality, these media visions bear little relationship to the actual human experience of dying in the United States.[1] In our society, the overwhelming majority of people who die are elderly. Typically, they die slowly of chronic diseases, over long periods of time, with multiple coexisting problems, progressive dependency on others, and heavy care needs met mostly by family members. They spend the majority of their final months and years at home but, in most parts of the country, actually die in the hospital or nursing home surrounded by strangers. Many of these deaths become protracted and negotiated processes, with health care providers and family members making difficult, often wrenching, decisions about the use or discontinuation of life-prolonging technologies such as feeding tubes, ventilators, and intravenous fluids. There is abundant evidence that the quality of life during the dying process is often poor, characterized by inadequately treated physical distress, fragmented care systems, poor to absent communication between doctors and patients and families, and enormous strains on family caregiver and support systems.

Demography of Dying and Death in the United States

The median age at death in the United States is now 77 years, associated with a steady and linear decline in age-adjusted death rates since 1940. In 1900, life expectancy at birth was less than 50 years, but a girl born today may expect to live to age 79 and a boy to age 75. Those of us reaching 75 years can expect to live another 10 (men) to 12 (women) years, average. By the year 2010, life expectancy is projected to increase to 86 years for women and 79 years for men.[2,3] This dramatic and unprecedented increase in life expectancy (equivalent to that occurring between the Stone Age and the year 1900) is due primarily to decreases in maternal and infant mortality, resulting from improved sanitation, nutrition, and effective control of infectious diseases. The result of these changes in demography has been an enormous growth in the number and health of the elderly, so that by the year 2030, 20% of the United States population will be over age 65, as compared to less than 5% at the turn of the last century. One of the results of this growth in the numbers of older adults is the financial impact of their medical and health care needs. Not only does the Medicare budget absorb much of these costs, but the out-of-pocket expenses for patients and their family caregivers themselves are enormous, and increase with longevity. It has been estimated that about half of all bankruptcies in persons over age 65 are attributable to high medical expenses.[4] Because of the growth in both numbers and longevity of older persons, the Centers for Medicare and Medicaid Services (formerly the Health Care Financing Administration)[5] and others[6] have projected a 73% increase in Medicare and long-term care expenditures in the next several decades.

Although death in the early part of the twentieth century was largely attributable to infectious diseases, today the leading causes of death are heart disease, cancer, and stroke. Advances in treatment of atherosclerotic vascular disease and cancer have turned these previously rapidly fatal diseases into chronic illnesses with which people often live for many years before death. In parallel, deaths that occurred at home in the early part of the twentieth century now occur primarily in institutions (53% in hospitals and 24% in nursing homes). The reasons for this shift in location of death are complex, but are related both to financial incentives, primarily Medicare reimbursement for hospital-based care, with the subsequent rise in the availability of hospitals and hospital beds, and to the care burdens of chronicity and functional dependency typically accompanying life-threatening disease in the elderly. The older the patient, the higher the likelihood of death in a nursing home or hospital, with an estimated 58% of persons over 85 spending at least some time in a nursing home in the last year of life.[7]

These statistics, however, hide the fact that the majority of an older person's last months and years is still spent at home in the care of family members, with hospitalization or nursing home placement occurring primarily near the very end of life. Additionally, national figures such as these hide the substantial regional variation in location of death. In Portland, Oregon, for example, only 35% of adult deaths occur in hospitals as compared to more than 50% in New York City,[8] a disparity associated at least in part with differences in regional hospital bed supply and availability of adequate community supports for the seriously ill and dying. Finally, national statistics also obscure the variability in the experience of dying that characterizes our highly diverse nation. For example, need for institutionalization or paid formal caregivers in the last months of life is significantly higher among the poor and women. Similarly, persons suffering from cognitive impairment and dementia are much more likely to spend their last days in a nursing home compared to cognitively intact elderly persons dying of nondementing illnesses.

The fiscal and care system incentives promoting an institutional death, as opposed to home death, persist despite evidence that many (although not all) patients prefer to die at home and despite the existence of the Medicare Hospice Benefit. The hospice benefit was designed to provide substantial professional and material support (medications, equipment) to families caring for the dying at home for their last 6 months of life. Reasons for the low rate of utilization of the Medicare Hospice Benefit (serving about 20% of adult deaths) vary by community but include the inhibiting requirements that patients must choose to give up disease-modifying treatments to access hospice services, that physicians must certify a prognosis of 6 months or less "if the disease follows its usual course," and that very few hours (usually 4 or less) of personal care home attendants are covered under the benefit. In addition, the fiscal structure of the Medicare Hospice Benefit lends itself well to the relatively predictable downward trajectory of late-stage cancers or AIDS, but not so well to the unpredictable, multiyear chronic course of other common causes of death in the elderly, such as congestive heart failure, chronic lung disease, stroke, and dementing illnesses.[2]

Experience of End of Life in Older Adults

Although death occurs far more commonly in the elderly than in any other age group, most research on the experience of dying has been done in younger populations.

Remarkably little is known about how death occurs in the oldest old, those over age 75. The largest and most detailed study of adult hospital deaths in the United States[9] focused on a relatively young population (the median age at death in the United States is 77 whereas the median age in the SUPPORT study was 66 years) and demonstrated a high rate of untreated pain in the last few days of life, poor doctor–patient communication about the goals of medical care, and frequent use of ventilators and intensive care.[9] There is some evidence that costly "aggressive" and potentially burdensome life-prolonging interventions are less frequently used among the oldest patients, independent of baseline functional measures,[10,11] which may represent a form of implicit rationing based on age. Others have shown consistently high levels of untreated or undertreated pain in the elderly. In one study of elderly cancer patients in nursing homes, 26% of patients with daily pain received no analgesic at all and 16% received only acetaminophen, a percentage that rose with increasing age and minority status.[12] Another study comparing pain management in cognitively intact versus demented elderly with acute hip fracture also found a high rate of undertreatment of pain in both groups, a phenomenon that worsened with increasing age and cognitive impairment.[13,14] Similarly, Cleeland's study of outpatients with cancer found that age and female sex were predictors of undertreatment, a disturbing observation given the dramatic rise in cancer prevalence and proportion of women with increasing age.[15,16] Finally, chronic pain caused by arthritis, other bone and joint disorders, and low back syndrome is probably the most common cause of distress and disability in the elderly, affecting 25% to 50% of community-dwelling older adults and, similar to cancer pain, consistently undertreated.[17] These data suggest that the time before death among elderly persons is often characterized by significant physical distress that is neither identified nor properly treated.

Impact of Serious Illness on Patients and Families

Aside from pain and other sources of physical distress, the key characteristic that distinguishes the dying process in the elderly from that experienced by younger groups is the nearly universal occurrence of long periods of functional dependency and need for family caregivers in the last months to years of life. SUPPORT, focusing on a younger age cohort, found that 55% of patients had persistent and serious family caregiving needs during the course of a terminal illness,[18] a figure that rises exponentially with increasing age. Estimates based on 1996 data suggest that more than 25 million Americans deliver care to a seriously ill relative at home, on average about 18 h per week. Assuming a conservative hourly rate of $8 for such services, this amounts to $194 billion in uncompensated care annually.[19]

Although the vast majority of caregiving is done by unpaid family members (transportation, homemaker services, personal care, and more skilled nursing care), paid care supplements or provides the sole source of care for 15% to 20% of patients, especially among poor elderly women living alone. Most family caregiving is provided by women (spouses and adult daughters and daughters-in-law), placing significant strains on the physical, emotional, and socioeconomic status of the caregivers.[20] More than 87% of caregivers say they need more help with transportation (62%), homemaking (55%), nursing (28%), and personal care (26%) for the patient. Caregiving in itself is a risk factor for death, major depression, and associated comorbidities.[21] Those ill and dependent patients without family caregivers, or those whose caregivers can no longer provide or afford needed services, are placed in nursing homes where 20% of the population over age 85 resides.[22,23] Thus, the dying process in the oldest old is characterized by a high prevalence of untreated pain and other symptoms due to chronic conditions, associated with progressive functional dependency, unpredictable disease course, and extensive family caregiver needs.

Mismatch Between Our Health Care "System" and the Needs

The current payment system is poorly matched to the needs of the chronically ill and dying elderly. Medicare fee-for-service promotes use of procedure-based payments, hospitalization, and associated specialization and discontinuity of care. Capitated managed care systems attempt to avoid seriously ill or dying patients with high-intensity service needs, focusing instead on healthier, lower-cost patient populations. The Medicare hospice benefit was designed for patients with cancer and predictably short (less than 6-month) life spans who are willing to give up efforts to prolong life and whose families can provide for the majority of their care needs at home. None of these payment systems addresses the long-term care needs (whether at home or in a nursing home) of chronically ill and functionally dependent individuals whose prognosis is uncertain and whose medical care usually requires simultaneous efforts to prolong life, palliate symptoms, and provide support for functional dependency. Neither paid personal care services at home nor nursing home costs for the functionally dependent elderly are covered by Medicare, but instead are paid for approximately equally from out-of-pocket and from Medicaid budgetary sources originally intended to provide care for the indigent. Even in nursing homes, standards of care focus on improvement of function and

maintenance of weight and nutritional status, and evidence of the decline that accompanies the dying process is typically regarded as a measure of substandard care. Thus, a death in a nursing home is often viewed as evidence, particularly by state regulators, of poor care rather than an expected outcome for a frail, chronically ill older person. Similarly, quality indicators required in long-term care settings fail to either assess or reward appropriate attention to palliative measures, including relief of symptoms, spiritual care, and promotion of continuity with concomitant avoidance of brink-of-death emergency room and hospitals.[24]

Good News and Bad News

Because of unprecedented improvements in maternal and infant mortality and successes in the control, if not cure, of common chronic diseases, most people who die in the United States are old and frail. They die of chronic, progressive illnesses (such as end-stage heart and lung disease, cancer, stroke, and dementia) with unpredictable clinical courses and prognoses. They have unrecognized and untreated symptoms and an extremely high prevalence of functional dependency and associated family caregiver burden. Current reimbursement systems are unresponsive to this patient population and their families, failing to provide primary care with continuity, support for family caregivers, and home care services, and instead promoting fragmented specialized care tied to procedures and hospitals for lack of any other coherent alternative financing mechanism. This phenomenon has prompted widespread calls[25,26] for change and reorganization that would ensure accountability for outcomes, processes, and costs of care for the growing population of frail, functionally dependent, and chronically ill elderly in their last phase of life.[27]

Because care for a dying person typically includes preventive, life-prolonging, rehabilitative, and palliative measures in varying proportion and intensity based upon the individual patient's needs and preferences, any new model of care must be responsive to this range of service requirements. For example, an 88-year-old woman with congestive heart failure and deconditioning after hospitalization for pneumonia typically requires life-prolonging measures (treatment of heart failure, oxygen, and antibiotics), preventive measures (annual influenza vaccination), rehabilitation (home physical therapy to restore independent bed-to-chair mobility), and palliative care (advance care planning, appointment of a health care proxy, treatment of depression, diuretics, oxygen, and low-dose opiates for dyspnea). Because her daughter works during the day, this woman also needs a 12-hour-a-day home health aide because she is unable to care for herself independently. Thus, the model of care needed provides simultaneous life-prolonging, palliative, and personal care (in this patient they are nearly one and the same) and, given the difficulty of prognosticating time of death in heart failure, will have to continue to do so for the remainder of the patient's life. This so-called mixed management model of care for the frail elderly has been tried in the PACE Demonstrations,[28] a capitated Medicare waiver program of full-service primary care for the elderly focusing on continuity, avoidance of hospitalization, and bringing needed services to the patient.

Another promising model, developed by Joanne Lynn and colleagues, is undergoing pilot evaluation in a chronically ill veterans' population with lung and heart disease. The MediCaring model will (1) define eligibility in terms of chronic disease severity (e.g., congestive heart failure with an ejection fraction of less than 30% and two hospitalizations in the last year), *not* by predicted time of death; (2) provide services that span the range of patient and family needs through use of interdisciplinary teams, consistent primary care providers across all care settings, and delivery of as much care as possible in the home setting, whether the focus be on life prolongation, palliation, rehabilitation, or, as is typical, all three; and (3) organize payment through a Medicare waiver combination of capitation (for team services, equipment) and fee-for-service or salary for participating physicians.[25–27]

Substantial change using approaches such as these will be necessary if the health care system is to bear any relationship to the needs of the patients seeking care: patients who are predominantly old and chronically ill and in urgent need of help truly fitted to their needs. Although the problem is daunting, the increase in attention to medical education, research, and clinical service delivery for patients near the end of life are indicators that the recognition necessary to begin the process of change has occurred. The next steps, testing new models and seeing what works, will define the new structure of health care services for future generations.

A century ago, virtually everyone died at home, surrounded by family and cared for by physicians whose primary role was the relief of suffering, whereas today the majority of Americans die within hospitals and nursing homes, surrounded by medical technology and physicians who believe there is nothing else that they can offer. Although the past 100 years have seen tremendous advances in the treatment of disease such that previously fatal illnesses (e.g., diabetes, congestive heart failure) have become chronic conditions, this progress has come at some substantial cost. We have transformed the culture of the dying process from an accepted part of life's experience to an unfamiliar and much-feared event. The majority of Americans have never witnessed a loved one die (a common experience at the turn of the century) and physicians are ill trained, ill equipped, and uncomfortable taking responsibility for the care of dying patients. It is clear that the time has come to restore the balance so that "relief of suffering and cure of disease are seen as twin obligations of a medical profession that is truly dedicated to the care of the sick."[29]

A New Section

This edition of *Geriatric Medicine* introduces a new section on palliative care. Palliative care is interdisciplinary medical care focused on the relief of suffering and achievement of the best possible quality of life for patients and for their family caregivers. It involves formal symptom assessment and treatment; aid with decision making and establishing goals of care; practical and moral support for patients and their family caregivers; mobilization of community supports and resources to assure a secure and safe living environment; and collaborative models of care (hospital, home, nursing home, hospice) for persons living with serious, complex, and eventually terminal illnesses.

These fundamentals bear a strong resemblance to the core precepts of geriatric medicine, and while it is true that not all older people suffer from multiple complex chronic illnesses that will ultimately lead to their death, most do, and all eventually will. As a result of the successes of modern medical care, dying and death is now a geriatric phenomenon—therefore, sophisticated management for patients and families entering this stage of their lives is the province of the geriatrician as well as all primary treating physicians. In this new section are chapters on practical approaches to communicating with older adults about prognosis, about the likelihood of death, and about patient preferences for how to use their remaining time; on management of diverse sources of suffering in older adults, including distress associated with transfer from home to a nursing home, with being dependent on others, and with being confused; on palliative approaches to caring for persons with dementia at all stages of the illness and regardless of how long the patient may have to live; and on the importance of the value of achieving a peaceful death and why physicians should care about and know how to help their patients ensure it. We hope our readers find these chapters useful as they accompany their patients and their families through one of the most difficult and important stages of late life.

References

1. Signorielli N. Physical disabilities, impairment and safety, mental illness, and death. In: *Mass Media Images and Impact on Health.* Westport, CT: Greenwood Press; 1993: 37–42.

2. Field MJ, Cassel CK. Approaching death: improving care at the end of life. In: Institute of Medicine. Washington, DC: National Academy Press; 1997.

3. Institute for the Future. *Health and Health Care 2010. The Forecast, The Challenge, vol. 2001, 2000.*

4. Warren E, Sullivan T, Jacoby M. Medical problems and bankruptcy filings. *Norton's Bankruptcy Advisor*, May. Jossey Bass, CA. 2000.

5. HCFA HCFA. *Highlights—National Health Expenditures, 1998, vol, 2001, 2000.*

6. Spillman B, Lubitz J. The effect of longevity on spending for acute and long term care. *N Engl J Med.* 2000;342: 1409–1415.

7. National Center for Health Statistics. *National Mortality Followback Survey: 1986 Summary, United States.* Vital and Health Statistics, series 20. Hyattsville, MD: National Center for Health Statistics; 1992.

8. Wennberg J. *Dartmouth Atlas of Health Care.* Center for the Evaluative Clinical Sciences, Dartmouth Medical School; 1999. *www.dartmouthatlas.org.*

9. SUPPORT Principal Investigators. A controlled trial to improve care for seriously ill hospitalized patients. The study to understand prognoses and preferences for outcomes and risks of treatments (SUPPORT). The SUPPORT Principal Investigators. *JAMA.* 1995;274:1591–1598.

10. Hamel M, Phillips R, Teno J, et al. Seriously ill hospitalized adults: do we spend less on older patients? *J Am Geriatr Soc.* 1996;44:1043–l048.

11. Perls T, Wood E. Acute care costs of the oldest old: they cost less, their care intensity is less, and they go to nonteaching hospitals. *Arch Intern Med.* 1996;156:754–760.

12. Bernabei R, Gambassi G, Lapane K, et al. Management of pain in elderly patients with cancer. *JAMA.* 1998;279: 1877–1882.

13. Feldt KS, Ryden MB, Miles S. Treatment of pain in cognitively impaired compared with cognitively intact older patients with hip-fracture. *J Am Geriatr Soc.* 1998;46: 1079–1085.

14. Morrison RS, Siu AL. A comparison of pain and its treatment in advanced dementia and cognitively intact patients with hip fracture. *J Pain Symptom Manage.* 2000;19:240–248.

15. Cleeland CS, Gonin R, Hatfield AK, et al. Pain and its treatment in outpatients with metastatic cancer. *N Engl J Med.* 1994:330:592–596.

16. Stein W. Cancer pain in the elderly. In: Ferrell BR, Ferrell BA, eds. *Pain in the Elderly.* Seattle: IASP Press; 1996.

17. AGS Panel on Chronic Pain in Older Persons. The management of chronic pain in older persons. *J Am Geriatr Soc.* 1998:46:635–651.

18. Covinsky K, Goldman L, Cook E, et al. The impact of serious illness on patients' families. *JAMA.* 1994;272:1839–1844.

19. Arno P, Levine C, Memmott M. The economic value of informal caregiving. *Health Affairs.* 1999;18:182–188.

20. Emanuel EJ, Fairclough DL, Slutsman J, Alpert H, Baldwin D, Emanuel L. Assistance from family members, friends, paid caregivers, and volunteers in the care of terminally ill patients. *N Engl J Med.* 1999;341:956–963.

21. Schulz R, Beach S. Caregiving as a risk factor for mortality: the Caregiver Health Effects Study. *JAMA.* 1999;282: 2215–2219.

22. Ferrell BA, Ferrell BR, Rivera LSO. Pain in cognitively impaired nursing home patients. *J Pain Symptom Manage.* 1995;10:591–598.

23. Ferrell B. Overview of aging and pain. In: Ferrell B, ed. *Pain in the Elderly.* Seattle: IASP Press; 1996.

24. Engle VF. Care of the living, care of the dying: reconceptualizing nursing home care. *J Am Geriatr Soc.* 1998;46: 1172–1174.

25. Lynn J, Wilkinson AM. Quality end of life care: the case for a MediCaring demonstration. *Hosp J.* 1998;13:151–163.

26. Lynn J. Serving patients who may die soon, and their families: the role of hospice and other services. *JAMA.* 2001;285:925–932.

27. Lynn J. Learning to care for people with chronic illness facing the end of life. *JAMA.* 2000;284:2508–2511.

28. Eng C, Pedulla J, Eleazer GP, McCann R, Fox N. Program of All-inclusive Care for the Elderly (PACE): an innovative model of integrated geriatric care and financing [see comments]. *J Am Geriatr Soc.* 1997;45:223–232.

29. Cassell EJ. The nature of suffering and the goals of medicine. *N Engl J Med.* 1982;306:639–645.

25
Doctor–Patient Communication Issues

James A. Tulsky

Why Worry About Communication?

Whether patient suffering is caused by pain, nausea, unwanted medical intervention, or spiritual crisis, the common pathway to treatment is through a provider who is able to elicit these concerns and is equipped to address them. In patients with cancer, the number and severity of unresolved concerns has been shown to predict high levels of emotional distress and future anxiety and depression.[1–3] Eliciting concerns requires skillful communication with the patient. Unfortunately, physicians and nurses tend to underestimate patients' concerns.[4] Even in a hospice setting, one study revealed that only 40% of concerns were elicited.[5] As elderly patients are less likely than younger patients to be proactive in the medical encounter, clinicians working with these patients must be particularly vigilant to elicit concerns and promote patient-centered care.[6]

A central goal of palliative care is to meet the disparate needs of patients and families. Everyone defines a good death differently.[7] Good communication is indispensable to uncovering these needs through empathic exploration and individually negotiated goals of care. Among the frequently articulated goals of patients at the end of life is the use or avoidance of particular medical treatments. Although patients generally wish to discuss even these most difficult issues, such discussions occur infrequently and late.[8–11] When they occur, the quality of communication has been found to be lacking.[12–18] Good communication is necessary to meeting patients' needs and to achieving good deaths.

Finally, considerable evidence suggests that improved physician–patient communication correlates with improved health outcomes, patient satisfaction, and emotional well-being.[19–23] In fact, primary care patients are more satisfied with their physicians if they discuss advance care planning.[24] The mechanisms for this impact are likely twofold. First, improved communication increases the likelihood that patient's needs will be recognized and addressed. Second, the communication itself may be therapeutic. Simply telling one's story may improve objective health outcomes.[25]

General Rules of Good Communication

Whether one is explaining the implications of hypertension or talking about impending death, the physician must adhere to basic principles of good communication. The primary difference between these communication tasks is the meaning of the conversation to the patient and the attendant level of emotional significance. When the situation is more likely to make the patient feel vulnerable, one should focus extra attention on the task.

Considerable data exist from the medical and psychologic literature to support certain general skills. For example, more accurate assessment of anxiety and depression is associated with good eye contact, clarifying of disclosures, responsiveness to cues of emotional distress, supportive comments, and explicit questions about psychologic content.[26] Disclosure of concerns is promoted by open-ended questions, focusing on psychologic aspects of illness, summarizing, educated guesses, and demonstrations of empathy. Likewise, disclosure is inhibited by closed-ended or leading questions, focusing on physical aspects of illness and offering of advice and premature reassurance.[27] Furthermore, short demonstrations of empathy can reduce patient anxiety.[28] Training programs that emphasize these sorts of skills have been able to demonstrate improvement in physician communication behaviors and decreased patient distress.[23,29,30]

The following sections identify and elaborate on general skills that are useful in all encounters with elderly patients. Practical advice for specific situations that arise in geriatric and palliative care follows.

Advance Preparation

A little effort spent on advance preparation can have a tremendous impact on the quality of the encounter with the elderly patient. Whenever possible, important medical information, particularly bad or sad news, should be delivered during a scheduled meeting. This plan allows patients to prepare themselves for the type of information they will hear and to ensure that appropriate family members or friends are present. It also allows the physician to allocate the necessary time to the encounter.

Communication best occurs face to face, particularly with elderly patients. Telephones accentuate physical communication difficulties, such as hearing loss and speech problems. There is no opportunity to employ the benefits of nonverbal communication. And, if the topic is emotionally threatening, it is more difficult to assess and ensure the patient's safety at the other end of the telephone.

If one is anticipating an emotionally charged conversation with a patient, as when expecting results of a biopsy of a suspicious lesion, it is best to schedule an office visit. Frequently, however, the physician is caught off guard, and unexpectedly discovers a bad result. In such cases, it is still best to try and schedule a time to discuss the results face to face. For example, one can call the patient and say, "I have received the results of your blood tests, and I would like to discuss these results with you in person. Can you come in tomorrow at lunchtime?" Most patients will understand that all is not well, however, will not ask further questions, and will come in for the visit where everything can be discussed. In effect, they have received a "warning shot" about the bad news and have begun to prepare themselves. Some patients, however, will respond by requesting to know the facts— "Is it cancer?" Even though it may seem evasive, it is worth trying to avoid delivering the news, even at this point, with a statement such as, "I can imagine that you are concerned about the results, and I will answer all your questions. There are a number of things we need to talk about, and I think I can help you better if we speak face to face." If the patient continues to insist on hearing the information, then one is obliged to answer directly, employing all the appropriate skills for delivering bad news. In such a case, it is valuable to inquire directly about the patient's support at home and their immediate plan of action.

One also needs to approach all such conversations prepared with basic medical information and anticipating the most likely questions regarding treatment options, prognosis, and resources for support and guidance. Finally, to the extent possible, such conversations are best held when both the physician and patient are well rested.

Sensory Issues and Control of the Environment

When speaking with older adults, choose a quiet, private room with good lighting to enhance the patient's ability to comprehend. The physician should sit at eye level and within reach of the patient. If possible, one's pager or cellular phone should be turned off, or at least on a quiet mode, and one should avoid interruptions. As presbycussis first affects higher sound frequencies, it is helpful to speak slowly in a clear, loud, low voice.[31] If patients wear hearing assistive devices, these devices should be in place.

Increasingly, we encounter non–English-speaking patients. One absolutely must employ the assistance of an interpreter in such settings. However, it is equally important to avoid using family members as interpreters. Not only does this run the risk of faulty translation or reinterpretation of the physician's statements, but it also places family members in the uncomfortable position of being both the physician's and patient's spokesperson. The common practice of using bilingual young children as translators is particularly problematic. Most hospitals and health care facilities in regions with high numbers of immigrants employ professional translators or maintain lists of language skills among facility staff members.

The Role of Affect in Communication

Most difficulties in communication are the result of inattention to affect. Affect refers to the feelings and emotions associated with the content of the conversation. Feelings such as anger, guilt, frustration, sadness, and fear modify our ability to hear, to communicate, and to make decisions. For example, after hearing bad news, most patients are so overwhelmed emotionally that they are unable to comprehend very much about the details of the illness or a treatment plan.[32,33] Conversations between doctors and patients often transpire only in the cognitive realm. Emotion is frequently not acknowledged or handled directly, and physicians miss opportunities to do so.[34,35] Consider the following conversations observed in a study of empathic communication and missed opportunities[36]:

MD: Does anybody in your family have breast cancer?
PT: No.
MD: No?
PT: . . . After I had my hysterectomy. I was taking estrogen, right?
MD: Yeah?
PT: You know how your breasts get real hard and everything? You know how you get sorta scared?
MD: How long were you on the estrogen?

PT: Oh, maybe about 6 months.
MD: Yeah, what, how, when were you, when did you have the, uh, hysterectomy?

In this exchange, the doctor ignores the patient's fears and proceeds with factual questions. Not only is this patient unlikely to feel supported, but she may also fail to give detailed information about her symptoms and hinder treatment. In contrast, in the following conversation, the physician recognizes the patient's expression of affect and delivers an empathic response. This is likely to continue the conversation in the realm of the emotions and leave the patient feeling supported.

MD: How do you feel about the cancer—about the possibility of it coming back?
PT: Well, it bothers me sometimes, but I don't dwell on it. But I'm not as cheerful about it as I was when I first had it. I just had very good feelings that everything was going to be all right, you know. But now I dread another operation.
MD: You seem a little upset; you seem a little teary-eyed talking about it.

It is important, as well, to be attentive to the physician's affect. When caring for dying patients, physicians are likely to experience many emotions; these include guilt ("If only I'd convinced him to get that screening colonoscopy"), impotence ("There's nothing I can do for her"), failure ("I messed up, I'm a bad doctor"), loss ("I'm really going to miss this person"), resentment ("This patient is going to keep me in the hospital all night"), and fear ("I know they're gonna sue me").[37] Such feelings are normal and common. However, they can affect one's ability to interact successfully with the patient. For example, feelings of failure may motivate one to avoid the patient, while feelings of loss may make discussions about dying too difficult. The first step toward managing such feelings is to acknowledge that they exist. The next step is to discuss them with colleagues or confidants. In most cases, however, patients do not benefit from hearing such thoughts. When considering sharing such feelings with a patient, a good rule of thumb is to ask oneself, "Am I doing this for me or for the patient?" If the answer is truly the latter, then it may be appropriate to share.

Emotion-Handling Skills

One barrier to eliciting patient affect is the fear of being unable to manage the patient's emotional response. This section describes an approach to handling emotions that is also likely to further elicit the sorts of concerns described earlier. The primary goal of emotion handling is to convey a sense of empathy. Empathy is the sense that "I could be you" and is what patients are usually

TABLE 25.1. NURSE-ing an emotion.

Name the emotion
Understand the emotion
Respect or praise the patient
Support the patient
Explore what underlies the emotion

Source: Fischer GS, Tulsky JA, Arnold RM. Communicating a poor prognosis. In: Portenoy RK, Bruera E, eds. Topics in Palliative Care, vol. 4. New York: Oxford University Press; 2000,[41] with permission.

feeling when they comment about a physician that really cared for them.[38] Robert Smith has created a useful mnemonic to recall four basic techniques to use when confronted by patient emotions: NURS (Name, Understand, Respect and Support).[39] This discussion adds a final "E" for Explore (Table 25.1).

Naming the emotion serves to acknowledge the feeling and to demonstrate that it is a legitimate area for discussion. Statements such as "that seems sad for you" can serve this purpose well, although one needs to be careful not to inappropriately label the patient. Therefore, naming is often best done in a quizzical fashion that does not presuppose the emotion (e.g., "Many people would feel angry if that happened to them. I wonder if you ever feel that way?").

Expressing a sense of understanding normalizes the patient's emotion and conveys empathy. However, expressing understanding must be done cautiously to prevent a response such as, "How can you possibly understand what I'm going through—have you ever had a stroke?" A typical statement might be, "Although I've never shared your experience, I do understand that this has been a really hard time for you."

Respect reminds us to praise patients and families for what they are doing and how they are managing with a difficult situation. Offering respect defuses defensiveness and makes people feel good about themselves and more capable of handling the future. A useful statement might be, "I am so impressed with how you've continued to provide excellent care for your mother as her dementia has progressed."

Support is essential to helping people in distress not feel alone. Simple statements, such as "I will be there with you throughout this illness," can be tremendously comforting. Health care providers ought not feel the entire support burden on their shoulders—support offered can include other members of a team. For example, "We will send a nurse to your home to check in on you in a couple of days, and if you'd like, I could ask the chaplain to pay you a visit."

Finally, patients will frequently make statements that deserve further exploration. For example, a patient may say, "After you gave me the results of the test, I thought that this is gonna be it." A simple response, such as "Tell me more," may help reveal the patient's fears and concerns about cancer that will be helpful in planning future treatment.

Communicating Bad News

Communicating bad news draws upon the skills discussed previously. Many protocols exist for the delivery of bad news; however, the behaviors tend to be grouped into several key domains that include preparation, content of message, dealing with patient responses, and ending the encounter (Table 25.2).[40,41] The primary elements of preparation (getting the setting right, getting needed information) have already been addressed.

Content of Message

Knowledge of what the patient already knows or believes is extremely valuable to have before revealing bad news to a patient.[41] This understanding allows the physician to begin their explanation from the patient's perspective, aligning oneself with the patient and making communication more efficient and effective. The time that a test is ordered is a good time to assess this. One might ask, "Is there anything that you are particularly concerned about?" If the patient mentions a serious illness that might be present, the physician can follow up by asking what the

TABLE 25.2. Key elements of delivering bad news.

Preparation
  Find out what patient knows and believes
  Find out what patient wants to know
  Suggest a supportive person accompany the patient
  Learn about the patient's condition
  Arrange the encounter in a private place with enough time
Content
  Get to the point quickly
  Fire "warning shot" (example: "I have bad news")
  State the news clearly, simply, and sensitively
  Allow silence
  Avoid false reassurance
  Make truthful, hopeful statements
  Provide information in small chunks
Handle patient's reactions
  Inquire about meaning of the condition for the patient
  NURSE (Name, Understand, Respect, Support, Explore) expressed emotions
  Assure continued support
Wrap-up
  Set up a meeting within the next few days
  Offer to talk to relatives/friends
  Suggest that patients write down questions
  Provide a written appointment and contact information and how to be reached in emergencies
  Assess suicidality

Source: Fischer GS, Tulsky JA, Arnold RM. Communicating a poor prognosis. In: Portenoy RK, Bruera E, eds. *Topics in Palliative Care*, vol. 4. New York: Oxford University Press; 2000,[41] with permission.

patient's specific fears and concerns are. Consider, for example, an elderly woman with a breast mass. Her doctor is concerned that it might be breast cancer. Here is how the physician might approach the patient[41]:

MD: Is there anything that you are particularly worried that this might be?
PT: I guess anyone would be scared that it is cancer.
MD: I'm afraid that it might be cancer. There are other things that it might be too, however. That's why we are going to do the biopsy—to find out. What worries you most about cancer?
PT: My mother died of colon cancer. She suffered terribly with it. In the end, she was so weak and thin ...she had to "do her business" in a bag—you know? And she always seemed to be in pain...

At the end of this exchange, note how the physician begins to find out what the patient's fears are in an effort to anticipate the patient's reactions to the news if the test result does turn out to be bad.

When prepared to deliver the content of the message, the physician should begin by firing a brief "warning shot" and then stating the news in clear and direct terms. One should avoid spending any time "beating around the bush" before sharing the news. For example:

MD: We have the test results back, and I'm afraid they don't look good.
PT: Oh no, what is it?
MD: The biopsy shows you have cancer.

Perhaps most important is what follows this exchange. The clinician should remain silent and allow the patient an opportunity for the news to sink in. One can strike an empathic stance, maintain comfortable eye contact, and perhaps use a nonverbal gesture, such as reaching out and touching the patient's hand. However, silence is imperative to allow the patient an opportunity to process the information, formulate a response, and experience his or her emotions. The clinician who feels uncomfortable during this silent phase needs to appreciate that the discomfort is rarely shared by the patient, who is engrossed in thought about the meaning of the news and thoughts about the future. Furthermore, very little that is said by the physician at this time will be remembered by the patient, so it is best not to say it at all. If the patient makes no verbal response after perhaps 2 minutes, it can be useful to check in: "I just told you some pretty serious news. Do you feel comfortable sharing your thoughts about this?"

Dealing with the Response

The remainder of the conversation should be spent primarily dealing with the patient's response, including using the NURSE skills to legitimize and empathize with the patient's experience. It is also important to explore the meaning the news has for the patient and to achieve a shared understanding of the disease and its implications. For example:

MD: What is most troubling to you about having cancer?

PT: It's a death sentence—my mother died from cancer; my brother died from cancer. I guess it's my turn now.

MD: Given your experience, I can see how this is really scary for you. And cancer can be very serious. However, in your case, there are a lot of treatment options, and you have a good chance of surviving with this disease.

PT: So this won't kill me?

MD: I certainly hope not. And I'll be there with you every step of the way fighting this illness.

The preponderance of literature stresses the importance of maintaining hope while remaining truthful.[40] Hopeful messages need to be tailored to patients' specific concerns, particularly addressing patient misconceptions and fears. Once patients' concerns have been explored, patients can be reassured more effectively. When effective treatment is available, this fact should be explained. When the treatment options are poor, hope may be found by alleviating patients' worst fears. Doctors may reassure patients that they will not be abandoned during their illness, that the doctor will remain available if things get worse, that everything will be done to maintain the patient's comfort, and that they will continue to watch for new treatment developments.[42] Often people find hope and strength from their religious or spiritual beliefs, from having their individuality respected, from meaningful relationships with others, and from finding meaning in their lives.[43] Exploring these with the patient over time may help to foster realistic hope. Although physicians may have a desire to make an overly reassuring statement to the patient right after revealing the diagnosis, hopeful statements that are truthful and that are made after taking the time to explore the patient's concerns first are more likely to be accepted by the patient.[44] One can offer a realistic sense of hope, whether biomedical ("We'll keep our eyes open for new treatments and discuss them as they become available") or psychosocial ("I look forward to talking with you more about how we can help you live every day as fully as possible, despite this illness").

Patients may have specific questions about further tests, treatment options, and prognosis. It is important to respond to these seriously. However, many patients suffer comprehension difficulties in such emotionally challenging situations. Give simple, focused bits of information, use nonvague language that patients can understand, carefully observe the patient's verbal and nonverbal reactions to what you say, and most importantly, avoid information-packed speeches.

Ending the Encounter

The clinician must end the encounter in a way that leaves the patient feeling supported and with some sense of hope. Support can be provided through meeting patients' immediate health needs and risks. One must treat pain and palliate other symptoms. Patients should be asked how they plan to cope with the news, and if their response raises any concerns about suicide, this should be asked about directly and addressed. One should try to minimize aloneness through statements of nonabandonment and referral to other resources, such as support groups, counselors, or pastoral care.

Last, one should provide a specific follow-up plan: "I'd like to you to keep a list of questions so I can answer them for you on our next visit this Tuesday. We'll talk about all your options again at that time ... Okay? And please feel free to call me." A legibly written phone number and date and time for the next appointment will provide concrete evidence of the ongoing connection to the physician and help a distressed patient to remember the plan. The physician needs to remember that the goal of this conversation is not to leave a happy patient. That is rarely possible (or even desirable) after delivering bad news. Instead, one hopes to leave a patient who feels supported and cared for and who can look forward to a specific plan of action.

Advance Care Planning

Discussions about advance care planning encompass many goals. These aims include preparing for death and dying, exercising control, relieving burdens placed on loved ones, helping patients make decisions consistent with their values, and leaving patients feeling supported and understood.[45] Unfortunately, frequently many of these goals are not met. Audiotape studies of actual discussions about advance care planning demonstrate that information is frequently presented in ways that may not be understood by patients, uncertainty is addressed insufficiently, empathic opportunities are missed, and the scenarios and treatments discussed do not reflect the most challenging situations confronted in real medical settings.[15,16] These data are not surprising. Patients struggle to understand the issues underlying hypothetical future treatment decisions while confronting the emotional impact of discussing their own mortality. Clinicians must respond to patients' cognitive and affective demands, yet few providers receive formal training in such communication.[46,47]

The first step in preparing to discuss advance care plans is deciding on the appropriate goals for the discussion.[48] What one hopes to accomplish will vary depending on the clinical situation.[49] Advance care planning includes many different tasks: informing the patient, eliciting preferences, identifying a surrogate decision maker, and providing emotional support. Frequently, one cannot accomplish all this in one conversation, and focusing on the goals of the discussion allows the physician to tailor the encounter. Advance care planning is completed as a process over time that allows patients and providers an opportunity for thoughtful reflection and interaction with others.

For a healthy, older patient, physicians might establish whom the patient would like to appoint as a health care surrogate. They might ask whether the patient already has a written advance directive and explore the patients' thoughts about dying and the general views about life-sustaining treatments. For an elderly patient with a serious chronic illness, the doctor might also discuss the patient's attitudes about specific interventions that are likely to occur. For example, the physician might ask about attitudes toward mechanical ventilation in a patient with severe chronic obstructive pulmonary disease (COPD). Finally, if the illness has progressed to the point where it seems that the patient will soon die, the doctor will shift the focus from future treatment in hypothetical scenarios to establishing what the goals should be for care provided in the present. In all cases, advance care planning can help patients prepare for death, discuss their values with their loved ones, and achieve a sense of control.[45] It can help build trust between doctors and their patients, so that when difficult treatment decisions arise, doctors, patients, and their loved ones can communicate openly and achieve resolution.

Despite considerable recent attention to the issue of advance care planning, advance directive discussions and completion rates remain low. Doctors may be uncomfortable discussing death because it evokes feelings of their own impotence and it calls to mind their own mortality. Doctors may also be concerned that the discussion will shock or trouble their patients.

Nevertheless, ample data demonstrate that many patients want to have discussions about advance directives with their physicians,[10,50] that they believe these discussions should occur before the onset of serious illness, and that they believe that physicians ought to initiate the discussions.[11,51] Most patients are not overly disturbed by these discussions and may actually have a positive emotional response to them because of increased sense of control.[10,52] Although some may have negative feelings of anxiety or sadness, patients who experience these emotions still want to discuss advance care plans.

Initiating the Conversation

There are a number of ways to begin the discussion.[48] Often physicians can relate the topic to a recent serious illness. For example, if the patient had been previously hospitalized for COPD, the doctor may begin an advance directive discussion this way:

MD: How have you been doing since you were discharged from the hospital?
PT: Pretty well. The breathing is pretty much back to normal . . . you know.
MD: Good. You know, I was pretty worried about you when the medics brought you to the ER.
PT: So was I. I was never that bad before. I really felt like I was suffocating.
MD: That sounds like it must have been awful.
PT: Yeah.
MD: Well, I realized that you and I have never had a chance to talk about what we should do if you were sicker, say so sick that you couldn't tell me what you wanted, and we had to do things like put you on a breathing machine . . .

Another way to begin is to ask about experiences with relatives or friends who have died. Elderly patients are no strangers to death. They have been to many funerals of family members and friends. They are likely to have observed serious illness closely and perhaps have had loved ones in some of the situations that the physician is describing. They are likely to have much information and misinformation about end-of-life care, and are likely to have thought about their own deaths. Opening a discussion in this manner can naturally lead to a discussion about how decisions were made and what the patient thought of that particular death. This will provide valuable insights into the patient's own values. Finally, when there is no such event to tie the discussion to, doctors can simply note that they discuss the topic with all their patients. One can reassure patients, when true, that one is not bringing the topic up because one believes that the patient's death is imminent or because the physician has information about the patient's condition that is not being shared.

Providing Information

Patients must have adequate information to make informed decisions. It helps to start by asking patients what they understand about their medical illness. ("Tell me what your understanding so far is of your illness. What have your other doctors told you?") If the patient's condition is more serious than he or she realizes, then the physician will need to shift focus. The physician will want to put off discussing advance care plan, focusing the discussion instead on explaining to the patient the seriousness of their condition.

Studies indicate that patients are more interested in what the expected health outcome will be than in details about the interventions themselves.[53,54] ("Many patients tell me they would not want their lives medically prolonged if they could not expect to recover to a point where they could recognize and interact with loved ones. Others say they want everything possible done to lengthen their life, no matter what. Which kind of person are you?") Furthermore, when elderly patients are provided with evidence-based outcome data about the prognosis after requiring CPR, they change their preferences for the intervention.[55,56] The primary reason for patients to consider withholding treatments is to avoid an outcome judged by them to be worse than death.[57] The other reason is that the burden of the treatment, on themselves or their loved ones, outweighs the potential benefit. Therefore, patients should achieve an understanding of the impact of common life-sustaining interventions on one's quality of life. In contrast, vivid descriptions of the nature of the treatments themselves (e.g., intubation, cardioversion, ICU care) may alarm patients but be less helpful.

Eliciting Preferences

Patients state preferences after learning about potential options and evaluating these in light of their personal values. Values refer to deeply held beliefs, such as a desire for personal independence or the importance of a religious practice. By exploring patients' values and goals, clinicians can help them clarify their specific preferences. Sometimes one can ask explicitly about such values (e.g., "What makes life worth living for you?"). Alternatively, values may be elicited in the process of asking about specific treatment preferences. For example, after a patient makes a statement about end-of-life care (e.g., "I'd never want to be on one of those machines."), the clinician may respond by simply asking, "Why?" The answer to this question (e.g., "Because I never want to be a burden on my family or society") may uncover a patient's core values that will impact greatly on treatment decisions.

Identifying what conditions the patient would find unacceptable can also help clarify a patient's preferences. A useful question is, "Can you imagine any situations in which life would not be worth living?"[58] Typically, patients mention persistent vegetative state or similar dire scenarios. This question can be followed by asking what the patient would be willing to forgo to avoid such states.

For many patients, dealing with uncertainty comprises the most difficult aspect of decision making. When doctors ask patients if they would want a particular treatment, like a ventilator, patients will often state that the treatment should be provided "if it will help me, but if it won't help me, don't do it." Statements like this ignore the reality that physicians are often uncertain about the outcome. Everyone responds to uncertainty differently, and the patient's approach to this issue should be discussed explicitly as well. For example, one may ask, "What if we are not sure whether we will be able to get you off the breathing machine?" Depending on the patient's answer to this question, the doctor can explore what the chance of success needs to be to pursue aggressive treatment. Some patients will state that any possibility of recovery is worth pursuing, whereas others will refuse curative treatment when the likelihood of recovery drops below a particular threshhold.[59] Some patients are comfortable using numbers talking about probabilities, others are less quantitatively facile.[60–62] The patient's preferences should dictate the extent to which numbers are used in this discussion. Many patients will be satisfied leaving it to the judgment of the physician and family members, with only general instructions. The option of a time-limited treatment trial is also a useful way to provide reasonable alternatives and clarity in the face of uncertainty.

It is impossible to elicit meaningful preferences for every intervention in every possible situation. By focusing on a patient's values and goals, the physician can then help the patient make decisions about future or current treatments that are consistent with those goals. Discussions should move back and forth from preferences to reasons and values to information and back again, ensuring that the patient understands the implications of their stated preferences and that the doctor understands the patients' values. In this way, when the physician is faced with an unanticipated clinical situation, he or she can use the patient's stated values and goals to help determine the appropriate course of action. In such discussions, it is frequently worthwhile to inquire specifically about some controversial treatments such as artificial nutrition and hydration; this is particularly true in states that require the patient's specific directive to withhold these treatments.

Patients and physicians often use vague terms that ought to be avoided. For example, a statement that a treatment should be continued so long as "quality of life is good" begs further clarification. How does the patient (or the surrogate or the physician) define a good quality of life? In fact, it is always important to ensure that the patient and physician have a shared understanding of the conversation and its implications. Similarly, medical jargon should be avoided, one should always define technical terms, and patients must be encouraged to ask questions.

Choosing Surrogate Decision Makers

Identifying who is to act as the patient's health care proxy may be the most important outcome of a conversation about advance care planning. Does the patient wish this to be a single individual or an entire family? Given the literature demonstrating poor concordance between patient preferences and surrogate perceptions of those preferences, the clinician would be wise to stress the need for the patient to communicate with the selected proxy decision maker.[63] Patients should also be asked how much leeway their proxies should have in decision making.[64] Should proxies adhere strictly to patients' stated preferences, or should they have more flexibility when making actual decisions?

These discussions can be emotionally difficult, even when they are welcome. It is important to draw upon the emotion-handling skills described earlier and to acknowledge the patient's feelings of sadness, fear, or anger when they arise and to validate those feelings by stating your understanding of their reaction. The physician can admit that the discussion can be difficult and support the patient by stating how helpful he or she has been in helping to understand his or her preferences. Another way doctors can provide support to the patient is to assure the patient that they will do whatever they can to meet their goals (such as comfort) and to articulate what some of those things might be. In this way, doctors can assure patients that they will continue to care for them, even if they are in a condition in which they would not want life-sustaining treatment.

Communicating about the Transition

It is possible that the greatest communication challenges face physicians and patients as they discuss progression of disease, the transition from a primary focus on life-prolonging therapy to a primary focus on palliation and the referral for hospice care. Such times of transition involve the recognition of loss, redefinition of self-concept and social role, and great emotional stress. Patients are likely to feel sadness, anger, and denial. Physicians frequently have difficulty with such discussions because they feel a sense of failure or are worried that patients will feel abandoned or that they will be overcome in the conversation by anxiety or despair.[41] Furthermore, they may have their own unresolved issues about mortality or fear the patient's anticipated emotional response.

Again, it is useful to identify the goals of these conversations, which include eliciting emotional, psychologic, and spiritual concerns and providing empathic and practical support. Of course, it is also important to help patients acknowledge their illness and to make appropriate health care decisions, such as enrolling in hospice. However, conversations should not be dominated by the physician's agenda, and patients must be given ample space to make decisions according to their own timetables. According to a recent study, patients facing terminal illness desire a physician who will talk in an honest and straightforward way, be willing to talk about dying, give bad news in a sensitive way, listen, encourage questions, and be sensitive to when they are ready to talk about death.[65] They also wish for physicians to maintain hope

TABLE 25.3. Open-ended questions to initiate conversations about dying.

"What concerns you most about your illness?"
"How is treatment going for you (your family)?"
"As you think about your illness, what is the best and the worst that might happen?"
"What has been most difficult about this illness for you?"
"What are your hopes (your expectations, your fears) for the future?"
"As you think about the future, what is most important to you (what matters the most to you)?"

Source: Lo B, Quill T, Tulsky J. Discussing palliative care with patients. *Ann Intern Med.* 1999;130:744–749, with permission.[69]

while being truthful. Easier said than done. As a general rule, it is important for physicians to employ behaviors that promote the sharing of concerns by patients and to avoid behaviors such as reassurance that inhibit such sharing. Table 25.3 provides useful open-ended questions with which one can initiate such conversations.

As patients respond to these questions, the physician should continue to focus on the psychosocial and spiritual aspects of their illness and not allow the biomedical issues to dominate. It is important to avoid false reassurance.[66] A particular form of response that can be extremely effective at these times is the "wish statement."[67] These are particularly effective in response to statements that appear to demonstrate significant denial of the severity of illness. For example:

PT: I'm going to get better. I know that this new chemotherapy they're offering at the university will make the difference.

MD: I wish that there was a treatment that would make this cancer go away.

PT: You mean that you don't think it will work.

MD: It's hard to come to terms with this, but unfortunately I don't believe it would help you overcome your cancer.

PT: I was afraid you might say that. What do we do now?

MD: There's a lot that we can do. Let's talk about what goals are most important for you right now.

The wish statement allows the doctor to demonstrate empathy toward the patient and to align herself with the patient's hopes. Yet, at the same time it implicitly conveys the message that certain goals are unrealistic. In this way, the physician can address the patient's denial without losing the therapeutic alliance.

Dreaded Questions

Finally, it is useful to consider several of the questions that many physicians find most difficult to answer. Responding to such questions draws upon the many skills described in this chapter, and it is useful to keep several additional points in mind.[68] Check the reason for the question (e.g., "Why do you ask that now?"), show interest in the patient's ideas, and empathize with their concerns. It is also important to be prepared to admit that you do not know.

Having anticipated replies can be useful, and several examples follow[69]:

PT: How long do I have to live?
MD: I wonder if it is frightening not knowing what will happen next, or when.

This response acknowledges that underlying such a question is tremendous emotion, most likely fear. It will be important for the physician to give a factual response to this question. However, the patient will not be prepared to hear this response until the doctor has addressed their emotional concerns. The suggested answer above allows patients to speak about their fears and worries. When the physician needs to use a more factual response, the following is a way of being honest while maintaining hope: "On average, a person in your situation lives 3 to 4 months, but some people have much less time, and others may live longer. I would take care of any practical or family matters now that you wish to have completed before you die but continue to hope that you are one of the lucky people who gets a bit more time."

FM: Does this mean you're giving up on him?
MD: Absolutely not. But tell me, what do you mean by giving up?

Suggesting that a patient receive palliative care risks conveying a sense of abandonment. Physicians must be emphatic that palliative care and hospice are active forms of care that meet patients' varying goals at the end of life. However, further exploration of a patient's or family's concerns about abandonment are important to understanding their perceptions and attitudes toward care at the end of life.

PT: Are you telling me that I am going to die?
MD: I wish that were not the case, but it is likely in the near future. I am also asking, how would you want to spend the remaining time if it were limited?

This wish statement helps the physician identify with the patient's loss. The following sentence is an attempt by the physician to reframe the patient's understanding of the situation. He has acknowledged that the patient is dying, but now he seeks to understand what the patient's goals might be in light of this new information. Creating new goals in this way provides an outlet for the patient's hope.

Bereavement

Caring for elderly patients means caring for bereaved patients. The loss of spouses, siblings, other family members, and close friends is extremely common among older persons. A full discussion of bereavement is beyond the scope of this chapter; however, it is useful to review several key elements of communication with patients after loss.[70] Patients should be encouraged to tell their stories of loss, including describing details of the days and weeks around the death of their loved one. Similarly, patients benefit by recalling earlier positive memories of the person. Physicians can explore how the patient has responded to the grief ("How have things been different for you since your husband died?") and identify the patient's social support and coping resources ("Has anyone been particularly helpful to you recently?" "What helps you get through the day?"). Last, one should not overlook the frequently enormous practical ramifications of loss, such as financial difficulties or the possible loss of a home and transportation.

Good communication skills provide the pathway to excellent care for elderly persons. The fundamentals of such communication are listening, attending to the patient's emotional needs, and achieving a shared understanding of the concerns at hand. Specific tasks such as delivering bad news, discussing advance care planning, helping patients through the transition to hospice care, and responding to bereavement require using these skills to ensure that patients' concerns are elicited and addressed, that they are informed, and that they feel supported.

References

1. Butow PN, Kazemi JN, Beeney LJ, Griffin AM, Dunn SM, Tattersall MH. When the diagnosis is cancer: patient communication experiences and preferences. *Cancer.* 1996;77: 2630–2637.
2. Heaven CM, Maguire P. The relationship between patients' concerns and psychological distress in a hospice setting. *Psycho-Oncology.* 1998;7:502–507.
3. Parle M, Jones B, Maguire P. Maladaptive coping and affective disorders among cancer patients. *Psychol Med.* 1996;26:735–744.
4. Goldberg R, Guadagnoli E, Silliman RA, Glicksman A. Cancer patients' concerns: congruence between patients and primary care physicians. *J Cancer Educ.* 1990;5:193–199.
5. Heaven CM, Maguire P. Disclosure of concerns by hospice patients and their identification by nurses. *Palliat. Med.* 1997;11:283–290.
6. Roter DL. The outpatient medical encounter and elderly patients. *Clin Geriatr Med.* 2000;16:95–107.
7. Steinhauser KE, Christakis NA, Clipp EC, McNeilly M, McIntyre L, Tulsky JA. Factors considered important at the

end of life by patients, family, physicians, and other care providers. *JAMA.* 2000;284:2476–2482.

8. Haas JS, Weissman JS, Cleary PD, et al. Discussion of preferences for life-sustaining care by persons with AIDS. Predictors of failure in patient-physician communication. *Arch Intern Med.* 1993;153:1241–1248.

9. Layson RT, Adelman HM, Wallach PM, et al. Discussions about the use of life-sustaining treatments: a literature review of physicians' and patients' attitudes and practices. *J Clin Ethics.* 1994;5:195–203.

10. Lo B, McLeod G, Saika G. Patient attitudes towards discussing life-sustaining treatment. *Arch Intern Med.* 1986; 146:1613–1615.

11. Shmerling RH, Bedell SE, Lilienfeld A, Delbanco TL. Discussing cardiopulmonary resuscitation: a study of elderly outpatients. *J Gen Intern Med.* 1988;3:317–321.

12. Ford S, Fallowfield L, Lewis S. Doctor-patient interactions in oncology. *Soc Sci Med.* 1996;42:1511.

13. Miles SH, Bannick-Mohrland S, Lurie N. Advance-treatment planning discussions with nursing home residents: pilot experience with simulated interviews. *J Clin Ethics.* 1990;1:108–112.

14. Miller DK, Coe RM, Hyers TM. Achieving consensus on withdrawing or withholding care for critically ill patients. *J Gen Intern Med.* 1992;7:475–480.

15. Tulsky JA, Chesney MA, Lo B. How do medical residents discuss resuscitation with patients? *J Gen Intern Med.* 1995; 10:436–442.

16. Tulsky JA, Fischer GS, Rose MR, Arnold RM. Opening the black box: how do physicians communicate about advance directives? *Ann Intern Med.* 1998;129:441–449.

17. Ventres W, Nichter M, Reed R, Frankel R. Do-not-resuscitate discussions: a qualitative analysis. *Fam Pract Res J.* 1992;12:157–169.

18. Ventres W, Nichter M, Reed R, Frankel R. Limitation of medical care: an ethnographic analysis. *J Clin Ethics.* 1993;4: 134–145.

19. Bertakis KD, Roter D, Putnam SM. The relationship of physician medical interview style to patient satisfaction. *J Fam Pract.* 1991;32:175–181.

20. Cohen SR, Mount BM, Tomas JJN, Mount LF. Existential well-being is an important determinant of quality of life: evidence from the McGill Quality of Life Questionnaire. *Cancer.* 1996;77:576–586.

21. Fakhoury W, McCarthy M, Addington-Hall J. Determinants of informal caregivers' satisfaction with services for dying cancer patients. *Soc Sci Med.* 1996;42:721.

22. Kaplan SH, Greenfield S, Ware JE Jr. Assessing the effects of physician-patient interaction on the outcomes of chronic disease. *Med Care.* 1989;27:S110–S127.

23. Roter DL, Hall JA, Kern DE, Barker LR, Cole KA, Rocxa RP. Improving physicians' interviewing skills and reducing patients' emotional distress: a randomized clinical trial. *Arch Intern Med.* 1995;155:1877.

24. Tierney WM, Dexter PR, Gramelspacher GP, Perkins AJ, Zhou XH, Wolinsky FD. The effect of discussions about advance directives on patients satisfaction with primary care. *J Gen Intern Med.* 2001;16:32–40.

25. Smyth JM, Stone AA, Hurewitz A, Kaell A. Effects of writing about stressful experiences on symptom reduction

in patients with asthma or rheumatoid arthritis: a randomized trial. *JAMA.* 1999;281:1304–1309.

26. Marks JN, Goldberg DP, Hillier VF. Determinants of the ability of general practitioners to detect psychiatric illness. *Psychol Med.* 1979;9:337–353.

27. Maguire P, Faulkner A, Booth K, Elliott C, Hillier V. Helping cancer patients disclose their concerns. *Eur J Cancer.* 1996;32A:78–81.

28. Fogarty LA, Curbow BA, Wingard JR, McDonnell K, Somerfield MR. Can 40 seconds of compassion reduce patient anxiety? *J Clin Oncol.* 1999;17:371–379.

29. Smith RC, Lyles JS, Mettler J, et al. The effectiveness of intensive training for residents in interviewing. *Ann Intern Med.* 1998;128:118–126.

30. Levinson W, Roter D. The effects of two continuing medical education programs on communication skills of practicing primary care physicians. *J Gen Intern Med.* 1993; 8:318–324.

31. Adelman RD, Greene MG, Ory MG. Communication between older patients and their physicians. *Clin Geriatr Med.* 2000;16:1–24.

32. Eden OB, Black I, MacKinlay GA, Emery AE. Communication with parents of children with cancer. *Palliat Med.* 1994;8:105–114.

33. Sell L, Devlin B, Bourke SJ, Munro NC, Corris PA, Gibson GJ. Communicating the diagnosis of lung cancer. *Respir Med.* 1993;87:61–63.

34. Levinson W, Gorawara-Bhat R, Lamb J. A study of patient clues and physician responses in primary care and surgical settings. *JAMA.* 2000;284:1021–1027.

35. Mishler EG. *The Discourse of Medicine: Dialectics of Medical Interviews.* Norwood: Aplex; 1984.

36. Suchman AL, Markakis K, Beckman HB, Frankel R. A model of empathic communication in the medical interview. *JAMA.* 1997;277:678–682.

37. Quill TE, Townsend P. Bad news: delivery, dialogue, and dilemmas. *Arch Intern Med.* 1991;151:463–468.

38. Spiro HM. What is empathy and can it be taught? In: Spiro HM, ed. *Empathy and Practice of Medicine: Beyond Pills and the Scalpel.* New Haven: Yale University Press; 1993; 7–14.

39. Smith RC, Hoppe RB. The patient s story: integrating the patient- and physician-centered approaches to interviewing. *Ann Intern Med.* 1991;115:470–477.

40. Ptacek JT, Eberhardt TL. Breaking bad news. A review of the literature. *JAMA.* 1996;276:496–502.

41. Fischer GS, Tulsky JA, Arnold RM. Communicating a poor prognosis. In: Portenoy RK, Bruera E, eds. *Topics in Palliative Care, vol 4.* New York: Oxford University Press; 2000.

42. Carnes JW, Brownlee HJ Jr. The disclosure of the diagnosis of cancer. *Med Clin North Am.* 1996;80:145–151.

43. Herth K. Fostering hope in terminally-ill people. *J Adv Nurs.* 1990;15:1250–1259.

44. Buckman R. Breaking bad news: why is it still so difficult? *Br Med J (Clin Res)* 1984;288:1597–1599.

45. Singer PA, Martin DK, Lavery JV, Thiel EC, Kelner M, Mendelssohn DC. Reconceptualizing advance care planning from the patient's perspective. *Arch Intern Med.* 1998;158:879–884.

46. Billings JA, Block S. Palliative care in undergraduate medical education. Status report and future directions. *JAMA*. 1997;278:733-738.

47. Tulsky JA, Chesney MA, Bernard L. See one, do one, teach one?—house staff experience discussing do-not-resuscitate orders. *Arch Intern Med*. 1996;156:1285–1289.

48. Fischer GS, Arnold RM, Tulsky JA. Talking to the older adult about advance directives. *Clin Geriatr Med*. 2000; 16:239–254.

49. Teno JM, Lynn J. Putting advance-care planning into action. *J Clin Ethics*. 1996;7:205–213.

50. Edinger W, Smucker DR. Outpatients' attitudes regarding advance directives. *J Fam Pract*. 1992;35:650–653.

51. Johnston SC, Pfeifer MP, McNutt R. The discussion about advance directives. Patient and physician opinions regarding when and how it should be conducted. End of Life Study Group. *Arch Intern Med*. 1995;155:1025–1030.

52. Smucker WD, Ditto PH, Moore KA, Druley JA, Danks JH, Townsend A. Elderly outpatients respond favorably to a physician-initiated advance directive discussion. *J Am Board Fam Pract*. 1993;6:473–482.

53. Frankl D, Oye RK, Bellamy PE. Attitudes of hospitalized patient toward life support: a survey of 200 medical in-patients. *Am J Med*. 1989;86:645–648.

54. Pfeifer MP, Sidorov JE, Smith AC. The discussion of end-of-life medical care by primary care patients and physicians: a multicenter study using structured qualitative interviews. *J Gen Intern Med*. 1994;9:82–88.

55. Murphy DJ, Burrows D, Santilli S, et al. The influence of the probability of survival on patients' preferences regarding cardiopulmonary resuscitation. *N Engl J Med*. 1994;330: 545–549.

56. Schonwetter RS, Walker RM, Kramer DR, Robinson BE. Resuscitation decision making in the elderly: the value of outcome data. *J Gen Intern Med*. 1993;8:295–300.

57. Patrick DL, Starks HE, Cain KC, Uhlmann RF, Pearlman RA. Measuring preferences for health states worse than death. *Med Decis Making*. 1994;14:9–18.

58. Pearlman RA, Cain KC, Patrick DL, et al. Insights pertaining to patient assessments of states worse than death. *J Clin Ethics*. 1993;4:33–41.

59. Weeks JC, Cook EF, O'Day SJ, et al. Relationship between cancer patients' predictions of prognosis and their treatment preferences. *JAMA*. 1998;279:1709–1714.

60. Mazur DJ, Hickam DH. Patients' interpretations of probability terms [see comments]. *J Gen Intern Med*. 1991; 6:237–240.

61. O'Connor AM. Effects of framing and level of probability on patients' preferences for cancer chemotherapy. *J Clin Epidemiol*. 1989;42:119–126.

62. Woloshin KK, Ruffin MT, Gorenflo DW. Patients' interpretation of qualitative probability statements. *Arch Fam Med*. 1994;3:961–966.

63. Seckler AB, Meier DE, Mulvihill M, Paris BE. Substituted judgment: how accurate are proxy predictions? *Ann Intern Med*. 1991;115:92–98.

64. Sehgal A, Galbraith A, Chesney M, Schoenfeld P, Charles G, Lo B. How strictly do dialysis patients want their advance directives followed? *JAMA*. 1992;267:59–63.

65. Wenrich MD, Curtis JR, Shannon SE, Carline JD, Ambrozy DM, Ramsey PG. Communicating with dying patients within the spectrum of medical care from terminal diagnosis to death. *Arch Intern Med*. 2001;161:868–874.

66. Maguire P. Barriers to psychological care of the dying. *Br Med J*. 1985;291:1711–1713.

67. Quill TE, Arnold RM, Platt F. Expressing wishes in response to loss, futility, and unrealistic hopes. Personal communication, 2001.

68. Faulkner A. ABC of palliative care. Communication with patients, families, and other professionals. *Br Med J*. 1998:316:130–132.

69. Lo B, Quill T, Tulsky J. Discussing palliative care with patients. *Ann Intern Med*. 1999;130:744–749.

70. Casarett D, Kutner JS, Abrahm J, for the End-of-Life Care Consensus Panel. Life after death: a practical approach to grief and bereavement. *Ann Intern Med*. 2001;134:208–215.

26
Care Near the End of Life

Sarah Goodlin

Advances in medical science during the past half century allow people to survive many acute illnesses that previously would have resulted in death. Yet, rather than curing illness, most medical interventions permit us to manage chronic disease. Most Americans age with one or more degenerative or disabling diseases and require daily assistance toward the end of life. It is difficult or impossible to identify a point at which a gradually worsening patient begins "dying" in many chronic disease states. In the process of ongoing care, physicians and patients often become aware that the likely benefits of certain treatments or diagnostic tests may be outweighed by their discomfort or other burdens. For some patients, no treatment offers hope for prolongation of life or restoration of function, and their care becomes focused on palliation of symptoms and enhancing the quality of their remaining life. Other patients with advanced illness may prefer to attempt to prolong life, but they will also benefit from efforts to reduce symptoms and address social, existential, and spiritual needs.

Because of the multitude of therapies and interventions available in current medical practice, caring for dying patients has been too often viewed as withdrawing or withholding treatment. Care near the end of life is better viewed as "shifting the emphasis" of treatment to an intensive focus on maintaining dignity, enhancing quality of life, supporting the family, and lessening the burden of illness. All patients with advanced illness will benefit from this focus, even when they are still receiving treatment directed at prolonging life. The provision of palliative care in settings such as the hospital or intensive care unit, associated with the acknowledgment that patients have a high likelihood of dying, will ease transition from life-prolonging efforts to palliation alone when such treatments are no longer appropriate.

Three-quarters of the 2.3 million deaths in the United States annually occur in persons over the age of 65 and 26% are in persons age 85 years or older.[1] The median age at death in the United States is 77 years. Hence, all physicians who care for elderly patients should know how to care for patients at the end of life. The interdisciplinary approach to patients with multiple medical, social, and functional problems utilized in all of geriatrics applies equally to all seriously ill and dying patients. This chapter reviews available data about death in elderly Americans and presents an approach to care for those nearing the end of life.

Dying in the United States

National data from 1998 death certificates indicate 33% of deaths were from heart disease, 23% from cancer or malignant neoplasm, and 7% from stroke. Evaluation of Medicare claims data for the last year of life shows multiple diagnoses in the majority of decedents. In that analysis, heart diseases are present in 66%, neoplasm in 31%, pneumonia and influenza in 29%, chronic obstructive pulmonary disease in 26%, cerebrovascular disease in 23%, and dementia in 14% (dementia is likely underrepresented, as Alzheimer's disease prevalence is 19% of individuals aged 75–84 years and up to 45% in those 85 years old and older[2]). Among Medicare beneficiaries receiving hospice care, 40% had malignant neoplasm, 10% had congestive heart failure, and 6% had other heart disease.[3] Only 23% of individuals dying in the United States received hospice care in 1998; more than 80% of those were white or Caucasian. Medicare was the source of hospice payment for two-thirds of individuals. Referrals from physicians to hospice programs often come very late in the course of the illness.[4] The median length of care in hospice in the United States in 1999 was 29 days and mean enrollment 48 days, suggesting that hospice services are not invoked until death is imminent for many patients.

In the United States, 50% to 60% of individuals die in hospitals, 25% in nursing homes, and 20% at home. After initiation of the "Diagnosis Related Group" prospective payment system for Medicare in the mid-1980s, the site of death for Medicare recipients shifted from the acute hospital toward nursing homes.[5] Predictors of death in the home include cancer or AIDS diagnosis, a caregiver or spouse in the home, younger age, type of health insurance, physician experienced in home death,[6] and geographic location. The regional number of hospital beds is inversely related to the likelihood of death at home. A fivefold difference among five geographically distinct hospitals in the rates of death at home correlated with hospital beds per capita when controlled for age, disease, income, preference for site of death, and family support.[7] The Dartmouth Atlas of Health Care documented wide geographic variation for Medicare recipients in location of death and care in the final 6 months of life. Death in the hospital varied for hospital referral region from 17.29% in Bend, Oregon, to 49% in Nevada in 1995 to 1996. In 1994 to 1995, the number of days in the hospital in the final 6 months of life was 4.4 days at the low end of the spectrum and 22.9 at the high end, with longest lengths of stay observed in the northeast and south. Similar variation was observed in intensive care use, visits by medical specialists, and visits to 10 or more physicians in the last 6 months of life.[8]

Death in the hospital often occurs without specific plans to meet patient and family needs and is frequently accompanied by interventions of uncertain value.[9] Inpatient palliative care and hospice units have been developed in several institutions[10] but are not the norm. Intensive care unit (ICU) deaths typically involve decisions to withhold or remove life-prolonging therapies.[11] The ICU brings unique challenges, including the dilemmas of attempting to prolong life for patients at high likelihood of dying and the obligation to ensure comfort in noncommunicative patients.[12]

Costs of care in the last year of life are greatest for those who die in the hospital, and Medicare payments for hospital care are five times the amount paid for home health and hospice care in the last year of life. Medicare annual reimbursement for decedents averaged $26,300, in contrast to $4400 for survivors.[13] The Dartmouth Atlas Project documented a bell-shaped curve by geographic region in Medicare-reimbursed inpatient care in the last 6 months of life. Very old persons receive less costly and less resource-intensive care than younger individuals.[14,15] Medicare expenditures in the final 2 years of life decrease with age above 75 and are significantly less for the oldest old.[16] Other costs may increase, however; individuals incur significant out-of-pocket expense for institutional and community-based long-term care services (unless they qualify for Medicaid) or receive nonreimbursed care from family.

Perversely, the reimbursement system for medical services favors in-hospital highly technical acute care and does not ensure payment for in-home supportive care.

Reducing highly technical or life-sustaining interventions for those who are very near death may yield only small effects on health care costs.[17,18]

The Process of Care

Care for patients near the end of life can be viewed as a series of steps. While each individual progresses toward death in his or her own way, the process of providing care should include certain fundamental steps, which are depicted in Figure 26.1.

Clarifying and Making Explicit the Goals of Care

Perhaps because of heterogeneity in disease course and patterns, physicians identify life expectancy and prognosis poorly in seriously ill persons.[19] Nonetheless, the clinician should employ relevant medical knowledge and experience to inform patients of their status, the likely course of their disease (including the fact that they will die of this disease at some point), and the benefits and burdens of interventions and treatments (Table 26.1). Physicians must talk with patients and their families about what is medically possible and reasonable in a given situation and elicit patients' values and preferences for care. Medical options and patient values and preferences should be integrated to form explicit goals of care. As disease and care progress, the goals may change; hence, decision making will be a dynamic process. The goals for care should be the foundation for planning and delivering care. Patients' status, their needs, and their family's needs should be continuously reevaluated relative to the goals.

Decision making about care near the end of life should occur as a shared process between the physician and patient. Family and other providers should be made aware of the decisions and included whenever appropriate. When the patient lacks decision-making capacity, an appointed proxy or surrogate can speak for the patient. A plan to meet the goals should follow. The plan should address interdisciplinary holistic care for the patient and family.

On occasion, patients or caregivers may request interventions for which the potential benefits would be significantly outweighed by probable burdens. Although a patient's right to refuse treatment is well established, patients have very limited legal or ethical authority to demand interventions that are not medically sound. Physicians are not obligated to provide futile therapy or treatments that are not medically appropriate.[20–22] Evaluating the interventions requested in relation to the goals of care can provide helpful insight for the patient or family.

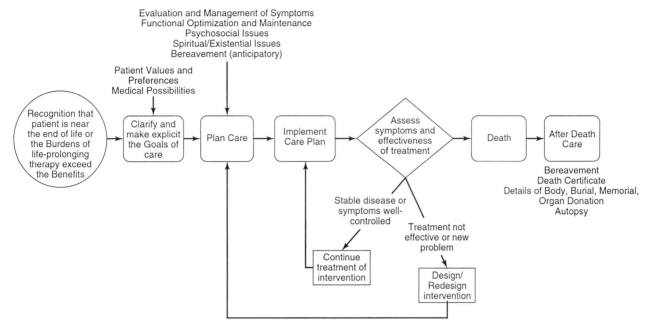

FIGURE 26.1. Care for patients near the end of life: core process.

Patient Preferences for the End of Life

Understanding what is and what was most important to the person facilitates a conversation about preferences for end-of-life care. Values help clarify how to structure goals and what interventions are acceptable. Discussion should review the potential desirable and undesirable outcomes and alternative approaches as they relate to the goals of care for the individual. Patients should be specifically asked if they wish life-prolonging treatments under circumstances of permanent loss of mental ability severe enough to keep them from recognizing and interacting with loved ones. For example, the alternative to attempted cardiopulmonary resuscitation (CPR) is to be kept comfortable and be allowed to die naturally when the heartbeat or breathing stop. As with other care decisions, conversations about preferences should involve the patient directly. Both physicians and surrogates do little better than random chance when predicting the patient's wishes about CPR.[23,24] Discussion with patients about preferences should ideally occur in advance of significant decline in cognitive status, although psychiatric or neurologic illness should not preclude a discussion with

TABLE 26.1. Issues to consider in decision making.

Capacity of patient to decide, and identification of surrogate
Likely course of illness, including impact on function and symptoms
The patient's values, concerns, and preferences
Alternative approaches that are possible to manage expected events
The good and bad effects likely from each alternative

the patient. Capacity is decision specific. Even patients who are mildly to moderately demented can usually state what they value and whom they trust to make decisions on their behalf. Mild to moderately impaired patients with Alzheimer's disease have the capacity to appoint a health care proxy and should be counseled to do so.[25] Depression does not mean that a patient has lost decisional capacity, although depressed persons may be more likely to decline life-sustaining interventions than others.[26,27]

Preferences and plans about attempted resuscitation must be integrated into the plan of care. Informing patients about their rights to make choices about treatment and about the use of advance directives, as required by the Patient Self-Determination Act (PSDA), has not been demonstrated to alter patient outcomes.[28,29] For hospitalized patients with serious illness, rates of attempted CPR varied significantly with geographic location and with diagnosis; CPR rates were more than threefold greater for patients with congestive heart failure than other diagnoses.[30] Orders to not attempt resuscitation (DNR) are more common for patients with more functional compromise and with increased age and vary by diagnosis, gender, race, and location.[31] In nursing homes[32] and in the community,[33] physicians, patients, and surrogates often choose to limit diagnostic and therapeutic interventions, limit hospitalization, and maintain comfort rather than prolong life. In one geriatric practice, a discussion of probability of survival reduced by approximately 50% the number of elderly patients who stated that they wished CPR attempted for a cardiac arrest.[34]

The topics of physician-assisted suicide and euthanasia are discussed in detail in Chapter 86. Requests for physician-assisted suicide center around patient fears of decline in function, suffocation, pain, suffering, and the desire to not be further dependent on others or to be a burden to others.[35] Aggressive management of physical and emotional symptoms and support for family caregivers may reduce fears of pain and suffering and obviate the demand for suicide. Allowing patients to refuse food and water in concert with pharmacologic treatment of any symptom distress has been proposed as an alternative to active physician aid in dying.[36]

Planning and Providing Care

The physician's willingness to listen to a patient's or family member's concerns and to discuss plans for care may be critical to satisfaction with their care.[37] Plans for the patient's care should address management of symptoms currently experienced and anticipated, likely medical events in the course of the illness, social and caregiver issues, existential issues, functional problems, and bereavement. An interdisciplinary team—either established or virtual (brought "together" via telephone or other communication for the specific patient)—can best address these varied issues based upon the explicit goals for the patient.[38] Specific issues confronted in care near the end of life require a perspective that may differ from general medical care.

Artificial Nutrition and Hydration

Artificial nutrition and fluids and the risks and benefits associated with them should be addressed with patients and their families, and specific plans should be made for the management of decreased oral intake in advance of its occurrence whenever possible.[39,40]

Dehydration and inadequate nutritional intake are typically not associated with discomfort when appropriate oral care is provided. Thirst decreases with advancing age. Elevated levels of tumor necrosis factor (TNF) that suppress appetite and may reduce the sensation of hunger are present in older persons in general, as well as in persons with advanced illness.[41] Other changes with age, such as decrease in growth hormone and vasopressin levels. may decrease sensations of hunger and thirst, and ketosis is believed to reduce the sensation of pain and other noxious stimuli. Concerns of patients and families about "starving" can often by assuaged by the knowledge that thirst and hunger are unusual during terminal illness and can be easily managed.[42] Understanding that the process of gradual dehydration leads to comfortable sleep and coma can ease fears about discomfort when the patient is not artificially supported. Often patients and family more easily accept decreased intake of food and fluids when they understand that comfort may be adversely effected by artificial or forced feeding. Several excellent patient and family guides may help with weighing the burdens and benefits of artificial nutrition and hydration and other treatments.[43,44] Hospice studies suggest that patient decisions to forego artificial nutrition and hydration do not lead to suffering.[45]

Nasogastric feeding tubes, restraints, and intravenous catheters are associated with moderate to severe discomfort[46] that may outweigh any benefits of improved hydration and nutritional status. In patients with progressive dementia, families can anticipate the loss of ability to eat and drink in the natural progression of advanced-stage illness. Decisions about tube feeding and other interventions can be made in advance, in the context of the goals of care (comfort and safety versus maximal possible life prolongation). When a decision is made not to employ artificial nutrition and hydration, patients should be offered food and fluids freely, and careful attention should be given to keeping the mouth and lips moist. Aspiration should be accepted as a consequence of late-stage dementia, with or without feeding. When aspiration is likely, the diet can be modified and caregivers can be coached in appropriate techniques (such as sitting up at 90°, tipping the chin forward), as there is not evidence that tube feeding reduces the risk of aspiration. Physically frail persons or those with advanced dementia frequently demonstrate aversion to food. Observing distress associated with feeding by mouth can help family reframe concerns about food and understand that forcing food may not be the most compassionate approach.

Functional Issues

Although the course toward death varies in length from hours to several years, most patients can benefit from efforts to maximize functional status. Improved function may enhance the patient's, and often the caregiver's, mood, sense of self-esteem, and quality of life. Aids in ambulation such as a walker, cane, or wheelchair make it possible for patients to interact in the community or move about in their environment as long as possible. Pain control should be directed at maintaining mobility. Analgesia before movement, other interventions such as nerve blocks, or a short course of palliative radiation therapy for cancer metastatic to bone may enhance mobility. Except in the final stages of life or when pain exacerbated by movement would require more sedation than desired, a range-of-motion program will prevent painful contractures. Occupational therapists can be particularly helpful in providing adaptive equipment to facilitate hygiene. When death is near, bathing and grooming should be directed at maintaining comfort.

Site of Care

The location of care while the person is ill and the place of death should be planned. Decisions may depend on resources available to the patient and family, their feelings about death in the home, and time available to organize care. Family caregivers suffer significant financial, psychologic, and health problems due to the stresses of providing care for their ill family member.[47] Volunteer hospice workers and other volunteer organizations may provide intermittent caregiver respite. Other emotional support and resources for family members are found through national programs run by the Alzheimer's and Related Disorders Society for patients with dementia, and Strength For Caring for patients with cancer.[48]

Care at Home

Home care services through visiting nurse agencies may provide "intermittent" care for up to 28 h per week or more under Medicare Part A, including skilled nursing, home health aide, physical, occupational, and speech therapy, and social work. The patient must be homebound and have a clear medical indication for skilled care. Health care providers in home care agencies do not have specific training in pain and symptom management or care for patients near the end of life. Home health agencies linked with hospice agencies may provide "prehospice" care.

The Medicare Hospice Benefit

The Medicare hospice benefit, available through certified visiting nurse agencies, allows patients to elect palliative care rather than usual (life-prolonging) care under Medicare Part A. Patients must sign a consent (drafted by each agency) to enroll in hospice care. The patient's attending physician and hospice medical director must sign a statement that life expectancy is 6 months or less, although hospice care may be recertified and provided indefinitely once a patient has enrolled. The National Hospice and Palliative Care Organization published guidelines for estimating prognosis in noncancer illnesses, although some Medicare intermediaries unfortunately apply these as criteria to determine appropriateness of hospice referral and reimbursement.

The Hospice benefit provides home care to meet patients' needs and covers the cost of all palliative medications (except a $5.00 co-pay), durable medical equipment, and any treatments and medical services (except for a 5% deductible) pertaining to the patient's terminal illness. Acute hospital stays are minimized (usually limited to periods of up to 5 days for acute symptom management or respite for caregivers). The "Continuous Care" level benefit provides intensive hospice services for a minimum of 8 h and up to 24 h per day for brief periods. Intravenous medications, transfu-

sions, artificial nutrition, radiation therapy, chemotherapy, and dobutamine infusions and other treatments may be provided in hospice care when the treatment is intended to palliate symptoms. In practice, such treatments are too expensive for all except for large hospice agencies to cover, given their Medicare per diem reimbursement of approximately $102 per day. (Reimbursement rates are higher for Continuous Care and for inpatient stays.) Hospice care under the Medicare Benefit may be provided to patients residing in nursing homes when the daily nursing home care is paid for privately or by Medicaid. Medicaid reimburses hospice care in 43 states and Washington, D.C. An individual may revoke hospice care and return to usual Medicare coverage at any time.

Symptom Management

A careful assessment of pain and other symptoms is crucial to good care of elderly dying patients. Patients may underreport symptoms, either because they assume symptoms are to be expected as they approach the end of life or because they wish to be a "good patient" and avoid "complaining" or admitting current treatment is not effective. Physicians should inquire about pain, dyspnea, constipation, nausea, insomnia, anxiety or worries, depression, and existential or spiritual concerns for all patients. An assessment should include the frequency, severity, character, duration, and location of the symptom, precipitating or exacerbating factors, and response to interventions or treatment. Numerical scales (e.g., a scale of 1 to 5)[49] help to assess severity of symptoms and to assess response to interventions. The particular scale or instrument chosen is less important than that symptoms are assessed routinely and reassessed in response to interventions.

Evaluation of symptoms will direct their management. For example, recognition that a patient with dyspnea has bronchospasm results in the use of inhaled bronchodilators to reduce shortness of breath. Excellent physical diagnosis skills may obviate the need for other diagnostic evaluation. In some locations, portable x-rays and other studies may be obtained at home without significant discomfort for the patient. The ability of diagnostic evaluations to change the plan of care should be weighed against the inconvenience and discomfort of the tests (Table 26.2). The effect or outcome of a treatment or intervention should be continuously reevaluated, and the intervention should be modified based on the ongoing assessment of symptoms.

Pain

Many people approaching death fear pain and physical suffering. Significant pain during cancer illness ranges from 50% to 75%.[50,51] Pain also accompanies advanced

TABLE 26.2. Approach to symptom management.

Identify symptoms through regular assessment
Evaluate the cause
Treat readily reversible causes
Address social, emotional, and spiritual issues
Weigh treatment options, including nonmedical interventions, with the patient
Prescribe around-the-clock palliative medications for constant symptoms and as-needed medications for episodic symptoms

neurologic illness, such as Parkinson's disease, or may be unrelated to the primary disease yet significantly impair quality of life, as with osteoarthritis or a compression fracture in patients with heart or lung disease. Primary care physicians can manage the majority of pain experienced by patients. Cognitive impairment should not deter providers from assessing pain, as even markedly impaired patients can describe pain and alternative assessments and standards can be applied to patients unable to communicate.[52] Sadly, nursing home residents with end-stage cancer and other serious illness often are not prescribed appropriate analgesia.[53] Appropriate treatment of pain demands that health care workers anticipate and aggressively try to reduce pain. The assessment and evaluation of pain in the elderly patient is addressed in detail in Chapter 29.

Respiratory Symptoms

Dyspnea or difficulty breathing is a subjective symptom and should be distinguished from tachypnea (increased rate of breathing), hyperpnea, and hyperventilation (increased ventilation).[54] Measurement of dyspnea relies on patient report of the sense of difficulty breathing using verbal descriptors, visual analogue scales, or numeric scales. One study of elderly dying patients found 50% experienced respiratory distress and fearfulness.[55] The prevalence of dyspnea in dying cancer patients is as high as 70%.[56] An underlying cause for dyspnea should be identified and treated specifically whenever possible. Oxygen may help alleviate symptoms of dyspnea even in those patients who are not significantly hypoxemic.[57] Benzodiazepines effectively relieve dyspnea, possibly by depressing the ventilatory response to carbon dioxide,[58] and relieve anxiety associated with dyspnea. Opioids relieve the sensation of air hunger and are the most effective and most commonly employed medications to treat shortness of breath.[59] Often patients with chronic dyspnea from congestive heart failure, lung disease, or degenerative neurologic disease can be well managed with moderate doses of sustained-release opioids. Parenteral opioids (morphine 0.5–1 mg i.v. or s.q., increasing by 1–2 mg q 10 min, then continuous dose at 50% of bolus dose or fentanyl beginning with 2–10 µg i.v. or s.q.,

increasing with 2 µg q 10 min, then continuous infusion) or sublingual opioids (morphine 2–10 mg s.l., or the fentanyl 200–800 µg Actiq "lollipop") are appropriate for patients who are otherwise unrelieved.[60] Respiratory suppression from opioids is rare when doses are begun low and titrated gradually to relieve dyspnea.

Suctioning may not decrease pulmonary congestion or increased secretions ("death rattle"). Glycopyrrolate (.1–.2 mg IV or SQ q 6–8 h) reduces secretions rapidly and effectively in most patients. Scopolamine (Transderm Scop 1–2 patches q 72 h or scopolamine 0.4 mg s.c. q 4 h) is also effective in reducing secretions.

Psychiatric Symptoms

Anxiety

Anxiety occurs commonly in dying patients, either independently or as a result of symptoms such as pain or dyspnea. Associated symptoms should be controlled whenever possible, but it may be necessary to initiate treatment for anxiety simultaneously. Identification of specific concerns and counseling by social workers, or by spiritual counselors, may effectively reduce anxiety. When anxiety relates to fear of being alone, it can be addressed by the companionship of family or volunteers.

The cornerstones of anxiolytic medication are the short- to moderate-acting benzodiazepines, such as lorazepam (Ativan) or oxazepam (Serax). Occasionally, buspirone (Buspar) or antidepressants [including paroxetine (Paxil), mirtazapine (Remeron), nortriptyline (Pamelor), nefazodone (Serzone), trazodone (Desyrel), or doxepin (Sinequan, Adapin)] may be employed to relieve anxiety. Some elderly individuals respond paradoxically to psychoactive medications, so medication effect must be closely monitored. Antipsychotic agents should be avoided as treatment for anxiety because of their side effect profiles, except in the case of terminal restlessness, apathetic or agitated delirium, paranoia, or hallucinations.

Depression

Approximately 25% of dying cancer patients are depressed.[61] In one study, more than half of terminally ill patients with a pervasive desire for death were depressed.[62] Depression is common in the elderly and is addressed in detail in Chapter 80. Patients may not have classic vegetative symptoms, yet they or their family will give a history of persistent sadness, guilt, or withdrawal from usual activities. Antidepressant therapy should be tried for these patients, with careful assessment of mood and status during the trial. Dysphoria, particularly when it relates to sadness or anticipatory grief, may also respond to counseling. Antidepressant medications are appropriate, even when the depressions "appropriate" to the related loss of function or when approaching the end of life. Methylphenidate (Ritalin) and other psychostimulants are effective in improving mood, alertness, and appetite and in reducing apathy in some patients and have the advantage of rapid onset of action. Antidepressants and psychostimulants have an adjuvant analgesic effect, and their use can lead to reduction in analgesic requirements. The tricyclic antidepressants have a lag to onset of action and significant anticholinergic side effects but may be quite effective for patients who need the anxiolytic or soporific effects or who have neuropathic pain. Doxepin and mirtazapine may also have the advantage of stimulating appetite.

Confusion and Delirium

Most individuals fear the loss of mental capacity. Except in cases of intractable symptoms, an effort should be made to titrate therapies to maintain alertness. Confusion and delirium are common at the end of life and should be considered whenever there is a change or decline in a patient's mental status. (The diagnosis and management of delirium are addressed in detail in Chapter 77.) Medications are often at fault. A patient may develop confusion with an increased or continued dose of an opioid, despite having done well previously, or develop a delirium on an H_2 blocker or other agent they previously tolerated. When caused by opioid analgesics, delirium may resolve with dose reduction change to a different opioid or addition of an antipsychotic agent.[63,64] Careful physical examination may reveal simply treated causes of delirium such as fecal impaction, hypoxemia, bladder outlet obstruction, or a urinary tract infection. When no clear etiology of delirium is identified, antipsychotic therapy (haloperidol, olanzepine, or resperidol) is appropriate to control distressing symptoms. Apathetic delirium is characterized by somnolence or decreased level of consciousness and is as distressing to the patient and family as an agitated delirium. Antipsychotic therapy is effective and is indicated in both apathetic and agitated delirium.

Dementia

Dementia may be the primary disease from which patients die or a problem in addition to the terminal illness.[65] Patients with late or end-stage dementia are at increased likelihood of dying following hospitalization for pneumonia or hip fracture compared to patients without cognitive impairment.[66] In one community, dementia patients with family caregivers most commonly died at home (42%) and in nursing homes (32%), with only 26% dying in the hospital. Of those at home, only a quarter had physician home visits and less than half had skilled nursing visits.[67] Recommendations for end-of-life care in dementia include advance care planning at the time of diagnosis of dementia and coordinated interdisciplinary care for patients and their families across the continuum.[68] Specific palliative care programs to care for severely demented individuals reduce measures of discomfort in these patients and reduce overall costs of care when compared with traditional long-term care.[69] The focus of care in Dementia Special Care Units is maintaining comfort, avoiding tube feeding and restraints, and minimizing the use of antibiotics and diagnostic testing.

Gastrointestinal Symptoms

Anorexia

Early in the course of the disease, encouraging adequate nutrition may enhance strength and a sense of well-being. Many dying patients become profoundly anorexic (92% of patients in one small series),[70] and the goal of feeding may shift to satisfying appetite and avoiding hunger, rather than providing adequate nutritional support. Allowing patients to eat preferred foods and relaxing dietary restrictions may help increase intake. Identifying and, when possible, treating causes of decreased oral intake, such as mouth pain from thrush or other processes, odynophagia, or dysphagia, can be helpful. Medical illnesses may present as anorexia or be associated with decrease food intake. For example, peptic ulcer disease may present as anorexia or nausea, and abdominal vascular disease or biliary disease may be associated with decreased food intake. Pharmacologic appetite stimulants such as megestrol (Megace) 40 to 400 mg qid, dronabinol (Marinol 2.5–10 mg before lunch and dinner), or cyproheptadine (Periactin 2–4 mg p.o. q 8 h) may be effective.

Nausea and Vomiting

Nausea is mediated through the chemoreceptor trigger zone (CTZ) on the floor of the fourth ventricle and the vomiting center (VC) in the medulla. Dopamine (D_2) receptors are the principal receptors in the CTZ, and muscarinic and histamine-1 are the most common receptors in the VC. Serotonin (5-HT3) receptors are present in both locations, and in vagal afferents. Metaclopramide (Reglan) speeds gastric emptying and has antidopaminergic action on the CTZ but rarely cause delirium, depression, and parkinsonism, so as low a dose as effective should be used, and side effects should be closely monitored. Prochlorperazine (Compazine) 5 mg i.v. or 25 mg p.o. or p.r. up to three times a day or other phenothiazines and butyrophenones (haloperidol 0.5–1 mg p.o. or i.m. q 8 h) act on the CTZ, but extrapyramidal and anticholinergic effects should be monitored. Serotonin antagonists such as ondansetron (Zofran) 8 mg p.o. or i.v. up to every 6 h are effective antiemetics, which do not have the antidopaminergic toxicity of the benzamides,

TABLE 26.3. Selected medications to treat nausea and vomiting.

Medication	Site of action	Dosage	Side effects
Prochlorperazine	Chemoreceptor trigger zone (CTZ)	5 mg p.o. or i.v./i.m. q 6–8 h	Anticholinergic[a] and extrapyramidal
Haloperidol		0.5–1 mg p.o./s.l./i.m. q 8 h	
Metaclopramide	Stomach (forward peristalsis), gastroesophagial junction (tone) at higher doses also CTZ	5–10 mg p.o. or i.v. 1/2 h before meals	Delirium, depression, and extrapyramidal
Cyclizine	Vomiting center in medulla	50 mg p.o. or i.m. q 4–8 h	Anticholinergic[a]
Dexamethasone	Unclear	4–10 mg p.o. or i.v. q 6–12 h	Hyperglycemia, delirium, and all common corticosteroid effects
Ondansetron	4HT$_3$ receptors on vagal nerve and in CTZ	4–8 mg p.o. or i.v. q 6 h	Expense

[a] Dry mouth, orthostatic hypotension, constipation, urinary retention.

but they are very expensive ($20 per tablet). Antihistamines (diphenhydramine or hydroxyzine PO or IV) act on the VC and may be quite effective with fewer potential side effects. Corticosteroids are also potent antiemetics.

Remediable causes of nausea or vomiting such as peptic disease and obstipation should be identified and treated (Table 26.3). Doses of H$_2$ blockers should be halved in the elderly, as they may precipitate delirium. Sucralfate (Carafate) or antacids may be effective in relieving dyspeptic symptoms. The proton pump inhibitors [omeprazole (Prilosec), lansoprazole (Prevacid), and others] are the most potent agents for decreasing gastric acid secretion and do not alter cognition.

Bowel Management

Constipation results in a myriad of other symptoms, including urinary retention, nausea and vomiting, delirium, and, if severe, intestinal perforation. Decreased mobility and bed rest predispose to constipation, so a bowel regimen should be initiated as patients become less mobile. Constipation occurs uniformly with opioid

analgesics. Any patient placed on opioids should simultaneously be started on stimulant laxatives. Osmotic stool softeners, such as lactulose, and milk of magnesia may be effective in maintaining bowel function for patients at bed rest (Table 26.4). A bowel regimen should be identified for all patients and followed routinely. Patients who develop constipation should be treated with saline, or mineral oil retention, or tap water enemas as needed to relieve the blockage in the lower gastrointestinal (GI) tract. Impaction should be resolved from below before giving oral laxatives. Bowel stimulants can be used once any lower GI tract obstruction is resolved. Patients often respond to regularly scheduled glycerin or bisacodyl suppositories (1–4 per rectum), after breakfast, daily.

Diarrhea

Although less common than constipation, diarrhea can be a particularly distressing symptom in dying patients, especially if mobility is impaired. When possible, the etiology of the diarrhea should be clarified, and processes amenable to treatment, such as *Clostridium difficile* colitis, or fecal impaction, should be treated aggressively.

TABLE 26.4. Selected agents to treat constipation.

Type of agent	Medication	Dose	Onset	Comments
Stimulant/ contact agents	Senna	1–3 tabs p.o. qd	6–12 h	Act by increasing fluid and electrolyte secretion in distal ileum and colon
	Bisacodyl	5–15 mg tabs p.o. or 10 mg suppository p.r.	6–8 h immediate	
	Docusate salts		3–5 days	Also have emollient action
Lubricants	Mineral oil	15–45 mL p.o. or 60–150 mL p.r.	6–8 h	Avoid p.o. in patients at risk for aspiration; can decrease absorption of fat-soluble vitamins
Osmotic agents	Polyethylene glycol (Miralax)	1–2 capsules q 8–12 h		
	Lactulose	15–60 mL p.o.		
	Magnesium citrate	mL		
	Milk of magnesia	15–60 mL p.o.		
	Sorbitol	15–60 mL p.o.		

First-line therapy for diarrhea should be Kaolin-pectin 60 mL p.o. q 2–3 h or bulk agents, such as cholestyramine (Questran) 4 g p.o. qid, because these agents may control diarrhea without systemic effects. Antispasmodic agents may be indicated to decrease frequency of bowel movements. Loperamide (Imodium) is preferable to diphenoxylate-atropine (Lomotil) combination, as the latter has greater potential for systemic and CNS toxicity.

Oral Care

As patients near death, they may increasingly need assistance moistening or lubricating mucous membranes (with moistened swabs or artificial saliva) and lips (with petrolatum or lip balm). Even when the patient is unresponsive, the mouth should be cleaned and moistened at regular intervals for patient comfort and to lessen family distress.

Urinary Symptoms

Urinary incontinence, dysuria, and frequency can be particularly disturbing symptoms for patients, especially if mobility is impaired. A urinalysis should be checked to identify an infection that could be treated. For symptoms of incontinence and frequency, a postvoid residual (PVR) volume should be documented. If the PVR is greater than 150 mL, an indwelling catheter should be left in place or intermittent catheterization performed regularly. Indwelling catheters may be used for easing caregiver burden or avoiding moving patients with severe pain; however, they are associated with urinary tract infections in all patients in whom they are in place for more than about 1 week. Some patients with urinary retention may respond to bethanechol (Urecholine) 5 to 10 mg bid to tid. In the absence of elevated PVR, tolterodine (Detrol) 1 to 2 mg daily or oxybutinin (Ditropan) 2.5 to 5 mg p.o. bid to tid may be effective in reducing frequency, urge symptoms, and incontinence. These agents may cause urinary retention, constipation, and changes in mental status. Dysuria can sometimes be reduced with a bladder anesthetic, such as pyridium 100 to 200 mg p.o. tid. Women with atrophic changes of the urethral meatus and external genitalia may have improved bladder function and reduction in irritative symptoms with small amounts of topical estrogen cream applied to the urethral meatus daily or several times per week.

Skin Care

Skin should be kept clean and dry and decubitus ulcers prevented, particularly in cachectic or malnourished patients. Prophylaxis includes avoiding friction, reducing prolonged pressure by turning every 2 h, or using an air or water mattress when patients become bedbound; however, in some situations, these interventions need to be weighed against the discomfort of frequent movement. Ulcers that develop should be treated to keep the area soft and clean to reduce discomfort. (See Chapter 66 on pressure ulcers and wound healing.)

Infectious Processes

Pneumonia and other infectious processes may still be "the old man's friend." In some dying patients, pneumonia or other infection is appropriately treated by relieving dyspnea and suppressing fever and discomfort, rather than administering antibiotics. Fever may be suppressed by round-the-clock acetaminophen orally or per rectum, or with cooling techniques such as bathing with cool water. When a decision is made to give antibiotics, a broad-spectrum oral antibiotic or once-daily injection will allow treatment at home. Other symptoms such as dyspnea associated with pneumonia, or dysuria and urinary frequency associated with urinary tract infection, should be addressed to relieve physical distress.

Bereavement

Anticipatory grieving, or sadness about the expected death, should be acknowledged and support offered to patients and family members. Communication before death between the patient and friends and family is important when possible. Hence, patients and their family members need to understand that death is likely, have adequate time to process that information, and spend time with each other. Information about what to expect as disease progresses and death approaches may dramatically reduce patient and family anxiety. When death seems imminent, the patient and family should be advised and given the opportunity to "say good-bye." Acknowledgment of our lack of precision in estimating the time course of what will transpire is imperative when counseling the patient and family about what to expect.

After death, the physician and other members of the caregiver team should participate in bereavement activities. Often a simple letter or telephone call may be adequate for the family to know that the physician recognizes their sense of loss. Some physicians maintain tickler files to call or to send a note to the patient's family on the anniversary of the patient's death. Hospice programs and clergy often open grief or bereavement programs or support groups to members of the community, and families should be made aware of these resources.

Conclusion

Care near the end of life focuses on optimizing quality of life for the patient and their family and minimizing symptoms. Excellent communication, management of symptoms, and maximizing patient function are essential. The process of caring for patients near the end of life should be learned by all health providers and improved within health systems.

References

1. Center for Disease Control and Prevention, *http://www.cdc.gov/nchs/fastats/deaths htm*.
2. Evans DA, Funkenstein HH, Albert MS, et al. Prevalence of Alzheimer's disease in a community population of older persons. Higher than previously reported. *JAMA*. 1989; 262:2551–2556.
3. Hogan V, Lynn J, Gabel J, et al. *Medicare Beneficiaries' Costs and Use of Care in the Last Year of Life*. Medicare Payment Advisory Commission; 2000.
4. Christakis NA. Timing of referral of terminally ill patients to an outpatient hospice. *J Gen Intern Med*. 1994;9:314–320.
5. Sanger MA, Easterling DE, Kindig DA, et al. Changes in the location of death after passage of Medicare's prospective payment system. *N Engl J Med*. 1989;320(7): 433–439.
6. Lubitz JD, Beebe J, Baker C. Longevity and Medicare expenditures. *N Engl J Med*. 1995;332(15):999–1003.
7. Pritchard RS, Fisher ES, Teno JM, et al., for the SUPPORT Investigators. Influence of patient preferences and local health system characteristics on the place of death. *J Am Geriatr Soc*. 1998;46:1242–1250.
8. Wennberg JE, Cooper MM. *The Dartmouth Atlas of Health Care in the United States*. Center for Central Evaluative Sciences, Dartmouth Medical School Hanover NH; 1998.
9. Goodlin SJ, Winzelberg GS, Teno JM, et al. Death in the hospital. *Arch Intern Med*. 1998(158):1570–1572.
10. Von Gunten CF, Martinez J. A program of hospice and palliative care in a private, nonprofit US teaching hospital. *J Palliat Med*. 1998;1(3):265–276.
11. Prendergast TJ, Classens MT, Luce JM. A national survey of end-of-life care for critically ill patients. *Am J Respir Crit Care Med*. 1998;158(4):1163–1167.
12. Truog RD, Burns JP, Mitchell C, et al. Pharmacologic paralysis and withdrawal of mechanical ventilation at the end of life. *N Engl J Med*. 2000;345(7):508–511.
13. Hogan V, Lynn J, Gabel J, et al. *Medicare Beneficiaries' Costs and Use of Care in the Last Year of Life*. Washington, DC: Medicare Payment Advisory Commission; 2000.
14. Hamel MB, Phillips RS, Teno JM, et al. Seriously ill hospitalized adults: do we spend less on older patients? *J Am Geriatr Soc*. 1996;44:1043–1048.
15. Perls TT, Wood ER. Acute care costs of the oldest old. *Arch Intern Med*. 1996;156:754–760.
16. Lubitz JD, Beebe J, Baker C. Longevity and Medicare expenditures. *N Engl J Med*. 1995;332(15):999–1003.
17. Emanuel EF, Emanuel LL. The economics of dying. The illusion of cost savings at the end of life. *N Engl J Med*. 1994;330(8):540–544.
18. Teno J, Murphy D, Lynn J, et al. Prognosis-based futility guidelines: does anyone win? *J Am Geriatr Soc*. 1994;42:1–6.
19. Christakis NA. *Death Foretold: Prophecy and Prognosis in Medical Care*. Chicago: University of Chicago Press; 1999.
20. The President's Commission for the Study of Ethics and Medicine. *Deciding to Forgo Life-Sustaining Treatment*. Washington, DC: US Government Printing Office; 1983.
21. *Guidelines on the Termination of Life-Sustaining Treatment and the Care of the Dying: A Report by the Hastings Center*. Bloomington: Indiana University Press; 1987.
22. *Current Opinions of the Council on Ethical and Judicial Affairs of the American Medical Association*. Chicago: American Medical Association; 1986.
23. Uhlmann RF, Pearlman RA, Cain KC. Physician's and spouses' predictions of elderly patients' resuscitation preferences. *J Gerontol*. 1988;43:M115–M121.
24. Seckler AB, Meier DE, Mulvihill M, et al. Substituted judgment: how accurate are proxy predictions? *Ann Intern Med*. 1991;115:92–98.
25. Marin DB, Rudin E, Fox B, et al. Feasibility of a healthcare proxy counseling program for patients with Alzheimer's disease. *J Palliat Med*. 1999;2(3):323–329.
26. Lee MA, Ganzini L. Depression in the elderly: the effect on patient attitudes toward life-sustaining therapy. *J Am Geriatr Soc*. 1992;40:983–988.
27. Freer JP. Depression and decision making. *J Am Geriatr Soc*. 1993;41:345.
28. Emanuel EJ, Weinberg DS, Gonin R, et al. How well is the Patient Self-Determination Act working? an early assessment. *Am J Med*. 1993;95(6):619–628.
29. Teno J, Lynn J, Wenger N, et al., for the SUPPORT Investigators. Advance directives for seriously ill hospitalized patients: effectiveness with the patient self-determination act and the SUPPORT intervention. *J Am Geriatr Soc*. 1997;45:500–507.
30. Goodlin SJ, Zhong Z, Lynn DJ, et al. Factors associated with use of cardiopulmonary resuscitation in seriously ill hospitalized adults. *JAMA*. 1999;282:2333–2339.
31. Wenger NS, Pearson ML, Desmond KA, et al. Epidemiology of do-not-resuscitate orders: disparity by age, diagnosis, gender, race, and functional impairment. *Arch Intern Med*. 1995;155:2056–2062.
32. Holtzman J, Pheley AM, Lurie N. Changes in orders limiting care and the use of less aggressive care in a nursing home population. *J Am Geriatr Soc*. 1994;42:275–279.
33. Fried TR, Gillick MR. Medical decision-making in the last six months of life: choices about limitation of care. *J Am Geriatr Soc*. 1994;42:303–307.
34. Murphy DJ, Burrows D, Santilli S, et al. The influence of the probability of survival on patients' preference regarding cardiopulmonary resuscitation. *N Engl J Med*. 1994;330(8): 545–549.
35. Mullen MT, van der Wal F, van Eijk JThM, et al. Voluntary active euthanasia and assisted suicide in Dutch nursing homes: are the requirements for prudent practice properly met? *J Am Geriatr Soc*. 1994;42:624–629.
36. Bernat JL, Gert B, Mogielnicki RP. Patient refusal of hydration and nutrition: an alternative to physician-assisted suicide or voluntary active euthanasia. *Arch Intern Med*. 1993;153:2723–2728.

37. Hanson LC, Danis M, Garrett J. What is wrong with end-of-life care: opinions of bereaved family members. *J Am Geriatr Soc.* 1997;45:1339–1244.

38. Last Acts Campaign Task Force on Palliative Care. Precepts of palliative care. *J Palliat Med.* 1998;1(2):109–112.

39. Rabeneck L, McCullough LB, Wray NP. Ethically justified, clinically comprehensive guidelines for percutaneous endoscopic gastrostomy tube placement. *Lancet.* 1997;349: 496–498.

40. The President's Commission for the Study of Ethical Problems in Medicine. *Deciding to Forgo Life-Sustaining Treatment.* Washington DC: USGPO; 1983.

41. Paolisso G, Rizzo MR, Mazziotti G, et al. Advancing age and insulin resistance: role of plasma tumor necrosis factor-alpha. *Am J Physiol.* 1998;275:E294–E299.

42. McCann RM, Hall WJ, Groth-Junker A. Comfort care for terminally ill patients: the appropriate use of nutrition and hydration. *JAMA.* 1994;272(16):1263–1266.

43. Dunn J. *Hard Choices for Loving People.* Herndon, VA: A&A Publishers; 1998.

44. Lynn J, Harrold J. *Handbook for Mortals.* New York: Oxford University Press; 1999.

45. Ellershaw JE, Sutcliffe JM, Saunders CM. Dehydration and the dying patient. *J Pain Symptom Manage.* 1995;10(3): 192–197.

46. Morrison RS, Ahronheim JC, Morrison GR, et al. Pain and discomfort associated with common hospital procedures and experiences. *J Pain Symptom Manage.* 1998;15(2):91–101.

47. Covinsky KE, Goldman L, Cook EF, et al. The impact of serious illness on patients' families. *JAMA.* 1994;272: 1839–1844.

48. Strength For Caring (888) ICARE80 Hotline, *www.oncolink.upenn.edu/sfc.*

49. Holtzman J, Pheley AM, Lurie N. Changes in orders limiting care & the use of less aggressive care in a nursing home population. *J Am Geriatr Soc.* 1994;42:275–279.

50. Coyle N, Adelhardt J, Foley KM, et al. Character of terminal illness in the advanced cancer patient: Pain and other symptoms during the last four weeks of life. *J Pain Symptom Manage.* 1990;5:83–93.

51. Bonica JJ. Treatment in cancer pain. Current status and future needs. In: Fields H, et al., eds. *Advances in Pain Research and Therapy.* New York: Raven Press; 1985;589–616.

52. Holtzman J, Pheley AM, Lurie N. Changes in orders limiting care and the use of less aggressive care in a nursing home population. *J Am Geriatr Soc.* 1994;42:275–279.

53. Bernabei R, Gambassi G, Lapane K, et al. Management of pain in elderly patients with cancer. *JAMA.* 1998;279: 1877–1915.

54. Ahmedzai S. Palliation of respiratory symptoms. In: *Oxford Textbook of Palliative Medicine.* New York: Oxford University Press; 1998.

55. Mogielnicki RP, Nelson WA, Dulac JA. A study of the dying process in elderly hospitalized males. *J Cancer Educ.* 1990; 5(2):135–145.

56. Reuben DB, Mor V. Dyspnea in terminally ill cancer patients. *Chest.* 1986;89:234–236.

57. Bruera E, de Stoutz N, Valasco-Leiva A, et al. Effects of oxygen on dyspnea in hypoxemic terminal-cancer patients. *Lancet.* 1993;342:13–14.

58. Jordan C. Assessment of the effects of drugs on respiration. *Br J Anesth.* 1982;54:763–782.

59. Bruera E, MacEachern T, Ripamonti C, et al. Subcutaneous morphine for dyspnea in cancer patients. *Ann Intern Med.* 1993;119:906–907.

60. Cohen MH, Anderson AJ, Krasnow SH, et al. Continuous intravenous morphine for severe dyspnea. *South Med J* 1991;84(2):229–234.

61. Massie MJ, Holland JC. Depression and the cancer patient. *J Clin Psychiatry.* 1990;51:12–17.

62. Chochinov HM, Wilson KG, Enns M, et al. Desire for death in the terminally ill. *Am J Psychiatry.* 1995;152(8):1185–1191.

63. Shuster JL. Delirium, confusion, and agitation at the end of life. *J Palliat Med.* 1998;1(2):177–186.

64. Maddocks I, Somogyi A, Abbott F, et al. Attenuation of morphine-induced delirium in palliative care by substitution with infusion of oxycodone. *J Pain Symptom Manage.* 1996;12:182–189.

65. Kukull WA, Renner DE, Speck CE, et al. Causes of death associated with Alzheimer disease: variation by level of cognitive impairment before death. *J Am Geriatr Soc.* 1994;42:723–726.

66. Morrison RS, Siu AL. Survival in end-stage dementia following acute illness. *JAMA.* 2000;284:47–52.

67. Collins C, Ogle K. Patterns of pre-death service use by dementia patients with a family caregiver. *J Am Geriatr Soc.* 1994;42:719–722.

68. Hurley AC, Volicer L, Blasi ZV. End of life care for patients with advanced dementia. *JAMA.* 2000;284(19):2449–2450.

69. Volicer L, Collard A, Hurley A, et al. Impact of special care unit for patients with advanced Alzheimer's disease on patients' discomfort and costs. *J Am Geriatr Soc.* 1994; 42:597–603.

70. Hockley JM, Dunlop R, Davies RJ. Survey of distressing symptoms in dying patients and their families in hospital and the response to a symptom control team. *B Med J.* 1988;296:1715–1717.

27
Sources of Suffering in the Elderly

Maria Torroella Carney and Diane E. Meier

The relief of suffering is one of the primary aims of medicine. The nature of suffering and what physicians can do to prevent or relieve it is poorly understood. Suffering is a global concept that must be distinguished from pain or other physical symptoms with which it may be associated. Although physicians, patients, and medical literature tend to link pain with suffering, these are distinct phenomena.[1]

Cassell describes suffering as it relates to personhood.[2] Personhood includes personality and character, the individual's past, the family's past, associations and relationships with family and others, work and social roles, body image, the unconscious mind, political affiliations, the secret life, the perceived future, and the transcendent or spiritual dimension. Suffering with sickness occurs when the illness or its symptoms not only threaten interference with some aspect of personhood, but when it destroys or is perceived to destroy the integrity of the person, as just define.[1]

Suffering often goes undiagnosed and unrelieved. Identification of suffering requires a high index of suspicion in the presence of serious disease and distressing symptoms.[3] Clinicians should ask both themselves and their patient whether there is suffering. Ask directly, "Are you suffering?" "I know you have pain, but are there things that are even worse than the pain?" "Are you frightened?"[3] The questions are purposely open-ended, telling patients that they have permission to talk about things that no one is likely to have wanted to hear before and conveying a sense of compassion and a willingness to listen from the person asking the questions. Intervening to try to relieve distress or suffering can only be accomplished once it has been identified, heard, and named.

The elderly often suffer from multiple acute disease processes superimposed on chronic and progressive illness, accompanied by an increased risk of sensory and cognitive impairment, and functional dependency.[4] This chapter attempts to address both physical and psychosocial sources of distress in elderly patients, as well as other factors associated with suffering often found in the elderly patient population.

Goals of Care

As symptoms are often interrelated with multiple concurrent medical problems, management can be challenging. As with any illness, the approach to treating symptoms requires a thorough history, physical examination, and laboratory or radiologic investigations appropriate to gain the best understanding of etiology and underlying pathophysiology. Once the cause and pathophysiology are known, intervention ideally includes therapy to relieve the symptoms as well as to treat underlying causes.

The goals of care may involve weighing the benefits and risks of treatments aimed at relief of suffering versus those aimed at prolongation of life. This approach is particularly important when symptom relief measures may either cause (or are perceived to cause) a higher risk of impairment or death. Many physicians fear that medications used to manage symptoms have an unacceptably high risk of an adverse event that may cause intolerable side effects or even shorten life, especially in the elderly. The fear of such consequences generally far outweighs their actual prevalence. It is extremely rare for opiate analgesics given at doses sufficient to relieve pain to simultaneously lead to respiratory depression. Nonetheless, the intent of the practitioner when offering a treatment is what determines whether it is ethical medical practice.[5] Education and involvement of the patient and family as partners in care are key to successful management of symptoms.

Symptoms and Their Treatment

Formal Assessment

Symptom control is an essential component of medical care. For most patients, physical pain is only one of several sources of distress. Symptom relief encompasses physical, psychologic, social, and spiritual aspects of suffering. Physical aspects of pain cannot be effectively treated in isolation from the emotional and spiritual components that contribute to it, nor can these sources of suffering be addressed adequately when patients are in physical distress. The various components of suffering must be addressed simultaneously. Many sources of distress and suffering are not visible and frequently are not spontaneously reported by patients. Formal and regular assessment is therefore critical to identification and appropriate treatment of diverse symptoms.[6]

Physical and psychologic symptoms have been assessed most frequently using simple, validated measures, often in the form of symptom checklists. The Edmonton Symptom Assessment Scale (ESAS) evaluates eight symptoms on visual analogue scales and has been extensively used in palliative care research.[7] The Memorial Symptom Assessment Scale (MSAS) is a validated patient-rated measure that provides multidimensional information about a diverse group of common symptoms.[8] It characterizes 32 physical and psychologic symptoms in terms of intensity, frequency, and level of distress.[8] Other frequently used symptom assessment instruments may be found on the web at *www.stoppain.org*, *www.growthhouse.org*, or *www.chcr.brown.edu/pcoc/toolkit.htm*.

Distressing symptoms addressed in this chapter include dyspnea, cough, nausea and vomiting, constipation, diarrhea, bowel obstruction, mouth symptoms, skin symptoms, odors, and dizziness. In addition, suffering caused by spiritual distress, developmental tasks faced at the end of life, the trauma of transferring or moving to hospital or nursing home, and the experience of being cared for by others is discussed. Pain is discussed separately in Chapter 29.

Respiratory Symptoms

Dyspnea

Dyspnea is a subjective sensation of shortness of breath[9] that is described in 70% of cancer patients during the last 6 weeks of life and in 50% to 70% of patients dying of other illnesses.[10] It is a common symptom associated with pneumonia, congestive heart failure exacerbations, and chronic obstructive pulmonary disease—all illnesses common to elderly adults. Nevertheless, dyspnea may be a subjective symptom that may not match any objective

TABLE 27.1. Dyspnea drug treatment.

Morphine 2.5–5 mg p.o. q 4 h while awake (opiate-naïve patient)
Morphine infusion 0.5 mg/h; titrate to relief of respiratory distress
Once dose requirement established, switch to long-acting opiate or fentanyl patch
Nebulized morphine or hydromorphone:
Injectable morphine 2.5–10 mg in 2 mL NS
or
Injectable hydromorphone 0.25–1 mg in 2 mL NS
Plus or minus
Albuterol 0.083% (3 mL)
Plus or minus
Solumedrol 10 mg
Corticosteroids:
Dexamethasone 16 mg initial, then
8 mg bid × 2 days, then 4 mg bid × 2 days, then 2 mg bid
Prednisone pulse
40 mg po bid × 5–7 days
Oxygen

Source: From Ref. 13, with permission.

signs of respiratory function,[9] and its management can be challenging. It is important to diagnose and treat the underlying reversible causes of dyspnea when possible. When therapy specific to the underlying cause is unavailable or ineffective, several techniques may alleviate breathlessness. Simple techniques include pursed-lip breathing and diaphragmatic breathing, leaning forward with arms on a table, cool air ventilation (fan or open window), and nasal oxygen. Opiates have been shown in numerous studies to be highly effective in the amelioration of dyspnea.[11,12] In one study of the effect of opiates on dyspnea and respiratory physiology, opiates sufficient to relieve dyspnea had no measurable adverse effect on respiratory rate, effort, oxygen saturation, and carbon dioxide concentration.[11] Along with treating the underlying cause, steroids and oxygen therapy may be of benefit. A list of some medications and dosages to alleviate refractory dyspnea can be found in Table 27.1.[13]

Cough

Cough is a normal but complex physiologic mechanism that protects the airways and lungs by removing mucus and foreign matter from the larynx, trachea, and bronchi. Cough is under both voluntary and involuntary control.[14] Management of cough should be determined by the type and the cause of the cough, as well as the patient's general condition and likely diagnosis. When possible, the aim should be to reverse or ameliorate the cause, combined with appropriate symptomatic measures. Exacerbating factors should be defined, and simple measures such as a change in posture can be very helpful. Breathlessness can trigger cough and vice versa. Persistent cough can also precipitate vomiting, exhaustion, chest or abdominal pain, rib fracture, syncope, and insomnia.

Cough suppressants are usually used to manage dry cough. The most effective antitussive agents are the opioids. Codeine is a mild antitussive, while other opioids (morphine, oxycodone, hydrocodone, hydromorphone) have a more pronounced effect. Methadone can be particularly effective at night, but due to its prolonged half-life, the risk of accumulation exists. Other useful measures include decongestants, antihistamines, and corticosteroids.

Gastrointestinal Symptoms

Nausea and Vomiting

Nausea and vomiting are present in up to 62% of cancer patients.[15] There are multiple potential causes for both nausea and vomiting, yet symptomatic relief is relatively easy to achieve with the appropriate use of medications. A thorough assessment is crucial to understanding the underlying etiology and, in turn, to providing the most beneficial form of treatment.

Two organ systems are particularly important in nausea and vomiting: the central nervous system and the gastrointestinal system.[16] The gastric lining, the chemoreceptor trigger zone in the base of the fourth ventricle, the vestibular apparatus, and the cortex are all involved in the physiology of nausea. Stimulation of the vomiting center from one or more of these areas is mediated through the neurotransmitters serotonin, dopamine, acetylcholine, and histamine. Serotonin seems to be important in the gastric lining and central nervous system, whereas acetylcholine and histamine are important in the vestibular apparatus. Cortical responses are mediated via neurotransmitters as well as through learned responses (e.g., nausea related to anxiety).

Table 27.2 describes the major causes of nausea and vomiting, classified by the mechanism's principal site of action. Dopamine-mediated nausea is probably the most common form of nausea and is the type most frequently targeted for initial symptom management. These medications are phenothiazines or butyrophenone neuroleptics (metoclopramide, prochlorperazine) and

TABLE 27.2. Management of nausea and vomiting.

Etiology	Pathophysiology	Therapy
Metastases		
Cerebral	Increased intracranial pressure	Steroids, mannitol
	Direct chemoreceptor trigger zone	Antidopamine, antihistamine
Liver	Toxin buildup	Antidopamine, antihistamine
Meningeal irritation	Increased intracranial pressure	Steroids
Movement	Vestibular stimulation	Antiacetylcholine
Mentation (e.g., anxiety)	Cortical	Anxiolytics
Medications		
Opioids	Chemoreceptor trigger zone, vestibular effect, gastrointestinal tract	Antidopamine, antiacetylcholine, prokinetic agents, stimulant cathartics
Chemotherapy	Chemoreceptor trigger zone, gastrointestinal tract	Antiserotonin, antidopamine, steroids
Others	Chemoreceptors	Antidopamine, antihistamine
Mucosal irriation		
NSAIDS	Gastrointestinal tract	Cytoprotective agents, antacids
Hyperacidity, gastroesophageal reflux		
Mechanical obstruction		
Intraluminal	Constipation, obstipation	Manage constipation
Extraluminal	Tumor, fibrotic stricture	Surgery, manage fluids, steroids, octreotide, scopolamine
Motility		
Opioids, ileus, other meds	Gastrointestinal tract	Prokinetic agents, stimulant laxatives
Metabolic		
Hypercalcemia	Chemoreceptor trigger zone	Antidopamine, antihistamine, rehydration, steroids
Hyponatremia		
Hepatic/renal failure		
Microbes		
Local irritation	Gastrointestinal tract	Antibacterials, antivirals, antifungals, antacids
Systemic sepsis	Chemoreceptor trigger zone	Antidopamine, antihistamine, antibacterials, antivirals, antifungals
Myocardial		
Ischemia	Vagal stimulation	Oxygen, opioids, antidopamine, antihistamine, anxiolytics
Congestive heart failure	Cortical, chemoreceptor trigger zone	

Source: From Ref. 5, with permission.

TABLE 27.3. Medications for Nausea and Vomiting.

Oral medications:
    Dexamethasone 2–8 mg q 6–12 h
    Diphenhydramine (Benadryl) 25–50 mg q 4–6 h
    Haloperidol (Haldol) 0.5–5 mg q 6–8 h
    Hydroxyzine (Atarax) 25–50 mg tid-qid
    Hyoscyamine (Levsin) 0.125–0.25 s.l. q 4 h
    Lorazepam 1–2 mg q 2–4 h
    Marinol 2.5–10 mg bid, tid
    Meclizine (Antivert) 12.5–25 mg bid-qid
    Metoclopramide (Reglan) 10–40 mg qid
    Ondansetron (Zofran) 8 mg p.o. tid-qid
    Prochlorperazine (Compazine) 5–10 mg q 4–6 h
    Prochlorperazine (Compazine) s.r. 10–15 mg bid
    Promethazine (Phenergan) 12.5–225 mg tid-qid
    Thiethylperazine (Torecan) 10 mg q d-tid
    Trimethobenzamide (Tigan) 250 mg tid-qid
Suppositories:
    Prochlorperazine (Compazine) 25 mg q 6 h
    Promethazine (Phenergan) 12.5, 25, 50 mg tid-qid
    Trimethobenzamide (Tigan) 200 mg tid-qid
Continuous infusion:
    Dexamethasone 8–100 mg/24 h
    Haloperidol 2.5–10 mg/24 h
    Hyoscyamine (Levsin) 1–2 mg/24 h
    Scopolamine 0.8–20 mg/24 h
    Metoclopramide (Reglan) 20–80 mg/24 h
    Ondansetron 0.45 mg/kg/24 h
I.V. medications:
    Dexamethasone 2–8 mg q 4–6 h
    Diphenhydramine (Benadryl) 25–50 mg q 6 h
    Dronabinol 5 mg/m^2 q 4 h; max, 6 doses/day 5 mg/m^2 (meter
squared)
    Granisetron (Kytril) 10 μg/kg q d
    Haloperidol 0.5–2 mg q 4–6 h
    Lorazepam 1–2 mg q 6–8 h
    Metoclopramide (Reglan) 10–20 mg q 6 h
    Ondansetron 4–8 mg q 8 h
    Prochlorperazine (Compazine) 5–10 mg q 4–6 h

Source: From Ref. 13, with permission.

have the potential to cause drowsiness and extrapyramidal symptoms. Haloperidol is a highly effective antinausea agent and may be less sedating. Antihistamines such as diphenhydramine can be used to control nausea but may cause sedation. Antihistamines also have anticholinergic properties covering two mechanisms of nausea. Serotonin has been implicated in chemotherapy-associated nausea. Serotonin blockers are effective but expensive. Other agents are listed in Table 27.3.

Nausea can also be caused by a slow gastric/intestinal motility, "squashed" stomach syndrome due to mechanical compression of the stomach or constipation, and thus prokinetic agents such as metoclpropamide should be considered as therapeutic modalities. Hyperacidity and mucosal erosion may be associated with significant nausea. Consider the use of antacids, H_2 bloekers, proton pump inhibitors, and misoprostol.

Constipation

Constipation can be defined as the passage of small hard feces infrequently and with difficulty.[17] Constipation is a common complaint among elderly patients. One study found 54% of its community-based elderly to report constipation.[18] Risk factors include immobility, depression, female sex, and polypharmacy.[19–23] Constipation also tends to be associated with illnesses and/or conditions such as diabetes mellitus, hypothyroidism, diverticular disease, irritable bowel syndrome, and hemorrhoids[24] (Table 27.4).

Inquiry should be made about the frequency and consistency of stools, nausea, vomiting, abdominal pain, distension and discomfort, mobility, diet, and any other symptoms.[17] As with any symptom, evaluation of a reversible cause is initial and paramount. A plain x-ray can be useful. Invasive evaluation with colonoscopy should be considered in difficult, refractory, or complicated cases. Many medications can contribute to constipation. First and foremost are opioid agents; many other medications, including beta-blockers, calcium channel blockers, anticholinergic agents, and diuretics, are also contributors[25] (Table 27.5).

Constipation is a universal side effect of opioid analgesic therapy, especially in the terminally ill and elderly, this can lead to serious, if not life-threatening, complications including bowel obstruction, ulceration or perforation, and delirium. Prevention of constipation must be accomplished by using stool softeners, rectal

TABLE 27.4. Constipation causes and risk factors.

Idiopathic
    Dietary factors: low residue, poor nutrition
    Motility disturbances: colonic inertia or spasm
    Sedentary living, weakness
    Depression
    Poor fluid intake
    Confusion
    Inability to reach the toilet
    Change in setting, travel
Structural abnormalities
    Anorectal disorders: fissures, thrombosed hemorrhoids
    Strictures
    Tumors
    Adhesions
Endocrine/metabolic
    Hypercalcemia
    Hypokalemia
    Hypothyroidism
Neurogenic
    Cerebrovascular events
    Spinal cord tumors
    Trauma
Smooth muscle/connective tissue disorders
    Amyloidosis
    Scleroderma

Source: From Ref. 17, with permission.

TABLE 27.5. Drugs and medications commonly associated with constipation.

Antacids: aluminum- and calcium-containing compounds
Antihistamines
Anticholinergics
Antidepressants
Barium sulfate
Beta-blocking agents
Calcium channel blockers
Calcium supplements
Cholestyramine
Cytotoxic agents
Iron supplements
Narcotics
Nonsteroidal anti-inflammatory drugs
Neuroleptics
Sympathomimetics: pseudoephedrine

Source: From Ref. 17, with permission.

suppositories, laxatives, and hyperosmotic agents, before and during opiate therapy. A multiple agent bowel regimen must be begun coincident with the initiation of opiates. Table 27.6 describes a seven-step suggested bowel regimen to avoid constipation in a patient receiving opioid therapy.[4] This regimen could also be utilized for anyone complaining of constipation once intestinal obstruction is ruled out. Operative management of severe constipation may be required in refractory cases.

Fecal impaction is stool impacted in the intestines, often causing "overflow" diarrhea. This disorder must be treated from below utilizing digital disimpaction and rectal laxatives (rectal suppositories, and/or enemas) before any forms of oral treatment are used.[17]

Various forms of laxatives exist. Rectal laxatives are available as suppositories or enemas. Table 27.7 lists stimulant, osmotic, and detergent laxatives, along with prokinetic agents, lubricant stimulants, and large-volume enemas. Clinicians should dose escalate a particular modality to a maximum therapeutic dose.

Polyethylene glycol solution (Golytely) or powder (Miralax) is often used as a precolonoscopic regimen but may be an effective means to treat constipation. It offers advantages over other laxatives in that it may cause less cramping. Mineral oil, is usually avoided in the elderly, as it may predispose to aspiration pneumonitis in people with swallowing problems.

Diarrhea

Diarrhea, potentially caused by fecal impaction, antibiotic-associated colitis, gastrointestinal bleeding, malabsorption, medications, or even stress, is a particularly distressing and exhausting symptom.[17] A general approach is to determine the patient's normal bowel habits. Once diarrhea is confirmed, the underlying cause must be evaluated and treated if possible. Initial therapy

for transient or mild diarrhea may respond to attapulgite or bismuth salts.[17] For persistent and bothersome diarrhea, kaolin-pectin of psyllium, loperamide, or tincture of opium may be effective. Octreotide is also an effective means of reducing gastrointestinal secretions.[26]

Bowel Obstruction

Symptoms of bowel obstruction include anorexia, confusion, abdominal distension, nausea and vomiting, constipation, and pain. Obstruction may be the presenting symptom that heralds the diagnosis of cancer or may occur later in the course of disease. Bowel obstruction can be caused by multiple and often coexisting etiologies, including intraluminal obstruction, infiltration of the bowel wall, external compression of the lumen, dysmotility, fecal impaction, and intra-abdominal adhesions. The prevalence of bowel obstruction is as high as 40% in bowel and pelvic cancers. Gastrointestinal obstruction can be particularly challenging to palliate if the cause of the obstruction cannot be removed. Therefore, investigation of the underlying cause of the obstruction is the first step in alleviating the distress. Furthermore, aggressive measures to prevent or treat constipation and impaction as previously described may be necessary. Treatment of bowel obstruction may involve the surgical relief of obstruction, nasogastric suction, and pharmacologic measures. Colicky or cramping pain may respond to dicyclomine, opiates (parenteral or rectal), and warm soaks to the abdomen. The obstruction and associated nausea and vomiting may respond to metoclopramide, haloperidol, or dexamethasone. Parenteral octreotide is also

TABLE 27.6. Bowel regimen.

With few exceptions, all patients on opioid therapy need an individualized bowel regimen. Start with the step 1 regimen. When an effective regimen is determined, it must be continued for the duration of the opioid therapy. If fecal impaction is present or suspected, rectal evacuation must occur (before any laxative agents are given orally), using digital disimpaction, enemas, high colonic enemas, and bisacodyl suppositories (2–4 at a time).

Step 1: Docusate 100 mg tid plus senna 1 tab q d or bid
Step 2: Docusate 100 mg tid plus senna 2 tab bid, plus bisacodyl rectal suppository 1–2 after breakfast
Step 3: Docusate 100 mg tid plus senna 3 tab bid, plus bisacodyl suppository 3–4 after breakfast
Step 4: Docusate 100 mg tid, senna 4 tab bid plus lactulose or milk of magnesia or polyethylene glycol powder or sorbitol 15–30 mL bid, plus bisacodyl suppository 3–4 after breakfast
Step 5: Sodium phosphate or oil retention enema; if no results add a high colonic tap water enema,[a] and continue until results

[a] High colonic enemas are given by warming 2-L bags of saline or water to body temperature, hanging bag at ceiling level, and infusing rectally over 30–60 min. May repeat continuously or until results.
Source: From Ref. 4, with permission.

TABLE 27.7. Treatments for constipation.

Stimulant laxatives: irritate the bowel and increase peristaltic activity
 Prune juice, 120–240 mL qd or bid
 Senna, 2 p.o. q h, titrate to effect (up to 9 or more per day)
 Casanthranol, 2 p.o. q h, titrate to effect (up to 9 or more per day)
 Bisacodyl, 5 mg p.o., p.r. q h, titrate to effect; bisacodyl
suppositories
  may be given per rectum, up to 4 at a time, preferably after
  breakfast

Osmotic laxatives: draw water into the bowel lumen, increase overall
stool volume
 Lactulose or sorbitol, 70%, 30 mL p.o. q 4–6 h, then titrate
 Milk of magnesia, 1–2 tablespoons 1–3 times per day
 Magnesium citrate, 1–2 bottles prn
 Polyethylene glycol (Golytely), 1–4 L p.o., drink 8 ounces every
  10 min until consumed
 Polyethylene glycol powder (Miralax), 17 g (1 tablespoon) powder
  q d in 8 ounces of water; 2–4 days may be required to produce a
  bowel movement; may increase dose as needed

Detergent laxatives (stool softeners): increase water content in stool
by facilitating the dissolution of fat
 Sodium docusate, 1–2 p.o. q d-bid, titrate to effect
 Calcium docusate, 1–2 p.o. q d-bid, titrate to effect
 Phosphosoda enema prn

Prokinetic agents: stimulate bowel's myenteric plexus and increase
peristaltic activity and stool movement
 Metoclopramide, 10–20 mg p.o. q 6 h

Lubricant stimulants: lubricate the stool and irritate the bowel,
increasing peristaltic activity and stool movement
 Glycerin suppositories
 Oil: mineral, peanut

Large-volume enemas: soften stool by increasing its water content,
distending the colon, and inducing peristalsis
 Warm water (addition of soap suds irritates bowel wall to induce
  peristalsis)

High colonic enemas
 Utilize gravity to bring fluid to more proximal parts of bowel; use
  2-L bags of water or saline warmed to body temperature, hang
  on intravenous pole at ceiling level and run in over 30 min,
  repeat q 1 h

Source: From Refs. 5 and 25, with permission.

useful in this setting to decrease the volume of bowel secretions.[26]

Mouth Symptoms

A patient's oral problems can be kept to a minimum by good hydration, brushing the teeth with a fluoride toothpaste twice daily, and daily observation of the oral mucosa. Oral problems can reduce intake of food and fluid due to altered taste, pain, and difficulty swallowing. The first step is managing local problems. Key questions to ask concerning mouth care include the following: Is the mouth dry? Is infection present? Is the mouth dirty? Is the mouth painful? Are oral ulcerations present?

Dry Mouth

The presence of saliva is hardly ever noticed, but the lack of it can seriously damage the quality of life for those experiencing a sensation of oral dryness. Xerostomia describes the subjective complaint of dry mouth. Xerostomia may have both salivary and nonsalivary causes.[27] More than 50% of elderly have been reported to have noticed oral dryness.[28–30] Table 27.8 lists principal causes of salivary gland dysfunction and xerostomia. Table 27.9 lists medications that have the potential to reduce salivary flow rates.

Almost all forms of xerostomia require symptomatic therapy irrespective of etiology. The goal of therapy is to moisten the oral mucosa, and the best, simplest aid is to sip water frequently. However, several mouth moisteners or artificial salivas have been designed that contain mucin

TABLE 27.8. Causes of salivary gland dysfunction and xerostomia.

Iatrogenic causes
 Medication
 Therapeutic irradiation
Systemic conditions
 Rheumatoid diseases (Sjögren's syndrome)
 Immunodeficiencies (AIDS)
 Hormonal disorders (diabetes mellitus)
 Neurologic disorders (Parkinson's disease)
 Dehydration
Diseases of the salivary gland
 Sialoadenitis
 Sialolithiasis
Psychogenic disorders
 Depression
Oral conditions
 Decreased mastication

Source: From Ref. 31, with permission.

TABLE 27.9. Medications that have potential to reduce salivary flow rate.

Anticholinergic agents
Medications with anticholinergic effects
 Antiarrhythmics
 Antihypertensives
 Antihistamines
 Antidepressants
 Antipsychotics
 MAO inhibitors
 Opiates
Psychotropic agents
 Benzodiazepines
Medications causing changes in fluid and electrolyte balance
 Diuretics
Antineoplastic agents
 Interleukin-2

Source: From Ref. 31, with permission.

TABLE 27.10. Local measures for oral problems.

Dry mouth
  Semifrozen fruit juice
  Frequent sips of cold water or water sprays
  Petroleum jelly rubbed on lips
Dirty mouth
  Regular brushing with soft toothbrush and toothpaste
  Pineapple chunks
  Cider and soda mouthwash
Infected mouth
  Topical corticosteroids: Betamethasone 0.5 mg in 5 mL water as
    mouthwash or triamcinolone in carmellose paste
  Tetracycline mouthwash, 250 mg every 8 h (one capful dissolved in
    5 mL water)
Painful mouth
  Coating agents: Sucralfate suspension as mouthwash, carmellose
    paste, carbenoxolone
  Topical anesthesia: Benzadymine mouthwash, choline salicylate,
    Mucasine, lozenges containing local anesthetics

Source: From Ref. 33, with permission.

and may be preferred by patients.[31,32] Pilocarpine tablets (Salagen) may be used (5–10 mg q 8 h) if these measures fail. Side effects may include nausea, diarrhea, urinary frequency, and dizziness.

Oral Ulcers/Mucositis

Oral infection can be due to multiple etiologies. Aphthous ulcers are common and can be helped by topical corticosteroids or tetracycline mouthwash. Oral candidiasis usually presents as adherent white plaques but can also present as erythema or angular cheilitis. Nystatin suspension is the usual treatment, but a 5-day course of oral ketoconazole 200 mg can be used as well. Severe viral infection (herpes simplex or zoster) requires acyclovir 200 mg every 4 h for 5 days. Malignant ulcers are often associated with anaerobic bacteria and may respond to metronidazole at 400–500 mg orally or rectally every 12 h or as a topical gel.[33] Table 27.10 lists other local measures.

Skin Symptoms

Pressure Sores

Pressure sores result from immobility, moisture, friction, shear (sliding movement), and pressure. Prevention and treatment require reduction in pressure (frequent turning and repositioning, foam or low-pressure mattresses), maintaining dryness and cleanliness, avoidance of shear, and friction. Patients at risk of pressure sores should be monitored regularly with daily visual inspection of pressure areas. How a patient moves or is moved by caregivers needs to be assessed and monitored. Even with regular turning and careful lifting and positioning, special pressure surfaces or mattresses are sometimes needed.[33] Good hydration, high-protein and -carbohydrate diets, and vitamin C supplements encourage healing.

Gel or colloid dressings that keep the area moist reduce pain and can be left in place for several days. Painful changing of dressings can be eased by extra analgesia before each change.[33]

Encourage family and caregivers to keep skin clean and dry. Absorbent surfaces, urinary catheters, and rectal tubes may be of assistance.[5] Cover fragile skin that is at risk for breakdown with clear, occlusive dressings. Cover pressure points with thin, hydrocolloid dressings.

Pressure ulcer management should be consistent with goals of care. If overall maintenance or improvement of function is the goal and prognosis is weeks to months, then treat the ulcer with expected management guidelines. If prognosis is limited, then the intent is to optimize quality of life.

For uncomplicated malignant ulcers, pain relief and wound care are managed in the same way as pressure sores. However, malignant wounds present special problems such as bleeding, odor, and disfigurement. A bleeding malignant ulcer should be treated with radiation therapy, topical sucralfate, or topical tranexamic acid. Dirty ulcers should be debrided, which can be accomplished chemically. Altered body image can be lessened with cavity foam dressings. Furthermore, empathetic listening is often therapeutic in itself, but anxiety, anger, or depression will need specific support.[33]

Foul-Smelling Wounds

Odors may be very distressing to patients, families, and caregivers and may lead to poor-quality care, as even professional caregivers avoid sickening smells. Odors are usually caused by anaerobic infections or poor hygiene or both. Treat superficial infections with topical metronidazole or silver sulfadiazine.[5] For soft tissue infections, add systemic metronidazole to topical management.

To control odors, place open kitty litter or activated charcoal in a pan under the patient's bed, provide adequate room ventilation, place an open cup of vinegar in the room, or burn a candle. Special charcoal-impregnated dressings placed over the odorous wound may also be helpful.[5]

Dizziness/Dysequilibrium

Dizziness is a well-recognized problem among older persons. The reported prevalence ranges from 13% to 38%.[34–38] Dizziness has been associated with increased risk for falls and with syncope, functional disability, nursing home placement, stroke, and death.[34,35,37,39–41] Dizziness and associated fear of falling often lead to progressive immobility and deconditioning. Given the fre-

TABLE 27.11. Potential causes and contributing factors of dizziness in geriatric patients.

Peripheral vestibular disorder
Vestibular neuronitis
Benign paroxysmal positional vertigo
Meniere's disease
Cardiovascular diagnoses
Orthostatic hypotension
Arrhythmia
Carotid sinus hypersensitivity
Vasovagal syncope
Central neurologic disorders
Cervical spondylosis
Drop attacks
Stroke disease
Migraine
Bilateral carotid stenosis
Associated diagnoses in patients in whom diagnosis remains unknown
Abnormal Romberg
Abnormal gait
Osteoarthritis of lower limbs
Medications

Source: From Ref. 45, with permission.

quency of dizziness and its associated morbidity, much attention has focused on identifying its causes.

In past studies, authors assumed that dizziness was a symptom of one or more discrete diseases. Investigators typically assigned the cause of the dizziness to specific diagnostic categories on the basis of clinical judgment or diagnostic algorithms. Vestibular disease, cerebrovascular disease, psychiatric disorders, and cervical spondylosis have all been identified as contributing causes[41,42] (Table 27.11). No diagnosis could be made in 8% to 22% of cases, and multiple diagnoses were assigned in 0% to 85% of cases.[43–45]

Due to the great variability in the prevalence of specific diagnoses and the frequency with which no diagnosis or multiple diagnoses were made, Tinetti et al. suggested the hypothesis that dizziness in elderly may result from multifactorial causes rather than being solely a symptom of a discrete disease, henceforth considering it a geriatric syndrome.[46] Dizziness is associated with an increased likelihood of self-reported worsening health, depressive symptoms, less involvement in social activities, and less participation in the activities of daily living.[47]

Treatment may be better directed toward strategy aimed at ameliorating the multiple contributing factors rather than focusing on diagnosing and treating discrete diseases.[46] Preliminary evidence suggests that factors including anxiety and depressive symptoms, hearing impairment, balance impairment, postural hypotension, and the use of multiple medications were additively associated with the likelihood of reporting chronic dizziness.[46] Chronic dizziness should be approached similarly to falls and amelioration of the symptoms—the physical, psy-

chologic, and social disability should be paramount. (See Chapter 68 for a more detailed discussion of dizziness.)

Spiritual Suffering

Patients who are living with life-threatening illness are frequently distressed by hopelessness, meaninglessness, remorse, anxiety, being worried, and disruption of personal identity.[2] These worries are universal and may result from past, present, or future concerns, independent of religious background or beliefs.[48] Facing a life-threatening illness brings to surface questions as to what life is all about.[49] People may suffer from an inability to find meaning in this last chapter of their lives, from an abbreviated future, from inability to relate meaningfully with family and loved ones at their final opportunity, from anger about being ill, and from isolation because of the reluctance of the healthy to broach the subject of dying.[49] These are all spiritual issues.

Yet patients do not suffer alone. Families and caregivers suffer, too. Family members may have to reshape their identities and redefine their basic commitments when their loved one is ill or dying. Long-unresolved family issues threaten to become permanently unresolvable. The family may suffer from guilt and a sense of abandonment.[49] Many turn to religious or spiritual beliefs for decision-making guidance and support when threatened by serious illness.[50,51]

Physicians are participants in their patient's life and have a distinctive role and responsibility to minimize patient and family suffering. Patients and families should be afforded the opportunity to explore issues relating to the nature of death and issues of afterlife.[48] Discussion of religious or spiritual beliefs might enhance physician–patient understanding and communication. Some patients may want to share their religious convictions with physicians.[52,53] In one study, two-thirds of patients surveyed would welcome a carefully worded inquiry about their spiritual or religious beliefs in the event that they became gravely ill. However, 16% would not. Therefore, spiritual guidance may be desired. When applicable, an appropriate religious chaplain or minister should be consulted for both patient and family.[48] Some appropriate questions for a physician to ask[54] are given in Table 27.12.

TABLE 27.12. Physician questions to explore patient's spiritual needs.

1. Are you a member of a faith community?
2. Does your community know you are ill?
3. Would you like them to be contacted?
4. Would you like me to call the priest (rabbi, minister, etc.) to come visit you?

Source: From Ref. 54, with permission.

Developmental Tasks at End of Life: Barriers and Associated Suffering

Throughout a person's life, the sense of who one is changes in the process of responding to the challenges and crises that define the developmental stages of infancy, childhood, adolescence, midlife, and late life. During each major life transition, there may be suffering. At times people may feel broken and never fully recover a sense of self, but most find a way to grow through these turning points. Many persons describe an experience of enhanced awareness and growth in the last stage of life. People who can be said to have grown in their dying are those who express satisfaction in personal change that occurred in response to the stresses of a disabling illness and for whom an enhanced subjective sense of self emerges during the process. Dying is surely among the most profound of life's challenges.[55]

Progressive illness offers an opportunity to reconcile previously strained relationships and achieve closure or resolution of unfinished tasks.[55] Byock describes developmental landmarks and tasks for the end of life that serve as diagnostic tools enabling clinicians to anticipate issues with which patients may struggle and from which struggling may arise (Table 27.13).

One of the central tenets of hospice care has been the need to discuss death openly with the patient; however, that is not possible for some individuals and in many cultures. Physicians, families, and perhaps patients from Native American, Asian, and other cultures may be reluctant to discuss the prospect of death openly. In the United States, there is more openness and emphasis on patient autonomy and the right to make decisions. The hospice movement, the work of Dr. Kubler-Ross, and the aging of the baby boom population have combined to cause a marked change in attitudes over the past two decades, so that it is now considered ethically appropriate for the patient to be given the news about a terminal illness directly. This approach increasingly tends to be the pattern in the United Kingdom. In Italy, a belief against

TABLE 27.13. Developmental landmarks and tasks for the end of life.

Sense of completion with worldly affairs
Sense of completion in relationships with one's community
Sense of meaning about one's individual life
Experienced love of self
Experienced love of others
Sense of completion in relationships with family and friends
Acceptance of the finality of life—of one's existence as an individual
Sense of a new self (personhood) beyond personal loss
Sense of meaning about life in general
Surrender to the transcendent, to the Unknown: "Letting Go"

Source: From Ref. 55, with permission.

speaking of cancer or terminal illnesses to the patient is strong, but this may be changing.[56] A reluctance to discuss death also seems to be prevalent in areas where there is no strong religious belief or ritual.[57] Traditional customs, religious beliefs, and ceremonies have typically helped patients come to terms with death and helped survivors deal with their loss. Cultural and religious variations should be explored and understood to optimally serve patients and their families.

Suffering Associated with Moving or Transferring to or from a Hospital or Nursing Home

Transfer anxiety is a term generally used only by nurses or social workers to describe anxiety experienced by the individual when he or she moves from a familiar, secure environment to an environment that is unfamiliar.[58] The nursing diagnosis of relocation stress syndrome was accepted in 1992 by the North American Nursing Diagnosis Association.[59] It is defined as a syndrome of physiologic or psychosocial disturbances as a result of transfer from one environment to another. The defining characteristics include increased confusion in the elderly, depression, anxiety, apprehension, and loneliness.[59] Relocation stress syndrome has been used to describe the experience of patients transferred from intensive care units to general hospital units and geriatric patients transferred from home or the hospital to a long-term care facility. Studies do not exist that demonstrate how to best limit the suffering associated with transfer, but common sense dictates that making the patient aware of possible location changes early, allowing for questions or preliminary visits, and having the family available for support and present during the transfer process may help to minimize the inevitable suffering associated with dislocation.

Suffering Associated with Being Cared for by Others

Physical disability is a substantial adverse outcome associated with aging.[60] Disability is reported by up to 40% of adults aged 65 and older and increases significantly after age 85.[61,62] Chronic disease is the major cause of long-term disability.[63–66] One of the major concerns patients repeatedly express with old age and end of life includes fear of being a burden on loved ones. Included in that fear may be not wanting to be cared for by others (family or strangers), being totally dependent, having loss of independent capabilities, being turned from a contributor into a burden on others, the humiliation and indignity of being unable to take care of even basic bodily functions, and feeling a sense of abandonment.[49] Patients often fear losing independence, living with disability, or dying without dignity. Such changes may interrupt an individual's sense of personhood. Approaches to the relief of suffering associated with humiliation and dependency include asking the patient how they feel about it, reminding patients that family members and other caregivers want to give care, and identifying and strengthening remaining areas of intact function.

Conclusion

Alleviation of suffering is the central tenet of the practice of medicine. However, because of multiple technical advances, medicine today—in its zealous striving to cure illness and prolong life—may, in fact, contribute to a patient's suffering.[67] It is critical to question patients about their sources of suffering, ranging from physical and psychosocial to spiritual. Regular formal assessment leads to identification of sources or suffering, and identification, in turn, leads to treatment and intervention trials.

Even when a patient's suffering admits of no cure, the act of listening and accompanying the patient on his journey is healing in itself. A physician's ability to hear about the patient's experience assures patients of their connection to a concerned physician who is not frightened to hear the truth and will not abandon them.

References

1. Cassell EJ. The relief of suffering. *Arch Intern Med.* 1983;143:522–523.
2. Cassell EJ. The nature of suffering and the goals of medicine. *N Engl J Med.* 1982;306:639–645.
3. Cassell EJ. Diagnosing suffering. *Ann Intern Med.* 1999;131:531–534.
4. Carney MT, Meier D. Palliative medicine and end of life care. *Anaesth Clin North Am.* 2000;18:183–209.
5. Emanuel LL, von Gunten CF, Ferris FD. The Education for Physicians on End-of-Life Care (EPEC) curriculum. Chicago: Institute for Ethics at the American Medical Association; 1999.
6. O'Neill B, Fallon M. Principles of palliative care. *Br Med J.* 1997;315:801–804.
7. Bruera E, Kuehn N, Miller M, et al. Symptom assessment system: a simple method for the assessment of palliative care patients. *J Palliat Care.* 1991;7:6–9.
8. Portenoy RK, Thaler HT, Kornblith AB, et al. Memorial Symptom Assessment Scale: an instrument for the evaluation of symptom prevalence, characteristics and distress. *Eur J Cancer.* 1994;30A:1326–1336.
9. Carrieri VK, Janson-Bjerklie S. The sensation of dyspnea: a review. *Heart Lung.* 1984;13:436.
10. Hockely JM, Dunlop R, Davies RJ. Survey of distressing symptoms in dying patients and their families in hospital and their response to a symptom control team. *Br Med J.* 1988;296:1715–1717.
11. Bruera E, MacMillan K, Pither J, et al. Effects of morphine on the dyspnea of terminal cancer patients. *J Pain Symptom Manage.* 1990;5:341.
12. Cohen MH, Anderson AJ, Krasnow SH, et al. Continuous infusion of morphine for severe dyspnea. *South Med J.* 1991;84:229.
13. Stegman MB. Non-pain symptoms. In: Stegman MB, ed. *Hope, Hospice Pain, and Symptom Control in Palliative Medicine, Part 6.* Fort Myers: Hospice Resources; 1997:6.1–6.38.
14. Davis C. ABC of palliative care: breathlessness, cough, and other respiratory problems. *Br Med J.* 1997;315:931–934.
15. Reuben DB, Mor V. Nausea and vomiting in terminally ill cancer patients. *Arch Intern Med.* 1986;146:2021–2023.
16. Baines MJ. ABC of palliative care: nausea, vomiting and intestinal obstruction. *Br Med J.* 1997;315:1148–1150.
17. Fallon M, O'Neill B. ABC of palliative care: constipation and diarrhea. *Br Med J.* 1997;315:1293–1296.
18. Harari D, Gurwitz JH, Avorn J, et al. How do older persons define constipation? *J Gen Intern Med.* 1997;12:63–66.
19. Donald IP, Smith RG, Cruikshank JG, Elton RA, Stoddard ME. A study of constipation in elderly living at home. *Gerontology.* 1985;31:112–118.
20. Campbell AJ, Busby WJ, Horwath CC. Factors associated with constipation in a community based sample of people aged 70 years and over. *J Epidemiol Community Health.* 1993;47:23–26.
21. Harari D, Gurwitz JH, Minaker KL. Constipation in the elderly. *J Am Geriatr Soc.* 1993;41:1130–1140.
22. Stewart RB, Moore MT, Marks RG, Hale WE. Correlates of constipation in an ambulatory elderly population. *Am J Gastroenterol.* 1992;87:859–864.
23. Whitehead WE, Drinkwater D, Chisken LJ, Heller BR, Shuster MM. Constipation in the elderly living at home: definition, prevalence and relationships to lifestyle and health status. *J Am Geriatr Soc.* 1989;37:423–429.
24. Meiring PJ, Joubert G. Constipation in elderly patients attending a polyclinic. *S Afr Med J.* 1998;88(7):888–890.
25. *Physician's Desk Reference, 55th Ed.* Montvale, NJ: Medical Economics Company; 2001:991.
26. Muir JC, von Gunten CF. Antisecretory agents in gastrointestinal obstruction. *Clin Geriatr Med.* 2000;16:327–334.
27. Fox PC, van der Ven PF, Sonies BC, et al. Xerostomia: evaluation of a symptom with increasing significance. *J Am Dent Assoc.* 1985;110(4):519–525.
28. Sreebny LM, Valdini A. Xerostomia. Part I: Relationship to other oral symptoms and salivary gland hypofunction. *Oral Surg Oral Med Oral Pathol.* 1988;66(4):451–458.
29. Narhi TO. Prevalence of subjective feelings of dry mouth in the elderly. *J Dent Res.* 1994;73(1):20–25.
30. Loesche WJ, Bromberg J, Terpenning MS, et al. Xerostomia, xerogenic medications and food avoidances in selected geriatric groups. *J Am Geriatr Soc.* 1995;43(4):401–407.
31. Narhi TO, Meurman JH, Ainamo A. Xerostomia and hyposalivation: causes, consequences and treatment in the elderly. *Drugs Aging.* 1999;15(2):103–116.

32. Visch LL. S-Gravenmade EJ, Panders AK, et al. A double-blind crossover trial of CMC- and mucin containing saliva substitutes. *Int J Oral Maxillofac Surg.* 1986;15(4):393–400.

33. Regnard C, Allport S, Stephenson L. ABC of palliative care: mouth care, skin care, and lymphoedema. *Br Med J.* 1997; 315:1002–1005.

34. Tilvus RJ, Hakula SM, Valvanne J, Erkinjuntti T. Postural hypotension and dizziness in a general aged population: a four-year follow-up of the Helsinki Aging Study. *J Am Geriatr Soc.* 1996;44:809–814.

35. Ensrud KE, Nevitt MC, Yunis C, Hulley SB, Grimm RH, Cummings SR. Postural hypotension and postural dizziness in elderly women. *Arch Intern Med.* 1992;152:1058–1064.

36. Colledge NR, Wilson JA, MacIntyre CC, MacLennan WJ. The prevalence and characteristics of dizziness in an elderly community. *Age Aging.* 1994;23:117–120.

37. Boult C, Murphy J, Sloane P, Mor V, Drone C. The relation of dizziness to functional decline. *J Am Geriatr Soc.* 1991; 39:858–861.

38. Sloane P, Blazer D, George LK. Dizziness in a community elderly population. *J Am Geriatr Soc.* 1989;37:101–108.

39. Grimley EJ. Transient neurological dysfunction and risk of stroke in an elderly English population: the different significance of vertigo and nonrotatory dizziness. *Age Aging.* 1990;19:43–49.

40. Sixt E, Landahl S. Postural disturbances in a 75-year-old population: I. Prevalence and functional consequences. *Age Aging.* 1987;16:393–398.

41. Kroenke K, Lucas CA, Rosenberg ML, et al. Causes of persistent dizziness. A prospective study of 100 patients in ambulatory care. *Ann Intern Med.* 1992;117:898–904.

42. Katsarkas A. Dizziness in aging: a retrospective study of 1194 cases. *Otolaryngol Head Neck Surg.* 1994;110:296–301.

43. Colledge NR, Barr-Hamilton RM, Lewis SJ, Sellar RJ, Wilson JA. Evaluation of investigations to diagnose the cause of dizziness in elderly people: a community-based controlled study. *Br Med J.* 1996;313:788–792.

44. Sloane PD, Baloh RW. Persistent dizziness in geriatric patients. *J Am Geriatr Soc.* 1989;37:4031–4038.

45. Lawson J, Fitzgerald J, Birchall J, Aldren CP, Kenny RA. Diagnosis of geriatric patients with severe dizziness. *J Am Geriatr Soc.* 1999;47:12–17.

46. Tinetti ME, Williams CS, Gill TM. Dizziness among older adults: a possible geriatric syndrome. *Ann Intern Med.* 2000; 132:337–344.

47. Tinetti ME, Williams CS, Gill TM. Health, functional, and psychological outcomes among older persons with chronic dizziness. *J Am Geriatr Soc.* 2000;48:417–421.

48. Fainsinger R, MacEachern T, Hanson J, et al. Symptom control during the last week of life on a palliative care unit. *J Palliat Care.* 1991;7:5–11.

49. Hardwig J. Spiritual issues at the end of life: a call for discussion. Hastings Center Rep. vol 30 2000:28–30.

50. Matthews D, McCullough M, Larson D, Koenig H, et al. Religious commitment and health status: a review of the research and implications for family medicine. *Arch Intern Med.* 1998;7:118–124.

51. Hamel R, Lysaught M. Choosing palliative care: do religious beliefs make a difference? *J Palliat Care.* 1994; 10:61–66.

52. Maugans T, Wadland W. Religion and family medicine: a survey of physicians and patients. *J Fam Pract.* 1991;32:210–213.

53. Daaleman T, Nease D. Patient attitudes regarding physician inquiry into spiritual and religious beliefs. *J Fam Pract.* 1994;39:564–568.

54. Pulschaski CM. Taking a spiritual history. In: *Spirituality and Medicine Connection*, vol 3. Washington, DC; FICA; 1999:1.

55. Byock IR. The nature of suffering and the nature of opportunity at the end of life. *Clin Geriatr Med.* 1996;12:237–252.

56. Cruciatti F, Monti M, Cunietti E. The first public hospice in Italy: socio-cultural, aspects and staff organization. *J Palliat Care.* 1995;11:33–37.

57. Rhymes JA. Barriers to effective palliative care of terminal patients. An international perspective. *Clin Geriatr Med.* 1996;12(2):407–417.

58. Roberts SL. Transfer anxiety. In: *Behavioral Concepts and the Critically Ill Patient.* Englewood Cliffs: Prentice-Hall; 1976:224–252.

59. Mallick MJ, Whipple TW. Validity of the nursing diagnosis of relocation stress syndrome. *Nurs Res.* 2000;49(2):97–100.

60. Williamson JD, Fried LP. Characterization of older adults who attribute functional decrements to "old age". *J Am Geriatr Soc.* 1996;44:1429–1434.

61. Jette A, Branch L. The Framingham Disability Study: II. Physical disability among the aging. *Am J Public Health.* 1981;71:211–216.

62. Havlick R, Liu B, Kovar M, et al. *Health Statistics in Older Persons, United States, 1986. Vital Statistics.* Hyattsville, MD: National Center for Health Statistics; 1987.

63. Guralnick J, Simonsick E. Physical disability in older Americans. *J Gerontol.* 1993;48:S3–S10.

64. Mor V, Murphy J, Masterson-Allen S, et al. Risk of functional decline among well elders. *J Clin Epidemiol.* 1989; 42:865–904.

65. Guralnick J, LaCroix A, Everett D, et al. Aging in the eighties: the prevalence of co-morbidity and its association with disability. In: *Advance Data from Vital Health Statistics 170.* Hyattsville, MD: National Center for Health Statistics; 1989.

66. Fried L, Ettinger W, Lind B, et al. Physical disability in older adults: a physiologic approach. *J Clin Epidemiol.* 1994;47:747–760.

67. Morrison RS, Ahronheim JC, Morrison GR, et al. Pain and discomfort associated with common hospital procedures and experiences. *J Pain Symptom Manage.* 1998;15(2): 91–101.

28
Acute and Chronic Pain

Bruce A. Ferrell

Pain is one of the most common symptoms of disease in older persons. Second only to symptoms of upper respiratory tract infections, it is one of the most common complaints in physicians' offices. The intensity of pain often correlates with the severity of disease and indicates the intensity of treatment needed for pain relief. Unrelieved pain, pain that persists, or pain out of proportion to tissue damage often results over time in complications that include physical disability and serious psychologic distress.

Pain assessment and management have reached a high level of sophistication over the last several years. The publication of clinical practice guidelines, the focus of quality review organizations, and moral outrage over suffering and unrelieved pain, especially in those near the end of life, have fueled rapid development of new strategies, products, and technology to improve pain management. Discovery and description of pathophysiologic mechanisms of pain have helped target existing pain management strategies more effectively and suggested new drugs and interventions with lower side effect profiles. Unfortunately, substantial barriers still exist, and pain often remains underrecognized and undertreated. Zealous regulation of opioid drugs and prejudicial attitudes about the patients who need them, health systems that still emphasize cure over care, and financial incentives that favor high-tech pain management strategies over other conventional approaches to pain management remain all too common.

The approach to pain assessment and management is different in elderly versus younger persons.[1] Older persons may underreport pain for a variety of reasons,[2] despite functional impairment, psychologic distress, and needless suffering related to pain. They often present with concurrent illnesses and multiple problems, making pain evaluation and treatment more difficult. Elderly persons have a higher incidence of side effects to medications and higher potential for complications and adverse events related to many treatment procedures.

Despite these challenges, pain can be effectively managed in most elderly patients. Moreover, clinicians have an ethical and moral obligation to prevent needless suffering and provide effective pain relief, especially for those near the end of life.[3]

Taxonomy of Pain

Pain is defined as an unpleasant sensory and emotional experience.[4] It is derived from complex physiologic processes that include elements of neural sensation and nerve transmission integrated with central nervous system processing of memory, expectations, and emotions. Unfortunately, there are no objective biologic markers of pain. There are no measurements in blood, or by electroencephalographic or other imaging devices that accurately reflect the intensity or character of pain experiences. The most accurate and reliable evidence for the existence and intensity of pain is the patient's description.[5] Pain complaints are quite variable in description, character, and intensity. For the purpose of understanding, predicting, and treating pain, a variety of classification schemes have been used. For clinical purposes, it may be helpful to categorize pain as acute or chronic.

Acute Pain

Acute pain is often defined by its distinct onset, obvious cause, and short duration. Trauma, burns, infarction, and inflammation are examples of pathologic processes that can result in acute pain. Acute pain is often associated with autonomic nervous system signs including tachycardia, diaphoresis, or elevation in blood pressure.[6] The presence of acute pain often indicates an acute injury or acute disease; and the intensity of acute pain often indicates the severity of injury or disease. Thus, acute pain should trigger an urgent search for an underlying cause that might be life-threatening or require immediate intervention.

The effective management of acute pain is important. The relief of acute pain can facilitate diagnostic tests by helping patients cooperate with prolonged radiographic or other procedures. Preoperative pain management makes anesthesia easier and postoperative pain control better. In some cases, management of acute pain can help prevent development of chronic pain syndromes.

Chronic Pain

Chronic pain is usually defined by its persistence beyond an expected time frame for healing. The International Association for the Study of Pain defines chronic pain as lasting more than 3 months.[5] Intensity of chronic pain is often out of proportion to the observed pathology and often associated with prolonged functional impairment, both physical and psychologic. Autonomic signs are often absent or exhausted. Underlying causes of chronic pain are often associated with chronic disease and are less curable.[5]

Chronic pain is often more difficult to manage because the underlying cause is less remedial and many treatment strategies are either short lived, difficult to maintain, or associated with long-term side effects. Chronic pain usually requires a multidimensional approach to treatment, including use of both analgesic drug and nondrug strategies with attention to sensory, emotional, and behavioral components of the pain experience.

Classification Based on Pathophysiology

The classification of pain by pathophysiologic mechanisms may help clinicians choose and target pain management strategies more effectively. Treatment aimed at specific pathophysiologic pain mechanisms may be more effective. The American Geriatrics Society Panel on Chronic Pain identified four basic pathophysiologic pain mechanisms that have important implications for choosing pain management strategies (Table 28.1).[7] Pain problems that result largely from stimulation of pain receptors are called nociceptive pain.[8] Nociceptive pain may arise from tissue injury, inflammation, or mechanical deformation. Examples include trauma, burns, infection, arthritis, ischemia, and tissue distortion. Pain from nociception usually responds well to common analgesic medications. Neuropathic pain results from pathophysiologic processes that arise in the peripheral or central nervous system.[9,10] Examples include diabetic neuralgia, postherpetic neuralgia, and posttraumatic neuralgia (postamputation or "phantom limb" pain). In contrast to nociceptive pain, neuropathic pain syndromes have been found to respond to nonconventional analgesic medications such as tricyclic antidepressants and anticonvulsant drugs. Mixed pain syndromes are often thought to have multiple or unknown pathophysiologic mechanisms. Treatment of

TABLE 28.1. Pain classification based on pathophysiology.

I. Nociceptive pain (somatic and visceral)
    a. Trauma (and burns)
    b. Ischemia
    c. Inflammation (e.g., infection, inflammatory diseases, arthritis)
    d. Mechanical deformity (e.g., tissue strain, swelling, tumor, physical distortion)
    e. Myalgias (e.g., myofascial pain syndromes)

II. Neuropathic pain
    a. Peripheral nerves
        i.   Diabetic neuralgia
        ii. Viral neuralgia (e.g., postherpetic neuralgia)
        iii. Traumatic neuralgia (e.g., postsurgical neuralgia, phantom limb)
        iv. Trigeminal neuralgia
    b. Central nervous system
        i.   Postthalamic stroke pain
        ii. Myelopathic pain (e.g., multiple sclerosis)
    c. Sympathetic nervous system
        i.   Reflex sympathetic dystrophy
        ii. Causalgia (e.g., complete regional pain syndromes)

III. Mixed or undetermined pathophysiology
     a. Chronic recurrent headaches
     b. Vasculopathic pain syndromes (e.g., vasculitic pain syndromes)

IV. Psychologically based pain syndromes (e.g., somatization disorders, hysterical reactions)

Source: Adapted from AGS Panel on Chronic Pain Management in Older Persons. The management of chronic pain in older persons. *J Am Geriatr Soc.* 1998;46:635–651, with permission.

these problems is more problematic and often unpredictable. Examples include recurrent headaches and some vasculitic syndromes. Finally, psychologically based pain syndromes are those with psychologic factors that play a major role in the pain experience.[11] Examples include somataform disorders and conversion reactions. These patients may benefit from specific psychiatric intervention, but traditional pain strategies are probably not indicated. It is important to remember that the pathophysiologic basis of pain may be multifactorial for many diseases. Cancer, for instance, may cause pain from tumor distension and deformation of surrounding tissues, invasion of peripheral nerves, or chronic inflammation. Arthritis may cause pain from inflammation, joint distortion with associated strain on muscles and connective tissue, and microfracture from eroded cartilage or bone. Unfortunately, for many diseases, the pathophysiologic basis of pain is only partially understood.

Age-Related Changes in Pain Perception

Age-related changes in pain perception have been a topic of interest for many years. Elderly persons have been observed to present with painless myocardial infarction

TABLE 28.2. Age-related changes in pain perception.

Component	Age-related change	Comments
Pain receptors	50% decrease in Pacini's corpuscles 10%–30% decrease in Meissner's/Merkle's disks Free nerve endings: no age change	Few studies, largely limited to skin

Peripheral nerves	Myelinated nerves
	  Decreased density
	  Increase abnormal/degenerating fibers
	  Slower conduction velocity
	Unmyelinated nerves
	  Decreased number of large fibers (1.2–1.6 μm)
	  No change in small fibers (0.4 μm)
	  Substance P content decreased
		Evidence of change in pain function is lacking; findings are not specific to pain

Central nervous system	Loss in dorsal horn neurons
	  Altered endogenous inhibition, hyperalgesia
	Loss of neurons in cortex, midbrain, brainstem
	  18% loss in thalamus
	  Altered cerebral evoked responses
	  Decreased catacholamines, acetylcholine, GABA, 5HT
	  Endogenous opioids: mixed changes
	  Neuropeptides: no change
		Findings not specific to pain

Source: Adapted from Gibson SJ, Helme RD. Age differences in pain perception and report: a review of physiological, psychological, laboratory and clinical studies. *Pain Rev.* 1995;2:111–137, with permission.

and painless intra-abdominal catastrophes. The extent to which these observations are attributable to age-related changes in pain perception remains uncertain.[12,13] Table 28.2 summarizes anatomic and neurochemical changes associated with pain perception in aging. Unfortunately, most of these findings are not specific to pain, and changes in pain perception related to these findings remain poorly defined. Studies of pain sensitivity across the life span have shown mixed results. A substantial number of studies of induced pain in normal volunteers have reported both increased and decreased pain threshold, as well as no change in pain threshold across the life span. Decreased pain sensitivity (increased threshold) with aging can be supported by evidence of decreased numbers of receptors and changes in nerve conduction. Increased pain sensitivity (decreased threshold) with aging can also be supported by evidence of alterations in spinal cord and central nervous system processing (poorer endogenous analgesia). If these observations are correct, overall pain perception may not change much with aging. Clearly, additional studies are needed to define age-related changes specific to nervous system function and pain perception.

Epidemiology of Pain Complaints in Older Persons

The precise incidence and prevalence of pain in older populations is not known. Pain is a universal sensation. Every individual has an occasional experience of pain, such as a headache or muscle or joint pain from overexertion. Epidemiology studies of pain in general populations have suffered from the lack of standard definitions for what might be considered "significant" pain. Nonetheless, studies have suggested that the prevalence of pain in community-dwelling older persons may be as high as 25% to 56%.[14] Sources of pain also vary from study to study. Prevalence of back pain has been reported from 21% to 49.5%; joint pain 20.5% to 71%; and headache 1.2% to 50% in persons over the age of 65 years.[15]

In 1997, a Louis Harris telephone poll reported 18% of elderly people take analgesic medications on a regular basis (several times a week or daily).[16] Of those who took analgesic drugs regularly, more than 70% reported taking over-the-counter analgesics, and more than 70% took prescription analgesics, suggesting that most patients took both sources of medication simultaneously. The study reported that most patients complained of musculoskeletal pain.

In general, the most common cause of pain in elderly persons is probably related to musculoskeletal disorders such as back pain and arthritis. Neuralgia is common, stemming from common diseases, such as diabetes or herpes zoster, and trauma, such as surgery, amputation, and other nerve injuries. Nighttime leg pain (e.g., cramps, restless legs) is also common, as is claudication. Cancer, although not so common as arthritis, is a cause of severe pain that is distressing to patients, families, and staff. The distress of cancer pain has brought attention to the moral, ethical, and recently legal obligation of clinicians to provide effective pain management near the end of life.[3]

Pain is also common in nursing homes. It has been suggested that 45% to 80% of nursing home residents may have substantial pain.[17] Many of these patients have multiple pain complaints and multiple potential sources of pain. Our studies have suggested that for 70% of nursing home patients pain results from arthritis and other musculoskeletal causes.[2,18]

Pain is associated with a number of negative outcomes in elderly people. Depression, decreased socialization, sleep disturbance, impaired ambulation, and increased health care utilization and costs have all been associated with the presence of pain in older people. Other outcomes less thoroughly explored include gait disturbances, slow rehabilitation, and adverse effects of analgesic medications.[19] Older patients rely heavily on family and other caregivers near the end of life. For these patients and their caregivers, pain can be especially distressing. Pain can have a substantial impact on caregiver strain and caregiver attitudes.[20]

Assessment of Pain in Elderly People

Pain assessment is the most important part of pain management. Accurate pain assessment is important to identify the underlying source and associated physiologic pain mechanisms to choose the most effective treatment and maximize patient outcomes. Pain management is most effective when the underlying cause of pain has been identified and treated definitively. Inherent in pain assessment is the need to evaluate acute pain that may indicate life-threatening injury and distinguish this from exacerbations of chronic pain. For chronic pain in which the cause is not reversible or only partially treatable, a multidimensional or multidisciplinary evaluation may be required. Among those with cognitive impairment or difficulty reporting pain, other clinicians, family, and caregivers may be helpful in providing a more accurate description.

Compared to younger patients, older persons often present with unique challenges to pain assessment. Elders may tend to underreport pain, despite substantial functional impairment. Multiple concurrent medical problems and multiple sources of pain make assessment more difficult. Finally, cognitive impairment, impaired sensory function, and denial and avoidance behaviors may all contribute to underreporting.

Pain History and Physical Examination

Assessment of pain should begin with a thorough history and physical examination to help establish a diagnosis of underlying disease and form a baseline description of pain experiences. The history should include questions to elicit: *when* the pain started; *what* events or illnesses coincided with the onset; *where* does it hurt (location) and *how* does it feel (character); *what* are the aggravating and relieving influences; and *what* treatments have been tried. Past medical and surgical history is important to identify coexisting disease and previous experience with pain and analgesic use. The review of systems should focus on the musculoskeletal and nervous system. Any history of trauma should be thoroughly investigated because falls, occult fractures, and other injuries are common in this age group. In this setting, care must be taken to avoid attributing acute pain to preexisting conditions. Complicating pain assessment is the fact that chronic pain does fluctuate with time. Injuries from minor trauma and acute disease, such as gout or calcium pyrophosphate crystal arthropathy, can be easily overlooked. Finally, many older persons do not use the word "pain" but may refer to their problems as "hurting," "aching," or some other description. It is important to probe for and identify pain in the patient's own words so that references for subsequent follow-up evaluations are clearly established.[21]

A physical examination should confirm any suspicions suggested by the history. Because of the frequency with which problems are often identified, the physical exam should concentrate on the musculoskeletal and nervous systems. Tender points of inflammation, muscle spasm, and trigger points should be sought. Observation of abnormal posture, gait impairment, and limitations in range of motion may trigger a need for physical therapy and rehabilitation. Evidence of kyphosis, scoliosis, and abnormal joint alignments should be identified. A systematic neurologic exam is also important to identify potential sources of neuropathic pain. Focal muscle weakness, atrophy, abnormal reflexes, or sensory impairments may indicate peripheral or central nervous system injury. Mottled skin in a denervated extremity, presence of a Charcot joint, orthostatic hypotension, impaired gastric emptying, or incontinence may indicate autonomic nervous system dysfunction that can imply sympathetically mediated pain or a complex regional pain syndrome.

It is important to assess functional status to identify self-care deficits and formulate treatment plans that maximize independence and quality of life. Functional status can also represent an important outcome measure of overall pain management. Functional status can be evaluated from information taken from the history and physical examination, as well as the use of one or several functional status scales validated in elderly people (see Chapter 17, Instruments to Assess Functional Status).

A brief psychologic and social evaluation is also important. Depression, anxiety, social isolation, and disengagement are all common in patients with chronic pain. There is a significant association between chronic pain and depression, even when controlling for overall health and functional status. Therefore, assessment should include routine screening for depression. Psychologic evaluation should also include consideration of anxiety and coping skills. Anxiety is common among patients with acute and chronic pain and requires extra time and frequent reassurance from health care providers. Chronic pain often requires effective coping skills for anxiety and other emotional feelings that can be learned.[22] For those with significant psychiatric symptoms, referral for formal psychiatric evaluation and management may be required. In these patients, specific counseling, supportive group therapy, biofeedback, or some psychoactive medications may be necessary for developing and maintaining effective coping strategies as well as management of major psychiatric complications. Social networks should also be explored for availability and involvement of family and other caregivers. It has been shown that the family's and informal caregivers' involvement can have a substantial impact on overall pain management.[23] Evaluation of caregivers is particularly necessary when complicated or high-tech pain management strategies are contemplated, such as continuous analgesic infusions. Need for frequent transportation, administration of pain treatments, and technical training may result in substantial stress for non-professional caregivers that can result in work absence or emotional and physical illness.

Pain Assessment Scales

A variety of pain scales are available to help categorize and quantify the magnitude of pain complaints. Results of these scales are also helpful in documenting and communicating pain experiences. It is helpful to evaluate pain using an appropriate pain scale initially and periodically to maximize treatment outcomes. Results can be recorded in flow chart or graph, making it easy to identify stability or changes in pain over time. Because there are no objective biologic markers or "gold standards," the validity of pain scales relies largely on face value, correlation with other known scales (concurrent validity), correlation with pain-related constructs (convergence), and experience in many populations over several years.

Pain scales can be grouped into multidimensional and unidimensional scales. In general, multidimensional scales with multiple items often provide more stable measurement and evaluation of pain in several domains. For example, the McGill Pain Questionnaire has been shown to capture pain in terms of intensity, affect, sensation, location, and several other domains that are not evaluable with a single question. At the same time, multidimensional scales are often long, time consuming, and can be difficult to score at the bedside, making them difficult to use in a busy clinical setting. Table 28.3 provides a description of several multidimensional scales for pain. Unfortunately, few data are available on the use of many of these scales specifically in elderly populations.

Unidimensional scales consist of a single item that usually relates to pain intensity alone. These scales are usually easy to administer and require little time or training to produce reasonably valid and reliable results. They have found widespread use in many clinical settings to monitor treatment effects and for quality assurance indicators. Table 28.4 describes some unidimensional scales that are commonly used, but a large number of variants are available that have similar characteristics and produce similar results. It is important to remember that unidimensional pain scales often require framing the pain question appropriately for maximum reliability. Subjects should be asked about pain in the present tense (here and now). For example, the interviewer should frame the question, "How much pain are you having right now?" Alternatively, the interviewer can ask, "How much pain have you had over the last week?" or "On average, how much pain have you had in the last month?" The latter questions require accurate memory and integration of pain experiences over time. Recent studies in those with cognitive impairment have shown that pain reports requiring recall are influenced by pain at the moment.[34] Thus, it may be more useful to use unidimensional scales to assess pain at the moment while evaluating changes in pain reports over time, much the way vital signs are used; this is especially true for those with some cognitive impairment.

Pain Assessment in Persons with Cognitive Impairment

Cognitive impairment, Alzheimer's disease, stroke, or dementia can present substantial challenges to pain assessment. Fortunately, it has been shown that pain reports from those with mild to moderate cognitive impairment are no less valid than other patients with normal cognitive function.[35] Weiner and associates have shown that these reports are also usually reliable (stable over time).[34] Our experience has shown that commonly available instruments, such as those in Table 28.5, are feasible for use in most patients with cognitive impairment.[18] Thus, most elderly patients with mild to moderate cognitive impairment appear to have the capacity to report pain accurately and reliably using commonly available methods.

Of particular interest is the Hurley Discomfort Scale.[31] This instrument was developed for the assessment of discomfort in patients with profound dementia. The scale consists of nine items scored by a trained examiner after observation of a noncommunicative patient. Behavioral observations such as breathing, vocalization, facial expression, body language, and restlessness are scored on Likert scales. Testing of the scale has demonstrated reasonable reliability and stability over time.[31,36] The scale

TABLE 28.3. Multidimensional scales for pain measurement.

Instrument	Description	Target	Validity	Reliability	Advantages	Disadvantages	References
McGill Pain Questionnaire	Subjects asked to identify words descriptive of individual pain from 78 words grouped in 20 categories; plus 4 other items (including a 5-point word descriptive scale of pain intensity at the moment [PPI] scored separately)	All pain	Good	Good	Multidimensional, extensively studied over a long time; may discriminate between types of pain	Long, difficult to score	Melzack[24]
Short-Form McGill Pain Questionnaire	15 words scored on Likert scale, plus a visual analogue and PPI scales	All pain	Good	Good	Shorter than original McGill; not studied as deeply as original	May not discriminate between pain types	Melzack[25]
Wisconsin Brief Pain Inventory	16-item scale; items scored separately	Cancer pain	Good	Good	Multidimensional	Studied largely in cancer pain	AHCPR Cancer Pain Guidelines[26]
Memorial Sloan–Kettering Pain Scale	Four word descriptor scales	Cancer pain	Good	Good	Multidimensional	Studied largely in cancer pain	Fishman et al.[27]
Geriatric Pain Measure	24-item questionnaire; 22 items scored dichotomously; 2 items scored 0–10	Ambulatory elderly	Good	Good	Multidimensional; tested in elderly	Limited experience; sensitivity to change unknown	Ferrell et al.[28]
Neuropathic Pain Scale	10 items each scored 1–10	Neuropathic pain			Specific for neuropathic pain	Individual item analysis may be more helpful than changes in total score	Galer and Dworkin[10]
WOMAC	41 items in 5 domains; pain, stiffness, physical function, social function, emotional function	Arthritis	Good	Good	Specific for arthritis	Difficult to use clinically	Bellamy et al. 1988[29]
Roland and Morris Disability Questionnaire	24 items scored yes or no	Back pain	Good	Good	Specific for back pain	May not be generalizable to other pain syndromes	Waddell et al.[30]
Hurley Discomfort Scale	Designed to score discomfort behaviors in patients with severe Alzheimer's disease	Acute pain	Probably fair	Reasonable	Does not rely on self-report	Relies on behavioral observation	Hurley et al.[31]
Osteoarthritis Pain Behavior Observation System	Designed to score position, movement, and behavior among adults	Osteoarthritis of knee	Compared to 0–10 scale, $r = 0.45$	Test-retest over 10 weeks, $r = 0.53$	Does not rely on verbal ability	Limited to osteoarthritis of knee	Keefe et al.[32]

Source: Adapted from Ferrell BA. Pain. In: Osterweil D, Brummel-Smith, K, Beck JB, eds. *Comprehensive Geriatric Assessment.* New York: McGraw-Hill; 2000:389, with permission.

TABLE 28.4. Unidimensional scales for pain measurement.

Scale	Description	Validity	Reliability	Advantages	Disadvantages	References
Visual Analog	100-mm line; vertical or horizontal	Good	Fair	Continuous scale	Requires pencil and paper	Clinical Practice Guidelines[5,7,26]
Present Pain Intensity	6-point 0–5 scale with word descriptors (subscale of McGill Pain Questionnaire)	Good	Fair	Easy to understand, word anchors decrease clustering toward middle of scale	Usually requires visual cue	Melzack[24]
Graphic pictures	Happy faces; others	Fair	Fair	Amusing	Requires vision and attention	Herr et al.[33]
Sloan Kettering Pain Card	7 words randomly distributed on a card	Good	Fair	Ease of administration	Requires visual cue	Ferrell et al.[18] Fishman[27]
Verbal 0–10 Scale	"On a scale of 0 to 10, if 0 means no pain and 10 means the worst pain you can imagine, how much is your pain now?"	Good	Fair	Probably easiest to use	Requires hearing	Ferrell et al.[18]

Source: Adapted from: Ferrell BA. Pain. In: Osterweil D, Brummel-Smith, K, Beck JB, eds. *Comprehensive Geriatric Assessment*. New York: McGraw-Hill; 2000:390, with permission.

requires some training and experience to administer, which may be problematic for some clinical settings.

Patients with severe cognitive impairment present substantial challenges for pain assessment. Although it has been assumed that those in deep coma do not experience pain, it is not clear that such brain damage necessarily results in complete anesthesia. Patients with "locked-in syndrome" (having intact perception and cognitive function but no purposeful motor function and no means of communication) may suffer severely. Unfortunately, no reliable methods exist to assess pain in these individuals. Health care providers must be aware of these situations and provide analgesia empirically, especially during procedures and conditions known to be uncomfortable or painful. More often, the majority with moderate to severe cognitive impairment can and do make their needs known in simple yes or no answers communicated in various ways. For example, those with profound aphasia can often provide accurate and reliable answers to yes and no questions when confronted by a sensitive and skilled interviewer. For these patients, it is important to be creative in establishing communication methods for the purpose of pain assessment.

Although pain is an individual experience, the use of family and caregivers in the assessment of pain can sometimes be helpful.[37] For patients with cognitive impairment, the history is often only obtainable from family or close caregivers. Family and caregivers are an excellent source of qualitative information about general behavior, medication usage, actions that seem to reduce pain, and actions that seem to aggravate pain. It is important to remember, however, that family and caregivers are limited in their interpretation of events and behaviors. In fact, evidence has suggested that when it comes to estimating pain intensity, proxies are not always very

TABLE 28.5. Acute pain control options.

Mild pain
    Administration of acetaminophen or NSAIDs
    Cognitive-behavioral strategies (relaxation, distraction, etc.)
    Physical agents (cold, heat, massage, etc.)
    Combined strategies

Moderate pain
    Low-dose or low-potency opioids
    Combinations of acetaminophen or NSAIDs with low-dose or low-potency opioids
    Combined strategies

Severe pain
    Potent opioid analgesics (intermittent or around the clock)
    Continuous infusions of opioid analgesics (e.g., PCA)
    Neural blockade (intermittent or continuous)
    Spinal anesthesia (e.g., epidural anesthesia, intermittent or continuous)
    Combined strategies

Source: Adapted from Acute Pain Management Guideline Panel. *Acute Pain Management: Operative or Medical Procedures and Trauma. Clinical Practice Guideline*. AHCPR Pub 92-0032. Rockville, MD: Agency for Health Care Policy and Research, Public Health Service, U.S. Department of Health and Human Services; 1992.

accurate or reliable. Our studies of elderly cancer patients suggest that caregivers may overestimate pain intensity and distress,[23] and both physicians and nurses have been found to underestimate pain, as well as provide inadequate pain medication.[38,39] In the final analysis, family and close caregivers can be valuable sources of qualitative information, but they probably should not be relied on entirely for quantitative assessment of pain intensity or distress, especially among those patients able to communicate their pain experiences.

Acute and Perioperative Pain Management

The treatment of acute pain relies largely on short-term use of analgesic medications and resolution of the underlying cause. A variety of nondrug strategies have also been shown to be helpful. The choice of analgesic medications and other strategies to be used may depend on the severity of pain, availability of technical equipment and expertise, expectations for resolution of underlying injury, and individual patient characteristics. Table 28.5 lists some options available for acute and postoperative pain control.

The most common approach to treating acute pain relies on the World Health Organization recommendations for choosing the intensity of treatment based on the intensity of pain.[6,40] Pain of mild intensity usually responds to nonopioid drugs used alone or in combination with other physical and cognitive-behavioral interventions. Pain of moderate intensity often requires more intensive efforts, such as weak opioids or low doses of more potent opioid drugs. Many of these drugs are compounded with NSAIDs or acetaminophen to achieve enhanced relief, with only modest exposure to the side effects of opioids. Severe pain usually requires potent opioid analgesic medications given alone or in combination with other analgesic strategies. For severe trauma or postoperative pain, intermittent intravenous, continuous intravenous, or spinal anesthesia may provide faster and more continuous pain relief. Table 28.5 provides an outline of acute pain control options for mild, moderate, and severe pain.

Although initially designed as a stepwise approach to cancer pain management, the WHO approach has become an acceptable approach to all pain with a few caveats. First, it is important to remember that the model does not require that strong opioids be withheld until after other treatments have failed. When patients present with severe pain, they should be treated initially with strong medications. Second, when pain rapidly escalates from mild to severe, analgesia should be rapidly escalated to strong opioids, with or without other combined strate-

gies. Third, adjuvant drugs and combined treatments should be used early for mild to moderate pain, especially those of the neuropathic type. Finally, when patients present with acute pain, even though establishing a diagnosis is a priority, symptomatic pain treatment should be initiated while investigations are proceeding. It is rarely justified to defer analgesia until a diagnosis is made. In fact, a comfortable patient is better able to cooperate with diagnostic procedures.

Acute and postoperative pain is dynamic. Without treatment, sensory input from damaged tissue causes alterations in spinal cord neurons that result in enhanced responses. Pain receptors also become more sensitive after injury. Studies have demonstrated long-lasting changes after brief painful stimuli.[5] These observations may explain why long-standing pain is more difficult to suppress. Thus, patients should be encouraged to take pain medications continuously or to prevent pain before it becomes severe and requires higher doses of medication to suppress. In general, it may be helpful to provide continuous analgesics initially, with intermittent or "prn" rescue doses reserved for breakthrough or intermittent pain as the injury resolves.

Aggressive pain prevention and control before, during, and after surgery can have both short- and long-term benefits. Good preoperative pain control has been shown to make postoperative pain easier to control.[41] Postoperative patients who use analgesia via a continuous infusion pump with self-administered boluses for breakthrough pain report less pain and are more satisfied with their pain control. These patients also use less medication, have fewer postoperative complications, and tend to be discharged earlier compared to similar patients who are given similar drugs on an intermittent or "as-needed" basis.[5,42]

The importance of preoperative patient education cannot be overemphasized. Studies have shown that preoperative patient education and preparation dramatically enhance postoperative outcomes and improved pain management.[43] Patients given complete information about specific procedures including detailed descriptions of expected discomfort postoperatively often have less pain, use less pain medication, and have earlier discharges.[5] Table 28.6 summarizes important preoperative information for patients and families.

Chronic Pain Management

Chronic pain management often requires a multimodal approach of drug and nondrug pain management strategies.[7] Although analgesic medications are the most common strategy employed, the concurrent use of cognitive behavior therapy and other nondrug strategies may be helpful to reduce long-term reliance on medications

TABLE 28.6. Preoperative patient education for pain control.

Discuss the patient's previous experiences with pain, beliefs, and
  preferences for pain control
Give detailed information about postoperative pain expectations
Give patient information about pain management strategies available
Develop with the patient a plan for pain assessment and management
Select a pain assessment method and teach the patient how to use it
Inform patients of the importance of pain prevention
Provide patient with suggestions and training for non–drug pain
  management activities such as breathing and relaxation techniques

Source: Adapted from Acute Pain Management Guideline Panel.
*Acute Pain Management in Adults: Operative Procedures. Quick Guide
for Clinicians*. AHCPR Pub 92-0019. Rockville, MD: Agency for Health
Care Policy and Research, Public Health Service, U.S. Department of
Health and Human Services; 1995.

alone. It is important to consider that chronic pain management is often a labor-intensive effort. Not unlike the effort required during warfarin anticoagulation, pain management requires frequent monitoring and adjustments. Indeed, elderly patients with chronic pain benefit particularly from physicians, nurses, and restorative personnel who are able to employ an interdisciplinary approach to complex problems.

In general, chronic pain is often more difficult to relieve that acute pain. Patients should be given an expectation of pain relief, but it unrealistic to suggest or sustain an expectation of complete relief for some patients with chronic pain. The goals and trade-offs of possible therapies need to be discussed openly. Sometimes a period of trial and error should be anticipated when new medications are initiated and titration occurs. Review of medications, doses, use patterns, efficacy, and adverse effects should be a regular process of care.[7] Ineffective drugs should be tapered and discontinued.

Economic issues are also important in the management of chronic pain. It is appropriate to consider economic issues and make balanced decisions while basic principles of assessment and treatment are followed. Health care professionals should be aware of the costs and economic barriers patients and families may encounter with the strategies often prescribed. These issues include lack of Medicare reimbursement, limited formularies, delays in referrals in some managed care environments, delays from mail-order pharmacies, and limited availability of opioid medications in some pharmacies.

Analgesic Medications

Any patient who has pain that impairs functional status or quality of life is a candidate for analgesic drug therapy.[7] Analgesic medications are safe and effective in elderly people. As with all pharmacotherapy, all analgesic interventions carry a balance of benefits and burdens. For some classes of pain-relieving medications (opioids, for example), elderly patients have been shown to have increased analgesic sensitivity.[44] Dosing for most patients requires beginning with low doses with careful upward titration, including frequent reassessment for optimum pain relief and management of side effects.

The least invasive route of drug administration should be used. Some drugs can be administered from a variety of routes, such as subcutaneous, intravenous, transcutaneous, sublingual, and rectal. Most drugs are limited to only a few safe routes of administration, but new delivery systems are being created each year. The oral route is preferable because of its convenience and relatively steady blood levels produced. Significant effects are often seen 30 min to 2 h after an oral dose, which may be a drawback in acute, rapidly fluctuating pain. Intravenous bolus provides the most rapid onset and shortest duration of action, which may require substantial labor, technical skill, and monitoring. Subcutaneous and intramuscular injection, although commonly used, has disadvantages of wider fluctuations in absorption and rapid falloff of action compared to oral routes. Transcutaneous, rectal, and sublingual routes are also more difficult to predict but may be essential for those with difficulty swallowing.[7]

Timing of medications is also important. Fast-onset, short-acting analgesic drugs should be used for episodic pain. Medications for intermittent or episodic pain can usually be prescribed as needed. For continuous pain, medications should be provided around the clock. In these situations, a steady-state analgesic blood level is more effective in maintaining comfort. Long-acting or sustained-release preparations should only be used for continuous pain. Most patients with continuous pain also need fast-onset short-acting drugs for breakthrough pain. Breakthrough pain includes (1) end-of-dose failure as the result of decreased blood levels of analgesic with concomitant increase in pain before the next scheduled dose; (2) incident pain, usually caused by activity that can be anticipated and pretreated; and (3) spontaneous pain, common with neuropathic pain that is often fleeting and difficult to predict.[7]

The use of placebos is unethical in clinical practice, and there is no place for their use in the management of acute or chronic pain. Placebos, in the form of inert oral medications, sham injections, or other fraudulent procedures are only justified in certain research designs in which patients have given informed consent and understand that they may be receiving a placebo as a part of the research design. In research, placebos help identify and measure random or uncontrollable events that may confound results of some research designs.[45] In clinical settings, placebo effects are common, but they are neither diagnostic of pain or indicative of a therapeutic response. The effects of placebos are short lived, and most patients eventually learn the truth, resulting in loss of patient trust and more needless suffering.

Acetaminophen

Acetaminophen is the drug of choice for elderly persons with mild to moderate pain, especially that of osteoarthritis and other musculoskeletal problems.[7] As an analgesic and antipyretic, acetaminophen acts in the central nervous system to reduce pain perception. Despite the lack of anti-inflammatory activity, studies have shown that acetaminophen is as effective as ibuprofen for chronic osteoarthritis of the knee.[46] It has also been suggested that acetaminophen may have deleterious effects on renal function (dose related over many years)[47] and may interfere with the concomitant administration of warfarin.[48] Nonetheless, given in a dose of 650 to 1000 mg four times a day, it remains the safest analgesic medication compared to traditional NSAIDs and other analgesic drugs for most patients. Unfortunately, acetaminophen overdose can result in irreversible hepatic necrosis. Therefore, the maximum daily dose should never exceed 4000 mg/day.[7]

Nonsteroidal Anti-inflammatory Drugs

Nonsteroidal anti-inflammatory drugs (NSAIDs) have analgesic activity both peripherally and centrally. They are potent inhibitors of prostaglandin synthesis, which have effects on inflammation, pain receptors, and nerve conduction and may have central effects as well.[49] It is now known that there are two major NSAID-sensitive cyclooxygenase enzymes (COX-1 and COX-2) synthesized in a variety of organs. COX-1 is present in most organ systems and plays a role in normal organ function such as gastric mucosal blood flow and barrier function, renal blood flow, hepatic blood flow, and platelet aggregation. COX-2, normally present in lower concentrations, is an inducible enzyme in response to injury or inflammation. It is now known that selective inhibition of COX-2 gives rise to analgesic and anti-inflammatory activity with less organ toxicity compared to the nonselective inhibition of both enzymes. These findings have resulted in new NSAIDs reaching the market that have substantially less gastric and platelet toxicity compared to older NSAID medications. In fact, clinical trials have found COX-2 inhibitors to be similarly effective to traditional NSAIDs in terms of peak pain relief, total pain relief, and in indices of joint inflammation in patients with arthritis. Safety profiles of these agents have been impressive in reduction of gastrointestinal injury and bleeding diathesis.[50] However, it is important to note that, like other NSAIDS, these drugs have ceilings to their effects and limited potency for patients with moderate to severe pain problems.

Nonspecific inhibitors of COX enzymes (most older NSAIDs) are still appropriate for short-term use in inflammatory arthritic conditions such as gout, calcium pyrophosphate arthropathy, acute flare-ups of rheumatoid arthritis, and other inflammatory rheumatic conditions. They have also been reported to relieve the pain of headache, menstrual cramps, and other mild to moderate pain syndromes. These drugs can be used alone for mild to moderate pain or in combination with opioids for more severe pain. They have the advantage of being nonhabit forming. Individual drugs in this class vary widely with respect to anti-inflammatory activity, potency, analgesic properties, metabolism, excretion, and side effect profiles. Moreover, it has been observed that failure of response to one NSAID may not predict the response to another. A disadvantage of NSAIDs is that, unlike opioids, they all demonstrate a ceiling effect, that is, a level at which increase dose results in no further increase in analgesia. A large number of NSAIDs are now available; however, there is no evidence to support a particular compound as the NSAID of choice. Several are available over the counter without a prescription. Table 28.7 lists COX-2 and other selected NSAIDs for pain.

High-dose NSAIDs for long periods of time should be avoided in elderly patients.[7] Of major concern is the high incidence of adverse reactions, including gastrointestinal bleeding,[51] renal impairment,[52] and bleeding diathesis from platelet disfunction. The concomitant use of mesoprostol, high-dose histamine-2 receptor antagonists, and proton pump inhibitors is only partially successful at reducing the risk of significant gastrointestinal bleeding associated with NSAID use.[53-55] Also, the side effect profiles of gastroprotective drugs in this population must be weighed against their limited benefits.[56] These gastroprotective medications do nothing to prevent the renal impairment and other side effects. For those with multiple medical problems, NSAIDs are associated with increased risk of drug–drug and drug–disease interactions. NSAIDs may interact with antihypertensive therapy.[57] Thus, the relative risks and benefits of NSAIDs must be weighed carefully against other available treatments for older patients with chronic pain problems. For some patients, chronic opioid therapy, low-dose or intermittent corticosteroid therapy, or other nonanalgesic drug strategies may have fewer life-threatening risks compared to long-term NSAID use.[7] (Also see Chapter 7, Principles of Pharmacology.)

Opioid Analgesic Medications

Opioid analgesic medications act by blocking receptors in the central nervous system (brain and spinal cord), resulting in a decreased perception of pain. Many opioids also act similar to local anesthetics and have recently found widespread use in epidural anesthesia.[58] Selected

TABLE 28.7. Selected nonsteroidal anti-inflammatory drugs for pain.

Drug	Maximum dose	Description	Comments
Celecoxib (Celebrex)	200 mg bid	Selective COX-2 inhibition; pain and anti-inflammatory activity similar to other NSAIDs	Less gastric toxicity; less platelet inhibition
Refocoxib (Vioxx)	50 mg q 24 h	Selective COX-2 inhibition; pain and anti-inflammatory activity similar to other NSAIDs	Less gastric toxicity; less platelet inhibition
Relafen (Nabumetone)	2000 mg/24 h (q 24 h dosing)	Partially COX-2 selective; gastric toxicity may be less; occasionally requires q 12 h dosing	Avoid maximum dose for prolonged periods
Aspirin	4000 mg/24 h (q 4–6 h dosing)	Prototype NSAID	Salicylate levels may be helpful in monitoring
Salsalate (Disalcid)	3000 mg/24 h (q 6–8 h dosing)	Hydrolyzed in small intestine to aspirin	Elderly may require dose adjustment downward to avoid salicylate toxicity; salicylate levels may be helpful in monitoring
Ibuprofen (Motrin by prescription; Advil, Nuprin, and others OTC)	2400 mg/24 h (q 6–8 h dosing)	Gastric, renal, and abnormal platelet function may be dose dependent; constipation, confusion, and headaches may be more common in older persons	Avoid high doses for prolonged periods of time
Diflunisal (Dolobid)	1000 mg/24 h maximim dose Loading = 1000 mg, then 500 q 12 h; or 750 mg then 250 mg q 8 h in small patients or frail elderly	Relatively good analgesic properties, but requires loading dose	Dose may need downward adjustment for small patients or frail elderly
Sulindac (Clinoril)	400 mg/24 h (q 12 h dosing)	Same as ibuprofen	Same as ibuprofen
Naproxen (Naprosyn by prescription; Aleve and others OTC)	1000 mg/24 h (q 8–12 h dosing)	Same as ibuprofen; may require a loading dose	Same as ibuprofen
Choline magnesium trisalicylate (Trilisate)	5500 mg/24 h (q 12 h dosing)	Lower effect on platelet function	Salicylate levels may be helpful to avoid toxicity
Indomethacin (Indocin)	200 mg/24 h (q 8–12 h dosing)	Extremely high toxicity in frail elderly; should be reserved for acute inflammatory conditions (e.g., gout)	Keep dose to a minimum (25 mg q 18 h) and for short-term use only; avoid use for osteoarthritis or other noninflammatory problems
Ketorolac (Toradol)	i.m., 120 mg/24 h (30–60 mg loading dose; followed by half the loading dose (15–30 mg q 6 h, limited to not more than 5 days) p.o., 60 mg/24 h (q 6 h dosing limited to not more than 14 days)	Substantial gastrointestinal toxicity as well as renal and platelet dysfunction; relatively high postoperative complications have been documented	Duration of treatment limited because of high toxicity; reduce dose in half for those <50 kg or >65 years of age

OTC, over the counter or available without prescription; i.m., intramuscular (injection); p.o., per oral route (by mouth).
Limited number of examples are provided. For comprehensive lists of other available NSAIDs and a host of brand names, clinicians should consult other sources.

opioid analgesic medications are listed in Table 28.8. Opioid drugs have no ceiling to their analgesic effects and have been shown to relieve all types of pain. Short-term studies have suggested that elderly people, compared to younger people, may be more sensitive to the analgesic properties of these drugs; this has been shown for acute postoperative pain, as well as chronic cancer pain.[59–61] One study noted enhanced analgesia in elderly women

TABLE 28.8. Selected opioid analgesic medications for pain.

Drug	Starting dose (oral)	Description	Comments
Morphine (Roxanol, MSIR)	30 mg (q 4 h dosing)	Short–intermediate half-life; older people are more sensitive than younger people to side effects	Titrate to comfort; continuous use for continuous pain; intermittant use for episodic pain; anticipate and prevent side effects
Codeine (plain codeine, Tylenol 3, other combinations with acetaminophen or NSAIDs)	30–60 mg (q 4–6 h dosing)	Acetaminophen or NSAIDs, limit dose; constipation is a major issue	Begin bowel program early; do not exceed maximum dose for acetaminophen or NSAIDs
Hydrocodone (Vicodin, Lortab, others)	5–10 mg (q 3–4 h dosing)	Toxicity similar to morphine, acetaminophen, or NSAID combinations; limit maximum dose	Same as above
Oxycodone (Roxicodone, Oxy IR; or in combinations with acetaminophen or NSAIDs such as Percocet, Tylox, Percodan, others)	20–30 mg (q 3–4 h dosing)	Toxicity similar to morphine, acetaminophen, or NSAID combinations; limit maximum dose; oxycodone is available generically as a single agent	Same as above
Hydromorphone (Dilaudid)	4 mg (q 3–4 h dosing)	Half-life may be shorter than morphine; toxicity similar to morphine	Similar to morphine
Sustained-release morphine (MS Contin, Oramorph, Kadian)	MS Contin, 30–60 mg (q 12 h dosing) Oramorph, 30–60 mg (q 12 h dosing) Kadian, 30–60 mg (q 24 h dosing)	Morphine sulfate in a wax matrix tablet or sprinkles; MS Contin and Oramorph should not be broken or crushed; Kadian capsules can be opened and sprinkled on food, but should not be crushed	Titrate dose slowly because of drug accumulation; rarely requires more frequent dosing than recommended on package insert; immediate-release opioid analgesic often necessary for breakthrough pain
Sustained-release oxycodone (Oxycontin)	15–30 mg (q 12 h dosing)	Similar to sustained-release morphine	Similar to sustained-release morphine
Transderm Fentanyl (Durgesic)	25-μg patch (q 72 h dosing)	Reservoir for drug is in the skin, not in the patch; equivalent dose compared to other opioids is not very predictable (see package insert); effective activity may exceed 72 h in older patients	Drug reservoir is in skin, not patch; titrate slowly using immediate-release analgesics for breakthrough pain; peak effect of first dose may take 18–24 h; not recommended for opioid-naive patients
Fentanyl lozenge on an applicator stick (Actiq)	Rub on bucal mucosa until analgesia occurs, then discard	Short half-life; useful for acute and breakthrough pain when oral route is not possible	Absorbed via bucal mucosa, not effective orally

Limited number of examples are provided. For comprehensive lists of other available opioids clinicians should consult other sources.

even when morphine was administered by the epidural route.[62] Advanced age is associated with a prolonged half-life and prolonged pharmacokinetics of opioid drugs. Thus, elderly people may achieve pain relief from smaller doses of opiate drugs than younger people.

Opioid drugs have the potential to cause cognitive disturbances, nausea, respiratory depression, constipation, and habituation in older people. Drowsiness, performance-based measures of cognitive impairment, and respiratory depression associated with opioids should be anticipated when opioids are initiated and doses are escalated rapidly. Central nervous system effects are dose dependent and can be used to judge rate of dose escalations. If patients have unrelieved pain with little drowsiness or cognitive impairment, doses may be escalated. Tolerance usually develops in a few days to central nervous system side effects, at which time patients usually return to a fully alert status and baseline cognitive function. Until tolerance develops, patients should be instructed not to drive and to take precautions against falls or other accidents. Once tolerance to these effects has developed, however, patients can return to normal activities, including driving and other demanding tasks, despite high doses of opioid drugs. In fact, cancer patients are often observed to improve physical and cognitive function once pain is adequately relieved on opioid analgesics.[7]

Constipation is a side effect of opioid drugs to which patients do not develop tolerance. The management of constipation must be preemptive and preventative and include increasing fluid intake, maintaining mobility, and regular use of cathartic medications. All patients require stool softeners and osmotic laxatives, such as milk of magnesia, lactolose, or sorbitol. For many patients, opioid-induced constipation also requires potent stimulant laxatives, such as senna or biscodyl. It should be remembered that stimulants should not be used until impactions have been removed and obstruction has been ruled out. Finally, some patients require regular enemas to ensure bowel evacuation during opioid administration for severe pain.

Nausea also occasionally complicates opioid therapy. Nausea from opioid medications may result from several mechanisms and typically wanes as tolerance develops over several days to a week. Traditionally, antiemetics such as prochlorperazine, chlorpromazine, and antihistamines have been the mainstay of treatment for nausea in younger patients. Recently, low-dose haloperidol and metaclopramide have been used, anecdotally noting a lower side effect profile compared to other neuroleptic drugs. It should be remembered that all these agents have high side effect profiles in elderly patients, including movement disorders, delirium, and anticholinergic effects. Thus, clinicians should choose antiemetic medications with the lowest side effects and continue to monitor patients frequently.[7]

It is important for clinicians who prescribe opioid analgesics to understand issues of tolerance, dependency, and addiction. Tolerance is a pharmacologic phenomenon that occurs with many drugs. Tolerance is defined by diminished effect of a drug associated with constant exposure to the drug over time. For opioid drugs, tolerance is difficult to predict. In general, tolerance to drowsiness and respiratory depression occurs much faster than tolerance to analgesic properties of the drug. Previous reports that described tolerance among cancer patients resulting in the need for massive doses of morphine to achieve adequate analgesia were probably misinterpreted because those patients also had rapidly advancing cancer.[63] More recent studies of opioid-managed arthritis pain have noted that tolerance was not often significant.[64] Many patients have been noted to remain on stable doses of opoids for many years without demonstrating significant tolerance to the analgesic effects. Tolerance develops quickly to central nervous system side effects and to nausea and never develops to constipation.

Dependency is also a pharmacologic phenomenon associated with many drugs, including corticosteroids and beta-blockers. Dependency is present when patients experience uncomfortable side effects when the drug is withheld abruptly. Drug dependence requires constant exposure to the drug for at least several days. The minimum dose and duration of drug exposure and development of withdrawal symptoms is not precisely known, but it appears to vary with individual opioid compounds. Symptoms associated with abrupt opioid withdrawal may include anorexia, restlessness, nausea, diaphoresis, tachycardia, mild hypertension, and mild fever. Worsening symptoms may include skin mottling, gooseflesh, and frank autonomic crisis. Fortunately, these symptoms can be completely prevented by tapering opioids over a few days. Opioid doses can be reduced by 50% every few days and safely discontinued within a week. In severe cases, clonidine given short term in titrated doses will usually control serious autonomic signs. It is important to remember that physiologic effects of opioid withdrawal are usually not life threatening compared to those common with alcohol, benzodiazepine, or barbiturate withdrawal.[65]

Addiction is a psychiatric and behavioral problem and is defined in such terms. Addictive behavior is defined by compulsive drug use despite negative physical and social consequences (harm to self and others) and the craving for effects other than pain relief. Addicted patients often have erratic behavior that can be observed in a clinical setting in the form of selling, buying, and procuring drugs on the street and using medication by bizarre means such as crushing or dissolving tablets for self-i.v. administration. It is now clear that drug use alone is not the major factor in the development of addiction. Other medical, social, and economic factors play immense roles in addictive behavior.[65] It is also important to not construe certain behaviors as necessarily addictive behaviors. Hoarding of medications, persistent or worsening pain complaints, frequent office visits, requests for dose escalations, and other behaviors associated with inadequately treated and unrelieved pain has coined the term pseudo-addiction. Laws, regulations, and unintentional behavior by prescribing clinicians may require patients to hoard medication and seek other physicians for additional help. In fact, true addiction is rare among patients taking opioid analgesic medications for medical reasons. This observation is not meant to imply that opioid drugs can be used indiscriminately, only that exaggerated fear of addiction and side effects do not justify failure to treat pain in elderly patients, especially those near the end of life.[63]

Fear of addiction has been identified as a major barrier to pain management in elderly people.[64] Unfortunately, fears by clinicians and patients have been overly influenced by social pressures to reduce illegal drug use among younger people and those who take narcotics for emotional rather than medical reasons. Regulation of controlled substances by state and federal authorities, as well as scrutiny of physician practices by state license boards, have intimidated many clinicians, who as a result may not prescribe potent analgesic medications, even for those with severe pain near the end of life. This hesitancy to treat symptom distress may actually contribute to patients who seek suicide rather than endure inadequately managed pain. More recently, many organizations, such as the American Medical Association, the American College of Physicians, and the American Geriatrics Society, have released position statements supporting comfort and the control of pain in patients near the end of life.[3,66,67] As emphasized by these organizations, clinicians have an obligation to provide comfort, pain relief, and dignity for patients.

Other Nonopioid Medications for Pain

A variety of other medications not formally classified as analgesics have been found to be helpful in certain specific pain problems. The term adjuvant analgesic drugs, although frequently used, is a misnomer in that some of these nonopioid drugs may be the primary pain-relieving pharmacologic intervention in certain cases. Table 28.9 provides some examples of nonopioid drugs that may help certain kinds of pain. The largest body of evidence available relates to the use of these drugs for neuropathic pain, such as diabetic neuropathies, postherpetic neuralgia, and trigeminal neuralgia. Tricyclic antidepressants, anticonvulsants, and local anesthetics are the nonopioid analgesics most frequently used for neuropathic conditions. In general, these drugs have had limited success in pain syndromes that are not associated with neuropathic mechanisms.[68,69] Most reports have found that these

agents are only partially successful. Typically, about 50% to 70% of patients subjects have a measurable response, and of those most experience only partial relief.[68–70] Thus, these drugs are often not panaceas and are rarely totally successful as single agents. One exception may be trigeminal neuralgia, where carbamazepine is probably the drug of choice.[7] Usually these agents work better in combination with other traditional drug and nondrug strategies in an effort to improve pain and keep other drug doses to a minimum. Failure of response to one particular class of drugs does not necessarily predict failure of another class of agents. In general, nonopioid medications for neuropathic pain should be chosen according to lowest side effects. Treatment should usually start with lower doses than recommended for younger patients, and doses should be escalated slowly based on known pharmacokinetics of individual drugs and appropriate knowledge of disease-specific treatment strategies. Unfortunately, most of the nonopioid medications for pain management have high side effect profiles in elderly people. Thus, these medications often must be monitored carefully.

Antidepressants have been the most widely studied class of nonopioid medications for pain. The mechanism of action for these drugs is not entirely known but probably has to do with interruption of norepinephrine and serotonin-mediated mechanisms in the brain.[68] For neuropathic pain, the major effect of these drugs is not their mood-altering capacity, although this may also be helpful in those with concurrent major depression. More is known about tricyclic antidepressants than the other subclasses. A randomized placebo-controlled trial of amitriptyline, desipramine, and fluoxitene indicated that desipramine may be as effective as amitriptyline, but fluoxetine is no better than placebo for the treatment of diabetic neuropathy.[62] Thus, desipramine may be a better choice because it has a lower side effect profile in elderly people than amitriptyline. Other studies of the serotonin reuptake inhibitors, which may have lower side effect profiles for elderly people, have had mixed reviews, and most have not been shown effective for pain management, with the exception of chronic headache and diabetic neuropathy (paroxetine).[68]

It has been known for many years that some medications with antiepileptic activity may relieve the pain of trigeminal neuralgia (tic douloureux).[71] Studies have shown that compounds such as diphenylhydantin, tegretol, and valproic acid may also help diabetic neuralgia and other neuropathic pains in some patients. In general, the usefulness of these drugs has been limited by their high side effect profiles in elderly people and the fact that most patients respond only partially, making the overall risk/benefit ratio large in this population. Indeed, these drugs are not simple analgesics and should not be used for the relief of trivial aches and pains.[7] Of recent interest has been the effectiveness of gabapentin for treatment

TABLE 28.9. Selected nonopioid medications for pain.

Drug	Description	Comments
Antidepressants: Amytriptyline, desipramine, nortriptyline, others	Older people are more sensitive to side effects, especially anticholinergic effects; desipramine or nortriptyline are better choices than amytriptyline	Complete relief unusual; used best as adjunct to other strategies; start low and increase slowly every 3–5 days
Anticonvulsants Clonazapam, carbamazepine	Carbamazepine may cause leukopenia, thrombocytopenia, and rarely aplastic anemia; clonazepam side effects may be similar to other benzodiazepines in the elderly	Start low and increase slowly; check blood counts on carbamazepine
Gabapentin (also an anticonvulsant) Neurontin	Less serious side effects than other anticonvulsants	Start with 100 mg and titrate up slowly; tid dosing; monitor for idiosyncratic side effects such as ankle swelling, ataxia, etc.; effective dose reported 100–800 mg q 8 h
Antiarrhythmics Mexiletine (Mexitil)	Common side effects include tremor, dizziness, paresthesias; rarely may cause blood dyscrasias and hepatic damage	Avoid use in patients with preexisting heart disease; start low and titrate slowly; monitor EKGs; q 6–8 h dosing
Local anesthetics Lidocaine (intravenous) Lidocaine transdermal patch (Lidoderm) Capsaicin	IV lidocaine associated with delirium. Transdermal patch has minimal systemic absorption Capsaicin depletes nerve endings of substance P	i.v. lidocaine may predict response to anticonvulsants and antiarrhythmics May apply up to three patches alternating 12-h interval to improve pain, reduce denervation hypersensitivity, and decrease systemic absorption May take 2 weeks to peak effect
Tramadol (Ultram)	Partial opioid and serotonin agonist; more of a norepinephrine antagonist; may cause drowsiness, nausea, vomiting, and constipation	Has ceiling effect; dose >300 mg/24 h usually not tolerated because of nausea; q 4–6 h dosing
Muscle relaxants (baclo Fen chlorzoxazone [Paraflex], cyclobenzaprine [Flexaril])	Sedation; anticholinergic effects; abrupt withdrawal of baclofen may cause CNS irritability	Mechanism of action not precisely known; monitor for sedation and anticholinergic effects; taper baclofen on discontinuation Poorly tolerated in older adults
Substance P inhibitors (capsaicin) available OTC; for topical use only	Burning pain during depletion of substance P may be intolerable by as many as 30% of patients; may take 14 days for maximum response; avoid eye contamination	Start with small doses; can be partially removed with vegetable oil
NMDA inhibitors	N-Methyl-D-aspartate antagonists (NMDA)	Ketamine only available i.v.
Ketamine Dextromethorphan	Ketamine: potent anesthetic Dextromethorphan: common cough suppressant	Both may cause delirium
Drugs for osteoporosis Calcitonin Bisphosphonates	Pain relief mechanisms unknown	Not effective on pain other than osteoporosis
Corticosteroids Prednisone Dexamethasone	Decrease inflammation in many tissues	Classic corticosteroid side effects limit overall usefulness in chronic pain

Limited number of examples are provided. For comprehensive lists of other available medications for pain, clinicians should consult other sources.

TABLE 28.10. Anesthetic or neurosurgical pain management techniques.

Procedure	Possible indications	Comments
Continuous infusion opioids (morphine, hydromorphone, fentanyl)	Perioperative pain; severe cancer pain when oral route has failed	Subcutaneous infusions are usually well tolerated by patients in nursing homes or home care; i.v. infusions may require more skilled monitoring
Epidural analgesia (intermittent local anesthetics or opioids, or continuous opioids)	Perioperative pain; severe cancer pain when oral route has failed	Can be supplied by external or internally implanted pumps; does not avoid constipation and occasional delerium; serious complications are rare but can be devastating
Nerve blocks	Mononeuropathies, postherpetic neuralgia, intercostal nerve pain (postthoracotomy or postherpetic neuralgia)	Usually temporary relief limited to a few days or weeks
Intrathecal analgesia	Perioperative pain	Can cause respiratory depression
Stellate ganglia blockade	Sympathetically mediated pain of the upper extremity	Not to be confused with complex regional pain syndromes
Lumbar sympathetic blockade	Sympathetically mediated pain of the lower extremity, peripheral vascular disease	
Celiac plexus blockade	Severe pain from carcinoma of pancreas	Requires substantial skill
Neuroablation (permanent nerve destruction)	Severe recalcitrant mononeuropathic pain	May recur after several years
Cordotomy	Severe recalcitrant cancer pain	May not relieve all pain
Neurostimulation (dorsal column or thalamic)	Severe recalcitrant pain, usually following thalamic stroke or spinal cord injury	Requires substantial skill

of diabetic neuralgia and postherpetic neuralgia.[72,73] Clinical observations suggest that this agent has a significant analgesic effect on neuropathic pain with a much lower side effect profile compared to other antiepileptic drugs and also most antidepressants.

Several local anesthetics have also been shown to relieve neuropathic pain when administrated systemically, in addition to their known local anesthetic effects. Intravenous lidocaine has been found to sometimes predict the response to other anticonvulsant and systemically administered local anesthetics.[71] Mexilitine (Mexitil), similar to lidocaine but active orally, has also shown some activity against neuropathic pain of diabetic neuralgia. Although this drug also has a high risk to benefit ratio, some studies have reported response rates at lower doses than are often recommended for cardiac arrhythmias.[74] Lidocaine transdermal patches have been effective for treatment of neuropathic pain.

Finally, chronic pain associated with osteoporosis has been shown to improve with calcitonin.[75] Most investigators of the effects of calcitonin on osteoporosis have reported anecdotally that pain improves significantly. These studies have not been designed as pain studies, but results thus far are encouraging.

Anesthetic and Neurosurgical Approaches to Pain Management

A wide variety of anesthetic and neurosurgical approaches to pain are available, and some require highly specialized skills.[76] Table 28.10 lists some common anesthesia and neurosurgical interventions for severe pain. Although it is beyond the scope of this chapter to review details of all these techniques, a few deserve mention.

Trigger-point injections have been used effectively for the treatment of myofascial pain syndromes. Trigger points may initiate a reflex mechanism that produces referred pain, tenderness, and muscle spasm. With local injection of the trigger point followed by stretching and reconditioning of the muscles, the myofascial pain syndrome may subside. More recently, similar results have been obtained using ice massage or vapocoolant spray applied topically, followed by specific muscle stretching and physical therapy techniques.[77] Trigger-point injection with dilute local anesthetics may be highly effective when combined with specific physical therapy for many myofascial pain syndromes.

Continuous drug infusions are effective for steady-state analgesic drug levels. Continuous infusions can be maintained by implantable pumps or external devices to deliver intravenous, subcutaneous, intrathecal, or epidural medications. Continuous infusions of opioid drugs have found widespread use in severe chronic cancer pain, especially among those nearing the end of life. Other uses have included continuous infusion of muscle relaxants for patients with muscle spasm from spinal injury, multiple sclerosis, or end-stage Parkinson's disease. Whether these invasive high-tech strategies are appropriate for patients with all kinds of chronic pain remains controversial. These techniques are expensive, but they are often reimbursed by third-party payors, including Medicare, raising ethical issues about the application of high-tech strategies for patients who might be equally well managed using oral medications that are not reimbursable.[78,79] In general, invasive methods carry risk and should be used only when oral medications become ineffective or the oral route of administration is no longer viable.

Nondrug Strategies for Pain Management

Nondrug strategies, used alone or in combination with appropriate analgesic medications, should be an integral part of the care plan for most elderly patients with significant pain problems. Nondrug strategies for pain management encompass a broad range of treatments and physical modalities, many of which carry low risks for adverse effects (Table 28.11). Used in combination with appropriate drug regimens, these interventions often enhance therapeutic effects while allowing medication doses to be kept low to prevent adverse drug effects.[7]

Among the nondrug interventions, the importance of patient education cannot be overstated. Studies have shown that patient education programs alone significantly improve overall pain management.[80,81] Such programs often include content about the nature of pain, how to use pain diaries and pain assessment instruments, how to use medications appropriately, and how to use

TABLE 28.11. Selected nondrug strategies for pain management.

Intervention	Comments	Limitations
Education	Content should include basic knowledge about pain (diagnosis, treatment, complications, and prognosis), other available treatment options, and information about over-the-counter medications and self-help strategies	May require substantial time
Exercise	Can be tailored for individual patient needs and lifestyle; moderate-intensity exercise should be maintained for 30 min or more 3–4 times a week and continued indefinitely	Maintenance is critical and difficult to continue indefinitely
Cognitive-behavioral therapy	Should be conducted by a trained therapist	Requires substantial cognitive function
Physical modalities (heat, cold, and massage)	A variety of techniques are available for application	Heat and cold should be used with caution in those with cognitive impairment to avoid thermal injuries
Physical or occupational therapy	Should be conducted by a trained therapist	Not appropriate for maintainence therapy; can be expensive if not reimbursed
Chiropractic	Has been shown to be as effective as Mackenzie exercises for acute back pain	Potential spinal cord or nerve root impingement should be ruled out before any spinal manipulation
Acupuncture	Should be provided only by a qualified acupuncturist	Effects may be short lived and require repetitive treatments
Transcutaneous electrical nerve stimulation (TENS)	Should initially be applied and adjusted by an experienced professional	Effects are often short lived; clear placebo effects have been observed
Relaxation and distraction techniques	Therapeutic modalities require individual acceptance and may require substantial training	Patients with cognitive impairment may not be good candidates

self-help nondrug strategies. Whether conducted in groups or individually, education should be tailored for individual patient needs and level of understanding. Written materials and methods of reinforcement are important to the overall success of the program.

Physical exercise is important for most patients with pain. A program of exercise can be tailored to most patients' needs and is extremely important for rehabilitation and the maintenance of strength and endurance. Clinical trials of older patients with chronic musculoskeletal pain have shown that moderate levels of exercise (aerobic and resistance training) on a regular basis are effective in improving pain and functional status.[82–84] Initial training for chronic pain patients usually requires 8 to 12 weeks with supervision by a professional who can focus on the needs of older people with musculoskeletal disorders. There is no evidence that one form of exercise is better than another, so programs can be tailored for the individual's needs, lifestyle, and preference. The intensity of exercise, along with frequency and duration, must be adjusted to avoid exacerbation of the underlying condition, while gradually increasing and later maintaining overall conditioning. It is important to remember that feeling better often gives rise to a false impression that the discipline of regular exercise is not necessary. Continued encouragement and reinforcement is often required. Unless complications arise, the program of exercise should be maintained indefinitely to prevent deconditioning and deterioration.

Psychologic strategies have also be shown to be helpful for some with significant pain. Cognitive therapies are strategies aimed at altering belief systems and attitudes about pain and suffering. Cognitive therapies include various forms of distraction, relaxation, biofeedback, and hypnosis. Behavioral therapies are strategies aimed at enhancing healthy behaviors and discouraging abnormal behavior that is unpredictable and self-defeating. Cognitive therapy can be combined with behavioral approaches, and together they are known as cognitive-behavioral therapy. Cognitive-behavioral therapy in its purest form includes a structured approach to teaching coping skills that might be used alone or in combination with analgesic medications and other nondrug strategies for pain control. Effective programs can be conducted by trained professionals with individual patients or in groups, and there is some evidence that the effect is enhanced with caregiver involvement. Although it may not be appropriate for those with significant cognitive impairment, there is evidence from randomized trials to support the use of cognitive-behavioral therapy for many patients with significant chronic pain.[85,86]

Finally, a variety of alternative therapies are also used by many patients. Many patients seek alternative medicine approaches with and without the knowledge or recommendation of their physician or other primary care provider. Alternative medicine approaches to chronic pain may include homeopathy, spiritual healing, or the growing market of vitamin, herbal, and natural remedies. Although there is little scientific evidence to support these strategies for pain control, it is important that health care providers not abandon or react to patients using these modalities, but rather educate both themselves and their patients about their benefits and risks.[87]

References

1. Ferrell BA. Overview of aging and pain. In Ferrell BR, Ferrell BA, eds. *Pain in the Elderly.* Seattle: IASP Press; 1996:1–10.
2. Ferrell BA, Ferrell BR, Osterweil D. Pain in the nursing home. *J Am Geriatr Soc.* 1990;38:409–414.
3. AGS Ethics Committee. The care of dying patients: A position statement. *J Am Geriatr Soc.* 1995;43:577–578.
4. Merskey H, Bogduk N, eds. *Classification of Chronic Pain, 2nd Ed.* Seattle: IASP Press; 1994:xi.
5. Acute Pain Management Guideline Panel. *Acute Pain Management: Post-operative or Medical Procedures and Trauma. Clinical Practice Guideline.* AHCPR pub 92-0032. Rockville, MD: Agency for Health Care Policy and Research, Public Health Service, U.S. Department of Health and Human Services; 1993.
6. Max B, et al. *Principles of Analgesic use in Treatment of Acute Pain and Cancer Pain, 4th Ed.* Glenview, IL: American Pain Society; 1999.
7. AGS Panel on Chronic Pain in Older Persons. The Management of chronic pain in older persons. *J Am Geriatr Soc.* 1998;46:635–651.
8. Myer RA, Campbell JN, Raja SN. Peripheral and neural mechanisms of nociception. In: Wall PD, Melzack R, eds. *Textbook of Pain, 3rd Ed.* New York: Churchill Livingstone; 1994:13–44.
9. Bennett GF. Neuropathic pain. In: Wall PD, Melzack R, eds. *Textbook of Pain, 3rd Ed.* New York: Churchill Livingstone; 1994:201–224.
10. Galer BS, Dworkin RH. *A Clinical Guide to Neuropathic Pain.* New York: McGraw-Hill; 2000:33–36.
11. Craig KD. Emotional aspects of pain. In: Wall PD, Melzack R, eds. *Textbook of Pain, 3rd Ed.* New York: Churchill Livingstone; 1994:261–274.
12. Gibson SJ, Helme RD. Age differences in pain perception and report: a review of physiological, psychological, laboratory and clinical studies. *Pain Rev.* 1995;2:111–137.
13. Gibson SJ, Helme RD. Age related differences in pain perception and report. *Clin Geriatr Med.* 2001;17:433–456.
14. Helm RD, Gibson SJ. Pain in older people. In: Cronbie IK, Croft R, Linton SJ, Leresche L, Von Dorff M, eds. *Epidemiology of Pain.* Seattle: IASP Press; 2000.
15. Helme RD, Gibson SJ. Epidemiology of pain in elderly people. *Clin Geriatr Med.* 2001;17:417–431.

16. Cooner E, Amorosi S. *The Study of Pain and Older Americans.* New York: Harris; 1997.

17. Ferrell BA. Pain evaluation and management in the nursing home. *Ann Intern Med.* 1995;123(9):681–687.

18. Ferrell BA, Ferrell BR, Rivera L. Pain in cognitively impaired nursing home patients. *J Pain Symptom Manage.* 1995;10:591–598.

19. Ferrell BA. Pain management in elderly people. *J Am Geriatr Soc.* 1991;39:64–73.

20. Herr KA, Mobily PR. Pain management in alternate care settings. In: Ferrell BR, Ferrell BA, eds. *Pain in the Elderly.* Seattle: IASP Press; 1996:101–109.

21. Nishikawa ST, Ferrell BA. Pain assessment in the elderly. *Clin Geriatr Issues Long Term Care.* 1993;1:15–28.

22. Keefe FJ, Beaupre PM, Weiner DK, Siegler IC. Pain in older adults: a cognitive behavioral perspective. In: Ferrell BR, Ferrell BA, eds. *Pain in the Elderly.* Seattle: IASP Press; 1996:11–19.

23. Ferrell BR, Ferrell BA, Rhiner M, et al. Family factors influencing cancer pain. *Postgrad Med J.* 1991;67(suppl 2): 654–669.

24. Melzack R. The McGill Pain Questionnaire: major properties and scoring methods. *Pain.* 1975;1:277–299.

25. Melzack R. The short-form McGill Pain Questionnaire. *Pain.* 1987;30:191–197.

26. Jocox A, Car DB, Payne R, et al. *Management of Cancer Pain. Clinical Practice Guideline no. 9.* AHCPR Publ 94-0592. Rockville, MD: Agency for Health Care Policy and Research, U.S. Department of Health and Human Services, Public Health Service; 1994.

27. Fishman B, Pasternak S, Wallenstein SL, Houde RW, Holland JC, Foley KA. The Memorial Pain Assessment Card: a valid instrument for the evaluation of cancer pain. *Cancer.* 1987;60(5):1151–1158.

28. Ferrell BA, Stein WM, Beck JC. The Geriatric Pain Measure: validity, reliability and factor analysis. *J Am Geriatr Soc.* 2000;48:1669–1673.

29. Bellamy N, Buchanan WW, Goldsmith GC, Stitt LW. Validation study of the WOMAC: a health status instrument for measuring clinically important patient relevant outcomes to antirheumatic drug therapy in patients with osteoarthritis. *J Rheumatol* 1988;15:1833–1840.

30. Waddell G, Turk DC. Clinical assessment of low back pain. In: Turk DC, Melzack R, eds. *Handbook of Pain Assessment.* New York: Guilford Press; 1992.

31. Hurley AC, Volicer BJ, Hanrahan PA, Houde S, Volicer V. Assessment of discomfort in advanced Alzheimer patients. *Res Nurs Health.* 1992;15:369–377.

32. Keefe FJ, Williams DA. Assessment of pain behaviors. In: Turk DC, Melzack R, eds. *Handbook of Pain Assessment.* New York: Guilford Press; 1992.

33. Herr KA, Mobily PR, Kohour FJ, et al. Evaluation of the faces pain scale for use with the elderly. *Clin J Pain.* 1998; 14:1–10.

34. Weiner DK, Peterson BL, Logue P, et al. Predictors of self-report in nursing home residents. *Aging Clin Exp Res.* 1998; 10:411–420.

35. Parmelee AP, Smith BD, Katz IR. Pain complaints and cognitive status among elderly institutional residents. *J Am Geriatr Soc.* 1993;41:517, 522.

36. Fabinszewiski KL, Volicer B, Volicer L. Effect of antibiotic treatment on outcomes of fevers in the institutionalized Alzheimer patients. *JAMA.* 1990;263:3168–3172.

37. O'Brien J, Francis A. The use of next-of-kin to estimate pain in cancer patients. *Pain.* 1988;35:171–178.

38. Von Roenn JH, Cleeland CS, Gonin R, Hatfield AK, Pandya KJ. Physician attitudes and practice in cancer pain management. A survey from the Eastern Cooperative Oncology Group. *Ann Intern Med.* 1993;119(2):121–126.

39. Camp DL. A comparison of nurses' assessments of pain as described by cancer patients. *Cancer Nurs.* 1988;11:237–243.

40. World Health Organization. *Cancer Pain Relief, 2nd Ed.* (With a guide to opioid availability, cancer pain relief and palliative care. Report of the WHO Expert Committee (WHO Technical Report Series no. 804). Geneva: WHO; 1996.

41. McQuay HJ, Carroll D, Moore RA. Post-operative orthopedic pain: the effect of opiate premedication and local anesthetic blocks. *Pain.* 1988;33:291–295.

42. Egbert AM, Parks LH, Shrot LM, Burnett ML. Randomized trial of postoperative patient controlled analgesia vs. intramuscular narcotics in frail elderly men. *Arch Intern Med.* 1990;150:1897–1903.

43. Egbert LD, Battit GE, Welch CE, Bartlett MK. Reduction in postoperative pain by encouragement and instruction of patients. *N Engl J Med.* 1964;270:825–827.

44. Foreman WB. Opioid analgesic drugs in the elderly. *Clin Geriatr Med.* 1996;12:489–500.

45. Turner JA, Deyo RA, Losser JD, et al. The importance of placebo effects in pain treatment and research. *JAMA.* 1994;271:1609–1614.

46. Bradley JD, Brandt KD, Katz BP, et al. Comparison of an anti-inflammatory dose of ibuprofen, an analgesic dose of ibuprofen and acetaminophen in treatment of patients with osteoarthritis of the knee. *N Engl J Med.* 1991;325: 87–91.

47. Perneger TV, Shelton PK, Klag MJ. Risk of kidney failure associated with use of acetaminophen, aspirin and non-steroidal antiinflammatory drugs. *N Engl J Med.* 1994;331: 1675–1679.

48. Shek, KL, Chan LN, Nutescu E. Warfarin-acetaminophen drug interaction revisited. *Pharmacotherapy.* 1999;19(10): 1153–1158.

49. Roth SH. Merits and liabilites of NSAID therapy. *Rheumatol Dis Clin N Am.* 1989;15:479–498.

50. Bell GM, Schnitzer TJ. COX-2 Inhibitors and other NSAIDs in the treatment of pain in the elderly. *Clin Geriatr Med.* 2001;17:489–502.

51. Griffin MR, Piper JM, Daugherty JR, et al. Nonsteroidal anti-inflammatory drug use and increase for peptic ulcer disease in elderly persons. *Ann Intern Med.* 1991;114:257–263.

52. Gurwitz JH, Avorn J, Ross-Degnan D, Sipsitz LA. Nonsteroidal anti-inflammatory drug associated azotemia in the very old. *JAMA.* 1990;264:471–475.

53. Graham DY, White RH, Foreland LW, et al. Duodenal and gastric ulcer prevention with misoprostol in arthritis patients taking NSAIDs: Misoprostol Study Group. *Ann Intern Med.* 1993;119:257–262.

54. Ehsanullah RS, Page MC, Tildesley G, Wood JR. Prevention of gastroduodenal damage induced by non-steroidal anti-inflammatory drugs: controlled trial of ranitidine. *Br Med J*. 1988;297:1017–1021.

55. Taha AS, Hudson N, Hawkey CJ, et al. Famotidine for the prevention of gastric and duodenal ulcers caused by nonsteroidal anti-inflammatory drugs. *N Engl J Med*. 1996; 334:1435–1449.

56. Stucki J, Hohannesson M, Liang MH. Use of misoprostol in the elderly: is the expense justified? *Drugs Aging*. 1996;8: 84–88.

57. Pope JE, Anderson JJ, Felson DT. A meta-analysis of the effects of nonsteroidal anti-inflammatory drugs on blood pressure. *Arch Intern Med*. 1993;153:477–484.

58. Morgan M. The rational use of intrathecal and extradural opioids. *Br J Anaesth*. 1989;63:165–188.

59. Kaiko RF. Age and morphine analgesia in cancer patients with postoperative pain. *Clin Pharmacol Ther*. 1980;28:823–826.

60. Bellville WJ, Forrest WH Jr, Miller E, Brown BW Jr. Influence of age on pain relief from analgesics: a study of postoperative patiets. *JAMA*. 1971;217:1835–1841.

61. Kaiko RF, Wallenstein SL, Rogers AG, et al. Narcotics in the elderly. *Med Clin North Am*. 1982;66:1079–1089.

62. Ready BL, Chadwick HS, Ross B. Age predicts effective epidural morphine dose after abdominal hysterectomy. *Anesth Analg*. 1987;66:1215–1218.

63. Melzack R. The tragedy of needless pain. *Sci Am*. 1990;262: 27–33.

64. Portenoy RK. Opiate therapy for chronic noncancer pain: can we get past the bias? *Am Pain Soc Bull*. 1991;1:4–7.

65. Jaffe JH. Drug addiction and drug abuse. In: Gilman AG, Goodman LS, Rall TW, Murad F, eds. *Goodman and Gillman's The Pharmacological Basis of Therapeutics, 7th Ed*. New York: Macmillian; 1985:532–581.

66. Council on Scientific Affairs. American Medical Association. Good care of the dying patient. *JAMA*. 1996;275: 474–478.

67. American College of Physicians and the ACP Ethics and Human Rights Committee: Ethics Manual 4th Ed. *Ann Intern Med*. 1998;128:576–594.

68. Max MB. Antidepressants and analgesics. In: Fields HL, Leibeskind JC, eds. *Progress in Pain Research and Management, vol. I*. Seattle: IASP Press; 1994:229–246.

69. Onghena P, Van Houdenhove B. Antidepressant-induced analgesia in chronic non-malignant pain: a metanalysis of 39 placebo-controlled studies. *Pain*. 1992;49:205–219.

70. Max MB, Lynch SA, Muir J, et al. Effects of desipramine, amytriptyline, and fluoxetine on pain in diabetic neuropathy. *N Engl J Med*. 1992;326:1250–1256.

71. Swerdlow M. The use of local anesthetics for relief of chronic pain. *Pain Clin*. 1988;2:3–6.

72. Backonja M, Beydoun A, Edwards KR, et al. Gabapentin for the symptomatic treatment of painful neuropathy in patients with diabetes mellitus: a randomized controlled trial. *JAMA*. 1998;280(21):1831–1836.

73. Rowbotham M, Harden N, Stacey B, Bernstein P, Magnus-Miller L. Gabapentin for the treatment of postherpetic neuralgia: a randomized controlled trial. *JAMA*. 1998;280(21):1837–1842.

74. Stracke H, Myer UE, Schumacher HE, Federlin K. Mexiletine in the treatment of diabetic neuropathy. *Diabetes Care*. 1992;15:1550–1555.

75. Gennari C, Agnusdei D, Camporeale A. Use of calcitonin in the treatment of bone pain associated with osteoporosis. *Calcif Tissue Int*. 1991;49(suppl 2):s9–s13.

76. Prager JP. Invasive modalities for the diagnosis and treatment of pain in the elderly. *Clin Geriatr Med*. 1996;12(3): 549–561.

77. McCain GA. Fibromyalgia and myofascial pain syndromes. In: Wall PD, Melzack R, eds. *Textbook of Pain, 3rd Ed*. New York: Churchill Livingstone; 1994:475–493.

78. Ferrell BR, Griffith H. Cost issues related to pain management: report from the Cancer Pain Panel of the Agency for Health Care Policy and Research. *J Pain Symptom Manage*. 1994;9:221–234.

79. Whedon M, Ferrell BR. Professional and ethical considerations in the use of high-tech pain management. *Oncol Nurs Forum*. 1991;18:1135–1143.

80. Ferrell BR, Rhiner M, Ferrell BA. Development and implementation of a pain education program. *Cancer* 1993; 72(suppl 11):3426–3432.

81. Rhiner M, Ferrell BR, Ferrell BA, Grant MM. A structured nondrug intervention program for cancer pain. *Cancer Pract*. 1993;1:137–143.

82. Ferrell BA, Josephson KR, Pollan AM, et al. A randomized trial of walking versus physical methods for chronic pain management. *Aging (Milano)*. 1997;9:99–105.

83. Ettinger WH Jr, Burns R, Messier SP, et al. A randomized trial comparing aerobic exercise and resistance exercise with a health education program in older adults with knee osteoarthritis: the Fitness Arthritis and Seniors Trial (FAST). *JAMA*. 1997;277:25–31.

84. Kovar PA, Allegrante JP, MacKenzie CR, et al. Supervised fitness walking in patients with osteoarthritis of the knee: a randomized trial. *Ann Intern Med*. 1992;116:529–534.

85. Keefe FJ, Caldwell DS, Williams DA, et al. Pain coping skills training in the management of osteoarthritic knee pain: a comparative study. *Behav Ther*. 1990;21:49–62.

86. Pruder RS. Age analysis of cognitive-behavioral group therapy for chronic pain outpatients. *Psychol Aging*. 1988; 3:204–207.

87. Eisenberg, Kessler RC, Foster C, et al. Unconventional medicine in the United States: prevalence, costs and patterns of use. *N Engl J Med*. 1993;328:246–252.

88. Ferrell BA. Pain, in *Comprehensive Geriatric Assessment*. Osterweil D, Brummel-Smith K, Beck JB, eds. New York: McGraw-Hill, 2000:389.

29
Palliative Care in Early, Moderate, and Advanced Dementia

Anna Monias and Diane E. Meier

Irreversible dementia is one of the most feared diagnoses in medicine. Patients with the disease face progressive deterioration of cognitive abilities, eventually resulting in loss of independence and inability to care for oneself. Prevalence of dementia increases with each decade of life over age 65.[1] Nineteen percent of the population suffers from dementia by age 80, 49% by age 90, and 60% among centenarians.[2,3] Alzheimer's disease (AD) is the most common cause of dementia, accounting for 50% of all cases. Over 4 million Americans are affected; this number is expected to increase to a minimum of 14 million by the middle of this century.[4,5] Worldwide, 22 million people are affected.[6] The second most common cause of dementia in the United States is vascular dementia, which accounts for another 20% to 40% of dementia cases.[7] Lewy body disease, Pick's disease, and Creutzfeldt–Jakob disease occur less often. Clinically, it is difficult to distinguish between different types of dementia, and many patients present with a "mixed" picture. In one study, the prevalence of "dementia of unknown etiology" increased with age and represented nearly 50% of dementia in those over age 90.[8]

Dementia is a chronic, terminal disease. All treatments are palliative, as there is no cure. The disease begins insidiously with mild decreases in memory, judgment, and spatial relationships. Care for the dementia patient should endeavor to preserve dignity and aggressively manage symptoms to sustain the best quality of life possible in patients with early, moderate, and end-stage dementia.

Each stage presents unique sources of suffering. In early dementia, patients may experience difficulties with word finding, driving, and learning new skills. Even in the early stages, patients require supervision. These patients may suffer depression, fear, and anxiety over their diagnosis and loss of independence. Over a period of time, on average 7 to 10 years, the disease progresses and patients suffer increased cognitive decline. Patients with moderate dementia lose the ability to perform previously routine tasks, such as balancing a checkbook or finding their way home from a neighborhood store. Family members or paid help begin to play a larger role in the patient's care. Often, behavioral disturbances including agitation, wandering, and paranoia develop, affecting both the patient and the caregiver. In advanced dementia, patients depend entirely on their caregivers for the activities of daily living, such as dressing, bathing, and toileting. They suffer from incontinence, gait instability, and decreased ability to chew and swallow. Eventually, they may be unable to remember their caregivers' names and cannot recognize members of their own family. Patients cannot verbally express emotions or describe pain and discomfort. Often, they are bedbound. By the end stages of dementia, most patients require nursing home care.

Caring for patients with dementing illness is physically, financially, and emotionally exhausting. Fifty percent of caregivers have financial difficulties and 66% have their own health problems.[9] Caregivers for dementia patients face different, and in some ways greater, stresses than caregivers in other terminal illnesses. The duration of family caregiving required often exceeds 10 years. In many cases, the disease affects the patient's personality. Paranoia and behavioral disturbances are common. In late stages, patients often can neither recognize nor appreciate their caregivers. In addition, the financial burden of this disease is staggering. In 1991, the direct costs of Alzheimer's disease were $20.6 billion, with indirect costs estimated at $67.3 billion.[9,10] The estimated 10-year direct cost for a man with Alzheimer's disease is $67,000. For women, who often have less support available in the home, the estimated 10-year direct cost is $100,900.[2] Indirect costs of Alzheimer's disease include unpaid hours that caregivers spend with patients, as well as lost wages secondary to hours missed from paid employment. Due to hospital and nursing home costs, Medicaid and Medicare expenditures on dementia patients are significantly more than age-matched patients without dementia.[11–14] When family labor is considered, the costs for caregiving at home in cases of advanced dementia exceed the costs of nursing home care.[15] The chronic stress associated with caring for a spouse with Alzheimer's disease has also been associated with decreased immunity and associated comorbidities, including depression.[16] Physicians can minimize caregiver burnout by letting caregivers know that they are available to talk with them during stressful times, simplifying medications and treatments, encouraging caregivers to take some time each day for their own needs, and providing information about support groups and community services, including hospice.

This chapter seeks to describe the medical and social issues that may become problems for dementia patients and their caregivers during the course of dementia and suggests appropriate interventions that will alleviate suffering. The needs of patients and caregivers change dramatically in each stage of the disease; therefore, this chapter is divided into three sections: early dementia, moderate dementia, and advanced dementia. Every dementia patient goes through all three stages; however, the disease affects each patient differently.

Physicians need to tailor care to the individual patient and caregiver. The patient with dementia may have or develop other chronic medical problems, including coronary artery disease, vascular ulcers, osteoarthritis, diabetes, renal insufficiency, and malignancy. A life-threatening illness, such as acute myocardial infarction, pneumonia, or urinary tract infection, could strike during any stage of dementia. Concurrent illnesses put additional stress on caregivers; the burdens of dressing changes, administering medications, and giving injections fall to them. The stage of dementia will affect the patient's ability to understand and comply with therapy. Physicians should continue to prescribe treatments that enhance comfort for demented patients with concurrent illness who do not undergo surgery, chemotherapy, and other invasive testing.

Early Dementia

D.G. is a 75-year-old retired businessman who was diagnosed with Alzheimer's dementia 3 months ago. He lives with his 70-year-old wife in a three-bedroom house. Before his diagnosis, Mr. G. had been repeating the same questions over and over, which was a source of irritation and concern to his wife of 47 years. Mr. G. was started on vitamin E and donepezil for Alzheimer's dementia, and both he and Mrs. G believe that his condition has been stable over the last few months. Mr. G. tells his physician that his grandmother was senile for a few years before her death. He fears losing control of his life and becoming a burden on his wife and two adult children.

After a medical evaluation to exclude reversible causes of dementia, physicians should implement evidence-based pharmacologic therapies to decrease the rate of cognitive decline. Treatment with cholinesterase inhibitors can modestly improve cognitive function and possibly improve activities of daily living in patients with mild to moderate Alzheimer's dementia.[6,17,18] These drugs may slow progression of the disease and help patients retain independence for a longer period of time. Although the first drug in this class, tacrine, was associated with liver toxicity, donepezil and rivastigmine are safe and well tolerated. There is less evidence to support using Hydergine, statins, nonsteroidal anti-inflammatory drugs, vitamin E, and dehydroepiandrosterone (DHEA) to delay cognitive decline.[19–21] Because the prevalence of AD is so high, much of the research on therapies has focused on AD rather than other types of dementia. Aggressive control of vascular risk factors may stabilize the rate of decline for patients with vascular dementia. Occupational therapy may also help patients with early and moderate dementia. Patients seem to derive both cognitive and behavioral benefits, at least in the short term, from reality orientation.[22]

In the early stages of dementia, it is important to inform both patients and caregivers of the diagnosis.[23] Educating patients and families about the course of the disease will help them make plans for medical care, financial affairs, and the way that they want to spend their remaining functional time. At this stage of the disease, patients can still make decisions for themselves. Physicians should ask them about their preferences for medical treatments in later stages of disease. Specifically, patients should be asked under what circumstances they would no longer wish life-prolonging technologies, such as a feeding tube. Many patients respond to this question by stating that if they are no longer able to recognize loved ones, then medical care should focus on comfort and quality of life, and they should be allowed to die peacefully. This is a more important and useful question than queries about desires for or against specific medical technologies, any one of which might be appropriate or inappropriate depending upon the details of the clinical context. Patients should also be asked to designate one or more primary decision makers in preparation for the time when they are no longer able to make medical decisions for themselves.

Early conversations about advance directives prepare family members for the burden of decision making in late dementia and may reduce later stress associated with surrogate decision making.[24] Goals of care should also be discussed early in the course of the disease. Patients and family members should be reassured that goals might change as the disease progresses. For example, early in the course of dementia, goals may be preserving autonomy, financial planning, continuing to participate in social activities and travel, ensuring safety, prolonging life, and forming a care plan for more advanced stages of disease.

Health care providers should advise patients and their families to speak with a financial advisor or attorney regarding their financial affair.[25] Physicians should remember that goals of care are likely to differ in relationship to individual belief systems and values.

Psychiatric disturbances are among the most frustrating problems of dementia. Early in the course of dementia, patients are aware of progressive memory loss and fear loss of identity. This fear can cause considerable anxiety and depression. Forty percent of patients with dementia experience anxiety.[26] Depressive symptoms are reported in 50% of patients with Alzheimer's dementia and may be more prevalent in vascular and Parkinson's dementia.[26] Depression in progressive dementia may be caused by anatomic damage to the brain.[27] Patients with AD are often diagnosed with depression as much as 2 years before the diagnosis of AD is made.[28] Antidepressants sometimes help these symptoms; however, therapies for classical depression may not be as efficacious in depression associated with dementia. Patient support groups may help in the early stages of disease. Euphoria is uncommon in AD but may be associated with frontal lobe dementias.[28] Depression is sometimes confused with personality changes in patients with AD. Frequently, Alzheimer's patients exhibit indifference, limited emotional engagement, and decreased motivation.[28] Therapy with cholinesterase inhibitors may improve psychiatric symptoms.

The period after diagnosis is also a time of great adjustment and grief for family caregivers. Before diagnosis, the patient may have been physically healthier and stronger than the caregiver. For many married couples, a diagnosis of dementia means that the healthier spouse will need to take on chores previously done by the patient, such as driving, financial planning and bill paying, housework, cooking, gardening, or shopping. Adult children may also have to play a caregiving role for the first time. Some family caregivers may find support groups helpful at this time.

Moderate Dementia

Despite treatment with donepezil, D.G., now 79, has faced progression of his dementia. He still lives with his wife, now 74. The couple moved to a smaller apartment a year ago after Mrs. G. was hospitalized for 1 week with a myocardial infarction. Mr. G.'s son, B.G., stayed with him during that hospitalization. Although he called frequently and visited one to two times per month, B.G. had not previously realized how forgetful his father had become. Night after night, he would wake up and begin looking for his wife. He tried to leave the house each night to look for Mrs. G. Although Mr. G. had stopped driving shortly after his diagnosis, on one occasion he tried to drive his son's car using a house key that he found on the kitchen table. When they went to the hospital, D.G. would

repeatedly ask where they were going and why. Although he still "read" the newspaper, he could no longer understand the articles. Mrs. G. had been doing all the shopping for several months because Mr. G. could no longer count change correctly. During meals, D.G. would eat minimally but put food in his pockets and take it to his bedroom. B.G. realized taking care of his father and a three-bedroom house was too much work for his mother. He helped his parents move to an apartment closer to his own home. Mrs. G. now has help with cleaning, cooking, and caring for her husband.

The middle stage of dementia is extremely challenging to health care providers and caregivers. Goals of care during this stage may focus on keeping the home environment safe and providing regular respite for caregivers. Patients suffer from increased paranoia and fear. This phase is marked by the need for greater supervision of patients due to safety concerns, decreased ability to perform the activities of daily living, and increased behavioral disturbances. These changes in patients are sources of immense caregiver stress; they may lead to nursing home placement. Patients with moderate dementia but without other medical comorbidities are difficult to place in nursing homes because reimbursement for this type of care is low. Families who choose to take care of dementia patients at home may access services such as adult day care and respite care, but availability is scarce and out-of-pocket costs are high. Palliative measures include modifying the diet and environment to meet nutritional and safety needs and improve behavior without compromising patient dignity. These changes require training family members and nursing home staff in behavioral management and feeding techniques as described in the following paragraphs.

Eating behaviors change in patients with moderate dementia. Decreased acuity of smell and taste and decreased sensitivity to thirst receptors predispose dementia patients to weight loss and dehydration. At this stage of disease, patients may also have difficulty using utensils. Caregivers can compensate by offering frequent, nutritious snacks. Patients may find finger foods more acceptable than more formal meals. Creating a pleasant dining setting and giving specially designed utensils, such as deep dishes and large spoons, may make feeding easier. Adding extra sweeteners or spices may also improve caloric intake. Health care providers should evaluate correctable causes of anorexia, such as medications, depression, odynophagia, constipation, and urinary retention, and physicians should try to eliminate medications that may cause anorexia. Common classes of medication that cause anorexia include diuretics, beta-blockers, digoxin, and statins.

Although neuropsychiatric disorders are intermittent and may occur at any stage of disease, they are associated with more rapid cognitive and functional decline.[28] Symptoms become more frequent as disease progresses.[28] In addition to anxiety and depression, patients with dementia suffer from paranoia, delusions, hallucinations, sleep disorders, agitation, and combativeness.[29] More than 50% of patients with Alzheimer's disease demonstrate aggressive behavior; nearly 20% physically assault their caregivers.[30] These symptoms affect quality of life for both patient and caregiver. Noncognitive features of dementia may have a greater impact on caregiver burden than decrease in cognitive function or decrease in activities of daily living.[31] In fact, neuropsychiatric disturbances, particularly aggressive behavior and paranoia, increase the likelihood of nursing home placement more than decline in cognitive function.[28,32]

Many pharmacologic and nonpharmacologic interventions have been studied to decrease behavioral disturbances. However, physicians should eliminate comorbid illnesses and pain as causes of behavioral disturbance before trials of neuroleptics or behavioral therapies. Treatment of medical illness leads to sustained improvement of cognition and behavior in a significant percentage of these patients.[26] When patients lose the ability to express themselves, they can only communicate through their actions. As with an infant, the caregiver needs to determine whether there is a reversible cause of agitation such as pain, hunger, thirst, or wet clothing, Identifying causes of discomfort may be difficult. Although patients with mild to moderate dementia can often complete a pain intensity scale, they may not verbally complain of pain in the same way as cognitively intact patients.[33,34] Behavioral symptoms such as restlessness, insomnia, pugnacity, tense body posture, grimacing, vocalization, withdrawal, and fear may all be symptoms of pain; therefore, before trying to stop these behaviors, physicians should look for their cause.

If there is no obvious physiologic reason for discomfort, modifying care practices may reduce behavioral disturbances. For many dementia patients, bathing and grooming are frightening assaults. Changing the routine by giving sponge baths and adjusting water temperature can make the experience less threatening. Also, research has suggested that encouraging patients to participate in grooming and bathing themselves decreases agitation.[35] Sleep disturbances affect up to 70% of patients with dementia. Daytime exercises, a consistent bedtime routine, and minimizing daytime napping can help improve sleep patterns.[36] A calm environment featuring favorite music from the patient's early adulthood and frequent social activities may also diminish disruptive behavior. Recordings of family members recounting favorite memories may also provide comfort to dementia patients.[37] When nonpharmacologic measures do not help, low doses of neuroleptics can alleviate nocturnal confusion, hallucinations, and delusions. At low doses, second-generation neuroleptics (risperidal, quetiapine, olanzapine) cause less extrapyramidal toxicity than

haloperidol.[32] Successful management of behavioral disturbances can prevent hospital admissions and nursing home placement.

Caregivers often begin to suffer from fatigue, emotional stress, and financial stress during this stage of Alzheimer's disease. Those who work return home and begin a second shift. Job performance may falter, secondary to lack of sleep and missed days resulting from caregiving demands. Often caregivers have to leave their jobs to care for loved ones. Hiring health aides and making safety modifications to the home is expensive. Day programs are also expensive. Unless the patient is on Medicaid, these services are not covered by health insurance. Caregivers may also feel unappreciated because patients may not be able to express appreciation or gratitude. During this stage, caregivers may begin to mourn the passing of the strong, independent people they once knew as they watch the patients gradually become shadows of their former selves. Health care providers should ask caregivers about fatigue, social isolation, depression, and physical symptoms. Caregivers should be given a list of local resources for adult day care, respite care, homemaker services, and support groups. Caregivers should be reminded to take breaks from patient care and encourage other family members or close friends to help care for the patient on a regular basis.

Advanced Dementia

D.G., now 85, was placed into a nursing home 1 year ago after Mrs. G. died. At first, he wandered frequently during the day and night. Four months ago, he fell while in the bathroom and suffered from a fracture to his left hip, requiring arthroplasty. Currently, he walks only with assistance. Although he has a walker, he does not remember to use it. He was unable to complete a physical therapy program after his surgery because he could not follow instructions. In the last few weeks, he has had decreased oral intake. Sometimes he seems to "pocket" food in his mouth without swallowing it. He often clamps his mouth shut or pushes the spoon away during feeding. He is incontinent of both urine and stool. His children visit frequently, but he does not seem to recognize them.

Patients with advanced dementia are at the end stage of a terminal disease. They are dying just as surely as patients with end-stage cancer, connective tissue disease, or heart failure are dying. Multiple studies have demonstrated a median 6-month mortality in persons with advanced dementia, with or without tube feeding, although the range of survival time is wide.[38] Advanced dementia patients may experience moments of lucidity; however, they do not consistently recognize caregivers or their own images in the mirror. Patients lose ambulation skills. They also experience weight loss as a result of forgetting how to chew and swallow. Family and physicians should pay close attention to managing symptoms of disease to keep patients as comfortable as possible. Although palliation of suffering and maximizing quality of life are the most appropriate treatment goals for patients with advanced dementia, many patients in the last days of life receive unwanted and largely ineffective nonpalliative interventions, such as artificial nutrition and hydration, cardiopulmonary resuscitation, and systemic antibiotics.[39]

At this stage, caregivers need to make difficult decisions about whether to proceed with potentially life-prolonging medical procedures, such as artificial nutrition and hydration, intravenous antibiotics, surgery, intubation, and cardiopulmonary resuscitation. If these decisions were made previously with advance directives, caregivers will have the heart-wrenching task of implementing them. These decisions should be based on two factors: (1) previously discussed wishes; and (2) the best interests of the patient, with particular regard to the benefits and burdens of the proposed medical intervention. In addition to the psychologic burden of making decisions for patients, caregivers continue to suffer from the escalating physical demands of caring for loved ones. Patients with advanced dementia are often placed in a nursing home due to increasing care demands. Regardless of whether the patient resides at home or in an institution, palliative measures include paying close attention to possible sources of pain and offering continued support to caregivers and family members with regular and repeated review of goals and expectations. At this stage, the goals of care should focus on reducing caregiver stress and relieving the patient's physical and emotional symptoms.

Advanced dementia patients suffer from chronic pain and discomfort from comorbid chronic diseases, such as osteoarthritis, congestive heart failure, chronic obstructive pulmonary disease, and decubitus ulcers, as well as pain secondary to acute illnesses, such as fractures or infection. Yet, this pain is often untreated secondary to the patient's inability to complain. Cognitively intact patients receive more analgesics than patients with advanced dementia after hip fracture.[40] Therefore, physicians should treat advanced dementia patients with pain medication preventively and empirically before procedures known to cause pain, such as dressing changes or postsurgical procedures. Physicians also need to remember that patients with advanced dementia may have increased pain from routine phlebotomy, blood pressure monitoring, fingersticks, and bladder cannulation because they do not understand what is being done to them.[41] Patients may view these minor procedures as assaults. Physicians can use topical anesthetic preparations to make needle sticks or catheter placement more comfortable.

Artificial Nutrition and Hydration

The development of dysphagia is a universal neurologic complication of advanced Alzheimer's disease and related dementias that puts patients at risk for aspiration pneumonia.[42] Initially, patients are given a pureed diet with thickened liquids to counteract swallowing dysfunction. Slow feeding of patients with small spoonfuls of a soft, pureed diet may also help prevent aspiration.[43] If these methods fail to deliver sufficient calories to maintain body mass, caregivers must make decisions about artificial nutrition. This is an emotional issue for many family members, as many may see withholding artificial nutrition as tantamount to starvation. Although tube feeding may provide psychologic comfort to caregivers, there is no evidence that it either prolongs or improves life in the long term for patients with advanced dementia.[38,44–46] Studies of mentally intact terminally ill patients with anorexia have shown that symptoms of thirst can be alleviated with small sips of water and oral hygiene.[47] Often tube feeding is initiated to increase protein stores to promote wound healing in dementia patients with decubitus ulcers, but studies have not shown that enteral feeding improves wound healing or albumin levels.[44,48] In fact, in one small study, 50% of nursing home patients had a decrease in albumin 13 to 18 months after beginning gastrostomy feeding.[48] One of the major reasons for starting artificial nutrition is to prevent aspiration pneumonia; however, there is no evidence that tube feeding reduces this risk and some evidence that it may actually increase risk of aspiration.[44,49]

The decision to proceed with tube feeding should be made only after the risk of operative complications and long-term adverse effects, such as need for restraints, diarrhea, and infection, are considered.[50] Patients who can no longer eat can be fed through parenteral or enteral nutrition. Parenteral nutrition is generally not offered to patients with an intact gastrointestinal tract because placement of long-term intravenous access predisposes patients to infection; furthermore, intestinal integrity may deteriorate without intraluminal fuels, predisposing patients to systemic infection from gut flora.[49]

Enteral feeding can be nasogastric, through gastrostomy tube, or through jejunostomy tube. Nasogastric feeding is recommended for temporary feeding, usually for a period of less than 30 days. This procedure may be appropriate if dysphagia occurs abruptly after a short illness and the patient is expected to recover. The most dangerous complications of nasogastric tube placement is inadvertent pulmonary intubation, chemical pneumonitis, and pneumothorax. Even when small-bore tubes are used, nasogastric feeding is uncomfortable. Patients often need to be restrained to prevent them from dislodging nasogastric tubes. Permanent placement of gastrostomy or jejunostomy tubes also has complications. The initial procedure causes pain, requires the patient to receive local anesthesia, or in some cases general anesthesia, and sedation. Patients often require restraints for the first 24 to 48 h after placement. The most common postoperative complication is local wound infection, but rarely perforation of a viscous, necrotizing fasciitis, and colocutaneous fistula can occur.[49] Once the tube is placed, common problems include aspiration, blockage of the tube, and diarrhea. Risk factors for aspiration include supine positioning during feeding, inability to clear oropharyngeal secretions, and bolus feeding. Diarrhea is multifactorial, and causes include formula composition, rate of infusion, hypoalbuminemia, and altered bacterial flora. *Clostridium difficile* infection rate is higher in patients receiving tube feeding than in similarly matched patients who are not tube fed.[51] The decision to proceed with artificial nutrition and hydration should be made only after considering the risks of operative complications and long-term adverse effects, such as infection, diarrhea, and aspiration.[50]

It is important to point out to family members that loss of appetite is a universal concomitant of the dying process, regardless of cause. Families should be encouraged to express their love and care through alternative means of nurturing when patients can no longer eat and drink. Mouth care with artificial saliva spray, moistened swabs, toothbrushing, ice chips, offers of small spoonfuls of ice cream, and hand and foot massage are all comforting and appropriate caregiving measures to suggest to family members.

Infection

Infection is the usual cause of death in patients with dementia.[52] Immobility, incontinence, and aspiration put dementia patients at higher risk of developing pneumonia, infected decubitus ulcers, and urinary tract infections than healthy elderly people. Furthermore, infection in advanced dementia patients may be detected later than in cognitively intact patients, secondary to atypical presentation and inability of the patient to express themselves. Patients may present with increased agitation or decreased appetite. Immunologic function may also be impaired in dementia patients. One study showed increased anergy in dementia patients when compared with other nursing home residents.[4]

Although infection in patients with advanced dementia is inevitable, risk factors can be reduced with careful attention to skin care and ambulation training. Incontinent patients should have diapers changed frequently; they should also be put on a toileting schedule. Turning on the sink while the patient is on the toilet sometimes stimulates micturition. Bedbound patients should be turned often and kept clean and dry to prevent decubiti.

When patients develop an infection, comfort measures should be implemented; these include antipyretics, pain medication, and oxygen. Atropine or glycopyrrolate can also be used to decrease tracheal secretions in an end-stage dementia patient. Physicians should avoid excess intravenous hydration, a cause of pulmonary and peripheral edema. Before starting antibiotics, risks and benefits should be weighed. Although there is no evidence that antibiotics improve survival in advanced dementia patients, they can provide comfort in some cases.[53] For example, antibiotics may alleviate dysuria, fever, sweats, shortness of breath, and cough. Antibiotic treatment can improve comfort by decreasing pain in patients with cellulitis and decreasing diarrhea in patients with *Clostridium difficile*. Drawbacks of antibiotic therapy include the risk of allergic reactions, development of infection with resistant organisms, the possible need to transfer the patient to the hospital for intravenous therapy, the need for repeat intravenous catheter placements, and frequent blood draws to monitor drug levels. Antibiotics can precipitate renal failure, diarrhea, rashes, bone marrow failure, seizures, nausea, and vomiting. These patients do not understand what is happening to them and may need to be restrained to tolerate placement and maintenance of intravenous lines, intramuscular injections, and other interventions and procedures.

The Hospice Benefit and Advanced Dementia

The Medicare Hospice Benefit requires that a physician certify an approximate prognosis of 6 months or less if the disease follows its usual course. Although multiple studies have shown a 6-month median survival in persons hospitalized with acute illness and advanced dementia, variability is high and prognostication unreliable.[38,54,55] As a result, hospice is rarely accessed for patients dying of advanced dementia.[56] Volicer and others have proposed that patients with end-stage dementia qualify for extra services through an extension of the Medicare hospice benefit. In addition to providing personal care attendants to assist family caregivers, the Medicare hospice benefit also provides critically needed grief and bereavement services for caregivers. Most family members and physician members of the Gerontological Society of America believe that care focusing on comfort and pain control is most appropriate for end-stage dementia patients.[57] Enhanced hospice care with more support for personal care services is appropriate for these patients because dementia patients and their often exhausted caregivers require more help at home in the last year of life than cancer patients.[58] In fact, end-stage dementia patients may be more appropriate for inpatient hospice within a nursing home or other institutional setting than other terminal patients. Research demonstrates that patients cared for in dementia support care units with a hospice approach experienced less discomfort and utilized fewer health care resources than similar patients treated in a traditional (usual care) long-term care unit.[59]

Conclusion

Caring for patients with progressive, irreversible dementia is challenging for physicians and caregiver. By focusing on quality of life as the primary goal of medical care in the later stages of dementia, health care providers may help patients and family members prepare for the degenerative course of the disease and plan for the future. Physicians should focus on preservation of independence and relief of physical and emotional suffering for both patients and their caregivers.

References

1. Fratiglioni L, De Ronchi D, Aguero-Torres H. Worldwide prevalence and incidence of dementia. *Drugs Aging*. 1999; 15(5):365–375.
2. Kinosian BP, Stullard E, Lee JH, Woodbury MA, Zbrozek AS, Glick HA. Predicting 10-year care requirements for older people with suspected Alzheimer's disease. *J Am Geriatr Soc*. 2000;48:631–638.
3. Fleming KC, Evans JM. Pharmacologic therapies in dementia. *Mayo Clin Proc*. 1995;70:1116–1123.
4. Small GW, Rabins PV, Barry PP, et al. Diagnosis and treatment of Alzheimer disease and related disorders. Consensus statement of the American Association for Geriatric Psychiatry, the Alzheimer's Association, and the American Geriatrics Society. *JAMA*. 1997;278(16):1363–1371.
5. Volicer L, Hurley A. *Hospice Care for Patients with Advanced Progressive Dementia*. New York: Springer; 1998.
6. Samuels SC. Alzheimer disease treatment: a focus on cholinesterase inhibitors. *Prim Psychiatry*. 2000;7(9):62–66.
7. Shuster JL. Palliative care for advanced dementia. *Clin Geriatr Med*. 2000;16(2):373–387.
8. Crystal HA, Dickson D, Davies P, Masur D, Grober E, Lipton RB. The relative frequency of "dementia of unknown etiology" increases with age and is nearly 50% in nonagenarians. *Arch Neurol*. 2000;57:713–719.
9. Kasuya RJ, Polgar Bailey PP, Takeuchi R. Caregiver burden and burnout. *Postgrad Med*. 2000;108(7):119–122.
10. Wimo A, Ljunggren G, Winblad B. Costs of dementia and dementia care: a review. *Int J Geriatr Psychiatry*. 1997; 12:841–856.
11. Gutterman EM, Markowitz JS, Lewis B, Fillit H. Cost of Alzheimer's disease and related dementias in managed Medicare. *J Am Geriatr Soc*. 1999;47:1065–1071.
12. Martin BC, Ricci JF, Kotzan JA, Lang K, Menzin J. The net cost of Alzheimer disease and related dementia: a population-based study of Georgia Medicaid recipients. *Alzheimer Dis Assoc Disord*. 2000;14(3):151–159.
13. Menzin J, Lang K, Friedman M, Neumann P, Cummings JL. The economic cost of Alzheimer's disease and related dementias to the California Medicaid Program in 1995. *Am J Geriatr Psychiatry*. 1999;7:300–308.
14. Taylor DH, Sloan FA. How much do persons with Alzheimer's disease cost Medicare? *J Am Geriatr Soc*. 2000;48:639–646.
15. Chiu L, Tang KY, Liu YH, Shyu WC, Chang TP. Cost comparisons between family-based care and nursing home care for dementia. *J Adv Nurs*. 1999;29:1005–1012.
16. Wu H. Chronic stress associated with spousal caregiving of patients with Alzheimer's dementia is associated with downregulation of B-lymphocyte GH mRNA. *J Gerontol Ser A Biol Sci Med Sci*. 1999;54(4):M212–M215.
17. Birks JS, Melzer D, Beppu H. Donepezil for mild and moderate Alzheimer's disease (Cochrane Review). Cochrane Library, Issue, 2, 2002. Oxford: Update Software.
18. Birks J, Grimley Evans J, Iakovidou V, Tsolaki M. Rivastigmine for Alzheimer's disease (Cochrane Review). In: *Cochrane Library*, Issue 4, 2000. Oxford: Update Software.
19. Huppert FA, Van Niekerk JK, Herbert J. Dehydro-epiandrosterone (DHEA) supplementation for cognition and well-being (Cochrane Review). In: *Cochrane Library*, Issue 4, 2000. Oxford: Update Software.
20. Olin J, Schneider L, Novit A, Luczak S. Hydergine for dementia (Cochrane Review). In: *Cochrane Library*, Issue 4, 2000. Oxford: Update Software.
21. Tabet N, Birks J, Grimley Evans J. Vitamin E for Alzheimer's disease (Cochrane Review). In: *Cochrane Library*, Issue 1, 2002. Oxford: Update Software.
22. Spector A, Orrell M, Davies S, Woods B. Reality orientation for dementia (Cochrane Review). In: *Cochrane Library*, Issue 4, 2000. Oxford: Update Software.
23. Post SG, Whitehouse PJ. Fairhill guidelines on ethics of the care of people with Alzheimer's disease: a clinical summary. *J Am Geriatr Soc*. 1995;43:1423–1429.
24. Tilden VP, Tolle SW, Nelson CA, Fields J. Family decision-making to withdraw life-sustaining treatments from hospitalized patients. *Nurs Res*. 2001;50:1–11.
25. Al-Adwani A, Nabi W. Financial management in patients with dementia; their adult children's knowledge and views. *Int J Geriatr Psychiatry*. 1998;13:462–465.
26. Carlson DL, Fleming KC, Smith GE, Evans JM. Management of dementia-related behavioral disturbances: a non-pharmacologic approach. *Mayo Clinic Proc*. 1995;70: 1108–1115.
27. Boland RJ. Depression in Alzheimer's disease and other dementias. *Curr Psychiatry Rep*. 2000;2(5):427–433.
28. Chung JA, Cummings JL. Neurobehavioral and neuropsychiatric symptoms in Alzheimer's disease. *Neurol Clin*. 2000;18(4):829–846.
29. Reisberg B, Borenstein J, Salob SP, et al. Behavioral symptoms in Alzheimer's disease: phenomenology and treatment. *J Clin Psychiatry*. 1987;48(suppl 5):9–15.
30. Eastley R, Wilcock GK. Prevalence and correlates of aggressive behaviours occurring in patients with Alzheimer's disease. *Int J Geriatr Psychiatry*. 1997;12:484–487.
31. Donaldson C, Tarrier N, Burns A. The impact of the symptoms of dementia on caregivers. *Br J Psychiatry*. 1997;170: 62–68.
32. De Deynl PP, Rabheru K, Rasmussen A, et al. A randomized trial of risperidone, placebo, and haloperidol for

behavioral symptoms of dementia. *Neurology*. 1999;53(5): 946–955.

33. Ferrell BA, Ferrell BR, Rivera L. Pain in cognitively impaired nursing home patients. *J Pain Symptom Manage*. 1995;10(8):591–598.

34. Krulewitch H, London MR, Skakel VJ, Lundstedt GJ, Thomason H, Brummel-Smith K. Assessment of pain in cognitively impaired older adults: a comparison of pain assessment tools and their use by nonpressional caregivers. *J Am Geriatr Soc*. 2000;48(12):1607–1611.

35. Wells DL, Dawson P, Sidani S, Craig D, Pringle D. Effects of an abilities-focused program of morning care on residents who have dementia and on caregivers. *J Am Geriatr Soc*. 2000;48(4):442–449.

36. Alessi CA, Yoon EJ, Schnelle JF, Al-Samarrai NR, Cruise PA. A randomized trial of a combined physical activity and environmental intervention in nursing home residents: do sleep and agitation improve? *J Am Geriatr Soc*. 1999;47(7): 784–791.

37. Camberg L, Woods P, Ooi WL, et al. Evaluation of simulated presence: a personalized approach to enhance well-being in persons with Alzheimer's disease. *J Am Geriatr Soc*. 1999;47(4):446–452.

38. Meier DE, Ahronheim JC, Morris J, Baskin-Lyons S, Morrison RS. High short-term mortality in hospitalized patients with advanced dementia: lack of benefit of tube-feeding. *Arch Intern Med*. 2001;161:594–599.

39. Ahronheim JC, Morrison RS, Baskin SA, Morris J, Meier DE. Treatment of the dying in the acute care hospital. *Arch Intern Med*. 1996;156(18):2094–2100.

40. Morrison RS, Siu AL. A comparison of pain and its treatment in advanced dementia and cognitively intact patients with hip fracture. *J Pain Symptom Manage*. 2000;19(4):240–248.

41. Morrison RS, Ahronheim JC, Morrison GR, et al. Pain and discomfort associated with common hospital procedures and experiences. *J Pain Symptom Management*. 1998;15(2): 91–101.

42. Martin BJW, Corlew MM, Wood H, et al. The association of swallowing dysfunction and aspiration pneumonia. *Dysphagia*. 1994;9:1–6.

43. Volicer L, Rheaume Y, Riley ME, Karner J, Glennon M. Discontinuation of tube feeding in patients with dementia of the Alzheimer type. *Am J Alzheimer's Care Relat Disord Res*. 1990;July/August:22–25.

44. Finucane TE, Christmas C, Travis K. Tube feeding in patients with advanced dementia. *JAMA*. 1999;282:1365–1370.

45. Fisman DN, Levy AR, Gifford DR, Tamblyn R. Survival after percutaneous endoscopic gastrostomy among older residents of Quebec. *J Am Geriatr Soc*. 1999;47:349–353.

46. Gillick MR. Rethinking the role of tube feeding in patients with advanced dementia. *N Engl J Med*. 2000;342: 206–210.

47. McCann RM, Hall WJ, Groth-Juncker A. Comfort care for terminally ill patients. The appropriate use of nutrition and hydration. *JAMA*. 1994;272:1263–1266.

48. Kaw M, Sekas G. Long-term follow-up of consequences of percutaneous endoscopic gastrostomy (PEG) tubes in nursing home patients. *Dig Dis Sci*. 1994;39(4):738–743.

49. Kirby DF, Delegse MH, Fleming CR. American Gastroenterological Association technical review on tube feeding for enteral nutrition. *Gastroenterology*. 1995;108(4):1282–1301.

50. Callahan CM, Haag KM, Buchanan NN, Nisi R. Decision-making for percutaneous endoscopic gastrostomy among older adults in a community setting. *J Am Geriatr Soc*. 1999;47:1105–1109.

51. Bliss DZ, Johnson S, Savik K, Clabots CR, Willard K, Gerding DN. Acquisition of *Clostridium difficile* and *Clostridium difficile*-associated diarrhea in hospitalized patients receiving tube feeding. *Ann Intern Med*. 1998; 129:1012–1019.

52. Beard CM, Kokmen E, Sigler C, Smith GE, Petterson T, O'Brien PC. Cause of death in Alzheimer's disease. *Ann Epidemiol*. 1996;6:195–200.

53. Fabiszewski KJ, Volicer B, Volicer L. Effect of antibiotic treatment on outcome of fevers in institutionalized Alzheimer patients. *JAMA*. 1990;263:3168–3172.

54. Hanrahan P, Luchins DJ. Feasible criteria for enrolling end-stage dementia patients in home hospice care. *Hospice J*. 1995;10(3):47–53.

55. Morrison RS, Siu AL. Survival in end-stage dementia following acute illness. *JAMA*. 2000;284:47–52.

56. Hanrahan P, Luchins DJ. Access to hospice programs in end-stage dementia: a national survey of hospice programs. *J Am Geriatr Soc*. 1997;43:56–59.

57. Luchins DJ, Hanrahan P. What is appropriate health care for end-stage dementia? *J Am Geriatr Soc*. 1993;41:25–30.

58. McCarthy M. The experience of dying with dementia: a retrospective study. *Int J Geriatr Psychiatry*. 1997;12(3): 404–409.

59. Volicer L, Collard A, Hurley A, Bishop C, Kern D, Karon S. Impact of special care unit for patients with advanced Alzheimer's disease on patients' discomfort and costs. *J Am Geriatr Soc*. 1994;42(6):597–603.

30
The Value of Achieving a Peaceful Death

Daniel Callahan

The ancient Greeks got the point long ago. At the core of human life is necessity. As the classical scholar William Arrowsmith nicely put it in explaining their perspective, "Call it destiny, call it fate, call it the gods, it hardly matters. Necessity is, first of all, death; but it is also old age, sleep, the reversal of fortune and the dance of life; it is thereby the fact of suffering as well as pleasure, for if we must dance and sleep, we also suffer, age and die."[1]

This is a hard wisdom for twenty-first-century ears. What else is modern medicine useful for if not to overcome and pacify that necessity? What is contemporary life all about if not to overcome fate, to put choice in our hands where destiny once prevailed? Why should we accept aging and death as fixed parts of life if perhaps we can do something about them? Why not fight back?

The Greeks were right the first time. Aging and death have not been conquered, and their necessity is still a fundamental part of the human condition. More than that, it is still an indispensable way of defining that condition.

Yet it is also true that aging and death are not what they used to be. What is? Lives are longer, death less omnipresent among the young, and old age perhaps a more hopeful time of life than it was for the Greeks. It is precisely the tension between the ancient but still real necessity of aging and death and the new possibilities for altering their circumstances that create the peculiar and troubling problem for geriatrics. In particular, what is an appropriate stance toward death, and how is a sensible, prudent balance to be struck between the need to recognize the necessity of death and, at the same time, to keep open the possibility of continued life?

That question should push itself on us when we try to think about the desire for, the need for, and the hope for a peaceful death. Every society has wanted such a death and, save possibly for the ideal of a heroic death in warfare, so too have most people. In his great work, *The Hour of Our Death*, the late French historian Philippe Ariès wrote movingly of what he called the "tame death" of earlier times, perhaps part myth but surprisingly well grounded in the human record.[2] It was a death that was tolerable and homely, expected with certainty, a common presence, and accepted without crippling fear.

There was, Ariès wrote, a "familiar simplicity" about death, in part because death came more quickly. It came across the life cycle, it was out in the open, and it was set within the context of religious and cultural rituals that tried, publicly and privately, to make sense of and give a meaning to death. For our part, he argued, we now have a "wild" death, drawn out by the chronic and degenerative diseases of aging societies, overshadowed and often dominated by technologies we barely control, and too often taking place within impersonal institutions, hospitals, or nursing homes, hidden from the public eye.

The struggle to move beyond a wild death has not been easy. It has seen the promotion of advance directives, the hospice movement, efforts to change the thinking and practice of clinicians, and, of late, a movement to introduce euthanasia and physician-assisted suicide. These are important developments (and dealt with elsewhere in *Geriatric Medicine*), but they need to be complemented by a clear idea of just what a decent death, an acceptable death—what might best be simply called a "peaceful death"—should encompass. It goes beyond having a choice about one's death, raising questions about the place of death in human life and the response of medicine and geriatrics to it.

Let it be understood at the outset that a peaceful death can only be an ideal toward which patients and their physicians can strive. There is no way that such a death can be ensured, no human stance toward death or medical tactic in coping with the dying of a person that can ensure a perfect absence of pain, suffering, anguish, and loss. Although there are occasions when death seems a merciful release for a patient, death is the end of a life and thus the end of hope and possibility. It is therefore always a kind of evil, the most profound symbol of human limits and finitude. There may be a "death with dignity," when everything comes together for a patient at the end, but there is also a profound sense in which death itself is the ultimate indignity of human life.[3] The idea of a peaceful death should always be in tension with that disturbing but abiding perception—as true for us as for the ancient Greeks.

I want to offer a preliminary notion of what might constitute a "peaceful death," move from there to some of the obstacles standing in its way, and then return to and fill out the concept still further.

A peaceful death might, as a first rough sketch, be defined as a death that is accepted and not unduly feared, a death which is not marked by excessive pain and suffering, and a death that takes place, so far as possible, in the presence of other people who are there to offer comfort, support, and love. If death itself is unacceptable, as it must be for most of us, there can still be an acceptance of its inevitability and its inescapable necessity. A peaceful death requires coming to terms with that necessity, on the part of the patient, the family, friends, and the medical staff. If there is to be peace, that acceptance will be at its heart.

For the physician or others responsible for the last days of a patient, the acceptance must be both stark and profound, coming down to an unavoidable truth: every patient will eventually die and the end of aging is death. This understanding means that the necessity of eventual death and a reconciliation to its inevitability must be an integral part of the care of all patients, but the elderly patient in particular, for whom death will be a more familiar figure than for the young. Biologically, death is no mishap but part of the human condition. A peaceful death should be as high on the agenda of the caretaker as the health and well-being of a patient. Just as the pursuit of good health is an enduring goal of medicine, so also should be the pursuit of a peaceful death when health is no longer possible. A peaceful death is not something to be sought at the last minute when all else has failed, but is to be thought about early and approached with care, out of a recognition that it lurks out of sight in all of us, just awaiting its final, dominant moment—if we are fortunate enough to bring it about, doctors and patients together.

Obstacles to a Peaceful Death

Many obstacles can stand in the way of a peaceful death, but three seem most important: chance and luck, the response of the physician to the threat of death, and the prior life and values that a patient brings to his or her dying.

Chance and Luck

It may seem trivial, self-evident, and unnecessary to mention the place of chance and luck in the making of a peaceful death. Yet it is there and must be taken account of. Some people will be fortunate in their dying, the victim of a condition that brings them a relatively benign death. Others will not be so blessed. We do not know, and can rarely know, which it is to be. Simply not knowing one's fate is, for many, part of the problem of dying: the fear of the unknown is as powerful a fear as any, sometimes all the worse because of the impossibility of preparing for it.

None of us can choose the disease from which we will die, and all of us might be likened to anxious spectators at a kind of poisonous feast, wondering which malady we will contract from those spread out on the medical table. Cancer? Stroke? Kidney failure? Perhaps it is just as well that we do not know in advance, although the uncertainty will itself be a source of anxiety. For those with a family history of a specific disease, there is often a special fear, not simply that they will themselves get the disease also, but that they will have to endure the suffering that they observed in others close to them. They may have an all-too-vivid image, an anxious foreshadowing of their final days from the memory of the last days of another. Their hope is that they will have the good luck to be spared the same fate. They may or they may not. And even if they contract the same disease, they may or may not have a peaceful death.

The physician is as helpless in the face of such fears as the patient. The physician can no more than the patient choose the fatal, final illness. There is no direct remedy that can be offered the patient at this point, with fears that are real but vagrant, with the utter certainty that death will come but matched by an utter uncertainty about how it will come. But when such fears surface, that is an occasion to begin the work of care and comfort, beginning with the recognition that the fear of dying, or of death itself (and they may, and probably will, run together in the patient's mind), can be as excruciating as anything that the dying itself might bring, if not worse. Fear should always be taken with utter seriousness. It can be lethal to the human spirit, as much so as any organic disease.

In the face of chance, luck, and uncertainty about death, the physician can only respond through talk and empathy, with the recognition that his or her ultimate fate is as open to the gratuitous play of chance as that of the patient. We are all in this together. Precisely because there is no medical remedy for this throw of the dice, the physician will be forced back on his or her own humanity—unable to give any more than his or her shared insight into the fragility of life, the defenselessness of all of us. Yet if that much can be done, then a decent foundation will have been laid for an ongoing conversation and relationship that can bear richer fruits as chance sooner or later reveals its hand. With luck, a peaceful death may be more readily attained—and with bad luck, more difficult.

The Response of the Physician

Why is it so hard to let a patient die, to give up in the face of the inevitability of death? And why is it that, once the physician has accepted the coming of death, there is too often a powerful temptation to turn away from this patient to those patients who are still amenable to improvement or cure? These are questions that have nagged at the conscience of medicine for some decades now, uncomfortably persistent, fretfully aware that it is by no means easy for a doctor in our day to accept death the way doctor a century ago could. That latter physician had a distinct advantage: he or she could do little or nothing about death. There was no choice but to accept it. This is no longer so. The means of struggling against death are considerable and compelling. Even so, of course, every patient will just as certainly die now as was the case then. It is the newfound power to keep death at bay longer which itself poses the greatest puzzle. When should that power be used, and when should it be relinquished?

Whether a person will have a peaceful death or not can hardly depend exclusively upon the behavior of the physician; chance and the patient's own response will be hardly less crucial. But if the physician is not able to relinquish the patient to death, then the patient's struggle is likely to be that much harder. The patient may well think that, in addition to the bad luck of the fatal illness itself, there is a double jeopardy in drawing a doctor who will not let go, even when that is the obvious thing to do.

There are three obstacles that physician attitudes can place in the way of a peaceful death: a tacit belief that individual deaths are accidental, a confusion between the value of life and the value of medical technology, and a failure to distinguish between killing and allowing to die.

Death as an Accident

Modern medicine is profoundly ambivalent about death. The clinician well understands that death is, as the saying goes, a part of life. Yet matters are otherwise with scientific research medicine, where death seems to remain the permanent enemy and the eradication of all fatal diseases the ultimate goal. Clinical medicine works, when it must, to accommodate itself to death, while scientific medicine always works to overcome death. Given these two stances, not easily reconciled, it is hardly a surprise that, even for the clinician, death can appear to be a kind of accident, a contingent event that, with enough skill, can be averted.[4]

Consider the paradox here. Death is understood well enough to be a biologic necessity, a part of all organic nature. But every known cause of death can be taken to be contingent, a matter of chance. By "contingent" and "chance," I mean that it need not exist, that in principle and in medical theory there is no reason why any partic-

ular fatal disease cannot be overcome. Put another way, although death in general is supposed to be accepted, none of the causes of death need be; each can be eliminated.

This paradox often surfaces at the bedside: this particular disease, with this particular patient, need not necessarily be the cause of death—so think many clinicians who want to struggle against an impending death. It is not that they disbelieve in the reality of an inevitable death for all, but that does not mean they must believe in this death at this time for this patient; that need not be. Yet there is a trap there, luring its victim into thinking that death is not a necessity, into evading its reality, its ineluctable force. There can be a kind of self-deceit when that happens, and an inadvertent deceit of patients and families as well, holding out meaningless hope and remote possibilities. A peaceful death, which requires an acceptance of death, is not possible if death is treated as an avoidable accident.

Valuable Life, Seductive Technology

Human life is of intrinsic value, a belief that is part of the traditional ethic of medicine and of every civilized society. Death is not a denial of the value of life or of its sanctity, to use the more religious term. Yet it is easy with a medicine dominated by science and technology to see in them a way of affirming the value of life—and thus turning to them to sustain life whatever this might mean to the patient as a person. It almost seems that technology has captured the value of life, giving the impression that life can only be respected by bringing the full force of technology to bear in the fight against death, as if it is our only way of acting upon our commitment to life.

Yet an ever-present hazard here is what might be termed "technologic brinkmanship," by which is meant an attempt to use technology up to the final moment out of some last, desperate hope that the hand of death can be stayed. It is an effort to go to the very edge of technologic possibility, but often naively assuming that technology can be mastered with the precision necessary to avoid overtreatment and the medical oppression of a patient. The brinkmanship itself is the danger—one more way of refusing to accept death, one more way of pretending that death need not take place.

While there has been much comment over the years about the "technologic imperative" in medicine, its full force has still to be grasped. Technology is seductive because it is, in truth, a potent way of extending and often improving life, sometimes all there is. It is no less seductive in its innovativeness, its promise to relieve burdensome uncertainty, and its attractiveness to patients and their families, who can be drawn to it no less than physicians.[5] The most troublesome technologies are not those that are useless, but those that may bring some marginal benefit, one last chance in the face of hopeless odds. Those are the technologies that both physicians and patients find seductive, and no less so sometimes than those elderly patients who had earlier insisted they did not want to battle death.

Yet medical technology that is deployed too compulsively, too optimistically, too unthinkingly can be a terrible impediment to a peaceful death. There is clearly a profound dilemma here between a desire to reject and struggle against death and an acceptance of death. There is no easy resolution of this dilemma, nor should there be, but it is a great help simply to approach technology with a sharp eye out for its capacity to interfere with a peaceful death. To get that far is already to make the dilemma more tractable.

Killing and Allowing to Die

Physicians are trained to be worried about making mistakes, about acting wrongly or incompetently. They are no less trained to preserve life, and in particular not to act in a way that would knowingly risk the life of a patient, or put that patient at greater risk than that already occasioned by illness. Yet it is unfortunately all too easy, with this kind of training in the background, reinforced by peer pressure and a fear of litigation, to feel excessively responsible for a patient's fate and welfare.

Nowhere is this possibility of excess more pronounced than in the anxiety that the cessation of treatment of a dying person is tantamount to killing that person. If something more could be done to extend life that remains undone, then many physicians feel that they and not the underlying disease are the real cause of death, and some philosophers would agree with them.[6] The source of this anxiety is understandable: a patient's life can often be extended for a short time, even a long time in some cases, by modern medical therapy, and it is easy to believe that a failure to pursue that possibility itself becomes the cause of death.

Yet the logic of this anxiety is mistaken. If treatment is terminated or abated out of a genuine conviction based on clinical evidence that no further benefit to a patient is possible, then it is nature and not the physician that bears the ultimate responsibility for death. Death is not a medical invention, to be turned on or off at will. At some point, nothing the physician can do will stop death from occurring. For the physician to judge that death is inevitable, that the patient has moved beyond the possibility of meaningful therapy and real benefit to the patient, is to do no more than recognize the transcendent sovereignty of death. It is irrelevant, morally and clinically, that a few more days or sometimes even weeks could be added to a life if, as a result of the underlying lethal pathology, the end is inevitable and reasonably foreseeable.

The physician did not create the fatal pathology, and a failure to stand against it any longer is not to kill a patient, but to let our human nature take its necessary course. A physician should not, in short, confuse his or her role with that of nature. The power of the physician to manipulate nature a bit, to hold off death for a time, does not mean that nature has been transcended. Most particularly, it does not mean that life and death have passed out of the hands of nature into those of the physician. Not at all. A physician can stay the hand of nature for a time without thereby having taken over nature. To be sure, a physician can be said to "kill" a patient if he or she acts directly to knowingly and with intent to shorten life, but it makes no sense to equate killing a patient with giving way to the power of nature as a force that can no longer be combated. A peaceful death can be impeded, even made impossible, by a wrong belief that death has become the ultimate responsibility of the physician—a matter only of choice and decision. Not only does that tempt technologic brinkmanship, it no less sets the stage for self-blame when death does occur, as it eventually must. A peaceful death can only be possible if it is understood that the power of death in the end triumphs over human science and artifice, and that only stepping aside to allow it to happen can be faithful to the force of nature and the respect owed to patients.

The Art of Dying

Although we hear less of it these days, most cultures have given a place of importance to the way people prepare themselves for death. *Ars moriendi*, the art of dying, was a long-standing part of life in the Middle Ages, but finds its counterpart in many parts of the world to this day. It has long been understood that the human response to mortality, pain, and suffering is not biologically fixed, and that the way people respond to them will be as much a function of their character and personality, and the culture of which they are a part, as it will be a characteristic of the disease that afflicts them. Michel de Montaigne wrote in the eighteenth century words that remain true to this day: "Fortune appears sometimes purposely to wait for the last year of our lives in order to show us she can overthrow in one moment what she has taken long years to build. . . . In this last scene between ourselves and death, there is no more pretense. We must use plain words, and display such goodness or purity as we have at the bottom of the pot."[7] The living of a life that is a preparation for a good death was understood then, and might well be understood now, as a wise counsel. How a patient dies will, in any case, reflect at least in part how that patient has lived a life and what kind of character is brought to the dying.

There is, of course, a problem here for the physician, who has had no hand in fashioning the earlier life of the patient and whose role in shaping or altering the personality of a patient is of necessity limited. Does this mean that the physician is thereby rendered helpless, unable to do more than stand by and watch as the patient works out his or her response to death? Not necessarily. Particularly with the elderly patient, who is often open to talking about death, it is possible to bring the problem of dying to the surface and to broach lines of exchange between doctor and patient that can touch on *ars moriendi*.

Here the imagination and empathy of the physician will be crucial. In that elderly dying patient before one's eyes, one can and should see one's own fate some day, however much one would like to avoid thinking about it. The self-protection of a therapeutic distance, the objective, scientific detachment so often held up as a medical ideal, should now give way to a supreme effort to understand what it must be like to know that death is on its way. This means grasping the fear, the uncertainty, the self-doubt and self-interrogation, that goes with such knowledge. It means understanding the terror of losing control of one's body, one's fate, one's life. At stake is the dissolution of the self, and with that everything that has made life worth living.[8]

Few patients are likely to be open, much less garrulous, about matters so deep and so personal, and few people will have had the opportunity to learn how to talk about them. It may be necessary to coax these thoughts out of a patient, to put into words for the patient ideas and feelings that are only half-formed or confusingly jumbled together. Simply helping someone articulate thoughts, giving words to a sense of loss, to fear and terror, is itself a great contribution to a peaceful death. How a patient dies, how a patient reacts to pain and suffering, is far more likely to be determined by what is happening to the patient's thinking and feeling than to what is happening to his or her body. What counts is not just what happens to people when they die—not just "how we die"—but what they make of that event.

There are some characteristic issues that are likely to arise with elderly dying people, stances toward illness and death that they bring with them and to which the physician should be prepared to respond.

Losing Control

A peculiar and disturbing feature of modern societies, particularly the United States, is that many people believe that their self-respect and integrity depend upon having a life under their control. But dying is the ultimate loss of control, and the physician should do whatever is possible to reassure the patient that the loss is inevitable, our common fate, and no negative mark against a person. Helping a patient cope with the sense of self-loss is critical to a peaceful death. Sometimes all that can be done is the expression of understanding and fellow-feeling, but that may be of great value.

Obsession with Pain and Suffering

People differ enormously in their capacity to bear pain and suffering, which in many cases will not bear a clear or direct relationship to their physical condition. They no less differ in their capacity to accept and understand their situation, which can make a great difference in their reaction to suffering. An obsession to overcome the suffering can itself exacerbate the strain. Nothing short of the most sensitive pain management and an awareness that suffering is not directly correlated with pain will do in these circumstances.[9] The goal, not easy to achieve, is that of reducing the obsessions and helping the patient to acquiesce to the suffering when it cannot be fully relieved. An imperfectly peaceful death is better than one that is not at all peaceful.

A Flexible Self

As the ultimate threat to the self, death and the process of dying invite a premature mourning for the self that will be lost and for the self that is no longer what it once was. Lurking in the wings here sometimes is a belief on the part of the elderly dying that there once existed in the past a kind of optimal or ideal self, which they now see falling away from them. It can be "destructive" to see all change and decline as loss. A better attitude, which the physician can help foster, is that all stages of life have their own demands and challenges, that aging and death are not some kind of fall from grace but instead a new demand on the self that can rise to the occasion. There is no ideal self or ideal stage of life. There is just life, and if the physician can help the patient see that, then a great contribution will have been made to the last days of a person.

Accepting Dependency

If self-control and self-determination are high on the list of Western cultural values, a desire not to be dependent or a burden on others is not far behind. Yet there is no inherent evil in being dependent upon others, or even in being an involuntary burden on them. The long decline that is now so often a part of the death of the elderly will no less often impose a period of dependency. Some will be lucky and not require the help of others. Many, however, will not be so fortunate. There are many kinds of reassurance the physician can offer in those circumstances: that the burden on others is often not as great or as damaging to others as they may think (if that can truthfully be said); that life with other human beings is a life of mutual interdependence; and that dependence does not necessarily rob a person of the respect of others or self-respect. It will be the response of the patient to dependency that will often matter far more than the actual fact of dependency. Physicians should help their patients to see this.

Death and Dignity

It is surely the case that others can treat us with indignity as if we count for little and are fit only for disposal. But real dignity is best understood as an interior virtue, the stance we take up within ourselves to confront what life—and death—throw in our path.[10] People cannot be deprived of that interior dignity, but whether they have it will have much more to do with the way they have lived and shaped their lives than with the way they have been treated by others. A physician can do many things to reduce the external indignities that medical treatments and medical institutions can unwittingly and haphazardly impose on patients, and it is important that they do so. They cannot as easily help the patient find the necessary inner dignity to cope with dying and the prospect of death. But even here there is a place for the sensitive, thoughtful physician who can help the patient to distinguish between external and internal dignity, cultivating the latter and not confusing the former with self-worth.

Pursuing a Peaceful Death

The idea of a peaceful death can now be filled out in greater detail. I have tried to suggest that it is not something any physician can guarantee to a patient. Chance and luck, not to mention the character of the patient, can always intervene and subvert the best intentions. But it also seems true that there is room to work with a patient—and for a patient to work with himself or herself—to enhance the possibility of a peaceful death. A peaceful death is rarely precluded altogether just as it is rarely guaranteed. There is thus considerable room for enhancing its possibility.

A first approach to the notion of a peaceful death encompasses an acceptance of death, the absence of excessive pain and suffering, and the presence of other people. That notion needs to be filled out and enriched. It is a starting point only. A full picture would include a sense of the meaning of death for a patient (a critical part of the acceptance of death); respectful and sensitive treatment by family and health care workers; a belief on the part of the dying that their deaths matter to others, a belief that their deaths signify a loss to the human community; a state of conscious awareness as close to the actual time of death as possible; a relatively quick death; and a sense of reassurance on the part of the dying person that he or she has not been an undue burden on others. (And sometimes they may be, so the truth may need to be hedged.)

By expanding the list of ingredients of a peaceful death, do I not thereby make it all the harder of achievement? Possibly so, but I would underline my earlier point that a peaceful death is an ideal, a goal toward which care should strive but may only rarely achieve with any degree of perfection. The expanded list touches, moreover, on most of those aspects of dying beyond pain and suffering that are most fearful for patients—an attenuated, drawn-out dying, loss of control, being a burden to others, despair and a feeling of meaninglessness, and the indifference of others to one's death. No physician can make others care that a person is dying, and no one may care. No physician can do much to relieve the burdens that a long illness and a slow dying may impose upon family members and friends. The point is to try to do what one can and to be aware that a peaceful death is multidimensional, with some of the dimensions more open to intervention and change than others. The point is to work as fully as possible with each of the dimensions, hoping at least for a partial success and maybe more than that.

The Presumption to Treat

A critical aspect of the goal of a peaceful death is that of the traditional presumption to treat a critically ill patient. When should that presumption be suspended, to be replaced by a presumption not to treat? By "treat," I mean the application of life-extending, life-preserving therapies, not the provision of comfort and palliation. The latter are always required, but not the former.[11] The presumption to treat should be suspended: (1) when there is a likely, although not necessarily certain, downward course of an illness, making death a strong probability (multiorgan failure in an elderly patient is an obvious example); (2) when the available treatments for a potentially fatal condition entail a significant likelihood of extended pain or suffering without compensatory benefits; (3) when successful treatment is more likely to bring extended unconsciousness or advanced dementia than cure or significant amelioration; and (4) when, whatever the medical condition, the available treatments increase the probability of a bad death, even if they also promise to extend life.

Obviously there can be no tidy algorithm for making these judgments. They all turn on probabilities that are often difficult to calculate, depend to a considerable degree upon clinical experience, and run the risk of error. Yet the fitting goal of a peaceful death justifies the risk. One way to think about the decision here is that of the need for and value of creating a strong struggle between two goals. One of them is the traditional medical goal of saving and extending life, certainly a dominant, usually overriding goal in modern medical culture. The other goal, no less traditional but easily pushed aside, is that of a peaceful death.

These two goals should, fittingly, be in tension with each other with critically ill, potentially dying patients. To allow a patient to die who could have genuinely benefited from treatment is a serious medical failure. But it is no less a medical failure when a person dies an avoidable bad death, the victim of insensitivity, medical timidity, technologic brinkmanship, or, that last refuge of evasion, fear of legal liability (almost always a non-issue, despite pervasive anxiety on the subject in treatment termination decisions with dying patients).[12] If there is to be fear, then there should be a fear of not preserving life pitted against the fear of increasing the possibility of a poor death. If there is to be optimism, then there should be the optimism that a peaceful death might be achieved pitted against the optimism that another round of disease–modifying treatment might benefit a patient.

Stages of Treatment Termination

A subtle error that can sometimes insinuate itself into medical decisions is to draw too sharp a line between getting sick and dying. Obviously not all sickness leads to death, and that is why it is struggled against. Yet there is another point, no less obvious but harder to face: every death will occur because of some fatal pathologic process, some final illness. In that sense, just as death will always sooner or later finally win, so will illness, each occasion of which can be avoided except the last one. Not only does this perception strengthen the case for the pursuit of a peaceful death, which will ordinarily in the elderly come with some illness, but it also brings to the foreground the value of taking a stance toward potentially fatal illness no less than a stance toward death. Here it is possible to work with patients to think about different stances toward illness and termination of treatment decisions. I will express these different stances in the language of stages that can be articulated and considered, and which range over a continuum:

Stage One: A patient can decide to refuse altogether to respond to health threats, even those potentially fatal, backing up this refusal by making no effort whatever to seek therapeutic medical treatment, accepting palliative care only.

Stage Two: A patient may be open to diagnosis or identification of a potentially lethal condition but refuse to undertake any curative efforts at all, embracing only palliation.

Stage Three: A patient can refuse to accept any medical treatment, for curative or ameliorative purposes, that does not promise a high probability of success and a minimum of unpleasant side effects in extending life.

Stage Four: A patient may be willing to accept any medical treatment that offers some probability, even if low, of success in preserving life.

Stage Five: A patient may be eager to pursue any medical treatment, established or experimental, that offers even a remote possibility of saving life.

One reason why it is worth considering these stages and trying to determine where a patient might psychologically be in relationship to them bears on an often-neglected aspect of advance directives. If the focus of an advance directive (or even informal discussions with patients) is on final decisions, when death is staring the patient in the face, then it becomes all too easy to avoid considering the full course of illness that leads to the threat or likelihood of death. Quite apart from what a patient says he or she wants done when death is imminent, what is the patient's attitude toward life-threatening illness in general? Here elderly patients may differ significantly from younger patients, depending in great part whether they have come to terms with the inevitability of death and are prepared to accept the illness and decline most likely to precede it.

Two patients can have exactly the same desires about what is to be done when they are indubitably dying—but one of them may be eager to avoid therapy when a critical illness occurs while the other may want maximum technologic brinkmanship in the face of illness. It is important, if possible, to unearth these different attitudes toward illness and not to let them get slighted in discussions of what is to be done at the last minute, when death is clearly on the way. It is, in short, just as important to determine how patients think about illness (and they may need help here if they have never given the subject much thought at all) as how they think about death and dying. They are inextricably tied together.

The Culture of Dying

All of us live our lives embedded in a culture that supplies us with our language, most of our values, and the social and political institutions within which we live out our lives. Our culture is enormously ambivalent about death, and the medicine that is part of that culture (and a shaper of it) is no less ambivalent. The clinical face of medicine lives day to day with death and works to remove its sting, acquiescing in its force when necessary. The scientific face of medicine, by contrast, continues to carry out unrelenting warfare against all the known causes of death, none of which it finds acceptable. These two faces are in endless conflict with each other, even if the conflict is rarely acknowledged in an open way. Scientific medicine tutors the physician to see death as a correctable accident, while clinical medicine counsels its inevitability and necessity.

The kind of a culture likely to enhance the possibility of a peaceful death requires a number of elements. It must be a culture that accepts the place of death in life and helps people find some meaning in death. It must be a culture that does not allow itself to become bemused with medical possibility and medical progress, as if a cure for death (or lethal cancer or heart disease) will be found just over the next hill. It must be a culture that no longer hides death, as if it is some kind of human scandal in a modern age. It must be a culture that supports physicians in their desire to foster peaceful death, not scaring them with lawsuits or treating them as failures when their patients die. It must be a culture that nurtures in its people the need to think about the kind of people they want to be and the kind of character they want to have when death comes near to them. It must be, in the end, a culture that understands death as part of the human condition, where patients and doctors work together, each doing what they can and must to make death as tolerable as possible. That goal should be understood as an achievement, not necessarily easy but possible and desirable.

Of course American culture, and increasingly other cultures as well, do not well fit those specifications. Human beings do not want to die. They did not in the past and they do not now. Yet medical progress, ambivalence about accepting the inevitability of death even when it is inevitable, and the love of last-chance technologic interventions throw great obstacles in the way of a peaceful death.

Can those obstacles be overcome? Perhaps not directly, and often not within a contemporary medical context at all. People come to their final days with the experience and reflection of a lifetime behind them, and by definition that is the situation of the elderly. But it is imperative that there be such reflection, and that is a task beyond the reach of medicine, even though it can help. Only if death is a more general topic for public education, for religious ministries, and for ordinary day-to-day discourse can progress be made. Only then will people come to their death ready and prepared. That is the larger cultural task. Getting there will be slow work, hard work, an uphill struggle as often as not. The good of a peaceful death makes it a necessary struggle, and even now movement can be seen. That is a start.

References

1. Arrowsmith W. The criticism of Greek tragedy. *Tulane Drama Rev*. 1959;3:55.
2. Ariès P. *The Hour of Our Death* (Weaver H, trans). New York: Knopf; 1981.
3. Ramsey P. The indignity of "death with dignity." *Hastings Cent Rep*. 1974;2(2):50–52.
4. Callahan D. Death and the research imperative. *N Engl J Med*. 2000;342:654–656.
5. Cassell E. The sorcerer's broom: medicine's rampant technology. *Hastings Cent Rep*. 1993;23(6):32–39.
6. Brock D. Taking human life. *Ethics*. 1985;95:851–865.
7. Montaigne M. That no man should be called happy until after his death. In: Cohen J, ed. *The Essays of Montaigne*. New York: Penguin; 1958:34–35.
8. Cassell E. *The Nature of Suffering and the Goals of Medicine*. New York: Oxford University Press; 1991.
9. Institute of Medicine. *Approaching Death: Improving Care at the End of Life*. Washington, DC: National Academy Press; 1997.
10. Kass L. Death with dignity and the sanctity of life. In: Kogan B, ed. *A Time to Be Born and a Time to Die*. New York: De Gruyter; 1991:133.
11. Wolf S. *Guidelines on the Termination of Treatment*. Briarcliff Manor, NY: The Hastings Center; 1987.
12. Meisel A. *The Right to Die*. New York: Wiley; 1989.

Part V
Medical Care

Section A
Cancer in the Elderly

Cancer in the Elderly: An Overview

Harvey Jay Cohen

Cancer is an important problem in the geriatric population because it occurs with increasing incidence throughout the middle and older years. In aggregate, it is the second leading cause of mortality in people age 55 and older. Moreover, 60% of all cancers occur in persons over 65.[1,2] It also produces a reservoir of older people living with the disease and its resultant morbidity. Of course, cancer is not one disease but many. Therefore, this section of the volume is organized to address some general issues, such as the biology of disease and approaches to prevention and screening (Chapters 31 and 32), and then to address those cancers responsible for the major portion of this mortality and morbidity (Chapters 33–38). In addition, cancers of the skin are addressed in Chapter 58.

In this overview, I want to add a general perspective on the approach to the older cancer patient. We still have much to learn about this interaction, as it has only recently become a subject of scientific investigation. An appropriate framework for the discussion is to consider the Biopsychosocial Model as applied to the elderly cancer patient, as we have previously described in the "Comprehensive Geriatric Model."[3] The concept is that in the setting of decreased hemostatic reserve of the elderly patient, the potential interactions of an emerging or established cancer well be impacted upon by changes in each part of the patient's hierarchy, that is, biologic, psychologic, and social, at the clinical interface. All must be considered if effective care for the older cancer patient is to be accomplished. Ways in which the model of comprehensive geriatric assessment can be applied to the older cancer patient are now being proposed.[4,5]

At the biologic level, as described in Chapter 31, issues relating to the reasons why cancer incidence increases with age are important to understand with regard to developing potential preventative approaches. This is a rapidly evolving area with new considerations arising regularly. Studies of cancer course in older people have shown variation, with some more and others less aggres-

sive, a situation paralleled in animal models. Finally, the knowledge of physiologic changes with age, well detailed throughout this volume, is applicable to the treatment of the cancer patient at many levels; for example, cardiopulmonary changes for surgery and cardiopulmonary toxic drugs, skin changes for wound healing, central nervous system (CNS) changes for patient communications and CNS toxic drugs, special senses for dealing with nutrition and radiation therapy, hematopoietic changes for chemotherapy and radiation therapy, immune system changes for infection, and hepatic and kidney changes for chemotherapeutic agent metabolism.[6] Recent work on the syndrome of frailty is of great relevance to the management of the older cancer patient. The vulnerability created by the combination of physiologic decline, comorbidities, and systems dysregulation must be addressed if appropriate management strategies are to be utilized.[7,8] Assessment of functional status and quality of life is an issue common to geriatricians and oncologists and may be useful in treatment planning, as well as determination of prognosis and response.[9,10]

Psychosocial issues can be as critical to the management of the older cancer patient as any of the biologic features. Thus, resistance to participation in screening programs and to responding to early warning signs and symptoms of cancer must be recognized and handled. Older people's fears about the dying process, misconceptions about the disease and about health care facilities, and concern of being a burden to family and friends can present problems. Communication issues, such as those presented by cognitive impairment, concerns about how much to tell, informed consent, and the involvement of caregivers are particularly prevalent in dealing with the older cancer patient. Assessing overall quality of life may be difficult. Although there are decrements in social support systems that can have adverse affects, older people, even with cancer, generally rate their quality of life better than do caregivers and health professionals, who thus do not always make good proxies. Moreover, specific side effects, such as nausea, vomiting, and pain, may be less in older cancer patients, and they and their caregivers seem to adapt and cope better with the disease than do younger patients.[11] Nevertheless, the caregiver for the older cancer patient faces a number of challenges that must be addressed.[12]

With respect to cancer management, because of the heterogeneity of the older population, care must be individualized and is complex.[13,14] Unfortunately, we do not have good biomarkers of treatment vulnerability, so we must use the aggregate of physiologic factors (noted above) and presence of comorbidities and functional disability to aid in decision making.[15,16] Thus, in decisions about cancer surgery, the physiologically intact elderly person without comorbidities appears to tolerate even extensive surgery well. Radiation therapy can be delivered effectively, but special attention must be paid to nutrition and hydration. Age-related chemotherapy responses and toxicities have only been critically examined over the past 15 years. Supportive and palliative care are discussed in Chapters 24 through 30 and are of particular relevance to the older cancer patient. Disease-specific therapy is addressed in the individual chapters, but patterns have arisen.

In treatment trials (information from which may not be applicable to all older cancer patients because they generally select the most physiologically fit),[17] single-agent and low-intensity therapy has generally been tolerated well and with equivalent outcomes in the elderly. Even here, particular attention must be paid to physiologic changes, which can impact upon toxicities (e.g., renal function for methotrexate use). As therapy complexity and intensity is increased, there is a progressive relative increase in toxicity in the elderly, in some cases with continued equivalent responses to the younger patient, but ultimately, in diseases such as acute leukemia and Hodgkin's disease, poorer outcomes as well. Newer approaches to these problems are being evaluated, including tailoring regimens with better effect, toxicity ratios, seeking new agents with better therapeutic profiles, and enhancing supportive care so that higher-intensity therapy can be delivered (e.g., bone marrow transplantation). These concerns should all be active areas for clinical research in the near future.

The overlapping concerns of oncology and geriatrics have led to a call for closer collaboration between the disciplines in patient care, research, and education.[18,19] We appear to be seeing the emergence of a combined discipline of gero-oncology.

References

1. Jemal A, Thomas A, Murray T, et al. Cancer statistics, 2002. *CA Cancer J Clin.* 2002;52:23–47.
2. Edwards BK, Howe HL, Ries LAG, et al. Annual report to the nation on the status of cancer, 1973–1999, featuring implications of age and aging on U.S. cancer burden. *Cancer.* 2002;94:2766–2792.
3. Cohen HJ. Geriatric principles of treatment applied to medical oncology. *Semin Oncol.* 1995;22(1):Suppl 1.
4. Bernabei R, Venturiero V, Tarsitani P, Gambassi G. The comprehensive geriatric assessment: when, where, how. *Oncology/Hematology* 2000;33:45–56.
5. Ingram SS, Seo PH, Martell RE, et al. Comprehensive assessment of the elderly cancer patient: the feasibility of self-report methodology. *J Clin Oncol.* 2002;20:770–775.
6. Cohen HJ. Biology of aging as related to cancer. *Cancer (Suppl)* 1994;74(7):2092–2100.
7. Cohen HJ. Editorial: In search of the underlying mechanisms of frailty. *J Gerontol Med Sci.* 2000;55A(12):M706–M708.
8. Balducci L, Stanta G. Cancer in the frail patient: a coming epidemic. *Hematol/Oncol Clin North Am.* 2000;14:235–250.
9. Cohen HJ. Cancer and functional status of the elderly. *Cancer.* 1997;80(10):1883–1886.
10. Extermann M, Overcash J, Lyman GH, Parr J, Balducci L. Comorbidity and functional status are independent in older cancer patients. *J Clin Oncol.* 1998;16(4):1582–1587.
11. Mor V, Allen S, Malin M. The psychosocial impact of cancer on older versus younger patients and their families. *Cancer (Suppl).* 1994;74(7):2118–2127.
12. Weitzner MA, Haley WE, Chen H. The family caregiver of the older cancer patient. Extermann M, Aapro M. Assessment of the older cancer patient. *Hematol Oncol Clin North Am.* 2000;14:269–282.
13. Cohen HJ, ed. Cancer and the older patient. *Semin Oncol* 1995;22(1):Suppl 1.
14. McKenna RJ. Clinical aspects of cancer in the elderly. *Cancer (Suppl).* 1994;74(7):2107–2117.
15. Extermann M, Aapro M. Assessment of the older cancer patient. *Hematol Oncol Clin North Am.* 2000;14:63–78.
16. Serraino D, Fratino L, Zagonel V for the GIOGer Study Group. Prevalence of functional disability among elderly patients with cancer. *Oncology/Hematology.* 2001;39:269–273.
17. Muss HB, Cohen HJ, Lichtman SM. Clinical research in the older cancer patient. *Hematol Oncol Clin North Am.* 2000; 14:283–472.
18. Cohen HJ. The oncology geriatric education retreat: commentary and conclusions. *Cancer* (Special Section: Aging and Cancer) 2000;80(7)1354–1356.
19. Lichtman SM. Integration of geriatrics in oncology training—the relationship between the academic center and the community. *Oncology/Hematology.* 2000;33:57–59.

31
The Science of Neoplasia and Its Relationship to Aging

Robert E. Martell and Harvey Jay Cohen

Demographics of Cancer in the Elderly

Cancer poses a significant health issue for the elderly. The incidence and mortality from cancer are progressively greater in older age groups. Sixty percent of all cancers exist in the 12% of the population over age 65. Even within the 65 to 84 age group, the incidence of cancer has increased steadily over the past 20 years. Furthermore, we are presently in the midst of a dramatic increase in the size of the older cohorts in our society due to increased longevity and the aging "baby boom" generation in the United States. Cancer is the second leading cause of death and is one of the most feared diseases in this age group. Indeed, the risk of dying from cancer increases exponentially with age.

The expanding incidence of cancer in the elderly is not uniform for all cancers. The incidence of lung, colon, breast, prostate, and B-cell hematologic malignancies, such as chronic lymphocytic leukemia and multiple myeloma, all increase with age. However, the incidence of many childhood cancers, as well as Hodgkin's disease, testicular cancer, and cervical cancer, do not show such a persistent increase with age and may even decrease in incidence in the elderly.

Biology of Cancer and Its Relationship to Aging

Given the striking increase in the incidence of cancer with age, it is prudent to consider relationships between aging biology and cancer biology.[1-3] Much of our understanding of cancer biology comes from pragmatic studies of physical and molecular forces that govern cell transformation and malignant progression without necessarily linking these findings to the reality of the age-related demographics of cancer. However, demographics reflect biology. In fact, much of cancer biology can be directly linked to characteristics of cellular aging. This chapter provides a systematic review of the major areas of study in cancer biology and, importantly, provides a scientific basis for a link with aging biology where relevant.

Factors That Impart Cancer-Causing Cellular Changes

Environmental and cellular factors have been identified as etiologic factors for cancer development. Many factors result in disruption of genetic integrity. The consequence of this disruption is altered expression of gene products critical for cell growth, which can lead to neoplasia. A distorted local cellular environment can also facilitate tumorigenesis (Fig. 31.1).

Disruption of Genetic Integrity

Disruption of genetic integrity is the cornerstone of cancer development.[4] Multiple sequential genetic changes are likely to be required for development of a tumor. Because acquisition of these changes is in part a time-dependent process, the elderly have had more time to acquire detrimental changes. Examples of disrupted genetic integrity include point mutations, frame shifts, chromosomal translocations, or deletions. Additionally, the body's ability to maintain genetic integrity is impaired at older ages. DNA repair is reduced in the elderly, whereas telomere shortening, formation of DNA adducts, DNA hypomethylation, and chromosomal breakage and translocation are more common in this age group. The most clearly studied example of the sequential accumulation of genetic change associated with development of cancer is the progression of colon cancer. A series of genetic changes have been defined that occur during the transformation of normal tissue to advanced colorectal carcinoma. In a variety of ways, this genetic change

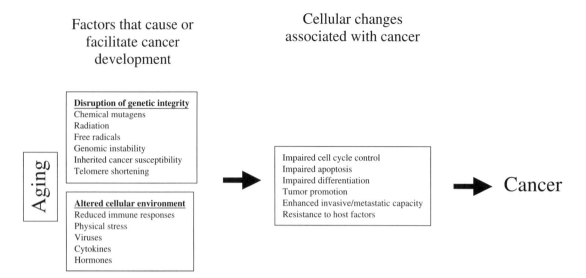

FIGURE 31.1. The etiology of cancer.

creates selective growth advantages for the affected cells. These advantages are often accomplished by a change that results in altered function of a protein end product, such as a factor that drives cell proliferation or impairs a cell's ability to undergo apoptosis.

Many genotoxic agents have been studied, and these can account for a subset of cancers, yet a large percentage of tumors harbor genetic alterations for which no clear link to a genotoxic agent can be made. Specific genotoxic modalities include chemical mutagens, radiation, and free radicals. In many cancers, the situation is compounded by disrupted DNA repair mechanisms, which accelerate accumulation of tumor-facilitating mutations. DNA mutations can also be acquired by inheritance of a mutant allele, the phenotype for which may be revealed at a later point by a subsequent mutation in the other allele.

Chemical Mutagens

The role of chemical mutagens in cancer[5–7] had been characterized initially by observing cancer rates in certain occupations and has been subsequently confirmed by experimental cell and animal studies. Agents that can cause genetic damage tend to have high chemical reactivity and form covalent adducts with DNA. Selectivity of the agents for tissue or cell type, nucleotide type, and DNA synthesis exists. The genetic damage involves base mispairings or small deletions, which result in missense or nonsense mutations. Other types of damage cause chromosomal breaks or large deletions. Examples of genotoxic substances include N-nitrosal compounds, aliphatic epoxides, aflatoxins, mustards, polycyclic aromatic hydrocarbons, combustion products of fossil fuel or vegetable matter, aryl aromatic amines, aminoazodyes, and hetero-

cyclic aromatic amines. Genetic polymorphisms of enzymatic pathways for carcinogen metabolism and activation are thought to play a significant role in cancer susceptibility.

Nongenotoxic carcinogens cause cancer in laboratory animals, but neither they nor their metabolites cause DNA damage. The mechanisms of carcinogenesis of these compounds are speculative but may involve regenerative hyperplasia in response to tissue damage, hormonal effects, induction of oxygen radicals, depurination, or deamination of 5-methylcytosine.

Radiation

Ionizing radiation and ultraviolet radiation have the capacity to invoke genetic damage. Many examples exist of association of cancer with ionizing radiation exposure. Potential sources of this type of radiation include natural radiation (cosmic rays or radioactivity from the earth), medical radiology, and nuclear power. Ionizing radiation releases large amounts of energy as it strikes a cell, sufficient to break chemical bonds in DNA. Solar ultraviolet (UV) radiation is highly associated with skin cancer, including malignant melanoma. UV radiation induces pyrimidine dimers, which are a unique form of DNA damage compared to other carcinogens. Efficient DNA repair is a critical factor in avoiding untoward effects from this damage. Additionally, UV radiation appears to impair local immune responses, which may result in greater permissiveness for tumor development.

Free Radicals

Reactive oxygen species and reactive nitrogen species are formed in conjunction with certain types of cell stress, including cell damage. Free radicals form initial chemical products with DNA itself or with other products to produce DNA-damaging agents, for example, oxidative activation of a procarcinogen. Free radicals are formed as a consequence of a variety of processes, such as radiation damage, exposure to cigarette smoke, exposure to asbestos, and even exposure to certain chemotherapy agents. They appear to play a role in the aging process per se as well.

Genomic Instability

Genomic instability implies increased propensity for developing DNA sequence changes (deletions, insertions, and point mutations) or chromosomal aberrations (gaps, breaks, translocations, and other chromosomal rearrangements).[8] At the level of the DNA sequence, important factors include the fidelity of DNA replication, detection of DNA damage, DNA damage repair, and mechanisms to discard cells that are badly damaged (e.g., cell cycle checkpoints and apoptosis). Genetic instability can be inherited or acquired. Cancer is highly associated with the impaired DNA repair seen with certain inherited genetic polymorphisms.

Acquired deficits in DNA repair appear to be the hallmark of progression of some types of cancer, including colon cancer. The gene for the p53 transcription factor is one of the most frequently mutated genes in cancers. The loss of functional p53 impairs the ability of the cell to recognize and repair DNA damage, thus enhancing the rate of selection of growth-facilitating mutations.

Inherited Cancer Susceptibility

In addition to the inherited cancer predispositions described involving DNA repair processes, several other familial cancer syndromes exist.[9,10] The breast and breast–ovarian cancer syndromes, involving inheritance of a mutant allele of the BRCA1 or BRCA2 tumor suppressor gene, are important examples. Other examples of inherited cancer susceptibility syndromes include adenomatous polyposis coli, retinoblastoma, Wilms' tumor, Li–Fraumeni syndrome, MEN 1 and 2, neurofibromatosis, and Beckwith–Wiedemann syndrome; these generally occur in younger individuals.

Telomere Shortening

The study of telomeres has revealed exciting links between aging biology and cancer.[11–18] Telomeres are specialized regions of reiterative DNA sequence found at chromosomal ends that play a role in chromosomal integrity. Due to the inability of DNA synthesis machinery to replicate DNA completely to the end, telomeres shorten incrementally during each cell division, presumably reducing the protective effect of telomeres. Indeed,

it has been shown that older individuals have shorter telomeres than younger individuals. Thus, the deterioration of these chromosomal ends in the elderly may make this group more susceptible to genetic damage.

It has been proposed that cells in the body have evolved a form of defense mechanism against this potential for genetic instability produced by telomere shortening. When grown in tissue culture, normal somatic human cells are able to replicate only a finite number of times before undergoing a cell cycle arrest. It appears that shortening of telomeres to a critical point induces some sort of signal, such as a DNA damage signal, causing cellular growth arrest. This growth arrest, or "replicative senescence," can be thought of as a tumor suppressive mechanism, whereby cells that have been driven to proliferate excessively will stop growing. Interestingly, normal germline cells express an RNA protein enzyme called telomerase, which adds telomeric repeats back on to chromosomal ends, giving these cells the capacity to replicated beyond a point that might normally be associated with replicative senescence. Unfortunately, cancer cells have evolved to express this same enzyme, giving them the ability to proliferate beyond a point at which they would normally senesce.

Links between telomere shortening and replicative senescence have been described in detail. One model describes replicative senescence as mortality phase 1, or M1. Early events in tumorigenesis, such as disruption of genes such as p53 or Rb, allow cells to have extended proliferative capacity. However, the population eventually again arrests in an M2 state, also called "crisis." In this state, chromosomal stability is substantially reduced, enhancing recombination events and genetic mutations. Ultimately, it is the acquisition of telomerase expression that allows cells to continue to proliferate and progress to an advanced malignant phase.

Alteration of Local Cellular Environment

In addition to agents that directly involve the genetic integrity of cells, there are several nongenotoxic modalities that affect cancer development and progression. These agents ultimately affect cell-signaling pathways. These agents range from physical stress to hormonal receptor agonists to viruses that actually enter and function within the cell.

Reduced Immune Response

Deficits in immunologic function have been observed in the aging population,[19–21] including deterioration of the ability of lymphocytes to proliferate in response to stimuli and a shift in T-cell and natural killer cell populations. Interestingly, the expression of cell-surface antigens by cells often mediates tumor cell growth. Human leukocyte antigen (HLA) molecules play a critical role in presentation of tumor antigens to cytotoxic T lymphocytes. The ability of the immune system to recognize these abnormal cells and deal with them appropriately is important in maintaining a low incidence of cancer and fighting existing tumors. The loss or downregulation of HLA class I molecules correlates with an invasive tumor phenotype. There is evidence that certain HLA determinants correlate with increased incidence of cancer. It is possible that these disease-associated alleles present antigens to T lymphocytes in a fundamentally different manner, resulting in an altered immune response. Finally, there are several clinical and experimental examples of an association between reduced systemic immune response and cancer. The variety of immune function changes that occur with age are covered in great depth in Chapter 53, Immunology of Aging.

Physical Stress

Tissue irritation and chronic inflammation are factors that can facilitate tumor promotion. For example, although the mechanism of asbestos carcinogenesis is not completely understood, it appears that cellular reactions to these nondegradable fibers activate tumor-promoting cell-signaling pathways. Additionally, inflammatory cell responses may produce carcinogenic by-products, such as oxygen radicals.[22–24]

Viruses

Viruses represent important agents in development of certain tumors and are thought to be responsible for one in seven cancers worldwide.[25] Studies of cancer-related viral mechanisms have provided vast insight to the mechanistic etiology of cancer. Tumor viruses function in a variety of ways to provide oncogenic stimuli for the cells they infect and for the surrounding tissue.

Retroviruses, including HTLV-I, HTLV-II, and HIV, all exhibit oncogenicity. Reverse-transcribed DNA from retroviruses is actually incorporated into the cellular genome. The oncogenic influence from these agents results from the virus providing cellular growth-related genes (virally transduced oncogenes) or by driving transcription of an existing cellular gene (proto-oncogene). Although the basic principle of these oncogenes is utilization of cellular or cell-derived genes to induce cell growth, they tend to have high mutation rates when present within the viral genome. This high mutation rate may contribute to evolution of further selective growth advantage.

DNA viruses, such as hepatitis B and C viruses, human papilloma virus (HPV), human herpesvirus 8 (HHV-8), and Epstein–Barr virus (EBV), are tumorigenic. These viruses may or may not become integrated into the host's genome. They can induce immunomediated injury and subsequent cellular proliferation that serves as an onco-genic force. Evidence suggests that these viruses can provide growth stimulatory signals, not only by activating genes adjacent to the viruses site of incorporation, but also by producing products that activate distant cellular genes.

Cytokines

Cytokines are soluble mediators of cell–cell communication and include interferons, interleukins, and colony-stimulating factors (CSF). Following interaction with their receptors, these factors initiate signaling cascades that activate or suppress transcription of various genes important for cell growth and survival.

Hormones

Hormone receptor/effector pathways appear to be important for growth of a variety of cancers.[26,27] Tumor cells may produce excess growth factors, such as platelet-derived growth factor (PDGF), transforming growth factor (TGF), fibroblast growth factor (FGF), hepatocyte growth factor-scatter factor (HGF-SF), or epidermal growth factor (EGF). Steroid hormone receptors are overexpressed in several cancers, such as breast, prostate, and endometrial cancer. Long-term estrogen replacement therapy is associated to some degree with increased incidence of breast cancer and, if unopposed by progesterone, with endometrial cancer. Steroid hormones act by binding their receptors and activating gene transcription in the nucleus. This process results in the expression of genes important in cell proliferation.

General Associations of Advanced Age with Cancer

As already described here, advanced age is highly associated with the development of cancer as well as the mortality from cancer. Because cancer is a multistep process, it has been proposed that time is required for accumulation of the requisite cellular and genetic changes to induce cancer, resulting in a frequent appearance later in life. Interestingly, the only known life span-prolonging intervention in animal models, dietary restriction, also reduces the incidence of cancer. Age is associated with a variety of cellular changes that could predispose to carcinogenisis, such as increased susceptibility to genetic change, telomere shortening, and impaired immune function.[28] These relationships are discussed in this chapter.

Cancer Cell Biology

The preceding section describes factors that have the ability to induce cancer-related change in cells. This section describes the nature of those changes. One of the

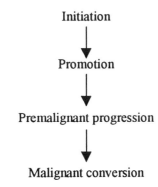

Initiation

↓

Promotion

↓

Premalignant progression

↓

Malignant conversion

FIGURE 31.2. Steps in carcinogenesis.

things that makes cancer so difficult to understand and treat is that there is no single unifying mechanism or genetic endpoint that explains malignancy. Many different types of cellular abnormalities can induce one type of cancer. Each individual tumor is relatively unique in its composite of genetic and cellular abnormalities. Indeed, a common characteristic of cancer is genetic instability, which creates an environment in which genetic change and evolution of a cell population occur in a somewhat random manner. These genetic and cellular changes exert their influences on cell functioning in several general and sometimes overlapping ways.[3]

At a very basic level, cancer-facilitating events impair a cell's ability to sense or respond to signals from the environment or signals from within itself. For example, a quiescent cell given altered environmental cues will proliferate and may induce vascular proliferation to support its proliferation. A damaged cell that should normally undergo apoptosis and die will continue to live. A cell that should remain compartmentalized will invade surrounding tissue. A cell that should develop a mature phenotype will remain poorly differentiated. The term checkpoint refers to specific phases in the cell cycle at which the cell in some way assesses the appropriateness of further progression in the cell cycle. If inappropriate signals or disruption of some aspect of cellular integrity is detected, the cell exits the cell cycle or undergoes apoptosis. Cancer cells often lose the ability to sense or heed checkpoint controls.

The events required for carcinogenesis can be thought of as a stepwise progression in which a normal cell undergoes transformation to a malignancy (Fig. 31.2). The first step, *initiation*, involves a genetic event, usually altering the activity of a growth-related signaling pathway. (Specific pathways are discussed in detail later in the chapter.) The second step is *promotion*, which is a nongenotoxic influence that provides a selective growth advantage to the initiated cell. Mechanistically, tumor promoters exert effects such as altering activity of cell-surface receptors,

cytosolic enzymes, and nuclear transcription factors. As a result, tumor promoters may stimulate cell proliferation or inhibit apoptotic cell death. The next step is *premalignant progression*, which involves acquisition of further genetic or chromosomal alterations. This progression is facilitated by genomic instability and is somewhat dependent on selection of cell clones that have acquired further selective growth advantage. Mutation of the p53 tumor suppressor gene is an example that may fall into this phase of carcinogenesis. The final step, *malignant conversion*, involves cell changes that facilitate migration and invasion.

Several general classes of cancer-related genes have been described. An "oncogene" refers to a gene whose activation is associated with development of cancer. An apposition is a "tumor suppressor gene," whose inactivation is associated with development of cancer. The following subsections describe different types of cellular changes associated with cancer.

Impairment of Cell Cycle Control

Cell cycle control has been one of the central icons in the study of cancer.[29-35] Changes in the cell cycle are also associated with cellular senescence, one of the important processes involved in the biology of aging. Because the mechanisms involved in cell cycle control are integral to both cancer cell growth and cellular senescence, detailed discussion of this topic is essential in this chapter.

The term cell cycle refers to a cyclic series of events through which a cell goes to replicate itself (Fig. 31.3). To proceed through the cell cycle, a normal diploid cell, existing in the "G_1" phase of the cycle, enters the "S" phase following the appropriate signals. In S phase, the cell replicates its entire genome and then enters the second gap phase, G_2. Next, the cell enters the mitosis or "M" phase, where it physically divides into two equal daughter cells. Each daughter cell is then considered to be back in the G_1 phase of the cell cycle. Cells can maintain a resting, or quiescent, state by exiting the cell cycle into a "G_0" state. There are also several checkpoints

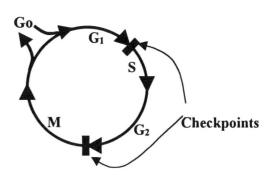

FIGURE 31.3. The cell cycle.

within the cell cycle where abnormal cells or cells lacking appropriate signals are prevented from proceeding further. The two primary checkpoints exist just before S phase and before M phase.

A key factor of most cancers is the presence of a force that promotes passage of cells abnormally through the cell cycle and usually influences entry into S phase. Importantly, this force does not necessarily require more rapid cell proliferation, just the inability to control it. Furthermore, this process can involve either lack of inhibitory signals (tumor suppressors) or the presence of cell cycle stimulatory signals (oncogenes).

Production of many of the enzymes and factors required for DNA synthesis and DNA replication is regulated by the E2F and Rb families of nuclear proteins. In fact, Rb, or retinoblastoma protein, derives its name because it is mutated in retinoblastomas, causing E2F to be deregulated in its action to initiate DNA synthesis. Several tumor-causing viruses, including human papilloma virus and SV40 virus, produce factors that bind to Rb, releasing E2F which then drives the cell cycle. Activity of the Rb family of proteins is in turn regulated by cyclins D and E and the cyclin-dependent kinases (cdk) cdk4 and cdk6. There are several examples of cancers where a priamry upregulation of these cyclins and/or kinases appears to be etiologic in the cancer, for example, in chronic lymphocytic leukemia or breast cancer.

Several signaling pathways regulate *cyclin/cdk* activity (Fig. 31.4). Ras and Ras-related pathways are very important in cellular growth signaling. Growth factors such as epidermal growth factor (EGF) utilize Ras pathways, involving activation of mitogen-activated protein kinases (MAPK) and ultimately the nuclear transcription factors,

c-*fos*, c-*jun*, and c-*myc*. Subsequent steps lead to mediation of the cdk/Rb/E2F pathway. Ras also activates other pathways that are involved in cell growth control. Another pathway, the Jak/STAT pathway, is initiated by binding of a cytokine such as interferon to its receptor, ultimately resulting in cell cycle advancement. A third pathway that is associated with tumor cell growth and differentiation is the inositol phosphate/protein kinase C (IP/PKC) pathway. Protein kinase C (PKC) is important for tumor promotion in some cells, and it can directly regulate the MAPK pathway. Another important pathway is associated with the adenomatous polyposis coli (APC) gene, which is mutated in familial adenomatous polyposis. This pathway, when APC is mutated, stimulates the cell cycle.

The following components of signaling pathways provide numerous examples of cancer-associated alterations.

Growth Factors

A variety of growth factors, including platelet-derived growth factor (PDGF), TGF-α, colony-stimulating factor 1 (CSF-1), fibroblast growth factor (FGF), and other polypeptide growth factors, are overexpressed in certain tumors.[36,37]

Growth Factor Receptors

Growth factor receptors can be activated by genetic mutations or overexpressed in certain human cancers.[38] Examples include TRK (nerve growth factor receptor), MET (hepatocyte growth factor/scatter factor receptor), ERB-B (epidermal growth factor receptor), ERBB-2/neu (orphan receptor), FMS (colony-stimulating factor-1),

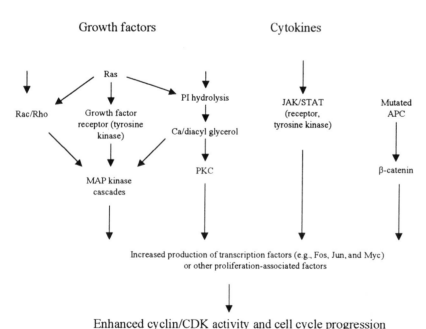

FIGURE 31.4. Signaling pathways that affect the cell cycle in cancer.

RET (orphan receptor), ROS (orphan receptor), and SEA (orphan receptor). The ERBB family, for example, is overexpressed in some breast, ovarian, and squamous carcinomas as well as in glioblastomas.

G Proteins

G proteins, or GTP-binding proteins, translate signals from cell-surface receptors to intracellular signaling cascades.[39] Activating mutations of the Ras family of G proteins are the most common dominant mutations in human cancer. The gene for neurofibromatosis produces a Ras-regulating protein.

Nuclear Oncogenes

Several transcription factors, including myc, fos, and jun, directly regulate gene expression that leads to cell proliferation, division, and differentiation.[40–47]

In addition to being unregulated by cyclins, cyclin-dependent kinases (cdk) are also inhibited by cdk inhibitors (cdki). There are two families of cdki: the first includes p21 and p27, and the second family, or INK4 family, includes p16, p15, p18, and p19. P15 and p16 are frequently mutated in human cancers. Additionally, p53, the most frequently mutated gene in cancer, conveys part of its activity through a cdki (p21).

Nutrient deprivations is yet another potential point of control over unregulated proliferation. If a cell population grows so rapidly that it outstrips its nutrient supply, the cells will enter a quiescent or G_0 state. Indeed, without additional vascularization, a tumor can grow no more than a few millimeters. Many tumors have adapted to this problem by secreting vascular growth factors that stimulate new vascular growth; this provides for the needed nutritional supply to support tumor growth.

Impairment of Apoptosis

An important cellular event that is often in apposition to cellular poliferation is apoptosis, or programmed cell death.[48–50] At a cellular level, this process involves an orderly, energy-requiring dismantling and processing of a cell, as opposed to necrosis, which is disorganized and probably more toxic to the organism. Apoptosis occurs naturally in a developing organism, with the coordinated loss of specific cell populations. It can also be induced by stress or cell damage. Cells arrested at cell cycle checkpoints (see Fig. 31.3), for example, with a certain level of DNA damage, will exit the cell cycle and undergo apoptosis. The number of cells in a tissue or tumor can be considered to represent a balance between proliferation and apoptosis.

The induction of apoptosis and inhibition of the cell cycle are closely linked. A central mediator of these processes is the p53 transcription factor, which is a recipient of cellular signals indicating damage or stress. Probably the most publicized and most frequently observed alteration in cancer is mutation of p53. In addition to inhibiting the cell cycle as already discussed, p53 appears to regulate a cascade of events resulting in apoptosis. Therefore, disruption of p53 in cancer results not only in disruption of the cell's ability to halt growth but also in impairment of its ability to carry out apoptosis.

The association of aging with apoptosis as it relates to cancer is more complex. Aging results in a generalized enhancement in apoptosis in a variety of organ systems. This increased tendency toward apoptosis is insufficient to result in reduced tumor development in the elderly. A malignant tumor clone has developed multiple mutations, some of which impair the cell's ability to recognize these apoptotic forces. Furthermore, the generalized increased apoptosis seen with aging may result in impaired organ fucntion that actually facilitates tumor growth. For example, greater apoptosis of specific T-cell subsets may reduce the body's ability to mount an adequate immunologic response to a tumor.

Impairment of Differentiation

A phenotype associated with many cancers is impaired cellular differentiation or maturation. Conceptually, all cells within the body derive from some form of stem or germ cell. This stem cell lacks phenotypic characteristics of mature tissues but has the capacity to produce daughter cells that undergo such maturation. Differentiation involves acquiring functional capabilities and expression of unique structural and functional components as well as loss of proliferative capacity in many cases. This process is thought of as an irreversible commitment. A common theme among cancers is the loss of this phenotypic differentiation, yet the molecular etiology for this change is understood in many fewer cases.

Tumor Promotion

The phorbol esters were the first class of compounds characterized as tumor promoters.[51,52] These compounds bind and activate protein kinase C (PKC). PKC regulation of the Ras/MAPK pathway may be its mechanism of tumor promotion. Dietary fat intake has been associated with increased cancer incidence, which may be the result of the direct tumor-promoting effects of certain lipids.

Enhanced Invasive/Metastatic Capacity

A critical issue in terms of a tumor's lethality is its ability to invade surrounding tissue and metastasize.[53–56] Cancer cells accomplish metastasis using several mechanisms. Rapid cellular growth results in mechanical pressure that may damage surrounding tissue or physically facilitate local invasion. Cancer cells acquire enhanced mobility, loss of cell-to-cell cohesive forces, and increased ability to degrade basement membranes and connective tissue extracellular matrix. Expression of enzymes such as metalloproteinases, collagenase, and heparinase correlates well with metastatic potential.

Resistance to Host Factors

Tumor cells exhibit immunogenic antigens. Although a tumor cell that is recognized by the immune system can be destroyed, certain tumor cells are actually stimulated to grow by cytokines involved in an immune response. Alternatively, certain tumor cells have developed reduced capacity to resist other factors that might result in the cell's demise.[57–59]

Tumor Biology

The biologic characteristics of individual tumors vary greatly depending on the tissue of origin, genetic makeup, and environmental stimuli. For example, leukemia, carcinomas, and sarcomas tend to have general growth and treatment-response factors that differ. Even tumors from the same organ can be vastly different; for example, basal cell carcinoma versus malignant melanoma, or chronic lymphocytic leukemia versus acute lymphocytic leukemia. These differences are largely a result of differing complements of genes being expressed. The tumor environment may also play a role in the tumor phenotype. The hormonal milieu or the presence of inflammatory cytokines may slow or hasten tumor growth. Tumors in the elderly may be less aggressive.

Biology of Cancer Therapy

Pharmacology of Therapeutics in the Elderly

A number of physiologic and pathophysiologic changes occur as people age that significantly affect the pharmacokinetics (the way in which drugs are absorbed, distributed, metabolized, and excreted) and pharmacodynamics (the body's response to the drug).[60,61] Pharmacokinetic changes include changes in body composition that result in decreased water content and increased lipid content. These changes affect the volume of distribution of drugs, depending on their polarity. A steady cross-sectional decline in renal function occurs as people age. This renal function decline can go unnoticed because of reduced muscle mass and deceptively low serum creatinine levels in the elderly. In addition, hepatic metabolism is reduced in the elderly because of an overall decline in hepatic blood flow. The expression of p-glycoprotein by resistant tumor cells represents a pharmacokinetic change at the cellular level.

Impaired responsiveness of the cardiovascular system in the elderly results from a series of pharmacodynamic changes, including reduced β-receptor sensitivity and increased vascular rigidity. These changes place the elderly at increased risk from events or treatments that produce hemodynamic compromise, including sepsis and cardiovascular-acting agents.

Chemoprevention

A number of agents are being studied that may reduce cancer-causing cellular events.[62–64] A reduction in development of contralateral breast cancer has been shown for patients taking the antiestrogen tamoxifen as an adjuvant therapy for breast cancer. This drug purportedly reduces the tumor-promoting effect of hormonal stimulation. Nonsteroidal anti-inflammatory agents have been proposed as a cancer-preventing intervention, particularly for colon carcinoma. Finally, a variety of antioxidants are being studied for their ability to reduce the incidence of cancer.

Cell Cycle-Directed Agents

The primary mechanism of action of most anticancer drugs currently in use is the disruption of the cell cycle.[65] Antimetabolites such as methotrexate interfere with DNA synthesis by inhibiting dihydrofolate reductase. Incorporation of modified pyrimidines, such as cytosine arabinoside during DNA synthesis, causes chain termination. Fluorinated pyrimidines, such as 5-fluorouracil, inhibit DNA and RNA synthesis. Platinum agents, such as cisplatin, and alkylating agents, such as nitrogen mustards and nitrosoureas, cross-link DNA and disrupt DNA repair. Topoisomerase inhibitors, like topotecan and etoposide, interfere with transcription, DNA synthesis, and mitosis. Microtubule-disrupting agents, such as vincristine and paclitaxel, impair cell division. Anthracyclines such as doxorubicin disrupt DNA synthesis, but also induce free radical formation and damage cell membranes. Regardless of the mechanism, the end result of a variety of chemotherapy agents is to inhibit cell proliferation of rapidly cycling cells, thus removing these cells from the cell cycle or delaying the cell cycle.

Apoptosis-Directed Agents

The initial effect of the chemotherapy agents previously described is inhibition of cell proliferation. As a result of these insults, a cell may undergo apoptosis. The action of many chemotherapeutic agents is also associated with apoptosis. In addition to cytotoxic chemotherapy, apoptosis can be induced by growth factor or hormone withdrawal and irradiation. As described, p53 is an important mediator of apoptosis. p53-defficient cells are resistant to the apoptosis-inducing effect of chemotherapy or radiation.

Receptor–Effector Antagonism

Because growth of many tumors depends on disrupted receptor activation, therapies have been developed to antagonize these receptors.[66] Hormonal agents, such as antiandrogens, antiestrogens, gonadotropin-releasing hormone analogues, and aromatase inhibitors, represent important classes of anticancer drugs currently widely in use for treatment of hormone-dependent tumors, such as breast, prostate, and endometrial cancer. Because G-protein farnesylation appears to be important in Ras signaling, an experimental approach currently being developed is the characterization of farnesylation inhibitors.

Angiogenesis-Directed Agents

Angiogenesis appears to be important for tumors that exceed several millimeters in size and has therefore become a target of intense investigation Endogenous peptide angiogenesis inhibitors have been identified, and one experimental approach has been to produce and administer these or similar peptides. Other agents such as thalidomide have been shown to inhibit angiogenesis and are currently being evaluated for their ability to stem tumor growth.

Differentiation-Directed Therapy

Cancer therapies can be directed at mediating cellular differentiation. An important example of this is the treatment of acute promyelocytic leukemia with all-trans-retinoic acid. Because the disease arises from inappropriate expression of the retinoic acid receptor, treatment of the leukemic blasts with retinoic acid results in rapid induction of differentiation of the cells. Retinoic acid has subsequently become an important agent for treatment of this disease.

Immunomediated Therapy

Enhancing immune function has been associated with antitumor responses in animal models and in humans. For example, interleukin-2 has antitumor efficacy in malignant melanoma and renal cell carcinoma. Interferon alpha also has efficacy in melanoma and renal cell carcinoma as well as in chronic myelogenous leukemia. It is believed that these agents stimulate the immune system's antitumor activity.[67]

Inhibitors of Basement Membrane-Degrading Enzymes

Still in the phase of discovery and development are agents that inhibit basement membrane-degrading enzymes such as matrix metalloproteinase.[53–56]

Resistance to Therapy

Genetic instability acquired by cancer cells during tumor progression increases the rate of tumor cell adaptation to specific stresses such as cancer therapy.[57–59] A related mechanism a cell may use is the development of the multidrug resistance (MDR) phenotype, which can be induced in acute leukemia in older patients. Upon exposure to chemotherapeutic agents, cancer cells increase expression of proteins that excrete the agent from the cell, maintaining low intracellular concentrations of drug. The best studied example of this involves cell-surface expression of p-glycoprotein (Pgp).

Conclusions

The biologic basis for cancer is clearly multidimensional and complex. This chapter systematically discusses the key elements of the development, progression, and treatment of cancer with a specific focus on the role of aging in these processes. Unfortunately, there is no unifying explanation that describes the essence of cancer. There are, however, many biologic and epidemiologic links to aging. Biologic changes that occur during aging probably increase the likelihood of developing cancer. Age-associated changes also impact significantly on cancer therapeutics. All these areas need more research, but understanding them can help the clinician at the forefront of cancer prevention, diagnosis, and treatment in an aging population.

References

1. Campisi J. Aging and cancer: the double-edged sword of replicative senescence. *J Am Geriatr Soc.* 1997;45:482–488.
2. Fernandez-Pol JA, Douglas MG. Molecular interactions of cancer and age. *Hematol Oncol Clin North Am.* 2000; 14:25–44.
3. Dunn BK, Longo DL. Molecular biology and biological markers. In: Hunter CD, Johnson KA, Muss HB, eds. *Cancer in the Elderly.* New York: Dekker; 2000.
4. Kinzler KW, Vogelstein B. Lessons from hereditary colorectal cancer. *Cell.* 1996;87:159–170.
5. Dipple A. DNA adducts of chemical carcinogens. *Carcinogenesis.* 1995;16:437–441.
6. Murray V. A survey of the sequence-specific interaction of damaging agents with DNA: emphasis on antitumor agents. *Prog Nucleic Acid Res Mol Biol.* 1999;63:367–415.

7. Yuspa SH. The pathogenesis of squamous cell cancer: lessons learned from studies of skin carcinogenesis. Thirty-third G.H.A. Clowes Memorial Award Lecture. *Cancer Res.* 1994;54:1178.

8. Vessey CJ, Norbury CJ, Hickson ID. Genetic disorders associated with cancer predisposition and genomic instability. *Prog Nucleic Acid Res Mol Biol.* 1999;63:189–221.

9. Fearon ER. Human cancer syndromes: clues to the origin and nature of cancer. *Science.* 1997;278:1043–1050.

10. Lynch HT, Smyrk TC. Hereditary colorectal cancer. *Semin Oncol.* 1999;26:478–484.

11. Wright WE, Shay JW. Telomere dynamics in cancer progression and prevention: fundamental differences in human and mouse telomere biology. *Nat Med.* 2000;6:849–851.

12. Buys CH. Telomeres, telomerase, and cancer. *N Engl J Med.* 2000;342:1282–1283.

13. Wynford-Thomas D. Replicative senescence: mechanisms and implications for human cancer. *Pathol Biol (Paris).* 2000; 48:301–307.

14. Campisi J. Cancer, aging and cellular senescence. *In Vivo.* 2000;14:183–188.

15. Vaziri H, Benchimol S. Alternative pathways for the extension of cellular life span: inactivation of p53/pRb and expression of telomerase. *Oncogene.* 1999;18:7676–7680.

16. Harley CB, Sherwood SW. Telomerase, checkpoints and cancer. *Cancer Surv.* 1997;29:263–284.

17. Smith JR, Pereira-Smith OM. Replicative senescence: implications for in vivo aging and tumor suppression. *Science.* 1996;273:63–67.

18. Hayflick L. How and why we age. *Exp Gerontol.* 1998;33: 639–653.

19. Bateman AC, Howell WM. Human leukocyte antigens and cancer: is it in our genes? *J Pathol.* 1999;188:231–236.

20. Ginaldi L, De Martinis M, D'Ostilio A, et al. The immune system in the elderly: II. Specific cellular immunity. *Immunol Res.* 1999;20:109–115.

21. Browning M, Dunnion D. HLA and cancer: implications for cancer immunotherapy and vaccination. *Eur J Immunogenet.* 1997;24:293–312.

22. Grisham MB, Jourd'heuil D, Wink DA. Review article: chronic inflammation and reactive oxygen and nitrogen metabolism—implications in DNA damage and mutagenesis. *Aliment Pharmacol Ther.* 2000;14(suppl 1):3–9.

23. Tselepis C, Perry I, Jankowski J. Barrett's esophagus: disregulation of cell cycling and intercellular adhesion in the metaplasia-dysplasia-carcinoma sequence. *Digestion.* 2000; 61:1–5.

24. Williams CS, Mann M, DuBois RN. The role of cyclooxygenases in inflammation, cancer, and development. *Oncogene.* 1999;18:7908–7916.

25. Blattner WA. Human retroviruses: their role in cancer. *Proc Assoc Am Physicians.* 1999;111:563–572.

26. Grady D, Gebretsadik T, Kerlikowske K, Ernster V, Petitti D. Hormone replacement therapy and endometrial cancer risk: a meta-analysis. *Obstet Gynecology.* 1995;85:304–313.

27. Cancer CGoHFiB. Breast cancer and hormone replacement therapy: collaborative reanalysis of data from 51 epidemiological studies of 52,705 women with breast cancer and 108,411 women without breast cancer. *Lancet.* 1997; 350:1047–1059.

28. Hursting SD, Kari FW. The anti-carcinogenic effects of dietary restriction: mechanisms and future directions. *Mutat Res.* 1999;443:235–249.

29. Sherr CJ. Cancer cell cycles. *Science.* 1996;274:1672–1677.

30. Nevins JR. E2F: a link between the Rb tumor suppressor protein and viral oncoproteins. *Science.* 1992;258:424–429.

31. Hanahan D, Weinberg RA. The hallmarks of cancer. *Cell.* 2000;100:57–70.

32. Campbell SL, Khosravi-Far R, Rossman KL, Clark GJ, Der CJ. Increasing complexity of Ras signaling. *Oncogene.* 1998;17:1395–413.

33. Lewis TS, Shapiro PS, Ahn NG. Signal transduction through MAP kinase cascades. *Adv Cancer Res.* 1998;74:49–139.

34. Morin PJ. Beta-catenin signaling and cancer. *Bioessays.* 1999;21:1021–1030.

35. Polakis P. The oncogenic activation of beta-catenin. *Curr Opin Genet Dev.* 1999;9:15–21.

36. Zumkeller W, Schofield PN. Growth factors, cytokines and soluble forms of receptor molecules in cancer patients. *Anticancer Res.* 1995;15:343–348.

37. Goustin AS, Leof EB, Shipley GD, Moses HL. Growth factors and cancer. *Cancer Res.* 1986;46:1015–1029.

38. Pinkas-Kramarski R, Alroy I, Yarden Y. ErbB receptors and EGF-like ligands: cell lineage determination and oncogenesis through combinatorial signaling. *J Mamm Gland Biol Neoplasia.* 1997;2:97–107.

39. Gutkind JS. Cell growth control by G protein-coupled receptors: from signal transduction to signal integration. *Oncogene.* 1998;17:1331–1342.

40. Sawyers CL, Callahan W, Witte ON. Dominant negative MYC blocks transformation by ABL oncogenes. *Cell.* 1992; 70:901–910.

41. Roussel MF, Cleveland JL, Shurtleff SA, Sherr CJ. MYC rescue of a mutant CSF-1 receptor impaired in mitogenic signalling. *Nature.* 1991;353:361–363.

42. Sklar MD, Thompson E, Welsh MJ, et al. Depletion of c-*myc* with specific antisense sequences reverse the transformed phenotype in *ras* oncogene-transformed NIH 3T3 cells. *Mol Cell Biol.* 1991;11:3699–3710.

43. Bhatia K, Huppi K, Spangler G, Siwarski D, Iyer R, Magrath I. Point mutations in the c-*Myc* transactivation domain are common in Burkitt's lymphoma and mouse plasmacytomas. *Nat Genet.* 1993;5:56–61.

44. Alitalo K, Schwab M. Oncogene amplification in tumor cells. *Adv Cancer Res.* 1986;47:235–281.

45. Hollstein M, Sidransky D, Vogelstein B, Harris CC. p53 mutations in human cancers. *Science.* 1991;253:49–53.

46. Oliner JD, Kinzler KW, Meltzer PS, George DL, Vogelstein B. Amplification of a gene encoding a p53-associated protein in human sarcomas. *Nature.* 1992;358:80–83.

47. Scheffner M, Werness BA, Huibregtse JM, Levine AJ, Howley PM. The E6 oncoprotein encoded by human papillomavirus types 16 and 18 promotes the degradation of p53. *Cell.* 1990;63:1129–1136.

48. Reed JC. Dysregulation of apoptosis in cancer. *J Clin Oncol.* 1999;17:2941–2953.

49. Wyllie AH, Bellamy CO, Bubb VJ, et al. Apoptosis and carcinogenesis. *Br J Cancer.* 1999;80(suppl 1):34–37.

50. Green DR. Apoptotic pathways: paper wraps stone blunts scissors. *Cell.* 2000;102:1–4.

51. Liu WS, Heckman CA. The sevenfold way of PKC regulation. *Cell Signal.* 1998;10:529–542.

52. Assembly of Life Sciences NRC. Diet, nutrition, and cancer. Executive summary of the report of the committee on diet, nutrition, and cancer. *Cancer Res.* 1983;43:3018–3023.

53. Matrisian LM. Cancer biology: extracellular proteinases in malignancy. *Curr Biol.* 1999;9:R776–R778.

54. Kleiner DE, Stetler-Stevenson WG. Matrix metalloproteinases and metastasis. *Cancer Chemother Pharmacol.* 1999;43(suppl):S42–S51.

55. Johnson LL, Dyer R, Hupe DJ. Matrix metalloproteinases. *Curr Opin Chem Biol.* 1998;2:466–471.

56. Leonard DM. Ras farnesyltrasferase: a new therapeutic target. *J Med Chem.* 1997;40:2971–2990.

57. Robert J. Multidrug resistance in oncology: diagnostic and therapeutic approaches. *Eur J Clin Investig.* 1999;29:536–545.

58. Kaye SB. Multidrug resistance: clinical relevance in solid tumours and strategies for circumvention. *Curr Opin Oncol.* 1998;10(suppl 1):S15–S19.

59. Volm M. Multidrug resistance and its reversal. *Anticancer Res.* 1998;18:2905–2917.

60. Vestal RE. Aging and pharmacology. *Cancer.* 1997;80:1302–1310.

61. Baker SD, Grochow LB. Pharmacology of cancer chemotherapy in the older person. *Clin Geriatr Med.* 1997;13:169–183.

62. Kelloff GJ, Crowell JA, Steele VE, et al. Progress in cancer chemoprevention. *Ann NY Acad Sci.* 1999;889:1–13.

63. Singh DK, Lippman SM. Cancer chemoprevention. Part 2: Hormones, nonclassic antioxidant natural agents, NSAIDs, and other agents. *Oncology (Huntingt).* 1998;12:1787–1800; discussion 1802, 1805.

64. Singh DK, Lippman SM. Cancer chemoprevention. Part 1: Retinoids and carotenoids and other classic antioxidants. *Oncology (Huntingt).* 1998;12:1643–1653, 1657–1658; discussion 1659–1660.

65. Chabner BA, Longo DL. *Cancer Chemotherapy and Biotherapy: Principles and Practice, 2nd Ed.* Philadelphia: Lippincott-Raven; 1996:824.

66. Rowinsky EK, Windle JJ, Von Hoff DD. Ras protein farnesyltransferase: a strategic target for anticancer therapeutic development. *J Clin Oncol.* 1999;17:3631–3652.

67. Jaffee EM. Immunotherapy of cancer. *Ann NY Acad Sci.* 1999;886:67–72.

32
Screening for Cancer

Eugene Z. Oddone, Mitchell T. Heflin, and John R. Feussner

When to Seek Early Diagnosis

Screening for cancer is an attractive and important component of comprehensive primary care. Clinicians understand and support this part of early disease detection because it may allow definitive and potentially curative therapy at a time when the patient's quality of life can be preserved, perhaps even prolonging their life. Patients also generally understand the concept of screening and, when questioned directly, place a high value on averting late-stage or metastatic cancer. Health care systems support the concept by using screening rates for certain cancers as markers of quality of care. Despite the generally accepted concept of screening for cancer, there are often wide gaps in the performance of screening for individual patients within practices and across health care systems. In some instances, conflicting or vague guidelines for particular screening tests lead to confusion for both clinicians and patients about what the suggested strategy should be. In other cases, the evidence for screening with a specific test is strong and mechanisms for payment exist, yet compliance with repeated screening is only average. The decision to screen for cancer in the elderly is even more difficult than for a younger population because the elderly were not included in many screening studies. Additionally, older patients face a high competing risk of dying from other causes, which reduces the potential effectiveness of any screening strategy.

As attractive as early detection of cancer may seem, certain principles should be considered to assure the appropriateness of any decision to seek early diagnosis. A paradigm upon which to evaluate the evidence for or against screening includes the importance or seriousness of the target disease; the presence of a detectable preclinical phase; the accuracy and acceptability of diagnostic tests used to detect cancer; the risk associated with the initial and any subsequent diagnostic tests necessary to confirm the diagnosis; and the efficacy, risk, cost, and availability of treatment for the cancer once it is uncovered. The absence of clear information about any one of these important considerations will diminish the potential value of a screening strategy.

The disease being considered as a potential target for early diagnosis should be an important problem. It should either occur frequently, be more readily treated when detected early, or be readily treated even though the prevalence may be low. Sackett and colleagues have succinctly summarized this point: the disease should be so common or so awful as to justify the effort and expense of early detection.[1] Cancer qualifies as an example of an important target disease that is both common and awful in the elderly.

For any screening strategy to be effective, knowledge about the natural history of the target disease should be apparent. Clinicians should know that early detection of disease is likely to be useful because the disease has a detectable preclinical phase. There must be evidence that detection of the disease at the presymptomatic stage matters. Finding and treating the disease at this point must result in either improved quality of life, reduced disability, or reduced mortality for screening to make a difference.

For a screening program to be feasible, diagnostic tests must be available that are accurate and acceptable to patients. The screening test should minimize false positives (healthy patients inaccurately identified by positive test results) and false negatives (patients with the disease of interest who have negative test results). The accuracy of most diagnostic tests is expressed in terms of the test sensitivity (patients with disease who are correctly identified by a positive test) and test specificity (patients without disease who are correctly identified by a negative test). Alternatively, these characteristics can be combined into likelihood ratios, which describe the odds that patients with positive or negative test results either do or do not have the target disease. The screening test should also be acceptable to patients in terms of risk, discomfort,

TABLE 32.1. Considerations in deciding to seek an early diagnosis.

1. Is the target disease an important clinical problem?
   a. Does the burden of disability warrant early action?
2. Is the natural history of the target disease understood?
   a. Is there a latent or early symptomatic period?
3. Is the screening diagnostic strategy effective?
   a. Is the accuracy of testing established?
   b. Is the test acceptable to patients, with little discomfort and low risks?
   c. If the screening test is positive, will patients accept subsequent diagnostic evaluation?
4. Is there a known treatment for the target disease at the detectable stage?
   a. Is the treatment effective and available?
   b. Is the cost of testing balanced by the benefit of treatment?

and cost. Patients must also understand that screening may involve a sequence of tests depending on results because additional definitive diagnostic tests are often required before definitive therapy.

Target diseases that meet the four criteria listed in Table 32.1 are often the focus of clinical studies that seek to establish the effectiveness of a particular screening strategy. In these studies, and unique to all clinical studies that seek to measure early diagnosis, the interpretation of the effectiveness of a specific strategy is susceptible to two specific biases. First, lead-time bias occurs when early detection establishes a diagnosis of cancer sooner than usual but without actually influencing the natural history, or survival time, of a given cancer. The duration of survival measured from the time of diagnosis to death will appear longer for the patient who underwent screening than for the patient whose cancer was detected when symptoms first appeared. Therefore, the screened patient did not actually live longer than the unscreened patient but appeared to live longer because the diagnosis of cancer was made earlier. Second, length-time bias describes a phenomenon whereby slower-growing cancers are more likely to be discovered by routine periodic screening than are faster-growing cancers. Faster-growing cancers, being more aggressive, grow and spread in the interval between screening events; this results in a longer average survival in the screened population because of the disproportionate detection of slower-growing cancers in the cohort.

Issues Specific to the Older Patient

The decision to offer cancer screening to the older patient is complex.[2] There are competing forces that simultaneously favor and dissuade clinicians from adopting screening for any individual. In addition to the traditional

inquiries about the strength of evidence supporting a given screening test, clinicians must consider other questions specific to the elderly (Table 32.2).

1. *What is the impact of the disease in older patients?* Sixty percent of persons affected by cancer are over age 65. Age-specific incidence rates for various cancers are severalfold higher in older patients when compared to their younger counterparts. Additionally, mortality rates rise dramatically as patients age into their eighth and ninth decades of life (Fig. 32.1). The burden of cancer is clearly significant in the elderly.

2. *Is cancer biology different in older patients?* In many cases, the detectable preclinical phase of a cancer changes with aging. For example, breast cancer in older women appears to evolve more slowly than in younger patients, whereas cervical cancer may become invasive in a shorter period. The specific biology of a cancer fundamentally determines its candidacy for screening.

3. *Do screening tests perform differently in older patients?* Often, screening tests perform differently in older patients due to factors such as comorbid illness or age-associated changes in anatomy or cellular biology. Mammography, for instance, performs better in older patients, whereas the Pap smear is less reliable.

4. *Will this patient or group of patients survive long enough to derive a benefit from screening?* Many groups making recommendations for screening in the elderly state that screening should be continued if the patient has "good health" or "a reasonable life expectancy." Because of a lack of clinical trial data in older patients, the answer often must be derived from the expected time to benefit projected from younger patients as well as the patient's estimated life expectancy. Estimated life expectancy is difficult to predict for individual patients. Current estimates from census life tables set the average life expectancy of a 75-year-old woman at 12.2 years and a 75-year-old man at 10 years. These numbers may be decreased, however, by the presence of comorbid illness. In fact, several studies have demonstrated that chronically ill patients diagnosed with early-stage cancer tend to die of a comorbid illness and not from cancer.[3,4]

TABLE 32.2. Questions specific to screening for cancer in the elderly.

What is the specific impact of the disease in older patients?
Is the biology of the cancer different in older patients?
Are the characteristics of the screening tests different in older patients?
Will this patient or group of patients survive long enough to benefit from screening?
What barriers exist to screening for this cancer in the patients?
How do patient preference and values impact the decision to offer screening in older patients?

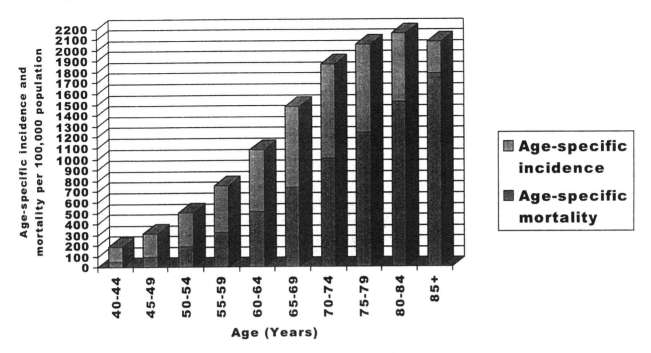

FIGURE 32.1. Age-specific incidence and mortality from cancer, 1993–1997. (Adapted from NCI SEER program data, online at *www.seer.cancer.gov/publications.*)

5. *What barriers exist to screening for cancer in the elderly?* Social factors such as race, access to health care, and socioeconomic status impact the receipt of screening. Likewise, provider knowledge and communication skills strongly influence patient understanding and compliance with recommended screening strategies.

6. *How do patient preference and quality of life impact screening decisions?* Consideration must be given not only to changes in survival associated with screening, but also to the stress associated with early diagnosis, the threat of disability with longer life, and the potential harm associated with treatment.

These questions must be answered separately for each cancer considered for screening and for each patient. This review attempts to identify the evidence available for screening for several cancers in the elderly and to provide clinicians with guides for decision making in each case.

Breast Cancer

Breast cancer is the leading cause of cancer and the second leading cause of cancer-related deaths among women in the United States. In 2002, although the number of new cases of breast cancer in the United States was expected to remain stable at approximately 203,500, the number of total deaths was expected to drop to fewer than 39,600 from more than 46,000 in 1994. Older women

continue to experience the majority of morbidity and mortality from breast cancer. The annual incidence among women over age 65 is nearly six times that of women under age 65 (441/100,000 versus 76/100,0000). Additionally, 67% of breast cancer deaths occur among women over age 60, and 24% occurred in those over age 80.[5,6]

In addition to advancing age, other well-established risk factors include personal or family history of breast cancer, a history of benign breast disease with atypical hyperplasia, and a longer duration of estrogen exposure, either endogenous or exogenous. The specific impact of these risk factors in older compared to younger women is not clear. Recent analyses of large populations of older women enrolled in studies of osteoporotic fractures have revealed marked decreases in breast cancer risk among those with the lowest bone mineral densities. Researchers speculate that bone mineral density may be a marker of lifetime estrogen exposure and, thereby, an indirect indicator of breast cancer risk.[7,8]

In addition to its high prevalence and mortality, breast cancer qualifies for screening due to its more favorable prognosis with early detection. For localized disease, 5-year survival rates in patients over 50 are 97.6%. With spread to regional lymph nodes at diagnosis, the 5-year survival in this group drops to 77.5% and with distant metastases to 20.1%.[5] These rates do not appear to change with advancing age, particularly for early-stage disease. Additionally, strong evidence exists that tumors diagnosed in the elderly appear to be more slow growing and therefore more amenable to screen detection and eradication with treatment.[9]

Screening strategies for the early detection of breast cancer include breast self-examination (BSE), clinical breast examination (CBE), and mammography. Breast self-examination has been studied in large, prospective, international trials. Although these trials have demonstrated a higher detection rate of smaller, more localized tumors, none of the studies has documented a mortality benefit for BSE.[10,11] Other studies indicate that BSE has a low sensitivity, between 20% and 30%, which may be even lower among older women.[12] Based on this evidence, BSE appears to have limited utility in screening for breast cancer.

Independent test characteristics for CBE are difficult to assess secondary to a lack of direct evidence. Clinical results from breast physical examination are likely to be variable and directly related to the skills of the health care professional performing the breast examination. Overall, the sensitivity of CBE has been estimated to be about 50%.[12] As with other screening modalities, specificity is difficult to determine because women with normal examinations do not receive the reference standard test, breast biopsy. Studies that use manufactured models to simulate breast examination show an average sensitivity of 65% for registered nurses and 87% for physicians.[13] CBE may augment screening with mammography but cannot stand alone as a screening maneuver.

The mammogram, on the other hand, remains the cornerstone of breast cancer screening. It detects smaller deeper breast masses and thereby allows the discovery of cancer earlier than physical exam alone. Overall, the sensitivity of mammography alone has been estimated to be approximately 75% to 90%, varying with age, breast density, and screening interval.[14] When combined with CBE, estimates have ranged from 75% to 88%; specificity ranges from 83% to 98.5%.[15] A significant body of evidence exists demonstrating that mammography has excellent test characteristics in elderly patients.[16] Researchers attribute the improved performance of mammography to a decrease in overall breast density and increased content of radiolucent fat with aging.

Several experimental trials have demonstrated that screening for breast cancer with mammography reduces disease-specific mortality. The standard trial establishing the efficacy of the combination of mammography and CBE was the Health Insurance Plan of Greater New York study that documented a 23% reduction in mortality at 18 years of follow-up.[17] This trial, however, excluded older women. Only the Swedish Two County trial and the Malmö trial included patients who were over age 65 years at the time of randomization. The Two County Trial reported a relative risk reduction of death from breast cancer between 25% and 44% for patients aged 50 to 74 years.[15] A subsequent subgroup analysis of patients aged 70 to 74 among *all* the Swedish trials, however, revealed an insignificant risk reduction of 0.94 (95% CI, 0.63–1.53) at 12 years of follow-up.[18] This analysis cast some doubt on the resilience of the mortality benefit from breast cancer screening in the elderly population. In addition, a recent metanalysis by the Cochrane Collaboration has highlighted methodologic flaws in several trials of screening mammography and, in so doing, has called into question the survival benefits described above.[19] However, this analysis is highly controversial, and its implications for decisions to offer breast cancer screening to older patients remain unclear. Additional evidence for benefit, however, may be found in observational studies, including a large case-control study from the Netherlands comparing patients responding to invitation to screen with those not responding. Among those aged 65 to 74, relative risk of death from breast cancer was 0.34 at 13 years follow-up and 0.45 at 18 years for biennial screening. Although this study demonstrated a strong effect, its validity is weakened by the bias inherent in its design.[20] More recently, in a retrospective analysis of information form the SEER program, McCarthy et al. found that older women with primary breast cancer who had not had screening mammograms within the previous 2 years were significantly more likely to have advanced-stage disease at diagnosis [stage II or greater, adjusted odds ratio (OR) 3.12 (2.74–3.58)] and were more likely to die of breast cancer [adjusted HR 2.28 (1.79–2.91)].[21] The clinician deciding whether or not to offer breast cancer screening to a woman over age 75 faces a clinical dilemma. On the one hand, the disease is highly prevalent and most deadly among this population. On the other hand, little direct evidence exists of the benefits of screening in this group. Further complicating the matter is the higher rate of comorbid illness and lower life expectancy among elderly women. Researchers have attempted to model such decisions. Mandelblatt and colleagues used a Markov decision model to evaluate screening elderly women with common comorbidities for breast cancer. They included four groups in the model: white and black women with average health, women with mild hypertension, and women with congestive heart failure. Assuming that women aged 65 to 85 would be screened with CBE and mammography, the model produced favorable but modest improvements in survival for all groups. The benefit was more pronounced for black women and women of average health.[22] Another model using a clinical database from the Netherlands compared the benefit of screening in terms of quality-adjusted life-years (QALYs) gained with the "excess burden" incurred by increased lead time in diagnosis without impact on survival. The authors concluded that the benefit from screening might extend to patients up to ages 75 to 80.[23,24]

In regard to the optimal frequency of screening with mammography, analyses indicate that no significant decrease in survival occurs with increasing the interval from 1 to 2 years.[16,23] Biennial screening is deemed appropriate for older women as the preclinical detectable phase in this group appears to exceed 2 years.

Utilization of breast cancer screening declines steadily as patients age. Several population studies in the mid-1990s of women over age 75 reported screening rates of 30% to 40%, values well short of national standards and goals.[25,26] In the latest statistics from the Centers for Disease Control, however, the overall rate of recent receipt of breast cancer screening in Americans over age 65 had reached 64% in 1998, up from 48% in the same population in 1991. Participation appears to be mediated by a number of patient- and physician-related factors. Family history of breast cancer and a personal history of benign breast disease both *increase* the likelihood of screening.[27] Age, comorbid illness, and functional decline *decrease* the likelihood of receiving screening.[25] In addition, a number of socioeconomic factors, including low income, knowledge deficits, low perceived benefit or susceptibility, lack of private insurance, and lack of access to a regular source of health care, negatively impact breast cancer screening.[28] For the provider, knowledge of current evidence and effective direct communication of recommendations have a strong positive impact on rates of receipt of screening among older women.

Most groups recommend screening with CBE and mammography or mammography alone every 1 to 2 years beginning at age 40 or 50. The American Cancer Society also recommends monthly BSE over age 40. They do not set a specific upper age limit but state that "as long as the woman is in good health" to continue to offer screening services.[29] The United States Preventive Services Task Force (USPSTF) recognizes the highest level of evidence exists to support screening for breast cancer between ages 50 and 69, and that convincing data is lacking outside this age range. They do acknowledge that women over age 70 with "reasonable life expectancy" might continue to warrant an offer of screening based on the high impact of the disease in the older population.[30]

The authors agree with the consensus of offering biennial screening mammography to women over 50 (Table 32.3). Additionally, if a woman has a life expectancy of greater that 5 to 7 years, regardless of age, she should continue to receive offers to screen. Routine exploration of potential barriers to screening should accompany each refused offer or missed appointment; these might include addressing misperceptions, economic concerns, transportation issues, or simply fear and uncertainty.

Cervical Cancer

Although cervical cancer has a lower overall prevalence than breast cancer, it remains an important, preventable cause of morbidity and mortality for women. In 2002, the estimated number of new cases of invasive cervical cancer in the United States was expected to be 13,000 with 4100 deaths.[5] Additionally, approximately 55,000 cases of carcinoma in situ (CIS) are diagnosed annually. As with most other malignancies, the incidence of invasive cancer increases with age, with 25% of all cases occurring in people over age 65. Importantly, 40% to 50% of deaths related to cervical cancer occurs in this same age group.[31]

Risk factors for cervical cancer are well recognized; these include early sexual intercourse, multiple sexual partners, and a history of human papilloma virus infection. For elderly patients, an additional consideration is the added risk associated with a lack of previous screening. In one case-control study, investigators found that 55% of women over the age of 65 diagnosed with cervical cancer reported never having a Pap smear versus 15% for cancer-free controls.[32]

The natural history of squamous cell cancer of the cervix involves the progression of cervical dysplasia or CIS to invasive cancer. The detectable preclinical phase associated with this change is estimated to last from 1 to 20 years, although most agree that the average duration is approximately 10 years. This period may shorten with aging, with estimates as brief as 4 years in those over 50 and 1 year in those over 65.[33] When discovered before invasion, however, local treatment with conization or cryotherapy confers a definite survival advantage. For localized cancer, 5-year survival is 90%, as opposed to 40% for more advanced disease. Successful early intervention also avoids the extensive surgery and radiation employed to treat invasive disease.

The Papanicolau test, or Pap smear, has been the standard method of screening for cervical cancer for more than three decades. Cervical cancer is not diagnosed with the Pap smear but rather is suggested by certain cellular abnormalities. Follow-up testing with colposcopy and biopsy is required to establish the presence of cancer. Sensitivity and specificity of the Pap smear have been difficult to gauge for reasons of variability in methods of specimen collection and pathologic analysis. A recent systematic review by Nanda and colleagues showed that Pap smear sensitivities ranged from 30% to 87% and specificities ranged from 86% to 100%.[34] The review also found that liquid-based monolayer preparations consistently outperformed traditional slide-based methods.[34] Further complicating matters, test characteristics change with aging. In older women, the target region for cell

TABLE 32.3. Recommendations for cancer screening in the elderly.

Cancer	Test(s)	ACS[a]	USPSTF[b]	CTFPHC[c]	Authors	Medicare reimbursement
Breast	Mammography ± CBE	Annual beginning at age 40, "as long as in good health"	Annual or biennial between 50 and 69; consider continuing if "reasonable life expectancy"	Annual or biennial between 50 and 69	Start biennial screening at age 50; continue to offer between 70 and 80 if life expectancy greater than 5–7 years, explain risks, explore barriers	Yes (1991); annually (2000)
Cervix	Pap test	Annual × 3, then "less frequently," no upper age limit	Biennial or triennial, may stop at 65 if has had regular, normal smears	Annual × 2, then triennial to age 69 Consider more frequently in higher-risk subjects	Biennial or triennial screening, stop at 65 if has had regular, normal smears; history of prior Pap smears and risk factors; initial speculum exam before excluding from screening for hysterectomy	Yes (1991); Pap smear and pelvic exam biennially (2001)
Colorectal	FOBT Flex sig Colonoscopy ACBE	Annual FOBT; or flex sig every 5 years; or both; or colonoscopy every 10 years; or ACBE every 5–10 years	Annual FOBT, flex sig every 3–5 years, or combination. Colonoscopy or ACBE also appropriate, but interval undetermined.	Annual or biennial FOBT, periodic flex sig, or combination. Insufficient evidence for colonoscopy or ACBE.	Annual FOBT ± flex sig every 5 years; assess risks/benefits in choosing invasive vs. noninvasive methods; consider one-time colonoscopy or combination of ACBE and flex sig	FOBT annually; flexible sigmoidoscopy q 48mo (1997); Colonoscopy q 10yr (2001)
Prostate	DRE PSA	Both annually starting at age 50	Not recommended	Not recommended	Discuss benefits and harms, assist in individual decisions	DRE (as part of office exam) and PSA annually (2000)
Lung	CXR Sputum cytology Spiral CT Fluoroscopy bronchoscopy	Not recommended	Not recommended	Not recommended	Not recommended	No
Ovary	Pelvic exam CA 125 TVS	Not recommended	Not recommended	Not recommended	Not recommended	No
Skin	Skin inspection	Annual	Not recommended	Not recommended	Annual only for high-risk patients	No
Oral	Mouth inspection and palpation	Annual	Not recommended	Not recommended	Annual only for high-risk patients	No

ACS, American Cancer Society; USPSTF, U.S. Preventive Services Task Force; CTFPHC, Canadian Task Force on Preventive Care; CBE, clinical breast examination; FOBT, fecal occult blood test; flex sig, flexible sigmoidoscopy; ACBE, air contrast barium enema; DRE, digital rectal exam; PSA, prostate-specific antigen; CXR, chest x-ray.
Source: (a) From Smith et al.,[59] with permission. (b) http://www.ahcpr.gov/clinic/uspstfix.htm (c) http://www.ctfphc.org

collection, the squamocolumnar junction, recedes into the cervical canal, making sampling more difficult and less reliable. A study of 50 asymptomatic older women with negative Pap smears found that 11 had positive findings on subsequent colposcopy.[35] Additionally, aging predisposes the cervix to inflammation and injury, conditions that can result in higher false-positive rates. No prospective, controlled trials have been performed to demonstrate the effectiveness of the Pap smear on improving survival in any age population. A large body of epidemiologic evidence, however, reveals that women dying of cervical cancer are eight to nine times less likely to have received a Pap smear in the past than those without the diagnosis. Few patients over 65 were included in these analyses.[36]

Human papilloma virus (HPV) testing may become an important adjunct of Pap smears in the future. Up to 99% of patients in whom cervical neoplasia is identified are infected with HPV. Subtypes 16 and 18 predict the most aggressive lesions. Widespread use of HPV testing will depend on the development of an affordable, easily performed test that identifies both the presence of infection and the subtype. At this time, such assays are still under development.[29]

Many recommendations from professional organizations disagree with regard to suggested intervals between screening Pap smears. A comprehensive review revealed little decrement in the diagnostic rate of invasive cervical cancer with triennial versus annual screening (93.5% reduction in rate of invasive cancer versus 90.8%).[36] Cost-effectiveness analysis predictably reveals that among women over age 65 triennial screening reduces mortality by 74% at a cost of $2254 per year of life saved. Continuing to screen women over age 65 who have had regular screening in the past (with normal cytologies) is not cost-effective, with little additional survival benefit.[37]

In addition to avoiding repeated screening in women over age 65, screening is also unnecessary in women who have never had sexual intercourse and those who have undergone total hysterectomy for benign lesions. The clinician must recognize, however, those patients who have undergone *partial* hysterectomies in which the cervical stump has not been removed continue to be at risk for cervical cancer. Providers should consider performing an initial speculum exam on newly encountered patients to clarify their anatomy.

The greatest challenge in the prevention of cervical cancer is compliance. In most cases, this involves overcoming socioeconomic and educational barriers. Several epidemiologic studies have established that rates of receipt of Pap smear are adversely impacted by lower income, lower level of education, and urban location. It is unclear if Medicare funding for the procedure has improved rates over the last decade. Additionally, once the procedure is performed, adequate follow-up is impeded by several factors, including older age.[38] Studies demonstrate that most of these barriers may be overcome by provider and patient education and improved social support.[28]

Groups issuing recommendations for cervical cancer screening generally agree on the performance of Pap smears at least every 3 years in women who have a uterine cervix and who have had sexual intercourse in the past. The American Cancer Society sets no specific upper age limit, whereas the Canadian Task Force recommends stopping at age 69. The USPSTF recommends suspending screening at age 65 if the woman has had repeatedly normal smears (see Table 32.3).

The authors concur with the recommendations of the USPSTF with the following amendments:

1. Take a careful history of prior Pap smears and potential risk factors in all women, regardless of age.
2. In women with a history of hysterectomy, perform initial speculum examination to clarify anatomy before excluding from screening.
3. If a woman is sexually active and has a life expectancy of greater than 5 to 7 years, consider offering continued screening beyond age 65.

Ovarian Cancer

Compared to other cancers covered in this chapter, the overall prevalence of ovarian cancer is low. An estimated 23,300 new cases of ovarian cancer and 13,900 deaths were expected in 2000.[5] The lifetime probability of developing ovarian cancer is about 1 in 60, and 46% of cases and 67% of deaths occur in women over age 65.[6] Ovarian cancer continues to be the most frequent cause of death from any gynecologic malignancy, excluding breast cancer, in the United States. The high case fatality to incidence ratio reflects the fact that less than 25% of patients who present with ovarian cancer have disease localized to the ovary.[5] Only lung and stomach cancer have lower proportions of patients who present with localized disease. Because a majority of women who present with ovarian cancer have either regional or distant metastases at the time of diagnosis, the 5-year survival rate is low, approximately 50% for all stages.[6] Five-year survival rates are particularly low for women who are over age 65 at initial diagnosis, that is, 31%, compared to 64% for women who are younger than age 65.[6] Despite new surgical and chemotherapeutic regimens, there has been almost no change in the age-adjusted death rate from ovarian cancer in the past 30 years. However, 5-year survival is excellent for women who present with localized disease, approximately 95%, and does not vary according to age at diagnosis.[6] This finding has perpetuated a search for new and more effective screening methods.

The major difficulty with ovarian cancer is that symptoms do not usually develop until patients experience complications of advanced disease, a stage for which therapy is only palliative. It is unlikely that any strategy that relies on symptom recognition or clinical examination will ever improve detection rates or change the 5-year survival rates in this disease. Thus, screening strategies that utilize more detailed radiologic or chemical assessment need to be developed. Due to the low incidence of disease, however, these screening strategies must be highly sensitive and specific before any strategy is considered for mass screening.

Three major screening tests are available for detecting early ovarian cancer: pelvic examination, ultrasound imaging, and monoclonal antibodies such as CA 125. There is no evidence that any frequency of pelvic examination leads to increased case-finding for early ovarian cancer. In the few studies that have evaluated the independent contribution of pelvic examination, the prevalence of ovarian cancer was too low to provide stable estimates of either sensitivity or specificity.[39]

Both abdominal and transvaginal ultrasonography have been studied extensively as screening tests. Both modes of ultrasonography are able to detect ovarian abnormalities in asymptomatic women with normal pelvic examinations. There is also more information from larger screening studies to calculate better estimates of the sensitivity and specificity of each of these tests. Carlson and colleagues reported an overall sensitivity for both ultrasound studies of 85% (95% CI, 80%–90%), based on a weighted average of all published studies.[39] The summary specificity for ultrasonography from the same studies was reported to be 93.8% (95% CI, 93.3%–94.3%). There does not appear to be a meaningful difference in either the sensitivities or specificities of these tests that would lead clinicians to prefer one above the other.

The development of monoclonal antibodies reactive to ovarian cancer-specific antibodies, particularly CA 125, was thought to be very promising with respect to ovarian cancer screening. CA 125 is elevated in 80% of women with epithelial ovarian cancer, but it is also elevated in some women with benign gynecologic conditions such as endometriosis, uterine fibroids, pelvic inflammatory disease, and ovarian cysts,[40] which lowers the sensitivity of the test compared to imaging studies such as ultrasonography. Carlson and colleagues[39] reported a summary sensitivity for CA 125 based on a reference value of 35 U/mL of only 78% (95% CI, 73%–83%) and a summary specificity of 98.9% (95% CI, 98.6%–99.2%). No information is available for any of these tests concerning the potential differential performance in young versus older women.

A recent randomized controlled trial evaluated the feasibility and potential effectiveness of a two-step screening strategy using first, CA 125 and second, pelvic ultrasound for women with CA 125 values of greater than or equal to 30 U/mL compared to no screening in approximately 22,000 women in the United Kingdom.[41] In this 3-year trial, women over age 45 were highly compliant with the screening strategy, with 86% completing at least one screen. Of the 29 women in the screening group who went on to surgical evaluation, 6 had a cancer (positive predictive value = 21%). In women who developed cancer, survival was longer in the screening group compared to the no screening group, but the overall mortality from index cancers did not differ between the two groups. The study, however, was not powered to detect a difference in overall mortality. This trial tells us that a screening strategy is feasible in a highly motivated group of women, but a much larger trial must be done before we can understand if this method of early detection reduces mortality from ovarian cancer.

The best evidence concerning the impact of screening tests is still derived from a decision model designed to evaluate both CA 125 antigen level and ultrasonography. Shapira et al. performed a decision analysis in which they modeled a screening strategy including transvaginal ultrasound and utilization of CA 125.[42] The combined sensitivity and specificity of this strategy were 81% and 99.95%, respectively. Even with this near perfect specificity, eight false-positive results are obtained for every early-stage cancer detected. Overall, the screening strategy resulted in a less than 1-day increase in the average life expectancy.

Ovarian cancer fulfills several of the important criteria for screening. It is an important disease that leads to premature mortality. The early-stage forms of the cancer can be treated effectively, and good screening tests exist. The main problem with advocating a mass screening strategy is that the disease has a relatively low overall prevalence. In diseases of low prevalence, high test specificity is crucial to minimize the ratio of false to true positives. A decision analysis model documented that the threshold value for test specificity below which a no-screening strategy would be preferred over screening was very high, 98.53%,[42] which implies that screening for ovarian cancer will never be feasible unless the specificity of the test is nearly perfect. A randomized controlled trial that enrolled 22,000 women has not added sufficient evidence to adopt this screening strategy.[41] Because of this lack of evidence, both the U.S. Preventive Services Task Force and the American College of Physicians state that routine screening for ovarian cancer is not recommended.[30,39] The American Cancer Society does not make a recommendation for routine screening for ovarian cancer for any aged population (see Table 32.3).[29]

Although ovarian cancer is more prevalent and more deadly than cervical cancer, there are no currently available screening tests or combination of tests that provide sufficiently high sensitivities and specificities to warrant mass screening. Until new screening tests are developed or until a more definitive trial evaluating the combination of CA 125 and ultrasonography is performed, it is not prudent to routinely screen women for ovarian cancer at any age.

Prostate Cancer

Prostate cancer is the most common cancer in men and the second leading cause of cancer mortality. Based on projections, 189,000 men are expected to be diagnosed with prostate cancer and 30,200 men are expected to die of the disease in 2002.[5] In the late 1990s, prostate cancer death rates began to decrease. Prostate cancer incidence rates are also dropping after a significant increase coincident with the rapid assimilation of prostate-specific antigen (PSA) testing that occurred in the early 1990s. As with many cancers that we have discussed, prostate cancer is a disease of older people. The incidence and mortality for men over age 65 is 1025 per 100,000 and 226 per 100,000 men, respectively. The incidence and mortality for men under age 65 is 50 per 100,000 and 2.6 per 100,000, respectively.[6] More than 80% of cases occur in men over age 65, and fully half of the deaths from prostate cancer occur in men over age 74. For men, the lifetime risk of being diagnosed with prostate cancer is 16%, and the lifetime risk of dying from the disease is 3.4%.[6]

Despite an incomplete understanding of the cause of prostate cancer, two factors identify patients as being at higher risk for developing and dying of the disease. First, advanced age is the dominant risk factor. Second, African-American men experience the highest rate of developing and dying of prostate cancer of any racial group; their risk is approximately twice that of white men and four times that of Asian men.[6] Having a family history of prostate cancer in a first-degree relative also confers an elevated risk.

Although the natural history of prostate cancer is not well understood, it is clear that patients diagnosed with localized disease have better survival rates. The 5-year survival rate for men diagnosed with local disease is 80%, compared to 8% for those with evidence of distant metastases at diagnosis.[6] Whether this favorable survival rate is due to effective treatment given for limited-stage disease or because of lead-time or length-time biases remains unclear. An additional confounder in the survival data is the fact that some men, particularly older men, may have less aggressive forms of prostate cancer and therefore may be much less likely to die of the disease. Autopsy studies have consistently shown that the majority of men over age 60 have evidence of prostate cancer at death, yet only a small percentage has clinically evident disease.[43]

The two principal screening tests used to detect early prostate cancer are the digital rectal examination (DRE) and the serum PSA. It is widely recognized that the DRE has limited usefulness in any early detection strategy. In the best of hands, the sensitivity of DRE for prostate cancer is only 33% with positive likelihood ratios of only 1.5 to 2.0 for organ-confined tumors.[44] Because of this poor sensitivity, a normal test does not significantly lower the odds of having prostate cancer. Serum PSA is an alternative method of screening that has become widely utilized. PSA is highly specific for the prostate, but elevated blood levels are not specific for prostate cancer. This fact significantly deteriorates its sensitivity. The normal range is taken to be 0 to 4 ng/mL, but several common prostatic disorders (e.g., prostatitis, benign hyperplasia) may raise PSA levels beyond this range. Likelihood ratios for different PSA cutpoints are shown in Table 32.4. Men whose PSA levels are elevated above 4.0 ng/mL have an approximate threefold increased odds of having organ-confined prostate cancer.

There is evidence that DRE and PSA may detect different prostate cancers, posterior lobe versus periuretheral cancers, respectively. Therefore, clinicians that advocate screening most often use both tests.[44] Because this strategy increases the number of men identified with abnormal findings, combined testing may increase subsequent testing, treatment, and the associated morbidity. Approximately one in four asymptomatic men have an elevated PSA or abnormal DRE.[44] Furthermore, there is no evidence that any screening or treatment strategy improves survival. Current trials and observational studies are underway.[45]

Until these studies are completed and improved information is available concerning the role of screening and treatment in this disease, no currently available test or combination of tests is sufficiently accurate for detecting localized prostate cancer. As with other cancers for which the evidence is either inconclusive or not available, there are discordant recommendations from the various professional societies. The American Cancer Society recom-

TABLE 32.4. Likelihood ratios for PSA at different cutpoints.

PSA level	Likelihood ratio[a]	
	Intracapsular Tumor	Extracapsular Tumor
<4.0 ng/ml	0.7 to 0.98	0.09 to 0.5
4.1–10 ng/ml	1.4 to 3.0	3.2 to 5.1
>10 ng/ml	0.4 to 3.0	23.7 to 49.6

PSA, prostate-specific antigen.
[a] Ranges derived from available studies where volunteers were included and submitted to reference standard test (biopsy) to allow calculation of likelihood ratios.
Source: Adapted from Coley CM, Barry MJ, Fleming C, Mulley AG. Early detection of prostate cancer. Part I: Prior probability and effectiveness of tests. *Ann Intern Med*. 1997;126:394–406,[44] with permission.

mends DRE plus PSA annually in men older than 50 years.[6] Their recommendation is similar to the American Urological Association. The U.S. Preventive Services Task Force does not recommend routine screening for prostate cancer with any available tests (see Table 32.3). An expert panel for the American College of Physicians has recently reviewed the evidence for prostate cancer screening and treatment.[46] They recommend that physicians should be prepared to discuss the benefits and harms of screening, diagnosis, and treatment and then assist men in making individual decisions. We concur with the recommendations of the American College of Physicians.

Colorectal Cancer

Colorectal cancer is the third leading cause of cancer and cancer-related death among both men and women in the United States. Recent projects estimated that 107,300 new cases would be diagnosed in 2002 and that more than 48,100 people would die of the disease.[5] Data from the surveillance, epidemiology, and end results (SEER) program, however, show that between 1985 and 1997 the overall incidence of colorectal cancer dropped by 9% to 43.9 cases per 100,000. Mortality has declined as well over the same period to 16.4 deaths per 100,000. Despite these trends, colorectal cancer continues to be a disease of late life. Age-adjusted incidence rates rise from 17.1 cases per 100,000 in patients under 65 to 287.8 cases per 100,000 in those over 65. This increase continues without plateau to 450 cases per 100,000 in patients over 85. Mortality, likewise, increases with age, from 5.7 deaths per 100,000 in those under 65 to 120 deaths per 100,000 in those over 65.[6]

Traditional factors that increase risk for colorectal cancer include inherited disorders such as familial polyposis, family history of colorectal cancer in a first-degree relative, and inflammatory bowel disease. For patients with colorectal cancer diagnosed over age 65, however, family history appears to play a less significant role.[47]

The natural history of colorectal cancer is well understood. The majority of cancers evolve from premalignant adenomas. The estimated time for progression from an adenomatous polyp to cancer is 5 to 10 years. Removal of these slowly growing lesions prevents the development of cancer. Predictably, the 5-year survival associated with an early lesion is very favorable compared with more advanced disease. For localized disease, 5-year survival is 90%, compared to 64% for regional spread and 8% for disease with distant metastases. Because of its prolonged detectable preclinical phase and responsiveness to therapy in early stages, colorectal cancer is an excellent candidate for screening.

For patients of average risk, digital rectal examination (DRE), fecal occult blood testing (FOBT), flexible sig-

moidoscopy, air contrast barium enema, and colonoscopy are commonly considered screening tests. Among these, DRE has the least supporting evidence. In retrospective analyses, less than 10% of colorectal cancers are within a finger's reach of the anus. In addition, a case-control study in patients with rectal carcinoma revealed no survival benefit with recent DRE.[48] It is still unclear if hemoccult of stool obtained via DRE is an adequate substitute for FOBT.

In contrast, FOBT boasts the strongest level of supporting evidence of any of the tests. The most commonly used is the Hemoccult test, but several other options now exist, including immunologic assays. Test utility relies on the fact that early cancers and some polyps bleed occultly, allowing early detection. In large trials with high rates of compliance, sensitivity is estimated to be 50% to 90%.[49] Specificity varies less, with estimates of 90% to 98%. The test characteristics appear dependent on a number of factors, including rehydration status of the sample and frequency of testing.[50] A recently proposed strategy initially screens patients with the traditional Hemoccult followed by confirmation of positive tests with an immunologic assay. Theoretically, this method would maintain sensitivity while maximizing specificity.[49] Standard follow-up for a positive screen with FOBT (one or more positive samples) is colonoscopy. The combination of flexible sigmoidoscopy and air contrast barium enema has been used frequently as an alternative in patients unable to tolerate colonoscopy.[51]

Five major prospective trials of FOBT have been conducted comparing screened versus unscreened populations. The trials unanimously demonstrate a mortality reduction in patients using FOBT (12%–43%).[49] This benefit appears to extend to the elderly, with similar reductions in mortality in subgroup analyses.[50] Inconsistencies in methods among the trials deserve note, however. The Minnesota trial examined rehydrated samples, resulting in a much higher positive rate compared with other studies (9% versus 1%–2%). This trial also reported a higher overall mortality reduction (33% versus 12%–18%). Critics speculate that the additional mortality reduction resulted from the "excess" number of colonoscopies performed due to "false" positives. Of note, the positivity rate among patients over 80 years old in this study was 16%. Nonetheless, in the remaining studies, a smaller but significant mortality benefit was found. Review of the optimal frequency of screening with FOBT using the trial data just cited reveals a significant survival advantage with annual versus biennial screening.[51]

Flexible sigmoidoscopy has become the other mainstay of colorectal cancer screening. Use of a 60-cm flexible scope allows direct visualization of the rectosigmoid and descending colon. Indications for follow-up colonoscopy include adenomatous polyps smaller than 1 cm, any polyp larger than 1 cm, or cancerous-appearing lesions. Its sensitivity, as estimated for only the portion of bowel within the reach of the scope, is 96.7% for cancers and large polyps and 73.3% for small polyps. Specificity is estimated to be 94% for cancers and 92% for small polyps.[51] The major complication is perforation, which occurs approximately once in every 10,000 procedures.

Two recent studies have also helped clarify the relationship between distal findings and proximal disease. Researchers performed colonoscopies in asymptomatic individuals and found that the presence of larger adenomas (>1 cm), adenomas with high-grade dysplasia, or invasive cancer in the distal colon predicated the presence of proximal colon lesions.[52,53] However, in half of those found to have advanced proximal neoplasia, no distal findings were present. Additionally, both studies found that increasing age predicted more advanced neoplasia in the lesions discovered through colonoscopy.

The best evidence supporting a mortality benefit from screening flexible sigmoidoscopy is a case-control study of 261 HMO members who died of cancer arising in the distal colon or rectum (case group) and 868 matched controls. Investigators observed that control patients were three times more likely than cases to have undergone screening with flexible sigmoidoscopy in the 10 years preceding the diagnosis of cancer. A subgroup analysis revealed that the survival benefit was limited to cancers within the reach of the sigmoidoscope. Further analysis found that the protective effect of this procedure extended up to 10 years.[54] Screening flexible sigmoidoscopy is currently under investigation in the PLCO trial, a 16-year randomized controlled trial of screening procedures for prostate, lung, colorectal, and ovarian cancer.

Most recommendations currently support a combination of annual FOBT and flexible sigmoidoscopy every 3 to 5 years. There is scant specific evidence for this schedule of screening, but many support the rationale that the combination provides improved surveillance of the entire colon.[51]

Considering the anatomic limitations of flexible sigmoidoscopy and the imperfect performance characteristics of FOBT, colonoscopy presents an attractive alternative for screening. Endoscopic visualization of the entire colon requires conscious sedation and has a somewhat higher complication rate (perforation in 1 of 1000 procedures), but it delivers a high sensitivity for small polyps (78.5%) and high specificity (98%) for all lesions.[51] The performance of colonoscopy in selected patients over 80 years of age resulted in a complication rate comparable to the younger population.[55] Direct evidence for its use as a screening tool is still lacking, but observational data from the National Polyp Study and a large VA case-control study indicate a significant mortality benefit. Major questions remain, however, regarding the cost-

effectiveness and feasibility of widespread screening with colonoscopy. Newer radiologic studies may afford the same views using computed tomography (CT) scanning. These virtual colonoscopies are currently under study as diagnostic tools but may offer older patients a safer means of screening for colorectal cancer.[56]

An alternative means of "total colonic" screening is air contrast barium enema. Although it has a lower complication rate than colonoscopy and comparable performance characteristics in large polyps (>1 cm) and cancers, its utility is limited by its insensitivity for small polyps (about 50% for polyps <1 cm) and lack of evidence for impact on mortality. Most experts feel that it is most appropriately employed in combination with flexible sigmoidoscopy for follow-up of positive FOBT in patients who cannot tolerate colonoscopy. This combination has achieved a sensitivity of 98%.[51]

Despite the available evidence that colorectal cancer is amenable to screening, compliance remains poor. Compliance with FOBT ranges from 30% to 90%. For flexible sigmoidscopy, rates are estimated to be 30% to 50%. Predictors of participation include family history of colorectal cancer, female gender, and higher level of education and, specifically, knowledge of risks of colorectal cancer.[57] For flexible sigmoidoscopy, although patients admit to experiencing pain and embarrassment, most state that they would undergo the procedure again, considering its potential benefit.[58]

Due to the different procedures available, recommendations for screening for colorectal cancer are varied. The American Cancer Society issued an updated set of recommendations in 2001. For adults over 50 years of age at average risk of colorectal cancer, one of the following maneuvers is recommended: (1) FOBT yearly, (2) flexible sigmoidoscopy every 5 years beginning at age 50, (3) a combination of annual FOBT and flexible sigmoidoscopy every 5 years (preferred to either test alone), (4) double-contrast barium enema every 5 years, or (5) colonoscopy every 10 years.[59] These guidelines set no upper age at which to suspend screening, suggesting instead that screening be continued as long as the elderly patient is in good health. Recent recommendations from the USPSTF and the Canadian Task Force strongly recommend screening for colorectal cancer in all average risk adults over age 50. Both organizations recognize that the strongest evidence exists supporting the use of annual or biennial FOBT and periodic flexible sigmoidoscopy. The USPSTF further indicates support for use of colonoscopy based on its superior diagnostic performance in examining the entire colon. (Table 32.3) A recent study also demonstrated the relative cost-effectiveness of all of these methods of colorectal cancer screening (less than $30,000 per life year gained).[91,92]

The authors recognize that screening for colorectal cancer has the potential to prevent an enormous amount of morbidity and mortality. Considering the evidence available at this time, options 1, 2, or 3 listed above are valid screening regimens. If the patient has a life expectancy of 5 to 7 years, a discussion of the potential risks and benefits of the various options should ensue. If the patient accepts screening, then the provider should guide him or her in selecting a specific screening regimen, taking into account preferences for the use of initially invasive versus noninvasive techniques. With the high rate of proximal neoplasia in older patients, studies of the efficacy, safety, and cost-effectiveness of screening colonoscopy should be monitored carefully by those providing primary care for the elderly, because this strategy may become preferred in subsequent years.

Lung Cancer

Lung cancer is the leading cause of cancer-related death for both men and women in the United States. Each year, more people die of lung cancer than breast, prostate, and colon cancer combined. Lung cancer, traditionally a disease of men, is increasingly prevalent in women, and deaths from lung cancer now exceed those from breast cancer among women.[6] In 2000, there were approximately 164,000 new cases of lung cancer, resulting in 157,000 deaths.[5,6] The incidence rates for lung cancer increase with age, beginning at 40 years and peaking at about age 70 to 75 years. The incidence rates of lung cancer for men aged 65 and older is 481 per 100,000 compared with a rate of 24 per 100,000 in men under age 64.[6] The incidence rate in women over age 65 is 253 per 100,000, a rate rapidly approaching the rate in men.[6]

Cigarette smoking is the major risk factor for developing lung cancer, and this risk dramatically increases with duration of tobacco use and the quantity of cigarettes smoked. Incidence rates for lung cancer are about 10 times higher in smokers versus nonsmokers.[60] Asbestos, radon gas, and several environmental agents (including chromate, nickel, polyhydrocarbons, and alkylating compounds) have also been demonstrated to increase lung cancer risk.[61,62] Advanced-stage lung cancer is particularly lethal, with 5-year survival remaining under 2%.[6] When lung cancer is localized at diagnosis, 5-year survival rate is 48%, a difference that affords a window of opportunity for screening. Surgical resection of localized cancer offers the only real potential for long-term cure.

Asymptomatic lung cancer can be detected by plain chest radiography or sputum cytology. Practically speaking, however, the discovery of "silent" lung cancer usually occurs during the investigation of a patient's nonspecific complaints (for example, cough, fatigue, weight loss). With both tests, there are problems of performance and interpretation that diminish their overall accuracy and usefulness. Screening chest radiographs are hampered by operational problems (radiographic technique, exposure) and by problems in the interpretation of the radiograph itself. In fact, significant disagreement between radiologists often occurs.[63] Similarly, screening with sputum cytology has the difficulties associated with obtaining adequate sputum samples and the problems of pathologic interpretation of the sputum cells. Finally, both chest radiography and sputum cytology require the "reference standard" of tissue biopsy to confirm the screening test result. With these inherent problems, determining the sensitivity of these tests is very difficult. Additionally, because patients with negative tests rarely receive further evaluation, specificity is difficult to estimate.

The high incidence rate and poor prognosis of lung cancer prompted three randomized trials of mass screening to detect and treat early-stage disease in the United States. In the Memorial Sloan-Kettering trial,[64] 10,040 male smokers over age 45 were randomized to receive either annual chest radiography plus sputum cytology every 4 months or annual chest radiographs alone. The trial at Johns Hopkins[65] was designed identically with more than 10,000 participants. Both trials followed study participants for 6 years. There were no differences in the lung cancer survival rates between the screened and control populations.

The Mayo Clinic trial[66] had a different design but similar results. The 10,900 study participants, relatively few of which were over 65, were assessed initially with chest radiography and sputum cytology to detect prevalent cases of lung cancers. All subjects who did not have lung cancer were then randomized. A screened group received chest radiography and sputum cytology every 4 months for 6 years. The control group was advised at baseline to obtain annual chest radiography and sputum cytology, but this advice was not repeated. About 50% of the control group obtained chest radiographs during the follow-up period. More cancers were discovered in the screened group, slightly more lung cancer deaths in the screened group, and no significant differences in mortality rates between the screened group (13.2 deaths per 1000 person-years) and the control group (13.0 deaths per 1000 person-years).

Despite the disheartening results from these trials, new advances in diagnostic testing are being evaluated. Currently, the "new" technology for early detection of lung cancer is low-dose spiral computed tomography (CT). Two recent studies suggested that spiral CT is more sensitive for the detection of noncalcified pulmonary nodules and early lung cancers.[67,68] Still, the test is not very specific, with a high false-positive rate. In the Early Lung Cancer Action Project, the positive predictive value of spiral CT was only 12% for detection of lung cancer.[67] These new studies have rekindled old controversies about the effectiveness of mass screening for lung cancer.

The full extent of the reemerging controversy for or against early detection of lung cancer was summarized in two recent papers.[69,70] Relying on essentially the same scientific evidence, Petty asserted that it is now time to embark on mass screening,[69] while Frame cautioned that the technology is not yet of proven value.[70] Fortunately, the National Cancer Institute (NCI) has supported the design of a multicenter, randomized, controlled trial of 7,000 persons at high risk for developing lung cancer.[71] The NCI is considering also an even larger trial with nearly 90,000 participants to evaluate whether these "new" technologies will reduce mortality from lung cancer.

Despite these recent studies, virtually all organizations (American Cancer Society, National Cancer Institute, U.S. Preventive Services Task Force, American College of Physicians, and the Canadian Task Force) concur that mass screening for lung cancer is not efficacious. However, elderly subjects were not adequately represented in the cancer screening trials even though they represent one of the highest risk groups. Whether selective screening for lung cancer in elderly smokers is useful remains to be established. Some studies suggest that lung cancer detected in older aged groups is more likely to occur at the local stage, and thus the possibility of surgical cure may be greater.[72] Additional research is needed to assess the efficacy of selective screening in this targeted high-risk group. At present, no advisory society or task force recommends screening for lung cancer in any group with any test at any frequency (see Table 32.3).

Oral Cancer

There were an estimated 28,900 new cases and 7400 deaths from oral cancer in the United States in 2002.[5] Two-thirds of the cases and 65% of the deaths occurred in men. The overall 5-year survival is poor and has not changed in the last 30 years. Five-year survival ranges from 21% for patients with distant spread at diagnosis to 81% for patients with localized disease.[6] As with all cancers we have reported in this chapter, oral cancer incidence increases with advancing age. The age effect in incidence and mortality, however, is not as steep as it is for other cancers; both rates plateau by age 65. Persons over age 65 account for approximately 50% of all cases and a majority of all deaths attributable to oral cancer.[73] In addition to advancing age as a risk factor for developing oral cancer, men experience approximately twofold increased incidence compared to women. This gender difference is most likely attributable to the increased prevalence of smoking in men, although this is diminishing as smoking becomes equally prevalent in men and women. Other risk factors include excessive alcohol intake, use of smokeless tobacco, and family history of oral cancer.

Approximately 96% of all oral cancers are squamous cell carcinomas, implying that the majority of these cancers begin on the mucosal surfaces.[74] However, the natural history of oral cancer is not as well described as it is for other cancers. Leukoplakia and erythroplakia are two precancerous lesions that may progress to squamous cell carcinoma, although not all oral cancer arises from one of these lesions. The prevalence of leukoplakia ranges from 0.2% to 11%, depending on the patient population, while erythroplakia is rare with an incidence of less than 0.1%.[75] Good evidence concerning the rates of transformation to oral cancer for either of these lesions is lacking.

Arguments for screening for oral cancer involve detecting and treating leukoplakia, erythroplakia, or early-stage squamous carcinoma before more extensive local spreading. Early detection does improve survival, a fact that provides the main argument for proponents of mass screening. A 2-cm tongue squamous cell carcinoma has a 90% cure rate with radiation therapy or local resection, with minimal treatment-associated morbidity. A lesion about twice that size may require total glossectomy and radiation with a cure rate of only 20%.[76]

Inspection and palpation of the oral cavity are the principal screening tests available for oral cancer. The reason that palpation is suggested in addition to inspection is that the majority of oral cancers arise on the lateral aspects of the tongue and on the floor of the mouth, making detection difficult with routine inspection. The recommended examination technique involves exploration of the oral cavity with a gloved hand using a gauze pad to retract the tongue and expose the ventral and posterolateral surfaces in addition to the floor of the mouth.[75] The sensitivity and specificity of this screening exam depend on the skill of the examiner and the criteria used to define a positive test. Maximum sensitivities have ranged from 71% to 81%, with specificity of 99% when screening is performed by dental practitioners.[77]

Several researchers have attempted to improve the performance of the clinical examination by visual enhancement of cancerous or precancerous lesions with vital staining agents such as toluidine blue. The use of this agent may improve the sensitivity of the oral examination (as high as 100% in one study) but at the expense of lower specificity.[75] No organization currently recommends use of toluidine blue or other agents until further research is conducted.

Because of an incomplete understanding of the natural history of the precancerous lesion, the utility of population screening for oral cancer is in question. If all patients with leukoplakia were classified as positive screenees, significant overdiagnosis and potentially overtreatment would occur. Most researchers require stronger levels of evidence before adopting screening for oral cancer. Unfortunately, as Rodrigues and colleagues have pointed out, a study designed to detect a 20% difference in mortality from oral cancer between a screened and unscreened group would require 1.4 million subjects.[75] It is unlikely that this large study will ever be done.

Until more definitive studies documenting the efficacy of the screening oral examination are published, there is insufficient evidence to warrant routine screening for all elderly patients, despite the increased risk in this population. Dentists should continue to examine elderly patients for evidence of oral cancer, although they will see only a minority of at-risk individuals. We believe that it is prudent for physicians to screen higher-risk elderly patients with a history of tobacco exposure or excessive amounts of alcohol. This recommendation mirrors the recommendation of the USPSTF. Despite the paucity of clinical evidence on the efficacy of oral examination, the American Cancer Society recommends a complete gloved oral examination as part of the routine cancer checkup (see Table 32.3).

Skin Cancer

Nonmelanoma skin cancer (NMSC), consisting of both basal and squamous cell cancers, is the most common cancer in the United States, with an estimated annual incidence of 800,000.[78] These cancers are readily diagnosed, highly treatable, and rarely metastasize. Basal cell carcinomas account for 80% of all NMSC.[79] They arise most commonly on the head and neck, although they can be found in sun-protected areas. Squamous cell carcinoma has a much higher proclivity for sun-exposed areas. Seventy-five percent of lesions are found on the face, 15% on the upper extremity, and 10% elsewhere.[80] Unlike basal cell carcinoma, squamous cell carcinoma has a higher tendency for metastasis (3%–11%). In a population-based study of NMSC, deaths from squamous cell carcinoma outnumbered deaths from basal cell carcinoma by 3:1.[81] The incidence of both NMSC increases markedly with age because they are thought to be associated with cumulative lifetime sun exposure.

Malignant melanoma is less common than NMSC, but it carries a much graver prognosis and, accordingly, accounts for 75% of all skin cancer deaths. In 2002, approximately 53,600 new cases of melanoma were diagnosed and 7400 people died of their disease.[5] The lifetime cumulative risk of developing melanoma is 1 in 90, making it the eighth most common cancer in the United States. More importantly, unlike many cancers, the incidence of melanoma has doubled in the past decade, and the incidence is not leveling off. Like many cancers, melanoma has a greater impact in older patients: 36% of cases and 54% of deaths from the disease occur in patients over age 65.[6]

Risk factors that increase the likelihood of developing both NMSC and melanoma have been established. For NMSC, older age, fair complexion, prior NMSC, poor ability to tan, and cumulative lifetime sun exposure are identified risk factors.[82] Similar risk factors increase the likelihood of developing melanoma. Recent research has extended risk factor assessment to develop personal risk factor scales that could be used in population-based screening. The MacKie risk factor flowchart has undergone the greatest degree of clinical evaluation.[83,84] This flowchart asks patients to answer four questions: (1) Does your skin have freckles or tendency to freckling? (2) Does you skin have moles? (3) Does your skin have any large moles with irregular borders? and (4) How many times in your life have you had a bad sunburn (0, 1 or 2, 3+)? Primary care patients have been shown to provide reliable answers when compared with dermatologists' examination. In primary care practices, approximately 4% of patients fall in a very high risk category.[84] However, it has not been established that widespread use of this or any risk stratification flowchart reduces morbidity or mortality from any skin cancer.

There is evidence that treatment of early-stage NMSC and melanoma confers improved outcomes for patients identified early. Early treatment of NMSC reduces disfigurement and may improve quality of life. In malignant melanoma, survival is closely linked to the thickness of the tumor, termed Breslow thickness. Approximately 40% of patients present with thin tumors (<1.5 mm); their 5-year survival is 93%. For the 30% who present with midthickness tumors (1.5–3.49 mm), 5-year survival drops to 67%. Last, for the 30% of patients who present with tumor thickness greater than 3.5 mm, 5-year survival is only 37%.[85] Unfortunately, no study has been published that establishes the efficacy of screening for skin cancer.

The primary screening test available for detecting early-stage skin cancer is physical examination of the skin by a clinician. However, no data from experimental studies support the efficacy of any frequency of screening by any clinician in any risk group. The primary problem is that the disease is rare and the sensitivity and specificity of the skin examination are poor. Estimates of sensitivity (30%–98%) and specificity (45%–95%) of screening by dermatologists vary widely across different studies.[86,87] Primary care clinicians who do not routinely evaluate skin lesions are no better than dermatologists: sensitivity, 57% and specificity, 88%.[88]

Despite the lack of evidence establishing efficacy for skin examination as a screening test for any skin cancer, the American Cancer Society recommends monthly skin self-examination for all adults and annual skin examination by clinicians for all people over 40 years old.[89] The USPSTF concludes that there is poor evidence to support screening for skin cancer with any currently available modality (see Table 32.3). The National Institutes of Health Consensus Development Panel recommends skill self-examination and skin as part of the periodic health examination.[90] Lastly the American College of Preventive Medicine issued a recent statement on skin cancer prevention and early screening. They state that high-risk individuals (based on family history, history of previous skin cancers, fair skin, or multiple nevi) should be screened periodically but that low-risk individuals cannot be recommended for screening.[79] They also state that physicians performing screening should receive adequate training to ensure high-quality examinations. The authors believe that the American College of Preventive Medicine's recommendation seems prudent for high-risk elderly. Until total skin examination is proven to be efficacious, the additional time and expense are not warranted. The frequency of any screening strategy has not been determined.

Summary

Screening for cancer has been an important component of comprehensive primary care for decades. Because most research projects designed to determine the efficacy of individual screening strategies require such large sample sizes and long follow-up periods, there is relatively little high-grade evidence to support specific screening strategies. Additionally, relatively few of the available studies enrolled a sufficient number of older patients to allow accurate generalization of efficacy to this population. Nevertheless, patients, providers, and health care systems are interested in screening. Additionally, there is epidemiologic evidence to support the importance of cancer as a leading killer in the elderly. In this chapter, we have summarized the evidence for or against screening for eight of the most common and deadly cancers. We find sufficient evidence to recommend screening for breast, cervical, and colorectal cancer. A decision to screen for prostate cancer requires individual discussions and cannot be justified in a blanket statement. We do not recommend screening for lung, ovarian, skin, or oral cancer at present. Providers should be encouraged to keep abreast of ongoing studies that will further direct the debate on screening for cancer in the elderly.

References

1. Sackett DL, Haynes RB, Guyatt GH, Tugwell P. *Clinical Epidemiology: A Basic Science for Clinical Medicine.* Boston: Little, Brown; 1991:153–170.
2. Walter LC, Covinsky KE. Cancer screening in elderly patients: a framework for individualized decision making. *JAMA.* 2001;285:2750–2756.
3. Satariano WA, Ragland DR. The effect of comorbidity on 3-year survival of women with primary breast cancer. *Ann Intern Med.* 1994;120:104–110.
4. Yancik R, Wesley MN, Ries LAG, et al. Comorbidity and age as predictors of risk for early mortality of male and female colon carcinoma patients: a population-based study. *Cancer.* 1998;82:2123–2134.
5. Jernal A, Thomas A, Murray T, et al. Cancer statistics, 2002. *CA Cancer J Clin.* 2002;52:23–47.
6. Ries LAG, Eisner MP, Dosary CL, et al., eds. *SEER Cancer Statistics and Review 1973–1997.* Bethesda, MD: National Cancer Institute; 2000.
7. Cauley AJ, Lucas FL, Kuller LH, Vogt MT, Browner WS, Cummings SR. Bone mineral density and risk of breast cancer in older women. *JAMA.* 1996;276:1404–1408.
8. Zhang Y, Kiel DP, Kreger BE. Bone mass and the risk of breast cancer among postmenopausal women. *N Engl J Med.* 1997;336:611–617.
9. Clark GM. The biology of breast cancer in older women. *J Gerontol.* 1992;47:19–23.
10. Semiglazov VF, Moiseyenko VM. Breast self examination for the early detection of breast cancer: a USSR/WHO controlled trial in Leningrad. *Bull WHO.* 1987;65:355–365.
11. Thomas D, Gao D, Self S, Allison C, Porter P. Randomized trial of breast self-examination in Shanghai: methodology and preliminary results. *J Natl Cancer Inst.* 1997;89:355–365.
12. O'Malley JS, Fletcher SW. Screening for breast cancer with breast self-examination. *JAMA.* 1987;257:2196.
13. Fletcher SW, O'Malley MS, Bunce LA. Physicians' abilities to detect lumps in silicone breast models. *JAMA.* 1985;253:2224–2228.
14. Kerlikowske K, Grady D, Barclay J, Sickles EA, Ernster V. Effect of age, breast density and family history on the sensitivity of first screening mammography. *JAMA.* 1996;276:33–38.
15. Fletcher SW, Black W, Harris R, Rimer BK, Shapiro S. Report of the international workshop on screening for breast cancer. *J Natl Cancer Inst.* 1993;85:1644–1656.
16. Kerlikowske K, Grady D, Barclay J, Sickles EA, Eaton A, Ernster V. Positive predictive value of screening mammography by age and family history of breast cancer. *JAMA.* 1993;270:2444–2450.
17. Shapiro S, Venet W, Strax P, et al. Ten to 14-year effect of screening on breast cancer mortality. *J Natl Cancer Inst.* 1982;69:349–356.
18. Nystrom L, Rutqvist LE, Wall S, et al. Breast cancer screening with mammography: overview of the Swedish randomised trials. *Lancet.* 1993;341:973–978.
19. Olsen O, Gotzsche PC. Screening for breast cancer with mammography. *Cochrane Database Syst Rev.* 2001;4:CD001877.
20. Van Dijk J, Broeders M, Verbeek A. Mammographic screening in older women: is it worthwhile? *Drugs Aging.* 1997;10:69–79.
21. McCarthy EP, Burns RB, Freund KM, et al. Mammography use, breast cancer stage at diagnosis, and survival among older women. *J Am Geriatr Soc.* 2000;48:1226–1233.
22. Mandelblatt JS, Wheat ME, Monane M, Moshief RD, Hollenberg JP, Tang J. Breast cancer screening for elderly women with and without comorbid conditions. *Ann Intern Med.* 1992;116:722–730.

23. Boer R, Koning HJ, van Oortmarssen GJ, van der Mass PJ. In search of the best upper age limit for breast cancer screening. *Eur J Cancer*. 1995;31A:2040–2043.

24. Jansen JTM, Zoetelief J. Assessment of lifetime gained as a result of mammographic breast cancer screening using a computer model. *Br J Radiol*. 1997;70:619–628.

25. Blustein J. Medicare coverage, supplemental insurance, and the use of mammography by older women. *N Engl J Med*. 1995;332:1138–1143.

26. Blustein J, Weiss LJ. The use of mammography by women aged 75 and older: factors related to health, functioning, and age. *J Am Geriatr Soc*. 1998;46:941–946.

27. Roetzheim F, Fox SA, Leake B, Houn F. The influence of risk factors on breast carcinoma screening of Medicare-insured older women. *Cancer*. 1996;78:2526–2534.

28. Fox SA, Roetzheim RG, Kington RS. Barriers to cancer prevention in the older person. *Clin Geriatr Med*. 1997;13: 79–95.

29. Smith RA, Cokkinides V, von Eschenbach AC, et al. American Cancer Society guidelines for the early detection of cancer. *CA Cancer J Clin*. 2002;52:8–22.

30. United States Preventive Services Task Force. *Guide to Clinical Preventive Services*. Baltimore: Williams & Wilkins; 1996.

31. Silverman MA, Zaidi U, Barnett S, et al. Cancer screening in the elderly population. *Hematol Oncol Clin North Am*. 2000;14:89–112.

32. Celentano DD, Shapiro S, Weisman CS. Cancer preventive screening behavior among elderly women. *Prev Med*. 1982; 11:454–463.

33. Mandelblatt J, Schecter C, Fahs M, Muller C. Clinical implications of screening for cervical cancer under Medicare. The natural history of cervical cancer in the elderly: what do we know? What do we need to know? *Am J Obstet Gynecol*. 1991;164:644–651.

34. Nanda K, McCrory DC, Myers ER, et al. Accuracy of the Papanicolaou test in screening for and follow-up of cervical cytologic abnormalities: a systematic review. *Ann Intern Med*. 2000;132:810–819.

35. Roberts AD, Denholm RB, Cordiner JW. Cervical intra-epithelial neoplasia in postmenopausal women with negative cervical cytology. *Br Med J*. 1985;290:281.

36. Eddy DM. Screening for cervical cancer. *Ann Intern Med*. 1990;113:214–226.

37. Fahs MC, Mandelblatt J, Schechter C, Muller C. *Ann Intern Med*. 1992;117:520–527.

38. Fox P, Arnsberger P, Zhang X. An examination of differential follow-up rates in cervical cancer screening. *J Community Health*. 1997;22:199–209.

39. Carlson KJ, Skates SJ, Singer DE. Screening for ovarian cancer. *Ann Intern Med*. 1994;121:124–132.

40. Bast RC Jr, Klug TL, St John E, et al. A radioimmunoassay using a monoclonal antibody to monitor the course of epithelial ovarian cancer. *N Engl J Med*. 1983;309:883–887.

41. Jacobs IJ, Skates SJ, MacDonald N, et al. Screening for ovarian cancer: a pilot randomised controlled trial. *Lancet*. 1999;353:1207–1210.

42. Schapira MM, Matchar DB, Young MJ. The effectiveness of ovarian cancer screening. A decision analysis model. *Ann Intern Med*. 1993;118:838–843.

43. Burack RC, Wood DP. Screening for prostate cancer. *Med Clin North Am*. 1999;83:1423–1442.

44. Coley CM, Barry MJ, Fleming C, Mulley AG. Early detection of prostate cancer. Part I: prior probability and effectiveness of tests. *Ann Intern Med*. 1997;126:394–406.

45. Wilt TJ. Uncertainty in prostate cancer care. *JAMA*. 2000; 283:3258–3260.

46. American College of Physicians. Screening for prostate cancer. *Ann Intern Med*. 1997;126:480–484.

47. Fuchs CS, Giovannucci EL, Colditz GA, Hunter DJ, Speizer FE, Willett WC. A prospective study of family history and the risk of colorectal cancer. *N Eng J Med*. 1994;331:1669–1674.

48. Herrington LJ, Selby JV, Friedman GD, Quesenberry CP, Weiss NS. A case-control study of digital-rectal screening in relation to mortality from cancer of the distal rectum. *Am J Epidemiol*. 1995;142:961–964.

49. Ransohoff DF, Lang CA. Screening for colorectal cancer with the fecal occult blood test: a background paper. *Ann Intern Med*. 1997;126:811–822.

50. Prindiville SA. Screening for colorectal cancer in the elderly. In: *Cancer in the Elderly*. New York: Dekker; 2000: 41–56.

51. Winawer SJ, Fletcher RH, Miller L, et al. Colorectal cancer screening: clinical guidelines and rationale. *Gastroenterology*. 1997;112:594–642.

52. Lieberman DA, Weiss DG, Bond JH, et al. Use of colonoscopy to screen asymptomatic adults for colorectal cancer. *N Engl J Med*. 2000;343:162–168.

53. Imperiale TF, Wagner DR, Lin CY, Larkin GN, Rogge JD, Ransohoff DF. Risk of advanced proximal neoplasms in asymptomatic adults according to the distal colorectal findings. *N Engl J Med*. 2000;343:169–174.

54. Selby JV, Friedman GD, Quesenberry CP, Weiss NS. A case-control study of screening sigmoidoscopy and mortality form colorectal cancer. *N Engl J Med*. 1992;326:653–657.

55. Bat L, Pines A, Shemesh E, et al. Colonoscopy in patients aged 80 or older and its contribution to the evaluation of rectal bleeding. *Postgrad Med J*. 1992;68:355–358.

56. Fenlon HM, Nunes DP, Schroy PC, Barish MA, Clarke PD, Ferrucci JT. A comparison of virtual and conventional colonoscopy for the detection of colorectal polyps. *N Engl J Med*. 1999;341:1496–1503.

57. Weinrich SP, Weinrich MC, Atwood J, Boyd M, Greene F. Predictors of fecal occult blood screening among older socioeconomically disadvantaged Americans: a replication study. *Patient Educ Counsel*. 1998;34:103–114.

58. McCarthy BD, Moskowitz MA. Screening flexible sigmoidscopy: patient attitudes and compliance. *J Gen Intern Med*. 1993;8:120–125.

59. Smith RA, von Eschenbach AC, Wender R, et al. American Cancer Society guidelines on screening and surveillance for the early detection of adenomatous polyps and cancer: update 2001. In: American Cancer Society Guidelines for the Early Detection of Cancer. Update of Early Detection Guidelines for Prostate, Colorectal, and Endometrial Cancers. Update 2001: Testing for Early Lung Cancer Detection. *CA Cancer J Clin*. 2001;51(1):38–75.

60. The Surgeon General's 1989 report on reducing the health consequences of smoking: 25 years of progress. *MMWR*. 1989;38(suppl 2):1–32.

61. Hammond EC, Selikoff IJ, Seidman H. Asbestos exposure, cigarette smoking and death rates. *Ann NY Acad Sci*. 1979; 330:473–490.

62. Roscoe RJ, Steenland K, Halperin WE, et al. Lung cancer mortality among nonsmoking uranium miners exposed to radon daughters. *JAMA*. 1989;262:629–633.

63. Herman PG, Gerson DE, Hessel SJ, et al. Disagreements in chest roentgen interpretation. *Chest*. 1975;68:278–282.

64. Melemed MR, Flehinger BJ, Zaman MB, et al. Screening for early lung cancer: results of the Memorial Sloan-Kettering study in New York. *Chest*. 1984;86:44–53.

65. Tockman MS. Survival and mortality from lung cancer in a screened population: the Johns Hopkins study. *Chest*. 1986; 89:324S–325S.

66. Fontana RS, Sanderson DR, Woolner LS, et al. Screening for lung cancer: a critique of the Mayo Lung Project. *Cancer*. 1991;67:1155–1164.

67. Henschke C, McCauley D, Yankelevitz D, et al. Early lung cancer action project: overall design and findings from baseline screening. *Lancet*. 1999;354:99–105.

68. Sone S, Takashima S, Li F, et al. Mass screening for lung cancer with mobile spiral computed tomography scanner: early reports. *Lancet*. 1998;351:1242–1245.

69. Petty TL. Screening strategies for early detection of lung cancer: the time is now. *JAMA*. 2000;284:1977–1979.

70. Frame PS. Routine screening for lung cancer? Maybe someday, but not yet. *JAMA*. 2000;284:1980–1983.

71. Hillman BJ, Gatsonis C, Sullivan DC. American College of Radiology Imaging Network: new national cooperative group for conducting clinical trials of medical imaging technologies. *Radiology*. 1999;213:641–645.

72. O'Rourke MA, Feussner JR, Feigel P, et al. Age trends of lung cancer stage at diagnosis: implications for lung cancer screening in the elderly. *JAMA*. 1987;258:921–926.

73. Fedele DJ, Jones JA, Niessen LC. Oral cancer screening in the elderly. *J Am Geriatr Soc*. 1991;39:920–925.

74. Silverman S. Precancerous lesions and oral cancer in the elderly. *Clin Geriatr*. 1992;8:529–541.

75. Rodrigues VC, Moss SM, Tuomainen. Oral cancer in the UK: to screen or not to screen. *Oral Oncol*. 1998;34:454–465.

76. Jacobs C. The internist in the management of head and neck cancer. *Ann Intern Med*. 1990;113:1771–1778.

77. Downer MC, Evans AW, Hughes Hallet CM, Jullien JA, Speight PM, Zakrzewska JM. Evaluation of screening for oral cancer and precancer in a company headquarters. *Community Dent Oral Epidemiol*. 1995;23:84–88.

78. Hill L, Ferrini RL. Skin cancer prevention and screening: summary of the American College of Preventive Medicine's practice policy statement. *CA Cancer J Clin*. 1998;48:232–235.

79. Ferrini RL, Perlman M, Hill L. American College of Preventive Medicine policy statement: screening for skin cancer. *Am J Prev Med*. 1998;14:80–82.

80. Pollack SV. Skin cancer in the elderly. *Clin Geriatr Med*. 1987;3:715–728.

81. Friedman RJ, Rigel DS, Silverman MK, et al. Malignant melanoma in the 1990s: the continued importance of early detection and the role of physician examination and self-examination of the skin. *CA Cancer J Clin*. 1991;41:201–226.

82. Karagas MR, Stukel TA, Greenberg ER, et al. Risk of subsequent basal cell carcinoma and squamous cell carcinoma of the skin among patients with prior skin cancer. *JAMA*. 1992;267:3305–3310.

83. MacKie RM, Preudenberger T, Aitchinson TC. Personal risk factor chart for cutaneous malignant melanoma. *Lancet*. 1989;ii:487–490.

84. Jackson A, Wilkinson C, Ranger M, Pill R, August P. Can primary prevention or selective screening for melanoma be more precisely targeted through general practice? A prospective study to validate a self-administered risk score. *Br Med J*. 1998;316:34–39.

85. Austoker J. Melanoma: prevention and early diagnosis. *Br Med J*. 1994;308:1682–1686.

86. Presser SE, Tailor FR. Clinical diagnostic accuracy of basal cell carcinoma. *J Am Acad Dermatol*. 1987;16:988.

87. Grin CM, Kipf AW, Welkovich B, et al. Accuracy in the clinical diagnosis of malignant melanoma. *Arch Dermatol*. 1990;126;763–766.

88. Whited JD, Hall RP, Simel DL, Horner RD. Primary care clinicians' performance for detecting actinic deratoses and skin cancer. *Arch Intern Med*. 1997;157:985–990.

89. Koh HK, Geller Ac, Miller DR, Lew RA. The early detection of and screening for melanoma. *Cancer*. 1995;75:674–683.

90. NIH Consensus Conference: diagnosis and treatment of early melanoma. *JAMA*. 1992;268:1314–1319.

91. U.S. Preventive Services Task Force. Screening for colorectal cancer: recommendations and rationale. *Ann Intern Med*. 2002;137:129–131.

92. Pignone M, Somnath S, Hoerger T, Mandelblatt, J. Cost-effectiveness analyses of colorectal cancer screening: a systematic review for the U.S. Preventive Services Task Force. *Ann Intern Med*. 2002;137:96–104.

33
Breast Cancer

Ann Partridge and Eric Winer

Breast cancer is the most common malignancy in women in the United States, with more than 180,000 reported cases yearly.[1] Despite recent advances,[2,3] more than 41,000 women per year die of breast cancer in the United States alone.[1] Other than female gender, age is the most important risk factor for the development of breast cancer. In the United States, women aged 65 years or older represent about 13% of the female population but account for nearly 50% of the newly diagnosed breast cancers.[4,5] More than 60% of breast cancer deaths occur among women over age 65.[5,6]

Despite the high prevalence of breast cancer among older women and the significant associated morbidity and mortality, researchers have only recently focused on treatment questions in this patient group. Most clinical trials and almost all randomized trials have included few women over age 65.[7–9] Extrapolation of results of many clinical trials to the geriatric population must be done with caution because of potential differences in tumor biology, host physiology, and problems common among older patients, including comorbidity, impaired functional status, and lack of social support.

This chapter examines the epidemiology, natural history, treatment, and care patterns of breast cancer in the elderly. Screening issues, discussed in Chapter 16, are not covered here.

Epidemiology

Incidence and Mortality

In 2000, an estimated 182,800 women were diagnosed with breast cancer in the United States.[1] This figure represents approximately 30% of cancer diagnoses in women, with breast cancer ranking as the most frequently diagnosed cancer and the second leading cause of cancer death among women in the United States. The average American woman has a 12% lifetime risk of a personal breast cancer diagnosis.[10] The longer a woman lives without cancer, the lower her future risk of breast cancer. For example, a 50-year-old woman who has not had breast cancer has an 11% chance of having breast cancer in her lifetime; a 70-year-old woman has a 7% chance of developing breast cancer during the remainder of her life.[10] However, these risks can increase dramatically depending on an individual's personal and family history. Although breast cancer can affect younger women, it is most commonly seen in women in their middle to later years. In women under age 30, breast cancer is extremely uncommon. The annual incidence rises precipitously with each decade until age 50, then more gradually as a woman enters her sixth, seventh, and eight decades. Data from the surveillance, epidemiology, and end results (SEER) Program at the National Cancer Institute, a population-based data system consisting of nine separate state and local cancer registries that cover about 10% of the U.S. population, clearly demonstrate the relationship between age and incidence of breast cancer[11] (Table 33.1).

Despite the estimate that a U.S. woman has a 1 in 8 chance of developing breast cancer in her lifetime, a woman only has a 3.4% risk of dying of breast cancer.[10,12] The majority of women diagnosed with breast cancer will not die of the disease. Approximately 80% of women with breast cancer can expect to survive at least 5 years following diagnosis. The survival rate has been increasing in recent years,[2,3] largely because of improvements in screening for early disease and the use of hormonal and cytotoxic treatments for early and advanced disease (Fig. 33.1). There is no question that the use of adjuvant systemic therapy has made a real, although modest, impact on mortality as demonstrated by multiple randomized controlled trials. Despite an increasing incidence of breast cancer from the 1970s to 1997, the annual breast cancer mortality per 100,000 from 1987 to 1997 decreased by 19% among U.S. women aged 20 to 49, 18% for women aged 50 to 69, and 9% for women aged 70 to 79.[2] In 1997, the annual breast cancer mortality rate per

TABLE 33.1. Age and incidence of breast cancer.

Age group	Cases/100,000 person-years
25–29	7.4
30–34	26.7
35–39	66.2
40–44	129.4
45–49	159.4
50–54	220.0
55–59	261.6
60–64	330.7
65–69	390.7
70–74	421.8
75–79	461.4
80–84	451.3
≥85	411.9

Source: Data are from the Surveillance, Epidemiology, and End Results (SEER) Program (1984–1988).[11]

100,000 U.S. women aged 70 to 79 was 112.5, compared to 10.8 and 65.0 among women aged 20 to 49 and 50 to 69, respectively.[2]

Conventionally, breast cancer in the elderly is thought to be a more indolent disease. However, several studies indicate that survival in older women (65 years of age and older) diagnosed with breast cancer is lower than in younger women.[2,3,13–26] The reasons for decreased survival may be related to differences in tumor characteristics and patient factors. There are also differences in health care services received by older women compared to younger women, including differential screening and treatment for breast cancer. Several recent studies have revealed that the negative effect of age has diminished significantly after adjustment for other prognostic factors, such as extent of disease and treatment.[27–31]

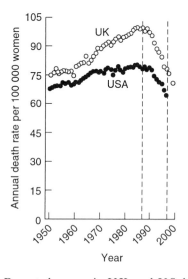

FIGURE 33.1. Recent decrease in U.K. and U.S. breast cancer mortality at ages 50–69 years. (From Peto et al., with permission.[2])

Risk Factors

Identification of risk factors is important in explaining the variation in breast cancer incidence across different populations. Risk factors can also identify women who may benefit from increased surveillance or preventive treatments. Table 33.2 outlines the major established risk factors for breast cancer, which include family history of breast cancer, early age at menarche, late age at birth of first child, nulliparity, late age at menopause, benign breast disease with proliferative changes, radiation exposure, and hormone replacement therapy.[10,12,32] Given the heightened risk of breast cancer with age, *all* older women should be considered at increased risk.

The relationship between exogenous hormone therapy and breast cancer risk may be of particular concern to older women and their physicians. Recent meta-analyses reveal small but statistically significant increases in risk (relative risks ranging from 1.02 to 1.35) of breast cancer among women exposed to hormone replacement therapy.[33–35] Risk appears to increase with current use and longer duration of use; it also appears to be reduced after cessation of hormone replacement therapy. These findings are consistent with the evidence that postmenopausal women with higher concentration of endogenous estrogen levels have a greater risk of developing breast cancer than women with lower estrogen levels.[36–38] Recent studies have also found statistically significant increases in risk in women taking both estrogen and progestin compared to those taking estrogen alone for hormone replacement therapy.[39,40] The decision to use hormone replacement therapy is complex and should entail careful consideration of the risks, including baseline breast cancer risk in an individual and potential benefits.

There are several other less well established risk factors for breast cancer that have also been studied

TABLE 33.2. Established risk factors for breast cancer.

Risk factor	Relative risk
Age (≥50 vs. <50 years old)	6.5
Family history of breast cancer	
First-degree relative	1.4–13.6
Second-degree relative	1.5–1.8
Age at menarche (<12 vs. ≥14 years old)	1.2–1.5
Age at menopause (≥55 vs. <55 years old)	1.5–2.0
Age at first live birth (>30 vs. <20 years old)	1.3–2.2
Benign breast disease	
Breast biopsy (any histologic finding)	1.5–1.8
Atypical hyperplasia	4.0–4.4
Hormone replacement therapy	1.0–1.5
Radiation	1.7–3.0

Source: Adapted from Armstrong et al. *The New England Journal of Medicine*. Massachusetts Medial Society, Boston, 2000;[10] Harris et al. *The New England Journal of Medicine*. Massachusetts Medical Society, Boston, 1992,[12] with permission.

extensively, including obesity, height, alcohol consumption, and oral contraceptive use.[12] Of these, moderate alcohol consumption has most consistently been associated with increased breast cancer risk.[41–43] The influence of diet on breast cancer risk has attracted great interest. The large variation in international breast cancer incidence rates suggests a possible relationship between breast cancer and diet.

Many studies have examined the effects of specific dietary components on breast cancer risk. Despite the lack of evidence that specific components such as fiber or individual vitamins and minerals confer any significant protective effect, a diet high in fruits and vegetables may decrease breast cancer risk.[44,45] Although national per capita fat consumption correlates with incidence and mortality from breast cancer, investigators have been unable to detect any relation between risk of breast cancer and total fat intake or consumption of specific types of fats.[46–48]

Studies of the relationship between energy balance and breast cancer have been more revealing. Although being overweight during early adult life has been associated with a lower incidence of premenopausal breast cancer, weight gain after age 18 is associated with a significantly increased risk of postmenopausal breast cancer.[49–51] The increased risk associated with weight gain and obesity in later adult life has been hypothesized to be due to the increased estrogen levels in these women secondary to increased production in adipose tissue.[49] Furthermore, these findings would appear to be consistent with the possible influence of physical activity on breast cancer risk. Limited evidence suggests that physical activity is protective against breast cancer.[52–54] This benefit may occur because exercise influences body fat stores, the principal source of estrogen in postmenopausal women. However, to date, the association of physical activity and decreased breast cancer risk is more pronounced among premenopausal women.[52]

With the exception of inherited susceptibility genes (see following), all the identified risk factors are associated with only weak to moderate increases in risk. Women without any identifiable risk factors still have a considerable lifetime risk of breast cancer (approximately 7% through age 80).[32] All women may improve their overall health, perhaps decreasing breast cancer risk, by maintaining a healthy weight, avoiding cigarettes, limiting alcohol consumption, getting regular exercise, and avoiding nondiagnostic ionizing radiation. Nevertheless, no lifestyle modifications have been proven to prevent or definitively lower the risk of breast cancer.

Genetics and Risk

For years, investigators have attempted to understand the clustering of breast cancer that occurs in certain families.

Familial breast cancer has been characterized by an earlier average age of onset, an increased risk of bilateral disease, and an increased risk of ovarian cancer.[55] Mutations in two genes, BRCA1 and BRCA2, have subsequently been found to confer an inherited predisposition to breast and ovarian cancer. An estimated 5% of breast cancer cases are thought to be due to such mutations, and the lifetime risk of cancer in mutation carriers is high. In women with BRCA1 mutations, cumulative risk of breast cancer is estimated to be 3.2% by age 30, 19.1% by age 40, 50.8% by age 50, 54.2% by age 60, and 85% by age 70.[56,57] Furthermore, BRCA1+ women who have had breast cancer have a 64% estimated cumulative risk of a contralateral breast cancer by age 70.[57] This risk is substantially increased from the estimated 1.0% annual risk of contralateral breast cancer for women with a history of sporadic breast cancer. In women with BRCA2 mutations, the risk of breast cancer appears to be similar to the risk among women with BRCA1 mutations.[57] More recent population-based studies[58,59] have demonstrated lower, although still substantial, breast cancer risk ranging from 55% to 85% for BRCA1 carriers and 37% to 85% for BRCA2 carriers.[60]

To date, no significant differences have been observed in terms of response to treatment between sporadic and inherited forms of breast cancer.[61–64] However, two recent studies have suggested that the presence of a BRCA1/2 mutation in women with breast cancer with a strong family history or of Ashkenazi Jewish ethnicity may portend a worse prognosis.[65,66] Further studies are necessary to confirm and extend these findings. As mutations of BRCA1 and BRCA2 have been identified, testing for these genetic mutations has become more common. This practice has led to recommendations for screening and prevention strategies for women with one of these mutations or with a high likelihood of having one.[57] These strategies, including more frequent and earlier screening, chemoprevention, or surgical prevention (prophylactic mastectomy), may make a substantial impact on the incidence and mortality of breast cancer in these populations. Ultimately, deciphering the functions of BRCA1 and BRCA2, which are assumed to have tumor suppressor functions, will lead to a better understanding of carcinogenesis and may lead to new strategies for therapy and prevention. Although known mutations of BRCA1 and BRCA2 are thought to account for only approximately 5% of all breast cancers, and an even smaller percentage among older women, this is still an important issue to consider in an older woman with breast cancer and a strong family history.

BRCA1 and BRCA2 are the first of what may be a series of breast cancer susceptibility genes. Other known although less common genetic syndromes that confer increased breast cancer risk include Li–Fraumeni syndrome, Cowden's disease, Peutz–Jeghers syndrome,

Muir–Torre syndrome, and ataxia telangiectasia.[60,67] These syndromes are associated with several other abnormalities and, in general, breast cancer appears earlier in life.

Biology and Natural History of Breast Cancer in the Elderly

Normal breast tissue changes with age. The dense fibrous and glandular breast tissue of early adulthood is replaced by increasing amounts of fat as a woman ages.[68] After menopause, there is further involution of the glandular structures. The fatty replacement simplifies mammographic screening in older women as there is better contrast between the density of a malignancy and the density of fatty tissue. With aging, there is also a decreased tendency to develop benign breast lesions.[68] The breast nodularity or fibrocystic change, occurring in response to cyclic hormonal changes in premenopausal women, rarely occurs in postmenopausal women unless they are receiving hormone replacement therapy. Gross cysts, which occur most commonly in women during the 15 years before menopause, are rare in the elderly. Fibroadenomas, most common between the ages of 20 and 35, are also rare in postmenopausal women. For these reasons, most newly developing breast masses in postmenopausal women are carcinomas.

Numerous studies have examined the relationship between age and extent of disease at time of breast cancer diagnosis. Stage at diagnosis is determined by two sets of factors: (1) tumor/host biology; and (2) patient/physician behavior surrounding the diagnostic process. Several studies have noted that older women have a higher likelihood of presenting with advanced disease.[14,20,31,69,70] The largest database is from the SEER program, which includes more than 125,000 women with breast cancer[14] (Table 33.3). These data indicate that a greater proportion of elderly women present with distant

TABLE 33.3. Stage distribution by age of breast cancer patients in the Surveillance, Epidemiology, and End Results (SEER) Program, 1973–1984.

Age group	Number	Localized disease, %	Regional disease, %	Distant disease, %	Stage unknown, %
<35	3,684	48.6	42.1	4.5	4.7
35–44	12,214	49.8	41.9	4.5	3.8
45–54	23,855	47.3	43.4	5.7	3.6
55–64	29,363	46.8	41.8	8.1	3.3
65–74	26,302	49.6	38.3	8.5	3.7
75–84	16,799	51.4	35.1	8.0	5.5
>84	5,770	45.6	34.3	8.9	11.2

Source: From Yancik et al.,[14] with permission of J.B. Lippincott Company.

TABLE 33.4. Established prognostic factors for breast cancer and risk of recurrence.

Prognostic factor	Effect on risk of recurrence
Axillary lymph node involvement present	Increased
Size of the primary tumor (large)	Increased
Tumor histologic and/or nuclear grade (higher)	Increased
Lymphatic and vascular channel invasion present	Increased
Estrogen and/or progesterone receptor positive	Decreased
Her-2/neu overexpressed	Increased
Measures of tumor proliferation (higher)	Increased

disease, although a smaller proportion present with regional disease. The proportion of patients who present with localized disease does not vary with age and remains about half in all age groups.

Although there is little evidence that biologic differences in tumor or host account for stage differences in older and younger patients at presentation, there is evidence that patient/physician behavior surrounding the diagnostic process is different for older women. Older women are less likely to practice breast self-examination, obtain regular breast examinations from their physicians, or undergo screening mammography.[71] Samet et al.[72] conducted a population-based study of 194 women with breast cancer, 65 years or older at diagnosis, to examine factors associated with stage at presentation. Factors associated with an advanced stage at presentation included longer delay between initial symptom and seeking medical care, older age, absence of breast self-examination, and poor performance on a short test of knowledge about cancer. Of the women who were symptomatic at time of diagnosis, 29% had delay of at least 3 months between symptom onset and seeking medical care. Delay in seeking care was associated with a lack of social support, a relatively common problem among the elderly.

Established prognostic factors for localized breast cancer include number of involved axillary lymph nodes, size of the primary tumor, tumor histologic and nuclear grade, lymphatic and vascular channel invasion, estrogen and progesterone receptor status, Her-2/neu overexpression, and measures of tumor proliferation such as mitotic index, Ki-67, and percent of cells in S phase of the cell cycle[73] (Table 33.4). In general, poor prognostic factors are less common in breast cancers of older women. Information from several large databases indicates that older women with localized disease have a higher proportion of estrogen and progesterone receptor-positive tumors[74–76] and a lower incidence of Her-2/neu overexpression.[77] The tumors of elderly women are more likely to be lower grade and have lower breast cancer cell proliferation rates.[78–81] Several groups have reported an increased proportion of mucinous and papillary carcinomas, histologic subtypes with a favorable prognosis, among older women.[14,68,82] These subtypes still account for less than 10% of breast cancers in older women, and the most common subtype in both older and younger women is infiltrating ductal carcinoma.

Age-related changes in the host may also have an effect on prognosis. In experimental animal models, some tumors behave less aggressively while others behave more aggressively in an older host.[83] Tumors that behave less aggressively tend to be those that are less immunogenic. Several investigators have proposed that immune senescence may be the cause of this altered tumor behavior with age. Cell-mediated and humoral immune responses to foreign antigens decrease with age. In experimental systems of less immunogenic tumors, manipulations that cause immunodeficiency actually inhibit tumor growth.[83] An intact immune system might actually be enhancing tumor growth, possibly through production of growth factors or tumor induction of suppressor T cells that block antitumor immunity. In contrast, highly immunogenic tumors in these same experimental models behave more aggressively in hosts with immune deficiencies and in older hosts. Most human tumors are thought to be relatively nonimmunogenic.

Although there is a subset of older women with early-stage disease who have exceptionally good survival,[80] older women have been found in general to have overall lower survival rates compared to younger women with breast cancer.[2,3,13–26] Adami et al.[16] examined the survival of 57,068 Swedish women diagnosed with breast cancer between 1960 and 1978. This database included about 98% of all cases diagnosed in Sweden during this period. The investigators found that relative survival declined markedly after age 49, and women over age 75 had the worst relative survival, although the results were not controlled for stage. Host and Lund examined the survival of 31,594 Norwegian women diagnosed with breast cancer between 1955 and 1980.[17] This database includes almost all cases diagnosed in Norway during this period. After controlling for stage, the worst relative survival was found in patients over the age of 74 and in patients under the age of 35. In their analysis of the SEER data, Yancik et al. found that stage-specific relative survival is worse only for women aged 85 years or older diagnosed with metastatic disease.[14]

In summary, examination of prognostic factors and tumor pathology indicates that older women, as a group, have slower-growing, more indolent, and more hormonally responsive tumors and should have a better prognosis. However, despite these findings, older women appear to have lower relative survival compared with younger women. Older women have a higher likelihood of presenting with metastatic disease, and differences in survival exist even after controlling for stage. Differences in the screening and treatment of older women may account for some of this discrepancy, and patterns of care are examined later in this chapter.

Prevention of Breast Cancer

Significant research over the past three decades has focused on the screening, early detection, and treatment of breast cancer. More recently, efforts have focused on primary prevention, particularly in women who are deemed to be at increased risk for the disease. Surgical prevention with bilateral mastectomy was the traditional approach, but there were no conclusive studies supporting the benefits of prophylactic mastectomy. More recently, Hartmann et al. have demonstrated, using a retrospective study design, that prophylactic mastectomies reduce the risk of breast cancer by approximately 90%.[84] A decision model suggests that prophylactic mastectomies could extend survival in young women with BRCA1 and BRCA2 mutations, but in older women prophylactic surgery will have little, if any, impact on survival.[85] Given the morbidity associated with prophylactic surgery, this is generally not an approach that should be considered in an older patient population.

In the National Surgical Adjuvant Breast and Bowel Project (NSABP) P1 trial,[86] tamoxifen significantly decreased the risk of both invasive and noninvasive breast cancer by approximately 50% compared to placebo at 55-month median follow-up. Eligibility for the trial was based on a breast cancer risk score calculated by the Gail Model,[32] and, given the increased risk of breast cancer with age, all women over the age of 60 were eligible to participate. The reduction in risk was seen in all groups regardless of age at enrollment; 30% of the participants were over 60 years of age and 6% were over 70. Unfortunately, tamoxifen therapy was associated with significantly increased risks of thromboembolic disease and endometrial cancer.[86] These risks are substantially higher in women over 50 than in women under the age of 50 and alter the therapeutic index of tamoxifen as a preventive agent in older women.[87] In moderate-risk white women, the risks associated with tamoxifen are greater than the benefits after age 60, and in moderate-risk black women, the risks exceed the benefits by age 50. In general, the risk/benefit analysis of tamoxifen for the prevention of breast cancer weighs strongly against recommending that older women take tamoxifen for primary prevention unless they are at extraordinary risk of breast cancer in the next 5 years.[87] Because the majority of breast cancer occurs in women over age 60, alternative chemoprevention strategies are desirable.

Other potential hormone-based strategies under consideration include newer selective estrogen receptor modulators (SERMs) and, for postmenopausal women, estrogen deprivation with agents that inhibit aromatase, the critical enzyme in conversion of androgen precursors to estrogen in adipose and breast tissue.[88–90] Currently underway is the NSABP-P2 trial, the STAR trial, which compares the efficacy and adverse effects of tamoxifen with raloxifene, another SERM not associated with an increased risk of endometrial cancer but with similar risk of thromboembolic disease.[91,92] Other studies are underway assessing the risks and benefits of aromatase inhibitors in the prevention of breast cancer in high-risk postmenopausal women.[93]

Treatment

Disease status, comorbidity, life expectancy, patient preferences, and goals of therapy should guide treatment of an older patient with breast cancer. These decisions should be made with an understanding of the treatment regimens that have been shown to improve survival or quality of life. Numerous advances have been made over the past 30 years in the treatment of breast cancer. Both local and systemic therapy have changed substantially during this time, guided by the results of large randomized clinical trials, often performed through large cooperative groups. Because most randomized clinical trials in breast cancer have not included patients over the age of 70, cautious extrapolation of the results to older women is often necessary.

A woman's likelihood of dying of breast cancer versus other causes can be assessed with competing risks analysis.[94] When devising rational treatment plans for an older woman with breast cancer, one must consider not only her risk of disease recurrence as influenced by disease stage, tumor grade, and hormone receptor status, but also her life expectancy as determined by age and comorbidity. Life expectancy for women in Western societies is approximately 15.5 years at age 70 and 9.2 years at age 80[95] (Table 33.5). As one might expect, comorbidity is a significant risk factor for shortened life expectancy in women with breast cancer.[96–100] Satariano and colleagues

revealed that among breast cancer patients identified through the Metropolitan Detroit Cancer Surveillance System, 3-year mortality was four times higher in women with three or more comorbid conditions when compared to women with no comorbid illness.[100] In women aged 55 to 84 years, those who died within 2 years after assessment of comorbidity were more likely to have reported one or more comorbid conditions than were survivors (62% versus 38%).[98] Furthermore, the greater the number of comorbid illnesses, the higher the risk of death from all causes, including breast cancer, independent of age and stage of disease.[98,101] Because the number of comorbid conditions tends to increase with age, older women with breast cancer are at increased risk of dying of nonbreast cancer-related causes. Fish et al.[94] analyzed 678 patients diagnosed between 1971 and 1990. Among women who died, 20% of women over age 65 died of causes other than breast cancer compared to 3% of women under age 65.

In the following sections, we review current breast cancer treatment recommendations, focusing on the data available regarding older patients and relevance of existing studies to breast cancer in the elderly.

Ductal Carcinoma In Situ (Intraductal Carcinoma)

Ductal carcinoma in situ (DCIS) in a noninvasive form of breast cancer in which tumor cells are confined to the ductolobular system and surrounded by an intact basement membrane. If left untreated, DCIS has a substantial risk of evolving into invasive ductal carcinoma of the breast. Currently in the United States at least 12% to 15% of newly diagnosed breast cancer cases annually are DCIS.[102] There was a marked increase in DCIS incidence beginning in the early 1980s, correlating with the widespread use of mammography for screening.[103,104] Average annual increases in rates between 1973 and 1983 and between 1983 and 1992 changed from 5.2% to 18.1% among women aged 50 years or older, compared to 0.3% to 12.0% among women aged 30 to 39 years and 0.4% to 17.4% among women aged 40 to 49 years.[103] Because DCIS cannot cause serious morbidity in and of itself, the major issue in the management of DCIS is the risk of progression to invasive breast cancer. Although many women with DCIS will ultimately develop invasive disease, not all untreated DCIS will go on to become invasive breast cancer in a woman's lifetime.[105] This issue is particularly important when considering the treatment of DCIS in an older woman with a potentially limited life expectancy.

In the past, mastectomy was the standard treatment for DCIS. In light of the success of breast-conserving surgery

TABLE 33.5. Average remaining life expectancy at age 55 years and beyond.

Age (year)	Life expectancy, males and females (years)	Life expectancy, females (years)
55–60	25.1	27.2
60–65	21.1	23.1
65–70	17.5	19.2
70–75	14.2	15.5
75–80	11.2	12.2
80–85	8.5	9.2
≥85	6.2	6.6

Source: Adapted from the U.S. Department of Health and Human Services,[95] with permission.

with radiation for invasive disease, there has been great interest in breast-conserving therapy with or without breast irradiation for the treatment of DCIS. NSABP protocol B-17 demonstrated that overall local recurrence rate for patients treated with excision alone was 27% at 8 years compared to 12% for those patients treated with excision plus radiotherapy.[106] Despite the improvement in local recurrence, there was no evidence that survival was compromised in the group that did not receive radiation. The use of tamoxifen as adjuvant therapy for DCIS has also been evaluated. In NSABP protocol B-24,[107] treatment with tamoxifen after breast-conserving therapy yielded a further reduction in breast cancer events (8.2% versus 13.4%; $p = 0.0009$) including recurrence of noninvasive disease and development of invasive disease. Once again, despite the decreased risk of breast recurrence, there was no impact of tamoxifen on survival. Several recent studies have revealed that older women with DCIS have a significantly decreased risk of recurrence than younger women after local therapy,[108,109] perhaps due to increased surgical margins obtained among older women.[109] Although radiation and tamoxifen are both considerations for the treatment of an older woman with DCIS, the option of wide excision alone remains a reasonable choice, particularly for patients with low- to intermediate-grade DCIS with clear margins.[110] Although tamoxifen is a consideration, the absence of a survival benefit and the increased risk of complications (thromboembolic disease and endometrial cancer) with tamoxifen mandate careful consideration of the risk and benefits of tamoxifen in an older woman with DCIS.

Invasive Breast Cancer: Early-Stage Disease

Local Therapy

Local treatment refers to treatment directed at the breast and regional lymph nodes. Local treatment alone can be curative in the majority of patients with stage I breast cancer and a substantial proportion of women with stage II and III disease. Table 33.6 presents breast cancer staging by the American Joint Committee on Cancer.

The two principal options for local treatment of early-stage breast cancer are mastectomy and breast-conserving surgery combined with breast irradiation. With either option, assessment of lymph node involvement is usually performed, either by full axillary node dissection or a sentinel lymph node biopsy. Several large randomized studies have compared mastectomy to breast-conserving surgery followed by radiation therapy.[111–114] These studies have revealed no difference in distant disease-free survival or overall survival between women who had a mastectomy compared to those who received breast-

TABLE 33.6. Breast cancer staging.

Stage	Definition
Stage I	Primary tumor ≤2 cm without axillary lymph node involvement
Stage II	Primary tumor >2 cm and ≤5 cm with or without axillary lymph node involvement Primary tumor ≤2 cm with axillary lymph node involvement Primary tumor >5 cm without axillary lymph node involvement
Stage III	Any primary tumor size with fixed axillary lymph nodes Primary tumor directly extending to chest wall or skin with or without axillary lymph node involvement Any primary tumor size with internal mammary lymph node involvement
Stage IV	Presence of distant metastases including supraclavicular lymph node involvement

Source: From the American Joint Committee on Cancer,[232] with permission.

conserving therapy. Based on these studies, the 1990 National Institutes of Health Consensus Development Conference on the Treatment of Early-Stage Breast Cancer concluded that, when possible, breast-conserving surgery combined with axillary lymph node dissection and postoperative radiation therapy is the preferred treatment for patients with early-stage breast cancer because it provides equivalent survival rates while preserving the breast.[115] No change was made in this recommendation at the 2000 Consensus Conference.[116] Although the four trials referenced above enrolled a total of 3947 patients, few of these women were over age 65 and none were over age 70. There are no compelling reasons, however, to believe that the relative efficacy of these two treatment strategies would be different in older compared to younger women.

In a retrospective study comparing women age 65 years and older to younger women, Merchant et al.[117] found that breast-conserving surgery plus radiation results in local failure rates at 10 years of 4% versus 13%, disease-free survival of 72% for both groups, and overall survival of 82% and 84%, respectively, despite significantly less aggressive adjuvant therapy among the older women in this study. In general, elderly patients tolerate breast surgery well and even with general anesthesia have little documented postoperative morbidity and mortality.[118–120] Furthermore, both breast-conserving surgery and mastectomy can be performed under local anesthesia with mortality rates approaching zero. Comorbid illness rather than age appears to be the main factor influencing surgical mobidity.[14,20,101]

Studies of quality of life and functional outcomes following breast cancer surgery have revealed that perceptions of body image are better among women who have undergone breast-conserving surgery rather than mastectomy. There does not appear to be excess concern about recurrence in women who opt for conservative surgery in lieu of a mastectomy.[121–124] Although these findings are largely from younger women, there is no reason to believe that this would be significantly different in older women. Investigators have shown that older women prefer and are more likely to choose breast conservation over mastectomy.[125,126] Sandison et al.[125] found that 34 of 38 women aged 70 or older who chose their own treatment had breast conservation and only 4 opted for mastectomy. Importantly, only 2 women in this study were unhappy with their choice of treatment at 12-month follow-up. Evaluating quality of life in a group of older women undergoing breast cancer surgery, Vinokur et al.[127] found that more extensive surgery was associated with greater physical impairments following surgery.

Radiation Therapy Following Breast-Conserving Surgery

Breast irradiation following breast-conserving surgery significantly decreases the risk of recurrence in the breast. In the NSABP B-6 trial, breast irradiation following breast-conserving surgery in women age 70 or younger decreased the local recurrence rate from 39% to approximately 10%.[114] The Milan group confirmed the risk reduction with breast irradiation, revealing that 0.3% of women in their study developed local recurrence after radiation compared to 8.8% of women who did not receive adjuvant radiation therapy with median follow-up of 39 months.[128] Despite the significant improvement in local recurrence rates, the omission of radiation therapy following conservative surgery does not appear to compromise survival. Among older women, there have been conflicting reports regarding the benefits of adjuvant breast irradiation. There is some evidence that the risk of recurrence in the breast decreases with age, with recurrence rates reported as less than 4% in older women after breast-conserving surgery without radiation.[128,129] Other studies have shown a risk of recurrence of more than 20% in elderly patients who do not receive adjuvant radiation after lumpectomy or partial mastectomy.[130–132] The Cancer and Leukemia Group B has completed accrual to a trial designed to test the value of radiation in older women, but there are no results available at this time. Although radiation therapy may provide only modest benefit in older women, breast irradiation should not be omitted based on advanced age alone in the absence of additional findings from clinical trials. Importantly, breast irradiation appears to be well tolerated in older women.[133] On the other hand, it is reasonable to consider omitting breast radiation in an individual of any age who has multiple comorbid conditions and is unlikely to survive more than a few years.

Axillary Lymph Node Assessment

Axillary nodal status is the single best predictor of overall survival in women with breast cancer. The presence or absence of lymph node involvement has been an important determinant for the use of systemic adjuvant treatment. An axillary dissection also reduces the risk of axillary recurrence as a result of removing lymph nodes that contain cancer.[134] Unfortunately, axillary lymph node dissection increases the risk of postoperative complications, including lymphedema, and increases the morbidity, hospital stay, recovery time, and cost of surgery.[135–137] Research to date has been conflicting regarding the impact of age at diagnosis on late complications after full axillary nodal dissection. Two studies[138,139] have reported older age at diagnosis to be a significant factor while a more recent study[140] found younger age to be a risk factor for lymphedema, and yet another study[135] revealed that age was unrelated to lymphedema incidence.

Using the newer sentinel node technique, a surgeon can identify patients with negative lymph nodes without performing a full axillary lymph node dissection. Sentinel lymph node biopsy entails injecting blue dye or radiolabeled colloid in the area of the breast lesion and following it out to the first lymph node that drains the cancerous area, the "sentinel" node. This lymph node, or a small group of nodes, is then assessed for tumor involvement. The status of the sentinel node can be used to predict the status of the remaining nodes in the axilla. However, the procedure can be technically challenging, and the success rate varies according to the surgeon and the characteristics of the patient.[141] When performed by experienced surgeons, the sentinel lymph node technique is minimally invasive and highly accurate. It can be performed successfully in more than 90% of eligible breast cancer patients, and the tumor status of the sentinel node accurately predicts the status of all axillary nodes in more than 95% of cases.[137,141–144] It should be noted that sentinel node biopsy is appropriate only for patients with a clinically negative axilla. Sentinel lymph node evaluation has been shown recently to provide accurate staging in elderly patients as well as younger women.[145]

The question of whether any form of axillary surgery (sentinel biopsy or a full dissection) is necessary has arisen based in part on studies assessing the utility and efficacy of node dissection in older women.[146–148] For an increasing number of patients, systemic treatment decisions will not be affected by nodal status. In older women with breast cancer, decisions about the use of tamoxifen or chemotherapy can often be made based on the size and characteristics of the primary tumor. Although some women desire axillary dissection to obtain prognostic information, others will be content without this information if they can be spared surgery to the axilla and the potential associated morbidity. In women who have had conservative surgery and have a clinically negative axilla, axillary irradiation can be administered at the same time as breast irradiation to prevent axillary recurrence.[134,146–149] The evaluation and management of the axilla has become increasingly complex in recent years. The options are varied, and physicians should carefully consider the treatment goals and a patient's preferences in the decision-making process.

Alternative Management Strategies for Local Disease

For most older women, treatments offered should be similar to those considered for younger women. However, alternative, less aggressive approaches to local therapy have been sought for older women, particularly for those in whom life expectancy is very limited or who are unable or unwilling to undergo standard therapy. Surgery or tamoxifen alone have been compared to each other and to combination therapy as the primary treatment for localized breast cancer in older women. Tamoxifen alone has been studied extensively as the initial treatment.[150–162]

In general, tamoxifen instead of surgery for localized breast cancer results in an initial response rate up to 70%. The median time to response is approximately 3 months (range, 5–124 weeks), and responses can be durable in a large number of patients.[101,156,157] Relapse rates with tamoxifen alone are high, however, and additional local therapy is necessary in more than 50% of patients. In a recent series, Ciatto and colleagues[162] reported on 120 women over age 69 treated initially with tamoxifen alone. After at least 6 months treatment, they report complete responses in 12 patients, partial response in 46 patients, and minor response or stable disease in 53 patients. Progressive disease was observed in 9 patients. Response duration was limited, and progression was observed increasingly over time. After 12 months, more than 50% of subjects were still showing response to treatment, which decreased to approximately 30% at 60 months follow-up. In a subset of 27 subjects, treatment response was strongly associated with tumor estrogen receptor content, progression being 100%, 43%, or 6% in subjects with 0%, 30% to 60%, or more than 60% immunostained cells, respectively.

When tamoxifen has been compared to surgery with or without tamoxifen,[153–155,160,161] survival rates are not significantly different among patients who did not undergo surgery (ranging from 66% to 88% after 2 to 6 years for both groups). However, local recurrence rates are more common among patients treated with tamoxifen only, up to 56% in one series compared to 44% with surgery alone after 6 years follow-up.[160] In the short term, tamoxifen

appears to provide an acceptable alternative to surgical therapy in the older patient with early-stage hormone receptor-positive breast cancer. With longer follow-up, however, tamoxifen only delays surgical therapy for the majority. Primary management of early-stage disease with tamoxifen alone should probably be reserved for patients who have a very limited life expectancy or for patients who refuse surgical intervention. However, limited surgery without axillary dissection plus adjuvant tamoxifen may achieve a local regional control rate in older women comparable to that obtained with more aggressive strategies.[126]

Alternative regimens of radiation therapy including weekly schedules have been considered for older patients who may be unable or unwilling to undergo daily radiation treatments or primary surgery. In two small retrospective analyses,[163,164] weekly high dose per fraction breast irradiation was well tolerated in older women and resulted in encouraging local control rates. Treating 70 older women (median age, 81 years) with all stages of disease with daily tamoxifen and weekly radiation, Maher et al.[164] reported an overall survival rate of 87%, disease-specific survival rate of 88%, and disease-free survival of 72% at a median follow-up of 36 months. The local control rate was 86% at 36 months. Based on such encouraging preliminary data, alternative radiation schedules should be explored further in clinical trials.

Adjuvant Systemic Therapy

Despite advances in local therapy, a substantial proportion of women with early-stage disease will not be cured with local treatment alone. Ten-year disease-free survival rates for patients treated with radical mastectomy alone are shown in Table 33.7. Despite optimal local therapy, many women develop distant disease over time, presumably because micrometastases have already spread to other parts of the body from the original breast tumor. Adjuvant systemic therapy attempts to eradicate this subclinical disease and improve disease-free and overall survival. The principal options for adjuvant therapy are hormonal treatment (tamoxifen) and cytotoxic chemotherapy.

Well over 100 randomized clinical trials examining adjuvant therapy for early-stage breast cancer have been

TABLE 33.7. Ten-year disease-free survival following radical mastectomy.

Study	Node negative	1 to 3 positive nodes	≥4 positive nodes
Fisher et al.[233]	76%	36%	14%
Valagussa et al.[234]	72%	34%	16%

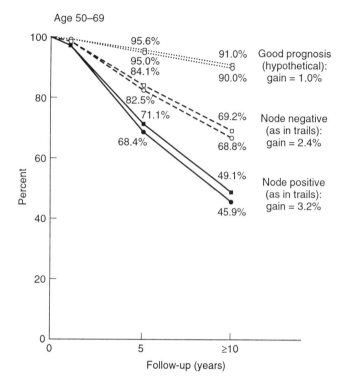

FIGURE 33.2. Estimated absolute survival advantages with prolonged polychemotherapy for women ages 50–69 years with good, intermediate, and poor prognosis. (Reproduced with permission from the Early Breast Cancer Trialists' Collaborative Group. Polychemotherapy for early breast cancer: an overview of the randomised trials.[166])

whose tumors were estrogen receptor-negative. Adjuvant chemotherapy also substantially reduced risk of recurrence and mortality in all age groups. Among women under 50, chemotherapy results in an proportional reduction in mortality of 15% to 27%, whereas among women age 50 or older, the proportional reduction was of the order of 8% to 14%. Thus, overall, adjuvant chemotherapy and hormonal treatments result in significant improvements in disease-free and overall survival (Fig. 33.2). Unfortunately, despite adjuvant therapy, a significant number of women will relapse and ultimately die of breast cancer. Thus, decisions about adjuvant therapy should be based on the risk of recurrence, and proportional risk reduction with specific therapies balanced with toxicities of therapy, life expectancy, and patient preferences.

Tamoxifen

Tamoxifen is an oral synthetic antiestrogen. It is believed to exert its antiestrogenic activity primarily by competitively blocking the binding of estradiol to the estrogen receptor.[167] When estrogen combines with the estrogen receptor in the cell nucleus, stimulation of cell growth occurs, as well as production of growth factors that function by autocrine and paracrine mechanisms. Breast cancer cells treated with tamoxifen accumulate in the G_0/G_1 stages of the cell cycle.[167] Tamoxifen is generally considered to be cytostatic rather than cytotoxic, although the significance of this distinction is often overemphasized. Tamoxifen also has nonestrogen receptor-mediated antitumor effects.[168,169] In the treatment of metastatic disease, tamoxifen has demonstrated substantial activity, particularly in patients with hormone receptor-positive tumors.

Most randomized trials of adjuvant tamoxifen have included some older women. Of the 37,000 women participating in the Oxford overview analysis of tamoxifen,[165] approximately 34% were age 60 or older and approximately 7% were over age 70. The proportional reductions in risk of recurrence and death with tamoxifen were similar across all age groups (Table 33.8), with

conducted worldwide. Large meta-analyses of adjuvant trials were updated in 1995.[165,166] The most recent publication of the Early Breast Cancer Trialists' Collaborative Group included 124 randomized trials beginning before 1990 from which primary data could be obtained, including data on more than 67,000 women. In general, tamoxifen treatment substantially reduced proportional mortality at 10 years by up to 26% among all women with estrogen receptor-positive (ER-positive) and ER-unknown tumors. Importantly, tamoxifen had essentially no impact on disease-free and overall survival in women

TABLE 33.8. Adjuvant tamoxifen in postmenopausal women (after exclusion of women with ER-poor disease): data from the 1998 overview analysis.

Age group (years)	Number of patients		Proportional reduction in recurrence (SD)	Proportional reduction in mortality (SD)
	5 years tamoxifen	Controls		
50–59	1285	1251	37% (6)	11% (8)
60–69	1606	1568	54% (5)	33% (6)
≥70	186	204	54% (13)	34% (13)
Overall (includes <50)	3738	3689	47% (3)	26% (4)

Source: From the Early Breast Cancer Trialists' Collaborative Group,[165] with permission.

benefits increasing with increasing duration of tamoxifen therapy up to 5 years. Based on the overview and randomized trials that have compared 5 years of tamoxifen treatment with a shorter duration,[165,170,171] 5 years of treatment has become the standard of care for patients with ER-positive breast cancer. There is also the suggestion that longer duration of therapy is of no additional benefit,[172–174] although two worldwide trials addressing this issue are ongoing.

The absolute benefits from tamoxifen are dependent on a patient's risk of recurrence and the proportional reduction in recurrence achievable with tamoxifen (up to 50% with 5 years of therapy). Two randomized trials have examined adjuvant tamoxifen therapy specifically in women 65 years of age or older who had one or more positive axillary nodes.[175,176] Both trials demonstrated significant improvements in disease-free survival in patients who received tamoxifen, despite competing causes of mortality in this older population. Among women with negative axillary lymph nodes, the benefits of tamoxifen have also been demonstrated,[177] although the absolute risk reduction is generally smaller because the risk of recurrence is lower in such women.

Tamoxifen may have beneficial effects apart from reducing the risk of breast cancer recurrence. Five years of tamoxifen has been shown to reduce the occurrence of contralateral breast cancers by up to 50%, consistent with its preventative effects in women at high risk for breast cancer.[86,165] The beneficial effects of tamoxifen on breast cancer prevention and risk reduction are thought to be secondary to the antiestrogenic effects of tamoxifen. Other antiestrogenic effects of tamoxifen include vasomotor symptoms and vaginitis.

Because it is a mixed estrogen antagonist and agonist, tamoxifen also has some estrogenic effects. The estrogenic activity is manifested as lowering of serum lipid levels, decreased rate of bone mineral loss, and stimulation of endometrial proliferation. It is not clear whether the effects on the bones and blood lipids can lead to clinically relevant improvements in fracture rates or cardiovascular mortality. It is clear that tamoxifen use leads to a significant although small increased risk of endometrial cancer, deep venous thrombosis, and pulmonary embolism. There is also some excess incidence of cataract development among tamoxifen users.[86,87] Thus, the benefits of tamoxifen must be balanced against the risks for a given individual. Although tamoxifen is generally well tolerated, common side effects include menopausal symptoms, such as hot flashes, and gynecologic symptoms, including vaginal discharge.[178] Importantly, many other symptoms commonly reported by women on tamoxifen, including psychologic symptoms, weight gain, and changes in overall quality of life, have been found to be not significantly different from placebo in large double-blinded studies.[86,178]

Chemotherapy

The role of adjuvant chemotherapy in older women is controversial. Although earlier trials showed minimal benefit in older women, recent larger trials and the Oxford overview analyses have revealed that adjuvant chemotherapy results in modest benefits in postmenopausal women (Table 33.9). In the most recently published overview analysis,[166] there were too few women in the 70 and older age group to draw conclusions about chemotherapy in this population, and few randomized trials have included many women over 70 years of age. Among women aged 50 to 69 years, chemotherapy for women with estrogen receptor-negative tumors resulted in a reduction in the risk of recurrence of 30% (±5%) compared to a reduction of 40% (±7%) in women less than 50 years of age. For women with estrogen receptor-positive tumors who will also benefit from tamoxifen, chemotherapy resulted in a decrease in the risk of recurrence of 18% (±4%) among women aged 50 to 69 years compared to 33% (±8%) proportional risk reduction in women less than 50 years of age.[166,179]

An important question for older women with ER-positive tumors is whether adjuvant chemotherapy adds anything to the benefits of tamoxifen. The overview analysis, as well as individual studies, have demonstrated that combination therapy with tamoxifen and chemotherapy is better than the use of either treatment alone in

TABLE 33.9. Adjuvant polychemotherapy for breast cancer: data from the 1998 overview analysis.

Age group (years)	Number of patients		Proportional reduction in recurrence (SD)	Proportional reduction in mortality (SD)
	Chemo group	Control group		
<40	694	675	37% (7)	27% (8)
40–49	1629	1531	34% (5)	27% (5)
50–59	3362	3411	22% (4)	14% (4)
60–69	3394	3413	18% (4)	8% (4)
≥70	307	302	—[a]	—[a]
Overall (including <50)	9386	9332	23.8% (2.2)	15.2% (2.4)

[a] So few women were aged 70 or over at presentation that they are excluded from the age-specific analysis.

Source: From the Early Breast Cancer Trialists' Collaborative Group,[166] with permission.

TABLE 33.10. Standard adjuvant chemotherapy regimens for breast cancer.

Regimen	Duration
CMF: cytoxan, methotrexate, 5-fluorouracil	6 months
CA: cytoxan and adriamycin	3 months
CA-T: cytoxan and adriamycin, followed by taxol	6 months
CAF: cytoxan, adriamycin, 5-fluorouracil	4–6 months
CEF: cytoxan, epirubicin, 5-fluorouracil	4–6 months

women with estrogen receptor-positive tumors.[166,180,181] In the overview, combination therapy resulted in an overall reduction in the risk of both recurrence and death of 19% (±3%) and 11% (±4%), respectively, among women aged 50 to 69 compared to tamoxifen alone. Because the benefits of chemotherapy appear to decrease with age,[166] however, the absolute incremental benefit of chemotherapy added to tamoxifen in older women with hormone receptor-positive tumors may be relatively small. In women with ER-positive disease of all ages, combination chemotherapy and tamoxifen resulted in a reduction in risk of recurrence and death of 52% (±8%) and 47% (±9%) respectively, compared to chemotherapy alone.[165,166,182] The overview analysis also suggested that anthracycline-containing chemotherapy regimens are superior to non–anthracycline-containing regimens.[166] However, concern about the inherent risk of cardiotoxicity with anthracycline-based chemotherapy mandates careful consideration of its use in older women in the adjuvant setting. Table 33.10 lists the standard adjuvant chemotherapy regimens for breast cancer.

The benefits of chemotherapy must also be weighed against the risks. The acute toxicities of standard chemotherapy regimens have been well studied, although largely in younger patient populations.[183] These toxicities are generally short term in nature. Some degree of nausea with or without vomiting is common but usually controllable with modern antiemetics. Mild mucositis is occasionally seen, although it is almost never severe. Myelosuppression is nearly universal; however, a systemic infection occurs in less than 5% of patients. Total alopecia will occur in almost all patients who receive an anthracycline-based regimen (including doxorubicin or epirubicin), compared to approximately 50% of patients who receive CMF (cyclophosphamide, methotrexate, and 5-fluorouracil). Weight gain is also not uncommon among women who receive adjuvant chemotherapy. Addition of paclitaxel to adjuvant chemotherapy results in an incidence of severe neuropathy of less than 5%. An increased risk of thromboembolic disease has been observed in patients receiving chemotherapy, particularly when it is given concurrently with tamoxifen. Long-term risks include a risk of less than 1% of cardiotoxicity resulting in congestive heart failure with anthracycline-based therapy, as well as a very small risk of treatment-related leukemia. It is unclear whether these risks are increased further among older women, although the risk of cardiotoxicity is increased in patients with cardiac disease, which is more common in older women.

The addition of the new biologic therapy, trastuzumab (Herceptin), to adjuvant regimens is currently being studied. Trastuzumab is a humanized monoclonal antibody to the Her-2/neu receptor, which is overexpressed in about one-third of breast cancers.[184] The use of trastuzumab alone and in combination with chemotherapy has resulted in significant disease responses and improvements in overall survival among women with Her-2/neu-overexpressing metastatic disease.[185] There is no reason to believe that trastuzumab would not benefit women of all age groups with Her-2/neu-positive tumors, and the treatment is generally well tolerated, although there may be an increased risk of cardiac problems in elderly.[186] However, older women have Her-2/neu-positive tumors much less frequently than younger women.[77]

It is widely assumed that older patients are less tolerant of chemotherapy than younger patients. Although a few small studies have reported significantly increased toxicity in the elderly, larger recent studies provide evidence to the contrary. Crivellari et al.[187] studied the burdens and benefits of adjuvant CMF and tamoxifen in elderly women. In this group, the 76 women aged 65 years or older had higher grades of toxicity, including hematologic and mucosal toxicity, than younger women. The subjective burdens of treatment, however, were similar for older and younger patients based on quality of life measures. Begg and Carbone[188] examined 19 Eastern Cooperative Oncology Group studies that included a total of 780 patients aged 70 years or older. These patients were compared with patients under age 70. Older patients had increased hematologic toxicity; otherwise, the incidence of severe toxicities was similar between groups. Giovanazzi-Bannon and colleagues[189] examined data from the Illinois Cancer Center database on the 672 patients treated in phase II trials, including 271 patients aged 65 or older. Except for experiencing slightly more hematologic toxicity, there were no differences in incidence of other toxicities, dose reductions, or length of treatment delays between the two groups.

In a more recent study, Dees and colleagues[190] treated 44 women ages 35 to 79 with early-stage breast cancer with four cycles of adjuvant AC (adriamycin and cyclophosphamide) chemotherapy. In this cohort, although myelosuppression was increased in older women, neither neutropenic complications, nor alteration in cardiac function, nor change in quality of life scores were significantly age-related. Pharmacokinetic analyses did not demonstrate age-related differences in the clearance of doxorubicin or cyclophosphamide. Although patients in these studies may represent a highly selected group, it is reassuring that the older patients appear to tolerate chemotherapy nearly as well as the younger patients.

Summary

Decisions regarding adjuvant therapy should take into account a woman's risk of disease recurrence, her life expectancy, the benefits and risks of each treatment, and her preferences. Adjuvant tamoxifen clearly reduces the risk of recurrence and death in older women, although the benefits are limited to women with hormone receptor-positive tumors. Five years of tamoxifen has a favorable side effect profile and should be considered for all older women with hormone receptor-positive tumors. Adjuvant chemotherapy appears to reduce the risk of recurrence and death in women under the age of 70. To date, there is not enough information about women age 70 and older to make definitive conclusions regarding the benefits of chemotherapy in this population. Chemotherapy should be considered in this age group if the tumor is hormone receptor negative or in the setting of a high risk of disease recurrence. In 1998, a panel of experts at the St. Gallen Breast Cancer Conference made recommendations for adjuvant therapy for women older than 70 years[191] (Table 33.11).

In addition to disease characteristics as outlined in the aforementioned recommendations, concern regarding toxicity of therapy, comorbidities, and life expectancy will weigh heavily on a decision to treat an elderly woman with adjuvant chemotherapy. Extermann and colleagues used a Markov model to determine the threshold risk of relapse for which women up to age 85 with or without comorbidity would derive benefit from adjuvant therapy.[192] For healthy women at age 65, the threshold risk of relapse was 11% for a 1% benefit in 10-year survival from tamoxifen. This threshold increased to 20% for women age 65 with significant comorbidity. For healthy women age 85, the threshold risk of relapse was 28% for a 1% benefit in 5-year survival, increasing to 35% for

sicker women in the same age group. Of note, no 10-year survival benefit was seen in the older age group. For chemotherapy, the threshold risk for a 1% benefit rose from 19% in a healthy 65-year-old to 62% in a sick 85-year-old. This model was sensitive to quality of life as well, a major consideration because of the relatively small impact of adjuvant therapy on survival in older women.

Future studies of adjuvant therapy should be designed to include more elderly women. These studies should measure quality of life as well as traditional endpoints. With its toxicities and modest benefits even in younger women, it is unlikely that adjuvant cytotoxic chemotherapy will ever be used extensively in women over age 70. Studies examining the benefits of new hormonal agents and other less toxic drugs, including trastuzumab, hold promise for the future adjuvant treatment in women of all age groups, including those age 70 or older.

Metastatic Breast Cancer

Metastatic breast cancer is incurable with currently available therapies. Median survival ranges from 2 to 3 years; however, there is substantial variability in survival, with as many as 10% of patients living more than 10 years. Factors associated with longer survival include disease involving soft tissue and bone only (rather than visceral organs), hormone receptor positivity in the tumor, a long disease-free interval from diagnosis to recurrence, and limited number of metastatic sites. Response to therapy is also quite variable. Patients with the better prognostic factors for survival as just described are more likely to respond well to hormonal therapy. The heterogeneity among breast cancer patients with metastatic disease must be considered carefully in the care of these patients.

The primary goals of treatment of metastatic breast cancer are palliation of symptoms, prolongation of survival, and improvement in quality of life. Only a few randomized studies have incorporated quality of life endpoints. Comparing a variety of treatments, each of these trials has shown that quality of life was better with the treatment that had the higher objective response rate, even if that treatment was more toxic.[193–195] Treatment of metastatic breast cancer may prolong survival, but proving that a survival benefit exists is difficult because trials have not randomized patients to a supportive-care-only arm. In a meta-analysis of 50 randomized chemotherapy trials comparing a more effective treatment to a lesser one, the more effective chemotherapy prolonged median survival by as much as 6 months.[194] This small improvement in average survival should not be used as routine justification to treat asymptomatic or minimally symptomatic patients with toxic therapy, particularly because there is no evidence that early initiation of therapy extends life.

TABLE 33.11. Consensus panel recommendations for adjuvant treatment of elderly breast cancer patients.

Risk category	Treatment
Minimal/low: (ER or PR positive, ≤1 cm, grade 1)	None or tamoxifen
Intermediate: (>1–2 cm, hormone receptor positive, grade 1–2)	Tamoxifen ± chemotherapy
High: (>2 cm, hormone receptor negative, grade 2–3, node positivity)	Tamoxifen (± chemotherapy) If hormone receptor negative, chemotherapy

Source: Adapted with permission from Goldhirsch et al.[191]

Management of metastatic disease involves the judicious use of local and systemic therapies that best palliate the patient's symptoms with the least toxicity. In certain clinical situations, local therapy may be preferable to systemic therapy, such as in the situation of an isolated local recurrence. Such a recurrence can often be managed with local excision, radiotherapy, or both. A small percentage of patients with local regional recurrence will do well without evidence of progressive disease for an extended period of time. Other situations when local therapy is preferable include impending fracture from a bone metastasis, spinal cord compression, and brain metastases. In each of these cases, radiation therapy can result in significant palliation. Surgery may also play an important role in these situations.

Systemic treatment for metastatic breast cancer includes hormonal therapy and chemotherapy. Hormonal therapy should be considered first as it is usually much better tolerated than cytotoxic chemotherapy and can result in long remissions. Patient characteristics that predict for response to hormonal therapy include estrogen or progesterone receptor positivity, a long disease-free interval (from time of diagnosis to recurrence), the absence of visceral disease, postmenopausal status, and prior response to hormonal therapy. The majority of elderly patients have hormone receptor-positive tumors, and hormonal therapy is usually the initial treatment of choice. Overall objective response rates to hormonal therapy are in the range of 20% to 40%, depending on the patient population, with higher response rates seen in patients with multiple characteristics as just listed. In most randomized trials comparing two different hormonal treatments, response rates and duration of response have been similar. Tamoxifen, which is one of the least toxic hormonal agents, has traditionally been the first agent administered, followed by an aromatase inhibitor (e.g., anastrozole, letrozole, or exemestane). Recent data also suggest that aromatase inhibitors are at least at active as tamoxifen in the first-line setting in postmenopausal women with metastatic breast cancer.[196,197] Table 33.12 lists the principally used hormonal therapies and their main toxicities. Patients who respond to one hormonal treatment should usually be treated with another hormonal agent at the time of disease progression, unless they have extensive visceral disease or rapid disease progression, in which case chemotherapy should be considered. Studying initial therapy for metastatic disease in elderly women, the Eastern Cooperative Oncology Group randomized 181 women over the age of 65 to receive either tamoxifen or cyclophosphamide, methotrexate, and 5-fluorouracil (CMF) with crossover to the other treatment at the time of progression.[198] Response rates were not significantly different between the two groups: initial response rates were 45% with tamoxifen and 38% with CMF, and response rates after

TABLE 33.12. Hormonal agents currently considered in postmenopausal women with breast cancer.

Class	Agents	Principal toxicities
Estrogen antagonists	Tamoxifen Toremifene	Hot flashes, vaginitis Rarely, endometrial cancer, venous thrombosis
Aromatase inhibitors	Anastrozole Letrozole Exemestane	Hot flashes, gastrointestinal distress
Progestins	Megestrol acetate	Weight gain, fluid retention Rarely, venous thrombosis
Androgens	Fluoxymesterone	Masculinizing effects

crossover were 29% with tamoxifen and 31% with CMF. Survival was slightly higher in the group treated initially with tamoxifen. Combined endocrine treatment (combinations of tamoxifen, aminoglutethamide, hydrocortisone, and fluoxymesterone) has been studied in older patients and thus far shown no significant benefit.[199] Newer specific aromatase inhibitors may show more promise, and combinations with them are currently being evaluated in clinical trials.

Older women should be offered chemotherapy when they are judged to be poor candidates for endocrine therapy (i.e., hormone receptor-negative tumors) or when their disease becomes refractory to hormonal treatment. Unfortunately, most trials evaluating chemotherapy in metastatic breast cancer have included few women over age 65. With combination regimens, approximately 40% to 50% of patients will have an objective response, and a small percentage will have a complete response (complete disappearance of disease). Patients with a good performance status, limited number of metastatic sites, and long disease-free interval (from diagnosis to recurrence) are most likely to respond to chemotherapy. Age and menopausal status have not been shown to predict for response. Response rates and toxicity profiles of standard regimens for metastatic breast cancer have not been found to be significantly different in older patients.[101] In a case comparison study of patients with metastatic breast cancer treated in five clinical trials,[200] 70 women aged 70 or older were compared to 60 patients aged 50 to 69 and 40 patients less than 50 years old. Evaluation of response rates, time to progression, survival, and toxicity revealed no significant differences between the three groups. Response rates were 40%, 30%, and 29%, respectively ($p = 0.53$) among the three groups. Estimates of time to progression and survival were 9.1 and 17.9 months, 6.2 and 12.8 months, and 7.2 and 14.2 months, respectively. Importantly, there were no significant differences in toxic effects, dose delivery, and dose delays among the three groups. Based on information from studies such as this, women age 70 or greater should not be excluded from chemotherapy clinical trials for advanced breast cancer based on age alone.

Combination chemotherapy has been compared to single-agent chemotherapy in women with advanced breast cancer.[201,202] Although response rates and duration of response tend to be increased, there is no significant difference in survival when combination chemotherapy is compared to single-agent sequential chemotherapy. Furthermore, treatment-related toxicity tends to be higher and quality of life worse with multiagent regimens. For these reasons, single-agent chemotherapy is used increasingly in the treatment of advanced breast cancer. In a patient who responds to therapy, physicians are often faced with the decision of how long to continue treatment. Therapy should be administered for at least 3 to 6 months. Continuing beyond that time will extend the time to disease progression but will not change overall survival.[193,203] The decision to continue treatment must be individualized based on the toxicity profile of the treatment regimen, disease-related symptoms, and patient preferences.

Concern regarding toxicity will weigh heavily on a decision to treat an elderly woman with cytotoxic chemotherapy. Although organ function and metabolism of drugs may be compromised in older patients, comparative studies show that chemotherapy-related toxicity is similar in older and younger patients.[200,204,205] Hematologic reserve is decreased in older individuals; therefore, hematologic toxicity from chemotherapy may be more severe in elderly patients. Cardiotoxicity, gastrointestinal effects, and neurotoxicity may also be more common in older patients. For chemotherapeutic agents that are primarily renally excreted, such as methotrexate and cyclophosphamide, dose adjustment based on creatinine clearance is recommended in older patients.[204,205] Agents such as vinorelbine and 5-fluoruracil derivatives such as capecitabine, which have favorable side effect profiles, are particularly suitable for treatment of elderly patients.[206,207] Although elderly women do not have a high proportion of Her-2/neu-positive tumors, the efficacy and favorable toxicity profile of traztuzumab make this a reasonable treatment option for older women with Her-2/neu-positive tumors. Future randomized trials evaluating these drugs in elderly women with metastatic breast cancer are warranted.

After failure of first-line chemotherapy, response rates to other regimens are lower in women of all ages. Second-line and subsequent chemotherapy regimens can be considered, but the potential toxicities of treatment must be weighed against potential benefits. Palliation of symptoms, pain management, other supportive care, and consideration of visiting nurse services and hospice care are of utmost importance. Bisphosphonate therapy (e.g., pamidronate) has resulted in significant reductions in skeletal complications, that is, pathologic fractures,

surgery for fracture or impending fracture, radiation, spinal cord compression, and hypercalcemia in women with metastatic breast cancer.[208,209] Intravenous (i.v.) pamidronate every 3 to 4 weeks is currently recommended in patients with metastatic breast cancer who have imaging evidence of lytic destruction of bone and who are concurrently receiving systemic therapy with hormonal therapy or chemotherapy.[210]

Quality of Life in Older Women with Breast Cancer

A number of studies suggest that older women adjust to breast cancer better than younger women.[211–214] In a study of 304 women immediately after completion of therapy for early-stage breast cancer, Wenzel et al.[214] compared quality of life (QOL) among women age 50 or younger to women over age 50. QOL was evaluated using standardized measures, including the Functional Assessment of Cancer Therapy—Breast instrument, the Center for Epidemiologic Studies Depression Scale, and the Impact of Event Scale. In this study, QOL was significantly worse for younger women globally ($p = 0.021$) and with regard to domains of emotional well-being ($p = 0.0002$) and breast carcinoma-specific concerns ($p = 0.022$). Furthermore, symptoms of depression ($p = 0.041$) and disease-specific intrusive thoughts ($p = 0.013$) were significantly worse for younger women. Of note, no significant sexual dysfunction or body image differences were noted between older and younger women. Although elderly women who survive breast cancer seem to cope better than their younger counterparts, their distress must not be overlooked. Older women are more likely to have decreased social support, limitations in physical and cognitive functioning, and significant comorbidity. Furthermore, rates of depression are high in elderly populations, particularly when faced with a serious illness. Interventions, such as use of social support, spirituality, and exercise, have demonstrated therapeutic benefits for older women with cancer and should be considered.[215]

Patterns of Care

Numerous studies have documented that there are significant treatment differences in older patients compared to younger patients.[14,18–20,70,117,216–225] Elderly women with early-stage breast cancer are less likely to undergo breast-conserving surgery than younger women, despite the increase in breast conservation over recent years among all age groups.[222,223,225] Older women are also more likely to have radiotherapy or lymph node dissection omitted after breast-conserving surgery.[18–20,117,219,220,222,225] Concerning systemic therapy, older women are more likely to be treated solely with adjuvant tamoxifen and are much less likely to undergo chemotherapy than younger women.[18-20,117,219,222,225]

Less aggressive care of elderly breast cancer patients may be associated with a poorer outcome. Studying 390 women ages 45 to 90, Lash et al.[226] found that patients who received a less than definitive prognostic evaluation had an adjusted relative hazard of recurrence of 1.7 [95% confidence interval (CI), 1.0–2.7] and an adjusted relative hazard for breast carcinoma mortality of 2.2 (95% CI, 1.2–3.9). Patients who received less than definitive therapy had an adjusted relative hazard of recurrence of 1.6 (95% CI, 1.0–2.5) and an adjusted relative hazard of breast carcinoma mortality of 1.7 (95% CI, 1.0–2.8). Women aged 75 to 90 were least likely to receive definitive care and had relative hazards associated with less than definitive care as great or greater than the relative hazards observed in the whole cohort. This finding has implications for older women with localized breast cancer who are not receiving standard evaluations and therapy, as they may be at excess risk for disease recurrence and mortality. Other authors have not found differences in survival between older women who receive standard treatment and those who receive less aggressive care, after controlling for age, stage, and other clinical factors.[18-20,76,117] Because elderly patients have more comorbidity, as well as functional limitations, less aggressive care may represent appropriate clinical judgment. Several studies indicate, however, that comorbidity or functional impairment cannot always explain less aggressive care. Furthermore, there is significant geographic variation in the care received by older breast cancer patients that cannot be explained by differences in functional status or comorbidity.[220,221,223,225] For example, Mandelblatt and colleagues found that, between 1995 and 1997, women with localized breast cancer from five regions in the United States were 3.3 times more likely to have a mastectomy if they lived in Texas than if they lived in Massachusetts.[225]

Other studies have shown that elderly patients with metastatic disease also appear to receive less aggressive care.[227,228] In a population-based study of the treatment of metastatic breast cancer, Fetting et al.[228] evaluated 132 cases of women who died of metastatic breast cancer in Washington County, Maryland, from 1984 to 1991. Sixty percent of women aged 75 years and older were referred to a medical oncologist, in contrast to 68% of women aged 65 to 74 years and 89% of women under age 65. Seventy-four percent of patients less than 65 years old received chemotherapy, compared to 42% of patients aged 65 to 74 years and 12% of women aged 75 years or older, despite the fact the there is not evidence that metastatic breast cancer responds differently to chemotherapy by age. Adjusting for other medical conditions and whether or not the patient saw a medical oncologist, there was still a significant effect of age on whether patients received chemotherapy. Of note, the different patterns of chemotherapy utilization were not associated with survival differences. Radiation therapy was also utilized significantly less frequently in older patients; however, there was no age effect on the utilization of hormonal therapy in this study. Less frequent utilization of palliative chemotherapy and radiation in older patients may be caused by a combination of patient and physician factors and may result in less effective palliation for older patients.

The specific reasons underlying these variations in care have not been studied extensively. Physician attitudes about appropriateness of therapy, patient comorbidity, and patient preferences, including body image and side effect concerns, have been found to influence the selection of treatment for elderly women with breast cancer.[216,219,222,225] In a recent study of 718 women with early-stage breast cancer aged 67 years and older, Mandelblatt et al.[225] found that women who were concerned with body image were 1.8 times more likely to receive breast-conserving surgery and radiotherapy compared to women without this concern. After controlling for other factors, women who preferred no therapy beyond primary surgery were 3.9 times more likely to undergo mastectomy than other women. In this study, women 80 years and older were 3.4 times less likely to undergo radiation therapy after breast-conserving surgery when compared to women ages 67 to 79 years, independent of comorbid illnesses, performance status, or women's treatment preferences. Furthermore, older women were 70% less likely to receive chemotherapy than women aged 67 to 79. However, women 80 years and older tended to receive tamoxifen more often than the younger women in this study. The finding that patient preferences were independent predictors of therapy among these women has implications for shared decision making and communication between elderly patients and their physicians.

Silliman et al.[219] surveyed physicians who did not recommend adjuvant therapy as part of a study in which women aged 75 years or older were significantly less likely to receive adjuvant therapy (including radiotherapy following breast-conserving surgery, chemotherapy, and hormonal therapy). Physicians' attitudes about appropriateness of therapy appeared to be the major determinant of what treatment was received. In the majority of cases, physicians believed that the treatment was not indicated on the basis of patient stage or treatment efficacy. Patient factors, such as age, comorbidity, functional status, ability to tolerate treatment, and patient preferences, were cited infrequently.

Goodwin and Samet[229] studied a population-based cohort of women 65 years or older with early-stage breast cancer in New Mexico. In this study, specific characteristics other than age that were associated with nonstandard treatment included impairments in activities of daily living, low physical activity, impaired mental status, poor access to transportation, and low social support. There was only a small, statistically nonsignificant relationship between comorbidity, based on patient self-report, and not receiving definitive treatment. It is likely that patient factors and preferences, as well as physician attitudes and beliefs, play an important role in explaining age-related variations in breast cancer care.

Elderly breast cancer patients (and elderly cancer patients in general) are substantially underrepresented in treatment protocols.[7–9,230] Some of the same physician and patient factors that contribute to less aggressive treatment of elderly patients probably contribute to this underrepresentation in clinical trials. Studies are necessary to better understand physician attitudes, patient preferences, and other barriers to standard care and protocol therapy for older women. Kemeny and colleagues studied barriers to participation in clinical trials among breast cancer patients.[231] After controlling for other conditions including comorbidity, older age was associated with whether a patient was offered participation in a clinical trial even when a patient met eligibility criteria. Reasons that physicians did not offer patients trial participation were similar for older and younger patients except for two factors: (1) the presence of comorbid conditions that was not excluded by the protocol but that the physician believed would have affected the patient's response was a factor in 17% of older patients and none of the younger patients; and (2) the opinion that the regimen was too toxic was a factor in 27% of the older patients and none of the younger patients. Patient difficulty in understanding, costs, transportation, and short life expectancy did not appear to influence physicians' decisions. Importantly, there was no evidence that age was associated with whether or not a patient accepted clinical trial participation when offered.

Conclusion

The incidence of breast cancer increases dramatically with age. Given the demographic changes occurring in the United States, the number of elderly women developing breast cancer will continue to rise. Older women as a group have more favorable prognostic factors but have lower relative survival compared with younger women. Older women have a higher likelihood of receiving nonstandard and less aggressive treatment compared to younger women, even after controlling for comorbidity. Treatment recommendations are based primarily on randomized trials of younger women. Extrapolation of these results is complicated by differences in tumor biology, host physiology, and problems common in the elderly, including comorbidity, impaired functional status, and lack of social support. Local treatment of early-stage breast cancer should be similar to that in younger women and consist of either mastectomy or breast-conserving surgery followed by breast irradiation. Most older women with hormone receptor-conserving surgery followed by breast irradiation. Most older women with hormone receptor-positive tumors should receive adjuvant tamoxifen. Some elderly patients may also benefit from adjuvant chemotherapy. Ongoing and future study results should be instructive in determining the relative efficacy of breast irradiation in older women, as well as the benefits and toxicities of different adjuvant chemotherapeutic regimens. In elderly women with advanced breast cancer, hormonal therapy will usually be the initial treatment of choice. Chemotherapy should be considered when a patient has symptomatic hormone receptor-negative disease, extensive visceral involvement, and rapid disease progression, with particular attention to the potential risks of therapy. Most importantly, patient preferences, comorbidities, disease status, and available evidence for improvement in survival and quality of life should guide treatment of older women with breast cancer of all stages.

References

1. Greenlee RT, Murray T, Bolden S, Wingo PA. Cancer statistics, 2000. *CA Cancer J Clin*. 2000;50:7–33.
2. Peto R, Boreham J, Clarke M, Davies C, Beral V. UK and USA breast cancer deaths down 25% in year 2000 at ages 20–69 years [letter] [see comments]. *Lancet*. 2000;355:1822.
3. Coleman MP. Trends in breast cancer incidence, survival, and mortality [letter; comment]. *Lancet*. 2000;356:590–591; discussion 593.
4. Parker SL, Davis KJ, Wingo PA, Ries LA, Heath CW. Cancer statistics by race and ethnicity. *CA Cancer J Clin*. 1998;48:31–48.
5. Soldo BJ, Agree EM. *America's Elderly*. Washington, DC: Population Reference Bureau, Inc.; 1998.
6. Parker SL, Davis KJ, Wingo PA, Ries LA, Heath CW Jr. Cancer statistics by race and ethnicity. *CA Cancer J Clin*. 1998;48:31–48.
7. Goodwin JS, Hunt WC, Humble CG, Key CR, Samet JM. Cancer treatment protocols. Who gets chosen? *Arch Intern Med*. 1988;148:2258–2260.
8. Kennedy BJ. Age-related clinical trials of CALGB. *Cancer Control*. 1995;2:14–16.
9. Hutchins LF, Unger JM, Crowley JJ, Coltman CA Jr, Albain KS. Underrepresentation of patients 65 years of age or older in cancer-treatment trials [see comments]. *N Engl J Med*. 1999;341:2061–2067.
10. Armstrong K, Eisen A, Weber B. Assessing the risk of breast cancer [see comments]. *N Engl J Med*. 2000;342:564–571.

11. *National Cancer Institute Statistics Review: 1975–1988.* NIH pub 91-2789. Bethesda, MD: National Cancer Institute; 1991.

12. Harris JR, Lippman ME, Veronesi U, Willett WC. Breast cancer. *N Engl J Med.* 1992;327:319–328.

13. Rutqvist LE, Wallgren A. Influence of age on outcome in breast carcinoma. *Acta Radiol Oncol.* 1983;22:289–294.

14. Yancik R, Ries LG, Yates JW. Breast cancer in aging women. A population-based study of contrasts in stage, surgery, and survival. *Cancer.* 1989;63:976–981.

15. Adami HO, Malker B, Meirik O, Persson I, Bergkvist L, Stone B. Age as a prognostic factor in breast cancer. *Cancer.* 1985;56:898–902.

16. Adami HO, Malker B, Holmberg L, Persson I, Stone B. The relation between survival and age at diagnosis in breast cancer. *N Engl J Med.* 1986;315:559–563.

17. Host H, Lund E. Age as a prognostic factor in breast cancer [published erratum appears in *Cancer* 1986;58(4):996]. *Cancer.* 1986;57:2217–2221.

18. Bergman L, Dekker G, van Kerkhoff EH, Peterse HL, van Dongen JA, van Leeuwen FE. Influence of age and comorbidity on treatment choice and survival in elderly patients with breast cancer. *Breast Cancer Res Treat.* 1991;18:189–198.

19. Bergman L, Dakker G, van Leeuwen FE, Huisman SJ, van Dam FS, van Dongen JA. The effect of age on treatment choice and survival in elderly breast cancer patients. *Cancer.* 1991;67:2227–2234.

20. Bergman L, Kluck HM, van Leeuwen FE, et al. The influence of age on treatment choice and survival of elderly breast cancer patients in south-eastern Netherlands: a population-based study. *Eur J Cancer.* 1992:1475–1480.

21. Sant M, Gatta G, Micheli A, et al. Survival and age at diagnosis of breast cancer in a population-based cancer registry. *Eur J Cancer.* 1991;27:981–984.

22. Levi F, Randimbison L, La Vecchia C. Breast cancer survival in relation to sex and age. *Oncology.* 1992;49:413–417.

23. La Rosa F, Patavino VM, Epifani AC, Petrinelli AM, Minelli L, Mastrandrea V. Ten-year survival and age at diagnosis of women with breast cancer from a population-based study in Umbria, Italy. *Tumori.* 1996;82:441–443.

24. Busch E, Kemeny M, Fremgen A, Osteen RT, Winchester DP, Clive RE. Patterns of breast cancer care in the elderly. *Cancer.* 1996;78:101–111.

25. Holli K, Isola J. Effect of age on the survival of breast cancer patients. *Eur J Cancer.* 1997;33:425–428.

26. Sant M, Capocaccia R, Verdecchia A, et al. Survival of women with breast cancer in Europe: variation with age, year of diagnosis and country. The EUROCARE Working Group. *Int J Cancer.* 1998;77:679–683.

27. Lethaby AE, Mason BH, Holdaway IM, Kay RG. Age and ethnicity as prognostic factors influencing overall survival in breast cancer patients in the Auckland region. Auckland Breast Cancer Study Group [published erratum appears in *N Z Med J.* 1993;106(954):166]. *N Z Med J.* 1992;105:485–488.

28. Thurfjell EL, Lindgren JA. Breast cancer survival rates with mammographic screening: similar favorable survival rates for women younger and those older than 50 years [see comments]. *Radiology.* 1996;201:421–426.

29. Ezzat A, Raja MA, Zwaan F, Brigden M, Rostom A, Bazarbashi S. The lack of age as a significant prognostic factor in non-metastatic breast cancer. *Eur J Surg Oncol.* 1998;24:23–27.

30. Masetti R, Antinori A, Terribile D, et al. Breast cancer in women 70 years of age or older. *J Am Geriatr Soc.* 1996;44:390–393.

31. Barchielli A, Balzi D. Age at diagnosis, extent of disease and breast cancer survival: a population-based study in Florence, Italy. *Tumori.* 2000;86:119–123.

32. Gail MH, Brinton LA, Byar DP, et al. Projecting individualized probabilities of developing breast cancer for white females who are being examined annually [see comments]. *J Natl Cancer Inst.* 1989;81:1879–1886.

33. Steinberg K, Thacker S, Smith S, et al. A meta-analysis of the effect of estrogen replacement therapy on the risk of breast cancer. *JAMA.* 1991;265:1985–1990.

34. Sillero-Arenas M, Delgado-Rodriguez M, Rodigues-Canteras R, et al. Menopausal hormone replacement therapy and breast cancer: a meta-analysis. *Obstet Gynecol.* 1992;79:286–294.

35. Collaborative Group on Hormonal Factors in Breast Cancer. Breast cancer and hormone replacement therapy: collaborative reanalysis of data from 51 epidemiological studies of 52,705 women with breast cancer and 108,411 women without breast cancer. *Lancet.* 1997;350:1047–1059.

36. Schairer C, Lubin J, Troisi R, et al. Menopausal estrogen and estrogen-progestin replacement therapy and breast cancer risk. *JAMA.* 2000;283:485–491.

37. Ross R, Paganini-Hill A, Wan P, Pike M. Effect of hormone replacement therapy on breast cancer risk: estrogen versus estrogen plus progestin. *J Natl Cancer Inst.* 2000;16:328–332.

38. Thomas HV, Reeves GK, Key TJA. Endogenous estrogen and postmenopausal breast cancer: a quantitative review. *Cancer Causes Control.* 1997;8.

39. Hankinson SE, Willett WC, Manson JE, et al. Plasma sex steroid hormone levels and risk of breast cancer in postmenopausal women. *J Natl Cancer Inst.* 1998:90:1292–1299.

40. Cauley JA, Lucas FL, Kuller LH, et al. Elevated serum estradiol and testosterone concentrations are associated with a high risk for breast cancer. *Ann Intern Med.* 1999;130:270–277.

41. Garfinkel L, Bofetta P, Stellman S. Alcohol and breast cancer: a cohort study. *Prev Med.* 1988;17:686–693.

42. Gapstur S, Potter J, Sellers T, et al. Increased risk of breast cancer with alcohol consumption in postmenopausal women. *Am J Epidemiol.* 1992;136:1221–1231.

43. Longnecker MP. A meta-analysis of alcohol consumption in relation to breast cancer risk. *JAMA.* 1994;260:73–82.

44. Freudenheim JL, Marshall JR, Vena JE, et al. Premenopausal breast cancer risk and intake of vegetables,

fruits, and related nutrients. *J Natl Cancer Inst.* 1996;88:340–348.

45. Fund AIfCR-WCR. *Food, Nutrition and the Prevention of Cancer: A Global Perspective.* Washington, DC: American Institute for Cancer Research; 1997.

46. Willett W, Stampfer M, Colditz G. Dietary fat and risk of breast cancer. *N Engl J Med.* 1987;316:22–28.

47. Hunter D, Spiegelman D, Adami H, et al. Cohort studies of fat intake and the risk of breast cancer—a pooled analysis. *N Engl J Med.* 1996;334:356–361.

48. Holmes MD, Hunter DJ, Colditz GA, et al. Association of dietary intake of fat and fatty acids with risk of breast cancer. *JAMA.* 1999;281:914–920.

49. Huang Z, Hankinson SE, Colditz GA, et al. Dual effects of weight and weight gain on breast cancer risk. *JAMA.* 1997;278:1407–1411.

50. Le Marchand L, Kolonel LN, Earle ME, Mi MP. Body size at different periods of life and breast cancer risk. *Am J Epidemiol.* 1988;128:137–152.

51. Ziegler RG, Hoover RN, Nomura AMY, et al. Relative weight, weight change, height, and breast cancer risk in Asian-American women. *J Natl Cancer Inst.* 1996;88:650–660.

52. Thune I, Brenn T, Lund E, Gaard M. Physical activity and the risk of breast cancer. *N Engl J Med.* 1997;336:1269–1275.

53. Rockhill B, Willett WC, Hunter DJ, et al. A prospective study of recreational physical activity and breast cancer risk. *Arch Intern Med.* 1999;159:2290–2296.

54. Levi F, Pasche C, Lucchini F, La Vecchia C. Occupational and leisure time physical activity and the risk of breast cancer. *Eur J Cancer.* 1999;35:775–778.

55. Claus EB, Risch N, Thompson WD. Genetic analysis of breast cancer in the cancer and steroid hormone study. *Am J Hum Genet.* 1991;48:232–242.

56. Easton DF, Ford D, Bishop DT, and the Breast Cancer Linkage Consortium. Breast and ovarian cancer incidence in BRCA1 mutation carriers. *Am J Hum Genet.* 1995;56:265–271.

57. Burke W, Daly M, Garber J, et al. Recommendations for follow-up care of individuals with an inherited predisposition to cancer. *JAMA.* 1997;277:997–1003.

58. Struewing JP, Hartge P, Wacholder S, et al. The risk of cancer associated with specific mutations of BRCA1 and BRCA2 among Ashkenazi Jews. *N Engl J Med.* 1997;336:1401–1408.

59. Thorlacius S, Struewing JP, Hartge P, et al. Population-based study of risk of breast cancer in carriers of BRCA2 mutation. *Lancet.* 1998;352:1337–1339.

60. Issacs CJD, Peshkin BN, Lerman C. Evaluation and management of women with a strong family history of breast cancer. In: Harris JR, ed. *Diseases of the Breast.* Philadelphia: Lippincott Williams & Wilkins; 2000.

61. Robson M, Gilewski T, Haas B, et al. BRCA-associated breast cancer in young women [see comments]. *J Clin Oncol.* 1998;16:1642–1649.

62. Robson M, Levin D, Federici M, et al. Breast conservation therapy for invasive breast cancer in Ashkenazi women

with BRCA gene founder mutations. *J Natl Cancer Inst.* 1999;91:2112–2117.

63. Robson M. Are BRCA1- and BRCA2-associated breast cancers different? Prognosis of BRCA1-associated breast cancer. *J Clin Oncol.* 2000;18:113S–118S.

64. Pierce LJ, Strawderman M, Narod SA, et al. Effect of radiotherapy after breast-conserving treatment in women with breast cancer and germline BRCA1/2 mutations. *J Clin Oncol.* 2000;18:3360–3369.

65. Chappuis PO, Kapusta L, Begin LR, et al. Germline BRCA1/2 mutations and p27 (Kip1) protein levels independently predict outcome after breast cancer. *J Clin Oncol.* 2000;18:4045–4052.

66. Stoppa-Lyonnet D, Ansquer Y, Dreyfus H, et al. Familial invasive breast cancers: worse outcome related to BRCA1 mutations. *J Clin Oncol.* 2000;18:4053–4059.

67. Offit K, Brown K. Quantitating familial cancer risk: a resource for clinical oncologists. *J Clin Oncol.* 1994;12:1724–1736.

68. Stewart JA, Foster RS. Breast cancer and aging. *Semin Oncol.* 1989;16:41–50.

69. Satariano WA, Belle SH, Swanson GM. Severity of breast cancer at diagnosis: a comparison of age and extent of disease in black and white women. *Am J Public Health.* 1986;76:779–782.

70. Golledge J, Wiggins JE, Callam MJ. Age-related variation in the treatment and outcomes of patients with breast carcinoma. *Cancer.* 2000;88:369–374.

71. Dawson DA, Thompson GB. *Breast Cancer Risks Factors and Screening: United States, 1987.* Series 10: Data from the National Health Interview Survey, No 172. Dept. of Health and Human Services pub 90-1550. Hyattsville, MD: National Center for Health Statistics; 1990.

72. Samet JM, Hunt WC, Lerchen ML, et al. Delay in seeking care for cancer symptoms: a population-based study of elderly New Mexicans. *J Natl Cancer Inst.* 1988;80:432–438.

73. Fitzgibbons PL, Page DL, Weaver D, et al. Prognostic factors in breast cancer. College of American Pathologists Consensus Statement 1999. *Arch Pathol Lab Med.* 2000;124:966–978.

74. McCarty KS, Silva JS, Cox EB, Leight GS, Wells SA. Relationship of age and menopausal status to estrogen receptor content in primary carcinoma of the breast. *Ann Surg.* 1983;197:123–127.

75. Clark GM, Osborne CK, McGuire WL. Correlations between estrogen receptor, progesterone receptor, and patient characteristics in human breast cancer. *J Clin Oncol.* 1984;2:1102–1109.

76. Diab SG, Elledge RM, Clark GM. Tumor characteristics and clinical outcome of elderly women with breast cancer. *J Natl Cancer Inst.* 2000;92:550–556.

77. Kallioniemi OP, Holli K, Visakorpi T, et al. Association of c-erbB-2 protein over-expression with high rate of cell proliferation, increased risk of visceral metastatic and poor long-term survival in breast cancer. *Int J Cancer.* 1991;49:650–655.

78. Gentili C, Sanfilippo O, Silvestrini R. Cell proliferation and its relationship to clinical features and relapse in breast cancers. *Cancer*. 1981;48:974–979.

79. Owens MA, Beardslee S, Wenger CR, et al. DNA ploidy and S-phase fraction by flow cytometry in a large breast cancer data base. *Proc Am Assoc Cancer Res*. 1990;31: 184.

80. Lyman GH, Lyman S, Balducci L, et al. Age and the risk of breast cancer recurrence. *Cancer Control*. 1996;3:421– 427.

81. Fisher CJ, Egan MK, Smith P, Wicks K, Millis RR, Fentiman IS. Histopathology of breast cancer in relation to age. *Br J Cancer*. 1997;75:593–596.

82. Schaefer G, Rosen PP, Lesser ML, et al. Breast carcinoma in the elderly woman: pathology prognosis, and survival. *Pathol Annu*. 1984;19:195–219.

83. Schwab R, Walters CA, Weksler ME. Host defense mechanisms and aging. *Semin Oncol*. 1989;16:20–27.

84. Hartmann LC, Schaid DJ, Woods JE, et al. Efficacy of bilateral prophylactic mastectomy in women with a family history of breast cancer. *N Engl J Med*. 1999;340:77–84.

85. Schrag D, Kuntz KM, Garber JE, Weeks JC. Decision analysis—effects of prophylactic mastectomy and oophorectomy on life expectancy among women with BRCA1 or BRCA2 mutations. *N Engl J Med*. 1997;336: 1465–1471.

86. Fisher B, Costantino JP, Wickerham DL, Redmond CK, et al. Tamoxifen for the prevention of breast cancer: report of the National Surgical Adjuvant Breast and Bowel Project P-1 Study. *J Natl Cancer Inst*. 1998;90:1371– 1388.

87. Gail MH, Costantino JP, Bryant J, Croyle R, et al. Weighing the risks and benefits of tamoxifen treatment for preventing breast cancer. *J Natl Cancer Inst*. 1999;91:1829– 1846.

88. Kelloff GJ, Lubet RA, Lieberman R, et al. Aromatase inhibitors as potential cancer chemopreventive. *Cancer Epidemiol Biomarkers Prev*. 1998;7:65–78.

89. Jordan VC. Estrogen receptor as a target for the prevention of breast cancer. *J Lab Clin Med*. 1999;133:408– 414.

90. Kelloff GJ. Perspectives on cancer chemoprevention research and drug development. *Adv Cancer Res*. 2000; 78:199–334.

91. Fuchs-Young R, Glasebrook AL, Short LL, et al. Raloxifene is a tissue-selective agonist/antagonist that functions through the estrogen receptor. *Ann NY Acad Sci*. 1995;761:355–360.

92. Cummings SR, Eckert S, Krueger KA, et al. The effect of raloxifene on risk of breast cancer in postmenopausal women—results from the MORE randomized trial. *JAMA*. 1999;281:2189–2197.

93. Haynes B, Dowsett M. Clinical pharmacology of selective estrogen receptor modulators. *Drugs Aging*. 1999;14:323– 336.

94. Fish EB, Chapman JA, Link MA. Competing causes of death for primary breast cancer. *Ann Surg Oncol*. 1998;5: 368–375.

95. US Department of Health and Human Services. *Health United States 1996–7 and injury chartbook; 1997*. DHHS

Publication No. 97–1232. National Center for Health Statistics. Hyattsville, Maryland: 1997.

96. Mueller CB, Ames F, Anderson GD. Breast cancer in 3558 women: age as a significant determinant in the rate of dying and causes of death. *Surgery*. 1978;83:123–132.

97. Manton KG, Wrigley JM, Cohen HJ, et al. Cancer mortality, aging, and patterns of comorbidity in the United States: 1968 to 1986. *J Gerontol*. 1991;46(4):S225–S234.

98. Santoriano WA, Ragheb NE, Dupuis MA. Comorbidity in older women with breast cancer: an epidemiologic approach. In: Yancik R, Yates J, eds. *Cancer in the Elderly: Approaches to Elderly Detection and Treatment*. New York: Springer; 1989:71.

99. Satariano WA. Comorbidity and functional status in older women with breast cancer: implications for screening, treatment, and prognosis. *J Gerontol*. 1992;47:24–31.

100. Satariano WA, Ragland DR. The effect of comorbidity on 3-year survival of women with primary breast cancer. *Ann Intern Med*. 1994;120:104–110.

101. Kimmick GG, Muss HB. Breast cancer in special populations. In: Harris JR, ed. *Diseases of the Breast*. Philadelphia: Lippincott Williams & Wilkins; 2000:945–954.

102. Winchester DJ, Menck HR, Winchester DP. National treatment trends for ductal carcinoma in situ of the breast. *Arch Surg*. 1997;132:660–665.

103. Ernster VL, Barclay J, Kerlikowske K, Grady D, Henderson C. Incidence of and treatment for ductal carcinoma in situ of the breast. *JAMA*. 1996;275:913–918.

104. Silverstein MJ, Gamagami P, Colburn WJ. Coordinated biopsy team: surgical, pathologic and radiologic issues. In: Silverstein MJ, ed. *Ductal Carcinoma In Situ of the Breast*. Baltimore: Williams & Wilkins; 1997:333–342.

105. Morrow M, Schnitt SJ, Harris JR. Ductal carcinoma in situ and microinvasive disease. In: Harris JR, ed. *Diseases of the Breast*. Philadelphia: Lippincott Williams & Wilkins; 2000:383–401.

106. Fisher B, Dignam J, Wolmark N, et al. Lumpectomy and radiation therapy for the treatment of intraductal breast cancer: findings from National Surgical Adjuvant Breast and Bowel Project B-17. *J Clin Oncol*. 1998;16:441–452.

107. Fisher B, Dignam J, Wolmark N, et al. Tamoxifen in treatment of intraductal breast cancer: National Surgical Adjuvant Breast and Bowel Project B-24 randomized controlled trial. *Lancet*. 1999;353:1993–2000.

108. Van Zee KJ, Liberman L, Samli B, Tran KN, et al. Long-term follow-up of women with ductal carcinoma in situ treated with breast-conserving surgery: the effect of age. *Cancer*. 1999;86:1757–1767.

109. Vincini FA, Kestin LL, Goldstein NS, et al. Impact of young age on outcome in patients with ductal carcinoma-in-situ treated with breast-conserving therapy. *J Clin Oncol*. 2000;18:296–306.

110. Silverstein MJ, Lagios MD, Groshen S, et al. The influence of margin width on local control of ductal carcinoma in situ of the breast [see comments]. *N Engl J Med*. 1999;340: 1455–1461.

111. Veronesi U, Saccozzi R, Del Vecchio M, et al. Comparing radical mastectomy with quadrantectomy, axillary dissection, and radiotherapy in patients with small cancers of the breast. *N Engl J Med*. 1981;305:6–11.

112. Sarrazin D, Le M, Rouesse J, et al. Conservative treatment versus mastectomy in breast cancer tumors with macroscopic diameter of 20 millimeters or less. The experience of the Institut Gustave-Roussy. *Cancer.* 1984;53:1209–1213.

113. Veronesi U, Banfi A, Del Vecchio M, et al. Comparison of Halsted mastectomy with quadrantectomy, axillary dissection, and radiotherapy in early breast cancer. *Eur J Cancer Clin Oncol.* 1986;22:1085–1089.

114. Fisher B, Redmond C, Poisson R, et al. Eight year results of a randomized clinical trial comparing total mastectomy and lumpectomy with or without irradiation in the treatment of breast cancer. *N Engl J Med.* 1989;320:822–828.

115. NIH Consensus Conference. Treatment of early-stage breast cancer. *JAMA.* 1991;265:391–395.

116. NIH Consensus Conference Statement on Adjuvant Therapy for Breast Cancer. From the NIH Consensus Development Conference on Adjuvant Therapy for Breast Cancer. Bethesda, MD: National Institutes of Health; 2000.

117. Merchant TE, McCormick B, Yahalom J, Borgen P. The influence of older age on breast cancer treatment decisions and outcome [see comments]. *Int J Radiat Oncol Biol Phys.* 1996;34:565–570.

118. Hunt KE, Fry DE, Bland KI. Breast carcinoma in the elderly patient: an assessment of operative risk, morbidity and mortality. *Am J Surg.* 1980;140:339–342.

119. Amsterdam E, Birkenfeld S, Gilad A, et al. Surgery for carcinoma of the breast in women over 70 years of age. *J Surg Oncol.* 1987;35:180–183.

120. Svastics E, Sulyok Z, Besznyak I. Treatment of breast cancer in women older than 70 years. *J Surg Oncol.* 1989; 41:19–21.

121. Schain W, Edwards BK, Gorrell CR, et al. Psychosocial and physical outcomes of primary breast cancer therapy: mastectomy vs. excisional biopsy and irradiation. *Breast Cancer Res Treat.* 1983;3:377–382.

122. de Haes JC, van Oostrom MA, Welvaart K. The effect of radical and conserving surgery on the quality of life of early breast cancer patients. *Eur J Surg Oncol.* 1986;12:337–342.

123. Lasry JC, Margolese RG, Poisson R, et al. Depression and body image following mastectomy and lumpectomy. *J Chron Dis.* 1987;40:529–534.

124. Kemeny MM, Wellisch DK, Schain WS. Psychosocial outcome in a randomized surgical trial for treatment of primary breast cancer. *Cancer.* 1988;62:1231–1237.

125. Sandison AJ, Gold DM, Wright P, Jones PA. Breast conservation or mastectomy: treatment choice of women aged 70 years and older. *Br J Surg.* 1996;83:994–996.

126. Martelli G, De Palo G. Breast cancer in elderly women (> or = 70 years): which treatment? *Tumori.* 1999;85:421–424.

127. Vinokur AD, Threatt BA, Vinokur-Kaplan, et al. The process of recovery from breast cancer for younger and older patients: changes during the first year. *Cancer.* 1990; 65:1242–1254.

128. Veronesi U, Luini A, Del Vecchio M, et al. Radiotherapy after breast-preserving surgery in women with localized cancer of the breast [see comments]. *N Engl J Med.* 1993; 328:1587–1591.

129. Nemoto T, Patel JK, Rosner D, et al. Factors affecting recurrence in lumpectomy without irradiation for breast cancer. *Cancer.* 1991;67:2079–2082.

130. Reed MW, Morrison JM. Wide local excision as the sole primary treatment in elderly patients with carcinoma of the breast. *Br J Surg.* 1989;76:898–900.

131. Kantorowitz DA, Poulter CA, Sischy B, et al. Treatment of breast cancer among elderly women with segmental mastectomy or segmental mastectomy plus postoperative radiotherapy. *Int J Radiat Oncol Biol Phys.* 1988;15:263–270.

132. De Csepel J, Tartter PI, Gajdos C. When not to give radiation therapy after breast-conserving surgery for breast cancer. *J Surg Oncol.* 2000;74:273–277.

133. Wyckoff J, Greenberg H, Sanderson R, et al. Breast irradiation in the older woman: a toxicity study. *J Am Geriatr Soc.* 1994;42:150–152.

134. Fisher B, Redmond C, Fisher ER, et al. Ten-year results of a randomized clinical trial comparing radical mastectomy and total mastectomy with or without radiation. *N Engl J Med.* 1985;312:674–681.

135. Kissin MW, Querci della Rovere G, Easton D, Westbury G. Risk of lymphoedema following the treatment of breast cancer. *Br J Surg.* 1986;73:580–584.

136. Ivens D, Hoe AL, Podd TJ, et al. Assessment of morbidity from complete axillary dissection. *Br J Cancer.* 1992;66:136–138.

137. Giuliano AE, Jones RC, Brennan M, Statman R. Sentinel lymphadenectomy in breast cancer. *J Clin Oncol.* 1997; 15:2345–2350.

138. Pezner RD, Patterson MP, Hill LR, et al. Arm lymphedema in patients treated conservatively for breast cancer: relationship to patient age and axillary node dissection technique. *Int J Radiat Oncol Biol Phys.* 1986;12:2079–2083.

139. Delouche G, Bachelot F, Premont M, Kurtz JM. Conservation treatment of early breast cancer: long term results and complications. *Int J Radiat Oncol Biol Phys.* 1987;13:29–34.

140. Warmuth MA, Bowen G, Prosnitz LR, et al. Complications of axillary lymph node dissection for carcinoma of the breast: a report based on a patient survey. *Cancer.* 1998; 83:1362–1368.

141. Krag D, Weaver D, Ashikaga T, et al. The sentinel node in breast cancer—a multicenter validation study [see comments]. *N Engl J Med.* 1998;339:941–946.

142. Hsueh EC, Hansen N, Giuliano AE. Intraoperative lymphatic mapping and sentinel lymph node dissection in breast cancer. *CA Cancer J Clin.* 2000;50:279–291.

143. Giuliano AE, Kirgan DM, Guenther JM, Morton DL. Lymphatic mapping and sentinel lymphadenectomy for breast cancer [see comments]. *Ann Surg.* 1994;220:391–398; discussion 398–401.

144. Morrow M, Harris JR. Primary treatment of invasive breast cancer. In: Harris JR, ed. *Diseases of the Breast.* Philadelphia: Lippincott Williams & Wilkins; 2000:515–560.

145. DiFronzo LA, Hansen NM, Stern SL, Brennan MB, Giuliano AE. Does sentinel lymphadenectomy improve staging and alter therapy in elderly women with breast cancer? *Ann Surg Oncol.* 2000;7:406–410.

146. Wazer DE, Erban JK, Robert NJ, et al. Breast conservation in elderly women for clinically negative axillary lymph nodes without axillary dissection. *Cancer.* 1994;74:878–883.

147. Feigelson BJ, Acosta JA, Feigelson HS, Findley A, Saunders EL. T1 breast carcinoma in women 70 years of age and older may not require axillary node dissection. *Am J Surg.* 1996;172:487–490.

148. Naslund E, Fernstad R, Ekman S, et al. Breast cancer in women over 75 years: is axillary dissection always necessary? *Eur J Surg.* 1996;162:867–871.

149. Recht A, Pierce SM, Abner A, et al. Regional nodal failure after conservative surgery and radiotherapy for early stage breast carcinoma. *J Clin Oncol.* 1991;74:878–883.

150. Preece PE, Wood RA, Mackie CR, Cuschieri A. Tamoxifen as initial sole treatment of localised breast cancer in elderly women: a pilot study. *Br Med J (Clin Res Ed).* 1982; 284:869–870.

151. Bradbeer JW, Kyngdon J. Primary treatment of breast cancer in elderly women with tamoxifen. *Clin Oncol.* 1983; 9:31–34.

152. Allan SG, Rodger A, Smyth JF, Leonard RC, Chetty U, Forrest AP. Tamoxifen as primary treatment of breast cancer in elderly or frail patients: a practical management. *Br Med J (Clin Res Ed).* 1985;290:358.

153. Bates T, Riley DL, Houghton J, Fallowfield L, Baum M. Breast cancer in elderly women: a Cancer Research Campaign trial comparing treatment with tamoxifen and optimal surgery with tamoxifen alone. The Elderly Breast Cancer Working Party. *Br J Surg.* 1991;78:591–594.

154. Robertson JF, Todd JH, Ellis IO, Elston CW, Blamey RW. Comparison of mastectomy with tamoxifen for treating elderly patients with operable breast cancer. *Br Med J.* 1988;297:511–514.

155. Gazet JC, Markopoulos C, Ford HT, Coombes RC, Bland JM, Dixon RC. Prospective randomised trial of tamoxifen versus surgery in elderly patients with breast cancer. *Lancet.* 1988;1:679–681.

156. Margolese RG, Foster RS Jr. Tamoxifen as an alternative to surgical resection for selected geriatric patients with primary breast cancer. *Arch Surg.* 1989;124:548–550; discussion 550–551.

157. Horobin JM, Preece PE, Dewar JA, Wood RA, Cuschieri A. Long-term follow-up of elderly patients with locoregional breast cancer treated with tamoxifen only. *Br J Surg.* 1991;78:213–217.

158. Akhtar SS, Allan SG, Rodger A, Chetty UD, Smyth JF, Leonard RC. A 10-year experience of tamoxifen as primary treatment of breast cancer in 100 elderly and frail patients. *Eur J Surg Oncol.* 1991;17:30–35.

159. Ciatto S, Bartoli D, Iossa A, Grazzini G, Cirillo A. Response of primary breast cancer to tamoxifen alone in elderly women. *Tumori.* 1991;77:328–330.

160. Gazet JC, Ford HT, Coombes RC, et al. Prospective randomized trial of tamoxifen vs. surgery in elderly patients with breast cancer. *Eur J Surg Oncol.* 1994;20:207–214.

161. Mustacchi G, Milani S, Pluchinotta A, De Matteis A, Rubagotti A, Perrota A. Tamoxifen or surgery plus tamoxifen as primary treatment for elderly patients with operable breast cancer: The G.R.E.T.A. Trail. Group for

Research on Endocrine Therapy in the Elderly. *Anticancer Res.* 1994;14:2197–2200.

162. Ciatto S, Cirillo A, Confortini M, Cardillo CL. Tamoxifen as primary treatment of breast cancer in elderly patients. *Neoplasma.* 1996;43:43–45.

163. Rostom AY, Pradhan DG, White WF. Once weekly irradiation in breast cancer. *Int J Radiat Oncol Biol Phys.* 1987;13:551–555.

164. Maher M, Campana F, Mosseri V, et al. Breast cancer in elderly women: a retrospective analysis of combined treatment with tamoxifen and once-weekly irradiation [see comments]. *Int J Radiat Oncol Biol Phys.* 1995;31:783–789.

165. Early Breast Cancer Trialists' Collaborative Group. Tamoxifen for early breast cancer: an overview of the randomized trials. *Lancet.* 1998;351:1451–1467.

166. Early Breast Cancer Trialists' Collaborative Group. Polychemotherapy for early breast cancer: an overview of the randomised trials. *Lancet.* 1998;352:930–942.

167. Love RR. Tamoxifen therapy in primary breast cancer: biology, efficacy, and side effects. *J Clin Oncol.* 1989;7: 803–815.

168. Jordan VC. Estrogen-receptor mediated direct and indirect antitumor effects of tamoxifen. *J Natl Cancer Inst.* 1990;82:1662–1663.

169. Lerner LJ, Jordan VC. Development of antiestrogens and their use in breast cancer: eighth Cain memorial award lecture. *Cancer Res.* 1990;50:4177–4189.

170. Swedish Breast Cancer Cooperative Group. Randomized trial of two versus five years of adjuvant tamoxifen for postmenopausal early stage breast cancer. [see comments]. *J Natl Cancer Inst.* 1996;88:1543–1549.

171. Current Trials Working Party of the Cancer Research Campaign Breast Cancer Trials Group. Preliminary results from the cancer research campaign trial evaluating tamoxifen during in women aged fifty years or older with breast cancer. [see comments] [published erratum appears in *J Natl Cancer Inst.* 1997;89(8):590]. *J Natl Cancer Inst.* 1996; 88:1834–1849.

172. Fisher B, Dignam J, Bryant J, et al. Five versus more than five years of tamoxifen therapy for breast cancer patients with negative lymph nodes and estrogen receptor-positive tumors [see comments]. *J Natl Cancer Inst.* 1996;88: 1529–1542.

173. Stewart HJ, Forrest AP, Everington D, et al. Randomised comparison of 5 years of adjuvant tamoxifen with continuous therapy for operable breast cancer. The Scottish Cancer Trials Breast Group. *Br J Cancer.* 1996;74:297–299.

174. Tormey DC, Gray R, Falkson HC. Postchemotherapy adjuvant tamoxifen therapy beyond five years in patients with lymph node-positive breast cancer. Eastern Cooperative Oncology Group [see comments]. *J Natl Cancer Inst.* 1996;88:1828–1833.

175. Castiglione M, Gelber RD, Goldhirsch A. Adjuvant systemic therapy for breast cancer in the elderly: competing causes of mortality. International Breast Cancer Study Group. *J Clin Oncol.* 1990;8:519–526.

176. Cummings FJ, Gray R, Tormey DC, et al. Adjuvant tamoxifen versus placebo in elderly women with node-positive breast cancer: long-term follow-up and causes of death [see comments]. *J Clin Oncol.* 1993;11:29–35.

177. Fisher B, Costantino J, Redmond C, et al. A randomized clinical trial evaluating tamoxifen in the treatment of patients with node-negative breast cancer who have estrogen-receptor-positive tumors. *N Engl J Med.* 1989; 320:479–484.

178. Love RR, Cameron L, Connell BL, Leventhal H. Symptoms associated with tamoxifen treatment in postmenopausal women. *Arch Intern Med.* 1991;151:1842–1847.

179. McCarthy NJ, Swain SM. Update on adjuvant chemotherapy for early breast cancer. *Oncology.* 2000;14:1267–1280.

180. Anonymous. Tamoxifen for early breast cancer: an overview of the randomised trials. Early Breast Cancer Trialists' Collaborative Group [see comments]. *Lancet.* 1998;351:1451–1467.

181. Fisher B, Redmond C, Legault-Poisson S, et al. Postoperative chemotherapy and tamoxifen compared with tamoxifen alone in the treatment of positive-node breast cancer patients aged 50 years and older with tumors responsive to tamoxifen: results from the National Surgical Adjuvant Breast and Bowel Project B-16 [see comments]. *J Clin Oncol.* 1990;8:1005–1018.

182. Goldhirsch A, Gelber RD. Adjuvant chemo-endocrine therapy or endocrine therapy alone in postmenopausal patients: Ludwig studies III and IV. In: Senn H, Goldhirsch A, Gelber RD, et al. eds. *Recent Results in Cancer Research: Adjuvant Therapy of Primary Breast Cancer.* Berlin: Springer-Verlag; 1989:153–162.

183. Winer E, Partridge AH, Burstein HJ. Influences of treatment-related side effects and quality-of-life issues on individual decision-making about adjuvant therapy: chemotherapy and combined chemohormonal therapy. NIH Consensus Development Conference on Adjuvant Therapy for Breast Cancer. Bethesda, MD: National Institutes of Heath; 2000.

184. Menard S, Tagliabue E, Campiglio M, et al. Role of HER2 gene overexpression in breast carcinoma. *J Cell Physiol.* 2000;182:150–162.

185. Tripathy D. Overview of recent clinical studies of trastuzumab alone or in combination with chemotherapy. *Biol Ther Breast Cancer.* 2000;2:2–8.

186. Hudis C, Seidman A, Paton V, et al. Characterization of cardiac dysfunction in the Herceptin (traztuzumab) clinical trials. *Breast Cancer Res Treat.* 1998;50:12a [abstract 24].

187. Crivellari D, Bonetti M, Castiglione-Gertsch M, et al. Burdens and benefits of adjuvant cyclophosphamide, methotrexate, and fluorouracil and tamoxifen for elderly patients with breast cancer: the International Breast Cancer Study Group Trial VII. *J Clin Oncol.* 2000;18:1412–1422.

188. Begg CB, Carbone PP. Clinical trials and drug toxicity in the elderly: the experience of the Eastern Cooperative Oncology Group. *Cancer.* 1983;52:1986–1992.

189. Giovanazzi-Bannon S, Rademaker A, Lai G, et al. Treatment tolerance of elderly cancer patients entered onto phase II clinical trials: an Illinois Cancer Center study. *J Clin Oncol.* 1994;12:2447–2452.

190. Dees EC, O'Reilly S, Goodman SN, et al. A prospective pharmacologic evaluation of age-related toxicity of adjuvant chemotherapy in women with breast cancer. *Cancer Investig.* 2000;18:521–529.

191. Goldhirsch A, Glick JH, Gelber RD, Senn HJ. Meeting highlights: International Consensus Panel on the Treatment of Primary Breast Cancer [see comments]. *J Natl Cancer Inst.* 1998;90:1601–1608.

192. Extermann M, Balducci GH, Lyman H. What threshold for adjuvant therapy in older breast cancer patients? *Proc Am Soc Clin Oncol.* 1998;17:102a.

193. Coates A, Gebski V, Bishop JF, et al. Improving the quality of life during chemotherapy for advanced breast cancer. A comparison of intermittent and continuous treatment strategies. *N Engl J Med.* 1987;317:1490–1495.

194. Tannock IF, Boyd NF, DeBoer G, et al. A randomized trial of two dose levels of cyclophosphamide, methotrexate, and fluorouracil chemotherapy for patients with metastatic breast cancer [see comments]. *J Clin Oncol.* 1988;6:1377–1387.

195. Baum M, Priestman T, West RR, et al. A comparison of subjective responses in a trial comparing endocrine with cytotoxic treatment in advanced carcinoma of the breast. In: Mouridsen H, Palshof T, eds. *Breast Cancer: Experimental and Clinical Aspects.* Oxford: Pergamon Press; 1980:223.

196. Buzdar A, Nabholtz JM, Robertson JF, et al. Anastrozole (Arimidex®) versus tamoxifen as first-line therapy for advanced breast cancer (abc) in postmenopausal (pm) women: combined analysis from two identically designed multicenter trials. *Proc Am Soc Clin Oncol.* 2000;19:154a [abstract 609d].

197. Smith R, Sun Y, Garin A, et al. Femara® (letrozole) showed significant improvement in efficacy over tamoxifen as first-line treatment in postmenopausal women with advanced breast cancer. *Breast Cancer Res Treat.* 2000;64:27 [abstract 8].

198. Taylor SGT, Gelman RS, Falkson G, Cummings FJ. Combination chemotherapy compared to tamoxifen as initial therapy for stage IV breast cancer in elderly women. *Ann Intern Med.* 1986;104:455–461.

199. Rose C, Kamby C, Mouridsen HT, Andersson M, et al. Combined endocrine treatment of elderly postmenopausal patients with metastatic breast cancer. A randomized trial of tamoxifen vs. tamoxifen + aminoglutethimide and hydrocortisone and tamoxifen + fluoxymesterone in women above 65 years of age. *Breast Cancer Res Treat.* 2000;61:103–110.

200. Christman K, Muss HB, Case LD, Stanley V. Chemotherapy of metastatic breast cancer in the elderly. The Piedmont Oncology Association experience. *JAMA.* 1992;268:57–62.

201. Chlebowski RT, Smalley RV, Weiner JM, Irwin LE, Bartolucci AA, Bateman JR. Combination versus sequential single agent chemotherapy in advanced breast cancer: associations with metastatic sites and long-term survival. The Western Cancer Study Group and The Southeastern Cancer Study Group. *Br J Cancer.* 1989; 59:227–230.

202. Joensuu H, Holli K, Heikkinen M, et al. Combination chemotherapy versus single-agent therapy as first- and second-line treatment in metastatic breast cancer: a

prospective randomized trial. *J Clin Oncol.* 1998;16: 3720–3730.

203. Muss HB, Case LD, Richards Fd, et al. Interrupted versus continuous chemotherapy in patients with metastatic breast cancer. The Piedmont Oncology Association [see comments]. *N Engl J Med.* 1991;325:1342–1348.

204. Gelman RS, Taylor SGT. Cyclophosphamide, methotrexate, and 5-fluorouracil chemotherapy in women more than 65 years old with advanced breast cancer: the elimination of age trends in toxicity by using doses based on creatinine clearance. *J Clin Oncol.* 1984;2:1404–1413.

205. Kimmick GG, Fleming R, Muss HB, Balducci L. Cancer chemotherapy in older adults. A tolerability perspective. *Drugs Aging.* 1997;10:34–49.

206. Bajetta E, Biganzoli L, Carnaghi C, et al. Oral doxifluridine plus levoleucovorin in elderly patients with advanced breast cancer. *Cancer.* 1998;83:1136–1141.

207. Vogel C, O'Rourke M, Winer E, et al. Vinorelbine as first-line chemotherapy for advanced breast cancer in women 60 years of age or older. *Ann Oncol.* 1999;10: 397–402.

208. Hortobagyi GN, Theriault RL, Porter L, et al. Efficacy of pamidronate in reducing skeletal complications in patients with breast cancer and lytic bone metastases. Protocol 19 Aredia Breast Cancer Study Group [see comments]. *N Engl J Med.* 1996;335:1785–1791.

209. Lipton A, Theriault RL, Hortobagyi GN, et al. Pamidronate prevents skeletal complications and is effective palliative treatment in women with breast carcinoma and osteolytic bone metastases: long term follow-up of two randomized, placebo-controlled trials. *Cancer.* 2000; 88:1082–1090.

210. Hillner BE. The role of bisphosphonates in metastatic breast cancer. *Semin Radiat Oncol.* 2000;10:250–253.

211. Ganz PA, Schag CC, Heinzich RL. The psychosocial impact of cancer on the elderly. A comparison with younger patients. *J Am Geriatr Soc.* 1985;33:429–435.

212. Ganz PA. Breast cancer in older women: quality-of-life considerations. *Cancer Control.* 1994;1:372–379.

213. Compas BE, Stoll MF, Thomsen AH, Oppedisano G, Epping-Jordan JE, Krag DN. Adjustment to breast cancer: age-related differences in coping and emotional distress. *Breast Cancer Res Treat.* 1999;54:195–203.

214. Wenzel LB, Fairclough DL, Brady MJ, et al. Age-related differences in the quality of life of breast carcinoma patients after treatment. *Cancer.* 1999;86: 1768–1774.

215. Kantor DE, Houldin A. Breast cancer in older women: treatment, psychosocial effects, interventions, and outcomes. *J Gerontol Nurs.* 1999;25:19–25; quiz 54–55.

216. Greenfield S, Blanco DM, Elashoff RM, Ganz PA. Patterns of care related to age of breast cancer patients. *JAMA.* 1987;257:2766–2770.

217. Samet J, Hunt WC, Key C, Humble CG, Goodwin JS. Choice of cancer therapy varies with age of patient. *JAMA.* 1986;255:3385–3390.

218. Chu J, Diehr P, Feigl P, et al. The effect of age on the care of women with breast cancer in community hospitals. *J Gerontol.* 1987;42:185–190.

219. Silliman RA, Guadagnoli E, Weitberg AB, Mor V. Age as a predictor of diagnostic and initial treatment intensity in newly diagnosed breast cancer patients. *J Gerontol.* 1989; 44:M46–M50.

220. Farrow DC, Hunt WC, Samet JM. Geographic variation in the treatment of localized breast cancer [see comments]. *N Engl J Med.* 1992;326:1097–1101.

221. Nattinger AB, Gottlieb MS, Veum J, Yahnke D, Goodwin JS. Geographic variation in the use of breast-conserving treatment for breast cancer [see comments]. *N Engl J Med.* 1992;326:1102–1107.

222. Newcomb PA, Carbone PP. Cancer treatment and age: patient perspectives. *J Natl Cancer Inst.* 1993;85:1580–1584.

223. Samet JM, Hunt WC, Farrow DC. Determinants of receiving breast-conserving surgery. The Surveillance, Epidemiology, and End Results Program, 1983–1986. *Cancer.* 1994;73:2344–2351.

224. Du X, Freeman JL, Freeman DH, Syblik DA, Goodwin JS. Temporal and regional variation in the use of breast-conserving surgery and radiotherapy for older women with early-stage breast cancer from 1983 to 1995. *J Gerontol A Biol Sci Med Sci.* 1999;54:M474–M478.

225. Mandelblatt JS, Hadley J, Kerner JF, et al. Patterns of breast carcinoma treatment in older women: patient preference and clinical and physical influences. *Cancer.* 2000;89:561–573.

226. Lash TL, Silliman RA, Guadagnoli E, Mor V. The effect of less than definitive care on breast carcinoma recurrence and mortality. *Cancer.* 2000;89:1739–1747.

227. Mor V, Masterson-Allen S, Goldberg RJ, Cummings FJ, Glicksman AS, Fretwell MD. Relationship between age at diagnosis and treatments received by cancer patients. *J Am Geriatr Soc.* 1985;33:585–589.

228. Fetting JH, Comstock GW, Eby S, et al. The effect of aging on the utilization of chemotherapy for metastatic breast cancer: a population-based study. *Cancer Investig.* 1997;15: 199–203.

229. Goodwin JS, Samet JM. Care received by older women diagnosed with breast cancer. *Cancer Control.* 1994;1: 313–319.

230. Benson ABD, Pregler JP, Bean JA, Rademaker AW, Eshler B, Anderson K. Oncologists' reluctance to accrue patients onto clinical trials: an Illinois Cancer Center study [see comments]. *J Clin Oncol.* 1991;19:2067–2075.

231. Kemeny M, Muss HB, Kornblith AB, Peterson B, Wheeler J, Cohen HJ. Barriers to participation of older women with breast cancer in clinical trials. *Proc Am Soc Clin Oncol.* 2000;19:602a (abstract 2371).

232. American Joint Committee on Cancer. In: Beahrs OH HD, Hutter RVP, et al., eds. *Manual for Staging of Cancer, 4th Ed.* Philadelphia: Lippincott; 1992:149–154.

233. Fisher B, Slack N, Katrych D, Wolmark N. Ten year follow-up results of patients with carcinoma of the breast in a co-operative clinical trial evaluating surgical adjuvant chemotherapy. *Surg Gynecol Obstet.* 1975;140:528–534.

234. Valagussa P, Bonadonna G, Veronesi U. Patterns of relapse and survival following radical mastectomy. Analysis of 716 consecutive patients. *Cancer.* 1978;41:1170–1178.

34
Colon Cancer and Other Gastrointestinal Malignancies

Peter C. Enzinger and Robert J. Mayer

In the year 2001, it was anticipated that 235,700 new cases of digestive tract cancer would be diagnosed in the United States,[1] accounting for just under one-fifth (19%) of all new cancers. The majority of these new gastrointestinal malignancies were colorectal cancers (57%), followed by pancreas (12%), stomach (9%), liver (7%), and esophagus (6%) cancers.[1] Digestive tract cancers tend to be highly aggressive tumors. Nearly one-quarter (24%) of all cancer deaths in the United States are caused by these malignancies.[1] Fortunately, diagnosis and treatment of these cancers is improving, and small but statistically significant improvements in survival have been documented for most digestive tract cancers during the past three decades.[1]

Age is clearly a risk factor for gastrointestinal malignancies. The majority (>65%) of these cancers occur in patients older than age 65 years (Fig. 34.1).[2,3] The incidence increases by 14- to 42 fold between the fourth and eighth decades of life. Survival is also reduced with increasing age. In a European study, 5 year survival rates for 170,000 elderly patients (65–99 years old) with colorectal, stomach, and pancreas cancer were obtained (Fig. 34.2).[4] Survival in these malignancies was 25% to 33% less in persons older than 80 years of age when compared to those younger than 70 years. Coexisting illnesses almost certainly contributed to this poorer outcome.

Although advanced age in itself is not a substantial risk factor for treatment-related morbidity and mortality, it is generally associated with a progressive decline in functional reserve of multiple organ systems and may reduce the tolerance of normal tissues to treatment complications.[5] Elderly patients often suffer from partial loss of organ function secondary to atherosclerosis, emphysema, diabetes, and other comorbidities. Further loss of tissue function from treatment-related stresses may lead to organ failure. Patients with multiple medical problems have a higher surgical complication rate and require more time to recover from their operations. Older patients, with decreased bone marrow and epithelial stem cell reserves, have an increased likelihood of developing myelosuppression and mucositis following radiation therapy.[6]

It appears that older patients generally tolerate chemotherapy as well as their younger counterparts.[7,8] With increasing age, however, the metabolism of cytotoxic drugs and the ability of normal cells to recover from damage caused by these drugs are diminished. Glomerular filtration rate is known to decline with increasing age, tending to reduce the excretion of certain chemotherapy agents. Hepatic function may also be impaired in older patients through decreased hepatic blood flow and a decline in the intracellular activity of P-450 cytochrome enzymes. Also, the elderly are more likely to require additional medications that can compromise hepatic functions. Many antitumor drugs are susceptible to these changes in hepatic metabolism. Older patients generally have decreased total body water and albumin levels, leading to increased free drug concentrations. Hematopoietic stem cell reserves are often compromised and lead to increased neutropenia, anemia, and fatigue. Anemia, in turn, may increase the free drug concentration of certain antitumor agents that are heavily bound to red blood cells. Decreased mucosal stem cell reserves in the elderly may lead to increased mucositis and diarrhea.[9]

Colorectal Cancer

Colorectal cancer is the third leading cause of cancer death in the world, after lung and gastric cancer.[10] Its highest incidence is in developed countries. In the United States, 98,200 cases of colon cancer and 37,200 cases of rectal cancer were diagnosed in 2001, leading to 48,100 and 8600 deaths, respectively.[1] Colorectal cancer has become the second leading cause of cancer-related death in the United States. At the time of diagnosis, approximately 40% of patients with colorectal cancer have

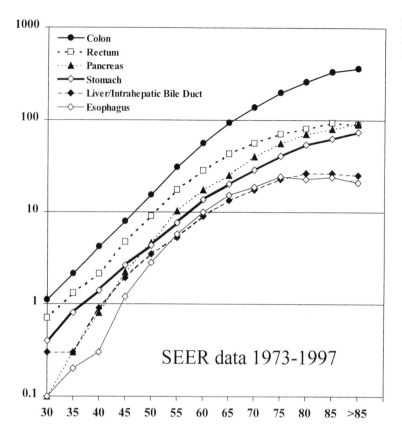

FIGURE 34.1. Age-specific incidence of gastrointestinal malignancies (per 100,000) in the United States. (From Ries et al.,[3] with permission.)

localized disease, 40% have lymph node involvement, and 20% have distant metastases.[3] The majority of colorectal cancers arise in the distal colon; however, a slight increase in the incidence of proximal colorectal cancer has been documented in the last decades.[11]

The probability of developing colorectal cancer increases from 0.05% in the first four decades of life to 3% to 4% in the sixth and seventh decades.[1] In women over 80 years of age, mortality from colorectal cancer significantly exceeds that of breast cancer and is nearly equal to that of lung cancer.[1] The mortality data vary

slightly in different countries. For instance, in the Netherlands, colorectal carcinoma has become the most common cancer in women and the second most common cancer (after prostate) in men aged 85 to 94 years.[12]

Older patients tend to have a higher frequency of right-sided colon cancers than do younger patients.[13,14] They generally present at diagnosis with the same percentages of localized and advanced disease as their younger counterparts.[2] Some studies, however, suggest that patients older than 80 years have earlier-stage disease than younger patients[11] and tend to have higher rates

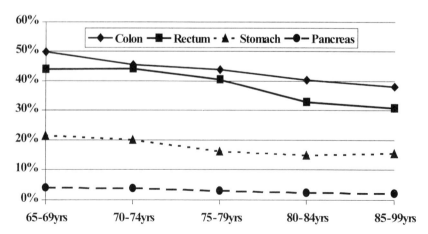

FIGURE 34.2. Age-specific 5-year survival (%) for 170,000 elderly patients with gastrointestinal malignancies from the EUROCARE II Project. (From Vercelli et al.,[4] with permission.)

of obstruction and perforation.[13] This, in turn, results in a higher likelihood of acute presentations, leading to a higher perioperative mortality rate in this older age group.[15,16] This trend is also suggested in a French series of 1734 patients (including 163 patients older than 80 years), in which 5-year survival was 35% for patients older than 80 years versus 46% for younger patients ($p < 0.05$).[17] However, this difference in survival no longer was significant if noncancer deaths were excluded from this series.

Comorbid conditions can have a significant impact on the outcome of older patients with colorectal cancer. In a population-based analysis, the National Institute on Aging stratified patients, listed in the surveillance, epidemiology, and end results (SEER) tumor registry, into three cohorts: 55 to 64 years, 65 to 74 years, and 75 years and over.[18] The number of comorbid conditions, such as hypertension, heart disease, and chronic obstructive pulmonary disease, was found to increase with age and was significant in predicting early mortality ($p = 0.0007$) in older patients.

Risk Factors

Approximately 75% of patients with colorectal cancer lack clearly defined risk factors for their disease.[19] Of the remaining patients, 15% to 20% have a history of inflammatory bowel disease or first-degree relatives with either colorectal cancer[20] or adenomatous polyps.[21] Patients with hereditary autosomal dominant colorectal cancer syndromes are rare. The two most common syndromes, hereditary nonpolyposis colorectal cancer (HNPCC) and familial adenomatosis polyposis (FAP), account for only 5% and 1% of all colorectal cancers, respectively.[22–24] These hereditary syndromes are even less important in the elderly, because 90% of persons with FAP and 68% to 75% of individuals with HNPCC are diagnosed before the age of 65 years.[23,24]

Other factors that have been suggested to increase the risk of colorectal cancer include physical inactivity, obesity, consumption of red meat or alcohol, tobacco use, and diets low in fruits and vegetables.[25] Contrary to prior beliefs, the consumption of coffee and tea or a diet low in fiber do not appear to increase risk.[26,27]

Prevention and Surveillance

Colon cancers are thought to develop from normal colonic epithelial cells through a series of pathologic changes that involve mutation or deletion of critical genes.[28] As these sequential genetic events occur, the epithelium first hyperproliferates and forms aberrant crypt foci.[29] Adenomatous polyps eventually develop in these areas of hyperproliferation. These premalignant lesions may become progressively larger and atypical until cancer evolves, usually within a period of 5 to 10 years.[30] Approximately one in three persons have an adenomatous polyp in their colon by the age of 50. By age 70, the incidence increases to approxiamtely 50%.[31]

Chemoprevention

Various dietary factors, supplements, and drugs have been proposed as chemopreventative agents for colorectal neoplasia (Table 34.1). Of these, aspirin and other nonsteroidal anti-inflammatory drugs (NSAIDs) are the most widely studied and appear to show the most conclusive benefit. These drugs are thought to induce apoptosis in abnormal colonic epithelial cells by cyclooxygenase-dependent and cyclooxygenase-independent mechanisms. The process by which cyclooxygenases increase apoptosis is unclear. Cyclooxygenase-independent pathways may inhibit the activation of nuclear factor-κB (NF-κB) or may interfere with the binding of peroxisome proliferator-activated receptor-δ (PPARδ) to DNA.[32,33] Cyclooxygenases may also act as angiogenesis inhibitors.[34]

Cycloxygenase-2 is elevated in 90% of sporadic colon cancers and in 40% of colonic adenomas, but is found at

TABLE 34.1. Chemoprevention trials of colorectal cancer.

Agent and author	Study design	Endpoint	No. of patients	Relative risk
Aspirin				
Thun et al.[39]	Prospective cohort	Death from colon cancer	666,424	0.77–0.73
Giovannucci et al.[40]	Prospective cohort	Colon cancer	47,900	0.68
Giovannucci et al.[41]	Prospective cohort	Colorectal cancer	89,446	0.56
Folate				
Giovannucci et al.[47]	Prospective cohort	Colon cancer	88,756	0.25
Calcium				
Baron et al.[50]	Randomized, placebo controlled	Colorectal adenomas	913	0.85
Estrogens				
Calle et al.[53]	Prospective cohort	Death from colon cancer	422,373	0.71
Grodstein et al.[54]	Prospective cohort	Colorectal cancer	59,002	0.65

normal levels in the unaltered colonic epithelium.[35] Inhibition of this enzyme can significantly reduce the number of colonic polyps in animal models[36] as well as in patients with hereditary polyposis syndromes.[37,38]

In the general population, multiple prospective cohort studies (but not randomized controlled trials or RCTs) have demonstrated that aspirin use reduces the risk of colon cancer. In the Cancer Prevention Study II, death rates from colon cancer decreased with increasing aspirin use.[39] Persons who used aspirin 16 or more times per month had the lowest risk of colorectal cancer death. In the Health Professionals Follow-Up Study, 25% of persons used aspirin more than twice per week.[40] In this group, the relative risk of colorectal cancer was only 0.68 compared to nonaspirin users. If regular aspirin use persisted for at least 6 years, this relative risk fell even further to 0.35. Moreover, in the group of patients who underwent regular screening sigmoidoscopies, regular aspirin use also reduced the development of distal colorectal adenomas (relative risk, 0.72). In the Nurses' Health Study, regular aspirin use two or more times per week for 20 years lowered the relative risk of colorectal cancer to 0.56. However, little or no reduction in risk was noted during the first 9 years of follow-up.[41]

Other anti-inflammatory drugs (NSAIDs) are also likely to reduce the risk of colorectal cancer in the general population; prospective studies examining this issue have not been completed. Recently, however, a large retrospective analysis of Medicaid patients who filled prescriptions for nonaspirin NSAIDs suggested that individuals who used these drugs for at least 2 of the past 5 years had a relative risk of colorectal cancer of 0.49.[42] In this study, the protective effect appeared to be most pronounced for right-sided colon lesions.

Fruits and vegetables, rich in folate and other micronutrients, are thought to lower the incidence of colorectal adenomas and cancer.[43,44] In fact, high intake of dietary folate has been shown to reduce the number of malignant and premalignant lesions in cohort and case-control studies.[45,46] In the Nurses' Health Study, long-term use (>15 years) of folate-containing multivitamins reduced the relative risk of colorectal cancer to 0.25.[47] Shorter periods (5–14 years) of folate supplementation had less impact (relative risk, 0.80–0.83). No benefit was noted when the duration of folate use was less than 5 years. These data suggest that folate may play a role in the early pathogenesis of colorectal cancer, although randomized trials are still needed.

There is also evidence that diets rich in red meat and animal fat are associated with a higher incidence of colorectal adenomas and cancer.[43] A fatty diet increases the production of bile acids, which in turn may cause hyperproliferation of the colonic epithelium.[48] Calcium, on the other hand, can bind bile acids and may therefore reduce the risk of colorectal cancer.[49] In a recent randomized double-blind placebo-controlled trial, patients with a history of colorectal adenoma received 3 g of calcium carbonate supplementation per day or a placebo. After only 1 year, the group allocated to calcium had a significant reduction in the number of recurrent colorectal adenomas compared to those patients who received placebo [relative risk (RR), 0.73].[50] The percentage of patients who were found to have no further adenomas at the time of follow-up colonoscopy increased from 62% to 69% following calcium supplementation.

Estrogens may also reduce the risk of colorectal cancer, but the exact mechanism of this effect is unclear. It has been hypothesized that this hormone acts by decreasing bile acid secretion or by a direct effect on the colonic epithelium.[51] Estrogens have been shown to reduce the risk of colorectal adenomas and carcinomas in multiple observational (non-RCT) studies.[52] The average risk reduction in these reports is approximately 20%. Similar benefits have been demonstrated in prospective cohort trials. Thus, women who used estrogen replacement therapy in the Cancer Prevention Study II had a significantly decreased risk of fatal colon cancer (RR, 0.71).[53] In the subgroup of active estrogen users, this reduction in risk was even more pronounced (RR, 0.55). Similar reductions in the incidence of colorectal cancer with estrogen use were also reported in the Nurses' Health Study.[54]

Vitamin supplementation with beta-carotene and vitamins A, C, D, or E does not appear to reduce the risk of colon cancer. Multiple prospective cohort studies and one randomized study have found no benefit for supplementation with these vitamins in the prevention of colorectal neoplasia.[47,55–57] Likewise, dietary fiber has not been found to be protective for primary or secondary prevention in various prospective cohort studies[27] and in several randomized trials.[58,59]

Screening

The rationale for surveillance screening of the colon and rectum is straightforward. Sporadic colorectal cancers typically evolve from adenomatous polyps over a 5- to 10-year period.[30] If these polyps can be identified and removed before they transform into a malignancy, the risk of colorectal cancer can be reduced by 50% to 90%.[60,61] Furthermore, if a colorectal cancer is discovered at an early stage, prognosis is dramatically improved. For a detailed discussion of screening for colorectal cancer, the reader is directed to Chapter 32, Screening for Cancer.

Diagnosis and Workup

Elderly patients tend to have similar symptoms at the time of presentation as those of younger patients.[62] Symp-

TABLE 34.2. American Joint Committee on Cancer (AJCC) and modified Dukes' classification of colorectal cancer.

AJCC (TNM)	Modified Dukes'	Pathologic description	Approximate 5-year survival
I (T1N0 M0)	A	Cancer limited to mucosa and submucosa	>90%
I (T2 N0 M0)	B1	Cancer extends into muscularis	85%
II (T3-4 N0 M0)	B2	Cancer extends into or through serosa	70%–85%
III (Any T N1-2 M0)	C	Cancer involves regional lymph nodes	30%–60%
IV (Any T Any N M1)	D	Distant metastases (i.e., liver, lung, etc.)	5%

TNM: T, depth of tumor invasion; N, lymph node involment; M, metastatic disease.

toms of occult bleeding, including fatigue, shortness of breath, and even angina, are most common. Blood studies in such patients may reveal a microcytic hypochromic anemia, indicative of iron deficiency. Changes in bowel habits or stool diameter are most characteristic of rectal lesions. Rectal lesions and distal colonic lesions most often present with frank bleeding. Tumors of the ascending colon may produce "mahogany stools," in which blood is admixed with feces. These right-sided lesions can grow quite large and are sometimes palpable on physical examination. Peritonitis or obstruction is indicative of locally advanced disease.

Such symptoms are frequently attributed to hemorrhoidal bleeding, diverticulitis, inflammatory bowel disease, or irritable bowel syndrome. Elderly patients with bleeding or changes in bowel habits should always be evaluated with colonoscopy. If a cancer or advanced polyp is found, a routine workup should be initiated; this includes a CT scan of the abdomen and pelvis, chest radiograph, and routine blood work. A carcinoembryonic antigen (CEA) level should also be measured before resection. Although this test is not diagnostic and cannot predict the resectability of colorectal cancer, elevated levels are associated with a poorer prognosis and may be an indication for postoperative therapy.[63–66] Patients considered unresectable for reasons of metastatic disease should undergo a confirmatory biopsy.

Patients with rectal cancers, in addition to undergoing a standard diagnostic evaluation, should also be assessed with endorectal ultrasound or magnetic resonance imaging. These studies can differentiate between relatively superficial tumors, which can often be treated with local excision, and more advanced disease, which may require radical srugery, excision of the anal sphincter, and a permanent colostomy (i.e., abdominoperineal resection).

Staging

Survival for patients with colorectal cancer is dependent on the stage of disease. The true stage of a colorectal cancer can only be determined by careful pathologic examination of the resected specimen. For many years,

the Dukes' staging system has been used to predict outcome and to determine treatment for individual patients (Table 34.2). Over the years, various modifications to this staging system have been made to improve its prognostic value. Currently, the TNM staging system, proposed by the American Joint Committee on Cancer, is employed. Prognosis worsens with depth of tumor invasion (T) and lymph node involvement (N); patients with metastatic disease (M) have the shortest survival.

Treatment

Surgery: Colon Cancer

Cancers of the colon are typically resected with a hemicolectomy. In this procedure, the cancer is removed with adjacent healthy bowel and mesentery, including blood vessels and lymphatics. The operative mortality is low and appears to decrease slightly (from 5.5% to 3.5%) when the resection is performed at a hospital at which such procedures are performed more often.[67] Such a high procedure volume is also associated with a modest increase in long-term survival, particularly for patients with stage II and III disease ($p < 0.001$). In patients between 70 and 79 years of age, the operative mortality rate may be as low as 2%;[68] this may rise to 7% to 9% in patients of 80 years or older.[68,69] Patients undergoing palliative resections, due to advanced disease, have higher mortality rates. In patients 70 to 79 years of age, the mortality may be as high as 21% and in octogenarians it may reach 38%. Age-related mortality is also evident in a series of 5586 patients from the Johns Hopkins Hospital in which the perioperative mortality rate was 9.3% in patients 85 years and older but only 3.3% in patients aged 66 to 69 years.[70]

Surgery: Rectal Cancer

The standard surgical procedure for cancer of the rectum is a radical resection with anastomosis. Most commonly, a low anterior resection is performed. Increasingly, colorectal surgeons are being trained to perform a total mesorectal excision. This procedure maximizes the volume of perirectal tissue removed and theoretically removes perirectal tumor deposits that would otherwise have remained in place.

Traditionally, rectal cancers close to the anal sphincter have required an abdominoperimeal resection. In this procedure, the anal sphincter is resected along with the rectum and a permanent colostomy is created. Morbidity is significant and includes urinary and male sexual dysfunction. For locally advanced disease, this procedure remains the standard of care. However, for minimally invasive, early-stage distal rectal cancers (T1–T2, stage I), transanal sphincter-sparing surgery and abdominoperineal resection appear to have similar local recurrence (5%–15%) and long-term survival (80%–90%) rates.[71–74] Patients with invasion of the muscularis propria or lymphovascular invasion benefit from postoperative chemoradiation.[74,75]

Postoperative Chemotherapy: Colon Cancer

Randomized studies have repeatedly demonstrated the value of 6 to 12 months of 5-fluorouracil-based (5-FU-based) chemotherapy given prophylactically after the resection of lymph node-positive (stage III/Dukes' C) colon cancer.[66,76] Postoperative chemotherapy can reduce the recurrence rate of colon cancer by 40% and mortality by 33%.[66] In absolute terms, chemotherapy can improve 5-year survival for lymph node-positive patients from 45% to more than 60%.

Such a clear benefit for postoperative chemotherapy has not been conclusively demonstrated in patients with fully resected, muscle-invasive, lymph node-negative (stage II/Dukes' B2) colon cancer.[77] In part, this is because the 5-year survival for this group is so favorable (75%–80%) that it is difficult to demonstrate a statistically significant improvement when chemotherapy is utilized without studying very large numbers of patients. Certain adverse prognostic factors, however, such as clinical obstruction,[77] perforation,[77] elevated preoperative plasma CEA levels,[66] poorly differentiated histology,[66] invasion of or adhesion to adjacent organs,[66]

TABLE 34.3. Poor prognostic predictors following total surgical resection of a colorectal cancer.

Tumor spread to regional lymph nodes
Tumor penetration through the bowel wall
Perforation
Obstruction
Poorly differentiated histology
Tumor adherence/invasion of adjacent organs
Lymphatic or vascular invasion
Preoperative elevation of CEA titer (>5.0 ng/mL)
Aneuploidy
Specific chromosomal deletion (allelic loss)

TABLE 34.4. Use of chemotherapy for colorectal cancer by age.

Age, years	Node positive		Metastatic	
	n	Treated, %	n	Treated, %
65–69	457	48	377	45
70–74	502	48	411	41
75–79	516	39	366	27
80–84	333	24	262	18
85+	249	6	214	5

Source: From Sundararajan et al.,[83] with permission.

lymphatic invasion,[78] and vascular invasion[79] (Table 34.3) increase the risk of recurrence substantially in this group. Therefore, many experts recommend postoperative chemotherapy to patients with these adverse prognostic factors.

Current postoperative chemotherapy for high-risk resected colon cancer is based on the combination of 5-FU and leucovorin. Fluorouracil is an antimetabolite that binds to the enzyme thymidylate synthase, thereby depleting thymidine pools and inhibiting DNA synthesis.[80,81] Leucovorin (also known as folinic acid) stabilizes the complex formed between 5-FU and thymidylate synthase, prolonging inhibition of this enzyme by more than 20 fold.[82]

Older patients receive adjuvant chemotherapy less often than their younger counterparts (Table 34.4).[13,83] Although chemotherapy has become the standard of care for high-risk resected colon cancer in the general population, some controversy remains regarding the relative benefit of this treatment in patients older than 70 years of age. Recently, an intention-to-treat meta-analysis was completed, pooling 3351 patients from seven randomized trials.[84] In these trials, patients with Dukes' B2 or C (stage II or III) colon cancer had been randomized to receive surgery alone or surgery followed by 5-FU-based chemotherapy. Patients were stratified by decade of life (<50, 50–60, 60–70, >70), with 15% of patients older than 70 years of age. Treatment effect (i.e., overall survival and disease-free survival) and toxicity were essentially the same for all age groups. It therefore appears that postoperative chemotherapy in high-risk colon cancer is as beneficial and tolerable in patients over age 70 years as it is for younger patients.

Adjuvant Chemotherapy and Radiation Therapy: Rectal Cancer

Chemoradiation after surgery reduces the local recurrence rate and increases disease-free survival in patients with deeply invasive (T3–T4) or lymph node-positive rectal cancer. In one study, 5-year disease-free survival increased from 46% to 70% in those patients who received chemoradiation after their surgery.[85] Similarly, regional recurrences were reduced from 24% to 11% with this approach. Radiation therapy is typically given over 5 to 6 weeks. Fluorouracil-based chemotherapy may be administered during this time either as a bolus[86] or as a continuous infusion.[87] Additionally, at least 4 months of 5-FU based chemotherapy is generally given.

Chemoradiation for rectal cancer may also be admin- sitered before surgery.[88,89] Preoperative chemoradiation is most often recommended if there is evidence by endo- scopic ultrasound or magnetic resonance imaging of lymph node involvement or deep invasion through the rectal wall. If this approach is undertaken, patients should still receive postoperative chemotherapy follow- ing surgical resection. If imaging studies reveal superfi- cial disease with no lymph node enlargement, surgery would seem to be the preferred initial treatment because patients with early-stage cancer do not require further therapy.

There are few data to suggest that elderly patients respond any differently to chemoradiotherapy than younger patients. Older patients, however, do appear to be at increased risk for radiation-related small bowel damage.[90] Therefore, particularly in this group, an effort should be made to limit the amount of small bowel in the radiation field.

Follow-Up

Prospective data have failed to show any survival benefit for the use of surveillance CT scans, chest radiographs, liver function tests, and fecal occult blood tests following the resection of a colorectal cancer.[91-93] However, a careful history and thorough physical examination every 3 to 6 months is recommended for the first 3 years fol- lowing resection and annually thereafter.[94]

The use of serial determinations of the plasma carci- noembryonic antigen (CEA) level as an early indication of clinically occult recurrent disease, although not uni- versally accepted, has been recommended at 3-monthly intervals for the first 3 postoperative years.[94] Such a rec- ommendation is based on evidence showing an elevated CEA level to be the initial indication of disease in 60% to 64% of cases and to be the most cost-effective approach to detect potentially resectable disease.[91,92,95]

Patients should undergo a colonoscopy within 1 year of the time of their diagnosis, with a goal of detecting other polyps or cancer within the large bowel. The purpose of this procedure is not to screen for recurrent cancer at the suture line, because such anastomotic recur- rences are exceedingly rare. Colonoscopy should be repeated yearly so long as further polyps are discovered. If no polyps are detected, the interval between future examinations may be extended to every 3 to 5 years.[94]

Advanced Colorectal Cancer

Surgery: Advanced Colorectal Cancer

Patients with anatomically isolated tumor recurrences may be candidates for an attempt at surgical resection, particularly if several years have elapsed since the time of the initial diagnosis. Five-year survival has been reported in 25% to 39% of selected patients who under- went the resection of liver or lung metastases.[96,97] In a series from the Memorial Sloan-Kettering Cancer Center, 128 patients 70 years of age or older underwent liver resection for metastatic colorectal cancer between 1985 and 1994.[98] Although these patients experienced a 4% perioperative mortality rate and a 42% complication rate, their median survival was 40 months and 5-year survival rate was 35%. These older patients had a similar outcome to 449 patients less than 70 years old who under- went comparable liver resections during the same time period. Similarly, studies have shown that appropriately selected octogenarians can tolerate lung resections with acceptable morbidity and mortality.[99]

Patients who did not initially receive postoperative 5- FU-based chemotherapy for their resected colon cancer should be considered for chemotherapy after complete resection of their recurrence. In patients who have received prior chemotherapy, the benefits of further treatment after reresection are uncertain.[97]

The merits of hepatic arterial infusion chemotherapy (delivered by an implanted abdominal pump) after resec- tion of hepatic metastases from colorectal cancer have been the source of debate. Such treatment clearly reduces the likelihood of recurrence in the liver but does not protect against extrahepatic recurrences and does not appear to prolong survival.[100,101]

Chemotherapy: Advanced Colorectal Cancer

For many years, the standard treatment for advanced col- orectal carcinoma has been the combination of 5-FU and leucovorin, given either for 5 consecutive days monthly or for 1 day per week. Small randomized studies have shown such chemotherapy to prolong survival when com- pared to best supportive care alone (11 versus 5 months; $p = 0.006$) and to improve quality of life.[102]

SEER data from 1992 demonstrated that the usage of chemotherapy in patients with advanced colorectal cancer falls with increasing age (see Table 34.4).[83] Furthermore, elderly patients are underrepresented in clinical trials. Although 72% of all advanced colorectal cancer patients are 65 years or older (1992–1994 SEER data), less than 50% of patients in clinical trials spon- sored by the National Cancer Institute (United States) were in this elderly age group.[103,104]

The reasons for this disparity in treatment remain unclear. In a review of major trials of advanced colorectal cancer, researchers from the Royal Marsden Hospital in London found no difference in the probability of disease regression (24% versus 29%), toxicity, failure-free survival, or 1-year overall survival (44% versus 48%) between patients older and younger than 70 years of age.[105] The median overall survival was shorter for the older patients (9.6 versus 11.5 months; $p = 0.04$), likely due to competing comorbidities.

Irinotecan (CPT-11, Camptosar) is a new antitumor agent that has been recently approved for the treatment of colorectal cancer. It acts primarily by inhibition of the topoisomerase I enzyme. Once bound to the topoisomerase I–DNA complex, irinotecan blocks reannealing of the parent DNA, thereby halting nucleic acid synthesis in the cell, leading to cell death. Severe diarrhea, neutropenia, and nausea may occur with this drug in approximately 25% to 33% of patients. The administration of irinotecan leads to disease regression in 13% to 23% of patients whose disease is refractory to 5-FU.[106] Compared to best supportive care alone in similar patients resistant to 5-FU, irinotecan therapy has been demonstrated to improve both survival duration and quality of life.[107] In patients who have received no prior chemotherapy, the probability of response to irinotecan is higher (29%) and is similar to that of 5-FU and leucovorin.[108]

Weekly irinotecan can safely be added to weekly 5-FU and low-dose leucovorin. Recently, this triple combination was compared to 5-FU and leucovorin alone in a randomized trial.[108] The response rate of the ironotecan/5-FU/leucovorin combination was superior to 5-FU and leucovorin (50% versus 28%; $p < 0.0001$) as was the median progression-free survival (7.0 months versus 4.3 months; $p = 0.004$). Overall toxicity and quality of life were similar with both regimens. Although these promising results have led some oncologists to consider this combination as initial therapy for patients with advanced colorectal cancer, only 40% of patients enrolled in the trial were 65 years of age or older, and the tolerance of treatment may well be poorer in the elderly. Conceivably, the same therapeutic effect may be achieved with less toxicity by giving 5-FU/leucovorin and irinotecan sequentially rather than concomitantly.

Fluorouracil may also be given as a continuous infusion. This form of administration offers a moderate improvement in response rate (22% versus 14%; $p = 0.0002$) and a small improvement in survival (13 versus 12 months; $p = 0.04$) compared to bolus 5-FU in patients with advanced colorectal cancer.[109] Infusional 5-FU causes less diarrhea, mucositis, and hematologic toxicity and may shrink colorectal cancers that no longer respond to bolus 5-FU therapy. The major side effect is palmar-plantar dysesthesia (burning, redness, and peeling of the hands and feet), which is severe in approximately one-third of patients. These advantages must be balanced by the inconvenience of continuous therapy and the complications that may arise from portacath placement.

To circumvent the complications and inconvenience of infusional 5-FU, orally administered forms of 5-FU have been developed. Of these, only capecitabine (Xeloda) is currently approved for use in the United States. In randomized studies, capecitabine and 5-FU/leucovorin appear to lead to equivalent outcomes.[110]

A number of antitumor agents are under active development for this disease. Among these, oxaliplatin[111] and IMC-C225[112] appear most promising. Both have demonstrated activity in 5-FU-refractory advanced colorectal cancer.

Pancreatic Cancer

In the United States, the number of expected new cases (29,200) and the number of expected deaths (28,900) for pancreas cancer in the year 2001 are almost identical.[1] In part, this dire prognosis is due to the advanced stage of disease at presentation. At the time of diagnosis, less than 10% of patients have localized disease.[3] The other patients have nodal (30%) or metastatic (60%) spread. Overall, the probability for 5-year survival for this cancer is less than 5%. For patients undergoing a potentially curative resection, this estimate rises to approximately 17%. The median survival for this group of resected patients is 12 to 18 months verus 3 to 6 months for patients with metastatic disease. The median age at presentation is 60 years, and thus a significant proportion of patients is elderly. Both genders are equally affected, and African-Americans have a slightly higher rate of disease.

Smoking appears to be the greatest risk factor for pancreas cancer. In one prospective study of 167,767 patients, the proportion of pancreatic cancers attributable to cigarette smoking was 25%.[113] Risk was reduced by 48% and then approached that of nonsmokers after 2 and 10 years of smoking cessation, respectively. Other risk factors are disputed. Pancreatitis and diabetes, among others, have been linked to this malignancy in some[114,115] but not all[116,117] studies.

Prevention and Surveillance

Smoking cessation is the most important preventative step for this disease. As indicated above, risk is reduced by nearly half within 2 years of quitting and drops to normal after less than 10 years of smoking cessation.[113] With the possible exception of those few individuals who have a strong family history of this cancer, serial imaging studies as a means of screening are not indicated.[118]

Diagnosis and Workup

Many patients seek medical attention because of jaundice, which may be unaccompanied by any pain. Several weeks or months of epigastric or back pain, as well as weight loss, are also common. Patients may recently have been diagnosed with glucose intolerance or malabsorption syndrome. The initial diagnostic evaluation usually includes a CT scan with contrast and endoscopic retrograde cholangiopancreatography (ERCP). Often, the latter procedure not only establishes the diagnosis of cancer but also can serve to relieve the jaundice (through endoscopic stent placement) with which the patient originally presented. Additionally, the blood tumor marker CA 19-9 should be obtained; although this marker is not diagnostic for pancreatic cancer, it has been shown to independently predict resectability.[119] Patients may be resectable if there is no evidence of distant disease or encasement or occlusion of the celiac axis or superior mesenteric artery. Those patients who appear resectable require further evaluation with magnetic resonance angiography (MRA) or laparoscopy but do not require a preoperative biopsy. Patients with metastatic lesions or unresectable tumors should undergo pathologic confirmation of their disease.

Such a pathologic diagnosis is often not established in older patients having a clinical suspicion of pancreatic cancer. In one series, tissue confirmation was established in 88% of persons in their sixties but only in 41% of persons in their nineties.[120] Patients with a clinical diagnosis of what appeared to be a locally confined pancreatic neoplasm had a 5-year survival of 27% compared to 4% for those with biopsy-proven cancer. Thus, a disproportionate number of elderly patients may be misdiagnosed with this malignancy and may be incorrectly given a poor prognosis in an attempt to spare them the discomfort of an accurate pathologic diagnosis. In experienced hands, the major complication rate for CT- or ultrasound-guided biopsy of pancreatic lesions is approximately 1%.[121]

Treatment

Patients with pancreas cancer can be divided into three groups. The first group, with resectable disease, usually receives postoperative chemoradiation. In the second group, who have a cancer that is unresectable but has not spread to other organs, slightly different regimens of chemoradiation are offered. The third group, having metastatic disease, may be treated with chemotherapy or may receive palliative care alone.

Surgery: Resectable Pancreas Cancer

Pancreaticoduodenectomy (the Whipple procedure) is the only potentially curative therapy for pancreas cancer. The resection includes the distal duodenum, the proximal jejunum, the neck, head, and uncinate process of the pancreas, the gallbladder, and the distal biliary tree. Historically, this procedure is associated with a high morbidity and mortality. In the last decade, however, mortality rates at hospitals at which the procedure is frequently performed have dropped to less than 3%.[122,123]

There is ample evidence that pancreaticoduodenectomy can be safely performed in geriatric patients. For instance, in 206 patients over 70 years of age treated at the Mayo Clinic from 1982 through 1987, operative mortality was 9% with a surgical morbidity of 28%.[124] Overall survival was 19 months and 5-year survival was 4%. Similarly, the operative mortality in 138 patients older than 70 years of age who underwent pancreatic resection at Memorial Sloan-Kettering Cancer Center was 6% and the major complication rate was 45%. These results were virtually identical to those of younger patients. However, 5-year survival was slightly lower in the group of older patients (21% versus 29%; $p = 0.03$).[98]

An even older cohort was reported from the Johns Hopkins Hospital.[125] At that institution, 46 patients older than 80 years of age who underwent pancreaticoduodenectomy had an operative mortality of 4.3%, compared to 1.6% for patients under 80 years ($p = NS$). The complication rate was 57% and 41%, respectively ($p = 0.05$). Other studies from Germany,[126] Sweden,[127] and Italy[128] provide further evidence that pancreatic surgery can be safely performed in the elderly with results akin to those of younger patients.

Postoperative Chemoradiation: Resectable Pancreas Cancer

Following the complete resection of pancreas cancer, the use of adjuvant postoperative chemoradiation should be considered. Trials have shown that such combined modality therapy can double the 2-year actuarial survival (43% versus 18%) and median survival (21 months versus 11 months) compared to surgery alone.[129,130] In one study, 19% of patients randomized to receive chemoradiation were alive 5 to 11 years following their surgery, whereas only 5% of patients randomized to surgery alone lived to the 5-year point.[130]

The results of these relatively small studies have recently come under question. Two large European trials have shown no statistical benefit for postoperative chemoradiation in pancreatic cancer.[131,132] It is too early to determine if these new studies will impact present practice patterns in the United States.

Some investigators have advocated preoperative chemoradiation[133] or intraoperative radiation therapy[134] for patients with localized pancreas cancer. There are theoretical advantages for these approaches, but the available data have emerged from small patient cohorts at single institutions in a setting where selection bias is likely. For these reasons, the use of preoperative or intra-operative therapy should be reserved for clinical trials only.

Advanced Pancreas Cancer

Patients who are found to be unresectable at the time of attempted pancreaticoduodenectomy may be candidates for surgical palliation for jaundice and pain. Typically, these patients undergo a retrocolic gastrojejunostomy, a hepatojejunostomy, and a chemical splanchnicectomy. In one series of 118 patients from the Johns Hopkins Hospital, the perioperative mortality for these procedures was 2.5%; only 3% subsequently developed gastric obstruction and only 1.6% developed jaundice.[122] In a randomized trial, chemical splanchnicectomy with 50% alcohol significantly reduced or prevented pain when compared to placebo injection with saline.[135]

Chemoradiation: Locally Unresectable Pancreas Cancer

It is unclear if chemoradiation is superior to chemotherapy alone or to supportive care in patients with locally unresectable pancreas cancer because no randomized trials have been performed in this clinical setting. However, promising results at single institutions[136,137] led investigators of the Gastrointestinal Tumor Study Group to randomize patients with unresectable pancreas cancer to chemotherapy plus radiation or to radiation therapy alone.[138] The median survival was 10 months for patients who received 5-FU in addition to radiation therapy versus 5.5 months for those who received radiation therapy alone ($p < 0.01$). Similarly, the 1-year survival was superior for the chemoradiation group (40% versus 10%). Therefore, chemoradiation is now commonly employed for this group of patients.

Chemotherapy: Metastatic Pancreas Cancer

Metastatic pancreas cancer has been treated with 5-FU since the early 1960s; disease regression rates have ranged from 7% to 19%, and the median survival has varied from 4.5 to 6.0 months. The addition of other anti-tumor agents to 5-FU, while sometimes increasing the response rate, has had no impact on survival.[139,140] In small, randomized trials, the use of these 5-FU-based regimens has, however, shown a significant survival advantage when compared to supportive care alone (30–33 weeks versus 7–15 weeks).[141,142]

More recently, gemcitabine, a nucleoside analogue, has been found to have antitumor activity in pancreas cancer.[143,144] Partial responses have been reported in 6% to 11% of patients, with an associated median survival of 5.6 to 6.3 months. Gemcitabine has been compared to weekly bolus 5-FU as initial therapy in patients with advanced pancreas cancer.[145] Although the improvements in response (5.4% versus 0%) and median survival (5.7 versus 4.4 months) for gemcitabine were modest, improvements in symptom control led to acceptance of the drug as standard therapy for this disease. Of note, patients up to 79 years of age were included in this trial, with a median age of 62 years. Efforts to combine gemcitabine with other agents are underway.

Palliation: Metastatic Pancreas Cancer

Neurolytic block of the celiac plexus and/or splanchnic nerves is an important adjunctive therapy to oral analgesia in pancreas cancer. In this procedure, ethyl alcohol is injected into the nerve via a small-gauge needle, guided by CT scan or other imaging technique. In experienced hands, this technique relieves pain in approximately 75% of patients.[146] Up to 50% of patients may have minimal or no pain 15 days following their procedure, without opioid therapy.[147] Effective pain relief is often attained for several months.

Gastric Cancer

Worldwide, gastric cancer is the second leading cause of cancer death (after lung cancer) in both men and women.[10] In East Asia, it is the most common cancer in men and the leading cause of cancer death in women. In the United States, the predicted number of new cases for 2001 was 21,700 with 12,800 deaths expected.[1] Symptoms occur relatively late in the development of the disease. Thus, more than 40% of patients present with metastatic cancer and only one-fifth of patients have localized disease.[3] The distribution of gastric cancers has changed over the past three decades, primarily due to an increase in the number of adenocarcinomas of the cardia and an even greater decline in cancers of the fundus, body, and antrum.[148]

Over the past decades, beginning in the early 1930s, the incidence of gastric cancer has shown a remarkable decline in the United States,[149] probably due to improvements in refrigeration and sanitation. Consumption of preserved, smoked, or cured foods has decreased and inversely intake of fresh fruits and vegetables has increased.[150] Infection with *Helicobacter pylori*, which increases the risk of gastric cancer by approximately twofold, has also declined.[151–153]

In general, it is thought that achlorhydria leading to dysplasia of the gastric mucosa, resulting from such etiologic causes as atrophic gastritis (occasionally accompanied by pernicious anemia), chronic active gastritis from *H. pylori* infection, and prior antrectomy for peptic ulcer disease, may lead to an increased risk of gastric cancer.[154–157] Less firm associations with this malignancy include cigarette smoking, blood group A, prior radiation exposure, family history, and Epstein–Barr virus infection.[149]

Prevention and Surveillance

Continued improvements in refrigeration and sanitation throughout the world will likely result in a further decrease in the prevalence of this disease. Although the eradication of *H. pylori* infection may further reduce the risks of this malignancy, such an appealing concept has not yet been validated in a clinical trial.[151,158] Endoscopic screening for gastric cancer may be justifiable in endemic areas, such as East Asia, but is not warranted in the United States.

Diagnosis and Workup

Generally, patients with epigastric pain and weight loss are first found to have a gastric cancer by the identification of an abnormality on upper GI series. Upper endoscopy usually reveals a malignant ulcer or suspicious rugal thickening. Biopsy, in most cases, demonstrates an adenocarcinoma. CT scan of the abdomen and pelvis and chest radiographs are utilized to determine the extent of disease. In contrast to colorectal cancer, which generally spreads initially to the liver, gastric cancer frequently metastasizes to the ovary ("Krukenberg tumor"), pelvic peritoneal cul-de-sac ("Blumer's shelf"), or periumbilical area ("Sister Mary Joseph node"). Operative candidates at many centers now undergo staging laparoscopy to "rule out" such intraperitoneal spread before attempting a surgical resection.

Treatment

Surgery: Resectable Gastric Cancer

Gastrectomy is the only curative treatment for gastric cancer. In patients who undergo the resection of all macroscopic and microscopic tumor (R0 resection), the long-term survival is approximately 35%.[159,160] Multivariate analysis reveals that the ratio of involved to removed lymph nodes, followed by depth of tumor invasion and postsurgical complications, are the most important prognostic factors for patients who have undergone a complete resection.

The extent of the surgical resection required to obtain an optimal clinical outcome has been the source of controversy. At a minimum, a so-called D-1 resection should be performed.[161] In this procedure, patients undergo an omentectomy and gastrectomy with complete removal of the perigastric lymph nodes. Such an operation generally results in the recovery of 17 lymph nodes on average.[162] In addition, many surgeons, particularly from Japan, advocate a D-2 resection, which adds the removal of the omental bursa portion of the transverse mesocolon, the removal of the left gastric, celiac, and splenic lymph nodes, and occasionally the spleen to the D-1 procedure. In the D-2 operation, approximately 30 lymph nodes are recovered in the resected specimen.[162] Proponents of the D-2 procedure have claimed a greater rate of surgical cure for this more radical approach while detractors have focused on a higher likelihood for perioperative morbidity and mortality. Consequently, two large prospective randomized trials have compared the D-1 and D-2 surgical procedures.[162,163] Neither demonstrated a survival benefit for the D2 operation, but both documented a significantly higher rate of complications (43% versus 25%; $p < 0.001$) and postoperative deaths (10% versus 4%; $p < 0.004$) for this more radical procedure.

Gastric surgery may be performed safely in patients older than 70 years of age. A prospective review of 310 elderly patients with gastric cancer found that surgery in this group was reasonably tolerated and led to a survival duration comparable to the results obtained in younger patients.[164]

Postoperative Chemotherapy: Gastric Cancer

Since the late 1960s, numerous randomized trials have attempted to demonstrate that postoperative chemotherapy reduces the rate of recurrence and prolongs survival after the resection of a gastric cancer. Most of these trials showed no significant survival benefit as summarized in a 1993 meta-analysis.[165] That review revealed a slight but nonsignificant improvement in survival for patients treated with postoperative chemotherapy (odds ratio, 0.88; 95% CI, 0.72–1.08). However, a more recent analysis, using stricter inclusion criteria and incorporating more current trials, showed a statistically significant 4% reduction in recurrence for postoperative chemotherapy in patients who had undergone R0 resections (odds ratio, 0.80; 95% CI, 0.66–0.97).[166] The greatest benefit was obtained in patients with tumor spread to regional lymph nodes.

Postoperative Chemoradiations: Gastric Cancer

Postoperative radiation therapy alone does not appear to offer a survival benefit in resectable gastric cancer.[167] Fluorouracil-based chemotherapy, however, has been shown to be a potent radiation sensitizer in this disease.[168] To explore the value of such radiosensitization, the impact of postoperative radiation therapy and 5-FU-based chemotherapy was recently compared to no postoperative therapy in a randomized trial involving more than 550 patients who had undergone a complete resection of a locally advanced adenocarcinoma of the stomach or the gastroesophageal junction.[169,170] The patient cohort randomly allocated to receive chemoradiation experienced a significant improvement in 3-year disease-free survival (49% versus 32%; $p = 0.001$) and 3-year overall survival (52% versus 41%; $p = 0.03$). The success of this combined modality treatment program required sophisticated radiation therapy planning.[171] At present, all patients with fully resected muscle-invasive or lymph node-positive gastric cancer should now be considered for postoperative chemoradiation.

Advanced Gastric Cancer

Surgery: Advanced Gastric Cancer

Radical surgery is not indicated for gastric cancer patients in whom tumor has spread within the peritoneum, to other organs, the omentum, or distant lymph nodes. However, a less extreme resection or a bypass procedure may be appropriate to provide more effective palliation.[172-175]

Chemotherapy: Advanced Gastric Cancer

The benefit of chemotherapy in the presence of unresectable or widely metastatic gastric cancer has been the topic of debate and the focus of several randomized trials. These studies, in which patients have been randomly allocated to received chemotherapy or supportive care alone, have consistently revealed a prolongation of survival[176,177] and an improvement in quality of life[178] in association with treatment.

The choice of chemotherapy regimens in this setting is difficult. Single-agent therapy generally has less toxicity than combination chemotherapy and may be better suited for older individuals. Chemotherapeutic compounds that have significant activity (15%–20% response rate) in gastric cancer include 5-FU, cisplatin, the anthracyclines (doxorubicin and epirubicin), irinotecan, and the taxanes (paclitaxel and docetaxel). Of these, 5-FU, irinotecan, and the taxanes are least toxic. The most widely studied is 5-FU, which forms the backbone of most combination regimens in this disease.

The use of chemotherapy combinations in gastric cancer has been characterized by response rates as high as 50% in uncontrolled studies that have not been confirmed in randomized trials.[139,179-181] A number of randomized trials have been completed during the past decade, comparing various antitumor combinations that have been developed for the treatment of advanced gastric cancer. The most promising among these is the combination of epirubicin, cisplatin, and continuous infusion 5-FU (ECF), which has had a response rate of 41% to 45% and a median survival of 8.9 to 9.4 months.[182,183] The treatment program is somewhat inconvenient because of the cumbersome administration of 5-FU as a prolonged continuous infusion and uncertainty about the contribution of epirubicin. As a result, some oncologists continue to consider a 5-FU and cisplatin combination as the standard of care.[184]

Esophageal Cancer

Cancers arising from the esophagus, including the gastroesophageal junction, are typically either squamous cell carcinomas or adenocarcinomas and are the sixth leading cause of cancer death worldwide.[10] Eighty percent of these deaths occur in developing countries, particularly South Africa and China, where squamous cell carcinomas predominate. In contrast, esophageal cancer is less common in the United States, although it has increased significantly during the past three decades. In 2001, 13,200 new cases and 12,500 deaths from this disease were anticipated.[1] Esophageal cancer is now the seventh leading cause of cancer death in American men. The rise in the incidence of esophageal cancer in the United States is primarily due to a significant increase in adenocarcinomas of the distal esophagus and, to a lesser extent, of the gastroesophageal junction. Between 1974 and 1994, adenocarcinomas of the esophagus increased dramatically in white males whereas squamous cell carcinomas of the esophagus declined slightly.[148] This trend is particularly evident in older men; the appearance of esophageal adenocarcinomas has doubled in white men younger than 55 years but has quadrupled in white men ages 65 to 74 years.

Smoking is thought to increase the risk of all esophageal cancers.[148,185,186] Significant alcohol intake, especially when combined with smoking, greatly enhances the risk of squamous cell carcinoma but has no impact on the development of adenocarcinoma.[185] The greatest risk for esophageal adenocarcinoma appears to be gastroesophageal reflux disease and the development of Barrett's esophagus. In Barrett's esophagus, the normal stratified squamous epithelium of the esophagus is replaced by columnar epithelium, presumably in response to chronic gastroesophageal reflux. Recurrent symptoms of reflux result in an eightfold increase in the risk of esophageal adenocarcinoma.[187] Patients with Barrett's esophagus are at even higher risk, with an annual rate of cancer development of approximately 0.8%.[188] Drugs that relax the gastroesophageal sphincter and increase reflux, such as anticholinergics and aminophyllines, may contribute to the development of as many as 10% of these cancers.[189,190] Obesity, which increases intra-abdominal pressure and gastroesophageal reflux, is also thought to add to the rising incidence of these tumors.[190,191]

The epidemiologic pattern of esophageal carcinoma does not appear different in elderly patients. In one series, 74% of patients 70 years or more of age were found to have adenocarcinoma and 26% had squamous carcinoma.[192] In another study, the incidence of Barrett's associated adenocarcinoma was lower in the patients 70 years or older compared to younger age groups (15.6% versus 24%; $p = 0.046$).[193] The location of tumors in the esophagus does not, however, differ between older and younger patients. A similar distribution in early- and late-stage cancers has also been reported.

The overall prognosis for this cancer is poor. More than half of all patients already have metastatic disease at the time of their diagnosis.[194] Five-year survival even with the earliest stages of cancer is only in the range of 60%.[195] With lymph node involvement, 5-year survival drops below 25%. Patients with metastatic disease have a median survival of less than 1 year.

Prevention and Surveillance

Smoking cessation and moderation of alcohol intake are important steps in reducing the appearance of squamous cell carcinoma of the esophagus. The risk for this cancer decreases substantially after a decade of smoking cessation.[186] In contrast, the risk for adenocarcinoma of the esophagus does not change appreciably even 30 years after exposure to cigarettes ceases.[185]

Patients with Barrett's esophagus who are otherwise in good health may be candidates for regular endoscopic surveillance. Endoscopic ablation therapy combined with proton pump inhibition may revert Barrett's esophagus to a normal squamous mucosa in some patients.[196] Small uncontrolled experiences have led to claims that endoscopic surveillance is cost-effective,[197] leads to the diagnosis of earlier-stage tumors,[198] and may improve survival.[199] Such observations remain anecdotal in the absence of randomized data. Some experts have recommended that endoscopy be performed every 2 years in patients with Barrett's esophagus in the absence of epithelial dysplasia and more frequently if mild dysplasia is discovered.[196,200] The identification of severe dysplasia (i.e., carcinoma in situ) has been considered an indication for an esophagectomy, because many of these patients have been found to have invasive cancer in their resection specimens.[201] Patients not considered surgical candidates may undergo mucosal ablation with photodynamic therapy or other techniques.[202,203]

Diagnosis and Workup

Patients with esophageal cancer usually experience dysphagia and often complain of odynophagia at the time of diagnosis. Weight loss is also common and is an independent poor prognostic indicator if greater than 10%. Barium swallow is often the first diagnostic study obtained and typically shows a stricture or erosion of the esophagus. Upper endoscopy reveals a friable, ulcerated mass; squamous cell carcinoma and adenocarcinoma appear visually similar and can only be distinguished histologically. A CT scan of the chest, abdomen, and pelvis should be performed as a means of detecting metastatic disease.

Patients with disease restricted to the esophagus may be further evaluated with endoscopic ultrasonography. This procedure is particularly effective in determining the depth of invasion of the tumor. Positron emission tomography is increasingly utilized to identify radiographically undetectable metastatic disease.[204] Scanning of the head or skeleton is not routine and should be reserved for symptomatic patients only.

Treatment

Surgery: Resectable Esophageal Cancer

Localized esophageal cancer may be resected either by a transthoracic or a transhiatal approach. Neither retrospective[205] nor prospective[206] trials have shown any difference in mortality or morbidity between these types of surgery. Patients who underwent surgery alone in recent, large randomized trials have had an operative mortality of 4% to 6% and perioperative morbidity of 26%.[207,208] In these trials, patients had a median survival of 16 to 19 months and 5-year survival probabilities of 20% to 26%. Age does not appear to be a limiting factor in surgery of the esophagus. Although elderly patients tend to have a higher incidence of respiratory and cardiovascular complications than younger patients, this does not appear to have a significant effect on operative mortality or survival.[193,209–213]

Chemoradiation: Localized Esophageal Cancer

Although radiation therapy alone cannot cure esophageal cancer,[214] the combination of radiation therapy with concurrent chemotherapy has led to long-term survival in about 25% of patients, similar to the results associated with surgery.[215–217] Such chemoradiation therapy appears equally effective in patients 70 years of age and older as in younger individuals.[215,216]

Adjuvant Therapy: Localized Esophageal Cancer

Preoperative radiation therapy does not appear to enhance the outcome associated with surgery.[218] However, the data assessing the value of preoperative chemotherapy are conflicting: a mature, randomized trial involving 440 American patients showed no benefit,[208] while the preliminary results from a seemingly similar study in 802 British patients suggested that the same treatment prolonged survival.[219]

With these uncertain results, attention has focused on the combination of chemotherapy and radiation therapy before surgery.[220–226] Of five randomized trials that have attempted to demonstrate a benefit for preoperative radiation therapy and concurrent chemotherapy in esophageal cancer, only one study from a single institution has shown a statistical improvement in survival.[227] More recently, a larger multi-institutional trial[207] demonstrated no difference in median overall survival. The other studies have had too few patients to give statistically meaningful results.[228–230]

Advanced Esophageal Cancer

Chemotherapy

Several forms of chemotherapy are effective in esophageal cancer.[194,231–236] Response durations are typically brief, lasting no longer than a few months, and survival is short, rarely exceeding more than 1 year. Although combination chemotherapy regimens tend to result in higher response rates, the therapeutic value of such intensive treatment must be balanced with a greater likelihood of toxicity. Cisplatin has become the cornerstone of combination chemotherapy in esophageal cancer, generally being combined with 5-FU, or more recently with paclitaxel,[237,238] irinotecan,[239] vinorelbine,[240] or gemcitabine.[241] The combination of weekly cisplatin and irinotecan appears particularly active, with objective disease regression occurring in more than half of patients.[239]

Hepatocellular Carcinoma

Hepatocellular carcinoma (or primary liver cancer) is the fourth most common cause of cancer death in the world, leading to almost half a million deaths annually.[10] More than half of these deaths are in China and Taiwan, where the condition represents the leading cause of cancer death in men.[242] In contrast, the annual incidence in the United States has been relatively low, with 16,200 cases expected in 2001.[1]

The incidence of hepatocellular carcinoma has nearly doubled in the United States in the past two decades, primarily due to a significant increase in hepatitis B and C infections, which, along with alcoholic cirrhosis, are the primary causes of this cancer in the developed world.[243] Eighty-five percent of patients infected with hepatitis C and 5% of patients infected with hepatitis B will develop persistent, chronic disease.[244,245] Cirrhosis develops in approximately 20% of chronic disease patients, and, in turn, hepatocellular carcinoma is diagnosed in 2% to 7% of patients with cirrhosis.[243]

Because the latency period for the development of hepatocellular carcinoma in patients infected with hepa-

titis B or C is one to three decades, it is thought that the rising incidence of this malignancy is a result of transfusion of unscreened blood and blood products, intravenous drug abuse, needle sharing, and unsafe sexual practices during the 1960s and 1970s.[243]

Other risk factors for this disease in the United States include alcoholic cirrhosis, inherited hemochromatosis, and the use of hormone supplements such as oral contraceptives and exogenous androgens. In the developing world, aflatoxin B_1 exposure (from the mold *Aspergillus flavus* on grain) and schistosomiasis are important additional etiologic factors.

Prevention and Surveillance

Important steps in reducing the incidence of this cancer in the United States include vaccination of all children and sexually active adults for hepatitis B and the recently implemented screening techniques of the blood supply for hepatitis B and C.

Approximately 75% of patients with hepatocellular carcinoma demonstrate an elevation in their serum alpha-fetoprotein level. Consequently, it has been proposed that patients at increased risk for the development of this tumor such as those with hepatitis B or C infections, alcoholic cirrhosis, or hemochromatosis undergo periodic alpha-fetoprotein testing as a form of surveillance screening.[246] This strategy has thus far been shown to be effective in Alaskan Native Americans with serologic evidence to hepatitis B exposure, in whom hepatocellular carcinomas were detected more frequently at a resectable stage than had occurred previously when such testing had not been performed.[247]

Prospective and retrospective studies of patients with hepatitis C, treated with short periods of interferon (3–6 months), have demonstrated a 50% to 34% reduction in the incidence of hepatocellular carcinoma.[248,249] Interferon therapy is less successful in the treatment of hepatitis B, and its efficacy in reducing the incidence of hepatocellular carcinoma has not been studied. The potential benefits of interferon therapy in this setting must be balanced by the numerous and often severe side effects (e.g., flu-like symptoms, fatigue, weight loss, depression, anemia, thrombocytopenia, cardiac toxicity) associated with this treatment, especially in older individuals.

Diagnosis and Workup

Patients most often seek medical attention for the development of an often painful abdominal mass in the right upper quadrant or epigastrium that is frequently accompanied by weight loss. In patients with cirrhosis, the development of hepatocellular carcinoma may be heralded by ascites, portal hypertension, and relatively abrupt clinical deterioration. Abnormal levels of serum transaminases and alkaline phosphatase on standard liver function testing are observed in most cases, but normal liver tests do not exclude the diagnosis. Alpha-fetoprotein is commonly elevated and is considered diagnostic when above 500 ng/mL.[250]

Ultrasonography and CT scan of the liver can determine the anatomic distribution of hepatocellular carcinoma and can also provide orientation for percutaneous needle biopsy. Patients with relatively small tumors and no evidence of distant disease or malignant ascites may be evaluated for resection. Magnetic resonance imaging, angiography, and laparoscopy can determine the resectability of the cancer. Contraindications to surgery include portal or hepatic vein invasion or portal vein thrombosis.[251] Relative contraindications include severe cirrhosis, active hepatitis, large or multifocal tumors, and comorbidities.

Treatment

Treatment options for hepatocellular carcinoma restricted to the liver include operative resection, orthotopic liver transplantation, nonsurgical tumor ablation, or transarterial hepatic chemoembolization. Patients treated with a partial hepatectomy at specialized medical centers have a 5-year survival rate of approximately 35% to 50% and an operative mortality rate less than 5%.[250] However, intrahepatic recurrences occur in up to 75% of patients[252]; spread to distant sites is also common. There is no evidence that postoperative treatment with chemotherapy is useful following the resection of a hepatocellular carcinoma.[253] Orthotopic liver transplantation is not tolerable in the geriatric population.

Localized tumor ablation with ethanol, cryotherapy, or radiofrequency has been increasingly utilized to eradicate small tumors and may be particularly appropriate for older patients, who are frequently considered poor candidates for surgery. Percutaneous ethanol injection (PEI) is the most commonly employed of these ablative techniques. Absolute or 95% ethanol is injected directly into the tumor either percutaneously or with direct visualization through a small incision. The probability of 5-year survival (32%–52%) and the rate of intrahepatic recurrence (60%–74%) are similar to those reported with surgical resection.[254–257] Surgical resection and PEI have not been compared in a randomized trial.

Transarterial chemoembolization (TACE) represents the most commonly used management strategy for patients with unresectable hepatocellular carcinoma.[250] The rationale for this treatment approach focuses on the observation that hepatocellular tumors derive nearly their entire blood supply from the hepatic artery while normal liver tissue is also oxygenated through the portal vein. In patients undergoing TACE, selective branches of the hepatic artery are occluded (often with gel foam), leading to tumor necrosis without destruction of adjacent normal tissues. Additional intrahepatic chemotherapy may also be given. Although this procedure often results in dramatic tumor shrinkage and transient symptomatic palliation, randomized trials have failed to show a survival advantage when compared to observation alone.[258,259]

Surgery and chemoembolization in the geriatric population have been found to be tolerable in most[260–262] but not all[261,263] experiences. In patients with advanced hepatocellular carcinoma, the use of chemotherapy has been disappointing[251]; randomized trials have not demonstrated a survival advantage for treated patients.[250,264]

Gallbladder Cancer

Cancers of the gallbladder occur infrequently in the United States.[1] The incidence increases with age and reaches its peak in the seventh decade of life. Women and Native Americans, who are more prone to gallstones, have a higher risk of gallbladder cancer.[265] Other risk factors include choledochal cysts, exposure to various carcinogens, gallbladder polyps, and calcification of the gallbladder ("porcelain gallbladder").[266] The 5-year probability for survival is favorable (>85%) only for those gallbladder cancers that do not invade beyond the muscular layer of the gallbladder.[266] Once the tumor invades the adjacent connective tissue, the probability of 5-year survival drops sharply (to <25%), falling to less than 10% in the presence of lymph node involvement or extension into the liver.

Prevention and Surveillance

Patients with sufficient symptoms attributable to gallstones to require medical attention have a fourfold increased risk of developing gallbladder cancer.[267] For these individuals, a cholecystectomy may represent cancer prophylaxis. However, there are no data to justify the morbidity and expense of such a surgical procedure as cancer prophylaxis in patients with asymptomatic gallstones.[265]

Diagnosis and Workup

Gallbladder tumors most frequently are detected because of symptoms indistinguishable from those of cholelithiasis and cholecystitis. Symptoms of bile duct obstruction, including jaundice, pruritis, clay-colored stools, and dark urine occur relatively late with this cancer and are associated with advanced disease. Evaluation of these tumors often includes ultrasound examination, CT scan, cholangiography, and magnetic resonance imaging. Extensive regional lymphadenopathy, hepatic artery or portal vein encasement, and liver or peritoneal metastases are contraindications to surgery.[268]

Treatment

Surgery is the only potentially curative treatment for this disease. Superficial tumors, which are usually incidental findings following routine cholecystectomy, are often cured with this surgical procedure. More deeply invasive tumors are sometimes approached with an extended or radical cholecystectomy, in which adjacent liver tissue and regional lymph nodes are removed,[269,270] occasionally followed by local radiation therapy.[271,272] Randomized data to support this aggressive approach are lacking.

Advanced Disease

Patients with unresectable gallbladder cancer and jaundice should be considered for either an endoscopic or percutaneous biliary stent. Patients with pain may benefit from a percutaneous celiac ganglion nerve block to reduce the need for narcotics.

Chemoradiation is often recommended for locally advanced, unresectable biliary tract cancer,[273–275] and chemotherapy may be considered for patients with metastatic disease.[276,277] It is uncertain whether such treatments prolong survival.

Conclusion

Gastrointestinal malignancies are diseases of the elderly. As the population continues to age and the proportion of elderly grows, these cancers will become more prevalent and a further public health problem. Changes in diet, smoking, and alcohol use, however, can reduce their incidence. Dysphagia, dyspepsia, weight loss, abdominal pain, and gastrointestinal bleeding should prompt a careful and thorough evaluation. Such symptoms should not be attributed simply to depression, hemorrhoids, or irritable bowel syndrome. Most elderly patients should be regularly screened for colorectal neoplasms. Such screening has been shown to reduce the risk of cancer and to uncover cancers at an earlier stage.

Although the majority of patients with gastrointestinal cancers are 65 years or older, treatments have been designed and tested mostly in younger patients. Nonetheless, treatment of the elderly is generally well tolerated. Surgical morbidity and mortality rates of older patients are now equivalent to those of younger patients a decade ago. Many procedures once thought too dangerous for young patients can now be performed safely in otherwise

healthy octogenarians. Likewise, radiation therapy is well tolerated in older individuals, perhaps with slight increases in bone marrow suppression and small bowel toxicity. Most chemotherapeutic agents do not cause increased toxicity in elderly patients. At present, too few elderly patients are enrolled in clinical trials. Prospective studies involving older patients should evaluate the efficacy, toxicity, and quality of life in this important and rapidly expanding age group.

Surgery remains the only effective curative modality for most gastrointestinal malignancies. Patients should be evaluated thoroughly before this option is dismissed. Based on randomized studies that have shown improved survival, postoperative chemotherapy or radiotherapy or both are currently given after the complete resection of locally advanced colorectal cancer, locally advanced stomach cancer, and resectable pancreas cancer. Patients with rectal and esophageal cancers may be considered for preoperative chemoradiation therapy. In the setting of disseminated disease, chemotherapy has demonstrated both palliative and survival advantages for many gastrointestinal malignancies. Particularly for the more aggressive cancers, however, the survival benefits are marginal, and the value of such treatment in elderly or infirm patients must be balanced with potential toxicities that may diminish their quality of life.

References

1. Greenlee R, Hill-Harmon M, Murray T, Thum M. Cancer Statistics, 2001. *CA Cancer J Clin.* 2001;51:15–36.
2. Yancik R, Ries L. Cancer in older persons. *Cancer.* 1994; 74:1995–2003.
3. Ries L, Eisner M, Kosary C, et al. *SEER Cancer Statistics Review, 1973–1997.* Bethesda, MD: National Cancer Institute; 2000.
4. Vercelli M, Capocaccia R, Quaglia A, Casella C, Puppo A, Coebergh J. Relative survival in elderly European cancer patients: evidence for health care inequalities. *Crit Rev Oncol Hematol.* 2000;35:161–179.
5. Balducci L, Extermann M. Management of cancer in the older person: a practical approach. *Oncologist.* 2000;5:224–237.
6. Farniok K, Levitt S. The role of radiation therapy in the treatment of colorectal cancer. Implications for the older patient. *Cancer.* 1994;74:2154–2159.
7. Giovanazzi-Bannon S, Rademaker A, Lai G, Benson A. Treatment tolerance of elderly cancer patients entered onto phase II clinical trials: an Illinois Cancer Center study. *J Clin Oncol.* 1994;12:2447–2452.
8. Cascinu S, DelFerro E, Catalano G. Toxicity and therapeutic response to chemotherapy in patients aged 70 years or older with advanced cancer. *Am J Clin Oncol.* 1996; 19:371–374.
9. Stein B, Petrelli N, Douglass H, Driscoll D, Arcangeli G, Meropol N. Age and sex are independant predictors of 5-

fluorouracil toxicity. Analysis of a large scale phase III trial. *Cancer.* 1995;75:11–17.

10. Pisani P, Parkin D, Bray F, Ferlay J. Estimates of the worldwide mortality from 25 cancers in 1990 [erratum: Int J Cancer 1999;83:870–873]. *Int J Cancer.* 1999;83:18–29.

11. Jessup J, McGinnis L, Steele G, Menck H, Winchester D. The National Cancer Data Base. Report on colon cancer. *Cancer.* 1996;78:918–926.

12. deRijke J, Schouten L, Hillen H, et al. Cancer in the very elderly Dutch population. *Cancer.* 2000;89:1121–1133.

13. Coburn M, Pricolo V, Soderberg C. Factors affecting prognosis and management of carcinoma of the colon and rectum in patients more than eighty years of age. *J Am Coll Surg.* 1994;179:65–69.

14. Zhang B, Fattah A, Nakama H. Characteristics and survival rate of elderly patients with colorectal cancer detected by immunochemical occult blood screening. *Hepatogastroenterology.* 2000;47:414–418.

15. Mulcahy H, Patchett S, Daly L, O'Donoghue D. Prognosis of elderly patients with large bowel cancer. *Br J Surg.* 1994;81:736–738.

16. Damhuis R, Wereldsma J, Wiggers T. The influence of age on resection rates and postoperative mortality in 6,457 patients with colorectal cancer. *Int J Colorectal Dis.* 1996;11:45–48.

17. Adloff M, Ollier J, Schloegel M, Arnaud J, Serrat M. Colorectal cancer in patients over the age of 80 years. *Ann Chir.* 1993;47:492–496.

18. Yancik R, Wesley M, Ries L, et al. Comorbidity and age as predictors of risk for early mortality of male and female colon carcinoma patients. *Cancer.* 1998;82:2123–2134.

19. Winawer S, Fletcher R, Miller L, et al. Colorectal cancer screening: clinical guidelines and rationale. *Gastroenterology.* 1997;112:594–642.

20. Fuchs C, Giovannucci E, Colditz G, Hunter D, Speizer F, Willett W. A propective study of family history and the risk of colorectal cancer. *N Engl J Med.* 1994;331:1669–1674.

21. Winawer S, Zauber A, Gerdes H, et al. Risk of colorectal cancer in the families of patients with adenomatous polyps. *N Engl J Med.* 1996;334:82–87.

22. Rustgi A. Hereditary gastrointestinal polyposis and non-polyposis syndromes. *N Engl J Med.* 1994;331:1694–1702.

23. Burt R. Hereditary aspects of the polyposis syndromes. *Hematol Oncol Annu.* 1994;2:163–170.

24. Burke W, Petersen G, Lynch P, et al. Recommendations for follow-up care of individuals with an inherited predisposition to cancer. I. Hereditary nonpolyposis colon cancer. Cancer Genetics Studies Consortium. *JAMA.* 1997;277:915–919.

25. Tomeo C, Colditz G, Willett W, et al. Harvard Report on Cancer Prevention. Volume 3: Prevention of colon cancer in the United States. *Cancer Causes Control.* 1999;10:167–180.

26. Baron J, Greenberg E, Haile R, Mandel J, Sandler R, Mott L. Coffee and tea and the risk of recurrent colorectal adenomas. *Cancer Epidemiol Biomarkers Prev.* 1997;6:7–10.

27. Fuchs C, Giovannucci E, Colditz G, et al. Dietary fiber and the risk of colorectal cancer and adenoma in women. *N Engl J Med.* 1999;340:169–176.

28. Kinzler K, Vogelstein B. Colorectal tumors. In: Vogelstein B, Kinzler K, eds. *The Genetic Basis of Human Cancer.* New York: McGraw-Hill; 1998:565–587.

29. Takayama T, Katsuki S, Takahashi Y, et al. Aberrant crypt foci of the colon as precursors of adenoma and cancer. *N Engl J Med.* 1998;339:1277–1284.

30. Fearon E, Vogelstein B. A genetic model for colorectal tumorigenesis. *Cell.* 1990;61:759–767.

31. Williams A, Balasooriya B, Day D. Polyps and cancer of the large bowel: a necropsy study in Liverpool. *Gut.* 1982;23:835–842.

32. Yamamoto Y, Yin M, Lin K, Gaynor R. Sulindac inhibits activation of the NF-kappaB pathway. *J Biol Chem.* 1999;274:27307–27314.

33. He T, Chan T, Vogelstein B, Kinzler K. PPARdelta is an APC-regulated target or nonsteroidal anti-inflammatory drug. *Cell.* 1999;99:335–345.

34. Tsujii M, Kawano S, Tsuji S, Sawaoka H, Hori M, DuBois R. Cyclooxygenase regulates angiogenesis induced by colon cancer cells. *Cell.* 1998;93:705–716.

35. Eberhart C, Coffey R, Radhika A, Giardiello F, Ferrenbach S, DuBois R. Up-regulation of cyclooxygenase 2 gene expression in human colorectal adenomas and adenocarcinomas. *Gastroenterology.* 1994;107:1183–1188.

36. Oshima M, Dinchuk J, Kargman S, et al. Suppression of intestinal polyposis in Apc delta 716 knockout mice by inhibition of cyclooxygenase 2 (COX-2). *Cell.* 1996;87:803–809.

37. Giardiello F, Hamilton S, Krush A, et al. Treatment of colonic and rectal adenomas with sulindac in familial adenomatous polyposis. *N Engl J Med.* 1993;328:1313–1316.

38. Steinbach G, Lynch P, Phillips R, et al. The effect of celecoxib, a cyclooxygenase-2 inhibitor, in familial adenomatous polyposis. *N Engl J Med.* 2000;342:1946–1952.

39. Thun M, Namboodiri M, Heath C. Aspirin use and reduced risk of fatal colon cancer. *N Engl J Med.* 1991;325:1593–1596.

40. Giovannucci E, Rimm E, Stampfer M, Colditz G, Asherio A, Willett W. Aspirin use and the risk for colorectal cancer and adenoma in male health professionals. *Ann Intern Med.* 1994;121:241–246.

41. Giovannucci E, Egan K, Hunter D, et al. Aspirin and the risk of colorectal cancer in women. *N Engl J Med.* 1995;333:609–614.

42. Smalley W, Ray W, Daugherty J, Griffin M. Use of nonsteroidal anti-inflammatory drugs and incidence of colorectal cancer: a population-based study. *Arch Intern Med.* 1999;159:161–166.

43. Giovannucci E, Stampfer M, Colditz G, Rimm E, Willett W. Relationship of diet to risk of colorectal adenoma in men. *J Natl Cancer Inst.* 1992;84:91–98.

44. Thun M, Calle E, Namboodiri M, et al. Risk factors for fatal colon cancer in a large prospective study. *J Natl Cancer Inst.* 1992;84:1491–1500.

45. Baron J, Sandler R, Haile R, Mandel J, Mott L, Greenberg E. Folate intake, alcohol consumption, cigarette smoking, and risk of colorectal adenomas. *J Natl Cancer Inst.* 1998;90:57–62.

46. Ferraroni M, LaVecchia C, D'Avanzo B, Negri E, Franceschi S, Decarli A. Selected micronutrient uptake

and the risk of colorectal cancer. *Br J Cancer*. 1994;70: 1150–1155.

47. Giovannucci E, Stampfer M, Colditz G, et al. Multivitamin use, folate, and colon cancer in women in the Nurses' Health Study. *Ann Intern Med*. 1998;129:517–524.

48. Nagengast F, Grubben M, vanMunster I. Role of bile acids in colorectal carcinogenesis. *Eur J Cancer*. 1995;31A:1067–1070.

49. Hyman J, Baron J, Dain B, et al. Dietary and supplemental calcium and the recurrence of colorectal adenomas. *Cancer Epidemiol Biomarkers Prev*. 1998;7:291–295.

50. Baron J, Beach M, Mandel J, et al. Calcium supplements for the prevention of colorectal adenomas. *N Engl J Med*. 1999;340:101–107.

51. McMichael A, Potter J. Reproduction, endogenous and exogenous sex hormones, and colon cancer: a review and hypothesis. *J Natl Cancer Inst*. 1980;65:1201–1207.

52. Grodstein F, Newcomb P, Stampfer M. Postmenopausal hormone therapy and the risk of colorectal cancer: a review and meta-analysis. *Am J Med*. 1999;106:574–582.

53. Calle E, Miracle-McMahill H, Thun M, Heath C. Estrogen replacement therapy and the risk of fatal colon cancer in a prospective cohort of postmenopausal women. *J Natl Cancer Inst*. 1995;87:517–523.

54. Grodstein F, Martinez E, Platz E, et al. Postmenopausal hormone use and risk for colorectal cancer and adenoma. *Ann Intern Med*. 1998;128:705–712.

55. Greenberg E, Baron J, Tosteson T, et al. A clinical trial of antioxidant vitamins to prevent colorectal adenoma. *N Engl J Med*. 1994;331:141–147.

56. Hennekens C, Buring J, Manson J, et al. Lack of effect of long-term supplementation with beta carotene on the incidence of malignant neoplasms and cardiovascular disease. *N Engl J Med*. 1996;334:1145–1149.

57. Albanes D, Malila N, Taylor P, et al. Effects of supplemental alpha-tocopherol and beta-carotene on colorectal cancer: results from a controlled trial. *Cancer Causes Control*. 2000;11:197–205.

58. Schatzkin A, Lanza E, Corle D, et al. Lack of effect of a low-fat, high-fiber diet on the recurrence of colorectal adenomas. *N Engl J Med*. 2000;342:1149–1155.

59. Alberts D, Martinez M, Roe D, et al. Lack of effect of a high-fiber cereal supplement on the recurrence of colorectal adenomas. *N Engl J Med*. 2000;342:1156–1162.

60. Muller A, Sonnenberg A. Prevention of colorectal cancer by flexible endoscopy and polypectomy. A case-control study of 32,702 veterans. *Ann Intern Med*. 1995;123:904–910.

61. Winawer S, Zauber A, Ho M, et al. Prevention of colorectal cancer by colonoscopic polypectomy. *N Engl J Med*. 1993;329:1977–1981.

62. Curless R, French J, Williams G, James O. Comparison of gastrointestinal symptoms in colorectal carcinoma patients and community controls with respect to age. *Gut*. 1994;35:1267–1270.

63. Wanebo H, Rao B, Pinsky C, et al. Preoperative carcinoembryonic antigen level as a prognostic indicator in colorectal cancer. *N Engl J Med*. 1978;299:448–451.

64. Moertel C, O'Fallon J, Go V, O'Connell M, Thynne G. The preoperative carcinoembryonic antigen test in the diagno-

sis, staging, and prognosis of colorectal cancer. *Cancer*. 1986;58:603–610.

65. American Society of Clinical Oncology. Clinical practice guidelines for the use of tumor markers in breast and colorectal cancer. *J Clin Oncol*. 1996;14:2843–2877.

66. Moertel C, Fleming T, Macdonald J, et al. Fluorouracil plus levamisole as effective adjuvant therapy after resection of stage III colon carcinoma: a final report. *Ann Intern Med*. 1995;122:321–326.

67. Schrag D, Cramer L, Bach P, Cohen A, Warren J, Begg C. Influence of hospital procedure volume on outcomes following surgery for colon cancer. *JAMA*. 2000;284:3028–3035.

68. Lewis A, Khoury G. Resection for colorectal cancer in the very old: are the risks too high? *Br Med J (Clin Res Ed)*. 1988;296:459–461.

69. Whittle J, Steinberg E, Anderson G, Herbert R. Results of colectomy in elderly patients with colon cancer, based on Medicare claims data. *Am J Surg*. 1992;163:572–576.

70. Whittle J, Steinberg E, Anderson G, Herbert R. Results of colectomy in elderly patients with colon cancer, based on Medicare claims data. *Am J Surg*. 1992;163:572–576.

71. McDermott F, Hughes E, Pihl E, Johnson W, Price A. Local recurrence after potentially curative resection for rectal cancer in a series of 1008 patients. *Br J Surg*. 1985;72:34–37.

72. Wilson S, Beahrs O. The curative treatment of carcinoma of the sigmoid, rectosigmoid, and rectum. *Ann Surg*. 1976;183:556–565.

73. Graham R, Garnsey L, Jessup J. Local excision of rectal carcinoma. *Am J Surg*. 1990;160:306–312.

74. Steele G, Herndon J, Bleday R, et al. Sphincter-sparing treatment for distal rectal adenocarcinoma. *Ann Surg Oncol*. 1999;6:413–415.

75. Bleday R, Breen E, Jessup J, Burgess A, Sentovich S, Steele G. Prospective evaluation of local excision for small rectal cancers. *Dis Colon Rectum*. 1997;40:388–392.

76. Haller D, Catalano P, Macdonald J, Mayer R. Fluorouracil (FU), leucovorin (LV) and levamisole (LEV) adjuvant therapy for colon cancer: four-year results of INT-0089. *Proc Annu Meet Am Soc Clin Oncol*. 1997;16:A940.

77. Moertel C, Fleming T, Macdonald J, et al. Intergroup study of fluorouracil plus levamisole as adjuvant therapy for stage II/Dukes' B2 colon cancer. *J Clin Oncol*. 1995;13:2936–2943.

78. Minsky B, Mies C, Rich T, Recht A. Lymphatic vessel invasion is an independant prognostic factor for survival in colorectal cancer. *Int J Radiat Oncol Biol Phys*. 1989;17:311–318.

79. Chapuis P, Dent O, Fisher R, et al. A multivariate analysis of clinical and pathological variables in prognosis after resection of large bowel cancer. *Br J Surg*. 1985;72:698–702.

80. Evans R, Laskin J, Hakala M. Assessment of growth-limiting events caused by 5-fluorouracil in mouse cells and in human cells. *Cancer Res*. 1980;40:4113–4122.

81. Santi D, McHenry C, Sommer H. Mechanism of interaction of thymidylate synthase with fluorodeoxyuridylate. *Biochemistry*. 1974;13:471–480.

82. Danenberg P, Danenberg K. Effect of 5,10-methylenetetrahydrofolate on the dissociation of 5-fluoro-2′-deoxy-

uridylate from thymidylate synthetase: evidence for an ordered mechanism. *Biochemistry.* 1978;17:4018–4024.

83. Sundararajan V, Grann V, Neugut A. Population-based variation in the use of chemotherapy for colorectal cancer in the elderly. *Proc Am Soc Clin Oncol.* 1999;18:A1598.

84. Sargent D, Goldberg R, MacDonald J, et al. Adjuvant chemotherapy for colon cancer (cc) is beneficial without significantly increased toxicity in elderly patients (pts): results from a 3351-pt meta-analysis. *Proc Am Soc Clin Oncol.* 2000;19:A933.

85. Gastrointestinal Tumor Study Group. Prolongation of the disease-free interval in surgically treated rectal carcinoma. *N Engl J Med.* 1985;312:1465–1472.

86. Tepper J, O'Connell M, Petroni G, et al. Adjuvant postoperative fluorouracil-modulated chemotherapy combined with pelvic radiation therapy for rectal cancer: initial results of Intergroup 0114. *J Clin Oncol.* 1997;15:2030–2039.

87. O'Connell M, Martenson J, Wieand H, et al. Improving adjuvant therapy for rectal cancer by combining protracted-infusion fluorouracil with radiation therapy after curative surgery. *N Engl J Med.* 1994;331:502–507.

88. Minsky B, Cohen A, Kemeny N, et al. Combined modality therapy of rectal cancer: decreased acute toxicity with the preoperative approach. *J Clin Oncol.* 1992;10:1218–1224.

89. Swedish Rectal Cancer Trial. Local recurrence rate in a randomised multicentre trial of preoperative radiotherapy compared with operation alone in resectable rectal carcinoma. *Eur J Surg.* 1996;162:397–3402.

90. Farniok K, Levitt S. The role of radiation therapy in the treatment of colorectal cancer. Implications for the older patient. *Cancer.* 1994;74:2154–2159.

91. Castells A, Bessa X, Daniels M, et al. Value of postoperative surveillance after radical surgery for colorectal cancer: results of a cohort study. *Dis Colon Rectum.* 1998;41:714–723.

92. Graham R, Wang S, Catalano P, Haller D. Postsurgical surveillance of colon cancer: preliminary cost analysis of physician examination, carcinoembryonic antigen testing, chest x-ray, and colonoscopy. *Ann Surg.* 1998;228:59–63.

93. Schoemaker D, Black R, Giles L, Toouli J. Yearly colonoscopy, liver CT, and chest radiography do not influence 5-year survival of colorectal cancer patients. *Gastroenterology.* 1998;114:7–14.

94. Benson A, Desch C, Flynn P, et al. 2000 update of American Society of Clinical Oncology colorectal cancer surveillance guidelines. *J Clin Oncol.* 2000;18:3586–3588.

95. Moertel C, Fleming T, Macdonald J, Haller D, Laurie J, Tangen C. An evaluation of the carcinoembryonic antigen (CEA) test for monitoring patients with resected colon cancer. *JAMA.* 1993;270:943–947.

96. Goldberg R, Fleming T, Tangen C, et al. Surgery for recurrent colon cancer: strategies for identifying resectable recurrence and success rates after resection. *Ann Intern Med.* 1998;129:27–35.

97. Fong Y, Blumgart L. Hepatic colorectal metastasis: current status of surgical therapy. *Oncology.* 1998;12:1489–1498.

98. Fong Y, Blumgart L, Fortner J, Brennan M. Pancreatic or liver resection for malignancy is safe and effective for the elderly. *Ann Surg.* 1995;222:426–434.

99. McKenna R. Thoracoscopic lobectomy with mediastinal sampling in 80-year-old patients. *Chest.* 1994;106:1902–1904.

100. Kemeny N, Huang Y, Cohen A, et al. Hepatic arterial infusion of chemotherapy after resection of hepatic metastases from colorectal cancer. *N Engl J Med.* 1999;341:2039–2048.

101. Kemeny M, Adak S, Lipitz S, Gray B, MacDonald J, Benson A. Results of Intergroup [Eastern Cooperative Group (ECOG) and Southwest Oncology Group (SWOG)] prospective randomized study of surgery alone versus continuous hepatic artery infusion of FUdR and continuous systemic infusion of 5FU after hepatic resection of colorectal liver metastases. *Proc Am Soc Clin Oncol.* 1999;18:A1012.

102. Scheithauer W, Rosen H, Kornek G, Sebesta C, Depisch D. Randomised comparison of combination chemotherapy plus supportive care with supportive care alone in patients with metastatic colorectal cancer. *Br Med J.* 1993;306:752–755.

103. Unger J, Hutchins L, Crowley J, Coltman C, Albain K. Southwest Oncology Group (SWOG) accrual by sex, race, and age, compared to US population rates. *Proc Am Soc Clin Oncol.* 1998;17:A1596.

104. Trimble E, Carter C, Cain D, Freidlin B, Ungerleider R, Friedman M. Representation of older patients in cancer treatment trials. *Cancer.* 1994;74:2208–2214.

105. Ross P, Popescu R, Cunningham D, Norman A, Parikh B. Adjuvant and palliative chemotherapy for colorectal cancer in patients aged 70 years or older. *Proc Am Soc Clin Oncol.* 1998;17:A1069.

106. Pitot H. US pivotal studies of irinotecan in colorectal carcinoma. *Oncology.* 1998;12:48–53.

107. Cunningham D, Pyrhoenen S, James R, et al. Randomized trial of irinotecan plus supportive care versus supportive care alone after fluorouracil failure for patients with metastatic colorectal cancer. *Lancet.* 1998;352:1413–1418.

108. Saltz L, Cox J, Blanke C, et al. Irinotecan plus fluorouracil and leucovorin for metastatic colorectal cancer. *N Engl J Med.* 2000;343:905–914.

109. Meta-analysis Group In Cancer. Efficacy of intravenous continuous infusion of fluorouracil compared with bolus administration in advanced colorectal cancer. *J Clin Oncol.* 1998;16:301–308.

110. Hoff P. Capecitabine as first-line treatment for colorectal cancer (CRC): integrated results of 1207 patients (pts) from 2 randomized, phase III studies. On behalf of the Capecitabine CRC Study Group. Presented at the 25th European Society for Medical Oncology Congress, Hamburg, Germany, 2000.

111. Machover D, Diza-Rubio E, deGramont A, et al. Two consecutive phase II studies of oxaliplatin (L-OHP) for treatment of patients with advanced colorectal carcinoma who were resistant to previous treatment with fluoropyrimidines. *Ann Oncol.* 1996;7:95–98.

112. Rubin M, Shin D, Pasmantier M, et al. Monoclonal antibody (MoAb) IMC-C225, an anti-epidermal growth factor receptor (EGFr), for patients (pts) with EGFr-positive tumors refractory to or in relapse from previous therapeutic regimens. *Proc Am Soc Clin Oncol.* 2000;19:A1860.

113. Fuchs C, Colditz G, Stampfer M, et al. Prospective study of cigarette smoking and the risk of pancreatic cancer. *Arch Intern Med.* 1996;156:2255–2260.

114. Lowenfels A, Maisonneuve P, Cavallini G, et al. Pancreatitis and the risk of pancreatic cancer. International Pancreatitis Study Group. *N Engl J Med.* 1993;328:1433–1437.

115. Silverman D, Schiffman M, Everhart J, et al. Diabetes mellitus, other medical conditions and familial history of cancer as risk factors for pancreatic cancer. *Br J Cancer.* 1999;80:1830–1837.

116. Karlson B, Ekbom A, Josefsson S, McLaughlin J, Fraumeni J, Nyren O. The risk of pancreatic cancer following pancreatitis: an association due to confounding? *Gastroenterology.* 1997;113:587–592.

117. Gullo L, Pezzilli R, Morselli-Labate A. Diabetes and the risk of pancreatic cancer. Italian Pancreatic Cancer Study Group. *N Engl J Med.* 1994;331:81–84.

118. Goggins M, Canto M, Hruban R. Can we screen high-risk individuals to detect early pancreatic carcinoma? [editorial]. *J Surg Oncol.* 2000;74:243–248.

119. Safi F, Schlosser W, Falkenreck S, Beger H. Prognostic value of CA19-9 serum course in pancreatic cancer. *Hepatogastroenterology.* 1998;45:253–259.

120. Nieman J, Holmes F. Accuracy of diagnosis of pancreatic cancer decreases with increasing age. *J Am Geriatr Soc.* 1989;37:97–100.

121. Brandt K, Charboneau J, Stephens D, Welch T, Goellner J. CT- and US-guided biopsy of the pancreas. *Radiology.* 1993;187:15–16.

122. Cameron J. The current management of carcinoma of the head of the pancreas. *Annu Rev Med.* 1995;46:361–370.

123. Nitecki S, Sarr M, Colby T, vanHeerden J. Long-term survival after resection for ductal adenocarcinoma of the pancreas. Is it really improving? *Ann Surg.* 1995;221:59–66.

124. Spencer M, Sarr M, Nagorney D. Radical pancreatectomy for pancreatic cancer in the elderly. Is it safe and justified? *Ann Surg.* 1990;212:140–143.

125. Sohn T, Yeo C, Cameron J, et al. Should pancreaticoduodenectomy be performed in octogenarians? *J Gastrointest Surg.* 1998;2:207–216.

126. Bottger T, Engelmann R, Junginger T. Is age a risk factor for major pancreatic surgery? An analysis of 300 resections. *Hepatogastroenterology.* 1999;46:2589–2598.

127. al-Sharaf K, Andren-Sandberg A, Ihse I. Subtotal pancreatectomy for cancer can be safe in the elderly. *Eur J Surg.* 1999;165:230–235.

128. DiCarlo V, Balzano G, Zerbi A, Villa E. Pancreatic cancer resection in elderly patients. *Br J Surg.* 1998;85:607–610.

129. Gastrointestinal Tumor Study Group. Adjuvant combined radiation and chemotherapy following curative resection. *Arch Surg.* 1985;120:899–903.

130. Gastrointestinal Tumor Study Group. Further evidence of effective adjuvant combined radiation and chemotherapy following curative resection of pancreatic cancer. *Cancer.* 1987;59:2006–2010.

131. Klinkenbijl J, Jeekel J, Sahmoud T, et al. Adjuvant radiotherapy and 5-fluorouracil after curative resection of cancer of the pancreas and periampullary region: phase III trial of the EORTC Gastrointestinal Tract Cancer Cooperative Group. *Ann Surg.* 1999;230:776–782.

132. Neoptolemos J, Dunn J, Mofitt D, et al. ESPAC-1 interim results: a European, randomized study to assess the roles of adjuvant chemotherapy (5FU + folinic acid) and adjuvant chemoradiation (40 Gy + 5FU) in resectable pancreatic cancer. *Br J Cancer.* 2000;83:CT1.

133. Evans D, Abbruzzese J, Lee J, et al. Preoperative chemoradiation for adenocarcinoma of the pancreas: M.D. Anderson experience. *Semin Surg Oncol.* 1995;11:132–140.

134. Cienfuegos J, Manuel F. Analysis of intraoperative radiotherapy for pancreatic carcinoma. *Eur J Surg Oncol.* 2000;26:S13–S15.

135. Lillemoe K, Cameron J, Kaufman H, Yeo C, Pitt H, Sauter P. Chemical splanchnicectomy in patients with unresectable pancreatic cancer: a prospective randomized trial. *Ann Surg.* 1993;217:447–455.

136. Haslam J, Cavanaugh P, Strapp S. Radiation therapy in the treatment of unresectable adenocarcinoma of the pancreas. *Cancer.* 1973;32:1341–1345.

137. Moertel C, Childs D, Reitemeir R, Colby M, Holbrook M. Combined 5-fluorouracil and supervoltage radiation therapy of locally unresectable gastrointestinal cancer. *Lancet.* 1969;2:865–867.

138. Moertel C, Frytak S, Hahn R, et al. Therapy of locally unresectable pancreatic carcinoma: a randomized comparison of high dose (6000 rads) radiation alone, moderate dose radiation (4000 rads + 5-fluorouracil), and high dose radiation + 5-fluorouracil. *Cancer.* 1981;48:1705–1710.

139. Cullinan S, Moertel C, Fleming T, et al. A comparison of three chemotherapeutic regimens in the treatment of advanced pancreatic and gastric carcinoma. Flurouracil vs fluorouracil and doxorubicin vs fluorouracil, doxorubicin, and mitomycin. *JAMA.* 1985;253:2061–2067.

140. Cullinan S, Moertel C, Wieand H, et al. A phase III trial on the therapy of advanced pancreatic carcinoma. Evaluations of the Mallinson regimen and combined 5-fluorouracil, doxorubicin, and cisplatin. *Cancer.* 1990;65: 2207–2212.

141. Mallinson C, Rake M, Cocking J, et al. Chemotherapy in pancreatic cancer: results of a controlled, prospective, randomized, multicentre trial. *Br Med J.* 1980;281:1589–1591.

142. Palmer K, Kerr M, Knowles G, Cull A, Carter D, Leonard R. Chemotherapy prolongs survival in inoperable pancreatic carcinoma. *Br J Surg.* 1994;81:882–885.

143. Casper E, Green M, Kelsen D, et al. Phase II trial of gemcitabine (2,2'-difluorodeoxycytidine) in patients with adenocarcinoma of the pancreas. *Investig New Drugs.* 1994;12:29–34.

144. Carmichael J, Fink U, Russell R, et al. Phase II study of gemcitabine in patients with advanced pancreatic cancer. *Br J Cancer.* 1996;73:101–105.

145. Burris H, Moore M, Anderson J, et al. Improvements in survival and clinical benefit with gemcitabine as first-line therapy for patients with advanced pancreas cancer: a randomized trial. *J Clin Oncol.* 1997;15:2403–2413.

146. Rykowski J, Hilgier M. Efficacy of neurolytic celiac plexus block in varying locations of pancreatic cancer: influence on pain relief. *Anesthesiology.* 2000;92:347–354.

147. Marra V, Debernardi F, Frigerio A, Menna S, Musso L, DiVirgilio M. Neurolytic block of the celiac plexus and

splanchnic nerves with computed tomography. The experience in 150 cases and an optimization of the technic. *Radiol Med (Torino)*. 1999;98:183–188.

148. Devesa S, Blot W, Fraumeni J. Changing patterns in the incidence of esophageal and gastric carcinoma in the United States. *Cancer*. 1998;83:2049–2053.

149. Neugut A, Hayek M, Howe G. Epidemiology of gastric cancer. *Semin Oncol*. 1996;23:281–291.

150. Palli D. Epidemiology of gastric cancer: an evaluation of available evidence. *J Gastroenterol*. 2000;35:84–89.

151. Stolet M, Meining A. *Helicobacter pylori* and gastric cancer. *Oncologist*. 1998;3:124–128.

152. Eslick G, Lim L, Byles J, Xia H, Talley N. Association of *Helicobacter pylori* infection with gastric carcinoma: a meta-analysis. *Am J Gastroenterol*. 1999;94:2373–2379.

153. You W, Zhang L, Hail M, et al. Gastric dysplasia and gastric cancer: *Helicobacter pylori*, serum vitamin C, and other risk factors. *J Natl Cancer Inst*. 2000;92:1607–1612.

154. Karlson B, Ekbom A, Wacholder S, McLaughlin J, Hsing A. Cancer of the upper gastrointestinal tract among patients with pernicious anemia: a case-cohort study. *Scand J Gastroenterol*. 2000;35:847–851.

155. Bajtai A, Hidvegi J. The role of gastric mucosal dysplasia in the development of gastric carcinoma. *Pathol Oncol Res*. 1998;4:297–300.

156. Hansson L, Nyren O, Hsing A, et al. The risk of stomach cancer in patients with gastric or duodenal ulcer disease. *N Engl J Med*. 1996;335:242–249.

157. Lundegardh G, Adami H, Helmick C, Zack M, Meirik O. Stomach cancer after partial gastrectomy for benign ulcer disease. *N Engl J Med*. 1988;319:195–200.

158. Uemura N, Mukai T, Okamoto S, et al. Effect of *Helicobacter pylori* eradication on subsequent development of cancer after endoscopic resection of early gastric cancer. *Cancer Epidemiol Biomarkers Prev*. 1997;6:639–642.

159. Wanebo H, Kennedy B, Chmiel J, Steele G, Winchester D, Osteen R. Cancer of the stomach. A patient care study by the American College of Surgeons. *Ann Surg*. 1993;218: 583–592.

160. Siewert J, Bottcher K, Stein H, Roder J. Relevant prognostic factors in gastric cancer: ten-year results of the German Gastric Cancer Study. *Ann Surg*. 1998;228:449–461.

161. Estes N, MacDonald J, Touijer K, Benedetti J, Jacobson J. Inadequate documentation and resection for gastric cancer in the United States: a preliminary report. *Am Surg*. 1998;64:680–685.

162. Bonenkamp J, Hermans J, Sasako M, vandeVelde C. Extended lymph-node dissection for gastric cancer. *N Engl J Med*. 1999;340:908–914.

163. Cuschieri A, Weeden S, Fielding J, et al. Patient survival after D1 and D2 resections for gastric cancer: long-term results of the MRC randomized surgical trial. Surgical Co-operative Group. *Br J Cancer*. 1999;79:1522–1530.

164. Schwarz R, Karpeh M, Brennan M. Factors predicting hospitalization after operative treatment for gastric carcinoma in patients older than 70 years. *J Am Coll Surg*. 1997;184:9–15.

165. Hermans J, Bonenkamp J, Boon M, et al. Adjuvant therapy after curative resection for gastric cancer: meta-analysis of randomized trials. *J Clin Oncol*. 1993;11:1441–1447.

166. Earle C, Maroun J. Adjuvant chemotherapy after curative resection for gastric cancer in non-Asian patients: revisiting a meta-analysis of randomized trials. *Eur J Cancer*. 1999;37:1059–1064.

167. Hallissey M, Dunn J, Ward L, Allum W. The second British Stomach Cancer Group trial of adjuvant radiotherapy or chemotherapy in resectable gastric cancer: five-year follow-up. *Lancet*. 1994;343:1309–1312.

168. Childs D, Moertel C, Holbrook M, Reitemeier R, Colby M. Treatment of unresectable adenocarcinomas of the stomach with a combination of 5-fluorouracil and radiation. *Am J Roentgenol Radium Ther Nucl Med*. 1968;102: 541–544.

169. Macdonald J, Smalley S, Benedetti J, et al. Postoperative combined radiation and chemotherapy improves survival in resected adenocarcinoma of the stomach and GE junction. Results of Intergroup Study INT-0116 (SWOG 9008). *Proc Am Soc Clin Oncol*. 2000;19:A1.

170. Macdonald JS, Smalley SR, Benedetti J. Chemoradiotherapy after surgery compared with surgery alone for adenocarcinoma of the stomach or gastroesophageal junction. *N Engl J Med*. 2001;345:725–730.

171. Smalley S, Benedetti J, Gunderson L, et al. Intergroup 0116 (SWOG 9008) phase III trial of postoperative adjuvant radiochemotherapy for high risk gastric and gastroesophageal junction adenocarcinoma: evaluation of efficacy and radiotherapy treatment planning. *Int J Radiat Oncol Biol Phys*. 2000;48:111–112.

172. Ekbom G, Gleysteen J. Gastric malignancy: resection for palliation. *Surgery*. 1980;88:476–481.

173. Bozzetti F, Bonfanti G, Audisio R, et al. Prognosis of patients after palliative surgical procedures for carcinoma of the stomach. *Surg Gynecol Obstet*. 1987;164: 151–154.

174. Boddie A, McMurtrey M, Giacco G, McBride C. Palliative total gastrectomy and esophagogastrectomy. A reevaluation. *Cancer*. 1983;51:1195–1200.

175. Meijer S, DeBakker O, Hoitsma H. Palliative resection in gastric cancer. *J Surg Oncol*. 1983;23:77–80.

176. Murad A, Santiago F, Petroianu A, Rocha P, Rodrigues M, Rausch M. Modified therapy with 5-fluorouracil, doxorubicin, and methotrexate in advanced gastric cancer. *Cancer*. 1993;72:37–41.

177. Pyrhonen S, Kuitunen T, Nyandoto P, Kouri M. Randomized comparison of fluorouracil, epidoxorubicin and methotrexate (FEMTX) plus supportive care with supportive care alone in patients with non-resectable gastric cancer. *Br J Cancer*. 1995;71:587–591.

178. Glimelius B, Ekstrom K, Hoffman K, et al. Randomized comparison between chemotherapy puls best supportive care with best supportive care in advanced gastric cancer. *Ann Oncol*. 1997;8:163–168.

179. Kulke M. The treatment of advanced gastric cancer: in search of the right combination. *J Clin Oncol*. 2000; 18:2645–2647.

180. Levi J, Fox R, Tattersall M, Woods R, Thomson D, Gill G. Analysis of a prospectively randomized comparison of doxorubicin versus 5-fluorouracil, doxorubicin, and

BCNU in advanced gastric cancer: implications for future sutdues. *J Clin Oncol.* 1986;4:1348–1355.

181. Cullinan S, Moertel C, Wieand H, et al. Controlled evaluation of three drug combination regimens versus fluorouracil alone for the therapy of advanced gastric cancer. North Central Cancer Treatment Group. *J Clin Oncol.* 1994;12:412–416.

182. Ross P, Hill M, Norman A, Cunningham D. ECF in gastric cancer [letter]. *J Clin Oncol.* 2000;18:3874–3875.

183. Webb A, Cunningham D, Scarffe J, et al. Randomized trial comparing epirubicin, cisplatin, fluorouracil versus fluorouracil, doxorubicin, and methotrexate in advanced esophagogastric cancer. *J Clin Oncol.* 1997;15:261–267.

184. Ajani J. Chemotherapy for gastric carcinoma: new and old options. *Oncology.* 1998;12:44–47.

185. Gammon M, Schoenberg J, Ahsan H, et al. Tobacco, alcohol, and socioeconomic status and adenocarcinomas of the esophagus and gastric cardia. *J Natl Cancer Inst.* 1997; 89:1277–1284.

186. Blot W, McLaughlin J. The changing epidemiology of esophageal cancer. *Semin Oncol.* 1999;25:2–8.

187. Lagergren J, Bergstrom R, Lindgren A, Nyren O. Symptomatic gastroesophageal reflux as a risk factor for esophageal adenocarcinoma. *N Engl J Med.* 1999;340:825–831.

188. Spechler S. Barrett's esophagus. *Semin Oncol.* 1994;21:431–437.

189. Vaughan T, Farrow D, Hansten P, et al. Risk of esophageal and gastric adenocarcinomas in relation to use of calcium channel blockers, asthma drugs, and other medications that promote gastroesophageal reflux. *Cancer Epidemiol Biomarkers Prev.* 1998;7:749–756.

190. Lagergren J, Bergstrom R, Adami H, Nyren O. Association between medications that relax the lower esophageal sphincter and risk for esophageal adenocarcinoma. *Ann Intern Med.* 2000;133:165–175.

191. Chow W, Blot W, Vaughan T, et al. Body mass index and risk of adenocarcinomas of the esophagus and gastric cardia. *J Natl Cancer Inst.* 1998;90:150–155.

192. Naunheim K, Hanosh J, Zwischenberger J, et al. Esophagectomy in the septuagenarian. *Ann Thorac Surg.* 1993;56:880–883.

193. Ellis F, Williamson W, Heatley G. Cancer of the esophagus and cardia: does age influence treatment selection and surgical outocmes? *J Am Coll Surg.* 1998;187:345–351.

194. Enzinger P, Ilson D, Kelsen D. Chemotherapy in esophageal cancer. *Semin Oncol.* 1999;26:12–20.

195. Reed C. Surgical management of esophageal carcinoma. *Oncologist.* 1999;4:95–105.

196. Morales T, Sampliner R. Barrett's esophagus: update on screening, surveillance, and treatment. *Arch Intern Med.* 1999;159:1411–1416.

197. Streitz J, Ellis F, Tilden R, Erickson R. Endoscopic surveillance of Barrett's esophagus: a cost-effectiveness comparison with mammographic surveillance for breast cancer. *Am J Gastroenterol.* 1998;93:911–915.

198. Lerut T, Coosemans W, Raemdonck D, et al. Surgical treatment of Barrett's carcinoma. Correlations between morphologic findings and prognosis. *J Thorac Cardiovasc Surg.* 1994;107:1059–1065.

199. Streitz J, Andrews C, Ellis F. Endoscopic surveillance of Barrett's esophagus. Does it help? *J Thorac Cardiovasc Surg.* 1993;105:383–387.

200. Beck I, Champion M, Lemire S, et al. The Second Canadian Consensus Conference on the management of patients with gastroesophageal reflux disease. *Can J Gastroenterol.* 1997;11:7B–20B.

201. Rusch V, Levine D, Haggitt R, Reid B. The management of high grade dysplasia and early cancer in Barrett's esophagus. A multidisciplinary problem. *Cancer.* 1994;74:1225–1229.

202. Corti L, Skarlatos J, Boso C, et al. Outcome of patients receiving photodynamic therapy for esophageal cancer. *Int J Radiat Oncol Biol Phys.* 2000;47:419–424.

203. Sharma P, Jaffe P, Bhattacharyya A, Sampliner R. Laser and multipolar electrocoagulation ablation of early Barrett's adenocarcinoma: long-term follow-up. *Gastrointest Endosc.* 1999;49:442–446.

204. Flamen P, Lerut A, VanCutsem E, et al. Utility of positron emission tomography for the staging of patients with potentially operable esophagela carcinoma. *J Clin Oncol.* 2000;18:3202–3210.

205. Pommier R, Vetto J, Ferris B, Wilmarth T. Relationships between operative approaches and outcomes in esophageal cancer. *Am J Surg.* 1998;175:422–425.

206. Goldminc M, Maddern G, LePrise E, Meunier B, Campion J, Launois B. Oesophagectomy by a transhiatal approach or thoracotomy: a prospective randomized trial. *Br J Surg.* 1993;80:367–370.

207. Bosset J, Gignoux M, Triboulet J, et al. Chemoradiotherapy followed by surgery compared with surgery alone in squamous-cell cancer of the esophagus. *N Engl J Med.* 1997;337:161–167.

208. Kelsen D, Ginsberg R, Pajak T, et al. Chemotherapy followed by surgery compared with surgery alone for localized esophageal cancer. *N Engl J Med.* 1998;339:1979–1984.

209. Alexiou C, Beggs D, Salama F, Brackenbury E, Morgan W. Surgery for esophageal cancer in elderly patients: the view from Nottingham. *J Thorac Cardiovasc Surg.* 1998;116:545–553.

210. Thomas P, Doddoli C, Neville P, et al. Esophageal cancer resection in the elderly. *Eur J Cardiothorac Surg.* 1996;10:941–946.

211. Jougon J, Ballester M, Duffy J, et al. Esophagectomy for cancer in the patient aged 70 years and older. *Ann Thorac Surg.* 1997;63:1423–1427.

212. Dalrymple-Hay M, Evans K, Lea R. Surgery for oesophageal carcinoma in the elderly. *Acta Chir Hung.* 1999;38:27–29.

213. Adam D, Craig S, Sang C, Cameron E, Walker W. Esophagectomy for carcinoma in the octogenarian. *Ann Thorac Surg.* 1996;61:190–194.

214. Earlam R, Cunha-Melo J. Oesophageal squamous cell carcinoma: II. A critical review of radiotherapy. *Br J Surg.* 1980;67:457–461.

215. Herskovic A, Martz K, Al-Sarraf M, et al. Combined chemotherapy and radiotherapy compared with radiotherapy alone in patients with cancer of the esophagus. *N Engl J Med.* 1992;326:1593–1598.

216. Al-Sarraf M, Martz K, Herskovic A, et al. Progress report of combined chemoradiotherapy versus radiotherapy alone in patients with esophageal cancer: an Intergroup study. *J Clin Oncol.* 1997;15:277–284.

217. Smith T, Ryan L, Douglass H, et al. Combined chemoradiotherapy vs radiotherapy alone for early stage squamous cell carcinoma of the esophagus: a study of the Eastern Cooperative Oncology Group. *Int J Radiat Oncol Biol Phys.* 1998;42:269–276.

218. Arnott S, Duncan W, Gignoux M, et al. Preoperative radiotherapy in esophageal carcinoma: a meta-analysis using individual patient data (Oesophageal Cancer Collaborative Group). *Int J Radiat Oncol Biol Phys.* 1998;41:579–583.

219. Clark P. Medical Research Council (MRC) randomized phase III trial of surgery with or without preoperative chemotherapy in resectable cancer of the oesophagus. *Br J Cancer.* 2000;83:CT2.

220. Forastiere A, Orringer M, Perez-Tamayo C, Urba S, Zahurak M. Preoperative chemoradiation followed by transhiatal esophagectomy for carcinoma of the esophagus: final report. *J Clin Oncol.* 1993;11:1118–1123.

221. Sauter E, Coia L, Keller S. Preoperative high-dose radiation and chemotherapy in adenocarcinoma of the esophagus and esophagogastric junction. *Ann Surg Oncol.* 1994; 1:5–10.

222. Stahl M, Wilke H, Fink U, et al. Combined preoperative chemotherapy and radiotherapy in patients with locally advanced esophageal cancer. Interim analysis of a phase II trial. *J Clin Oncol.* 1996;14:829–837.

223. Adelstein D, Rice T, Becker M, et al. Use of concurrent chemotherapy, accelerated fractionation radiation, and surgery for patients with esophageal carcinoma. *Cancer.* 1997;80:1011–1020.

224. Ganem G, Dubray B, Raoul Y, et al. Concomitant chemoradiotherapy followed, where feasible, by surgery for cancer of the esophagus. *J Clin Oncol.* 1997;15:701–711.

225. Wright C, Wain J, Lynch T, et al. Induction therapy for esophageal cancer with paclitaxel and hyperfractionated radiotherapy: a phase I and II study. *J Thorac Cardiovasc Surg.* 1997;114:811–816.

226. Forastiere A, Heitmiller R, Kleinberg L, et al. Long follow-up of patients with esophageal cancer treated with preoperative cisplatin/5-FU and concurrent radiation. *Proc Am Soc Clin Oncol.* 1999;19:A1036.

227. Walsh T, Noonan N, Hollywood D, Kelly A, Keeling N, Hennessy T. A comparison of multimodal therapy and surgery for esophageal adenocarcinoma. *N Engl J Med.* 1996;335:462–467.

228. LePrise E, Etienne P, Meunier B, et al. A randomized study of chemotherapy, radiation therapy, and surgery versus surgery for localized squamous cell carcinoma of the esophagus. *Cancer.* 1994;73:1779–1784.

229. Apinop C, Puttisak P, Preecha N. A prospective study of combined therapy in esophageal cancer. *Hepato-Gastroenterology.* 1994;41:391–393.

230. Urba S, Orringer M, Turrisi A, Iannettoni M, Forastiere A, Strawderman M. Randomized trial of preoperative chemoradiation versus surgery alone in patients with locoregional esophageal carcinoma. *J Clin Oncol.* 2001;19:305–313.

231. Bleiberg H, Conroy T, Paillot B, et al. Randomized phase II study of cisplatin and 5-fluorouracil (5-FU) versus cisplatin alone in advanced squamous cell oesophageal cancer. *Eur J Cancer.* 1997;33:1216–1220.

232. Ajani J, Ilson D, Daugherty K, Pazdur R, Lynch P, Kelsen D. Activity of Taxol in patients with squamous cell carcinoma and adenocarcinoma of the esophagus. *J Natl Cancer Inst.* 1994;86:1086–1091.

233. Kelsen D, Ilson D, Wadleigh R, Leichmann L. A phase II multi-center trial of paclitaxel (P) [Taxol] as a weekly one-hour infusion in advanced esophageal cancer (EC). *Proc Am Soc Clin Oncol.* 2000;19:A1266.

234. Slabber C, Falkson C, Musi N, Burger W. A phase II study of docetaxel in advanced, inoperable squamous carcinoma of the esophagus. *Proc Am Soc Clin Oncol.* 1999;18:A1511.

235. Enzinger P, Kulke M, Clark J, et al. Phase II trial of CPT-11 in previously untreated patietns with advanced adenocarcinoma of the esophagus and stomach. *Proc Am Soc Clin Oncol.* 2000;19:A1243.

236. Conroy T, Etienne P-L, Adenis A, et al. Phase II trial of vinorelbine in metastatic squamous cell esophageal carcinoma. *J Clin Oncol.* 1996;14:164–170.

237. Costa F, Ilson D, Forastiere A, et al. Phase II study of paclitaxel and cisplatin in patients with advanced adenocarcinoma (A) and squamous cell (S) carcinoma of the esophagus. *Proc Am Soc Clin Oncol.* 1997;16:A930.

238. Petrasch S, Welt A, Reinacher A, Graeven U, Konig M, Schmiegel W. Chemotherapy with cisplatin and paclitaxel in patients with locally advanced, recurrent or metastatic oesophageal cancer. *Br J Cancer.* 1998;78:511–514.

239. Ilson D, Saltz L, Enzinger P, et al. Phase II trial of weekly irinotecan plus cisplatin in advanced esophageal cancer. *J Clin Oncol.* 1999;17:3270–3275.

240. Etienne P-L, Conroy T, Adenis A, et al. Vinorelbine and cisplatin in metastatic epidermoid carcinoma of the esophagus (MECE). An EORTC phase II study. *Proc Am Soc Clin Oncol.* 1999;18:A1037.

241. Kroep J, Peters G, Giacone G, Pinedo H, vanGroeningen C. Phase II study of cisplatin (CDDP) preceding gemcitabine (GEM) in patients with advanced gastric and esophageal cancer. *Proc Am Soc Clin Oncol.* 2000;19:A1033.

242. Ou L, Chau G, Tsay S, et al. Clinicopathological comparison of resectable hepatocellular carcinoma between the young and the elderly patients. *Chung Hua I Hsueh Tsa Chih (Taipei).* 1997;60:40–47.

243. El-Serag H, Mason A. Rising incidence of hepatocellular carcinoma in the United States. *N Engl J Med.* 1999;340:745–750.

244. McQuillan G, Townsend T, Fields H, Carroll M, Leahy M, Polk B. Seroepidemiology of hepatitis B virus infection in the United States: 1976 to 1980. *Am J Med.* 1989;87:5S–10S.

245. McQuillan G, Alter M, Everhart J. Viral hepatitis. In: Everhart J, ed. *Digestive Diseases in the United States: Epidemiology and Impact.* NIH pub 94–1447. Washington, DC: Government Printing Office; 1994:127–156.

246. Peng Y, Chan C, Chen G. The effectiveness of serum alpha-fetoprotein level in anti-HCV positive patients for screening hepatocellular carcinoma. *Hepatogastroenterology.* 1999;46:3208–3211.

247. McMahon B, Bulkow L, Harpster A, et al. Screening for hepatocellular carcinoma in Alaska natives infected with chronic hepatitis B: a 16-year population study. *Hepatology.* 2000;32:842–846.

248. Yoshida H, Shiratori Y, Moriyama M, et al. Interferon therapy reduces the risk for hepatocellular carcinoma: national surveillance program of cirrhotic and noncirrhotic patients with chronic hepatitis C in Japan. *Ann Intern Med.* 1999;131:174–181.

249. Nishiguchi S, Kuroki T, Nakatani S, et al. Randomized trial of effects of interferon-alpha on incidence of hepatocellular carcinoma in chronic active hepatitis C with cirrhosis. *Lancet.* 1995;346:1051–1055.

250. Nakakura E, Choti M. Management of hepatocellular carcinoma. *Oncology.* 2000;14:1085–1098.

251. Carr B, Flickinger J, Lotze M. Hepatobiliatry cancers. In: DeVita V, Hellman S, Rosenberg S, eds. *Cancer: Principles and Practice of Oncology.* Philadelphia: Lippincott-Raven; 1997:1087–1114.

252. Nagasue N, Uchida M, Makino Y, et al. Incidence and factors asociated with intrahepatic recurrence following resection of hepatocellular carcinoma. *Gastroenterology.* 1993;105:488–494.

253. Chan E, Chow P, Tai B, Machin D, Soo K. Neoadjuvant and adjuvant therapy for operable hepatocellular carcinoma. *Cochrane Database Syst Rev.* 2000;2: CD001199.

254. Shiina S, Tagawa K, Niwa Y, et al. Percutaneous ethanol injection therapy for hepatocellular carcinoma: results in 146 patients. *Am J Roentgenol.* 1993;160:1023–1028.

255. Lencioni R, Bartolozzi C, Caramella D, et al. Treatment of small hepatocellular carcinoma with percutaneous ethanol injection. Analysis of prognostic factors in 105 Western patients. *Cancer.* 1995;76:1737–1746.

256. Livraghi T, Giorgio A, Marin G, et al. Hepatocellular carcinoma and cirrhosis in 746 patients: long-term results of percutaneous ethanol injection. *Radiology.* 1995;197:101–108.

257. Livraghi T, Lazzaroni S, Meloni F, Torzilli G, Vettori C. Intralesional ethanol in the treatment of unresectable liver cancer. *World J Surg.* 1995;19:801–806.

258. Group d'Etude et de Traitement du Carcinome Hepatocellulaire. A comparison of lipiodol chemoembolization and conservative treatment for unresectable hepatocellular carcinoma. *N Engl J Med.* 1995;332:1256–1261.

259. Pelletier G, Ducreux M, Gay F, et al. Treatment of unresectable hepatocellular carcinoma with lipiodol chemoembolization: a multicenter randomized trial. Groupe CHC. *J Hepatol.* 1998;29:129–134.

260. Poon R, Fan S, Lo C, et al. Hepatocellular carcinoma in the elderly: results of surgical and nonsurgical management. *Am J Gastroenterol.* 1999;94:2460–2466.

261. Takenaka K, Shimada M, Higashi H, et al. Liver resection for hepatocellular carcinoma in the elderly. *Arch Surg* 1994;129:846–850.

262. Hoshida Y, Ikeda K, Saito S, et al. The efficacy and prognosis of transcatheter chemoembolization for hepatocellular carcinoma in the elderly. *Nippon Shokakibyo Gakkai Zasshi.* 1999;96:142–146.

263. Lui W, Chau G, Wu C. Surgical resection of hepatocellular carcinoma in elderly cirrhotic patients. *Hepatogastroenterology.* 1999;46:640–645.

264. Pignata S, Izzo F, Farinati F, et al. Role of tamoxifen (TM) in the treatment of hepatocellular carcinoma (HCC). Results from the CLIP-01 randomized trial. *Proc Am Soc Clin Oncol.* 1998;17:A986.

265. Lowenfels A, Maisonneuve P, Boyle P, Zatonski W. Epidemiology of gallbladder cancer. *Hepatogastroenterology.* 1999;46:1529–1532.

266. Pitt H, Dooley W, Yeo C, Cameron J. Malignancies of the biliary tree. *Curr Probl Surg.* 1995;32:1–90.

267. Zatonski W, Lowenfels A, Boyle P, et al. Epidemiologic aspects of gallbladder cancer: a case-control study of the SEARCH Program of the International Agency for Research on Cancer. *J Natl Cancer Inst.* 1997;89:1132–1138.

268. DeGroen P, Gores G, LaRusso N, Gunderson L, Nagorney D. Biliary tract cancers. *N Engl J Med.* 1999;341:1368–1378.

269. Fong Y, Heffernan N, Blumgart L. Gallbladder carcinoma discovered during laparoscopic cholecystectomy: aggressive reresection is beneficial. *Cancer.* 1998;83:423–427.

270. Donohue J, Nagorney D, Grant C, Tsushima K, Ilstrup D, Adson M. Carcinoma of the gallbladder. Does radical resection improve outcome? *Arch Surg.* 1990;125:237–241.

271. Bosset J, Mantion G, Gillet M, et al. Primary carcinoma of the gallbladder. Adjuvant postoperative external irradiation. *Cancer.* 1989;64:1843–1847.

272. Mahe M, Stampfli C, Romestaing P, Salerno N, Gerard J. Primary carcinoma of the gall-bladder: potential for external radiation therapy. *Radiother Oncol.* 1994;33:204–208.

273. Foo M, Gunderson L, Bender C, Buskirk S. External radiation therapy and transcatheter iridium in the treatment of extrahepatic bile duct carcinoma. *Int J Radiat Oncol Biol Phys.* 1997;39:929–935.

274. Bowling T, Galbraith S, Hatfield A, Solano J, Spittle M. A retrospective comparison of endoscopic stenting alone with stenting and radiotherapy in non-resectable cholangiocarcinoma. *Gut.* 1996;39:852–855.

275. Kuvshinoff B, Armstrong J, Fong Y, et al. Palliation of irresectable hilar cholangiocarcinoma with biliary drainage and radiotherapy. *Br J Surg.* 1995;82:1522–1525.

276. Falkson G, MacIntyre J, Moertel C. Eastern Cooperative Oncology Group experience with chemotherapy for inoperable gallbladder and bile duct cancer. *Cancer.* 1984;54:965–969.

277. Lozano R, Patt Y, Hassan M, et al. Oral capecitabine (Xeloda) for the treatment of hepatobiliary cancers (hepatocellular carcinoma, cholangiocarcinoma, and gallbladder cancer). *Proc Am Soc Clin Oncol.* 2000;19:A1025.

35
Lung Cancer

Eric B. Haura, Susan A. Blackwell, and Jeffrey Crawford

Epidemiology and Risk Factors

In the United States, the leading cause of cancer death in men is lung cancer, with lung cancer continuing to surpass breast cancer as the leading cause of cancer death in women. In men, the overall incidence of lung cancer currently approximates 80 per 100,000 men;[1] this escalates to nearly 600 per 100,000 for men aged 60 to 79 years. In women, the overall incidence of lung cancer is approximately 50 per 100,000 women; lung cancer incidence rates are approximately 400 per 100,000 women aged 60 to 79. The number of older persons who will develop lung cancer is expected to increase as the smoking exposure time effects on birth cohorts become more apparent[2] (Fig. 35.1).

There is a dose–response relationship for smoking and lung cancer, and the risk for lung cancer increases with smoking duration, number of cigarettes smoked, age at onset of smoking, use of unfiltered cigarettes, tar and nicotine content, and degree of inhalation.[1] The pivotal trial by Doll and Hill in 1956 showed that smoking cessation reduces the risk of lung cancer compared to those who continue to smoke.[3] This finding was reproduced by Pathak et al. in 1986 in a case control study of lung cancer in New Mexico, which compared cases and controls less than 65 years of age to those more than 65 years of age[4] and additionally showed that one decline in lung cancer risk that occurs with smoking cessation in the older person is comparable to that of the young. This same study showed that the number of years of smoking is relatively less important than the number of cigarettes smoked per day in determining the risk for lung cancer in those persons 65 and older.[5]

In a reanalysis of the 1986 Adult Use of Tobacco Survey (AUTS), Orleans et al. found that older smokers smoked cigarettes with a slightly higher nicotine content than younger smokers.[6] The number of cigarettes smoked per day was similar: 21.3 for smokers aged 21 to 49 and 29.1 for smokers aged 50 to 74. In this reanalysis, it was estimated that 53% of Americans aged 21 to 49 years were ever smokers, including 31% who were current smokers and 22% former smokers. In the 50- to 74-year-old group, 58% were ever smokers, including 23% current smokers and 35% former smokers. Although the older smokers had smoked for more than twice as many years as the younger group (mean, 39 years versus 16 years), the AUTS survey showed very little difference between the older and younger smokers in either smoking habits or quitting history. Even though the older smokers had smoked longer, they did not report an increased number of quitting attempts. The AUTS did suggest that older smokers underestimate both the risk of smoking and the benefits of stopping smoking (Table 35.1).

A recent American Cancer Society study clarified the risk of lung cancer mortality in smokers and former smokers. Halpern et al. examined and compared absolute and relative lung cancer death risk in former smokers as a function of age at cessation.[7] In a prospective cohort study with 6 years of follow-up, the absolute risk of lung cancer mortality was compared in individuals who had never smoked and current and former smokers. As expected, there was a lower lung cancer death risk seen for those patients who quit smoking earlier in life, and the risk for those who were former smokers was significantly lower than for those who continued to smoke. However, the influence of age was profound (Fig. 35.2A,B). The lung cancer death risk for persons who stopped smoking between the ages of 30 and 49 rose gradually with age at a rate slightly greater than for those persons who had never smoked. If one quit between the ages of 50 and 64, the lung cancer death risk leveled off at the risk attained at the time of quitting until around age 75, when it increased significantly.

For current smokers at age 75, the annual lung cancer mortality is estimated at 1 per 100 for males and 1 per 200 for females. Table 35.2 demonstrates the relative risk reductions as a function of age of smoking cessation.

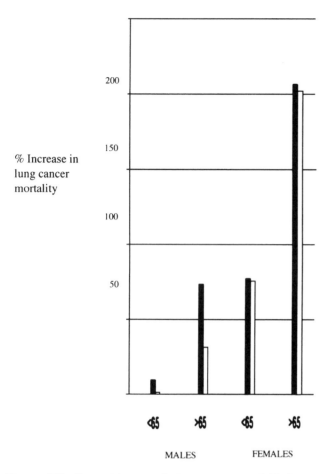

FIGURE 35.1. Percent increase in lung cancer mortality by age group, sex, and race. SEER data, 1973–1990. ■, black; □, white.

Former smokers had a relative risk of lung cancer death of approximately 0.45 if they had quit in their early sixties, 0.20 if they had stopped smoking in their early fifties, and 0.10 for those who had stopped smoking in their thirties, compared with nonsmokers who had a relative risk of 0.05 or less. Therefore, in terms of reduced risk of lung cancer mortality, stopping smoking at any age is beneficial, but much more beneficial for those quitting at a younger age. The authors showed that even though the absolute lung cancer risk can plateau following smoking cessation, the lung cancer risk for former smokers is still consistently greater than that of those who have never smoked.

In their model in Figure 35.2, the authors have shown that there is a rise in lung cancer risk seen after age 75, and this is consistent over several cohorts. This biologic difference in the older patient may reflect decline in cellular DNA repair activity with age, or perhaps the cumulative exposure to smoking and other carcinogens combined with decreased repair mechanisms late in life may have a synergistic effect on lung cancer risk. It is, however, also possible that this late rise is a reflection in the differing smoking characteristics of older and younger smokers, as mentioned earlier.

Although this study demonstrated that a greater reduction in lung cancer risk by smoking cessation at a young age, it also confirmed that stopping smoking is beneficial at any age, even in those patients beyond age 60.[7] Because smokers benefit from quitting smoking and because one in four persons will be age 55 and older by the year 2010, it is important that health care providers counsel all

TABLE 35.1. Perceived benefits and harms of smoking by age among 4835 AUTS smokers 21 to 74 years of age.

Variable	Age 21–49 years (n = 3151)	Age 50–74 years (n = 1234)
Perceived benefits (pros) of smoking		
Smoking reduces tension	65.65	75.91±
Smoking helps me cope	49.18	55.86±
Smoking controls weight	49.12	55.08±
Smoking is less harmful than being 20 lb overweight	28.44	47.0±
Perceived harms (cons) of smoking		
How concerned about personal health effects		
[% fairly/very (vs. not at all/slightly)]	45.43	35.45±
How much connection is there between smoking and illness?		
[% very strong (vs. some or none)]	33.48	27.18±
How much more likely are smokers to get these diseases?		
[% somewhat or much more (vs. no more)]		
Heart disease	79.53	69.64±
Lung cancer	91.19	80.27±
Bladder cancer	33.80	26.87±
Emphysema	91.21	86.83±
Coughs	92.23	86.72±
Larynx cancer	89.81	81.14±
Bronchitis	82.05	72.81±
Belief that smokers get more diseases (mean score)	1.40	1.23±

AUTS, Adult Use of Tobacco Survey.
Source: From Orleans et al.,[6] with permission.

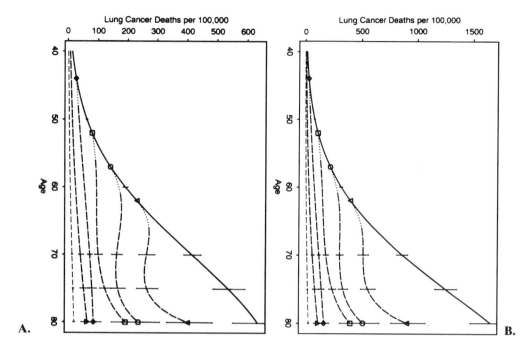

FIGURE 35.2. (A) Lung cancer death rates by age for men, current, former, and nonsmokers, starting smoking at age 17.5 and smoking 26 cigarettes/day. (B) Estimated lung cancer death rates for women current, former, and never smokers. Starting smoking at age 18.5 smoking 22 cigarettes/day. Plotted are current smokers (*solid lines*), never smoked (*dotted line*), former smokers (*dashed lines*). Age-at-quitting cohorts are distinguished by the following symbols at the age of quitting and also at age 80: △, 30–39; ◇, 40–49; □, 50–54; ○, 55–59; ▽, 60–64. (From Halpern et al.,[7] with permission.)

patients on stopping smoking. Specifically, older patients are an important target for smoking cessation because they tend to be long-term, heavier smokers and are more likely to have chronic diseases that can be aggravated by smoking.[8]

Pathogenesis

Because of the difference in natural history, survival, and type of treatment, primary bronchogenic carcinomas are commonly divided into two groups, non–small cell lung cancer and small cell lung cancer. Histologically, non–small cell lung cancer can be subdivided into squamous cell carcinoma, large cell carcinoma, and adenocarcinoma, with bronchoalveolar cell being a subtype of adenocarcinoma. Non–small cell lung cancer accounts for approximately 75% to 80% of all lung cancers. Squamous cell carcinoma was once the most common type of non–small cell lung cancer in this country; however, there has been an increase in adenocarcinoma, now accounting for approximately 40% of all lung cancer. Squamous cell carcinoma and small cell carcinoma are highly associated with smoking, although cigarette smoking has been linked with all histologic subtypes. Although there are some differences in the clinical behavior of subtypes of non–small cell lung cancer, they are generally grouped together because of their similar natural history and

response to treatment and because histology and cytology often overlap between these subtypes.[1]

Small cell lung cancer can generally be distinguished from non–small cell lung cancer by histology or cytology alone in 95% of cases. Small cell lung cancer also tends

TABLE 35.2. Estimated relative risk (RR) of lung cancer death following smoking cessation: never and former smokers compared with current smokers.

	Relative risk		
	Age 55	Age 65	Age 75
Men:			
Never smokers	0.05	0.03	0.03
Quit 30–39	0.14	0.09	0.07
Quit 40–49	0.36	0.18	0.12
Quit 50–54	—	0.29	0.19
Quit 55–59	—	0.56	0.27
Quit 60–64	—	—	0.45
Current smokers	1.0	1.0	1.0
Women:			
Never smokers	0.07	0.05	0.04
Quit 30–39	0.17	0.11	0.10
Quit 40–49	0.40	0.22	0.15
Quit 50–54	—	0.33	0.23
Quit 55–59	—	0.60	0.31
Quit 60–64	—	—	0.49
Current smokers	1.0	1.0	1.0

Source: From Halpern et al.,[7] with permission.

to be detected at a more advanced stage because it grows rapidly and metastasizes early, with very few cases being surgically resectable. Non–small cell lung cancers, in contrast, tend to grow more slowly and are often detected at a stage where surgery may be curative.

The relative proportion of squamous cell cancer increases with increasing age and is particularly prevalent in older males. Squamous cell carcinoma was also found to be the subtype most likely to be detected at an early stage and with the best 5-year survival rate in the National Cancer Institute Early Lung Cancer Detection Program. Large cell carcinoma and adenocarcinoma are intermediate in their growth rate between squamous cell and small cell lung cancer. Adenocarcinoma is particularly prominent in females and is increasing in incidence. Importantly, adenocarcinoma and large cell carcinoma, like squamous cell carcinoma, may also present at a localized stage at which surgery is an option.

Clinical Presentation

Most patients with lung cancer are symptomatic at the time of diagnosis. Unfortunately, their symptoms are often associated with locally advanced or distant disease, which may render them inoperable (Table 35.3).

TABLE 35.3. Lung cancer symptoms and signs.

Asymptomatic
Primary
  Cough
  Wheeze and stridor
  Chest pain
  Shortness of breath
  Hemoptysis
  Fever, chills, or sweats (associated pneumonia)
Systemic
  Anorexia
  Weight loss
  Fatigue
  Weakness
  Finger clubbing
  Paraneoplastic endocrine syndromes
Metastatic
  Regional
    Hoarseness
    Superior vena cava syndrome
    Dysphagia
    Horner's syndrome
    Brachial plexus pain
    Chest wall pain
  Distant
    Bone pain (bone metastases)
    Altered mental status (brain metastases)
    Palable lymph nodes
    Jaundice (liver metastases)
    Abdominal pain (liver metastases)

Source: From Crawford et al.,[5] with permission.

TABLE 35.4. Lung cancer symptoms that may be confused with noncancer symptoms in the elderly.

Lung Cancer Symposium	Cormorbid disease or "aging explanation"
Cough	Chronic bronchitis
Dyspnea	Emphysema, old age
Fever (postobstructive pneumonia)	Cold, flu
Weight loss	Depression, inactivity
Bone pain (bone metastases)	Arthritis, old age
Altered mental status (brain metastases, hypercalcemia)	Dementia, old age

Source: From Crawford et al.,[5] with permission.

Specific signs and symptoms depend on the location of the tumor, its locoregional spread, and the presence of metastatic disease. In addition, paraneoplastic syndromes occur more frequently in lung cancer than in any other tumor. Also, some patients are totally asymptomatic and for unrelated reasons undergo incidental chest x-ray and are found to have an asymptomatic lesion.[1] Unfortunately, many of the symptoms of lung cancer are nonspecific and in the elderly may be attributed to comorbid illness. This may result in a delay in diagnosis, which may have profound effects on the treatment options available for the patient (Table 35.4).

A study by DeMaria and Cohen showed that patients at all ages had a similar prevalence of cough, hoarseness, dysphasia, and weight loss, but patients older than 70 years of age presented more frequently with dyspnea but less frequently with chest pain than did younger patients.[9]

Although mass screening for lung cancer has not been recommended, high-risk patients over age 65 might benefit from screening to detect earlier-stage squamous cell carcinomas with favorable prognosis.[5] It would seem logical that patients presenting with early-stage lung cancer are far more likely to be cured than those patients with advanced disease. However, over the past 30 years, the percentage of localized disease and resectability rates has remained unchanged at approximately 20%, indicating that screening and early detection programs have been unsuccessful.

Several prospective randomized studies using serial chest x-rays and sputum cytologies to complement each other in early lung cancer diagnosis did not result in detection of lung cancers at a curable stage or demonstrate that intensive screening led to a lower death rate from lung cancer. However, a study conducted by O'Rourke et al. suggested that lung cancer may present at a less advanced stage with increasing age.[10] Information from the centralized cancer patient data system with a total of 22,874 cases showed that the percentage of lung cancer patients with local stage disease increased from 15.3% for patients aged 54 years or younger to 25.4% of those 75 years or older. An additional 6,332 patients who underwent surgical staging were analyzed and showed a greater likelihood of presenting with local disease with an increase in age. Therefore, in addition to having a higher age-specific incidence, older cancer patients may have a higher likelihood of local stage lung cancer. Thus, the older high-risk patient, smoker or former smoker, should be followed carefully for the development of lung cancer. In the absence of an official recommendation for routine screening, the physician should have a low threshold for obtaining a chest x-ray in these patients as symptoms develop.[11]

The case for screening for lung cancer has recently resurfaced with the results of the Early Lung Cancer Action Project (ELCAP) group, who examined the usefulness of annual helical low-dose computed tomography (CT) scanning compared to chest x-ray in heavy smokers over the age of 60.[12] Cancers were detected in 2.7% of patients by CT scan compared to 0.7% by chest x-ray; 85% of the CT-detected tumors were stage I and all but one were resectable. The overall rate of detection by CT scanning was six times higher than by chest x-ray. To prevent a large number of questionable biopsies, recommendations were made by the ELCAP investigators to initially biopsy only nodules with nonsmooth edges or noncalcified nodules 10mm or larger. For smaller nodules, documented growth by high-resolution CT was recommended before biopsy. Biopsies were done on 28 of 233 patients with noncalcified lesions, with 27 having malignant disease and 1 having a benign nodule.

Despite these encouraging results, a number of problems still remain. First, the 27 cancers detected by CT scanning represented only one-quarter of all nodules found on CT scans, potentially necessitating a large number of follow-up scans. The need for biopsies, however, was maintained at a reasonable level, possibly because of recommendations offered by the investigators. Issues regarding cost also remain unclear although the investigators claim that the CT scan costs are only slightly higher than that of a chest x-ray and that only 20 s of CT time are required to obtain the images. Finally, the ability of annual screening CT scans to improve overall survival in smokers remains to be determined.

Diagnosis and Differential Diagnosis

Once a patient is suspected of having lung cancer, a diagnosis should be confirmed by obtaining adequate specimens for pathologic analysis. Diagnosis is most commonly made from sputum cytology, bronchoscopy with bronchial washings, and biopsy or transthoracic needle aspiration. It has been shown that elderly patients

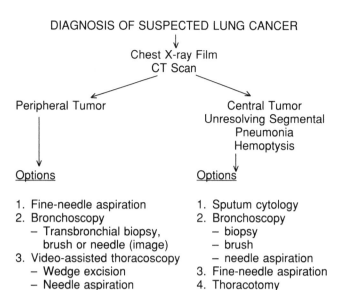

FIGURE 35.3. Indicated procedures for diagnosis of lung cancer depending on location of lesion. (From Yancik et al.,[2] with permission.)

tolerate such diagnostic procedures well, unless they have significant comorbid pulmonary conditions.[5]

Figure 35.3 outlines a strategy based on location of the lung mass. Approximately two-thirds of neoplastic lesions can be seen through the fiber optic bronchoscope. In addition, those lesions that cause extrinsic narrowing of a bronchus can be biopsied transbronchially. The complications of bronchoscopy are minimal in experienced hands. The sensitivity for diagnosis when a lesion is visible is approximately 90%, and the specificity is excellent, with false positives occurring less than 1% of the time.

Bronchoscopy has essentially replaced the once common repeated samples of sputum for cytology because of the greater sensitivity of bronchoscopy. Washing and brushings are routinely obtained during bronchoscopy, and occasionally the cytology is diagnostic although the biopsy specimen is nondiagnostic. For more peripheral lung lesions or when the diagnosis cannot be made by bronchoscopy, transthoracic fine-needle aspiration (TTNA) and biopsy can be performed under fluoroscopic or CT guidance. This procedure, however, carries a much higher complication rate than bronchoscopy, with pneumothorax occurring in approximately 27% of patients and hemoptysis in 2% to 5%. It is, however, an alternative to more invasive procedures. TTNA may also be useful in aspiration of mediastinal structures, with no higher complication rate in the mediastinum than in a peripheral lung lesion. The incidence of false negatives with transthoracic needle aspiration and biopsy ranges from 11% to 69%.[13] This rate can be improved by the presence of a pathologist at the time of the procedure to assure that an adequate sample has been obtained, and often a diagnosis can be made immediately in this setting.

The differential diagnosis for patients who present with abnormalities on chest x-ray includes lung cancer, as well as other nonmalignant conditions. These conditions include infectious etiologies such as tuberculosis or bacterial pneumonias, or inflammatory conditions such as sarcoidosis that can result in mediastinal lymphadenopathy and sometimes mimic locally advanced lung cancers. Patients with widely metastatic disease to the lungs are rarely mistaken to have other illnesses, and usually the major problem is confirming the primary source of malignancy.

Prognosis and Course of Illness

Once a tissue diagnosis has been made, staging becomes an important factor in the treatment of patients with lung cancer. Appropriate staging is critical to the prognosis and optional for treatment, as well as to compare results from different clinical treatment series and experimental clinical trials and to develop multimodality treatment regimens.

Mediastinoscopy, mediastinotomy, thoracotomy, and, more recently, video-assisted thoracoscopy (VATS) have been incorporated into the diagnosis and staging of lung cancer. Although video-assisted thoracoscopy remains an investigative tool, prospective studies are currently ongoing. It has proven to be useful in biopsing or excising peripheral nodules and sampling mediastinal nodes and is less invasive than standard thoracotomy (see Fig. 35.3). All these techniques are useful adjuncts in staging lung cancer in appropriate patients. However, many patients present with signs of distant disease, such as distant lymph nodes, skin lesions, liver, adrenal, or bone involvement. Needle-directed biopsies in these patients can often confirm both the cell type and metastatic spread of the cancer and limit further need for evaluation.[11]

Several studies have suggested that lung cancer presents at a less advanced stage in the elderly patient. Ershler et al., in a review of 157 lung cases in Vermont, showed that the percent of cases with metastatic disease decreased from 80% at age 40 to 40% at age 70.[14] In a review of a centralized cancer patient data system, Crawford et al. analyzed 20,000 lung cancer cases registered between 1977 and 1982. There was an increase in the percent with local stage from 15.3% at age 54 and younger to 25.4% of those 75 or older. In those with distant disease, there was a decrease from 48.7% age 54 or younger to 36.7% age 75 or older.[5]

In 1985, a new international staging system for lung cancer was adopted. The TNM classification groups patients according to the size and extent of their tumor (T), the lymph node involvement (N), and the presence or absence of metastatic disease (M). A patient's clinical stage is the best estimate of TNM before surgery, with the surgical stage of TNM determined after surgery and with pathologic review of surgical specimens (Table 35.5).

The TNM classifications can then be grouped into four stages of non–small cell lung cancer, with a significant difference in the 5-year survival depending on the stage at which the disease is diagnosed. Stages I and II represent surgically resectable disease, with stage III representing regionally advanced disease and stage IV distant metastatic disease (Table 35.6).

The TNM staging classification can be used in small cell lung cancer, but because of the more advanced stage at

TABLE 35.5. TNM classification of lung cancer.

Primary tumor (T):

TX   Primary tumor cannot be assessed, or tumor proven by the presence of malignant cells in sputum or bronchial washings but not visualized by imaging or bronchoscopy

T0   No evidence of primary tumor

Tis   Carcinoma in situ

T1   Tumor 3cm or less in greatest dimension, surrounded by lung or visceral pleura, without bronchoscopic evidence of invasion more proximal than the lobar bronchus (i.e., not in the main bronchus)

T2   Tumor with any of the following features of size or extent: more than 3cm in greatest dimension, involves main bronchus, 2cm or more distal to the carina; invades the visceral pleura; associated with atelectasis or obstructive pneumonitis that extends to the hilar region but does involve the entire lung

T3   Tumor of any size that directly invades any of the following: chest wall (includes superior sulcus tumors), diaphragm, mediastinal pleura, parietal pericardium, tumor in the main bronchus less than 2cm distal to the carina but without involvement of the carina; or associated atelectasis or obstructive pneumonitis of the entire lung

T4   Tumor of any size that invades any of the following: mediastinum, heart, great vessels, trachea, esophagus, vertebral body, carina; or tumor with a malignant pleural effusion

Regional lymph nodes (N):

NX   Regional lymph nodes cannot be assessed

N0   No regional lymph node metastasis

N1   Metastasis in ipsilateral peribronchial and/or ipsilateral hilar lymph nodes, including direct extension

N2   Metastasis in ipsilateral mediastinal and/or subcarinal lymph node(s)

N3   Metastasis in contralateral mediastinal, contralateral hilar, ipsilateral or contralateral scalene, or supraclavicular lymph node(s)

Distant metastasis (M):

MX   Presence of distant metastasis cannot be assessed

M0   No distant metastasis

M1   Distant metastasis

T, primary tumor; N, regional lymph nodes; M, distant metastasis.
Source: From Crawford et al.,[5] with permission.

TABLE 35.6. Stage grouping.

Occult carcinoma	T	N	M
Stage 0	Tis	N0	M0
Stage I	T1	N0	M0
	T2	N0	M0
Stage II	T1	N1	M0
	T2	N1	M0
	T3	N0	M0
Stage IIIA	T1	N2	M0
	T2	N2	M0
	T3	N1, N2	M0
Stage IIIB	Any T	N3	M0
	T4	Any N	M0
Stage IV	Any T	Any N	M1

presentation, small cell carcinoma is generally classified as limited or extensive disease, similar to stage III or IV disease. In small cell lung cancer, limited disease is confined to one hemithorax and capable of being encompassed in a single radiation therapy port; this allows for mediastinal or supraclavicular nodal involvement and does not make a distinction between local and regional disease. Extensive disease is defined as metastatic spread beyond the limits of one hemithorax. Extensive disease occurs in two-thirds of small cell lung cancer cases. In small cell lung cancer, the distinction between limited and extensive disease is important in determining combined modality approaches with curative intent versus palliative chemotherapy. In addition, occasional patients present with a peripheral stage I small cell lung cancer and may undergo surgery.[5]

It is important to stage all lung cancer patients before treatment and after therapy. A comprehensive history and physical examination are important to obtain symptoms suggesting regional spread, such as chest pain, hoarseness to suggest recurrent laryngeal nerve palsy, or evidence of obstruction. In addition, symptoms such as bone pain, weight loss, or neurologic symptoms can suggest metastatic disease. Examination of the head and neck for lymphadenopathy may reveal lymphagitic spread.

The chest x-ray remains probably the most valuable tool in diagnosing lung cancer. However, CT plays an important role in staging of lung cancer, often detecting abnormalities that cannot be adequately evaluated on chest x-ray. The mediastinal structures, chest wall, and vertebrae can be evaluated with small pleural nodules or small pleural effusions often not seen on plain films shown on CT scans. In addition, the CT scan can detect metastatic disease to the liver or adrenals. It is important in staging a patient with lung cancer to include the upper abdomen to the level of the kidneys to evaluate for liver or adrenal gland abnormalities.[1]

A CT scan can be helpful in selecting patients who should undergo mediastinoscopy. If the CT reveals mediastinal nodes greater than 1.5 cm in diameter, it should not be assumed that this indicates metastatic node involvement with tumor; histologic proof by thoracotomy or mediastinoscopy is indicated. This information is critical for patients with non–small cell lung cancer (NSCLC) being considered for surgery. Developed some 30 years ago to facilitate staging of superior mediastinal lymph nodes, mediastinoscopy remains the most accurate lymph node staging technique to assess superior mediastinal lymph nodes that are frequently involved with disease. In a large study by Luke et al., the mortality rate of mediastinoscopy was zero with major morbidity rate less than 1%.[15] In this study, it was reported that patients who were mediastinoscopy negative but found to have mediastinal lymph node involvement at thoracotomy had better 5-year survivals, compared with patients who were found at mediastinoscopy to have positive lymph nodes, who had much poorer survival.[1,13]

In patients with small cell lung cancer, staging is important to determine if a patient has limited versus extensive stage disease. In addition to differences in prognosis, those patients with limited disease may also receive chest radiation and possibly prophylactic cranial irradiation. Thus, patients with small cell lung cancer should undergo brain CT or MRI to evaluate the presence or absence of CNS metastases. A CT scan including the upper abdomen to evaluate the liver and the adrenals as well as a bone scan are also important. Pretreatment staging will detect metastatic disease to the bone in approximately 38% of patients, metastases to the liver in 34% of patients, and CNS disease in 14% of patients. If these studies reveal no evidence of metastatic disease, bone marrow aspirate and biopsy should be done because approximately 5% of patients have bone marrow involvement as the only site of metastatic disease.[1]

Treatment and Management of Illness

Once the patient has a tissue diagnosis and has been accurately staged, the treatment plan can be determined. The patient's ability to tolerate treatment is of utmost importance, whether the planned therapy is surgery, radiation therapy, chemotherapy, or multimodality therapy. A patient's performance status has consistently been the single most prognostic factor for treatment planning. Patients who are asymptomatic with a Karnofsky performance status of 100% or symptomatic but normally active with a performance status of 80% to 90% generally tolerate therapy better and live longer than patients

TABLE 35.7. Karnofsky performance status.

100%	Normal, no complaints, no evidence of disease
90%	Able to carry on normal activity; minor signs or symptoms of disease
80%	Normal activity with effort; some signs or symptoms of disease
70%	Cares for self, unable to carry on normal activity or do active work
60%	Requires occasional assistance, but is able to care for most personal needs
50%	Requires considerable assistance and frequent medical care
40%	Disabled; requires special care and assistance
30%	Severly disabled; hospitalization is indicated, although death not imminent
20%	Very sick; hospitalization necessary; active support treatment is necessary
10%	Moribund; fatal processes progressing rapidly
0%	Dead

who have decreased performance status (Table 35.7). In addition, weight loss is also an important prognostic variable, with weight loss greater than 5% of body weight being an adverse predictor of survival.

Cancer is no less devastating to an elderly person than to a younger person. Older patients have the same right as younger patients to take part in the decision-making process about their treatment. Quality of life is equally important to older patients, and often they will prefer improved quality over quantity of life, with less interest in a trade-off of months or years of life in exchange for the side effects of treatment. Even though cancer is a disease of the elderly, older patients are often treated less aggressively; this can be explained somewhat by the presence of comorbid conditions that often exist in the elderly.[16]

It may be that many physicians are uncertain about subjecting older patients to aggressive chemotherapy. Studies of the psychosocial impact of cancer treatments upon the elderly have shown that older patients are able to cope with the impact of chemotherapy as well if not better than younger patients. Older patients report no greater frequency of toxic side effects and often experience lower levels of emotional distress and life disruption than younger patients.[17]

Treatment of Non–Small Cell Lung Cancer

The treatment of non–small cell lung cancer is highly dependent on accurate staging regimens, as already discussed. The following discussion delineates treatment plans based on accurate clinical staging.

Stages I and II

Surgical resection is the treatment of choice for those patients with non–small cell lung cancer presenting with surgically resectable disease, that is, stages I, II, and possibly IIIa. Five-year survival for stage I is 60% to 80% and for stage II, 40%. In the elderly, extensive preoperative planning is necessary to determine the best surgical procedure for a complete resection of tumor with preservation of as much normal lung tissue as possible. If a pneumonectomy is being considered, the patient's pulmonary status must be adequately evaluated before surgery.

In the past, many physicians have viewed age greater than 70 as an independent risk factor for thoracotomy. However, because surgical resection remains the only potentially curative form for treatment for lung cancer and the life expectancy of patients age 70 is approximately 15 years, surgery should never be denied solely on the basis of a patient's age.

Massard et al.[18] reviewed 1616 patients who underwent thoracotomy for lung cancer from January 1983 to December 1992, with 233 patients aged 70 years or more, at the University Hospital in Strasbourgh, France. Of these patients, 29% had no medical history, 26% had a history of cardiovascular disease, and 19% had a previous history of malignancy that was in complete remission; 48% of patients were stage I, 17% stage II, and 30% stage III. Of these, 210 patients were able to undergo resection, with 60 receiving pneumonectomies and 150 lobectomies. A total of 16 patients died postoperatively: 7.2% for the whole series, 10% after pneumonectomy, and 6.6% after lobectomy. The mortality was similar below and above 75 years of age. The 5-year survival for stage I was 45%, 36.3% for stage II, and 13.8% for stage III, with an overall 5-year survival of 39.9%. Survival was not influenced by age.

Patients who have complete resections are sometimes considered for adjuvant therapy with either chemotherapy or radiation therapy. These strategies attempt to reduce the risk of recurrence by treating presumed remaining tumor cells, either still in the chest (radiation) or disseminated to other sites (chemotherapy). Pre- and postoperative radiation therapy has not been shown to benefit survival in two large randomized trials. In addition, a recent meta-analysis also failed to demonstrate improvement in overall survival in completely resected patients who then went on to receive radiation therapy.[19]

Despite advances in the treatment of breast and colon carcinomas with adjuvant chemotherapy, there continues to be no strong proof of survival benefit of adjuvant chemotherapy in lung cancer, despite occasional trials that suggest a benefit. However, clinical trials involving newer agents are ongoing in the adjuvant setting and should be considered if available. In one study, patients with stage IB non–small cell lung cancers are being randomized to either observation alone or four cycles of chemotherapy with carboplatin and paclitaxel. Another large intergroup study is randomizing patients with completely resected stage II or stage III disease to either observation alone or four cycles of cisplatin and vinorelbine chemotherapy. Results from these studies are not expected to be available for a number of years, so until then, no firm recommendation of adjuvant chemotherapy can be given.

Operable Stage III

Surgery alone for stage III disease is associated with 5-year survival of less than 10%. In an attempt to improve long-term outcome of patients with this stage of disease, investigators have added chemotherapy preoperatively before a curative resection is attempted. In one study by Rosell et al., patients with IIIA disease (N_2-ipsilateral node involvement) disease had improved survival after three courses of preoperative chemotherapy with mitomycin, ifosfamide, and cisplatin.[20] Another study by Roth et al. demonstrated a 3-year survival of 56% for patients treated with preoperative chemotherapy compared with 15% for patients treated with surgery alone.[21] Although these studies were not designed specifically for the geriatric population, nonetheless elderly patients were not excluded (in fact, the Rosell study had a patient aged 78 years in the combined treatment arm). The applicability of these studies to elderly patients remains questionable; however, elderly patients with good performance status and absence of other significant comorbidities should be considered for this treatment.

Inoperable Stage III

Radiation therapy has been the most common treatment in inoperable regional non-small cell lung cancer. It has also been considered an alternative treatment for those patients with underlying medical problems who cannot undergo surgery or those patients who decline surgical resection. The median survival for patients undergoing primary radiation therapy for unresectable disease is less than 1 year. Five-year survival data, however, show approximately 6% of patients alive and well with radiation therapy alone. This finding should not be compared with surgical results, because patients who are selected for radiation alone are usually patients with decreased performance status or other less favorable prognostic factors. Radiation therapy can be very useful in the palliation of symptoms resulting from thoracic tumor growth, such as intractable cough, hemoptysis, dyspnea, and chest pain. The major toxicity encountered is esophagitis, which is usually easily managed with patients who received radiation therapy without chemotherapy. Pneumonitis and pulmonary fibrosis are also important toxicities and, although rare, can result in significant morbidity in a patient population that already has preexisting pulmonary compromise.

Lung cancer may be one of the most common tumors treated with primary radiation therapy in the over-65 age group. There are several advantages to radiation therapy. There is no appreciable acute mortality associated with the treatment, and underlying comorbid conditions other than severe pulmonary disease do not often preclude radiation treatments. The normal healthy lung parenchyma can be preserved while relief of endobronchial obstruction is achieved, and the risk of a second malignancy is of less concern than in a younger patient. Relative disadvantages of radiation include the length of time involved in the course of treatment (often 4 to 6 weeks or more) and the side effects associated with radiation treatment, such as fatigue, loss of appetite, nausea and vomiting, dysphagia, and lowered blood counts.[22]

Because of the poor survival rates with radiation alone in stage III NSCLC and the frequent development of metastatic disease at distant sites, the role of chemotherapy in combination with radiotherapy has been evaluated. In one study in which vinblastine and cisplatin chemotherapy plus radiation therapy was given, survival rates in years 1 to 7 were 54%, 26%, 24%, 19%, 17%, 13%, and 13%, respectively, in chemotherapy- and radiation-treated patients compared with 40%, 13%, 10%, 7%, 6%, and 6% for patients treated with radiation alone.[23,24] The benefit of chemotherapy before radiation treatment has been confirmed by other studies as well. Another pivotal trial demonstrated that the concomitant treatment of inoperable NSCLC with cisplatin and radiation leads to improved local control of tumor as well as survival benefit.[25] Thus, for good performance status patients with minimal weight loss, the combination of chemotherapy with radiation therapy should be strongly considered. What remains to be determined are the optimal chemotherapy agents used, as well as how they should be combined with radiation therapy.

Stage IV Metastatic Disease

Unlike small cell lung cancer, chemotherapy in advanced (stage IV) non-small cell lung cancer has shown marginal benefit. With the introduction of platinum-based chemotherapy, a modest survival benefit has been seen in patients. However, these benefits are usually brief and have been accompanied by a relatively high incidence of treatment-related toxicity. Best supportive care over chemotherapy remains a frequent choice, although there have been several studies that have shown a statistically significant survival advantage for combination chemotherapy over best supportive care.[26,27] Much of the debate relates to the lack of quality of life studies in this setting to assess whether the modest improvement in survival is associated with improved quality of life as well.

Recent studies have actually suggested that elderly patients with NSCLC may have a better prognosis with treatment. Albain et al. analyzed 2531 patients with advanced-stage (IIIB/IV) NSCLC in the Southwest Oncology Group from 1974 to 1988 to assess the interactions of host- or tumor-related prognostic factors in therapy to determine whether each independently predicts outcome and define prognostic subsets with different survival potentials.[28] It was found that a good performance status, female sex, and age greater than 70 years were significant independent predictors. Giovanazzi-Bannon et al., in an analysis from the Illinois Cancer Center, determined that there were no major differences between patients 65 years of age or more and patients less than 65 years of age when treated on phase II clinical trials.[29] It was concluded that elderly patients should not be denied access to cancer clinical trials because of age alone. In this review, the older patients received slightly more courses of therapy with no significant difference between the two groups for treatment interruptions, days of delay, or number of dose reductions. When best response to therapy was analyzed, the elderly patients had more stable disease and less progressive disease than the younger patients. Older patients experienced only slightly more grade III or greater hematologic toxicities with no significant differences in other severe toxicities.

These results support the concept that at least some elderly patients can receive chemotherapy with similar benefit and side effects, if carefully selected based on good performance status and lack of comorbid disease, which are eligibility-applied to most clinical trials. However, application of these regimens to more dependent elderly populations requires further study, and very intensive regimens must be used with caution even in the well elderly. The importance of performance status as a predictor for the ability to tolerate polychemotherapy was most recently demonstrated by the Eastern Cooperative Oncology Group. Patients with performance status two suffered more toxicity and had inferior survival compared with patients with better performance status.[30]

More recently, the choice of chemotherapy agents useful for the treatment of non-small cell lung cancer has increased; these include the cisplatin analogue carboplatin, the taxanes paclitaxel and docetaxel, the vinca alkaloid vinorelbine, the camphothecin irinotecan, and gemcitabine. In addition to being more effective compared with prior drugs, these compounds are also better tolerated and more easily delivered to patients. Furthermore, formal testing of these agents in elderly patients has now been undertaken.

The Elderly Lung Cancer Vinorelbine Italian Study Group (ELVIS) investigators designed and executed a study to compare best supportive care in elderly patients with good performance status to single-agent chemotherapy with vinorelbine.[31] Patients aged 70 years or older who had good performance status (defined as spending no more than 50% of the waking day in bed) were enrolled in the study. All patients had biopsy-proven non-small cell lung carcinoma, either stage IV or stage IIIB (malignant pleural effusions or metastatic disease to the supraclavicular lymph nodes). Treatment consisted of either best supportive care or vinorelbine $30\,mg/m^2$ given on days 1 and 8. The chemotherapy was repeated every 3 weeks for a maximum of six cycles. Supportive care treatments were at the discretion of the physicians, and radiotherapy was allowed. No crossover was allowed. The major endpoints of the study included toxicity and response evaluations, a quality of life assessment, and overall survival. Baseline characteristics of the patients were well balanced in both arms. The median age was 74 years, with the majority of patients being men and having stage IV disease. Patients treated with vinorelbine demonstrated a clear survival benefit, with median survival increasing from 21 to 28 weeks; 1-year survival was extended from 14% in the best supportive care arm to 32% in the arm of patients receiving chemotherapy with vinorelbine. The overall response rate (complete and partial responses) was 19.7%. Results of the quality of life assessments were complicated by missing data (resulting from patient death and noncompliance) but nonetheless demonstrated a benefit of chemotherapy. Notable findings include benefits of vinorelbine in dyspnea, pain, and pain medicine consumption. Negative effects of chemotherapy included constipation, nausea and vomiting, hair loss, and peripheral neuropathy. However, only five patients discontinued therapy because of serious side effects, four due to severe constipation and one due to atrial arrhythmia.

This trial is of great importance as it is the first randomized trial of chemotherapy versus best supportive care in the elderly patient population. The results of this trial, as well as others, will make it difficult if not impossible for future trials to include a best supportive care arm. It is important to point out that the survival benefit of chemotherapy was not at the expense of high levels of toxicity and poor quality of life. The safety of this regimen is further suggested by a low level of hematologic toxicities and no treatment-related episodes of neutropenic fever or sepsis.

Vinorelbine has been approved by the Food and Drug Administration (FDA) for treatment of patients with non–small cell lung cancer and was the first of the "modern" chemotherapy drugs approved for lung cancer in the United States in more than 20 years. The combination of vinorelbine with cisplatin has been shown to be superior to single-agent vinorelbine, with single-agent vinorelbine chemotherapy producing a 1-year survival of 30% and a median survival of 31 weeks, whereas the combination led to a 35% 1-year survival rate with median survival time increasing to 40 weeks.[32]

The effect and tolerability of monotherapy with gemcitabine has recently been examined in a series of patients over the age of 70 years who had good performance status.[33] Patients received gemcitabine 1000 mg/m^2 given every week for 3 weeks, followed by a 1-week rest period; the cycle was then repeated every 4 weeks for a maximum of six cycles. Dose reductions and delays were made for hematologic toxicities. Forty-six patients were treated on the study, with the majority of patients being men with stage IV disease. The overall response rate including partial and complete responses was 22.2%. Ten patients who had symptoms demonstrated an improvement in their performance status on therapy. No WHO grade IV toxicities were demonstrated, there were no episodes of neutropenic fever, and no patients died due to complications of therapy. Two patients required discontinuation of therapy due to skin rash. Although this study does not demonstrate a meaningful benefit of single-agent gemcitabine on overall survival, it does suggest that the drug has activity, can improve the performance status of some patients receiving therapy, and has minimal toxicity. Furthermore, gemcitabine may be able to replace cisplatin-based chemotherapy in the elderly, given results of recent trials that demonstrate similar efficacy and better toxicity than the older standard regimen of cisplatin and etoposide.

Preliminary evidence also suggests that paclitaxel given weekly to elderly patients has efficacy and is well tolerated. One study treated patients over 70 years of age with paclitaxel and found a near 30% response rate coupled with symptom relief and minimal or absent side effects.[34] Future studies will be needed to determine if a survival benefit exists similar to that seen in the ELVIS trial.

It is hoped that these new agents will lead to more substantial gains in both quality of life and survival for patients with advanced NSCLC.

Treatment of Small Cell Lung Cancer

Surgery is rarely thought to be an option in small cell lung cancer. However, approximately 3% of small cell lung cancer patients present with a solitary peripheral nodule. Surgical resection of the tumor in these patients has been associated with a 5-year survival rate greater than 30%. In those patients presenting with a stage I small cell lung cancer, surgery should be considered as primary treatment with adjuvant chemotherapy, with or without radiation therapy postresection. Chemotherapy is the most important component of small cell lung cancer treatment because of the sensitivity of small cell lung cancer to chemotherapy and the systemic nature of the disease. Patients with limited-stage disease treated with combination chemotherapy have a median survival of approximately 14 to 15 months and 9 months for extensive-stage disease. There is a 2-year disease-free survival of approximately 13% in patients with limited-stage disease, with only 2% long-term survival in patients with extensive-stage disease. The development of tumor resistance to chemotherapy appears to be a major factor contributing to relapse. Small cell lung cancer cells are quite sensitive to radiation therapy, and therefore radiotherapy is best used early in treatment in combination with chemotherapy in patients with limited-stage disease and good performance status, with the potential to increase the curability of this disease.[11] In the elderly, however, the benefits of combined modality therapy must be balanced against the increased toxicities, particularly myelosuppression, pulmonary toxicity, fatigue, and anorexia. Thus, supportive care is critical in the success of combined modality approaches in this population.

The management of limited-stage small cell lung cancer continues to consist of a treatment plan combining chemotherapy and radiation therapy. A meta-analysis of trials comparing chemotherapy with chemotherapy plus radiotherapy demonstrated a small, albeit significant, improvement in overall survival in patients who received a combined approach. However, questions still remain on the best way to combine chemotherapy with radiotherapy, especially given the increased toxicity with the combination. One recent study has suggested that twice-daily radiotherapy improved survival in patients with limited-stage small cell lung cancer.[35] Patients with limited-stage small cell lung cancer were treated with four cycles of cisplatin and etoposide chemotherapy given every 21 days. Patients were randomized to receive a standard dose of 45 Gy of concurrent radiation given either twice daily over a 3-week period or once daily over a 5-week period. The median age of the patient population was 62 years, with patients aged over 65 years comprising 31% and 40% of the two arms. At 5 years, 26% of patients receiving twice-daily radiotherapy were alive compared with 16% of patients receiving once-daily radiotherapy. The improvement in survival was at the expense of increased esophageal toxicity in the twice-daily treated group, but no differences in hospitalization or esophageal perforation, and no strictures, were noted. Whether the results of this trial can be generalized to the geriatric population remains to be determined.

One controversial area in the management of small cell lung carcinoma concerns the use of prophylactic cranial irradiation (PCI) for patients with complete responses to chemotherapy. Advances in radiotherapy techniques have reduced the rate of recurrent disease in the chest; however, these patients continue to be at high risk for the development of systemic metastasis, mainly to liver, bone, adrenal glands, and brain. At diagnosis, only 10% to 20% of patients have brain metastasis, while at 2 years postdiagnosis nearly 50% of patients developed brain metastasis. Because of the blood–brain barrier inhibiting chemotherapy effects, the brain has been believed to be a sanctuary site for subclinical metastasis. Investigators over the years have thought that giving radiotherapy to the whole brain may prevent the development of brain metastasis and positively impact on quality of life and overall survival. Randomized trials have demonstrated a clear reduction in the development of brain metastasis; however, an impact on survival was unclear given the low numbers of patients randomized. Coupled with this enthusiasm, however, came the worry about a deleterious effect on neuropsychologic functioning. Subsequently, studies have demonstrated that a high proportion of patients with limited-stage SCLC had preexisting cognitive dysfunction before receiving PCI, which might have influenced previous studies.[36,37] To get a better idea of whether PCI can impact patient survival, a meta-analysis was performed on individual data from studies that randomized patients demonstrating a complete response to chemoradiotherapy, to PCI, or to no PCI.[38] PCI decreased the cumulative incidence of brain metastasis by nearly 50%, which translated to a 5% increase in the rate of survival at 3 years. The median age of patients in this trial was 59 years, with a range up to 80 years. Again, whether this trial can be generalized to elderly patients remains in question. Subgroup analysis, despite its known limitations, did not demonstrate any difference in benefit as a function of age.

Controversy continues over the benefit of treating elderly patients with chemotherapy, given commonly held views that they are less tolerant compared with younger patients. Elderly patients may be at increased risk of myelosuppression because of less marrow cellularity, as well as impaired renal and hepatic function that alters drug metabolism and excretion. Comorbid disease, often the result of years of smoking, also limits the enthusiasm of oncologists to treat elderly patients. Indeed, in elderly small cell lung carcinoma patients, nearly three-quarters had comorbid disease, including coronary artery disease, chronic obstructive pulmonary disease, and second malignancies. Biases against the treatment of small cell lung cancer in the elderly may not be justified. For example, Shepherd et al. found that elderly patients can tolerate chemotherapy and derive a survival benefit.[39] The delivery of chemotherapy was impaired, however, with most patients requiring dose reductions, and less than half of the patients completed six cycles of chemotherapy. These and other studies that have demonstrated similar response rates and overall survival in young and old SCLC patients have made the oncology community reevaluate its view of treating elderly patients with SCLC. Even single-agent chemotherapy, such as with etoposide, can result in high response rates and improvements in survival. Finally, the addition of colony-stimulating factors such as G-CSF and erythropoietin may allow for more aggressive treatment of these patients. We believe that all elderly patients with small cell lung cancer should receive oncology consultation and those that are medically fit and interested in the palliation and survival benefits offered by chemotherapy should receive treatment.

Supportive Care

Just as elderly patients are often not treated aggressively for lung cancer, the associated side effects of their diseases or treatment may not sufficiently be addressed. Elderly patients with cancer require substantial supportive care. The goal of all supportive therapy should be to maximize the ability of the patient to tolerate both the disease and its treatment.[40] (Cancer pain is addressed in Chapter 28; also see other Palliative Care chapters in Part IV.)

Patients may present to their physician complaining of unexplained weight loss and loss of appetite and may subsequently be diagnosed with cancer. Cancer cachexia is common in patients with advanced metastatic disease but may also occur in patients with localized disease. Anorexia with abnormalities in taste perception, such as intolerance for sweets, sour, or salty flavors, as well as an aversion for meats, may exist before initiation of treatment and subsequently be exacerbated by the initiation of chemotherapy or radiation therapy.[41] Substantial weight loss, which is progressive, and a malnourished state often prevent a patient from being treated. Treatment should include counseling of the patient and family members as to why the symptoms are present, consultation with a dietician to discuss meal planning and preparation, and often treatment with medications such as megestrol acetate or prednisone that may stimulate the appetite.

Improvements in antiemetics with the use of serotonin antagonists, as well as the use of colony-stimulating factors to ameliorate neutropenia and its complications when appropriate, have had a major impact on the supportive care of the cancer patient receiving chemotherapy. These agents may particularly be useful in the elderly and assist the physician in the decision to use chemotherapy in the elderly lung cancer patient. Recently, the benefit of recombinant erythropoietin on quality of life was described in patients receiving chemotherapy for nonmyeloid malignancies.[42] In this study, patients were treated with erythropoetin-alpha 10,000 units three times weekly, which could be increased to 20,000 units three times weekly depending on the hematologic response. This therapy was associated with improvements in quality of life scores that were well correlated with levels of hemoglobin. A large number of patients had cancer of the lung and were being treated with modern chemotherapy regimens, including carboplatin/paclitaxel, carboplatin/etoposide, paclitaxel, and cisplatin/etoposide. The mean increase in hemoglobin was approximately 2 g/dL with nearly two-thirds of patients responding to erythropoetin-alpha. Tumor type, tumor response to chemotherapy, performance status, chemotherapy regimen, baseline hemoglobin, and baseline erythropoietin levels were not found to correlate with quality of life responses. Although not specifically targeting the elderly population, nonetheless the median age of lung cancer patients was 65 years.

Of increasing importance in patients with lung cancer is the coexistence of depression, which can serve as a predictor of quality of life. Recently, the rates of depression were reported in patients with both small and non–small cell lung cancer.[43] Depression existed in one-third of patients before the initiation of treatment and persisted in more than 50% of patients. Multivariate analysis revealed that functional impairment was the most important risk factor for the development of depression, along with physical symptom burden and fatigue. Age was not a risk factor for the development of depression; rather, there was a nonsignificant trend toward lower rates of depression in older patients.

Conclusions

The epidemic of lung cancer continues in the United States, and the elderly remain the major target. Despite a decline in smoking by men in the United States, antismoking campaigns have not been successful in preventing teenage smoking or in decreasing the percent of women who smoke, so the epidemic will continue.

Despite the high mortality of lung cancer, however, long-term survival is now possible, not only for surgically resected patients but also for some patients with stage III non–small cell lung cancer or limited-stage small cell lung cancer. Even in advanced disease, significant improvement have been made by the use of chemotherapy and supportive care in appropriate patients. Elderly patients with lung cancer deserve careful evaluation of treatment options in a multidisciplinary setting.

References

1. Ginsberg RJ, Vokes EE, Rosenzweig K. Cancer of the lung. In: Devita VT, Hellman S, Rosenberg SA, eds. *Cancer Principles and Practice of Oncology, 6th Ed.* Philadelphia: Lippincott Williams & Wilkins; 2001:925–983.
2. Yancik R, Reis LA. Cancer in older persons—magnitude of the problem. How do we apply what we know? *Cancer.* 1994; 74(suppl 1):1995–2003.
3. Doll R, Hill AB. Lung cancer and other causes of death related to smoking: a second report on the mortality of British doctors. *Br Med J.* 1956;2:1071–1081.
4. Pathak DR, Samet JM, Humble CG, et al. Determinants of lung cancer risk in cigarette smokers in New Mexico. *JNCI.* 1994;76:597–604.
5. Crawford J, O'Rourke MA, Cohen HJ. Age factors in the management of lung cancer. In: Yancik R, Yates JW, eds. *Cancer in the Elderly.* New York: Springer; 1989:177–203.
6. Orleans TC, Jepson C, Resch N, et al. Quitting motives and barriers among older smokers; the 1987 Adult Use of Tobacco Survey revisited. *Cancer (Suppl).* 1994;74:2055–2061.
7. Halpern M, Gillespie B, Warner K. Patters of absolute risk of lung cancer: mortality in former smokers. *JNCI.* 1993; 85:457–464.
8. Rimer BK, Orleans TC. Tailoring smoking cessation for older adults. *Cancer (Suppl).* 1994;74:2051–2054.
9. DeMaria LC, Cohen HJ. Characteristics of lung cancer in the elderly patients. *J Gerontol.* 1987;42:540–545.
10. O'Rourke MA, Feussner JR, Ferge P, et al. Age trends of lung cancer at diagnosis. *JAMA.* 1987;258:921–926.
11. Rimer BK, Heman D, Crawford J, et al. Lung cancer in North Carolina. *NC Med J.* 1993;54:334–341.
12. Henschke C, McCauley D, Yankelevitz D, et al. Early Lung Cancer Action Project: overall design and findings from baseline screening. *Lancet.* 1999;354:99–105.
13. Vaporciyan AA, Nesbitt JC, Lee JS, et al. Cancer of the Lung. In: Bast RC, Kufe DW, Pollock RE, Weichselbaum RR, Holland JF, Frie E, eds. Cancer Medicine, 5th ed. Ontario: BC Decker, Inc. 2000:1227–1292.
14. Ershler EB, Socinski MA, Greene CJ. Bronchogenic cancer, metastases and aging. *J Am Geriatr Soc.* 1994;31:673–676.
15. Luke WP, Pearson FG, Todd TFJ, et al. Prospective evaluation of medianstinoscopy for assessment of carcinoma of the lung. *J Thorac Cardiovasc Surg.* 1986;91:53–56.
16. McKenna RJ. Clinical aspects cancer in the elderly. Treatment decisions, treatment choices, and follow up. *Cancer.* 1994;74:2107–2117.
17. Walsh SJ, Begg CB, Carbone PP. Cancer chemotherapy in the elderly. *Semin Oncol.* 1989;16:66–75.
18. Massard G, Moog R, Wihlm JM, et al. Bronchogenic cancer in the elderly: operative risk and long-term prognosis. *Thorac Cardiovasc Surg.* 1996;44:40–45.
19. PORT Meta-analysis Trialists Group. Postoperative radiotherapy in non-small cell lung cancer: systemic review and meta-analysis of individual patient data from nine randomized controlled trials. *Lancet.* 1998;352:257–263.
20. Rosell R, Gomez-Codina J, Cmaps C, et al. A randomized trial comparing preoperative chemotherapy plus surgery with surgery alone in patients with non-small cell lung cancer. *N Engl J Med.* 1994;330:153–158.
21. Roth J, Rossella F, Komaki R, et al. A randomized trial comparing perioperative chemotherapy and surgery with surgery alone in resectable non-small cell lung cancer. *JNCI.* 1994;86:673–680.
22. Crocker I, Prosnitz L. Radiation therapy of the elderly. In: *Clinics in Geriatric Medicine, vol III.* Philadelphia: Saunders; 1987:473–478.
23. Dillman RO, Seagren SL, Propert KJ, et al. A randomized trial of induction chemotherapy plus high dose radiation versus radiation alone in stage III non small cell lung cancer. *N Engl J Med.* 1990;323:989–990.

24. Dillman R, Herndon J, Seagren S, Eaton W, Green M. Improved survival in Stage III non-small cell lung cancer: seven-year follow-up of Cancer and Leukemia Group B (CALGB) 8433 Trial. *JNCI.* 1996;88:1210–1215.

25. Schaake-Koning C, van den Bogert W, Dalesio O, et al. Effects of concomitant cisplatin and radiotherapy on inoperable non-small cell lung cancer. *N Engl J Med.* 1992; 326:524–530.

26. Souquet PJ, Chauvin F, Boissel R, et al. Polychemotherapy in advanced non–small cell lung cancer: a metaanalysis. *Lancet.* 1993;342:19–21.

27. Grilli R, Oxman A, Julian JJ. Chemotherapy for advanced non–small cell lung cancer: how much benefit is enough? *J Clin Oncol.* 1993;11:1966–1972.

28. Albain KS, Crowley JJ, LeBlanc M, et al. Survival determinants in extensive stage non–small cell lung cancer: The Southwest Oncology Group experience. *J Clin Oncol.* 1991; 9:1618–1626.

29. Giovanazzi-Bannon S, Rademake A, Lai G, et al. Treatment tolerance of elderly cancer patients entered onto Phase II clinical trials: an Illinois cancer center study. *J Clin Oncol.* 1994;12:2447–2452.

30. Johnson DH, Zhu J, Schiller J, et al. E1494: a randomized phase III trial in metastatic non-small cell lung cancer (NSCLC)—outcome of performance status 2 patients: an Eastern Cooperative Group Trial (ECOG). *Proceedings American Society of Clinical Oncology.* 1999;18:461a [abstract 1779].

31. The Elderly Lung Cancer Vinorelbine Italian Study Group. Effects of vinorelbine on quality of life and survival of elderly patients with advanced non-small cell lung cancer. *JNCI.* 1999;91:66–72.

32. LeChevalier T, Brisgand D, Douillard J-Y, et al. Randomized study of vinorelbine and cisplatin alone in advanced non-small cell lung cancer: results of a European multicenter trial including 612 patients. *J Clin Oncol.* 1994;12:360–367.

33. Shepherd FA, Abratt RP, Anderson H, et al. Gemcitabine in the treatment of elderly patients with advanced non-small cell lung cancer. *Semin Oncol.* 1997;24(2):S7–S50.

34. Fidias P, Supko J, Martins R, et al. A phase II clinical and pharmacokinetic study of weekly paclitaxel in elderly patients with non-small cell lung cancer. *Lung Cancer.* 2000;29(1):57 [abstract 184].

35. Turrisi A, Kim K, Blum R, et al. Twice-daily compared with once-daily thoracic radiotherapy in limited small-cell lung cancer treated concurrently with cisplatin and etoposide. *N Engl J Med.* 1999;340:265–271.

36. Komaki R, Meyers C, Shin D, et al. Evaluation of cognitive function in patients with limited small cell lung cancer prior to and shortly following prophylactic cranial irradiation. *Int J Radiat Oncol Biol Phys.* 1995;33:179–182.

37. Lishner M, Feld R, Payne D, et al. Late neurological complications after prophylactic cranial irradiation in patients with small-cell lung cancer: the Toronto Experience. *J Clin Oncol.* 1990;8:215–221.

38. Auperin A, Arriagada R, Pignon J, et al. Prophylactic cranial irradiation for patients with small-cell lung cancer in complete remission. *N Engl J Med.* 1999;314:476–484.

39. Shepherd FA, Amdemicheal E, Evans WK. Treatment of small cell lung cancer in the elderly. *J Am Geriatr Soc.* 1994; 42:64–70.

40. Foley KM. Supportive care and the quality of life in the cancer patient. In: Devita VT, Hellman S, Rosenberg SA, eds. *Cancer Principles and Practice of Oncology, 4th Ed.* Philadelphia: Lippincott; 1993:2417–2448.

41. Daly JM, Torosian MH. Nutritional support. In: Devita VT, Hellman S, Rosenberg SA, eds. *Cancer Principles and Practice of Oncology, 4th Ed.* Philadelphia: Lippincott;1993: 2480–2501.

42. Demetri G, Kris M, Wade J, Degos L, Cella D, for the Procrit Study Group. Quality-of-life benefit in chemotherapy patients treated with Epoetin Alfa is independent of disease response or tumor type: results from a prospective community oncology study. *J Clin Oncol.* 1998;16: 3412–3425.

43. Hopwood P, Stephens RJ, Fletche I, Lee A. The impact of depression on quality of life and survival in patients with inoperable lung cancer. *Lung Cancer.* 2000;29(1):272 [abstract 931].

36
Prostate Cancer

Khalid Matin and Donald L. Trump

Prostate cancer is second only to lung cancer as a cause of cancer mortality in men; in 2000, 31,900 deaths were estimated to occur.[1] Among males, no cancer is more prevalent than prostate cancer. Cancer is second only to heart disease as a cause of death in adults; prostate cancer accounts for 20% of the cancer deaths in men over the age of 75. One of every eight men in the 60- to 79-year-old age group will be diagnosed with prostate cancer; by comparison, 1 in 15 women of the same age will be diagnosed with breast cancer. Although many older men who are found to have prostate cancer do not die of prostate cancer, many require treatment of symptoms such as pain, bleeding, and urinary obstruction. Prostate cancer is a major cause of mortality, morbidity, and expenditure of health care resources in older men.

The single greatest risk factor for the development of prostate cancer is age.[2] As demonstrated in Figure 36.1, the incidence of prostate cancer increases exponentially with age. The underlying biologic cause of this increased incidence is not clear. As the population of the United States ages, the incidence of prostate cancer will likely continue to increase.[3]

Other risk factors for the development of prostate cancer include family history and race. Men with a first-degree relative (father or brother) with prostate cancer have a twofold increase in the risk of developing the disease, and the risk increases with the number of involved relatives.[4,5] The risk of prostate cancer is also increased in men with a first-degree female relative with breast or ovarian carcinoma.[6,7] This latter observation suggests a link between these hormone-related carcinomas. This association is an area of active investigation, and attention is currently focused on the long arm of chromosome 17, also the reported site of the BRCA1 gene. Linkage analysis suggests that alterations at this locus may be associated with prostate, ovarian, and breast cancer in some families.[8]

Considerable work has been done to define a gene or genes associated with prostate cancer. At the broad struc-

tural level the clues are limited. Studies have shown almost 77% of specimens to have a normal karyotype.[9–11] Careful family and detailed linkage studies indicate that familial aggregation of this disease occur in one-quarter of men (two first-degree relatives); however, linkage studies revealing a susceptibility, some inherited with a Mendelian pattern, seem only to account for 9% of hereditary prostate cancer.[12,13] Genes located on two regions of chromosome 1q, the HPC 1, have been implicated as predisposing to the development to prostate cancer.[14] There is also a report of a second susceptibility gene, Xq (27–28), seen mainly in families of North American and Scandinavian origin.[15] Although other loci including *myc* and *erb* B2/*neu* proto-oncogenes have been implicated because structural abnormalities or abnormal expression sometimes are seen, data supporting a causative or primary genetic role for these loci are lacking. Alterations in loci on chromosomes 8, 10, and 16 have also been identified as potential markers for the development of prostate cancer.[16,17]

The racial distribution of prostate cancer also offers the potential for exploring causal relationships. Autopsy studies reveal that blacks, whites, and Asians have essentially the same prevalence of "clinically silent" or latent prostatic carcinoma.[18] Blacks, however, have a higher rate of clinically significant prostate cancer, as compared with whites and Asians.[19] There is evidence that African and Asian immigrants to the United States have increasing risk in successive generations. The risk gradually approaches that seen in African-Americans and whites born in the United States.[20–22] This finding suggests that environmental factors may play a role in the progression from latent to clinically significant prostate cancer. Several hypotheses for these observations, including quantity and quality of dietary fat intake, vitamin A, and vitamin D metabolism have been suggested.[23–25] Androgens are *clearly* important in prostate cancer. Men who are hypogonadal rarely, if ever, develop prostate cancer. There are data indicating that polymorphisms in

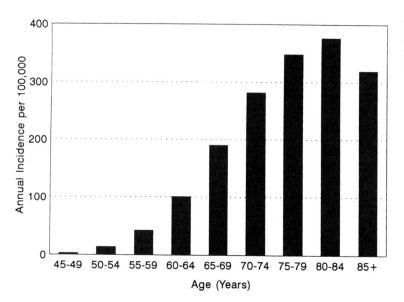

FIGURE 36.1. Annual incidence of prostate cancer in the United States. (Data from the Surveillance, Epidemiology, and End Results [SEER] Program Staff.[2])

both androgen receptor structure as well as the androgen-metabolizing enzyme, 5-alpha reductase, confer increased risk of prostate cancer. Certain polymorphisms in these moieties can enhance androgen effects on target cells, and this may contribute to enhanced prostate cancer risk.[26,27]

Although age is a major risk factor for developing prostate cancer, the effect of age on the course of the disease is less clear. Many clinicians have argued that the disease is more indolent in older patients and requires no active therapy. This perception is likely based on the observation that older patients often die of diseases other than prostate cancer. This perception results in less aggressive diagnostic and therapeutic approaches in older patients.[28] Data documenting the effect of age on the course of prostate cancer are lacking. Studies that have been carried out provide conflicting data.[28–32] Multivariate analysis of patients enrolled in a large Scandinavian trial showed that older patients with metastatic disease had a longer time to progression and cause-specific survival.[33] Similar findings were reported for overall survival of patients entered in the National Prostate Cancer Project (NPCP) chemotherapy trials.[34] These large studies suggest that if age has any effect, it is a positive one. Decisions about therapy should be based primarily on clearly defined prognostic factors, such as performance status, tumor grade, and extent of disease. Data do suggest that prostate cancers in older men may progress more slowly than in younger men. A critical factor to be taken into consideration in evaluating therapy options is the life expectancy of the patient.

Screening for Prostate Cancer

The basic principles of screening for disease in an elderly population are covered in Chapter 17, Prevention.

However, there are several issues concerning prostate cancer that warrant special mention. Two of the fundamental aspects of a successful screening strategy are the identification of significant cases and the delivery of effective therapy.[35] Despite the multiple studies in this area, current diagnosis and therapy of prostate cancer remains controversial in these two aspects. Although measurement of the serum level of prostate-specific antigen (PSA) provides an early indicator of the presence of prostatic disease, this may not necessarily be due to prostate cancer. PSA levels may reflect abnormalities in the prostate that are benign, for example, hypertrophy, infection, or infarction. Until recently, it was unclear whether men who are diagnosed with prostatic malignancy using a PSA-based strategy have clinically significant disease that will result in morbidity and mortality. Data from the Physician's Health Study indicate that an elevated PSA level on a single blood draw is predictive of clinically significant prostate cancer with a low false-positive rate.[36] This finding argues strongly that PSA-based screening detects clinically important cancers.

A more difficult problem is that clear proof that the definitive therapies applied to the treatment of prostate cancer improve quality of life or overall survival is lacking. Identifying a patient with prostate cancer may lead to significant diagnostic and therapeutic morbidity and cost for the patient and family because treatment decisions often seem inevitable once the diagnosis is made. Thus, before obtaining a screening serum PSA level, a frank and open discussion about the use of the information and the consequences of the various options is required. For a man with a life expectancy of less than 10 years, even the most ardent therapist is hard pressed to suggest an advantage to diagnosing and subsequently treating prostate cancer.

Diagnosis of Prostate Cancer

Prostate cancer has a long and highly variable natural history. Patients may present with any of several manifestations of the disease, which range from the patient presenting with symptoms of bladder outlet obstruction and a normal PSA in whom cancer is discovered as an incidental finding at transurethral resection of the prostate, to the patient who presents with debilitating bone pain secondary to metastatic disease. In all cases, the diagnosis of prostate cancer should be established by biopsy. A typical scenario in current practice is the patient who presents with an elevated PSA, with or without a palpable abnormality on digital rectal examination. If treatment would be pursued, these patients usually undergo transrectal ultrasound-guided biopsy of the prostate. If treatment is considered, the importance of this biopsy cannot be overstated, particularly because there are benign conditions that can result in a mild to moderate elevation in the serum PSA.[37] Furthermore, histologic examination of the biopsy in cases of malignancy yields prognostic information that can have a significant impact on future management. Once the diagnosis of prostate cancer has been established, a limited staging evaluation, typically consisting of a bone scan and routine laboratory studies, is often performed. There are data indicating that a bone scan is unnecessary for asymptomatic patients with PSA less than 20 ng/mL.[38] More intensive and invasive staging procedures, such as computed tomography or magnetic resonance imaging, are reserved for special situations and do not impact routinely on clinical decisions.

The clinical stage of prostate cancer is based on extent of disease determined by these data. Histologic description of the biopsy specimen also offers important prognostic information. Although relatively simple staging descriptions have been used for years,[39,40] the most widely accepted system is that based on the tumor-node-metastasis (TNM) assessment.[41] The TNM system takes into account the patients whose disease is detected by PSA alone without palpable abnormality, reflecting the advances in diagnosis over the past few years (Table 36.1).

Another important prognostic factor is the histologic description of the tumor. This aspect is particularly important in early-stage lesions. The information derived from the histologic evaluation includes the extent of involvement of the resected specimen and the extent of differentiation of the tumor. This latter characteristic is best described in terms of the Gleason grade.[42] The Gleason grade ranges from 2 to 10 and is derived by the pathologist. Gleason scores (1 through 5) are assigned to the *two* most common histologic patterns seen in the prostate specimen. A well-differentiated tumor is scored as 1 or 2, while a poorly differentiated tumor receives

TABLE 36.1. Comparison of staging systems.

AUA	Entity	TNM
A	Diagnosed incidentally at transurethral resection	T1
A1	≤5% Of tissue involved	T1a
A2	>5% Of tissue involved	T1b
	Diagnosed by needle biopsy, elevated PSA only	T1c
B	Palpable nodule	T2
B1	≤Half of a lobe	T2a
B1	>Half lobe, not both	T2b
B2	Both lobes	T2c
C	Tumor penetrates capsule	T3
	Unilateral	T3a
	Bilateral	T3b
	Seminal vesicle invasion	T3c
	Tumor fixed or invades adjacent structures	T4
	Bladder neck, sphincter, rectum	T4a
	Levator muscles or fixed to pelvic sidewall	T4b
D1	Regional nodes (true pelvis)	N
	One node ≤ 2 cm	N1
	One node > 2 ≤ 5, multiple nodes	N2
	Any node > 5 cm	N3
D2	Metastases	M1
	Nonregional nodes	M1a
	Bone	M1b
	Other	M1c

AUA, American Urologic Assoiation; TNM, tumor-node-metastasis.

a 4 or 5 score. These two scores are added together and expressed as a Gleason score; for example, $4 + 3 = 7$. This grade is useful in predicting the biologic aggressiveness of a tumor and correlates with prognosis and extent of disease.[43–45]

Management of the Patient with Prostate Cancer

Once a histologic diagnosis and clinical stage have been established, patients and their physicians face several major decisions. These decisions are complicated by the variable natural history of this disease and the lack of randomized prospective trials to guide therapeutic decisions. Particularly in the older patient, the primary care physician can and should play a crucial role in this decision making because the past medical history and current condition of the patient will have a significant impact on the options to be considered. The decisions to be made differ widely based on the extent of the disease. In general, patients can be grouped into three categories: (1) those with organ-confined disease; (2) those with regionally advanced disease; and (3) those with metastatic disease.

Organ-Confined Disease

This category is composed of patients with localized prostate cancer (T_{1-2c}, N_0, M_0). There is controversy about the management of patients in this broad category. These patients range from those with well-differentiated, incidentally detected tumors involving less than 5% of the gland (T_{1a}), to those with palpable tumor diffusely involving both lobes (T_{2c}). These tumors have widely variable natural histories, but the unifying characteristic is that they are potentially curable by definitive therapy. Whether such therapy has an impact on overall survival, particularly for the population of men with T_{1a} or T_{1b} disease, is not known. Thus, there is debate as to how these patients should be managed. This debate is particularly relevant in an elderly population where life expectancy and tolerance of morbidity have considerable impact on treatment decisions.

Consideration of the natural history of prostate cancer is crucial. The overall survival for patients with organ-confined disease who are not treated is numbered in terms of several years.[46] The two definitive therapeutic modalities that have been utilized to treat this disease are radical prostatectomy and irradiation. There are several techniques for administering irradiation: external beam irradiation administered via an increasing number of techniques that allow increase in dose intensity of irradiation [three-dimensional (3-D), conformal field treatment planning, intensity-modulated radiation therapy (IMRT), brachytherapy using intra prostatic implantation of 1^{125} or palladium-impregnated seeds or high-dose-rate, afterloading techniques]. It is beyond the scope of this chapter to discuss the variety of irradiation techniques. The greatest experience and longest follow-up data for irradiation are derived from a series of patients treated by external beam irradiation.

After surgical treatment for T_1 and T_2 prostate cancer, the cancer-specific survival rate is 90% to 94% at 10 years and 82% to 90% at 15 years.[47–49] If the PSA level is considered as an indicator of disease progression, the reported progression rate for the foregoing group is 17% to 31% at 5 years and 23% to 53% at 10 years.[50,51] Treatment of localized prostate cancer with irradiation yields similar results. In a study of 313 patients with T_1 disease by Hanks et al.[52] with external beam radiation alone, survival was 77% at 5 years and 51% at 10 years (comparing well with 81% and 62% survival for age-matched normal males). Another study[53] of 500 men mostly with T_1 and T_2 disease treated with irradiation revealed 80% survival at 5 years with 72% surviving without clinical evidence of any disease. The rate went down to 51% when the PSA was taken into account as an indicator of recurrence. (*NB*: The surgery data represent cancer-specific mortality and the radiation data overall mortality.) It is critical to realize, when examining outcomes of irradiation and prostatectomy, that surgical series usually include younger men and report results by pathologic stage. By contrast, irradiation series generally are composed of older men and results are reported as the clinical stage, which notoriously underestimates the local and regional extent of tumor.

Improved results have been obtained in localized prostate cancer using a combination of external beam radiation and goserelin [a gonadotropin-releasing hormone agonist (GnRHa)].[54] Bolla and colleagues[54] studied 415 patients with T_1–T_4 prostate cancer, randomly assigned to irradiation versus radiation and goserelin. The survival in the combined therapy arm was 79% at 5 years versus 62% in the radiation-only group ($p < 0.001$). Eighty-five percent of the surviving patients were free of disease at 5 years. When comparing these data with those for surgery, it should be noted that the Bolla study included patients with T_3 and T_4 prostate cancer, which are not included in the surgery data. The Radiation Therapy Oncology Group (RTOG) has several such ongoing trials in which short-term or long-term therapy with GnRHa + antiandrogen + irradiation is being studied with respect to local control and time to progression in comparison to irradiation alone.

Prostatectomy and irradiation have complications that may have a significant impact on quality of life.[55] The major complications of these approaches are listed in Table 36.2. Acute radiation proctitis and cystitis are seen often in men receiving external beam radiotherapy; infrequently, chronic cystitis or proctitis may result. Following radical prostatectomy, impotence and incontinence are the complications with the most significant impact on quality of life. In addition, this procedure is associated with 1 to 2 units of blood loss and a 0.1% to 2% risk of perioperative mortality. Reported series from major centers with large experiences note impotence and incontinence rates of 30% to 40% and 5% to 10% respectively. However, a more population-based survey of Medicare patients who had undergone radical prostatectomy revealed that the vast majority were impotent and more than 40% had some problem with continence.[56] Nearly one-fourth of the patients reported that they required further therapy for recurrent cancer. This survey suggests that the published estimates for the efficacy and complication rates of this procedure may be overly optimistic. There are no satisfactory trials comparing prostatectomy

TABLE 36.2. Complications of prostate cancer treatments.

Treatment	Complications
External beam radiotherapy	Acute cystitis, proctitis: 30%–40%
	Urinary retention: 3%–5%
	Chronic prostitis: cystitis 4%–7%
	Impotence: 40%–60%
Radical prostatectomy	Blood loss: 1–2 units
	Impotence: 40%–60%
	Incontinence: 5%–15%
	Anastomotic stricture: 1%–25%
	Thromboembolism: 1%–12%
	Mortality: 0.1%–2%

with radiation that has been completed.[57] At this time, there is little compelling evidence to support either irradiation or prostatectomy as superior.

The debate regarding radical prostatectomy and radiotherapy takes on particular significance in men with competing morbidities, particularly when there are data suggesting that no treatment at all is an acceptable approach for some men. There are published series that suggest the survival of men with localized prostate cancer who are not treated is comparable to that of men who undergo radical prostatectomy,[58,59] but methodologic problems, including the lack of statistical power, limit the conclusions to be drawn from these trials. A larger trial designed to address this question is now underway in the Veterans Administration System. There are no randomized trials comparing radiation therapy with observation.

Observation-only is an option for some men with organ-confined prostate cancer, and this is especially true in the elderly population with reduced life expectancy. Several studies have shown that most men with small tumors and well- or moderately differentiated cancer will have long survival without major interventions.[60–66] A pooled analysis of more than 800 men with localized disease identified tumor grade as the major factor in predicting disease-specific and metastasis-free survival.[46] The 10-year, disease-specific survival is 87% for men with histologic grade 1 and 2 tumors (Gleason ≤ 7) and 34% for men with grade 3 (Gleason >7) tumors. This disease-specific survival for men with well- and moderately differentiated tumors compares favorably with the reported survival for both radical prostatectomy and external beam radiotherapy.[67,68]

A recent development in the therapy of localized prostate cancer is the use of ultrasound-guided cryoablation of the prostate. A preliminary report on this technique showed that 82% of the 55 men who underwent the procedure had no residual disease at 3 months of follow-up.[69] The procedure is associated with significantly shortened hospital stays and overall morbidity when compared with prostatectomy. However, it has been studied in a relatively small number of men, and short- and long-term efficacy is unknown. Currently, cryoablation for localized prostate cancer is an experimental procedure.

Clinical decision making in older patients with organ-confined disease is largely an issue of how much and which risks patients are willing to tolerate. With observation alone, there is the risk of developing widespread metastatic disease, whereas each of the treatments has risk of side effects. In the older patient, the risk of developing metastatic disease must be weighed against the life expectancy and comorbid conditions that may limit that life expectancy and raise the risk associated with therapy. An open and frank discussion of these risks with each individual is required.

Regionally Advanced Disease

These patients have cancer that is no longer confined to the prostate gland but has not spread to the soft tissue structures or lymph nodes in the pelvis (T_3,N_0 or T_x,N_{1-3}). Patients with clinical T_3 tumors have 5-year survival of 64% to 72% following radical prostatectomy, external beam radiotherapy, or hormonal therapy, and 10-year survival of 29% to 47%.[70–72] Recognizing the increased risk for local recurrence and development of progressive disease, most investigators do not believe that patients in this disease category are curable by either radical prostatectomy or external beam radiotherapy alone. In general, however, these patients do appear to have the potential for prolonged survival with median survival greater than 5 years in most studies no matter what therapy is given.

Intuitively, pathologic stage T_3 disease (microscopic penetration of the prostatic capsule or invasion of the seminal vesicles) should have a better prognosis than clinical stage T_3 disease (palpable involvement of the seminal vesicles). Unfortunately, the data to support this assumption are lacking. Patients with T_3 prostate cancer have been treated with radical prostatectomy, with or without additional (adjunctive) irradiation or hormonal therapy,[70,73] definitive radiotherapy,[71] immediate hormonal therapy,[72] or observation with hormonal therapy on progression.[74] Adjuvant radiotherapy has been the primary modality of treatment for patients with extracapsular spread after prostatectomy (pathologic stage C disease).[75] In most studies, the 5-year survival rates range from 60% to 75% regardless of therapy. Thus, there are no convincing data to specifically recommend any of these approaches.

Patients with regional nodal involvement (N_1) have a much worse prognosis. Median survival is reported to be as low as 39.5 months.[76] In this small study (44 patients), radical prostatectomy, adjuvant hormonal therapy, and radiotherapy seemed indistinguishable with regard to survival. However, in a large consecutive series of 120 patients with D_1 disease, the 5-year prostate cancer-specific survival was 61% in a group followed with expectant management alone.[77] The group at the Mayo Clinic has argued that the high risk of recurrence in N_1 patients justifies adjuvant hormonal therapy. This group has reviewed data from 631 patients who underwent pelvic node dissection and were found to have D_1 disease.[78] Of these patients, 251 went on to radical prostatectomy and orchiectomy, with 97 receiving radiation and orchiectomy and 60 orchiectomy alone. Prostate cancer-specific survival was markedly improved in the prostatectomy patients at 5 and 10 years when compared with the orchiectomy-alone patients (5 year, 90% versus 66%; 10 year, 78% versus 39%). As with many prostate cancer studies, however, these are retrospective data; unknown, unrecognized, or unstated selection bias leading to treatment decisions prevent firm conclusions from such data.[77]

Adjunctive Androgen Deprivation

Considerable data have emerged in the past 5 years regarding the use of androgen deprivation therapies (ADT) (usually GnRHa ± antiandrogen) in conjunction with irradiation and surgery for localized disease. Already referred to are the data of Bolla et al.,[54] which demonstrated a substantial survival advantage for patients with T_3–T_4 primary tumors treated with irradiation + LHRHa compared to irradiation alone. The RTOG is conducting trials of T_3, T_4 and T_1, T_2 tumors evaluating pen-irradiation as well as prolonged androgen deprivation compared to irradiation alone. Freedom from local progression and freedom from PSA progression occur significantly more often when irradiation is accompanied by ADT in RTOG studies. In a multi-institutional randomized trial, Messing et al.[79] reported an improved survival in men with N+ disease following prostatectomy if ADT was employed. D'Amico[80] and colleagues note improved survival when irradiation is combined with ADT in a retrospective, case-control study. Taken together, these data suggest that adjunctive ADT improves survival in certain subsets of patients. Although considerably more work is required to clearly define the role of "early" ADT, these observations call into question the long-held dictum that ADT does not affect survival in prostate cancer. No data are available examining the role of ADT as sole therapy for clinically localized prostate cancer. Studies demonstrating superiority of ADT + irradiation versus irradiation alone raise the question of the role of ADT *alone* in men with localized disease, especially, perhaps, men with competing causes of morbidity or mortality.

Metastatic Disease

Approximately 30% of patients diagnosed with prostate cancer have metastatic disease at presentation.[81] An additional 30%, who initially present with organ-confined or regionally advanced disease, manifest evidence of metastasis at some point in the course of their disease. Metastatic prostate cancer is a significant cause of morbidity and mortality in the elderly male population.

Hormonal therapy of patients with metastatic prostate cancer is one of the most effective therapies available for the treatment of disseminated malignancy. Based on the Nobel Prize-winning work of Huggins and Hodges[82] in the 1940s, ADT had been utilized with great palliative benefit in patients with disseminated prostate cancer. Response rates of 80% to 90% are reported with each of the currently available therapies: estrogens, orchiectomy, and the LHRHa.[83,84] Diethylstilbestrol (DES) is the primary estrogen used in the therapy of prostate cancer. This agent is clearly effective in treating metastatic prostate cancer; clinical responses following DES occur as often as with orchiectomy. Unfortunately, even with low-dose regimens, this agent is associated with a significant incidence of cardiovascular side effects, including cardiovascular death.[85]

Orchiectomy is the "gold standard" for ADT, particularly for men at high risk for complications as indicated by extensive bony involvement, obstructive uropathy, or cord compression. Surgical castration results in a rapid, 95% reduction in circulating testosterone and is not associated with the cardiovascular complications of DES.[86] GnRH analogues require 2 to 3 weeks to produce castrate levels of testosterone.[81] Nonetheless, the GnRHa analogues are effective therapy for prostate cancer. The major limitations to their use are compliance and cost. The currently available analogues require monthly or every 3- or 4-month injections. The cost of these injections is approximately $400 and $1400, respectively. A once-yearly implantable form of leuprolide (Viadur) has been developed and is being tested for efficacy and safety.[87] In a cost comparison analysis with the GnRHa analogues, orchiectomy is clearly more cost effective.[88] In addition, GnRHa initially induces an increase in circulating levels of testosterone, which may result in tumor flare.[82,89,90] This surge in testosterone can cause a significant exacerbation of bone pain, increased urinary obstruction, and potentially significant spinal cord compression in some patients. The effects of this flare can be controlled using antiandrogens such as flutamide, bicalutamide, or nilutamide.[91]

The antiandrogens are combined with the GnRHa analogues or orchiectomy in a strategy known as total androgen blockade (TAB). This therapeutic approach seeks to improve outcome through "totally" blocking androgen-stimulated growth of prostate cancer by reducing the circulating androgens and blocking receptor binding by any remaining androgens. In uncontrolled studies, response rates as high as 97% with 2-year survival of 89% were reported.[92] There are currently three antiandrogens in use in this country: flutamide (Eulexin), bicalutamide (Casodex), and nilutamide (Nilandron). Numerous trials have explored TAB with either orchiectomy or GnRHa + antiandrogens compared to orchiectomy or GnRHa alone. Flutamide was studied in a randomized controlled trial in which previously untreated patients with metastatic prostate cancer were randomized to receive the GnRHa analogue leuprolide (Lupron, daily subcutaneous injection) with or without flutamide.[93] This trial enrolled more than 600 patients and demonstrated a statistically significant benefit for the combination therapy in terms of both progression-free survival and overall survival. In a subset analysis, these differences seemed particularly prominent in the patients with good performance status and minimal disease. In contrast, a European study of 571 patients randomized to goserelin with or without flutamide showed no advantage for the combination in terms of response rate, time to progression, or overall survival.[94] Thus, the efficacy of this combination remains controversial. Metanalyses reveal either no or limited benefit of TAB versus testicular androgen suppression.

An important U.S. trial randomized 1200 men to receive orchiectomy alone or orchiectomy + flutamide. No benefit of TAB was seen in this trial. Benefits of TAB, if any, seem to be limited to TAB employing LHRHa + antiandrogen. This finding may reflect the benefits of antiandrogen antagonism of the initial androgen surge that accompanies initiation of LHRHa or conceivably antiandrogens offsetting a small, but perhaps important, frequency of failure of LHRHa to completely suppress testicular androgen secretion.

Orchiectomy alone an be a highly effective form of androgen suppression. If LHRHa are employed, we routinely initiate antiandrogens simultaneously and continue antiandrogens for at least 6 to 10 months. The major drawbacks to total androgen blockade are the costs and the side effects of antiandrogens. Flutamide is associated with diarrhea (possibly due to the lactose filler in the capsules) and occasional cases of hepatic toxicity.[95]

Preliminary preclinical and limited clinical data suggest that intermittent androgen deprivation (IAD) may have merit in prostate cancer treatment. In androgen-dependent animal tumor models, IAD appears to delay the emergence of androgen-independent tumor growth. In a number of pilot clinical trials IAD appears to be better tolerated than continuous androgen suppression and may be associated with a delay in development of androgen-independent disease progression. A large randomized national trial is underway comparing IAD to continuous androgen deprivation. If IAD is equivalent or superior to continuous therapy in terms of disease control, it will clearly be the preferred approach, because suppressed libido, hot flashes, and loss of bone mineralization should be less frequent with IAD.

The timing of ADT has always been a controversial topic. In a randomized study of 938 patients with either locally advanced (T_{2-4}) or asymptomatic metastatic prostate cancer, done in the United Kingdom, a significant benefit in morbidity and mortality from prostate cancer was seen in the patients who received immediate ADT (orchiectomy or LHRHa) versus the patients who did not receive ADT until clinically indicated.[96]

Despite the success of androgen deprivation therapy as measured by "response," palliation of symptoms, improvement in bone scan, and reduced PSA, the median duration of response for men with metastatic prostate cancer is approximately 18 to 24 months, no matter what therapy they receive. Eventually, in all men, cells emerge that are able to grow despite androgen deprivation.[83] Median survival, once this hormone-"independent" state is established, is approximately 1 year. It is these patients who are destined to die of their prostate cancer. To date, no therapy has been shown to improve overall survival in men with androgen-independent disease. With the increased use of PSA levels to monitor the status of disease in men with prostate cancer, evidence of tumor activity despite androgen deprivation can be ascertained earlier than symptomatic recurrence, radiographic, or physical exam would reveal. By defining survival from the date of increasing PSA, survival in the androgen-independent phase of disease may appear to be increasing; this is an artifact of earlier definition of androgen independence.

Recent studies indicate that the first intervention in patients with androgen-independent prostate cancer should be withdrawal of antiandrogens in those who are taking them. Declines in PSA and decreases in the size of soft tissue masses have been documented following cessation of therapy with flutamide and bicalutamide.[97–99] These responses occur primarily in men treated for a prolonged period with total androgen blockade and are usually short lived (6–9 months), but some patients may have extended periods of disease stabilization.

Secondary hormonal therapy has been utilized for many years in the treatment of men with androgen-independent disease.[100] Unfortunately, unlike breast cancer, a prior response to hormonal therapy does not predict for response to secondary hormonal therapy in prostate cancer. Numerous agents have been tested. A partial listing is included in Table 36.3. Objective responses (primarily reduction in PSA) occur in 15% to 20% of patients and are typically of short duration. Appetite stimulation has been demonstrated as a side effect of megestrol acetate.[100,101] These agents may improve the cachexia seen in these patients but have limited benefit in treating prostate cancer.

TABLE 36.3. Agents used in hormonal therapy.

Reduction in androgen levels
  Orchiectomy
  Adrenal suppression
    Aminoglutethimide
    Ketoconazole
Direct cytotoxicity
  Ketoconazole
  Diethylstilbestrol
  Megestrol acetate
Androgen receptor antagonists
  Flutamide
  Bicalutamide
  Nilutamide
Multiple mechanisms
  PC-SPES
  Megestrol acetate

Two secondary "hormonal approaches" merit special mention.

1. Several randomized trials have employed glucocorticoids alone as the "standard" therapy for androgen independent prostate cancer. These studies consistently reveal a 15% to 20% frequency of 50% or greater decrease in PSA and a similar rate of pain reduction and an improved sense of well-being. These data suggest that relatively low dose glucocorticoids provide real, albeit relatively infrequent, and temporary benefit in men with androgen-independent prostate cancer.

2. The agent PC-SPES is a commercially available, Chinese combination of eight herbs. The active component or components in PC-SPES are unclear, but preclinical studies and clinical trials indicate that PC-SPES suppresses the growth of prostate cancer cells in vitro, reduces PSA levels in men with no prior hormonal therapy, and, most intriguingly, results in subjective improvement and a 50% or greater decrease in PSA in approximately 50% of men with androgen-independent prostate cancer. This activity of PC-SPES is dependent, at least in part, on the fact that PC-SPES contains phytoestrogen compounds that suppress testicular androgen synthesis and likely have direct antiproliferative effects against prostate cancer. The toxicity of PC-SPES is the toxicity of estrogen: thromboembolic disease, fluid retention, congestive heart failure. There are no data comparing PC-SPES to other first- or second-line approaches to androgen deprivation.

Cytotoxic chemotherapy has been studied extensively in men with hormone-refractory prostate cancer.[102–104] Despite numerous studies, there is no evidence that cytotoxic therapy provides survival benefit. This result has led some investigators to question whether any patient with prostate cancer should receive cytotoxic chemotherapy.[105] Two carefully conducted, randomized trials evaluated the role of mitoxantrone and glucocorticoids. Both studies revealed a significant improvement in palliation of bone pain and greater reduction in serum PSA in those who received the combination compared to the arm receiving only glucocorticoids. Mitoxantrone has been approved by the FDA for use in metastatic prostate cancer. Although no impact in survival has been seen with mitoxantrone therapy, these studies do indicate that limited, but real, palliative benefit is achieved with a very safe and well-tolerated cytotoxic therapy.[106,107]

Several other studies show that taxanes (paclitaxel or docetaxel), with or without estramustine, have antitumor effects in men with androgen-independent prostate cancer. Ketoconazole + doxorubicin alternating with vinblastine + estramustine also has clear antitumor effects. Although "effective" systemic cytotoxic therapy for androgen-independent prostate cancer remains to be defined, considerable data suggest that we have entered an era in the care of prostate cancer patients in which the use of cytotoxic therapy will be increasingly employed.[108–112]

Supportive Care of the Patient with Prostate Cancer

Prostate cancer is a significant cause of morbidity in elderly men, even in those destined to die of other causes. The primary care physician plays a crucial role in the management of problems with metastatic prostate cancer. The major cause of morbidity in advanced prostate cancer is bone metastasis. These metastases often involve critical structures such as the vertebral bodies and weight-bearing bones, as well as the marrow cavity itself. These patients are at risk for cord compression, major fractures, and bony pain.

Spinal Cord Compression

Spinal cord compression is a true oncologic emergency that occurs in 10% to 15% of patients with prostate cancer.[113] The key to the management of this complication is early recognition. Most patients develop back pain before the onset of neurologic symptoms, and any evidence of neurologic impairment consistent with either nerve root or cord compression is an indication for careful evaluation. Motor abnormalities are usually the initial neurologic manifestation, followed by sensory loss. Once motor or sphincter function in impaired, improvement is relatively uncommon. Approximately 50% of patients who are paraparetic at presentation are able to regain the ability to walk, whereas patients who present with frank paraplegia rarely regain ambulatory function. A high index of suspicion of spinal cord compression must be maintained. High-dose intravenous corticosteroid therapy (dexamethasone 6 mg q 6 h) should be instituted in cases of suspected cord compression.[114] Contrast-enhanced magnetic resonance imaging or computed tomographic (CT) myelography are the diagnostic tools of choice in assessing this condition. The thoracic spine is the most commonly involved site, and multiple levels of compression are not unusual. Once the diagnosis has been established, therapy is directed at relieving the pressure on the cord exerted by the tumor mass either with external beam radiotherapy or surgery.[115,116] Currently, there is no evidence that surgery yields superior results when compared with radiotherapy alone in terms of preservation or recovery of neurologic function.

Bone Metastases

Impending Fracture

The management of bony metastases in patients with advanced prostate cancer presents a major challenge. Not only can these metastases result in cord compression as already noted, but they are a significant cause of morbidity and contribute to mortality, particularly when they involve the long bones. Pathologic fracture involving the femurs and hips have an even more ominous prognosis than traumatic fractures do in the healthy elderly. Pathologic fractures are relatively rare in men with prostate cancer, despite the high rate of bone involvement,[117,118] likely because of the propensity for these metastases to be osteoblastic rather than osteolytic. The development of pain on weightbearing is often the first sign of an impending fracture and should be investigated promptly in patients with known metastatic disease. External beam radiotherapy and prophylactic orthopedic procedures often prevent the development of debilitating fractures and preserve function. Once a pathologic fracture has developed, the outlook for regaining function is markedly decreased, and an aggressive approach to preventing fractures is clearly waranted.[119]

Pain

Pain due to bone metastases is a common and vexing clinical problem; effective management is often difficult.[120] Pain may be a major cause of functional limitation and suffering. Several surveys have indicated that patients are extremely fearful of cancer pain and that our current approaches to pain management are marked by an underutilization of appropriate medication.[121,122] Narcotic analgesics are the mainstay of the management of cancer pain.[123] Sustained-release morphine preparations with shorter-acting opioids for breakthrough pain are effective in most patients. Elderly patients are reported to have a higher risk of cognitive impairment with narcotics, but they can be used safely in this population. In the case of bony metastases, narcotics are often supplemented with nonsteroidal anti-inflammatory drugs to good advantage.[124] These agents were typically associated with side effects including gastric erosions and bleeding and must be used with care in an elderly population.[125] (Also see Chapter 28, Acute and Chronic Pain.)

External beam radiotherapy should be utilized frequently in the management of painful bone metastases.[126,127] Irradiation has the advantage of providing rapid and often complete relief of pain. However, it is not unusual for patients to develop multiple areas of involvement with new areas of bony pain occurring during a course of radiotherapy. This complication often results in expansion or addition to previously existing radiotherapy ports with a resultant exposure of significant amounts of marrow to the toxicity of radiotherapy, which may contribute to the anemia associated with marrow infiltration by prostate cancer, thus having a significant negative impact on quality of life.

Newer approaches to the management of painful bone metastases include the use of bisphosphonates and radiolabeled compounds that are incorporated into bone, including radioisotopes of strontium, samarium, and rhenium.[128–130] These agents are preferentially taken up in bone and appear to have significant activity in terms of ameliorating bone pain; up to 70% to 80% of patients report decreased pain. The bisphosphonates may be useful in prostate cancer involving the bone. These agents inhibit osteoclast activity and erosion of bone. Several bisphosphonates have undergone clinical trials to assess their effect on bone pain. Encouraging results have been seen. Bisphosphonates decrease indices of bone resorption that are above normal in 50% to 80% of cancer patients.[131] Recent data indicate that these drugs may also inhibit the adhesion of tumor cells to bone, thereby preventing or delaying the development of new bony, as well as extraosseus, metastases.[132] The precise role of bisphosphonates in men with prostate cancer is uncertain. In patients with either breast cancer or multiple myeloma, initiation of bisphosphonates early in the evolution of metastatic disease is associated with reduced skeletal morbidity and even improved survival. Some have argued that the primarily osteoblastic nature of bone metastases in patients with prostate cancer means that bisphosphonates will have a limited role. However, osteolysis does accompany even markedly osteoblastic bone metastases. The role of bisphosphonates in men with this disease remains to be determined.

Conclusion

Prostate cancer is a major health problem in the elderly male population, causing significant morbidity, mortality, and expenditure of health care dollars. This problem will only increase as the population ages. Currently, controversy exists in several key areas of prostate cancer management, including screening and treatment of localized, advanced, and androgen-independent disease. These areas are under active investigation, and new approaches to this disease are emerging.

References

1. Greenlee RT, Murray T, Bolden S, et al. Cancer Statistics 2000. *CA Cancer J Clin.* 2000;50(1):7–33.
2. Data from the Surveillance, Epidemiology, and End Results (SEER) program staff. Section III: Incidence. In:

Cancer Statistics Review 1973–1986. Bethesda, MD: NIH; 1989:III.45.

3. Carter HB, Coffey DS. The prostate: an increasing medical problem. *Prostate.* 1990;16:39–48.

4. Carter BS, Bova GS, Beaty TH, et al. Hereditary prostate cancer: epidemiologic and clinical features. *J Urol.* 1993; 150:797–802.

5. Spitz MR, Currier RD, Fueger JJ, et al. Familial patterns of prostate cancer: a case-control analysis. *J Urol.* 1991; 146:1305–1307.

6. Tulinius H, Egilsson V, Olafsdottir GH, et al. Risk of prostate, ovarian, and endometrial cancer among relatives of women with breast cancer. *Br Med J.* 1992;305:855–857.

7. Thiessen EU. Concerning a familial association between breast cancer and both prostatic and uterine malignancies. *Cancer.* 1974;34:1102–1107.

8. Arason A, Barkardottir RB, Egilsson V. Linkage analysis of chromosome 17q markers and breast-ovarian cancer in Icelandic families, and possible relationship to prostatic cancer. *Am J Hum Genet.* 1993;52:711–717.

9. Brothman AR, Peehl DM, Patel AM, et al. Frequency and pattern of karyotypic abnormalities in human prostate cancer. *Cancer Res.* 1990;50:3795–3803.

10. Arps S, Rodewald A, Schmalenberger B, et al. Cytogenetic survey of 32 cancers of the prostate. *Cancer Genet Cytogenet.* 1993;66:93–99.

11. Jones F, Zhu SL, Rohr LR, et al. Aneusoury of chromosomes 7 and 17 detected by FISH in prostate cancer and the effects of selection in vitro. *Genes Chromosomes Cancer.* 1994;11:163–170.

12. Cooney KA. Hereditary prostate cancer in African-American families. *Semin Urol Oncol.* 1998;16:202–206.

13. Walsh PC, Partin AW. Family history facilitates the early diagnosis of prostate carcinoma. *Cancer.* 1997;80:1871–1874.

14. Berthon P, Valeri A, Cohen-Akenine A, et al. Predisposing gene for early onset prostate cancer, localized on chromosome lq 24, 2–43. *Am J Hum Genet.* 1998;62:1416–1424.

15. Xu J, Meyers D, Freije D, et al. Evidence for a prostate cancer susceptibility locus on the x chromosome. *Nat Genet.* 1998;20:175–179.

16. Trapman J, Sleddens HF, van der Weiden MM, et al. Loss of heterozygosity of chromosome 8 microsatellite loci implicates a candidate tumor suppressor gene between the loci D8S87 and D8S133 in human prostate cancer. *Cancer Res.* 1994;54:6061–6064.

17. Gray IC, Phillips SM, Lee SJ, et al. Loss of the chromosomal region 10q 23–25 in prostate cancer. *Cancer Res.* 1995; 55:4800–4803.

18. Pienta KJ, Esper PS. Risk factors for prostate cancer. *Ann Intern Med.* 1993;118:793–803.

19. Waterhouse J, Muir C, Shanmugaratnam K, et al. Cancer incidence in five continents. In: *Anonymous Cancer Incidence.* Lyon, France: International Agency for Research in Cancer; 1989.

20. Dunn JE. Cancer epidemiology in populations of the United States with emphasis on Hawaii and California—and Japan. *Cancer Res.* 1975;35:3240–3245.

21. Shimizu H, Ross RK, Bernstein L, et al. Cancers of the prostate and breast among Japanese and white immigrants in Los Angeles county. *Br J Cancer.* 1991;63:963–966.

22. Meikle AW, Smith JA Jr. Epidemiology of prostate cancer. *Urol Clin North Am.* 1990;17:709–718.

23. Giovannucci E, Rimm EB, Colditz GA, et al. A prospective study of dietary fat and risk of prostate cancer. *J Natl Cancer Inst.* 1993;85:1571–1579.

24. Hayes RB, Bogdanovicz JF, Schroeder FH, et al. Serum retinol and prostate cancer. *Cancer.* 1988;62:2021–2026.

25. Schwartz GG, Hulka BS. Is vitamin D deficiency a risk factor for prostate cancer? (hypotheses). *Anticancer Res.* 1990;10:1307–1312.

26. Palmberg C, Koivisto P, Hyytinen E, et al. Androgen receptor gene amplification in recurrent prostate cancer after monotherapy with the nonsteroidal potent antiandrogen Casodex (bicalutamide) with a subsequent favorable response to maximal androgen blockade. *Eur Urol.* 1997; 31(2):216–219.

27. Edwards SM, Badzioch MD, Minter R, et al. Androgen receptor polymorphisms: association with prostate cancer risk, relapse and overall survival. *Int J Cancer.* 1999;84(5): 458–465.

28. Bennett CL, Greenfield S, Aronow H, et al. Patterns of care related to age of men with prostate cancer. *Cancer.* 1991;67:2633–2641.

29. Cook GB, Watson FR. A comparison by age of death rates due to prostate cancer alone. *J Urol.* 1968;100:669–671.

30. Smedley HM, Sinnott M, Freedman LS, et al. Age and survival in prostatic carcinoma. *Br J Urol.* 1968;100:669–671.

31. Ishigawa S, Soloway MS. Van Der Zwaag R, et al. Prognostic factors in survival free of progression after androgen deprivation therapy for treatment of prostate cancer. *J Urol.* 1988;141:1139–1142.

32. Chodak GW, Vogelzang NJ, Caplan RJ, et al. Independent prognostic factors in patients with metastatic (stage D2) prostate cancer. *JAMA.* 1991;265:618–621.

33. Johansson JE, Andersson SO, Holmberg L, et al. Prognostic factors in progression-free survival and corrected survival in patients with advanced prostatic cancer: results from a randomized study comprising 150 patients treated with orchiectomy or estrogens. *J Urol.* 1991;146:1327–1333.

34. Emrich U, Priore RL, Murphy GP, et al. Prognostic factors in patients with advanced stage prostate cancer. *Cancer Res.* 1985;45:5173–5179.

35. Kramer BS, Brown ML, Prorok PC, et al. Prostate cancer screening: what we know and what we need to know. *Ann Intern Med.* 1993;119:914–923.

36. Gann PH, Hennekens CH, Stampfer MJ. A prospective evaluation of plasma prostate-specific antigen for detection of prostatic cancer. *JAMA.* 1995;273:289–294.

37. Stamey TA, Yang N, Hay AR, et al. Prostate-specific antigen as a serum marker for adenocarcinoma of the prostate. *N Engl J Med.* 1987;307:909–916.

38. Chybowski FM, Keller JJ, Bergstralh EJ, et al. Predicting radionuclide bone scan findings in patients with newly diagnosed, untreated prostate cancer: prostate specific antigen is superior to all other clinical parameters. *J Urol.* 1991;145:313–318.

39. Whitmore WF. Hormone therapy in prostatic cancer. *Am J Med.* 1956;21:697–713.

40. Jeweft HJ. The present status of radical prostatectomy for stage A and B prostatic cancer. *Urol Clin North Am.* 1975; 2:105–124.

41. Montie JE. 1992 staging system for prostate cancer. *Semin Urol.* 1993;11:10–13.

42. Gleason DF. Classification of prostatic carcinomas. *Cancer Chemother Rep.* 1966;50:125.

43. Partin AW, Steinberg GD, Pitcock RV, et al. Use of nuclear morphometry, Gleason histologic scoring, clinical stage, and age to predict disease-free survival among patients with prostate cancer. *Cancer.* 1992;70:161–168.

44. Partin AW, Yoo J, Carter HB, et al. The use of prostate specific antigen, clinical stage and Gleason score to predict pathological stage in men with localized prostate cancer. *J Urol.* 1993;150:110–114.

45. McGowan DG, Bain GO, Hanson J. Evaluation of histological grading (Gleason) in carcinoma of the prostate: adverse influence of highest grade. *Prostate.* 1983;4:111–118.

46. Chodak GW, Thisted RA, Gerber GS, et al. Results of conservative management of clinically localized prostate cancer. *N Engl J Med.* 1994;330:242–248.

47. Gibbons RP, Cornea RJ, Brannen GE. Total prostatectomy for clinically localized prostate cancer: long-term results. *J Urol.* 1989;141:564–566.

48. Zincke H, Oesterling JE, Blute ML, et al. Long-term (15 years) results after radical prostatectomy for clinically localized (stage T2c or lower) prostate cancer. *J Urol.* 1994; 152:1850–1857.

49. Paulson DF. Impact of radical prostatectomy in the management of clinically localized disease. *J Urol.* 1994;152: 1826–1830.

50. Catalona WJ, Smith DS. Five years tumor recurrence rates after anatomical radical prostatectomy for prostate cancer. *J Urol.* 1994;152:1837–1842.

51. Trapasso JG, de Kernion JB, Smith RB, et al. The incidence and significance of detectable levels of serum PSA after radical prostatectomy. *J Urol.* 1994;152:1821–1825.

52. Hanks GE, Krall JM, Martz KL, et al. The outcome of treatment of 313 patients with T_1 (UICC) prostate cancer treated with external beam radiation. *Int J Radiat Oncol Biol Phys.* 1988;14:243–248.

53. Lee WR, Hanks GE, Shaltheiss TE, et al. Localized prostate cancer treated by external beam radiotherapy alone: serum PSA-driven outcome analysis. *J Clin Oncol.* 1995;13:464–469.

54. Bolla M. Improved survival in patients with locally advanced prostate cancer treated with radiotherapy and goserelin. *N Engl J Med.* 1997;337:295–300.

55. Catalona WJ. Management of cancer of the prostate. *N Engl J Med.* 1994;331:996–1004.

56. Fowler FJ Jr, Barry MJ, Lu-Yao G, et al. Patient reported complications and follow-up treatment after radical prostatectomy: the National Medicare Experience: 1988–1990. *Urology.* 1993;42:622–629.

57. Paulson DF, Lin GH, Hinshaw W, et al. Radical surgery versus radiotherapy for adenocarcinoma of the prostate. *J Urol.* 1981;128:502–503.

58. Byar DP, Corle DK. VACURG randomized trial of radical prostatectomy for stages I and II prostate cancer. *Urology (Suppl).* 1981:17:7–11.

59. Madsen PO, Graversen PH, Gasser TC, et al. Treatment of localized prostatic cancer. Radical prostatectomy versus placebo. A 15-year follow-up. *Scand J Urol Nephrol (Suppl).* 1988;110:95–100.

60. Epstein JI, Paull G, Eggleston JC, et al. Prognosis of untreated stage Al prostatic carcinoma: a study of 94 cases with extended follow-up. *J Urol.* 1986;136:837–839.

61. George NJR. Natural history of localized prostatic cancer managed by conservative therapy alone. *Lancet.* 1988;1: 494–497.

62. Adolfsson J, Ronstrom L, Carstensen J, et al. The natural course of low grade, non-metastatic prostatic carcinoma. *Br J Urol.* 1990;65:600–614.

63. Zhang G, Wasserman NF, Sidi AA, et al. Long-term follow-up results after expectant management of stage Al prostatic cancer. *J Urol.* 1991;146:99–103.

64. Whitmore WF Jr, Warner JA, Thompson IM. Expectant management of localized prostatic cancer. *Cancer.* 1991; 67:1091–1096.

65. Adolfsson J, Carstensen J, Lowhagen T. Deferred treatment in clinically localized prostatic carcinoma. *Br J Urol.* 1992;69:183–187.

66. Johansson JE. Expectant management of early stage prostatic cancer. Swedish experience. *J Urol.* 1994;152:1753–1756.

67. Paulson DF, Moul JW, Walther PJ. Radical prostatectomy for clinical stage T1-2N0M0 prostatic adenocarcinoma: long-term results. *J Urol.* 1994;152:1753–1756.

68. Hanks GE. External beam radiation treatment for prostate cancer: still the gold standard. *Oncology.* 1992;6: 79–94.

69. Onik GM, Cohen JK, Reyes GD, et al. Transrectal ultrasound-guided percutaneous radical cryosurgical ablation of the prostate. *Cancer.* 1993;72:1291–1299.

70. Schroeder FH, Belt E. Carcinoma of the prostate: a study of 213 patients with stage C tumors treated by total perineal prostatectomy. *J Urol.* 1974;114:257–260.

71. Zagars GK, von Eschenback AC, Johnson DE, et al. Stage C adenocarcinoma of the prostate. An analysis of 551 patients treated with external beam radiation. *Cancer.* 1987;60:1489–1499.

72. Gee WF, Cole JR. Symptomatic stage C carcinoma of the prostate. Traditional therapy. *Urology.* 1980;15:335–337.

73. Zincke H, Utz DC, Taylor WF. Bilateral pelvic lymphadenectomy and radical prostatectomy for clinical stage C prostatic cancer: role of adjuvant treatment for residual cancer and in disease progression. *J Urol.* 1985;135:1199–1205.

74. Paulson DR, Hodge GB Jr, Hinshaw W. Radiation therapy versus delayed androgen deprivation for stage C carcinoma of the prostate. *J Urol.* 1984;131:901–902.

75. Gibbons RP, Cole BS, Richardson RG, et al. Adjuvant radiotherapy following radical prostatectomy: results and complications. *J Urol.* 1986;135:65–68.

76. Kramer SA, Cline WA, Farnham R, et al. Prognosis of patients with stage D1 prostatic adenocarcinoma. *J Urol.* 1981;125:817–819.

77. Steinberg GD, Epstein JI, Piantadosi S, et al. Management of stage D1 adenocarcinoma of the prostate: the Johns Hopkins experience 1974 to 1987. *J Urol.* 1990;144:1425–1431.

78. Cheng CW, Bergstralh EJ, Zincke H. Stage D1 prostate cancer. A nonrandomized comparison of conservative treatment options versus radical prostatectomy. *Cancer.* 1993;71:996–1004.

79. Messing EM, Manola J, Sarosdy M, et al. Immediate hormonal therapy compared with observation after radical prostatectomy and pelvic lymphadenectomy in men with node positive prostate cancer. *N Engl J Med.* 1999; 341:1781–1788.

80. D'Amico AV, Schultz D, Loffredo M, et al. Biochemical outcome following external beam radiation therapy for clinically localized prostate cancer. JAMA 2000;284(10): 1280–1283.

81. Scardino PT, Weaver R, Hudson MA. Early detection of prostate cancer. *Hum Pathol.* l992;23:211–222.

82. Huggins C, Hodges CV. Studies on prostatic cancer: the effect of castration, of estrogen and of androgen injection on serum phosphatases in metastatic carcinoma of the prostate. *Cancer Res.* 1941;1:293–297.

83. The Leuprolide Study Group. Leuprolide versus diethylstilbestrol for metastatic prostate cancer. *N Engl J Med.* 1984;311:1281–1286.

84. Peeling WB. Phase III studies to compare goserelin (Zoladex) with orchiectomy and with diethylstilbestrol in treatment of prostatic cancer. *Urology.* 1989;33:45–52.

85. De Voogt HJ, Smith PH, Pavone-Macaluso M, et al. Cardiovascular side effects of diethylstilbestrol, cyproterone acetate, medroxyprogesterone acetate and estramustine phosphate used for the treatment of advanced prostatic cancer: results from European organization for research on treatment of cancer trials 30761 and 30762. *J Urol.* 1986; 135:303–307.

86. Lin BJ, Chen KK, Chen MT, et al. The time for serum testosterone to reach castrate level after bilateral orchiectomy or oral estrogen in the management of metastatic prostatic cancer. *Urology.* 1994;43:834–837.

87. Fowler JE Jr, Gottesman JE, Reid CF, et al. Safety and efficacy of an implantable leuprolide delivery system in patients with advanced prostate cancer. *J Urol.* 2000;164(3 pt 1):730–734.

88. Bennett CL, McLeod DG, Hillner BE. Estimating the cost-effectiveness of total androgen blockade (TAB) for stage D-2 prostate cancer (meeting abstract). *Proc Annu Meet Am Soc Clin Oncol* 1994;13.

89. Ahmann FR, Citrin DL, De Haan HA, et al. Zoladex: a sustained-release, monthly luteinizing hormone-releasing hormone analogue for the treatment of advanced prostate cancer. *J Clin Oncol.* 1987;5:912–917.

90. Warner B, Worgul TJ, Drago J, et al. Effect of very high dose D-leucine^6-gonadotropin-releasing hormone proethylamide on the hypothalamic-pituitary testicular axis in patients with prostatic cancer. *Clin Investig.* 1983;71:1842–1853.

91. Schulze H, Senge T. Influence of different types of antiandrogens on luteinizing hormone-releasing hormone analogue-induced testosterone surge in patients with metastatic carcinoma of the prostate. *J Urol.* 1990;144:934–941.

92. Labrie F, Dupont A, Belanger A, et al. New approach in the treatment of prostate cancer: complete instead of partial withdrawal of androgens. *Prostate.* 1983;4:579–594.

93. Crawford ED, Eisenberger MA, McLeod DG, et al. A controlled trial of leuprolide with and without flutamide in prostatic carcinoma. *N Engl J Med.* 1989;321:419–424.

94. Tyrrell CJ, Altwein JE, Lippel F, et al. A multicenter randomized trial comparing the luteinizing hormone-releasing hormone analogue goserelin acetate alone and with flutamide in the treatment of advanced prostate cancer. *J Urol.* 1991;146:1321–1326.

95. Wysowski DK, Freiman JP, Tourtelot JB, et al. Fatal and nonfatal hepatotoxicity associated with flutamide. *Ann Intern Med.* 1993;118:860–864.

96. The Medical Research Council Prostate Cancer Writing Party Investigators Group. Immediate versus deferred treatment for advanced prostatic cancer: initial results of the Medical Research Council trial. *Br J Urol.* 1997;79: 235–246.

97. Kelly WK, Scher HI. Prostate specific antigen decline after antiandrogen withdrawal: the flutamide in advanced prostate cancer in progression under combination therapy. *J Urol.* 1993;150:908–913.

98. Dupont A, Gomez JL, Cisan L, et al. Response to flutamide withdrawal in advanced prostate cancer in progression under combination therapy. *J Urol.* 1993;150: 908–913.

99. Small EJ, Carroll PR. Prostate-specific antigen decline after Casodex withdrawal: evidence for an antiandrogen withdrawal syndrome. *Urology.* 1994;43:408–410.

100. Smith DC, Bahnson RR, Trump DL. Secondary hormonal manipulation (prostate cancer). In: Vogelzang NJ, Scardino PT, Shipley WU, et al., eds. *Comprehensive Textbook of Genitourinary Oncology.* Baltimore: Williams & Wilkins; 1996;885–919.

101. Loprinzi CL, Ellison NM, Goldberg RM, et al. Alleviation of cancer anorexia and cachexia: studies of the Mayo Clinic and the North Central Cancer Treatment Group. *Semin Oncol.* 1990;17:8–12.

102. Eisenberger M. How effective is cytotoxic chemotherapy for disseminated prostatic cancer? *Oncology.* 1987;1:59.

103. Eisenberger MA, Simon R, O'Dwyer PJ, et al. A reevaluation of nonhormonal cytotoxic chemotherapy in treatment of prostatic carcinoma. *J Clin Oncol.* 1985;3:827–841.

104. Yagoda A, Petrylak D. Cytotoxic chemotherapy for advanced hormone-resistant prostate cancer. *Cancer.* 1993; 71:1098–1109.

105. Tannock IF. Is there evidence that chemotherapy is of benefit to patients with carcinoma of the prostate? *J Clin Oncol.* 1985;3:1013–1021.

106. Tannock IF, Osoba D, Stockler MR, et al. Chemotherapy with mitoxantrone plus prednisone or prednisone alone for symptomatic hormone resistant prostate cancer: a Canadian randomized trial with palliative endpoints. *J Clin Oncol.* 1996;14:1756–1764.

107. Kantoff PW, Halabi S, Conaway M, et al. Hydrocortisone with or without mitoxantrone in men with hormone-refractory prostate cancer: results of the cancer and

leukemia group B9182 study. *J Clin Oncol.* 1999;17(8): 2506–2513.

108. Oh WK. Chemotherapy for patients with advanced prostate carcinoma: a new option for therapy. *Cancer.* 2000; 88:3015–3021.

109. Trivedi C, Redman B, Flaherty LE, et al. Weekly 1-hour paclitaxel clinical feasibility and efficacy in patients with hormone-refractory prostate cancer. *Cancer.* 2000;89(2): 431–436.

110. Bracarda S, Tonato M, Bosi P, et al. Oral estramustine and cyclophosphamide in patients with metastatic hormone refractory prostate carcinoma: a phase II study. *Cancer.* 2000;88(6):1438–1444.

111. Petrylak DP. Chemotherapy for advanced hormone refractory prostate cancer. *Urology.* 1999;54(suppl 6A): 30–35.

112. Millikan RE. Chemotherapy of advanced prostatic carcinoma. *Semin Oncol.* 1999;26(2):185–191.

113. Pienta, KJ. Pain management in patients with advanced prostate cancer. *Oncology.* 1999;13:1537–1546.

114. Vecht CJ, Haaxma-Reiche H, van Putten WLJ, et al. Initial bolus of conventional versus high-dose dexamethasone in metastatic spinal cord compression. *Neurology.* 1989;39: 1255–1257.

115. Smith EM, Hampel N, Ruff RL, et al. Spinal cord compression secondary to prostate carcinoma: treatment and prognosis. *J Urol.* 1993;149:330–333.

116. Shoskes DA, Perrin RG. The role of surgical management for symptomatic spinal cord compression in patients with metastatic prostate cancer. *J Urol.* 1989;142:337–339.

117. Dijstra S, Wiggers T, van Geel BN, et al. Impending and actual pathological fractures in patients with bone metastases of the long bones. A retrospective study of 233 surgically treated fractures. *Eur J Surg.* 1994;160:535–542.

118. Nielsen OS, Munro AJ, Tannock IF. Bone metastases: pathophysiology and management policy. *J Chin Oncol.* 1991;9:509–524.

119. Hardman PD, Robb JE, Kerr GR, et al. The value of internal fixation and radiotherapy in the management of upper and lower limb bone metastases. *Clin Oncol (R Coll Radiol).* 1992;4:244–248.

120. Ashburn MA, Lipman AG. Management of pain in the cancer patient. *Anesth Analg.* 1993;76:402–416.

121. Cleeland CS, Gonin R, Hatfield AK, et al. Pain and its treatment in outpatients with metastatic cancer. *N Engl J Med.* 1994;330:592–596.

122. Cherny NI, Portnoy RK. The management of cancer pain. *CA Cancer J Clin.* 1994;44:263–303.

123. Hammack JE, Loprinzi CL. Use of orally administered opioids for cancer-related pain. *Mayo Clin Proc.* 1994;69: 384–390.

124. Eisenberger E, Berkey CS, Carr DB, et al. Efficacy and safety of nonsteroidal antiinflammatory drugs for cancer pain: a meta-analysis. *J Clin Oncol.* 1994;12:2756–2765.

125. Kantor TG. Control of pain by nonsteroidal antiinflammatory drugs. *Med Clin N Am.* 1982;66:1053–1059.

126. Benson RC Jr, Hasan SM, Jones AG, et al. External beam radiotherapy for palliation of pain from metastatic carcinoma of the prostate. *J Urol.* 1981;127:69–71.

127. Gilbert HA, Kagan AR, Nussbaum H, et al. Evaluation of radiation therapy for bone metastases: pain relief and quality of life. *Am J Roentgenol.* 1977;129:1095–1096.

128. Robinson RG, Preston DF, Spicer JA, et al. Radionuclide therapy of intractable bone pain: emphasis on strontium-89. *Semin Nucl Med.* 1992;22:28–32.

129. Maxon FR III, Schroder LE, Hertzberg VS, et al. Rhenium-186(Sn)HEDP for treatment of painful osseous metastases: results of a double-blind crossover comparison with placebo. *J Nucl Med.* 1991;32:1844–1881.

130. Collins C, Eary JF, Donaldson G, et al. Samarium-153-EDTMP in bone metastases of hormone refractory prostate carcinoma: a phase I/II trial. *J Nucl Med.* 1993;34:1839–1844.

131. Bishop M, Fellow G. Urinary hydroxyproline excretion—a matter of bony metastases in prostatic carcinoma. *Br J Urol.* 1997;49:711–718.

132. Boissier S, Magnetto S, Frappart L, et al. Bisphosphonates inhibit prostate and breast carcinoma cell adhesion to unmineralized and mineralized bone extracellular matrices bone extracellular matrices. *Cancer Res.* 1997;57:3890–3894.

37
Gynecologic Cancers

Angeles A. Alvarez and Daniel L. Clarke-Pearson

Genital tract cancer afflicts a significant portion of postmenopausal women. These malignancies account for 13% of all cancers in women. Approximately 75,400 new cases were diagnosed and 24,700 deaths resulted from gynecologic malignancies in 1999.[1] Risk of developing a gynecologic cancer increases with age.[2] Figures 37.1 and 37.2 show the age-related incidence and mortality, respectively, of these malignancies. As with other cancers, early detection provides the best opportunity for successful management. Therapeutic strategies include surgery, chemotherapy, and radiation treatment. Integration of these diverse modalities is best coordinated by a gynecologic oncologist who has the skills necessary to accomplish surgical and medical treatment of these women, as well as the knowledge of appropriate circumstances for the use of radiotherapy.

Endometrial Cancer

Endometrial cancer is the most common invasive gynecologic cancer, representing 5.4% of all malignancies of women, and one of the 10 most frequent cancers.[3] The incidence is 72 cases per 100,000 women per year, yielding a lifetime risk of 1 in 45. Approximately 37,400 new cases and 6,470 deaths occurred in 1999.[1] An estimated 39,300 cases will occur in 2002.[1] Seventy-five percent of endometrial cancer patients are postmenopausal, and the average age of onset is 60 years.[2]

Several risk factors for endometrial cancer have been identified.[4] Obesity increases the risk threefold for women 21 to 50 pounds overweight; risk is heightened to 10 fold for individuals exceeding ideal body weight by 50 pounds. Risk for nulliparous women is two times higher than primiparas and three times that of multiparous women. Late menopause (age 52 versus age 49) leads to a 2.4-fold increased incidence of endometrial cancer.

Hormones significantly alter the risk of endometrial neoplastic disorders.[5] "Unopposed" estrogen replacement therapy in postmenopausal patients increases endometrial cancer risk 4- to 15 fold; risk is related to dose and duration of therapy.[6] On the other hand, cyclic or continuous supplementation with progestins provides protection against endometrial cancer, reducing risk to below that of women without postmenopausal hormonal support.[5] Tamoxifen, an antiestrogen used in the therapy of breast cancer patients, increases the risk of endometrial cancer two- to threefold. Despite this unwanted side effect of tamoxifen, it is generally accepted that the benefits of tamoxifen therapy outweigh the risks and that therapy should not, in general be halted because of fears of endometrial cancer.[7] Estrogen-secreting tumors (granulosa cell tumors of the ovary) and polycystic ovarian disease increase the risk of endometrial cancer.[8] Oral contraceptives decrease the risk of endometrial cancer by approximately 50%, and this effect persists for about 10 years after discontinuation of the pill.[9] Hypertension has been reported to increase endometrial cancer risk onefold, and diabetes elevates the risk threefold. Ironically, smoking one pack of cigarettes a day decreases risk by about 30%, presumably due to enhanced estrogen metabolism in smokers.[10]

Symptoms of endometrial cancer include abnormal uterine bleeding, vaginal discharge, pelvic pressure, and manifestations of metastatic disease. Abnormal uterine bleeding is the most common clinical feature and is present in approximately 80% of women with endometrial cancer. The differential diagnosis of a postmenopausal woman who presents with abnormal vaginal bleeding includes endometrial atrophy, endometrial hyperplasia, endometrial polyps, cervical cancer, and vaginal cancer, in addition to endometrial carcinoma.

Patients with suspicious symptoms should be carefully evaluated with a detailed history, with emphasis on the risk factors already discussed.[11] A thorough physical examination should also be performed. The pelvic examination should include a careful assessment of uterine size and an endometrial biopsy.[12] A Pap smear should

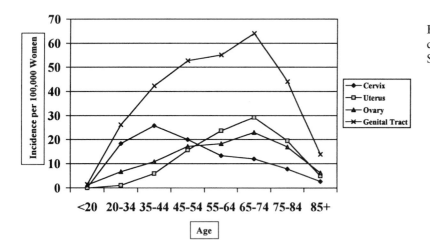

FIGURE 37.1. Annual incidence of genital tract cancers by age per 100,000 women in the United States, 1992–1996. (Adapted from Ries et al.[108])

also be done as well; however, Pap smears lack sufficient sensitivity for the diagnosis of endometrial cancer and must not be substituted for biopsy of the endometrial cavity. Transvaginal ultrasound, with measurement of the endometrial stripe thickness, is a useful adjunct. Using a "normal" endometrial stripe measurement of 4mm or less for women less than 5 years since menopause and 3 mm or less for those 5 years or more since menopause, transvaginal ultrasound demonstrated a 97% sensitivity, 76% specificity, and 99.7% negative predictive value in the detection of endometrial cancer.[13] For patients receiving tamoxifen, the endometrial stripe may measure up to 10mm and is not a reliable measurement for the detection of endometrial cancer compared to patients not receiving tamoxifen.[14] Dilatation and curettage are recommended if office biopsy cannot be performed or if the clinical suspicion of cancer remains high in the face of a negative biopsy and transvaginal ultrasound. Hysteroscopy may also be performed, allowing visual inspection of the endometrial cavity, and may identify small foci of tumor missed on routine biopsy.

Screening for endometrial cancer has not proven to be of much clinical value. Methods such as routine endometrial biopsy and pelvic sonography have been explored. Given that a high percentage of endometrial cancer patients become symptomatic early in the course of their disease and that endometrial biopsy is readily available, screening does not improve outcome significantly if practitioners keep in mind the risk factors and diligently biopsy the endometrium in suspicious cases.[15]

Endometrial cancers are initially treated and staged using a surgicopathologic evaluation to document the extent of spread.[16] Preoperative medical assessment should search for metastases (physical exam and chest x-ray), as well as assure that the patient is medically fit to undergo surgery. Table 37.1 outlines the current staging system. Standard therapy comprises exploratory laparotomy, total abdominal hysterectomy, bilateral salpingo-

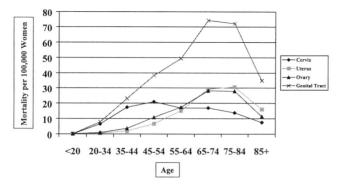

FIGURE 37.2. Annual mortality of genital tract cancers by age per 100,000 women in the United States, 1992–1996. (Adapted from Ries et al.[108])

TABLE 37.1. FIGO staging of endometrial cancer.

Stage[a]		Definition
IA	Grade 1,2,3	Carcinoma confined to the endometrium
IB	Grade 1,2,3	Invasion of less than one-half myometrial thickness
IC	Grade 1,2,3	Invasion of equal to or more than one-half myometrial thickness
IIA	Grade 1,2,3	Spread to endocervical glands
IIB	Grade 1,2,3	Invasion of cervical stroma
IIIA	Grade 1,2,3	Invasion of serosa and/or adnexa and/or positive peritoneal cytology
IIIB	Grade 1,2,3	Vaginal metastases
IIIC	Grade 1,2,3	Pelvic and/or para-aortic lymph node involvement
IVA	Grade 1,2,3	Invasion of bowel and/or bladder mucosa
IVB	Grade 1,2,3	Distant metastases including spread to abdominal viscera or inguinal lymph nodes

FIGO, International Federation of Gynecology and Obstetrics.
[a]Grade 1, 5% of less of a nonsquamous or nonmorular solid growth pattern; grade 2, 6%–50% of a nonsquamous or nonmorular solid growth pattern; grade 3, more than 50% of a nonsquamous or nonmorular solid growth pattern.

oophorectomy, washings from the abdomen and pelvis to assess for cytologic evidence of tumor extension, and pelvic and para-aortic lymphadenectomies if poor prognostic or adverse histologic features are present.[17] Clinical staging was employed before 1988 and is still utilized in the fewer than 5% of cases in which the patient is unfit to undergo surgery.[18]

Increased risk of recurrence and decreased survival are associated with high-grade histology, cervical extension, deep myometrial invasion, extrauterine extension, and malignant peritoneal cytology.[16,19] The presence of estrogen and progesterone receptors is associated with a better prognosis and a higher response rate to progestational therapy. Progestational therapy is usually reserved for recurrent disease, salvage therapy, or the medically infirm who are poor surgical candidates.[20]

Postoperative management of patients with endometrial cancer varies according to the stage and grade of their tumor. Women at low risk for recurrence (stage IA, grade 1 and 2) require no additional therapy. A recent phase III randomized study of surgery versus surgery plus adjunctive radiation therapy in intermediate-risk individuals [stage IB, IC, IIA (occult) and IIB (occult)] demonstrated that the use of adjuvant pelvic radiation therapy decreased the risk of pelvic recurrence but had no significant effect on overall survival. Patients randomized to the radiotherapy group had a higher incidence of adverse effects, including hematologic, gastrointestinal (with and without obstruction), genitourinary, and cutaneous toxicities.[21] Patients with stage IIB or IIIA should receive tailored treatment, which may include vaginal cuff irradiation, pelvic radiotherapy, or intraperitoneal ^{32}P.[22] Patients at high risk for persistent, recurrent, or progressive disease (stages IIIB, IIIC, IVA, and IVB, all grades) usually receive postoperative radiation treatment to the vaginal cuff, pelvic, or para-aortic regions.[23,24] Whole abdominal radiation is sometimes employed in cases of intraabdominal tumor spread.[25] Currently, a randomized prospective trial comparing whole abdominal radiation versus doxorubicin-cisplatin chemotherapy for patients with advanced disease is under way. Radiation as a primary means of therapy is usually reserved for poor surgical candidates. When utilized, external beam technique followed by uterine intracavitary placement of a radiation source is the usual strategy.[26]

Hormonal therapy is sometimes used for metastatic or recurrent endometrial cancer.[8] Progestational agents have proven to be most effective, although responses to tamoxifen have been described.[27] Tumors that express progesterone receptor are more sensitive to the growth-suppressive effects of progestins that those lacking receptors (70% versus 16% response rate).[28] Cytotoxic chemotherapy may be used for palliation in advanced or recurrent disease.[29] Doxorubicin and cisplatin are the best agents available. Response rates of 31% to 81%

have been achieved, but long-term survivors are rare. Paclitaxel combined with platinum-based chemotherapy has demonstrated a partial response rate of 63% in recurrent disease, and this agent is currently being evaluated in phase III trials.[30]

Prognosis varies according to clinical stage. Five-year survival according to stage is as follows: I, 93%; II, 73%; III, 48%; IV, 25%.[31] Patients with stage IA endometrial cancer have a 5-year survival of more than 95%. Multivariate analysis has demonstrated that age at diagnosis is an independent prognostic factor; survival decreases from 93% to 71% as age increased from 30 to 70+[20,31] Recurrence is most likely in the first 3 years after treatment. About half of recurrences are in the vagina or pelvis. Patients should be seen every 3 to 4 months in follow-up and should be asked about spotting, bleeding, pain, or any other unusual symptoms that may portend relapse. A careful physical examination including Pap smear and pelvic assessment should be performed. Chest x-ray may be valuable for screening for pulmonary metastases. CA 125 is not routinely used to follow these patients but can be useful in isolated cases.[32]

Recurrent endometrial cancer is treated on an individual basis. Strategies include radiation therapy (depending on prior treatment), surgery for resection of isolated tumor, pelvic exenteration for recurrence after radiotherapy, or systemic therapy with hormonal or cytotoxic agents. Some patients with recurrent endometrial cancer, especially those localized to the vaginal cuff, can be treated successfully with radiotherapy, surgery, or a combination of the two. Patients who have metastatic recurrent disease generally have a poor survival. Hormonal therapy and chemotherapy may provide palliative benefit.

Although it is labeled as contraindicated by the U.S. Food and Drug Administration (FDA), estrogen replacement given after definitive cancer treatment does not appear to influence survival for patients with early-stage disease. Provision of hormonal support for women with advanced disease must be decided on an individual basis and should be done in close consultation with a gynecologic oncologist.[33]

Ovarian Cancer

Ovarian cancer is the leading cause of death among gynecologic malignancies. In 1999, there were 25,200 new ovarian cancers diagnosed and 14,000 deaths from this disease.[1] Women have a 1 in 70 lifetime risk of developing ovarian cancer, and 1 in 100 will die of this disease.[34] More than 48% of ovarian cancers occur in women over the age of 65. Age-adjusted incidence rates increase as age advances. For women under 40, the incidence is 1.4 per 100,000 women; the incidence is between 40 and 50 per 100,000 for women over age 60,[2] and peaks at

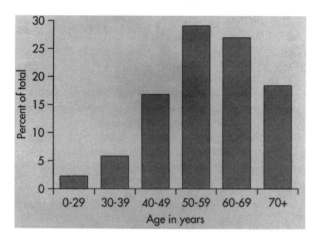

FIGURE 37.3. Age distribution of patients with epithelial ovarian cancer, based on data from the International Federation of Gynecology and Obstetrical (FIGO) 1988 Annual Report. (Reprinted with permission from Morley G, Reynolds RK. *Gynecologic, Obstetric, and Related Surgery, 2nd Ed.* Mosby, Boston, 2000.)

57.0 per 100,000 for women 70 to 74 years old[35] (Fig. 37.3). Most ovarian cancers are diagnosed at advanced stage, with extensive intraabdominal spread present at the time of initial diagnosis.

Many risk factors have been identified for ovarian cancer.[36] The best documented of these is the relationship between the number of lifetime ovulatory cycles and ovarian cancer risk. Events or conditions that suppress ovulation protect women against this malignancy. Thus, multiparity, oral contraceptive use, and a history of breastfeeding are protective. Conversely, women who are nulliparous or who undergo a late menopause are at increased risk. Women who have undergone ovulation induction therapy for infertility may have a higher risk, but this has not yet been firmly established.[37] High dietary fat consumption, use of talc in perineal regions, and mumps infections before menarche have also been implicated as factors that elevate ovarian cancer risk.

Genetic influences are also important. About 5% of ovarian cancer patients have a family history of significance.[38] Three familial ovarian cancer syndromes have been identified.[39] Women who fall into these categories often develop ovarian cancer at a younger age than those who develop sporadic tumors. Site-specific ovarian cancer afflicts families by causing ovarian cancer in the affected kindred. In familial breast/ovarian cancer syndrome, female family members develop early-onset breast or ovarian cancers. Cancer family syndrome (Lynch type II) is characterized by nonpolyposis colon cancer and either breast, ovarian, or endometrial adenocarcinoma. All these syndromes are transmitted in an autosomal dominant pattern with variable degrees of penetrance.

Several pathologic categories of ovarian tumors exist.[40] Epithelial cancer (adenocarcinoma) accounts for more than 80% of ovarian tumors and has an average age of onset over 40. These malignancies arise from coelomic epithelium; histologic subtypes of epithelial tumors include serous, mucinous, transitional cell, clear cell, and undifferentiated. Epithelial cancers are assigned grades of 1 to 3; the higher the grade, the less well differentiated the tumor. It is important to recognize tumors of low malignant potential (borderline tumors). These tumors are also of epithelial origin and are characteristically indolent and slow growing. They have cellular features of both malignancy and benignity. Because of their torpid nature, low malignant potential tumors have a more favorable prognosis than frankly invasive ovarian cancer. Another malignancy commonly misdiagnosed as ovarian cancer is primary peritoneal serous carcinoma. This cancer, arising from the peritoneum, spreads like ovarian cancer, looks histologically similar, yet minimally involves the ovary.

Sex cord/stromal tumors arise from mesenchymal tissues and account for about 5% of ovarian cancers. These tumors may occur at any age; subtypes consist of granulosa cell, thecoma, fibroma, and Sertoli–Leydig histologies. Germ cell tumors make up another category. They typically afflict children and adolescents and are relatively rare in postmenopausal women. These tumors account for approximately 15% to 20% of ovarian cancers. Ovarian metastases may arise from other primary cancers such as breast, endometrial, lymphoma, colon, and stomach and may present with signs and symptoms similar to de novo ovarian cancer. Because the majority of ovarian cancers in the geriatric population are of epithelial origin, our discussion focuses on this category. Other issues specifically related to the care of elderly ovarian cancer patients are addressed next.

Ovarian cancer often has an insidious onset with nonspecific symptoms, which often results in a delay in diagnosis. Gastrointestinal symptoms are common including dyspepsia, nausea, early satiety, altered bowel habits, eructation, abdominal discomfort, pain, and distension. Patients are often initially misdiagnosed with stress, depression, irritable bowel syndrome, or gastritis.[41] The correct diagnosis of ovarian cancer requires a high index of suspicion.

A carefully detailed history and physical examination are essential. Symptoms, family history, and risk factors should be assessed. Physical examination should include meticulous abdominal, pelvic, and lymph node examinations. Omission of the pelvic exam at the first visit is an important factor associated with delay of diagnosis.[41] Examination frequently reveals a significant abdominopelvic mass accompanied by ascites. Radiographic studies are sometimes useful in securing the diagnosis and triaging patients for appropriate treatment. Ultrasound can help differentiate benign from malignant lesions. Benign tumors often appear as simple cysts under 10 cm in diameter with septations less than 3 mm thick. Malignant lesions often are complex with solid and cystic components or are completely solid. Other malignant features include bilaterality, multiple septations greater than 3 mm, papillations, mural nodules, excrescences, and ascites. Doppler flow studies of malignant tumors show increased vascularity, enhanced blood flow, and decreased blood flow resistance. Computed tomography (CT) scans may be helpful, especially in the evaluation of retroperitoneal structures and the upper abdomen. Magnetic resonance imaging (MRI) is expensive and thus far unproven in the evaluation of the adnexa. Barium enema is useful in cases where gastrointestinal symptoms suggestive of a colonic neoplasia are present. Abdominal plain films are beneficial for demonstrating small bowel obstruction in symptomatic patients. In cases of undiagnosed abdominopelvic masses, radiographic studies cannot replace surgical exploration for definitive diagnosis and treatment.

Standard laboratory studies include complete blood count, electrolyte screen, and BUN–creatinine. Liver function analysis and coagulation panels are not usually informative in the absence of symptoms. The tumor marker CA 125 may be useful in the diagnosis and therapy of ovarian cancer.[32] If serum CA 125 is elevated in postmenopausal women with a pelvic mass, cancer should be strongly suspected. However, there are many other causes of elevated CA 125, and this test should not be considered a definitive verification of the presence or absence of cancer. CA 125 is most helpful for monitoring disease status (tumor burden) during therapy.[42] Paracentesis for analysis of ascitic fluid for diagnosis should be avoided. Risks of this procedure are (1) rupture of a cyst, which could release cancer cells or viscous mucoid material; (2) seeding of the needle tract with tumor; and (3)

false reassurance may be acquired if cytology studies prove to be falsely negative. However, if the patient is experiencing intolerable symptoms, such as dyspnea due to ascites, a therapeutic paracentesis may be indicated.

Spread of ovarian cancer occurs by capsular invasion, peritoneal seeding and lymphatic infiltration.[40] Peritoneal spread is the most common pattern and includes most peritoneal surfaces with frequent involvement of the omentum and diaphragm. Carcinoma of the uterus and cervix usually disseminate through pelvic lymphatics, whereas ovarian cancer drains to the para-aortic nodal tissue. Distant spread to intrathoracic regions or liver parenchyma may occur when malignant cells are transported via hematogenous routes. Extraovarian spread worsens prognosis. Another prognostic factor is tumor grade, which is usually more important than histologic subtype when forecasting outcome for women with early-stage ovarian epithelial cancers.

Staging of ovarian cancer employs a surgicopathologic system and is outlined in Table 37.2. Surgical staging is best accomplished by a gynecologic oncologist.[43] Patients usually undergo preoperative antibiotic and mechanical bowel preparation. Exploratory laparotomy, comprehensive abdominal exploration, hysterectomy, bilateral adnexectomy, omentectomy, and tumor debulking are performed. Peritoneal washings or ascites fluid is obtained for cytology. Random peritoneal or lymph node biopsies are performed in apparent early-stage cases to uncover occult microscopic tumor foci and document their locations. Pelvic and para-aortic lymph node dissections are completed to document extent of tumor spread or to "debulk" the cancer. Bowel surgery is performed in appropriate cases to relieve obstruction or to reduce tumor volume.[44] Surgical cytoreduction is performed to remove macroscopic tumor deposits because prognosis is directly related to the volume of residual disease before the initiation of adjuvant therapy. Bristow

TABLE 37.2. FIGO staging of ovarian cancer.

Designation	Definition
Stage I	Cancer limited to the ovaries
IA	Growth limited to one ovary, capsule intact, no malignant ascites, no tumor on external surface
IB	Growth limited to both ovaries, capsule intact, no malignant ascites, no tumor on external surface
IC	As for IA or IB but with surface growth, ruptured capsule (before or during surgery), positive washings, or malignant ascites
Stage II	Growth involving one or both ovaries with pelvic extension
IIA	Extension and/or metastases to the uterus and/or tubes
IIB	Extension to other pelvic organs
IIC	As for IIA or IIB but with surface growth, ruptured capsule (before or during surgery), positive washings, or malignant ascites
Stage III	Tumor involving one or both ovaries with peritoneal implants outside the pelvis and/or positive retroperitoneal or inguinal nodes; liver capsule involvement
IIIA	Tumor grossly limited to the true pelvis with negative nodes but microscopic seeding of abdominal peritoneal surfaces
IIIB	Abdominal peritoneal implants, but none exceeding 2 cm; nodes negative
IIIC	Abdominal peritoneal implants larger than 2 cm and/or positive retroperitoneal or inguinal nodes
Stage IV	Tumor involving one or both ovaries with distant metastases; pleural effusions must be demonstrated to harbor malignant cells; liver parenchymal involvement

et al. demonstrated that even patients with stage IV disease benefited from aggressive cytoreduction. Median survival was 50 months for patients in whom both extra- and intrahepatic optimal cytoreduction had been accomplished versus only 7 months for patients who were suboptimally debulked.[45] The full extent of tumor spread and amount of residual disease is documented so that appropriate therapeutic decisions can be made. Clearly surgical judgement is necessary to achieve optimal surgical and medical outcome, especially in elderly women who may have underlying medical problems.

Patients with stage IA grade 1 epithelial ovarian cancer have such an excellent prognosis that postoperative adjuvant therapy is unnecessary. For those with more advanced cancers, postoperative treatment usually consists of six courses of platinum-based multiagent chemotherapy, usually cisplatin or carboplatin combined with paclitaxel. Paclitaxel and platinum-based therapy has been demonstrated in prospective randomized clinical trials to improve progression-free survival and overall survival for patients with advanced suboptimally debulked ovarian cancer.[46] Carboplatin is just as efficacious as cisplatin and is associated with an improved adverse effect profile.[47] Intraperitoneal chemotherapy is also under investigation, and currently clinical trials are evaluating intravenous versus intraperitoneal cisplatin and paclitaxel for patients with optimally debulked stage III ovarian cancer. Novel therapeutic agents (such as antiangiogenic agents and gene therapies) are currently being evaluated in the treatment of ovarian cancer in clinical trials. Herceptin, anti-Her2*neu* antibody, is available to patients with recurrent or refractory ovarian cancer who overexpress Her2*neu*.

Chemotherapeutic treatment spawns many side effects; elderly women particularly have an elevated risk of complications with some regimens.[48] Cisplatin causes nausea, irreversible renal damage, and peripheral neuropathy (which is the dose-limiting toxicity). Administration of cisplatin requires extensive hydration and antiemetic therapy but can be safely used in the elderly.[49] Carboplatin differs from its congener, cisplatin, in that it is much less emetogenic, nephrotoxic, and neurotoxic. Debilitated patients tolerate carboplatin therapy better than cisplatin treatment, owing to different toxicity profiles of these agents.[50] Carboplatin is better tolerated by the elderly because it does not cause renal injury or nausea. Furthermore, because aggressive hydration is not required, carboplatin administration is less likely to exacerbate congestive heart failure or cause other side effects related to volume overload. The predominant side effects of paclitaxel are neutropenia and alopecia. Age alone is an insufficient criterion to alter the dose of either carboplatin or paclitaxel.[51]

Radiation therapy (RT) has a limited role in treatment of ovarian cancer. Intraperitoneal ^{32}P has sometimes been used to treat stage IC disease or for patients with persistent microscopic tumor deposits after chemotherapy. However, there are conflicting data regarding the efficacy of ^{32}P therapy, and one study has even demonstrated that cisplatin significantly prevented relapse in stage IC patients compared to ^{32}P therapy.[52]

External beam radiation therapy is sometimes useful for local control of sizable tumor foci, or residual disease, or for treatment of extremely poor surgical candidates. Treatment of the entire peritoneal cavity with teletherapy with curative intent is impractical in most cases. However, lower-dose whole abdominal radiation may be employed in selected cases to control small-volume disease.[53]

Survival of patients treated for ovarian cancer varies according to the stage of their disease. Five-year survival for women with epithelial ovarian cancer has improved and is as follows: stage I, 93%; stage II, 70%, stage III, 37%; stage IV, 25%.[54] Survival in ovarian cancer patients is influenced by age.[31] Multivariate analysis has revealed age to be an independent predictor of outcome. Overall, 5-year survival for elderly women over the age of 75 is only 20%, compared to 70% for women under 45 years of age.[35] This trend toward decreasing survival with advancing age holds true for patients with the same stage of ovarian cancer, even when adjustments for life expectancy are included.[55] Older women are more likely to be diagnosed with advanced-stage disease.[35] Older women are also less likely to undergo complete surgical staging, extensive debulking, or receive multimodality therapy because of overriding comorbities.[35,55] Bulky residual disease often remains after surgery due to the patient's otherwise poor health or because of limited experience of the surgeon in managing ovarian cancer patients.[56] More than 40% of women 85 years or older, according to a review of hospital records, did not receive any definitive therapy.[55] Older women with ovarian cancer, in general, are treated less aggressively than their younger counterparts.[55] Optimal therapy should not be withheld in elderly patients unless there are overriding medical contraindications.

Analysis of outcomes for patients involved with six randomized Gynecologic Oncology Group (GOG) trials revealed that those over age 69 had poorer survival rates than younger women, even after correcting for stage, residual disease, and performance status.[57] A retrospective case-control investigation has confirmed this finding.[58] Other studies have shown that more conservative surgery and less aggressive adjuvant therapy are contributing factors that may lead to decreased survival in elderly patients with epithelial ovarian cancer,[55] which was demonstrated to be due, in part, to these women receiving their care from obstetrician-gynecologists, general surgeons, and other nononcologists who persuaded them not to seek aggressive treatments. This bias against elderly women has been shown in another report documenting decreased specialist referral and use of physician influence to dissuade these cancer victims from obtaining optimum therapy.[59] Thus, although advanced age presages a poorer prognosis, in appropriate candidates maximal surgical debulking and aggressive chemotherapy may partially mollify the effect of age.

Follow-up involves serial physical and pelvic examinations, CA 125 levels, and sometimes CT imaging. Today, "second-look" surgery is infrequently performed after initial chemotherapy to determine the status of the tumor, that is, whether microscopic or grossly evident foci exist.[60] Although somewhat controversial,[61] and with no evidence that this surgery improves overall survival, this procedure is generally limited to those participating in research protocols to assess the effectiveness of new treatment modalities. About 55% of patients who are clinically free of disease will have a positive (i.e., persistent tumor) second-look operation. Debate regarding second-look operation exists because of its fallibility in predicting survival. There is a 25% to 45% recurrence rate after a negative second-look procedure, and some argue that the information gained does not justify the expense and morbidity of the surgery.[62]

Recurrence risk is increased with advanced-stage disease, high tumor grade, and large tumor volume.[31] A number of strategies may be employed to control tumor recurrences, although most are aimed at palliation rather than "cure." Treatment with secondary surgical debulking, multiagent chemotherapy, radiation therapy, biologic response modifiers, or chemotherapy with monoclonal antibody-directed agents, intraperitoneal instillation, or systemic administration with experimental compounds have all been utilized. Therapy must be individualized based upon the site(s) of recurrence, the biology of the tumor, the patient's performance status, her medical comorbidities, and her wishes regarding how aggressively she wants the cancer treated.[63]

Refractory cancer carries with it a very poor prognosis.[64] Death usually occurs within 18 to 36 months as the cancer propagates and sprawls out on the splanchnic bed, causing bowel obstruction, nausea, and vomiting. Sepsis often follows bowel or ureteral obstruction. Severe electrolyte abnormalities may result from nutritional deficiencies, renal dysfunction following cisplatin treatment, and accumulation of massive peritoneal or pleural effusions. Decisions regarding management of persistent, progressive disease must be made with care and with the participation of the patient and her family.[44] Relevant issues include support with total parenteral nutrition (which often can be administered at home by the patient or a family member), medical or surgical relief of bowel obstruction, intravenous hydration or antibiotics, hospice care, and pain management. It is imperative that maintaining quality of life and assuagement of pain be goals of therapy.

Epithelial ovarian cancer is not generally considered an estrogen-dependent neoplasia and, therefore, hormonal replacement therapy is not contraindicated. In fact, estrogen may augment the patient's quality of life and be an important part of her treatment.

Cervical Cancer

Cervical cancer accounts for about 20% of all gynecologic cancers. This cancer is largely preventable through screening and treatment of premalignant lesions. However, there were about 12,800 new cases and 4,200 deaths related to cervical cancer in 1999.[1] More than 50,000 new cases of cervical carcinoma in situ are diagnosed each year. The incidence is 8 to 10 cases per 100,000 women per year. Average age of onset is 45 to 55, but there is a wide variation in the ages of those afflicted.

Several epidemiologic risk factors have been identified.[2,65–71] Advanced age increases risk twofold. Black, Hispanic, and Native American women have a two- to threefold elevation in risk. A risk about three times that of the general female population is found in women of low socioeconomic status, multiparas, those engaging in sexual activity at a young age or with multiple partners, and chronic smokers. Women with a history of sexually transmitted disease (especially herpes or genital warts) are 2 to 10 times more likely to develop cervical cancer. Lack of regular Pap screening increases risk two- to sixfold. Immunosuppressed patients have a higher risk of cervical carcinoma. Dietary deficiency of ascorbic acid and carotene has been reported to augment the development of cervical neoplasia, although this is less well documented than the other risk factors. Screening is vital for diagnosis and treatment of cervical cancer in its earliest phases.[72,73] A more detailed discussion of cancer screening may be found in Chapter 32.

Pathogenesis of cervical cancer has received immense scrutiny in recent years. Molecular analysis has demonstrated that the etiology of cervical cancer in older women is similar to younger women.[74] Human papillomavirus is regarded as the vector that confers susceptibility to neoplastic conversion or that directly incites transmutation to a malignant phenotype in some infected epithelial cells.[70,75] Neoplastic tranformation usually originates at the squamocolumnar junction of the cervix. Varying degrees of cervical intraepithelial neoplasia (CIN) exist; these are graded from 1 to 3 on the basis of increasing severity of the lesion. Carcinoma in situ designates the condition in which all epithelial layers consist of neoplastic cells that are abutting the basement membrane, poised for invasion through this delimitation. It usually takes 10 to 20 years for intraepithelial neoplasia to progress to invasive disease. Most tumors (80%–90%) exhibit squamous histology; adenocarcinoma is the other predominant category. Other morphologies are rare.

Women with early invasive cervix cancer may have a cervix that appears normal to the naked eye, or they may have a small, ulcerated lesion that may seem to represent a benign inflammatory process. In such cases, cervical smears may be particularly effective in detecting preinvasive or early-stage disease. Most of these women are asymptomatic. On the other hand, patients with advanced cancer often experience symptoms. The most common abnormality is irregular vaginal bleeding. Postcoital spotting has long been considered a warning sign, but metrorrhagia or menorrhagia may occur as well. Some patients have a serosanguinous or yellow vaginal discharge that frequently is malodorous. Another symptom attributable to advanced cervical cancer is pain in the lower abdomen, pelvis, or back. Hematuria or rectal bleeding may occur if bladder or rectal invasion exists.

Invasive cancers display two primary modes of extension: local spread and metastasis via lymphatic and hematogenous routes. Cervical cancer may exhibit an ulcerative or exophytic appearance. Local expansion usually involves extension to the endocervix or vaginal fornices, followed by progressive infiltration of parametrial tissues, uterine corpus, bladder, or rectum. Lymphatic dissemination typically occurs in a stepwise progression. Pelvic nodes become involved before common iliac and para-aortic lymph node chains. Hematogenous spread may give rise to distant implants of cancer in lungs, bones, liver parenchyma, or other tissue. In general, the likelihood of metastasis rises with increasing size and expanse of tumor.[76] Spread to the pelvic nodes is present in 15%, 30%, or 47%, respectively, for tumors confined to the cervix, in the parametrium, or involving the pelvic side-

wall. The corresponding para-aortic nodal involvement for these situations is 6%, 16%, or 29%.

Cervical cancer is evaluated using a clinical staging system that is shown in Table 37.3. A pelvic examination should include a through evaluation of the cervix, vagina, parametria, and pelvic sidewalls. Extrapelvic regions that should receive extra attention include the abdomen, chest, and supraclavicular lymph nodes. Chest x-ray and intravenous urography are allowable radiographic techniques (under the clinical staging guidelines) for documenting the extent of tumor spread. Cystoscopy and proctoscopy are also permitted. General or conduction anesthesia is often employed to facilitate pelvic examination, procurement of biopsies, and cystoscopic and proctoscopic evaluations. Other studies that are sometimes helpful for diagnosis and treatment planning include lymphangiography, computed tomography (CT) scan, CT-directed lymph node aspiration, magnetic resonance imaging (MRI), positive emission tomograghy (PET) scan, blood count, serum chemistry profile, and urinalysis.

Treatment for cervical carcinoma may include surgery, radiotherapy and chemotherapy.[77,78] The most commonly utilized modality is radiotherapy, which ideally employs one or both of two techniques. (1) Teletherapy, or external beam application, is directed to cervical, parametrial, and pelvic nodal regions (Fig. 37.4A). The field may be extended superiorly if there is suspected or documented involvement of the common iliac or para-aortic nodes.[79] (2) Brachytherapy, or intracavitary treatment, is commonly done with intrauterine placement of cesium over a time period calculated to deliver a standard dose (Fig. 37.4B). The advantage of this technique is that extremely high doses of radiation can be applied to the tumor with less penetration of surrounding normal tissue. Recently, the utility of radiotherapy with concurrent cisplatin-

TABLE 37.3. FIGO staging of cervical cancer.

Designation	Definition
Stage 0	Carcinoma in situ
Stage I	Cancer confined to the cervix (corpus extension is disregarded)
IA	Preclinical cancer, i.e., diagnosed by microscopy only
IA$_1$	Measured depth of stromal invasion no greater than 3.0 mm
IA$_2$	Microscopically measurable lesion with depth of invasion <5 mm and horizontal spread <7 mm
IB	Clinical lesions confined to the cervix or preclinical lesions greater than stage IA$_2$
IB$_1$	Clinical lesions no greater than 4.0 cm in size
IB$_2$	Clinical lesions greater than 4.0 cm in size
Stage II	Parametrial extension, but not to the sidewall; involvement of the upper two-thirds of the vagina
IIA	No evidence of parametrial involvement
IIB	Obvious parametrial extension
Stage III	Extension of cancer to the pelvic sidewall or lower one-third of the vagina; hydronephrosis or nonfunctioning kidney secondary to cancer
IIIA	No pelvic sidewall extension
IIIB	Extension to the sidewall and/or hydronephrosis or nonfunctioning kidney
Stage IV	Spread beyond the reproductive tract
IVA	Infiltration of bladder or rectal mucosa
IVB	Metastases to distant organs or disease outside the true pelvis

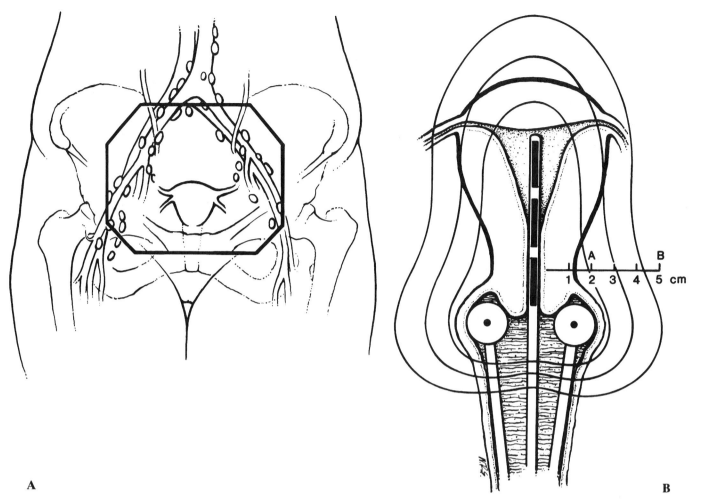

A

B

FIGURE 37.4. (A) External beam radiation therapy (teletherapy) is usually delivered to the pelvis through anterior and posterior portals covering the area *outlined*. Pelvic lymph nodes, parametria, cervix, uterus, and upper vagina are incorporated in this port. (B) Intracavitary Flecher-Suit applicator system. Intracavitary radiation therapy (brachytherapy) is usually given by placing cesium in an intrauterine tandem and contracervical applicators. The cesium sources are placed in a tandem fashion in the uterus, and a single source of cesium is placed in each vaginal applicator. The isodose curve from this application is depicted as three concentric lines. The dose to various pelvic sites is calculated (dosimetry) and depends on the strength of the cesium sources placed, the amount of time the sources remain in place, and the distance from the sources to the tissue in question. Two arbitrary points are usually calculated. *Point A* is found 2 cm cephalad and 2 cm lateral from the external cervical os. This point is where the ureter crosses underneath the uterine artery. *Point B*, which is 3 cm more lateral to point A, represents approximately the pelvic sidewall and pelvic lymph nodes. (Reprinted with permission from Clarke-Pearson D, Dawood Y. *Green's Gynecology, 4th Ed.* Little, Brown, Boston, 1990.)

based chemotherapy has been evaluated in several randomized trials. Patients with locally advanced (stage IIB–IVA) and bulky stage IB$_2$ cervical cancers who were treated with combined radiation and chemotherapy had significantly improved progression-free and overall survival rates.[80–82] Of the chemotherapy regimens available, single-agent cisplatin was shown to be just as efficacious as cisplatin/fluorouracil and better than regimens containing hydoxyurea.[82]

Surgical strategies vary according to the extent of the lesion. Cervical conization or simple hysterectomy (abdominal or vaginal) may effectively treat carcinoma in situ and microinvasive cervical cancers.[76] A radical hysterectomy involves removal of the uterus along with parametrial and paravaginal tissues; this is a treatment option for patients with Stage IA$_2$–IIA disease. The upper portion of the vagina and the pelvic and para-aortic lymph nodes are excised as well (Fig. 37.5). In premenopausal women, ovaries are not removed unless other indications necessitate their removal; however, in the postmenopausal patient a bilateral salpingo-oophorectomy is routinely performed.

The decision of whether to use surgery or RT for early-stage disease turns on several issues. Patients who are

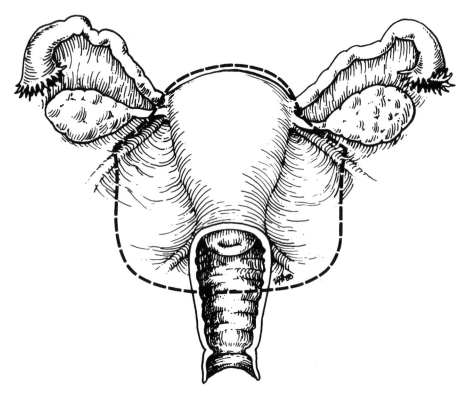

FIGURE 37.5. Radical hysterectomy. This operation is usually performed for the treatment of cervical carcinoma. Therefore, the goals include resection of the parametria and upper vagina to achieve a clear surgical margin around the cancer. Radical hysterectomy does not imply removal of the tubes and ovaries, which may often be preserved in young women. The cardinal ligament and major portions of the uterosacral and vesicouterine ligaments are resected as part of the radical hysterectomy. (Reprinted with permission from Clarke-Pearson D, Dawood Y. *Green's Gynecology, 4th Ed.* Little, Brown, Boston, 1990.)

frail or have serious comorbidities may be poor surgical candidates. Recovery from surgery and most of its potential complications occurs within a narrow time frame, whereas radiation has both acute and chronic effects.[77,83] Radiation-induced fibrosis is a lifetime process that is set in motion by the endarteritis provoked by RT. Ovarian function is obliterated by RT unless the ovaries have been positioned out of the pelvis. Sexual function is usually better preserved in women who have had surgery, as radiotherapy leads to agglutination of the vaginal tissues.

Advanced age has traditionally been considered a relative contraindication to radical pelvic surgery. The belief that such procedures in the elderly yield unacceptable morbidity has led to treatment of many older cervical cancer patients with radiotherapy rather than radical hysterectomy. Three retrospective studies have shown that, in properly selected older women, application of radical hysterectomy with modern surgical and postoperative care leads to complication rates comparable to those of younger women.[84,85] Thus, radical hysterectomy should not be withheld as a treatment option for older patients who are otherwise good surgical candidates.

Choice of therapy is based on the clinical stage. Patients with stage IA_1 cervical cancer may be treated by simple hysterectomy or, in selected cases, with conization. Women with stage IA_2 cancer are treated the same as those with stage IB disease if there is more than 3mm of invasion or lymphocapillary space involvement.[76] Stage IB and stage IIA cancer is treated similarly; cure rates are comparable regardless whether radical hysterectomy or RT is employed.[86] Cervical carcinoma of stages IIB, III, or IVA should be treated with radiation therapy. If ureteral obstruction is present, urinary diversion via nephrostomy or insertion of ureteral stents may be necessary to preserve renal function.[87] Palliative RT may be used in individuals with stage IVB disease to control pain and bleeding from the pelvic tumor. Chemotherapy with agents such as cisplatin, 5-fluorouracil, bleomycin, vincristine, and ifosfamide is often given in hopes that some therapeutic benefit may be derived in cases of metastatic disease.[88,89] "Cures," however, are unlikely with currently available chemotherapy.

Exenteration is an ultraradical procedure that is typically used for treatment of central tumor recurrence or persistence after radiotherapy.[90] This procedure entails removal of pelvic organs, including the bladder and rectosigmoid colon. Exenteration obviously leads to disfigurement and has profound psychologic impact on the patient. Significant potential for morbidity attends this procedure. Therefore, this technique is reserved for patients who are medically fit to undergo an extended procedure and in whom there is a substantial prospect for cure.

Five-year survival figures are given in Table 37.4.[31] These data highlight the importance of early detection and treatment of this cancer. Influence of age on treatment and survival related to cervical cancer has been

TABLE 37.4. Cervical cancer 5-year survival.

Stage	Survival (%)
0	99+
1A	97
1B	79
IIA	55
IIB	52
IIIA	40
IIIB	27
IVA	14
IVB	2

examined. Five-year survival decreases as age increases; this holds true both for global comparison of age groups and for relationships within stage.[31] Interestingly, a study from Japan has demonstrated that, when matched with respect to depth of invasion, patients over 60 had a lower incidence of lymph node metastases than their younger counterparts.[91] Despite the lower frequency of lymphatic involvement, the older women still demonstrated a worse prognostic trend. Another study found that overall survival in women 85 years and older was only 23.8%.[92] The 5-year survival rates for women 85 years and older were 37.5% for stage II and 22.2% for stage III. There were no stage I or stage IV survivors.[92] Survival is worse in older women, in part because cervical cancer is diagnosed at more advanced stages in this age group.[76,92]

Interval evaluation of the cervical cancer patient after therapy is imperative. Recurrent cervical cancer detected at its earliest stages might be successfully treated with surgery, radiation, chemotherapy, or a combination of the three. Thirty-five percent of patients with invasive cervical cancer will have persistent or recurrent disease following treatment.[76] The patient should be seen every 3 months for follow-up for 2 years, then visits should be at the discretion of the practitioner. In addition to focused history and physical examination, a Pap smear should be done. Chest x-rays, intravenous urograms, and CT scans may be ordered if circumstances dictate.

Recurrent cervical cancer carries a poor prognosis.[76] Seventy-five percent of recurrences occur in the first 2 years after treatment; by the 5-year milestone, 90% of recurrences have developed. Fewer than 15% of patients with recurrent disease survive 1 year, and 5-year survival is less than 5%. Pain control is an extremely important aspect of caring for women with relapses. Therapeutic approaches include RT if the primary treatment was surgical. Cure is sometimes possible for patients with central recurrence following RT if they are candidates for pelvic exenteration. Palliative chemotherapy may be administered.[88]

Death occurs by several mechanisms in cervical cancer patients. Extension of the tumor to the pelvic sidewall may cause ureteral obstruction and uremia. If the patient has received all available treatment for her cancer, usually no attempt is made at placing ureteral stents or percutaneous nephrostomies because uremic coma is not an unpleasant means of death in these women, who would otherwise often experience severe pain. Hemorrhage from the tumor bed or from erosion into pelvic vessels may lead to exsanguination and death. Hypercoagulability may precipitate pulmonary embolism. Sepsis occurs in many of these women and can be fatal if not promptly recognized. Physical external compression of the rectosigmoid colon may cause large bowel obstruction and the attendant consequences. Radiation enteritis, cystitis, and pelvic fibrosis may all contribute to or directly induce the patient's demise.[93]

Hormone replacement is not contraindicated in women with cervical cancer. Estrogen therapy may be especially important for maintenance of healthy vaginal tissue following castration or RT. To prevent endometrial hyperplasia or carcinoma, a progestin should be added to the estrogen if the uterus remains intact. Because many women treated for carcinoma of the cervix are relatively young, hormonal therapy affords the same advantages that would otherwise apply if they did not have cancer.

Vulvar Cancer

Vulvar cancer is an uncommon malignancy, responsible for only 5% of all gynecologic neoplasms, but its incidence is on the rise. Although the age of onset of vulvar cancer varies widely, most cases occur in women over age 50. Peak incidence occurs between the ages of 65 to 70.[83]

Epidemiologic studies have shown associations between vulvar cancer and genital warts, abnormal Pap smears, and smoking.[76,94] Molecular analysis of vulvar neoplasias has revealed the presence of human papillomavirus (HPV) genomic material.[95] These findings support an etiologic relationship between papillomavirus and vulvar cancer. Vulvar intraepithelial neoplasia (VIN) predisposes to vulvar cancer. Lichen sclerosis is not generally considered to be a premalignant condition. Squamous cell hyperplasia is often found in regions adjacent to vulvar cancer, but the relationship of this lesion to invasive cancer is unclear.[40] Advanced age and race (white) have been shown to be independent predictors of poor outcome.[31]

Although it seems intuitive that vulvar cancer would be relatively easy to diagnose because of the accessibility of the vulva to visual inspection, clinical findings may be subtle. Most patients experience a delay in diagnosis; this happens for a variety of reasons. Women may dismiss symptoms as mild or unimportant and delay seeking medical attention. Alternatively, many physicians treat patients on the basis of their symptoms without performing a biopsy of the lesion. About 50% of vulvar

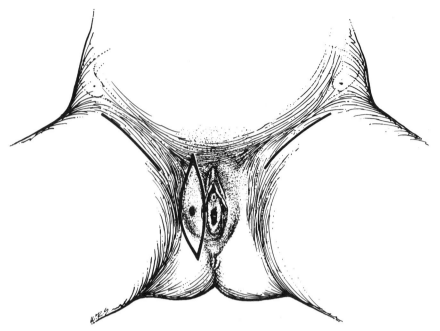

FIGURE 37.6. Modified radical vulvectomy with inguinal lymphadenectomy. Small unilateral (stage I) lesions may be adequately treated by a modified radical vulvectomy. Shown here are the lines of incision. The depth of the excision is carried down to the pelvic floor fascia and pubic ramus, as for a complete radical vulvectomy. The inguinal incisions shown allow inguinal lymphadenectomy through separate portals. (Reprinted with permission from Clarke-Pearson D, Dawood Y. *Green's Gynecology, 4th Ed.* Little, Brown, Boston, 1990.)

cancer patients experience prolonged pruritis or have an ulcerated or palpable mass on their vulva.

Vulvar cancer is easily mistaken for other conditions. There is no absolute consistency in the appearance of vulvar lesions such as VIN, lichen sclerosis, or squamous cell hyperplasia that allows them to be easily distinguished from vulvar cancer. Therefore, it is best to advise that any suspicious areas should be biopsied. Examination of the vulva should include a thorough inspection of the perineal area, including areas around the clitoris and urethra. Palpation of the Bartholin's glands should be performed as well. Biopsies may be guided by use of toluidine blue dye (1%) or dilute acetic acid. Uptake of blue dye is increased in neoplastic cells with enlarged nuclei. This increased nuclear to cytoplasmic ratio is also responsible for the altered appearance of neoplastic cells treated with acetic acid (causing them to appear more white than surrounding tissues). Abnormally pigmented lesions suspicious for melanoma should be biopsied by a gynecologist or gynecologic oncologist familiar with the anatomy of the region because wide excisional margins are required.

More than 85% of vulvar malignancies are of squamous histology. About 5% of vulvar cancers are melanomas.[76] Squamous cell cancer of the vulva is usually indolent, growing slowly and metastasizing late in its course. Local extension of the tumor occurs first, followed by lymphatic invasion. In general, lymphatic spread occurs in an organized, progressive fashion with superficial inguinal nodes affected before deeper (inguinofemoral and pelvic) nodal chains become involved.

Staging and therapy are primarily surgical, and the extent of resection is related to the stage of the tumor and the likelihood of nodal metastases. For lesions with less than 1 mm of invasion, radical wide local excision will suffice. Stage I lesions (≤2 cm) can be treated effectively with modified radical hemivulvectomy and ipsilateral superficial inguinal node dissection (Fig. 37.6).[96] Larger tumors usually require radical vulvectomy and inguinal lymphadectomy (Fig. 37.7). Larger tumors may also be treated primarily with radiotherapy and concurrent chemotherapy followed by surgical resection of residual disease.[97] Pelvic exenteration is sometimes employed for women with extensive disease or as a salvage strategy for patients with recurrent cancer.[98] Postoperative morbidity is related to the extent of the surgery. Therefore, the most conservative operation that can effectively treat the patient's condition is performed.[99] As with the cancers previously discussed here, elderly patients with vulvar cancer should be allowed to receive the full benefit of optimal surgical therapy, as age alone is a poor determinant of surgical risk.[100]

Survival is related to clinical stage and the extent of nodal involvement. Five-year survival for stages I and II vulvar cancer treated by standard surgical means is of the order of 90%. Survival (for all stages) still exceeds 70% in the absence of lymph node metastasis. However, lymphatic spread portends a worse outcome. Patients found to have inguinal lymph node metastases are usually treated with inguinal and pelvic radiation therapy postoperatively. Only one-third of patients survive 5 years if nodal metastasis is present. Involvement of the deeper, pelvic nodes results in a 20% 5-year survival rate. Approximately 80% of recurrences occur in the first 2 years after treatment. The majority of recurrences occur near the site of the primary lesion. Seventy-five percent

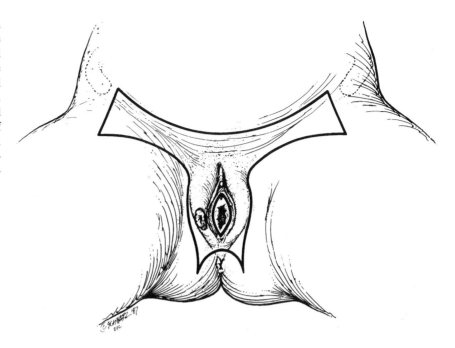

of patients with locally recurrent disease (limited to the vulva) can be salvaged with radical wide local excision.[101] In contrast, patients who develop a groin recurrence are rarely curable, and palliative surgical resection is associated with a high risk of complications.

The most common complications of treatment are related to wound breakdown and infection and occur in approximately 15% of patients. Other complications that arise in the early postoperative period include urinary tract infection, hematomas, seromas, venous thromboembolic disorders, femoral nerve injury manifestations, and osteitis pubis. Late complications may include lymphangitis, stress urinary incontinence, lymphocyst formation, introital stenosis, vaginal fistula, femoral hernia, and sexual dysfunction, but the most common late complication is intractable leg edema (lymphedema).

Estrogen replacement can usually be given to these patients. Hormonal treatment may help to maintain the health of surrounding perineal and vaginal tissues postoperatively.

Additional Issues for the Geriatric Patient

Since 1990, Medicare coverage for Pap smears has been available.[102] Presently, Medicare pays only the cost of laboratory analysis; the physician visit is covered only if Medicare-eligible services are rendered. Screening interval has been set at every 3 years under the current guidelines. The law permits provisions for more frequent Pap smears in high-risk women. However, no such benefits have been enacted to date.

Given that elderly women are at particularly high risk of developing malignancies, they should be entitled to receive adequate screening for these cancers. Older women are often uninformed about the importance of screening, and physicians are often reluctant to put elderly patients through the discomfort of a pelvic examination if they are asymptomatic.[103] Geriatric patients usually can safely undergo radical surgery, dose-intense chemotherapy, and radiotherapy after thorough medical evaluation.[100,104] Decisions to withhold optimum therapy should be made in conjunction with the patient and should be based on intercurrent medical conditions rather than on age alone.[105,106]

Treatment for gynecologic cancer commonly influences a woman's image of herself and her sexuality. It is imperative that physicians caring for these patients be sensitive to their concerns. Frank discussions about how treatment for cancer will affect appearance and sexuality must be conducted with the patient and her partner before initiation of therapy. Remediable causes of dysfunction should be corrected and referral for counseling considered if problems persist. It is important that sexual apprehensions be taken seriously and that practitioners recognize the importance of sexual issues to older individuals.[107]

Summary

As with other malignancies, gynecologic cancers are best managed if they are detected and treated early. Tumor biology varies substantially for each of the cancers reviewed. Stage for stage, elderly patients tend to have poorer survival rates than their younger cohorts. Appropriate attention to detail during annual or problem-related examinations and diligence in following screening protocols should allow prompt diagnosis. Age does not preclude aggressive management of cancer. Referral to a gynecologic oncologist is important if the patient is to receive the benefit of the most effective therapy and the option of participation in randomized research protocols involving novel treatments. Hormone replacement therapy, sexuality, and other quality of life issues should be considered when caring for individuals with gynecologic cancer.

References

1. Ries LAG, Eisner MP, Kosary CL, Hankey BF, Miller BA, Clegg L, Edwards BK: SEER Cancer Statistics Review, 1973–1999, National Cancer Institute. Bethesda, MD. http://seer.cancer.gov/csr/1973_1999/, 2002.

2. Ries LAG, Hankey BF, Miller BA, et al. *Cancer Statistics Review.* NIH pub 91-2789. Bethesda, MD: National Cancer Institute, 1991.

3. Edwards BK, Howe HL, Ries LA, Thun MJ, et al. Annual report to the nation on the status of cancer, 1973–1999: featuring implications of age and aging on U.S. cancer burden. *Cancer.* 2002;94:2766–2792.

4. Parazzini F, La Veccia C, Bocciolone L, et al. The epidemiology of endometrial cancer. *Gynecol Oncol.* 1991;41:1–16.

5. Gambrell RDJ, Bagnell CA, Greenblatt RB. Role of estrogens and progesterone in the etiology and prevention of endometrial cancer. *Am J Obstet Gynecol* 1983;146:696–707.

6. Smith DC, Prentice R, Thompson DJ, et al. Association of exogenous estrogen and endometrial carcinoma. *N Engl J Med.* 1975;293:1164–1167.

7. Seoud MA, Johnson J, Weed JCJ. Gynecologic tumors in tamoxifen-treated women with breast cancer. *Obstet Gynecol.* 1993;82:165–169.

8. Quinn MA, Cauchi M, Fortune D. Endometrial carcinoma: steroid receptors and response to medroxyprogesterone acetate. *Gynecol Oncol.* 1985;21:314–319.

9. Centers for Disease Control. Oral contraceptive use and the risk of endometrial cancer. The Centers for Disease Control Cancer and Steroid Hormone Study. *JAMA.* 1983;249:1600–1604.

10. Lawrence C, Tessaro I, Durgerian S, et al. Smoking, body weight, and early-stage endometrial cancer. *Cancer.* 1987;59:1665–1669.

11. Smith EM, Anderson B. Symptomatology, delay, and stage of disease in endometrial cancer. *Cancer Detect Prev.* 1987;10:247–254.

12. Walters D, Robinson D, Park RC, et al. Diagnostic outpatient aspiration curettage. *Obstet Gynecol.* 1975;46:160–164.

13. Tsuda H, Kawabata M, Yamamoto K, et al. Prospective study to compare endometrial cytology and transvaginal ultrasonography for identification of endometrial malignancies. *Gynecol Oncol.* 1997;65:383–386.

14. Cohen I, Beyth Y, Tepper R. The role of ultrasound in the detection of endometrial pathologies in asymptomatic postmenopausal breast cancer patients with tamoxifen treatment. *Obstet Gynecol Surv.* 1998;53:429–438.

15. Hall KL, Dewar MA, Perchalski J. Screening for gynecologic cancer. Vulvar, vaginal, endometrial, and ovarian neoplasms. *Prim Care.* 1992;19:607–620.

16. Creasman WT, Morrow PC, Bundy BN, et al. Surgical pathologic spread patterns of endometrial cancer. A Gynecologic Oncology Group Study. *Cancer.* 1987;60:2035–2041.

17. Sant CL, Weppelmann B, Shingleton H, et al. Management of early endometrial carcinoma. *Gynecol Oncol.* 1989;35:362–366.

18. Cowles TA, Magrina JF, Masterson BJ, et al. Comparison of clinical and surgical-staging in patients with endometrial carcinoma. *Obstet Gynecol.* 1985;66:413–416.

19. Sutton GP, Geisler HE, Stehman FB, et al. Features associated with survival and disease-free survival in early endometrial cancer. *Am J Obstet Gynecol.* 1989;160:1385–1391.

20. Palmer DC, Muir IM, Alexander AI, et al. The prognostic importance of steroid receptors in endometrial carcinoma. *Obstet Gynecol.* 1988;72:388–393.

21. Roberts JA, Brunetto VL, Keys HM, et al. A phase III randomized study of surgery versus surgery plus adjunctive radiation therapy in intermediate risk endometrial adenocarcinoma (GOG 99). Presented at Society of Gynecologic Oncologists, 28th Annual Meeting, Orlando, FL, 1998.

22. Soper JT, Creasman WT, Clarke-Pearson DL, et al. Intraperitoneal chromic phosphate P32 suspension therapy of malignant peritoneal cytology in endometrial carcinoma. *Am J Obstet Gynecol.* 1985;153:191–196.

23. Martinez A, Podratz K, Schray M, et al. Results of whole abdominopelvic irradiation with nodal boost for patients with endometrial cancer at high risk of failure in the peritoneal cavity. A prospective clinical trial at the Mayo Clinic. *Hematol Oncol Clin North Am.* 1988;2:431–446.

24. Potish RA, Twiggs LB, Adcock LL, et al. Paraaortic lymph node radiotherapy in cancer of the uterine corpus. *Obstet Gynecol.* 1985;65:251–256.

25. Martinez A, Schray M, Podratz K, et al. Postoperative whole abdomino-pelvic irradiation for patients with high risk endometrial cancer. *Int J Radiat Oncol Biol Phys.* 1989;17:371–377.

26. Ahmad K, Kim YH, Deppe G, et al. Results of treatment in locally advanced carcinoma of the endometrium. *Acta Oncol.* 1990;29:203–209.

27. Bonte J, Ide P, Billiet G, et al. Tamoxifen as a possible chemotherapeutic agent in endometrial adenocarcinoma. *Gynecol Qncol.* 1981;11:140–161.

28. Kauppila A. Oestrogen and progestin receptors as prognostic indicators in endometrial cancer. A review of the literature. *Acta Oncol.* 1989;28:561–566.

29. Thigpen T, Vance RB, Balducci L, et al. Chemotherapy in the management of advanced or recurrent cervical and endometrial carcinoma. *Cancer.* 1981;48:658–665.

30. Price FV, Edwards RP, Kelley JL, et al. A trial of outpatient paclitaxel and carboplatin for advanced, recurrent, and histologic high-risk endometrial carcinoma: preliminary report. *Semin Oncol.* 1997;24:S15–S15.

31. Kosary CI. FIGO stage, histology, histologic grade, age and race as prognostic factors in determining survival for cancers of the female gynecological system: an analysis of 1973–87 SEER cases of cancers of the endometrium, cervix, ovary, vulva, and vagina. *Semin Surg Oncol.* 1994; 10:31–46.

32. Olt G, Berchuck A, Bast RC Jr. The role of tumor markers in gynecologic oncology. *Obstet Gynecol Surv.* 1990;45: 570–577.

33. Creasman WT. Recommendations regarding estrogen replacement therapy after treatment of endometrial cancer. *Oncology.* 1992;6:23–26.

34. Ozols RF, Rubin SC, Thomas GM, et al. Epithelial ovarian cancer. In: Hoskins WJ, Perez CA, Young RC, eds. *Principles and Practice of Gynecologic Oncology, 2nd Ed.* Philadelphia: Lippincott-Raven; 1996:919–986.

35. Yancik R. Ovarian cancer. Age contrasts in incidence, histology, disease stage at diagnosis, and mortality. *Cancer.* 1993;71:517–523.

36. Heintz APM, Hacker NF, Lagasse LD. Epidemiology and etiology of ovarian cancer: a review. *Obstet Gynecol.* 1985;66:127–135.

37. Rossing MA, Daling JR, Weiss NS, et al. Ovarian tumors in a cohort of infertile women. *N Engl J Med.* 1994;331: 771–776.

38. Piver MS, Baker TR, Jishi MF, et al. Familial ovarian cancer. A report of 658 families from the Gilda Radner Familial Ovarian Cancer Registry 1981–1991. *Cancer.* 1993; 71:582–588.

39. Lynch HT, Watson P, Lynch JF, et al. Hereditary ovarian cancer. Heterogeneity in age at onset. *Cancer.* 1993;71: 573–581.

40. Kurman RJ. *Blaustein's Pathology of the Female Genital Tract, 4th Ed.* New York: Springer-Verlag; 1994.

41. Goff BA, Mandel LS, Muntz HG, et al. Ovarian cancer diagnosis: results of a national cancer survey. Presented at Society of Gynecologic Oncologists, 31st Annual Meeting, San Diego, CA 2000.

42. Podczaski E, Whitney C, Manetta A, et al. Use of CA 125 to monitor patients with ovarian epithelial carcinomas. *Gynecol Oncol.* 1989;33:193–197.

43. McGowan L. Patterns of care in carcinoma of the ovary. *Cancer.* 1993;71:628–633.

44. Clarke-Pearson DL, DeLong ER, Chin N, et al. Intestinal obstruction in patients with ovarian cancer: variables associated with surgical complications and survival. *Arch Surg.* 1988;123:42–45.

45. Bristow RE, Montz FJ, Lagasse LD, et al. Survival impact of surgical cytoreduction in stage IV epithelial ovarian cancer. *Gynecol Oncol.* 1999;72:278–287.

46. McGuire WP, Hoskins WJ, Brady MF, et al. Cyclophosphamide and cisplatin compared with paclitaxel and cisplatin in patients with stage III and stage IV ovarian cancer. *N Engl J Med.* 1996;334:1–6.

47. Ozols RF, Bundy BN, Fowler JM, et al. Randomized phase III study of cisplatin (CIS)/paclitaxel (PAC) versus carboplatin (CARBO)/PAC in optimal stage III epithelial ovarian cancer: a Gynecologic Oncology Group trial. Presented at Society of Gynecologic Oncologists, 31st Annual Meeting, San Diego, CA 2000.

48. Ozols RF, Young RC. Ovarian cancer. *Curr Probl Cancer.* 1987;11:57–122.

49. Thyss A, Saudes L, Otto J, et al. Renal tolerance of cisplatin in patients more than 80 years old. *J Clin Oncol.* 1994;12:2121–2125.

50. Alberts DS, Dahlberg S, Green SJ, et al. Analysis of patient age as an independent prognostic factor for survival in a phase III study of cisplatin-cyclophosphamide versus carboplatin-cyclophosphamide in stages III (suboptimal) and IV ovarian cancer. A Southwest Oncology Group study. *Cancer.* 1993;71:618–627.

51. Bicher A, Sarosy G, Kohn E, et al. Age does not influence taxol dose intensity in recurrent carcinoma of the ovary. *Cancer.* 1993;71:594–600.

52. Bolis G, Colombo N, Pecorelli S, et al. Adjuvant treatment for early epithelial ovarian cancer: results of two randomised clinical trials comparing cisplatin to no further treatment or chromic phosphate (32P). G.I.C.O.G.: Gruppo Interregionale Collaborativo in Ginecologia Oncologica. *Ann Oncol.* 1995;6:887–893.

53. Dembo AJ. Abdominopelvic radiotherapy in ovarian cancer. A 10-year experience. *Cancer.* 1985;55:2285–2290.

54. Trimble EL, Kosary CL, Cornelison TL, et al. Temporal trends in ovarian cancer survival. Presented at Society of Gynecologic Oncologists, 30th Annual Meeting, San Francisco, CA 1999.

55. Ries LA. Ovarian cancer. Survival and treatment differences by age. *Cancer.* 1993;71:524–529.

56. Gershenson DM, Mitchell MF, Atkinson N, et al. Age contrasts in patients with advanced epithelial ovarian cancer. The M.D. Anderson Cancer Center experience. *Cancer.* 1993;71:638–643.

57. Steiner M, Rubinov R, Borovik R, et al. Multimodal approach (surgery, chemotherapy, and radiotherapy) in the treatment of advanced ovarian carcinoma. *Cancer.* 1985;55: 2748–2752.

58. Marchetti DL, Lele SB, Priore RL, et al. Treatment of advanced ovarian carcinoma in the elderly. *Gynecol Oncol.* 1993;49:86–91.

59. Newcomb PA, Carbone PP. Cancer treatment and age: patient perspectives. *J Natl Cancer Inst.* 1993;85:1580–1584.

60. Podczaski ES, Stevens CWJ, Manetta A, et al. Use of second-look laparotomy in the management of patients with ovarian epithelial malignancies. *Gynecol Oncol.* 1987; 28:205–214.

61. Potter ME. Secondary cytoreduction in ovarian cancer: pro or con? *Gynecol Oncol.* 1993;51:131–135.

62. Friedman JB, Weiss NS. Second thoughts about second-look laparotomy in advanced ovarian cancer. *N Engl J Med.* 1990;322:1079–1082.

63. Hightower RD, Nguyen HN, Averette HE, et al. National survey of ovarian carcinoma. IV: Patterns of care and related survival for older patients. *Cancer.* 1994;73:377–383.

64. Sutton GP, Stehman FB, Einhorn LH, et al. Ten-year follow-up of patients receiving cisplatin, doxorubicin, and

cyclophosphamide chemotherapy for advanced epithelial ovarian carcinoma. *J Clin Oncol.* 1989;7:223–229.

65. Brinton LA, Herrero R, Reeves WC, et al. Risk factors for cervical cancer by histology. *Gynecol Oncol.* 1993;51:301–306.

66. Vermund SH, Kelley KF, Klein RS, et al. High risk of human papillomavirus infection and cervical squamous intraepithelial lesions among women with symptomatic human immunodeficiency virus infection. *Am J Obstet Gynecol.* 1991;165:392–400.

67. Brinton LA, Hamman RF, Huggins GR, et al. Sexual and reproductive risk factors for invasive squamous cell cervical cancer. *J Natl Cancer Inst.* 1987;79:23–30.

68. La Vecchia C, Decarli A, Fasoli M, et al. Dietary vitamin A and the risk of intraepithelial and invasive cervical neoplasia. *Gynecol Oncol.* 1988;30:187–195.

69. Beral V, Hannaford P, Kay C. Oral contraceptive use and malignancies of the genital tract. Results from the Royal College of General Practitioners' Oral Contraception Study. *Lancet.* 1988;2:1331–1335.

70. Reeves WC, Rawls WE, Brinton LA. Epidemiology of genital papillomaviruses and cervical cancer. *Rev Infect Dis.* 1989;11:426–439.

71. Schneider V, Kay S, Lee HM. Immunosuppression as a high-risk factor in the development of condyloma acuminatum and squamous neoplasia of the cervix. *Acta Cytol.* 1983;27:220–224.

72. Benedet JL, Anderson GH, Matisic JP. A comprehensive program for cervical cancer detection and management. *Am J Obstet Gynecol.* 1992;166:1254–1259.

73. Runowicz CD, Goldberg GL, Smith HO. Cancer screening for women older than 40 years of age. *Obstet Gynecol Clin North Am.* 1993;20:391–408.

74. Gostout BS, Podratz KC, McGovern RM, et al. Cervical cancer in older women: a molecular analysis of human papillomavirus types, HLA types, and p53 mutations. *Am J Obstet Gynecol.* 1998;179:56–61.

75. Taylor RR, Teneriello MG, Nash JD, et al. The molecular genetics of gyn malignancies. *Oncology.* 1994;8:63–70.

76. DiSaia PJ, Creasman WT. *Clinical Gynecologic Oncology, 5th Ed.* St. Louis: Mosby; 1997.

77. DiSaia PJ. Surgical aspects of cervical carcinoma. *Cancer.* 1981;48:548–559.

78. Stehman FB, Bundy BN, DiSaia PJ, et al. Carcinoma of the cervix treated with radiation therapy. I. A multi-variate analysis of prognostic variables in the Gynecologic Oncology Group. *Cancer.* 1991;67:2776–2785.

79. Brookland RK, Rubin S, Danoff BF. Extended field irradiation in the treatment of patients with cervical carcinoma involving biopsy proven para-aortic nodes. *Int J Radiat Oncol Biol Phys.* 1984;10:1875–1879.

80. Keys HM, Bundy BN, Stehman FB, et al. Cisplatin, radiation, and adjuvant hysterectomy compared with radiation and adjuvant hysterectomy for bulky stage IB cervical carcinoma. *N Engl J Med.* 1999;340:1154–1161.

81. Rose PG, Bundy BN, Watkins EB, et al. Concurrent cisplatin-based radiotherapy and chemotherapy for locally advanced cervical cancer. *N Engl J Med.* 1999;340:1144–1153.

82. Whitney CW, Sause W, Bundy BN, et al. Randomized comparison of fluorouracil plus cisplatin versus hydroxyurea as an adjunct to radiation therapy in stage IIB-IVA carcinoma of the cervix with negative para-aortic lymph nodes: a Gynecologic Oncology Group and Southwest Oncology Group study. *J Clin Oncol.* 1999;17:1339–1348.

83. Magrina JF. Complications of irradiation and radical surgery for gynecologic malignancies. *Obstet Gynecol Surv.* 1993;48:571–575.

84. Fuchtner C, Manetta A, Walker JL, et al. Radical hysterectomy in the elderly patient: analysis of morbidity. *Am J Obstet Gynecol.* 1992;166:593–597.

85. Geisler JP, Geisler HE. Radical hysterectomy in patients 65 years of age and older. *Gynecol Oncol.* 1994;53:208–211.

86. Hopkins MP, Morley GW. Radical hysterectomy versus radiation therapy for stage IB squamous cell cancer of the cervix. *Cancer.* 1991;68:272–277.

87. Carter J, Ramirez C, Waugh R, et al. Percutaneous urinary diversion in gynecologic oncology. *Gynecol Oncol.* 1991;40:248–252.

88. Sorbe B, Frankendal B. Bleomycin-adriamycin-cisplatin combination chemotherapy in the treatment of primary advanced and recurrent cervical carcinoma. *Obstet Gynecol.* 1984;63:167–170.

89. Giannone L, Brenner DE, Jones HW, et al. Combination chemotherapy for patients with advanced carcinoma of the cervix: trial of mitomycin-C, vincristine, bleomycin, and cisplatin. *Gynecol Oncol.* 1987;26:178–182.

90. Morley GW, Hopkins MP. Pelvic exenteration. In: Thompson JD, Rock JA, eds. *Te Linde's Operative Gynecology, 7th Ed.* Philadelphia: Lippincott; 1992:1329–1345.

91. Kodama S, Kanazawa K, Honma S, et al. Age as a prognostic factor in patients with squamous cell carcinoma of the uterine cervix. *Cancer.* 1991;68:2481–2485.

92. Chapman GW. Patterns of cervical carcinoma in women of advanced age. *J Natl Med Assoc.* 1997;89:801–804.

93. Jolles CJ, Freedman RS, Hamberger AD, et al. Complications of extended-field therapy for cervical carcinoma without prior surgery. *Int J Radiat Oncol Biol Phys.* 1986;12:179–183.

94. Brinton LA, Nasca PC, Mallin K, et al. Case-control study of cancer of the vulva. *Obstet Gynecol.* 1990;75:859–866.

95. Rusk D, Sutton GP, Look KY, et al. Analysis of invasive squamous cell carcinoma of the vulva and vulvar intraepithelial neoplasia for the presence of human papillomavirus DNA. *Obstet Gynecol.* 1991;77:918–922.

96. Stehman FB, Bundy BN, Dvoretsky PM, et al. Early stage I carcinoma of the vulva treated with ipsilateral superficial inguinal lymphadenectomy and modified radical hemivulvectomy: a prospective study of the Gynecologic Oncology Group. *Obstet Gynecol.* 1992;79:490–497.

97. Berek JS, Heaps JM, Fu YS, et al. Concurrent cisplatin and 5-fluorouracil chemotherapy and radiation therapy for advanced-stage squamous carcinoma of the vulva. *Gynecol Oncol.* 1991;42:197–201.

98. Hopkins MP, Morley GW. Pelvic exenteration for the treatment of vulvar cancer. *Cancer.* 1992;70:2835–2838.

99. Farias-Eisner R, Berek JS. Current management of invasive squamous carcinoma of the vulva. *Clin Geriatr Med.* 1993;9:131–143.

100. Lawton FG, Hacker NF. Surgery for invasive gynecologic cancer in the elderly female population. *Obstet Gynecol.* 1990;76:287–289.

101. Piura B, Masotina A, Murdoch J, et al. Recurrent squamous cell carcinoma of the vulva: a study of 73 cases. *Gynecol Oncol.* 1993;48:189–195.

102. Power EJ. Pap smears, elderly women, and Medicare. *Cancer Investig.* 1993;11:164–168.

103. List ND, Kucuk O. Approaches to and effectiveness of current cancer interventions in the elderly. *Oncology.* 1992;6: 31–38.

104. McGonigle KF, Lagasse LD, Karlan BY. Ovarian, uterine, and cervical cancer in the elderly woman. *Clin Geriatr Med.* 1993;9:115–130.

105. McKenna RJS. Clinical aspects of cancer in the elderly. Treatment decisions, treatment choices, and follow-up. *Cancer.* 1994;74:2107–2117.

106. Ganz PA. Does (or should) chronologic age influence the choice of cancer treatment? *Oncology.* 1992;6:45–49.

107. Ganz PA. Age and gender as factors in cancer therapy. *Clin Geriatr Med.* 1993;9:145–155.

108. Ries LAG, Kosary CL, Hankey BF, Miller BA, Clegg L, Edwards BK. *SEER Cancer Statistics Review, 1973–1996.* Bethesda, MD: National Cancer Institute; 1999.

38
Hematologic Malignancies

Marc Gautier, Elizabeth M. Bengtson, Edward M. Liebers, and Harvey Jay Cohen

The hematologic malignancies are a diverse group of disorders that are frequently considered together because they consist of clonal expansions of hematopoietic cells. The cell of origin of many of the hematologic malignancies is known. The stage of differentiation of the transformed cell essentially determines the phenotype of the disorder. Before considering the types of hematologic malignancies, we review the normal differentiation pathway of hematopoietic cells.

Figure 38.1 shows a version of the differentiation pathway from the lymphopoietic stem cell to the lymphoid lineages (T and B). There is also a stem cell (not shown) that matures to the myeloid lineages, giving rise to neutrophils, platelets, red cells, monocytes, eosinophils, and basophils. Steps of the differentiation pathway can be blocked, resulting in a clonal expansion of malignant cells. Thus, multiple myeloma represents as accumulation of the terminally differentiated B cell, whereas pre-B acute lymphocytic leukemia (ALL) represents a less differentiated B lymphocyte. Characteristic cell surface markers including the CD antigen system determine the immunophenotype of the malignant cell and assists in the diagnosis; this helps to differentiate morphologically similar entities. Thus, ALL can be differentiated from acute myelocytic leukemia (AML) by the presence of typical lymphoid cell-surface markers, such as CD10 and CD19. In many cases such distinctions have important therapeutic implications.

Hematologic malignancies disproportionately affect elderly patients. The disorders AML, chronic lymphocytic leukemia (CLL), and multiple myeloma all have characteristic patterns of increasing incidence with advancing age, such that the average age of onset of these diseases is 60 years of age or older. Additionally, other than with the acute leukemias, the clinical onset of hematologic malignancies is typically insidious, mimicking many other disease processes and frequently going unrecognized. As the name implies, many of the chronic malignancies can have an indolent or prolonged course.

Elderly patients are frequently compromised from other comorbid diseases and in the past have not always benefited from interventions such as chemotherapy and radiotherapy because of the associated toxicities. More recently, we have made advances in tailoring therapy to the geriatric patient. More importantly, new approaches to treatment, such as immunotherapy and molecular-targeted therapy, have revolutionized our ability to successfully treat the elderly patient while avoiding significant toxicity.

This chapter examines the acute leukemias (AML and ALL). Myelodysplastic syndromes that frequently evolve into leukemia are also considered. We discuss myeloproliferative disorders and lymphoproliferative disorders, including the lymphomas, the chronic leukemias, and the plasma cell dyscrasias. We emphasize new therapy developments that may impact responses and survival while offering less toxic and more tolerable treatment for the elderly patient.

Acute Leukemias

Acute leukemia, now more accurately referred to as acute nonlymphocytic leukemia (ANLL), is the more common form of leukemia in adults. Acute lymphoblastic leukemia is predominantly a disease of children that accounts for approximately 20% of all acute leukemias in adults.[1] ANLL occurs with increasing frequency with advancing age and frequently is preceded by a more chronic hematologic disorder. Multiple myeloma, polycythemia vera, paroxysmal nocturnal hemoglobinuria (PNH), chronic myeloid leukemia (CML), and the myelodysplastic syndromes all have a high propensity to culminate in acute leukemia. When acute leukemia follows these disorders, the prognosis is significantly poorer than de novo leukemia.

Clinical manifestations of the acute leukemias are similar regardless of the cell of origin (lymphocytic or

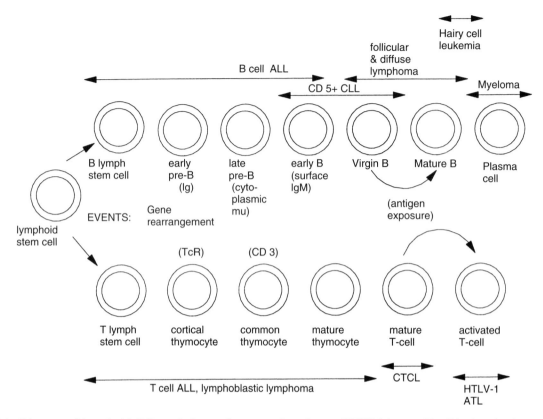

FIGURE 38.1. Diagram of lymphoid differentiation and corresponding disease states. *ALL*, acute lymphocytic leukemia; *CLL*, chronic lymphocytic leukemia; *CTCL*, cutaneous T cell lymphoma; *HTLV-1*, human T-cell leukemia virus 1; *ATL*, adult T-cell leukemia–lymphoma.

myelogenous). Typically there is an abrupt onset of nonspecific complaints, including fatigue, anorexia, weight loss, and weakness. Hematologic abnormalities frequently lead to the presenting symptoms; thus, anemia contributes to fatigue, thrombocytopenia leads to bleeding and bruising, and lack of mature neutrophils can lead to serious infections and concomitant fevers. Those patients who evolve into AML from a preceding hematologic disorder tend to have a more chronic evolution in their symptoms. The presence of anemia, thrombocytopenia, and granulocytopenia with circulating blast cells are the hallmark of acute leukemia. The marrow, when examined, is hypercellular with a lack of differentiation and a predominance of blasts.

The etiology of the acute leukemias is not completely understood but is thought to be the result of multiple genetic aberrations to a clone of hematopoietic cells. Many genetic defects have been associated with both acute myelogenous leukemia and acute lymphocytic leukemia. These genetic defects tend to be chromosomal translocations and frequently when characterized have involved so-called oncogenes.[2] Many of these abnormalities are thought to be etiologically involved in the evolution of leukemia.

Classification

The acute leukemias are broken down into acute nonlymphocytic leukemia, of which there are seven types, and the acute lymphocytic leukemias, of which there are three types. The lymphocytic leukemias and their subtypes are differentiated from the nonlymphocytic leukemia by the combination of morphology, immunophenotype, and cytogenetics. In some cases, the distinction can be very difficult. Nonetheless, it is important because therapy is directly related to the cell of origin of the leukemia. The most characteristic morphologic features distinguishing acute nonlymphocytic from acute lymphocytic leukemias are the presence of Auer rods and peroxidase stain positivity, which defines the leukemia as acute nonlymphocytic.

Treatment

Acute leukemias have a fulminant course if left untreated, with a median survival of less than 4 months. Death secondary to cytopenias is the rule, with bleeding and infections being very common. The goal of treatment is to induce remission, and currently that requires intensive chemotherapy for both ALL and ANLL. The initial induction chemotherapy is intended to be myeloablative, and thus a prolonged period of cytopenia follows the initiation of therapy.

The chemotherapeutic agents used for remission induction depend on the classification of the leukemia. AML is usually treated with a combination of two drugs, usually cytarabine and an anthracycline such as daunorubicin, given over several days to 1 week. The likelihood of attaining a complete response (CR) with this regimen in patients over 60 is approximately 50% as compared to 70% for younger patients.[3] Factors playing a role in the inability of this group of patients to achieve remission is the high incidence of preexisting hematologic disorders, such as myelodysplastic syndrome, chromosomal abnormalities, and chemotherapy resistance. All of these are poor prognostic factors for achieving remission at any age. In addition to difficulty attaining CR, treatment-related mortality associated with induction can be as high as 25% to 50% in patients over 60 years old as compared to 5% to 15% in younger patients.[3]

The requirements for supportive care through the period of induction are enormous, and in general only hematologists experienced in the care of leukemic patients with adequate blood bank support should treat these patients. Although it has been suggested that a reduced dose of induction therapy is more effective in elderly patients, this remains a controversial area. Several trials have studied the use of hematopoietic growth factor support (G-CSF or GM-CSF) during induction. The growth factors shorten the time of neutropenia but did not impact on early mortality or long-term survival.[4]

Once remission is achieved, additional postremission or consolidation chemotherapy is administered to maximize the odds for a prolonged remission. Several trials support the use of less intense chemotherapy for the elderly during this period without jeopardizing long-term survival.[5]

Much of the effort to have impact on the acute leukemias has been centered on intensification of induction therapy and consolidation therapy with bone marrow transplantation support. This strategy is generally not available to patients over the age of approximately 60 and thus remains of limited value to those patients most commonly affected by these diseases. A more promising approach is the use of molecular targeted therapy. Acute promyelocytic leukemia (APL), a subtype of acute myeloid leukemia, is defined by a t(15:17) chromosomal translocation.[6] This translocation involves one of the retinoic acid receptor genes. All-*trans* retinoic acid (ATRA) induces differentiation of leukemic blasts and results in a significant remission. With the use of ATRA, induction doses of chemotherapy in APL have been reduced and the prolonged cytopenia following induction has been significantly decreased. In the future,

we may know enough about the pathophysiology of the various forms of leukemia that therapy can be tailored in a much more specific manner, sparing the normal hematopoietic clones.

ALL, which is less common in adults, is treated with multiple drugs. Four drugs are frequently used for induction: vincristine, prednisone, L-asparaginase, and daunorubicin. ALL has rapidly become a curable disease in children, but results in adults are less favorable. Central nervous system treatment is required in all patients. In ALL, once remission is achieved, approximately 2 years of maintenance and consolidation therapy is currently the standard.

Future Directions

As mentioned, most of the progress to date in treating leukemia has centered on optimizing myeloablative approaches. Bone marrow transplantation, which represents the extreme of this approach, was not previously an option in older patients. However, a new approach, the submyeloablative bone marrow transplant, offers a potential cure for some patients over 60 as well. The basis of this approach involves lower doses of chemotherapy with reliance on graft versus leukemia effect to ultimately clear the malignant clone. We need to await results of early trials before we can judge the long-term success of this approach.

Research in immunotherapy is advancing rapidly and offers effective therapy with isolated toxicity. Gemtuzumab ozogamicin (Mylotarg) is an anti-CD33 antibody conjugated with a cytotoxic antitumor antibiotic. CD33 is an antigen found on the surface of myeloblasts. This approach specifically targets the myeloblast and spares other hematologic differentiation pathways. How this cytotoxic antibody will be used in the treatment of acute myeloid leukemia is yet to be determined. Aggressive research and development of molecular-targeted therapy and immunotherapy offers hope for effective treatment options with less toxicity in the future.

Myelodysplasia

The myelodysplastic syndromes (MDS) are a collection of disorders that predominately affect older patients with the median age of 63 at diagnosis. MDS is a heterogenous group of disorders characterized by abnormal growth of the myeloid bone marrow components. This section examines the common mechanism believed to underlie the MDS and then relates that to the propensity of these conditions to evolve into acute leukemia. In addition, we discuss the classification, natural history, and treatment options for MDS.

Pathogenesis

The pathogenesis of MDS is complicated. Current theory holds that MDS results from chromosomal injury that occurs in stepwise progression. Beginning with an initial predisposition to genomic instability, progressive insults result in chromosomal damage that culminates in MDS and can further progress to AML. Common chromosomal alterations involve 5, 7, 8, and 20. The involved chromosome areas are usually rich in hematopoietic genes. In addition to gross chromosome alterations, submicroscopic DNA mutations result in abnormal oncogene expression. Because of secondary DNA damage, exposure to chemicals or prior chemotherapy increases the risk for developing MDS. Although these genes may play a pathologic role in the development of MDS, we still do not understand the critical molecular events that lead to these diseases. The progression of MDS to leukemia is likely the result of additional genetic mutations that provide the evolving clone further growth advantages.

The biology of the disease is further complicated by other abnormalities, including aberrant cytokine production and responsiveness, altered stem cell adhesion, abnormal marrow microenvironment, early cell death secondary to accelerated apoptosis, and immuno-mediated marrow suppression. With all these contributing factors, MDS is ultimately a clonal hematopoietic stem cell disorder characterized by ineffective hematopoiesis and peripheral cytopenias.

Classification

The WHO classification system was recently proposed to replace the previous FAB classification system.[7] Some of the subsets are listed here. The distinction among these groups is based on the appearance of the bone marrow. The clinical presentation, however, can be very similar. Low blood counts (cytopenias) are the hallmark, and anemia occurs in the majority of patients. Isolated neutropenia or thrombocytopenia also occurs, but the usual picture is trilineage cytopenias. On examination of the peripheral blood, abnormal morphology is usually apparent. The findings in the marrow are more obvious, with hypercellularity, bizarre nuclear morphology, abnormal iron granules (sideroblasts), and nuclear/cytoplasmic maturation dysynchrony evident. All lines are affected, although frequently one lineage is more markedly dysplastic. An important determinant of overall prognosis is the percentage of blast cells in the bone marrow.

Some of the major types of MDS are (1) refractory anemia (RA); (2) refractory anemia with ringed sideroblasts (RARS); (3) refractory anemia with excess of blasts (RAEB); and (4) chronic myelomonocytic leukemia (CMML). CMML has features of both the dysplastic syndromes and the myeloproliferative disorders

(discussed in the next section). There is usually a significant increase in circulating monocytes, as well as trilineage dysplasia in CMML. This classification system is dependent on the percentage of blast cells in the marrow and also stratifies the risk of progression to leukemia. The risk of leukemia is low (5%–15%) in RA and RARS and higher (20%–40%) in RAEB. Still, up to 50% of patients with MDS die of complications of cytopenias rather than leukemia. The classification system also predicts median survivals, ranging from about 60 months for RA to less than 2 years for RAEB.

The International Prognostic Scoring System (IPSS) has been proposed, which identified significant prognostic indicators;[8] these include the number of cytopenias, percentage of blasts, and cytogenetic features. This system may be more useful in comparing results of interventions across clinical trials.

Treatment

Treatment of MDS remains problematic. For younger patients with high-grade disease, intensive chemotherapy and bone marrow transplant have been successful. Autologous and submyeloablative allogeneic bone marrow transplants are now being offered to older patients; however, the majority of older patients are still excluded because of either age or comorbid illness. Acute myelocytic leukemia (AML)-type treatment has produced some improvement in patients with severe disease, but this is usually transient and not generally applicable to elderly patients.

Less aggressive treatment options are actively being developed. Most are not of curative intent, but hematologic response and overall survival can be influenced. Use of recombinant growth factors to stimulate an increase in specific lineages has been explored recently. The use of myeloid growth factors has been approached cautiously because of fear of increasing the risk of leukemia. Trials of granulocyte colony-stimulating factor (G-CSF) and granulocyte-macrophage colony-stimulating factor (GM-CSF) were effective in improving peripheral neutropenia but did not influence leukemic transformation, hemoglobin levels, or overall survival. G-CSF and GM-CSF are not recommended for routine therapy.

Erythropoietin can improve anemia in MDS with an overall response rate of 16%. However, subgroup analysis reports response rates as high as 40% in patients with RA (versus RARS and RAEB) and low serum erythropoietin levels. The addition of G-CSF to erythropoietin can induce erythroid responses in erythropoietin-resistance patients. The mechanism of synergy is unknown. A predictive model for treatment with G-CSF and erythropoietin found the highest response in patients who have low serum erythropoietin levels and low RBC transfusion requirements.

Low-dose chemotherapy has met some success in older patients. Low-dose Ara-C induces a response in 30% of patients. Whether this translates to a survival advantage is unclear. More recently, melphalan has emerged as a well-tolerated oral chemotherapy regimen, with response rates as high as 40% and a significant improvement in survival. Additionally, 5-azacytidine trials report a response rate of 50% to 60% with tolerable toxicity and improved survival.

Future Directions

Research is opening new frontiers in treatment of MDS. Thalidomide, an immunosuppresant and angiogenesis inhibitor, shows promise in preliminary trials. Antithymocyte globulin and cyclosporin are being explored as immunosuppressive agents capable of modulating disease. Finally, cytokine inhibition trials with amifostine and pentoxifylline are underway. As we learn more about the pathophysiology of MDS, we will be able to better tailor therapy to effectively treat the disease with less toxicity.

Myeloproliferative Disorders

The myeloproliferative disorders are a group of diseases characterized by excessive proliferation of the myeloid elements secondary to a defect in the hematopoietic stem cell. As discussed earlier, the myeloid elements consist of erythrocytes, platelets, and the granulocytes, and there are disorders associated with the proliferation of each of these lines. These diseases are chronic in nature but tend to culminate in a more acute picture, such as acute leukemia. We consider four clinical expressions of the myeloproliferative disorders:

1. Chronic myelogenous leukemia (CML), with a predominant increase in the granulocytes
2. Polycythemia vera (PV), with a predominant increase in the red cells
3. Essential thrombocythemia (ET), with a predominant increase in the platelets
4. Myeloid metaplasia with myelofibrosis (MMMF), with a progressive fibrosis of the bone marrow with relocation of hematopoietic tissues to extramedullary sites

Chronic Myelogenous Leukemia

CML is a clonal stem cell disorder, characterized by increased proliferative capacity in the myeloid lineage, that is almost universally associated with a typical chromosomal translocation known as the Philadelphia chromosome. This is an acquired disorder, and although no specific etiologic agent has been identified, radiation exposure does lead to a significant increase in risk. There is an increasing incidence with advancing age, but the average age remains in the fifth and sixth decades of life.

The characteristic Philadelphia chromosome is a result of translocation of genetic material from chromosome 9 to chromosome 22. The gene on chromosome 9 has been identified as the Abelson proto-oncogene (abl). The region on chromosome 22 has been defined as the breakpoint cluster region (bcr). The rearrangement creates a bcr/abl fusion gene, which is believed to be pathophysiologically involved in the development of leukemia. Depending on the sensitivity of the detection method for the presence of the bcr/abl rearrangement, upward of 95% of all cases of CML demonstrate this very typical 9:22 translocation.[9]

The clinical characteristics of CML involve a standard triphasic course of the disease, with an initial chronic phase followed by an accelerated phase and culminating in a blast phase, with the entire course of the disease spanning an average of approximately 3 years. The typical findings at the time of diagnosis include an elevated white blood cell (WBC) count, which may be mild or can exceed 200,000 cells/mL. Anemia or thrombocytopenia may contribute to the presenting symptoms. The most frequent complaints include fatigue, anorexia, abdominal discomfort, and early satiety related to splenomegaly and are generally gradual in onset. Splenomegaly is the most common physical finding, with more than 90% of the cases demonstrating an enlarged spleen. The accelerated phase of CML is heralded by progressive leukocytosis, despite therapy with worsening cytopenia and progressive splenomegaly. Blast crisis has the same clinical presentation as acute leukemia.

The diagnosis of CML is confirmed by the presence of a marked increased in granulocytes with the presence of immature myeloid cells in the peripheral blood. There is usually not a significant peripheral blast count. Eosinophils and basophils in the peripheral blood are common. Leukocyte alkaline phosphatase is typically low or zero in CML. The bone marrow shows hypercellularity with predominantly granulocytic differentiation. The presence of splenomegaly is further evidence for the diagnosis of CML. Chromosomal evidence of the Philadelphia chromosome is confirmatory; however, a rare case of Philadelphia chromosome-negative CML exists.

Treatment

The treatment of CML is beginning to reap the benefit of decades of research into the pathophysiology of the disease. Until recently, there were no curative therapeutic strategies, and the therapeutic goal was to maintain controlled myelopoiesis in the chronic phase and accelerated phase; however, no therapy was known to delay the conversion to the accelerated phase (or blastic phase) of CML. Standard therapy has consisted of hydroxyurea delivered at 1 to 3 g per day by mouth, with a goal of maintaining the WBC count between 10,000 and 20,000. Direct inhibitors of the *bcr/abl* fusion protein are now able to impact on the disease with minimal toxicity.

Interferon-alpha has been shown to improve the survival of patients with CML compared with treatment with hydroxyurea. Interferon-alpha is generally initiated at 3 to 5 million units subcutaneously per day, and the response is maintained with a 3- to 5-day per week treatment schedule. Flu-like symptoms are common but frequently can be managed with acetaminophen.

Interferon-alpha improved the rate of karyotypic response, as well as the time of progression from chronic phase to accelerated or blastic phase, and was associated with a significant improvement in overall survival (72 months versus 52 months for hydroxyurea).[10] Addition of chemotherapy can improve the percentage of patients achieving a cytogenetic remission. Unfortunately, few older patients have been included in the reported trials.

Bone marrow transplant has been an attractive option for younger patients; in fact, preliminary results suggest early transplant in the chronic phase is associated with the best outcome for those patients who have a human leukocyte antigen- (HLA-) compatible sibling. Unfortunately, two-thirds of the patients diagnosed with CML are either considered too old to undergo this intensive therapy or do not have HLA-compatible siblings.

The development of compounds to directly inhibit the *bcr/abl* fusion product has been a promising area of research. The fusion protein is a unique tyrosine kinase, and the first FDA-approved inhibitor of this kinase has recently been approved for patients with CML who cannot tolerate or have not responded to interferon. Initial results of the oral drug suggest excellent activity with minimal toxicity,[11] which may be particularly important to elderly patients who tend to tolerate high doses of interferon poorly. A randomized trial comparing the oral kinase inhibitor (Gleevec) to interferon plus chemotherapy for newly diagnosed patients with CML is ongoing. It is possible that the payoff for years of research will be realized soon.

Polycythemia Vera

Polycythemia vera (PV) is a myeloproliferative disorder with excessive proliferation of red cells, megakaryocytes, and myelocytes. It is usually an insidious disease with gradual onset and can be associated with prolonged survival if the cytosis is controlled. Splenomegaly is common and is frequently one of the presenting features. The clinical course of PV can be quite varied. With uncontrolled proliferation of red cells and platelets, an increase in whole blood viscosity can occur, leading to impairment

of blood flow to critical organs. Central nervous system and cardiovascular symptoms, including confusion, angina, and claudication, can occur as a result of insufficient oxygen delivery. Thrombotic complications are a significant cause of morbidity and mortality, with strokes, myocardial infarctions, arterial occlusions, and thromboembolic complications being common. There is also an increased risk of hemorrhage.

The long-term course of PV can include distinct phases. Initially, an asymptomatic phase may be associated with only mild elevation of the red cell mass and mild splenomegaly; this gives way to an erythrocytic phase associated with pancytosis, with complications such as thrombosis and hemorrhage. An inactive phase may ensue in which no therapy is required to control the proliferative cells, and eventually a postpolycythemic myeloid metaplasia phase can develop with evidence of marrow fibrosis and extramedullary hematopoiesis. A significant percentage of patients with PV will culminate in acute nonlymphocytic leukemia. The ongoing management of patients during the erythrocytic phase affects the risks of developing this devastating outcome.

Although PV increases in incidence with advancing age, there is a wide range of ages, including some childhood cases. There is no known cause, and surprisingly there is no link to radiation exposure. In mice, the friend erythroleukemia virus causes a similar disease, but no viral infection has been found associated with PV in humans.

The diagnosis of PV rests on a combination of clinical and laboratory findings. The polycythemia study group established the diagnostic criteria shown in Table 38.1. The most important step is to confirm that the red cell mass is actually increased using chromium-51 red cell labeling and a plasma volume study. In many patients with apparently elevated hematocrit, the red cell mass is normal and the plasma volume is below normal or reduced, giving a spuriously increased hematocrit without true polycythemia; this effect can be seen in

TABLE 38.1. Criteria for diagnosis of polycythemia vera.[a]

Category A
  (1) Significantly elevated red cell mass
  (2) Arterial blood oxygen saturation ≥92%
  (3) Splenomegaly

Category B
  (1) Thrombocytosis >400,000 μL
  (2) Leukocytosis >12,000 μL
  (3) Increased leukocyte alkaline phosphatase score in absence of fever or infection
  (4) Serum vitamin B_{12} level greater than 900 pg/mL or vitamin B_{12}-binding capacity greater than 2200 pg/mL

[a] Diagnosis of polycythemia vera if A1 + A2 + A3 or A1 + A2 + any two factors from category B.

patients on a diuretic or patients known to have spurious erythrocytosis.

Once the red cell mass is confirmed to be elevated, other primary causes must be evaluated. Hypoxia either from lung disease or as a result of an abnormal hemoglobin variant, as well as erythropoietin-producing renal tumors, needs to be evaluated. The leukocyte alkaline phosphatase score is frequently elevated as opposed to the situation in CML.

Treatment for the patient with PV needs to be individualized. Phlebotomy can reduce the hematocrit quickly. However, in elderly patients, one has to be careful to avoid inducing significant hemodynamic changes that could further compromise the circulation. Very few patients are managed with phlebotomy alone.

The PV study group evaluated three common treatments: phlebotomy, ^{32}P, and chlorambucil. None of these treatments was without shortcomings.[12] Patients who were managed with phlebotomy alone had a significantly increased risk of thrombotic complications, which appears to be independent of the level of hematocrit or platelet count. Patients treated with ^{32}P or chlorambucil had a markedly increased risk of developing acute leukemia. Hydroxyurea has emerged as a primary option for many patients. It is well tolerated, and, although not devoid of mutagenic risks, it appears to have significantly less risk than alkylating therapy for the development of acute leukemia.

The goal of therapy should be to maintain the hematocrit in the range of 42% to 45%. There is a direct relationship between the level of hematocrit and the risk of vascular occlusive episodes. Other goals of therapy include control of the frequently associated pruritis with histamine antagonists. Elective surgical procedures should be delayed until counts have been controlled for at least 2 months to reduce the risk of hemorrhage or thrombosis. Aspirin and other antiplatelet agents have not been proven to reduce the risk of thrombotic events and may, in fact, increase the risk of hemorrhage and are not routinely recommended. The prognosis for patients with controlled PV is excellent as compared with the other hematologic malignancies. Long-term survival is common.

Future directions for patients with polycythemia vera include the use of interferon-alpha. In early studies, it appears to be active in reducing the red cell mass and platelet counts.[13] Although side effects of interferon continue to limit its use in older patients, it can be useful in patients with extreme thrombocytosis.

Essential Thrombocythemia

Essential thrombocythemia (ET) is a myeloproliferative disorder defined as a persistent isolated platelet count above 600,000/mL. It is frequently accompanied by a marked increase in megakaryocytes in the bone marrow, and on physical examination splenomegaly is common. Patients frequently develop complications with both thrombosis and hemorrhage.

The exact incidence of ET is unknown, although it is not a rare disorder. There is no known etiology. The major clinical manifestations are related to the elevated platelet count, resulting in either hemorrhagic or thrombotic episodes. Elderly patients can be particularly prone to these additional thrombohemorrhagic complications because of other comorbid conditions. The platelets in patients with ET are qualitatively abnormal, and this may explain why the frequency of thrombohemorrhagic complications is not directly related to the absolute number of circulating platelets.

The diagnosis is made on the basis of a sustained and unexplianed increase in the platelet count. It is important to distinguish primary thrombocythemia from reactive thrombocytosis, as well as to consider the possibility of another myeloproliferative disorder associated with an elevated platelet count. Some of the important causes of secondary thrombocytosis that should be considered in a differential diagnosis include iron deficiency anemia, occult carcinoma, chronic inflammatory conditions such as rheumatoid arthritis and inflammatory bowel disease, and acute or chronic infections. Treatment for patients who have reactive thrombocytosis should be directed at the underlying etiology regardless of the platelet count because these patients rarely develop thrombohemorrhagic complications despite markedly elevated platelet counts.

Treatment

The treatment of ET is usually with hydroxyurea, and the goal is to control the platelet count to around 500,000/mL. The important point is that many patients can be observed without therapy until the platelet count approaches 1 million. Older patients may need to be treated somewhat earlier because of their otherwise increased risk for thrombohemorrhagic complications. Previous studies using busulfan and ^{32}P have demonstrated increased toxicities, and these therapies are no longer standard for ET. The prognosis is similar to that of PV, with prolonged survival possible. Hemorrhage or thrombotic complications frequently contribute to morbidity and mortality. Some patients will evolve to myelofibrosis or acute leukemia.

Future Directions

The new antiplatelet agent anagrelide can inhibit platelet aggregation and platelet production. Interferon-alpha has some activity in this disorder. Combinations of these agents, with or without hydroxyurea, may represent an improvement in the management of patients with ET.

Carefully controlled trials are needed to assess these issues.

Myeloid Metaplasia with Myelofibrosis (MMMF)

MMMF is an unusual clonal disorder sometimes also known as idiopathic myelofibrosis. Gradual fibrosis of the marrow space with extramedullary hematopoiesis is the typical course. Splenomegaly is common. An examination of the peripheral blood film shows the presence of nucleated red blood cells and teardrop forms that are the characteristic leukoerythroblastic findings. The incidence of MMMF is unknown, but it tends to be a disease of the elderly, with an average age of approximately 60 years.

The malignant transformation appears to occur at the level of the stem cells, with a dense collagen fibrosis developing in the marrow space. There is no known etiology. The clinical manifestations relate to either the presence of splenomegaly or the consequences of anemia or other cytopenia. Rarely, sites of extramedullary hematopoiesis appearing in the pulmonary, gastrointestinal, central nervous, or genitourinary systems have been the presenting finding for occult MMMF.

As noted, the peripheral blood smear typically shows teardrop poikilocytes, confirming the leukoerythroblastic blood picture. Nucleated red blood cells and immature myeloid elements are also frequently seen. There are variable effects on circulating white cells and platelets. The diagnosis is made on the basis of the characteristic clinical findings and the presence of fibrotic marrow, which can be more accurately assessed histologically with the aid of a reticulin stain. Many conditions can lead to secondary fibrosis of the marrow, including lymphoma, carcinoma, and chronic diseases such as TB and histoplasmosis, as well as some of the other myeloproliferative syndromes as previously mentioned, and these need to be ruled out before a primary diagnosis is made.

Therapy for MMMF is unsatisfactory. In general, a conservative management strategy is adopted, although some authors have suggested that chemotherapy early in the course of disease can be beneficial. Symptomatic patients generally require symptom-directed therapy. Thus, anemia is treated with transfusion, as well as complete evaluation for other coexistent disorders such as nutrient deficiencies. Androgen stimulation is also frequently used.

Symptoms of splenomegaly, such as early satiety, are treated with measures to induce reduction in splenic size. Chemotherapy with hydroxyurea, ^{32}P, and other agents has been used with some, at least short-term, success. Interferon has been used successfully to shrink splenomegaly but has frequently resulted in worsened cytopenias. Splenic radiation has also been used, but usually a short duration of response is seen. Splenectomy is a controversial issue.[14] It is indicated for patients with severe thrombocytopenia, uncontrolled hemolysis, or painful splenomegaly that is refractory to other methods of control. However, there is a significant perioperative mortality rate. The prognosis for MMMF is worse than that for essential thrombocythemia and polycythemia vera. Average survival is approximately 5 years.

Lymphoproliferative Disorders

Chronic Lymphocytic Leukemia

Chronic lymphocytic leukemia (CLL) is the most common form of leukemia in the United States. This prevalence is due to two factors. First, the incidence of CLL rises with advancing age with the median age in the sixties. As noted previously, the population over the age of 60 continues to grow. Second, patients with CLL can experience a long survival, with median survival approaching 6 years. Thus, the prevalence of the disease is quite high.

CLL is generally a neoplasm of activated B lymphocytes. The leukemic cell morphologically resembles mature small lymphocytes normally seen in the peripheral blood. A sustained blood lymphocyte count that is greater than $10 \times 10^3/\text{mL}$ has been required to diagnose CLL. Additionally, 30% of nucleated cells in the bone marrow should be lymphocytes, and the peripheral blood lymphocytes should be positive for B-cell markers. In some clinical situations, CLL can be diagnosed with fewer total lymphocytes if surface markers confirms a monoclonal population of typical lymphocytes.

The exact cell of origin in CLL is unknown. Although 95% of patients have a B-cell phenotype, T-cell CLL can rarely occur. The typical B-cell CLL does stain positive with antibody to CD5, which is normally a T-cell antigen, and this has been taken to imply that the malignant cell is arrested at an intermediate stage of B-cell differentiation. Other diseases, such as hairy cell leukemia, to be considered later, are thought to result from the malignant transformation of a lymphocyte at a different stage of development.

The etiology of CLL is also unknown. Retroviruses and ionizing radiation, which lead to other forms of leukemia, apparently do not increase the risk for CLL. Interestingly, the incidence of CLL is far less in Japan than in Western populations. In addition, there is an increased risk of a variety of autoimmune disorders in relatives of patients with CLL, implying a genetic predisposition to the development of lymphocytic disorders.[15]

The lymphocytes in CLL usually express a specific surface immunoglobulin, although at low intensity. Normal control of antibody production in patients with

TABLE 38.2. Staging systems for chronic lymphocytic leukemia (CLL).

	Rai	Binet	Expected median survival (years)
Lymphocytosis	O	A	8–10
Lymphadenopathy	I	BI[a]	5–6
Hepatomegaly/splenomegaly	II	BII	5–6
Anemia	III	C	2.5
Thrombocytopenia	IV	C	2.5

[a] Three or more groups of lymph nodes must be positive.

CLL is disrupted. There is a marked reduction in normal antibody production manifested as a diffuse hypogammaglobulinemia, resulting in a high incidence of infections. On the other hand, there is a paradoxical increase in autoimmune complications, including hemolytic anemias. This dysregulation is an exaggeration of the phenomena seen in normal aging.

The diagnosis and staging of CLL has produced two excellent classification systems, one by Binet and one by Rai. Recently, these two staging systems have been combined and are represented in Table 38.2, along with the expected median survivals. There are a few points worth making regarding the stage of CLL at the time of diagnosis.

Approximately 25% of patients present with only a lymphocytosis in the peripheral blood and the marrow but no evidence of lymphadenopathy, organomegaly, or other cytopenias. These patients have an exceedingly good prognosis and in general should not undergo any therapy unless their disease progresses. The development of multiple enlarged lymph nodes, hepatomegaly, or splenomegaly mark progression to stage B disease. The development of either anemia or thrombocytopenia on the basis of marrow compromise portends a significantly worse prognosis.

The treatment of CLL has, in general, been aimed at controlling the disease rather than curing it. Therapy is withheld until significant cytopenias or symptomatic lymphadenopathy or organomegaly develops. In general, treatment is initiated with an alkylating agent. Most frequently chlorambucil is used, in either low daily doses or pulses from 2 to 4 weeks. Fludarabine is an active agent for the treatment of CLL. It produces a higher rate of complete remissions and a longer duration of response than chlorambucil.[16] This agent has response rates of 50% to 80% in both previously untreated as well as treated patients. Overall survival is not improved, and because fludarabine is associated with increased toxicity, especially for older patients with renal impairment, many clinicians use it only after failure of chlorambucil. Other alkylating agents such as cyclophosphamide are also effective. Prednisone is usually given with the alkylating agent and sometimes alone for patients with manifestations of autoimmune phenomena.

Unfortunately, the course of CLL is progressive despite initiation of therapy. Several attempts have been made to predict the course of patients with CLL more accurately than the current staging system. At least two criteria appear to suggest rapid progression of disease. The rate of increase of blood lymphocytes has long been recognized to be a useful indicator of prognosis. Most authors recommend a period of observation before initiating cytotoxic therapy in an effort to evaluate the pace of the disease. A doubling of lymphocytes in the peripheral blood in less than 1 year is associated with a worse prognosis. Investigators have also reported that the pattern of bone marrow infiltration with lymphocytes is prognostic. Patients with a diffuse lymphocytic infiltration have more rapid progression of their disease than patients with nodular involvement of the bone marrow.

Future Direction

Recently, there has been renewed interest in immunotherapy of CLL. Recombinant monoclonal antibodies have demonstrated activity against this disease. Campath 1-H is approved for patients with CLL who have failed fludarabine. This modified antibody recognizes the CD-52 antigen on the surface of CLL lymphocytes and can initiate antibody-dependent cell-mediated cytotoxicity (ADCC), as well as activate the complement cascade causing death of CLL cells.[17] There is a considerable infusion-related reaction with the drug, and patients can be immunosupressed because of the resultant lymphopenia resulting in reactivation of latent CMV. Nonetheless, this new avenue of attack may prove quite beneficial to elderly patients.

Supportive therapy is very important for patients with CLL because of the many associated clinical phenomena. Autoimmune phenomena, such as anemia or thrombocytopenia, can be treated with a steroid alone without cytotoxic therapy. Pure red cell aplasia, which occasionally occurs, may respond to either cyclosporin or antithymocyte globulin (ATG). Recurrent infections with encapsulated organisms frequently result from the hypogammaglobulinemia that occurs in these patients. The mainstay of therapy is prompt initiation of appropriate antibiotics. However, intermittent intravenous gamma globulin can be effective in reducing the frequency of infections, especially in those patients with very low levels of serum immunoglobulin G (IgG).[18]

Hairy Cell Leukemia

Hairy cell leukemia is another chronic lymphoproliferative disorder that is now known to be a clinical entity distinct from CLL. Similar to CLL, it is a proliferation of neoplastic B lymphocytes. Hairy cell leukemia cells also expresses the receptor for interleukin 2 known as CD-25; this suggests that the arrest in differentiation for these lymphocytes occurs later than that for CLL but earlier than that of the lymphocytes in myeloma.

Most patients with hairy cell leukemia present with pancytopenia. Circulating hairy cells are seen in approximately 90% of the cases. The typical hairy cell is a large lymphocyte with an eccentric nucleus, and the cytoplasm typically has fine irregular projections. The tartaric acid-resistant acid phosphatase (TRAP) stain, although not specific, is usually positive because of increased levels of an isoenzyme in these cells. The majority of patients present with complications of cytopenia, and 80% will have splenomegaly.

Treatment

Therapy for hairy cell leukemia has undergone a rapid change over the last few years. In fact, the hematologist is now confronted with choosing from more than one highly effective therapy. Historically, initial therapy was splenectomy. This intervention usually improved the cytopenias but only provided transient benefits. Subsequently, interferon-alpha demonstrated significant activity with a response rate of close to 80%.[19] Some patients (about 10%) achieved complete responses. Once interferon was stopped, relapses were common, but frequently patients would respond to another course of treatment with interferon.

Most recently, deoxycoformycin and chlorodeoxyadenosine (2-CDA) have demonstrated remarkable activity.[20] Deoxycoformycin appears to be active even in those patients who fail interferon, whereas 2-CDA has an extremely high complete response rate and, in fact, may be curative after a single course of therapy.

With such impressive therapy, the indications for initiation of therapy have been reevaluated. In general, up to 20% of patients with hairy cell leukemia have a very indolent form of the disease and may never require therapy. It is important to spare these patients the potential morbidity of treatment. The indications to consider therapy include significant cytopenias, repeated infections, massive or painful splenomegaly or lymphadenopathy, or vasculitis. Close observation for those patients without these indications is warranted.

Plasma Cell Dyscrasias

The lymphoproliferative disorders are malignant transformations of lymphocytes. The clinical syndromes corresponding to each diagnostic category result from the characteristic behavior of the transformed cell. The end stage of B-lymphocyte development is the plasma cell producing large amounts of immunoglobulin. The malignant transformation of cells with this degree of differentiation represents a group of diseases termed the plasma cell dyscrasias or plasma cell proliferative disorders.

A spectrum of clinical conditions exists from monoclonal gammopathy of uncertain significance to multiple myeloma, Waldenstrom's macroglobulinemia, and amyloidosis. However, it is the production of immunoglobulin by a plasma cell that ties these diseases together.

Normal B-cell development involves production of one of the five classes of immunoglobulins. The earliest event in B-cell development involves rearrangement of the germline immunoglobulin genes to produce a unique immunoglobulin. Ultimately, a specific immunoglobulin of the IgM class is made. Subsequently, the cell is able to alter the class of immunoglobulin (IgG, -A, -D, -E) while retaining the unique antigenic recognition sites. Each clone of cells produces only one immunoglobulin with one heavy chain (G, A, M, E, D) and one light chain (kappa, lambda). Protein electrophoresis and immunoelectrophoresis can detect the production and secretion of these immunoglobulins or their components (a light chain or heavy chain). The abnormal accumulation of monoclonal immunoglobulin in the serum is frequently called an M spike and is usually one of the early clues to the diagnosis of plasma cell dyscrasias.

Monoclonal Gammopathy of Uncertain Significance

Monoclonal gammopathy of uncertain significance (MGUS) is a relatively common condition that increases in older patients. The definition of monoclonal gammopathy of uncertain significance is somewhat problematic. In essence, it represents the presence of an M spike without an underlying diagnosis of multiple myeloma, Waldenstrom's macroglobulinemia, or amyloidosis. Formerly known as benign monoclonal gammopathy, it is no longer called this because a significant proportion of patients ultimately will develop one of the aforementioned diseases. In this way, it can be considered one step in the multistep pathway to oncogenesis.

MGUS is defined as having an M spike of IgG less than 3.5 g/dL or IgA less than 2 g/dL or the presence of a small amount of urinary light chain in the urine in 24 h. The plasma cells in the marrow cannot exceed 10%, and there can be no lytic bone lesion or other symptoms related to a lymphoproliferative disorder. Finally, a stable level of monoclonal protein characterizes MGUS. MGUS is common and, like myeloma, shows an increasing incidence with advancing age. As many as 10% to 14% of those over the age of 70 may have a detectable M spike.[21]

The course of monoclonal gammopathy has been well characterized by the Mayo Clinic Group. They followed 241 patients for a median of 19 years and found that only

24% of them had a stable or "benign" monoclonal gammopathy; 22% of them developed myeloma, macroglobulinemia, or amyloidosis, and 51% died of unrelated causes. Only 3% of the patients had a progressive rise of their M protein without the development of an underlying disorder.[22]

The evaluation of a patient who has been found to have an M spike should be aimed at discovering a potential underlying lymphoproliferative disorder. In a report of more than 800 cases of monoclonal protein seen at a referral center during 1988, 64% were related to MGUS, with myeloma, amyloid, lymphoma, Waldenstrom's macroglobulinemia, and CLL accounting for the remainder.[23] However, it should be remembered that the incidence of MGUS far exceeds the incidence of myeloma in the general population. This referral population is markedly enriched for patients with documented lymphoproliferative disorders.

A complete history and physical examination, routine CBC, electrolytes, and renal function with a serum calcium and uric acid should be obtained. Quantitative immunoglobulin, a 24-h urine for electrophoresis, and total skeletal x-rays may be required to evaluate the significance of a monoclonal gammopathy. A bone marrow aspirate and biopsy or a biopsy of a single soft tissue mass or lytic bone lesion may also be required.

In the absence of identifying an underlying lymphoproliferative disorder, the patient should be diagnosed with MGUS. Follow-up electrophoresis in 3 to 6 months and then yearly should be adequate for those patients who show no progression in their M spike. Patients who have an M protein in the urine should be followed more closely.

Multiple Myeloma

Multiple myeloma is a common malignancy with about 12,000 cases each year in the United States and 9000 deaths. The incidence of the disease increases dramatically with advancing age. The incidence is approximately 2 per 100,000 under the age of 50, but 20 to 25 per 1000,000 of those in the seventies. The mean age of diagnosis is in the upper sixties. Given the increase in the geriatric population in the United States, we should continue to see an increasing incidence of multiple myeloma.

The etiology of myeloma is unknown, but there are genetic as well as environmental factors. Controversy exists regarding the role of viral factors in the development of myeloma. Specifically, human herpesvirus 8 (HHV-8) has been associated with some patients with myeloma. The disease occurs more frequently in blacks than whites and more frequently in males than in females. Radiation exposure, as well as occupational exposure to asbestos and petroleum products, is associated with increased risk for the development of myeloma. Multiple myeloma can evolve from a monoclonal gammopathy of uncertain significance (MGUS).

The cell of origin in multiple myeloma remains unknown. Plasma cells themselves have little proliferative potential. It is likely that clonogenic pre-B cells account for the majority of proliferation in multiple myeloma. Thus, it is at the level of the pre-B cell or earlier that the transformation to malignancy occurs.

Karyotypic alteration is frequently seen in myeloma, with 30% to 50% of patients having abnormalities of their chromosomes. Oncogenes and tumor suppressor gene abnormalities, such as *ras*, *myc*, *bcl*-1/PRAD-1/cyclin D-1, *bcl*-2, Rb, and P53, have recently been implicated in the development of myeloma. The low proliferative potential of plasma cells has hampered the elucidation of genetic events in this disease.

Clinically, the manifestations of the disease are usually caused by one or a combination of the following factors: (1) proliferation of the malignant clone causing replacement of normal structures; (2) elaboration of cytokines by the malignant plasma cells; and (3) accumulation of the M component in plasma and in tissue.

The most common findings include fatigue, anemia, renal failure, hypercalcemia, hypogammaglobulinemia, and infections. Rarely, hyperviscosity or complications of amyloid infiltration of tissues can occur. The diagnosis of multiple myeloma requires a significant M spike (3.5 g/dL of IgG or 2.0 g/dL of IgA), plasmacytosis greater than 30% in the marrow, or plasmacytoma on tissue biopsy. Additionally, the presence of lytic bone lesions or low residual immunoglobulins can provide supportive evidence in the diagnosis of myeloma.

Pathophysiology

We now understand the pathophysiology of many of the characteristic clinical manifestations of multiple myeloma. Skeletal complications occur quite commonly. Because the lesions are typically osteoclastic with minimal osteoclastic activity, bone scans are typically negative. Plain x-ray and magnetic resonance imaging (MRI) of the bone are more sensitive than a bone scan.

The excessive bone resorption that occurs has been the subject of much research. The plasma cells in the marrow secrete tumor necrosis factor (TNF) and interleukin 1 (IL-1), among other cytokines. These cytokines contain most of the activity previously referred to as osteoclast-activating factor (OAF). Further, the TNF and IL-1 secreted by the plasma cells stimulate secretion of IL-6 by marrow stromal cells. IL-6 not only adds to the osteoclastic activity but also is one of the major growth factors for the myeloma cell clone. A cascade of bone resorption and myeloma cell growth with continued secretion of cytokines can quickly result in clinical hypercalcemia.

The hypercalcemia associated with multiple myeloma usually is multifactorial, with increased bone turnover, dehydration commonly found in the elderly, and renal insufficiency all playing a role. Inactivity secondary to debilitation or bone pain also adds to the progression of hypercalcemia.

The anemia of multiple myeloma is also a multifactorial process. The major influence, however, remains the proliferation of the myeloma cell clone within the bone marrow. Renal insufficiency, chemotherapy, and shortened red cell survival also play a role. Renal insufficiency in the setting of myeloma is a bad prognostic indicator. Monoclonal light chains (known as Bence–Jones proteinuria) accounts for more than 90% of the renal dysfunction. However, amyloid, infection, Fanconi's syndrome, and hyperuricemia can be other mechanisms for renal insufficiency.

Hypogammaglobulinemia is common and frequently results in recurrent infection by encapsulated organisms. Amyloid may develop in the setting of myeloma, with light chain deposition in susceptible organs. Hyperviscosity typically occurs in the setting of IgM production but can occur with very high levels of IgG or IgA. Transfusion in the setting of subclinical hyperviscosity can precipitate symptomatic hyperviscosity because the increased hematocrit after transfusion can adversely affect the whole blood viscosity.

Staging

The Durie and Salmon staging system combines easily obtainable clinical parameters and divides patients into three groups with significantly different expected survival (Table 38.3). More recently, additional prognostic factors have been evaluated. Of these, beta-2-microglobulin and plasma cell labeling index appear to be useful individual parameters. Overall, the median survival is 2 to 3 years with treatment.

Treatment

Treatment for myeloma has shown marked improvements over the last several years, but cure remains elusive. In the 1960s, melphalan and prednisone were first used and improved survival from about 7 months to the current level of about 3 years.

Multiple regimens combining alkylating agents, nitrosourea, doxorubicin, vincristine, and prednisone, as well as interferon, have been studied over the last 15 years. An overview analysis comparing melphalan/prednisone versus several other combination chemotherapy (CCT) regimens demonstrated there was no improvement in overall survival for those patients who received the CCT regimen.[24]

Although melphalan/prednisone remains an option, particularly for the majority of patients who are over the

TABLE 38.3. Durie and Salmon staging system for multiple myeloma.

Stage	Criteria	Survival (months)
I	All the following:	
	1. Hemoglobin >10 g/dL	
	2. Serum calcium <12 mg/dL	
	3. Normal bones or single plasmacytoma	46
	4. Low M component:	
	a. IgG <5 g/dL	
	b. IgA <3 g/dL	
	c. Urinary M component: <4 g/24 h	
II	Neither stage I nor III	32
III	At least one of following:	
	1. Hemolobin <8.5 g/dL	23
	2. Serum calcium >12 g/dL	
	3. Advanced bone disease	
	4. High M component:	
	a. IgG >7 g/dL	
	b. IgA >5 g/dL	32
	c. Urinary M component: >12 g/24 h	11

Subclassification: A, serum creatinine <2.0 mg/dl; B, serum creatinine >2.0 mg/dl.

age of 65, high-dose therapy with bone marrow transplantation has been explored for younger patients as well as older patients with good performance status. A randomized study confirmed a survival advantage for those patients who underwent bone marrow transplant compared to those patients who received multiagent chemotherapy.[25] Many of the patients who were over the age of 60 were unable to proceed on to their planned high-dose chemotherapy program. Nonetheless, a significant improvement in survival was noted with a dose-intense strategy.

The group in Arkansas has further explored the value of a high-dose strategy in older patients. In a separate report, among 49 patients over the age of 65 who underwent autotransplant for multiple myeloma, outcomes were identical to a matched-pair group of younger patients receiving the same therapy.[26] This finding suggests that age alone is not sufficient to deny a high-dose strategy to the patient with multiple myeloma. The group further explored the value of an intermediate dose of melphalan (100 mg) in patients over the age of 60 compared to an historic control group of matched patients who received melphalan and prednisone. Overall survival was 56 months for the Mel 100 versus 48 months for MP. These studies suggest that every patient needs to be evaluated for a high-dose strategy regardless of the age of the patient.

Although high-dose strategies can improve duration of survival, they do not appear to induce a high rate of long-term control. Thus, relapses continue to be a problem both for the patients treated with standard dose chemotherapy as well as for those who have been through a high-dose program. For patients who either develop resistance or are refractory to melphalan/prednisone, there are a variety of therapeutic choices. However, response rates are on the order of 25% to 30%. Pulse high-dose steroids appear to be as effective as more toxic combination regimens.

Recently, enthusiasm has been generated for the use of thalidomide in patients with myeloma. The initial reports suggested that as many as 30% of patients who had failed high-dose chemotherapy programs would have a significant response to the use of oral thalidomide.[27] Multiple reports have confirmed significant activity of this compound. Continued clinical trials are evaluating the optimal role of thalidomide with consideration for both upfront therapy as well as therapy of relapsed disease. Combinations of thalidomide with dexamethasone appear to be particularly active even in patients who had failed dexamethasone regimens previously.[28]

Resistance to chemotherapy that frequently develops in the setting of myeloma is caused by multiple mechanisms. One important mechanism is expression of the multidrug resistance (MDR) gene product. The MDR acts as an energy-dependent pump that can remove cytotoxic agents from the cytoplasm. This pump also transports other substances, such as cyclosporin. Trials have aimed at providing a molecule that will be transported by the pump and allow increased concentrations of cytotoxic agents to accumulate in the cell. Attempts at reversing the MDR phenotype have been promising in patients previously resistant to therapy.[29] Overcoming resistance to treatment may be a valuable therapeutic tool in the future.

The typical response to therapy is the achievement of a plateau phase where the level of tumor, as reflected by the M spike, remains stable. Further therapy during this period has been termed maintenance, and many studies have attempted to evaluate the role of maintenance therapy. The most promising agent for maintenance therapy has been interferon. Studies have produced mixed results, but, for some patients who have a significant reduction in the M spike level, interferon given three times per week may prolong a stable plateau phase. The side effects of interferon include a flu-like syndrome, and this can be very bothersome for elderly patients. Newly available pegylated interferon may generate more enthusiasm for maintenance because this formulation is more convenient and has fewer side effects.

Future Direction

Thalidomide has been the most encouraging new drug to become available for the treatment of patients with myeloma. Optimal use of this drug continues to be explored. Unfortunately, it does not seem to induce a high rate of complete remission or to induce cures. Likewise, high-dose therapy with bone marrow transplant support has not been able to induce elimination of the malignant clone in most patients and has only been applied to older patients with excellent performance status.

Increased understanding of the biology of the disease, highlighted by the important role played by IL-6, has prompted studies aimed at interrupting the IL-6 cytokine loop with a variety of strategies. Although the initial reports were promising, this therapy has not produced a significant impact. Immunotherapy continues to be attractive. Several reports have demonstrated the feasibility of idiotype vaccine development in patients with myeloma. While the studies are early in development, they may prove particularly useful for older patients.

Supportive care measures have improved for patients with multiple myeloma. The anemia associated with multiple myeloma, although multifactorial, frequently responds to erythropoietin.[30] The skeletal complications, including hypercalcemia, can be impacted on with bisphosphonates. These agents act as analogues of pyrophosphatases and are incorporated into the hydroxyapatite, subsequently inhibiting osteoclastic bone resorption. These compounds may exert some outright antimyeloma activity. Newer, more potent, and more convienient formulations of bisphosponates will be available soon. Last, bacterial infection is a major cause of morbidity and mortality. Prompt recognition and initiation of appropriate antibiotics are required. Intravenous gamma globulin may be helpful, although expensive.

Waldenstrom's Macroglobulinemia

This disorder also involves a proliferation of neoplastic B cells, which produce an M protein of the IgM class. The disease is similar to other lymphocytic malignancies, with a median age of approximately 63 years. It is an uncommon disease, with an incidence of approximately one-tenth that of myeloma.

Clinically, the manifestations of the disease are frequently the result of the very high viscosity resulting from an increased level of IgM in the plasma. Visual changes, neurologic symptoms, congestive heart failure, and recurrent infections frequently occur. Bone pain and lytic lesions are rare in macroglobulinemia. Hepatosplenomegaly and lymphadenopathy are common. Retinal hemorrhaging and vascular segmentation (sausage links) are characteristic. A chronic demyelinating polyneuropathy can be seen in 10% of the patients.

The serum protein electrophoresis demonstrates a protein peak of gamma mobility (IgM), and frequently a monoclonal light chain is present in the urine. The bone marrow demonstrates extensive infiltration with so-called plasmacytoid lymphocytes. In one series, the measured serum viscosity related well with development of symptoms; six of eight patients with a serum viscosity higher than 5 cp (normal is 1.8 or lower) had symptoms, whereas no patients had symptoms if viscosity was below 3 cp.[31]

The prognosis for patients with Waldenstrom's macroglobulinemia can be quite variable. About one-third of patients will die of unrelated causes and one-third will die of infectious complications. The remainder will die of complications of their illness including the conversion to a higher-grade lymphoma, conversion to AML, renal failure, or other complications.

Treatment

Treatment for complications of the M protein, including hyperviscosity, cryoglobulin, or peripheral neuropathy, should be a course of plasmapheresis. The emergent treatment of symptomatic hyperviscosity is effected with plasmapheresis. It is recommended that daily plasma exchanges of 3 to 4 L occur until the patient is asymptomatic.

Reducing further M protein excretion by the lymphocytic clone requires cytotoxic chemotherapy. Chlorambucil is the most frequently used alkylating agent for Waldenstrom's macroglobulinemia. However, regimens similar to those used for myeloma are also successful. Recently, nucleoside analogues 2-CDA and fludarabine have produced a significant number of responses for untreated patients (80% response rate), as well as those patients refractory to standard alkylating agent therapy.

Amyloidosis

Amyloidosis is a group of disorders of varying etiology. The consistent pathologic event is the deposition of a characteristic insoluble protein in tissues and structures causing organ impairment. The most susceptible organs are the kidney, gastrointestinal tract, myocardium, and peripheral nerve. Amyloid is detectable by tissue biopsies where the characteristic apple-green fluorescence using the Congo red stain is seen. Rectal biopsies or subcutaneous fat biopsies have 80% to 90% sensitivity in confirming the presence of amyloid.

Primary amyloid is generally considered among the plasma cell dyscrasias, although an extremely low order of plasma cell proliferation is noted. Primary amyloid, or so-called AL amyloid. results from the deposition of immunoglobulin light chain in the susceptible organs. Secondary amyloid, also known as the AA type, is derived from "serum amyloid precursor protein" and is not associated with immunoglobulins. Secondary amyloid is associated with chronic conditions such as rheumatoid arthritis or chronic infections such as tuberculosis (TB).

Therapy for primary AL amyloid is generally directed at the presumed underlying lymphoproliferative cellular elements. Thus, melphalan and prednisone have been used most frequently. Unfortunately, response to therapy is difficult to follow because the total body burden of amyloid is unmeasurable.

In several studies from the Mayo Clinic, there appears to be an improvement in survival for those patients who take melphalan/prednisone versus placebo or colchicine.[32] However, the studies have been complicated by design flaws and small numbers of patients. Most responses have been seen in patients with predominately renal, splenic, or hepatic involvement. The management of organ dysfunction remains important. Once patients develop symptomatic congestive heart failure, survival is poor. Those patients who have only a peripheral neuropathy have a median survival of more than 5 years.

Based on the success of high-dose strategies with the treatment of myeloma, high-dose strategies are also being applied to patients with amyloidosis. The initial results suggest that in selected patients there may be substantial benefit to this strategy.

Malignant Lymphomas

The malignant lymphomas are a group of lymphoproliferative disorders that are usually divided into Hodgkin's disease and the non-Hodgkin's lymphomas. These two disease entities have markedly different clinical characteristics. For instance, Hodgkin's lymphomas commonly occur as localized areas of lymph node enlargement. They tend to spread to contiguous lymph node groups and do not commonly involve extranodal sites of disease. Further, they are cured in more than 75% of the cases. Non-Hodgkin's lymphomas tend to be disseminated at presentation, will spread in a discontinuous fashion, and frequently involve extranodal areas. Further, the cure rates remain in the 30% to 40% range. The cell of origin in the non-Hodgkin's lymphomas is usually a B cell but occasionally a T cell. The cell of origin in Hodgkin's disease remains unknown.

An experienced hematopathologist is required to distinguish some forms of non-Hodgkin's lymphoma from Hodgkin's disease. However, the importance of the subclassification of the non-Hodgkin's lymphomas is critical, as is detailed later.

Non-Hodgkin's Lymphomas

The non-Hodgkin's lymphomas occur commonly. There are more than 40,000 new cases of non-Hodgkin's lymphoma each year in the United States. Recently, it has become clear that there is an increasing incidence of the non-Hodgkin's lymphomas. There are several components to this increasing incidence. First, non-Hodgkin's lymphomas occur more frequently in the elderly, and as the elderly population has increased in the United States, so has the incidence of NHL. However, the rates of non-Hodgkin's lymphomas seem to be going up for all age groups, with the largest increase occurring in the elderly. HIV infections account for a proportion of the increase but in general has added only to the incidence in young single males. The possibility of environmental exposures such as chemicals, pesticides, solvents, and infectious etiologies adding to the increased incidence of lymphoma needs to be considered.[33]

There is no clear etiology of the non-Hodgkin's lymphomas. However, there are several known factors that increase the risk. Chief among these are immunodeficient states, either acquired, iatrogenic, or genetic. Concomitant Epstein–Barr virus (EBV) infection appears to markedly increase the risk of non-Hodgkin's lymphoma in immunosuppressed populations. Environmental factors as noted may be involved, and several viruses are closely associated with development of non-Hodgkin's lymphoma. EBV is strongly associated with the development of Burkitt lymphomas in Africa (but not in the United States). The human T-cell leukemia virus 1 (HTLV-1) has been associated with adult T-cell leukemia–lymphoma. The hepatitis C virus has been linked to a variety of B-cell malignancies, including indolent lymphomas and cryoglobulinemia. Bacterial infections seem to play a role in some non-Hodgkin's lymphomas. For example, not only is the *Helicobacter pylori* infection associated with the development of gastric mucosal-associated lymphoid tissue (MALT) lymphoma, but its eradication through antibiotic therapy leads to tumor regression in a majority of cases.

A host of genetic alterations have been reported in the non-Hodgkin's lymphomas.[34] One example of a translocation seen frequently in follicular lymphomas is the t(14:18) translocation. When this occurs, the gene for *bcl-2* is juxtaposed to the immunoglobulin heavy chain locus with subsequent overexpression of *bcl-2*, which is normally involved in control of programmed cell death or apoptosis. The process of planned death of a cell, known as apoptosis, is an important mechanism for maintaining homeostasis in all organisms. Prevention of apoptosis provides a survival advantage to the clone of cells. The increased levels of *bcl-2* prevent the programmed death of the cell from occurring. This translocation appears to be present in at least 85% of follicular lymphomas.

Classification

The classification of the non-Hodgkin's lymphomas can be confusing and has been controversial. Multiple classification systems have been introduced and used over the past 40 to 50 years. The various classification schemes differ in their primary guiding principles of classification from cell morphology, to cell lineage and differentiation, to clinical response to treatment and survival. Over time, as advances in immunophenotyping and molecular genetics have been made, classification based primarily on a single guiding principle has proven inadequate, failing to recognize many distinct, clinically relevant disease entities. This realization led to the introduction of the Revised European-American Classification of Lymphoid Neoplasms (REAL) by the International Lymphoma Study Group in 1994. This classification scheme attempts to include immunophenotype, genetic information, morphology, and clinical features in defining a specific disease entity. Nonetheless, for the purposes of treatment and development of new therapies for the non-Hodgkin's lymphomas, many clinicians find it useful to distinguish those diseases with a more indolent natural history from those with a more aggressive course.

The indolent lymphomas frequently present with few symptoms but disseminated disease. Survival is quite long, but there is no known curative therapy. Aggressive lymphomas frequently present with more localized disease and can be cured with multiagent chemotherapy, even in advanced stages.

Clinical Manifestations and Treatment

The indolent lymphomas, which make up 20% to 40% of all the non-Hodgkin's lymphomas, tend to occur with advancing age. The median age is approximately 50 to 60 years. The majority of patients have advanced-stage disease, and bone marrow involvement is common. The t(14:18) translocation is seen in most patients with follicular lymphomas. Fevers, sweats, and weight loss (B symptoms) are uncommon.

The staging evaluation of indolent lymphomas is not as critical as in the aggressive lymphomas or in Hodgkin's disease. Typically, physical examination, routine laboratory tests, chest x-ray, computed tomography (CT) scans, and bone marrow biopsy provide sufficient information to evaluate prognosis and plan of treatment.

Physicians treating indolent lymphomas must recognize that although these diseases are slow to progress and frequently respond to chemotherapy, they are as yet incurable. The median survival approaches 7 to 8 years. However, ultimately the disease progresses and frequently transforms to a more aggressive lymphoma.

The goals of therapy are generally palliative. Rarely, a patient with localized disease can obtain long-term remission with involved field radiation. For the majority of patients who present with advanced-stage disease, there is a wide range of treatment options. Most studies have shown no survival benefit for early treatment, and, in fact, a watch-and-wait approach may be optimal for many patients. However, in these circumstances patients should be monitored closely to prevent complications such as renal failure secondary to ureteral obstruction. In reported series when watchful waiting is applied to a cohort of patients, overall survival is equivalent to those treated at presentation. The median time to instituting therapy is 2 to 3 years.[35] This strategy may be particularly appropriate for older individuals with significant comorbidities that might further adversely affect therapy.

Other treatment strategies, including immediate chemotherapy or aggressive chemotherapy, have also been attempted. Cyclophosphamide and chlorambucil have been used alone, with response rates in the 50% to 80% range. Cyclophosphamide, vincristine, and prednisone frequently have been combined, showing higher response rates. Nonetheless, a continuous relapse pattern is observed. When more aggressive chemotherapy is used, such as the CHOP regimen containing cyclophosphamide, hydroxydaunomycin, Oncovin (vincristine), and prednisone, a higher percentage of responses and complete responses is seen. However, it does not appear to change the rate of recurrence. The purine analogues such as fludarabine have shown activity in indolent lymphomas alone and in combination. Fludarabine, when combined with mitoxantrone, has demonstrated significant response rates.

As an alternative to chemotherapy, the option of monoclonal antibody therapy for indolent, B-cell non-Hodgkin's lymphoma has become available. The human–mouse chimeric anti-CD20 monoclonal antibody, rituximab, was initially shown to be effective in the setting of recurrent indolent lymphoma, with a response rate of 48% and a favorable toxicity profile.[36] The median time to progression for those responding was approximately 1 year. More recently, rituximab has been studied as initial therapy for indolent lymphoma and has shown high levels of activity, mild toxicity, and excellent progression-free survival.[37] Rituximab's activity as a single agent, in addition to its favorable toxicity profile and specifically the lack of significant hematologic toxicity, has led to the investigation of its use in combination with conventional chemotherapy. Czuczman et al. have reported an overall response rate of 95% and a complete response rate of 55% in patients with indolent B-cell lymphomas treated with a combination of CHOP and rituximab.[38] The study suggests additive activity with the combination without a significant increase in toxicity, which may be particularly pertinent for some elderly patients who have a limited ability to tolerate more toxic therapies. Interestingly, the *bcl-2* t(14:18) translocation could not be detected in the follicular lymphoma patients who demonstrated a complete response.

The indolent lymphomas tend to be radiosensitive, and frequently symptomatic areas of adenopathy can be treated with palliative radiotherapy. This sensitivity to radiation has also been utilized through radiolabeled monoclonal antibodies. Anti-CD20 monoclonal antibodies radiolabeled with yttrium-90 or iodine-131 have shown superior CR and overall response rates to those of rituximab alone in trials looking at recurrent or refractory indolent lymphomas. Toxicity is greater when compared with rituximab, with the primary toxicity being myelosuppression.

The aggressive lymphomas tend to present with diffuse adenopathy but rarely involve the bone marrow. When the bone marrow is involved, there is a high correlation with involvement of the central nervous system, and this portends a bad prognosis. Extranodal sites such as the gastrointestinal tract are frequent areas of origin of the intermediate-grade lymphomas. They are predominantly B-cell, although as many as 20% of them may be T-cell immunophenotype, which has identical behavior.

The prognosis for patients with aggressive lymphoma has improved markedly with the advent of multiagent chemotherapy, as is detailed here. Nonetheless, many patients do not either obtain or maintain a complete remission (CR). The prognostic factors that predict the likelihood of response have recently been more fully characterized.[39]

Age remains an important prognostic factor. Patients under the age of 60 have a significantly better prognosis than those patients over the age of 60. Serum levels of lactate dehydrogenase (LDH), performance status, and stage of disease, as well as the number of extranodal sites, are also important prognostic factors, as detailed in the international index recently reported.[39] Other important parameters of prognosis include the rapidity of response, usually measured as the time to achieve a CR. Those patients who achieve a CR quickly (fewer than three to four cycles of therapy) have an improved long-term survival compared with those patients who have not achieved a CR by this time. There appears to be a significant dose–response relationship in the treatment of these lymphomas. Patients who receive dose-reduced therapy appear to achieve CR less frequently and relapse from CR more frequently than those who receive full-dose therapy.

The dose intensity of therapy has been studied specifically in the elderly. The Southwest Oncology group studied CHOP chemotherapy in elderly patients.[40] There were several interesting results of this study. The rate of complete response was 65% in those under 40 years of age and 37% in those 65 years and older. The median survival for the younger group was 101 months but only 16 months in the older group. This protocol called for initial dose reduction for patients 60 years of age and older; however, some patients received full doses of chemotherapy in violation of the protocol. When these patients were examined separately, the rates of CR and survival were markedly better than those receiving reduced doses of chemotherapy. This finding suggests that full doses of chemotherapy are important in elderly patients as well as in younger patients. Toxicity, however, remains a major problem.

Other investigators have sought to develop regimens specifically for the elderly. In one prospective, randomized, phase III trial, CHOP was compared to CNOP (cyclophosphamide, mitoxantrone, vincristine, and prednisone) in patients 60 years of age and older with aggressive lymphomas. CHOP was found to be superior in achieving complete responses in 49% versus 31% in the CNOP group. Three-year survival was also superior in the CHOP group, and toxicity was comparable.[41]

Rituximab therapy in elderly patients with aggressive lymphomas has been studied with some promising results. In a recent report, previously untreated patients aged 60 to 80, with aggressive B-cell lymphomas, were treated with a combination of CHOP plus rituximab versus CHOP therapy alone. At 1 year, the combination of CHOP plus rituximab was found to demonstrate superior overall survival and event-free survival as compared with CHOP alone, with comparable toxicity.[42]

In general, it would appear that, for elderly patients with aggressive lymphoma who have good performance status and normal organ function, attempting full-dose chemotherapy with a curative intent seems reasonable. Patients with poor performance status or impaired cardiopulmonary or renal reserves are unlikely to tolerate these aggressive therapies without significant morbidity. There may also be a role for hematopoietic growth factors in mitigating hematologic toxicity for elderly patients. The physician needs to balance the risks and benefits of these aggressive regimens.

For patients who do not achieve a CR or who relapse from CR, the overall prognosis is poor. Several aggressive regimens are available for the treatment of relapsed and refractory lymphoma, and high-dose therapy with bone marrow transplant support has also been used. In general, elderly patients are unlikely to significantly benefit from these aggressive interventions. Continued effort to define optimal initial treatment regimens that may be curative for elderly patients seems warranted.

Hodgkin's Disease

As noted previously, Hodgkin's disease is a group of disorders with a characteristic clinical course. The early studies by Henry Kaplan defined the typical pattern of spread of Hodgkin's disease. As opposed to the non-Hodgkin's lymphomas, Hodgkin's disease tends to spread to contiguous lymph node groups. Thus, intricate staging at the time of diagnosis is critical for developing a plan of treatment. The incidence of Hodgkin's disease demonstrates a bimodal age-specific pattern. There is an early peak between the ages of 20 and 30. Some have suggested that there is an infectious etiology for this form of Hodgkin's disease as there is increasing risk for Hodgkin's disease with higher socioeconomic status. The later peak, occurring about age 50, is not related to socioeconomic status. There are many reasons to think that the etiology of the early peak of Hodgkin's diseases is different from the etiology of the cases that occur in elderly individuals.

Classification and Clinical Presentation

All forms of Hodgkin's disease have demonstrable Reed–Sternberg cells, which are large binucleated cells with prominent nucleoli, and although not pathognomic for Hodgkin's disease these are typical. The debate regarding the origin of this cell continues. There are four subtypes of Hodgkin's disease. In decreasing frequency, they are nodular sclerosing, mixed cellularity, lymphocyte predominant, and lymphocyte depleted.

Most patients present with an enlarged lymph node; however, there is some difference in the clinical presentation from older to younger patients. Older patients are more likely to have systemic symptoms and abdominal disease, especially bulky abdominal disease. The most common histologic pattern in all age groups is nodular sclerosing, but it appears from a multitude of studies that with advancing age there is decreasing nodular sclerosis and increasing mixed cellularity.

The clinical presentation of Hodgkin's disease as noted is typically with adenopathy, with more than 70% of people presenting with palpable lymph node enlargement. Rarely, the lymph nodes become painful after consumption of alcoholic beverages. As many as a third of patients will develop so-called B symptoms with fevers, night sweats, and weight loss of more than 10% of body weight. Other symptoms such as fatigue, weakness, and pruritus occur commonly but are not officially considered B symptoms. Presence of true B symptoms has adverse prognostic implications.

Staging

An important point to differentiate between the Hodgkin's lymphomas and the non-Hodgkin's lymphomas is the relative importance of histologic classification and staging. The treatment plan for Hodgkin's disease is critically dependent on accurate staging, whereas the histologic subtype is less important. Conversely, in the non-Hodgkin's lymphomas, the histologic subtype is the critically important determinant of therapy, and, while staging is important, it is not as critically important as in Hodgkin's disease.

The Ann Arbor classification is the most commonly used staging system for Hodgkin's disease (Table 38.4). The suffix E represents the presence of extralymphatic involvement with disease, and the suffix A or B denotes

TABLE 38.4. Ann Arbor staging system for Hodgkin's disease.

Stage	Involved lymph nodes	Extralymphatic organ
I	One region (I)	Or localized involvement of single site (Ie)
II	Two or more regions on same side of diaphragm (II)	With localized involvement of one site (IIe)
III	Regions on both sides of diaphragm (III)	With localized involvement of one site (IIIe) or spleen (IIIs)
IV		Diffuse or disseminated involvement of one or more organs (liver, bone marrow)

Subdesignations: A, asymptomatic; B, fever, sweats, weight loss; CS, clinical staging; PS, pathologic staging (usually laparotomy).

presence or absence of B symptoms, as noted in the previous section.

The optimal staging procedures for Hodgkin's disease continue to be an area of debate. Given that therapy is dependent on stage, accurate staging is essential. CT scans of the chest, abdomen, and pelvis can accurately search for enlarged lymph nodes. Bone marrow biopsy should also be obtained. Routine laboratory studies, including liver and renal function, uric acid level, and the erythrocyte sedimentation rate (ESR), are useful. Specialized staging studies for patients with otherwise localized disease are important. A lymphangiogram to evaluate periaortic and iliac abnormalities is better than CT scans at detecting normal-size lymph nodes that are involved with Hodgkin's disease.[43] Staging laparotomy and splenectomy at one time were a standard intervention for all patients with stage I, II, or III Hodgkin's disease. However, this continues to be evaluated, and clearly those patients who will be receiving chemotherapy for other indications should be spared laparotomy and splenectomy. Gallium scan is useful both at the initial diagnosis and in follow-up of patients. It is recommended that it be obtained before initiating therapy to determine if the lymphoma is gallium uptake positive because treatment with chemotherapy can produce false-negative results in the gallium scan.

Treatment

Hodgkin's disease is a curable malignancy, and treatment should be initiated with curative intent. Both radiotherapy and combination chemotherapy can cure Hodgkin's disease. The choice of therapy modality is dependent on the stage of disease. Localized disease (stage IA, IIA, IB, and IIB) is typically treated with radiotherapy. Abbreviated courses of chemotherapy before radiation treatment may improve outcome in early-stage Hodgkin's disease.

The principles of radiation treatment were established by Henry Kaplan. Although doses less than 4000 centigray (cGy) were effective in inducing responses, 4000 centigray was required for curative therapy. Because of the typical contiguous pattern of spread of Hodgkin's disease, radiation treatment ports could be devised to cover all known involved regions of disease plus one additional nodal group. Using current radio-

therapy, patients with localized disease (stage IA and IIA) have a cure rate greater than 80%. B symptoms reduce the cure rate to approximately 70%.

More advanced disease requires combination chemotherapy. DeVita developed the regime MOPP [nitrogen mustard, Oncovin (vincristine), procarbazine, and prednisone] and for the first time demonstrated long-term disease-free survival for patients with advanced-stage Hodgkin's disease. Over the past 20 years, attempts at refining MOPP therapy have concentrated on improving the response rates, as well as limiting toxicity. Most recently, ABVD (adriamycin, bleomycin, velban, and dexamethasone) has been shown to be more effective than MOPP, with less toxicity.[44] Hybrid regimens combining MOPP and ABVD are also an improvement over MOPP alone. Toxicity from chemotherapy includes acute side effects such as bone marrow suppression and a high incidence of sterility. Secondary malignancies, including leukemia and solid tumors, have been recognized as a late toxicity from these therapies.

Using both chemotherapy and radiotherapy together has been referred to as combined modality therapy. The rationale for combined modality therapy in advanced-stage Hodgkin's disease rests with documentation that recurrence frequently occurs in the site of previous bulk adenopathy. Thus, in retrospective studies, radiotherapy to areas of previous bulk disease once chemotherapy has been completed has been associated with improved survival rates. Nonetheless, no randomized trial has demonstrated superior results with combined modality therapy. There is concern regarding increased toxicity when combining chemotherapy and radiotherapy. Despite the controversy, patients with bulky mediastinal adenopathy are routinely treated with combined modality therapy because they fare less well with single modality therapy. As mentioned earlier, there is support for combined treatment for early-stage disease as well.

Salvage

Patients who relapse with Hodgkin's disease need to be accurately restaged. The prognosis for those who never achieved a CR or relapse within 12 months of obtaining a CR is significantly worse than for those who remain in complete remission for a significant duration of time. Patients who relapse after curative radiotherapy should be treated with chemotherapy and have a high likelihood of response and long-term disease-free survival. Patients who relapse with localized disease after chemotherapy can be treated with salvage radiotherapy. For those patients relapsing in less than 12 months, a salvage regimen that is noncross-resistant with their induction regimen should be considered. High-dose therapy with autologous or allogenic bone marrow support can also be considered for younger patients. There is little evidence that older patients can undergo these aggressive regimens.

Prognosis and Survival

Many studies have evaluated the prognostic factors associated with surviving Hodgkin's disease. Increasing age is a poor prognostic factor. Different investigators have used different age cutoffs, but typically survival worsens for patients over the age of about 40 to 50. In the recent study reported by Canellos et al., 5-year survival for patients under the age of 40 was 80%; for those 40 to 60, it was was 63%; and for those over 60 survival was 31%.[45]

It has been suggested that the inability to tolerate chemotherapy has been a factor in the poor prognosis for elderly patients. Although this may be true, other factors may also play a role in the worse outcome for elderly patients. Given the different epidemiologic phenomena and the response to therapy for this age group, patients over the age of 60 with Hodgkin's disease probably have a different disease from younger patients.[45] Other prognostic factors, including bulky disease, high LDH, and extranodal site involvement, may be as important as age.

Summary

The hematologic malignancies are a diverse group of disorders that vary in clinical severity and response to treatment. Some are compatible with a long life expectancy, and others can produce a fulminant course rapidly leading to death. Treatment strategies generally result in significant morbidity, and for elderly patients with comorbid conditions, a careful analysis of options, including no treatment, is appropriate. Supportive care is improving, and elderly patients should benefit from improved understanding of the biology of many of these diseases. Molecularly targeted and immunologically targeted treatment may improve the ratio of benefit to toxicity for older patients.

Reference

1. Perti A, Kantarjin HM. Management of adult acute lymphocytic leukemia: present issues and key challenges. *J Clin Oncol.* 1994;12:1312–1322.

2. Hoelzer DF. Therapy of the newly diagnosed adult with acute lymphoblastic leukemia. *Hematol Oncol Clin N Am.* 1993;7:139–160.

3. Mayer RJ, Davis RB, Schiffer CA, et al. Intensive postremission chemotherapy in adults with acute myeloid leukemia. Cancer and Leukemia Group B. *N Engl J Med.* 1994; 331(14):896–903.

4. Larson RA, Dodge RK, Linker CA, et al. A randomized controlled trial of filgrastim during remission induction and consolidation chemotherapy for adults with acute lymphoblastic leukemia: CALGB study 9111. *Blood.* 1998; 92(5):1556–1564.

5. Appelbaum FR, Baer MR, Carabasi MH, et al. National Comprehensive Cancer Network. NCCN Practice Guidelines for Acute Myelogenous Leukemia. *Oncology (Hunting).* 2000;14(11A):53–61.

6. Tallman MS, Rowe JM. Acute promyelocytic leukemia: a paradigm for differentiation therapy with retinoic acid. *Blood Rev.* 1994;8:70–78.

7. Harris NL, Jaffe ES, Diebold J, et al. World Health Organization classification of neoplastic diseases of the hematopoietic and lymphoid tissues: report of the Clinical Advisory Committee meeting, Airlie House, Virginia, November 1997. *J Clin Oncol.* 1999;17(12):3835–3849.

8. Greenberg P, Cox C, Le Beau MM, et al. International scoring system for evaluating prognosis in myelodysplastic syndromes. *Blood.* 1997;89:2079.

9. Kantarjian HM, Deisseroth A, Kurzrock R, et al. Chronic myelogenous leukemia: a concise update. *Blood.* 1993;82: 691–703.

10. Tura S, Baccarani M, Zuffa E, et al. Interferon alpha-2a as compared with conventional chemotherapy for the treatment of chronic myeloid leukemia. *N Engl J Med.* 1994;330: 820–825.

11. Druker BJ, Sawyers CL, Kantarjian H, et al. Activity of a specific inhibitor of the BCR-ABL tyrosine kinase in the blast crisis of chronic myeloid leukemia and acute lymphoblastic leukemia with the Philadelphia chromosome. *N Engl J Med.* 2001;344(14):1038–1042.

12. Berk PD, Wasserman LR, Fruchtman SM, et al. Treatment of polycythemia vera: a summary of trials conducted by the Polycythemia Vera Study Group. In: Wasserman LR, Berk PD, Berlin NI, eds. *Polycythemia Vera and the Myeloproliferative Disorders.* Philadelphia: Saunders; 1995:166–194.

13. Sacchi S, Leoni P, Riccardi A, et al. A prospective comparison between treatment with phlebotomy alone and with interferon-alpha in patients with polycythemia vera. *Ann Hematol.* 1994;68:247–250.

14. Benblassat J, Gilon D, Penchas S. The choice between splenectomy and medical treatment in patients with advanced agnogenic myeloid metaplasia. *Am J Hematol.* 1990;33:128–135.

15. Oscier DG. Cytogenetic and molecular abnormalities in chronic lymphocytic leukemia. *Blood Rev.* 1994;8:88–97.

16. Rai KR, Peterson BL, Appelbaum FR, et al. Fludarabine compared with chlorambucil as primary therapy for chronic lymphocytic leukemia. *N Engl J Med.* 2000;343(24):1750–1757.

17. Flynn JM, Byrd JC. Campath-1H monoclonal antibody therapy. *Curr Opin Oncol.* 2000;12(6):574–581.

18. Cooperative Group for the Study of Immunoglobulin in Chronic Lymphocytic Leukemia. Intravenous immunoglobulin for the prevention of infection in chronic lymphocytic leukemia. A randomized controlled clinical trial. *N Engl J Med.* 1988;319:902.

19. Smalley RV, Conners J, Tuttle RL, et al. Splenectomy vs. alpha interferon: a randomized study in patients with previously untreated hairy cell leukemia. *Am J Hematol.* 1992; 41:13–18.

20. Saven A, Piro L. Newer purine analogues for the treatment of hairy-cell leukemia. *N Engl J Med.* 1994;330:691–697.

21. Crawford J, Eye MK, Cohen HJ. Evaluation of monoclonal gammopathies in the "well" elderly. *Am J Med.* 1987;82:39–45.

22. Kyle RA. Monoclonal gammopathy of undetermined significance. *Curr Top Microbiol Immunol.* 1996;210:375.

23. Kyle RA. Current concepts on monoclonal gammopathies. *Aust N Z J Med.* 1992;22:291–302.

24. Alexanian R, Dimopoulos M. The treatment of multiple myeloma. *N Engl J Med.* 1994;330:484–489.

25. Attal M, Harousseau JL, Stoppa AM, et al. A prospective, randomized trial of autologous bone marrow transplantation and chemotherapy in multiple myeloma. *N Engl J Med.* 1996;335:91–97.

26. Siegel DS, Desikan KR, Mehta J, et al. Age is not a prognostic variable with autotransplants for multiple myeloma. *Blood.* 1999;93:51–54.

27. Singhal S, Mehta J, Desikan R, et al. Antitumor activity of thalidmide in refractory multiple myeloma. *N Engl J Med.* 1999;341:1565–1571.

28. Rajkumar S, Fonseca R, Dispenzieri A, et al. Thalidomide in the treatment of relapsed mutliple myeloma. *Mayo Clin Proc.* 2000;75:897–901.

29. Sonneveld P, Durrie BGM, Lokhorst HM, et al. Modulation of multidrug-resistant multiple myeloma by cyclosporine. *Lancet.* 1992;340:255–259.

30. Ludwig H, Fritz E, Kotzmann H, et al. Erythropoietin treatment of anemia associated with multiple myeloma. *N Engl J Med.* 1990;322:1693–1699.

31. Crawford J, Cox EB, Cohen HJ, Evaluation of hyperviscosity in monoclonal gammopathies. *Am J Med.* 1985;79:13.

32. Gertz MA, Kyle RA, Greipp PR. Response rates and survival in primary systemic amyloidosis. *Blood.* 1991;77:257–262.

33. Weisenburger DD. Epidemiology of non-Hodgkin's lymphoma: recent findings regarding an emerging epidemic. *Ann Oncol.* 1994;5(suppl 1):19–24.

34. Gaidano G, Dalla-Favera R. Biologic and molecular characterization of non-Hodgkin's lymphoma. *Curr Opin Oncol.* 1993;5:776–784.

35. Young RC, Longo DL, Glatsein E, et al. The treatment of indolent lymphomas: watchful waiting vs. aggressive combined modality treatment. *Semin Hematol.* 1988;25:11.

36. McLaughlin P, Grillo-Lopez AJ, Link BK, et al. Rituximab chimeric anti-CD20 monoclonal antibody therapy for relapsed indolent lymphoma: half of patients respond to four dose treatment program. *J Clin Oncol.* 1998;16:2825–2833.

37. Hainsworth JD, Burris HA III, Morrissey LH, et al. Rituximab monoclonal antibody as initial systemic therapy for patients with low-grade non-Hodgkin's lymphoma. *Blood.* 2000;95:3052–3056.

38. Czuczman MS, Grillo-Lopez AJ, White CA, et al. Treatment of patients with low-grade B-cell lymphoma with the combination of chimeric anti-CD20 monoclonal antibody and CHOP chemotherapy. *J Clin Oncol.* 1999;17:268–276.

39. Shipp MA. Prognostic factors in aggressive non-Hodgkin's lymphoma: who has "high-risk" disease? *Blood.* 1994;83:1165–1173.

40. Dixon DO, Neilan B, Jones SE, et al. Effect of age on therapeutic outcome in advanced diffuse histiocytic lymphoma: the Southwest Oncology Group experience. *J Clin Oncol.* 1986;4:295–305.

41. Sonneveld P, de Ridder M, van der Lelie H, et al. Comparison of doxorubicin and mitoxantrone in the treatment of elderly patients with advanced diffuse non-Hodgkin's lymphoma using CHOP versus CNOP chemotherapy. *J Clin Oncol.* 1995;13:2530–2539.

42. Coiffier B, Lepage E, Herbrecht R, et al. Mabthera (Rituximab) plus CHOP is superior to CHOP alone in elderly patients with diffuse large B-cell lymphoma (DLCL): interim results of a randomized GELA trial. *Blood.* 2000; 96: abstract 950.

43. Kaufman D, Longo DL. Hodgkin's disease. *Clin Rev Oncol Hematol.* 1992;13:135–187.

44. Canellos GP, Anderson JR, Propert KJ, et al. Chemotherapy of advanced Hodgkin's disease with MOPP, ABVD, or MOPP alternating with ABVD. *N Engl J Med.* 1992;327:1478–1484.

45. Mir R, Anderson J, Strauchen J, et al. Hodgkin's disease in patients 60 years of age or older. *Cancer.* 1993;71:1857–1866.

Part V
Medical Care

Section B
Organ System Diseases and Disorders

39
Cardiovascular Disease

Nanette Kass Wenger

Thirteen percent of the U.S. population is currently 65 years or older, and about half of these 25 million people have cardiovascular disease. By the year 2030, 1 in 5 Americans will be older than 65 years, with the subset older than 85 years increasing most prominently in size. Data are limited regarding cardiovascular disease in the octogenarian and beyond, compromising optimal clinical care for such patients.[1]

Cardiovascular disease increases dramatically with aging and is the major cause of mortality and disability in elderly persons; 83% of all cardiovascular deaths in the United States occur in patients older than 65 years of age.[2] Cardiovascular disease is also a major contributor to the need for hospital, ambulatory, and custodial care. In 1987, two-thirds of the U.S. health care expenditures for cardiac disease (totaling $22.3 billion) was for patients older than age 65.[3] Elderly patients are intensive users of emergency medical services[4] and of medical services in general. However, because most elderly cardiovascular patients entering hospitals are discharged, the majority of elderly patients appear to benefit from active treatment rather than using the hospital for custodial care. The aim of ongoing care should be to return elderly patients to independent living in their home setting for so long as is reasonable. Coronary heart disease is the most prevalent cardiac problem, followed by hypertensive cardiovascular disease,[5] with valvular and pulmonary heart disease other important etiologies. Despite these statistics, the scarcity of scientific studies involving very elderly patients is striking. Age-based exclusions from most clinical trials limit the generalizability of data to the characteristically high-risk geriatric population. Review of databases can provide added information about efficacy and safety of interventions and identify priority areas for future study.[6] Cardiovascular disease at elderly age is additionally complicated by its frequent association with multiple other comorbid illnesses. Moreover, data from the Cardiovascular Health Study define a substantial decline in functional status between persons aged 75 to 84 years and those 85 years and older.[7] Physical disability independently predicted coronary mortality in the established populations for epidemiologic studies of the elderly (EPESE) cohort.[8]

Recent data suggest that the management and outcomes for most patients aged 65 to 75 years are comparable to their younger counterparts, but that cardiovascular diagnosis and therapy must be highly individualized beyond this age.

Cardiovascular Changes of Aging

The presentation of cardiovascular disease in elderly patients is complicated by its superimposition on the physiologic and structural cardiovascular changes of aging. These variables influence the response of elderly patients both to specific cardiac illnesses and to their therapies. Both the physiologic and the structural changes that occur in the cardiovascular system with aging decrease cardiac functional reserve capacity, limit the performance of physical activity, and lessen the ability to tolerate a variety of stresses, including cardiovascular disease.[9]

Maximal heart rate and maximal aerobic capacity decrease progressively with age,[10] independent of habitual physical activity status, owing in part to decreased catecholamine responsiveness. Although maximal oxygen uptake decreases with aging, the decline is less prominent than previously described when corrected for the decreased lean body mass of aging. Nonetheless, the maximal oxygen uptake of sedentary elderly individuals is 10% to 20% less than that of their physically active counterparts, with maximal work capacity comparably decreased. Peak exercise cardiac output and peak exercise ejection fraction also decrease at elderly age. Cardiac dilation, enabling an increase in stroke volume, compensates for the diminished heart rate response to maintain the increase in cardiac output required for exercise.

Aortic and large artery thickness and vascular stiffness increase with aging, with a resultant increase in arterial systolic pressure and impedance to left ventricular ejection. This increased afterload of aging is likely the stimulus for left ventricular hypertrophy, even in normotensive elderly persons. Both systolic blood pressure and mean blood pressure increase with aging with widening of the pulse pressure.

Aging changes in the heart also include the following features:[11] an altered geometric contour; a decrease in ventricular compliance with substantial reduction in the early diastolic filling rate, the diastolic dysfunction of aging, with increased dependence on the contribution of atrial contraction to late left ventricular filling to maintain cardiac output; a prolonged duration of myocardial contraction and relaxation times; and lessened chronotropic and inotropic responses to sympathetic (catecholamine) stimulation. Cardiac filling pressures at rest vary little with increasing age, but end-diastolic pressure with exercise is prominently greater as an adjustment to the decreased left ventricular distensibility. Combined with the increase in left ventricular mass, this places the aged heart at a mechanical disadvantage. Cardiac dilation with exercise (using the Frank–Starling mechanism) enables the ventricles to increase stroke volume and cardiac output; this differs from the exercise response at younger age, when an increase in heart rate effects the increase in exercise cardiac output.

Baroreceptor responsiveness decreases with aging, due in part to loss of vascular distensibility. Although consequences of postural hypotension, particularly falls, have been attributed to the sluggish baroreceptor reflex of aging, recent studies in community-dwelling elderly individuals show that they have preserved baroreceptor responsiveness.[12] Nevertheless, more than 18% of community-dwelling elderly individuals in the Cardiovascular Health Study[13] had orthostatic hypotension, with the prevalence increasing with increasing age.

The number of pacemaker cells in the sinoatrial (SA) node and number of bundle branch fibers decrease with age, with loss of SA pacemaker cells more pronounced.[14] The sick sinus syndrome is caused by loss of sinus node pacemaker cells and fatty infiltration around the sino-atrial node with aging. Atrioventricular block, intraventricular conduction delay, and bundle branch blocks may be caused by fibrosis and calcium deposition in the cardiac skeleton. These problems may be accentuated by drugs used to treat hypertension and coronary disease, such as beta-blockers and calcium antagonist drugs. The combination of atrial dilation and atrial fibrosis may underlie the increased prevalence of atrial arrhythmias.

Thickening of the aortic and mitral valve leaflets and the circumference of all four cardiac valves increase at elderly age. Collagen degeneration and secondary calcium deposition are common at elderly age; one-third of patients aged 70 and older have calcium deposition in either the aortic or mitral valve.[15] Calcific degeneration is the major cause of aortic valve disease in elderly patients. Mitral annular calcification, appearing initially in the submitral position, also increases in frequency with age. Mean pulmonary artery pressures and pulmonary vascular resistance are also increased at elderly age.

These myriad changes require that the cardiovascular manifestations of aging be differentiated from those of disease.

Limitations of the History and Physical Examination in the Diagnosis of Cardiovascular Disease in Elderly Patients

Limitations in obtaining information from the clinical history include the potential altered mental acuity with aging; cognitive disturbances related to illness, medications, or effects of depression; or a combination of these features. The coexistence of multiple diseases also hinders the accurate evaluation of symptoms. Because these variables may obscure or complicate the patient's clinical history, confirmatory data often must be obtained from family members or medical records. Habitual activity levels differ substantially but often decrease with progressive aging, so that many symptoms do not retain their activity-precipitated characteristics.

Because orthostatic hypotension is common in elderly persons, it is essential to document the effect of postural change when measuring blood pressure. Disease and medications, rather than aging per se, account for the preponderance of postural hypotension. However, in frail elderly nursing home residents, orthostatic hypotension is often encountered postprandially and when first arising in the morning.[16] Reduced heart rate variability, a measure of cardiac autonomic function, predicted an increased mortality risk among the elderly cohort of the Framingham Heart Study.[17]

The increased vascular stiffness of aging causes the upstroke of the arterial pulse to appear more brisk than usual, potentially masking the slowly rising carotid pulse of aortic stenosis. Frequent findings in elderly individuals include the early-peaking basal systolic murmur of aortic sclerosis, typically accompanied by a fourth heart sound at the cardiac apex as evidence of reduced ventricular compliance. Aortic sclerosis, potentially as a marker for atherosclerosis, is associated with an approximate 50% increase in cardiovascular mortality risk and risk of myocardial infarction (MI).[18] Dilation of the ascending aorta as well as decreased aortic compliance may also produce basal systolic murmurs. Neither the S_4 nor the increased ventricular filling pressure reflect ventricular systolic dysfunction, whose counterpart is an S_3. S_2 may be single at elderly age or the inspiratory splitting may be less prominent. A combination of dorsal kyphosis, emphysema, or chest wall alterations may limit palpation of the apical impulse, even when left ventricular hypertrophy is present. Data from the Cardiovascular Heath Study suggest the importance of the ankle–arm index, a noninvasive assessment for peripheral arterial disease; a normal value is inversely related to the risk of cardiovascular disease.[17]

Importance of Noninvasive Diagnostic Tests and Their Limitations

Because of difficulties in obtaining a clinical history and in interpreting findings at physical examination, diagnostic tests assume greater importance. Noninvasive methods should initially be selected in that elderly patients are at increased risk for complications of most diagnostic procedures. However, many noninvasive tests have limitations unique to an elderly population.

Resting Electrocardiogram

About 50% of elderly individuals have abnormalities of the resting electrocardiogram (ECG). Aging changes in the cardiac conduction system and the age-related increase in left ventricular mass underlie the ECG changes, most commonly PR and QT interval prolongation, intraventricular conduction abnormalities, reduction in QRS complex and T-wave voltage, nonspecific ST-segment and T-wave changes, and a leftward shift of the frontal plane QRS axis. QT prolongation is more common in elderly women than elderly men.[19] QTc dispersion in the Rotterdam Study predicted cardiac mortality at an elderly age.[20] Both lung hyperinflation and dorsal kyphosis accentuate the diminution in QRS voltage, despite the increase in left ventricular mass. ECG criteria are unreliable for the detection of left ventricular hypertrophy at an elderly age.[21] These changes occur in addition to the arrhythmias described next. Elderly men more frequently have major electrocardiographic abnormalities than elderly women, and the prevalence of these abnormalities increases with older elderly age. Electrocardiographic evidence of myocardial infarction occurs far more frequently than reported in the clinical history.[22]

Long-Term (24-h) Ambulatory Electrocardiogram

The 24-h ambulatory electrocardiogram or use of an event recorder is the most useful diagnostic technique

TABLE 39.1. Ambulatory ECG findings in elderly subjects with no clinical heart disease.

Variable	Finding
Heart rate, beats/min	34–180
Longest sinus pauses, s	1.8–2
Supraventricular premature complexes (>20/h), %	66
Paroxysmal supraventricular tachycardia, %	13–28
Ventricular premature complexes (>10/h), %	32
Ventricular couplets, %	8–11
Ventricular tachycardia, %	2–4

Source: Modified from Marcus et al. ECG indicates electrocardiographic. Reprinted with permission from American College of Cardiology (*J Am Coll Cardiol.* 1987;10:67A–72A), with permission.

to identify symptomatic arrhythmias, particularly when diary evidence is available to correlate symptoms with these spontaneously occurring arrhythmias. The test is indicated to identify cardiac rhythm disturbances as etiologic of otherwise unexplained lightheadedness, dizziness, giddiness, falls, frank syncope, or uncomfortable palpitations. The limitation of utility of this study is the high prevalence of both supraventricular and ventricular arrhythmias in the absence of cardiac disease or cardiac symptoms, even arrhythmias as potentially serious as nonsustained ventricular tachycardia[23] (Table 39.1). Most asymptomatic arrhythmias in the absence of cardiac disease do not warrant therapy. Importantly, syncope may result from orthostatic hypotension, significant aortic stenosis, carotid sinus hypersensitivity, and age- and disease-related impairments of cerebral blood flow, as well as arrhythmias. Specific arrhythmia identification is needed to guide pharmacologic or pacemaker therapy.

The increase in both supraventricular and ventricular ectopic beats with aging is more likely a consequence of aging changes in the aorta and ventricles than of intrinsic abnormalities of the conduction system.

Echocardiogram

The echocardiogram is far more accurate than the chest roentgenogram in the assessment of cardiac chamber size because the kyphoscoliotic chest deformity and sternal depression common in elderly persons may cause a factitious increase in heart size on the chest roentgenogram. The echocardiogram is also more accurate for the determination of left ventricular hypertrophy, a powerful marker for coronary risk, than is the electrocardiogram; in addition to identifying left ventricular wall thickness and mass, cardiac chamber size, and valvular abnormalities, wall motion abnormalities and ventricular ejection fraction can be determined, as can pericardial effusion. However, a technically adequate echocardiogram cannot be recorded in some elderly patients because of their chest configuration.

Doppler echocardiography is reliable for determining the aortic valve area and estimating the pressure gradient in elderly patients with significant aortic stenosis; there is a good correlation of the calculated echocardiographic valve area with cardiac catheterization data.[24]

Dobutamine stress echocardiography to detect myocardial ischemia has not been systematically assessed in an elderly population.

Exercise Tests and Exercise Radionuclide Studies

Exercise testing can be undertaken with comparable safety and efficacy in elderly patients as in younger patients, that is, among elderly patients able to perform an adequate exercise test. Treadmill exercise testing in elderly individuals provided prognostic information incremental to clinical data.[25] A normal response to exercise testing has the same favorable prognosis as in a younger population, and an abnormal response to exercise imparts comparable risk as in younger individuals; the high predictive accuracy of an abnormal exercise test at elderly age reflects the high prevalence and severity of coronary heart disease in this population.[26] Few data are available regarding exercise testing in patients older than 75 years of age. Careful explanation of the test procedure, a practice session on the bicycle or treadmill before the actual test, meticulous skin preparation and electrode placement, and selection of an appropriately low-intensity exercise protocol increase the likelihood of a satisfactory exercise test. The Naughton protocol or a modification of the standard Bruce protocol is preferable for treadmill exercise testing of elderly patients with limited exercise capability. Arm ergometry can be considered for elderly patients who are unable to perform treadmill or bicycle exercise because of arthritis, claudication, or cerebrovascular or musculoskeletal disorders. The exercise test can help determine if the chest discomfort represents myocardial ischemia, can characterize risk status in the patient with angina pectoris or following myocardial infarction, can guide recommendations for a physical activity regimen, and can assess the suitability for return to work when appropriate.

Exercise thallium scintigraphy is helpful when conduction abnormalities or repolarization changes on the resting ECG limit the interpretation of the exercise ECG. The presence and extent of exercise-induced reversible thallium-201 or technetium-99m scintigraphic abnormalities permit effective risk stratification in elderly patients.[27,28] Exercise-induced evidence of cardiac dilation and abnormal radioisotope lung uptake indicate a high-risk status. Myocardial perfusion scintigraphy after intravenous administration of dipyridamole (Persantine) is well tolerated by aged patients and may help identify myocardial ischemia in elderly patients who are unable to exercise. The sensitivity, specificity, and safety appear comparable in populations older and younger than 70 years of age.[29]

Ventricular function can be assessed by radionuclide ventriculography; although it is more expensive than echocardiography, it is applicable to elderly patients in whom adequate echocardiographic images cannot be obtained. Contrast-enhanced computed tomography (CT), positron emission tomography (PET) scanning, and magnetic resonance imaging (MRI) require systematic study in elderly populations.

Because of the progressive nonuniformity of lung function with aging, perfusion defects may occur in the absence of pulmonary embolism, rendering this test somewhat less reliable in an elderly population. Spiral CT imaging appears valuable to identify pulmonary embolism.

Invasive Diagnostic Tests

Transesophageal echocardiography, used to evaluate for aortic dissection, infective endocarditis, and valvular heart disease, among others, appears well tolerated at elderly age.

Cardiovascular catheterization and coronary arteriography are also well tolerated in elderly patients. Precise diagnosis may enable more successful medical and surgical therapies. Procedure-related morbidity and mortality, although relatively infrequent, are increased two- to threefold at elderly age.[30,31] The number of coronary arteriograms performed annually on patients older than age 65 continues to escalate in the United States; arterial tortuosity increases the difficulty of the procedure.

Manifestations of Cardiovascular Disease

Heart Failure

Most of the 5 million patients with heart failure in the United States[32] are elderly, and heart failure is the most frequent hospital discharge diagnosis for patients older than 65 years of age.[33] Seventy-five percent of heart failure hospitalizations occur in individuals older than 65 years and 50% in patients 75 years and older. Heart failure is more common in men than in women until about age 80; an eightfold increase in heart failure among men in the seventh decade of life compared with the fifth decade was noted in the Framingham population.[34] In a Medicare cohort, one-third of patients died within 1 year of initial hospitalization for heart failure.[35] During the past two decades, heart failure deaths have almost doubled in the over-75 population. Most of the 400,000 new cases of heart failure diagnosed annually in the

United States are in the geriatric population. With the continuing dramatic increases in the size of the elderly population, comparable dramatic increases in heart failure incidence and prevalence can be anticipated. The prevalence of heart failure increases with increasing age and is estimated to involve 5% of the population aged 65 to 74 years and 10% of those older than 75 years.

Heart failure tends to be both underdiagnosed and overdiagnosed in elderly patients. Many elderly patients fail to report progressive easy fatigability, dyspnea, cough, and ankle edema, considering these a consequence of aging. Early manifestations of heart failure may be masked by the sedentary lifestyle of many elderly patients, whereas exertional dyspnea may reflect another common problem, chronic pulmonary disease, rather than cardiac failure. Deconditioning may also cause breathlessness. Pulmonary changes associated with aging may decrease exercise tolerance, even in the absence of heart failure. Basal lung rales and relatively large heart volumes, normal in an older population, may be mistakenly ascribed to heart failure. Owing to activity limitations, profound fatigue rather than exertional dyspnea may be the presenting feature. However, comparable fatigue, as well as exhaustion, confusion, and altered mentation, may result from excessive diuresis. Ankle edema may reflect venous stasis, decreased tissue turgor, or be a consequence of treatment with vasodilator drugs, rather than evidence for heart failure. On occasion, only anorexia, insomnia, nocturnal cough, or frequent nocturnal urination may herald heart failure. Many elderly patients with heart failure may have disordered mental function and behavior consequent to diminished cerebral blood flow.

Coronary atherosclerotic heart disease, hypertensive cardiovascular disease, and hemodynamically significant calcific aortic stenosis are the most prevalent causes. Mitral regurgitation is also contributory. Pooled data from hypertension trials in elderly patients showed a 52% reduction in incident heart failure with antihypertensive therapy.[36] Because of its high prevalence, occult coronary disease must be considered with otherwise unexplained systolic heart failure.[32] Cardiac amyloidosis increases in prevalence with aging; the initial diastolic dysfunction is often accompanied by arrhythmias and conduction disturbances. Heart failure is more frequently precipitated or exacerbated by associated medical problems than in younger patients. These problems include atrial fibrillation and other arrhythmias, acute myocardial infarction, uncontrolled hypertension, intercurrent infections and fever, fluid overload,[37] acute blood loss, pulmonary embolism, anemia, occult thyrotoxicosis, renal insufficiency, acute lower urinary tract obstruction in men, and major dietary indiscretions. Drugs causing myocardial depression (β-blocking drugs, calcium-blocking drugs, and a number of antiarrhythmic agents) and/or poor compliance with the medical regimen are also contributory. Frequent use of nonsteroidal inflammatory agents by elderly patients, often as nonprescription drugs, can precipitate heart failure by a combination of sodium and water retention and the induction of renal dysfunction. Iatrogenic heart disease, often related to inappropriate pharmacotherapy, in hospitalized frail elderly patients portends a poor prognosis.[37] Given the limited cardiac reserve and the frequent multifactorial etiology of heart failure in an elderly patient, remediable factors should be carefully identified and corrected. The occurrence of heart failure adversely affects the prognosis of most cardiovascular disorders and is an important contributor to the excessive mortality among elderly patients in the early months after myocardial infarction.

Echocardiography has substantially improved the recognition of heart failure in elderly patients and is the most useful noninvasive test to differentiate systolic and diastolic ventricular dysfunction.[38] Echocardiography is also useful in defining an otherwise inapparent cause of the heart failure; it can assess the characteristics of the heart valves, the size and function of the cardiac chambers, the presence of pericardial effusion, and focal wall motion abnormalities.

Although ventricular systolic dysfunction with cardiac enlargement is a frequent finding in elderly patients with heart failure, diastolic dysfunction is a prominent cause of heart failure in this population; this is the case in more than half of octogenarians with heart failure.[39] Among octogenarians, the predominant presentation of heart failure is in women with systolic hypertension and diastolic dysfunction with preserved ventricular systolic function. Clues to diastolic dysfunction as the mechanism for heart failure include a normal or near-normal heart size and a cause for left ventricular hypertrophy such as hypertension or hypertrophic cardiomyopathy. The characteristics of the aging heart and associated diabetes mellitus may impair ventricular diastolic distensibility. Ventricular diastolic dysfunction may be present in as many as half of all elderly patients with clinical manifestations of heart failure and has a more favorable prognosis than systolic dysfunction when correctly treated.[40] The earlier descriptions of adverse outcomes of diastolic heart failure may reflect suboptimal or inappropriate therapies.[41] About 40% of patients hospitalized with a diagnosis of heart failure have preserved ventricular systolic function, and this percentage increases dramatically at elderly age.

The decreased ventricular compliance of aging is an important contributor to age-related exertional dyspnea, even with exercise of low to moderate intensity. Decreased ventricular compliance results in elevated left atrial and pulmonary capillary pressures and may produce pulmonary congestion, pulmonary edema, and other classic manifestations of heart failure. Differentiation from predominant systolic dysfunction is important in that therapies differ markedly. Diuretic and venodilator drugs alone may reduce ventricular filling volume and potentiate diastolic dysfunction; in one study, withdrawal of furosemide improved postprandial hypotension in elderly patients with heart failure and intact ventricular systolic function.[42] The positive inotropic effect of digitalis may also be deleterious in diastolic dysfunction. Alleviation of heart failure symptoms in patients with ventricular diastolic dysfunction occurs with treatment with calcium channel-blocking drugs, beta-blocking drug, and angiotensin-converting enzyme (ACE) inhibitors.[43,44] With verapamil, diltiazem, and beta-blocking drugs, surveillance is needed for adverse effects, including slowing of atrioventricular conduction and serious bradyarrhythmias.

Patients with left ventricular systolic decompensation present with cardiac enlargement, tachycardia, gallop sounds, lung rales or pulmonary edema; dependent edema, jugular venous distension, hepatomegaly, and ascites occur when right-sided heart failure supervenes. Weight gain may be evident. The skin, particularly of the extremities, may be cool as a result of peripheral vasoconstriction. Restlessness and agitation are due, in part, to increased sympathetic activity; control of heart failure more effectively limits these symptoms than does sedation. Pulsus alternans and Cheyne–Stokes respiration are evidence for severe cardiac decompensation.

As in younger patients, the major components of therapy for ventricular systolic dysfunction include restriction of dietary sodium, activity limitation until compensation is achieved, digitalis, diuretic drugs, vasodilator drugs, beta-blocking drugs, and spironolactone. These agents improve cardiac function by decreasing the cardiac workload, limiting sodium and water retention, and enhancing myocardial contractility.

Vasodilator therapy, beta blockade, and spironolactone have improved the outlook for elderly patients with ventricular systolic dysfunction. Vasodilator drugs—ACE inhibitors, angiotensin receptor-blocking drugs, and hydralazine plus nitrates[45–48]—favorably alter the loading conditions of the heart, improve symptoms of reduced cardiac output, improve functional status, retard the spontaneous worsening of heart failure, and improve survival.

Some controlled clinical trials documenting the benefits of vasodilator therapy have included elderly patients.[45,49,50] In the Veterans Administration Cooperative Study of hydralazine and nitrates that randomized patients as old as 75 years,[51] comparable benefit occurred in patients older and younger than 60 years. ACE inhibitor benefit has also been demonstrated at very old age.[52] ACE inhibitors are superior to hydralazine plus nitrates,[47] which can be used for patients intolerant to ACE inhibitors. Although a pilot study[53] suggested superior survival benefit with angiotensin II receptor blockade with losartan compared with ACE inhibition with captopril at elderly age, this was not subsequently substantiated.[54] Comparable benefit of ACE inhibitor

therapy in improving exercise tolerance and left ventricular ejection fraction occurred in patients older and younger than 65 years. As in younger patients, ventricular ejection fraction correlates poorly with symptoms and with exercise tolerance in the elderly. Although experience with beta-blocking drugs in elderly patients is less extensive than at younger age, with trials excluding patients over age 75 to 80 years, both carvedilol and metoprolol given to patients with class II and III heart failure improved ventricular systolic function, exercise tolerance, and survival.[55–57] Spironolactone in patients up to age 80 with severe heart failure improved symptoms and prognosis.[58] These data suggest that newer therapies for heart failure should be applied to elderly patients, with careful attention to dose titration. However, these pharmacologic agents are currently underutilized in elderly patients hospitalized for heart failure.[59]

Digitalis improves myocardial contractility and remains an important component of management of ventricular systolic dysfunction, even when sinus rhythm is present;[60] digitalis may limit the ventricular response to supraventricular tachyarrhythmias. In the DIG Trial,[61] although survival was not altered, the combined endpoint of heart failure death or hospitalization was reduced in patients treated with digitalis. Lower doses are appropriate for elderly patients, such as 0.125 mg digoxin daily; because of the reduced glomerular filtration rate at elderly age that lessens drug excretion and because of the decrease in lean body mass, the volume in which digitalis is distributed, which causes an increase in plasma concentration. Dosage should be further reduced if quinidine, verapamil, or amiodarone are given concomitantly or if renal function is compromised. Digitalis overdosage should be suspected when confusion, bizarre behavior, altered mental status, fatigue, or anorexia occur, in addition to the usual nausea and vomiting. Digitalis given for heart failure precipitated by an acute problem that has resolved can be safely discontinued.

Common complications of excessive diuretic therapy include dehydration and electrolyte abnormalities that often are manifest as altered mental status, increased likelihood of digitalis toxicity, and orthostatic hypotension that may result in orthopedic complications. The expected reflex tachycardia response to hypotension and hypovolemia is delayed and decreased at elderly age because of attenuation of baroreceptor reflexes.

Sodium restriction improves diuresis and limits the resultant hypokalemia; however, major dietary alterations require assistance and encouragement in elderly patients. Difficulties with food purchasing and preparation, lack of interest in meals when eating alone, dental problems that impair chewing, and financial constraints often hamper dietary alterations. Preprocessed "convenience foods," which have high sodium content, are often a sizeable component of the diet of elderly individuals.

Although physical activity limitation is advisable when heart failure is decompensated, protracted immobilization predisposes to deep vein thrombosis and pulmonary embolism. When activity levels are increased after initial control of heart failure, the patient should be carefully observed for fatigue, breathlessness, edema, and weight gain as evidence of recurrent decompensation.

Deconditioning of skeletal muscles and impaired skeletal muscle vasodilator response to exercise result in a greater impairment of functional capacity in elderly than in younger patients with systolic heart failure. Resumption of a regular physical activity regimen is recommended once compensation is achieved;[38] functional capacity improves without apparent deterioration of ventricular function,[62] predominantly due to adaptations of the intact skeletal musculature. Improvement in functional capacity can decrease dependency and disability.[63] Functional capacity, as gauged by a 6-min walk test, is an independent marker of prognosis.[64]

Elderly patients with severe systolic dysfunction, particularly in association with atrial fibrillation, are candidates for oral anticoagulant therapy to limit thromboembolic complications.

Reversion of atrial fibrillation or atrial flutter to sinus rhythm can substantially augment the cardiac output and improve heart failure because of the importance of the atrial contribution to ventricular filling in the poorly compliant aged ventricle.

Because of the significant morbidity and mortality from cardiac failure at elderly age, patients require frequent and meticulous surveillance. An intensive multidisciplinary treatment strategy for heart failure involving specialized education, assessment, and management in a randomized clinical trial decreased readmissions and improved medication compliance. This approach has proved cost-effective in elderly populations by limiting rehospitalizations.[65,66] Intensive home care surveillance resulted in improved functional status.[67] Absence of emotional support was a strong independent predictor of fatal and nonfatal cardiovascular events after hospitalization in older women.[68]

Cardiac transplantation is uncommon in elderly patients but has been accomplished using older donor hearts. Rejection is less frequent, but the risk of infection and malignancy is higher in older than younger transplant patients.[69]

Arrhythmias and Conduction Abnormalities

Both arrhythmias and conduction abnormalities increase in prevalence with increasing age.[70–72] Reflecting age-related changes in specialized conducting tissue and in atrial and ventricular myocardium.[14]

Although arrhythmias may present as syncope or altered consciousness, many elderly patients have significant arrhythmias in the absence of these symptoms or of palpitations. Syncope may result from either tachyarrhythmias or bradyarrhythmias. Because of the age- and disease-related decreases in cerebral blood flow, a lesser severity of bradyarrhythmia or tachyarrhythmia than required in younger patients may cause an alteration of consciousness or true syncope at elderly age. Because syncope of cardiovascular origin entails an enormous 1-year mortality rate, 24%, identification of its mechanism is urgent to enable appropriate therapy; elderly patients with syncope of a noncardiac cause have a more favorable outlook, with their annual mortality approximating 3%.[73,74]

The prevalence of single supraventricular premature beats increases with aging. These beats are present in virtually all individuals older than 80 years of age, even in the absence of heart disease, are typically asymptomatic, and do not require treatment. There was no gender difference in the Cardiovascular Health Study.[75]

Atrial fibrillation also increases in prevalence with increasing age, being present in almost 10% of the population older than 80 years;[76] it is a major contributor to stroke in elderly patients, even in the absence of valvular disease.[77] Atrial fibrillation was present in 5% to 6% of patients in the Cardiovascular Health Study,[78] predominantly in association with cardiovascular disease. In this study,[78] a history of heart failure, valvular heart disease, or stroke; left atrial enlargement on echocardiogram; abnormal mitral or aortic valve function; treated hypertension, and advanced age all were independently associated with an increased prevalence of atrial fibrillation in community-dwelling elderly men and women. In the Framingham Heart Study,[79] atrial fibrillation was associated with an increased risk of mortality, more so for women than for men (odds ratio of 1.5 and 1.9, respectively). The major issues relate to rate control, cardioversion, and stroke prevention. Success of cardioversion, in a prospective study, was comparable for patients older and younger than age 65.[80]

Chronic atrial fibrillation is associated with an increased incidence of stroke that accelerates with age. Anticoagulation[81] can reduce stroke risk by almost 70%. Warfarin anticoagulation appears particularly warranted when atrial fibrillation is associated with heart failure.[82] Reduction in stroke and stroke mortality has been documented with warfarin treatment, even in patients older than 75 years so treated. However, elderly patients remain undertreated with warfarin based on clinical practice guidelines for atrial fibrillation.[83] Antiplatelet agents have not been effective in preventing stroke in elderly patients with nonvalvular atrial fibrillation.

Ambulatory electrocardiography in elderly persons who are presumably free of cardiac disease shows that ventricular arrhythmias are pervasive (see Table 39.1), including frequent multiform ventricular ectopic complexes (PVCs)[84] and nonsustained ventricular tachycardia (VT).[72] Asymptomatic ventricular arrhythmias do not impart excess risk in healthy elderly patients and rarely require treatment in the absence of significant myocardial ischemia or ventricular dysfunction. Ventricular arrhythmias on 24-h ambulatory ECG were more common in elderly men than elderly women in the Cardiovascular Health Study.[75] Nonsustained VT on 24-h ambulatory ECG in the Bronx Longitudinal Aging Study[84] independently predicted death and MI. Very frequent ventricular premature beats, in excess of 1000 per 2 h, signify a poor prognosis in very old people with coronary heart disease.[23]

Older age independently predicted increased ventricular arrhythmia following MI in the cardiac arrhythmia suppression trial (CAST) Registry.[85] Hourly PVCs increased from 0.4 in patients younger than 50 to 4.0 at 75 to 80 years, with VT prevalence increasing from 7.3% to 15.3% respectively. Electrophysiologic testing or signal-averaged ECGs offer little benefit in identifying high risk status in asymptomatic elderly patients with ventricular arrhythmias.[86]

Adverse antiarrhythmic drug reactions are more common in elderly patients due to their altered metabolic function and drug elimination, as well as to the frequent polypharmacy; antiarrhythmic drugs also are more likely to potentiate conduction abnormalities and ventricular dysfunction in an elderly population. In one study of antiarrhythmic drug therapy for asymptomatic complex ventricular arrhythmias in a geriatric population, the high incidence of adverse drug effects necessitated frequent discontinuation of therapy, and therapy did not improve survival, with or without ventricular systolic dysfunction.[87] Elderly patients with symptomatic, refractory life-threatening ventricular tachyarrhythmias tolerate electrophysiologic testing well; this procedure can identify patients who require drug therapy or surgical intervention including Coronary Artery Bypass Graft (CABG) surgery, endocardial resection, aneurysmectomy, or cardioverter-defibrillator implantation.[88] The pharmacologic management of supraventricular and ventricular arrhythmias is comparable in elderly and younger patients, except that lower doses of medication are usually indicated. Radiofrequency catheter ablation therapy is effective and safe to treat tachyarrhythmias at elderly age.[89,90]

Bradyarrhythmias, both the sick sinus syndrome and complete atrioventricular block, occur frequently in an elderly population; symptomatic bradyarrhythmias are the major indications for pacemaker implantation. Sick sinus syndrome does not generally require treatment in the absence of symptoms or extreme bradycardia. Digitalis and calcium- and β-blocking drugs, used to treat coronary disease and hypertension, may accentuate the bradycardia of the sick sinus syndrome; in elderly patients with the bradycardia-tachycardia subset of the sick sinus syndrome, pacemaker implantation may be required to permit pharmacologic treatment of the tachyarrhythmias with digitalis, β-blocking drugs, or calcium-blocking drugs.

Pacemaker implantation is appropriate at all ages, because pacemakers can improve symptoms and both the length and quality of life.[91] Currently the median patient age of pacemaker recipients in the United States is approximately 70 years, rendering the geriatric population the major beneficiary of this therapy. Before permanent pacing, more than half of all patients with complete atrioventricular block died within 2 years. Pacemaker implantation, even at an elderly age, entails minimal morbidity and mortality. Even in octogenarians and nonagenarians, normal relative survival occurred in those without other heart disease.[92] Coexisting heart disease and, in particular, preexisting heart failure adversely affect long-term survival.[92]

Although ventricular demand pacemakers remain the most common units in use, rate-responsive dual-chambered pacemakers have advantages in alert and active elderly patients with underlying sinus rhythm in that atrial contraction contributes importantly to ventricular function when ventricular compliance is abnormal, and that the cardiac rate is proportional to the activity need.[93] Disadvantages of these complex pacemakers are their higher cost and the increased skill of the physician needed for implantation and surveillance. However, dual-chamber pacemaker use in the Medicare national hospital database was associated with increased survival,[94] even after controlling for potentially confounding patient characteristics.

Pacing mode should be determined not by patient age but by the etiologic electrophysiologic problem. Sinus bradycardia is a common rhythm in elderly patients; when asymptomatic, it is not an indication for pacemaker implantation or other intervention. Similarly, asymptomatic complete atrioventricular block does not warrant pacing. A consensus guideline for indications for pacemaker implantation prepared by the American College of Cardiology/American Heart Association is equally appropriate for older and younger patients.[95] In elderly patients with limited mobility, transtelephonic pacemaker surveillance may be helpful.

Limited data are available about use of implantable cardioverter-defibrillators in elderly patients. Although these devices can be placed with minimal risk and are equally effective in preventing sudden death in older as in younger patients, nonsudden cardiac death was increased three times in one series of patients older than 75 years.[96]

A review of the success of cardiopulmonary resuscitation in elderly patients shows it to be less effective than in younger individuals. Characteristics associated with a favorable outcome include ventricular tachycardia or fibrillation as etiologic versus asystole or electromechanical dissociation and the symptom of chest pain versus that of dyspnea. Survival after cardiopulmonary resuscitation among elderly nursing home residents is extremely low.[97]

Atherosclerotic Coronary Heart Disease

Atherosclerotic coronary heart disease (CHD) is the most prevalent cardiac disease at elderly age, involving an estimated 3.6 million patients.[98] Coronary disease is responsible for more than two-thirds of all cardiac deaths among the elderly U.S. population, and morbidity and mortality from CHD increase progressively with age. In the United States, most patients with CHD, with new episodes of acute myocardial infarction, and with chronic heart failure secondary to CHD are older than 65 years of age.[99] About 60% of patients hospitalized in the United States for acute myocardial infarction are older than 65 years,[100] and the incidence of MI increases prominently with increasing older age.[101] Not only is coronary disease highly lethal at elderly age, but disability is prominent; 50% of men and 20% of women aged 55 to 64 years with CHD have activity limitation, versus 85% and 55%, respectively, at 75 years and older. Nevertheless, there is a wide variation in the severity of coronary illness and in the functional status of elderly coronary patients. The male preponderance among younger coronary patients lessens at elderly age and gender difference in MI incidence virtually disappears by the eighth decade; clinical evidence of CHD is present in about 20% of both men and women by age 80. Although coronary atherosclerosis is almost uniformly present at autopsy examination of elderly patients, many have never had clinical manifestations of myocardial ischemia.

Angina Pectoris

A recent study of nonhospitalized patients with angina pectoris[102] revealed a mean age of 69 years, with 75% of the population women; although 90% described effort angina, 47% had rest angina, and 35% had angina precipitated by mental stress.

The presentation of angina pectoris, both as an isolated event and following myocardial infarction, is more likely to be atypical, owing to a combination of a habitually decreased activity level, associated diseases, and possibly an altered sensitivity to pain in elderly persons. Angina is less likely to be activity induced in that arthritis, claudication, or musculoskeletal problems limit activity for many elderly patients before angina occurs. This angina

may be misinterpreted as unstable because it occurs at rest in predominantly inactive patients. Furthermore, angina is more likely to be precipitated by a concurrent medical or surgical problem such as infection, blood loss, hypertension or hypotension, thyrotoxicosis, or arrhythmia. Dyspnea and fatigue may be the prominent manifestations of myocardial ischemia, and eating may precipitate angina. Additionally, patients with memory loss may not remember transient chest pain and those with chronic brain syndromes may not appreciate, describe, or express the occurrence of chest discomfort. Silent ischemia is highly prevalent at elderly age,[103] with the risks greatest in the early morning hours or on awakening; standard anti-ischemic therapy is appropriate. Despite this high prevalence of silent ischemia, exertional chest pain independently predicts coronary death at elderly age,[104] with comparable prognostic significance for men and women, although anginal severity does not define risk status.

Therapy is as for younger patients, but attention must be directed to identification and remediation of precipitating or exacerbating factors. Elderly patients with stable angina, without evidence of early ischemia at exercise testing, who have a satisfactory symptomatic response to medical management are best suited for this approach. Elderly age is associated with increased fatal and nonfatal coronary events in patients with both stable and unstable angina; suboptimal pharmacologic and revascularization therapies likely contribute to the less favorable outcome.[105]

Severe unstable angina is common in elderly persons. When unresponsive or poorly responsive to intravenous nitroglycerin, oral aspirin, heparin, β- and calcium-blocking drugs as tolerated, and IIb/IIIa glycoprotein inhibitor therapy, urgent coronary arteriography is indicated to evaluate suitability for myocardial revascularization.

Myocardial Infarction

Elderly patients have a significantly different presentation, clinical course, and prognosis of MI than is the case at younger ages.[99] There is a marked increase in morbidity and mortality,[106] with 80% of all MI deaths occurring after age 65. Mortality from acute MI is increased 6-fold at ages 75 to 84 years and 15-fold after 85 years, compared with that at ages 55 to 64 years.[107] Functional disability before MI importantly predicts MI severity and postinfarction survival.[108] Although age adversely affects MI survival in part because prior MI, hypertension, and heart failure all increase with increasing age,[109] the contribution of less aggressive therapies requires study.[110] In the Myocardial Infarction Triage and Intervention (MITI) project, MI mortality was increased 10-fold in elderly patients (17.8% at 75 years or more versus 2% at less than 55 years).[111] The prognosis was worse for elderly women than elderly men,[112] although data from the U.S. National Registry of Myocardial Infarction-2 suggest otherwise.[113]

Chest pain as the presenting manifestation of acute MI is less frequent in elderly individuals.[114,115] Classic chest pain is reported by only one-third of patients older than 85 years of age. Elderly patients have an increased prevalence of comorbid illness associated with painless infarction such as diabetes and hypertension. Additionally, there may be lesser or altered sensitivity to pain with aging. Although the myocardial infarction may be painless, the clinical presentation is often not asymptomatic and may include acute dyspnea, exacerbation of heart failure, or pulmonary edema; and syncope, cerebrovascular accident, vertigo, palpitations, peripheral arterial embolism, nausea and vomiting, or acute renal failure; more subtle changes involve altered mentation, including acute confusion or agitation, profound weakness or fatigue, and changes in eating pattern or in other usual behaviors. The onset of symptoms of MI is more likely to occur at rest or during sleep in elderly patients, likely reflecting their more sedentary lifestyle. Unrecognized MI has as serious a prognosis as identified episodes of MI.[114] Based on Framingham data, unrecognized MI is more common in elderly women than in elderly men. Twenty-three percent and 38% of elderly men and women, respectively, with ECG evidence of MI in the Cardiovascular Health Study[6] did not report a history of MI. In the Goteborg Study, 60% of patients with ECG evidence of MI gave no history of an acute episode.[116]

Asymptomatic or atypical presentations of MI commonly exclude elderly patients from the potential benefits of thrombolytic therapy or acute coronary angioplasty. Acute MI in elderly patients is often a non-Q-wave MI and, as is the case with angina pectoris, is more often precipitated by an intercurrent medical or surgical problem associated with hypovolemia, blood loss, infection, hypotension, and the like (Table 39.2). Atypical symptoms may partly explain the delayed hospital presentation at elderly age.[117] Acute myocardial infarction, because of its atypical presentation, is more often unrecognized in aged patients, despite the fact that infarction in elderly persons characteristically is of increased severity, has a greater occurrence of complications, entails a longer hospital stay, and results in a higher mortality than in a younger age group. Elderly patients are more likely to be female; to have associated hypertension, diabetes mellitus, and cerebrovascular accident; and to have a history of prior infarction and of heart failure.

In addition to the atypical presentation, the diagnosis of MI may be further obscured in that the electrocardiographic diagnosis is limited by the increased occurrence of non-Q-wave infarction,[118] and elevated myocardial

TABLE 39.2. Atypical manifestations: acute myocardial infarction (MI) in elderly patients.

Presentation
  Painless infarction more common
  Acute symptoms
    Dyspnea
    Exacerbation of heart failure
    Pulmonary edema
    Syncope
    Stroke
    Vertigo
    Acute confusion
    Palpitations
    Peripheral arterial emboli
    Nausea and vomiting
    Acute renal failure
Subtle manifestations
  Altered mentation
  Excessive weakness or fatigue
  Changes in eating pattern
  Changes in other usual behaviors
Common precipitating factors
  Hypovolemia
  Blood loss
  Infection
  Hypotension

band (MB) fractions of creatine kinase (CK) are common in the presence of a normal total CK level because of decreased lean body mass with aging.[119]

Pooled data from large randomized placebo-controlled trials of thrombolytic therapy for acute MI, involving more than 58,600 patients, have shown comparable benefit at young and older ages up to age 75 years, with comparable efficacy of all thrombolytic drugs tested in elderly patients.[120–122] Advanced age alone (up to age 75) should not exclude patients from treatment with thrombolytic therapy.[123] The ACC/AHA clinical practice guidelines for acute MI cite a class I recommendation for this treatment for patients up to age 75 and a class IIa for those 75 and older.[124] Statistically significant reduction in mortality was more prominent at older than at younger age, despite the increased risk of bleeding, and in particular intracerebral bleeding, in the elderly.[125–128]

Improvement in ventricular function occurred at all ages studied. Because the absolute risk of MI mortality is greater at 65 to 75 years than for younger patients, the absolute benefit of successful coronary thrombolysis is also greater.[129] However, even with successful thrombolysis, patients older than 75 years in GUSTO-I had more left ventricular (LV) dysfunction and greater mortality than those younger than age 75.[130] Lesser use of thrombolytic therapy at advanced age is due, in part, to the later arrival at hospital of elderly patients.[111,131,132] Even in elderly patients known to have CHD, delay in accessing medical care was substantially greater than at younger age.[133] Elderly female patients and those with diabetes were treated later in the GUSTO-I trial, adding to their already substantial risk.[134] Since 1990, however, data suggest increased use of thrombolytic therapy for elderly patients, particularly elderly women.[135] Robust data are lacking for patients older than 75 years of age[136] because these patients typically have been excluded from earlier studies of these interventions.

Caution is warranted regarding coronary thrombolysis beyond age 75. An observational study derived from the Medicare database suggested significant survival disadvantage, without benefit in any clinical subgroup.[137] Clearly randomized trial data are needed, given the limitations of observational studies.[138] In particular, the contribution of higher-dose, nonweight-based heparin therapy to bleeding risk at elderly age was not ascertained. In GUSTO V, thrombolysis with half-dose reteplase plus abciximab (a IIb/IIIa platelet glycoprotein inhibitor) was associated with increased intracranial bleeding beyond age 75.[139]

In the Cooperative Cardiovascular Project, primary percutaneous transthoracic coronary angioplasty (PTCA) was associated with modestly lower short- and long-term mortality rates than coronary thrombolysis;[140] there was a 16% reduction in 30-day mortality risk. Among the 80 patients older than age 80 in GUSTO-IIB,[141] there was no 30-day mortality difference between coronary thrombolysis and acute angioplasty, with high mortality rates in both groups. Acute coronary angioplasty (PTCA) should also be considered for elderly patients for whom coronary thrombolysis is contraindicated; up to a 90% procedural success rate was described for patients age 70 years and older,[142] with favorable outcomes also described in octogenarians.[143] Risk of cerebral hemorrhage is dramatically less with acute PTCA than with coronary thrombolysis in elderly patients.

In-hospital mortality is greater in patients older than 70 years of age; the 30% to 40% mortality is about twice that of younger patients. Complications including hypotension and cardiogenic shock, atrioventricular block, atrial arrhythmias, heart failure, pulmonary edema, and cardiac rupture occur with increased frequency in elderly patients. In the SHOCK trial, emergency revascularization did not benefit patients with MI and cardiogenic shock older than age 75.[144] Cardiac rupture during the first week after MI occurs, particularly in elderly women with hypertension. In one series, MI mortality was doubled with the occurrence of atrial fibrillation. Right ventricular infarction substantially increases hospital mortality.[145] Severe mitral regurgitation due to papillary muscle infarction and cardiac rupture of either the ventricular septum or a papillary muscle usually are heralded by recurrent chest pain, pulmonary edema, and/or cardiogenic shock. Use of intraaortic balloon counterpulsation enables survival until cardiac catheterization and surgical repair can be performed. In patients with these surgically correctable lesions, favorable responses to surgical intervention have been described.[146] Despite the high operative mortality, survivors have a satisfactory long-term outcome. Not surprisingly, elderly patients often have a more protracted hospital stay for MI.

Although survival of elderly patients improved substantially from 1987 to 1990, particularly for those younger than 85 years, the decline in CHD mortality has been less prominent in elderly than in younger patients. Concomitant changes included the increased use of acute pharmacologic and invasive interventions to limit infarct size and revascularize myocardium.[147,148] In one study,[149] hospital complications and 30-day and 1-year mortality rates declined approximately 30% in patients aged 75 and older, with the most marked benefit in reperfused patients. Major differences still persist in the application of beneficial therapies to patients older than 75 versus younger than 55: 5% versus 39% thrombolytic therapy, 7% versus 29% PTCA, 5% versus 11% CABG, and 57% versus 82% aspirin use.[111,150,151] Early beta-blocker therapy was not used for 51% of elderly patients hospitalized for acute MI in the Cooperative Cardiovascular Project,[152] although this therapy was associated with a 19% reduction in mortality risk across all age groups in the Medicare cohort. Posthospital mortality is also increased following MI, due to the increased severity of infarction, often superimposed on prior infarction; this also accounts for the increased residual invalidism and increase in late deaths at elderly age.

In the early years of acute coronary care, elderly patients were arbitrarily excluded from coronary or intensive care facilities on the basis of age alone. However, elderly patients benefit equally from intensive coronary care, ECG monitoring, and arrhythmia prevention and reversion. In particular, they have an equally favorable response to defibrillation as younger patients. The increased occurrence of heart failure at elderly age and other complications of infarction and frequent complicating illnesses warrant meticulous surveillance. Elderly patients with heart failure more often require monitoring of cardiac output and intracardiac pressures through a pulmonary artery catheter to guide therapy. Other problems encountered more frequently in the elderly patient with MI include difficulty with urination, particularly in men with prostatic enlargement who receive diuretic therapy; constipation and a variety of nonspecific gastrointestinal symptoms; and the precipitation of glaucoma, urinary retention, or confusion when atropine is used to reverse sinus bradycardia. The early mortality of elderly patients after MI has been reduced from an estimated 43% to 79% to as low as 25% to 27% with coronary care unit management; this difference probably is related to increased intensity of coronary care unit therapy.[153]

Drug management of acute MI is comparable with that of a younger population. There is an increased propensity to adverse effects from narcotic analgesic medications; half the dosage usual for younger individuals is recommended. In general, adverse responses to drug therapy are more likely to occur and can be exacerbated by coexisting medical illnesses and related multiple-drug therapy. All drugs should be introduced at lower doses than in younger patients, with gradual dosage increases as tolerated. Intravenous administration of beta-blocking drugs in acute MI improved survival only in older patients,[154–158] although data are not available for patients older than 75 years. Long-term oral beta-blocking drugs provide equal or greater long-term survival benefit and reduction of reinfarction after MI in elderly as in younger patients,[159] particularly for patients with anterior MI, with data available to age 75 years.[155,160,161] Contemporary data suggest underutilization of beta-blocking drugs in elderly patients after acute MI,[162] with only 21% of eligible patients receiving this therapy[163] in one study and 50% in another.[164] Beta-blocker use was associated with a 43% decreased mortality rate and 22% decreased rehospitalizations in a Medicare cohort, with benefit also evident in patients older than age 75.

Diltiazem and verapamil appear to provide comparable benefits in younger and older patients with non-Q-wave MI and preserved ventricular function, although calcium channel-blocking drugs have not improved survival and may worsen outcome in patients with ventricular dysfunction.[165] However, most studies of calcium channel-blocking drugs in patients with non-Q-wave MI did not provide aged-based analysis, despite inclusion of elderly patients.

Comparable reduction in mortality occurred in patients with MI older and younger than 70 years treated with aspirin during acute MI in the international study of infarct survival (ISIS-2) trial.[166] Virtually no patients older than 75 years were enrolled in other clinical trials of aspirin use. Of concern is that about one-third of elderly patients with acute MI without contraindications to aspirin use failed to receive aspirin during the first 2 days of MI hospitalization.[167] Aspirin use was associated with a 22% decrease in 30-day mortality risk in this Medicare population. Aspirin was not prescribed at discharge to 24% of eligible elderly patients in the Cooperative Cardiovascular Project.[168]

Angiotensin-converting enzyme (ACE) inhibitors likely provide comparable benefit in elderly and younger patients, particularly those with large infarctions and ventricular dysfunction. ACE inhibitor therapy in patients with a decreased ejection fraction following MI decreased fatal and nonfatal cardiovascular events, including the development of heart failure and recurrent infarction; relative risk reduction was greater for the 35% of patients older than 65 years.[49] Elderly patients in the GISSI-3 trial also had decreased mortality and severe ventricular dysfunction associated with ACE inhibitor therapy.[169]

Long-term warfarin anticoagulation after acute MI reduced reinfarction in elderly patients in the Sixty-Plus Reinfarction Trial, without significant deleterious bleeding risk. The Warfarin Re-Infarction Study[170] showed survival, reinfarction, and cerebrovascular benefits in patients up to age 75 randomized to warfarin, although a post hoc analysis showed attenuated benefit with increasing age.[171]

Data from the Cardiac Arrhythmia Suppression Trial (CAST) discourage use of antiarrhythmic drugs for MI survivors of all ages without symptomatic arrhythmia, even those with complex ventricular arrhythmia, owing to increased mortality risk from drug proarrhythmic effects.[172] In CAST, ambulatory ECG data showed that age was an important independent predictor of ventricular ectopy in postinfarction patients.[173]

Nitrate drug use requires attention to orthostatic hypotension because of diminished baroreceptor responsiveness; elderly patients must be cautioned to sit when taking sublingual nitroglycerin for relief of angina.

Among eligible patients recently hospitalized for MI, lipid-lowering drugs were used by only one-third. Age greater than 74 years was independently related to lack of lipid-lowering drug use.[174]

A substantial number of elderly patients have an essentially uncomplicated MI with an excellent prognosis for recovery and rehabilitation. They are ideal candidates for early ambulation to prevent the deleterious effects of prolonged immobilization. Education and counseling are important components of care. At discharge, there should be a careful review of medications, with written recommendations for diet, activity, and coronary risk reduction.

Predischarge exercise testing appears safe for appropriately selected elderly patients who remain asymptomatic and offers prognostic data comparable to that reported for younger patients.[175] Inability to undergo exercise testing 1 month after MI is a marker of unfavorable prognosis.[176] As is the case in younger patients, the lower the exercise intensity at which ischemic ST segment abnormalities appear, the greater their severity, and the longer their persistence after cessation of exercise, the greater the risk. Failure of SBP to increase with exercise or exercise-induced hypotension also indicates a high-risk status. Evidence of residual ischemia at exercise testing, with and without radionuclide studies, or with dipyridamole-thallium imaging in elderly patients with non-Q-wave MI is associated with an increased risk of mortality and warrants consideration for invasive intervention.[177,178] Elderly patients with non-Q-wave MI have greater mortality risk in the year after hospital discharge than do patients with Q-wave MI; aggressive diagnostic and therapeutic interventions may be of particular benefit in these patients.[179] (See p. 530 for coronary risk reduction.)

Lack of emotional support independently predicts mortality risk after MI.[180] Although many male coronary patients 80 years and older have a spouse for social support and to assist as a caregiver, women with CHD of comparable age often have no such companion and may forfeit their independent lifestyle.

Exercise test data can be used to recommend the intensity of physical activity that can be performed with safety following discharge from the hospital. Many elderly patients can exercise safely without supervision; predischarge exercise testing can identify the high-risk subset of patients for whom initially supervised exercise is appropriate. Exercise test results can also guide recommendations for return to preinfarction physical activities, including resumption of remunerative work when appropriate. Many physicians underestimate the habitual physical activity level of their older cardiac patients and inappropriately recommend restriction of physical activity.[181] Excessive immobilization is associated with detrimental physical and psychologic consequences. In contrast, many elderly individuals decrease their activity levels because any submaximal task is perceived as requiring increased work; this is because of the increase in relative energy cost caused by the lessened aerobic capacity that occurs with aging. Even with usual daily activities, there is a greater increase in heart rate in elderly people. Additionally, combinations of musculoskeletal instability, emotional problems (particularly depression), and often inappropriate admonitions from family members and friends further decrease activity levels.

Rehabilitative exercise training can limit the high risk of disability of elderly patients after a coronary event[181] and encourage coronary risk reduction.[182] The goal of rehabilitation is restoration, maintenance, and extension of a reasonably independent and active lifestyle. Although an increasing percentage of elderly patients after MI or myocardial revascularization procedures are currently enrolled in supervised exercise rehabilitation programs or prescribed an independent exercise regimen by their physicians, elderly patients (particularly elderly women) are less likely to be referred than younger patients.[63] Comparable improvements in physical work capacity and in endurance occur in elderly as in younger men and women, and appropriate exercise entails no greater risk.[63,183,184] Walking is an ideal exercise regimen after discharge from the hospital, with gradual increases in the pace and distance of walking. Because the energy expenditure of walking often entails a significant proportion of the aerobic capacity of elderly patients, walking even as slowly as 3.5 miles per hour is an excellent physical conditioning stimulus. The major physio-

logic effect is a decrease in the heart rate response to submaximal work. Additional benefits of exercise training include improved neuromuscular coordination, joint mobility, coordination, and flexibility, and the potential to limit bone demineralization. Exercise testing for exercise prescription is recommended before embarking on a more intensive physical activity regimen. High-impact aerobic activities are inappropriate at elderly age as they are associated with an increase in musculoskeletal complications.[185]

Myocardial Revascularization

Elderly patients with chronic angina unresponsive or poorly responsive to medical management, or those with persisting chest pain following MI, are candidates for coronary arteriography to assess their suitability for myocardial revascularization. Older patients with evidence of myocardial ischemia at low work loads at exercise testing also constitute a high-risk group for early recurrent coronary events and should be evaluated for myocardial revascularization. Because a high percentage of posthospital deaths in very elderly patients are either sudden or due to recurrent MI, risk stratification testing should routinely be considered for patients older than 75 years as at ages 65 to 75[150] to identify the subset for whom myocardial revascularization is appropriate.

Elderly patients are more likely to have multivessel coronary disease and left main coronary stenosis, and coronary lesions are more likely to be diffuse and calcified. It is thus not surprising that elderly patients undergoing CABG are more likely to have unstable angina, prior MI, and New York Heart Association class IV heart disease than younger patients. Elderly patients are also characterized by a higher percentage of women and a greater likelihood of comorbid conditions including diabetes, hypertension, heart failure, renal insufficiency, and PVD.

Older age patients now constitute more than half the population undergoing cardiac catheterization, PTCA, and CABG surgery.[100] CABG surgery in patients 80 years and older increased 67% between 1987 and 1990,[186] providing a Medicare database of almost 25,000 such patients; in recent years, mortality rates for elderly patients undergoing revascularization procedures decreased in this Medicare database. In nonrandomized but comparable elderly patients older than 70 years undergoing myocardial revascularization procedures, there was substantially less hospital mortality, stroke, and MI with PTCA than with CABG; in the ensuing 5 years, however, PTCA patients required more repeat procedures, but 5-year mortality was comparable for PTCA and CABG patients, about 30%.[187] Elderly patients (≥70 years) with unstable angina at high risk for CABG who were treated successfully with PTCA had long-term mortality comparable to that of age-matched subjects without diagnosed CHD.[188]

Recent series have described outcomes of CABG surgery in selected octogenarians and nonagenarians, usually with highly symptomatic and unstable coronary disease, who were unresponsive or poorly responsive to medical management.[189–192] In addition to the more likely left main and triple-vessel coronary disease, often with ventricular dysfunction, and substantial comorbidity in elderly patients, older age is an independent risk factor for morbidity and mortality from CABG, with elderly women at highest risk.[193] A recent report describes a 10% hospital mortality rate in octogenarians, with diabetes and ventricular dysfunction adversely affecting outcome.[189] Despite the initial high risk and significant hospital expenses, survivors were pain-free, often with restored performance status, and with 5-year survival rates comparable to that of the general octogenarian population in the United States.[186] Evaluation of elderly patients with diabetes in the CASS Registry[194] showed surgical benefits comparable to those in nondiabetic elderly patients, a 44% reduction in mortality compared with medical therapy. As in younger populations, use of at least one internal mammary artery graft improved symptoms and event-free survival in patients 70 years and older.[195] The symptomatic improvement and favorable late sustained improvement and quality of life among elderly survivors of CABG suggest that an optimistic approach to the management of symptomatic elderly patients with advanced obstructive CHD is reasonable,[196] even for selected octogenarians and nonagenarians.[190,191]

Patients older than 70 years of age sustain a higher operative mortality from elective CABG than do younger individuals, as well as higher rates of postoperative cardiac and noncardiac complications, which occur in as many as 30% to 50%. These complications include greater need for prolonged ventilatory support for respiratory failure; for implanted pacemakers; for inotropic support and use of the intra-aortic balloon pump; greater reoperation for bleeding; stroke; delirium; renal failure; perioperative infarction; and sepsis. Complications are most frequent in elderly women.[197] Atherosclerotic emboli from aortic atheromatous disease contribute importantly to complications; intraoperative transesophageal echocardiography can identify protruding atheromas that require modification of aortic manipulation.[198] Increased age predisposes to impaired cognition after cardiac surgery unrelated to changes in cerebral blood flow autoregulation.[199] Elderly patients can be anticipated to have a longer hospital stay following CABG, with more time spent in an intensive care setting.[189] Emergency CABG in elderly patients entails a substantially increased mortality risk, 14.9% versus 3.6% for elective surgery in one series.[200]

In elderly patients with preserved ventricular function and without major associated medical problems, 5-year survival following successful CABG approximates 90%. In the CASS, 81% of elderly patients were free of recurrent angina, MI, requirement for repeat CABG surgery, or death at 1 year, and 40% were free of such events at 5 years. These results were comparable to those in patients younger than age 65. High-risk patients older than age 65 years in the CASS[201] had better survival and freedom from chest pain with surgical management than with medical management. Nevertheless, operative morbidity and mortality is greater, hospitalization is more protracted, and overall survival is less than that for younger patients.[202] However, because elective CABG in patients older than 75 years resulted in an operative mortality of 3.6% in one series versus 14.9% mortality for urgent or emergency CABG surgery,[200] early evaluation and referral for elective revascularization of symptomatic elderly patients may avert the excess mortality of emergency revascularization. In a study comparing CABG in patients older and younger than 75 years, actuarial 5-year cardiac event-free survival rates were comparable.[203] As myocardial revascularization procedures are increasingly undertaken in highly symptomatic octogenarians and nonagenarians, the outcomes appropriate for assessment include restoration of comfort, self-sufficiency, and improved functional status, that is, meaningful long-term survival.[204] Early ambulation and gradually progressive physical activity after CABG can help limit complications and improve the functional status at discharge from the hospital.

Although direct comparison of the results of PTCA with those of CABG is not available, because of the increased risk of CABG at elderly age and because catheter-based interventions often are better tolerated than surgery, there has been increased application of PTCA to elderly patients. There is an equal or greater increase in PTCA application among elderly women than elderly men. However, often the coronary anatomy is unsuitable for transcatheter revascularization. The incidence of left main coronary artery disease has been estimated to be 13% to 35% in different series. Recent reports of PTCA at elderly age documented angiographic success rates of 80% to 90%, even with multivessel PICA, without excess occurrence of procedural complications and with functional improvement and patency rates comparable to those at younger age.[205–207]

If complete revascularization is achieved, freedom from recurrent angina and cardiac death is comparable to that in younger patients.[208] Incomplete revascularization is associated with poorer long-term survival.[209] In the Mayo Clinic experience, despite improved technical success and decreased short-term PTCA complication rates, event-free survival rates continued to be influenced by baseline characteristics.[210] Restenosis rates, even among octogenarians, are comparable to those in younger patients.[211]

Age remains an important predictor for procedural mortality and late survival in PTCA, particularly for patients older than 80 years.[206,212] However, almost three-fourths of elderly survivors of PTCA do not require CABG surgery and remain free of MI at 4 to 5 years. Compared with patients 65 to 74 years, patients older than 75 years were more symptomatic, more likely to have heart failure, and more likely to require multivessel PICA.[213] The increased incidence of vascular site complications reflects the high prevalence of PVD. Despite a high rate of procedural success, PTCA in patients older than 90 years involved a high rate of inhospital complications and limited clinical benefit.[214]

Limited data from elderly patients with high-risk lesion morphology at coronary arteriography suggest that coronary angioplasty using new devices and stenting may be a therapeutic alternative.[215] Substantial changes in both surgical and transcatheter revascularization techniques mandate comparison of these contemporary approaches in the elderly population.

Systemic Arterial Hypertension and Cardiovascular Risk

Hypertension is highly prevalent at elderly age, occurring in more than half of the U.S. population older than 65 years.[216] Hypertension and its consequences comprise the major reason for which patients in the United States consult their physicians. In most populations, systolic blood pressure (SBP) increases into the eighth and ninth decades, whereas diastolic blood pressure (DBP) levels off in the fifties and sixties; thus, isolated systolic hypertension (ISH) is prominent in geriatric populations.[217] Both reduced arterial compliance and increased cardiac output appear to contribute to ISH at elderly age.[218] Pulse pressure widens in old age as a result of a continued increase in SBP and a decrease in DBP. Low DBP, particularly in association with a wide pulse pressure, appears to reflect widespread atherosclerosis at elderly age.[219] The age-related increase in SBP is not invariable and is infrequent in most nonindustrialized societies. Lower rates of hypertension are described in physically active elderly women, with blood pressure progressively lower at higher levels of activity.[220] The World Health Organization (WHO) definition of hypertension is a blood pressure in excess of 160/95 mmHg. Isolated systolic hypertension is defined as a SBP in excess of 150 mmHg with a DBP below 90 mmHg, and accounts for approximately two-thirds of hypertension in persons older than 65 years. In the United States, approximately one-third of elderly women and one-fifth of elderly men have ISH. Either ISH or combined sys-

tolic and diastolic hypertension occurs in 63% of whites and more than 75% of blacks older than 65 years.[216] Major elevation in DBP in excess of 110 mmHg is three times as common in elderly black patients as in elderly white patients. Hypertension remains a powerful predictor of cardiovascular mortality at all ages; even borderline systolic or diastolic hypertension doubles the risk of cardiovascular events at elderly age. Although the increase in risk is related to the severity of hypertension, systolic hypertension is more closely correlated with cardiovascular and cerebrovascular morbidity and mortality at elderly age than is diastolic hypertension.[221,222] Systolic blood pressure, determined by ambulatory blood pressure monitoring, significantly predicted cardiovascular risk over and above conventional blood pressure monitoring in the Systolic Hypertension in Europe trial.[223] Development of left ventricular hypertrophy (LVH), a potent independent risk factor for cardiovascular mortality, is highly correlated with systolic hypertension. In the Framingham Heart Study, even borderline ISH at elderly age was associated with increased LV wall thickness and impaired diastolic filling.[224] Antihypertensive agents that can effect regression of LVH may contribute to decreasing cardiovascular complications. Elevated SBP, which increases ventricular afterload and myocardial oxygen demand, may depress cardiac function, particularly with coincident CHD. Blood pressure should be measured annually even in previously normotensive elderly persons. Because blood pressure measurements are highly variable at elderly age, two or three baseline readings on separate occasions are recommended before treatment is initiated.[225]

Hypertension contributes importantly to accelerated CHD, heart failure, cerebrovascular accident, renal failure, aortic dissection, and aortic aneurysm rupture in the elderly, as well as in younger populations. Although only 20% of patients in the Veterans Administration Cooperative Study on Antihypertensive Agents were older than 60 years, half of all morbidity, heart failure, and stroke occurred in this age group.[226] Control of hypertension decreases the risk of complications: cardiovascular death, fatal MI, heart failure, and stroke in elderly patients.[216,227] Control of isolated systolic hypertension in the Systolic Hypertension in the Elderly Program (SHEP)[228] using low-dose chorthalidone as initial therapy, with low-dose beta blockade added as needed, reduced stroke by 36% and fatal and nonfatal cardiovascular events by 32%, the latter largely due to decreased fatal MI. Occurrence of heart failure was reduced approximately 50%, particularly among patients with prior MI,[229] with comparable benefits in patients with and without baseline ECG abnormalities and with or without noninsulin-treated diabetes.[230] In the SHEP cohort, depression was associated with a significant substantial increase in risk of death and stroke or MI.[231] In the

Swedish Trial in Old Patients with Hypertension-2 (STOP-2) study,[232] outcomes were comparable with conventional drugs (beta blockers and diuretics) and the newer ACE inhibitors and calcium channel-blocking drugs. However, elderly patients receiving ACE inhibitor compared with calcium channel-blocking drugs had fewer MIs and less heart failure.

Particularly in elderly patients with mild hypertension, nonpharmacologic approaches including reduction of sodium intake, weight reduction, moderation of alcohol consumption, and regular modest-intensity physical activity[225] should be initially considered. In the randomized Trial of Nonpharmacologic Intervention in the Elderly (TONE), the best results were associated with combined sodium restriction and weight loss.[233] Elderly patients should be cautioned that nonsteroidal anti-inflammatory drugs can decrease the efficacy of antihypertensive drug treatment.[234]

Based on results of major randomized clinical trials that enrolled elderly patients,[217,235] comparable or greater benefit of pharmacotherapy to that at younger age was documented, at least to age 80 years. The European Working Party on Hypertension in the Elderly (EWPHE) trial,[222] in which 70% of patients were women, showed a favorable effect of antihypertensive therapy on cardiac mortality, fatal MI, heart failure, and overall cardiovascular mortality. In these clinical trials, there were no increased rates of therapy discontinuation resulting from adverse effects in elderly patients, and study medication adherence was comparable to younger patients. In one study, calcium antagonist drugs, compared with beta-blockers, increased the risk of gastrointestinal hemorrhage in hypertensive patients over age 67.[236] Meta-analysis of antihypertensive therapy trials involving more than 15,000 patients older than 60 years showed comparable reduction in stroke risk and cardiac morbidity as in younger patients.[237]

Goal blood pressure should be 140/90mmHg, with avoidance of postural hypotension and maintenance of renal function; this should be accomplished without adverse symptomatic side effects and at reasonable cost. Goal blood pressure of less than 130/85 is a cost-effective intervention in elderly diabetic hypertensive patients.[238] Initiation of drug therapy should involve half the usual adult dose, with gradual increments in drug dosage. However, few elderly patients achieve goal blood pressure levels with monotherapy; low doses of two drugs are often necessary. Because of impaired baroreflex control of blood pressure at elderly ages, blood pressure should be checked in the sitting and standing positions when therapy is instituted. The drugs chosen, in addition to lowering blood pressure, should be those that effect regression of left ventricular hypertrophy. Hypertension and its therapy are discussed in more detail in Chapter 40.

Valvular Heart Disease, Congenital Heart Disease, Infective Endocarditis, and Nonvalvular Cardiovascular Infections

Aortic Stenosis

Hemodynamically significant symptomatic calcific aortic stenosis is the most frequent valvular heart disease that requires surgical correction in elderly patients.[239] One in four patients who undergo aortic valve replacement are 70 years or older. Although more common in men in younger age groups, calcific aortic stenosis predominates in women after age 80. Frequent underdiagnosis of hemodynamically significant aortic stenosis is of concern because correct diagnosis and valve replacement surgery are associated with a favorable long-term prognosis, that is, improved symptoms and survival.

Aortic stenosis in elderly patients is typically caused by calcification of a tricuspid aortic valve; 90% of aortic valves in elderly patients with calcific aortic stenosis are tricuspid.

Symptomatic hemodynamically important aortic valvular stenosis is characterized by the same presentations in the elderly as in a younger population: angina pectoris, exertional dizziness or syncope, and dyspnea or heart failure; however, these symptoms are often misinterpreted as being caused by other cardiac problems, such as CHD, or by neurologic disease when the presentation is with syncope.[240] Significant aortic stenosis is one of the most common anatomic causes of syncope at elderly age. Symptoms are less often activity precipitated than in younger patients because a relatively sedentary lifestyle more frequently occurs with aging. Progression of the severity and symptoms of aortic stenosis at elderly age is characteristic and often rapid. Aortic valve replacement is indicated, in that fewer than 50% of patients with hemodynamically significant symptomatic calcific aortic stenosis survive for more than 5 years after symptom onset; sudden death is common.[241] Differentiation is required from the benign, but pervasive, short early-peaking basal systolic murmur of aortic sclerosis, present in one-half to one-third of elderly patients.

The classic slow-rising small-volume carotid pulse of a younger patient with aortic stenosis, occasionally associated with a thrill, may be masked by sclerosis and decreased elasticity of the carotid vessels in an elderly patient; these may also mask the usual narrow pulse pressure. The carotid bruit may be erroneously attributed to primary vascular disease. Systemic arterial hypertension, rarely seen in younger individuals with severe aortic stenosis, is not uncommon in elderly persons because of vascular stiffening. The late-peaking, harsh basal systolic murmur that radiates into the neck often has high-frequency components that are heard along the lower left sternal border and toward the cardiac apex throughout most of systole, mimicking the murmur of mitral regurgitation. The apical systolic murmur of associated mitral annular calcification may further complicate recognition. Hyperexpansion of the lungs and dorsal kyphosis may limit the palpatory evidence of the forceful sustained apex impulse of left ventricular hypertrophy and, at times, the basal systolic thrill; the harsh basal systolic murmur may become softer and the thrill no longer palpable as the cardiac output lessens. Lack of commissural fusion of the calcified aortic valve in elderly persons further mutes the harsh characteristics of the murmur and also explains the absence of an ejection sound. S_2 is soft with occasional reversal of splitting, and an S_4 is prominent when sinus rhythm is present. Atrial fibrillation rarely occurs in younger patients with aortic stenosis, but often precipitates heart failure in elderly patients, due to a loss of the atrial contribution to ventricular filling in a poorly compliant ventricle in combination with the lessened ventricular filling resulting from the rapid heart rate. Atrial fibrillation may be present in as many as one-fourth of elderly patients with severe aortic valvular stenosis. There is frequently a coexisting basal early diastolic decrescendo murmur of aortic regurgitation, but aortic regurgitation of hemodynamic significance is unusual.

The ECG has characteristic changes of left ventricular hypertrophy, although concomitant emphysema may mask the increased voltage. The heart size on chest radiograph is usually normal; aortic valvular calcification may be evident and can be confirmed by echocardiography. Critical aortic stenosis virtually never occurs in the absence of echocardiographically detectable calcium deposition. An increased left ventricular wall thickness is evident in most patients.

Echocardiography with Doppler studies can noninvasively assess the severity of aortic valvular obstruction. The aortic valvular pressure gradient at Doppler echocardiography correlates reasonably with the aortic valve area at cardiac catheterization. Hemodynamically severe aortic stenosis as evaluated by Doppler echocardiography in the Helsinki Aging Study[242] markedly increased 4-year mortality risk. Cardiac catheterization and coronary arteriography are warranted, nonetheless, because coexistent coronary disease is frequent[243] and concomitant myocardial revascularization may be required if aortic valve replacement is undertaken.[244] Exercise testing is hazardous if critical aortic stenosis is suspected because syncope and sudden death have been precipitated.

Aortic valve replacement for symptomatic critical aortic stenosis is indicated at virtually all ages in otherwise functional elderly patients[244] because of their excessive mortality after the onset of angina pectoris, heart failure, or syncope. Asymptomatic elderly patients with reasonable exercise tolerance with severe aortic stenosis do not warrant surgery; sudden death is very rare without antecedent symptoms.[245] Symptomatic geriatric patients with severe aortic stenosis have mortality rates as high as 50% in the first year.[246] Although angina and heart failure symptoms may respond to medical management, clinical deterioration is frequent, leading to urgent surgery with its increased operative mortality. Aortic valve replacement can be performed at an acceptable risk, even in octogenarians and in patients with class III and class IV disease,[247] because left ventricular function is often well preserved even after the onset of heart failure. CHD, prior MI, heart failure, and atrial fibrillation all increase surgical risk.[248] Aortic valve replacement dramatically improves survival, hemodynamic status, and the patient's quality of life. However, neurologic complications are more common than at younger age. In one series, actuarial survival at 1, 3, and 5 years was 90.8%, 84.2%, and 76.0%, respectively, although concomitant surgical procedures increased the operative risk.[249] In another series, perioperative mortality was 2.5% in patients below 70 years, 7.3% in those beyond 70 years, and 12.5% in those older than 80 years; among patients older than age 70, 1-year survival was 83%, and 5-year survival 52%.[250] There was a favorable 10-year postoperative survival with maintenance of functional status. About 10% of patients will require permanent pacemaker implantation for perioperative heart block.

Comparison of valve replacement for aortic stenosis in another series among patients older and younger than 75 years showed a surgical mortality of 12.4% versus 6.6% in the two groups.[251] In another report of aortic valve replacement in octogenarians where half had concomitant CABG surgery, operative mortality was 9.8%.[252] In a more recent series,[253] isolated aortic valve replacement beyond age 70 entailed a perioperative mortality of 4.3%, which increased to 10% with concomitant CABG surgery. Of equal importance to survival is the resultant functional status and life quality. Among an octogenarian group with 69% of patients class III or IV preoperatively, 81% were class I or II at follow-up.[254] Formal quality of life assessment in patients 70 to 89 years after aortic valve replacement showed comparable scores to age-matched population norms in most domains.[255] Bioprosthetic rather than mechanical valves are often chosen for very elderly patients to avoid problems of anticoagulation and because these valves deteriorate more slowly in elderly patients.[256] Concurrent CABG surgery decreased early mortality in elderly patients with significant associated CHD.[244]

Aortic balloon valvotomy is rarely undertaken because of the high rates of restenosis and of posthospital mortality, but it may offer limited palliation for highly symptomatic elderly patients who are not candidates for valve replacement.[257–259] Despite modest decreases in peak pressure gradient and increases in valve area, hospital mortality was 4% to 9%, one-fourth of patients had died by 6 months, and their event-free 1-year survival was 43%.[258] Balloon valvotomy may be used to improve the status of elderly patients with severe aortic stenosis and heart failure, increasing the likelihood of subsequent successful valve replacement.[260]

Aortic Regurgitation

Aortic regurgitation, caused by myxomatous or other valvular degeneration, congenital bicuspid aortic valve, rheumatic heart disease, infective endocarditis, rheumatoid disease, aortic dissection, trauma, syphilis, systemic arterial hypertension, and a number of other disorders, is the most common cause of a diastolic murmur at old age and can usually be diagnosed by clinical examination. Echocardiography and Doppler studies can help to assess the hemodynamic severity.

Aortic regurgitation is typically managed medically with dietary sodium restriction, diuretics, vasodilator drugs, and digitalis to control cardiac failure. Nifedipine therapy in asymptomatic patients with severe aortic regurgitation and normal left ventricular function may avert or delay the need for valve replacement.[261] Exercise tolerance, as in younger patients, is often preserved even with advanced disease. Decrease in left ventricular contractility (ejection fraction below 50%–55%) or progressive increase in ventricular volumes (end-systolic volume greater than 55%) warrant valve replacement; surgical mortality is excessive once clinical heart failure supervenes.[245] The results of aortic valve replacement for aortic regurgitation are less satisfactory than for aortic stenosis, at least in part because of the frequently severe ventricular dysfunction.

Acute aortic regurgitation, as may occur with trauma or infective endocarditis, typically presents with acute pulmonary edema and requires urgent valve replacement. Patients may be misdiagnosed as having MI. The diagnosis is often overlooked because of the lack of the characteristic wide pulse pressure and cardiac enlargement and the brief or inaudible murmur due to overwhelming cardiac failure. Diagnosis is often made by echocardiography.

Mitral Regurgitation

Mitral regurgitation is more common than mitral stenosis at elderly age. Common causes of mitral regurgitation in elderly patients include rheumatic heart disease, myxomatous mitral leaflet degeneration, mitral valve prolapse, mitral annular calcification, and papillary muscle dysfunction or chordal rupture, secondary to CHD. Mitral annular calcification is more frequent in women than men and can often be diagnosed by the character-

istic C-shaped roentgenographic calcification or at echocardiography. Myxomatous degeneration of the mitral valve may cause mitral valve prolapse. Many elderly patients with chronic mitral regurgitation and sinus rhythm are asymptomatic, with the onset of atrial fibrillation precipitating hemodynamic decompensation. The diagnosis of mitral regurgitation usually can be made by clinical examination, but echocardiographic examination often suggests the cause. Medical therapy is usually appropriate unless mitral regurgitation is of major hemodynamic importance; Doppler echocardiography may help to quantify the severity of the mitral regurgitation. Assessment of exercise capacity and noninvasive documentation of left ventricular systolic function can identify symptomatic patients for whom cardiac catheterization is appropriate to assess suitability for operative intervention. Outcomes are improved with operation before deterioration of ventricular function.[262]

The prevalence of mitral valve prolapse in elderly patients is not well established. Mitral valve prolapse may be asymptomatic in some elderly patients and be diagnosed only by the classic auscultatory findings. In others, however, disabling chest pain occurs.[263] Because of the frequently associated nonspecific repolarization abnormalities on the electrocardiogram, an erroneous diagnosis of angina pectoris may be made. Palpitations should suggest an associated arrhythmia. In contrast to younger patients, mitral valve prolapse in elderly patients, particularly elderly men, may result in severe mitral regurgitation and symptomatic heart failure. There may be complicating infective endocarditis or ruptured chordae tendineae; again, in contrast to the female predominance in the younger population, heart failure secondary to mitral valve prolapse predominates in elderly men.

Mitral valve replacement in elderly patients is less satisfactory than aortic valve replacement,[264] with a surgical mortality rate of 10% to 14%. This difference is due in part to urgent or emergency surgery as with MI-related severe acute mitral regurgitation, prior limited attention to papillary muscle preservation, and almost uniform associated left ventricular dysfunction. Papillary muscle integrity seems especially important in elderly patients to prevent progressive ventricular failure.

Mitral regurgitation secondary to myocardial ischemia is also more frequent in elderly patients. The mortality rate of combined mitral valve replacement and CABG surgery may average 30% for patients in the eighth and ninth decades, and residual cardiac dysfunction and symptoms are more likely to be present than after aortic valve replacement. Mitral valve repair entails both lower mortality and fewer thromboembolic complications, but data are limited on mitral valve reconstruction in elderly patients.[197,202,265] Extensive mitral annular calcification may complicate surgery. Requirement for anticoagulation must be considered with decision for mechanical valve implantation. Although bioprosthetic valves may enable freedom from anticoagulation in patients in sinus rhythm, bioprosthetic valve degeneration may necessitate reoperation at even older age.

Education of elderly patients, attention to drug interactions, and contemporary lower-dose regimens can minimize bleeding complications of ambulatory anticoagulation. Antibiotic prophylaxis against infective endocarditis is needed for the frequent invasive diagnostic or surgical procedures performed in hospitalized elderly patients; recommendations apply comparably to older and younger patients.[266]

Acute massive mitral regurgitation, as occurs with chordal rupture or flail mitral leaflet associated with infective endocarditis or papillary muscle rupture in the setting of acute MI, typically presents with acute pulmonary edema with hypotension or cardiogenic shock and requires emergency valve replacement. Transesophageal echocardiography is valuable for clinical decision making.[267] Intraaortic balloon counterpulsation support may be needed to enable cardiac catheterization and induction of anesthesia.

Mitral Stenosis

Mitral stenosis, usually rheumatic in origin, rarely becomes newly symptomatic in elderly patients, except at the development of atrial fibrillation. Control of the ventricular response rate typically restores compensation. Rarely, mitral stenosis is caused by progressive mitral annular calcification. Mitral balloon commissurotomy is increasingly used for symptomatic elderly patients because of its long-term beneficial effects on symptoms, functional status, hemodynamic measurements, and exercise capacity.[257,268,269] However, calcification of the mitral valve and valve apparatus limits the suitability for balloon valvuloplasty.

Congenital Heart Disease

Congenital cardiac lesions rarely cause de novo hemodynamic problems in the elderly population. Most congenital cardiac lesions of hemodynamic significance have been corrected in childhood or young adulthood.[270] Too few patients with corrected congenital heart disease have yet reached a very old age for determination to be made regarding their risk of arrhythmia, ventricular dysfunction, and other abnormalities.

Uncorrected secundum atrial septal defect is the most frequent congenital cardiac lesion in elderly patients; these patients are characteristically asymptomatic in the absence of complicating pulmonary hypertension or supraventricular tachyarrhythmias. In patients symptomatic with dyspnea and fatigue who do not have elevated pulmonary vascular resistance, shunt closure improves symptoms and entails only a modestly greater risk than in a younger age group. Surgical correction is not indicated for a small calcified persistent ductus arteriosus because of the unacceptably high surgical risk without defined benefit.

Infective Endocarditis and Nonvalvular Cardiovascular Infections

Although one-third of all cases of infective endocarditis occur in elderly patients, its recognition is often delayed or missed in this age group because of fewer and atypical symptoms[271] and an absent or minimal febrile response. A cardiac murmur may not be prominent; the major presentations may be anemia, renal failure, hemiplegia, or unexplained coma. A high index of suspicion for endocarditis is warranted in elderly patients with otherwise unexplained fever, weight loss, embolic episodes, or confusion. Earlier recognition associated with the high diagnostic sensitivity of transesophageal echocardiography is credited in a recent report with improving clinical outcomes at elderly age, making them comparable to those for younger patients.[271] Elderly individuals constitute an increasing percentage of patients with infective endocarditis, and the problem is likely to increase further in prevalence as more elderly patients are hospitalized and undergo complex invasive diagnostic and therapeutic procedures. Endocarditis is associated with a higher mortality than in younger patients,[272] in part because of the delay in diagnosis and in the initiation of appropriate therapy. Invasive vascular procedures are the most common sources of infection; almost one-fourth of all episodes are nosocomially acquired. In addition to the organisms usually encountered in a younger population, enterococci, *Streptococcus bovis*, and coagulase-negative staphylococci occur with excess frequency in elderly patients.[272] Coagulase-negative staphylococci are typically traceable to invasive vascular or skin sources. *Streptococcus bovis* appears due to gastrointestinal problems, and enterococcal endocarditis appears related to the increase in genitourinary procedures performed in elderly men.

Aortic valve endocarditis is most common, with mitral regurgitation the second most frequent predisposing valvular lesion. Infective endocarditis often occurs in elderly patients with intracardiac prosthethic devices.[273]

Dosages of antibiotics may require reduction due to abnormalities of renal function and comorbid illness. Valve replacement must be addressed with hemodynamically significant abnormalities. Use of prophylactic antibiotics for appropriate invasive procedures can limit the occurrence of infective endocarditis in susceptible elderly patients.[266]

Nonvalvular cardiovascular infections are also more common in elderly patients, reflecting frequent use of implantable devices and prosthetic materials in a geriatric population. The subtle presentations warrant a high index of suspicion to initiate diagnostic measures.[274]

Cardiomyopathy

Hypertrophic cardiomyopathy occurs relatively frequently and is commonly underdiagnosed in elderly patients;[275] it may be incorrectly labeled as aortic valvular stenosis, mitral regurgitation, or the papillary muscle dysfunction of CHD. Incorrect diagnosis, with resultant inappropriate drug therapy (e.g., digitalis and other positive inotropic drugs, diuretics, nitroglycerin, and vasodilator drugs), may exacerbate the outflow obstruction and result in serious complications. Although about one-third of individuals with hypertrophic cardiomyopathy are older than age 60, little is known about the natural history of hypertrophic cardiomyopathy in elderly patients. In some series, women predominate among elderly patients with hypertrophic cardiomyopathy. The prognosis appears to be better than in a younger population, as serious arrhythmias or sudden cardiac death are unusual.[276] This prognosis may represent survival of a low-risk population, decreased physical activity with aging that limits risk, or this may be a different disease; disproportionate septal thickening and alteration in ventricular configuration occur with aging.[277] It remains uncertain whether hypertension is etiologic;[278] anterior displacement of the mitral valve due to mitral annular calcification may also be contributory. Left ventricular hypertrophy is described as more modest in elderly patients, involving predominantly the ventricular septum, with outflow obstruction caused by a combination of systolic anterior motion of the anterior mitral leaflet and posterior motion of the ventricular septum.[279]

Elderly patients characteristically have onset of symptoms late in life.[279] Clinical symptoms include dizziness, palpitations, syncope, chest pain, fatigue, and dyspnea, with the latter often the prominent complaint. Severe dyspnea portends an unfavorable prognosis.[276] It is uncertain whether symptoms differ from those of younger patients. Onset of atrial fibrillation may produce rapid hemodynamic deterioration, owing to dependence of the poorly compliant hypertrophied ventricle on the atrial contribution to ventricular filling to maintain stroke volume.

Physical examination may pose diagnostic problems in that brisk carotid pulsations are erroneously ascribed to decreased vascular elasticity, and an S_4 and nonspecific systolic murmurs are common in elderly patients. A bisferiens carotid pulse or a double cardiac apex impulse may be the clue to perform appropriate maneuvers. The left sternal border systolic murmur increases with a Valsalva maneuver and decreases on squatting. An aortic regurgitant murmur may be caused by coexisting calcific aortic valve disease.

The electrocardiogram is that of left ventricular hypertrophy; Q waves of septal hypertrophy may mimic MI. Echocardiography can confirm the diagnosis. Free wall myocardial hypertrophy may equal that of the ventricular septum.

Prophylaxis against infective endocarditis is appropriate. The majority of symptomatic elderly patients benefit from medical therapy. Calcium- or beta-blocking drug therapy can alleviate symptoms of angina and dyspnea. Hypovolemia increases risk and should be avoided. Occasionally, severely symptomatic elderly patients with a significant ventricular outflow gradient and an unsatisfactory response to medical management warrant surgical correction.[280]

Dilated cardiomyopathy is infrequent in an elderly population, as the majority of patients with this problem do not survive to an elderly age. Hypertension and lower educational levels are associated with dilated cardiomyopathy at elderly age.[281] The management is as for ventricular systolic dysfunction and includes digitalis, diuretics, angiotensin-converting enzyme (ACE) inhibitors, and other vasodilator drugs; anticoagulation is recommended, particularly when there is associated atrial fibrillation, to prevent embolic events.[282]

Restrictive cardiomyopathy is unusual in elderly patients. Although senile cardiac amyloidosis has a high prevalence among the oldest old patients, atrial fibrillation, rather than restrictive cardiomyopathy, seems to be the more frequent manifestation. ECG voltage is low in patients with cardiac amyloidosis, and echocardiography may demonstrate a "sparkling" appearance to the myocardium. Hemochromatosis is another, although uncommon, cause of restrictive cardiomyopathy. Restrictive cardiomyopathy is increasingly encountered as a consequence of CABG surgery and postoperative pericarditis, as well as of radiation therapy to the chest.

Cardiac Disease Secondary to Pulmonary Disease

Pulmonary embolism is a frequent and often unrecognized complication of many systemic illnesses in elderly patients.[283] The combination of prolonged bed rest, a sedentary lifestyle, cardiopulmonary diseases, heart failure, and frequent surgical procedures are the major predisposing factors, as is atrial fibrillation. It is often misdiagnosed as pneumonia or heart failure. An estimated 107,000 hospitalizations annually in the Medicare population result from deep vein thrombosis and pulmonary embolism.[284]

The clinical presentation varies from an acute cardiovascular emergency characterized by dyspnea, orthopnea, chest discomfort, syncope, or shock, or at times may be manifest only as increased cough, mild chest discomfort, transient dyspnea, or a worsening of heart failure. Sudden unexplained dyspnea should be considered to be caused by pulmonary embolism until proved otherwise. A high index of suspicion is warranted to search for evidence of deep vein thrombosis of the leg and evidence of acute cor pulmonale. Pulmonary ventilation-perfusion scanning is the initial screening procedure. However, isotopic perfusion lung scanning abnormalities may occur in the absence of pulmonary embolism because of the nonuniform perfusion of the aged lung. Spiral CT scanning appears to provide comparable diagnostic accuracy and greater safety. Pulmonary angiography, if needed, does not entail substantially greater risk than at younger age, save for the more frequent complicating renal failure.[283]

Clinical findings include tachypnea, tachycardia, often a low-grade fever, an accentuated pulmonic component of S_2 with wide splitting, a prominent parasternal impulse, an accentuated a wave in the jugular venous pulse, and at times evidence of right ventricular decompensation. Deep vein thrombosis of the leg also may be evident.

In a Medicare population, the 30-day case-fatality rates increased with increasing age. The risk of fatality was very high (25%–40%) when pulmonary embolism complicated cardiac problems, including heart failure, stroke, MI, and chronic pulmonary disease, and after CABG surgery or hip or knee replacement. These data highlight the need for deep vein thrombosis prophylaxis in these populations.[285]

Anticoagulation, initially with heparin and subsequently with warfarin, is the treatment of choice. Thrombolytic therapy may be indicated for massive pulmonary embolism with hemodynamic instability; the risk of bleeding is increased at elderly age. Vena caval obstruction with a transvenously inserted filter device is appropriate when anticoagulation is contraindicated.

Pulmonary heart disease in elderly patients is superimposed on the decreased elastic properties of the aged lung, as well as the loss of pulmonary vascular reserve and the decrease in ventilatory function and pulmonary diffusing capacity of aging. The most common form of chronic pulmonary heart disease that causes cor pulmonale and right ventricular failure at elderly age is chronic obstructive pulmonary disease due to chronic bronchitis and emphysema. The mortality from this problem among elderly patients is related, at least in part, to their coexisting cardiovascular disease, predominantly CHD and hypertensive cardiovascular disease. Recurrent pulmonary embolism is an important etiology, especially with prolonged immobilization at bed rest. Primary pulmonary hypertension has also been described in old age.[286] Smoking is a chronic contributor to the increased severity of cardiac decompensation; environmental pollutants and respiratory infections cause intermittent exacerbations.

An accentuated pulmonic component of S_2, often with wide splitting; jugular venous distension with prominent a and v waves; a parasternal cardiac impulse; a right-sided S_3; the holosystolic murmur of tricuspid regurgitation that increases with inspiration; hepatomegaly and peripheral edema; and right axis deviation of the frontal plane QRS axis and evidence of right ventricular hypertrophy and right atrial abnormality on the ECG are the clinical findings of pulmonary hypertension and right ventricular decompensation.

Echocardiography or radioisotope angiography may help differentiate pulmonary hypertension due to pulmonary vascular obstruction with right-sided heart failure from left-sided heart disease, pulmonary hypertension, and right-sided heart failure.

Therapy includes smoking cessation, bronchodilator drugs, liquefaction of sputum, and treatment of respiratory infections. Sodium restriction and diuretic therapy may lessen heart failure. Digitalis use is controversial except for control of the ventricular response rate to supraventricular tachyarrhythmias. Digitalis toxicity is common in elderly patients with chronic lung disease.

Compensation of the pulmonary status best controls supraventricular arrhythmia. There is no evidence that any pulmonary vasodilator drugs have a beneficial effect on a long-term basis, despite the demonstration of acute hemodynamic improvement. Similarly, phlebotomy to reduce blood viscosity in patients with moderate erythrocytosis remains controversial in that the oxygen-carrying capacity of the blood is reduced and little hemodynamic benefit is attained. Low- to moderate-intensity regular aerobic exercise can improve functional status in patients with a compensated pulmonary status.

Therapeutic problems are accentuated with concomitant cardiac and pulmonary disease, in that the nonselective beta-blocking drugs used to treat CHD or hypertension may induce bronchospasm and worsen chronic lung disease; conversely, theophylline and beta-agonist drugs used as bronchodilators to manage chronic obstructive pulmonary disease may worsen angina and hypertension and induce arrhythmias. Corticosteroid therapy for chronic obstructive pulmonary disease may exacerbate hypertension and heart failure. When significant hypoxemia is present, elderly patients have a favorable response, comparable with that of younger patients, to continuous low-flow oxygen therapy, if respiratory depression does not occur.

Noncardiac Surgery in Elderly Patients with Cardiovascular Disease

The increasing numbers of elderly persons and the success of surgical procedures at geriatric age have increased the number of surgical interventions in this population. More than one-fifth of all noncardiac surgical procedures currently involves elderly patients. Cardiac complications are the major contributors to perioperative morbidity and mortality. Emergency surgery entails the highest cardiovascular risk, as cardiac problems cannot be optimally managed preoperatively or cardiac risk status is unknown.

There is more heterogeneity in an elderly population than within any other age group; chronologic age poorly predicts either a patient's physiologic age or functional capabilities. Negative stereotypes of elderly persons as being seriously ill and disabled often inappropriately bias recommendations and decisions about medical care and particularly surgical interventions for elderly cardiac patients. Age alone should not constitute a contraindication to surgical therapy; the increased complications in elderly patients relate predominantly to their associated diseases; these should prominently influence clinical decisions. Mental status, cognitive ability, and expectations from medical care are other attributes to be considered. Both overt and occult cardiovascular disease, but particularly CHD, contribute to the increased risk of perioperative cardiovascular complications. In addition to cardiac disease, noncardiovascular surgery in elderly patients is often complicated by cerebrovascular and peripheral vascular disease, atherosclerosis of the aorta and great vessels, impaired renal function, prostatic obstruction, pulmonary disease, and malnutrition. In addition to cardiac status, cardiac risk for anesthesia and surgery encompasses the baseline physiologic changes of aging and the comorbid illnesses. As with cardiac surgery, overall recovery from noncardiac surgery at elderly age is protracted, with increased needs for nursing care and more time spent in an intensive care setting.

Perioperative MI is the major cause of postoperative mortality at elderly age owing to the high prevalence of known and unrecognized CHD.[287] The highest risk for noncardiac surgery is within 6 months of MI; only emergency or urgent surgery should be undertaken in this period. Unstable angina, residual myocardial ischemia, uncontrolled hypertension, and decompensated heart failure also entail an adverse prognosis. Because of the high prevalence of significant CHD in asymptomatic or minimally symptomatic elderly patients, preoperative exercise or pharmacologic thallium scintigraphy or echocardiography helps evaluate CHD status, assessing the extent of myocardial ischemia and consequent risk status, suggesting the need for further evaluation.[288] A normal study identifies low risk status, abnormalities in one vascular territory intermediate risk status, and reversible defects in more than one vascular territory (suggesting multivessel CHD) high risk status. Determination of anaerobic threshold at exercise testing is described to precisely assess cardiovascular reserve and surgical risk at elderly age.[289] Coronary arteriography can define the need and suitability for myocardial revascularization before noncardiac surgery. High-risk patients with a varied age range who had CABG surgery before noncardiac surgery had a mortality risk comparable to that of patients without significant CHD.[290] Risk stratification is particularly indicated before elective peripheral vascular surgery because of the substantial concordance of known and unrecognized but correctable CHD with peripheral arterial disease.[291,292]

Intraoperative and postoperative surveillance should highlight adequate oxygenation, electrolyte balance, and control of cardiac failure and arrhythmia. Pulmonary artery catheter monitoring is warranted for severe heart failure or suspected myocardial ischemia. Prophylactic digitalis administration and prophylactic pacemaker insertion are not indicated. Most patients with known suspected CHD should have continuous intraoperative ECG monitoring. Evaluation for an acute event by cardiac enzymes and ECG daily for at least 3 days postoperatively shows the highest occurrence of acute coronary events on postoperative days 2 and 3.

Preventive and Rehabilitative Approaches to Care

As increased numbers of reasonably healthy and active individuals enter old age, more precise assessment of their functional capabilities will be required to determine suitable vocational, as well as recreational and leisure, activities. Remunerative work, continuing into the eighth decade, may soon be usual. This elderly population can be anticipated to have greater interest in and requirements for both primary and secondary preventive cardiovascular care. At the same time, an overriding concern among elderly persons is maintenance of a self-sufficient and independent lifestyle, to which loss or deterioration of functional capability is viewed as a threat.

Preventive strategies are increasingly applied to the elderly population, as modifiable coronary risk factors are highly prevalent in elderly patients[293] and continue to predict the occurrence and recurrence of coronary events and mortality in old age[294] (Table 39.3). Elderly persons are health conscious, as shown by their disproportionate representation in most health screening programs. Given the estimated U.S. life expectancy of 16.9 years at age 65 and 10.7 years at age 75, coronary risk reduction strategies are appropriate. However, data from a Canadian study[295] show that even among hospitalized patients at high risk for cardiovascular events, risk factor assessment and modification was suboptimal, particularly for women and elderly patients. Because of continued progression of coronary atherosclerotic lesions even in old age, risk intervention may arrest the progression or induce regression of atherosclerosis. Because preventive data are less

TABLE 39.3. Impact of risk factors on cardiovascular disease incidence by age in men and women at 30-year follow-up: Framingham Study.

| Risk factor | Multivariate logistic regression coefficients[a] at age: | | | |
| | 35–64 years[b] | | Age, 65–94 years[b] | |
	Men	Women	Men	Women
Systolic pressure	0.341*	0.361*	0.410*	0.207*
Diastolic pressure	0.302*	0.288**	0.259*	0.089*
Serum cholesterol level	0.230***	0.202*	0.091****	0.040*
Blood glucose level	0.087***	0.176***	0.146*	0.173*
Relative weight	0.080****	0.134**	0.044*	0.052*
Vital capacity	−0.089****	−0.252*	−0.109*	−0.216*
Cigarettes	0.333*	0.183*	0.045*	0.083*
ECG-LVH	0.121*	0.112*	0.142*	0.229*
Intraventricular block	0.049***	0.075****	0.096****	0.096****
NSA-ST-T	0.053*	0.130*	0.187*	0.147*

ECG-LVH, electrocardiographic evidence of left ventricular hypertrophy; NSA-ST-T, nonspecific ST segment and T-wave abnormalities.
[a] Covariates for each variable cited in "Risk Factor" column: blood pressure, cholesterol, cigarettes, and electrocardiographic evidence of left ventricular hypertrophy.
[b] Age at biennial examination.
* $p < 0.001$; ** $p < 0.01$; *** not significant; **** $p < 0.05$.
Source: Modified from Kannel et al. Coronary events, stroke, cardiac failure, and peripheral arterial disease. Reprinted with permission from American College of Cardiology (*J Am Coll Cardiol*. 1987;10:25A–28A), with permission.

robust than for younger patients, interventions should entail few risks, involve few adverse effects, and have reasonable cost. Preventive approaches include control of hypertension, weight reduction or control, dietary sodium and fat restriction, regular modest-intensity physical activity, and emphasis on smoking cessation. Although the relative importance of coronary risk factors decreases somewhat with age, the absolute or attributable risk is greater due to the excess coronary morbidity and mortality in elderly patients. In the Honolulu Heart Study smoking, hypertension, diabetes, and hypercholesterolemia conferred a comparable relative risk for CHD at middle and old age.[296]

In the Cardiovascular Health Study (CHS),[297] noninvasively detected subclinical disease was associated with a very high risk of clinical disease, with systolic hypertension and diabetes the most powerful traditional risk factors.[101] Noninvasively detected subclinical disease, that is, abnormal echocardiographic ejection fraction, increased internal carotid intima-medial thickness, and low ankle–arm index, also was an independent predictor for 5-year mortality.[298] Aggressive preventive interventions appear warranted for elderly persons with subclinical disease.

Higher levels of fibrinogen and factor VIII[299] were associated with an increased risk for cardiovascular events and mortality in CHS, and C-reactive protein was associated with incident cardiovascular events, especially in elderly individuals with subclinical disease.[300]

The lesser risk relationship of cholesterol levels to coronary disease in older adults is offset by the greater occurrence of CHD in elderly persons.[301] Elevated total

cholesterol levels increase risk of coronary death at elderly age; risk for coronary death decreased as cholesterol levels decreased.[302] In the Zutphen Elderly Study,[303] both total and HDL cholesterol were important predictors of CHD in elderly men. Vegetarians, who have lower cholesterol levels than nonvegetarians, also show lower CHD rates even in the 75- to 84-year-old age group.[304] Women constitute a greater proportion of the elderly population, where the occurrence of MI is comparable in elderly men and women, so that detection and management of CHD must intensively involve elderly women. Although mean blood cholesterol levels are higher in men before the fifth decade, women subsequently have higher mean total cholesterol levels, which continue to increase at least to age 80, due to progressive increases in low-density (LDL) cholesterol, which exceeds that for men at elderly age.

Recommendations for recognition and management of hyperlipidemia are comparable in younger and elderly populations, as hypercholesterolemia continues to confer increased coronary risk at elderly age. The Adult Treatment Panel of the National Cholesterol Education Program (NCEP) recommends that all adults with total blood cholesterol values above 200 mg/dL be evaluated and that those with elevated LDL cholesterol levels be treated.[305] About one-third of elderly men and one-half of elderly women have elevated cholesterol levels warranting intervention, based on NCEP guidelines.[306] Recommendations for cholesterol lowering in the elderly population are based predominantly on extrapolation of data derived from younger populations, although one study of postinfarction patients that included a sizeable elderly cohort[307] described a 28% reduction in total mortality in patients treated with lipid-lowering agents. Nevertheless, few elderly patients were enrolled in most secondary prevention studies, and virtually none older than 75 years. Although intervention outcome data are limited for geriatric populations, statin drugs appear to have similar efficacy and safety in nonelderly and elderly populations.[308–311] Dietary therapy is recommended for the aged adult; this consists of a diet restricted in saturated fat and cholesterol and high in fruits, vegetables, and grains; additional dietary components include lean meats, fish, and low-fat dairy products. A trained nutritionist or dietitian can often help elderly individuals initiate appropriate dietary management, while assuring adequate nutrition. This diet may confer other health benefits as well.

Cigarette smoking continues to be associated with an increased risk of sudden cardiac death and fatal reinfarction,[312] and smoking cessation decreases cardiovascular risk to that of nonsmoking individuals, independent of the age at smoking cessation.[313] Smoking cessation decreased the risk of mortality or MI in older men and women with angiographically documented coronary disease in the Coronary Artery Surgery Study (CASS) Registry.[314]

Because deconditioning from inactivity occurs more rapidly at elderly age, a physically active lifestyle should be encouraged for elderly patients, incorporating a planned regimen of modest-intensity physical activity, designed to improve functional status and minimize or delay subsequent disability and dependency. A physical activity regimen, even in previously sedentary elderly patients, can enhance endurance and functional capacity. Resistance training improved walking endurance in healthy elderly individuals.[315] Although the effect of exercise on coronary risk has not been examined systematically in elderly populations, high-level physical activity (>2000 Kcal weekly) in persons 65 to 79 years was associated with improved survival compared with individuals with lower physical activity levels.[316] Moderate- and high-intensity walking lowered blood pressure in normotensive elderly subjects;[317] lower rates of hypertension are described in physically active elderly women.[220]

Both the physiologic characteristics of aging and the superimposed limitations due to cardiovascular disease must be addressed in formulating physical activity recommendations. Exercise recommendations must be individualized, avoiding excessive fatigue or exhaustion and limiting musculoskeletal injuries by restriction of running, jumping, and other high-impact activities.[185] Brisk walking is generally recommended. Both physical activity[318] and correct nutrition, including weight control, contribute importantly to the maintenance of cardiovascular function at elderly age. High-intensity resistance exercise can effectively counteract muscle weakness and physical frailty in very elderly people.[319]

Hypertension, elevation of both the systolic and the diastolic blood pressures, is the dominant cardiovascular risk factor in the elderly population, with its incidence increasing with advancing age; it continues to impart risk in elderly persons. Control of blood pressure limits cerebrovascular complications and facilitates the management of angina and of heart failure. Dietary sodium restriction is important in blood pressure control. Electrocardiographic evidence of left ventricular hypertrophy, intraventricular conduction disturbances, and nonspecific repolarization abnormalities all independently predict future cardiovascular events.

Control of obesity, in addition to decreasing cardiac work and cardiovascular risk, favorably affects glucose tolerance, blood pressure, and serum lipid levels. Diabetes mellitus or glucose intolerance remains an independent predictor of cardiovascular risk in old age. Postmenopausal estrogen use by women in the Cardiovascular Health Study[320] was associated with a more favorable cardiovascular risk profile well into the eighth decade. Whether this improvement reflects hormone effect or the baseline characteristics of women who continue hormone therapy or both is unknown. The role of dietary and pharmacologic antioxidants remains uncertain.[321] The decline in coronary mortality in the United States from 1963 to 1981 affected all ages, but was less prominent in the elderly population; because most cardiovascular risk factors can be modified in elderly persons, attention to this aspect seems to be appropriate. Based on Framingham data,[99] the 10% of individuals aged 65 to 74 years with the highest multivariate coronary risk scores had a twofold greater occurrence of coronary events among men and fourfold greater occurrence among women. In the elderly Framingham cohort, elevated risk levels for cardiovascular disease were associated with increased Medicare costs.[322] Benefits of risk reduction, however, must be extrapolated from intervention trials in younger-aged patients; however, conventional risk modification may favorably affect other health aspects as well.

Risk status can be ascertained by standard clinical examinations and simple laboratory tests. Most preventive measures that are appropriate for older individuals constitute reasonable and relatively simple modifications of existing habits; unfavorable lifestyle behaviors can be modified to favorably affect cardiovascular risk.

Conclusion

In planning for health care in the twenty-first century, the increased proportion of elderly patients, who often will have cardiovascular disease and often will require advanced technology diagnostic and therapeutic interventions, must be addressed.[323] Comparison must be made of the resources required for and outcomes of palliative care if sophisticated techniques are not undertaken. The use of health care resources will increase not only with increasing age but with the improved expectations of older persons about their health status.

At the same time, it will be necessary to avoid overzealous and redundant diagnostic and therapeutic measures. Data are needed to define interventions at old and very old age that favorably affect morbidity and mortality, functional status, and other meaningful quality of life attributes. Preventive aspects will increasingly become important components of care for elderly cardiac patients, and require the development of cost-effective preventive strategies, although it remains uncertain how much extension of years of health and decrease in disability can be anticipated in later life. The decline in premature cardiovascular mortality in recent decades appears an important component in the longevity of the elderly population; however, it is not certain whether the effect of preventive efforts in limiting or delaying cardiovascular disease will ultimately decrease overall health care costs.

Acknowledgments. With appreciation to Julia Wright and Jeanette Zahler for assistance in the preparation of the manuscript.

References

1. Wenger NK, ed. *Cardiovascular Disease in the Octogenarian and Beyond*. London: Dunitz, 1999.
2. National Center for Health Statistics. *Advance Report of Final Mortality Statistics, 1988. Monthly Vital Statistics Report, vol 39, no. 7 (suppl).* Hyattsville, MD: Public Health Service; 1990:1–48.
3. Riley G, Lubitz J, Prihoda R, et al. The use and costs of Medicare services by cause of death. *Inquiry.* 1987;24:233–244.
4. Gerson LW, Skvarch L. Emergency medical service utilization by the elderly. *Ann Emerg Med.* 1982;11:610–612.
5. Mittelmark MB, Psaty BM, Rautaharju PM, et al. Prevalence of cardiovascular diseases among older adults: the Cardiovascular Health Study. *Am J Epidemiol.* 1993;137:311–317.
6. Cheitlin MD, Gerstenblith G, Hazzard WR, et al. Do existing databases answer clinical questions about geriatric cardiovascular disease and stroke? *Am J Geriatr Cardiol.* 2001;10:207–223.
7. Bild DE, Fitzpatrick A, Fried LP, et al. Age-related trends in cardiovascular morbidity and physical functioning in the elderly: The Cardiovascular Health Study. *J Am Geriatr Soc.* 1993;41:1047-1056.
8. Corti M-C, Salive ME, Guralnik JM. Serum albumin and physical function as predictors of coronary heart disease mortality and incidence in older persons. *J Clin Epidemiol.* 1996;49:519–526.
9. Sollott SJ, Lakatta EG. Normal aging changes in the cardiovascular system. *Cardiol Elderly.* 1993;1:349–358.
10. Fleg JL, Lakatta EG. Role of muscle loss in the age-associated reduction in VO_2 max. *J Appl Physiol.* 1988;65: 1147–1151.
11. Lernfelt B, Wikstrand J, Svanborg A, et al. Aging and left ventricular function in elderly healthy people. *Am J Cardiol.* 1991;68:547–549.
12. Mader SL, Josephson KR, Rubenstein LZ. Low prevalence of postural hypotension among community-dwelling elderly. *JAMA.* 1987;258:1511–1514.
13. Rutan GH, Hermanson B, Bild DE, et al. Orthostatic hypotension in older adults. The Cardiovascular Health Study. *Hypertension.* 1992;19(part 1):508–519.
14. Bharati S, Lev M. Pathologic changes of the conduction system with aging. *Cardiol Elderly.* 1994;2:152–160.
15. Lindroos M, Kupari M, Heikkilä J, et al. Prevalence of aortic valve abnormalities in the elderly: an echocardiographic study of a random population sample. *J Am Coll Cardiol.* 1993;21:1220–1225.
16. Ooi WL, Barrett S, Hossain M, et al. Patterns of orthostatic blood pressure change an their clinical correlates in a frail, elderly population. *JAMA.* 1997;277:1299–1304.
17. Newman AB, Siscovick DS, Manolio TA, et al., for the Cardiovascular Health Study (CHS) Collaborative Research Group. Ankle-arm index as a marker of atherosclerosis in the Cardiovascular Health Study. *Circulation.* 1993;88: 837–845.
18. Otto CM, Lind BK, Kitzman DW, et al., for the Cardiovascular Health Study. Association of aortic-valve sclerosis with cardiovascular mortality and morbidity in the elderly. *N Engl J Med.* 1999;341:142–147.
19. Rautaharju PM, Manolio TA, Psaty BM, et al., for the Cardiovascular Health Study Collaborative Research Group. Correlates of QT prolongation in older adults (the Cardiovascular Health Study). *Am J Cardiol.* 1994;73: 999–1002.
20. de Bruyne MC, Hoes AW, Kors JA, et al. QTc dispersion predicts cardiac mortality in the elderly. The Rotterdam Study. *Circulation.* 1998;97:467–472.
21. Casiglia E, Maniati G, Daskalakis C, et al. Left-ventricular hypertrophy in the elderly: unreliability of ECG criteria in 477 subjects aged 65 years or more: the CArdiovascular STudy in the ELderly (CASTEL). *Cardiology.* 1996;87: 429–435.
22. Furberg CD, Manolio TA, Psaty BM, et al., for the Cardiovascular Health Study Collaborative Research Group. Major electrocardiographic abnormalities in persons aged 65 years and older (the Cardiovascular Health Study). *Am J Cardiol.* 1992;69:1329–1335.
23. Ingerslev J, Bjerregaard P. Prevalence and prognostic significance of cardiac arrhythmias detected by ambulatory electrocardiography in subjects 85 years of age. *Eur Heart J.* 1986;7:570–575.
24. Come PC, Riley MF, McKay RG, et al. Echocardiographic assessment of aortic valve area in elderly patients with aortic stenosis and of changes in valve area after percuta-

neous balloon valvuloplasty. *J Am Coll Cardiol.* 1987;10: 115–124.

25. Goraya TY, Jacobsen SJ, Pellikka PA, et al. Prognostic value of treadmill exercise testing in elderly persons. *Ann Intern Med.* 2000;132:862–870.

26. Deckers JW, Simoons ML, Fioretti P. The value of exercise testing in elderly patients. *Geriatr Cardiovasc Med.* 1988;1: 89–93.

27. Iskandrian AS, Heo J, Decoskey D, et al. Use of exercise thallium-201 imaging for risk stratification of elderly patients with coronary artery disease. *Am J Cardiol.* 1988; 61:269–272.

28. Hilton TC, Shaw LJ, Chaitman BR, et al. Prognostic significance of exercise thallium-201 testing in patients aged ≥70 years with known or suspected coronary artery disease. *Am J Cardiol.* 1992;69:45–50.

29. Lam JYT, Chaitman BR, Glaenzer M. Safety and diagnostic accuracy in dipyridamole-thallium imaging in the elderly. *J Am Coll Cardiol.* 1988;11:585–589.

30. Gersh BJ, Kronmal RA, Frye RL, et al. Coronary arteriography and coronary artery bypass surgery: morbidity and mortality in patients age 65 years or older. A report from the Coronary Artery Surgery Study. *Circulation.* 1983;67:483–491.

31. Clark VL, Khaja F. Risk of cardiac catheterization in patients age ≥80 years without previous cardiac surgery. *Am J Cardiol.* 1994;74:1076–1077.

32. Williams JF, Bristow MR, Fowler MB, et al. Guidelines for the evaluation and management of heart failure: report of the American College of Cardiology/American Heart Association Task Force on Practice Guidelines (Committee on Evaluation and Management of Heart Failure). *Circulation.* 1995;92:2764–2784.

33. Smith WM. Epidemiology of congestive heart failure. *Am J Cardiol.* 1985;55:3A–8A.

34. McKee PA, Castelli WP, McNamara PM, et al. The natural history of congestive heart failure: the Framingham Study. *N Engl J Med.* 1971;285:1441–1446.

35. Croft JB, Giles WH, Pollard RA, et al. Heart failure survival among older adults in the United States. A poor prognosis for an emerging epidemic in the Medicare population. *Arch Intern Med.* 1999;159:505–510.

36. Moser M, Hebert PR. Prevention of disease progression, left ventricular hypertrophy and congestive heart failure in hypertension treatment trials. *J Am Coll Cardiol.* 1996; 27:1214–1218.

37. Rich MW, Shah AS, Vinson JM, et al. Iatrogenic congestive heart failure in older adults: clinical course and prognosis. *J Am Geriatr Soc.* 1996;44:638–643.

38. Konstam MA, Dracup K, Baker D, et al. *Heart Failure: Evaluation and Care of Patients with Left-Ventricular Systolic Dysfunction. Clinical Practice Guideline No. 11.* AHCPR Pub 94-0612. Rockville, MD: Agency for Health Care Policy and Research, Public Health Service, U.S. Department of Health and Human Services; June 1994.

39. Vasan RS, Benjamin EJ, Levy D. Prevalence, clinical features and prognosis of diastolic heart failure: an epidemiologic perspective. *J Am Coll Cardiol.* 1995;26:1565–1574.

40. Wong WF, Gold S, Fukuyama O, et al. Diastolic dysfunction in elderly patients with congestive heart failure. *Am J Cardiol.* 1989;63:1526–1528.

41. Senni M, Tribouilloy CM, Rodeheffer RJ. Congestive heart failure in the community. A study of all incident cases in Olmsted County, Minnesota, in 1991. *Circulation.* 1998;98: 2282–2289.

42. van Kraaij DJW, Jansen RWMM, Bouwels LHR, et al. Furosemide withdrawal improves postprandial hypotension in elderly patients with heart failure and preserved left ventricular systolic function. *Arch Intern Med.* 1999; 159:1599–1605.

43. Kessler KM. Heart failure with normal systolic function. Update of prevalence, differential diagnosis, prognosis and therapy [editorial]. *Arch Intern Med.* 1988;148:2109–2111.

44. Cody RJ, Torre S, Clark M, et al. Age-related hemodynamic, renal, and hormonal differences among patients with congestive heart failure. *Arch Intern Med.* 1989;149: 1023–1028.

45. The CONSENSUS Trial Study Group. Effects of enalapril on mortality in severe congestive heart failure: results of the Cooperative North Scandinavian Enalapril Survival Study (CONSENSUS). *N Engl J Med.* 1987;316:1429–1435.

46. The SOLVD Investigators. Effect of enalapril on survival in patients with reduced left ventricular ejection fractions and congestive heart failure. *N Engl J Med.* 1991;325:293–302.

47. Cohn JN, Johnson G, Ziesche S, et al. A comparison of enalapril with hydralazine-isosorbide dinitrate in the treatment of chronic congestive heart failure. *N Engl J Med.* 1991;325:303–310.

48. Chapman D, Wang T, Gheorghiade M. Therapeutic approaches to heart failure in elderly patients. *Cardiol Elderly.* 1994;2:89–97.

49. Pfeffer MA, Braunwald E, Moyé LA, et al. Effect of captopril on mortality and morbidity in patients with left ventricular dysfunction after myocardial infarction. *N Engl J Med.* 1992;327:669–677.

50. The Acute Infarction Ramipril Efficacy (AIRE) Study Investigations. Effect of ramipril on mortality and morbidity of survivors of acute myocardial infarction with clinical evidence of heart failure. *Lancet.* 1993;342:821–828.

51. Cohn JN, Archibald DG, Ziesche S, et al. Effect of vasodilator therapy on mortality in chronic congestive heart failure: results of a Veterans Administration Cooperative Study. *N Engl J Med.* 1986;314:1547–1552.

52. De Bock V, Mets T, Romagnoli M, et al. Captopril treatment of chronic heart failure in the very old. *J Gerontol.* 1994;49:M148–M152.

53. Pitt B, Segal R, Martinez FA, et al., on behalf of the ELITE Study Investigators. Randomised trial of losartan versus captopril in patients over 65 with heart failure. Evaluation of Losartan in the Elderly Study, ELITE. *Lancet.* 1997; 349:747–752.

54. Pitt B for the ELITE II Investigators. Randomized evaluation of losartan compared to captopril in elderly patients with heart failure: ELITE II. Presented at the American

Heart Association 72nd Annual Scientific Sessions, Atlanta, GA, November 1999.

55. Packer M, Bristow MR, Cohn JN, et al. The effect of carvedilol on morbidity and mortality in patients with chronic heart failure. *N Engl J Med.* 1996;334:1349–1355.

56. CIBIS-II Investigators and Committees. The Cardiac Insufficiency Bisoprolol Study II (CIBIS II): a randomised trial. *Lancet* 1999;353:9–13.

57. Effect of metoprolol CR/XL in chronic heart failure: Metoprolol CR/XL Randomised Intervention Trial in Congestive Heart Failure (MERIT-HF). *Lancet.* 1999;353: 2001–2007.

58. Pitt B, Zannad F, Remme WJ, et al. The effect of spironolactone on morbidity and mortality in patients with severe heart failure. Randomized Aldactone Evaluation Study Investigators. *N Engl J Med.* 1999;341:709–717.

59. Krumholz HM, Wang Y, Parent EM, et al. Quality of care for elderly patients hospitalized with heart failure. *Arch Intern Med.* 1997;157:2242–2247.

60. Packer M, Gheorghiade M, Young JB, et al. Withdrawal of digoxin from patients with chronic heart failure treated with angiotensin-converting-enzyme inhibitors. RADIANCE Study. *N Engl J Med.* 1993;329:1–7.

61. The Digitalis Investigation Group. The effect of digoxin on mortality and morbidity in patients with heart failure. *N Engl J Med.* 1997;336:525–533.

62. Giannuzzi P, Tavazzi L, Temporelli PL, et al., for the EAMI Study Group. Long-term physical training and left ventricular remodeling after anterior myocardial infarction: Results of the Exercise in Anterior Myocardial Infarction (EAMI) Trial. *J Am Coll Cardiol.* 1993;22:1821–1829.

63. Wenger NK, Froelicher ES, Smith LK, et al. *Cardiac Rehabilitation.* Clinical Practice Guideline No. 17. AHCPR Pub 96-0672. Rockville, MD: U.S. Department of Health and Human Services, Public Health Service, Agency for Health Care Policy and Research and the National Heart, Lung, and Blood Institute; October 1995.

64. Pearson AC, Gudipati CV, Labovitz AJ. Systolic and diastolic flow abnormalities in elderly patients with hypertensive hypertrophic cardiomyopathy. *J Am Coll Cardiol.* 1988;12:989–995.

65. Rich MW, Beckham V, Wittenberg C, et al. A multidisciplinary intervention to prevent the readmission of elderly patients with congestive heart failure. *N Engl J Med.* 1995; 333:1190–1195.

66. Rich MW, Gray DB, Beckham V, et al. Effect of a multidisciplinary intervention on medication compliance in elderly patients with congestive heart failure. *Am J Med.* 1996;101:270–276.

67. Kornowski R, Zeeli D, Averbuch M, et al. Intensive home-care surveillance prevents hospitalization and improves morbidity rates among elderly patients with severe congestive heart failure. *Am Heart J.* 1995;129:762–766.

68. Krumholz HM, Butler J, Miller J, et al. Prognostic importance of emotional support for elderly patients hospitalized with heart failure. *Circulation.* 1998;97:958–964.

69. Kobashigawa JA. Early and late complications in the elderly heart transplant recipient. *Cardiol Elderly.* 1996;4: 15–21.

70. Martin A, Benbow LJ, Butrous GS. Five-year follow-up of 101 elderly subjects by means of long-term ambulatory cardiac monitoring. *Eur Heart J.* 1984;5:592–596.

71. Fleg JL, Kennedy HL. Cardiac arrhythmias in a healthy elderly population: detection by 24-hour ambulatory electrocardiography. *Chest.* 1982;81:302–307.

72. Kantelip JP, Sage E, Duchene-Marullaz P. Findings on ambulatory electrocardiographic monitoring in subjects older than 80 years. *Am J Cardiol.* 1986;57:398–401.

73. Lipsitz LA, Wei JY, Rowe JW. Syncope in an elderly, institutionalized population: prevalence, incidence, and associated risk. *Q J Med.* 1985;55:45–54.

74. Gordon M, Huang M, Gryfe CI. An evaluation of falls, syncope, and dizziness in prolonged ambulatory cardiographic monitoring in a geriatric institutional setting. *J Am Geriatr Soc.* 1982;30:6–12.

75. Manolio TA, Furberg CD, Rautaharju PM, et al., for the Cardiovascular Health Study (CHS) Collaborative Research Group. Cardiac arrhythmias on 24-h ambulatory electrocardiography in older women and men. The Cardiovascular Health Study. *J Am Coll Cardiol.* 1994;23: 916–925.

76. Ryder KM, Benjamin EJ. Epidemiology and significance of atrial fibrillation. *Am J Cardiol.* 1999;84:131R–138R.

77. Wolf PA, Abbott RD, Kannel WB. Atrial fibrillation: a major contributor to stroke in the elderly. *Arch Intern Med.* 1987;147:1561–1564.

78. Furberg CD, Psaty BM, Manolio TA, et al., for the Cardiovascular Health Study (CHS) Collaborative Research Group. Prevalence of atrial fibrillation in elderly subjects (the Cardiovascular Health Study). *Am J Cardiol.* 1994;74:236–241.

79. Benjamin EJ, Wolf PA, D'Agostino RB, et al. Impact of atrial fibrillation on the risk of death: the Framingham Heart Study. *Circulation.* 1998;98:946–952.

80. Carlsson J, Tebbe U, Rox J, et al., for the ALKK-Study Group. Cardioversion of atrial fibrillation in the elderly. *Am J Cardiol.* 1996;78:1380–1384.

81. Stroke Prevention in Atrial Fibrillation Investigators. Stroke prevention in atrial fibrillation study: final results. *Circulation.* 1991;84:527–539.

82. Petersen P, Boysen G, Godtfredsen J, et al. Placebo-controlled, randomised trial of warfarin and aspirin for prevention of thromboembolic complications in chronic atrial fibrillation: the Copenhagen AFASAK study. *Lancet.* 1989;1:175–179.

83. White RH, McBurnie MA, Manolio T, et al. Oral anticoagulation in patients with atrial fibrillation: adherence with guidelines in an elderly cohort. *Am J Med.* 1999;106:165–171.

84. Frishman WH, Heiman M, Karpenos A, et al. Twenty-four-hour ambulatory electrocardiography in elderly subjects: prevalence of various arrhythmias and prognostic implications. Report from the Bronx Longitudinal Aging Study. *Am Heart J.* 1996;132:297–302.

85. Josephson RA, Papa LA, Brooks MM, et al., for the CAST Investigators. Effect of age on postmyocardial infarction ventricular arrhythmias (Holter registry data from CAST I and CAST II). *Am J Cardiol.* 1995;76:710–713.

86. Mercando AD, Aronow WS, Epstein S, et al. Signal-averaged electrocardiography and ventricular tachycardia as predictors of mortality after acute myocardial infarction in elderly patients. *Am J Cardiol.* 1995;76:436–440.

87. Aronow WS, Mercando AD, Epstein S. et al. Effect of quinidine or procainamide versus no antiarrhythmic drug on sudden cardiac death, total cardiac death, and total death in elderly patients with heart disease and complex ventricular arrhythmias. *Am J Cardiol.* 1990;66: 423–428.

88. Tresch DD, Troup PJ, Thakur RK, et al. Comparison of efficacy of automatic implantable cardioverter defibrillator in patients older and younger than 65 years of age. *Am J Med.* 1991;90:717–724.

89. Zado ES, Callans DJ, Gottlieb CD, et al. Efficacy and safety of catheter ablation in octogenarians. *J Am Coll Cardiol.* 2000;35:458–462.

90. Kalusche D, Ott P, Arentz T, et al. AV nodal re-entry tachycardia in elderly patients: clinical presentation and results of radiofrequency catheter ablation therapy. *Coronary Artery Dis.* 1998;9:359–363.

91. Shen W-K, Hayes DL. Pacing the octogenarians and nonagenarians: should age be a consideration for pacing and outcome analysis of pacing in the very elderly? *Cardiol Elderly.* 1994;2:161–170.

92. Shen W-K, Hayes DL, Hammill SC, et al. Survival and functional independence after implantation of a permanent pacemaker in octogenarians and nonagenarians. A population-based study. *Ann Intern Med.* 1996;125:476–480.

93. Channon KM, Hargreaves MR, Cripps TR, et al. DDD vs VVI pacing in patients aged over 75 years with complete heart block: a double-blind crossover comparison. *Q J Med.* 1994;87:245–251.

94. Lamas GA, Pashos CL, Normand S-LT, et al. Permanent pacemaker selection and subsequent survival in elderly Medicare pacemaker recipients. *Circulation.* 1995;91: 1063–1069.

95. Gregoratos G, Cheitlin MD, Conill A, et al. ACC/AHA guidelines for Implantation of Cardiac Pacemakers and Antiarrhythmia Devices: A Report of the American College of Cardiology/American Heart Association Task Force on Practice Guidelines (Committee on Pacemaker Implantation). *J Am Coll Cardiol.* 1998;31:1175–1209.

96. Panotopoulos PT, Axtell K, Anderson AJ, et al. Efficacy of the implantable cardioverter-defibrillator in the elderly. *J Am Coll Cardiol.* 1997;29:556–560.

97. Tresch DD. CPR in the elderly: when should it be performed? *Geriatrics.* 1991;46:47–56.

98. Dawson DA, Adams PF. *Current Estimates from the National Health Interview Survey, United States, 1986. Vital and Health Statistics, Series 10, No 164.* Department of Health and Human Services Publication PHS 87-1592. Hyattsville, MD: National Center for Health Statistics, Public Health Service; 1987:98.

99. Wenger NK, Furberg CD, Pitt E. *Coronary Heart Disease in the Elderly. Working Conference on the Recognition and Management of Coronary Heart Disease in the Elderly, National Institutes of Health, Bethesda 1985.* New York: Elsevier; 1986.

100. Graves EJ. *Summary, 1989 National Hospital Discharge Survey: Advance Data from Vital and Health Statistics No 199.* Hyattsville, MD: National Center for Health Statistics; 1991:1–12.

101. Psaty BM, Furberg CD, Kuller LH, et al. Traditional risk factors and subclinical disease measures as predictors of first myocardial infarction in older adults: the Cardiovascular Health Study. *Arch Intern Med.* 1999;159:1339–1347.

102. Pepine CJ, Abrams J, Marks RG, et al., for the TIDES Investigators. Characteristics of a contemporary population with angina pectoris. *Am J Cardiol.* 1994;74:226–231.

103. Umachandran V, Ranjadayalan K, Ambepityia G, et al. Aging, autonomic function, and the perception of angina. *Br Heart J.* 1991;66:15–18.

104. LaCroix AZ, Guralnik JM, Curb JD, et al. Chest pain and coronary heart disease mortality among older men and women in three communities. *Circulation.* 1990;81:437–446.

105. Stone PH, Thompson B, Anderson HV, et al., for the TIMI III Registry Study Group. Influence of race, sex, and age on management of unstable angina and non-Q-wave myocardial infarction: the TIMI III Registry. *JAMA.* 1996; 275:1104–1112.

106. Marcus FI, Friday K, McCans J, et al. Age-related prognosis after acute myocardial infarction (the Multicenter Diltiazem Postinfarction trial). *Am J Cardiol.* 1990;65:559–566.

107. American Heart Association National Center. *Vital Statistics of the United States.* Dallas, TX: American Heart Association; 1995.

108. Vaccarino V, Berkman LF, Mendes de Leon CF, et al. Functional disability before myocardial infarction in the elderly as a determinant of infarction severity and postinfarction mortality. *Arch Intern Med.* 1997;157:2196–2204.

109. Devlin W, Cragg D, Jacks M, et al. Comparison of outcome in patients with acute myocardial infarction aged >75 years with that in younger patients. *Am J Cardiol.* 1995;75: 573–576.

110. Krumholz HM, Murillo JE, Chen J, et al. Thrombolytic therapy for eligible elderly patients with acute myocardial infarction. *JAMA.* 1997;277:1683–1688.

111. Weaver WD, Litwin PE, Martin JS, et al., the MITI Project Group. Effect of age on use of thrombolytic therapy and mortality in acute myocardial infarction. *J Am Coll Cardiol.* 1991;18:657–662.

112. Wolinsky FD, Wyrwich KW, Gurney JG. Gender differences in the sequelae of hospitalization for acute myocardial infarction among older adults. *J Am Geriatr Soc.* 1999; 47:151–158.

113. Vaccarino V, Parsons L, Every NR, et al., for the National Registry of Myocardial Infarction 2 Participants. Sex-based differences in early mortality after myocardial infarction. *N Engl J Med.* 1999;341:217–225.

114. Nadelmann J, Frishman WH, Ooi WL, et al. Prevalence, incidence and prognosis of recognized and unrecognized myocardial infarction in persons aged 75 years or older: the Bronx Aging Study. *Am J Cardiol.* 1990;66:533–537.

115. Solomon CG, Lee TH, Cook EF, et al., for the Chest Pain Study Group. Comparison of clinical presentation of acute myocardial infarction in patients older than 65 years of age

to younger patients: the Multicenter Chest Pain Study experience. *Am J Cardiol.* 1989;63:772–776.

116. Svanborg A, Bergstrom G, Mellstrom D. *Epidemiological Studies on Social and Medical Conditions of the Elderly. European Reports and Studies 62.* Copenhagen: WHO Regional Office for Europe; 1982.

117. Gurwitz JH, McLaughlin TJ, Willison DJ, et al. Delayed hospital presentation in patients who have had acute myocardial infarction. *Ann Intern Med.* 1997;126:593–599.

118. Paul SD, O'Gara PT, Mahjoub ZA, et al. Geriatric patients with acute myocardial infarction: cardiac risk factor profiles, presentation, thrombolysis, coronary interventions, and prognosis. *Am Heart J.* 1996;131:710–715.

119. Hong RA, Licht JD, Wei JY, et al. Elevated CK-MB with normal total creatine kinase in suspected myocardial infarction: associated clinical findings and early prognosis. *Am Heart J.* 1986;111:1041–1047.

120. Gruppo Italiano per lo Studio della Streptochinasi nell'Infarto Miocardico (GISSI). Long-term effects of intravenous thrombolysis in acute myocardial infarction: final report of the GISSI study. *Lancet.* 1987;ii:871–874.

121. Wilcox RG, Von der Lippe G, Olsson CG, et al., for the Anglo-Scandinavian Study of Early Thrombolysis. Effects of alteplase in acute myocardial infarction: 6-month results from the ASSET study. *Lancet.* 1990;335:1175–1178.

122. AIMS Trial Study Group: Long-term effects of intravenous anistreplase in acute myocardial infarction: final report of the AIMS study. *Lancet.* 1990;335:427–431.

123. Fibrinolytic Therapy Trialists' (FTT) Collaborative Group. Indications for fibrinolytic therapy in suspected acute myocardial infarction: collaborative overview of early mortality and major morbidity results from all randomised trials of more than 1000 patients. *Lancet.* 1994;343:311–322.

124. Ryan TJ, Anderson JL, Antman EM, et al. ACC/AHA guidelines for the management of patients with acute myocardial infarction: a report of the American College of Cardiology/American Heart Association Task Force on Practice Guidelines (Committee on Management of Acute Myocardial Infarction). *J Am Coll Cardiol.* 1996;28:1328–1428.

125. Chaitman BR, Thompson B, Wittry MD, et al. The use of tissue-type plasminogen activator for acute myocardial infarction in the elderly: results from Thrombolysis in Myocardial Infarction Phase I, open label studies, and the Thrombolysis in Myocardial Infarction Phase II pilot study. *J Am Coll Cardiol.* 1989;14:1159–1165.

126. The International Study Group. In-hospital mortality and clinical course of 20,891 patients with suspected acute myocardial infarction randomised between alteplase and streptokinase with or without heparin. *Lancet.* 1990;336: 71–75.

127. Gruppo Italiano per lo Studio della Sopravvivenza nell'Infarto Miocardico. GISSI-2: a factorial randomised trial of alteplase versus streptokinase and heparin versus no heparin among 12,490 patients with acute myocardial infarction. *Lancet.* 1990;336:65–71.

128. Gore JM, Sloan M, Price TR, et al. Intracerebral hemorrhage, cerebral infarction, and subdural hematoma after acute myocardial infarction and thrombolytic therapy in the Thrombolysis in Myocardial Infarction Study: Thrombolysis in Myocardial Infarction, Phase II, pilot and clinical trial. *Circulation.* 1991;83:448–459.

129. White HD, Barbash GI, Califf RM, et al., for the GUSTO-I Investigators. Age and outcome with contemporary thrombolytic therapy. Results from the GUSTO-I trial. *Circulation.* 1996;94:1826–1833.

130. Lesnefsky EJ, Lundergan CF, Hodgson JMB, et al. Increased left ventricular dysfunction in elderly patients despite successful thrombolysis: the GUSTO-l angiographic experience. *J Am Coll Cardiol.* 1996;28:331–337.

131. Pfeffer MA, Moye LA, Braunwald E, et al. Selection bias in the use of thrombolytic therapy in acute myocardial infarction. The SAVE Investigators. *JAMA.* 1991;266:528–532.

132. McLaughlin TJ, Gurwitz JH, Willison DJ, et al. Delayed thrombolytic treatment of older patients with acute myocardial infarction. *J Am Geriatr Soc.* 1999;45:1222–1228.

133. Tresch DD, Brady WJ, Aufderheide TP, et al. Comparison of elderly and younger patients with out-of-hospital chest pain: clinical characteristics, acute myocardial infarction, therapy, and outcomes. *Arch Intern Med.* 1996;156:1089–1093.

134. Newby LK, Rutsch WR, Califf RM, et al., for the GUSTO-I Investigators. Time from symptom onset to treatment and outcomes after thrombolytic therapy. *J Am Coll Cardiol.* 1996;27:1646–1655.

135. Gurwitz JH, Gore JM, Goldberg RJ, et al., for the Participants in the National Registry of Myocardial Infarction. Recent age-related trends in the use of thrombolytic therapy in patients who have had acute myocardial infarction. *Ann Intern Med.* 1996;124:283–291.

136. Maggioni AP, Maseri A, Fresco C, et al., on behalf of the Investigators of the Gruppo Italiano per lo Studio della Sopravvivenza nell'Infarto Miocardico (GISSI-2). Age-related increase in mortality among patients with first myocardial infarctions treated with thrombolysis. *N Engl J Med.* 1993;329:1442–1448.

137. Thiemann DR, Coresh J, Schulman SP, et al. Lack of benefit for intravenous thrombolysis in patients with myocardial infarction who are older than 75 years. *Circulation.* 2000;101:2239–2246.

138. Ayanian JZ, Braunwald E. Thrombolytic therapy for patients with myocardial infarction who are older than 75 years. Do the risks outweigh the benefits? [editorial]. *Circulation.* 2000;101:2224–2226.

139. The GUSTO V Investigators. Reperfusion therapy for acute myocardial infarction with fibrinolytic therapy or combination reduced fibrinolytic therapy and platelet glycoprotein IIb/IIIa inhibition: the GUSTO V randomised trial. *Lancet.* 2001;357:1905–1914.

140. Berger AK, Schulman KA, Gersh BJ, et al. Primary coronary angioplasty vs thrombotysis for the management of acute myocardial infarction in elderly patients. *JAMA.* 1999;282:341–348.

141. Holmes DR Jr, White HD, Pieper KS, et al. Effect of age on outcome with primary angioplasty versus thrombolysis. *J Am Coll Cardiol.* 1999;33:412–419.

142. Forman DE, Bernal JLG, Wei JY. Management of acute myocardial infarction in the very elderly. *Am J Med*. 1992; 93:315–326.

143. Laster SB, Rutherford BD, Giorgi LV, et al. Results of direct percutaneous transluminal coronary angioplasty in octogenarians. *Am J Cardiol*. 1996;77:10–13.

144. Hochman JS, Sleeper LA, Webb JG, et al. Early revascularization in acute myocardial infarction complicated by cardiogenic shock. SHOCK (Should We Emergently Revascularize Occluded Coronaries for Cardiogenic Shock). *N Engl J Med*. 1999;341:625–634.

145. Bueno H, López-Palop R, Bermejo J, et al. In-hospital outcome of elderly patients with acute inferior myocardial infarction and right ventricular involvement. *Circulation*. 1997;96:436–441.

146. Weintraub RM, Wei JY, Thurer RL. Surgical repair of remediable postinfarction cardiogenic shock in the elderly: early and long-term results. *J Am Geriatr Soc*. 1986;34:389–392.

147. McClellan M, McNeil BJ, Newhouse JP. Does more intensive treatment of acute myocardial infarction in the elderly reduce mortality? Analysis using instrumental variables. *JAMA*. 1994;272:859–866.

148. Pashos CL, Newhouse JP, McNeil BJ. Temporal changes in the care and outcomes of elderly patients with acute myocardial infarction, 1987 through 1990. *JAMA*. 1993; 270:1832–1836.

149. Gottlieb S, Goldbourt U, Boyko V, et al., for the SPRINT and Thrombolytic Survey Groups. Improved outcome of elderly patients (≥75 years of age) with acute myocardial infarction from 1981–1983 to 1992–1994 in Israel. *Circulation*. 1997;95:342–350.

150. Smith SC Jr, Gilpin E, Ahnve S, et al. Outlook after acute myocardial infarction in the very elderly compared with that in patients aged 65 to 75 years. *J Am Coll Cardiol*. 1990;16:784–792.

151. Rogers WJ, Bowlby LJ, Chandra NC, et al., for the Participants in the National Registry of Myocardial Infarction. Treatment of myocardial infarction in the United States (1990–1993): observations from the National Registry of Myocardial Infarction. *Circulation*. 1994;90: 2103–2114.

152. Krumholz HM, Radford MJ, Wang Y, et al. Early β-blocker therapy for acute myocardial infarction in elderly patients. *Ann Intern Med*. 1999;131:648–654.

153. Daida H, Kottke TE, Backes RJ, et al. Are coronary-care unit changes in therapy associated with improved survival of elderly patients with acute myocardial infarction? *Mayo Clinic Proc*. 1997;72:1014–1021.

154. The First International Study of Infarct Survival (ISIS-I) Collaborative Group. Randomised trial of intravenous atenolol among 16,027 cases of suspected acute myocardial infarction. *Lancet*. 1981;2:823–827.

155. Hjalmarson A, Elmfeldt D, Herlitz J, et al. Effect on mortality of metoprolol in acute myocardial infarction: a double-blind randomised trial. *Lancet*. 1981;2:823–827.

156. The MIAMI Trial Research Group. Metoprolol in acute myocardial infarction (MIAMI): a randomised placebo-controlled international trial. *Eur Heart J*. 1985;6: 199–226.

157. The International Collaborative Study Group. Reduction of infarct size with the early use of timolol in acute myocardial infarction. *N Engl J Med*. 1984;310:9–15.

158. The TIMI Study Group. Comparison of invasive and conservative strategies after treatment with intravenous tissue plasminogen activator in acute myocardial infarction: results of the Thrombolysis in Myocardial Infarction (TIMI) phase II trial. *N Engl J Med*. 1989;320:618–627.

159. Gundersen T, Abrahamsen AM, Kjekshus J, et al., for the Norwegian Multicentre Study Group. Timolol-related reduction in mortality and reinfarction in patients ages 65–75 years surviving acute myocardial infarction. *Circulation*. 1982;66:1179–1184.

160. Pederson TR, for the Norwegian Multicenter Study Group. Six-year follow-up of the Norwegian multicenter study on timolol after acute myocardial infarction. *N Engl J Med*. 1985;313:1055–1058.

161. Beta-Blocker Heart Attack Trial Research Group. A randomized trial of propranolol in patients with acute myocardial infarction. I. Mortality results. *JAMA*. 1982; 247:1707–1714.

162. Gurwitz JH, Goldberg RJ, Chen Z, et al. β-Blocker therapy in acute myocardial infarction: evidence for underutilization in the elderly. *Am J Med*. 1992;93:605–610.

163. Soumerai SB, McLaughlin TJ, Spiegelman D, et al. Adverse outcomes of underuse of β-blockers in elderly survivors of acute myocardial infarction. *JAMA*. 1997;277: 115–121.

164. Krumholz HM, Radford MJ, Wang Y, et al. National use and effectiveness of β-blockers for the treatment of elderly patients after acute myocardial infarction. National Cooperative Cardiovascular Project. *JAMA*. 1998;280:623–629.

165. Held PH, Yusuf S, Furberg CD. Calcium channel blockers in acute myocardial infarction and unstable angina: an overview. *Br Med J*. 1989;299:1187–1192.

166. ISIS-2 (Second International Study of Infarct Survival) Collaborative Group. Randomised trial of intravenous streptokinase, oral aspirin, both, or neither among 17,187 cases of suspected acute myocardial infarction: ISIS-2. *Lancet*. 1988;ii:349–360.

167. Krumholz HM, Radford MJ, Ellerbeck EF, et al. Aspirin in the treatment of acute myocardial infarction in elderly Medicare beneficiaries: patterns of use and outcomes. *Circulation*. 1995;92:2841–2847.

168. Krumholz HM, Radford MJ, Ellerbeck EF, et al. Aspirin for secondary prevention after acute myocardial infarction in the elderly. Prescribed use and outcomes. *Ann Intern Med*. 1996;124:292–298.

169. Gruppo Italiano per lo Studio della Sopravvivenza nell'Infarto Miocardico. GISSI-3: effects of lisinopril and transdermal glyceryl trinitrate singly and together on 6-week mortality and ventricular function after acute myocardial infarction. *Lancet*. 1994;3443:1115–1122.

170. Smith P, Arnesen H, Abdelnoor M. Effect of long-term anticoagulant therapy in subgroups after acute myocardial infarction. *Arch Intern Med*. 1992;152:993–997.

171. Second Report of the Sixty-Plus Reinfarction Study Research Group. Risk of long-term anticoagulant therapy

in elderly patients after myocardial infarction. *Lancet.* 1982;1:64–68.

172. Echt DS, Liebson PR, Mitchell LB, et al. Mortality and morbidity in patients receiving encainide, flecainide, or placebo: The Cardiac Arrhythmia Suppression Trial. *N Engl J Med.* 1991;324:781–788.

173. Josephson RA, Papa LA, Brooks MM, et al., for the CAST Investigators. Effect of age on postmyocardial infarction ventricular arrhythmias (Holter Registry Data from CAST I and CAST II). *Am J Cardiol.* 1995;76:710–713.

174. Majumdar SR, Gurwitz JH, Soumerai SB. Undertreatment of hyperlipidemia in the secondary prevention of coronary artery disease. *J Gen Intern Med.* 1999;14:711–717.

175. Ciaroni S, Delonca J, Righetti A. Early exercise testing after acute myocardial infarction in the elderly: clinical evaluation and prognostic significance. *Am Heart J.* 1993; 126:304–311.

176. Maggioni AP, Turazza FM, Tavazzi L. Risk evaluation using exercise testing in elderly patients after acute myocardial infarction. *Cardiol Elderly.* 1995;3:88–93.

177. Nicod P, Gilpin E, Dittrich H, et al. Short- and long-term clinical outcome after Q wave and non-Q wave myocardial infarction in a large patient population. *Circulation.* 1989;79:528–536.

178. Camerieri A, Picano E, Landi P, et al., on behalf of the Echo Persantine Italian Cooperative (EPIC) Study Group. Prognostic value of dipyridamole echocardiography early after myocardial infarction in elderly patients. *J Am Coll Cardiol.* 1993;22:1809–1815.

179. Chung MK, Bosner MS, McKenzie JP. Prognosis of patients ≥70 years of age with non-Q-wave acute myocardial infarction compared with younger patients with similar infarcts and with patients ≥70 years of age with Q-wave acute myocardial infarction. *Am J Cardiol.* 1995;75: 18–22.

180. Berkman LF, Leo-Summers L, Horwitz RI. Emotional support and survival after myocardial infarction: a prospective, population-based study of the elderly. *Ann Intern Med.* 1992;117:1003–1009.

181. Wenger NK. Populations with special needs for exercise rehabilitation. Elderly coronary patients. In: Wenger NK, Hellerstein HK, eds. *Rehabilitation of the Coronary Patient*, 3rd Ed. New York: Churchill Livingstone, 1992: 415–420.

182. Lavie CJ, Milani RV. Effects of cardiac rehabilitation programs on exercise capacity, coronary risk factors, behavioral characteristics, and quality of life in a large elderly cohort. *Am J Cardiol.* 1995;76:177–179.

183. Ades PA, Waldmann ML, Poehlman ET, et al. Exercise conditioning in older coronary patients: submaximal lactate response and endurance capacity. *Circulation.* 1993;88:572–577.

184. Lavie CJ, Milani RV. Benefits of cardiac rehabilitation and exercise training in elderly women. *Am J Cardiol.* 1997;79:664–666.

185. Pollock ML, Carroll JF, Graves JE, et al. Injuries and adherence to walk/jog and resistance training programs in the elderly. *Med Sci Sports Exerc.* 1991;23:1194–1200.

186. Peterson ED, Cowper PA, Jollis JG, et al. Outcomes of coronary artery bypass graft surgery in 24,461 patients aged 80 years or older. *Circulation.* 1995;92(suppl II): 85–91.

187. O'Keefe JH Jr, Sutton MB, McCallister BD, et al. Coronary angioplasty versus bypass surgery in patients >70 years old matched for ventricular function. *J Am Coll Cardiol.* 1994;24:425–430.

188. Morrison DA, Bies RD, Sacks J. Coronary angioplasty for elderly patients with "high risk" unstable angina: Short-term outcomes and long-term survival. *J Am Coll Cardiol.* 1997;29:339–344.

189. Weintraub WS, Clements SD, Ware J, et al. Coronary artery surgery in octogenarians. *Am J Cardiol.* 1991;68: 1530–1534.

190. Glower DD, Christopher TD, Milano CA, et al. Performance status and outcome after coronary artery bypass grafting in persons aged 80 to 93 years. *Am J Cardiol.* 1992; 70:567–571.

191. Ko W, Gold JP, Lazzaro R, et al. Survival analysis of octogenarian patients with coronary artery disease managed by elective coronary artery bypass surgery versus conventional medical treatment. *Circulation.* 1992;86(suppl II): II-191–II-97.

192. Tsai TP, Denton TA, Chaux A, et al. Results of coronary artery bypass grafting and/or aortic or mitral valve operation in patients ≥90 years of age. *Am J Cardiol.* 1994;74: 960–962.

193. Gersh BJ, Kronmal RA, Schaff HV, et al. Long-term (5-year) results of coronary bypass surgery in patients 65 years or older: a report from the Coronary Artery Surgery Study. *Circulation.* 1983;68(suppl II):II-190–II-199.

194. Barzilay JI, Kronmal RA, Bittner V, et al. Coronary artery disease and coronary artery bypass grafting in diabetic patients aged ≥65 years (report from the Coronary Artery Surgery Study [CASS] Registry). *Am J Cardiol.* 1994;74: 334–339.

195. Noyez L, van der Werf T, Remmen GHJ, et al. Importance of the internal mammary artery for coronary bypass grafting in patients aged ≥70 years. *Am J Cardiol.* 1995;75: 734–736.

196. Eagle KA, Guyton RA, Davidoff R, et al. ACC/AHA guidelines for coronary artery bypass graft surgery: a report of the American College of Cardiology/American Heart Association Task Force on Practice Guidelines (Committee to Revise the 1991 Guidelines for Coronary Artery Bypass Graft Surgery). *J Am Coll Cardiol.* 1999;34: 1262–1347.

197. Naunheim KS, Dean PA, Firoe AC, et al. Cardiac surgery in the octogenarian. *Eur J Cardiothorac Surg.* 1990;4: 130–135.

198. Katz ES, Tunick PA, Rusinek H, et al. Protruding aortic atheromas predict stroke in elderly patients undergoing cardiopulmonary bypass: experience with intraoperative transesophageal echocardiography. *J Am Coll Cardiol* 1992;20:70–77.

199. Newman MF, Croughwell ND, Blumenthal JA, et al. Effect of aging on cerebral autoregulation during cardiopulmonary bypass: association with postoperative cognitive dysfunction. *Circulation.* 1994;90(suppl II): II-243–II-249.

200. Horvath KA, DiSesa VJ, Peigh PS, et al. Favorable results of coronary artery bypass grafting in patients older than 75 years. *J Thorac Cardiovasc Surg.* 1990;99:92–96.

201. Gersh BJ, Kronmal RA, Schaff HV, et al., and participants in the CASS Study. Comparison of coronary artery bypass surgery and medical therapy in patients 65 years of age or older: a nonrandomized study from the Coronary Artery Surgery Study (CASS) Registry. *N Engl J Med.* 1985;313: 217–224.

202. Freeman WK, Schaff HV, O'Brien PC, et al. Cardiac surgery in the octogenarian: perioperative outcome and clinical follow-up. *J Am Coll Cardiol.* 1991;18:29–35.

203. Hirose H, Amano A, Yoshida S, et al. Coronary artery bypass grafting in the elderly. *Chest.* 2000;117:1262–1270.

204. Jaeger AA, Hlatky MA, Paul SM, et al. Functional capacity after cardiac surgery in elderly patients. *J Am Coll Cardiol.* 1994;24:104–108.

205. Kelsey SF, Miller DP, Holubkov R, et al. Results of percutaneous transluminal coronary angioplasty in patients ≥65 years of age (from the 1985 to 1986 National Heart, Lung, and Blood Institute's Coronary Angioplasty Registry). *Am J Cardiol.* 1990;66:1033–1038.

206. Bedotto JB, Rutherford BD, McConahay DR, et al. Results of multivessel percutaneous transluminal coronary angioplasty in persons aged 65 years and older. *Am J Cardiol* 1991;67:1051–1055.

207. Jackman JD, Navetta FI, Smith JE, et al. Percutaneous transluminal coronary angioplasty in octogenarians as an effective therapy for angina pectoris. *Am J Cardiol.* 1991; 68:116–119.

208. ten Berg JM, Voors AA, Suttorp MJ, et al. Long-term results after successful percutaneous transluminal coronary angioplasty in patients over 75 years of age. *Am J Cardiol.* 1996;77:690–695.

209. Tan KH, Sulke N, Taub N, et al. Percutaneous transluminal coronary angioplasty in patients 70 years of age or older: 12 years' experience. *Br Heart J.* 1995;74:310–317.

210. Thompson RC, Holmes DR Jr, Grill DE, et al. Changing outcome of angioplasty in the elderly. *J Am Coll Cardiol.* 1996;27:8–14.

211. Macaya C, Alfonso F, Iniguez A, et al. Long-term clinical and angiographic follow-up of percutaneous transluminal coronary angioplasty in patients ≥65 years of age. *Am J Cardiol.* 1990;66:1513–1515.

212. Taddei CFG, Weintraub WS, Douglas JS Jr, et al. Influence of age on outcome after percutaneous transluminal coronary angioplasty. *Am J Cardiol.* 1999;84:245–251.

213. Thompson RC, Holmes DR Jr, Gersh BJ, et al. Percutaneous transluminal coronary angioplasty in the elderly: early and long-term results *J Am Coll Cardiol.* 1991;17: 1245–1250.

214. Weyrens FJ, Goldenberg I, Mooney JF, et al. Percutaneous transluminal coronary angioplasty in patients aged ≥90 years. *Am J Cardiol.* 1994;74:397–398.

215. Popma JJ, Satler LF, Mintz GS, et al. Coronary angioplasty and new device therapy. *Cardiol Elderly.* 1993;1:62–70.

216. National High Blood Pressure Education Program Working Group. National High Blood Pressure Education Program Working Group Report on Hypertension in the Elderly. *Hypertension.* 1994;23:275–285.

217. Staessen J, Amery A, Fagard R. Editorial review. Isolated systolic hypertension in the elderly. *J Hypertens.* 1990;8: 393–405.

218. Pasierski T, Pearson AC, Labovitz AJ. Pathophysiology of isolated systolic hypertension in elderly patients: Doppler echocardiographic insights. *Am Heart J.* 1991;122:528–534.

219. Bots ML, Witteman JCM, Hofman A, et al. Low diastolic blood pressure and atherosclerosis in elderly subjects: the Rotterdam Study. *Arch Intern Med.* 1996;156:843–848.

220. Reaven PD, Barrett-Connor E, Edelstein S. Relation between leisure-time physical activity and blood pressure in older women. *Circulation.* 1991;83:559–565.

221. Applegate WB. Hypertension in elderly patients. *Ann Intern Med.* 1989;110:901–915.

222. Amery A, Birkenhäger W, Brixko R, et al. Efficacy of antihypertensive drug treatment according to age, sex, blood pressure, and previous cardiovascular disease in patients over the age of 60. *Lancet.* 1986;2:589–592.

223. Staessen JA, Thijs L, Fagard R, et al., for the Systolic Hypertensions in Europe Trial Investigators. Predicting cardiovascular risk using conventional vs ambulatory blood pressure in older patients with systolic hypertension. *JAMA.* 1999;282:539–546.

224. Sagie A, Benjamin EJ, Galderisi M, et al. Echocardiographic assessment of left ventricular structure and diastolic filling in elderly subjects with borderline isolated systolic hypertension (the Framingham Heart Study). *Am J Cardiol.* 1993;72:662–665.

225. Joint National Committee on Prevention, Detection, Evaluation, and Treatment of High Blood Pressure. The sixth report of the Joint National Committee on Prevention, Detection, Evaluation, and Treatment of High Blood Pressure. *Arch Intern Med.* 1997;157:2413–2446.

226. Veterans Administration Cooperative Study Group on Antihypertensive Agents. Effects of treatment on morbidity in hypertension. III: Influence of age, diastolic pressure, and prior cardiovascular disease: further analysis of side effects. *Circulation* 1972;45:991–1004.

227. Amery A, Birkenhager W, Brixko P, et al. Mortality and morbidity results from the European Working Party on High Blood Pressure in the Elderly Trial. *Lancet.* 1985;1: 1349–1354.

228. SHEP Cooperative Research Group. Prevention of stroke by antihypertensive drug treatment in older persons with isolated systolic hypertension: final results of the Systolic Hypertension in the Elderly Program (SHEP). *JAMA.* 1991;265:3255–3264.

229. Kostis JB, Davis BR, Cutler J, et al., for the SHEP Cooperative Research Group. Prevention of heart failure by antihypertensive drug treatment in older persons with isolated systolic hypertension. *JAMA.* 1997;278:212–216.

230. Curb JD, Pressel SL, Cutler JA, et al., for the Systolic Hypertension in the Elderly Program Cooperative Research Group. Effect of diuretic-based antihypertensive treatment on cardiovascular disease risk in older diabetic patients with isolated systolic hypertension. *JAMA.* 1996;276:1886–1892.

231. Wassertheil-Smoller S, Applegate WB, Berg K, et al., for the SHEP Cooperative Research Group. Change in

depression as a precursor of cardiovascular events. *Arch Intern Med.* 1996;156:553–561.

232. National Intervention Cooperative Study in Elderly Hypertensives Study Group. Randomized double-blind comparison of a calcium antagonist and a diuretic in elderly hypertensives. *Hypertension* 1999;34:1129–1133.

233. Whelton PK, Appel LJ, Espeland MA, et al., for the TONE Collaborative Research Group. Sodium reduction and weight loss in the treatment of hypertension in older persons: a randomized controlled Trial of Nonpharmacologic Interventions in the Elderly (TONE). *JAMA.* 1998; 279:839–846.

234. Gurwitz JH, Everitt DE, Monane M, et al. The impact of ibuprofen on the efficacy of antiyhypertensive treatment with hydrochlorothiazide in elderly persons. *J Gerontol* 1996;51A:M74–M79.

235. Mulrow CD, Cornell JA, Herrera CR, et al. Hypertension in the elderly: implications and generalizability of randomized trials. *JAMA.* 1994;272:1932–1938.

236. Pahor M, Guralnik JM, Furberg CD, et al. Risk of gastrointestinal haemorrhage with calcium antagonists in hypertensive persons over 67 years old. *Lancet.* 1996;347: 1061–1065.

237. MacMahon S, Rodgers A. The effects of blood pressure reduction in older patients: an overview of five randomized controlled trials in elderly hypertensives. *Clin Exp Hypertens.* 1993;15:967–978.

238. Elliott WJ, Weir DR, Black HR. Cost-effectiveness of the lower treatment goal (of JNC VI) for diabetic hypertensive patients. *Arch Intern Med.* 2000;160:1277–1283.

239. Culliford AT, Galloway AC, Colvin SB, et al. Aortic valve replacement for aortic stenosis in persons aged 80 years and over. *Am J Cardiol.* 1991;67:1256–1260.

240. Nylander E, Ekman I, Marklund T, et al. Severe aortic stenosis in elderly patients. *Br Heart J.* 1986;55:480–487.

241. Horstkotte D, Loogen F. The natural history of aortic valve stenosis. *Eur Heart J.* 1988;9(suppl E):57–64.

242. Iivanainen AM, Lindroos M, Tilvis R, et al. Natural history of aortic valve stenosis of varying severity in the elderly. *Am J Cardiol.* 1996;78:97–101.

243. Lombard JT, Selzer A. Valvular aortic stenosis: a clinical and hemodynamic profile of patients. *Ann Intern Med* 1987;106:292–298.

244. Lund O, Nielsen TT, Magnussen K, et al. Valve replacement for calcified aortic stenosis in septuagenarians infers normal life-length. *Scand J Thorac Cardiovasc Surg.* 1991; 25:37–44.

245. Bonow RO, Carabello B, de Leon AC Jr, et al. ACC/AHA guidelines for the management of patients with valvular heart disease: executive summary. A report of the American College of Cardiology/American Heart Association Task Force on Practice Guidelines (Committee on Management of Patients with Valvular Heart Disease). *Circulation.* 1998;98:1949–1984.

246. Turina J, Hess O, Sepulcri F, et al. Spontaneous course of aortic valve disease. *Eur Heart J.* 1987;8:471–483.

247. Aranki SF, Rizzo RJ, Couper GS, et al. Aortic valve replacement in the elderly. Effect of gender and coronary artery disease on operative mortality. *Circulation.* 1993; 88(part 2):17–23.

248. Verheul HA, van den Brink RBA, Bouma BJ, et al. Analysis of risk factors for excess mortality after aortic valve replacement. *J Am Coll Cardiol.* 1995;26:1280–1286

249. Elayda MacAA, Hall RJ, Reul RM, et al. Aortic valve replacement in patients 80 years and older: operative risks and long-term results. *Circulation.* 1993;88(part 2): 11–16.

250. Craver JM, Weintraub WS, Jones EL, et al. Predictors of mortality, complications, and length of stay in aortic valve replacement for aortic stenosis. *Circulation.* 1988; 78(suppl I):I-85–I-90.

251. Logeais Y, Langanay T, Roussin R, et al. Surgery for aortic stenosis in elderly patients: a study of surgical risk and predictive factors. *Circulation.* 1994;90:2891–2898.

252. Glock Y, Faik M, Laghzaoui A, et al. Cardiac surgery in the ninth decade of life. *Cardiovasc Surg.* 1996;4:241–245.

253. Zaidi AM, Fitzpatrick AP, Keenan DJM, et al. Good outcomes from cardiac surgery in the over-70s. *Heart.* 1999;82:134–137.

254. Kolh P, Lahaye L, Gerard P, et al. Aortic valve replacement in the octogenarians: perioperative outcome and clinical follow-up. *Eur J Cardiothorac Surg.* 1999;16:68–73.

255. Tseng EE, Lee CA, Cameron DE, et al. Aortic valve replacement in the elderly: risk factors and long-term results. *Ann Surg.* 1997;225:793–804.

256. Cohen G, David TE, Ivanov J, et al. The impact of age, coronary artery disease, and cardiac comorbidity on late survival after bioprosthetic aortic valve replacement. *J Thorac Cardiovasc Surg.* 1999;117:273–284.

257. McKay CR, Waller BF. Current status of balloon valvuloplasty. *Cardiol Elderly.* 1993;1:77–85.

258. O'Neill WW, for the Mansfield Scientific Aortic Valvuloplasty Registry Investigators. Predictors of long-term survival after percutaneous aortic valvuloplasty: report of the Mansfield Scientific Balloon Aortic Valvuloplasty Registry. *J Am Coll Cardiol.* 1991;17:193–198.

259. Otto CM, Mickel MC, Kennedy JW, et al. Three-year outcome after balloon aortic valvuloplasty: insights into prognosis of valvular aortic stenosis. *Circulation.* 1994;89: 642–650.

260. Cheitlin MD. Valve disease in the octogenarian. In: Wenger NK, ed. *Cardiovascular Disease in the Octogenarian and Beyond.* London: Dunitz; 1999:255–266.

261. Scognamiglio R, Rahimtoola SH, Fasoli G, et al. Nifedipine in asymptomatic patients with severe aortic regurgitation and normal left ventricular function. *N Engl J Med.* 1994;331:689–694.

262. Lee EM, Porter JN, Shapiro LM, et al. Mitral valve surgery in the elderly. *J Heart Valve Dis.* 1997;6:22–31.

263. Kolibash AJ, Bush CA, Fontana MB, et al. Mitral valve prolapse syndrome: analysis of 62 patients aged 60 years and older. *Am J Cardiol.* 1983;52:534–539.

264. Nair CK, Biddle P, Kaneshige A, et al. Ten-year experience with mitral valve replacement in elderly. *Am Heart J.* 1992; 124:154–159.

265. Bolling SF, Deeb M, Bach DS. Mitral valve reconstruction in elderly, ischemic patients. *Chest.* 1996;109:35–40.

266. Dajani AS, Taubert KA, Wilson W, et al. Prevention of bacterial endocarditis: recommendations by the American Heart Association. *JAMA.* 1997;277:1794–1801.

267. Ofili EO, Rich MI, Brown P, et al. Safety and usefulness of transesophageal echocardiography in persons aged ≥70 years. *Am J Cardiol.* 1990;66:1279–1280.

268. Le Feuvre C, Bonan R, Lachurie M-L, et al. Balloon mitral commissurotomy in patients aged ≥70 years. *Am J Cardiol.* 1993;71:233–236.

269. Meneveau N, Schiele F, Seronde M-F, et al. Predictors of event-free survival after percutaneous mitral commissurotomy. *Heart.* 1998;80:359–364.

270. Cheitlin MD. Congenital heart disease in the adult. *Mod Conc Cardiovasc Dis.* 1986;55:20–24.

271. Werner GS, Schulz R, Fuchs JB, et al. Infective endocarditis in the elderly in the era of transesophageal echocardiography: clinical features and prognosis compared with younger patients. *Am J Med.* 1996;100:90–97.

272. Terpenning MS, Buggy BP, Kauffman CA. Infective endocarditis: clinical features in young and elderly patients. *Am J Med.* 1987;83:626–634.

273. Selton-Suty C, Hoen B, Grentzinger A, et al. Clinical and bacteriological characteristics of infective endocarditis in the elderly. *Heart.* 1997;77:260–263.

274. Kearney RA, Eisen HJ, Wolf JE. Nonvalvular infections of the cardiovascular system. *Ann Intern Med.* 1994;121:219–230.

275. Krasnow N, Stein RA. Hypertrophic cardiomyopathy in the aged. *Am Heart J.* 1978;96:326–336.

276. Fay WP, Taliercio CP, Ilstrup DM, et al. Natural history of hypertrophic cardiomyopathy in the elderly. *J Am Coll Cardiol.* 1990;16:821–826.

277. Lever HM, Karam RF, Currie PJ, et al. Hypertrophic cardiomyopathy in the elderly: distinctions from the young based on cardiac shape. *Circulation.* 1989;79:580–589.

278. Pearson AC, Gudipati CV, Labovitz AJ. Systolic and diastolic flow abnormalities in elderly patients with hypertensive hypertrophic cardiomyopathy. *J Am Coll Cardiol.* 1988;12:989–995.

279. Lewis JF, Maron BJ. Clinical and morphologic expression of hypertrophic cardiomyopathy in patients ≥65 years of age. *Am J Cardiol.* 1994;73:1105–1111.

280. Koch J-P, Maron BJ, Epstein ES, et al. Results of operation for obstructive hypertrophic cardiomyopathy in the elderly: septal myotomy and myectomy in 20 patients 65 years of age or older. *Am J Cardiol.* 1980;46:963–966.

281. Coughlin SS, Tefft MC, Rice JC, et al. Epidemiology of idiopathic dilated cardiomyopathy in the elderly: pooled results from two case-control studies. *Am J Epidemiol.* 1996;143:881–888.

282. Shah PM, Abelmann WH, Gersh BJ. 18th Bethesda Conference: Cardiovascular Disease in the Elderly. Cardiomyopathies in the elderly. *J Am Coll Cardiol.* 1987;10(suppl A):77A–79A.

283. Stein PD, Gottschalk A, Saltzman HA, et al. Diagnosis of acute pulmonary embolism in the elderly. *J Am Coll Cardiol.* 1991;18:1452–1457.

284. Kniffin WD Jr, Baron JA, Barrett J, et al. The epidemiology of diagnosed pulmonary embolism and deep venous thrombosis in the elderly. *Arch Intern Med.* 1994;154:861–866.

285. Siddique RM, Siddique MI, Connors AF Jr, et al. Thirty-day case-fatality rates for pulmonary embolism in the elderly. *Arch Intern Med.* 1996;156:2343–2347.

286. Braman SS, Eby E, Kuhn C, et al. Primary pulmonary hypertension in the elderly. *Arch Intern Med.* 1991;151:2433–2438.

287. Mangano DT. Perioperative cardiac morbidity. *Anesthesiology.* 1990;72:153–184.

288. Eagle KA, Brundage BH, Chaitman BR, et al. Guidelines for perioperative cardiovascular evaluation for noncardiac surgery: report of the American College of Cardiology/American Heart Association Task Force on Practice Guidelines (Committee on Perioperative Cardiovascular Evaluation for Noncardiac Surgery). *Circulation.* 1996;93:1278–1317.

289. Wasserman K. Preoperative evaluation of cardiovascular reserve in the elderly. *Chest.* 1993;104:663–664.

290. Foster ED, David KB, Carpenter JA, et al. Risk of noncardiac operation in patients with defined coronary disease: the Coronary Artery Surgery Study (CASS) Registry experience. *Ann Thorac Surg.* 1986;41:42–50.

291. Gersh BJ, Rihal CS, Rooke TW, et al. Evaluation and management of patients with both peripheral vascular and coronary artery disease. *J Am Coll Cardiol.* 1991;18:203–214.

292. Towne JB, Weiss DG, Hobson RW II. First phase report of Cooperative Veterans Administration asymptomatic carotid stenosis study: operative morbidity and mortality. *J Vasc Surg.* 1990;11:252–259.

293. World Health Organization Study Group. *Epidemiology and Prevention of Cardiovascular Diseases in Elderly People.* WHO Technical Report Series 853. Geneva: World Health Organization; 1995.

294. Tervahauta M, Pekkanen J, Nissinen A. Risk factors of coronary heart disease and total mortality among elderly men with and without preexisting coronary heart disease: the Finnish Cohorts of the Seven Countries Study. *J Am Coll Cardiol.* 1995;26:1623–1629.

295. The Clinical Quality Improvement Network (CQIN) Investigators. Low incidence of assessment and modification of risk factors in acute care patients at high risk for cardiovascular events, particularly among females and the elderly. *Am J Cardiol.* 1995;76:570–573.

296. Masaki KH, Petrovitch H, Rodriquez BL, et al. The value of risk factor modification in old age. *Cardiol Elderly.* 1993;1:391–397.

297. Kuller L, Borhani N, Furberg C, et al. Prevalence of subclinical atherosclerosis and cardiovascular disease and association with risk factors in the Cardiovascular Health Study. *Am J Epidemiol* 1994;139:1164–1179.

298. Fried LP, Kronmal RA, Newman AB, et al., for the Cardiovascular Health Study Collaborative Research Group. Risk factors for 5-year mortality in older adults: the Cardiovascular Health Study. *JAMA.* 1998;279:585–592.

299. Tracy RP, Arnold AM, Ettinger W, et al. The relationship of fibrinogen and factors VII and VIII to incident cardiovascular disease and death in the elderly: results from the Cardiovascular Health Study. *Arterioscler Thromb Vasc Biol.* 1999;19:1776–1783.

300. Tracy RP, Lemaitre RN, Psaty BM, et al. Relationship of C-reactive protein to risk of cardiovascular disease in the elderly: results from the Cardiovascular Health Study and the Rural Health Promotion Project. *Arterioscler Thromb Vasc Biol.* 1997;17:1121–1127.

301. Kannel WB, Doyle JT, Shephard RJ, et al. 18th Bethesda Conference: Cardiovascular Disease in the Elderly. Prevention of cardiovascular disease in the elderly. *J Am Coll Cardiol.* 1987;10(suppl A):25A–28A.

302. Corti M-C, Guralnik JM, Salive ME, et al. Clarifying the direct relation between total cholesterol levels and death from coronary heart disease in older persons. *Ann Intern Med.* 1997;126:753–760.

303. Weijenberg MP, Feskens EJM, Kromhout D. Total and high density lipoprotein cholesterol as risk factors for coronary heart disease in elderly men during 5 years of follow-up: the Zutphen Elderly Study. *Am J Epidemiol.* 1996;143:151–158.

304. Snowdon DA, Phillips Rl, Fraser GE. Meat consumption and fatal ischemic heart disease. *Prev Med.* 1984;13:490–500.

305. The Expert Panel on Detection, Evaluation and Treatment of High Blood Cholesterol in Adults. Summary of the Second Report of the National Cholesterol Education Program (NCEP) Expert Panel on Detection, Evaluation, and Treatment of High Blood Cholesterol in Adults (Adult Treatment Panel II). *JAMA.* 1993;269:3015–3025.

306. Denke MA, Grundy SM. Hypercholesterolemia in elderly persons: resolving the treatment dilemma. *Ann Intern Med.* 1990;112:780–792.

307. Carlson LA, Rosenhamer G. Reduction of mortality in the Stockhom Ischaemic Heart Disease Secondary Prevention Study by combined treatment with clofibrate and nicotinic acid. *Acta Med Scand.* 1988;223:405–418.

308. Pacala JT, McBride PE, Grady SL. Management of older adults with hypercholesterolaemia. *Drugs Aging.* 1994;4: 366–378.

309. Santinga JT, Rosman HS, Rubenfire M, et al. Efficacy and safety of pravastatin in the long-term treatment of elderly patients with hypercholesterolemia. *Am J Med.* 1994;96: 509–515.

310. Hulley SB, Newman TB. Cholesterol in the elderly: is it important? *JAMA.* 1994;272:1372–1374.

311. Scandinavian Simvastatin Survival Study group. Randomised trial of cholesterol lowering in 4444 patients with coronary heart disease: the Scandinavian Simvastatin Survival Study (4S). *Lancet.* 1994;344:1383–1389.

312. Jajich CL, Ostfeld AM, Freeman DH Jr. Smoking and coronary heart disease mortality in the elderly. *JAMA.* 1984;252:2831–2834.

313. LaCroix AZ, Lang J, Scherr P, et al. Smoking and mortality among older men and women in three communities. *N Engl J Med.* 1991;324:1619–1625.

314. Hermanson B, Omenn GS, Kronmal RA, et al., and participants in the Coronary Artery Surgery Study. Beneficial six-year outcome of smoking cessation in older men and women with coronary artery disease. Results from the CASS Registry. *N Engl J Med.* 1988;319:1365–1369.

315. Ades PA, Ballor DL, Ashikaga T, et al. Weight training improves walking endurance in healthy elderly persons. *Ann Intern Med.* 1996;124:568–572.

316. Paffenbarger RS Jr, Hyde RT, Wing AL, et al. Physical activity, all-cause mortality, and longevity of college alumni. *N Engl J Med.* 1986;314:605–613.

317. Braith RW, Pollock ML, Lowenthal DT, et al. Moderate- and high-intensity exercise lowers blood pressure in normotensive subjects 60 to 79 years of age. *Am J Cardiol.* 1994;73:1124–1128.

318. Wenger NK. Physical inactivity and coronary heart disease in elderly patients. *Clin Geriatr Med.* 1996;12:79–88.

319. Fiatarone MA, O'Neill EF, Ryan ND, et al. Exercise training and nutritional supplementation for physical frailty in very elderly people. *N Engl J Med.* 1994;330: 1769–1775.

320. Manolio TA, Furberg CD, Shemanski L, et al., for the CHS Collaborative Research Group. Associations of postmenopausal estrogen use with cardiovascular disease and its risk factors in older women. *Circulation.* 1993;88(part 1):2163–2171.

321. Hertog MGL, Feskens EJM, Hollman PCH, et al. Dietary antioxidant flavonoids and risk of coronary heart disease: the Zutphen Elderly Study. *Lancet.* 1993;342:1007–1011.

322. Schauffler HH, D'Agostino RB, Kannel WB. Risk for cardiovascular disease in the elderly and associated Medicare costs: the Framingham Study. *Am J Prev Med.* 1993;9: 146–154.

323. Wenger NK, ed. Proceedings from the Millennium Symposium: Heart disease in the octogenarian, March 11, 2000. *Am J Geriatr Cardiol.* 2000;9:1–112.

40
Hypertension

Mark A. Supiano

Classification and Epidemiology

Results from cross-sectional studies have shown that blood pressure, particularly systolic blood pressure (SBP), increases with increasing age.[1] No age adjustment is made in setting the threshold value that defines high blood pressure. The classification of blood pressure outlined by the Joint National Committee on Detection, Evaluation, and Treatment of High Blood Pressure (JNC-VI), shown in Table 40.1, is the same for all adults irrespective of age.[2] There were several minor modifications made in the JNC-VI revision of blood pressure classification that have major significance with respect to geriatric hypertension. The former category of isolated systolic hypertension [i.e., SBP > 160 mmHg and diastolic blood pressure (DBP) < 90 mmHg] was removed. In addition, the conjunction linking the systolic and diastolic blood pressure columns that define each stage was changed from "and" to "or." As a consequence of this new approach to classification and because isolated diastolic hypertension is so uncommon in older individuals, the correct categorization of blood pressure among those above age 60 may be made by using the level of SBP alone in 99% of cases.[3] Thus, the SBP level matters for the purposes of classification. Finally, as is discussed, treatment recommendations are stratified, based in large part on the classification strategy shown in Table 40.1.

Contrary to a former point of view that held that high blood pressure is an expected normal aspect of aging, it is now evident that hypertension in older individuals defined according to these blood pressure levels should be viewed as a disease state that is associated with an increased risk for adverse outcomes [e.g., coronary heart disease, congestive heart failure (CHF), stroke, peripheral vascular disease, and renal disease) and mortality. Therefore, although common, high blood pressure in older individuals is not benign. It is also important to note that, for any level of diastolic blood pressure, the risk for

these adverse events is progressively greater at higher levels of systolic blood pressure.[4,5] Thus, systolic blood pressure matters as a risk factor for cardiovascular disease. In addition, it is increasingly being recognized that a major predictor of cardiovascular risk is the pulse pressure—the difference between systolic and diastolic blood pressure.[6] An analysis of data from the Systolic Hypertension in the Elderly Program (SHEP) identified that pulse pressure was a significant predictor of stroke and total mortality independent of the influence of mean arterial blood pressure.[7] Therefore, the age-associated increases in systolic blood pressure and in pulse pressure are important contributors to the morbidity and mortality associated with hypertension in older individuals.

Epidemiologic studies such as the National Health and Nutrition Examination Surveys have shown that the overall prevalence of hypertension in noninstitutionalized individuals above the age of 65 is between 50% and 70%. The prevalence is highest among African-Americans relative to whites and Mexican-Americans. Unlike the younger hypertensive population in which there is a male predominance, there is no marked gender difference in the overall prevalence of hypertension in the elderly. Moreover, the age-associated increase in the prevalence of isolated systolic hypertension appears to be greater for women than for men.[8]

Pathophysiology

Many age-related changes in physiology contribute to the increase in blood pressure. Lifestyle factors, such as diet, obesity, and physical activity, and the presence of comorbidities are also important contributors. A multitude of pathophysiologic mechanisms interact in the dynamic and complex regulation of arterial blood pressure. The maintenance of blood pressure homeostasis and the provision of adequate cerebral perfusion in the response to such hypotensive stimuli as volume depletion, upright

TABLE 40.1. Classification of blood pressure.

Category	Systolic (mmHg)		Diastolic (mmHg)
Normal	<130	and	<85
High normal	130–139	and	85–89
Hypertension			
Stage 1	140–159	or	90–99
Stage 2	160–179	or	100–109
Stage 3	≥180	or	≥110–119

Source: Adapted from JNC-VI. *Arch Intern Med*. 1997;157:2413–2446,[2] with permission.

posture, vasodilating medications, or a meal is an important physiologic challenge facing the aging individual. As is the case in younger individuals, the etiology of essential hypertension in older humans is not known. An increase in peripheral vascular resistance is one pathognomonic feature of hypertension in the elderly. Several mechanisms contribute to the increase in peripheral vascular resistance. Table 40.2 summarizes those mechanisms that appear to be associated with aging and are discussed in detail here. A rational approach to therapy of hypertension in older individuals requires an understanding of this pathophysiologic context. Although not all the following mechanisms have been convincingly proven to be primary age-associated changes (i.e., independent of the effects of disease or lifestyle factors), they may be important contributors to hypertension in the elderly. It is also quite possible that the age-associated increase in blood pressure is secondary to age-related disease or lifestyle factors, because in some populations the increase in blood pressure with aging is either absent or less marked.[9]

An age-associated increase in arterial vascular stiffness has been demonstrated, particularly in the larger arteries.[10,11] Several alterations in vessel structure contribute to the decrease in distensibility, such as an increase in smooth muscle cell size and number, an increase in medial collagen deposition, and a decrease in elastin content.[9] Arterial compliance and stroke volume are the major determinants of pulse pressure. Because stroke volume does not vary significantly with age, the decline in arterial compliance produces an increase in pulse pressure, which contributes to a disproportionate increase in systolic pressure. This finding may account for the age-associated increase in the prevalence of isolated systolic hypertension, as well as an increase in pulse pressure. Another consequence of the decrease in arterial compliance with aging is an increase in arterial pulse wave velocity.[12] The increase in arterial pulse wave velocity has been shown to lead to an early return of wave reflection, which alters the aortic pressure wave contour, increasing the pressure in late systole.[13] The wave reflection further accentuates the increase in pulse pressure between central and peripheral arteries.

In addition to changes in vascular structure, the dynamic regulation of vascular tone by the autonomic nervous system, as well as by the vascular endothelium, is an important determinant of peripheral vascular resistance. A decrease in baroreceptor sensitivity with age has been described,[14,15] perhaps as a manifestation of the decrease in arterial distensibility already discussed. The decline in baroreceptor sensitivity alters the central nervous system (CNS) control of sympathetic nervous system (SNS) outflow, resulting in two important manifestations. First, having an insensitive baroreceptor means that a larger change in blood pressure is needed to activate the baroreceptor and produce the appropriate compensatory response. Attenuated baroreceptor sensitivity is believed to contribute to the greater blood pressure variability in older individuals.[16] Second, attenuated baroreceptor sensitivity results in enhanced SNS activity for a given level of arterial blood pressure.[17,18] Many studies have demonstrated an age-associated increase in the activity of the SNS measured by an increase in plasma norepinephrine levels,[19,20] rates of norepinephrine release determined from tracer kinetics studies,[18,21,22] and muscle sympathetic nerve activity.[23] The increase in the rate of norepinephrine release would be expected to result in increased cardiovascular adrenergic responses if it were not for the corresponding downregulation of adrenergic receptor function. Indeed, there is evidence to suggest an age-associated decrease in adrenergic responsiveness for β-adrenergic receptor chronotropic,[24] inotropic,[25] and vascular[26] responses, as well as for α-adrenergic vasoconstrictor responses.[22,27] As a result of the decrease in arterial α-adrenergic receptor response, it appears that overall arterial α-adrenergic tone is similar in older normotensive compared with younger normotensive subjects[22] and that an increase in peripheral vascular resistance cannot be accounted for solely by age-associated changes in SNS function. Hypertensive older individuals, however, have been characterized by having greater arterial α-adrenergic receptor responsiveness relative to their level of SNS activity in comparison to older normotensive subjects.[28]

Another important modulator of vascular tone is the vascular endothelium, which synthesizes a number

TABLE 40.2. Pathophysiologic alterations that may contribute to or are associated with elevated blood pressure in aging.

Increased arterial stiffness
Decreased baroreceptor sensitivity
Increased sympathetic nervous system activity
Decreased α- and β-adrenergic responsiveness
Decreased endothelial cell-derived relaxing factor function
Sodium sensitivity
Low plasma renin activity
Insulin resistance

of vasoactive substances. Endothelial-derived relaxing factor (EDRF) is a potent vasodilator that has been extensively investigated since being identified as nitric oxide.[29,30] Several studies have demonstrated that there is an age-associated decrease in EDRF-mediated vasocilation,[11,31] and there may also be endothelial dysfunction with hypertension.[32] Impaired function of this important regulator of vasodilator tone could lead to an increase in peripheral vascular resistance if not met by appropriate compensatory alterations in other vasoactive systems. The extent to which impaired endothelial function contributes to an increase in blood pressure in aging remains to be defined.

Several age-associated changes in renal function (e.g., decreased renal blood flow and glomerular filtration rate) combine to result in an age-associated inability to rapidly excrete a sodium load.[33] The net result of these alterations is a tendency for sodium retention by the aging kidney and an increase in total body sodium.[34] It has been observed that a greater proportion of older hypertensives demonstrate an increase in mean arterial blood pressure in response to challenge with a sodium load or demonstrate sodium sensitivity.[35,36] These renal changes in sodium balance may contribute to the increased prevalence for sodium sensitivity among older individuals.

The renin-angiotensin system represents another blood pressure regulatory system that may be altered with advancing age. The evidence in this instance is for an age-associated decline in plasma renin activity.[33] There is a corresponding low prevalence of older hypertensives with high renin levels.[37] The decrease in plasma renin activity may be related to a decrease in the number of glomeruli, as well as an increased delivery of sodium to the macula densa.[37]

Several studies have identified an age-associated impairment in glucose tolerance.[38,39] Decreased sensitivity to the peripheral effects of insulin on carbohydrate metabolism, or insulin resistance, with aging may contribute to the decline in glucose tolerance.[40–42] Insulin resistance and an associated increase in fasting insulin levels have been shown to be a characteristic of some hypertensive groups,[43,44] including older hypertensives.[45] Although a mechanistic causal link between insulin resistance and hypertension has not yet been identified, if such a mechanism exists, an age-associated decline in insulin sensitivity could contribute to hypertension. However, based on the results of a study performed to determine predictors of insulin sensitivity, it appears that age is not an independent predictor of insulin sensitivity after accounting for the confounding effects of higher body mass index and blood pressure.[46] Thus, although there is a clear association between blood pressure and insulin resistance and many older hypertensives are insulin resistant, there are no data to indicate that an age-associated decline in insulin sensitivity independently contributes to hypertension in older adults.

Diagnosis and Evaluation

Measurement Issues

In light of the greater variability in blood pressure among older individuals (due, in part, to the decrease in baroreceptor sensitivity), it s critically important to make an accurate diagnosis of hypertension in this population. To do so requires careful attention to correct measurement of blood pressure with respect to utilizing the proper cuff size, measuring the blood pressure in both arms, having the patient appropriately positioned (sitting comfortably following 5 min of quiet rest with the arm supported at heart level), palpating the systolic blood pressure level at the radial artery to avoid the auscultatory gap, and taking two blood pressure measurements separated by at least 2 min (more if there is greater than 5 mmHg difference between the first two readings) at each of three visits. The average of these measurements is used to define an individual's blood pressure, which determines the presence or absence of hypertension according to the classification scheme given in Table 40.1. The statement that "hypertension should not be diagnosed on the basis of a single measurement"[2] is especially relevant to the older patient. It has been observed that, when antihypertensive medication is withdrawn from some older individuals, a significant number do not manifest a blood pressure high enough to be classified as hypertensive, suggesting that some older individuals are at risk for overtreatment of their blood pressure.[47] Careful adherence to these measurement techniques will minimize the likelihood that older individuals are misdiagnosed as hypertensive and inappropriately placed on an antihypertensive medication.

Given the age-associated increase in arterial vascular stiffness, there have been concerns that indirect (cuff) blood pressure measurement may not accurately reflect actual intra-arterial blood pressure in older individuals. This overestimation of true blood pressure by the indirect method secondary to the incompressibility of the brachial artery is referred to as pseudohypertension. Despite these concerns, it has been demonstrated that indirect blood pressure measurement is as accurate among older (at least up to age 80 years) as it is in younger individuals; the indirect measurement tends to underestimate systolic and overestimate diastolic blood pressure to similar degrees in both age groups.[48] Similar findings have been observed in a group of 26 subjects from age 50 to 80 years who had isolated systolic hypertension.[49] There remains some uncertainty as to the true frequency of pseudohypertension in the elderly population;

prevalence estimates vary from 2% to 70% among the published descriptions.[50] Some investigators have suggested that the presence of a positive Osler's sign, the ability to palpate the radial artery when the radial pulse is obliterated by inflating an arm cuff to above the systolic blood pressure, increases the likelihood of pseudohypertension.[51] The utility of identifying a positive Osler's sign has been questioned, however, due to its poor reproducibility[52] and low positive predictive value.[53] The possibility of pseudohypertension should be entertained in the presence of a discrepancy between the severity of the blood pressure and evidence of target organ damage, a wide pulse pressure, or perhaps a positive Osler's sign. In these situations, other measurement techniques, such as oscillometric or plethysmography of the digital blood pressure (Finapres) methods, or in some cases direct intra-arterial blood pressure monitoring, may be utilized to make the definitive diagnosis.

Another clinical situation in which overestimation of blood pressure may occur is office or "white coat" hypertension. Ambulatory home blood pressure monitoring or patient self-monitoring may provide additional information needed to evaluate the patient's blood pressure when concern for white coat hypertension arises, in borderline situations where there is uncertainty about the diagnosis of hypertension, or when there is extreme variability in blood pressure readings. In a substudy reported from the Systolic Hypertension in Europe Trial, results from 24-h ambulatory blood pressure readings provided a better predictor of subsequent cardiovascular events than did the standard blood pressure readings, suggesting another potential benefit of ambulatory blood pressure monitoring.[54]

Although not directly pertinent to the diagnosis of hypertension, another critically important aspect of blood pressure measurement in the older hypertensive patient is obtaining baseline postural or orthostatic blood pressure measurements. Orthostatic hypotension is usually defined as a decline in blood pressure from the supine baseline of greater than 20 mmHg systolic and/or 10 mmHg diastolic after 1 to 2 min of standing. This definition is supported by a careful study of the postural blood pressure response of normal individuals that determined that this extent of decline exceeded the 95% confidence limits for the postural change in blood pressure.[55] Aging per se is not associated with an increased prevalence of orthostatic hypotension.[56,57] The supine systolic blood pressure has been identified as the best predictor of the postural decrease in systolic blood pressure.[58,59] Accordingly, the presence of supine hypertension is an important risk factor for orthostatic hypotension.[57] Baseline orthostatic blood pressure readings are therefore required in every patient to avoid adverse events related to further declines in postural blood pressure that may result from antihypertensive therapy.

Secondary Causes

The approach to the evaluation for secondary and potentially reversible factors that may account for the increase in blood pressure in older individuals is similar to that recommended for younger hypertensive patients. Thus, a standard clinical evaluation consisting of a complete history and physical exam, chemistry profile (to assess electrolytes, renal function, and glucose), ECG, and chest x-ray is recommended to identify these factors. Further evaluation is normally not needed unless there are abnormal symptoms or signs elicited from this evaluation that would be consistent with renal disease (elevated serum creatinine or abnormal urinalysis), renovascular disease (e.g., presence of abdominal bruit), hyperaldosteronism (hypokalemia), hypercortisolism (hyperglycemia, cushingoid appearance), hyperparathyroidism (hypercalcemia), or pheochromocytoma (symptoms of headache, palpitations, diaphoresis, and paroxysmal elevations of blood pressure). A careful review of medications is warranted to determine if medication-related increases in blood pressure (e.g., due to corticosteroids or nonsteroidal anti-inflammatory drugs) could be contributing to the elevated blood pressure. Other clinical situations that might lead to an evaluation for secondary hypertension in the older patient include malignant hypertension, the abrupt development of diastolic hypertension (which is unusual in light of the general decrease in diastolic blood pressure with age above the age of 60 years), worsening of blood pressure control, or blood pressure that remains uncontrolled on a regimen of three antihypertensive medications.

As is the case in younger hypertensive populations, the overwhelming majority (greater than 90%) of older hypertensive patients have essential or primary hypertension. Secondary forms of hypertension may be even more rare in the older population. Renal disease and renovascular hypertension are the most frequent cause of secondary hypertension in the elderly; endocrinologic causes are generally less common. The only possible exception to this is a suggestion that the incidence rate for pheochromocytoma, although still exceedingly rare (incidence less than 1% among patients with hypertension), may increase progressively with age.[60]

Target Organ Damage and Risk Factor Assessment

Once the diagnosis of hypertension has been appropriately made and secondary causes considered, the remainder of the evaluation should be directed toward the identification of target organ damage, an assessment of other cardiovascular risk factors, and identification of comorbid conditions that may influence the therapeutic decision-making process. In the older hypertensive patient, it may be more difficult to detect the manifestations of target organ damage that are directly attributable to elevated blood pressure because of concurrent age- or disease-associated changes in organ function. With this proviso, it is useful to determine if there is any previous history consistent with coronary artery disease, cardiac failure, cerebrovascular disease (transient ischemic attack or stroke), or peripheral vascular disease. The patient should be assessed for any physical signs consistent with these conditions, as well as for evidence of hypertensive retinopathy or left ventricular hypertrophy. In addition to identifying the presence of hyperlipidemia or diabetes mellitus, information concerning smoking history, dietary intake of salt and fat, alcohol intake, and level of physical activity should be obtained to aid in a determination of overall cardiovascular risk. This information will affect the patient's risk stratum assignment and the approach to his or her treatment and is also needed to advise the patient about lifestyle modifications that may be recommended as nonpharmacological approaches to blood pressure control. Finally, knowledge of comorbid conditions is necessary to identify special clinical situations where a given class of antihypertensive medication would be either recommended or contraindicated (see Table 40.2).

Treatment

Results from Clinical Trials

There is now no question that a significant reduction in cardiovascular and cerebrovascular morbidity and mortality results from treatment to reduce blood pressure in older hypertensive patients. Several randomized clinical trials of antihypertensive therapy in older populations have provided compelling evidence that treatment is effective in reducing cardiovascular (e.g., chronic congestive heart failure) and cerebrovascular (e.g., stroke) morbidity and mortality. A meta-analysis of outcome trials in systolic hypertension demonstrated that treatment was associated with significant reductions in overall mortality, cardiovascular events, and stroke.[61] The treatment effect was largest in men, in those over the age of 70 years, and in those who had larger pulse pressures. Similarly, another meta-analysis of nine treatment trials[62–70] confirmed that treatment of hypertension in the older population is associated with significant benefits: the treatment group had significant reductions in all-cause mortality [odds ratio, 0.88; 95% confidence interval (CI), 0.80–0.97], stroke mortality (0.64; CI, 0.49–0.82), and morbidity (0.65; CI, 0.55–0.76), as well as cardiac mortality (0.75; CI, 0.64–0.88) and morbidity (0.85; 0.73–0.99).[71] Based in part on these data, an analysis of the effectiveness of antihypertensive therapy utilizing data derived

from the NHANES I survey suggested that the number needed to treat (assuming a 12 mmHg reduction in SBP for 10 years) to prevent cardiovascular events and deaths or all-cause mortality decreased as a function of the initial blood pressure reading and of increasing risk strata (derived from JNC-VI definitions); the prevention of 1 all-cause death required that 81 patients in the lowest risk grouping be treated compared to 9 patients in the highest risk group.[72]

In addition to the demonstrated efficacy of antihypertensive therapy with respect to cardiovascular and stroke outcomes, it is worth noting that there may be other benefits. An analysis of data from the SHEP study identified that the relative risk of developing congestive heart failure among the treatment group was approximately one-half that of the control group.[73] Other studies have focused on a possible relationship between hypertension and the risk of developing cognitive impairment. Results from a vascular dementia project designed as part of the Syst-Eur trial suggest that the rate of the development of dementia was significantly lower (approximately one-half) in the active treatment compared with the control group.[74] It should be noted, however, that the dementia incidence was small (7.7 and 3.8 cases per 1000 patient-years in control and treated groups, respectively), and this observation has not yet been replicated.

Although the results from these randomized clinical trials have provided convincing support for the beneficial effects of treatment of hypertension in older patients, there nevertheless are several unanswered questions. The majority of these trials focused on those with simple hypertension and, for example, excluded those with significant comorbidities such as diabetes or a history of prior stroke or heart disease. The extent to which these results are applicable to frail older patients with multiple coexisting diseases is not known. Another issue is whether these beneficial results extend to the old-old, individuals over the age of 85 years. One report has identified an inverse association between blood pressure and mortality in a group of individuals over the age of 85 years.[75] This study reported the entry blood pressure measurements (separately grouped by systolic and diastolic) and 5-year survival rates of a group of 561 individuals over the age of 85 years who resided in the community, as well as in nursing homes and hospitals, in Tampere, Finland. The lowest survival rate was in the lowest systolic and lowest diastolic groups. Because 80% of individuals in these groups resided in either hospital or nursing home settings, it is not certain whether other confounding disease-related factors might have accounted for their decreased survival. However, a subsequent report whose study population was restricted to community-dwelling elderly aged 84 to 88 years demonstrated increased mortality in those with either very low or very high blood pressure.[76] Another report utilizing data obtained from the Established Populations for Epidemiological Studies of the Elderly (EPESE) determined the mortality risk associated with blood pressure in community-dwelling older people.[77] This study found an increasing risk of death with increasing systolic blood pressure in men and women between age 65 and 84 years, but in men above the age of 85 years, an inverse relationship between systolic blood pressure and mortality risk was observed.

Very limited numbers of subjects over the age of 80 years have been included in the controlled clinical trials of hypertension treatment. Results from the European Working Party on High Blood Pressure in the Elderly (EWPHE) Trial suggested that no significant benefits of drug treatment occurred in those 80 years and older (group size, $n = 155$).[63] A similar trend for a reduction in treatment benefit with age was noted in the meta-analysis of the nine studies already cited (including the EWPHE); however, this difference was not statistically significant.[71] For isolated systolic hypertension, comparable treatment benefits were observed in the 649 subjects 80 years and older who were enrolled in the SHEP study.[62] Finally, a meta-analysis of data from subjects older than 80 years enrolled in randomized controlled studies suggests that significant reductions in the development of stroke (34%), cardiovascular events (24%), and congestive heart failure (42%) occurred in the treatment compared to the control group.[78] However, in this analysis a slight, although statistically nonsignificant, 6% increase in all-cause mortality was identified in the treatment group. Ultimately, results from the Hypertension in the Very Elderly trial should help to resolve this matter.

Another still unanswered question is a concern that reduction in blood pressure below a certain level may be associated with increased rather than decreased mortality, or a J-shaped curve. This relationship has been most often identified between the level of diastolic blood pressure and cardiovascular mortality. The knowledge that blood flow to the myocardium occurs primarily during diastole provides a potential physiologic mechanism to account for a relationship between low diastolic blood pressure and cardiovascular mortality. The J-shaped curve has been raised as a concern in some treatment studies in which reduction in cerebrovascular but not cardiovascular mortality has been identified. Results from several longitudinal studies have identified an increased risk for stroke and overall mortality in individuals in the lowest systolic and, particularly, diastolic blood pressure levels. The relationship between the diastolic blood pressure achieved in subjects enrolled in the Systolic Hypertension in the Elderly Program with respect to their relative risk for developing cardiovascular disease has been shown to be inverse; namely, the relative risk increased as diastolic blood pressure decreased below

70 mmHg.[79] Thus, until additional prospective data are available to provide guidance in this therapeutic dilemma, it is prudent to use caution in lowering blood pressure in older individuals with hypertension. Excessive reductions in blood pressure (e.g., diastolic levels below 70 mmHg) and the development of treatment-induced postural hypotension should be avoided.

General Approach to Therapy and Monitoring

As is the case in the approach to treatment of other chronic diseases in an older patient, it is important to define goals of antihypertensive therapy that are individualized to a given patient. In this context, the benefits as well as the potential risks of any therapeutic intervention need to be balanced to achieve, on the one hand, an overall goal of preventing the morbidity and mortality associated with high blood pressure without adversely affecting the patient's functional performance or quality of life on the other. A therapeutic approach directed toward reduction of systolic blood pressure to below 135 to 140 mmHg and diastolic blood pressure to less than 85 to 90 mmHg should be developed utilizing treatments least likely to produce adverse effects. For individuals with markedly elevated systolic blood pressure, an intermediate target, such as 160 mmHg, may be appropriate. The major focus of treatment should be on the systolic blood pressure and pulse pressure because, among older hypertensive individuals, these are stronger predictors of adverse outcomes than is the diastolic blood pressure. In view of the concerns about the J-shaped curve, it is important not to overtreat with an intervention that produces an excessive reduction in diastolic blood pressure. With the exception of hypertensive urgencies and emergencies (discussed next), it is unnecessary and perhaps deleterious to attempt rapid reductions in blood pressure to achieve this target level of control. In light of the age-associated pathophysiologic changes that result in impaired blood pressure homeostasis, too rapid a reduction in blood pressure may be associated with the development of symptomatic hypotension in some situations (e.g., postural or postprandial hypotension). Likewise, it is advisable to not make dosage adjustments or additions of other therapies too rapidly to avoid overtreatment. Once the patient's blood pressure has been controlled to an optimal level, it is appropriate to reevaluate the need for continued therapy. A reduction in dose or in some cases a trial period without antihypertensive medication (with close monitoring of the patient's home and office blood pressure) will help to minimize the possibility of overtreatment of blood pressure.

Another general approach to therapy is to continuously assess not only the response to therapy, but also the development of adverse effects of treatment. The development of orthostatic hypotension is an adverse effect that may occur with any antihypertensive medication, although central-acting agents and vasodilators are more commonly implicated in this regard. The symptoms of orthostatic hypotension may be atypical; rather than providing a history of postural unsteadiness, the older patient may cite generalized weakness or fatigue. Because orthostatic hypotension is common in hypertensive patients (its frequency increasing in parallel with the supine systolic blood pressure level[58,59]), and given the often occult nature of its presenting symptoms, it is essential to determine supine and upright blood pressure measurements as part of routine monitoring of all older hypertensive patients.

Nonpharmacologic Treatment Modalities

There are several reasons to review the role of nonpharmacological treatment modalities in treating geriatric hypertension. The older hypertensive population may in general be characterized as overweight, sedentary, and salt sensitive. Lifestyle modifications targeted toward these characteristics may therefore be of particular benefit in older hypertensive patients. Nonpharmacological therapies may be effective initial therapy; individuals with stage 1 hypertension (systolic blood pressure less than 160 mmHg) who do not have diabetes should complete a 6-month trial of nonpharmacologic therapy before adding an antihypertensive medication if the target blood pressure is not achieved. In addition, these therapies may be adjunctive in combination with pharmacologic treatments, they may result in concurrent improvements in other cardiovascular risk factors, and there are minimal associated risks (as well the benefit of possibly avoiding adverse side effects associated with antihypertensive medications). A number of lifestyle modifications may be recommended: weight reduction; an aerobic exercise program; dietary alterations to decrease sodium, saturated fat, and cholesterol while maintaining adequate intake of potassium, calcium, and magnesium; smoking cessation; and moderation of alcohol intake.

A randomized trial of nonpharmacologic interventions in older hypertensive subjects that evaluated the effects of dietary sodium restriction and weight loss (the TONE study) demonstrated that relatively modest reductions in dietary sodium intake (~40 mmol/day) and in body weight (~4 kg) were accompanied by a 30% decrease in the need to reinitiate pharmacologic treatment.[80] A meta-analysis of randomized trials assessing the effects of dietary sodium restriction demonstrated that there is a significant reduction in systolic (a mean decrease of 3.7 mmHg for each 100 mmol/day decrease in sodium intake) but not in diastolic blood pressure.[81] Consistent with these results, a follow-up study to the dietary approaches to stop hypertension (DASH) trial[82] that added a sodium restriction component identified that the DASH diet in combination with sodium restriction (~65 mmol/day intake) resulted in a decrease in SBP of 11.5 mmHg in hypertensive patients in comparison to the control, high-sodium diet.[83] Although diastolic blood pressure was also lower, the magnitude of the effect was less than that for systolic BP. The differential reduction in systolic pressure in response to dietary sodium restriction observed in these studies is particularly well suited for the older hypertensive patient.

There is a high prevalence of obesity in the older population: 26% of black and white men, 36% of white women, and 60% of black women between the ages of 65 and 74 years were characterized as overweight (defined by body mass index $\geq 27.8 \, kg/m^2$ for men and $\geq 27.3 \, kg/m^2$ for women) in the National Health and Nutrition Examination Survey.[84] There is increasing evidence that the distribution of body weight is an important determinant of cardiovascular risk. In particular, central adiposity has been shown to be associated with hypertension, hyperlipidemia, and insulin resistance.[85] Weight reduction is recommended for hypertensive individuals who are more than 10% above their ideal body weight, and weight loss of the order of 5 kg has been shown to result in small (generally less than 5 mmHg), but significant, decreases in blood pressure.[86–88] There are likely additive antihypertensive effects of lower extremity aerobic exercise programs.[89] Although there are special considerations in an older hypertensive patient with regard to screening for the presence of underlying cardiovascular disease and attention to the prevention of injuries, the safety and efficacy of aerobic exercise has been identified in studies of older hypertensive individuals.[90]

Overview of Pharmacologic Treatments

The general approach to pharmacologic treatment of hypertension is outlined in JNC-VI.[2] Treatment is stratified as a function of blood pressure stage (high normal: 130–139/85–89; stage 1: 140–159/90–99; and stage 2 and 3: $\geq 160/\geq 100$ mmHg) and three levels of risk. Because age greater than 60 years is considered as one component of cardiovascular risk, all older hypertensive patients fall into the middle risk group (risk group B) at a minimum. For those with high-normal and stage 1 hypertension with no additional cardiovascular risk factors, 6-month trial of nonpharmacologic therapy is warranted. If a 6-month trial of nonpharmacologic treatment fails to produce the desired reduction in blood pressure, pharmacologic therapy should be initiated while nonpharmacologic treatments are continued. Older patients who initially present with more severe hypertension (stage 2 or 3), as well as those with diabetes or additional cardiovascular risk factors or evidence of target organ damage (risk group C), should receive pharmacologic therapy initiated concurrently with nonpharmacologic methods.

The choice of initial antihypertensive drug class should be based on an individualized patient assessment. One should consider whether the patient has simple hypertension or if their hypertension is complicated by the coexistence of other conditions (e.g., diabetes, coronary artery disease, heart failure, or prostatism) that may influence drug selection. Each of the antihypertensive drug classes have been shown to be effective in reducing blood pressure in the older patient population. For those with simple hypertension, the initial drug selection based on the evidence available to date is either a thiazide diuretic or a long-acting dihydropyridine calcium channel antagonist.[2] Beyond this general recommendation, selection of a particular antihypertensive drug needs to be an individualized decision for each patient, taking into account the drug's potential advantages and disadvantages (see Table 40.2), together with the patient's comorbidities. Irrespective of the initial agent that is selected, in general, the starting dose should be reduced and dose titration done more gradually in an older hypertensive patient. If the target blood pressure goal is not obtained at a maximal dose of the initial agent following several months of treatment, therapy may either be switched to an alternate class or a second drug from another class may be added. A brief overview of the major classes of antihypertensive drugs that are currently recommended for initial therapy follows, focusing on their potential benefits and side effect profiles.

Diuretics

Therapy with low-dose thiazide diuretics (e.g., hydrochlorthiazide dose <50 mg daily, or equivalent) has demonstrated significant benefits in mortality, stroke, and coronary events in randomized clinical trials in older hypertensive patient populations. These beneficial effects combined with their relative safety, favorable side effect profile (their adverse metabolic effects—hypokalemia, hyperuricemia, and glucose intolerance—are attenuated at lower doses), once-daily dosing, and low cost have led to the recommendation that thiazide diuretics are preferred for initial therapy.[91] Another advantage is that diuretic therapy leads to a disproportionate reduction in systolic relative to diastolic blood pressure and is better at achieving a reduction in systolic blood pressure compared to other agents.[91,92] Thiazide diuretics are also well suited for use in combination therapies because of synergistic effects with other antihypertensive drug classes. It is worth nothing that, despite these recommendations, only 23% of the subjects who were on monotherapy at the time of their entry into the TONE study were treated with diuretics,[80,93] suggesting that this class of therapy is being underutilized.[94]

Calcium Channel Antagonists

Each of the three chemical classes of calcium channel antagonists, that is, phenylalkylamines, dihydropyridines, and benzothiazepines, has been shown to be effective in treating hypertension in older patient populations.[95–97] There are significant age-associated alterations in the pharmacokinetics of each of the three classes of calcium channel antagonists (a decrease in clearance and an increase in plasma levels) such that lower doses of these agents should be used in older patients.[98,99] Based on their mechanism of action, which leads to a reduction in peripheral vascular resistance and their lack of significant CNS or metabolic effects, the calcium channel antagonist family of medications is well matched to the pathophysiology of the older hypertensive patient. The dihydropyridine class (e.g., nifedipine) has more potent direct vasodilator effects and may be more likely to produce peripheral edema and reflex tachycardia. Members of the phenylalkylamine (e.g., verapamil) and benzothiazepine (e.g., diltiazem) classes have more potent effects on suppressing atrioventricular (AV) conduction and may produce heart block, and also these appear to be more commonly associated with the development of constipation.

Several randomized controlled trials of the efficacy of long-acting dihydropyridine calcium channel antagonists (nicardipine or amlodipine) in the treatment of older hypertensive patient populations have been reported. The Systolic Hypertension in Europe (Syst-Eur) trial identified that active treatment was associated with a significant decrease in cardiovascular complications, including a 44% reduction in nonfatal stroke.[100] No significant benefits were observed in all-cause mortality. The conclusions were similar in a subsequent per protocol analysis of these data.[101] The benefits of treatment on total and cardiovascular mortality were less in those older than 80 years. From the per protocol analysis, it was estimated that treating 1000 patients for 5 years would prevent 24 deaths, 54 major cardiac events, and 29 strokes.[101] To address concerns that calcium antagonist therapy may be deleterious in those with diabetes, a subgroup analysis of the Syst-Eur population found similar beneficial effects in the diabetic population as had been noted in nondiabetics.[102] Finally, a Japanese Intervention Cooperative Study followed older hypertensive patients randomized to the dihydropyridine calcium channel antagonist nicardipine or a thiazide diuretic and reported similar benefits in decreasing the risk of cardiovascular events between groups.[103]

β-Adrenergic Antagonists

Beta-receptor antagonists are recommended in the JNC-VI report as another option for initial drug therapy for uncomplicated hypertension.[2] The primary mechanism of action of β-adrenergic antagonists is a reduction in

TABLE 40.3. Potential advantages, disadvantages, and special clinical considerations in the older hypertensive related to the major antihypertensive classes recommended for initial treatment.

Antihypertensive class	Potential advantages	Potential disadvantages	Clinical situations to recommend use	Clinical situations to recommend against use, or that require monitoring
Diuretics	Benefit documented in clinical trials Produce greater reduction in SBP than DBP Inexpensive	Metabolic abnormalities Urinary incontinence	Systolic hypertension	Glucose intolerance, gout, hyperlipidemia
Calcium antagonists	Benefit documented in clinical trials Absence of CNS or metabolic effects	Peripheral edema, constipation, heart block	Systolic hypertension Coronary artery disease	Left ventricular dysfunction
β-Antagonists	Benefit documented in clinical trials	May increase peripheral vascular resistance Metabolic abnormalities CNS effects	Coronary artery disease and postmyocardial infarction	COPD, peripheral vascular disease, heart block, glucose intolerance, type 2 DM, hyperlipidemia, depression
ACE inhibitors	Absence of CNS or metabolic effects	Hyperkalemia, renal insufficiency, cough	Congestive heart failure, type 2 DM	Renal insufficiency or renal artery stenosis

SBP, systolic blood pressure; DBP, diastolic blood pressure; ACE, angiotensin-converting enzyme; COPD, chronic obstructive pulmonary disease; DM, diabetes mellitus; CNS, central nervous system.

cardiac output without significant reduction in peripheral vascular resistance (and less reduction in systolic blood pressure compared to other agents). Based on the physiologic characteristics of the older hypertensive (Table 40.3), there are several reasons to question whether β-adrenergic antagonists would be the appropriate choice for the older hypertensive patient. Indeed, one report that analyzed evidence from recent randomized controlled trials has questioned whether β-adrenergic antagonists are effective therapy for older hypertensive individuals.[104] This report analyzed results from 10 randomized controlled trials that evaluated morbidity and mortality outcomes in hypertensive patients above the age of 60 years following β-adrenergic antagonist therapy. These results suggested that β-receptor antagonist therapy is less effective as monotherapy with respect to blood pressure reduction and in the prevention of cardiovascular events and death in comparison with low-dose thiazide diuretics. In addition, there was a higher discontinuation rate due to adverse side effects. This report concluded with a recommendation that β-receptor antagonists not be considered as first-line monotherapy for simple hypertension in older patients. Because of their effectiveness in the management of symptomatic coronary artery disease, in secondary prevention following myocardial infarction, and in certain congestive heart failure settings, β-receptor antagonists should be considered in older patients whose hypertension is complicated by these comorbid conditions. Glucose and lipid profile monitoring should be done in patients who are treated

with β-receptor antagonists. In addition, depression and lethargy may develop during β-receptor antagonist therapy, particularly with those who are more lipophilic.

Angiotensin-Converting Enzyme (ACE) Inhibitors

Because older hypertensive individuals are in general characterized as having low renin levels (see Table 40.3), one might predict that ACE inhibitors would not be effective therapeutic agents in this population. Nevertheless, this antihypertensive class has been shown to be effective in treating the older hypertensive.[96,97] ACE inhibitors are generally well tolerated by older patients (with the exception of cough), and their lack of CNS and metabolic (glucose, electrolyte, and lipid) effects may be a particular advantage. Although postural hypotension is not common, an exaggerated hypotensive effect may develop in volume-depleted patients receiving concurrent therapy with diuretics; particular attention to this possibility is required with the initiation of ACE inhibitor therapy. There are compelling indications to use ACE inhibitor therapy in patients with coexisting left ventricular systolic dysfunction as well as in diabetic patients who have microalbuminuria.

The major limitations to the use of ACE inhibitors in older hypertensive patients are the development of hyperkalemia (especially in those with renal insufficiency) and the potential for development of renal failure in the setting of bilateral renal artery stenosis. Fortunately, ACE inhibitor-mediated renal failure is not a common occurrence and is generally reversible. The use of ACE inhibitors with short duration of action and frequent monitoring of renal function will aid in the detection and prevention of this adverse outcome. Although it may seem paradoxical, despite these potential adverse effects on renal function, there appears to be a role for ACE inhibitors in treating hypertensive patients with chronic renal insufficiency.[105] Close monitoring of potassium levels and renal function is necessary when ACE inhibitors are utilized in these patient groups. Other potential adverse effects of ACE inhibitors are the development of a nonproductive cough (occurring in up to 10% of patients), rash, or angioneurotic edema.

α₁-Adrenergic Receptor Antagonists

Although the reduction in peripheral vascular resistance that occurs with α-receptor antagonist therapy is particularly appropriate for the pathophysiologic profile of geriatric hypertension, and although these agents are effective in blood pressure reduction,[106,107] the development of postural hypotension has limited the widespread use of this class of antihypertensive in the geriatric population. Further, a preliminary report from the currently ongoing Antihypertensive and Lipid Lowering Treatment to Prevent Heart Attack Trial (ALLHAT) identified that subjects randomized to therapy with the α-receptor antagonist doxazosin had similar outcomes to those receiving a diuretic but had a twofold greater likelihood to be hospitalized for CHF. Consequently, this arm of the ALLHAT study was closed. Until additional information is available from the ALLHAT and other ongoing trials, monotherapy with α-adrenergic receptor antagonists to treat simple hypertension is not advised. One clinical situation in which α-receptor antagonist therapy may be considered is in older hypertensive men with prostatism, because these drugs have been shown to be efficacious in improving obstructive urinary symptoms.[99]

Patient Adherence and Resistant Hypertension

Effective management of hypertension in an older individual requires an approach that promotes the patient's adherence to its long-term treatment. The role of patient education cannot be overlooked with regard to explaining the goals of a therapeutic program and the importance of adherence to this program. There are several specific methods to enhance adherence to the long-term medical therapy of this condition. Written information describing the specific treatment and an agreed-upon blood pressure goal should be given to the patient. In general, a simpler regimen promotes patient adherence. The use of calendar or pillbox systems may be recom-

mended to further assist patient adherence. Blood pressure self-monitoring by the patient is another approach to involve the patient in the management of their hypertension and perhaps enhance adherence to therapy. Patient education regarding the significant benefits to be gained from adequate blood pressure control is of particular importance because hypertension is usually asymptomatic. The interdisciplinary geriatric team is well suited to promoting this approach. To this end, it may be useful to involve nurses to provide reinforcement and feedback on the degree of blood pressure control during visits for blood pressure monitoring, dietitians to review dietary information and adherence, pharmacists to promote adherence to the medical regimen, and social workers to solicit the assistance of family members, if needed, and to review the financial burden associated with the cost of medical therapy.

The frequency of follow-up visits should be adjusted to reflect the patient's degree of blood pressure elevation at presentation with closer follow-up indicated for those with stage 3 hypertension (i.e., a systolic blood pressure greater than 180mmHg). With the exception of hypertensive urgencies (discussed next), attempts to reduce the patient's blood pressure to target levels too rapidly are unnecessary and likely deleterious. For most patients, an interval of 1 to 2 months is appropriate between visits to determine the need for dose titration. Given the age-related changes in systems that regulate blood pressure and impaired blood pressure homeostasis, overtreatment of hypertension may result in situational (postural or postprandial) hypotension. At all follow-up visits, it is imperative to determine the supine and standing blood pressure. It is good practice to titrate antihypertensive drug doses to achieve the target (seated) blood pressure only with the knowledge of whether this increase in dose could exacerbate preexisting postural hypotension. It is also prudent to assess the patient's adherence to his or her antihypertensive medication before recommending an increase in its dosage or considering switching to an alternative medication. For some patients, it will be important to obtain additional information derived from home or nonoffice setting blood pressure measurements.

Patients who fail to achieve adequate control of their blood pressure (failure to reach a target of 140/90) despite the use of three antihypertensive medications at maximal doses should be evaluated for causes of resistant hypertension. This evaluation should include an assessment of their adherence to the medical therapy, a review focused on potential drug interactions (e.g., nonsteroidal anti-inflammatory agents, corticosteroids, sympathomimetics, and alcohol), and an assessment for volume overload. Other potential explanations for resistant hypertension are the presence of a secondary cause (renovascular hypertension in particular) or pseudohypertension, which should be evaluated as already outlined.

Special Clinical Situations

Hypertensive Urgencies and Emergencies

Hypertensive urgencies and emergencies are defined by the necessity to reduce blood pressure quickly to prevent target organ damage, not by an absolute blood pressure level. Elevated blood pressure in and of itself without symptoms or signs of target organ damage does not usually require aggressive therapy. Aggressive blood pressure reduction in a patient who presents with incidentally noted elevated blood pressure is inappropriate in the absence of a true urgency or emergency. It is of particular importance to obtain an accurate blood pressure measurement to avoid overdiagnosis of a hypertensive emergency when none is present (e.g., to consider the possibility of pseudohypertension as just discussed). It is possible to produce complications such as orthostatic hypotension or coronary or cerebral hypoperfusion syndromes resulting from treating an elderly patient with elevated blood pressure too aggressively.

Hypertensive urgencies are more common than true hypertensive emergencies.[108] These are defined as situations in which blood pressure should be lowered within 24h to prevent the risk of target organ damage, such as accelerated or malignant hypertension without symptoms or evidence of ongoing target organ damage.[109] The majority of these situations may be managed as with oral administration of antihypertensive medications but generally necessitate a hospitalized setting for frequent blood pressure monitoring. The medications recommended for this situation include nifedipine, clonidine, labetalol, and captopril. Because no additional benefit has been noted with the use of sublingual administration of any of these agents and the more rapid onset of action may unpredictably produce a deleterious reduction in blood pressure, the oral dosage forms, which are effective within 15 to 30min, are recommended.[110] It should be noted that the blood pressure need not be reduced to normal levels within 24h; indeed, an attempt to do so carries with it the risks of complications from coronary or cerebral hypoperfusion.

Examples of true hypertensive emergencies in older patients include hypertensive encephalopathy, intracranial hemorrhage, acute heart failure with pulmonary edema, dissecting aortic aneurysm, and unstable angina. These situations present with symptoms and signs of vascular compromise of the affected organs: brain (symptoms of severe headache, altered vision, altered mental status, and severe hypertensive retinopathy including papilledema, or focal neurologic signs), heart (symptoms

and signs of left ventricular failure or angina), or kidney (presenting as acute renal failure). The goal of treatment in these emergent clinical situations is immediate reduction in blood pressure, although again not necessarily to a normal level. The management of these conditions usually requires an acute hospital setting to permit the parenteral administration of an antihypertensive agent and continuous blood pressure monitoring by either arterial line, automatic cuff, or oscillometric (Finapres) devices. Intravenous nitroprusside has been the most widely utilized of these medications. Its onset of action is essentially immediate, it has a very short duration of action, and its rate of infusion may be titrated to result in a carefully controlled reduction in blood pressure over a 30- to 60-min period. Prolonged nitroprusside administration is limited by the accumulation of a thiocyanate metabolite and the risk of cyanide toxicity. Intravenous nitroglycerine is an alternative for longer duration of therapy. Additional parenteral alternatives include labetalol, enalaprilat, and hydralazine. In addition, for patients with evidence for fluid overload, parenteral loop diuretics may aid in achieving blood pressure control. Once the hypertensive emergency or urgency has been managed, the next steps are an evaluation to attempt to determine an explanation for the increase in blood pressure (i.e., a workup for secondary causes paying particular attention to the possibility of renovascular hypertension, assessment of adherence with the antihypertensive regimen, and evaluation of resistant hypertension) and developing a plan to achieve effective blood pressure control with appropriate close patient follow-up and monitoring.

Hypertension in Long-Term Care Center Residents

Information concerning the prevalence and management of hypertension in residents of long-term care (LTC) facilities is beginning to emerge.[111,112] The prevalence of hypertension in this population ranges from approximately one-third to two-thirds. Special considerations are warranted in LTC residents with respect to making the correct diagnosis and defining the goals of therapy and its effects on quality of life. Blood pressure measurements in LTC settings may not be accurate.[113] Inaccuracies result from measurement errors and from the temporal variability in blood pressure, particularly in relation to meals. Blood pressure appears to be highest in the morning before breakfast.[111] Postprandial hypotension is common among LTC residents, affecting about one-third of this population.[114,115] The presence of postprandial hypotension has been associated with otherwise unexplained syncope and has been found to be a significant independent risk factor for falls, syncope, stroke, and overall mortality.

There are several factors to consider in the management of hypertension in the LTC population. First, the advanced average age and multiple comorbidities in this population raises several questions surrounding the beneficial effects of antihypertensive therapy. The beneficial effects of treatment must be carefully balanced against the potential adverse effects of therapy, and the goals of therapy must be defined within the context of the patient's overall clinical situation. Even an intervention as seemingly innocuous as a sodium-restricted diet needs to be evaluated in the context of the high prevalence of protein-energy malnutrition among nursing home residents. Second, the medication list of the average LTC resident includes seven medications, and most have three or more comorbid conditions. The addition of an antihypertensive medication increases the possibility of an adverse drug event in this frail, at-risk group. Third, several studies have identified antihypertensive medications, particularly vasodilators, as a risk factor for falls in this high-risk population who experience an average of two falls each year.[116–118] Consequently, it is appropriate to assess both postural and prandial blood pressure in this population. Randomized controlled trials have not yet been conducted in the LTC population to provide clear risk–benefit evidence to support an approach to antihypertensive management. The available data suggest that diuretic therapy is effective in controlling systolic blood pressure elevations and that blood pressure reduction with diuretics lowered the prevalence of postural hypotension.[111]

References

1. Kannel WB, Gordon T. Evaluation of cardiac risk in the elderly. *Bull N Y Acad Med.* 1978;54:573–591.
2. Sheps SG. The sixth report of the Joint National Committee on Prevention, Detection, Evaluation and Treatment of High Blood Pressure. *NIH Pub.* 1997;98–4080.
3. Lloyd-Jones DM, Evans JC, Larson MG, O'Donnell CJ, Levy D. Differential impact of systolic and diastolic blood pressure level on JNC-VI staging. *Hypertension.* 1999;34: 381–385.
4. Kannel WB, Cupples LA, Vokonas PS. Epidemiology and risk of hypertension in the elderly: the Framingham study. *J Hypertens.* 1986;6(suppl 1):S3–S9.
5. Alli C, Avanzini F, Betelli G, Colombo F, Torri V, Tognoni G. The long-term prognostic significance of repeated blood pressure measurements in the elderly: SPAA (Studio sulla Pressione Arteriosa nell' Anziano) 10-year follow-up. *Arch Intern Med.* 1999;159:1205–1212.
6. Benetos A, Rudnichi A, Safar M, Guize L. Pulse pressure and cardiovascular mortality in normotensive and hypertensive subjects. *Hypertension.* 1998;32:560–564.
7. Domanski MJ, Davis BR, Pfeffer MA, Kastantin M, Mitchell GF. Isolated systolic hypertension: prognostic information by pulse pressure. *Hypertension.* 1999;34:375–380.
8. Wilking SVB, Belanger A, Kannel WB, D'Agostino RB, Steel K. Determinants of isolated systolic hypertension. *JAMA.* 1988;260(23):3451–3455.
9. Lakatta E. Mechanisms of hypertension in the elderly. *J Am Geriatr Soc.* 1989;37:780–790.
10. Hallock P, Benson I. Studies on the elastic properties of human isolated aorta. *J Clin Investig.* 1937;16:595–602.
11. Cooper LT, Cooke JP, Dzau VJ. Minireview: The vasculopathy of aging. *J Gerontol Biol Sci.* 1994;49(5):B191–B196.
12. Nichols W, O'Rourke M, Avolio A, et al. Effects of age on ventricular-vascular coupling. *Am J Cardiol.* 1985;55: 11789–11184.
13. O'Rourke MF, Kelly RP. Wave reflection in the systemic circulation and its implications in ventricular function. *J Hypertens.* 1993;11:327–337.
14. Gribbin B, Pickering TG, Sleight P. Effect of age and high blood pressure on baroreflex sensitivity in man. *Circ Res.* 1971;29:424–420.
15. Shimada K, Kitazumi T, Sadakane N, Ogura H, Ozawa T. Age-related changes of baroreflex function, plasma norepinephrine, and blood pressure. *Hypertension.* 1985;7: 113–117.
16. Lipsitz LA. Minireview: Altered blood pressure homeostasis in advanced age: clinical and research implications. *J Gerontol Med Sci.* 1989;44(6):M179–M183.
17. Hajduczok G, Chapleau MW, Johnson SL, Abboud FM. Increase in sympathetic activity with age. I. Role of impairment of arterial baroreflexes. *Am J Physiol.* 1991;260: H1113–H1120.
18. Pfeifer MA, Weinberg CR, Cook D, Best JD, Reenan A, Halter JB. Differential changes of autonomic nervous system function with age in man. *Am J Med.* 1983;75:248–258.
19. Linares OA, Halter JB. Sympathochromaffin system activity in the elderly. *J Am Geriatr Soc.* 1987;35:448–453.
20. Ziegler MG, Lake CR, Kopin IJ. Plasma noradrenaline increases with age. *Nature.* 1976;261:333–335.
21. Supiano MA, Linares OA, Smith MJ, Halter JB. Age-related differences in norepinephrine kinetics: effect of posture and sodium-restricted diet. *Am J Physiol.* 1990; 259:E422–E431.
22. Hogikyan RV, Supiano MA. Arterial α-adrenergic responsiveness is decreased and sympathetic nervous system activity is increased in older humans. *Am J Physiol.* 1994; 266:E717–E724.
23. Iwase S, Mano T, Watanabe T, Saito M, Kobayashi F. Age-related changes of sympathetic outflow to muscles in humans. *J Gerontol.* 1991;46:M1–M5.
24. Vestal RE, Wood AJJ, Shand DG. Reduced beta-adrenoreceptor sensitivity in the elderly. *Clin Pharmacol Ther.* 1979;26:181–186.
25. Guarnieri T, Filburn CR, Zitnik G, Roth GS, Lakatta EG. Contractile and biochemical correlates of beta-adrenergic stimulation of the aged heart. *Am J Physiol.* 1980;239: H501–H508.
26. Hoffman BB, Blaschke TF, Ford GA. Beta adrenergically medicated cardiac chronotropic and vascular smooth

muscle responses during propranolol therapy and with-drawal in young and elderly persons. *J Gerontol.* 1992; 47(1):M22–M26.

27. Supiano MA, Hogikyan RV, Stoltz AM, Orstan N, Halter JB. Regulation of venous α-adrenergic responses in older humans. *Am J Physiol.* 1991;260:E599–E607.

28. Supiano MA, Hogikyan RV, Sidani MA, Galecki AT, Krueger JL. Sympathetic nervous system activity and α-adrenergic responsiveness in older hypertensive humans. *Am J Physiol.* 1999;276:E519–E528.

29. Lowenstein CJ, Dinerman JL, Snyder SH. Nitric oxide: a physiologic messenger. *Ann Intern Med.* 1994;120:227–237.

30. Vallance P, Collier J, Moncada S. Effects of endothelium-derived nitric oxide on peripheral arteriolar tone in man. *Lancet.* 1989;2:997–1000.

31. Egashira K, Inou T, Hirooka Y, et al. Effects of age on endothelium-dependent vasodilation of resistance coronary artery by acetylcholine in humans. *Circulation.* 1993; 88:77–81.

32. Panza JA, Casino PR, Kilcoyne CM, Quyyumi AA. Role of endothelium-derived nitric oxide in the abnormal endothelium-dependent vascular relaxation of patients with essential hypertension. *Circulation.* 1993;87:1468–1474.

33. Meyer BR. Renal function in aging. *J Am Geriatr Soc.* 1989;37:791–800.

34. Lever AF, Berretta-Piccoli C, Brown JJ, Davies DL, Fraser R, Robertson JIS. Sodium and potassium in essential hypertension. *Br Med J.* 1981;283:1–15.

35. Luft FC, Weinberger MH, Fineberg NS, Miller JZ, Grim CE. Effects of age on renal sodium homeostasis and its relevance to sodium sensitivity. *Am J Med.* 1987;82(suppl 1B):9–15.

36. Dengel DR, Hogikyan RV, Brown MD, Glickman SG, Supiano MA. Insulin sensitivity is associated with blood pressure response to sodium in older hypertensives. *Am J Physiol.* 1998;274:E403–E409.

37. Hall JE, Coleman TG, Guyton AC. The renin-angiotensin system: normal physiology and changes in older hypertensives. *J Am Geriatr Soc.* 1989;37:801–813.

38. Shimokata H, Muller DC, Fleg JL, Sorkin J, Ziemba AW, Andres R. Age as independent determinant of glucose tolerance. *Diabetes.* 1991;40:44–51.

39. Reaven GM, Chen N, Hollenbeck C, Chen Y-DI. Effect of age on glucose tolerance and glucose uptake in healthy individuals. *J Am Geriatr Soc.* 1989;37:735–740.

40. Rowe JW, Minaker KL, Pallotta JA, Flier JS. Characterization of the insulin resistance of aging. *J Clin Investig.* 1983;71:1581–1587.

41. Chen M, Bergman R, Pacini G, Porte D. Pathogenesis of aging-related glucose intolerance in man: insulin resistance and decreased β-cell function. *J Clin Endocrinol Metab.* 1984;60:13–20.

42. Fink RI, Kolterman OG, Griffin J, Olefsky JM. Mechanisms of insulin resistance in aging. *J Clin Investig.* 1983;71: 1523–1535.

43. Ferrannini E, Buzzigoli G, Bonadonna R, et al. Insulin resistance in essential hypertension. *N Engl J Med.* 1987; 317:350–357.

44. Swislocki ALM, Hoffman BB, Reaven GM. Insulin resistance, glucose intolerance and hyperinsulinemia in patients with hypertension. *Am J Hypertens.* 1989;2:419–423.

45. Supiano MA, Hogikyan RV, Morrow LA, et al. Hypertension and insulin resistance: role of sympathetic nervous system activity. *Am J Physiol.* 1992;263:E935–E948.

46. Supiano MA, Morrow LA, Hogikyan RV, et al. Aging and insulin resistance: role of sympathetic activity and blood pressure. *J Gerontol Med Sci.* 1993;48:M237–M243.

47. Applegate W. High blood pressure treatment in the elderly. *Clin Geriatr Med.* 1992;8(1):103–117.

48. O'Callaghan WG, Fitzgerald DJ, O'Malley K, O'Brien E. Accuracy of indirect blood pressure measurement in the elderly. *BMJ.* 1983;286:1545–1546.

49. Vardan S, Mookherjee S, Warner R, Smulyan H. Systolic hypertension: direct and indirect BP measurements. *Arch Intern Med.* 1983;143:935–938.

50. Zweifler AJ, Shahab ST. Pseudohypertension: a new assessment. *J Hypertens.* 1993;11(1):1–6.

51. Messerli FH. Osler's maneuver, pseudohypertension, and true hypertension in the elderly. *Am J Med.* 1986;80:906–910.

52. Taapatsatis NP, Napolitana GT, Rothchild J. Osler's maneuver in an outpatient clinic setting. *Arch Intern Med.* 1991;151:2209–2211.

53. Oliner CM, Elliott WJ, Gretler DD, Murphy MB. Low predictive value of positive Osler manoeuvre for diagnosing pseudohypertension. *J Hum Hypertens.* 1993;7:65–70.

54. Staessen JA, Thijs L, Fagard R, et al. Predicting cardiovascular risk using conventional vs. ambulatory blood pressure in older patients with systolic hypertension. *JAMA.* 1999;282:539–546.

55. Streeten DHP, Anderson GH, Richardson R, Thomas FD. Abnormal orthostatic changes in blood pressure and heart rate in subjects with intact sympathetic nervous function: evidence for excessive venous pooling. *J Lab Clin Med.* 1988;111(3):326–335.

56. Mader SL. Aging and postural hypotension: an update. *J Am Geriatr Soc.* 1989;37:129–137.

57. Mader SL, Josephson KR, Rubenstein LZ. Low prevalence of postural hypotension among community-dwelling elderly. *JAMA.* 1987;258(11):1511–1514.

58. Harris T, Lewis A, Kleinman JC, Cornoni-Huntley J. Postural change in blood pressure associated with age and systolic blood pressure. *J Gerontol Med Sci.* 1991;46(5): M159–M163.

59. Lipsitz LA, Storch HA, Minaker KL, Rowe JW. Intra-individual variability in postural blood pressure in the elderly. *Clin Sci.* 1985;69:337–341.

60. Stenstrom G, Svardsudd K. Pheochromocytoma in Sweden 1959–1981: an analysis of the national cancer registry data. *Acta Med Scand.* 1986;220:225–232.

61. Staessen JA, Gasowski JG, Thijs L, et al. Risks of untreated and treated isolated systolic hypertension in the elderly: meta-analysis of outcome trials. *Lancet.* 2000;355:865–872.

62. SHEP Cooperative Research Group. Prevention of stroke by antihypertensive drug treatment in older persons with isolated systolic hypertension: final results of the systolic hypertension in the elderly program (SHEP). *JAMA.* 1991; 265(24):3255–3264.

63. European Working Party. Mortality and morbidity results from the European Working Party on high blood pressure in the elderly trial. *Lancet.* 1985;i:1349–1354.

64. MRC Working Party. Medical research council trial of treatment of hypertension in older adults: principal results. *Br Med J.* 1992;304:405–412.

65. National Heart Foundation of Australia. Treatment of mild hypertension in the elderly. *Med J Aust.* 1981;2:398–402.

66. Veterans Administration Cooperative Study Group on Antihypertensive Agents. Effects of treatment on morbidity in hypertension. *Circulation.* 1972;45:991–1004.

67. Dahlof B, Lindholm LH, Hannson L, Schersten B, Ekbom T, Wester P-O. Morbidity and mortality in the Swedish trial in old patients with hypertension (STOP-hypertension). *Lancet.* 1991;338:1281–1285.

68. Sprackling ME, Mitchell JR, Short AH, Watt G. Blood pressure reduction in the elderly: a randomised controlled trial of methyldopa. *Br Med J (Clin Res Ed).* 1981;283:1151–1153.

69. Coope J, Warrender TS. Randomized trial of treatment of hypertension in the elderly patients in primary care. *Br Med J (Clin Res Ed).* 1986;293:1145–1148.

70. Maxwell MH, Ford CE. Cardiovascular morbidity and mortality in HDFP patients 50–69 years old at entry. *J Cardiovasc Pharmacol.* 1985;7(suppl 2):S5–S9.

71. Insua JT, Sacks HS, Lau T-S, et al. Drug treatment of hypertension in the elderly: a meta-analysis. *Ann Intern Med.* 1994;121:355–362.

72. Ogden LG, He J, Lydick E, Whelton PK. Long-term absolute benefit of lowering blood pressure in hypertensive patients according to the JNC VI risk stratification. *Hypertension.* 2000;35:539–543.

73. Kostis JB, Davis BR, Cutler J, et al. Prevention of heart failure by antihypertensive drug treatment in older persons with isolated systolic hypertension. *JAMA.* 1997;278:212–216.

74. Forette F, Seux ML, Staessen JA, for the Syst-Eur Investigators. Prevention of dementia in randomised double-blind placebo-controlled Systolic Hypertension in Europe (Syst-Eur) trial. *Lancet.* 1998;352:1347–1351.

75. Mattila K, Haavisto M, Rajala S, Heikinheimo R. Blood pressure and five year survival in the very old. *Br Med J.* 1988;296:887–889.

76. Heikinheimo RJ, Haavisto MV, Kaarela RH, Kanto AJ, Koivunen MJ, Rajala SA. Blood pressure in the very old. *J Hypertens.* 1990;8:361–367.

77. Satish S, Freeman DH, Ray L, Goodwin JS. The relationship between blood pressure and mortality in the oldest old. *J Am Geriatr Soc.* 2001;49:367–374.

78. Gueyffier F, Bulpitt C, Boissel J-P, et al. Antihypertensive drugs in very old people: a subgroup meta-analysis of randomised controlled trials. *Lancet.* 1999;353:793–796.

79. Somes GW, Pahor M, Short RI, Cushman WC, Applegate WB. The role of diastolic blood pressure when treating isolated systolic hypertension. *Arch Intern Med.* 1999;159:2004–2009.

80. Whelton PK, Appel LJ, Espeland MA, et al. Sodium reduction and weight loss in the treatment of hypertension in older persons: a randomized controlled trial of nonphar-

macologic interventions in the elderly (TONE). *JAMA.* 1998;279:839–846.

81. Midgley JP, Matthew AG, Greenwood CM, et al. Effect of reduced dietary sodium on blood pressure: a meta-analysis of randomized controlled trials. *JAMA.* 1996;275:1590–1597.

82. Appel LJ, Moore TJ, Obarzanek E, et al. A clinical trial of the effects of dietary patterns on blood pressure. *N Engl J Med.* 1997;336:1117–1123.

83. Sacks FM, Svetkey LP, Vollmer WM, Appel LJ, Bray GA, for the DASH-Sodium Collaborative Research Group. Effects on blood pressure of reduced dietary sodium and the dietary approaches to stop hypertension (DASH) diet. *N Engl J Med.* 2001;344:3–10.

84. Plan and operation of the second National Health and Nutrition Examination Survey, 1976–1980. *Vital and Health Statistics, Series 1, No. 15.* Hyattsville, MD: National Center for Health Statistics; 1981.

85. Landsberg L. Pathophysiology of obesity-related hypertension: role of insulin and the sympathetic nervous system. *J Cardiovasc Pharm.* 1994;23(suppl 1):S1–S8.

86. The Trials of Hypertension Prevention Collaborative Research Group. Reducing blood pressure by nonpharmacologic interventions. *JAMA.* 1992;267:1213–1220.

87. Cutler JAK. Combinations of lifestyle modification and drug treatment in management of mild-moderate hypertension: a review of randomized clinical trials. *Clin Exp Hypertens.* 1993;15(6):1193–1204.

88. Schotte DE, Stunkard AJ. The effects of weight reduction on blood pressure in 301 obese patients. *Arch Intern Med.* 1990;150:1701–1704.

89. Kelley G, McClellan P. Antihypertensive effects of aerobic exercise: a brief meta-analytic review of randomized controlled trials. *Am J Hypertens.* 1994;7:115–119.

90. Hagberg JM, Montain SJ, Martin WHI, Ehsani AA. Effect of exercise training in 60- to 69-year-old persons with essential hypertension. *Am J Cardiol.* 1989;64:348–353.

91. Wright JM, Lee C-H, Chambers GK. Systematic review of antihypertensive therapies: does the evidence assist in choosing a first-line drug? *Can Med Assoc J (CMAJ).* 1999;161:25–32.

92. Ekbom T, Dahlof B, Hansson L, Lindholm LH, Schersten B, Wester P-O. Antihypertensive efficacy and side effects of three beta-blockers and a diuretic in elderly hypertensives: a report from the STOP-Hypertension study. *J Hypertens.* 1992;10:1525–1530.

93. Espeland MA, Kumanyika S, Kostis JB, et al. Antihypertensive medication use among recruits for the trial of non-pharmacologic interventions in the elderly (TONE). *J Am Geriatr Soc.* 1996;44:1183–1189.

94. Moser M. Why are physicians not prescribing diuretics more frequently in the management of hypertension? *JAMA.* 1998;279:1813–1816.

95. Vidt DG, Borazanian RA. Calcium channel blockers in geriatric hypertension. *Geriatrics.* 1991;46:28–38.

96. Materson BJ, Reda DJ, Cushman WC, et al. Single-drug therapy for hypertension in men. *N Engl J Med.* 1993;328:914–921.

97. Applegate WB, Phillips HL, Schnaper H, et al. A randomized controlled trial of the effects of three antihyperten-

sive agents on blood pressure control and quality of life in older women. *Arch Intern Med.* 1991;151:1817–1823.

98. Donnelly R, Reid JL, Meredith PA, Ahmed JH, Elliott HL. Factors determining the response to calcium antagonists in hypertension. *J Cardiovasc Pharmacol.* 1988;12(suppl 6):S109–S113.

99. Oesterling JE. Benign prostatic hyperplasia: medical and minimally invasive treatment options. *N Engl J Med.* 1995; 332:99–109.

100. Staessen JA, Fagard R, Thijs L, et al. Randomised double-blind comparison of placebo and active treatment for older patients with isolated systolic hypertension. *Lancet.* 1997;350:757–764.

101. Staessen JA, Fagard R, Thijs L, et al. Subgroup and per-protocol analysis of the randomized European trial on isolated systolic hypertension in the elderly. *Arch Intern Med.* 1999;158:1681–1691.

102. Tuomilehto J, Rastenyte D, Birkenhager WH, et al. Effects of calcium-channel blockade in older patients with diabetes and systolic hypertension. *N Engl J Med.* 1999;340: 677–684.

103. National Intervention Cooperative Study in Elderly Hypertensives Study Group. Randomized double-blind comparison of a calcium antagonist and a diuretic in elderly hypertensives. *Hypertension.* 1999;34:1129–1133.

104. Messerli HF, Grossman E, Goldbourt U. Are beta-blockers efficacious as first-line therapy for hypertension in the elderly? a systematic review. *JAMA.* 1998;279:1903–1907.

105. Weder AB. The renally compromised older hypertensive: therapeutic considerations. *Geriatrics.* 1991;46:36–48.

106. Eisalo A, Virta P. Treatment of hypertension in the elderly with labetalol. *Acta Med Scand.* 1984;65(suppl 6):129–133.

107. Neaton JD, Grimm RHJr, Prineas RJ, et al. Treatment of mild hypertension study; final results. *JAMA.* 1993;270: 713–724.

108. Thacker HL, Jahnigen DW. Managing hypertensive emergencies and urgencies in the geriatric patient. *Geriatrics.* 1991;46:26–37.

109. Joint National Committee on Detection Evaluation, and Treatment of High Blood Pressure. The Fifth Report of The Joint National Committee on Detection, Evaluation, and Treatment of High Blood Pressure. *Arch Intern Med.* 1993;153:154–183.

110. Zeller KR, Kuhnert LV, Matthews C. Rapid reduction of severe asymptomatic hypertension: a prospective, controlled trial. *Arch Intern Med.* 1989;149:2186–2189.

111. Auseon A, Ooi WL, Hossain M, Lipsitz LA. Blood pressure behavior in the nursing home: implications for diagnosis and treatment of hypertension. *J Am Geriatr Soc.* 1999;47:285–290.

112. Gambassi G, Lapane K, Sgadari A, et al. Prevalence, clinical correlates, and treatment of hypertension in elderly nursing home residents. *Arch Intern Med.* 1998;158:2377–2385.

113. Stoneking HT, Hla KM, Samsa GP, Feussner JR. Blood pressure measurements in the nursing home: are they accurate. *Gerontologist.* 1992;32(4):536–540.

114. Jansen RWMM, Lipsitz LA. Postprandial hypotension: epidemiology, pathophysiology, and clinical management. *Ann Intern Med.* 1995;122:286–295.

115. Vaitkevicius PV, Esservein DM, Maynard AK, O'Connor FC, Fleg JL. Frequency and importance of postprandial blood pressure reduction in elderly nursing-home patients. *Ann Intern Med.* 1991;115(11):865–870.

116. Myers AH, Baker SP, Van Natta ML, Abbey H, Robinson EG. Risk factors associated with falls and injuries among elderly institutionalized persons. *Am J Epidemiol.* 1991; 133(11):1179–1190.

117. Granek E, Baker SP, Abbey H, et al. Medications and diagnoses in relation to falls in a long-term care facility. *J Am Geriatr Soc.* 1987;35:503–511.

118. Lipsitz LA, Jonsson PV, Kelley MM, Koestner JS. Causes and correlates of recurrent falls in ambulatory frail elderly. *J Gerontol Med Sci.* 1991;46(4):M114–M122.

41
Peripheral Arterial Disease

William R. Hiatt and Mark R. Nehler

Peripheral arterial disease (PAD) involves the atherosclerotic occlusion of the arterial circulation to the lower extremities. The disease may be asymptomatic (identified only by a reduced blood pressure in the ankle), or it may manifest symptoms of intermittent claudication or severe chronic leg ischemia. The typical patient with PAD presents a decade later than the patient with coronary artery disease and experiences a profound limitation in exercise capacity and quality of life. In addition to affecting the limbs, PAD is a manifestation of systemic atherosclerosis affecting other major circulations involving the cerebral and coronary circulations. Thus, all patients with PAD are at an increased risk of cardiovascular morbidity and mortality. The treatment goals are directed at providing symptom relief and at reducing the risk of systemic cardiovascular morbidity and mortality.

Epidemiology

In the Framingham study, subjects were assessed for PAD using a history of claudication as a marker of the disease. Men and women had a similar incidence of intermittent claudication, which increased with age.[1] However, symptoms underestimate the true incidence and prevalence of the disease. Using the ankle–brachial index (ABI; described later), the prevalence of PAD is quite high, affecting 12% of the adult population and 20% of individuals over the age of 70.[2] These figures extrapolate to approximately 8 million persons affected with PAD in the United States.

The natural history of PAD has been evaluated in several studies.[3–7] These studies have shown that elderly control subjects had an all-cause mortality rate of 1.6% per year. This rate was increased to 4.8% per year in patients with PAD, a 2.5-fold increased risk. Cardiovascular mortality rates are similarly affected, with 3- to 4-fold increased risk for patients with PAD. Importantly,

women are at approximately the same risk as men, and even asymptomatic individuals, who are identified solely based on an abnormal ankle–brachial index (ABI), have a markedly increased risk of cardiovascular events. The mortality risk in patients with PAD is maintained after adjustment for other cardiovascular risk factors and even in patients with known coronary artery disease.[8]

Risk Factors

The risk factors for PAD are those that are expected for any patient population with atherosclerosis. The most potent risk factors for PAD are age, diabetes mellitus, and cigarette smoking. In addition, hyperlipidemia, hypertension, and elevations in plasma homocysteine levels play an important role in promoting peripheral atherosclerosis.

Age

All forms of cardiovascular disease become more prevalent with age, and PAD is particularly prevalent in the elderly. In several studies, the risk of PAD increased approximately twofold for every 10-year increase in age.[2,9]

Diabetes Mellitus

Diabetes is a major risk factor for PAD; persons with diabetes were four to five times more likely to develop claudication than nondiabetics.[2] The major risk for PAD due to diabetes appears to be the association of smoking, hypertension, and byperlipidemia with diabetes, and not the degree of glycemic control per se.[10] Thus, diabetes is a critical risk factor in the development of PAD, particularly in conjunction with other risk factors.

Cigarette Smoking

Cigarette smoking is associated with an approximate three- to fourfold increase in risk for peripheral atherosclerosis.[11] In addition, current cigarette smoking also significantly affects PAD outcomes. For example, progression from intermittent claudication to ischemic rest pain with risk of amputation occurs significantly more frequently in patients who continue to smoke than those who are abstinent.[12,13]

Hyperlipidemia

Independent risk factors for PAD include a reduced HDL cholesterol level, and elevations of total cholesterol, LDL cholesterol, triglycerides, and lipoprotein(a).[2,11] For every 10 mg/dL increase in total cholesterol concentration, the risk of PAD increases approximately 10%.[2]

Hypertension

The presence of hypertension increases risk of PAD approximately two- to threefold.[2,11]

Homocysteine

Alterations in homocysteine metabolism are a recognized independent risk factor for PAD.[14,15] Homocysteine promotes the formation of oxidized LDL cholesterol, endothelial dysfunction, and the proliferation of vascular smooth muscle cells.[16] Perhaps the most common cause of elevations in homocysteine levels are nutritional deficiencies of B vitamins, particularly folic acid and vitamins B_6 and B_{12}.

Additional Risk Factors

An elevated fibrinogen level is an independent predictor of PAD and also for the severity of claudication.[17] Hypercoagulable states have not been extensively evaluated as risk factors in PAD. The lupus anticoagulant has been associated with peripheral atherosclerosis, as have markers of platelet activation such as increases in beta thromboglobulin levels.[18,19] However, the frequency of these abnormalities is low and not fully substantiated and therefore does not warrant screening.

Pathogenesis

The underlying disease process in PAD is the result of atherosclerosis in the arterial circulation of the lower extremity, caused by similar pathogenic mechanisms as for coronary and cerebral atherosclerosis. Arterial occlusive disease results in reduced blood flow, particularly to the calf muscles during exercise in patients with claudication, but with critical leg ischemia, blood flow is inadequate to meet the resting metabolic demands of the limb. Importantly, altered hemodynamics do not completely explain the pathophysiology of claudication. Work from several laboratories has demonstrated secondary changes in the skeletal muscle of patients with PAD that are consistent with motor nerve injury and loss of type II muscle fibers leading to muscle weakness.[20,21] In addition, these patients acquire a metabolic myopathy characterized by the presence of somatic mutations in the mitochondrial genome, alteration in the expression of mitochondrial enzymes, and the accumulation of metabolic intermediates that have functional significance.[22–24] These abnormalities are associated with specific defects in the activity of complex I and complex III of the electron transport chain that provide further evidence of a chronic, ischemia-induced myopathy in PAD.[25]

Clinical Presentation and Diagnosis

Clinical Assessment

PAD is associated with two very characteristic types of limb symptoms, intermittent claudication and ischemic rest pain. Claudication is derived from the Latin word meaning to limp, which is the type of gait observed when a patient with PAD develops symptoms of claudication. The discomfort most commonly involves the calf or buttocks during walking exercise and is resolved within 10 min of rest. These patients commonly can walk no more than two to three blocks (200–300 m) before they must stop to relieve the claudication pain. Peak exercise capacity is reduced 50% compared to healthy elderly subjects, and there is a profound limitation in daily activities.[26]

Patients with chronic critical limb ischemia often present with rest pain in the distal foot that occurs at night and is relieved with dependency. Patients with more severe disease develop ischemic ulcers that are usually found at the distal points of the foot (toes, etc.) and are painful. In general, any patient with an open foot wound needs to have adequate arterial circulation confirmed by vascular studies.

The differential diagnosis in patients with leg symptoms includes PAD, diabetic sensory neuropathy, reflex sympathetic dystrophy, vasculitis, spinal stenosis, and arthritis. Patients with diabetic neuropathy may present with normal pedal pulses, but symptoms consistent with ischemic pain, and nonhealing neuropathic ulcers (these ulcers are usually on the plantar surface of the foot at pressure points—metatarsal heads). Reflex sympathetic dystrophy may present after surgical or other forms of trauma and leads to a painful, discolored, swollen extremity. Although this disorder is most likely caused by an autonomic neuropathy, arterial perfusion is typically normal. Patients with vasculitis may present with Buerger's disease (thromboangitis obliterans) and a strong smoking history. Claudication-like symptoms may also arise from spinal stenosis, which is due to osteophytic narrowing of the lumbar neurospinal canal. These symptoms include numbness and weakness in the lower extremity that is produced by standing or increasing lumbar lordosis rather than just ambulation. The symptoms are relieved not simply by rest, but also by sitting down or leaning forward to straighten out the lumbar spine. Patients with arthritis of the knee or hip may also have not only pain in the joint with ambulation, but also pain at rest or with weightbearing.

Hemodynamic Assessment

An ankle–brachial index (ABI) should be performed in patients suspected of having PAD, which would include persons at risk who are over the age of 70 years or younger patients between the age of 50 to 69 years who smoke or have diabetes. The estimated prevalence of PAD in this population at risk is more than 25%.[27] In addition, patients with exertional leg symptoms should also be evaluated with an ABI. The ABI test can be performed in the office setting using a routine sphygmomanometer and a handheld, continuous-wave Doppler to determine the systolic blood pressure in the arms and posterior tibial and dorsalis pedis arteries of each ankle. The ABI calculation is based on the higher of the two arm pressures and the higher pressure of the two vessels in each ankle. There is not a single cutoff value to define an abnormal ABI, but a ratio of 0.90 or less should be considered diagnostic for PAD.[28] ABI values of 0.40 or less are consistent with critical leg ischemia. In addition to obtaining the ABI, occlusive lesions can be further localized by taking pressure measurements in the upper and lower thigh and calf (segmental limb pressures). In patients with iliac occlusive disease, the thigh pressures are reduced, whereas patients with disease more distal in the leg may have a normal thigh pressure but reduced calf and ankle pressures.

Functional Assessment

Patients with claudication have a severe limitation in exercise performance and walking ability. Thus, determining functional status is an important aspect of the overall evaluation of the patient with PAD. In patients with claudication, treadmill testing can be used to define the distance at which claudication pain begins (initial claudication distance) and the maximal walking distance. Claudication therapies typically increase both the initial and maximal walking distances.[29]

In addition to treadmill testing, several questionnaire measures of functional status have been developed and validated in this patient population. The walking impairment questionnaire (WIQ) is a disease-specific instrument that asks a series of questions regarding the patient's claudication severity and ability to walk defined distances, speeds, and stairs.[29] This questionnaire is simple to administer and has been shown to predict the response to claudication therapies.[30] The Medical Outcomes Short Form-36 instrument is a nondisease-specific questionnaire that assesses a variety of functional status domains. This questionnaire has also been sensitive in detecting treatment effect, particularly in the physical functioning realm.

Figure 41.1 provides an approach to the diagnosis of PAD in elderly populations.

Medical Therapy

The primary initial goals of medical therapy in patients with PAD are to treat the systemic atherosclerosis by risk modification and antiplatelet drugs in an attempt to reduce cardiovascular morbidity and mortality. Once that has been accomplished, the physician can then address the relief of symptoms and limb preservation.

Smoking Cessation

Several studies have suggested that smoking cessation will decrease the risk of critical leg ischemia and even reduce mortality in patients with PAD.[12,13] All patients with PAD should be referred to a smoking cessation program and prescribed nicotine replacement and antidepressants.[32] Nicotine replacement therapies, in addition to behavior modification, are slightly more effective than behavior modification alone. A recent meta-analysis of several placebo-controlled trials revealed cessation rates of 23% to 27% over 6 to 12 months using a nicotine patch as compared to placebo, where the quit rates ranged from 13% to 18%.[33] Also, in patients with medical diseases, transdermal nicotine patches have been shown to be safe even in high-risk populations. Thus, this is a strategy that should be considered for patients with PAD.

Diabetes

Patients with diabetes should first undergo intensive blood glucose control to target a hemoglobin A_1C less than 7.0%. Obtaining this goal may have favorable effects on the risk of cardiovascular events in both type 1 and type 2 diabetes.[34,35] However, intensive glycemic control had no effect on the risk of amputation from PAD.[35] In addition to intensive blood sugar control, patients with atherosclerosis and diabetes also need

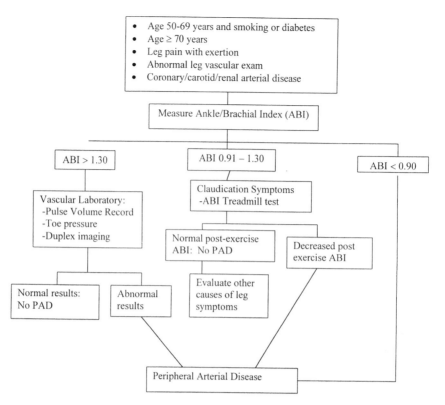

FIGURE 41.1. Evaluation of patients suspected to have peripheral arterial disease (PAD). Patients should be evaluated for peripheral arterial disease if they if they are at increased risk because of their age or presence of atherosclerotic risk factors, have leg symptoms on exertion, or have distal limb ulceration for which history and examination do not provide an obvious explanation. Additional vascular studies can be obtained in patients with an ankle–brachial index (ABI) above 1.30, including pulse volume recordings (PVR), and pressure in the first toe, or by duplex imaging of the peripheral vessels to determine if peripheral arterial disease is present. Patients with leg symptoms on exertion who have an ankle–brachial index of 0.91 to 1.30 should be considered for an exercise test. An ankle–brachial index that is above 0.90 at rest but decreases by 20% after exercise is diagnostic of peripheral arterial disease.[96] If the initial ankle–brachial index is 0.90 or less at rest, then the patient likely has peripheral arterial disease and no additional tests are necessary.

aggressive risk factor modification; this may be particularly true in the treatment of hypertension when an angiotensin-converting enzyme (ACE) inhibitor may be a preferable agent.[36] Given the lack of specific trials, drug therapy for patients with diabetes and PAD should follow general published recommendations.[37]

Hyperlipidemia

Several effective therapies have been developed to treat patients with hyperlipidemia. Dietary restriction of cholesterol and saturated fats has only a modest effect on LDL cholesterol levels, but a more substantial decrease in triglyceride levels, important in the management of PAD. The statin drugs have become a well-established means of reducing LDL cholesterol levels. In addition to statin drugs, gemfibrozil has been shown to lower LDL cholesterol concentration, with the added benefit of increase in HDL cholesterol concentrations. Additional means to modify HDL cholesterol concentration is the use of niacin, which in a recent study was found to be safe in patients with PAD and diabetes.[38]

In patients with PAD, a meta-analysis of randomized trials of lipid-lowering therapies showed a nonsignificant reduction in reducing mortality (odds ratio, 0.21; 95% CI, 0.03–1.17). This analysis also concluded that lipid reduction therapies favorably altered angiographic disease progression and symptoms of claudication.[39] Limitations of the analysis were a relatively small sample size and the fact that there have been no clinical trials in PAD of lipid therapy to prevent ischemic events.

Patients with PAD are at high risk for systemic ischemic events but at less risk for progression of their leg arterial disease. Based on evidence from the lipid trials in coronary artery disease, the National Cholesterol Education Program guidelines include PAD as a patient population at the highest risk for future coronary heart disease events and therefore in need of aggressive secondary prevention therapies.[40] The current recommendation for lipid therapy in the PAD population is to achieve an LDL cholesterol level less than 100mg/dL and a triglyceride level less than 150mg/dL.[41] The LDL cholesterol goals often require the use of HMG-coenzyme A reductase inhibitors, and achieving the HDL cholesterol goals often requires the use of niacin.

Hypertension

All patients with PAD and hypertension should undergo aggressive lowering of their blood pressure according to the Joint National Committee VI guidelines.[42] All classes of antihypertensive agents can be used in patients with PAD, including beta-adrenergic blockers, which are safe in patients with claudication.[43,44] In addition, beta-adrenergic blockers are routinely used in the perioperative setting to decrease the risks of vascular surgery.[45] Another class of drugs, the ACE inhibitors, may be protective against cardiovascular events in PAD patients. In the Heart Outcomes Prevention Evaluation Study, 44% of the population had evidence of PAD.[46] The study demonstrated that ramipril was associated with a reduced risk for vascular death, nonfatal myocardial infarction, or stroke in patients with PAD. This study suggests that ACE inhibitors may be important agents in reducing the risk of ischemic events in the PAD population.

Additional Approaches to Risk Modification

Elevated homocysteine levels can be reduced by supplementing the diet with B vitamins and folate.[47] Despite the ease of therapy with vitamin supplements, there are no clinical trials that demonstrate a clinical benefit in reducing homocysteine levels.

Estrogen therapy in postmenopausal women may also favorably influence several cardiovascular risk factors.[48] However, the Heart and Estrogen/Progestin Replacement Study showed no overall benefit of hormone therapy for reduction of cardiovascular events or peripheral arterial endpoints.[49] Thus, at the present time, there are no recommendations for this therapy in PAD patients.

Antioxidant vitamins such as vitamin E have been advocated to prevent ischemic events. However, the HOPE trial showed no benefit of vitamin E on prevention of cardiovascular events.[46] Thus the use of antioxidant vitamins in patients with PAD may not result in any clinical benefits.

Antiplatelet Therapy

In addition to risk factor modification, other therapies have been targeted to slow the progression of peripheral atherosclerosis, as well as to decrease the risk of cardiovascular morbidity and mortality. The role of platelets in thrombus formation has led to many studies in the effectiveness of various antiplatelet agents, particularly aspirin, in the prevention of ischemic events. The meta-analysis by the Antiplatelet Trialists' Collaboration concluded that, in patients with a history of myocardial infarction or stroke, antiplatelet therapy reduced the risk of ischemic events by approximately 25%.[50,51] In patients with PAD treated with bypass surgery, the Antiplatelet Trialists' Collaboration also found that antiplatelet therapy significantly promoted graft patency following vascular surgery.[52] Thus, it would seem prudent to treat patients with PAD with low-dose aspirin.

In patients with PAD, ticlopidine has been shown to be more effective than placebo at reducing the risk of fatal and nonfatal myocardial infarction and stroke.[53,54] This observation has led to the development of other drugs including clopidogrel, which lacks many of the side effects of ticlopidine. The clopidogrel versus aspirin for the prevention of ischemic events (CAPRIE) trial demonstrated that PAD patients showed a 24% risk reduction on clopidogrel as compared to aspirin in terms of reducing risk for ischemic events.[55]

In summary, patients with PAD frequently have a history of coronary artery disease and stroke, and even in the absence of this history, PAD remains an independent predictor of cardiovascular morbidity and mortality. Aspirin should be considered as the primary antiplatelet agent for preventing ischemic events in PAD. Aspirin is also effective in maintaining vascular graft patency and may prevent thrombotic complications of PAD. Clopidogrel has FDA approval for the prevention of ischemic events in PAD, and, although based on a subgroup analysis, clopidogrel may be more effective than aspirin in PAD patients.

Claudication Medical Therapy

Exercise Training

The use of a formal exercise program to treat claudication has been studied over the past 30 years. Exercise therapy for claudication had demonstrated efficacy in terms of improving exercise performance, quality of life, and functional capacity.[56] Numerous types of exercise programs have been devised, but the most successful employ a supervised exercise setting. Patients should also undergo an exercise test to maximal claudication pain. A typical supervised exercise program is 60min in duration and is monitored by a skilled nurse or technician. Patients should be encouraged to walk primarily on a treadmill because this most closely reproduces walking in the community setting. The initial workload of the treadmill is set to a speed and grade that brings on claudication pain within 3 to 5min. Patients walk at this work rate until they achieve claudication of moderate severity. They then rest until the claudication abates and then resume exercise. This repeated on-and-off form of exercise is continued throughout the supervised rehabilitation setting. On a weekly basis, patients should be reassessed as they are able to walk farther and farther at their chosen workload; this then will necessitate an increase in speed or grade or both to allow patients to successfully work at harder and harder workloads. This scenario then induces a training benefit. The duration of an exercise program is 3 to 6 months. The typical benefits include a 100% to 200% improvement in peak exercise performance on the treadmill and significant improvements in functional status.[30]

Drug Therapy for Claudication

Vasodilators were an early class of agents used to treat claudication but have not been shown to have clinical efficacy.[57] In 1984, pentoxifylline was approved for the treatment of claudication. In early controlled trials, the drug produced a 12% improvement in the maximal treadmill walking distance.[58] However, in a recent study, pentoxifylline was no more effective than placebo on improving treadmill walking distance or functional status assessed by questionnaires.[59] A meta-analysis concluded that the drug produced modest increases in treadmill walking distance over placebo, but the overall clinical benefits were questionable.[60]

Cilostazol is currently the most effective drug for claudication. Approved in 1999, the primary action of cilostazol is to inhibit phosphodiesterase type 3, which results in vasodilation and inhibition of platelet aggregation, arterial thromboses, and vascular smooth muscle proliferation.[61–63] In four trials of 1534 patients, cilostazol 100mg twice daily improved both pain-free and maximal walking distance as compared with placebo.[59,64–66] In one trial, cilostazol 100mg twice daily was superior to both placebo and pentoxifylline.[59] In three of the trials, cilostazol also improved several aspects of physical functioning and quality of life as assessed by questionnaires.[64–66] The most common side effects of cilostazol are headache, transient diarrhea, palpitations, and dizziness. Cilostazol should not be given to patients with claudication who also have heart failure.

Additional drugs are in clinical trials for treating claudication. Propionyl-L-carnitine is a metabolic agent that has been shown to improve treadmill performance and quality of life in patients with claudication.[67–69] Prostaglandins have been extensively studied in patients with PAD, but with mixed results. In a recent study, beraprost, an oral prostaglandin, had positive effects on treadmill walking distance and quality of life.[70] However, these drugs are still under study and their utility needs further evaluation. Very few studies have addressed the issue of combined drug plus exercise therapy for claudi-

cation. However, the available data suggest at least an additive effect of exercise training plus a drug for claudication.[71,72]

Interventional Therapy for PAD

Claudication

In patients with claudication, the natural history of the limb disease is relatively benign in that the risk of progression to critical limb ischemia and limb loss is quite small.[73,74] Therefore, the decision to proceed with interventional therapy in patients with claudication is typically based on lack of response to medical therapy and a suitable lesion for angioplasty or surgery.

Angioplasty with or without stenting has been evaluated in both the iliac and femoral arteries. Although the initial technical success is high (>90% for both), the durability of angioplasty with stenting is far greater in the iliac vessels.[75] The Trans-Atlantic Inter-Society Consensus (TASC) document provides summary recommendation for lesions that are appropriately treated with angioplasty.[76] In the iliac arteries, a single stenosis of 10 cm or less, two stenoses less than 5 cm, and unilateral common iliac occlusion are best treated initially with angioplasty. In the femoral arteries, a single stenosis of 10 cm or less and multiple lesions each less than 3 cm may also be approached with angioplasty, typically without a stent.

Surgery for claudication generally involves two operations, the aortofemoral bypass and the femoral above-knee popliteal bypass. Aortofemoral bypass has good patency in older patients (80% patent at 10 years).[77] However, these procedures have a 3% to 5% mortality risk and a 1% incidence of graft infection.[78] Aortic surgery is a morbid operation from which an older patient frequently requires months to recover completely. Femoral popliteal bypass is less durable, with patencies of 50% to 60% at 5 years.[79,80] Operative mortality rates up to 3% are typical when operating for claudication.[81] In addition, femoral popliteal bypass is more likely to lead to limb threat following graft failure. The TASC recommendations for aortoiliac surgery are for more diffuse disease,[76] which would include bilateral stenoses of 5–10 cm, diffuse, multiple unilateral stenoses greater than 10 cm, bilateral occlusions, and diffuse disease involving the aorta and iliac arteries. In the femoral vessels, similar criteria apply for surgery, including multiple stenoses or occlusions, each 3 to 5 cm, and complete common or superficial artery occlusions.

Critical Leg Ischemia

The initial management of patients with critical leg ischemia involves pain relief including narcotics. Patients with more severe disease including ischemic ulceration or gangrene also need wound care to control infection and prevention of further trauma to the extremity. Specific medical treatments for critical leg ischemia have been limited. Numerous trials have been performed in Europe using prostaglandin drugs. These trials have met with marginal success using a variety of agents. Antiplatelet therapy is critical to maintain graft patency, whereas the use of anticoagulation to maintain graft patency is empiric and done only in selected cases.

Definitive evaluation and management requires arteriography and revascularization, or primary amputation. Revascularization operations for critical limb ischemia use the patient's own veins (greater saphenous, lesser saphenous, and arm veins) as the optimal bypass conduit. Current 5-year patency rates for below-knee popliteal (distal anastomosis to a modest-sized artery just below the knee) and tibial (distal anastomosis to smaller arteries at the calf level or below) bypass of 60% to 70% and 50% to 60%, respectively, have been reported by multiple centers.[80] Limb salvage (prevention of amputation) rates of 80% or better for the same time interval are also the rule,[80] which is due to success in second bypass surgeries when the first operation eventually fails. Operative mortality is 5% in most series but may reach 10% in patients over 80 years of age.[82] Hospital stays of 10 or more days are common due to slow healing and frequent complications and comorbidities. About one-quarter to one-third of patients need to go to some sort of rehabilitation facility on discharge, although the majority will stay for only a few weeks.[82] The decision to use surgery or angioplasty as the initial treatment option follows the TASC guidelines described earlier.

Despite these impressive patency data, 23% of bypasses will need some sort of operative revision (usually within the first year) to repair a stenotic area that develops in the vein graft.[83] Twenty percent of patients will require at least one readmission for wound care issues, usually associated with an operative incision.[84] The majority of patients develop significant lymphedema in the operated leg. Constant graft ultrasound surveillance to locate the asymptomatic stenoses before graft occlusion and limb threat (every 3 months for the first year and every 6 months for life) and potential revision needs lead to a substantial amount of patient anxiety.

In patients who progress to amputation, below-knee amputations are performed in patients with ambulatory potential. However, despite many different techniques, there is no guaranteed method to assure healing of below-knee amputations. Issues that complicate healing include poor circulation, chronic edema, and skin changes consistent with chronic venous disease. This difficulty is reflected in a reamputation rate to attempt below-knee salvage from 4% to 30%.[85–87] Importantly, half of all below-knee amputees who fail primary healing ulti-mately require above-knee amputation.[88] Primary above-knee amputation is considered the best option for patients without any ambulatory potential (dementia, stroke, obesity, etc).

More below-knee amputees achieve ambulation than above-knee amputees,[89–91] although overall the number of major amputees who achieve meaningful independent ambulation is small. Initial rehabilitation can require 9 months or longer. By 2 years, 30% of amputees who were walking are no longer using their prostheses.[89] Advanced age and female gender bode poorly for ambulation.[92] Fifteen percent of amputees require contralateral amputation, and another 20% to 30% have died by 2 years.[89,93,94]

An overall approach to the treatment of PAD is presented in Figure 41.2.

Conclusions

Peripheral arterial disease is a prevalent manifestation of atherosclerosis that is associated with significant risk of morbidity and mortality and also a marked reduction in ambulatory capacity and quality of life. Unfortunately, PAD is undertreated with regard to risk factor modification, use of antiplatelet therapies, and management of symptoms.[95] The data to support intensive risk modification in PAD patients have not been as extensively established as is the case for patients with coronary artery disease. Clinical trials specifically in the PAD population are needed to address the benefits of the treatment of hyperlipidemia (including not only LDL cholesterol reduction, but also modification of other lipid fractions), diabetes, elevated homocysteine levels, and other prevalent risk factors in PAD. Despite these limitations, patients with PAD should be considered candidates for secondary disease prevention strategies. Target goals for the management of atherosclerotic risk factors should be achieved in all PAD patients. The use of ACE inhibitors may confer additional benefits in terms of a reduction in the risk of fatal and nonfatal ischemic events. The data are better in support of the use of antiplatelet therapies to prevent ischemic events in PAD. Aspirin should be considered in all PAD patients, with clopidogrel an alternate (and potentially more effective) agent. Studies evaluating the combination of clopidogrel with aspirin or aspirin with other antiplatelet agents are needed.

Medical therapies to treat the symptoms of claudication and limited mobility are now well established. A supervised walking exercise program should first be considered in all patients, given the low risk and marked improvements seen in functional capacity. Pharmacologic therapies are also available that offer meaningful improvements in functional status. Pentoxifylline has limited utility, but cilostazol has been shown to improve both

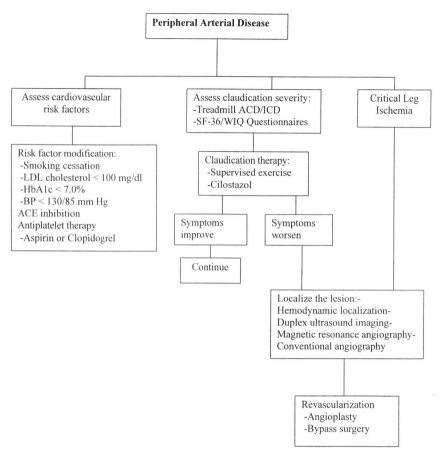

FIGURE 41.2. Evaluation and treatment of patients with proven peripheral arterial disease. All patients with peripheral arterial disease, regardless of symptom severity, should undergo risk factor modification to achieve the listed treatment goals and receive antiplatelet drug therapy with aspirin, but clopidogrel is an acceptable alternative drug. Angiotensin-converting enzyme inhibitors should be considered because of the potential for prevention of ischemic events that is independent of blood pressure lowering. A treadmill test to define the absolute claudication distance (*ACD*) and the initial claudication distance (*ICD*) can provide an objective assessment of the severity of claudication and response to therapy. The functional limitations of claudication and response to therapy can also be quantified by the physical function scales of the nondisease-specific Medical Outcomes Short Form 36 questionnaire (*SF-36*) and the disease-specific Walking Impairment Questionnaire (*WIQ*).

Treatment of claudication should begin with exercise therapy or drugs such as cilostazol. Patients who do not improve and remain disabled, or who have worsening symptoms, should have additional localization of the occlusive lesions to plan endovascular or surgical intervention. Noninvasive disease localization can be done with hemodynamic tests such as segmental limb pressures or pulse volume recordings. In addition, duplex ultrasound and magnetic resonance angiography (MRA) both have a high sensitivity and specificity for localization of lesions (with MRA having the highest sensitivity), but conventional angiography is still required in most patients before a surgical or angioplasty procedure. Patients with critical leg ischemia typically have an ankle–brachial index less than 0.40 and should initially be considered for localization of their occlusive disease in anticipation of the need for revascularization.

treadmill walking capacity and quality of life. A number of other compounds such as propionyl-L-carnitine, prostaglandins, L-arginine, lipid-lowering drugs, and angiogenic growth factors are under investigation for both claudication and critical leg ischemia. Future studies may confirm the benefits of combining treatments for claudication, including exercise following angioplasty or exercise plus a medication.

Patients who do not respond to medical therapies for their claudication symptoms should be considered for

angioplasty if they have a lesion amenable to the procedure. Patients with critical leg ischemia should be initially considered for vascular surgery and/or angioplasty.

References

1. Kannel WB, McGee DL. Update on some epidemiologic features of intermittent claudication: the Framingham Study. *J Am Geriatr Soc.* 1985;33:13–18.

2. Hiatt WR, Hoag S, Hamman RF. Effect of diagnostic criteria on the prevalence of peripheral arterial disease. The San Luis Valley diabetes study. *Circulation.* 1995;91:1472–1479.

3. Criqui MH, Langer RD, Fronek A, et al. Mortality over a period of 10 years in patients with peripheral arterial disease. *N Engl J Med.* 1992;326:381–386.

4. Vogt MT, Cauley JA, Newman AB, Kuller LH, Hulley SB. Decreased ankle/arm blood pressure index and mortality in elderly women. *JAMA.* 1993;270:465–469.

5. Newman AB, Tyrrell KS, Kuller LH. Mortality over four years in SHEP participants with a low ankle-arm index. *J Am Geriatr Soc.* 1997;45:1472–1478.

6. Leng GC, Fowkes FG, Lee AJ, et al. Use of ankle brachial pressure index to predict cardiovascular events and death: a cohort study. *Br Med J.* 1996;313:1440–1444.

7. Leng GC, Lee AJ, Fowkes FG, et al. Incidence, natural history and cardiovascular events in symptomatic and asymptomatic peripheral arterial disease in the general population. *Int J Epidemiol.* 1996;25:1172–1181.

8. Eagle KA, Rihal CS, Foster ED, Mickel MC, Gersh BJ. Long-term survival in patients with coronary artery disease: importance of peripheral vascular disease. The Coronary Artery Surgery Study (CASS) Investigators. *J Am Coll Cardiol.* 1994;23:1091–1095.

9. Vogt MT, Cauley JA, Kuller LH, Hulley SB. Prevalence and correlates of lower extremity arterial disease in elderly women. *Am J Epidemiol.* 1993;137:559–568.

10. Beach KW, Strandness DE. Arteriosclerosis obliterans and associated risk factors in insulin-dependent and non-insulin-dependent diabetes. *Diabetes.* 1980;29:882–888.

11. Murabito JM, D'Agostino RB, Silbershatz H, Wilson WF. Intermittent claudication. A risk profile from The Framingham Heart Study. *Circulation.* 1997;96:44–49.

12. Quick CRG, Cotton LT. The measured effect of stopping smoking on intermittent claudication. *Br J Surg.* 1982; 69(suppl):S24–S26.

13. Stewart CP. The influence of smoking on the level of lower limb amputation. *Prosthet Orthot Int.* 1987;11:113–116.

14. Malinow MR, Kang SS, Taylor LM, et al. Prevalence of hyperhomocyst(e)inemia in patients with peripheral arterial occlusive disease. *Circulation.* 1989;79:1180–1188.

15. Hoogeveen EK, Kostense PJ, Beks PJ, et al. Hyperhomocysteinemia is associated with an increased risk of cardiovascular disease, especially in non-insulin-dependent diabetes mellitus: a population-based study. *Arterioscler Thromb Vasc Biol.* 1998;18:133–138.

16. Welch GN, Loscalzo J. Homocysteine and atherothrombosis. *N Engl J Med.* 1998;338:1042–1050.

17. Lee AJ, Lowe GDO, Woodward M, Tunstall-Pedoe H. Fibrinogen in relation to personal history of prevalent hypertension, diabetes, stroke, intermittent claudication, coronary heart disease, and family history: the Scottish Heart Health Study. *Br Heart J.* 1993;69:338–342.

18. Donaldson MC, Weinberg DS, Belkin M, Whittemore AD, Mannick JA. Screening for hypercoagulable states in vascular surgical practice: a preliminary study. *J Vasc Surg.* 1990; 11:825–831.

19. Catalano M, Russo U, Libretti A. Plasma beta-thromboglobulin levels and claudication degrees in patients with peripheral vascular disease. *Angiology.* 1986;37:339–342.

20. England JD, Regensteiner JG, Ringel SP, Carry MR, Hiatt WR. Muscle denervation in peripheral arterial disease. *Neurology.* 1992;42:994–999.

21. Regensteiner JG, Wolfel EE, Brass EP, et al. Chronic changes in skeletal muscle histology and function in peripheral arterial disease. *Circulation.* 1993;87:413–421.

22. Hiatt WR, Wolfel EE, Regensteiner JG, Brass EP. Skeletal muscle carnitine metabolism in patients with unilateral peripheral arterial disease. *J Appl Physiol.* 1992;73:346–353.

23. Bhat HK, Hiatt WR, Hoppel CL, Brass EP. Skeletal muscle mitochondrial DNA injury in patients with unilateral peripheral arterial disease. *Circulation.* 1999;99:807–812.

24. Brass EP, Hiatt WR. Acquired skeletal muscle metabolic myopathy in atherosclerotic peripheral arterial disease. *Vasc Med.* 2000;5:55–59.

25. Brass EP, Hiatt WR, Gardner AW, Hoppel CL. Decreased NADH dehydrogenase and ubiquinol-cytochrome *c* oxidoreductase in peripheral arterial disease. *Am J Physiol.* 2001;280:H603–H609.

26. Bauer TA, Regensteiner JG, Brass EP, Hiatt WR. Oxygen uptake kinetics during exercise are slowed in patients with peripheral arterial disease. *J Appl Physiol.* 1999;87:809–816.

27. Hirsch AT, Criqui MH, Treat-Jacobson D, et al. Peripheral arterial disease detection, awareness, and treatment in primary care. *JAMA.* 2001;286(11):1317–1324.

28. Carter SA. Clinical measurement of systolic pressures in limbs with arterial occlusive disease. *JAMA.* 1969;207:1869–1874.

29. Hiatt WR, Hirsch AT, Regensteiner JG, Brass EP. Clinical trials for claudication. Assessment of exercise performance, functional status, and clinical end points. Vascular Clinical Trialists. *Circulation.* 1995;92:614–621.

30. Regensteiner JG, Steiner JF, Hiatt WR. Exercise training improves functional status in patients with peripheral arterial disease. *J Vasc Surg.* 1996;23:104–115.

31. Jonason T, Bergstrom R. Cessation of smoking in patients with intermittent claudication. *Acta Med Scand.* 1987;221:253–260.

32. Jorenby DE, Leischow SJ, Nides MA, et al. A controlled trial of sustained-release bupropion, a nicotine patch, or both for smoking cessation. *N Engl J Med.* 1999;340:685–691.

33. Joseph AM, Norman SM, Ferry LH, et al. The safety of transdermal nicotine as an aid to smoking cessation in patients with cardiac disease. *N Engl J Med.* 1996;335:1792–1798.

34. Effect of intensive diabetes management on macrovascular events and risk factors in the Diabetes Control and Complications Trial. *Am J Cardiol.* 1995;75:894–903.

35. Intensive blood-glucose control with sulphonylureas or insulin compared with conventional treatment and risk of complications in patients with type 2 diabetes (UKPDS 33). UK Prospective Diabetes Study (UKPDS) Group. *Lancet.* 1998;352:837–853.

36. Estacio RO, Jeffers BW, Hiatt WR, et al. The effect of nisoldipine as compared with enalapril on cardiovascular outcomes in patients with non-insulin-dependent diabetes and hypertension. *N Engl J Med.* 1998;338:645–652.

37. DeFronzo RA. Pharmacologic therapy for type 2 diabetes mellitus. *Ann Intern Med*. 1999;131:281–303.

38. Elam MB, Hunninghake DB, Davis KB, et al. Effect of niacin on lipid and lipoprotein levels and glycemic control in patients with diabetes and peripheral arterial disease: the ADMIT study: a randomized trial. Arterial Disease Multiple Intervention Trial. *JAMA*. 2000;284:1263–1270.

39. Leng GC, Price JF, Jepson RG. Lipid-lowering for lower limb atherosclerosis (Cochrane Review). In: *The Cochrane Library*. Oxford: Update Software; 1999.

40. Summary of the second report of the National Cholesterol Education Program (NCEP) expert panel on detection, evaluation, and treatment of high blood cholesterol in adults (Adult Treatment Panel II). *JAMA*. 1993;329:3015–3023.

41. Ansell BJ, Watson KE, Fogelman AM. An evidence-based assessment of NCEP Adult Treatment Panel II guidelines. National Cholesterol Education Program. *JAMA*. 1999;282:2051–2057.

42. The sixth report of the Joint National Committee on prevention, detection, evaluation, and treatment of high blood pressure. *Arch Intern Med*. 1997;157:2413–2446.

43. Hiatt WR, Stoll S, Nies AS. Effect of β-adrenergic blockers on the peripheral circulation in patients with peripheral vascular disease. *Circulation*. 1985;72:1226–1231.

44. Radack K, Deck C. Beta-adrenergic blocker therapy does not worsen intermittent claudication in subjects with peripheral arterial disease. A meta-analysis of randomized controlled trials. *Arch Intern Med*. 1991;151:1769–1776.

45. Poldermans D, Boersma E, Bax JJ, et al. The effect of bisoprolol on perioperative mortality and myocardial infarction in high-risk patients undergoing vascular surgery. *N Engl J Med*. 1999;341:1789–1794.

46. The Heart Outcomes Prevention Evaluation Study Investigators. Effects of an angiotensin-converting-enzyme inhibitor, ramipril, on cardiovascular events in high-risk patients. *N Engl J Med*. 2000;342:145–153.

47. Jacques PF, Selhub J, Bostom AG, Wilson PW, Rosenberg IH. The effect of folic acid fortification on plasma folate and total homocysteine concentrations. *N Engl J Med*. 1999;340:1449–1454.

48. The Writing Group for the PEPI Trial. Effects of estrogen or estrogen/progestin regimens on heart disease risk factors in postmenopausal women. The Postmenopausal Estrogen/Progestin Interventions (PEPI) Trial. *JAMA*. 1995;273:199–208.

49. Hulley S, Grady D, Bush T, et al. Randomized trial of estrogen plus progestin for secondary prevention of coronary heart disease in postmenopausal women. Heart and Estrogen/Progestin Replacement Study (HERS) Research Group. *JAMA*. 1998;280:605–613.

50. Antiplatelet Trialists' Collaboration. Secondary prevention of vascular disease by prolonged antiplatelet treatment. *Br Med J*. 1988;296:320–331.

51. Antiplatelet Trialists' Collaboration. Collaborative overview of randomised trials of antiplatelet therapy. I: Prevention of death, myocardial infarction, and stroke by prolonged antiplatelet therapy in various categories of patients. *Br Med J*. 1994;308:81–106.

52. Antiplatelet Trialists' Collaboration. Collaborative overview of randomised trials of antiplatelet therapy. II: Maintenance of vascular graft or arterial patency by antiplatelet therapy. *Br Med J*. 1994;308:159–168.

53. Bokissel JP, Peyrieux JC, Destors JM. Is it possible to reduce the risk of cardiovascular events in subjects suffering from intermittent claudication of the lower limbs? *Thromb Haemostasis*. 1996;62:681–685.

54. Arcan JC, Blanchard J, Boissel JP, Destors JM, Panak E. Multicenter double-blind study of ticlopidine in the treatment of intermittent claudication and the prevention of its complications. *Angiology*. 1988;39:802–811.

55. CAPRIE Steering Committee. A randomised, blinded, trial of clopidogrel versus aspirin in patients at risk of ischaemic events (CAPRIE). *Lancet*. 1996;348:1329–1339.

56. Gardner AW, Poehlman ET. Exercise rehabilitation programs for the treatment of claudication pain. A meta-analysis. *JAMA*. 1995;274:975–980.

57. Coffman JD. Vasodilator drugs in peripheral vascular disease. *N Engl J Med*. 1979;300:713–717.

58. Porter JM, Cutler BS, Lee BY, et al. Pentoxifylline efficacy in the treatment of intermittent claudication: multicenter controlled double-blind trial with objective assessment of chronic occlusive arterial disease patients. *Am Heart J*. 1982;104:66–72.

59. Dawson DL, Cutler BS, Hiatt WR, et al. A comparison of cilostazol and pentoxifylline for treating intermittent claudication. *Am J Med*. 2000;109:523–530.

60. Girolami B, Bernardi E, Prins MH, et al. Treatment of intermittent claudication with physical training, smoking cessation, pentoxifylline, or nafronyl: a meta-analysis. *Arch Intern Med*. 1999;159:337–345.

61. Kohda N, Tani T, Nakayama S, et al. Effect of cilostazol, a phosphodiesterase III inhibitor, on experimental thrombosis in the porcine carotid artery. *Thromb Res*. 1999;96:261–268.

62. Igawa T, Tani T, Chijiwa J, et al. Potentiation of anti-platelet aggregating activity of cilostazol with vascular endothelial cells. *Thromb Res*. 1990;57:617–623.

63. Tsuchikane E, Fukuhara A, Kobayashi T, et al. Impact of cilostazol on restenosis after percutaneous coronary balloon angioplasty. *Circulation*. 1999;100:21–26.

64. Beebe HG, Dawson DL, Cutler BS, et al. A new pharmacological treatment for intermittent claudication: results of a randomized, multicenter trial. *Arch Intern Med*. 1999;159:2041–2050.

65. Money SR, Herd JA, Isaacsohn JL, et al. Effect of cilostazol on walking distances in patients with intermittent claudication caused by peripheral vascular disease. *J Vasc Surg*. 1998;27:267–274.

66. Dawson DL, Cutler BS, Meissner MH, Strandness DEJ. Cilostazol has beneficial effects in treatment of intermittent claudication: results from a multicenter, randomized, prospective, double-blind trial. *Circulation*. 1998;98:678–686.

67. Brevetti G, Perna S, Sabba C, Martone VD, Condorelli M. Propionyl-L-carnitine in intermittent claudication: double-blind, placebo-controlled, dose titration, multicenter study. *J Am Coll Cardiol*. 1995;26:1411–1416.

68. Brevetti G, Diehm C, Lambett D. European multicenter study on propionyl-L-carnitine in intermittent claudication. *J Am Coll Cardiol*. 1999;34:1618–1624.

69. Brevetti G, Perna S, Sabba C, et al. Effect of propionyl-L-carnitine on quality of life in intermittent claudication. *Am J Cardiol*. 1997;79:777–780.

70. Lievre M, Morand S, Besse B, et al. Oral beraprost sodium, a prostaglandin I(2) analogue, for intermittent claudication: a double-blind, randomized, multicenter controlled trial. *Circulation*. 2000;102:426–431.

71. Mannarino E, Pasqualini L, Innocente S, et al. Physical training and antiplatelet treatment in stage II peripheral arterial occlusive disease: alone or combined? *Angiology*. 1991;42:513–521.

72. Scheffler P, de la Hamette D, Gross J, Mueller H, Schieffer H. Intensive vascular training in stage IIb of peripheral arterial occlusive disease. The additive effects of intravenous prostaglandin E1 or intravenous pentoxifylline during training. *Circulation*. 1994;90:818–822.

73. Dormandy JA, Murray GD. The fate of the claudicant: a prospective study of 1969 claudicants. *Eur J Vasc Surg*. 1991;5:131–133.

74. O'Riordain DS, O'Donnell JA. Realistic expectations for the patient with intermittent claudication. *Br J Surg*. 1991; 78:861–863.

75. Wilson SE, Wolf GL, Cross AP. Percutaneous transluminal angioplasty versus operation for peripheral arteriosclerosis. *J Vasc Surg*. 1989;9:1–8.

76. Dormandy JA, Rutherford RB. Management of peripheral arterial disease (PAD). TASC Working Group. *J Vasc Surg*. 2000;31:S1–S296.

77. Poulias GE, Doundoulakis N, Prombonas E, et al. Aortofemoral bypass and determinants of early success and late favourable outcome. Experience with 1000 consecutive cases. *J Cardiovasc Surg*. 1992;33:664–678.

78. Lorentzen JE, Nielsen OM, Arendrup H, et al. Vascular graft infection: an analysis of sixty-two graft infections in 2411 consecutively implanted synthetic vascular grafts. *Surgery*. 1985;98:81–86.

79. Veith FJ, Gupta SK, Ascer E, et al. Six-year prospective multicenter randomized comparison of autologous saphenous vein and expanded polytetrafluorethylene grafts in infrainguinal arterial reconstructions. *J Vasc Surg*. 1986; 3:104–114.

80. Dalman RL, Taylor LM. Basic data related to infrainguinal revascularization procedures. *Ann Vasc Surg*. 1990;4:309–312.

81. Samson RH, Veith FJ, Janko GS, Gupta SK, Scher LA. A modified classification and approach to the management of infections involving peripheral arterial prosthetic grafts. *J Vasc Surg*. 1988;8:147–153.

82. Nehler MR, Moneta GL, Edwards JM, et al. Surgery for chronic lower extremity ischemia in patients eighty or more years of age: operative results and assessment of postoperative independence. *J Vasc Surg*. 1993;18:618–626.

83. Nehler MR, Moneta GL, Yeager RA, et al. Surgical treatment of threatened reversed infrainguinal vein grafts. *J Vasc Surg*. 1994;20:558–565.

84. Nicoloff AD, Taylor LMJ, McLafferty RB, Moneta GL, Porter JM. Patient recovery after infrainguinal bypass grafting for limb salvage. *J Vasc Surg*. 1998;27:256–263.

85. Yamanaka M, Kwong PK. The side-to-side flap technique in below-the-knee amputation with long stump. *Clin Orthop*. 1985;201:75–79.

86. Robinson KP. Long posterior flap amputation in geriatric patients with ischaemic disease. *Ann R Coll Surg Engl*. 1976;58:440–451.

87. Silverman DG, Roberts A, Reilly CA, et al. Fluorometric quantification of low-dose fluorescein delivery to predict amputation site healing. *Surgery*. 1987;101:335–341.

88. Tripses D, Pollak EW. Risk factors in healing of below-knee amputation. Appraisal of 64 amputations in patients with vascular disease. *Am J Surg*. 1981;141:718–720.

89. Kihn RB, Warren R, Beebe GW. The "geriatric" amputee. *Ann Surg*. 1972;176:305–314.

90. Rigdon EE, Monajjem N, Rhodes RS. Criteria for selective utilization of the intensive care unit following carotid endarterectomy. *Ann Vasc Surg*. 1997;11:20–27.

91. Gregg RO. Bypass or amputation? Concomitant review of bypass arterial grafting and major amputations. *Am J Surg*. 1985;149:397–402.

92. Cameron HC. Amputations in the diabetic: outcome and survival. *Lancet*. 1964;ii:605–607.

93. Rush DS, Huston CC, Bivins BA, Hyde GL. Operative and late mortality rates of above-knee and below-knee amputations. *Am Surg*. 1981;47:36–39.

94. Whitehouse FW, Jurgensen C, Block MA. The later life of the diabetic amputee: another look at the fate of the second leg. *Diabetes*. 1968;17:520–521.

95. McDermott MM, Mehta S, Ahn H, Greenland P. Atherosclerotic risk factors are less intensively treated in patients with peripheral arterial disease than in patients with coronary artery disease. *J Gen Intern Med*. 1997;12:209–215.

96. Orchard TJ, Strandness DE, Cavanagh PR, et al. Assessment of peripheral vascular disease in diabetes. Report and recommendations of an international workshop. *Circulation*. 1993;88:819–828.

42
Rheumatologic Diseases

Daniel J. Brauner, Leif B. Sorensen, and Michael H. Ellman

Old age superbly rising! O welcome, ineffable grace of dying days.

—Walt Whitman, *Song of Myself*

Part of the ineffable grace of growing older involves living with and overcoming the travails of rheumatic diseases, especially osteoarthritis (OA), which becomes increasingly common with age. The projected growth of people aged 65 years and older in the United States has focused attention on preserving and improving their quality of life; important among the factors determining this are the prevention and treatment of musculoskeletal conditions. Arthritis and other rheumatic conditions, and chronic back conditions, are the leading causes of disability in the United States, affecting approximately 43 million people.[1] Given current population projections, arthritis will affect nearly 60 million people in the year 2020 and will limit the major activities of nearly 11.6 million. Arthritis has a sizable economic impact, as it is the source of at least 44 million visits to a health care provider, 744,000 hospitalizations, and 4 million days of hospital care per year. In 1992, the estimated medical care cost for persons with arthritis was $15 billion, and total cost (medical care plus lost productivity) was $65 billion, the latter amount being equal to 1.1% of the gross domestic product.[2] Arthritis is a leading health problem among all demographic groups, but it is especially important in the elderly; the prevalence of common types of arthritis increases with age, with as many as 50% of people aged 65 years and older affected by some type of arthritis.[3]

The older patient with rheumatologic disease presents a unique opportunity for the astute clinician to untangle diagnostic puzzles and offer treatments that can improve function and relieve pain and suffering in very meaningful ways, but diagnosis of rheumatic disease in the elderly can be especially challenging for several reasons (Table 42.1). Besides presenting important diagnostic and therapeutic demands because of its almost ubiquitous presence in the older patient, osteoarthritis, the most common rheumatic disease, also provides the substrate on which other rheumatic diseases are superimposed in this group, complicating their diagnosis.

The presentation of other rheumatic diseases in the older patient is further altered by immune, endocrine, and vascular changes associated with aging, modulating their expression and making their diagnosis more difficult. The well-described higher rate of false-positive serology in older patients is among the changes that complicate the diagnosis of rheumatic disease in this group. The commonly held misconception that "other" rheumatic diseases are rare or nonexistent in this age group is another factor that often delays or precludes the diagnosis of rheumatic diseases in the older patient. As we show here, incidence rates of diseases such as rheumatoid arthritis and systemic lupus in older patients are high enough to warrant more consideration than they are presently given. Some, such as temporal arteritis and polymyalgia rheumatica, occur almost exclusively in the older patient. Because unifying diagnoses to explain multiple symptoms are less common in the older patient, multisystem rheumatic diseases such as systemic lupus and temporal arteritis are less often considered in this group and are often diagnosed late or possibly not at all.

Inflammatory conditions, such as rheumatoid arthritis, can "burn out" in older patients who may still have pain and decreased function from osteoarthritis, which is more common in previously damaged joints. There may even be some inflammation in these joints from crystal-induced arthritis that is also common in this group, further complicating the diagnosis. We begin this chapter with an in-depth review of osteoarthritis, the most important rheumatic disease in the older patient, and then go on to cover the other rheumatic diseases, with special emphasis on their altered manifestations in this group.

TABLE 42.1. Factors complicating diagnosis of rheumatic diseases in the elderly.

1. High prevalence of underlying osteoarthritis
2. Immune, endocrine, and vascular changes
3. Higher rates of false-positive serology
4. Misconceptions about incidences of rheumatic diseases
5. Lower incidence of "unifying" diagnoses
6. Inflammatory conditions may "burn out"

Source: Adapted from Stevens MB. Connective tissue disease in the elderly,[4] with permission.

Osteoarthritis

Osteoarthritis (OA), once the poor stepchild of the more esoteric and "interesting" rheumatic diseases, with patients often systematically "weeded out" of standard rheumatology clinics, is finally getting the attention it deserves as one of the most prevalent conditions of humankind and the one that causes the most disability. The commonly held notions that OA is an inevitable consequence of aging because of the normal "wear and tear" of the joint is much too simplistic. Cartilage does not simply wear out like the soles of one's shoes. Rather, the changes seen in OA involve the complex interaction of genetic susceptibility, joint mechanics and injury, chondrocytes that live a robust metabolic existence, biochemical alterations, and the complex interplay of mediators, as well as structures that surround the joint.

Perhaps more than any other condition, the changes associated with OA are most strongly associated with images of aging, as in the gnarled hands and antalgic or painful, noisy gait of the old person with arthritis. But although OA is common in older people, it is not universal or inevitable. Teasing out the normal changes of aging from those associated with OA and their interplay has been a major area of inquiry and is discussed in detail later. Definitions of OA are problematic because they are so dependent on what tools, modalities, or scales one chooses to consider: clinical symptoms, functional impairment, findings on physical examination, x-ray changes, gross or microscopic structural changes, biochemical alterations including cytokines and enzymes, and cellular alterations. One useful way of understanding OA is as a final common pathway, a clinical and pathologic outcome of a range of disorders resulting in similar alterations in articular anatomy and function.[5] OA occurs when the dynamic equilibrium between the breakdown and repair of joint tissues is overwhelmed. Factors that have been implicated include occupation, body weight, trauma, recreational activities, developmental abnormalities, collagen gene mutations, muscle weakness, alterations in proprioception, denervation of joints, and inherited and acquired errors of metabolism.

Epidemiologic studies have shown that the prevalence of OA increases progressively with age. Autopsy surveys have shown that, by age 40, 90% of all persons have histologic evidence of OA, while in the tenth decade the process has become universal. In a survey of roentgenograms of hands and feet, 37% of all adults in the United States had some evidence of OA. The prevalence rose from 4 per 100 among persons 18 to 24 years of age to 85 per 100 at age 75 to 79. In the Framingham study,[6] radiographic evidence of knee OA increased with age, from 27% in subjects younger than age 70 to 44% in subjects aged 80 and older. Anatomic and radiologic examinations define disease earlier than do clinical studies based on symptoms and signs. In two studies, the prevalence of symptomatic knee OA was only 29%[7] and 43%[8] of radiologically defined disease. Until middle age, OA occurs with the same frequency in men and women, but after age 50, symptomatic osteoarthritis is more common in women, and this difference in prevalence widens with increasing age. Women are also more likely to have multiple joint involvement.

Presentation of the Older Patient with Osteoarthritis

When presented with an older patient with mobility problems or pain that appears to be musculoskeletal in origin, the geriatrician should take a broad perspective that includes evaluation of the involved joints and the surrounding tendons, bursae, bones, and, importantly, muscles. Very often, by the time the patient comes to the physician's attention several of these structures have been affected. The clinician needs to consider the "functional unit" composed of articulating bones, cartilage, ligaments, capsule, the muscles that affect movement and the nerves that control movement, and sense position and movement, that is, proprioception. Pain is the classic symptom that brings the patient to see a physician. However, aches and pains of joints and muscles, especially with prolonged or increased use, are so common among older people and often expected as a part of aging that many patients do not seek medical care or complain of pain unless specifically probed. This pattern, of course, varies with patients and is dependent on psychologic factors, the presence of other medical problems often deemed more serious, access to health care, pain threshold, and impact on function.

The most common pain described with OA is an achy type associated with use of the particular joint. Occasionally, the pain is described as sharp and fleeting, especially in the knees, where it can be associated with certain movements during weightbearing. When osteoarthritis involves the lower back or hips, the pain is often poorly localized. The pain is typically related to activity, but rest pain is present in approximately 50% and night pain in about 30%. The origin of the pain experienced in OA is a complex phenomenon, as the primary tissue that is involved, cartilage, contains no nerve input. Other structures in and around the joint have been implicated. The impact of psychosocial factors is poorly understood but may help explain difficulties correlating pain with other measures of disease such as radiologic findings. In one study, women with knee pain who did not have radiographic evidence of knee OA had higher anxiety scores than those without pain.[9]

Stiffness is another commonly described symptom of OA. The stiffness associated with OA may be described as difficulty initiating movement in a joint or decreased or painful movement in a joint. Morning stiffness, commonly seen in the more inflammatory types of arthritis such as rheumatoid arthritis, may be present but is usually of shorter duration (less than 30 min) and limited to fewer joints. More commonly, patients describe a gelling phenomenon in which particular joints, most commonly the knees and hands, become stiff after periods of inactivity. This discomfort is usually quite short lived, lasting minutes, and improves after the joint is "worked out."

As opposed to the younger patient with OA who commonly presents with one affected joint, frequently associated with a history of trauma, the older patient is more likely to have involvement of multiple joints in characteristic patterns. Even though trauma may have initiated problems in a joint in an older patient, OA is such an insidious condition that the trauma is usually not reported or remembered, as it may have occurred 20 to 30 years previously. Even if the mind can forget an insult, however, the body is tenacious when it comes to remembering old traumas.

An attractive explanation of the patterns of joint involvement in OA and one that helps track the joints commonly involved in older patients comes from an evolutionary theory first elaborated by Hutton. Our human ancestors have only been walking upright for about 3 million years, starting with *Australopithecus aferensus*. The bulk of the evolution of our joints, therefore, probably occurred while our ancestors were brachiating (swinging through the trees by their arms) and knuckle-walking. According to this theory, certain joints that are more prone to OA may be underdesigned for the stresses of modern life, with little functional reserve. Underdesigned joints include those required for pincer grip, such as the distal interphalangeal and proximal interphalangeal joints, as well as those stressed by upright walking such as the knees and lower back. Overdesigned joints, the shoulders (for brachiating) and metacarpophalangeal joints (for knuckle-walking), are rarely involved in primary OA.[10]

The joints most commonly involved in osteoarthritis are the distal and proximal interphalangeal joints of the hands, the first carpometacarpal joint, the first metatarsophalangeal joint, the knee, the hip, and the spine. As the clinical manifestations of OA are dependent on which joints are involved, they are discussed individually.

Heberden's nodes, characterized by bony enlargement of the dorsolateral and dorsomedial aspects of the distal interphalangeal (DIP) joints of the fingers, are extremely common in older patients. Flexor and lateral deviation of the distal phalanx are common. They may be single, but they usually are multiple. In most patients, they develop slowly over months or years, usually around the time of the menopause, giving rise to little or no pain. In a few patients, they evolve rapidly with redness and tenderness. Small gelatinous cysts sometimes appear over the dorsal aspects of the joint. These cysts, which morphologically resemble ganglia, may disappear spontaneously or persist indefinitely. Similar nodes at the proximal interphalangeal (PIP) joints are known as *Bouchard's nodes*. Involvement of the *first carpometacarpal (CMC) joint* is common and is frequently symptomatic. Marked osteophytosis at this site leads to a characteristic squaring appearance of the hands. The radiographic patterns of hand OA assessed in the older Framingham subcohort found women with a much higher incidence than men. However, the relative frequency of joint involvement was similar in both sexes: DIPs, followed by the first CMC, PIPs, and rarely metacarpophalangeal joints (MCPs). Isolated involvement of any one or two MCP joints can occur as a result of trauma or in association with crystal disease. Once established, OA of the hands is usually not very painful, but a weaker grip and some functional impairment involving fine motor skills with increasing clinical severity of hand OA are common complaints.

Erosive inflammatory osteoarthritis is a variant of OA of the hands. This entity, which most often affects postmenopausal women, involves the distal and proximal interphalangeal joints and less often the metacarpophalangeal joints. Painful inflammatory episodes eventually lead to joint deformities and sometimes to ankylosis. After years of intermittent acute flares, the joints become quiescent. The clinical picture may be confused with rheumatoid arthritis. Radiographic findings include loss of joint cartilage, spur formation, subchondral sclerosis, and bony erosions, usually in the central portion of the joints. Rheumatoid factor tests are negative, and the sedimentation rate is normal or only slightly elevated. The presence of immune complexes in the synovium and a frequent association with the sicca syndrome suggest that immune mechanisms may be at work in this subset of OA.

Osteoarthritis of the knee, although not the most common site, probably has the greatest impact in terms of disability. Knee pain severity is the strongest risk factor for self-reported difficulty in performing tasks of upper and lower extremity function.[11] The knee joint is composed of three compartments, the medial and lateral tibiofemoral and the patellofemoral. The medial compartment bears the greatest load during walking and is most commonly involved, followed by the patellofemoral and last, the lateral compartment. Persons affected with knee OA commonly complain of pain on walking, stiffness of the joint, and difficulty with ascending steps. Involvement of the medial compartment will eventually lead to varus deformity secondary to loss of joint space (cartilage) from this compartment. Bony deformities are further compounded by osteophyte production at the medial and lateral joint margins. Crepitations caused by cartilage irregularities, eburnated or exposed subchondral bone, or thickened joint capsule or tendons are frequently felt and occasionally heard with flexing and extending the joint. Not uncommonly, joint effusions can be appreciated either by a positive bulge sign in which fluid is milked from the medial compartment and then seen to flow back when pressure is placed on the lateral compartment, or when more fluid is present by ballotment of the patella. When testing for ballotment, care needs to be taken to milk the fluid out of the suprapatellar joint compartment by gentle pressure applied above the patella, as this pushes the fluid, if present, under the patella. Otherwise, fluid will simply flow upward and produce a falsely negative test. Assessment for quadriceps atrophy and strength is important with consideration that obese patients may have proportionally decreased strength and still appear fairly strong.[12]

A common complaint associated with knee OA is a feeling that the knee is about to "give out." A thorough assessment for ligament stability should be performed. Laxity of the collateral ligaments is documented by increased varus-valgus movement. However, on examination, many of these patients do not have grossly unstable knees, and it is thought that the perceived instability is more related to muscle weakness and fatigue. The neighboring joints should be carefully examined, as they often exhibit decreased range of motion despite not being primarily involved with OA. The physical examination should include observation of the gait, checking for an antalgic gait that is characterized by a short stance phase on the affected side, but when subtle, more easily recognized by a fast swing phase on the opposite side. Patients with cognitive impairment may not complain of pain but may instead present with antalgic gait, falls, or decreased mobility, causing them to spend more time in bed.

Spontaneous osteonecrosis of the knee must be considered in the differential diagnosis of an acutely painful knee in the elderly. In a study of 68 patients with spontaneous osteonecrosis of the knee, the mean age of onset was 68 years and the majority were female.[13] The structural changes alter biomechanics of the joint and may lead to the rapid development of severe osteoarthritis.

Osteoarthritis of the *hip* is less common but primarily confined to older individuals. It may be unilateral or bilateral. Hip joint pain is usually localized to the groin or along the inner aspect of the thigh. It may be referred to the buttock or along the obturator nerve to the knee. At times, the pain in the knee dominates the clinical presentation, and the diagnosis may be missed. Conversely, in the evaluation of pain in the hip area, other causes must be considered. Disorders of the lumbar spine at the L2–L3 level may refer pain into the groin, and at the L5–S1 level into the buttock. Trochanteric bursitis also may be confused with intra-articular hip disease. Physical examination shows loss of internal rotation and abduction early in the disease process. Flexion contracture may be determined by using the Thomas test, in which the knee of the uninvolved leg is drawn to the chest to flatten the lumbar lordosis. If a flexion contracture exists, the involved leg will flex off the examining table. On gait examination, the patient may demonstrate an antalgic gait limp or a gluteus medius lurch, in which the torso leans over the involved weightbearing hip. This move reflects an unconscious attempt to place the center of gravity over the painful hip, thereby decreasing the forces across that joint. In advanced disease, the leg is often held in external rotation, with the hip flexed and adducted. Functional shortening of the leg may result in a short-limb limp.

Osteoarthritis involving the back is a complex and poorly understood syndrome. Back pain or discomfort is an extremely common symptom in older people. As part of the Framingham Study, Felson et al. studied back symptoms in their elderly cohort aged 68 to 100 years.[14] In their study group, 22.3% reported back symptoms on most days. Lower back pain was more common than mid- or upper back complaints. Age did not affect the prevalence of back symptoms within this elderly cohort. Symptoms were more common in women than men. Older people confined mostly to their homes had an especially high prevalence of back symptoms.

Degenerative joint disease of the spine results from involvement of the intervertebral disks, vertebral bodies, and/or the posterior apophyseal articulations. Narrowing of the disks may cause subluxation of the posterior apophyseal joints. The term *spinal osteoarthritis* describes the changes in the apophyseal joints, whereas *degenerative disk disease* applies to the changes in the invertebral synchondrosis.

Impingement on the nerve roots by spurs that compromise the intervertebral foramina is particularly common in the neck because of the small size of foraminal spaces in this location. In patients with involvement of the lower cervical spine, pain in the neck radiates to the shoulder and sometimes to the arm and hand. Paresthesias and reflex changes are common in the distribution of the involved nerve root.

Osteophytes in the uncovertebral (Luschka) joints may compress the neighboring vertebral arteries as they traverse the transverse processes of the cervical spine, leading to signs and symptoms of basilar artery insufficiency. Narrowing of the vascular lumen is most marked during rotation of the head. Symptoms that frequently present in an intermittent pattern include vertigo, headache, blurring of vision, diplopia, and defects in visual field. Other symptoms include sudden loss of strength in an extremity, as well as nystagmus and ataxia, which may be seen on examination. Angiographic studies serve to confirm the diagnosis.

Large spurs arising anteriorly from the vertebral bodies are prevalent. They rarely give rise to symptoms, but dysphagia due to external compression of the esophagus and respiratory symptoms in the form of coughing and hoarseness have been reported. Large posterior spurs protruding into the spinal canal may compress the spinal cord, leading to upper motor neuron and other long tract signs. Compression of the anterior spinal artery may produce a central cord syndrome.

Nerve root compression in the dorsal spine causing radicular pain around the chest wall is less common. Involvement of the nerve roots in the lumbosacral area is associated with low back pain and neurologic signs and symptoms in the distribution of the involved roots. Neurologic symptoms that are secondary to spinal OA must be differentiated from those that result from primary neurologic disorders. Neurologic complications of osteoarthritis of the cervical spine may be confused with amyotrophic lateral sclerosis, spinal cord tumors, and basilar artery disease. The differential diagnosis is also complicated by the high prevalence of asymptomatic x-ray evidence of OA in the elderly.

Acquired spinal stenosis is an important cause of low back symptoms in the older patient rarely seen in those under 50 years. Symptoms consist of back, buttock, or leg pain that usually worsens with ambulation, occasionally in combination with lower limb sensory and motor deficits and rarely with problems with bowel and bladder control. Classically, pseudoclaudication is present, with pain and discomfort worsened with walking and relieved with stopping, sitting, or lying down and with symptoms eased in positions of flexion (bending forward, e.g., on a grocery cart) and exacerbated by positions of lumbar extension (walking uphill). The volume of the lumbar canal tends to decrease with age with most individuals having at least an anatomic lumbar stenosis by age 80 relative to the volume of a younger population. With the development and progression of OA involving the lower back, the facet joints and ligamentum flavum hypertrophy, diminishing the spinal cord volume and purportedly reducing the blood supply to the nerve roots, thus causing symptoms.

A variant form of spinal osteophytosis seen in the elderly is the *ankylosing hyperostosis of Forestier*. This condition is characterized by large spurs or marginal proliferations that fuse to form flowing ossifications along the anterolateral aspects of vertebral bodies. The process extends to the connective tissue surrounding the spine, including the anterior longitudinal ligament. The distal thoracic spine is the site of predilection, but other levels of the spine may be affected. Radiographic criteria include the presence of flowing calcifications and ossifications along the anterolateral aspects of at least four contiguous vertebral bodies, relative preservation of the intervertebral disk height, and absence of ankylosis of the sacroiliac and apophyseal joints. It is estimated that 5% to 10% of persons over 65 years meet the radiologic criteria for establishing a diagnosis of Forestier's disease. Despite extensive anatomic abnormalities, the patients are either free of symptoms or they complain of modest pain and stiffness and mild restriction of motion.

The term *diffuse idiopathic skeletal hyperostosis* is applied when the vertebral condition is accompanied by extraspinal manifestations. Those changes include irregular new bone formation or "whiskering" commonly seen in the paraacetabular, tarsal, and metatarsal areas, large bone spurs on the olecranon process, calcaneus, and patella, and ligamentous calcification and ossification, particularly of the sacrotuberous and ileolumbar ligaments. Heel pain may be a prominent symptom. Dysphagia related to cervical osteophytosis has been reported.

Commonly Associated Conditions: Bursitis and Tendinitis

Part of the assessment of a painful joint in the older patient should include evaluation of periarticular bursae and tendons, irritation of which can mimic joint involvement. Inflammation of the anserine bursa, which is situated just inferior to the knee joint on the medial aspect of the tibia, can produce fairly significant juxta-articular pain that is difficult to distinguish from primary knee OA. Tenderness over the bursa that reproduces the pain the patient experiences may indicate that the anserine bursa is the culprit. Injection of a crystalline corticosteroid preparation into the bursa may relieve the discomfort. When evaluating the painful hip, one should always check for tenderness over the greater trochanter. Trochanteric bursitis causes pain, often aggravated by stair climbing, over the lateral aspect of the hip whereas hip joint pain is usually experienced more in the groin.[15]

Fibromyalgia

Fibromyalgia is a poorly characterized, poorly understood clinical syndrome whose main characteristic is pain in various locations without any clear underlying pathology. The American College of Rheumatology guidelines for fibromyalgia is the presence of 11 or more tender points and widespread pain.[16] Associated symptoms include fatigue, sleep disturbance, anxiety, and depression. Geriatricians need to have a good understanding of this syndrome because the prevalence increases with age, with the highest prevalence attained between 60 and 79 years (>7.0% in women).[17] Fibromyalgia may be a primary or secondary disorder related to other rheumatic diseases. In the older patient, it is most commonly seen as secondary problem related to OA.

Besides presenting a treatment dilemma, it appears that the presence of fibromyalgia may have important implications on how patients will experience and report other medical problems. Data suggest that patients with fibromyalgia appraise medical symptoms and their importance differently from patients with other rheumatic conditions. Wolfe et al. found patients with fibromyalgia reported more conditions (4.5 versus 3.1) than those with RA or OA, and in 20 of the 23 conditions, the importance attached to the conditions by patients with fibromyalgia exceeded that of the importance attributed by RA and OA patients without fibromyalgia.[18] Although fibromyalgia is a recognizable clinical entity, there seems to be no rationale for treating fibromyalgia as a discrete disorder, and it would seem appropriate to consider the entire range of tenderness and distress with the tender point count potentially functioning as a "sedimentation rate" for distress.[19]

Laboratory and Radiographic Findings

Although the diagnosis of OA can be made without x-ray, the plain x-ray is still the most important imaging tool for investigating OA. The classic x-ray findings of OA include osteophytosis, joint space narrowing, subchondral sclerosis, and cysts. Cysts, varying in size from a few millimeters to several centimeters, are seen as translucent areas in juxta-articular bone. Small age-related marginal osteophytes associated with some squaring of the joint margin should be differentiated from OA, in which the osteophytes are larger and have a more abnormal shape.[20] X-rays are useful for confirming the diagnosis, assessing progression of disease, and timing for joint replacement. It is important to remember that x-rays often do not correlate well with symptoms. However, when joint space narrowing, sometimes with "bone-on-bone" appearance, large osteophytes, and subchondral sclerosis, are present on a knee x-ray, there is little doubt that such changes represent severe OA. Proper positioning is important. In the case of the knee, loading the joint by standing is necessary to adequately assess the extent of cartilage wear.

Radiographic changes of OA of the spine are common in the older patient and are notorious for their lack of correlation with actual symptoms. Abnormal findings include decreased intervertebral space, endplate sclerosis, osteophyte formation, and spondylolithesis, which is a slipping of one vertebra forward on the one below. The sclerotic bony changes associated with OA of the spine can give falsely elevated readings of bone mineral density.[21]

As mentioned, there are large discrepancies between radiologic incidence of OA and clinical complaints. In the Framingham Study[22] of elderly subjects, the prevalence of radiographic changes of OA in the knee was 34% in women and 31% in men. Yet, only 11% of all women and 7% of all men had symptomatic disease. The discordance between symptoms and radiographic findings of OA in the lumbar spine is striking. At age 50, 87% of adults have radiographic evidence of lumbar spondylosis, and almost 70% of asymptomatic persons have degenerative disk disease on spine films.[23] Because of the high frequency of osteoarthritic changes on radiologic examination of the lower spine, the main utility of plain x-rays in older patients is to rule out other processes such as infection, fracture, or malignancy.

Tailored magnetic resonance imaging (MRI) producing high spatial or contrast resolution images is proving to be an important tool in the early detection and surveillance of OA progression, as well as assessment of surrounding soft tissues. MRI, with its unique ability to noninvasively image and characterize soft tissue, has shown promise in assessment of cartilage integrity. MRI imaging of knee cartilage correlates well with arthroscopy for quantification of chondropathy.[24] Conventional radiographs are unreliable for evaluating articular cartilage loss in patients with early OA. Interestingly, initial joint space narrowing by conventional knee radiographs has been shown by MRI to be caused mostly by meniscal extrusion rather than thinning of articular cartilage.[25] Meniscal subluxation seen on MRI is highly associated with symptomatic knee OA, and increasing meniscal subluxation on MRI correlates with the severity of joint space narrowing.[26] This finding has important implications for evaluating therapies that may have a disease-modifying effect, because actual narrowing may not reflect cartilage damage but movement of menisci.

The need for better evaluation of OA and its progression, from a clinical perspective as well as for assessing possible disease-modifying osteoarthritis drugs (DMOADs), has prompted substantial effort to develop markers that accurately evaluate the progression of joint damage; this is especially important in evaluating early disease, as standard radiographs and even MRI detect relatively advanced disease. Earlier excitement was generated when serum levels of cartilage-derived keratin sulfate appeared to reflect the magnitude of articular cartilage breakdown in OA, but subsequent studies found the correlation to be weak. Serum concentrations of cartilage oligomeric protein is considered the current main contender for a serum marker of OA, but some argue that no serum marker can adequately reflect what is going on in specific joints.[27] The C-reactive protein level, but not the erythrocyte sedimentation rate, was found to be associated with clinical severity in patients with OA of the knee, probably reflecting an inflammatory component to the disease.[28] Interest has shifted to searching for possible synovial fluid markers. A "daunting" number of matrix proteins, enzymes, cytokines, and other macromolecules are detectable in OA synovial fluid. Altered concentrations of chondroitin sulfate and keratan sulfate can be detected in OA with characteristics that differ from those seen in RA.[29] One problem with this approach relates to the changing clearance kinetics with progression of disease that can lead to misleading levels. As yet, there is no synovial fluid marker that has been shown to reflect disease activity accurately and consistently.[30]

Risk Factors

Knowledge of risk factors is important in understanding OA to help identify those with higher likelihood of getting the disease, as well as for developing preventive strategies, both primary and secondary, and for therapeutic interventions. Factors that place increased stress on joints appear to be important risk factors for the later development of OA. This stress can take the form of repetitive stress and trauma as occurs in certain occupations. Probably the oldest evidence of occupation-related OA was reported in a 7000-year-old skeleton of a prehistoric man with bilateral scapholunate advanced collapse, the most common form of OA of the wrist.[31] Ligamentous rotary subluxation of the scaphoid is the most common cause of scapholunate advanced collapse. Bilateral ligamentous distension caused by repeated microtrauma, possibly from the manufacture of stone tools, was suspected to have been responsible for these lesions. Many classic studies have implicated various occupations such as coal miners, pneumatic drillers, cotton operatives, iron workers, and elite athletes.

Large longitudinal health studies have identified several important risk factors associated with OA. Heavy physical activity in general has been implicated in the development of OA, and it appears that modulating factors such as type of activity, presence of obesity, and at what point in the life cycle the activity took place are all important. In a subcohort analysis of the Framingham Heart Study, heavy physical activity was found to be a risk factor for incident knee OA in a dose-dependent fashion in both men and women.[32] Although activities such as moderate running appear to be well tolerated in younger people, a stronger association of knee OA with physical activity has been found in women over the age of 50, compared with younger women. Increasing age is an important factor in determining the development of OA after a joint injury such as to the anterior cruciate ligament.[33]

There is a well-described association between obesity and OA, established mostly from cross-sectional studies, but the question of whether obesity is a true causative factor or whether OA predisposed individuals to obesity because of decreased activity was until recently uncertain. Longitudinal studies have since found obesity to be a predictor for the development of OA. This association has been found to be the strongest for knee OA, less so for OA of the hands, and inconsistent for OA of the hip. The risk appears to be much stronger in women, although it also is present in men with severe obesity (highest quintile).[34,35] Even mild obesity (BMI > 25) has been found to put women at increased risk for the development of OA of the knee.[36] Obesity appears to provide an additive risk when combined with heavy physical activity. As yet unknown metabolic factors, possibly related to estrogen, are theorized to explain the differences in risk associated with sex, as well as the increased risk for hand OA with obesity. Because of the markedly increased prevalence of OA in women, as well as the appearance of generalized OA around the time of the menopause, several studies have addressed a possible protective role of estrogen replacement on OA. One cross-sectional study showed an association between postmenopausal estrogen replacement therapy and a reduced risk of radiographic evidence of OA of the hip, with greatest reduction among those who had taken estrogen for 10 or more years.[37] The first prospective cohort study to address this question was performed on a subcohort from the Framingham Study.[38] Only a modest and not statistically significant protective effect of estrogen replacement therapy on OA of the knee was observed in this particular study.

Ever since orthopedic surgeons began noticing that patients undergoing surgery for hip fractures seemed to have a lower than expected prevalence of OA, the possibility of an inverse relationship between OA and osteoporosis has been suspected. The theoretical underpinning for this relationship is that subchondral bone acts as a shock absorber for overlying cartilage and that osteoporotic or softer bone may be acting as a better shock absorber and thus protect against the development of OA.[39] This observation has been strengthened in epidemiologic studies, which have verified an inverse correlation between OA and osteoporosis. Women with radiographically defined knee OA had greater bone mineral density (BMD), as measured by dual-energy x-ray absorptiometry at the femoral neck, than did women without knee OA.[40] An inverse relationship between OA and osteoporosis of the spine was found when comparing normal subjects with those with OA or osteoporosis of the spine.[41] Radiographic hip OA was associated with increased BMD in the femoral neck compared with control subjects in a large prospective study in a cohort from the Study of Osteoporotic Fractures.[42] Interestingly, the increase in BMD was not associated with a decreased risk of hip fractures, possibly related to the numbers and types of falls sustained by subjects with OA. This relationship seemingly pertains to OA involving the hand joints as well.[43] Osteoarthritis was associated not only with increased BMD but with an increased rate of bone loss as well, suggesting an increased turnover.[44]

Crystals that are known to cause acute arthritis and periarthritis also play an important role in mediating the expression of OA. The class of crystals most commonly found in osteoarthritic joints is the calcium-containing crystals, of which calcium pyrophosphate and basic calcium phosphate are the best studied.[45] Osteoarthritis is both more common and more severe in joints in which chondrocalcinosis or crystals have been demonstrated. The distribution of joints is altered in those with crystal-associated OA. Involvement of the carpus, elbow, and shoulder is significantly more common in crystal-associated OA than in primary OA. The presence of multiple knee compartment involvement is also more common in crystal-associated OA than in the absence of crystal deposition. In the only prospective study to systematically evaluate knee synovial fluid for the presence of calcium pyrophosphate crystals, the presence of crystals was found to be associated with progressive cystic changes, progressive bone attrition, and poor symptomatic and functional outcome.[46] However, chondrocalcinosis was not found to be a risk factor for the development of knee OA in a subanalysis of the Framingham Study.[34] Importantly, the true prevalence of crystals is probably underestimated by both x-ray and routine synovial fluid analysis as more sensitive methods have demonstrated one or both crystal types in the majority of cases of severe OA of the knee.[45]

The Role of Joint Instability in the Pathogenesis of OA

OA is not merely a disease of cartilage but of all the tissues of the diarthrodial joint, as well as surrounding structures. There is now increasing interest in the changes that take place in the periarticular skeletal muscles, as well as other factors involved in maintaining joint stability and proprioception. Ligaments, essential components of joint stability, become more compliant with increasing age, but whether this is clinically important and related to the increasing prevalence of OA with age is not known. Ligamentous laxity is a cause of OA in animal models but

has been less well studied in humans, although the hypermobility syndromes are known to be a risk factor for OA. Increased ligamentous laxity, as evidenced by increased varus-valgus movement, has been found to be correlated with the degree of radiologic OA of the knee.[47] In patients with unilateral OA of the knee, the uninvolved knee had greater varus-valgus laxity compared with control knees. This finding supports the concept that ligamentous laxity may predate the disease and may increase the risk of knee OA, as well as contributing to its progression.

The role of periarticular muscle weakness in the pathogenesis and progression of OA has sparked recent interest. Reduced quadriceps strength relative to body weight is found in women with OA of the knee compared to those without OA.[48] Although it had been previously assumed that decreased quadriceps strength in OA of the knee was related to decreased use of the painful joint, recent studies point to a possible pathogenic role of quadriceps weakness. Comparing a community-based cohort of older persons (average age, 71 years), researchers found quadriceps weakness was greater in participants with radiographic knee OA compared with those without it, even in the absence of joint pain. This finding suggests that knee extensor weakness may be a risk factor for the initiation and progression of knee OA.[49] Complaints referable to quadriceps weakness are one of the most common and early symptoms reported by patients with OA and are a better determinant of pain than radiographic changes.[50] Muscle weakness may play a large role in the age-related increase in incidence of OA, as aging is also frequently associated with generalized weakness related to deconditioning. The phenomenon of arthrogenous muscle dysfunction (AMD) describes the decreased strength of voluntary contraction of muscle acting across a joint with OA and may, in part, explain knee extensor weakness in OA.[51]

The relationship between muscle weakness and OA is receiving increasing interest. Skeletal muscles are essential components of the neuromuscular protective mechanisms that provide shock absorption for the joint. Coordinated joint movement and muscle activity control joint loading so that loads applied across joints are dissipated. A well-described example of this occurs with normal gait when the knee is loaded during heel strike. Eccentric quadriceps contraction, which involves muscle lengthening but maintaining tension, cushions the impact. Weak muscles are fatigued more readily, and their voluntary and reflex motor control is slower than those of well-conditioned muscles; this compromises the neuromuscular protective mechanisms of the muscle and leads to excessive joint movement and instability that stresses innervated tissues, elicits pain, and gives rise to rapid jarring loading of the joint. This rapid loading results in microtrauma to articular cartilage and subchondral bone.

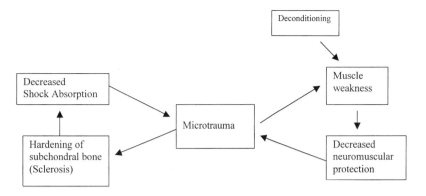

FIGURE 42.1. The relationship between muscle weakness, subchondral bone, and osteoarthritis.

Subchondral bone becomes harder and less able to act as a shock absorber, which then creates an amplification loop in which mild trauma can result in severe joint destruction (Fig. 42.1).

Problems with proprioception, the conscious and unconscious perception of limb position and movement in space, have been implicated as a risk factor for OA. In a canine model of anterior cruciate ligament (ACL) transection, OA was more severe and developed earlier when performed in combination with either a dorsal root ganglionectomy or articular neurectomy than with ACL transection alone.[52] In humans, this question has been studied most extensively in the knee where proprioception derives from integration of afferents from receptors in muscles, tendons, joint capsule, ligaments, meniscal attachments, and skin. The hypermobility syndrome, a well-known risk factor for precocious OA, is associated with impaired proprioception, especially near full extension, and may result in mechanically unsound joint positions that could predispose to OA.[53] Cross-sectional studies show that knee proprioception is worse in patients with knee OA than in controls. Proprioception was found to be worse in older subjects and even worse in the elderly subjects with knee OA.[54]

Theoretically, proprioceptive inaccuracy may contribute to gait characteristics associated with increased stress across joints that predispose toward OA. However, it is not clear whether the proprioceptive problems predispose to OA or if changes associated with OA themselves contribute to worsening in proprioception. Proprioception in older patients with unilateral knee OA was found to be worse in both the involved knee as well as the uninvolved knee compared with older control subjects.[55] This finding implies that impaired proprioception is not exclusively a result of local disease in knee OA, but the relative importance of impaired proprioception in the development and progression of knee OA requires longitudinal study.

Inactivity is an important risk factor for OA that has been incompletely explored in humans, although there are excellent animal models that demonstrate immobi-

lization leading to OA. Prolonged bed rest with lack of joint loading is a theoretical risk for the development of OA that should be included on the long list of adverse consequences of bed rest.

Acetabular dysplasia, a very important risk factor for hip OA in younger people, is responsible for only a very small percentage of incident hip OA in the elderly.[56]

Genetics of OA

Since the familial occurrence of Heberden's nodes was documented 60 years ago, there has been an appreciation that genetic factors play a major role in OA. Because of the complex nature of this role and the multifactorial nature of OA, the genetics of OA is poorly understood. Primary generalized OA is the most common form of OA that is clearly associated with genetic influences. About 20% of those patients describe a positive family history. Multiple studies suggest that the inheritance is probably polygenic. Family aggregation of OA among siblings involving the DIP, PIP, and first CMC joints in a cohort from the Baltimore Longitudinal Study on Aging contributes to evidence of inheritability.[57] Study of hand and knee radiographs of families from the Framingham Study cohort and Framingham Offspring Study suggests a mixed model in a Mendelian mode with a major recessive gene and a residual multifactorial component in generalized OA.[58] Mutations of the genes that code for type II collagen are probably responsible for small groups of families with precocious OA. The Arg519-Cys mutation in type II collagen results in severe, precocious familial OA in 100% of carriers within the first three decades of life.[59] Another area of possible genetic influence is in control of mediators such as IGF-1 that may be important in cartilage formation during development stages and remodeling of adult cartilage.[60]

Pathophysiology of OA

Knowledge of the physiology of cartilage and the pathophysiology of OA is becoming increasingly important to appreciate risk factors and institute preventive measures, as well as to understand new treatment modalities.

Cartilage

Hyaline articular cartilage, the main tissue of interest in OA, is composed mainly of a protein matrix and chondrocytes, which live scattered in normal cartilage in isolation. The "effete" chondrocyte comprises less than 5% by volume of the cartilage but is extremely metabolically active and responsible for maintaining the extracellular matrix (ECM). The two major components of the ECM are proteoglycans and collagen fibers. The collagen fibers (90% type II collagen) provide the tensile strength and structural integrity of the cartilage, and the proteoglycans, extremely complex glycoconjugates, are responsible for its ability to undergo reversible deformation or elasticity. The predominant proteoglycan of articular cartilage is aggrecan, which is composed largely of glycosaminoglycans. Glycosaminoglycans are long-chained, repeating, sulfated, disaccharide units (the most common ones being keratin sulfate and chondroitin sulfate) that are attached to a core protein. Aggrecan molecules are synthesized and secreted into the ECM by the chondrocyte, where they form aggregates of up to 200 aggrecans attached to a hyaluronic acid core, a linear,

high molecular weight glycosaminoglycan, via a link protein. Aggrecans are highly concentrated in the ECM and compressed to approximately 20% of their extended volume by the collagen fibers that form a three-dimensional network, preventing further expansion of the proteoglycans. The proteoglycans carry a high concentration of negatively charged anions at physiologic conditions and thus are highly hydrophilic, providing a swelling pressure that is restrained by the stiffness and tensile strength of the collagen fibers so that only a fraction of their hydrodynamic domain is exposed.

When cartilage is loaded, it is deformed by the expulsion of fluid, which tends to move toward the load into the synovial cavity, carrying the waste products of the cells with it. As water is released from the aggrecans, negative charges are exposed. As aggrecan molecules are forced closer together by the load, increases in the density of negative charges and in the repulsive forces tend to resist further deformation. Ultimately equilibrium is reached, in which the external loading force is balanced by internal forces. When the load is removed, water, along with nutrients, is forced back into the ECM and the cartilage regains its original shape[61] (Fig. 42.2).

The fact that cartilage is both avascular and aneural has important clinical ramifications. Nutrients diffuse into the cartilage via the synovial fluid, but this requires

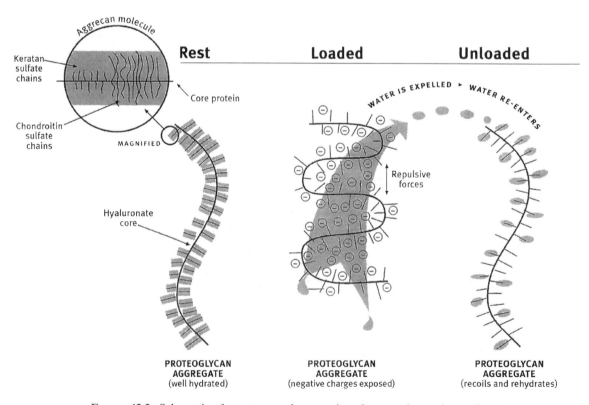

FIGURE 42.2. Schematic of structure and properties of proteoglycans in cartilage.

TABLE 42.2. Changes in cartilage proteoglycans with aging.

1. Progressive decrease in the average length of the core protein of the aggrecan molecule
2. Decreased hydrodynamic size of the aggrecan molecule via decreased length of chondroitin sulfate chains and increase in number of keratin sulfate chains
3. Decreased proportion of aggrecans able to form aggregates with hyaluronic acid
4. Decreased size of aggregates from reduction of length of the hyaluronic acid molecule and smaller size of the aggrecan molecules

joint loading, as already described. A well-described model for inducing OA in animals involves unloading limb joints by casting for several weeks, thus disrupting the flow of nutrients to the chondrocyte. When the cast is removed and the joint is reloaded, premature cartilage damage and OA quickly ensue. Importantly, because of the lack of neural input when damage is isolated to the cartilage, there will be no associated sensation or warning.

Many changes have been found to occur in cartilage with aging. The changes in cartilage proteoglycans are summarized in Table 42.2. These changes lead to a decrease in the hydration of the articular cartilage with aging, which causes a thinning and increased stiffness of the articular cartilage. Articular cartilage show a marked age-related enrichment in a different type of cross-linking product produced by nonenzymatic means (browning) that tends to stabilize it and retain its properties. Collagen has an extremely long half-life, of the order of 100 years; thus, tensile integrity should remain despite aging.

Changes in Matrix in OA

Under normal physiologic conditions, chondrocytes regulate a dynamic metabolic steady state in which anabolism is balanced by catabolism. The earliest change of OA observed from animal models and ex vivo analysis of human cartilage involves increased hydration of the cartilaginous matrix; this is in distinction to the normal changes of aging, which involve a decrease in the water content of cartilage, as just described. This increase in hydration is thought to be associated with clipping of collagen fibers and consequent release of the physical restraint to the hydrophilic proteoglycans that swell with water. Early on in the process there is an increase in the rate of proteoglycan synthesis by the chondrocyte, which may be an attempt to compensate for an increase in catabolism of the matrix, causing an early hypertrophic phase preceding the later degenerative phase. The subsequent degenerative phase is associated with extensive depletion of matrix proteoglycans via digestion of their core proteins by proteases released from chondrocytes. In later stages, chondrocytes synthesize less matrix than normal. Matrix synthesis varies by regions, being strongly suppressed in the superficial layers of cartilage but less so in the deeper layers.[62]

Because chondrocytes lack cell-to-cell contact, communication between them must occur across the ECM via cytokines. Elucidating the complex interactions and effects of these cytokines in OA has been an important area of recent investigation. A number of mediators that influence chondrocyte metabolism have been elucidated, including interleukin-1-alpha and -beta (IL-1), tumor necrosis factor (TNF), and nitric oxide (NO). The cytokine IL-1 is the prototypic inducer of cartilage catabolism. IL-1 inhibits collagen production and causes collagen degradation through the induction of matrix metalloproteinases, a variety of which have been described.[63]

Chondrocytes are probably the major site of production of mediators of inflammation in OA showing high expression of IL-1, TNF, and NO.[64] IL-1-alpha and -beta have been demonstrated in chondrocytes at the articular surface, as well as distributed throughout cartilage demonstrating OA changes.[65] Cartilage exhibiting the early changes of OA had the highest intensity of staining and the highest frequency of positive cells, suggesting a role in pathogenesis.

The free radical nitric oxide also appears to occupy an important mediator role. In the joint, chondrocytes are the major cell source of NO. One of the major functions of NO in cartilage is its role in the suppression of matrix synthesis. NO is at least partly responsible for IL-1-induced suppression of glycosaminoglycan and collagen synthesis. Interestingly, production of NO by normal cartilage in response to IL-1 decreases with advancing age. NO may also be involved as a mediator of IL-1-induced expression of matrix metalloproteinase mRNA and protein and may contribute as an activator of the latent forms of the enzymes. NO also regulates chondrocyte metabolism in response to mechanical loading.[66] NO may also to have some protective effects in cartilage; it is probably involved in antimicrobial defense and may have anabolic effects stimulating proteoglycan production under certain conditions, as well as participating in wound healing and stimulating collagen production.

Another response of the chondrocyte to cartilage damage is the production of matrix molecules such as type X collagen, not found in normal articular cartilage but found in developing growth plate cartilage. Although this is interpreted as a repair response, it results in the production of a mixture of fibrocartilage-like and hyalin cartilage-like matrix, in addition to matrix calcification.

Besides alterations in chondrocyte metabolism, there are also changes in their growth characteristics. In normal mature human articular cartilage, there are no detectable levels of chondrocyte proliferation, although very low levels of proliferation are probably needed to maintain cartilage cellularity. With increasing age, there is a decline in cellularity. In osteoarthritis, once the continuity of the surface of cartilage is disrupted, the cells can divide, forming clusters of chrondrocytes, the so-called brood capsules. Another response of chondrocytes found in OA cartilage is to undergo morphologic changes characteristic of apoptosis, possibly as a result of NO production.

Fibrillation is the earliest gross change of cartilage in OA seen in association with increased hydration and depletion of proteoglycan. As fibrillated cartilage is abraded, focal erosions and vertical clefts are formed. These erosions coalesce with progressive denudation of underlying sclerotic bone. Proliferation of bone occurs at the joint margins to form osteophytes and in subchondral bone, especially in areas denuded of cartilage. The term eburnation applies to the glistening appearance of the polished sclerotic bone surface.

The classic morphologic changes of subchondral sclerosis in OA are thought by some to have a role in the pathogenesis of the condition. Although many authorities believe that the earliest events in OA occur in cartilage, an alternate view suggests that changes in subchondral bone precede measurable changes in the cartilage. It is postulated that the earliest lesions are trabecular fractures in cancellous bone. The healing of these fatigue fractures results in thickening of the trabeculae, leading to an increase in the density of bone with a consequent reduction in its ability to absorb energy. With loss of this functional role of bone, energy absorption is shifted toward the overlying cartilage whose collagen fibers sustain fatigue fractures, eventually leading to deterioration of cartilage. Cyst formation is commonly seen in the juxta-articular bone, probably a result of tissue breakdown related to focal areas of microfracture in the ischemic subchondral bone. Although several studies have shown evidence of increased subchondral bone turnover in early OA, there is still disagreement about whether these changes are concurrent with, primary to, or secondary to cartilage deterioration.[67]

Focal, chronic synovitis, characterized by lymphocyte and mononuclear cell infiltration, is frequently seen in OA; this is probably due to secretion of inflammatory mediators initiated by the release of hydroxyapatite or calcium pyrophosphate crystals or by cartilage breakdown components, or the presence of immune complexes in the surface of the cartilage.

Prevention

As with other chronic diseases for which there is no cure, priority needs to be given to measures that can prevent the condition. Although OA is commonly thought of as a disease of older people, consideration needs to be given

to events that occurred earlier in life. Studies have shown associations between recreational physical activity performed years ago and radiographic OA.[68] The level of activity appears to correlate with risk; however, it is also well known that some loading, as well as maintenance of muscle strength, is also important in preventing OA. The ideal level of activity to minimize OA development has not been established and probably is quite variable between individuals. In a 9-year longitudinal study of recreational runners compared with nonrunners (average age, 66 at the end of the study), Lane et al. found no increase in the rate of development of hip or knee OA.[69] Much more attention should be paid to the activities, especially sports, in which even very young children are participating, and the potential risks they pose for later development of OA. Well-designed long-term studies of programs to determine if prophylactic exercises can prevent OA or diminish its severity are needed to answer these questions.

Although obesity is an important risk factor, from a prevention perspective, early intervention is important because it appears that cumulative exposure is important, with increased body mass index (BMI) in young men 20 to 29 being more predictive of subsequent knee OA than at ages 30 to 39 or 40 to 49.[70] Observational data from the Framingham OA Study suggest that weight loss of approximately 5 kg will reduce a person's risk for the development of knee OA over the subsequent 10 years by 50%.[71] The role of micronutrients in prevention is a frequently asked question. An analysis of the Framingham data found no significant association of incident radiographic knee OA with any micronutrient.[72] However, a threefold reduction in risk for progression of radiographic OA was noted for those in the middle and upper thirds of vitamin C intake; those in the upper third for vitamin C intake also had a reduced risk of developing knee pain during the course of the study. The theoretical explanation for the possible effects of vitamin C on OA comes from its involvement in collagen metabolism. Vitamin C acts as an electron donor in the synthesis of type II collagen and is involved in the hydroxylation of proline to form hydroxyproline. It also plays a role in glycosaminoglycan synthesis through its role as a carrier of sulfate groups. Its role as an antioxidant may also have some effect.[73] Interest in vitamin D increased when investigators reported that a relative deficit of vitamin D intake predisposes to progression of preexisting OA.[74] Both lower intake of vitamin D and decreased serum levels have been well documented in older people.

Treatment

The goals of therapy for OA are to reduce pain, slow progression, and improve function and quality of life. As for many other chronic diseases, lifestyle modifications play an important part of the therapeutic approach of OA. Nonpharmacologic approaches are by far the most important therapies for OA. An important goal of therapy is to reduce stress on joints by weight reduction if indicated, strengthening of the muscles around involved joints, improving flexibility and proprioception, and joint protection strategies, including improving joint mechanics and the use of assistive devices and orthotics. In managing osteoarthritis, it is important to establish and communicate realistic objectives for each patient. It is critical to focus the patient's attention on enhancement and preservation of functional ability, such as walking, dressing, and living independently. Many patients who present with hand involvement need only reassurance that the disease process is not likely to become generalized or crippling.

Exercise in the Treatment of OA

"Exercise may be the most effective, malleable, and inexpensive modality available to achieve optimal outcomes for people with OA."[75]

There is a growing recognition that health and fitness are achievable with less intense regimens than previously thought and that these regimens are feasible for people with a variety of chronic and disabling conditions. For more information on this subject, the interested reader is referred to the American College of Sports Medicine Guide to Exercise Testing and Prescription for People with Chronic Diseases and Disabilities.[76]

Rehabilitation that increases muscle strength has been shown to be associated with decreased joint pain and disability without exacerbation of knee OA pain. Reeducation of neuromuscular skills can decrease reaction times and improve functional joint stability and proprioception, which are important in restoring shock absorption function of muscle and protecting against further joint damage.

OA changes found in one joint frequently affect other joints with range of motion and strength deficits generally found in adjacent joints and bilaterally. A poorly appreciated but consistent finding in people with unilateral knee OA is not only decreased range of motion of the involved knee, but of the hip and ankle as well, and significant limitation of motion of all three joints of the uninvolved contralateral limb. Older people with knee OA have been found to decrease range of motion in all the major joints of the lower extremities.[77] Decreased range of motion of the hip and knee increases the risk for injury and falls, in part because it becomes much more difficult to recover balance from a stumble. To prevent a fall after a stumble, one must produce rapid changes in hip and knee flexion angles while weightbearing.[78] Maintaining or improving the compliance of periarticular soft tissue is also thought to protect joints from damaging

peak forces as part of the neuromuscular protective system. Stretching and flexibility exercises are therefore key elements in exercise programs for people with OA. In the first large multicenter controlled study of its kind, investigators sought to answer several important questions about the potential benefits of exercise for people with OA. They found that both aerobic and resistance exercise programs over an 18-month period resulted in modest but consistent improvement in self-reported pain and disability and better scores on performance measures of function compared with controls participating in a health education program. Importantly, they found that the subgroup of older participants, those over 70, experienced the same beneficial effects. They also showed that moderate exercise did not worsen the disease in terms of either pain or x-ray scores.[79]

Improved proprioceptive accuracy has also been demonstrated following muscle training. Knee orthoses have been shown to improve knee proprioception. Use of an elastic knee bandage improves proprioception, probably because the bandage stimulates superficial skin receptors, free nerve endings, and hair end organs that would react strongly to bandage movement on skin.[80] This increase in proprioception may, in part, explain the improvement, especially the sense of safety patients report with elastic bandages, which do not provide significant mechanical support. A modality intimately linked with exercise but also found to be an important adjunct in itself for the treatment of OA is education. Self-care education for OA resulted in notable preservation of function and control of resting knee pain in one large study.[81] The cost of such a program was shown to be defrayed by a drop in the number of clinic visits but had no significant effects on the utilization and cost of pharmaceutical, laboratory, or radiology services.[82]

Biomechanical Approaches to Therapy

Simple interventions directed toward reducing the load in affected joints include the use of walking aids, wedged insoles that change the angle of the legs, shock-absorbing footwear that reduces impact, and a heel lift if one leg is shorter than the other. Viscoelastic inserts may be effective in relieving pain and disease progression or even prevention, as they have been found to reduce the amplitude of the shock waves at heel strike with walking by 42%.[83] If hip or knee involvement is unilateral, a cane held in the contralateral hand is helpful. If involvement is bilateral, crutches or a walker are more desirable. Biomechanical principles provide a rationale for prescribing adaptive devices such as an elevated toilet seat and high chairs. Knee cages around the knee may provide some stability when ligamentous laxity is pronounced. Pillows should never be placed under the knees at night because of the risk of devloping flexion contracture.

Flexion contracture of the hip may be prevented and mild contractures may be corrected by having the patient lie prone for 30 min twice daily. Occupational therapy to modify activities of daily living can reduce unnecessary overloading of the joints of the upper and lower extremities. Other nonpharmacologic approaches include thermal modalities, transcutaneous electrical nerve stimulation (TENS), exercise programs, weight loss programs, patellar taping, tidal irrigation, and programs to improve coping skills and social support.

Sexual function is often affected in persons with arthritis. It is important for the physician to evaluate problems in this area and to advise the patient of measures aimed at overcoming handicaps. Patients with osteoarthritis of the hips, knees, or spine frequently have problems with sexual intercourse due to pain or mechanical problems. Despite these limitations, sexual activity can be undertaken with the use of analgesics beforehand. Patients should be encouraged to try a variety of positions that allow the successful, pain-free performance of intercourse. The Arthritis Foundation's pamphlet "Living and Loving with Arthritis" describes a variety of sexual problems and suggested solutions.

Drug Therapy

Although the future holds promise for the development of disease-modifying modalities for the treatment of OA, the current pharmacologic approach to treating OA is palliative rather than curative. The primary objective of drug therapy is to reduce pain. Pain is generally undertreated in older patients, and the pain of OA is no exception. On the other hand, pain may be an important signal to prevent certain types of use that might result in further damage to the joint. Analgesic arthropathy, in which the relief of pain causes accelerated joint damage because of increased joint loading, needs to be kept in mind with any successful therapy.

Guidelines for management of OA suggest a stepwise approach, starting with simple analgesic medication, which is usually acetaminophen. Despite its lack of antiinflammatory properties, acetaminophen has been shown to perform well in double-blind placebo-controlled trials against the nonsteroidal anti-inflammatory drug, ibuprofen.[84] These data suggest that pure analgesics should be considered as first-line drugs in OA much more frequently than is the case today. For patients without liver disease, doses of 1 g acetaminophen up to four times daily are recommended. For the management of moderately severe pain, viz., acute radicular pain of spinal osteoarthritis, tramadol HCl (Ultram) has comparable efficacy to acetaminophen with codeine #3. Ultram is a centrally acting agent with low potential for addiction. For pain associated with acute or chronic conditions, the dose is one or two 50-mg tablets every 4 to 6 h, as needed,

to a maximum of 400 mg/day. For patients over 75 years of age, the maximum dose should not exceed 300 mg/day. Individualization of dose is necessary for patients who have renal or hepatic impairment. Propoxyphene is no better than acetaminophen and should be avoided in older patients.

For patients not receiving adequate relief, the addition or switch to a nonsteroidal anti-inflammatory drug (NSAID) is the next step. NSAIDs are among the most widely used therapeutic agents today, with nearly $2 billion spent in the United States yearly on prescription NSAIDs alone.[85] These agents provide analgesia and suppress inflammation by inhibiting the cyclooxygenase enzymes that catalyze the formation of prostaglandins from arachidonic acid. Cyclooxygenase (COX) exists in two distinct isoforms, which display important differences in their patterns of distribution as well as their regulation. COX-1 is constitutively expressed in virtually all tissues. COX-1-mediated prostaglandins regulate renal and platelet function, protect the gastric mucosa, and promote hemostasis. COX-2-mediated prostaglandins play a role in pain, inflammation, and fever, and in the regulation of cell growth, apoptosis, and angiogenesis. COX-2 is constitutively found in small amounts in such dissimilar tissues as the brain, endometrium, and the kidneys, as well as in certain neoplasms. A characteristic feature of the COX-2 enzyme is its presence in an inducible form and its upregulation at sites of inflammation and in some tumors. Stimulation by inflammatory cytokines, endotoxin, or growth factor leads to a 10- to 80-fold increase in COX-2 levels in such cells as macrophages, fibroblasts, chondrocytes, synovial cells, and endothelial cells.

It is a widely held view that the anti-inflammatory properties of NSAIDs are mediated through COX-2 inhibition, whereas most of their adverse effects occur as a result of the inhibiting effects on COX-1. Conventional or traditional NSAIDs, such as ibuprofen and naproxen, suppress both COX-1- and COX-2-mediated prostaglandins. More recently, a new class of NSAIDs, termed coxibs, has been added to the therapeutic armamentarium. The actions of coxibs are more specific to COX-2. The traditional NSAIDs include the time-honored aspirin and other salicylates, and a large number of NSAIDs that have been developed over the past 30 years in the hope of enhancing efficacy and reducing side effects. These drugs have in common analgesic effects at a lower dosage and anti-inflammatory effects at a higher dosage. At therapeutically equivalent dosages, most traditional NSAIDs have not proven to be much safer than aspirin. No significant differences in efficacy or side effects are apparent among the different classes of traditional NSAIDs. The choice between the various traditional NSAIDs becomes largely empirical, and it is often necessary to go through a sequential trial of several different NSAIDs to arrive at the one that best suits the patient. Intermittent rather than continuous use of NSAIDs is preferable. In the elderly, compounds with a short biological half-life, such as ibuprofen and ketoprofen, are preferable to those with prolonged half-lives. Concomitant administration of two NSAIDs is not generally recommended because of the potential for added adverse effects. If the decision has been made to prescribe a traditional NSAID to an older patient, it is important to keep in mind that the starting dose should be lower than that recommended for younger adults, and stepwise adjustments should be made until an optimal therapeutic response is obtained. Patients with OA generally obtain effective analgesia at about half the daily dose given to patients with rheumatoid arthritis.

There is a vast body of literature on the evils of NSAIDs for older patients who are more prone to their side effects, especially gastrointestinal toxicity and renal dysfunction. Serious gastrointestinal toxicity such as bleeding, ulceration, and perforation can occur at any time, with or without warning symptoms, in patients treated chronically with conventional NSAIDs. Gastroduodenal ulcers can be demonstrated by endoscopy in 10% to 20% of patients who take NSAIDs on a regular basis, and the annual incidence of clinically important GI complications approaches 2%.[86] It has been conservatively estimated that 16,500 NSAID-related deaths occur among patients with rheumatoid arthritis and osteoarthritis every year in the United States. If deaths from gastrointestinal toxic effects of NSAIDs were tabulated separately in the National Vital Statistics reports, these effects would constitute the fifteenth most common cause of death in the United States. Advanced age has been consistently found to be a primary risk factor for adverse gastrointestinal (GI) events. The risk increases linearly with age.[87] The very essence of this debate, especially as regards GI side effects, has been altered by the recent release of the new class of NSAIDs, the selective COX inhibitors.

At the time of this writing, two specific COX-2 inhibitors are available, rofecoxib and celecoxib. Additional coxibs are currently undergoing clinical trials. The recommended daily dose of rofecoxib is 12.5 to 25 mg and that of celecoxib 100 to 200 mg. Several investigators have concluded that rofecoxib 12.5 mg qd is equipotent to celecoxib 200 mg qd. Although rofecoxib is the more selective of the two, both agents appear to be as effective as traditional NSAIDs in suppressing inflammation and providing analgesia, while reducing the incidence of endoscopic ulcers to levels similar to those seen with placebo.[86] In a double-blind, placebo-controlled study, specific inhibition of COX-2 by rofecoxib, administered once daily, resulted in clinically meaningful improvements in patients with OA, confirming that COX-2-derived prostanoids are important mediators of pain and

other symptoms of knee OA and that inhibition of COX-1 is not required for clinical benefit.[88] Celecoxib has similarly been shown to be associated with a lower incidence of upper GI ulcer complications in a recent randomized controlled study.[89] Another important benefit of the coxibs is that, in contrast to the nonselective NSAIDs, they do not inhibit thromboxene B2 levels or the antiplatelet effects of low-dose acetylsalicylic acid (ASA), nor do they increase bleeding time.[90]

Although coxibs do reduce the risk of ulcers, a cost–benefit analysis is useful for putting the benefits into perspective. Peterson and Cryer considered patients at higher risk for ulcer complications, such as those aged 75 years or older with a prior history of ulcer and gastrointestinal tract bleeding, who have about a 5% risk of developing a complicated ulcer while taking a traditional NSAID. Assuming that COX-1-sparing agents reduce the risk by approximately 50% (i.e., to 2.5%), 40 patients would need to be treated with a COX-1-sparing NSAID instead of a nonselective NSAID to prevent one ulcer complication. The yearly incremental cost of this approach to preventing one complicated ulcer would be about $30,000, a cost that was thought to justify switching such patients to COX-1-sparing NSAIDs. This approach also would be less costly than prescribing cotherapy for a generic NSAID with misoprostol or a proton pump inhibitor, although the occurrence rate of complicated ulcers with these two strategies has not been compared in a head-to-head study.[85]

Because COX-2 is expressed in both a constitutive and inducible fashion in the kidney, it is not surprising that renal adverse effects may result from treatment with coxibs as they do with nonselective NSAIDs. In general, renal adverse effects of NSAIDs include reductions in glomerular filtration rate (GFR) and renal blood flow, sodium retention, and increases in serum potassium. These effects can lead to fluid retention, edema, mild elevations of the blood pressure, and hyperkalemia. Obviously, these effects are more likely seen in frail patients, such as the elderly and those with chronic illnesses. Supportive of this notion is a study in elderly subjects demonstrating that COX-2 inhibition resulted in renal effects similar to those observed with nonselective NSAIDs.[91]

Systemic adrenal corticosteroid analogues are not usually recommended in the management of osteoarthritis. Clinical results with these drugs are equivocal and are outweighed by their potential side effects. However, in the patient with severe debilitating pain in whom other therapies have not helped sufficiently, a brief course of low-dose prednisone (5 mg A.M.) may give remarkable palliation.

Topical application of creams containing a NSAID or capsaicin appears to have analgesic effects. Local application of capsaicin, which depletes substance P from sensory nerve endings, caused a 30% reduction in pain in OA of the knee.[92]

If pain relief is still not adequate, then Tylenol with codeine or oxycodone, which has been shown to be effective in OA, should be tried in carefully selected patients. Controlled-release oxycodone or in fixed combination with acetaminophen added to NSAIDs have been compared in patients with OA with similar significant effectiveness in reducing pain and improving sleep found over placebo. The controlled-release preparation was found to produce fewer side effects with significantly less nausea and dry mouth.[93]

Nutraceuticals as Therapeutic Agents in OA

Two compounds that are receiving increasing attention are the nutraceuticals glucosamine and chondroitin sulfate. These compounds have been used in various forms for OA in continental Europe for more than a decade and have recently acquired substantial popularity in this country because of several lay publications. The medical community in the United Kingdom and the United States, on the other hand, has paid little attention to the potential benefits of these compounds, largely due to concerns about the validity of clinical trials.

The theoretical considerations for the possible effectiveness of glucosamine in OA stems from its status as a principal component of glycosaminoglycan (GAG), a key constituent of the matrix of all connective tissues. It is formed by the addition of an amino group to glucose that is then acetylated to acetyl-glucosamine. More than 50% of the glucosamine is nonionized at a pH of the small intestine, thus allowing significant and rapid absorption. Glucosamine has a special tropism for cartilage and is incorporated by the chondrocyte into proteoglycans, which are secreted into the extracellular matrix. In rats, ^{14}C-labeled glucosamine appears in rat cartilage 4h after ingestion. When glucosamine is added to cultured human chondrocytes from osteoarthritic cartilage, a dose-dependent increase in proteoglycan synthesis occurs.[94]

Most clinical studies have been conducted on glucosamine. In some preparations glucosamine is combined with chondroitin sulfate. Glucosamine and chondroitin are prepared by extraction from animal products, including bovine and calf cartilage. More than 90% of ingested glucosamine is absorbed, while less than 10% of chondroitin sulfate is absorbed. In short-term studies, glucosamine and chondroitin preparations have proven to be safe, but long-term toxicity studies remain to be done. The concern about the quality of clinical trials led McAlindron et al. to perform a meta-analysis combined with systematic quality assessment of 15 double-blind, placebo-controlled clinical trials of these preparations in knee and/or hip OA.[95] In summing up the results, the

authors found that the clinical trials of glucosamine and chondroitin preparations for OA symptoms demonstrate moderate to large effects but exhibit methodologic problems that have been associated with exaggerated estimates of benefit. The overall impression was that the compounds did show some benefit in treating OA symptoms. Given their excellent safety profile, glucosamine and chondroitin are likely to be useful in the treatment of OA even though they may be only modestly effective. Glucosamine and chondroitin are available in pharmacies and health food stores. The amounts generally administered are glucosamine 1500 mg/day and chondroitin sulfate 1200 mg/day, with an average cost of about $30 to $45 per month.

Joint and Bursa Injections

Aspiration and joint injections with corticosteroids have been one of the mainstays for the palliative therapy of painful joints. When effusions are large, especially in the knee, relief of symptoms often occurs with simple aspiration of the joint fluid. However, the fluid will quickly reaccumulate unless corticosteroids are also injected. A singe intra-articular injection of triamcinolone hexacetonide in knee OA provides short-term pain relief compared with placebo, with best results seen in those with clinical evidence of joint effusion and successful aspiration of synovial fluid at the time of injection.[96] The mechanism for alleviating pain besides decreasing inflammation, which is usually minimal in OA, is unclear. Because of earlier experience with frequent injections of corticosteroids leading to an accelerated rate of joint damage, it is recommended to limit the frequency of joint injections to once every 3 months and not to exceed three injections in a given joint per year. The joint damage seen with multiple corticosteroid injections over shorter periods of time has been attributed to a direct effect of steroids on chondrocyte metabolism, possibly combined with a component of analgesic arthropathy. In weightbearing joints, decreased loading should be recommended for at least 2 days. Response to steroid injections is highly variable, and repeat injections should be limited to those who have a significant response that lasts several months.

Steroid injections are also useful adjuncts in the treatment of inflamed bursae. Observational studies have demonstrated both short- and long-term response to steroid injection, with a majority of patients showing improvement when assessed 26 weeks after injection.[97]

Viscosupplementation

In recent years, viscosupplementation has begun to emerge as an alternative or supplement to analgesics and NSAIDs in the management of patients with OA of the knee. Viscosupplementation for the management of OA was first used and tested on race horses in the early 1970s and shortly thereafter in people with OA of the knee. The rationale for this therapy stems from the unique properties of hyaluronic acid (HA).

The synovial lining of the diarthrodial joint is composed of one to two layers of cells that produce a highly viscous lubricating fluid, which contains high molecular weight substances, such as HA and lubricin. These substances coat the surface of the articular cartilage, providing lubrication as the articular cartilage surfaces move across each other during movement. The highly viscous nature of the synovial fluid is important for normal joint function, providing a nearly frictionless surface for joint movement.

Arthritis is associated with elaboration of enzymes and free radicals that degrade both HA and lubricin. Breakdown of HA leads to a decrease in the viscosity of the synovial fluid with loss of smooth movement of the articular surfaces, leading to further joint deterioration. It has been known for many years that synovial fluid from OA joints is lower in elasticity and viscosity than that from normal joint joints. This decrease in rheologic properties of the synovial fluid is due to reductions in the molecular size and concentration of hyaluronan and results not only from increased degradation but also from decreased synthesis and an inferior quality of synthesized hyaluronan.

In early clinical studies with hyaluronan products (1–2 million in molecular weight), viscosupplementation was shown to be a safe treatment in osteoarthritis. However, 6 to 10 injections were often required to show any efficacy because the elastoviscous properties of the early hyaluronan preparations were inadequate and the injected hyaluronan was eliminated too quickly. Because of this limitation, hylans were developed to produce a more highly elastoviscous fluid with rheologic properties similar to those of synovial fluid in the knee joint of healthy young persons.[98] Hylans are cross-linked forms of purified hyaluronan to form polymers of high molecular weight (6 million). Hylan preparations have a longer residence time in the joint space, and because of cross-links, they become more resistant to free radical degradation. A treatment regimen consisting of three injections of hylan given 1 week apart has been shown to provide optimal pain relief in people with OA of the knee. In one study comparing hylan G-F 20 with a lower molecular weight hyaluronon, hylan was found to yield significantly better results at 12 weeks in all the primary outcome measure, which included weightbearing pain and overall treatment response.[99] Systemic adverse events have been reported rarely with viscosupplementation and have not occurred with repeat injection, but mild to moderate transient local pain and swelling occur in 2% to 3% of intra-articular injections of hylan G-F 20.

There is some speculation that hylan may act as a DMOAD, but no studies are yet available to confirm this. Theoretically, the introduction of replacement HA preparations of sufficiently high molecular weight might delay, if not halt, the progression of OA. More studies are needed to assess long-term effects of this therapy. Some skepticism is warranted in view of recent findings in a canine model of OA. In this study, a series of intra-articular injections of HA did not alter the development of osteophytosis or fibrillation, and, in addition, prostaglandin concentration in the cartilage of treated knees was significantly reduced, suggesting that HA therapy may adversely affect cartilage.[100]

Joint Replacement

Surgical intervention, mostly in the form of total knee and hip arthroplasty, is recommended for patients in whom pain and disability cannot be controlled by other means. Many recent studies have established the effectiveness and safety of total joint arthroplasty. However, these studies have tended to include mostly younger patients. Brander et al. looked specifically at subjects 80 years of age and older who were undergoing either hip or knee arthroplasty and compared their outcome with a younger, otherwise matched control group. They found that the older group had similar dramatic improvements in pain and function, as well as similar complication rates and length of stay in acute care facilities, compared with the younger group. The most dramatic postoperative functional gains were seen in the most disabled people.[101] The decision to perform a total hip arthroplasty (THA) for patients with OA is based largely on patient reports of pain and disability and not on the radiographic findings of OA. Fox et al. reviewed the x-rays of elderly patients who had undergone unilateral THA and found that this group tended to have the contralateral THA performed with less severe x-ray findings.[102] This finding suggests that if patients had a better understanding of the procedure and its benefits, they would opt for earlier surgical intervention. Besides alleviating pain and improving function, elective THA has consistently resulted in improved health-related quality of life, which was often dramatic and was most likely to occur within the first 3 to 6 months after THA.[103]

Loosening remains a major complication following total joint replacement. Infection needs to be ruled out whenever loosening occurs. However, the rate of prosthetic joint infection has decreased to less than 1% with improvements in the operating room environment and the use of prophylactic antibiotics. Recent studies suggest inflammatory reactions directed against the implanted materials may contribute to aseptic loosening. Elevated immune cell proliferation responses to both acrylic and cobalt/chromium were observed in patients with aseptically loosened prostheses.[104] Like many other procedures, the outcome of elective hip replacement bears a relationship to the volume of procedures performed by surgeons and hospitals, with low-volume providers tending to have higher rates of adverse events and serious complications.[105]

Treatment of Low Back Pain

Besides the usual therapies already discussed, therapy for low back pain may include a course of physical therapy, with special attention to body mechanics, and epidural injections in selected cases. Osteopathic manual therapy (i.e., spinal manipulation) is a frequently used method of treatment for patients with chronic and subchronic back pain that has only recently been systematically studied. A randomized controlled trial comparing standard allopathic therapies with osteopathic manual therapy, albeit in subjects between 20 and 59 years of age with low back pain that had lasted at least 3 weeks but less than 6 months, found that both groups improved similarly during the 12-week follow-up. The allopathic treatment included analgesics, anti-inflammatory medication, active physical therapy, or therapies such as ultrasonography, diathermy, hot or cold packs (or both), use of a corset, or TENS. The osteopathic group required significantly less medication and used less physical therapy.[106]

Surgical and Nonsurgical Treatment of Spinal Stenosis

Conservative treatment of lumbar spinal stenosis consisting of exercise programs and pain medication is recommended for those with tolerable symptoms or in whom surgery is too risky or not desired. Caudal epidural blocks are a reasonable therapeutic option in some patients with lumbar stenosis, especially those who are poor surgical risks or have refused surgery. For those with progressive neurologic impairment, decompressive lumbar laminectomy with or without posterior spinal fusion may be indicated. A prospective cohort study assessed 4-year outcomes for patients with lumbar stenosis treated surgically or nonsurgically.[107] For the patients with severe lumbar spinal stenosis, surgical treatment was associated with greater improvement in patient-reported outcomes than nonsurgical treatment at 4-year evaluation, even after adjustment for differences in baseline characteristics among treatment groups. The relative benefit of surgery declined over time but remained superior to nonsurgical treatment. Outcomes for the nonsurgically treated patients improved modestly and remained stable over 4 years. In a study with a longer evaluation period, Amundsen et al. followed a cohort of 100 patients with symptomatic stenosis for 10 years who received either surgical or conservative treatment.[108] Those patients selected for surgery had better outcomes than those treated conservatively. Importantly, Amundsen et al. found that many improved with conservative therapy and, in those who did not, that a delay in surgery of from 3 to 27 months did not appreciably alter their outcomes compared with those who had surgery initially, suggesting that an initial conservative approach is prudent. There has been limited systematic study of surgical outcomes in older patients; however, two recent studies evaluated the efficacy of surgical treatment in patients who were older than 70 and 75 years of age, respectively.[109,110] These studies found that with appropriate preoperative selection and evaluation, the surgical treatment of elderly patients with lumbar spinal stenosis can produce significant improvement with acceptable levels of morbidity. Katz et al. found that the most powerful predictors for positive outcomes after surgery for degenerative lumbar stenosis was the patient's report of good or excellent health before surgery.[111]

Role of Acupuncture

Acupuncture appears to be a safe and effective adjunctive therapy for short-term relief of symptoms of OA involving the knee. The benefit of treatment shows some decline at 4 weeks after cessation.[112] The response to acupuncture appears to be quite variable among patients. Efforts to relate differences in response to psychosocial factors have not been rewarding in predicting response.

Experimental Therapies

The recent appreciation of the active metabolic life of the chondrocyte has led to an interest in biologically based therapies for OA. The potential use of doxycycline in the treatment of OA is based on its inhibition of protease activity against collagen in vitro at concentrations achieved in serum after oral dosing.[113] Oral administration of doxycycline significantly inhibited collagenase and gelatinase activity in human OA cartilage that was removed for THA.[114] Much more work is needed before therapy with doxycycline can be recommended for OA. Other potential biologic agents include inhibitors of IL-1 and NO, which are known to suppress synthesis of cartilage matrix. The administration of NO synthase inhibitors in experimentally induced arthritis have resulted in reduction of both synovial inflammation and destruction of cartilage and bone. Another avenue of future potential treatment is gene therapy, specifically manipulation of those genes whose products stimulate chondrogenesis or inhibit breakdown of cartilaginous matrix.[115]

Crystal Deposition Disease

Deposition of crystals in and around joints may be associated with acute or chronic arthritis. Crystals implicated in arthritis include monosodium urate monohydrate (MSU), calcium pyrophosphate dihydrate (CPPD), and HA and other basic calcium phosphates. The prevalence of crystal deposition diseases increases with age. Deposits of calcium pyrophosphate and hydroxyapatite are often seen in association with OA. Articular manifestations of this group of diseases are extremely common in the geriatric population, presenting a wide range of clinical responses.

Deposition of Crystals: Relationship to Aging and Osteoarthritis

The precise mechanisms by which crystals are deposited are imperfectly understood, but increased concentrations of metastable calcium salts and sodium urate, the unmasking of activators of crystal nucleation and crystal growth, or a decrease in concentration of inhibitors of crystal nucleation may act singly or together to promote crystal formation. In idiopathic or sporadic CPPD deposition disease seen in the elderly, isolated elevation of pyrophosphate in synovial fluid is due to local abnormalities. Increased pyrophosphate production has been demonstrated in osteoarthritic cartilage and probably results from enhanced breakdown of nucleotides mediated by the chondrocytic ectoenzymes, 5'-nucleotidase and nucleoside triphosphate pyrophosphohydrolase. The increased activity of these metabolic processes is an attempt by chrondrocytes to repair damaged cartilage. Ultrastructural studies have demonstrated deposits of CPPD in chondrocyte lacunae in areas of damaged matrix and activated chondrocytes. Aggregated proteoglycans are potent inhibitors of crystal formation. Deaggregation of proteoglycans in aged and osteochondritic cartilage would lead to a loss of natural calcium crystal inhibitor.

It would appear that deposits of CPPD and MSU can form in the absence of osteoarthritis. The familial cases of chondrocalcinosis and gout in younger persons are examples of deposition of crystals in seemingly normal cartilage. On the other hand, biochemical changes in osteoarthritic cartilage may predispose to crystal deposition, which in turn may contribute to further joint deterioration. In this latter setting, crystal deposition is a secondary, opportunistic process in damaged cartilage. Aging alone appears to be the major factor leading to formation of CPPD in fibrocartilaginous structures. The simultaneous finding of mixtures of crystal deposits in the same joints of elderly patients is further evidence of their susceptibility to intraarticular and periarticular crystal deposition. A positive association exists between gout and CPPD deposition disease and between CPPD and hydroxyapatite formation.

Crystal-Induced Synovitis

It is generally believed that preformed microcrystals are shed from cartilage or synovium. Crystals that are associated with arthritis possess a negative surface charge and avidly bind proteins, including immunoglobulins, albumin, lysosomal enzymes, complement, and lipoproteins. Urate crystals have a strong affinity for IgG. The molecular orientation of IgG on the crystal surface leaves the Fc portion exposed and free to interact with Fc cell membrane receptors on leukocytes, monocytes, synoviocytes, and platelets. The interaction between cells and crystals causes the cells to become activated with release of a host of inflammatory mediators. Coating of the crystal surface with IgG greatly enhances phagocytosis and complement activation. Monocytes and polymorphonuclear leukocytes release a potent chemotactic factor that causes rapid accumulation of polymorphonuclear leukocytes. Phagocytosis induces release of oxygen radicals and lysosomal enzymes. MSU crystals induce release of interleukin-1 from monocytes, an observation that may explain the fever of acute gouty arthritis.

Some crystals, for example, MSU, are membranolytic. After digestion of their protein coating in the phagolysosome, the uncoated crystal causes rupture of the phagolysosome with release of its enzymes into the cytoplasm, resulting in cellular autolysis, increased permeability of the cell wall, and release of intracellular enzymes into the surrounding medium. Coating of the crystals with hyaluronic acid and certain proteins, such as albumin or lipoprotein, may inhibit or prevent crystal-induced inflammation, which may explain the occurrence of crystals in joint fluid after the inflammatory reaction has subsided or even in the absence of any detectable inflammation.

Study of synovial fluid by polarized light microscopy provides clinicians with a precise method of identifying MSU and CPPD when the crystals are more than $1\,\mu m$ in size. Using a first-order red plate compensator allows one to determine the sign of birefringence and further differentiate between crystal types. Nonbirefringent apatite and other basic calcium phosphate crystals are so minute that they cannot be identified by ordinary light microscopy; they tend to aggregate into nonbirefringent microspherules that are difficult to distinguish from cell detritus and fat droplets. Definitive identification of apatite and other basic calcium phosphates requires sophisticated techniques.

Plain radiographs identify macroscopic deposits of radiopaque calcium containing salts. Hydroxyapatite deposits are frequently seen in periarticular and capsular distribution, whereas CPPD deposition disease is associated with characteristic punctate and linear calcifications in fibrocartilaginous and hyaline cartilage.

Gout

New onset of gouty arthritis is common among the elderly. Most of these patients have hyperuricemia on the basis of decreased urinary excretion of uric acid, related to the effects of diuretic therapy, mild renal failure, hypertension, or hypertriglyceridemia. It has been estimated that about half of all patients who present with their initial attack of acute gouty arthritis are taking a diuretic. With the widespread use of these drugs in the elderly population, it is hardly a surprise that diuretic use is a major cause of gout in this age group. Less commonly, gout is secondary to overproduction of uric acid due to increased turnover of cells, as in myeloproliferative disorders.

The presentation of gout in the elderly differs from the more classic picture in younger men. The pattern is frequently polyarticular, subacute or chronic, and men and women appear to be affected with the same frequency. In women, the first manifestations of gout may be acute arthritis in finger joints, sometimes presenting as inflamed Heberden's or Bouchard's nodes. Elderly women are particularly prone to develop diuretic-induced polyarticular gout. Many have underlying osteoarthritis, and concomitant tophi and osteoarthritic changes in the same joint have been described. The appearance of asymptomatic tophi in Heberden's and Bouchard's nodes in elderly women as the initial manifestation of gout has been highlighted in several recent reports.[116,117]

Chronic polyarticular gout with tophi can be misdiagnosed as rheumatoid arthritis with rheumatoid nodules, resulting in improper treatment and otherwise preventable disability. To add to the confusion, rheumatoid factor tests are positive in about 30% of patients with tophaceous gout, a finding that relates to the coating of urate crystals by IgG.

The diagnosis of gout can be readily established by studying synovial fluid or tophaceous material by polarized light microscopy. Needle-shaped negatively birefringent crystals of MSU are seen in 95% of patients with acute gouty arthritis and are a sine qua non for establishing a definitive diagnosis. Hyperuricemia, common in the elderly, is less reliable as a diagnostic test. Furthermore, serum urate levels are within normal limits at the time of the acute attack in 7% of the cases. Calcium pyrophosphate dihydrate crystals can coexist with urate crystals, and isolated cases of bacterial arthritis superimposed on gouty arthritis have been reported. If the clinical picture is suspicious of a septic joint, synovial fluid must be cultured.

The management of gout in the elderly is guided by the same principles that apply to a younger age group. The acute attack is treated with colchicine or one of the NSAIDs. The cautious use of NSAIDs has been discussed under osteoarthritis. A patient with decreased renal function, whose gout is precipitated by administration of a diuretic, is at risk of developing renal insufficiency if a NSAID is used to treat acute gouty arthritis. Colchicine has a low therapeutic margin and should be administered with caution. It is given in hourly doses of 0.6 mg, for a total of four to eight doses with decreases in dosage for hepatic or renal disease. The drug must be stopped promptly at the first sign of loose stools to avoid the consequences of dehydration and potassium loss. Renal, hepatic, and myocardial impairment, and the presence of cardiac arrhythmias, enhance the risk for colchicine toxicity. Chronic usage in patients with renal insufficiency has been associated with myoneuropathy syndrome. Colchicine may be administered slowly into a large vein in a dose of 2 mg. Great caution must be exercised to avoid extravasation, which may result in tissue necrosis and sloughing of the skin. Intra-articular injection of corticosteroid is helpful when gout involves an accessible joint. Oral administration of corticosteroids is also useful in older patients, but because of a tendency of gouty arthritis to rebound, concomitant administration of a maintenance dose of colchicine or a NSAID is necessary.

Drugs to lower serum urate should be initiated once the acute attack has subsided. Because acute gouty arthritis may occur during the initial treatment with a hypouricemic drug, it is advisable to use colchicine prophylactically in a dose of 0.6 mg twice daily for several weeks. Uricosuric drugs are effective so long as the creatinine clearance exceeds 50 mL/min. Probenecid and sufinpyrazone are the principal uricosuric drugs. Diflunisal in a dose of 500 mg two times daily is weakly uricosuric and may be worth trying in a patient who also requires an analgesic drug for symptomatic OA. Aspirin abolishes the effect of uricosuric drugs and should not be given concomitantly. Allopurinol is the drug of choice for patients with overproduction of uric acid or with significant reduction in renal function or those who require continuous treatment with aspirin, diuretics, or other drugs that interfere with the tubular secretion of urate. The dose of allopurinal in elderly patients with diminished uric acid excretion is smaller than in overproducers of uric acid. The goal is to prescribe the lowest dose of allopurinol that will maintain serum urate between 5 and 6 mg/dL. Frequently, 100 or 200 mg allopurinol given in a single morning dose will suffice. Serious toxicity includes agranulocytosis, granulomatous hepatitis, and exfoliative dermatitis. Many cases of prolonged hypersensitivity reactions characterized by an erythematous maculopapular rash, eosinophilia, fever, liver function abnormalities, and progressive renal failure have been recorded. Another concern in using allopurinol is the observation of an increased incidence of severe hypersensitivity reactions from coadministered drugs, for example, penicillin and ampicillin. Asymptomatic hyperuricemia is not an indication for long-term urate-lowering therapy; the risks of drug toxicity outweigh any benefit.

Calcium Pyrophosphate Dihydrate Deposition Disease

Calcium pyrophosphate dihydrate (CPPD) causes the most common crystal-associated arthritis in the elderly. In 1962, McCarty reported an acute arthritis mimicking gout, and therefore termed pseudogout, in elderly patients with chondrocalcinosis.[118] He further identified the crystals in synovial fluid and cartilage as calcium pyrophosphate dihydrate ($Ca_2P_2O_7 \cdot 2H_2O$). CPPD crystal deposition disease is a heterogenous disorder. Familial or hereditary cases have been reported from several countries. A small fraction are associated with underlying metabolic disorders, including hyperparathyroidism, hypothyroidism, hypophosphatasia, hypomagnesemia, hemochromatosis, ochronosis, gout, Wilson's disease, and senile amyloidosis. CPPD crystal deposition disease associated with genetic disorders has an early onset. In the elderly, the idiopathic or sporadic form is by far the most common type of CPPD deposition disease. The prevalence increases in stepwise fashion with age. It is rare before age 50 and increases from 10% to 15% in those aged 65 to 75 to 30% to 60% in those over 85 years. Ellman et al. studied the prevalence of knee chondrocalcinosis in hospital and clinic patients older than 50 years and found an overall prevalence of 9.6%.[119] In a representative sample of 79-year-olds in Gothenburg, radiographic evidence of chondrocalcinosis in knees or hands was present in 16%.[120]

The majority of patients with chondrocalcinosis are free of symptoms. Radiopaque densities are noted in fibrocartilage (especially menisci, radiocarpal joint, symphysis pubis, shoulders, and hips and in the midzonal layer of hyaline cartilage), giving rise to punctate of linear calcification. Acute synovitis, or pseudogout, is the most dramatic clinical manifestation. It presents as an acute monoarthritis, most often located to the knee, but also commonly seen in the wrist, shoulder or ankle. As in gout, surgery, trauma or serious medical illness may trigger an acute attack. About 10% of patients have oligoarticular involvement or a migratory pattern involving several joints successively, sometimes over a course of many weeks or months. About half of symptomatic patients present with clinical and radiographic features that are reminiscent of low-grade osteoarthritis, except that joint involvement is that of pseudogout rather than generalized OA. The patients complain of chronic pain, stiffness and restricted movement of knees, wrists, shoulders, elbows, metacarpophalangeal joints, hips, and ankles. Minor acute attacks may be superimposed on chronic symptoms. Acute and chronic tenosynovitis may be present. Wrist involvement may produce a carpal tunnel syndrome. The chronic polyarticular arthropathy seen in 5% of the patients may be confused with rheumatoid arthritis. A number of reports have described a severe destructive arthropathy similar to a Charcot joint and affecting almost exclusively elderly women in association with calcium pyrophosphate deposition, involving the shoulder, elbow, or wrist, in addition to knees or hips.[121] In addition to the typical x-ray findings of calcifications in articular cartilage already described, calcifications may be seen in the joint capsule, synovium, and bursae and in tendons, especially the Achilles, triceps, quadriceps, and supraspinatus tendons.

The diagnosis is confirmed by presence of weakly positively birefringent calcium pyrophosphate crystals in synovial fluid and characteristic radiologic findings. In acute arthritis, polymorphonuclear leukocytes predominate. Total synovial fluid WBC counts range from 4000 to 50,000/mm^3. Triclinic (crystals with three axes, all unequal and none at right angles), rhomboid crystals are found within leukocytes and extracellularly. In chronic arthritis, the leukocyte count is lower and mononuclear cells are more numerous. CPPD synovitis is a prevalent disease, and one should always keep in mind the possible coexistence of another joint disease. The screening for rare metabolic disorders is unrewarding in the elderly, but measurement of serum calcium, iron, and iron-binding capacity should be obtained, and screening for hypothyroidism in a geriatric population is always worthwhile.

Treatment of acute synovitis is with nonsteroidal anti-inflammatory drugs, aspiration of joint fluid, and intra-articular injection of corticosteroid. The effect of colchicine is less reliable than in acute gouty arthritis. Chronic CPPD arthritis is managed in much the same way as osteoarthritis. The principles and potential hazards of using NSAIDs have been discussed in the section on OA.

Hydroxyapatite Deposition Disease

Hydroxyapatite (HA) and other basic calcium phosphates, which comprise the mineral phase of bone and teeth, make up the majority of ectopic or extraskeletal calcifications. Ectopic calcifications can be divided into dystrophic types, which occur in tissue that has been injured, and metastatic calcifications, which are related to increased calcium and phosphate concentration. Examples of dystrophic lesions are calcifications, which may occur in scleroderma, dermatomyositis, ochronosis, and tophi and following local injections of corticosteroids. Metastatic calcifications may be seen in hyperparathyroidism, sarcoidosis, and end-stage renal disease managed with chronic hemodialysis.

Idiopathic periarticular HA deposition occurs commonly in bursae and tendons. More recently, HA crystals have been found in synovial fluid in a high percentage of patients with osteoarthritis, and less often in patients with other types of arthritis. Because of their minute size (75–250 Å in diameter), individual HA crystals cannot be identified by ordinary or polarized light microscopy. Their precise identification requires electron microscopic techniques or microprobe or x-ray diffraction analysis.

HA crystals can cause acute inflammation of tendons and bursae. The common rotator tendon is one typical site. The etiology of calcific tendinitis is unknown; presumably trauma leads to tissue damage with calcium deposition in the form of HA occurring at the site of tissue injury. In calcific periarthritis, the skin is often warm and red over the affected joints and the tissues are boggy and tender, but effusion is absent. Periarthritic calcification is visible on radiographs.

HA crystals, detected by electron microscopy, were present in synovial fluid from more than half of patients with OA of the knee.[122] The crystals were associated with more severe disease but did not correlate with the concentrations of putative markers of cartilage such as keratan sulfate. HA crystals have been shown to have phlogistic properties and have been implicated as a cause of the flares of synovitis seen in osteoarthritis, in which cases there is a tendency to higher synovial fluid cell count and a more severe course.

HA-associated destructive arthritis is an unusual form of rapidly progressive destructive OA of the large joints in elderly patients that is associated with HA crystals in the synovial fluid. Although the shoulder is a typical site (so-called Milwaukee shoulder),[123] it is well recognized that similar destructive changes can occur in other larger joints such as the knee, hip, and ankle and even in small joints. The overwhelming majority of patients with HA-associated destructive arthritis have been elderly women. Rapid joint destruction leading to instability and large, noninflammatory, often hemorrhagic effusions, containing large amounts of HA particles and joint detritus, are cardinal clinical features. Radiographs show characteristic changes, such as marked attrition of bone and cartilage on both sides of the joint, scalloping pressure defects, and periarticular calcifications. Osteophytosis, subchondral sclerosis, and cyst formation are either absent or are minor findings. The pathogenesis of this destructive arthropathy has not been fully delineated, but activated collagenase and neutral protease play a major role in accelerating chondrolysis and joint destruction.

Other Crystals and Particles

A variety of other birefringent materials may occasionally cause synovitis. Calcium oxalate crystal deposition can be seen in elderly patients with end-stage renal disease who are receiving chronic hemodialysis. Positively birefringent bipyramidal and polymorphic calcium oxalate crystals have been demonstrated in cartilage, synovium, and synovial fluid. Radiographically, deposits in cartilage cannot be distinguished from calcium pyrophosphate deposition. Involvement of metacarpophalangeal and proximal interphalangeal joints is common. Joint disease in chronic renal failure may be associated with either HA or calcium oxalate deposition.

Cryoglobulins found in essential cryoglobulinemia and multiple myeloma can precipitate in crystalline form in a variety of tissues, including the synovium. Rare cases of cryoglobulin crystal-associated arthritis have been reported. Cholesterol crystals are mainly seen in chronic inflammatory effusions. Crystalline depot corticosteroid preparations may occasionally induce a transient inflammation hours after intra-articular injection (postinjection flare). Corticosteroid crystals can appear as positively or negatively birefringent rods, similar in size to urate or CPPD, as granules, or as irregular debris. Finally, particles of wearing surgical articular implants can be associated with a chronic detritic synovitis in elderly patients who have undergone partial or total joint replacement.

Polymyalgia Rheumatica and Giant Cell Arteritis

Temporal arteritis and polymyalgia rheumatica are closely related diseases that primarily affect the elderly, frequently occur in the same individual, and usually are associated with constitutional symptoms in the form of malaise, fatigue, weight loss, anemia, and elevated levels of acute-phase reactants. Furthermore, in both syndromes, a rapid response to glucocorticoids is seen regularly. Temporal arteritis and polymyalgia rheumatica are nosologic terms used to define typical clinical syndromes, whereas giant cell arteritis denotes a specific pathologic process. The question of the relationship between temporal arteritis and polymyalgia rheumatica is still a valid one. Some consider the two to be syndromes at either end of the spectrum of one disease, with temporal arteritis the more severe and polymyalgia rheumatica the less severe expression of an underlying giant cell arteritis. Others believe that a common etiologic agent produces either a proximal synovitis leading to symptoms of polymyalgia rheumatica, or a giant cell arteritis leading to symptoms of vasculitis and occlusion of elastic arteries originating from the aortic arch.

The association of polymyalgia rheumatica with giant cell arteritis is striking. Most series have shown that 40% to 60% of patients with giant cell arteritis have symptoms of polymyalgia rheumatica, which may be the initial presentation in one-third of patients. Conversely, biopsy of the temporal artery has demonstrated giant cell arteritis in 15% to 30% of patients with polymyalgia rheumatica who had no symptoms or signs of arteritis.

The term *polymyalgia rheumatica* was coined by Barber in 1957 to describe a syndrome characterized by myalgias and stiffness of the shoulder and pelvic girdles, neck, or torso for a duration of 1 month or more, accompanied by constitutional symptoms and an elevated erythrocyte sedimentation rate in patients who have no underlying disease to explain the symptoms. The syndrome is extremely rare in people under the age of 50 years. Despite widespread awareness of the condition in the United States, the first report in the American literature did not appear until 1963.

Giant cell arteritis, clinically also known as temporal arteritis or cranial arteritis, is a form of granulomatous vasculitis, typically containing giant cells, that most often causes occlusion of the branches of the external and internal carotids but may involve many medium- and large-sized arteries throughout the body, including the aorta.

Epidemiology

Polymyalgia rheumatica and giant cell arteritis are relatively common diseases in the elderly. The incidence rate has been shown to be highest in northern Europe and in populations of the same ethnic background in the northern United States. Epidemiologic studies of these entities have been conducted in Olmstead County, Minnesota, which comprises an urban population in Rochester and a surrounding rural population.[124,125] The mean annual incidence of polymyalgia rheumatica over a 10-year span (1970–1979) was 53.7 per 100,000 population 50 years of age and older; this may be compared to an incidence of rheumatoid arthritis of 77 per 100,000 in the same age group. The prevalence of polymyalgia rheumatica was estimated at 550 per 100,000 aged 50 and older. The average annual incidence of giant cell arteritis in the period between 1950 and 1983 was 16 per 100,000 population 50 years and over, with a slightly higher figure of 21.7 for the period between 1975 and 1983. The age-specific incidence rate rose, from 1.4 per 100,000 population aged 50 to 59 years, to a maximum of 44.7 per 100,000 population older than 80 years. In 1984, the prevalence of persons with a history of temporal arteritis was 234 per 100,000 population aged 50 and older. Two prospective studies from Denmark and Norway found incidence rates that were higher than those reported in prior retrospective studies;[126,127] the annual incidence of giant cell arteritis, which was the term used to encompass temporal arteritis and polymyalgia rheumatica, occurring either together or alone, was 76.6 and 141.7 per 100,000 population aged 50 years or more, respectively. The annual incidence of biopsy-proven giant cell arteritis in persons 50 years and older was 23.3 and 29.0 per 100,000, respectively. All studies have found the incidence rates of polyalgia and giant cell arteritis to be significantly higher for women than for men. Autopsy studies suggest that giant cell arteritis may be even more prevalent. In a prospective study, Östberg examined sections of the temporal arteries and two transverse sections of the aorta and found giant cell arteritis in 1.6% of 889 consecutive postmortem cases.[128]

Etiology and Pathogenesis

The causes of polymyalgia rheumatica and giant cell arteritis is not known, nor has its striking prevalence in older people been elucidated. However, during the past few years, remarkable progress has been achieved in the understanding of the pathogenic mechanisms that lead to inflammation and damage of the vessel wall in giant cell arteritis.[129,130] The cellular infiltrate is dominated by macrophages, a heterogenous population of CD-4+ T lymphocytes, a smaller number of CD-8+ T cells, and nucleated giant cells. B lymphocytes are usually absent. The CD-4+ T lymphocytes accumulate preferentially in the adventitia of the artery in close proximity to TGF-β_1- and IL-1-producing macrophages. A small population of CD-4+ T cells takes on the phenotype of an activated T-cell blast and undergoes clonal expansion with associated production of interferon-γ. These findings suggest recognition of an antigen that resides in the adventitia. This location is apart from the internal elastic membrane and adjoining tissue that bears the brunt of injury and which is characterized by infiltration by a population of macrophages that have undergone functional differentiation to produce collagenase and inducible nitric oxidase synthase. The nature of the antigen in giant cell arteritis has not been identified. The fragmentation of the elastic lamina observed in pathologic specimens has long led to speculation that elastic fibers represent a target antigen. Support for this view has come from a recent report suggesting release of elastase-derived elastin peptides that serve as the putative autoimmune targets in this disease.[131] On the other hand, the sudden onset of giant cell arteritis in some patients and the finding that the peaks of incidence of giant cell arteritis correlate with peaks of incidence of respiratory diseases have raised questions of an infectious agent triggering the autoimmune process. A viral etiology has been suspected but never proven.

Two recent studies have suggested that a virus may play a role in the pathogenesis of giant cell arteritis. The Mayo group found a statistically significant association between histologic evidence of giant cell arteritis and the presence of parvovirus B19 DNA in temporal artery biopsies.[132] A strong association of IgM directed against parainfluenza virus type 1 and biopsy-verified temporal arteritis, with a significant rise in positivity rate between the onset of symptoms and diagnosis, was found in a multicenter, prospective study.[133] This finding suggested that reinfection with parainfluenza virus type 1 is linked to the onset of giant cell arteritis in a subset of patients. Although vasculitic lesions are absent in polymyalgia rheumatica, it may nevertheless represent a forme fruste of arteritis. Analysis of tissue cytokines by molecular techniques has demonstrated the presence of proinflammatory cytokines such as $TGF-\beta_1$, IL-1, and IL-6 in temporal artery specimens from patients with polymyalgia rheumatica who had no obvious findings for arteritis on histologic examination.[134]

Epidemiologic evidence supports a genetic role in the pathophysiology of the disease. Although no association with class I HLA antigens has been detected, susceptibility and disease severity appear to be linked to certain class II antigens. Studies of northern European populations have shown an association with the HLA-DR4 haplotype, but not as strong as that observed in rheumatoid arthritis. The incidence of HLA-DR4 in patients with giant cell arteritis seen at the Mayo Clinic was 60% compared with 24% for a normal control group. An analysis of the functionally most important locus of the HLA class II complex, the HLA-DRB1 locus, in patients with biopsy-proven giant cell arteritis revealed an overrepresentation of three allelic variants of the HLA-DRB1 *04 family.[135] In this particular study, the clinical findings were similar in DR4+ and DR4– patients. Relapses occurred in both subsets, and associated polymyalgia rheumatica was observed with similar frequency. The frequency of molecularly defined HLA alleles varies greatly among different ethnic groups. The lower incidence of polymyalgia rheumatica and giant cell arteritis among blacks and in southern Europe can be explained, at least in part, by the lower prevalence of the HAL-DR4 haplotype in these populations. In addition, recent studies from Spain and Italy show that susceptibility and severity of these diseases are more closely associated with other, non-DR4, HLA class II alleles.

Pathology

The pathologic diagnosis of giant cell arteritis is based on the presence of typical histology changes in each arterial layer. The changes tend to affect the arteries in a patchy fashion with abnormal segments of the artery interspersed with normal segments. A distinctive fibromyxoid

intimal proliferation causing variable degrees of luminal compromise with or without thrombus formation is seen in almost all patients. Giant cells are often closely associated with elastic lamina fragmentation. The media shows patchy degeneration, dropout of smooth muscle cells, and granulomas containing lymphocytes, histiocytes, epithelioid cells, and multinucleated giant cells. Giant cells are not seen in all sections, and their presence is not required to make the diagnosis if other histologic findings are characteristic.

Giant cell arteritis has a predilection for elastic arteries that originate from the arch of the aorta, but involvement of almost every medium- and large-sized artery has been reported. The intracranial arteries are involved less often. It has been suggested that the relative sparing of the intracranial arteries is related to the small amount of internal elastic lamina in this vascular bed.

In polymyalgia rheumatica, muscle biopsies have been normal or at most have shown nonspecific type II muscle atrophy, but a number of ultrastructural abnormalities have been observed. Arthroscopy and biopsy of shoulder and knee joint have demonstrated synovitis, characterized histologically by mild inflammation with lymphocytes and a few polymorphonuclear leukocytes, but without vasculitis. Granulomatous myocarditis and hepatitis have also been reported.

Clinical Picture

The mean age of onset of both giant cell arteritis and polymyalgia rheumatica is about 70 years. Both diseases occur twice as often in women as they do in men. In terms of diagnosis and treatment, it is useful to recognize four patient groups: (1) patients with polymyalgia rheumatica; (2) patients with temporal arteritis; (3) patients with symptoms of both polymyalgia rheumatica and temporal arteritis; and (4) patients without local symptoms of arteritis or muscular symptoms but with systemic symptoms such as fever, malaise, and weight loss.

The onset of polymyalgia rheumatica usually is insidious but can be abrupt. The most common symptoms are aches and stiffness involving the proximal muscle girdles and the neck. The discomfort usually extends to the proximal portion of the arms and thighs and to the axial musculature. The stiffness is prominent in the morning and after prolonged inactivity. Pain is accentuated by movements of the joints. Pain and stiffness may be so incapacitating that the patient cannot get out of bed in the morning without the assistance of another person. Generalized systemic complaints may include low-grade fever, night sweats, anorexia, weight loss, and depression. Peripheral musculoskeletal symptoms occur in approximately half the cases of polymyalgia rheumatica; these include a mild, usually asymmetric arthritis that predominantly involves wrists and knees, and inflammatory involvement of distal tenosynovial structures that may cause a carpal tunnel syndrome or swelling of the distal extremities, with and without pitting edema. In the absence of peripheral manifestations, physical signs are conspicuously few. Muscular strength is not impaired. Tenderness, when present, is felt mostly around the shoulders. Active range of motion may be limited due to elicitation of pain, but passive motion is normal.

Giant cell arteritis is also often insidious in onset and is associated with symptoms and signs that are dictated by the anatomic involvement. Most of the clinical features can be related to vasculitis and occlusion of the cranial branches of arteries originating from the aortic arch. The most common symptom is a headache, which is usually boring or lancinating in nature. Scalp tenderness along the course of the superficial temporal, posterior auricular, or occipital arteries is a telltale sign. The temporal artery may be swollen and pulseless. Tender nodules are sometimes felt. Rarely, occlusion leads to areas of gangrene of the scalp. Jaw claudication is often considered pathognomonic but occurs in less than half of patients. Giant cell arteritis may present with unusual manifestations, and the diagnosis should be considered in elderly patients who complain of pain with deglutination, throat or tongue pain, hoarseness, cough, ear pain, or sudden loss of hearing when no obvious cause for these symptoms can be found.

A well-recognized and serious complication of giant cell arteritis is ocular involvement, leading to partial or complete visual loss in 15% to 20% of the patients. An even lower incidence rate of permanent loss of vision (8%) was found in the Mayo Clinic series of 166 patients with biopsy-proven giant cell arteritis.[136] This incidence is lower than the incidence found in older studies and may reflect earlier recognition and treatment of the disease. Even though the dramatic manifestations of ocular involvement may appear abruptly, most patients have various complaints relating to the eyes for some time before loss of vision occurs, that is, transient blurring, amaurosis fugax, and diplopia, ptosis, or other manifestations of ophthalmoplegia. Both eyes can be affected, but loss of vision in one eye usually precedes loss of vision in the other by 1 to 12 days. Impaired visual acuity is caused by ischemic optic neuritis that is secondary to involvement of the opthalmic or the posterior ciliary arteries that supply the optic nerve. Occlusion of the central retinal artery is rarely a cause of blindness in temporal arteritis. Opthalmoplegia is a common ocular manifestation, and, as mentioned, it may precede more classical symptoms of giant cell arteritis. Occasionally, patients may complain of diplopia in the absence of detectable opthalmoplegia. Other opthalmologic complications of giant cell arteritis include episcleritis and scleritis.

Clinical evidence of involvement of large arteries occurs in 15% of cases. Arteritic lesions of the aorta may lead to aortic valve incompetence or a dissection aneurysm and rupture of the aorta. Several reports have called attention to the increased incidence of aortic aneurysm and dissection in patients with giant cell arteritis. A population-based study from Olmsted County, Minnesota, revealed aneurysm of the thoracic aorta in 11.5% of their cases, a 17-fold higher rate than observed in the general population.[137] Aortic aneurysm rupture was the cause of death in 8% of their patients. Upper extremity claudication, Raynaud's phenomenon, paresthesias, bruits over the large proximal arteries, and decreased or absent pulses and blood pressure are common manifestations of vasculitis of the large arteries to the upper extremities. Lower extremity involvement, when it occurs, presents as leg claudication. Rare cases of involvement of the vasculature of the foot, leading to pedal gangrene, have been reported. Visceral manifestations include myocardial infarction, abdominal angina, and neurologic symptoms due to vertebral arteritis. Fever and high erythrocyte sedimentation rate in patients with myocardial infarction, cerebrovascular accident, or aortic aneurysm may signal giant cell arteritis. Acute neurologic problems were observed in 51 of 166 patients with biopsy-proven giant cell arteritis.[136] This group excluded patients with opthalmologic problems and large artery abnormalities on physical examination. Of these 51 patients, 23 had peripheral neuropathies and 12 had transient ischemic attacks or strokes related to carotid or vertebral artery involvement. A multitude of neurologic manifestations can be seen when the vertebrobasilar artery system is involved, including ataxia, lateral medullary syndrome, hemianopsia, hearing loss, and dementia.

Instead of the classic symptoms of arteritis, patients may present with prominent constitutional symptoms, such as fever, weight loss, malaise, and depression. In a retrospective study of 100 patients with biopsy-proven temporal arteritis, 15 fulfilled the criteria for fever of unknown origin.[138] In 11 of the 15 patients, manifestations suggesting giant cell arteritis were eventually recognized, but in 4 patients the giant cell arteritis was discovered only after a random temporal artery biopsy. Therefore, temporal artery biopsy must be considered strongly in an elderly patient who presents with fever or unexplained anemia.

The prognosis for giant cell arteritis is generally favorable once the condition has been recognized and treatment is under way. In most studies, the survival rate for patients with giant cell arteritis was found to be the same as for the general population of the same age. A recent follow-up study of the more than 200 patients in the 1990 American College of Rheumatology giant cell arteritis classification criteria cohort found survivorship to be virtually identical to that of the general population.[139] However, large artery involvement resulting in a fatal outcome does occur,[140] and a study from Sweden showed an increase in mortality during the first 4 months after diagnosis in 284 patients with biopsy-proven giant cell arteritis.[141] Thereafter, the death rate was equal to that of the general population. Fatal outcome was usually seen in patients who were insufficiently treated with corticosteroids. It is important that all patients with giant cell arteritis be examined carefully for large artery lesions, because early recognition and treatment may prevent arterial occlusion, rupture, and death.

Diagnostic Studies

Polymyalgia rheumatica and giant cell arteritis characteristically are associated with a very high erythrocyte sedimentation rate and elevation of other acute-phase reactants, such as C-reactive protein, fibrinogen, platelet count, and complement level. Westergren's sedimentation rate in giant cell arteritis is frequently more than 100 mm in 1 h. It should be appreciated that a normal sedimentation rate does not completely rule out a diagnosis of polymyalgia rheumatica. A subgroup of polymyalgia rheumatica with low sedimentation rate (<40 mm/h) at the initial presentation has been recognized over the past 15 years. The frequency of a normal sedimentation rate has varied between 7% and 20% in several retrospective studies. It is not clear whether patients in this subgroup have a more benign disease. The levels of C-reactive protein (CRP) increase and decrease more rapidly than does the erythrocyte sedimentation rate, and diagnostic specificity is enhanced by the use of CRP in conjunction with the sedimentation rate. The Mayo group has used IL-6 serum levels as a measure of disease activity in polymyalgia rheumatica and giant cell arteritis. A moderate normochromic, normocytic anemia is a characteristic finding. The leukocyte count is generally normal. Abnormal liver function tests, especially elevation of alkaline phosphatase, are present in one-third of the cases. Rates of positive rheumatoid factor and antinuclear antibody tests do not differ from those in control populations of elderly patients. Antithyroid antibodies are found in about 10% of the patients. The synovial fluid is mildly inflammatory, with a cell count between 1000 and 8000/mm[3], of which 40% to 50% are polymorphonuclear leukocytes. Synovial fluid complement level is normal. In patients with polymyalgia rheumatica, technetium-99[m] diphosphonate scintigrams show increased uptake in central joints, such as shoulders and hips.

The diagnosis of giant cell arteritis may be confirmed by superficial temporal artery biopsy, but because this condition is segmental and often has skip areas, it is necessary to remove a 2- to 3-cm segment of the artery and perform serial sections. If the first biopsy is normal, and suspicion of giant cell arteritis remains strong, a contralateral biopsy should be carried out. The posterior auricular or the occipital arteries may be chosen for biopsy when tenderness is marked along their distribution. Miniarteriography and Doppler flow studies have been used to locate a suitable area of the temporal artery for biopsy, but these methods are nonspecific and inconsistent and are not advocated for routine use. In patients with aortic arch syndrome, angiographic studies should be performed because temporal artery biopsy is not always diagnostic of giant cell arteritis. Angiographic features of arteritis include segments of smooth-walled constrictions, alternating with areas of normal caliber or aneurysmal dilatation, smooth-tapered occlusions of affected large arteries, and absence of irregular plaques and ulcerations. These lesions are characteristically found in the subclavian, axillary, and brachial arteries.

The need for temporal artery biopsy in all cases of polymyalgia is debatable. An acceptable course of action would be to follow carefully, without biopsy, those patients who show a rapid response to corticosteroid treatment in terms of symptomatic relief and normalization of the sedimentation rate. On the other hand, biopsy should be performed in cases where clinical evidence for giant cell arteritis is present. It is well recognized that symptoms of giant cell arteritis may occur suddenly in a patient who was originally thought to have pure polymyalgia and who is being treated with small doses of prednisone sufficient to control all symptoms of polymyalgia and to normalize the sedimentation rate.

Differential Diagnosis

When the typical clinical features of polymyalgia rheumatica occur in an elderly person, the diagnosis is usually easy. The clinical picture may at times be obscured by musculoskeletal symptoms related to underlying degenerative joint disease and neurologic conditions that are prevalent among the elderly. The differential diagnosis includes other inflammatory and noninflammatory rheumatic diseases, malignancy, and occult infections. About a quarter of patients with elderly-onset rheumatoid arthritis present with synovitis involving shoulder and hip, absence of rheumatoid nodules, an erythrocyte sedimentation rate greater than 50 mm/h, and a negative test for rheumatoid factor. This presentation resembles that of polymyalgia rheumatica, and it may not be until later in the course that a clear differentiation between the two can be made. Conversely, the occurrence of peripheral arthritis or carpal tunnel syndrome may pose diagnostic difficulties between polymyalgia rheumatica and elderly-onset seronegative rheumatoid arthritis. Associated peripheral manifestations of polymyalgia rheumatica respond dramatically to corticosteroid treatment. Any evidence of erosive arthropathy suggests an alternative diagnosis.

Polymyositis can be distinguished from polymyalgia rheumatica by its characteristic muscular weakness, elevated muscle enzymes, and abnormal electromyogram. Prolonged viremia or chronic bacterial infection, such as subacute bacterial endocarditis, may present with polymyalgia-like symptoms. The elevated sedimentation rate in polymyalgia rheumatica is helpful in differentiating noninflammatory rheumatic diseases, such as fibromyositis, tendonitis, and capsulitis. Patients with hyperparathyroidism or hypothyroidism may present with musculoskeletal symptoms that may be mistaken for polymyalgia rheumatica. One study found a higher prevalence of hypothyroidism (4.9%) and antithyroid antibodies (37 of 367 patients) in polymyalgia rheumatica and giant cell arteritis than in the general population.[142] Occult cancer may be associated symptoms similar to polymyalgia rheumatica. Search for malignancy should be considered if patients fail to improve clinically with corticosteroid treatment. These are several case report of polymyalgia rheumatica associated with malignancies, but compared with age- and sex-matched controls, the incidence of neoplasia does not appear to be increased.

The diagnosis of giant cell arteritis is not difficult in the presence of classic symptoms. It is important to keep this diagnosis in mind when an elderly patient presents with fever and marked constitutional symptoms. Likewise, it is important to recognize cases of giant cell arteritis with typical clinical features of the disease, but with a normal erythrocyte sedimentation rate, to prevent vascular catastrophies of untreated vasculitis. Patients with giant cell arteritis and a low sedimentation rate are more likely to have a history of polymyalgia rheumatica or to have received prior corticosteroid treatment.

Treatment

Pure polymyalgia rheumatica is best treated with 10 to 15 mg prednisone given in the morning. Usually, the patient obtains dramatic, symptomatic relief within a few days. A prompt response to corticosteroids can be regarded as additional confirmation of the diagnosis. In contrast, polymyalgia-like symptoms of a paraneoplastic syndrome respond poorly to corticosteroid treatment. Prednisone dosage should be slowly tapered in parallel with symptomatic relief and the decrease in the erythrocyte sedimentation rate or serum C-reactive protein. When the daily dose level has reached 10 mg, we recommend that further reduction be done in 1-mg decrements. Relapses accompanied by new elevation of the sedimentation rate are usually caused by too rapid reduction of corticosteroid dosage. In such a situation, prednisone dosage will have to be increased temporarily, and subsequent reductions may have to be made in smaller decrements at longer intervals. Polymyalgia rheumatica shows considerable variability in its course. Several studies have noted that patients differ in their initial response to prednisone as well as in their long-term steroid requirements,[143,144] a finding that suggests the existence of patient subsets differing in disease course and prognosis. In one study, patients treated with a defined schedule of prednisone could be subdivided into three groups on basis of clinical response and laboratory parameters.[144] An earlier study found two populations of patients, one with a self-limited illness requiring prednisone for 1 to 2 years, and another with a more persistent process requiring long-term therapy;[143] 40% of the patients in the latter group required treatment for more than 4 years.

A debate is ongoing in regard to the ideal initial dosage and the optimal tapering schedule. Mild cases of polymyalgia rheumatica have been treated with aspirin or nonsteroidal anti-inflammatory drugs, but the response has been less dramatic, and many patients initially treated in this way have had to be switched to prednisone. The risk of diabetes mellitus, vertebral fractures, and femoral neck fractures was found to be two to five times greater among patients with polymyalgia rheumatica compared with age- and sex-matched individuals. Other drugs such as methotrexate and azathioprine have been tried as corticosteroid-sparing agents, but the results have not been convincing. These drugs should be reserved for patients with severe comorbid conditions, such as uncontrolled diabetes mellitus or severe osteoporosis.

The manifestations of giant cell arteritis respond favorably to high-dose corticosteroid. Treatment should begin with 60 to 80 mg prednisone in divided daily doses. Constitutional symptoms resolve within 24 to 48 h after initiation of treatment. Localized symptoms of arteritis usually improve after 2 to 4 weeks. However, visual loss, once it occurs, is rarely reversible. In patients with threatening vascular complications, corticosteroid therapy should be initiated while awaiting arterial biopsy. Changes of inflammation of the arterial wall can be recognized for at least a week after corticosteroid treatment has been started. Once reversible symptoms have subsided and laboratory tests have reverted to normal, the dose of prednisone may be tapered slowly to a maintenance dose of 7.5 to 10 mg daily, with careful attention to readjustment of dosage if symptoms recur. Stepwise reduction of the corticosteroid dose should be done in decrements of 10%. Treatment should be continued for at least 2 years. In general, the prognosis is quite good with optimal corticosteroid treatment. Most patients achieve complete remission that is often maintained after withdrawal of treatment.

Patients should be made aware that adverse effects of corticosteroid treatment, including cushingoid appearance, symptomatic vertebral compression fractures, proximal muscle weakness, subcapsular cataracts, and, in patients with diabetes mellitus, increased insulin resistance, occur in one-third of the patients. Corticosteroids continue to be first-line therapy for giant cell arteritis. The addition of methotrexate with gradual tapering of corticosteroids is a reasonable alternative to reduce the potential adverse events seen with chronic administration of glucocorticoids. A recent study found methotrexate to be effective in the treatment of giant cell arteritis.[145] In this 2-year clinical trial to determine safety and efficacy of combined therapy with prednisone plus methotrexate versus prednisone alone, the group who was treated with combined therapy had fewer relapses (45%) compared with the group who received prednisone alone (84%).

Rheumatoid Arthritis

Rheumatoid arthritis (RA) is the most common inflammatory arthritis and second only to osteoarthritis as the most common type of arthritis. The disease affects about 1% of the adult population with a peak incidence between the 35th and 45th year; however, new onset of disease is not uncommon in older people. Several surveys have shown that the incidence of rheumatoid arthritis in the 60 or older age group amounts to 10% to 20% of the total population with RA. As a result of new cases being added to those carrying residua from prior onset, the prevalence of RA rises with age. The prevalence among 537 79-year-olds in Gothenburg, Sweden, was 10%.[146] Other surveys have found the prevalence to be even higher. In all age groups, women have the disease more often than men do. At any age, the disease needs to be diagnosed promptly and treatment started early as joint damage occurs early in the course of the disease, although in some patients there is continuous progression of joint damage.[147]

The disease is characterized by synovial thickening in the involved joints, and this soft tissue swelling can be readily palpated allowing diagnosis and separation from OA. Normal synovium is only one or two cell layers thick and cannot normally be appreciated on examination. In OA, bony overgrowth rather than soft tissue swelling causes the joint enlargement. The pattern of joint involvement in RA is quite different than in OA. There is usually sparing of the distal interphalangeal joints, and the axial skeleton, and wrist, elbow, and shoulder involvement is common in RA and uncommon in OA. However, it is very common to encounter OA in the older patient with RA because of the high prevalence of OA in this group as well as the increased prevalence of OA in previously damaged joints. In patients with earlier onset of RA, the articular disease may "burn out" in old age, but others have argued that once established the disease will likely require treatment for that patient's life-

time.[148] The disease can shorten the patient's life span and is a major cause of disability. Even disease that begins very late in life (median age, 73 years) is associated with marked increased morbidity and mortality compared to an age-matched general population.[149] It reduces the quality of life in almost all patients. On an optimistic note, there has been an explosion in successful treatment options in the past several years that has created an excitement among rheumatologists that has probably not been experienced since the disease was first named by Alfred Baring Garrod in 1876.

Epidemiology

Rheumatoid arthritis is present worldwide, but the incidence varies widely in different populations. Women are two- to threefold more likely than men to develop RA. The explanation for this has not been fully elucidated. Estrogen and pregnancy mitigates against the development of RA, and pregnancy improves the symptoms of RA in about 75% of patients. Postpartum flares of RA are common. Prolactin has a likely role in rheumatoid inflammation stimulating T-cell activity and promoting inflammation, with new evidence suggesting a paracrine effect of prolactin because of its production by T lymphocytes infiltrating synovium.[150] However, no consistent association between postmenopausal estrogen therapy and disease activity in RA has been demonstrated.[151] The phenotype of rheumatoid arthritis may be different in men and women. Erosive arthritis is more common in men, but structural consequences requiring joint surgery was more common in women. In one study, arthroplasties and arthrodesis of hand and foot joints were performed 34 times in women and once in men (the study had 110 women and 55 men with RA).[152] Nodules and rheumatoid lung disease were more common in men, and the sicca syndrome was more common in women.

There is a strong genetic basis for the development of rheumatoid arthritis. In most but not all populations, there is an association between the MHC class II HLA-DR1 and -DR4 genes and seropositive (rheumatoid factor-positive) RA. This HLA association influences the severity and persistence of the disease more than the absolute predisposition to the development of RA. A 5-amino-acid sequence is present in position 70 to 74 in the third hypervariable region of DR-beta-1 molecules that is present in the haplotypes associated with RA. HLA-DR molecules encode nonpolymorphic alpha (A) chains and polymorphic beta (B) chains. The subtypes of the beta chains of HLA-DR1 and -4 are now designated B1*0101, B1*0401, etc. Patients expressing two DR haplotypes carrying the shared epitope in position 70 to 74 have the highest risk of developing severe disease.

Etiology

Joints have unique qualities that may predispose them to damage in the presence of immune inflammation. The cartilage is avascular and has limited ability for repair. Chondrocytes are able to produce proinflammatory cytokines and toxic oxygen species when appropriately stimulated, leading to cell death and irreversible cartilage damage. Antigens that penetrate into the joint may be able to persist on cartilage for prolonged periods of time while inducing an inflammatory reaction that may be difficult to extinguish. There is a sense that once inflammation starts in the confines of the joint with release of self-antigens and persistence of the inciting antigen, it becomes self-sustaining. Once joint damage ensues, the joint may become unstable, leading to further joint deterioration.

The inflamed synovial membrane becomes infiltrated with activated lymphocytes and macrophages. Most investigations have focused on activated T lymphocytes, suggesting that presentation of antigen to effector T cells is involved in the pathogenesis of RA. However, B lymphocytes, mast cells, and especially macrophages are enriched in rheumatoid synovium and contribute to the soup of activated cells, chemokines, cytokines, lytic enzymes, etc., that makes up the pannus and synovial fluid.

Rheumatoid factors are autoantibodies, classically IgM but of any isotype, reacting to epitopes in the Fc portion of IgG. These autoantibodies may be present in the sera of patients with a variety of inflammatory diseases, and they are present in putatively normal subjects, especially those over the age of 60 years. However, in one recent study, the prevalence of rheumatoid factor was only increased in older subjects with chronic illnesses and not in healthy elderly subjects.[153] This finding raises the possibility that the presence of rheumatoid factor is related more to global health status than to the effects of aging. Rheumatoid factor, although not specific for RA, is nevertheless an important serologic test supporting a diagnosis of RA. Seropositivity is associated with more aggressive joint destruction, the presence of nodules, and extra-articular manifestations. Rheumatoid factors are prominent constituents of immune complexes, enhancing complement activation and influencing the processing of the complexes. Rheumatoid factor can interfere with phagocytosis of IgG complexes and directly activate natural killer cells.

Clinical Features

The clinical course and prognosis of RA in adults varies widely, ranging from a mild pauciarticular disease to a progressive destructive symmetric polyarthritis associated with systemic vasculitis. The pattern is influenced by sex, rapidity of onset, presence of rheumatoid factor, and genetic and endocrine factors. In general, patients whose sera contain high titers of rheumatoid factor fare less well. Insidious onset and slow progression are usual but sudden onset of RA occurs and the latter is generally associated with a better prognosis. Age is of significance, and when onset occurs before the age of 16 years, the difference in clinical presentation is recognized by its separate classification of juvenile rheumatoid arthritis. Changes in the pattern of disease in old age are less well recognized. Nevertheless, the few studies that have addressed onset of RA after age 60 have noted a greater frequency of acute onset, systemic symptoms, and large joint involvement, as well as less rheumatoid factor seropositivity, than in younger patients, and a better prognosis for seronegative elderly-onset rheumatoid arthritis.

Most elderly patients with RA have lived with their disease since youth or middle years. In many cases, the disease is no longer active, and the patient presents with functional deficits from deformities or with symptoms and signs of superimposed osteoarthritis. However, some patients continue to show evidence of active synovitis, or they develop serious extra-articular and systemic complications such as vasculitis presenting as skin ulcers or mononeuritis multiplex.

When rheumatoid arthritis has its onset after the age of 60 years, the clinical picture conforms more often than not to the pattern seen in younger patients. Constitutional symptoms such as fatigue, weight loss, and generalized stiffness may precede or accompany the insidious onset of arthritis in the small joints of hands and feet, wrists, and knees. Symmetric swelling of the second and third metacarpophalangeal joints (MCP), fusiform swelling of the fingers, and prolonged morning stiffness of the inflamed joints are characteristic. Later, arthritis may spread to involve more central joints. As the disease progresses, erosions of bone of the MCP and PIP joints, the wrists, and the metatarsophalangeal (MTP) joints become visible on radiographic examination. Progressive joint damage leads to the development of characteristic deformities. This presentation is usually associated with rheumatoid factor positivity, and rheumatoid nodules are seen in approximately 25% of the patients. Unlike early-onset RA, vasculitis is uncommon in RA that has its onset in later years. A retrospective review of the natural history and clinical features of RA in 129 patients with onset after age 60 years had some disquieting findings.[154] Forty-eight patients had abrupt onset, with illness occurring in less than 2 months; 69 had indolent onset, with illness occurring from 2 to 6 months; and 12 had a polymyalgia rheumatica-like syndrome. Of the 129 patients, 91% were rheumatoid factor positive, and 83% had erosive disease. Secondary Sjögren's syndrome was present in 63% of the patients. Most of the patients had progressive erosive joint disease. Over the 6-year follow-up period, there were eight deaths, three directly attributable to active RA.

Several medical reports indicate that about a quarter of patients with elderly-onset RA (EORA) exhibit a clinical picture that is less often seen in younger age groups. This subgroup is characterized by the acute and florid onset of arthritis, early and more severe involvement of large joints, especially the shoulder joint, prominent constitutional symptoms, very high sedimentation rates, and a near equal sex distribution.[154] Three small studies that included a younger onset rheumatoid arthritis (YORA) group for direct comparison[155–157] found abrupt onset arthritis occurred nearly twice as often in the EORA group.[157] Younger patients were twice as likely to have small joint disease, whereas elderly patients tended to have more arthritis in hips and shoulders. Patients with EORA had a higher initial sedimentation rate and were more likely to be negative for rheumatoid factor. A polymyalgia rheumatica-like presentation was observed in 23% of the EORA group, compared with only 5% of the YORA group. Both groups received nearly identical treatment. Patients with EORA had significantly better outcomes than younger patients after a disease duration of 2.5 years and at the end of the study, some 5 years after disease onset. These outcome differences persisted when patients with polymyalgia-like presentations were excluded from the analysis.

Although RA is often associated with systemic features and extra-articular organ involvement, it is first and foremost an arthritis, characterized by synovial thickening and inflammation. Some patients, especially those with rheumatoid factor and those with more severe disease, have nodules that are prominent over pressure sites such as the forearm. These patients more often experience extra-articular inflammation such as rheumatoid lung disease. Morning stiffness that represents pain with joint motion may last for hours and often makes morning activities of daily living very difficult to perform. Hand involvement is the bellwether of the disease. Foot involvement usually mirrors the hand arthritis. Flexion contractures can develop early, although in the wrist it is the loss of extension that may occur rapidly and contribute to hand weakness. The subtalar joint, the joint that provides inversion and eversion of the foot, is often involved with inflammation early in the disease, and limited motion commences quickly. Fatigue is common.

Atlantoaxial subluxation happens frequently in patients with chronic RA. The odontoid process is normally surrounded by synovium, and as this synovium proliferates, it can rupture the transverse ligament that normally keeps the odontoid process snug to the posterior portion of C1. Over time, the odontoid shifts becomes more posterior in position as C1 slips forward on C2, with the odontoid compressing the cervical cord.

Pyramidal tract findings may be detected on examination. Deep tendon reflexes usually decrease with age, but with high cord compression, the reflexes may be hyperactive and Hoffman's sign may be positive and the toes upgoing with the Babinski maneuver. Remembering the possibility of atlantoaxial subluxation is important if neck manipulation is planned, for instance, when inducing general anesthesia or with physical therapy or chiropractic treatment. It is also important to remember that older patients with "burnt-out" RA can harbor asymptomatic atlantoaxial subluxation that may become symptomatic with manipulation. Plain cervical spine radiographs in flexion and extension usually detect the cervical instability and atlantoaxial subluxation, although MRI best demonstrates the cervical cord compression.

The joint fluid is always inflammatory in RA and has a predominance of neutrophils on examination. Anemia is common, and the acute-phase reactant proteins are usually elevated. Renal and liver involvement are uncommon, although the medications used to treat RA can induce abnormalities in those organs. Pulmonary involvement occurs more frequently than renal or liver involvement and can have a variety of manifestations that include interstitial fibrosis and pleural inflammation. Cardiovascular disease may be more common in RA and is a cause of 40% of the increased mortality seen in the disease.[158,159] Male sex, rheumatoid factor positivity, and late age of RA onset predicted premature death due to cardiovascular disease.[160]

Differential Diagnosis

Rheumatoid arthritis is usually easy to diagnose at the bedside, but symmetric small joint synovitis may be seen in other diseases. Systemic lupus erythematosus with predominantly joint involvement and polymyalgia rheumatica may be difficult to differentiate from early RA. Even sarcoid and certain viral infections can mimic early RA. However, once RA is established, the disease is quite unique having exuberant pannus formation, nodules, and characteristic hand changes including prominent ulnar deviation of the fingers.

The clinical overlap between RA, especially seronegative disease, and polymyalgia rheumatica can be quite striking.[161] When a patient presents with constitutional symptoms, marked shoulder synovitis, and a high erythrocyte sedimentation rate (ESR), it is often difficult to differentiate polymyalgia rheumatica (PMR) from EORA. The two diseases have many manifestations in common. PMR is usually an axial synovitis, primarily of hips and shoulders, but peripheral synovitis is seen in a third of the patients, most frequently involving knees, wrists, carpal tunnels, and metacarpophalangeal joints. It is not unusual to diagnose polymyalgia rheumatica and find the disease "progressing" to RA as the arthritis persists.[162] The difficulty in separating these two diseases poses a challenge to geriatricians and rheumatologists.

Amyloid arthropathy may be mistaken for RA. Primary amyloid and that which occurs in association with multiple myeloma may infiltrate the synovium of joints and periarticular structures, causing joint swelling and sometimes carpal tunnel syndrome. Prolonged morning stiffness is not a feature of amyloid arthritis. Other conditions that need to be excluded include erosive osteoarthritis of the hands, polyarticular gout and other crystal diseases, and cancer-related syndromes, including pulmonary osteoarthropathy.

Treatment

The treatment of a chronic disease of unknown etiology can be difficult. However, a standardized approach to the treatment of RA has become generally accepted although there is wide latitude about the timing and type of medication use. Early diagnosis is extremely important because significant joint damage occurs early in RA. The treatment of RA arising de novo in the elderly follows the same guidelines as in younger patients. The main objectives are to reduce or suppress inflammation, relieve pain, and preserve muscle and joint function. Appropriate drug treatment in concert with systemic and local rest, good nutrition, physical and occupational therapy, use of appropriate appliances and special equipment, and orthopedic evaluation and corrective surgery are the mainstays of the management program. Every patient with RA should have a physical exercise program tailored for optimum activity and rest. Patients must learn that both excessive rest and excessive exercise can lead to increased joint stress. Prescribed individual exercises alternating with specific rest periods are required to maintain good muscle tone and avoid fatigue.

Treatment is needed at every stage of the disease. Patient education and effective communication between the medical and nursing personnel and the patient and family are crucial. Physical and occupational therapies are needed in most patients.

Drug Treatment

Three major classes of drugs are available in the treatment of rheumatoid arthritis: nonsteroidal anti-inflammatory drugs, corticosteroids, and disease-modifying drugs. Until recently, it was customary to start a patient with newly diagnosed rheumatoid arthritis on aspirin or one of the newer NSAIDs. These drugs are quick in their action, provide symptomatic relief, and often reduce joint swelling, but they do not prevent progression of rheumatoid arthritis. Because there is only a narrow window between disease onset and the beginning of irreversible joint destruction, a more vigorous approach to treatment is essential. In recent years, several new disease-modifying drugs with proven and prompt efficacy in the majority of patients have been added to the treatment armamentarium. These drugs have not been studied extensively in the elderly, and their interactions with other medications and concurrent illnesses have also not been well studied.

The cautious use of NSAIDs and the new selective cyclooxygenase inhibitors has been discussed under osteoarthritis. A key difference in treating RA is that to obtain the anti-inflammatory effect of NSAIDs they must be administered in a higher dosage than is required for relief of pain. The principles guiding the use of these drugs in the older patient with inflammatory arthritis dictate that the starting dose should be low, that adjustments are made stepwise until optimal therapeutic response is obtained, and that the maximum tolerated dose may well be lower than that for younger individuals. Physiologic changes that occur with aging may profoundly alter patient response to therapy. Most NSAIDs are bound to plasma proteins. In elderly patients with low serum albumin concentration and in patients who are treated with other drugs that bind to plasma proteins, concomitant treatment with an NSAID may require a reduction in its dose. Drug interactions are more likely in the elderly, who frequently take multiple medications. Potential drug interactions of NSAIDs with some of the most commonly used drugs in the elderly (anticoagulants, hypoglycemic drugs, digoxin, antihypertensives, and diuretics) should be kept in mind.

Most patients who develop joint erosions do so within 2 years of onset of joint symptoms. It is important to identify these patients early on in the course of RA. The indications for commencing second-line or disease-modifying antirheumatic drugs (DMARDs) are not different in elderly patients. Experience to date suggests that second-line drugs are as effective in the older age groups as in younger patients but that the elderly are at increased risk of developing adverse effects, in part as a consequence of altered pharmacokinetics and reduced functional reserve of organ systems. In the study of late-onset RA, 77% of the patients required continued use of disease-modifying drugs to maintain disease control.[154] Overall, methotrexate was the most efficacious second-line drug in EORA, with clinical improvement being noted in 33 of 37 cases.

Methotrexate

Methotrexate has become the drug treatment of choice of rheumatoid arthritis in patients with progressive disease and disease that is or likely will be destructive. It is administered in pulse fashion, usually orally once weekly in divided doses, with 7.5mg being the current standard starting dose. In the elderly, starting at lower doses may reduce the incidence of stomatitis and gastrointestinal symptoms. We prescribe daily folic acid (1 mg) as it likely reduces some of the gastrointestinal and hepatic side effects. Liver and bone marrow monitoring should be performed bimonthly, and renal function should be assessed periodically. In patients with diabetes mellitus or heart disease, renal testing should be more frequent. Methotrexate is almost completely cleared by the kidney and should not be used in patients with renal insufficiency. The original concern with methotrexate use in RA was with its liver toxicity; that complication has proved uncommon with pulse use as just described, although regular liver testing is recommended. Hypersensitivity reactions involving the lungs are uncommon although often serious. If cough or shortness of breath develops in patients receiving methotrexate, drug cessation and complete evaluation of the patient for causation are warranted.

Hydroxychloroquine, Sulfasalazine, and Minocycline

Hydroxychloroquine has been used to treat inflammatory arthritis for many years. The drug is safe but generally less effective than the other disease-modifying medications. There is concern about retinal toxicity after long-term use, although that is uncommon. Ophthalmologic evaluations should be performed twice yearly. Skin rash occurs occasionally and can be severe. Hydroxychloroquine is most often used early in the course of mild RA and in combination with other medications (see following). The dose is 200 mg twice daily, often reduced to 200 mg daily when a good response has been obtained. We never hesitate to use it in older patients, even those with ophthalmologic disorders, but always in consultation with ophthalmologists.

Sulfasalazine has been used to treat RA since the 1940s. It is more widely used in Europe than in the United States, where it is often used in combination with methotrexate and hydroxychloroquine. We start with 1.0 g daily and increase the dosage slowly to 3.0 g daily in older patients. Sulfa allergy needs to be excluded before its use. Extra fluids need to be administered to prevent renal stones, and serial blood testing monitoring the bone marrow and liver should be performed.

Minocycline is another modestly effective disease-modifying drug that can slow the progression of RA.[163]

Newer Agents

Tumor Necrosis Factor Inhibitors. It appears that the cytokine TNF plays a central role in chronic inflammation. Early on after its identification, TNF was thought to primarily play a role in defending the body from gram-negative infections; it is produced by macrophages and activated T lymphocytes and is found in excess in rheumatoid arthritis and other inflammatory states. TNF stimulates the production of other proinflammatory cytokines, activates neutrophils and endothelial cells, is a pyrogen, and at higher levels causes cachexia and even hypotension and decreased cardiac contractility. Receptors for TNF are present on almost all cells.

Two biologic agents are available to decrease TNF-α. Etanercept is the soluble recombinant receptor protein for the p75 TNF-α protein combined with immunoglobulin G. This agent is self-injected subcutaneously twice weekly. Infliximab is a recombinant humanized antibody to TNF. It is administered intravenously on a regular schedule and has been successfully used in the treatment of Crohn's disease and for its complications of fistula formation. Both drugs, when administered concomitantly with methotrexate, are setting new standards for effectiveness in suppressing the inflammation in rheumatoid arthritis and delaying or stopping the progression of x-ray changes. Etanercept has recently been approved for use alone after being studied as the sole disease-modifying agent in early RA. Both etanercept and infliximab work quickly and to date are associated with few side effects. There is, however, great concern about the patient's ability to handle bacterial infections with their chronic use. As of now, the benefits of this therapy seem to greatly outweigh this concern. The medications should be stopped when infection is present.

Leflunomide. Leflunomide is a reversible inhibitor of dihydroorotate dehydrogenase, a key enzyme in pyrimidine synthesis.[164] It provides a novel approach to the treatment of RA and may be as effective as methotrexate. It has also been used in combination with methotrexate. The drug can cause diarrhea, hair loss, and elevation of liver enzymes.

Azathioprine. Azathioprine should be restricted to patients with severe, active, and erosive disease that has not responded to other DMARDs. The initial dose should be approximately 1.0 mg/kg. Therapeutic response usually occurs after 6 to 8 weeks of treatment. The dose may be increased after several weeks if there are no toxicities and the initial response is suboptimal. Dose increments should be 0.5 mg/kg daily up to a maximum dose of 2.0 mg/kg/day. Patients who have no improvement after 12 weeks should be considered refractory.

Corticosteroids. The use of high-dose corticosteroids administered orally or parenterally in RA can be lifesaving in elderly patients with serious systemic complications such as vasculitis. In smaller doses, corticosteroids are helpful in maintaining mobility and reducing long-term disability. This beneficial effect of corticosteroids is particularly useful in the elderly who may have other conditions affecting ambulation and for whom superimposed RA might become the final event leading to a sedentary existence. The ability to remain ambulatory and active will generally offset the risk of osteoporosis and compression fracture due to steroid therapy. From a purely practical standpoint, the ease of administration, low cost, and relative safety of low doses make corticosteroids a reasonable alternative for the elderly with persistent disabling systemic manifestations refractory to other therapeutic modalities. The recommended dose is 5 to 10 mg of prednisone given once daily in the morning. Alternate-day regimens are usually not effective in RA. Prednisone also is useful as a therapeutic bridge between aspirin and other nonsteroidal anti-inflammatory drugs and the DMARDs, which may not become effective for several months. Finally, it is reasonable to treat the subgroup of elderly-onset RA with constitutional symptoms and proximal joint involvement in the same way as one would polymyalgia rheumatica, that is, an initial dose of prednisone of 10 to 15 mg/day. As constitutional symptoms subside and the erythrocyte sedimentation rate falls, prednisone is tapered slowly to the lowest dose that will control symptoms. The side effects of corticosteroids are legion. Adverse reactions that pertain particularly to the elderly include compression fractures, osteonecrosis, skin changes of steroid atrophy and purpura, electrolyte disturbances and fluid retention, glaucoma, and increased risk of sepsis. Osteoporosis, however, can be preempted in part with the concomitant use of bisphosphonate medications.[165]

Combination Therapy

Most patients with rheumatoid arthritis respond best to a combination of drugs. It is usual in the United States to combine low doses of prednisone with initial treatment of RA. Reduction of the drug should start when the disease improves or stabilizes. The addition of hydroxychloroquine and sulfasalazine to methotrexate is frequently employed in patients not responding to methotrexate alone. Today, we more often add etanercept or infliximab to methotrexate if the RA is progressing or not adequately suppressed. We are using leflunomide in recalcitrant disease, often in combination with the medications already mentioned.

The potential oncogenic effects of immunosuppressive drugs have been assessed. Even in the absence of immunosuppressive treatment, patients with rheumatoid arthritis have a twofold increased risk of developing non-Hodgkin's lymphoma. This risk increases in patients treated with azathioprine or cyclophosphamide.

Intra-articular injection of "depot" corticosteroids is a useful adjunct for synovitis limited to a few joints. Repeat injections into the same joint can be associated with necrosis and collapse of bone. For this reason, injections into one joint should be spaced not less than 3 months apart, and no joint should be injected repeatedly.

Prognosis

Rheumatoid arthritis is not thought of as a fatal disease. Nonetheless, these patients have a reduced life expectancy. Patients with a more severe disease at baseline, manifested by many involved joints and poor functional status, are those at greatest risk of premature death. Most patients die of the same causes as the general population but at an earlier age. Patients with RA have an increased susceptibility to bacterial infections, and all studies have shown an increased death rate from infections. In a carefully conducted study of more than 1000 patients with RA in the Canadian province of Saskatchewan, Mitchell et al. identified 233 deaths over a mean period of 12 years, 79 more than expected in a matched control population.[166] Survival in rheumatoid arthritis was diminished by 4 years in men and by 10 years in women. Of the 79 excess deaths, 18 were caused by infection, particularly pneumonia and sepsis; 20 were directly related to rheumatoid arthritis, including vasculitis, rheumatoid lung disease, and cervical subluxation, whereas 8 could be attributed to complications of drug therapy, mainly gastrointestinal bleeding and perforation. Only 1 death was caused by drug-induced blood dyscrasia. Amyloidosis and renal failure appear to cause death in rheumatoid arthritis patients four to five times more frequently in Finland than in North America.[167]

Conclusion

The diagnosis and treatment of rheumatoid arthritis should be made in concert with a rheumatologist. In the elderly, concomitant osteoarthritis can cloud the physical findings of RA, and the similarity of early RA and systemic lupus erythematosus and polymyalgia rheumatica can be striking. Treatment should be appropriately aggressive with awareness of all the complicating features of aging and diseases that occur with older age. Modification of medication regimes should always be considered. Lower doses of drugs and less frequent administration of the tumor necrosis factor antagonists may be needed in many older patients. Laboratory testing for possible drug side effects may have to be performed more often than customary in selected older patients. Close collaboration between the primary care physician, the geriatrician, the rheumatologist, and the patient will provide for the best treatment decisions.

Sjögren's Syndrome

Introduction and Demographics

It is common to attend an older patient with complaints of mucosal dryness. Tears and saliva decrease with age, although salivary and presumably lacrimal gland function is well preserved in the healthy older population. Saliva does become thicker and more viscous with aging. Medications that patients take for concurrent medical disorders are frequently associated with mucosal dryness. The diuretic, antihistamine, antidepressant, anticholinergic, and beta-blocker medications are especially associated with dryness of the oral, nasal, and eye mucosal surfaces. Chronic mouth breathing can diminish saliva, as can many systemic illnesses such as diabetes mellitus because of autonomic neuropathy and renal insufficiency. Approximately 27% of individuals aged 65 to 84 years report dry eye or dry mouth symptoms to be present often or all the time.[168]

Sjögren's syndrome, a frequently underdiagnosed autoimmune disorder, should be considered in patients presenting with the sicca complex (xerophthalmia and xerostomia), especially if systemic features of illness are present.[168] Sjögren's syndrome, estimated to be the second most common autoimmune rheumatic disease after rheumatoid arthritis, affects about 2% of the adult population. This disorder may occur alone (primary Sjögren's syndrome) or in association with other autoimmune diseases, primarily rheumatoid arthritis and systemic lupus erythematosus. Secondary Sjögren's syndrome parallels the age distribution of the associated diseases whereas primary Sjögren's syndrome predominates in the older age group. More than 90% of the patients are women. Age does not modify the clinical picture; however, it does complicate the diagnosis because of the common complaint of dryness in older patients.

Henrik Sjögren was a Swedish ophthalmologist who described the syndrome bearing his name in 1933. He reported 19 adult women with sicca symptoms and systemic manifestations of illness, especially arthritis, and emphasized the systemic nature of the illness. The illness is worldwide in distribution and runs the gamut from simple xerostomia to systemic features including brain and peripheral nerve inflammation.

Pathogenesis

Sjögren's syndrome occurs more frequently in families than would be expected. There is an association between the disease and the major histocompatibility haplotype HLA-DR3 in Caucasians. There are different associations with the major histocompatability locus in different ethnic populations. These differences may reflect influences on autoantibody production rather than disease susceptibility. The underlying process is a lymphocyte-mediated destruction of exocrine glands that leads to diminished or absent glandular secretions and mucosal dryness. Biopsies of salivary and lacrimal tissue reveal damaged acini and lymphoid infiltrates with a predominance of CD4+ T-helper cells. B-cell activation accounts for the local production of immunoglobulin and autoantibodies, including rheumatoid factor. Blocked apoptosis may be present in the lymphocytes residing in the salivary gland periductal aggregates,[169] and the activated T cells may induce apoptosis of the acinar cells.[170] In addition to lacrimal and salivary glands, other exocrine glands may be affected. In about a quarter of the patients, there is evidence of extension of lymphoproliferation to extraglandular sites, such as lymph nodes, lung, kidney, the central nervous system, and bone marrow. The lymphoid infiltrates may be benign or malignant. The term pseudolymphoma describes tumor-like clusters of lymphoid cells that do not meet the histologic criteria for malignancy. In the kidney, the histopathologic lesion is interstitial lymphocytic infiltration with tubular atrophy and fibrosis, which clinically presents as hyposthenuria and renal tubular acidosis. Involvement of the lungs leads to diffuse interstitial pneumonitis or fibrosis. There is an association between Sjögren's syndrome and lymphoma, especially lymphomas of mucosa-associated lymphoid tissue.

Clinical Presentation

Xerostomia and xerophthalmia are the most common complaints in patients with Sjögren's syndrome. Many patients present with other manifestations of the disease such as arthritis or neurologic abnormalities ranging from peripheral neuropathy to central nervous system involvement. In patients with primary Sjögren's syndrome, Raynaud's phenomenon and a nondeforming, nonerosive polyarthritis are the most common extraglandular manifestations. Sjögren's syndrome should be considered in any elderly patient with unexplained systemic features, even disorders as common as peripheral neuropathy. Asking patients about oral or lacrimal dryness or a gritty sensation in the eyes may elicit the clues that will help make the diagnosis. The lack of saliva pooling under the tongue and obvious nasal and lacrimal dryness are usually present on examination. A parched tongue on examination, complaints of fatigue, and interruptions of the patient's narrative history by frequent drinking of water may also be clues to the diagnosis. Dry skin due to immunologic injury of the exocrine glands is a common complaint. The dry throat, nose, and trachea lead to a chronic nonproductive cough and hoarseness. Upper gastrointestinal involvement may cause dysphagia and atrophic gastritis with achlorhydria. Vaginal involvement causes dyspareunia and pruritus. Pulmonary and renal involvement with inflammation are common occurrences, leading to shortness of breath and cough and hyposthenuria and mild renal insufficiency, respectively.

Neurologic manifestations are common and protean. Peripheral nervous system involvement with sensory neuropathy are most common, followed by cranial nerve palsies, especially trigeminal sensory neuropathy. Carpal tunnel manifestations may be seen in many patients. In some small studies, the majority of patients were found to have neurologic deficits.[171,172] Spinal cord involvement can result in neurogenic bladder and paraparesis secondary to transverse myelitis or chronic progressive myelopathy. Central nervous system involvement is more difficult to assess. Focal high dense cerebral white matters lesions are seen on MRI examinations,[173] and Sjögren's patients may present with chronic or acute CNS disturbances ranging from cognitive loss and depression to strokes and neurologic findings mimicking multiple sclerosis.

About 20% of patients with primary Sjögren's syndrome develop vasculitis, which presents with purpura and other cutaneous manifestations, myositis, or mononeuritis multiplex. Histopathologic studies have shown this to be mononuclear cell or less often a neutrophilic vasculitis. A strong association exists between vasculitis and active CNS disease. An immune complex glomerulonephritis has also been reported.

Diagnosis

Sjögren's syndrome is more common than previous estimates. This diagnosis should be considered in elderly patients with unexplained neuropsychiatric dysfunction, interstitial lung disease, or polyarthritis. Patients with Sjögren's syndrome can fall anywhere along a spectrum ranging from benign sicca syndrome with local involvement of exocrine glands to extracellular spread of benign lymphoproliferation and symptoms secondary to various organ involvement. Lymphoreticular malignancy may occur.

The combination of sicca symptoms, systemic illness, and abnormal laboratory testing will establish the diagnosis in most patients. Saliva production can usually be assessed by visual inspection. The Schirmer test is easily performed at the bedside. If the Whatman no. 41 filter paper hanging from the lower conjunctival sac has less than 5 mm of wetting within 5 min, it is considered abnormal. Other important diagnostic aids in the sicca syndrome are rose bengal or fluorescein staining of the cornea to document filamentary keratitis. However, dryness does not always mean the presence of Sjögren's syndrome, as xerophthalmia has a wide diagnostic base (see following). Laboratory testing for inflammation (the Westergren sedimentation rate, C-reactive protein, nor-

TABLE 42.3. Serologic laboratory testing for Sjögren's syndrome.

Antinuclear antibodies (ANA): almost always positive
Rheumatoid factor: 60%–80% of patients
Cryoglobulins: 15% of patients
Antineutrophil cytoplasmic antibodies (ANCA): approximately 11%, especially in cutaneous vasculitis and peripheral neuropathy
Anti-Ro/SS-A[a]: found in 50%–80% of patients with primary disease
Anti-La/SS-A[a]: found in 30%–60% of patients with primary disease

[a]These antibodies are not specific for Sjögren's syndrome; they can be present in systemic lupus erythematosus, are almost always present in subacute cutaneous lupus, and are found in other autoimmune disorders.

mocytic, and normochromic anemia) is usually abnormal. Rheumatoid factor may also be positive. The incidence of anti-Ro(SS-A) and anti-La(SS-B) antibodies is very high and serves as a reliable diagnostic marker for Sjögren's syndrome in its primary form or when it occurs in association with systemic lupus erythematosus (Table 42.3). Lip or gingival biopsy may allow for a specific diagnosis. The findings of focal lymphocytic sialadenitis in the minor salivary glands can establish the diagnosis and provide a rough estimation about the severity of the disease. Parotid gland biopsy can be performed in selected patients who have parotid gland enlargement. Salivary gland enlargement can sometimes be difficult to assess because of the commonly seen benign enlargement caused by adipose cell infiltration in older patients. The cerebrospinal fluid findings in CNS disease may include a mild mononuclear cell pleocytosis, elevated total protein and IgG, and oligoclonal bands on agarose gel electrophoresis. In contrast to multiple sclerosis, which usually has between 2 and 10 bands, patients with Sjögren's syndrome generally have only 1 or 2 bands.

Prognosis and Treatment

The course of Sjögren's syndrome is variable. Many patients just need treatment and advice regarding the sicca symptoms, but others will have life-threatening vasculitis and neuropathy that require intervention with major medications. There is always a concern about the development of lymphoma. In one study, there was increased risk for the development of lymphoma in patients with swollen salivary glands, lymphadenopathy, and leg ulcers.[174] In three large series, lymphomas, usually of a non-Hodgkin's, B-cell type, were diagnosed in 2.3%, 4.7%, and 5.8% of the patients. The interval between the onset of symptoms of the sicca syndrome and the diagnosis of malignancy ranged from 18 months to 12 years. The development or progression of neuropathy has not been well defined and needs to await future studies.

The symptomatic treatment (there is no curative treatment) of Sjögren's syndrome include artificial tears and adequate oral intake. Consultation with an ophthalmologist and oral hygienist is mandatory. Local measures for relief of sicca symptoms include artificial tears for keratoconjunctivitis, oral lubricants containing a carboxymethyl cellulose base (Xero-lube, Saliva Substitute), and K-Y jelly for sicca vaginitis. Oral pilocarpine is effective in increasing saliva and is well tolerated, although excessive sweating is a common adverse effect. Recently, cevimeline, a cholinergic agonist that binds to muscarinic receptors, has been approved for use in Sjögren's syndrome. Hydroxychloroquine is used frequently by rheumatologists in the treatment of Sjögren's syndrome. The drug has proved to have salutary effects in other autoimmune diseases and may benefit some patients. There is reduction of erythrocyte sedimentation rates and other measures of inflammation.[175] Low-dose prednisone therapy increases saliva production,[176] but whether that improvement outweighs the deleterious effects of prednisone on the elderly patient remains to be determined.

Treatment of the vasculitis components of the disease includes use of all the major immunosuppressive and chemotherapy medications. Lymphoma is treated with the standard antitumor protocols.

Systemic Lupus Erythematosus

Systemic lupus erythematosus (SLE) is a distinctive chronic inflammatory disorder of unknown cause that can affect any tissue and organ but predominantly affects the skin, joints, and kidney. It is the prototype for the autoimmune diseases, representing a dysregulated immune system producing autoantibodies that can damage tissues. There are variants of lupus erythematosus that involve only the skin (discoid lupus erythematosus), or predominantly the skin (subacute cutaneous lupus erythematosus), or occur because of reactions to drugs (drug-induced lupus erythematosus). There are also disorders that overlap a variety of the autoimmune disorders, such as mixed connective tissue disease and undifferentiated connective tissue disease, the latter an entity that includes SLE-like clinical or laboratory findings but with overlap of other diseases making the exact diagnosis uncertain. The antiphospholipid syndrome has been better defined, and with its considerable overlap with SLE is discussed later.

The diagnosis of SLE in older patients may present a challenge to the geriatrician. Clinical findings may be subtle or unrepresentative of the "classic" lupus-like findings, and symptoms and signs of disease may suggest a variety of other illnesses or be as nonspecific as unexplained fever or arthralgia. Laboratory testing can be helpful in establishing a diagnosis but also can be confusing if interpreted incorrectly.

Demographics and Clinical Presentation

Lupus is mainly a disease of younger women, and the late development of SLE after menopause is not common (but it is not rare by any means). In established SLE, lupus flares are less frequent and less severe after menopause.[177] In unselected series, elderly-onset SLE comprises from 6% to 18% of the SLE population; however, SLE is often not considered in the differential diagnosis of a debilitating illness in an elderly patient. Several studies of "late-onset SLE" have addressed age-related differences in the clinical picture at onset, course, survival, and serologic characteristics.[178–182] In these studies, the division between "old" and "young" was set at either 50 or 55 years and defined either as onset of symptoms or time of clinical diagnosis. Difficulties in comparing these series arise from differences in geographic region, racial distribution, age-related entry, and case selection of a relatively small number of patients in each study. Despite these variances, there is convincing evidence that age modifies the clinical expression of SLE.

Most studies indicate that female predominance is less marked in elderly patients. One study found that the sex ratio between women and men was 2:1 in the older age group compared to 7:1 in younger patients.[183] The mean age at diagnosis was almost 10 years higher for white men than for white women, and almost one-half of white men were diagnosed at age 55 years and older. This difference in age of onset is thought to be related to hormonal factors. The clinical onset of SLE in older patients may be more insidious with less typical SLE manifestations, and an increased time interval between onset of symptoms and establishment of diagnosis is frequently reported.[180,184,185] In one series, the interval from onset of symptoms to time of diagnosis was 4 years when SLE developed after age 55 compared to 2 years in the younger age group.[180]

Age also influences the pattern of organ involvement. Severe renal disease, neurologic complications, mesenteric vasculitis, cutaneous vasculitis, Raynaud's phenomenon, and alopecia are less common in the older group, whereas polyserositis, especially as a presenting syndrome, interstitial lung disease, and peripheral neuropathy occur more commonly. Some authors have likened the expression of SLE in the elderly to the clinical picture of drug-induced lupus. Two studies have identified increased frequency of secondary Sjögren's syndrome and of antibodies to SS-A and SS-B in white patients with late-onset SLE.[180,181] These antibodies are found in approximately one-third of patients with SLE and in a much higher percentage of patients with primary Sjögren's syndrome. Cattogio et al. found that 38% of the patients who had onset of SLE after age 55 developed keratoconjunctivitis sicca, 88% had anti-SS-A antibodies, and 62% had anti-SS-B antibodies compared to only 36% in younger patients.[180]

Late-onset lupus is generally considered less severe.[186] This impression is partly based on the reduced steroid requirement in patients with older-onset SLE and the longer time lag between onset of symptoms and diagnosis. The perception of SLE being a more benign disease in older individuals may have to be revised in view of data on the survival of individuals with SLE. Studenski et al. could not show evidence of improved outcome with age.[183] These authors examined the effects of age, race, sex, and socio-economic status on clinical outcome and survival utilizing multivariate analytic techniques in 411 patients with SLE, almost equally divided between whites and blacks. Black race and low economic status had independent negative effects on survival. The authors suggested that previously reported findings of improved survival rate with age may have been confounded by racial differences in age and mortality; viz., if younger groups were heavily weighted with blacks and older age groups were weighted with whites, age would appear, incorrectly, to be related to improved survival in pooled groups. Comparing 102 patients with late-onet SLE with an early-onset group in a predominantly Chinese population, researchers found no differences in all major organ involvement as well as steroid requirements between the two groups.[184]

Fatigue and malaise are the most common symptoms of SLE. Arthritis and rash are the most common findings on physical examination, although the disease has such protean manifestations and presentations that almost any clinical abnormality can be due to SLE. The arthritis of SLE is similar in presentation to that of early RA. There is generally symmetric involvement of the small joints of the hand and the wrists. The distal interphalangial joints are usually spared, but in older patients those joints are typically abnormal from involvement with OA. Sjögren's syndrome is more common in the elderly patient, and sometimes separating the two disorders, SLE and Sjögren's, is difficult. In patients with the antiphospholipid syndrome, stroke, thrombophlebitis, or peripheral arterial occlusion can be early manifestations of the disease.

Younger women with SLE are 50 times more likely to develop a myocardial infarction in later life than women without SLE of the same age. Older age at lupus diagnosis, longer duration of corticosteroid use, hypercholesterolemia, and postmenopausal status are more common in women presenting with a cardiovascular event.[187] The implications of this problem are underrecognized and require added vigilance in older patients with a history of lupus for cardiovascular disease.

Pathogenesis

The immunologic basis of SLE is complex and multi-faceted. The pieces of the puzzle that include heredity, the role of hormones, age, immune complex injury, abnormalities in B and T cells, and apoptosis have not yet all been found or pieced together. Apoptosis has assumed an increasingly important role in the understanding of autoimmune disorders. The process of programmed cell death includes both the killing and removal of dead cells. Apoptotic cells are characterized by translocation of autoantigens such as nucleosomes (the only way to generate nucleosomes in vivo is by the process of apoptosis) to the surface of the cell—these antigens become the targets of autoantibody production. In mice, this process produces transient hypergammaglobulinemia, anti-DNA and anticardiolipin antibody production, and glomerular deposits of protein.[188] Sturfelt et al. suggested that complement deficiency enhances the pathogenic properties of the immune complexes generated by antibody production to the exposed antigens on the apoptotic cells.[189] They also speculated that the immune complex-induced injury accelerates apoptosis and enhances tissue damage. The apoptotic "waste" itself may serve as immunogens for the induction of autoreactive lymphocytes.[190] Abnormalities in the regulation of apoptotic cells can lead to a breakdown in tolerance.[191,192]

Laboratory Diagnosis

The laboratory testing for SLE is very helpful (Table 42.4; also see Table 42.3 for Sjögrens). The absence of antinuclear antibodies (ANA) makes the diagnosis unlikely, as ANAs are present in almost all patients with SLE. These autoantibodies may react with nucleoprotein, denatured and native DNA, Smith antigen, nuclear RNP, SS-A and SS-B antigens, histones, and other basic proteins. Most

TABLE 42.4. Laboratory testing for systemic lupus erythematosus (SLE).

1. Antibodies to nuclear antigens (ANA) are almost always positive. In "seronegative SLE" (no ANA), antibodies to SS-A may be present.
2. The speckled pattern of immunofluorescence is the most common pattern encountered in SLE.
3. The speckled pattern should be followed up with testing for antibodies to RNP (usually seen in mixed connective tissue disease), Smith (Sm), SS-A, and SS-B (the latter two are seen in both SLE and Sjögren's syndrome). The Sm antigen is extremely specific for SLE.
4. The homogenous pattern of immunofluorescence is seen in SLE and other illnesses such as rheumatoid arthritis and is the pattern usually encountered in drug-induced lupus erythematosus.
5. Antibodies to double-stranded DNA are usually specific for the diagnosis of SLE and are associated with kidney involvement. Rarely antibodies to double-stranded DNA can be seen in autoimmune liver disease.
6. Decreased levels of complement proteins are often found in active SLE but may be low in any immune complex disease, e.g., hepatitis B or C.

patients seen in a medicine clinic with positive antibodies to nuclear antigens do not have SLE. It can be demonstrated in 70% of patients with other autoimmune diseases in an assortment of other clinical entities, especially chronic inflammatory disorders involving the liver or lung, and be present in a low titer in about one-third of all "normal" elderly persons. False positivty increases with age. However, antibodies to double-stranded DNA and the Smith antigen are almost only found in SLE. Because antibodies to SS-A and SS-B are found with high frequency in elderly-onset SLE, they become useful in the diagnosis as well, although they cannot serologically distinguish SLE from primary Sjögren's syndrome. Antibodies to double-stranded (ds) DNA and to SS-A and SS-B do not occur with increased frequency in the normal elderly population. Some studies have reported a lower frequency of antibodies to ds DNA in elderly patients with SLE, but this has not been substantiated in other studies. Hypocomplementemia is more common in younger patients with SLE. In the extremely rare patient with SLE and a negative ANA, antibodies to SS-A or SS-B are usually present. Similar to any chronic disease, anemia, and elevation of acute-phase reactants are usual findings.

HLA-DR2 and -DR3 are weakly associated with SLE, HLA-DR2 occurring more frequently in young-onset SLE than in older-age onset and HLA-DR3 showing the reverse relationship. Further analysis has shown that the association between HLA phenotypes and antibodies to Ro and La are stronger than HLA correlation with SLE itself.[181] In fact, when SS-A and SS-B antibody populations were removed from a group of 113 white SLE patients, the frequencies of HLA-DR2 and -DR3 were similar to those in normal Caucasians. SLE is more common in African-Americans, Latinos, and Asians (especially Filipinos and Chinese). The HLA-DR2 haplotype is significantly increased among Chinese patients with SLE. The Caucasian allele of HLA-DR3 present in African-Americans may be a factor in the higher prevalence and apparent more aggressive nature of SLE in African-Americans.[193]

Drug-Induced Lupus

In contrast to idiopathic SLE, the incidence of drug-induced lupus (DIL) increases with age, in part reflecting the increased usage in the elderly of drugs that can produce a lupus-like syndrome. The incidence of DIL is probably decreasing from previous estimates of 50,000 cases, or 10% of all patients with SLE, because the two most responsible drugs, procainamide and hydralazine, are used far less frequently than they once were. More than 50 drugs have been reported to be associated with drug-induced autoimmunity or symptomatic lupus. Drug-induced autoimmunity refers to induction of ANA, which is much more common than symptomatic DIL.

Two categories of drugs can be recognized: an unambiguous group that includes procainamide, hydralazine, phenytoin, quinidine, isoniazid, methyldopa, and chlorpromazine; and an ambiguous group of drugs for which anecdotal reporting has suggested a possible association. Recently reported drugs in the latter category include sulfasalazine and carbamazepine,[194,195] although a prospective study of 200 patients with RA treated with sulfasalazine over 5 years showed no association.[196] Other drugs in this latter group include lovastatin and recombinant human interferon. Patients treated with the recombinant antibody to TNF-alpha, infliximab, have a relatively high incidence of generating ANA and ds DNA, and some of these patients develop clinical SLE. Drugs that induce lupus have widely dissimilar chemical features. The common denominator appears to depend on metabolic transformation to reactive metabolites that are cytotoxic. Jiang et al. have shown that the chemical transformation to reactive products requires the enzymatic action of myeloperoxidase in activated neutrophils and that the ability of drugs to induce lupus in vivo depends on their capacity to serve as substrates for myeloperoxidase in vitro.[197]

Procainamide and hydralazine pose the greatest risk of inducing both ANA and DIL. Use of procainamide will generate a positive ANA in 80% of the patients. About a quarter of this group will manifest clinical symptoms. Women are at greater risk of developing procainamide- and hydralazine-induced lupus. The male-to-female ratio of 2:1 in symptomatic procainamide-treated patients is accounted for by the disproportionate use of procainamide in men. Approximately one-fifth of patients treated with isoniazid, methyldopa, or chlorpromazine develop positive ANA during treatment, but the incidence of a lupus-like syndrome induced by these drugs is less than 1%.

To make a diagnosis of DIL, it is necessary to exclude preexisting SLE. Symptoms typically occur after several months or years of drug therapy. Antinuclear antibodies are invariably present and usually in the homogenous pattern. Following withdrawal of the offending drug, there should be rapid improvement in the clinical symptoms and a gradual fall in the antinuclear antibodies. The most common features of DIL include fever, myalgias, arthralgias, and polyserositis. CNS and renal involvement is highly unusual. Severe cytopenias, butterfly rash, discoid lesions, and mucosal ulcerations are observed less often than in idiopathic SLE. A strong association between acetylator phenotype and the incidence of autoantibodies and DIL has been noted for procainamide and hydralazine. ANA appear more quickly in slow acetylators, and clinical symptoms occur earlier and predominantly in patients with this phenotype. However, slow acetylator phenotype is not a general predisposing factor underlying autoimmunity, as indicated by a lack of association between acetylator phenotype and induction of ANA by isoniazid or by captopril, as well as in idiopathic SLE.

Antihistone antibodies occur in more than 90% of the DIL patients. Different drugs are associated with different antihistone profiles. Antihistone antibodies are not specific for DIL, as they are also found in idiopathic systemic lupus, although usually in a lower titer. Antibodies to denatured DNA are seen less often. Hypocomplementemia is rare in DIL, but in vivo complement activation can often be detected by measuring the cleavage products of C4.

The Antiphospholipid Antibody Syndrome

The antiphospholipid antibody syndrome has become a frequently diagnosed entity. It can be part of SLE, as approximately 25% of SLE patients have antibodies to phospholipid,[198] or the disease may exist alone or be associated with other autoimmune disorders. Historically it was seen in patients with SLE who had a false-positive test for syphilis or a prolonged partial thromboplastin time that was not corrected with normal serum (the lupus anticoagulant). Evaluation is now performed by the detection of antibodies to cardiolipin and beta$_2$ glycoprotein 1 as well as the lupus anticoagulant. It is of special importance to geriatricians as it is a cause of preventable arterial vascular disease, including cerebrovascular accidents. The syndrome is associated with heart valve lesions, including Libman–Sacks endocarditis, thrombocytopenia, lower extremity cutaneous ulcers, livedo reticularis, thrombophlebitis, and other disorders such as retinal thrombosis.[199] It is associated with recurrent fetal loss, and such history in an older woman with SLE should make the antiphospholipid syndrome suspect as an additional diagnosis.

The use of estrogen in SLE has always been controversial. Estrogen use is associated with thrombosis and reactivation of disease.[200] The combination of estrogen use and the antiphospholipid syndrome may pose additional risks for the occurrence of thrombosis and thus estrogen must be used with great caution.

Treatment

The management of SLE has become relatively uniform during the past 5 years. Basic measures such as rest and sun avoidance are needed in selected patients. The control of hypertension is important in maintaining renal function in patients with renal disease. There is concern about the routine use of nonsteroidal anti-inflammatory medications in patients because of resultant decreased renal blood flow. This result can be especially striking if there is preexisting renal insufficiency or cardiac failure. These drugs can all raise blood pressure in patients with renal insufficiency because of sodium retention. The antimalarial hydroxychloroquine is effective in the treatment of the arthritis and the rash of SLE. It may also be effective in preventing flares of disease.[201] (See hydroxychloroquine in the rheumatoid arthritis section.) Corticosteroids remain the drug of choice in treating patients with life-threatening illness, although the side effects of these medicines are magnified in older patients. High doses of corticosteroid are almost inevitably associated with deleterious events in the older patient. Osteoporosis, however, can be preempted in part with the concomitant use of a bisphosphonate medication.

Corticosteroid-sparing medication is used frequently and early in older patients with severe SLE. Azathioprine and methotrexate[202] can be very effective in allowing reduction of the corticosteroid. Cyclosporine may be effective as treatment in patients with or without renal disease,[203,204] and mycophenolate mofetil,[205] another transplant rejection drug, may be an important newer drug for the treatment of SLE. We are awaiting testing of some of the newer medications that have proved effective in rheumatoid arthritis, such as the tumor necrosis factor inhibitors and the pyrimidine antagonist leflunomide. Autologous stem cell transplantation may be useful in conventional treatment-resistant patients, although to date it is limited to experimental use and in younger patients.

Renal disease needs to be always suspected and assessed thoroughly in the older patient as it is in the younger SLE patient, and kidney biopsies should be performed if needed to help define the extent of the disease. Cyclophosphamide has remained the treatment of choice for diffuse proliferative glomerulonephritis. We have never withheld aggressive management for major organ involvement because of the patient's age. Renal transplantation in older patients with end-stage renal disease has been beneficial in selected patients. As in all the chronic diseases, consultation among specialists such as the nephrologist and rheumatologist will help the geriatrician and primary care doctor offer the best available treatment options to the patient.

Dermatomyositis and Polymyositis

Dermatomyositis and polymyositis are uncommon chronic idiopathic inflammatory disorders that affect muscle, skin, and other organs throughout the life span. The criterion for diagnosis include proximal symmetric muscle weakness, an elevated serum level of muscle enzyme, an abnormal electromyogram, an abnormal muscle biopsy, and characteristic rash for dermatomyositis (heliotrope rash and Gottron's papules). Dermatomyositis and polymyositis have long been considered to be accompanied by a higher incidence of malignancy than in the general population. The association is much stronger with dermatomyositis than polymyositis, and it increases with age. The rate of malignant disease in dermatomyositis in most population-based studies is reported at 20% to 25%.[206] Although patients with polymyositis have been found to have a slightly increased rate of cancer, the increase is not highly significant and may be related to a diagnostic suspicion bias causing a more aggressive search for cancer. In general, no unusual concentration of one type of cancer has been observed, although gynecologic malignancies, in particular ovarian carcinoma and rectal adenocarcinoma, are thought by some to be overrepresented.[207,208] The site of malignancy reflects the most common tumor types for any given age and sex, so that in the older population these would include breast, lung, ovary, colon, stomach, and uterus, in that order. The temporal relationship of malignancy and myositis is such that in about one-third of the cases myositis precedes the tumor by several years; in one-third, they occur concomitantly, and in another one-third myositis follows tumor by many years. Concurrent improvement of dermatomyositis with tumor therapy and relapse with recurrence of the tumor suggests a causal relationship. Because the association of dermatomyositis and cancer is high in the elderly, a search for cancer is justified in this age group. The most common malignancies occur in areas that can be evaluated by physical examination or fairly simple radiologic procedures such as chest x-ray and mammography. Finally, a lack of response of myositis to treatment with prednisone or other modalities should result in a more extensive search for malignancy.

Recent studies have found some important differences besides increased malignancies in older patients presenting with polymyositis and dermatomyositis. One study found that the lag time from onset of symptoms to diagnosis was significantly longer in older patients and that they tended to experience a more chronic form of the disease.[208] In another large retrospective study comparing younger and older patients, dysphagia with abnormal esophageal manometry as well as the incidence of bacterial pneumonia were significantly higher in the older group.[209]

Amyloidosis

Amyloidosis is a syndrome characterized by extracellular deposits of insoluble proteinaceous amyloid fibrils in tissues that result in pressure atrophy with dysfunction of the affected organs. Despite their very different protein components, all amyloid deposits have the following in common: fibrillar structure when examined by electron microscopy; a green birefringence when observed with Congo red stain under polarization microscopy; and an unusual beta pleated structure when examined by x-ray diffraction. The modern classification of amyloidosis is based on the biochemical composition of the amyloid fibrils. The fibrils of primary amyloidosis and of amyloidosis associated with multiple myeloma consist of portions of immunoglobulin light chains and are called AL. Amyloid deposits of secondary amyloidosis, associated with chronic inflammatory and infectious diseases, show immunochemical homology with portions of the acute-phase reactant serum amyloid A, and are called AA. In some of the familial forms of amyloidosis, such as AF, the fibrils are immunologically identical to prealbumin. Several different types of senile amyloid found in the heart and brain of elderly patients are designated AS. Amyloid deposits of endocrine origin (AEO), occurring in or adjacent to endocrine glands, are closely related to polypeptide hormones, their precursors or breakdown products.

Amyloidosis is relevant to rheumatic disease for two reasons: (1) it occurs as a potentially fatal complication of long-standing chronic inflammatory disease, such as RA; and (2) amyloid may be deposited in periarticular and synovial tissues, causing joint pain and restricted motion.

In secondary amyloidosis, deposits of amyloid AA accumulate predominantly in the kidneys, spleen, adrenal gland, and liver, resulting in dysfunction of the organs. Death as a consequence of amyloidosis, secondary to rheumatoid arthritis, is not uncommon in Europe. Although this type of amyloidosis is found at postmortem examination in 10% of RA cases in the United States, it is rarely of clinical significance.

Amyloid arthropathy is caused by deposition of amyloid AL and occurs, therefore, in multiple myeloma and in a disorder of immunoglobulin, previously known as primary amyloidosis. Amyloid arthropathy can affect any joint. Small and large joints are involved with equal frequency. When the small joints are involved, amyloidosis can be easily mistaken for RA, but joint inflammation is less conspicuous and the swelling distinctly firmer on palpation. Flexion contractures of the hand joints may appear early in the illness. Subcutaneous amyloid deposits may be mistaken for rheumatoid nodules. Amyloid arthropathy may present as massive deposition at an isolated site; an example is the so-called Hercules look, in which amyloid deposition in or around the shoulder joint produces the characteristic "shoulder pad sign." Occasionally, amyloidosis results in punched-out lytic lesions in bone; large tumefactions in bone may be complicated by pathologic fractures.

Synovial fluid analysis reveals a noninflammatory fluid with mononuclear cells predominating. Examination of centrifuged Congo red-stained sediment from synovial fluid under polarization microscopy may reveal the typical apple-green birefringence of amyloid fibrils.

Carpal tunnel syndrome occurs in approximately 25% of the cases. When elderly men present with idiopathic carpal tunnel syndrome, the possibility of amyloidosis should be entertained. The diagnostic yield from biopsy of the carpal ligament approaches 100%.

Progressive systemic sclerosis and polyarteritis nodosa have their peak onset earlier in life but may occur in the older age group. There are no data in the literature to support age-related modulation of the clinical expression of these diseases.

Paraneoplastic Syndromes

Certain musculoskeletal syndromes have a close temporal relationship to the onset of a malignancy. Hypertrophic pulmonary osteoarthropathy is perhaps the best known entity. This condition is most often associated with pleuropulmonary disease, in particular lung cancer and mesothelioma. The term pulmonary is somewhat misleading, because certain extrathoracic diseases such as nonneoplastic liver diseases and inflammatory bowel disease may be associated with hypertrophic osteoarthropathy.

The age distribution of hypertrophic pulmonary osteoarthropathy coincides with that of lung cancer, about one-half of which occurs above the age of 60 years. Approximately 10% of patients with lung cancer develop symptoms and signs of hypertrophic osteoarthropathy. Patients complain of pain in the ankles, knees, and wrists. On examination, the most conspicuous but also the least specific sign is clubbing of the fingers and toes. Diffuse periarticular tenderness is present on palpation, and knee effusion is not unusual. The skeletal symptoms may precede clinical manifestastions of lung cancer by many months. When this occurs, hypertrophic osteoarthropathy may be mistaken for RA. The diagnosis is confirmed by bone scan or x-ray examination, which demonstrates periostitis with subperiosteal new bone formation along the distal or proximal ends of long bones.

Carcinomatous polyarthritis is characterized by a close temporal relationship between onset of seronegative arthritis and the discovery of malignancy. Most cases occur in the elderly age group. Clinically, it has certain similarities with rheumatoid arthritis, but is less likely to be symmetric. The onset may be explosive or insidious. Characteristically, the arthropathy remits when the tumor has been resected and reappears with recurrence of the neoplasm. In contrast to hypertrophic pulmonary osteoarthropathy, the association with carcinomatous arthritis is not limited to intrathoracic solid tumors. Women with this syndrome have a high incidence of breast cancer. The association of palmar fasciitis and polyarthritis with ovarian carcinoma in postmenopausal women has been reported.[210] Because of prominent shoulder and hand involvement, this syndrome has a certain similarity to reflex sympathetic dystrophy; however, arthritis may involve elbows, wrists, knees, and ankles, joints that are not affected in reflex sympathetic dystrophy. Palmar fasciitis and tendon sheath thickening leading to flexion contractures of the fingers is a prominent feature.

A variety of miscellaneous musculoskeletal syndromes have been described as a manifestation of underlying malignancy. The Eaton–Lambert syndrome that commonly presents with weakness of the pelvic girdle musculature has a strong association with small cell carcinoma of the lung. Carcinomatous neuromyopathy is characterized by symmetric proximal muscular weakness out of proportion to the loss of muscle mass. Involvement of pelvic girdle muscles causes gait disturbances and difficulty in climbing stairs. These syndromes must be distinguished from polymyositis and polymyalgia rheumatica. The diagnosis is best established by electromyography.

Dermatomyositis/polymyositis that has a close temporal relationship in onset and a parallel course with a malignancy can be considered a paraneoplastic syndrome. Rarely, malignancy may present as a lupus-like syndrome. In at least some of these cases, autoantibodies are directed against nuclear antigens that are distinct from those recognized in patients with idiopathic SLE.[211]

Conclusion

Rheumatologic disease in older people, perhaps more than any other area of geriatrics, presents an opportunity to apply principles from two different disciplines in novel and exciting ways. The sheer numbers and vast amount of disability caused by rheumatic disease in older patients makes knowledge of these two fields important for physicians who care for this group of patients. Because of the nexus between these two fields, many rheumatologists have developed interest in geriatrics and many academic programs are now offering joint fellowships in geriatrics and rheumatology.

References

1. CDC. *MMWR (Morb Mortal Wkly Rep)*. 1999;48(17): 349–353.
2. Yetlin E, Callahan LF, for the National Arthritis Data Workgroup. The economic cost and social and psycho-

logical impact of musculoskeletal conditions. *Arthritis Rheum.* 1995;38:1351–1362.

3. Lawrence RC, Helmick CG, Arnett FC, et al. Estimates of prevalence of arthritis and selected musculoskeletal disorders in the United States. *Arthritis Rheum.* 1998;41: 778–799.

4. Stevens, MB. Connective tissue disease in the elderly. *Clin Rheum Dis.* 1986;12:11–32.

5. Nuki G. Osteoarthritis: a problem of joint failure. *Z Rheumatol.* 1999;58:142–147.

6. Felson DT, Naimark A, Anderson J, et al. The prevalence of knee osteoarthritis in the elderly: the Framingham Osteoarthritis Study. *Arthritis Rheum.* 1987;30:914–918.

7. Felson DT. The epidemiology of knee osteoarthritis: results from the Framingham study. *Semin Arthritis Rheum.* 1990;20:42–50.

8. Davis MA, Ettinger WH, Neuhaus JM. Obesity and osteoarthritis of the knee: evidence from the National Health and Nutrition Examination Survey (NHANES I). *Semin Arthritis Rheum.* 1990;20:34–41.

9. Creamer P, Lethbridge-Cejku M, Costa P, et al. The relationship of anxiety and depression with self-reported knee pain in the community: data from the Baltimore Longitudinal Study of Aging. *Arthritis Care Res.* 1999;12:3–7.

10. Hutton CW. Generalized osteoarthritis: an evolutionary problem? *Lancet.* 1987;1:1463–1465.

11. Jordan J, Luta G, Renner J, et al. Knee pain and knee osteoarthritis severity in self-reported task specific disability: the Johnson County Osteoarthritis Project. *J Rheum.* 1997;24:1344–1349.

12. Slemenda C, Heilman DK, Brandt KD, et al. Reduced quadriceps strength relative to body weight: a risk factor for osteoarthritis in women? *Arthritis Rheum.* 1998;41: 1951–1959.

13. Houpt JB, Pritzker KPH, Alpert B, et al. Natural history of spontaneous osteonecrosis of the knee (SONK): a review. *Semin Arthritis Rheum.* 1983;13:212–227.

14. Felson DT. Prevalence of back symptoms in elders. *J Rheum.* 2000;27:220–225.

15. Shbeeb MI, Matteson EL. Trochanteric bursitis (greater trochanter pain syndrome). *Mayo Clin Proc.* 1996;71:565–569.

16. Wolfe F, Smythe HA, Yunus MB, et al. The American College of Rheumatology 1990 Criteria for the Classification of Fibromyalgia: report of the Multicenter Criteria Committee. *Arthritis Rheum.* 1990;33:160–172.

17. Wolfe F, Ross K, Anderson J, Russell IJ, Hebert L. The prevalence and characteristics of fibromyalgia in the general population. *Arthritis Rheum.* 1995;38(1):19–28.

18. Wolfe F, Hawley DJ. Evidence of disordered symptom appraisal in fibromyalgia: increased rates of reported comorbidity and comorbidity severity. *Clin Exp Rheumatol.* 1999;17(3):297–303.

19. Wolfe F. The relation between tender points and fibromyalgia symptom variables: evidence that fibromyalgia is not a discrete disorder in the clinic. *Ann Rheum Dis.* 1997;56(4):268–271.

20. Dieppe P, Peterfy C, Watt I. Osteoarthritis and related disorders: imaging. In: Klippel JH, Dieppe PA, eds. *Rheumatology.* London: Mosby; 1998:8.4.1–8.4.10.

21. Liu G, Peacock M, Eilam O, et al. Effect of osteoarthritis in the lumbar spine and hip on bone mineral density and diagnosis of osteoporosis in elderly men and women. *Osteoporosis Int.* 1997;7:564–569.

22. Felson DT, Naimark A, Anderson J, et al. The prevalence of knee osteoarthritis in the elderly: the Framingham Osteoarthritis Study. *Arthritis Rheum.* 1987;30:914–918.

23. Hult L. Cervical, dorsal and lumbar spinal syndromes. A field investigation of a non-selected material of 1200 workers in different occupations with special reference to disc degeneration and so-called muscular rheumatism. *Acta Orthop Scand.* 1954;Suppl17:1–102.

24. Drape JL, Pessis E, Auleley GR, et al. Quantitative MR imaging evaluation of chrondropathy in osteoarthritic knees. *Radiology.* 1998;208:49–55.

25. Adams JG, McAlindon T, Dimasi M, et al. Contribution of meniscal extrusion and cartilage loss to joint space narrowing in osteoarthritis. *Clin Radiol.* 1999;54:502–506.

26. Gale DR, Chaisson CE, Totterman SM, et al. Meniscal subluxation: association with osteoarthritis and joint space narrowing. *Osteoarthritis Cartil.* 1999;7:526–532.

27. Wollheim FA. Serum markers of articular cartilage damage and repair. *Rheum Dis Clin N A.* 1999;25:417–431.

28. Wolfe F. The C-reactive protein but not erythrocyte sedimentation rate is associated with clinical severity in patients with osteoarthritis of the knee or hip. *Source J Rheumatol.* 1997;24(8):1486–1488.

29. Belcher C, Yaquab R, Fawthrop F, et al. Synovial fluid chondroitin and keratan sulphate epitopes, glycoaminoglycans, and hyaluronan in arthritic and normal knees. *Ann Rheum Dis.* 1997;56:299–307.

30. Myers SL. Synovial fluid markers in osteoarthritis. *Rheum Dis Clin N A.* 1999;25:433–449.

31. Masmejean E, Dutour O, Touam C, et al. Bilateral SLAC (scapholunate advanced collapse) wrist: an unusual entity. Apropos of a 7000-year-old prehistoric case. *Ann Chir Main Membre Super.* 1997;16:207–214.

32. McAlindon TE, Wilson PW, Aliabadi P, et al. Level of physical activity and the risk of radiographic and symptomatic knee osteoarthritis in the elderly: the Framingham Study. *Am J Med.* 1999;106:151–157.

33. Roos H, Adalberth T, Dahlberg L, et al. Osteoarthritis of the knee after injury to the anterior cruciate ligament or meniscus: the influence of time and age. *Osteoarthritis Cartil.* 1995;3:261–267.

34. Felson DT, Zhang Y, Hannan MT, et al. Risk factor for incident radiographic knee osteoarthritis in the elderly: the Framingham Study. *Arthritis Rheum.* 1997;40:728–733.

35. Oliveria SA, Felson DT, Cirillo PA, et al. Body weight, body mass index, and incident symptomatic osteoarthritis of the hand, hip and knee. *Epidemiology.* 1999;10:161–166.

36. Sahyoun NR, Hochberg MC, Helmick CG, et al. Body mass index, weight change, and incidence of self-reported physician-diagnosed arthritis among women. *Am J Public Health.* 1999;89:391–394.

37. Nevitt MC, Cummings SR, Lane NE, et al. Association of estrogen replacement therapy with the risk of osteoarthritis in elderly white women. Study of Osteoporotic Fractures Research Group. *Arch Intern Med.* 1996;156: 2073–2080.

38. Zhang Y, McAlindon TE, Hannan MT. Estrogen replacement therapy and worsening of radiographic knee osteoarthritis: the Framingham Study. *Arthritis Rheum.* 1998;41:1867–1873.

39. Radin EL, Paul IL. Does cartilage compliance reduce skeletal impact loads. *Arthritis Rheum.* 1970;13:199–144.

40. Sowers M, Lachance L, Jamadar D, et al. The associations of bone mineral density and bone turnover markers with osteoarthritis of the hand and knee in pre- and perimenopausal women. *Arthritis Rheum.* 1999;42:483–489.

41. Dai LY. The relationship between osteoarthritis and osteoporosis in the spine. *Clin Rheum.* 1998;17:44–46.

42. Arden NK, Nevitt MC, Lane NE, et al. Osteoarthritis and risk of falls, rates of bone loss, and osteoporotic fractures. Study of Osteoporotic Fractures Research Group. *Arthritis Rheum.* 1999;42:1378–1385.

43. Sowers MF, Hochberg M, Crabbe JP, et al. Association of bone mineral density and sex hormone levels with osteoarthritis of the hand and knee in premenopausal women. *Am J Epidemiol.* 1996;143:38–47.

44. Bruger H, van Daele PL, Odding E, et al. Association of radiographically evident osteoarthritis with higher bone mineral density and increased bone loss with age. The Rotterdam Study. *Arthritis Rheum.* 1996;39:81–86.

45. Ryan LM, Cheung HS. The role of crystals in osteoarthritis. *Rheum Dis Clin N A.* 1999;25:257–267.

46. Ledingham J, Regan M, Jones A, et al. Factors affecting radiographic progression of knee osteoarthritis. *Ann Rheum Dis.* 1995;54:53–58.

47. Sharma L, Lou C, Felson DT, et al. Laxity in healthy and osteoarthritic knees. *Arthritis Rheum.* 1999;42:861–870.

48. Slemenda C, Heilman DK, Brandt KD, et al. Reduced quadriceps strength relative to body weight: a risk factor for knee osteoarthritis in women? *Arthritis Rheum* 1998;41:1951–1959.

49. Slemenda C, Brandt KD, Heilman DK, et al. Quadriceps weakness and osteoarthritis of the knee. *Ann Intern Med.* 1997;127:97–104.

50. Hurley MV. The role of muscle weakness in the pathogenesis of osteoarthritis. *Rheum Dis Clin N A.* 1999;25:283–298.

51. Hurley MV, Newham DJ. The influence of arthrogenous muscle inhibition on quadriceps rehabilitation of patients with early, unilateral osteoarthritis. *Br J Rheum.* 1993;32:127–131.

52. Sharma L. Proprioceptive impairment in knee osteoarthritis. *Rheum Clin N A.* 1999;25:299–314.

53. Hall MG, Ferrell WR, Sturrock RD, et al. The effect of the hypermobility syndrome on knee joint proprioception. *Br J Rheum.* 1995;34:121–125.

54. Pai YC, Rymer WZ, Chang RW, Sharma L. Effect of age and osteoarthritis on knee proprioception. *Arthritis Rheum.* 1997;40:2260–2265.

55. Sharma L, Pai YC, Holtkamp K, Rymer WZ. Is knee joint proprioception worse in the arthritic knee versus the unaffected knee in unilateral knee osteoarthritis? *Arthritis Rheum.* 1997;40:1518–1525.

56. Lane NE, Lin P, Christiansen L, Gore LR, et al. Association of mild acetabular dysplasia with an increased risk of incident hip osteoarthritis in elderly white women: the study of osteoporotic fractures. *Arthritis Rheum.* 2000;43:400–404.

57. Hirsch R. Lethbridge-Cejku M, Hanson R, et al. Familial aggregation of osteoarthritis: data from the Baltimore Longitudinal Study on Aging. *Arthritis Rheum.* 1998;41:1227–1232.

58. Felson DT, Couropmitree NN, Chaisson CE, et al. Evidence for a mendelian gene in a segregation analysis of generalized radiographic osteoarthritis: the Framingham Study. *Arthritis Rheum.* 1999;42:1068–1070.

59. Bleasel JF, Poole AR, Heinegard D, et al. Changes in serum cartilage marker levels indicate altered cartilage metabolism in families with osteoarthritis-related type II collagen gen COL2A1 mutation. *Arthritis Rheum.* 1999;42:39–45.

60. Meulenbelt I, Bijkerk C, Miedema HS, et al. A genetic association study of the IGF-1 gene and radiological osteoarthritis in a population-based cohort study (the Rotterdam Study). *Ann Rheum Dis.* 1998;57:371–374.

61. Kuettner KE, Thonar J-MA. Cartilage integrity and homeostasis. In: Klippel JH, Dieppe PA, eds. *Rheumatology.* London: Mosby; 1998:8.6.1–8.6.16.

62. Aligner T, Vornehm SI, Zeiler G, et al. Suppression of cartilage matrix gene matrix expression in upper zone chondrocytes of osteoarthritic cartilage. *Arthritis Rheum.* 1997;40:562–569.

63. Mehraban F, Lark MW, Ahmed FN, et al. Increased secretion and activity of matrix metalloproteinase-3 in synovial tissues and chondrocytes from experimental osteoarthritis. *Osteoarthritis Cartil.* 1998;6:286–294.

64. Melchiorri C, Meliconi R, Frizziero L, et al. Enhanced coordination in vivo expression of inflammatory cytokines and nitric oxide synthase by chondrocytes from patients with osteoarthritis. *Arthritis Rheum.* 1998;41:2165–2174.

65. Towle CA, Hung HH, Bonassar LJ, et al. Detection of interleukin-1 in the cartilage of patients with osteoarthritis: a possible autocrine/paracrine role in pathogenesis. *Osteoarthritis Cartil.* 1997;5:293–300.

66. Lotz M. The role of nitric oxide in articular cartilage damage. *Rheum Clin N A.* 1999;25:269–282.

67. Mansell JP, Tarlton JF, Bailey AJ. Biochemical evidence for altered subchondral bone collagen metabolism in osteoarthritis of the hip. *Br J Rheum.* 1997;36:16–19.

68. Lane NE, Hochberg MC, Pressman A, et al. Recreational physical activity and the risk of osteoarthritis of the hip in elderly women. *J Rheum.* 1999;26:849–854.

69. Lane NE, Oehlert JW, Bloch DA, Fries JD. The relationship of running to osteoarthritis of the knee and hip and bone mineral density of the lumbar spine: a 9 year longitudinal study. *J Rheumatol.* 1998;26:334–341.

70. Sahyoun NR, Hochberg MC, Helmick CG. Body mass index, weight change, and incidence of self-reported physician-diagnosed arthritis among women. *Am J Public Health.* 1999;89:391–394.

71. Felson DT, Zhang Y, Anthony JM, et al. Weight loss reduces the risk for symptomatic knee osteoarthritis in women. *Ann Intern Med.* 1992;116:535–539.

72. McAlindon T, Felson DT. Nutrition: risk factors for osteoarthritis. *Ann Rheum Dis.* 1997;56:397–400.

73. Sowers MF, Lachance L. Vitamins and arthritis: the roles of vitamins A, C, D, and E. *Rheum Clin N A*. 1999;25:315–332.

74. McAlindon TE, Felson DT, Zhang Y, et al. Relation of dietary intake and serum levels of vitamin D to progression of osteoarthritis of the knee among participants in the Framingham Study. *Ann Intern Med*. 1996;125:353–359.

75. Minor MA. Exercise in the treatment of osteoarthritis. *Rheum Clin N A*. 1999;25:397–415.

76. Pate RR, Pratt M, Blair SN, et al. Physical activity and public health. A recommendation from the Centers for Disease Control and Prevention and the American College of Sports Medicine. *JAMA*. 1995;273:402–407.

77. Messier SP, Loeser RF, Hoover JL, et al. Osteoarthritis of the knee: effects of gait, strength and flexibility. *Arch Phys Med Rehabil*. 1992;11:29–36.

78. Grabiner MD, Koh TJ, Lundin TM, et al. Kinematics of recovery from a stumble. *J Gerontol*. 1993;48:M97–M102.

79. Ettinger WH, Burns R, Messier SP, et al. A randomized trial comparing aerobic exercise and resistance exercise with a health education program in older adults with knee osteoarthritis: the fitness arthritis and seniors trial (FAST). *JAMA*. 1997;277:25–31.

80. Perleau R, Frank C, Fick G. The effect of elastic bandages on human knee proprioception in the uninjured population. *Am J Sports Med*. 1995;23:251–255.

81. Mazzuca SA, Brandt KD, Katz BP, et al. Effects of self-care education on the health status of inner-city patients with osteoarthritis of the knee. *Arthritis Rheum*. 1997;40:1466–1474.

82. Mazzuca SA, Brandt KD, Katz BP, et al. Reduced utilization and cost of primary care clinic visits resulting from self-care education for patients with osteoarthritis of the knee. *Arthritis Rheum*. 1999;42:1267–1273.

83. Voloshin A, Wosk J. Influence of artificial shock absorbers on human gait. *Clin Orthop Relat Res*. 1981;160:52–56.

84. Bradly JD, Brandt KD, Katz BP. Comparison of an antiinflammatory dose of ibuprofen, an analgesic dose of ibuprofen, and acetaminophen in the treatment of patients with osteoarthritis of the knee. *N Engl J Med*. 1991;325:1807–1809.

85. Peterson WL, Cryer B. COX-1-sparing NSAIDs—is the enthusiasm justified? [editorial; comment]. *JAMA*. 1999;282:1961–1963.

86. Lichtenstein DR, Wolfe MM. COX-2 selective NSAIDs: new and improved? [editorial]. *JAMA*. 2000;284:1297–1299.

87. Wolfe MM, Lichtenstein DR, Singh G. Gastrointestinal toxicity of nonsteroidal antiinflammatory drugs. *N Engl J Med*. 1999;340:1888–1899.

88. Ehrich EW, Schnitzer TJ, McIlwain H, et al. Effect of specific COX-2 inhibition in osteoarthritis of the knee: a 6-week double-blind, placebo-controlled pilot study of rofecoxib. Rofecoxib Osteoarthritis Pilot Study Group. *J Rheum*. 1999;26:2438–2447.

89. Silverstein FE, Faich G, Goldstein JL, et al. Gastrointestinal toxicity with Celecoxib vs. nonsteroidal anti-inflammatory drugs for osteoarthritis and rheumatoid arthritis. The CLASS study: a randomized controlled trial. *JAMA*. 2000;284:1247–1255.

90. Golden BD, Abramson SB. Selective cyclooxygenase-2 inhibitors. *Rheum Dis Clin N A*. 1999;25:359–378.

91. Swan SK, Rudy DW, Lasseter KC, et al. Effect of cyclooxygenase-2 inhibition on renal function in elderly person receiving a low-salt diet. A randomized, controlled trial. *Ann Intern Med*. 2000;133:1–9.

92. Deal CL, Schnitzer TJ, Lipstein E. Treatment of arthritis with topical capsaicin: a double-blind trial. *Clin Ther*. 1991;13:383–395.

93. Caldwell JR, Hale ME, Boyd RE, et al. Treatment of osteoarthritis pain with controlled release oxycodone or fixed combination oxycodone plus acetaminophen added to nonsteroidal antiinflammatory drugs: a double blind, randomized, multicenter, placebo controlled trial. *J Rheum*. 1999;26:862–869.

94. Deal CL, Moskowitz RW. Nutraceuticals as therapeutic agents in osteoarthritis: the role of glucosamine, chondroitin sulfate and collagen hydrolysate. *Rheum Dis Clin N A*. 1999;25:379–395.

95. McAlindon TE, LaValley MP, Gulin JP, Felson DT. Glucosamine and chondroitin for treatment of osteoarthritis: a systematic quality assessment and meta-analysis. *JAMA*. 2000;283:1469–1475.

96. Gaffney K, Ledingham J, Perry JD. Intra-articular triamcinolone hexactonide in knee osteoarthritis: factors influencing the clinical response. *Ann Rheum Dis*. 1995;54:379–381.

97. Shbeeb MI, O'Duffy JD, Michet CJ Jr, et al. Evaluation of glucocorticosteroid injection for the treatment of trochanteric bursitis. *J Rheum*. 1996;23:2104–2106.

98. Wobig M, Dickhut A, Maier R, Vetter G. Viscosupplementation with hylan G-F 20: a 26-week controlled trial of efficacy and safey in the osteoarthritic knee. *Clin Ther*. 1998;20:410–423.

99. Wobig M, Bach G, Beks P, et al. The role of elastoviscosity in the efficacy of viscosupplementation for osteoarthritis of the knee: a comparison of hylan G-F 20 and a lower-molecular-weight hyaluronan. *Clin Ther*. 1999;21:1549–1562.

100. Smith GN Jr, Myers SL, Brandt KD. Effect of intraarticular hyaluronan injection in experimental canine osteoarthritis. *Arthritis Rheum*. 1998;41:976–985.

101. Brander VA, Malhotra S, Jet J, et al. Outcome of hip and knee arthroplasty in persons aged 80 years and older. *Clin Orthop Relat Res*. 1997;345:67–78.

102. Fox KM, Hochberg MC, Resnik CS, et al. Severity of radiographic findings in hip osteoarthritis associated with total hip arthroplasty. *J Rheum*. 1996;23L:693–697.

103. Towheed TE, Hochberg MC. Health-related quality of life after total hip replacement. *Semin Arthritis Rheum*. 1996;26:483–491.

104. Toumbis CA, Kronick JL, Wooley PH, Nasser S. Total joint arthroplasty and the immune response. *Semin Arthritis Rheum*. 1997;27:44–47.

105. Kreder HJ, Deyo RA, Koepsell T, et al. Relationship between the volume of total hip replacements performed

by providers and the rates of postoperative complications in the state of Washington. *Bone Joint Surg Am Vol* 1997;79:485–494.

106. Andersson GBJ, Lucente T, Davis AM, Kappler RE, Lipton JA, Leurgans G. A comparison of osteopathic spinal manipulation with standard care for patients with low back pain. *N Engl J Med.* 1999;341:1426–1431.

107. Atlas SJ, Keller RB, Robson D, et al. Surgical and nonsurgical management of lumbar stenosis: four-year outcomes from the Maine lumbar spine study. *Spine.* 2000;25:556–562.

108. Amundsen T, Weber H, Nordal HJ, et al. Lumbar spinal stenosis: conservative or surgical management? A prospective 10-year study. *Spine.* 2000;25:1424–1435.

109. Kalbarczyk A, Lukes A, Seiler RW. Surgical treatment of lumbar spinal stenosis in the elderly. *Acta Neurochir.* 1998; 140:637–641.

110. Vitaz TW, Raque GH, Shields CB, et al. Surgical treatment of lumbar spinal stenosis in patients older than 75 years of age. *J Neurosurg.* 1999;91:181–185.

111. Katz JN, Stucki G, Lipson SJ, et al. Predictors of surgical outcome in degenerative lumbar spinal stenosis. *Spine.* 1999;24:2229–2233.

112. Berman BM, Singh BB, Lao L, et al. A randomized trial of acupuncture as an adjuvant therapy in osteoarthritis of the knee. *Rheumatology.* 1999;38:346–354.

113. Smith GN, Mickler EA, Hasty KA, Brandt KD. Specificity of inhibition of matrix metalloproteinase activity by doxycycline: relationship to structure of the enzyme. *Arthritis Rheum.* 1999;42:1140–1146.

114. Smith GN, Yu LP, Brandt KD. Oral administration of doxycycline reduces collagenase and gelatinase activities in extracts of human osteoarthritic cartilage. *J Rheum.* 1998;25:532–535.

115. Evans CH, Robbins PD. Potential treatment of osteoarthritis by gene therapy. *Rheum Dis Clin N A.* 1999;25: 333–344.

116. Hollingworth P, Scott JT, Burry HC. Nonarticular gout: hyperuricemia and tophus formation without gouty arthritis. *Arthritis Rheum.* 1983;26:98—101.

117. Wernick R, Winkler C, Campbell S. Tophi as the initial manifestation of gout: report of six cases and review of the literature. *Arch Intern Med.* 1992;152:873–876.

118. McCarty DJ, Kohn NN, Faires JS. The significance of calcium phosphate crystals in the synovial fluid of arthritic patients: The "Pseudogout Syndrome". I. Clinical Aspects. *Ann Int Med.* 1962;56:711–737.

119. Bergström G, Bjelle A, Sorensen LB, et al. Prevalence of rheumatoid arthritis, osteoarthritis, chondrocalcinosis and gouty arthritis at age 79. *J Rheumatol.* 1986;13:527–534.

120. Menkes CJ, Simon F, Delrieu F, et al. Destructive arthropathy in chondrocalcinosis. *Arthritis Rheum.* 1976;19(suppl): 329–348.

121. Carroll GJ, Stuart RA, Armstrong JA, et al. Hydroxyapatite crystals are a frequent finding in osteoarthritic synovial fluid, but are not related to increased concentrations of keratan sulfate or interleukin 1β. *J Rheumatol.* 1991;18: 861–866.

122. McCarty DJ, Halverson PB, Carrera GF, et al. Milwaukee shoulder association of microspheroids containing hydrox-

yapatite crystals, active collagenase and neutral protease with rotator cuff defects. I. Clinical aspects. *Arthritis Rheum.* 1981;124:464–473.

123. Chuang T-Y, Hunder GG, Ilstrup DM, et al. Polymyalgia rheumatica: a 10-year epidemiologic and clinical study. *Ann Intern Med.* 1982;97:672–680.

124. Machado EB, Michet CJ, Ballard DJ, et al. Temporal arteritis: an epidemiologic and clinical study. *Arthritis Rheum.* 1987;30(suppl 4):S50.

125. Boesen P, Sørensen SF. Giant cell arteritis, temporal arteritis, and polymyalgia rheumatica in a Danish county: a prospective investigation, 1982–1985. *Arthritis Rheum.* 1987;30:294–299.

126. Gran JT, Myklebust G. The incidence of polymyalgia rheumatica and temporal arteritis in the county of Aust Agder, south Norway: a prospective study 1987–94. *J Rheumatol.* 1997;24:1739–1743.

127. Östberg G. On arteritis with special reference to polymyalgia arteritica. *Acta Pathol Microbiol Scand.* 1973; 237(suppl A):1–59.

128. Weyand CM, Schönberger J, Oppitz U, et al. Distinct vascular lesions in giant cell arteritis share identical T cell clonotypes. *J Exp Med.* 1994;179:951–960.

129. Weyand CM, Wagner AD, Björnsson J, et al. Correlation of topographical arrangement and the functional pattern of tissue-infiltrating macrophages in giant cell arteritis. *J Clin Investig.* 1996;98:1643–1649.

130. Gillot J-M, Masy E, Davril M, et al. Elastase derived elastin peptides: putative autoimmune targets in giant cell arteritis. *J Rheumatol.* 1997;24:677–682.

131. Gabriel SE, Espy M, Erdman DD, et al. The role of parvovirus B19 in the pathogenesis of giant cell arteritis: a preliminary evaluation. *Arthritis Rheum.* 1999;42:1255–1258.

132. Duhaut P, Bosshard S, Calvet A, et al. Giant cell arteritis, polymyalgia rheumatica, and viral hypotheses: a multicenter, prospective case-control study. *J Rheumatol.* 1999;26: 361–369.

133. Weyand CM, Hicok KC, Hunder GG, et al. Tissue cytokine patterns in patients with polymyalgia rheumatica and giant cell arteritis. *Ann Intern Med.* 1994;121:484–491.

134. Weyand CM, Hicok KC, Hunder GG, et al. The HLA-DRB1 locus as a genetic component in giant cell arteritis. Mapping of a disease-linked sequence motif to the antigen binding site of the HLA-DR molecule. *J Clin Investia* 1992;90:2355–2361.

135. Caselli RJ, Hunder GG, Whisnant JP. Neurologic disease in biopsy-proven giant cell (temporal) arteritis. *Neurology.* 1998;38:352–359.

136. Evans JM, Bowles CA, Björnsson J, et al. Thoracic aortic aneurysm and rupture in giant cell arteritis. *Arthritis Rheum.* 1994;37:1539–1547.

137. Calamia KT, Hunder GG. Giant cell arteritis (temporal arteritis) presenting as fever of undetermined origin. *Arthritis Rheum.* 1981;1414–1418.

138. Matteson EL, Gold KN, Bloch DA, et al. Long-term survival of patients with giant cell arteritis in the American College of Rheumatology giant cell arteritis classification criteria cohort. *Am J Med.* 1996;100:193–196.

139. Säve-Söderbergh J, Malmvall B-E, Andersson R, et al. Giant cell arteritis as a cause of death: report of nine cases. *JAMA*. 1986;255:493–496.

140. Nordborg E, Bengtsson BÄ. Death rates and causes of death in 284 consecutive patients with giant cell arteritis confirmed by biopsy. *Br Med J*. 1989;299:549–550.

141. Bowness P, Shotliff K, Middlemiss A, et al. Prevalence of hypothyroidism in patients with polymyalgia rheumatica and giant cell arteritis. *Br J Rheum*. 1991;30:349–351.

142. Ayoub WT, Franklin CM, Torretti T. Polymyalgia rheumatica: duration of therapy and long-term outcome. *Am J Med*. 1985;79:309–315.

143. Weyand CM, Fulbright JW, Evans JM, et al. Corticosteroid requirements in polymyalgia rheumatica. *Arch Intern Med*. 1999;159:577–584.

144. Jover JA, Hernandez-Garcia C, Morado IC, et al. Combined treatment of giant-cell arteritis with methotrexate and prednisone. A randomized double-blind placebo-controlled trial. *Ann Intern Med*. 2001;134:106–114.

145. Bergström G, Bjelle A, Sorensen LB, et al. Prevalence of rheumatoid arthritis, osteoarthritis, chondrocalcinosis and gouty arthritis at age 79. *J Rheumatol*. 1986;13:527–534.

146. Kaarela K, Kautiainen H. Continuous progression of radiological destruction in seropositive rheumatoid arthritis. *J Rheumatol*. 1997;24:1285–1287.

147. Eberhardt K, Fex E. Clinical course and remission rate in patients with early rheumatoid arthritis: relationship to outcome after 5 years. *Br J Rheumatol*. 1998;37:1324–1329.

148. Glennas A, Kvien TK, Andrup O, et al. Recent onset arthritis in the elderly: a 5 year longitudinal observational study. *J Rheumatol*. 2000;27:101–108.

149. Nagafuchi H, Suzuki N, Kaneko A, et al. Prolactin locally produced by synovium infiltrating T lymphocytes induces excessive synovial cell functions in patients with rheumatoid arthritis. *J Rheumatol*. 1999;29:1890–1900.

150. Barrett-Conner E. Postmenopausal estrogen therapy and selected (less-often-considered) disease outcomes. *Menopause*. 1999;6(1):14–20.

151. Weyand CM, Schmidt D, Wagner U, Goronzy JJ. The influence of sex on the phenotype of rheumatoid arthritis. *Arthritis Rheum*. 1998;41:817–822.

152. Juby AG, Davi P. Prevalence and disease associations of certain autoantibodies in elderly patients. *Clin Investig Med*. 1998;21:4–11.

153. Lance NJ, Curran JJ. Late-onset, seropositive, erosive rheumatoid arthritis. *Semin Arthritis Rheum*. 1993;23:177–182.

154. Schmidt KL, Frencl V. Die rheumatoide Arthritis mit Beginn im höheren Lebensalter. *Dtsch Med Wochenschr*. 1982;107:1506–1510.

155. Terkeltaub R, Esdaile J, Décary F, et al. A clinical study of older age rheumatoid arthritis with comparison to a younger onset group. *J Rheum*. 1983;10:418–424.

156. Deal CL, Meenan RF, Goldenberg DL, et al. The clinical features of elderly-onset rheumatoid arthritis. *Arthritis Rheum*. 1985;28:987–994.

157. Myllykangas-Luosujari R, Aho K, Kautiainen H, Isomaki H. Shortening of life span and causes of excess mortality in a population-based series of subjects with rheumatoid arthritis. *Clin Exp Rheumatol*. 1995;13:149–153.

158. Myllykangas-Luosujari R, Aho K, Kautiainen H, Isomaki H. Cardiovascular mortality in women with rheumatoid arthritis. *J Rheumatol*. 1995;22:1065–1067.

159. Wallberg-Jonsson S, Ohman ML, Dahlqvist SR. Cardiovascular morbidity and mortality in patients with seropositive rheumatoid arthritis in Northern Sweden. *J Rheumatol*. 1997;24:445–451.

160. Brooks RC, McGee SR. Diagnostic dilemmas in polymyalgia rheumatica. *Arch Intern Med*. 1997;157:162–168.

161. Bahlas S, Ramos-Remus C, Davis P. Clinical outcome of 149 patients with polymyalgia rheumatica and giant cell arteritis. *J Rheumatol*. 1998;25:99–104.

162. O'Dell JR, Paulsen G, Haire CE, et al. Treatment of early seropositive rheumatoid arthritis with minocycline: four-year follow-up of a double-blind, placebo controlled trial. *Arthritis Rheum*. 1999;42:1691–1695.

163. Emery P. Disease modification in rheumatoid arthritis with leflunomide. *Scand J Rheumatol (Suppl)*. 1999;112:9–14.

164. Himik J, Cranney A, Shea B, et al. Bisphosphonates for steroid induced osteoporosis. *Cochrane Database Syst Rev*. 2000;2:CD001347 [computer file].

165. Mitchell DM, Spitz PW, Young DY, et al. Survival, prognosis, and causes of death in rheumatoid arthritis. *Arthritis Rheum*. 1986;29:706–714.

166. Laakso M, Mitru O, Isomäki H, et al. Mortality from amyloidosis and renal disease in patients with rheumatoid arthritis. *Ann Rheum Dis*. 1986;45:663–667.

167. Schein OD, Hochberg MC, Munoz B, et al. Dry eyes and dry mouth in the elderly: a population-based assessment. *Arch Intern Med*. 1999;159:1359–1363.

168. Nakamura H, Kawakami A, Tominaga M, et al. Expression of CD40/CD40 ligand and Bcl-2 family proteins in labial salivary glands of patients with Sjogren's syndrome. *Lab Investig* 1999;79:261–269.

169. Tabbara K, Sharara N. Sjogren's syndrome: pathogenesis. *Eur J Ophthalmol*. 1999;9:1–7.

170. Mauch E, Volk C, Kratzsch G, et al. Neurological and neuropsychiatric dysfunction in primary Sjögren's syndrome. *Acta Neurol Scand*. 1994;89:31–35.

171. Tajima Y, Mito Y, Owada Y, et al. Neurological manifestations of primary Sjogren's syndrome in Japanese patients. *Intern Med*. 1997;36:690–693.

172. Coates T, Slavotinek JP, Rischmueller M, et al. Cerebral white matter lesions in primary Sjögren's syndrome: a controlled study. *J Rheumatol*. 1999;26:1301–1305.

173. Sutcliffe N, Inanc M, Speight P, Isenberg D. Predictors of lymphoma development in primary Sjögren's syndrome. *Semin Arthritis Rheum*. 1998;28:80–87.

174. Tishler M, Yaron I, Shirazi I, Yaron M. Hydroxychloroquine treatment for primary Sjögren's syndrome: its effects on salivary and serum inflammatory markers. *Ann Rheum Dis*. 1999;58:253–256.

175. Miyakawi S, Nishiyami S, Matoba K. Efficacy of low-dose prednisone maintenance for saliva production and serological abnormalities in patients with primary Sjögren's syndrome. *Intern Med*. 1999;38:938–943.

176. Mok CC, Lau CS, Ho CT, Wong RW. Do flares of systemic lupus erythematosus decline after menopause. *Scand J Rheumatol*. 1999;28:357–362.

177. Dimant J, Ginzler EM, Schlesinger M, et al. Systemic lupus erythematosus in the older age group: computer analysis. *J Am Geriatr Soc.* 1979;27:58–61.

178. Ballou SP, Khan MA, Kushner I. Clinical features of systemic lupus erythematosus. Differences related to race and age of onset. *Arthritis Rheum.* 1982;25:55–60.

179. Catoggio LJ, Skinner RP, Smith G, et al. Systemic lupus erythematosus in the elderly: clinical and serological characteristics. *J Rheum.* 1984;11:175–181.

180. Hochberg MC, Boyd RE, Ahearn JM, et al. Systemic lupus erythematosus: a review of clinico-laboratory features and immunogenetic markers in 150 patients with emphasis on demographic subsets. *Medicine.* 1985;64:285–295.

181. Baer AN, Pincus T. Occult systemic lupus erythematosus in elderly men. *JAMA.* 1983;249:3350–3352.

182. Studenski S, Allen NB, Caldwell DS, et al. survival in systemic lupus erythematosus. A multivariate analysis of demographic factors. *Arthritis Rheum.* 1987;30:1326–1331.

183. Mak SK, Lam EK, Wong AK. Clinical profiles of patients with late-onset SLE: not a benign subgroup. *Lupus.* 1998;7:23–28.

184. Baker SB, Rovira JR, Campion EW, Mills JA. Late onset systemic lupus erythematosus. *Am J Med.* 1979;66:727–732.

185. Formiga F, Moga I, Pac M, et al. Mild presentation of systemic lupus erythematosus in elderly patients assessed by SLEDAI. SLE Disease Activity Index. *Lupus.* 1999;8:462–465.

186. Manzi S, Meilahn EN, Rairie JE, et al. Age-specific incidence rates of myocardial infarction and angina in women with systemic lupus erythematosus: comparison with the Framingham Study. *Am J Epidemiol.* 1997;145:408–415.

187. Mevorach D. The immune response to apoptotic cells. *Ann N Y Acad Sci.* 1999;887:191–198.

188. Sturfelt G, Bengtsson A, Klint C, et al. Novel roles of complement in systemic lupus erythematosus: hypothesis for a pathogenetic vicious circle. *J Rheumatol.* 2000:27:661–663.

189. Herrman M, Voll RE, Zoller OM, et al. Impaired phagocytosis of apoptotic cell material by monocyte derived macrophages from patients with systemic lupus erythematosus. *Arthritis Rheum.* 1998;41:1241–1250.

190. Levine JS, Koh JS. The role of apoptosis in autoimmunity: immunogen, antigen, and accelerant. *Semin Nephrol.* 1999;19:34–47.

191. Ring GH, Lakkis FG. Breakdown of self-tolerance and the pathogenesis of autoimmunity. *Semin Nephrol.* 1999;19:25–33.

192. Arnett FC, Bias WB, Reveille JD. Genetic studies in Sjögren's syndrome and systemic lupus erythematosus. *J Autoimmun.* 1989;2:403–413.

193. Gunnarrsson I, Kanerud L, Pettersson E, et al. Predisposing factors in sulphasalazine-induced systemic lupus erythematosus. *Br J Rheum.* 1997;36:1089–1094.

194. Sunil VP, Nidal Y, Lekos A, et al. Carbamazepine-induced systemic lupus erythematosus presenting as cardiac tamponade. *Chest.* 2000;117:597–598.

195. Gordon MM, Porter DR, Capell HA. Does sulphasalazine cause drug-induced systemic lupus erythematosus? No effect evident in a prospective randomised trial of 200 rheumatoid patients treated with sulphasalazine or auranofin over five years. *Ann Rheum Dis.* 1999;58:288–290.

196. Jiang X, Khursigara G, Rubin RL. Transformation of lupus-inducing drugs to cytotoxic products by activated neutrophils. *Science.* 1994;266:810–813.

197. Sebastiani GD, Galeazzi M, Tincani A, et al. Anticardiolipin and anti-beta2GP1 antibodies in a large series of European patients with systemic lupus erythematosus. Prevalence and clinical associations. European Concerted Action on the Immunogenetics of SLE. *Scand J Rheumatic.* 1999;28:344–351.

198. Cobo-Soriano R, Sanchez-Ramon S, Aparico MJ, et al. Antiphospholipid syndrome antibodies and retinal thrombosis in patients without risk factors: a prospective case-control study. *Am J Ophthalmol.* 1999;128:725–732.

199. Rood MJ, Van Der Velde EA, Ten Cate R, et al. Female sex hormones at the onset of systemic lupus erythematosus affect survival. *Br J Rheumatol.* 1998;39:1008–1010.

200. Tsakonas E, Joseph L, Esdaile JM, et al. A long-term study of hydroxychloroquine withdrawal on exacerbations in systemic lupus erythematosus. The Canadian Hydroxychloroquine Study Group. *Lupus.* 1998;7:80–85.

201. Carneiro JR, Sato EI. Double blind, randomized, placebo controlled clinical trial of methotrexate in systemic lupus erythematosus. *J Rheumatol.* 1999;26:1275–1279.

202. Dostal C, Tesar V, Rychlik I, et al. Effect of 1 year cyclosporine A treatment on the activity and renal involvement of systemic lupus erythematosus: a pilot study. *Lupus.* 1998;7:29–36.

203. Tam LS, Li EK, Leung CB, et al. Long-term treatment of lupus nephritis with cyclosporin A. *Q J Med.* 1998;91:573–580.

204. Dooley MA, Cosio FG, Nachman PH, et al. Mycophenolate mofetil therapy in lupus nephritis: clinical observations: *J Am Soc Nephrol.* 1999;10:833–839.

205. Callen JP. Dermatomyositis. *Lancet.* 2000;355:53–57.

206. Whitmore SE, Rosenshein NB, Povost TT. Ovarian cancer in patients with dermatomyositis. *Medicine.* 1994;73:153–160.

207. Pautaus E, Cherin P, Piette JC, et al. Features of polymyositis and dermatomyositis in the elderly: a case control study. *Clin Exp Rheum.* 2000;18:241–244.

208. Marie I, Hatron PY, Levesque H. Influence of age on characteristics of polymyositis and dermatomyositis. *Medicine.* 1999;78:139–147.

209. Medsger TA, Dixon JA, Garwood VF. Palmar fasciitis and polyarthritis associated with ovarian carcinoma. *Ann Intern Med.* 1982;96:424–431.

210. Freundlich B, Makover D, Maul GG. A novel antinuclear antibody associated with a lupus-like paraneoplastic syndrome. *Ann Intern Med.* 1988;109:295–297.

43
Skeletal Fragility in the Elderly

Angela Inzerillo, Jameel Iqbal, Bruce Troen, and Diane E. Meier

Osteoporosis, the leading cause of serious morbidity and functional loss in old age, was once thought to be a natural part of the aging process. Although at times it is difficult to distinguish between the disease and normal skeletal aging per se in the clinical approach to osteoporosis management, progress in the scientific understanding of the underlying disease process has made it largely a preventable disease. Defining the point at which these age-related skeletal changes require intervention presents a major challenge to researchers and clinicians alike. There are several reasons for these difficulties. There is a long latent period of bone loss before the onset of clinically apparent disease. Although current diagnostic procedures have been shown to distinguish those at risk of fracture from those not at risk, there is a large overlap in bone density between persons who fracture and persons who do not. Research efforts directed at these issues have increased dramatically as a result of demographic changes leading to a large aging female population at high risk for osteoporosis and because of rapidly developing technologies in the measurement and screening of decreased bone mineral. Additionally, ongoing advances in the therapeutic modalities have allowed us to treat this disorder.

Osteoporosis is a skeletal disorder in which bone strength is compromised by loss of bone density and quality. This chapter describes the mechanisms responsible for osteoporosis, modalities used to screen and diagnose this common disorder, and current and experimental modalities.

Anatomy and Physiology of Bone

Bone consists of cells and extracellular matrix. Cell types include osteoblasts, osteoclasts, stromal cells, and osteocytes. The extracellular matrix is composed of collagen and noncollagenous proteins. Histologically there are two varieties of bone: immature or woven bone and mature or lamellar bone. Woven bone is formed during growth and fracture repair. It is replaced by lamellar bone. Collagen fibers are found in bundles that are oriented in a specific direction and contain spindle-shaped hydroxyapatite or calcium phosphate. The direction of these fibers alternates from layer to layer, giving adult bone its characteristic lamellar structure and imparting strength to bone.

Observation of bone reveals dense areas (compact) or cortical bone and areas with connecting cavities (cancellous) or trabecular bone. There are two types of bone composing the skeleton: flat bone and long bone. Long bones of the extremities are predominantly cortical type whereas the axial skeleton is composed of trabecular bone.

The cellular organization of bone is similar for both cortical and trabecular bone. Bone is constantly undergoing a process of remodeling through the processes of resorption and formation throughout life. To understand the pathogenesis of osteoporosis, one must consider the function of normal bone cells and their activities. Bone is resorbed by osteoclasts and is formed through the action of osteoblasts. Osteoblasts can either undergo apoptosis or become buried into the matrix they form and differentiate into osteocytes, the transducers of mechanical loading. In addition, bone has continuously replicating lining cells, the osteoprogenitor cells and osteoclast precursors.

Osteoprogenitor cells are pluripotent stem cells capable of differentiation into osteoblasts upon stimulation by transcription factors. Osteoblasts are found in clusters along the surface of bone. They express receptors for estrogen and vitamin D in their nucleus, as well as integrin and cytokine receptors on their surface. Endogenous stimulants of osteoblastic activity include fibroblast growth factor (FGF), platelet-derived growth factor (PDGF), insulin-like growth factor (IGF), and transforming growth factor-β (TGF-β).

In contrast, osteoclasts are derived from hematopoietic progenitor cells. They are giant multinucleated cells found alone or in a cluster. An excessive level of osteo-clast activity causes inappropriate bone destruction in several bone and joint diseases including osteoporosis, Paget's disease, tumor-induced osteolysis, hyperparathyroidism, and rheumatoid arthritis.

Receptor activator of NE–κB ligand (RANK-L or osteoprotegerin ligand) is now considered to be the single most important cytokine that is both necessary and sufficient for bone formation. In addition, a variety of other factors modulate bone formation at various stages: these include interleukin-1 (IL-1), IL-3, IL-6, IL-11, tumor necrosis factor (TNF), vitamin D_3, granulocyte-macrophage colony-stimulating factor (GM-CSF), and macrophage colony-stimulating factor (M-CSF).

The resorptive process includes osteoclast formation, polarization with creation of a ruffled border, induction of resorption through acidification and release of enzymes, resulting release of molecules from the matrix, and finally apoptosis of the osteoclast (Fig. 43.1). Note that bone matrix digestion releases important molecules that are stored within the matrix, including a variety of growth factors, such as IGF and TGF-β, and cytokines.

During resorption, osteoclasts generate and are consequently exposed to very high levels of ionized Ca^{2+} as a result of hydroxyapatite dissolution. A high Ca^{2+} concentration can inhibit resorption through the action of Ca^{2+} on a cell-surface receptor, the Ca^{2+} receptor; this is one

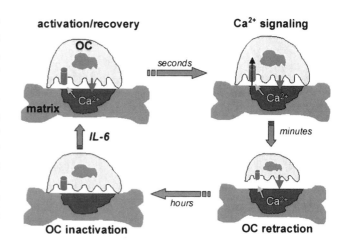

FIGURE 43.2. Inactivation of mature osteoclasts (OC): Ca^{2+} receptor.

mechanism for feedback control of resorption. Resorption can continue in spite of high $[Ca^{2+}]$ through the actions of IL-6, which is released from the cell in response to a high extracellular Ca^{2+}. IL-6 inhibits the effect of high extracellular Ca^{2+} on the osteoclast (Fig. 43.2).

Once resorption is completed, the resorptive cavity is refilled by osteoblasts with matrix. Thus, resorption is closely coupled to formation. It is known that osteoblasts migrate to the site of resorption responding to likely chemotactic signals, which are possibly secreted by osteoclasts or released from the bony matrix during resorption. After migration into the resorptive cavity, new osteoblasts lay down "osteoid" (or protein matrix) that is later mineralized and becomes new bone.

Defining the Types of Bone loss

Osteoporosis, as defined by the World Health Organization (WHO) Consensus Conference, is characterized not only by low bone mass but also by microarchitectural deterioration of bone tissue with a consequent increase in bone fragility and susceptibility to fractures.[1] The bone mass of an individual depends not only on the amount lost as a function of age, but also upon the peak bone mass attained during growth and development. Thus, osteoporosis can occur either when there is a failure to reach peak bone mass or when resorption exceeds formation after peak bone mass is achieved.

Osteoporosis is essentially a disease in which formation and resorption become decoupled. Overall, there is either an absolute or relative increase in osteoclastic activity. There is an absolute osteoclast overactivity (possibly with increased numbers of cells) in *high turnover* osteoporosis, including the postmenopausal bone variety. In contrast, in *low-turnover* osteoporosis, such as occurs with aging, bone formation lags behind resorption; hence,

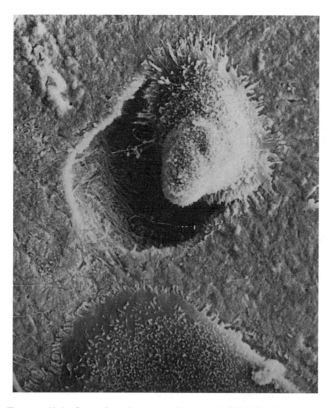

FIGURE 43.1. Scanning electron micrograph (SEM) of an osteoclast after bone resoprtion.

TABLE 43.1. Pathophysiology of osteoporosis.

Involutional	Postmenopausal	Secondary
Remodeling normal or decreased	Remodeling increased	Etiology-dependent changes in remodeling
Formation less than resorption	Resorption greater than formation	
Osteoblastic defect	Osteoclastic overactivity	

the rate of resorption is relatively higher than that of formation with net bone loss.

There are a variety of causes of osteoporosis, meriting a classification into primary and secondary forms. Primary osteoporosis occurs in association with menopause or with aging. It is traditionally subdivided into types I and II (Table 43.1). Type I is referred to as postmenopausal osteoporosis and is due to estrogen deficiency. Estrogen deficiency leads to increased numbers of osteoblasts and osteoclasts, resulting in a high bone turnover state with resorption exceeding formation and consequent acceleration in bone loss. The exact cellular mechanism by which estrogen exerts this effect is not entirely known. However, with estrogen loss there is upregulation of cytokines, particularly IL-6 and M-CSF, leading to enhanced osteoclast formation and activity, which then results in bone loss (Fig. 43.3).

Type II primary osteoporosis, often called senile or involutional osteoporosis, is associated with aging. In contrast to type I, there is decreased bone turnover with a primary defect in osteoblastic activity and decreased bone formation. Again the precise cellular details remain unclear. However, certain osteoblastic genes have been found to be up- or downregulated as a function of aging, for example, IGF-1, FGF, and their intracellular binding proteins. Normal coupling between formation and resorption is lost, with a net decrease in bone formation resulting in a relative increase in resorption. Another hypothesis is that bone loss, even in men, is caused by reductions in estrogen that occur with aging.

Other age-related factors could contribute to osteoporosis. Aging is associated with a number of disorders of vitamin D metabolism as well as with diminished intestinal calcium absorption. Dietary calcium also decreases with age, further exacerbating this calcium-deficient state. It is important to clarify the difference between osteoporosis and osteomalacia. Osteoporosis results from abnormalities in bone remodeling, whereas osteomalacia results from defects in bone mineralization caused by calcium deficiency.

Secondary osteoporosis is osteoporosis resulting from conditions other than aging or menopause. It may arise from a variety of causes (Table 43.2). All patients with unexplained bone loss should be considered candidates for laboratory evaluation for secondary causes that may also be superimposed on primary bone loss. To exclude common secondary causes, basic laboratory tests, thyroid function tests, immunoprotein electrophoresis (IPEP), 25-(OH) vitamin D_3, 24-h urine free cortisol, testosterone and/or estrogen, 24-h urinary calcium, and intact parathyroid hormone (PTH) may be obtained. If these tests are negative or if further testing is warranted, a bone biopsy may be performed.

The most common cause of secondary osteoporosis is hypercortisolism, endogenous as in Cushing's syndrome, or more commonly iatrogenic from chronic glucocorticoid administration. Osteoporosis induced by glucocorticoid excess is characterized by decreased bone formation causing a relative increase in resorption and bone loss. Trabecular bone (as seen predominantly in the lumbar spine) is more affected than cortical bone. Research has shown that decreased bone formation results from reduced osteoblast proliferation, reduced bone matrix protein secretion, and increased osteoblast apoptosis. In addition, there is a negative calcium balance due to decreased gastrointestinal calcium absorption and increased urinary calcium loss. Secondary hyperparathyroidism can ensue with further increases in net bone resorption. Steroids may also induce hypogonadotrophic hypogonadism, again with negative results on bone homeostasis.

Another common cause of secondary osteoporosis is hyperthyroidism. In hyperthyroidism, similarly to postmenopausal osteoporosis, there is increased bone remodeling with resorption exceeding formation and, hence, net bone loss. This state is mostly reversible with treatment of the hyperthyroid state. Postmenopausal women with significant hyperthyroidism are at the greatest risk

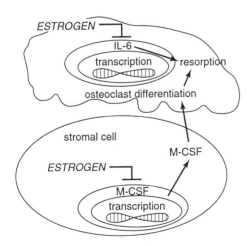

FIGURE 43.3. Cellular mechanism of estrogen on the regulation of bone remodeling.

TABLE 43.2. Secondary causes of systemic osteoporosis.

Endocrine
  Hypogonadism
  Cushing's syndrome
  Hyperthyroidism
  Type 1 diabetes
  Hyperparathyroidism

Malignancy
  Multiple myeloma
  Lymphoma
  Leukemia
  Malignancy-induced
    PTHrP secretion
  Mastocytosis

Gastrointestinal
  Low vitamin D intake
  Malabsorption
  Celiac disease
  Crohn's disease
  Lactase deficiency
  Hepatic failure
  Small bowel resection
  Anorexia nervosa
  Gastrectomy

Lifestyle
  Smoking

Drugs
  Anticonvulsants
  Heparin
  Glucocorticoids
  FK 506
  Levothyroxine excess
  Vitamin A excess
  Methotrexate
  Cyclosporin A
  Alcohol

Immobilization
  Hip fracture
  Paralysis

Genetic and other
  Osteogenesis imperfecta
  Homocystinuria
  Marfan's syndrome
  Rheumatoid arthritis
  Ehler–Danlos syndrome

Renal disease
  Renal Failure
  RTA
  Idiopathic hypercalciuria

because they have increased bone loss and fracture risk. This category also includes women on suppressive doses of levothyroxine for the treatment of thyroid diseases. Several studies have shown that markers of bone turnover are often increased in patients with asymptomatic hyperthyroidism. The use of these markers in the diagnosis of pretoxic goiter has yet to be substantiated.

As transplantation medicine advances, more patients with end-stage organ failure are able to live longer after successful organ transplantation. Pretransplanta-tion bone loss can be seen in patients with end-stage renal, hepatic, and pulmonary diseases. For cardiac transplant patients, unless there is concomitant renal failure, liver disease, or hypogonadism, the majority have normal pretransplant bone mineral density. As our aging population increasingly undergoes organ transplantation, the prevalence of low pretransplant bone mineral density (BMD) will increase.

Many of the data on transplantation osteoporosis are derived from cardiac transplant patients. These patients suffer from a dramatic severe bone loss, particularly in the first 6 months to 1 year following transplantation.[2,3] The cause of accelerated bone loss is multifactorial, but it is principally a result of immunosuppressive therapy, primarily glucocorticoids, cyclosporine A (CsA), and tacrolimus (FK 506).[4,5]

Epidemiology of Osteoporosis

Osteoporosis is the most common bone disease. The prevalence of low bone mass is dependent on a number of variables, including the study population utilized, diagnostic thresholds, densitometric techniques, and the skeletal sites measured. The prevalence of low bone mass increases with increasing age in both men and women, reflecting age-associated bone loss. It is higher for women (approximately 80% of all cases) than men because accelerated bone loss occurs in the immediate post-menopausal period.[6] The differences between men and women are partially related to the achievement of higher peak bone mass and absence of an accelerated phase of bone loss in men. Low bone mass is also more prevalent in Caucasians than in blacks.[6]

Based on data from the National Health and Nutrition Examination Survey III (NHANES), 10 million people in the United States have osteoporosis at the hip and nearly 18 million more have low bone mass at the hip, placing them at risk for future hip fractures. It is anticipated that the prevalence of osteoporosis will increase as the population ages.[7] The occurrence of osteoporotic fractures is even more striking. In the United States alone, the incidence approximates 1.5 million per year, including 700,000 spine fractures, 300,000 hip fractures, 250,000 wrist fractures, and 300,000 other fractures. One in 2 women and 1 in 8 men over age 50 will have an osteo-porotic fracture in their lifetime.[8]

Although the incidence of osteoporotic fractures is high, when viewed in perspective to other common chronic ailments in the United States, the figures appear even more dramatic. For instance, after the age of 65, the incidence of hip fracture in white women is greater than the incidence of stroke, breast cancer, and diabetes.[9] Among other chronic ailments, 28 million are affected with osteopenia and osteoporosis compared with 52 million and 42 million affected with hypercholesterolemia and hypertension, respectively.[10] These figures are staggering and will increase as the population ages.

The economic burden this places on society is self-evident. The cost of all fractures in the United States is between $35 and $41 billion per year. The cost of all osteoporotic fractures totals between $10 and $15 billion per year. Hip fractures alone total between $4 and $6 billion per year.[11] Expected costs for the year 2025 are $64 billion.[12]

Male Osteoporosis

Osteoporosis in men is a significant but understudied problem. According to the National Osteoporosis Foundation, approximately 2 million American men have osteoporosis. Although men are less likely to fracture, the lifetime risk of fracture is 13% to 25%.[13] The prevalence of osteoporosis in men will increase as the population ages.

Recent studies suggest a higher prevalence of secondary causes of osteoporosis in men than in women. Specifically, more than one-third of men presenting with osteoporotic vertebral fractures have a secondary cause (such as glucocorticoid administration, hypogonadism, gastrectomy, and hypercalciuria with nephrolithiasis) and a high incidence of cigarette smoking, alcoholism, and low body weight.[14] Careful evaluation for secondary and potentially remediable causes of osteoporosis is mandatory in male patients.[15]

There is some controversy in the diagnosis of osteoporosis in men. Currently there are no established guidelines for the use of BMD in male patients. The Rotterdam Study, a prospective cohort study, suggested the risk of hip fracture may be estimated on the basis of BMD and age in both men and women.[16] Males over the age of 65 and males under the age of 65 with one or more risk factors for osteoporosis and males with fragility fractures should have BMD measurement by dual-energy x-ray absorptiometry (DEXA).

Therapeutic intervention in male osteoporosis has been poorly studied. Controlled trials utilizing available treatment modalities are few. One controlled trial of calcium (1000 mg/day) with vitamin D (1000 IU/day) failed to reduce radial or spinal bone loss in men.[17] Replacement of testosterone in hypogonadal patients has led to increased bone mass, but there is no experimental basis for such therapy in eugonadal osteoporotic men. Routine calcium, low-dose vitamin D supplementation, and weightbearing exercise are reasonable and safe measures but are not yet supported by controlled studies. Bisphosphonates have been shown to increase BMD and decrease fracture rates in males on chronic glucocorticoid treatment.[18,19] A recent 2-year clinical trial of alendronate in osteoporotic men revealed increases at the lumbar spine (7.1%), femoral neck (2.5%), and total body (2%).[20] More prospective long-term controlled trials are

required to establish the fracture reduction efficacy of these therapeutic options in osteoporotic men.[21]

Risk Factors for Osteoporosis

Although the presence of risk factors associated with osteoporosis is of clinical utility, their ability to predict bone mineral density is poor.[22] However, the ability of clinical risk factors to predict fracture risk is good.[23] According to the 1998 National Osteoporosis Foundation (NOF) guidelines, family history, age, history of fracture, smoking, female sex, Caucasian race, estrogen deficiency, and low body weight are risk factors for the development of osteoporosis.[24] Smoking poses a major risk for the development of osteoporosis. Specifically, it increases the relative incidence of hip fracture by 1.5 to 2.0.[25] This incidence may increase by as much as 15% over the next several decades. Low calcium intake, below the recommended daily allowance (RDA) of 800 mg/day, has been observed in about 75% of U.S. women.[26] Even if the increased relative risk of hip fracture due to this factor were small, the very large numbers of women affected could ultimately lead to a high percentage of fractures due to low calcium intake.[27] Other major risk factors associated with hip fracture are maternal history of hip fracture, past fracture, particularly after age 50, use of glucocorticoids and anticonvulsants, and hyperthyroidism (Tables 43.2, 43.3).

Fracture Risk

Although clinical risk factors for osteoporosis are of limited use in the identification of women with higher than average chance of fracture,[28] low bone mass has now been shown in a number of prospective studies to accurately predict fracture risk.[29-31] For every standard deviation decrease in bone density measured at any site, the odds ratio for a fracture at any site is 1.6 to 2.4.[32-35] This relationship holds for both men and women.[35] Other

TABLE 43.3. Risk factors for osteoporotic fractures.

Age
Female sex
Caucasian
Low bone density
Prior fracture after age 50
Hypogonadism
Smoking
Inactivity
Falls
Anticonvulsant therapy
Glucocorticoids
Hyperthyroidism
Alcoholism
Excess dietary protein
Family history

factors clearly predictive of risk are the type of fall (falls directly on the hip or wrist increase fracture risk at that site),[36] greater hip axis length (defined as the distance from the lower lateral aspect of the greater trochanter to the inner pelvic brim (each standard deviation decrease in hip axis length doubles hip fracture odds ratio),[33] and history of prior fractures at any site.[34,35] A combination of low bone density plus one or more prior vertebral fractures increases relative risk of fracture by fourfold.[34,35] Fracture risk increases progressively and exponentially with decreasing bone density (see Table 43.3 for other risk factors for osteoporotic fractures).

Genetics of Osteoporosis

A family history of osteoporosis, particularly a maternal history, is considered a risk factor for osteoporosis.[24] The occurrence of osteoporosis within families suggests some level of genetic etiology that manifests its phenotype in the elderly. Bone mass is a complex trait with multiple external influences; it has become difficult to separate external from genetic influences.[37]

Genetic factors are increasingly becoming of interest in determining a contribution to osteoporosis and the possibility of novel therapeutic strategies. Unfortunately, progress in identifying genetic etiologies in osteoporosis has been slow. Several approaches have been used, including association studies where a certain gene allele is found at a higher frequency in those with a particular phenotype. The candidate gene approach has been the most widely employed. In this approach, DNA from families, first-degree relative, or siblings is analyzed with respect to polymorphic markers in genes thought to be related to a particular trait. Positive correlations have been noted between polymorphisms of several candidate genes and bone mass; these include the vitamin D receptor (VDR), collagen type I (COL1AI), estrogen receptor, transforming growth factor-beta (TGF-β), and IL-6.[37] These studies are limited by variable reproducibility in different study populations.

Although the potential implications for treatment and diagnosis are vast, because bone mass is a complex trait, it is unlikely that a monogenetic cause of osteoporosis will be found. More linkage studies are needed to attempt unravel the genetic predisposition to this complex trait.

Clinical Presentation

The clinical presentation of osteoporosis can vary from a symptomatic vertebral compression fracture to the observation of low bone mineral density on a baseline DEXA, screening ultrasound, or plain radiograph.

Vertebral fractures are the most common type of osteoporotic fracture. Their prevalence increases with age. Vertebral fractures often are asymptomatic and are detected on routine chest radiography. The most common sites for fractures are the lower thoracic and upper lumbar spine. Fractures occurring in the cervical and upper thoracic (above T6) vertebrae should suggest a secondary or pathologic cause, such as tumor or infection (see Table 43.2).

An acute vertebral compression fracture may present with sudden onset of pain at the site of the fracture with associated radiation of pain laterally, paravertebral muscle spasm, and signs and symptoms of spinal cord compression. Vertebral fractures may occur in clusters of five or six over short time periods. New crush fractures may result in substantial short-term pain and disability, but many patients with vertebral osteoporosis have either chronic back discomfort, height loss, postural changes, or no symptoms at all.[38,39] In the absence of radiographic evidence of fracture or bone scan evidence of microfracture, back pain should not be attributed to a diagnosis of osteoporosis.

Sufficient numbers of wedge or crush fractures may lead to height loss and kyphosis with attendant back pain and impaired functional capacity.[38] Associated abdominal distension, discomfort, and pulmonary restriction also may occur in severe cases of thoracic kyphosis.

Hip fractures are second in frequency, are associated with substantial morbidity and mortality, and occur primarily in persons over age 75. Morbidity is between 30% and 50%, as most of those affected are unable to return to their previous level of function. Mortality is estimated to be between 10% and 20% and increases with age and comorbid conditions.[40] Hip fractures are almost always associated with a fall, but whether the fracture precedes or follows the fall is not always clear. Occasionally, a patient with an impacted hip fracture retains the ability to walk, but most hip fracture patients are unable to stand. The involved limb may appear shorter and externally rotated.

Patients with osteoporosis generally suffer one of two types of hip fracture, intracapsular or intertrochanteric. In the former, fracture occurs within the joint capsule and frequently results in interruption of the vascular supply to the femoral head, with a high rate of non-union and avascular necrosis. Intertrochanteric fractures are extracapsular, occur between the greater and lesser trochanter, and are not associated with non-union or avascular necrosis. (Refer to Chapters 45 and 46 for further discussion of hip fracture.)

Distal radial fractures (Colle's fracture), the third most common osteoporotic fracture, usually occur in middle-aged women who attempt to break a fall with outstretched arms and hands (parachute reflex). Some elderly patients experiencing this type of fracture with concomitant medical problems may require hospitalization. Presentation with pain and deformity usually is straightforward. Rehabilitation exercises of the hand and forearm may be necessary.

Diagnosis of Osteoporosis

Bone mass measurements have now been shown in multiple prospective studies to accurately predict fracture risk.[28-33] Potential uses of bone densitometry include screening of asymptomatic persons to assess their risk of future fracture, diagnostic density measurements in persons with known risk factors for osteopenia, and repeat measurements for purposes of following bone mass changes over time in response to disease or anti-resorptive treatments.[41]

Screening Guidelines

Screening patients with suspected osteoporosis is clearly important. The criteria for utility of a screening test for osteoporosis require that (1) the disorder causes sufficient morbidity, mortality, and cost to warrant screening; (2) the screening test is safe and affordable; (3) treatment in an asymptomatic phase would reduce fractures; (4) screening would affect a patient's decision to accept treatment; and (5) the screening test can accurately predict the risk of fracture. Densitometry has been generally acceptable to patients and involves low radiation doses.

Therapeutic interventions have been shown to decrease the risk of hip and vertebral fractures by up to 50%. Thus, a patient's decision to be treated could be substantially influenced by a low bone mass measurement.[42] Furthermore, prospective data have demonstrated bone mass measurement as predictive of fracture risk, regardless of the site measured. The hip measurement is the best predictor of hip fracture and vertebral measurement is the best predictor of vertebral fracture.[43]

The National Osteoporosis Foundation (NOF) has recommended densitometry for women at menopause in whom estrogen decisions would be influenced by knowledge of bone mass.[44] Other recommended indications for densitometry (Tables 43.4, 43.5) include densitometry

TABLE 43.5. Additional indications for BMD testing.

H:	Hypogonadal states in both men and women
I:	Incidental (= radiographic evidence of osteopenia, incidental discovery of fracture, or fracture with minimal trauma)
P:	Prednisone
P:	Parathyroid disease

in patients with radiographic evidence of osteopenia, patients on chronic glucocorticoids, or those with other conditions such as asymptomatic primary hyperparathyroidism for whom knowledge of bone density will influence management.[41,44]

Increasingly utilized for screening are peripheral measurements of bone density; these are useful for screening because of low cost, little to no ionizing radiation exposure, and portability. However, results are difficult to determine because different normative databases are utilized and T scores (see diagnostic guidelines below) do not correspond to the WHO criteria applicable to central DEXA measurements.

Diagnostic Guidelines

The World Health Organization (WHO) has defined osteoporosis in terms of boue mineral density in postmenopausal Caucasian women. A bone density measurement of more than 2.5 SD below the mean for young adult women, without fractures, is osteoporosis.[45] Table 43.6 outlines these criteria for diagnosis. Note that these criteria identify approximately 30% of postmenopausal women as having osteoporosis, using DEXA of spine, hip, or forearm. This diagnosis approximates equivalent lifetime fracture risk for spine, hip, and forearm as approximately 17% and lifetime fracture risk for any of the three fractures as about 40%.[45]

The WHO diagnostic criteria are not appropriate for groups other than postmenopausal Caucasian women, sites other than spine, hip, or forearm, or modalities other than DEXA, partly because of the different normative databases utilized. Diagnostic criteria for osteoporosis in groups other than postmenopausal women are controversial. In these groups, the presence of fracture, second-

TABLE 43.4. 1998 National Osteoporosis Foundation (NOF) recommendations for bone mineral density (BMD) testing.

1. All postmenopausal women under age 65 who have one or more additional risk factors for osteoporosis (besides menopause)
2. All women age 65 and older regardless of additional risk factors
3. Postmenopausal women who present with fractures
4. Women who are considering therapy for osteoporosis, if BMD testing would facilitate the decision
5. Women who have been on hormone replacement therapy for prolonged periods

TABLE 43.6. World Health Organization (WHO) diagnostic criteria for postmenopausal Caucasian women.

Normal: Bone density no lower than 1 SD below the mean for young adult women (T score ≥ -1)

Osteopenia: Bone density between 1 and 2.5 SD below the mean for young adult women (T score between -1 and -2.5)

Osteoporosis: Bone density more than 2.5 SD below the mean for young adult women, without fractures (T score ≤ -2.5)

Established osteoporosis: Bone density below the mean for young adult women, with a history of fragility fracture (T score ≤ -2.5)

ary causes of bone loss, or the presence of low BMD may indicate the need to treat.

Serial Measurements to Assess Bone Loss Rates

Serial densitometry can help to determine need for treatment in patients with normal baseline bone mass, but who are at risk for rapid loss, as in the immediate postmenopausal period or with the initiation of glucocorticoid therapy. Similarly, bone mass changes over time may be used to assess effectiveness of therapy. The measurement of rates of change of bone mass is dependent on the actual in vivo change in bone density, the reproducibility of the densitometric technique used, the number of measurements taken, and the type of antiresorptive therapy initiated.

Currently only serial measurements utilizing DEXA have been substantiated. Presently available methods are sufficiently precise for measurement of bone mass changes if multiple measurements are taken or expected changes in bone mass is large. The short-term precision of commonly used densitometric techniques varies from 1% to 5%, even in research settings with stringent quality control requirements. Precision is dependent on the equipment utilized in the assessment and the skill of the technologist. Long-term precision and precision in non-research settings is less defined. Because bone loss rates in humans generally do not exceed 1% per year, except during the immediate postmenopausal years or in pathologic states, the potential for error in bone loss rate assessment in individuals is obvious. Increasing the number of measurements will improve the accuracy of the estimate but at the expense of increased cost to the patient and treatment time lost while attempting to assess the true rate of bone loss.

When patients undergo treatments expected to produce large (>10%) losses or gains of bone mineral density, serial measurements may help identify non-responders or patients requiring a change in therapy. Serial measurements over relatively short intervals are not useful in assessing bone mass response to preventive measures such as estrogen replacement, because expected rates of change are small by comparison with the precision variability of the technique. There are no prospective data supporting the ability of serial measures of bone loss rates to predict fracture risk.

When a serial measurement fails to show a significant increase, or reveals a decrease in BMD, should this finding institute a change in therapy? A recent study attempted to address the question of regression to the mean.[46] This principle predicts that patients with unusual responses to treatment are likely to have more typical responses if treatment is continued.[47] The study groups consisted of patients from the Fracture Intervention Trial (FIT) and Multiple Outcomes of Raloxifene Evaluation Trial (MORE) trials who appeared to lose BMD after the first year of active treatment. The study demonstrated that those who lost more during the first year of treatment with alendronate or raloxifene were more likely to gain in the second year of treatment. Therefore, treatment should be continued in patients who appear to lose BMD early in treatment.

Techniques Commonly Used

Dual-Energy X-Ray Absorptiometry (DEXA)

DEXA utilizes a beam of x-ray photons passing through the bone region of interest. The amount of beam passing through the bone and detected by the scintillation counter is inversely proportional to the bone mass. This technique measures the sum of cortical and trabecular bone at the midradius (95% cortical bone), lumbar spine, femoral neck, total hip, and total body with a precision of approximately 1% to 3%, depending on the operator and skeletal site measured.[44] Radiation exposure is low (1–3 µSv per site), and patient acceptability is high. The high reproducibility and low radiation dose of DEXA, and freedom from the error introduced by radioisotopic decay seen with older photon absorptiometry techniques, have resulted in virtual elimination of the photon absorptiometric method in recent years (Table 43.7).

For the diagnosis of osteoporosis with DEXA, measurement of at least two skeletal sites is preferable, usually PA spine and hip (Fig. 43.4 A,B). Falsely elevated bone mineral density on DEXA is important to recognize while interpreting results. Reasons for such artifacts include degenerative joint or disk disease, compression fractures, vascular calcifications, or scoliosis occurring in the path of the measurement beam. Use of femoral neck, total hip, and forearm measurement sites is usually preferable under these clinical circumstances.[44] Lateral spine measurement may also be useful in this clinical circumstance. A midradius measurement, which consists primarily of cortical bone, may be useful in hyperparathyroidism, as these patients tend to have greater cortical bone loss.

DEXA values are reported by comparison to age and gender reference groups with T scores (standard deviations above or below values for young normals) and Z scores (standard deviations above or below age-matched values).[44] A T score more than 2 SD below young normals indicates an increased risk of fracture and should lead to consideration of antiresorptive therapy to prevent further bone loss. A Z score of more than 1 to 2 SD below the age-matched mean value should prompt a thorough evaluation for secondary causes of bone loss (see Tables 43.2, 43.3).

TABLE 43.7. Comparison of modalities in bone mass measurement.

Method	Major site	Precision error (%)	Benefits	Problems	Serial Exams	Radiation[a]
DXA	PA lumbar spine Lateral lumbar spine Hip Distal 1/3 forearm Total body	1–2 5–15 1.5–3 1 1	1. Low radiation 2. Expensive 3. Precise	1. Requires a skilled technician 2. Subject to artifacts, particularly the spine	Yes	1–3 μSv
pDXA	Radius Phalanges Calcaneus	1–2	1. Portable 2. Screening 3. Low radiation 4. Easy to operate 5. Shorter scan times 6. Inexpensive	1. Able to scan one site only 2. Different normative database 3. False negative 4. Measure site unresponsive to treatment	No	<1 μSv
QCT	L1–L3 spine	1.5–4	1. Precise 2. Volumetric BMD (mg/cm³) 3. Useful in large-size individuals 4. Useful for spine abnormalities 5. Most feasible technique for postmenopausal bone loss	1. Expensive 2. High radiation exposure 3. No data for serial measurements 4. Marrow fat can underestimate BMD 5. Different normative database	No	50–60 μSv
pQCT	Radius	1–2	1. Volumetric BMD (mg/cm³) 2. Portable 3. Screening 4. Easy to use 5. Lower radiation than qCT	1. Different normative database 2. Requires dedicated scanner 3. Measure site unresponsive to treatment	No	1–30 (10) μSv
QUS	Radius Phalanges Calcaneus Tibia	1–2	1. Portable 2. Screening 3. Low radiation 4. Easy to operate 5. Shorter scan times 6. Inexpensive	1. Peripheral measurement only 2. Affected by amount of soft tissue 3. Different normative database 4. Measure site unresponsive to treatment	No	None
LVA	Lateral spine	N/A	1. Morphology 2. Better image	1. Different normative database 2. No data for serial measurements	No	1–3 μSv

DXA, dual-energy x-ray absorptiometry; pDXA, peripheral dual-energy x-ray absorptiometry; qCT, qualitative computerized axial tomography; pQCT, peripheral qualitative computerized axial tomography; QUS, quantitative ultrasound; LVA, lateral vertebral assessment.
[a] 1 Sv = 100 rem (for comparison, chest x-ray = 50–150 μSv).

Peripheral DEXA (pDEXA)

Compared to central DEXA, peripheral DEXA (pDEXA) is smaller, portable, easier to operate, and the radiation exposure is less. It requires shorter scan times and its decreased expense make it particularly suitable for screening. Sites measured include the radius, calcaneus, or phalanges. Because different normative databases are utilized, these are not used for serial measurements (see Table 43.7).

Quantitative Computed Tomography (qCT)

Because of the wide availability of CT scanners, vertebral bone densitometry by qCT is an attractive alternative to DEXA. The technique is the only method available that is able to separately quantitate cortical and trabecular bone and potentially detect signs of bone loss occurring earliest in the trabecular skeletal compartment, that is, postmenopausal. qCT allows volumetric BMD measurement (reported in g/cm³). It is useful in degenerative disease in the spine and individuals at extremes for size and weight. Short-term precision in vivo is about 4% in research settings,[44] limiting its applicability for serial determinations of bone loss rates. Radiation dose per scan is also substantial (50–60 μSv) and patient acceptability is accordingly limited (see Table 43.7).

In theory, measurement of pure trabecular bone in the centrum of the vertebrae should result in clearer separation of at-risk from low-risk subjects.[48] However, accuracy error, due to marrow fat, which increases with age, is high, making quality assurance technically more difficult. In most hospital computed tomography centers, radiation dose is substantial and artifactual errors due to lumbar spine abnormalities do limit its regular use. Thus, DEXA is generally preferable to qCT in terms of precision, accuracy, radiation exposure, quality control, and logistics in the clinical radiology setting.[44]

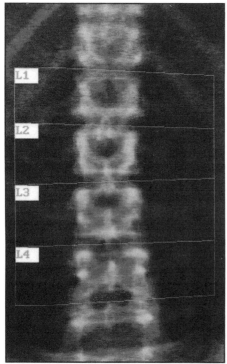

Hologic QDR-4500C (S/N 47303)
Lumbar Spine V8.26a:5

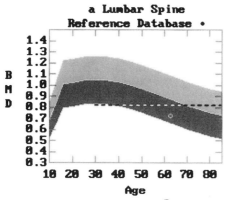

BMD(L1-L4) = 0.717 g/cm^2

Region	BMD	T(30.0)		Z	
L1	0.590	-3.04	64%	-1.62	77%
L2	0.766	-2.38	75%	-0.80	90%
L3	0.696	-3.52	64%	-1.86	77%
L4	0.789	-2.98	71%	-1.26	85%
L1-L4	0.717	-3.00	69%	-1.40	82%

• Age, sex, and ethnicity matched
T = peak BMD matched
Z = age matched

A

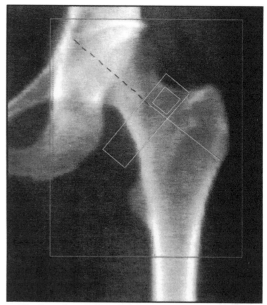

Hologic QDR-4500C (S/N 47303)
Left Hip V8.26a:5

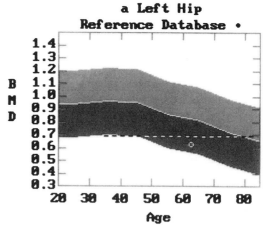

BMD(Total[L]) = 0.627 g/cm^2

Region	BMD	T		Z	
Neck	0.490	-3.26 (35.0)	56%	-1.91	68%
Troch	0.459	-2.32 (35.0)	65%	-1.37	76%
Inter	0.737	-2.38 (45.0)	65%	-1.48	75%
TOTAL	0.627	-2.50 (35.0)	65%	-1.48	76%
Ward's	0.319	-3.28 (25.0)	43%	-1.56	62%

• Age, sex, and ethnicity matched
T = peak BMD matched
Z = age matched

B

FIGURE 43.4. (A) DEXA scan of PA lumbar spine demonstrating L1–L4 *T* score of –3.00 consistent with WHO criteria for osteoporosis. (B) DEXA scan of the total hip demonstrating a *T* score of –2.50 consistent with WHO criteria for osteoporosis.

Quantitative Ultrasound (QUS)

Newer measures of bone strength, such as quantitative ultrasound (QUS), have been introduced. Currently only peripheral sites can be measured, including radius, phalanges, calcaneus, and tibia. Correlation with calcaneal BMD is moderately high, and correlation with spine or hip BMD is at best modest.[49] The poor correlation between QUS T scores and central DEXA is partly explained by the different reference population utilized.[50] Recent prospective studies using QUS of the heel have predicted hip and nonvertebral fractures nearly as well as DEXA at the femoral neck.[50] QUS or DXA at the femoral neck predict hip fracture better than DEXA at the lumbar spine.[51] QUS precision is less than DEXA, other artifacts can affect measurements, and controversy exists as how to express precision of QUS devices[49] (see Table 43.7).

Other Modalities

Advances in bone density measurement include lateral vertebral assessment (LVA) using DEXA as well as magnetic resonance imaging (MRI). LVA is useful in its ability to demonstrate actual bone morphology as an interpretable image in contrast with central DEXA, which merely provides quantitative information on bone mineral density. The lateral view of LVA is useful when severe kyphosis or degenerative changes falsely elevate lumbar spine BMD measurement on a PA central DEXA image; this, in addition to a low radiation exposure, makes LVA an attractive option for future use. MRI is being utilized in research settings for microarchitectural bone morphology (see Table 43.7).

Biochemical Markers of Bone Turnover

Biochemical markers of bone turnover may be used as an adjunct in the management of osteoporosis. Although serial DEXA measurements are useful in monitoring clinical response to treatment, most antiresorptive therapies require long-term administration with little to modest increase in BMD, necessitating 2-year or more intervals before repeat determinations are obtained. High bone turnover, which can be measured by biochemical markers, is an independent predictor of increased fracture risk.[52–58] Biochemical markers are useful in assessing rapid bone loss, risk of fracture, and monitoring therapy.[59] Common markers of bone formation available for clinical use include alkaline phosphatase, bone-specific alkaline phosphatase, and osteocalcin. Resorption markers include pyridinoline, deoxypyridinoline, and N- and C-telopeptides. The latter are collagen breakdown products that enter the circulation following bone resorption; their clinical usefulness in individual patients needs to be determined.[59]

Prevention and Treatment of Osteoporosis

Osteoporosis therapy should ideally be aimed at the underlying type of osteoporosis, that is, involutional, postmenopausal, or due to secondary causes. The majority of agents available today are antiresorptive, exerting the most beneficial effect in high-turnover osteoporosis; these include estrogen, selective estrogen receptor modulators (SERMs), bisphosphonates, and calcitonins. Agents that increase formation would be most advantageous in age-related osteoporosis where the primary defect is decreased osteoblastic bone formation; these include parathyroid hormone (PTH), vitamin D analogues, fluoride, and new osteoblastic stimulatory agents.

Calcium

The physiologic roles of calcium in the body are twofold. First, calcium provides structural integrity of the skeleton. In the extracellular fluids and in the cytosol, the Ca^{2+} concentration is critical to a number of biochemical processes, and its levels are tightly regulated.[60] In high bone turnover states, as with estrogen deficiency, there is an elevation in PTH levels. The rationale for the administration of calcium in this setting is partly because calcium inhibits PTH secretion and further bone loss.

Multiple placebo-controlled studies[61,62] have demonstrated the importance of adequate calcium intake for both primary and secondary prevention of osteoporosis. Chronic calcium deficiency inevitably leads to skeletal demineralization and enhanced fracture risk.[61] The effects of calcium supplementation are maximized in patients in whom baseline intake is low, especially in the elderly.[61] Nevertheless, there is continued controversy whether calcium supplementation can prevent bone loss or restore bone mass.

Premenopausal[61,62] and menopausal women[63,64] as well as middle-aged and older men[61] and frail female nursing home residents[65] respond to calcium supplementation in terms of small to modest increases in bone mineral density. Women in early menopause, presumably because of the dominant effect of gonadal hormone loss, do not show such an effect.[61,62] A large, randomized, placebo-controlled study of 1.2g calcium per day and 800IU vitamin D_3 per day in frail female nursing home residents revealed significantly fewer nonvertebral and hip fractures after an 18-month trial.[65] No other controlled studies have shown an effect of calcium supplements on fracture rate. These data, together with other studies on vitamin D-deficient residents in nursing homes,[66] suggest that the use of calcium and vitamin D supplementation in institutionalized elderly should be routine, particularly in those who have subclinical secondary hyperparathyroidism.

How much calcium is enough? The 1994 Consensus Development Conference on optional calcium intake recommended increases in the RDA for calcium in most age groups, particularly during childhood and adolescence when 40% of total adult bone mineral is formed. Total, that is, diet plus supplemental, intakes of 1.5 to 2 g of "elemental" calcium per day are recommended in postmenopausal women,[67] although intake must be individualized. There is little evidence that one form of calcium supplementation is superior to another. Older persons have a high prevalence of gastric achlorhydria and should take their supplements with meals. Patients must be informed that calcium supplementation alone is not sufficient to prevent either menopausal or age-related bone loss. Risks of calcium supplementation are minimal, but persons with a personal or family history of nephrolithiasis must be screened with 24-h urinary calcium determination. In addition, some older patients suffer from constipation and/or rebound gastric hyperacidity. Calcium citrate or calcium glubionate may be better tolerated in persons unable to tolerate other forms of calcium supplementation.

Some experts recommend that a routine urinary 24-h calcium level corrected for creatinine is a useful and inexpensive tool for a regular evaluation of the adequacy of dietary calcium intake. With the recommended intake, the 24-h urine calcium should remain in the 150 to 250 mg range. Calcium supplements should be prescribed with care in patients with end-stage renal disease, mainly for phosphate control. Notably, calcium citrate should be avoided in renal failure as it enhances the absorption of aluminum, the excessive absorption of which could worsen the bone disease secondary to renal failure.

Exercise

It is evident from multiple studies that immobility and disuse lead to accelerated bone loss. This conclusion is supported by animal studies in rats and turkeys, as well as cellular studies that have investigated the consequences of cellular loading. There is increasing evidence that mechanotransduction through osteocytes and bone-lining cells play a key role in bone formation. The accelerated bone loss that accompanies immobilization correlates significantly with cellular hypoxia due to reduced blood flow in bone canaliculi.[68]

Active individuals have higher bone mass than inactive individuals,[69] as has been shown in several cross-sectional studies. Correlations have been shown between muscle mass and bone density. For example, athletes have higher bone mass in skeletal regions of greatest exertion, and some prospective controlled studies in menopausal

women have demonstrated increases in bone mass, total body calcium, and improved calcium balance in the exercising groups.[69,70] A nonrandomized study in white postmenopausal women of walking more than 7.5 miles per week demonstrated higher bone density and slower rate of bone loss in the lower extremities in the long-distance group or runners.[71] It is also clear that exercise is less critical than gonadal hormone sufficiency in the prevention of bone loss because excessive weight loss in premenopausal female marathoners leads to amenorrhea, bone loss, and fractures.[72] Similarly, only a small percentage of the variability in bone density over a broad range of ages can be accounted for by differences in physical activity.[69,73] In addition, compliance with exercise recommendations is difficult to achieve in clinical practice, and there is some evidence that exercise-induced gains in bone mass are lost within months of discontinuation of the regimen.[70]

Questions regarding timing, age at onset, frequency, duration, and type of exercise most beneficial to bone remain to be answered. Many have proposed that the principal benefit of exercise in reducing fracture is its enhancement of muscle strength, balance, and coordination and the associated reduction in fall risk.[73] Elderly patients may require preexercise stress testing before initiation of a new exercise program.

In summary regarding exercise, prescriptions have been developed at the Institute on Aging at the University of Pennsylvania (Table 43.8). General recommenda-

TABLE 43.8. Exercise intervention for osteoporosis based on T scores.[a]

<1 SD below mean	Encourage weightbearing activity; low to moderate impact or loading activities: walking, jogging, running, hiking, stair climbing, stair-step machines, dancing, aerobics, weight training, ski machines
1–2.5 SD below mean	Low to moderate activities with low risk of falling or collision: stair-step machines, walking, ski machines Education on posture, fall prevention Recommend referral to physical therapy and occupational therapy
>2.5 SD below mean	Low- or no-impact exercise, risk of falling minimal: walking, water aerobics, deep-water walking, swimming, stationary cycle Education on posture and falls prevention Avoidance of activities that have a high degree of twisting or unbalancing movement, such as golf, bowling, tennis, or racquetball Recommend referral to physical therapy and occupational therapy

[a] Exercise prescriptions developed at the Institute on Aging at the University of Pennsylvania.

tions include duration of 30 min per day, 5 to 6 days per week, and maintenance of a high level of daily activity with adaptation according to age, lifestyle, strength, and agility.

Bisphosphonates

Bisphosphonates (BPs) are stable analogues of pyrophosphate that inhibit bone resorption. Their main effects include decreased osteoclast progenitor development, decreased osteoclast recruitment, and induction of osteoclast apoptosis leading to inhibition of bone resorption.[74,75] In BPs, the oxygen atom of the P-O-P (pyrophosphate) is replaced with a carbon atom, resulting in a P-C-P bond (Fig. 43.5). Drug variations of BPs are possible by changing the lateral carbon side chains. The R_1

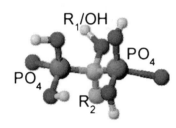

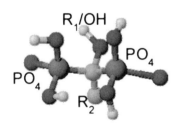

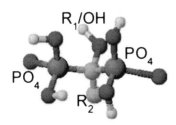

FIGURE 43.5. Biochemical structure of the bisphosphonates.

side chain is usually a hydroxyl group to enhance the affinity of the compound for bone, whereas variations in the structure and conformation of the R_2 side chain determine the antiresorptive potency.[76–78] Early BPs are less potent than later bisphosphonates, which have an amino-containing R_2 side chain[78] (Table 43.9).

The drug is tightly bound to the hydroxyapatite crystal and is retained in bone for many years. Only a small percentage of an oral dose is absorbed, mandating avoidance of food and other medications for several hours before and after a dose.

Previously etidronate was the only bisphosphonate available for oral use in the United States in the management of resorptive bone disease (see Table 43.9). It is FDA approved for the treatment of Paget's disease, heterotopic ossification, and hypercalcemia of malignancy, although not FDA approved for treatment of osteoporosis.[79] Etidronate inhibits bone mineralization at a dose similar to that required to inhibit bone resorption (see Table 43.9). Therefore, it is usually given cyclically, 400 mg daily for 2 weeks every 3 months, in concert with daily calcium supplementation to prevent osteomalacia.[80]

Short-term controlled trials of etidronate in postmenopausal and elderly patients have yielded slower rates of bone loss at the spine and hip, slight improvement or no change in radial cortical bone mass, and in two studies a trend toward diminished vertebral fracture rate.[81,82] Additionally, long-term clinical trials including more than 3 years and up to 7 years of treatment with etidronate demonstrate efficacy of cyclic etidronate therapy in increasing BMD and reducing vertebral fractures.[83,84]

Pamidronate is an intravenous BP presently FDA approved for the treatment of hypercalcemia of malignancy, Paget's disease, multiple myeloma, and breast

TABLE 43.9. Bisphosphonate generations and their potency ratios.[a]

First generation:
  Etidronate, 1
  Clodronate, 10

Second generation:
  Tiludronate, 10
  Pamidronate, 100
  6-Amino-1-hydroxyhexylidene, 100
  Alendronate, >100, <1,000
  Dimethyl-APD, >100, <1,000
  EB-1053, >100, <1,000
  YM 175, >100, <1,000

Third generation:
  Ibandronate, >1,000, <10,000
  Risedronate, >1,000, <10,000
  Zolendronate, >1,000, <10,000

[a] Potency ratios refer to the ratio of dose required to inhibit resorption to the dose required to inhibit bone mineralization.

cancer metastatic to bone (see Table 43.9). It is not FDA approved for the treatment of osteoporosis and is not currently reimbursable by Medicare for the treatment of osteoporosis. A number of studies have shown the efficacy of pamidronate infusions in increasing BMD at the hip and spine and reducing vertebral fractures.[85,86] It can be utilized as an alternative therapy in patients with osteoporosis who are intolerant of other forms of therapy. Treatment with pamidronate is usually well tolerated. Side effects are rare and may include fever, thrombophlebitis, and gastrointestinal symptoms. Hypocalcemia, hypophosphatemia, hypokalemia, and hypomagnesemia can occur, necessitating monitoring of these parameters. The dosage needs to be decreased in renal failure. Rapid intravenous administration has been associated with renal failure. Because of this they must be administered by slow i.v. infusion.[87]

Alendronate sodium, a second-generation aminobisphosphonate, has been FDA approved for the prevention and treatment of postmenopausal osteoporosis as well as the treatment of glucocorticoid-induced osteoporosis and Paget's disease (see Table 43.9). The dose of alendronate required to inhibit bone mineralization is 1000 times greater than that required to inhibit bone resorption, allowing daily administration. The recommended dose of alendronate for treatment of osteoporosis is 10 mg and that for prevention of osteoporosis is 5 mg. It is to be taken daily in the morning on an empty stomach with 8 oz plain water. Patients are instructed to delay eating or taking other medications for a minimum of 30 min. Calcium supplements, at a different time of day, at least 1500 mg per day must be given with bisphosphonates to reduce the risk of mineralization defects. A once-weekly 70-mg dose of alendronate sodium (for the treatment of osteoporosis) and 35-mg dose (for prevention) has recently been FDA approved. Randomized controlled trial data using alendronate in postmenopausal women have demonstrated significant reductions in both vertebral and nonvertebral fractures in association with significant gains in bone mineral density.[88-92]

A new BP, risedronate sodium, is a potent third-generation bisphosphonate that was recently FDA approved for the prevention and treatment of postmenopausal osteoporosis and treatment of glucocorticoid-induced osteoporosis in men and women. The current dose is 5 mg by oral administration daily (see Table 43.9).

Several other BPs (i.e., ibandronate) are currently undergoing phase III clinical trials. These BPs also inhibit osteoclastic bone resorption at doses much lower than that which impairs mineralization, allowing continuous daily administration. This group of drugs has been shown to inhibit bone loss in early menopause, in immobilized patients. and in corticosteroid-treated patients.[80,93]

Side Effects

Side effects, which have been generally minimal with both alendronate and etidronate, include abdominal and musculoskeletal pain. Although tolerability profiles of alendronate are similar to placebo in the literature, there is a rare association of alendronate with erosive esophagitis. More commonly patients experience nausea, dyspepsia, and other nonspecific gastrointestinal side effects, prompting their discontinuation. Recent short-term studies revealed similar increases in BMD with once- and twice-weekly dosing of alendronate to minimize GI side effects and maximize compliance.[94-96] Long-term efficacy studies are needed to document increased BMD and decreased fracture rates.

Patients with renal failure or hypocalcemia of any etiology should not receive BP therapy, and active upper gastrointestinal disease poses a relative contraindication to the use of this class of drugs. Because of the potent and long-term suppression of bone turnover effected by BPs, concern about impaired remodeling, diminished ability to repair microfractures, and progressively worsening bone fragility has been expressed. Bone biopsies in subjects treated with cyclical intermittent etidronate or daily alendronate have not shown a mineralization defect, nor has suppression of bone formation been observed. Biomechanical competence of bone after BP treatment has also been maintained or improved in animal studies.

Combination Therapy

The effects of combination therapy in the treatment of osteoporosis have been studied. One study evaluated 72 postmenopausal women in a 4-year study evaluating the efficacy of etidronate plus hormone replacement therapy (HRT), HRT alone, etidronate alone, and placebo. Patients on combination therapy experienced a significant increase in hip BMD compared with monotherapy with etidronate or estrogen, although there was no statistically significant decrease in fracture rates among groups.[97] Patients on combination therapy with alendronate 10 mg and continued HRT versus placebo with HRT were studied for 12 months. The BP plus estrogen group demonstrated significant increase in BMD at the lumbar spine (3.6% versus 1.0%; $p < 0.001$) and trochanter (2.7% versus 0.5%; $p < 0.001$).[98]

Estrogen

Evidence for the role of estrogen loss in osteoporosis is severalfold: bone loss is accelerated as ovarian function ceases,[99] such loss is inhibited with initiation of estrogen replacement therapy,[100,101] and bone loss resumes when estrogen replacement is terminated.[102]

At the cellular level, estrogens bind to nuclear receptors present in both osteoblasts and osteoclasts.[103–107] Estrogen acts on osteoblasts to produce a spectrum of different effects including enhanced procollagen production and increased alkaline phosphatase expression.[105,106,108,109] Estrogen also modulates the synthesis of certain growth factors and cytokines. For example, in osteoclast precursors, estrogen inhibits the production of interleukin-1 (IL-1), tumor necrosis factor-α (TNF-α), and interleukin-6 (IL-6).[103,110,111,112]

Estrogen deficiency causes increased osteoclast formation (see Fig. 43.3) by increasing production of the osteoclast-forming cytokine, M-CSF, from supporting stromal cells.[113] Estrogen application inhibits osteoclast formation. Estrogen inhibits transcription of the gene for an osteoclast-forming molecule, RANk-L (receptor activator for NFκB ligand).[114] Therefore, in addition to modulating molecules such as M-CSF, osteocalcin, osteonectin, and osteopontin, estrogen can directly suppress RANk-L-induced osteoclast differentiation and thus bone resorption.

When estrogen treatment is begun early in menopause (i.e., within the first 5 years) and continued for at least 10 years, hip fracture incidence is reduced by 50%,[115–121] and significant reductions in distal radial and vertebral fracture also occur. Optimally, hormone therapy for purposes of preventing bone loss should therefore begin as soon after menopause as possible to inhibit this accelerated loss, which ensues within 4 to 6 years of menopause. When estrogens are given during this phase, some patients may in fact gain new bone, as bone formation during this phase of intense remodeling can transiently exceed bone resorption.[100] Thereafter, bone mass is stabilized or the rate of loss is slowed until treatment is discontinued, whereupon rapid loss once again begins. Thus, although estrogens theoretically should be given indefinitely, every year of use delays the onset of clinically important osteopenia, as demonstrated by the reduced hip fracture incidence seen in elderly women treated in the distant past with several years of hormone replacement.[100,116,118,119] Even in older women with established bone loss, estrogen replacement has been shown to significantly increase bone mass.[122,123]

Studies of estrogen replacement in the elderly or in women with established osteoporosis have yielded conflicting results. Several trials have shown stabilization or improved bone density in estrogen-treated women after more than 10 years of menopause,[122–124] but at least 7 years of treatment seems necessary to maintain any benefit in the over-75-years age group.[125,126] This loss of benefit with shorter treatment durations may be due to resumption of rapid bone loss for several years after hormones are discontinued. Some argue that initiation of hormone replacement after age 70 might result in a substantial decrease in fracture risk and suggest that osteopenic elderly women are, contrary to widespread assumption, good candidates for estrogen treatment for fracture risk reduction.

Dosing Regimens

A number of dosing regimens of estrogen are currently utilized, including continuous and cyclic progestins to prevent endometrial hyperplasia and cancer. The most commonly used combination is equine estrogen (Premarin) 0.625 mg plus medroxyprogesterone 2.5 mg daily. Alternatively, estrogen is administered on days 1 to 30 plus medroxyprogesterone 5 or 10 mg on days 1 to 12. The former minimizes the risk of bleeding. Estrogen alone is utilized in women without a uterus. Several studies have concluded that the minimum effective daily dose of oral conjugated estrogens is 0.625 mg or its equivalent. A recent randomized, double-blind placebo-controlled study of 128 white postmenopausal women with low BMD (T score < 1.3) evaluated the efficacy of low-dose estrogen 0.3 mg per day plus medroxyprogesterone 2.5 mg per day.[127] This study revealed an increase in spinal BMD of 3.5% but with no significant change at the hip after 3.5 years of treatment. Additionally, the availability of transdermal estrogen formulations (which avoid the first-pass effect of oral estrogens on hepatic protein synthesis) may prove useful in patients with hepatic disease, coagulopathies, hypertension, or congestive heart failure. The minimum transdermal estrogen dose necessary to inhibit bone loss has not yet been determined, although one study showed fracture reduction at a daily dose of 0.1 mg estradiol in a 20-cm^2 transdermal patch.[123]

Other Effects

Some of the other benefits of estrogen replacement therapy include amelioration of mood disturbances, prevention of vasomotor symptoms including flushes and night sweats, and relief of symptoms of vaginal atrophy.

Estrogen replacement therapy has been associated in several prospective and case-control studies with a reduction in cardiovascular morbidity and mortality and in all-cause mortality. There is an associated increase in HDL levels.[128–130] The mechanism of the cardiovascular benefit of estrogen is not known, but direct action on vascular endothelium as well as favorable changes in plasma lipoproteins have been noted. Of some concern is the adverse effect of progestational agents on HDL. The only prospective, randomized controlled trial of estrogen and progesterone in women with coronary disease indicated an early increased risk of cardiovascular mortality.[131] These findings may, in part, result from the androgenic effects of medroxyprogesterone. These findings raise concern about the possible deleterious cardiovascular effects of estrogen, but the results must be interpreted with caution. The results can only be applicable to women with preexisting coronary disease. More prospective randomized trials are under way. Additionally, epidemiologic evidence suggests estrogen may confer protection against Alzheimer's disease[132] and colon cancer.[133] Prospective randomized studies are under way to determine the efficacy of estrogens in prevention of dementia.

Unopposed estrogen poses an increased risk of endometrial hyperplasia and carcinoma.[134] Cycling or continuous oral medroxyprogesterone reduces this risk.[135,136] Other common side effects of estrogen include breast tenderness, thrombosis, weight gain, irregular bleeding, fluid retention, and worsening of hypertension.

There is widespread concern regarding the risk of breast cancer from menopausal estrogen replacement, which has not been consistently corroborated by available evidence. A recent meta-analysis reported a summary risk estimate of 1.3 (confidence interval, 1.2–1.6) in women treated with estrogen for more than 15 years compared with nonusers.[136,137] The Nurses' Health Study showed a higher risk in current as opposed to past users or never users, independent of dose or duration.[138,139] Notable is that in one of these studies[138] the increased risk of breast cancer associated with 5 or more years of postmenopausal hormone use was greater among older than younger postmenopausal women [relative risk (RR), 1.7 versus 1.3 among all current users].

The addition of progesterone to the regimen has unknown effects on breast cancer risk but is at least theoretically likely to increase mitotic activity in breast tissue.[136,138] Recent data regarding estrogen and breast cancer, however, cannot be overlooked. Data from the Breast Cancer Demonstration Project included 46,355 postmenopausal women showed increased risk, 1.2 (confidence interval, 1.0–1.4), for estrogen users and 1.4 (1.0–1.8) in estrogen–progestin users.[140] The relative risk of breast cancer increased by 0.01 per year of estrogen replacement and by 0.08 per year for combination therapy. The relative risk was further increased in women with low body weight with body mass indices (BMI) of 24.4 or less. Additionally, a population-based case-control study on 3500 postmenopausal women also similarly concluded that the addition of a progestin increased the risk of breast cancer relative to estrogen use.[141]

The long-term effects of estrogen and progestin use on total mortality are unknown. Large-scale prospective randomized studies are required to clarify the ultimate effect of menopausal hormone replacement on overall morbidity and mortality, coronary heart disease, breast and uterine cancer, and osteoporotic fracture.[138] Physician and patient alike must balance her risk of osteoporosis and coronary heart disease against the risk of breast cancer in deciding for or against menopausal hormone replacement.[136] Despite the current knowledge of potential benefits of estrogen to inhibit bone loss, many women discontinue treatment within 1 year due to side effects, such as bleeding, and more commonly, fears of breast cancer and thrombosis.[142,143]

There are certain contraindications to estrogen replacement therapy, which include previous history of breast or uterine cancer, active thrombotic disorders, and liver or gallbladder disease. A positive family history in a first-degree relative of breast cancer, coagulopathy, or hypertriglyceridemia must also lessen the enthusiasm for estrogen therapy. Smoking is not a contraindication to HRT.

Selective Estrogen Receptor Modulators

An important addition to our armamentarium of osteoporosis treatment is the development of selective estrogen receptor modulators (SERMs). Raloxifene has been shown to bind with high affinity to estrogen receptors. By binding differently from parent estrogens to the same receptor, SERMs can confer a conformation that enables the receptor to interact with a different second messenger. Thus, raloxifene is an agonist at bone and with respect to lipoproteins, but in contrast to estrogen is an antagonist at the breast and uterus. Its mechanism of action in bone may involve the upregulation of TGF-β_3 expression, thus inhibiting osteoclast formation and bone.[144,145]

The SERMs currently include tamoxifen, raloxifene, and draloxifene. Raloxifene is U.S. Food and Drug Administration (FDA) approved for the prevention and treatment of osteoporosis at a 60-mg dosage. The clinical effects of raloxifene on BMD and antifracture efficacy have been shown by a number of prospective placebo-controlled trials. Studies have demonstrated a BMD increase of 2.4% at the spine and the hip at 3 years.[146] Results from the Multiple Outcomes of Raloxifene Evaluation (MORE) study demonstrated a significant reduction, about 30% to 50%, in vertebral fractures but no change in nonvertebral fractures.[147] Additional benefits of raloxifene include its favorable lipoprotein profile and a 76% reduction in invasive breast cancer.[148] Its side effects include venous thromboembolism and lack of relief of postmenopausal vasomotor symptoms. More long-term studies are needed to evaluate hip fracture efficacy as well as possible side effects on the uterus and breast.

Calcitonin

Calcitonin is a 32-amino-acid peptide hormone synthesized and secreted from the C cells of the thyroid. The main action of calcitonin is on bone, although it may, at pharmacologic concentrations, increase renal calcium and phosphate excretion and 1,25-dihydroxycholecalciferol production. In bone sections, calcitonin application results in a rapid loss of ruffled borders. When applied for a longer term, there is a reduction in the number of osteo-

FIGURE 43.6. Light microscopy of an osteoclast before (A) and after the addition of calcitonin (B).

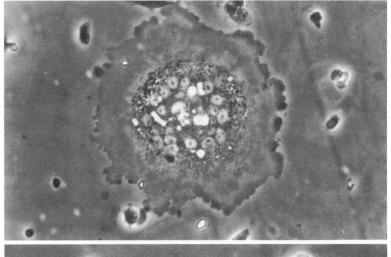

A

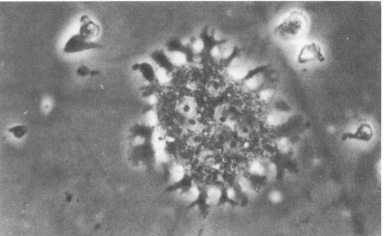

B

clasts in bone (see Fig. 43.6). In osteoclasts, calcitonin inhibits bone resorption, which occurs by the inhibition of cell motility and enzyme secretion.[149–156]

Salmon calcitonin has a 40-fold greater potency than human calcitonin, but long-term use is associated with a high rate of development of neutralizing antibodies.[157] Resistance to human calcitonin has also been observed, presumably due to receptor downregulation. Resistance can be minimized by use of lower doses, intranasal or rectal administration, or intermittent administration of the drug.

The utility of calcitonin as a therapeutic agent in disease states of accelerated bone resorption has been clearly demonstrated in Paget's disease and hypercalcemia of malignancy. Several prospective controlled trials have also documented stabilization of, and in some cases modest short-term increases in, bone mass in osteoporotic patients treated for 5 years or less.[158–160] Much of this benefit has been observed in trabecular bone; the benefit of calcitonin in reducing cortical bone loss has not been clearly demonstrated.[160,161] Similar effects have been demonstrated utilizing calcitonin as a preventive treatment for menopausal trabecular bone loss.[160,162] Three

studies directly evaluating the impact of calcitonin on fracture reduction have all shown significant reduction in hip fracture, vertebral compression fracture, and peripheral limb fractures. This benefit was observed both in postmenopausal and elderly women.[161,163,164] Long-term studies using calcitonin reveal a 1.2% increase in BMD at the posteroanterior (PA) spine over 5 years.[165] Preliminary data from the PROOF trial (Prevent Recurrence of Osteoporotic Fractures), a 5-year double-blind, randomized, placebo-controlled study of 1255 postmenopausal women with osteoporosis, demonstrate that 200 IU salmon calcitonin nasal spray reduced the relative risk of vertebral fractures by 36% versus placebo.

Compromised trabecular microarchitecture is an important and independent causal factor in the pathogenesis of vertebral fractures in both men and women.[166] It is now emerging that there is a temporal dissociation between reduction in fracture risk that can occur in 12 to 18 months, bone markers, and long-term effects on BMD. Notably, a benefit in fracture risk occurs before a change in BMD. Recent clinical trials with antiresorptives, such as calcium plus vitamin D, calcitonin, and raloxifene, indicate significant protection from fracture despite only modest increases in BMD. This finding has led to the belief that antiresorptives conserve bone microarchitecture by preventing osteoclastic resorption.[167]

The major drawbacks of calcitonin therapy include its high cost and the need for parenteral, nasal, or rectal administration; as of 1996 both parenteral and nasal calcitonin have been FDA approved for treatment of osteoporosis in the United States. Analgesic effects of calcitonin have also been documented in multiple studies of vertebral fracture patients, but these results are compromised by failure to utilize appropriate control groups.[160]

The major side effect of parenteral calcitonin therapy, the use of which is now restricted to acute vertebral compression syndrome, is transient nausea and vomiting, which are both self-limited. Nasal calcitonin is generally well tolerated; its use may be associated with local irritation and rhinitis, which usually subside with continued therapy. There is no evidence of any serious or long-term side effects in studies of up to 5 years duration.

Treatment of Secondary Osteoporosis

With the exception of glucocorticoid-induced osteoporosis, few studies of therapeutic measures for primary osteoporosis have assessed their utility in treatment of secondary osteoporosis. Wherever possible the underlying primary disease process leading to bone loss should be treated. When this is not possible, routine calcium and vitamin D supplementation, as well as treatment of hypogonadism in women and men, may be of benefit. Similarly, it is reasonable to utilize other antiresorptive agents (such as calcitonin or bisphosphonates) in an effort to minimize bone loss.

Osteoporosis is among the most serious consequences of long-term glucocorticoid treatment, leading to a 50% increase in risk of hip and other fractures. Glucocorticoids inhibit osteoblastic bone formation, increase osteoclastic bone resorption, and inhibit intestinal calcium absorption. In this setting calcitriol therapy has been associated with a very high incidence (25%) of hypercalcemia.[168] Alendronate has been shown to increase BMD on oral glucocorticoids at a daily dose of prednisone at 7.5 mg or greater. The dosage of alendronate for the prevention of glucocorticoid induced osteoporosis is 5 mg, except in postmenopausal women not receiving estrogen, for whom the dosage is 10 mg once daily. There are no data on fracture efficacy due to insufficient number of patients.[18] Risedronate has also been shown to be efficacious in the treatment of glucocorticoid-induced osteoporosis.[19]

Currently, there are insufficient clinical data on the prevention of osteoporosis in patients who undergo transplantation. In a pilot study, two groups of cardiac transplant patients were studied for 1 year.[169] After transplantation, all patients received 500 mg elemental calcium twice daily and 400 IU vitamin D. The intervention group (n = 18 subjects) were given calcitriol and bisphosphonate therapy in addition to calcium and vitamin D during the first year after transplantation (intravenous pamidronate, 60 mg administered within 10 days after transplantation, followed by four courses of oral etidronate, 400 mg daily for the first 14 days of every third month). Forty-one control patients in the calcium and vitamin D only group were observed for 1 year. The bisphosphonate-treated group had no lumbar spine bone loss (0.2%) versus 6.8% loss per year ($p < 0.0001$) in the untreated group. Significantly less bone loss was also observed at the femoral neck in the treated group. There were 3 incident vertebral fractures in the treated group versus 30 in the untreated group. This study demonstrates the potential treatment benefits in cardiac transplant patients of preventative therapy with bisphosphonates.

Other Treatments for Osteoporosis

Sodium Fluoride

Fluoride is an agent capable of stimulating new bone formation by increasing osteoblastic activity. Bone biopsies demonstrate increased trabecular volume and thickness and increased osteoid surfaces. Initially, the new bone formed may be poorly mineralized woven bone, which is eventually replaced by a lamellar bone structure. Prospective controlled clinical trials have demonstrated linear increases in spine and hip bone mass but decreased radial cortical bone mass.[170,171] No significant decreases in vertebral fractures and a significant increase in nonvertebral fractures at sites high in cortical bone were observed in these studies.[170,171] This finding suggests that fluoride therapy may preferentially cause new trabecular bone formation but at the expense of appendicular cortical bone. Fluoride remains an experimental drug, has not been shown to decrease fracture risk, and is not approved for treatment of osteoporosis by the FDA.[170–172] Because of its substantial side effects, fluoride is best used only in clinical trials.[172]

Parathyroid Hormone

Parathyroid hormone (PTH) acts on osteoblasts to modulate the expression of a variety of growth factors, including IGF-1, TGF-β_1, and TGF-β_2, as well as certain cytokines.[173,174] The precise mechanism underlying the anabolic effects of PTH on bone is just beginning to be unraveled.[175–177]

When administered at a low dose, intermittently, PTH stimulates bone formation. Several clinical trials have demonstrated increases in bone mass and volume with low intermittent doses of PTH.[178] One study evaluated the use of PTH administration daily in a randomized clinical trial for 12 months in women treated with gonadotropin-releasing hormone (GnRH) antagonists for endometriosis. PTH administration increased BMD at the AP spine by 2.1% and lateral spine by 7.5% and prevented bone loss at the hip and total body.[179] Although results to date show promise, PTH(1–34) remains experimental until larger controlled clinical trials evaluating fracture rate are completed. The major drawback to utilizing PTH is its need to be given parenterally and in achieving the pulses in the circulation necessary to enable bone formation.

To modulate the endogenous secretion of PTH, antagonists of the parathyroid Ca^{2+}-sensing receptor called calcilytics have been developed. Antagonizing the Ca^{2+} receptor imitates a state of hypocalcemia and stimulates PTH secretion. Animal studies with such compounds found that bone turnover increased, unless estrogen was coadministered.[180] Another way of inducing PTH anabolic effects on bone is by using Ca^{2+}-sensing receptor agonists (calcimimetics) to intermittently decrease PTH levels. Animal studies have shown an increase in bone mineral density and cancellous bone volume using such a technique.[181]

Vitamin D

Gastrointestinal calcium absorption diminishes with age and is abnormally low in patients with osteoporosis, in association with diminished calcitriol levels and decreased responsiveness of the 1α-hydroxylase enzyme to parathyroid hormone stimulation.[182,183] Although vitamin D may indirectly stimulate bone resorption, it also enhances gastrointestinal calcium absorption, pro-

motes mineralization, and inhibits PTH-induced bone resorption.[183]

One clinical trial utilizing cholecalciferol (800 IU daily) in combination with calcium supplements (1200 mg daily) significantly reduced hip and other fractures in a nursing home population.[65] Another controlled trial of annual injection of 150,000 IU of vitamin D alone also demonstrated a significant reduction in fracture rate in an elderly population.[184] However, results from multiple trials of calcitriol (1,25-dihydroxyvitamin D) have been contradictory, with four showing increased bone mass or fewer fractures, three showing lower bone mass or more fractures, and three showing no effect.[183] Because of the risk of hypercalcemia and hypercalciuria with calcitriol, regular monitoring of calcium intake and serum and 24-h urinary calcium is required. Given the risks and the contradictory findings of available clinical trials, pharmacologic doses of active vitamin D metabolites must be considered experimental. However, physiologic replacement of vitamin D (800 IU per day) has demonstrated efficacy in reducing fractures in the elderly and should now be considered routine treatment.

HMG-Co A Reductase Inhibitors

Recent animal studies have shown that the inhibition of HMG-Co A reductase by the lipid-lowering statins activates osteoclast apoptosis, reduces osteoclast recruitment, and promotes osteoblastic bone formation.[185,186] In vitro and in vivo evidence has demonstrated that amino bisphosphonates inhibit the biosynthetic pathway from mevalonate to cholesterol, resulting in decreased farnesyl or geranylgeranyl pyruvate.[185] Decreased prenylation of GTP-binding proteins resulted in osteoclast apoptosis (see flow diagram in Fig. 43.7).

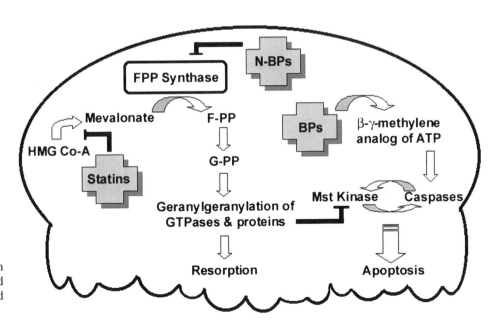

FIGURE 43.7. Cellular mechansim of bisphosphonates (*BP*) and statins in the mevolonic acid pathway.

Promising clinical trials have become recently become available. Patients with type II diabetes mellitus exhibited significant increases in BMD at the lumbar spine and the hip in those treated with lovastatin, pravastatin, or simvastatin compared to controls.[187] Other studies document a decreased fracture risk in those treated with statins.[188,189] Further controlled studies are necessary to determine the clinical applicability in the treatment of osteoporosis.

Other Treatment Strategies

Growth factors [insulin-like growth factor (IGF) I and II and transforming growth factor-β (TGF-β)] act to increase proliferation of osteoblasts and are currently undergoing evaluation for methods of localizing their effects to the skeleton. Anabolic steroids are potent antiresorptives, but androgenic side effects, adverse lipid changes, and hepatotoxicity limit their use. Flavinoids[183] are common plant metabolites with some indirect estrogenic properties, and ipriflavone has been shown in animal and human studies to prevent bone loss or increase bone mass in diverse research settings. It has not yet been shown to reduce fracture rates, and long-term evaluation of both efficacy and toxicities is needed.

Primary Hyperparathyroidism

Primary hyperparathyroidism is a metabolic bone disorder caused by excess secretion of parathyroid hormone from hyperplastic or, more commonly, adenomatous parathyroid glands and manifested by hypercalcemia. Increased use of multichannel autoanalyzers has led to greater and earlier detection of asymptomatic hypercalcemia due to hyperparathyroidism. From 25% to 50% of cases occur between age 60 and 90 years, and the distinction between the myriad manifestations of the disease versus other concomitants of old age presents a major clinical challenge.[190,191]

Clinical Manifestations

The skeletal manifestations of primary hyperparathyroidism include primarily osteoporosis with loss of cortical bone and increased risk of fracture. The classic findings of osteitis fibrosa cystica are only rarely seen today. Additionally, dental problems with tooth loss and generalized arthralgias may be manifested. Gastrointestinal signs and symptoms include peptic ulcer disease, pancreatitis, constipation, and nausea and vomiting. The latter are observed in those with severe elevations of serum calcium or hypercalcemic crisis, generally when serum calcium is greater than 14 mg/dL. Renal effects include polyuria due to hypercalciuria-induced osmotic diuresis, nephrolithiasis, nephrocalcinosis, and diminished glomerular filtration rate.[192] Although hypertension is more prevalent among patients with hyperparathyroidism, the underlying mechanism is not well defined. Neuromuscular manifestations include muscle weakness, paresthesias, and fatigue, although the typical neuromuscular findings are uncommon today. Finally, and of great importance in the elderly, primary hyperparathyroidism may become manifest with memory loss, delirium, personality changes, or depression.[191,193] Thus, while as many as 50% of hyperparathyroid patients are reported to be asymptomatic, many manifestations of the disease may have been inappropriately attributed to the aging process alone.

Diagnosis

The diagnosis requires the presence of hypercalcemia, which may be intermittent, in association with an elevated or inappropriately normal parathyroid hormone concentration. Other laboratory findings may include hypophosphatemia, hyperchloremia, hypercalciuria, and elevated measures of bone turnover including serum or bone-specific alkaline phosphatase, osteocalcin, and other measures of bone turnover.[192,194] Classic bone densitometry findings include decreased BMD at the distal one-third radius, which is composed principally of cortical bone.

It is necessary to obtain complete laboratory evaluation in a patient presenting with hypercalcemia, particularly in those presenting with hypercalcemic crisis; this includes intact PTH, $1,25(OH)_2$ vitamin D_3, 25OH vitamin D_3, and PTH-related protein (PTH rp). The differential diagnosis of hypercalcemia includes various neoplasms (especially lung, breast, GI tract, kidney, lymphoma, and multiple myeloma), vitamin D intoxication, milk alkali syndrome, hyperthyroidism, sarcoidosis, tuberculosis, drugs (lithium and thiazides), and immobilization (especially in active Paget's disease). Thiazide diuretics and lithium may cause small elevations in serum calcium levels that should resolve upon discontinuation of the drug.

An important entity to exclude before consideration of surgery in patients with hypercalcemia would be familial hypocalciuric hypercalcemia (FHH), where serum PTH and calcium are elevated but urinary calcium is depressed. The underlying mechanism is an inactivating mutation of the calcium-sensing receptor in the parathyroid glands. Normally, elevated ionized calcium levels should inhibit PTH synthesis and secretion from the parathyroid gland. However, these individuals have a higher "set point" for calcium recognition; thus, PTH is inappropriately elevated for their level of ionized calcium. This fact should be considered in patients with a family history of hypercalcemia. It may also be necessary to obtain previous laboratory data on the patient if they have a lifelong history of hypercalcemia; in the setting of low urinary calcium excretion, the diagnosis of FHH is more likely. This is a clinically important entity to recognize as one would not expose a patient to unnecessary surgical treatment.

Severe elevations in serum calcium with associated suppressed parathyroid hormone concentrations suggest a diagnosis of neoplasm with increased PTH rp or granulomatous disorder with increased 1α-hydroxylase activity and increased $1,25(OH)_2$ vitamin D levels, as opposed to primary hyperparathyroidism. Because primary hyperparathyroidism is an increasingly recognized disease entity, it would not be rare to find concomitant hypercalcemia of malignancy and primary hyperparathyroidism in the same individual.

Treatment

In those affected, who have definite signs and symptoms of the disease or severe hypercalcemia, appropriate management requires surgical neck exploration and removal of the adenomatous or hyperplastic tissue. The risk of neck exploration is greatly reduced when performed by a highly experienced surgeon. Postoperative hypocalcemia and tetany occur rarely, caused by hypoparathyroidism or hungry bone syndrome, primarily in patients with severe bone disease or hyperplastic glands, mandating frequent monitoring and replacement of calcium, magnesium, and vitamin D as needed to restore normocalcemia. Marked improvement in subtle symptoms of fatigue or memory loss may follow surgery, especially in the elderly.

Treatment of asymptomatic hyperparathyroidism remains controversial. A 1991 NIH Consensus Conference set forth recommendations for surgical intervention in patients with asymptomatic hyperparathyroidism; these include hypercalcemia (greater than 1–1.6 mg/dL over the upper limit of normal), a 30% decrease in creatinine clearance compared to age-matched normals, a 24-h urinary calcium determination of greater than 400 mg, and a Z score on bone densitometry of less than −2.0. Additionally, surgery is preferable for those patients who request surgery, where consistent follow-up would be unlikely, when coexistent illness complicates management, and if the patient is less than 50 years of age.[195]

In asymptomatic patients with milder hypercalcemia, general recommendations include appropriate hydration, exercise, and avoidance of diuretics. Restriction of dietary calcium has not been shown to be of clear benefit and should not be employed unless this measure results in reduced serum and urine calcium levels without a concomitant rise in parathyroid hormone concentration.

In one 10-year study, 23% of untreated asymptomatic patients ultimately required surgery because of development of clinical manifestations of disease.[196] Indications for consideration of surgery in these patients include declining renal function, hypercalciuria, nephrolithiasis, poorly controlled hypertension, a rise in serum calcium (more than 1 mg above the upper limit of normal), rapid decline in bone density or appearance of osteoporotic fractures, peptic ulcer disease, or altered mental status. In the absence of these manifestations, continued conservative management, including hydration, regular bone densitometry, and careful observation, is a reasonable alternative.

Some have argued that most of the osseous complications of hyperparathyroidsm could be prevented and bone loss reversed if parathyroidectomy were performed early in the course of the disease. A 10-year prospective cohort study of patients with symptomatic and asymptomatic hyperparathyroidism defined the natural history of disease and assessed the differences between surgical versus nonsurgical patients.[197] During the course of the study, 121 patients were followed, 61 patients underwent parathyroidectomy, and 60 patients were followed without surgery. Parathyroidectomy in patients with or without symptoms led to normalization of biochemical parameters and significantly increased lumbar spine and femoral neck bone mineral density. In 52 asymptomatic patients followed without surgery, none had changes in biochemical parameters; however, 27% had progression of disease or development of at least one indication for parathyroidectomy.

The conservative approach to management of asymptomatic hyperparathyroidism may undergo transformation, based on the findings that parathyroidectomy leads to normalization of biochemical parameters and increases in BMD, as well as the advent of new surgical techniques and imaging studies. Minimally invasive parathyroidectomy[198,199] under local anesthesia with a skilled surgeon demonstrates a high success rate and decreased surgical risks compared to general anesthesia. This approach is a relatively new technique available only in a few centers; more long-term studies are necessary before general recommendations can be made. There may be a shift toward early surgical intervention before bone loss ensues and renal function declines, with the ultimate goal of preservation of bone mass and subsequent decrease in fracture rates. Prospective long-term data on fracture prevention have not been established.

Patients who refuse or are poor candidates for surgery should be considered for efforts to inhibit the effect of parathyroid hormone on bone. Possible agents for this purpose include oral phosphate, which is used rarely because it requires careful monitoring due to the risk of ectopic calcification. Oral bisphosphonates, because of their poor absorption and short half-life, are ineffectual and may further exacerbate an autonomously functioning gland. Estrogen in the treatment of postmenopausal women with primary hyperparathyroidism shows promise. A higher bone density and biochemical evidence of diminished bone turnover and decreased serum and urinary calcium without change in parathyroid hormone concentration has been observed in estrogen-treated patients.[200,201]

A new promising treatment possibility is calcimimetic drug therapy. The search for an effective medical therapy has been stimulated in part by the discovery of a calcium-sensing receptor in the parathyroid and the kidney that regulates the synthesis and secretion of PTH. R-568 or phenylalkylamine (R)-N-(3-methoxy-alpha-phenylethyl)-3-(2-chlorophenyl)-1-propylamine is a calcimimetic compound that increases cytoplasmic calcium and decreases parathyroid hormone secretion. In a randomized placebo-controlled trial, single doses of the drug decreased serum PTH and ionized calcium in post-menopausal women with mild primary hyperparathyroidism.[202] More long-term controlled studies are needed to determine the implications in the medical treatment of hyperparathyroidism.

Paget's Disease of Bone

Paget's disease of bone is a chronic focal disorder of the skeleton that is asymptomatic in most affected individuals. It is characterized by an early period of sharply demarcated areas of bone resorption, followed by rapid formation of disorganized new bone, resulting in histologically abnormal bone, skeletal deformity, and increased fracture risk.

Epidemiology

Paget's disease of bone affects 1% to 4% of persons over age 40 and greater than 10% of those over age 80. It is common in Northern European (except Scandinavia) and North American temperate regions and rare in tropical and Asian nations. A slight predominance of males has been observed and some familial clustering disease has been reported, suggesting a genetic susceptibility to the disease.[203]

Etiology

Although the etiology of Paget's disease is unknown, the osteoclasts in pagetic bone contain typical nuclear and cytoplasmic inclusions in a random or paracrystalline microfilament array, suggestive of a slow viral etiology. However, no infectious agents have been found. No single etiologic agent has been identified to date. In situ hybridization studies have yielded conflicting results, including paramyxovirus, respiratory syncitial virus, measles, and canine distemper.

Pathology

The early pagetic lesion is characterized by a well-defined focal area of osteolytic bone resorption, resulting from the proliferation of large multinucleated osteoclasts, each containing more than 100 nuclei. Increased osteoclastic activity is associated with greatly increased osteoblast activity with enlarged osteoblasts lining the bony lacunae. Pagetic bone has a mosaic pattern resulting from the simultaneous appearance of disordered and accelerated bone resorption and formation and replacement of displaced hematopoietic marrow with fibrovascular connective tissue. "Burned-out" lesions or areas in which accelerated osteoclastic and osteoblastic activity have ceased can be seen. This bone is poor quality due to disorganized collagen deposition and poor mineralization.[203]

Clinical Presentation

Paget's disease is rare in persons under 45 years of age. It is typically asymptomatic, requiring treatment in less than 1% of affected individuals affected. It is commonly detected by an incidental elevation of serum alkaline phosphatase or an abnormal X-ray. The disease may be mild or severe, occur in single or in multiple skeletal locations, and result in a variety of possible clinical presentations.[203] Deformity of skull and clavicle, bowing and fracture of weightbearing bones, and associated mild to moderate bone pain are typical signs and symptoms. Severe bone pain in a patient with Paget's disease should suggest coexisting arthritis, acute fracture, neurologic impairment, or sarcomatous degeneration of a bone lesion. Enlargement of skull structures may lead to headache, cranial nerve deficits (vertigo, tinnitus, and hearing loss) and, if pressure on the base of skull occurs, diplopia, incontinence, abnormal gait, slurring of speech, and abnormal swallowing may result. Involvement of spinal vertebrae with subsequent spinal cord compression may also be observed.

Neoplastic transformation occurs in less than 1% of patients and is characterized by rapid increase in alkaline phosphatase, severe bone pain, or accelerated deformity. It requires bone biopsy for diagnosis. Other complications include ectopic calcification (of vessels, heart valves, joints, and Bruch's membrane with angioid streaks), high-output congestive heart failure from increased shunting of blood flow through bone, and hyperuricemia and gout from increased cell turnover. Hypercalcemia and hypercalciuria with nephrolithiasis secondary to immobilization after a pathologic fracture or neurologic complication may also occur. These symptoms and complications are indications for aggressive therapy.[203]

Diagnosis

Laboratory Studies

Elevation in serum alkaline phosphatase is an early herald of the disease, correlates well with extent of bony involvement, and is a reliable indicator of disease activity and response to therapy. Urinary hydroxyproline elevation is a measure of increased osteoclastic activity and is also a useful guide to response to therapy. Serum osteocalcin, bone-specific alkaline phosphatase, urinary pyridinoline cross-links, and other biochemical markers of bone turnover are increasingly utilized in diagnosis and management of Paget's disease. Serum and urinary calcium and phosphorus are normal unless immobilization of a patient with active disease occurs or a neoplasm supervenes.[203]

Radiologic Studies

Radiographic appearance of bone typically reflects the stage and extent of disease. Early well-defined lucent areas (osteoporosis circumscripta) may be adjacent to areas of dense or sclerotic bone in later stages of disease. Osteoblastic bone metastases may have a similar radiographic appearance. Bowed and thickened cortex of long bones with an advancing V-shaped osteolytic front, thickened iliopectineal line, sclerotic vertebral margins, and honeycomb or cotton wool-like mottling of the skull also may occur. Radioisotope bone scans are highly sensitive, but not specific, for Paget's disease and are useful to define the activity and skeletal distribution of the disease.[203] These scans may also be useful in monitoring disease activity during the course of treatment.

Differential diagnosis requires consideration of diseases resulting in substantial elevations of serum alkaline phosphatase that include metastatic prostate carcinoma, osteogenic sarcoma, and recent fracture. Osteoporotic fractures and accompanying pain may present some difficulties in differential diagnosis. However, the postfracture elevation in alkaline phosphatase is usually mild and transient, and the radiographic characteristics of simple osteopenia are not typical of Paget's disease. The two diseases may occur simultaneously in the elderly. Distinguishing osteoarthritis from Paget's disease is also difficult because of the frequent coexistence of these conditions. Appropriate radiographic and laboratory studies usually clarify the etiology of the pain. Treatment may require use of both anti-inflammatory agents for the arthritis and specific therapy of Paget's disease.

Treatment

Indications for treatment of Paget's disease include skeletal pain, bony deformity, neurologic complications, presence of medical complications (such as high-output congestive heart failure, hypercalcemia, and hypercalciuria), and preparation for orthopedic surgery. With the exception of skull or facial bone involvement, preventive intervention in asymptomatic patients with active disease is of uncertain utility. However, given the advent of newer high-potency bisphosphonates and greater tolerability, this approach may change.

Efficacy of therapy depends on reducing osteoclast and osteoblast activity. Response is evaluated by reduction in pain and other symptoms, reduced alkaline phosphatase, reduction in urinary hydroxyproline levels or other measures of bone turnover, and improved radiographic findings. Surgical intervention may be required in patients with symptoms of bone pressure on brain or spinal cord, severe hip dysfunction, and long bone bowing sufficient to precipitate fracture.[203]

Bisphosphonates

This class of drugs constitutes the choice of therapy in patients with Paget's disease of bone. Etidronate previously was most commonly used to induce remission. With the advent of second- and third-generation bisphosphonates with greater antiresorptive specificity, etidronate, although efficacious, is rarely used today. Alendronate, risedronate, and tiludronate are oral bisphosphonates FDA approved for use in the treatment of Paget's disease[204-206] (see Table 43.10 for dosing schedules of bisphosphonates).

The clinical effects of bisphosphonates are dose related and include relief of bone pain and complications of disease, as well as about a 50% reduction in biochemical indices of disease after a standard treatment course. Calcium supplementation should be given in an effort to reduce the risk of clinically significant osteomalacia. Because of poor gastrointestinal absorption, oral bisphosphonates should be taken daily first thing in the morning with water, 30 min before food, other pills, or other

TABLE 43.10. Treatment regimens for Paget's disease of bone.

Alendronate sodium: 40 mg p.o. daily for 6 months
Risedronate sodium: 30 mg p.o. daily for 2 months
Tiludronate: 400 mg p.o. daily for 3 months
Pamidronate[a]: 30–60 mg in normal saline i.v. infusion over 4–6 h[b]
Etidronate: 400 mg p.o. daily for a 14-day course cycled every 3 months for a 6-month course
Salmon calcitonin: 0.25–1.0 mL (50–200 MRC units) i.m. or s.q. at bedtime every other day or every day
Human calcitonin: 0.25–1.0 mL (50–200 MRC units) i.m. or s.q. at bedtime every other day or every day

[a] Lower doses must be used in renal insufficiency. Monitoring of serum calcium, phosphorus, and renal function is required.
[b] No standardized dosing regimen; this allows for individualized dosing depending on disease extent.

liquids. Treatment for 3 to 6 months is usually sufficient to achieve remission or biochemical plateau, and symptoms may not recur for variable periods thereafter. A drug-free interval of 6 months is recommended. Recurrent signs and symptoms of disease are indications for a repeat course of therapy.

Side effects are seen more often with bisphosphonates than with calcitonin and include abdominal pain, muscle or skeletal pain, diarrhea, nausea, and, in patients treated at high doses, hyperphosphatemia and mineralization defects. High-dose etidronate or alendronate are more effective than lower doses in reducing disease activity but may be associated with more serious mineralization defects, worsening of osteolysis, and pathologic fracture. Thus, high-dose bisphosphonate should be used only if a poor response to lower doses is obtained and then only for short (1- to 3-month) intervals.

During periods of immobilization, Paget's disease may lead to accelerated bone resorption. Treatment with bisphosphonates may be useful in reducing hypercalciuria, stone formation, and bone loss under these clinical circumstances.

Calcitonin

Experience with calcitonin in the treatment of Paget's disease is extensive. Treatment with calcitonin is followed by a rapid decrease in urinary hydroxyproline and a slower decline of serum alkaline phosphatase, healing of bone lesions, and reduction in symptoms and complications of the disease. Treatment may be discontinued after 1 year of therapy, and symptoms may not recur for months to years thereafter. Response to calcitonin appears to plateau after approximately a 50% reduction in disease activity in most patients, for reasons that are not well understood. More than half of treated patients develop antibodies to salmon calcitonin, which may result in resistance to therapy. Human calcitonin therapy does not appear to result in antibody formation and may be utilized if responsiveness to salmon calcitonin is lost; however, a similar plateau effect of uncertain cause has also been observed with human calcitonin treatment[207] (see Table 43.10 for dosing schedules of calcitonin).

Calcitonin is extremely costly and must be administered by subcutaneous or intramuscular injection. Side effects occur in 10% to 20% of patients and include nausea and vomiting, flushing, polyuria, hypercalciuria, paresthesias, nasal irritation, and local injection site irritation. Continuation at a reduced dose usually resolves these symptoms. Hypersensitivity reactions are rare, but a dilute initial test dose is recommended by the manufacturer for parenteral use. Combination therapy with etidronate and calcitonin has been reported to prevent progression and permit healing of osteolytic areas. Dosage and administration are listed in Table 43.10.

Other Therapies

Aspirin or other nonsteroidal anti-inflammatory agents may relieve bone pain. Surgical intervention for decompression of neurologic deficits, total hip replacement, tibial and fibular osteotomy, or fracture fixation may be complicated by hemorrhage. Presurgical treatment is usually recommended with intravenous pamidronate or calcitonin to decrease the vascularity of bone. A 50% reduction in biochemical indices of disease is usually sufficient to prevent major bleeding. Fracture and postoperative healing in Paget's disease is generally excellent.[203]

References

1. Anonymous. Consensus development conference: diagnosis, prophylaxis, and treatment of osteoporosis. *Am J Med.* 1993;94:646–650.
2. Shane E, Rivas M, Staron MB, et al. Fracture after cardiac transplantation: a prospective longitudinal study. *J Clin Endocrinol Metab.* 1996;81:1740–1746.
3. Shane E, Rivas M, McMahon DJ, et al. Bone loss and turnover after cardiac transplantation. *J Clin Endocrinol Metab.* 1997;82:1497–1506.
4. Epstein S. Post transplantation bone disease: the role of immunosuppressive agents on the skeleton. *J Bone Miner Res.* 1996;11:1–7.
5. Adebanjo OA, Blair H, Moonga BS, et al. Osteoclastic overactivity, cortical bone loss, reduced bone formation and muscle dysfunction in calcineurin A α deficient mice [abstract]. *Proc Annu Meet Am Soc Bone Miner Res.* 2000; 22:S189 (1203).
6. Looker AC, Orwoll ES, Johnston CC Jr, et al. Prevalence of low femoral bone density in older US adults from NHANES III. *J Bone Miner Res.* 1997;12:1761–1768.
7. NIH Consensus Conference. Osteoporosis prevention, diagnosis and therapy. *JAMA* 2001;285:785–795.
8. Cooper C. Epidemiology of osteoporosis. *Osteoporos Int* 1999;Suppl 2:S2–S8.
9. Melton LJ III. Epidemiology of hip fractures: implications of the exponential increase with age. *Bone.* 1996;18(suppl 3):121S–125S.
10. Melton LJ III. How many women have osteoporosis now? *J Bone Miner Res.* 1995;10:175–177.
11. Ray NF, Chan JK, Thamer M, et al. Medical expenditures for the treatment of osteoporotic fractures in the United States in 1995: report from the National Osteoporosis Foundation. *J Bone Miner Res.* 1997;12:24–35.
12. Cooper C, Campion G, Melton LJ III. Hip fractures in the elderly: a worldwide projection. *Osteoporosis Int.* 1992; 2:285–289.
13. Bilezikian JP. Osteoporosis in men. *J Clin Endocrinol Metabol.* 1999;84:3431–3434.
14. Seeman B, Melton LJ, O'Fallon WM, et al. Risk factors for spinal osteoporosis in men. *Am J Med* 1983;75:977–983.
15. Kelepouris N, Harper KD, Gannon F, et al. Severe osteoporosis in men. *Ann Intern Med.* 1995;123:452–460.

16. DeLaet CEDH, VanHout BA, Burger H, et al. Hip fracture prediction in elderly men and women: validation in the Rotterdam Study. *J Bone Miner Res.* 1998;13:1587–1593.

17. Orwoll ES, Oviatt SK, McClung MR, et al. The rate of bone mineral loss in normal men and the effects of calcium and cholecalciferol supplementation. *Ann Intern Med.* 1990;112:29–34.

18. Saag KG, Emkey R, Schnitzer TJ, et al. Alendronate for the prevention and treatment of glucocorticoid-induced osteoporosis. *N Engl J Med.* 1998;339:292–299.

19. Reid DM, Hughes RA, Laan R, et al. Efficacy and safety of daily risedronate in the treatment of corticosteroid-induced osteoporosis in men and women: a randomized trial. *J Bone Miner Res.* 2000;15:1006–1013.

20. Orwoll E, Ettinger M, Weiss, et al. Alendronate for the treatment of osteoporosis in men. *N Engl J Med.* 2000;343:604–610.

21. Seeman E. Osteoporosis in men: epidemiology, pathophysiology, and treatment possibilities. *Am J Med.* 1993;95 (suppl 5A):25S–28S.

22. Ribot C, Tremollieres F, Pouilles JM. Can we detect women with low bone mass using clinical risk factors? *Am J Med.* 1995;98:52S–55S.

23. Cummings SR, Nevitt MC, Browner WS, et al. Risk factors for hip fracture in white women. Study of Osteoporotic Fractures Research Group. *N Engl J Med.* 1995;332:767–773.

24. Fulton JP. New guidelines for the prevention and treatment of osteoporosis. National Osteoporosis Foundation. *Med Health R I.* 1999;82:110–111.

25. Williams AR, Weiss NS, Ure CL, et al. Effect of weight, smoking, and estrogen use on the risk of hip and forearm fractures in post-menopausal women. *Obstet Gynecol.* 1982;60:695–699.

26. Heaney RP, Gallagher IC, Johnston CC, et al. Calcium nutrition and bone health in the elderly. *Am J Clin Nutr.* 1982;36:986–1013.

27. Cummings SR. Epidemiology of osteoporotic fractures: selected topics. In: Roche AF, ed. *Osteoporosis: Current Concepts.* Report of the 7th Ross Conference on Medical Research. Columbus, OH: Ross Laboratories; 1987:3–8.

28. Slemenda CW, Hui SL, Longcope C, et al. Predictors of bone mass in perimenopausal women. *Ann Intern Med.* 1990;112:96–101.

29. Hui SL, Slemenda CW, Johnston CC. Baseline measurement of bone mass predicts fracture in white women. *Ann Intern Med.* 1989;111:355–361.

30. Cummings SR, Black DM, Nevitt MC, et al. Appendicular bone mass and age predict hip fracture in women. *JAMA.* 1990;263:665–668.

31. Wasnich RD, Ross PD, Heilbrun LK, et al. Prediction of postmenopausal fracture risk with use of bone mineral measurements. *Am J Obstet Gynecol.* 1985;153:745–751.

32. Cummings SR, Black DM, Nevitt MC, et al. Bone density at various sites for prediction of hip fractures. The Study of Osteoporotic Fractures Research Group. *Lancet.* 1993;341:72–75.

33. Faulkner KG, Cummings SR, Black D, et al. Simple measurement of femoral geometry predicts hip fracture: the study of osteoporotic fractures. *J Bone Miner Res.* 1993;8:1211–1217.

34. Ross PD, Davis JW, Epstein R, et al. Pre-existing fractures and bone mass predict vertebral fracture incidence in women. *Ann Intern Med.* 1991;114:919–923.

35. Wasnich R. Bone mass measurement: prediction of risk. *Am J Med.* 1993;95(suppl 5A):6S–10S.

36. Nevitt MC, Cummings SR, and Study of Osteoporotic Fractures Research Group. Type of fall and risk of hip and wrist fractures. *J Am Geriatr Soc.* 1993;41:1226–1234.

37. Nguyen TV, Blangero J, Eisman JA. Perspective: genetic epidemiologic approaches to the search for osteoporosis genes. *J Bone Miner Res.* 2000;15:392–401.

38. Ryan PJ, Blake G, Herd R, et al. A clinical profile of back pain and disability in patients with osteoporosis. *Bone.* 1994;15:27–30.

39. Kanis JA, Pitt FA. Epidemiology of osteoporosis. *Bone.* 1992;13:S7–S15.

40. Cooper C, Atkinson EJ, Jacobsen SJ, et al. Population-based study of survival after osteoporotic fractures. *Am J Epidemiol.* 1993;137:1001–1005.

41. Riggs BL, Wahner HW. Bone densitometry and clinical decision-making in osteoporosis [editorial]. *Ann Intern Med.* 1988;108:293–295.

42. Johnston CC Jr, Slemenda CW, Melton LJ III. Clinical use of bone densitometry. *N Engl J Med.* 1991;324:1105–1109.

43. Mazess RB, Barden H, Ettinger M, et al. Bone density of the radius, spine, and proximal femur in osteoporosis. *J Bone Miner Res.* 1988;3:13–18.

44. Chestnut CH. The imaging and quantitation of bone by radiographic and scanning methodologies. In: Coe FL, Favus MJ, eds. *Disorders of Bone and Mineral Metabolism.* New York: Raven Press; 1992:447–448.

45. Kanis JA, Melton LJ III, Christiansen C, et al. The diagnosis of osteoporosis. *J Bone Miner Res.* 1994;9:1137–1141.

46. Gardener MJ, Hardy JA. Some effects of within-person variability in epidemiologic studies. *J Chronic Dis.* 1973:781–795.

47. Cummings SR, Palermo L, Browner W, et al. Monitoring osteoporosis therapy with bone densitometry: misleading changes and regression to the mean. *JAMA.* 2000;283:1318–1321.

48. Pacifici R, Rupich R, Griffin M, et al. Dual energy radiography vs. quantitative computer tomography for the diagnosis of osteoporosis. *J Clin Endocrinol Metab.* 1990;70:705–710.

49. Gluer CC. Quantitative ultrasound techniques for the assessment of osteoporosis: expert agreement on current status. The international quantitative ultrasound consensus group. *J Bone Miner Res.* 1997;12:1280–1288.

50. Faulkner KG, Von Stetten E, Miller P. Discordance in patient classification using T scores. *J Clin Densitom.* 1999;2:343.

51. National Institutes of Health Consensus Development Conference Statement. *Osteoporosis Prevention, Diagnosis and Therapy, vol 17, no. 1.* Bethesda: National Institutes of Health; 2000.

52. Riis BJ, Hansen MA, Jensen AM, et al. Low bone mass and fast rate of bone loss at menopause: equal risk factors

for future fracture: a 15 year follow-up study. *Bone.* 1996; 19:9–12.

53. van Daele PLA, Seibel MJ, Burger H, et al. Case control analysis of bone resorption markers, disability, and hip fracture risk: the Rotterdam study. *Br Med J.* 1996; 312:482–483.

54. Garnero P, Hausherr E, Chapuy MC, et al. Markers of bone resorption predict hip fracture in elderly women: the EPIDOS prospective study. *J Bone Miner Res.* 1996; 11:1531–1538.

55. Riggs BL, Melton LJ III, O'Fallon WM. Drug therapy for vertebral fractures in osteoporosis: evidence that decreases in bone turnover and increases in bone mass both determine antifracture efficacy. *Bone.* 1996;18:197S– 201S.

56. van Daele PLA, Seibel MJ, Burger H, et al. Evidence for uncoupling of bone formation and bone resorption in women with hip fractures: a prospective study. *Osteoporosis Int.* 1996;6(suppl 1):S199.

57. Melton LJ III, Khosla S, Atkinson EJ, et al. Relationship of bone turnover to bone density and fractures. *J Bone Miner Res.* 1997;12:1083–1091.

58. Garnero P, Dargent-Molina P, Hans D, et al. Do markers of bone resorption add to bone mineral density and ultra-sonographic heel measurement for the prediction of hip fracture in elderly women? The EPIDOS prospective study. *Osteoporosis Int.* 1998;8:563–569.

59. Miller PD, Baran DT, Bilezikian JP, et al. Practical clinical application of biochemical markers of bone turnover. *J Clin Densitom.* 1999;2:323–342.

60. Broadus AE. Mineral balance and homeostasis. In: Favus MJ III, ed. *Primer on the Metabolic Bone Diseases and Disorders of Mineral Metabolism.* Philadelphia: Lippincott-Raven; 1996:57–63.

61. Heaney RP. Nutritional factors in osteoporosis. *Annu Rev Nutr.* 1993;13:287–316.

62. Dawson-Hughes B. Calcium supplementation and bone loss: a review of controlled clinical trials. *Am J Clin Nutr.* 1991;54:274S–280S.

63. Reid IR, Ames RW, Evans MC, et al. Effect of calcium supplementation on bone loss in postmenopausal women. *N Engl J Med.* 1993;328:460–464.

64. Aloia JF, Vaswani A, Yeh JK, et al. Calcium supplementation with and without hormone replacement therapy to prevent postmenopausal bone loss. *Ann Intern Med.* 1994; 120:97–103.

65. Chapuy MC, Arlot ME, Duboeuf F, et al. Vitamin D$_3$ and calcium to prevent hip fractures in elderly women. *N Engl J Med.* 1992;327:1637–1642.

66. McKenna MJ. Differences in vitamin D status between countries in young adults and elderly. *Am J Med.* 1992; 93:69–77.

67. Heaney RP, Rocker RR, Saville PD. Calcium balance and calcium requirement in middle aged women. *Am J Clin Nutr.* 1977;30:1603–1611.

68. Srinivasan S, Gross TS. Canalicular fluid flow induced by bending of a long bone. *Med Engl Phys.* 2000;22:127–133.

69. Chestnut CH. Bone mass and exercise. *Am J Med.* 1993; 95(5A):34S–36S.

70. Dalsky GP, Stocke KS, Ehsani AA, et al. Weight bearing exercise training and lumbar bone mineral content in postmenopausal women. *Ann Intern Med.* 1988;108:824–828.

71. Krall EA, Dawson-Hughes B. Walking is related to bone density and rate of bone loss. *Am J Med.* 1994;96:20–26.

72. Drinkwater BD, Nilson KC, Chestnut CH. Bone mineral content of amenorrheic and eumenorrheic athletes. *N Engl J Med.* 1984;311;277–281.

73. Drinkwater BL. Exercise in the prevention of osteoporosis. *Osteoporosis Int.* 1993;1:S169–S171.

74. Boonekamp PM, Lowik CW, van der Wee-Pals LJ, et al. Enhancement of the inhibitory action of APD on the transformation of osteoclast precursors into resorbing cells after dimethylation of the amino group. *J Bone Miner Res.* 1987;2:29–42.

75. Hughes DE, Wright KR, Uy HL, et al. Bisphosphonates promote apoptosis in murine osteoclasts in vitro and in vivo. *J Bone Miner Res.* 1995;10:1478–1487.

76. van Beek E, Hoekstra M, van de Ruit M, et al. Structural requirements for bisphosphonate actions in vitro. *J Bone Miner Res.* 1994;9:1875–1882.

77. Rogers MJ, Xiong X, Brown RJ, et al. Structure-activity relationships of new heterocycle-containing bisphosphonates as inhibitors of bone resorption and as inhibitors of growth of *Dictyostelium discoideum* amoebae. *Mol Pharmacol.* 1995;47:398–402.

78. Benford HL, Frith JC, Auriola S. et al. Farnesol and geranylgeraniol prevent activation of caspases by amino-bisphosphonates: biochemical evidence for two distinct pharmacological classes of bisphosphonate drugs. *Mol Pharmacol.* 1999;56:131–140.

79. Watts NB, Harris ST, Genant HK, et al. Intermittent cyclical etidronate treatment of postmenopausal osteoporosis. *N Engl J Med.* 1990;332:75–79.

80. Papapoulos SE. The role of bisphosphonates in the prevention and treatment of osteoporosis. *Am J Med.* 1993;95(suppl 5A):48S–52S.

81. Harris ST, Watts NB, Jackson RD, et al. Four-year study of intermittent cyclic etidronate treatment of post-menopausal osteoporosis: three years of blinded therapy followed by one year of open therapy. *Am J Med.* 1993;95: 557–567.

82. Storm T, Thamsborg G, Steiniche T, et al. Effect of intermittent cyclical etidronate therapy on bone mass and fracture rate in women with postmenopausal osteoporosis. *N Engl J Med.* 1990;332:1265–1271.

83. Miller PD, Watts NB, Licata AA, et al. Cyclic etidronate in the treatment of postmenopausal osteoporosis: efficacy and safety after seven years of treatment. *Am J Med.* 1997; 103:468–476.

84. Watts NB. Treatment of osteoporosis with bisphosphonates. *Endocrinol Metab Clin N Am.* 1998;27:419–439.

85. Thiebaud D, Burckhardt P, Melchior J, et al. Two years' effectiveness of intravenous pamidronate (APD) versus oral fluoride for osteoporosis occurring in postmenopause. *Osteoporosis Int.* 1994;4:76–83.

86. Peretz A, Body J, Dumon JC, et al. Cyclic pamidronate infusions in postmenopausal osteoporosis. *Maturitas.* 1996; 25:69–75.

87. Pecherstorfer M, Ludwig H, Schlosser, et al. Administration of the bisphosphonate ibandronate (BM21.0955) by intravenous bolus injection. *J Bone Miner Res.* 1996;11: 587–1593.

88. Liberman UA, Weiss SR, Bröll J, et al. Effect of treatment with oral alendronate on bone mineral density and fracture incidence in postmenopausal osteoporosis. *N Engl J Med.* 1995;333:1437–1444.

89. Eastell R. Treatment of postmenopausal osteoporosis. *N Engl J Med.* 1998;338:736–746.

90. Black DM, Cummings SR, Karpf DB, et al. Randomized trial effect of alendronate on risk of fracture in women with existing vertebral fractures. *Lancet.* 1996;348:1535–1541.

91. Hosking D, Chilvers CE, Christiansen C, et al. Prevention of bone loss with alendronate in postmenopausal women under 60 years of age. Early postmenopausal intervention study group. *N Engl J Med.* 1998;338;8:485–492.

92. Tonino RP, Menunier PJ, Emkey RD, et al. Long-term (seven year) efficacy and safety of alendronate in the treatment of osteoporosis in postmenopausal women. *Osteoporos Int.* 2000;11(suppl 2):S202.

93. Struys A, Snelder AA, Mulder H. Cyclical etidronate reverses bone loss of the spine and proximal femur in patients with established corticosteroid-induced osteoporosis. *Am J Med.* 1995;99:235–242.

94. Luckey M, Insogna K, Gilchrist N, et al. Therapeutic equivalence of alendronate 35 mg once weekly and 5 mg daily in the prevention of postmenopausal osteoporosis. *Osteoporos Int.* 2000;11(suppl 2):S209.

95. Schnitzer T, Bone HG, Crepaldi G, et al. Therapeutic equivalence of alendronate 70 mg once-weekly and alendronate 10 mg daily in the treatment of osteoporosis. Alendronate once-weekly study group. *Aging (Milano).* 2000;12:1–12.

96. Rossini M, Gatti D, Braga V, et al. Effects of two intermittent alendronate regimens in the treatment of postmenopausal osteoporosis. *Osteoporos Int.* 2000;11(suppl 2):S170.

97. Wimalawansa SJ. A four-year randomized controlled trial of hormone replacement and bisphosphonate, alone or in combination, in women with postmenopausal osteoporosis. *Am J Med.* 1998;104:219–226.

98. Lindsay R, Cosman F, Lobo RA, et al. Addition of alendronate to ongoing hormone replacement therapy in the treatment of osteoporosis: a randomized, controlled clinical trial. *J Clin Endocrinol Metab.* 1999;84:3076–3081.

99. Heaney RE, Recker RR, Saville PD. Menopausal changes in bone remodeling. *J Lab Clin Med.* 1978;92:964–970.

100. Lindsay R. Osteoporosis. *Clin Geriatr Med.* 1988;4:411–430.

101. Nachtigall LE, Nachtigall RH, Nachtigall RD. Estrogen replacement therapy. I: A 10 year prospective study in the relationship of osteoporosis. *Obstet Gynecol.* 1979;53:277–284.

102. Lindsay R, Hart DM, MacLean A, et al. Bone response to termination of estrogen treatment. *Lancet.* 1978;1:1325–1327.

103. Rickard DJ, Subramaniam M, Spelsberg TC. Molecular and cellular mechanisms of estrogen action on the skeleton. *J Cell Biochem.* 1999;Suppl 32–33:123–132.

104. Oursler MJ, Osdoby P. Pyfferoen J, et al. Avian osteoclasts as estrogen target cells. *Proc Natl Acad Sci USA.* 1991; 88:6613–6617.

105. Gray TK, Flyn TC, Gray KM. et al. 17β-Estradiol acts directly on the clonal osteoblast line UMR 106. *Proc Natl Acad Sci USA.* 1987;84:6267–6271.

106. Eriksen EF, Colvard DS, Berg NJ, et al. Evidence of estrogen receptors in normal human osteoblast-like cells. *Science.* 1988;241:84–86.

107. Komm BS, Terpening CM, Benz DJ, et al. Estrogen binding, receptor mRNA, and biologic response in osteoblast-like osteosarcoma cells. *Science.* 1988;241: 84.

108. Ernst M, JK Heath, Rodan GA. Estradiol effects on proliferation, messenger ribonucleic acid for collagen and insulin-like growth factor-i, and parathyroid hormone-stimulated adenylate cyclase activity in osteoblastic cells from calvariae and long bones. *Endocrinology.* 1989;125: 825–833.

109. Lin HY, Harris TL, Flannery NS, et al. Expression cloning of an adenylate cyclase-coupled calcitonin receptor. *Science.* 1991;254:1022–1024.

110. Tabizzadeh S. Santhanan U, May L, et al. Cytokine-induced production of IFN-α_2/IL-6 by freshly explanted human endometrial stroma cells: modulation by estradiol-17β. *J Immunol.* 1989;142:3134–3139.

111. Girasole G, Jilka RL, Passeri G, et al. 17β-Estradiol inhibits interleukin-6 production by bone marrow stromal derived stromal cells and osteoblasts in vitro: a potential mechanism for the anti-osteoporotic effect of estrogen. *J Clin Investig.* 1992;89:883–891.

112. Horowitz MC. Cytokines and estrogen in bone antiosteoporotic effects. *Science.* 1993;206:626–627.

113. Cenci S, Weitzmann MN, Gentile MA, et al. M-CSF neutralization and egr-1 deficiency prevent ovariectomy-induced bone loss. *J Clin Investig* 2000;105:1279–1287.

114. Shevde NK, Bendixen AC, Dienger KM, et al. Estrogens suppress RANK ligand-induced osteoclast differentiation via a stromal cell independent mechanism involving c-Jun repression. *Proc Natl Acad Sci USA.* 2000;97:7829–7834.

115. Kiel D, Felson D, Anderson J, et al. Hip fracture and the use of estrogens in postmenopausal women: the Framingham Study. *N Engl J Med.* 1987;317:1169–1174.

116. Ettinger B, Genant HK, Cann CE. Long term estrogen therapy prevents bone loss and fracture. *Ann Intern Med.* 1985;102:319–324.

117. Hutchinson TA, Polansky JM, Feinstein AR. Postmenopausal oestrogens protect against fracture of the hip and distal radius. *Lancet.* 1979;2:705–709.

118. Kreiger N, Kelsey JL, Holford TR. An epidemiological study of hip fracture in postmenopausal women. *Am J Epidemiol.* 1982;116:141–148.

119. Smith DM, Khairi MRA, Johnston CC. The loss of bone mineral with aging and its relationship to risk of fracture. *J Clin Investig.* 1975;56:311–318.

120. Weiss NS, Ure CL, Ballard JH, et al. Decreased risk of fractures of the hip and lower forearm with postmenopausal use of estrogen. *N Engl J Med.* 1980;303: 1195–1198.

121. Maxim P. Ettinger B, Spitalny GM. Fracture protection provided by long term estrogen treatment. *Osteoporosis Int.* 1995;5:23–29.

122. Lindsay R, Thome JF. Estrogen treatment of patients with established osteoporosis. *Obstet Gynecol.* 1990;76:290–295.

123. Lufkin EG, Wahner HW, O'Fallon WM, et al. Treatment of postmenopausal osteoporosis with transdermal estrogen. *Ann Intern Med.* 1992;117:1–9.

124. Marx CW, Daily GE, Cheney C, et al. Do estrogens improve bone mineral density in osteoporotic women over age 65? *J Bone Miner Res.* 1992;7:1275–1279.

125. Ettinger B, Grady D. The waning effect of postmenopausal estrogen therapy on osteoporosis. *N Engl J Med.* 1993;329: 1192–1193.

126. Felson DT, Zhang Y, Hannan MT, et al. Effect of postmenopausal estrogen therapy on bone density in elderly women. *N Engl J Med.* 1993;329:1141–1146.

127. Recker, RR, Davies M, Dowd R, et al. The effect of low dose continuous estrogen and progesterone therapy with calcium and Vitamin D on bone in elderly women. *Ann Intern Med.* 1999;130:897–904.

128. Lobo RA. Cardiovascular complications of estrogen replacement therapy. *Obstet Gynecol.* 1990;75(suppl):18S–25S.

129. Barrett-Connor E, Bush TL. Estrogen and coronary heart disease in women. *JAMA.* 1991;265:1861–1867.

130. Stampfer MJ, Colditz GA, Willett WC, et al. Postmenopausal estrogen therapy and cardiovascular disease: ten year follow-up from the Nurses' Health Study. *N Engl J Med.* 1991;325:756–762.

131. Hulley S, Grady D, Bush T, et al. Randomized trial of estrogen plus progestin for secondary prevention of coronary heart disease in postmenopausal women. *JAMA.* 1998;208:605–613.

132. Yaffe K, Sawaya G, Lieberburg I, Grady D. Estrogen therapy in postmenopausal women: effects on cognitive function and dementia. *JAMA.* 1998;279:688–695.

133. Grodstein F, Newcomb PA, Stampfer MJ. Postmenopausal hormone therapy and the risk of colorectal cancer: a review and meta-analysis. *Am J Med.* 1999;106:574–582.

134. Shapiro S, Kelley JP, Rosenberg L. Risk of localized and widespread endometrial cancer in relation to recent and discontinued use of conjugated estrogens. *N Engl J Med.* 1985;313:969–972.

135. Gambrell RD, Massey FM, Castaneda TA, et al. Reduced incidence of endometrial cancer among postmenopausal women treated with progestogens. *J Am Geriatr Soc.* 1979; 27:389–394.

136. Grady D, Rubin SM, Petitti DB, et al. Hormone therapy to prevent disease and prolong life in postmenopausal women. *Ann Intern Med.* 1992;117:1016–1037.

137. Steinberg KK, Thacker SB, Smith SJ, et al. A meta-analysis of the effect of estrogen replacement therapy on the risk of breast cancer. *JAMA.* 1991;265:1985–1990.

138. Colditz GA, Hankinson SE, Hunter DJ, et al. The use of estrogens and progestins and the risk of breast cancer in postmenopausal women. *N Engl J Med.* 1995;332:1589–1593.

139. Colditz GA, Stampfer MJ, Willett WC, et al. Postmenopausal hormone use and the risk of breast cancer: 12 year follow-up of the Nurses' Health Study. In: Mann RD, ed. *Hormone Replacement Therapy and Breast Cancer Risk.* Carnforth, England: Parthenon; 1992:63–77.

140. Schairer C, Lubin J, Troisi R, et al. Menopausal estrogen and estrogen-progestin replacement therapy and breast cancer risk. *JAMA.* 2000;283:485–491.

141. Ross RK, Paganini-Hill A, Wan PC, et al. Effect of hormone replacement therapy on breast cancer risk: estrogen versus estrogen plus progestin. *J Natl Cancer Inst.* 2000;92(4):328–332.

142. Ettinger B, Pressman A. Effect of age on reasons for initiation and discontinuation of hormone replacement therapy. *Menopause.* 1999;6:282–289.

143. Bjorn I, Backstrom T. Drug-related negative side effects is a common reason for poor compliance in hormone replacement therapy. *Maturitas.* 1999;32:77–86.

144. Balfour JA, Goa KL. Raloxifene. *Drugs Aging.* 1998;12: 335–341.

145. Spencer CP, Morris EP, Rymer JM. Selective estrogen receptor modulators: women's panacea for the next millenium? *Am J Obstet Gynecol.* 1999;180:763–770.

146. Delmas PD, Bjarnason NH, Mitlak BH, et al. Effects of raloxifene on bone density, serum cholesterol concentrations, and uterine endometrium in postmenopausal women. *N Engl J Med.* 1997;337:1641–1647.

147. Ettinger B, Black D, Mitlak B, et al. Reduction of vertebral fracture risk in postmenopausal women with osteoporosis treated with raloxifene. *JAMA.* 1999;282:637–645.

148. Cummings SR, Black D, Barrett-Connor E, et al. The effect of raloxifene on risk of breast cancer in postmenopausal women: results from the MORE randomized trial. Multiple outcomes of raloxifene evaluation. *JAMA.* 1999;281:2189–2197.

149. Anderson RE, Schraer H, Gay CV. Ultrastructural immunocytochemical localization of carbonic anhydrase in normal and calcitonin-treated chick osteoclasts. *Anat Rec.* 1982;204:9–20.

150. Akisaka T, Gay CV. Ultracytochemical evidence for a proton-pump adenosine triphosphatase in chick osteoclasts. *Cell Tissue Res.* 1986;24:507–512.

151. Chambers TJ, Fuller K, Darby JA. Hormonal regulation of acid phosphatase release by osteoclasts disaggregated from neonatal rat bone. *J Cell Physiol.* 1987;132:92–96.

152. Moonga BS, Moss DW, Patchell A, et al. Intracellular regulation of enzyme release from rat osteoclasts and evidence for a functional role in bone resorption. *J Physiol.* 1990;429:29–45.

153. Yumita S, Nicholson GC, Rowe DJ, et al. Biphasic effect of calcitonin on tartrate-resistant acid phosphatase activity in isolated rat osteoclasts. *J Bone Miner Res.* 1991;6: 591–597.

154. Offermanns S, Iida-Klein A, Segre GV, et al. G alpha q family members couple parathyroid hormone (PTH)/PTH-related peptide and calcitonin receptors to phospholipase C in COS-7 cells. *Mol Endocrinol.* 1996;10:566–574.

155. Zaidi M. Calcium "receptors" on eukaryotic cells with special reference to the osteoclast. *Biosci Rep.* 1990;10: 493–507.

156. Moonga BS, Alam AS, Bevis PJR, et al. Regulation of cytosolic free calcium in isolated osteoclasts by calcitonin. *J Endocrinol.* 1992;132:241–249.

157. Muff R, Dambacher MA, Fischer IA. Formation of neutralizing antibodies during intranasal synthetic salmon calcitonin treatment of postmenopausal osteoporosis. *Osteoporosis Int.* 1991;1:72–75.

158. Gruber HE, Ivey IL, Bayhuk DL, et al. Long term calcitonin therapy in postmenopausal osteoporosis. *Metabolism.* 1984;33:295–303.

159. Mazzuoli GF, Passeri M, Gennari C, et al. Effects of salmon calcitonin in postmenopausal osteoporosis: a controlled double-blind clinical study. *Calcif Tissue Int.* 1986;38:3–8.

160. Reginster JY. Calcitonin for prevention and treatment of osteoporosis. *Am J Med.* 1993;95(suppl 5A):44S–47S.

161. Overgaard K, Hansen MA, Jensen SB, et al. Effect of salmon calcitonin given intranasally on bone mass and fracture rates in established osteoporosis: a dose–response study. *Br Med J.* 1992;305:56–61.

162. McDermott MT, Kidd GS. The role of calcitonin in the development and treatment of osteoporosis. *Endocr Rev.* 1987;8:377–390.

163. Kanis IA, Johaell O, Gullberg B, et al. Evidence for efficacy of drugs affecting bone metabolism in preventing hip fracture. *Br Med J.* 1992;305:1124–1128.

164. Rico H, Hernandez ER, Revilla, et al. Salmon calcitonin reduces vertebral fracture rate in post-menopausal crush fracture syndrome. *J Bone Miner Res.* 1992;16:131–138.

165. Silverman SL, Chestnut C, Andriano K, et al. Salmon calcitonin nasal spray reduces risk of vertebral fracture(s) in established osteoporosis and has continuous efficacy with prolonged treatment accrued 5 year world wide data of the PROOF study. *Bone.* 1998;23(suppl 5):S174.

166. Legrand E, Chappard D, Pascaretti C, et al. Trabecular bone microarchitecture, bone mineral density, and vertebral fractures in male osteoporosis. *J Bone Miner Res.* 2000;15:13–19.

167. Dempster DW. The contribution of trabecular architecture to cancellous bone quality. *J Bone Miner Res.* 2000;15:20–23.

168. Sambrook PB, Ingham J, Kelly P. Prevention of corticosteroid osteoporosis: a comparison of calcium, calcitriol and calcitonin. *N Engl J Med.* 1993;328:1747–1752.

169. Shane E, Rodino MA, McMahon DJ, et al. Prevention of bone loss after heart transplantation with antiresorptive therapy: a pilot study. *J Heart Lung Transplant.* 1998;17:1089–1096.

170. Riggs BL, Hodgson SF, O'Fallon WM, et al. Effect of fluoride treatment on the fracture rate in postmenopausal women with osteoporosis. *N Engl J Med.* 1990;322:802–809.

171. Kleerekoper M, Peterson EL, Nelson DA, et al. A randomized trial of sodium fluoride as a treatment for postmenopausal osteoporosis. *Osteoporosis Int.* 1991;1:155–161.

172. Pak CYC, Sakhaee K, Adams-Huet B, et al. Treatment of postmenopausal osteoporosis with slow-release sodium fluoride: final report of a randomized controlled trial. *Ann Intern Med.* 1995;123:401–408.

173. Wu Y, Kumar R. Parathyroid hormone regulates transforming growth factor beta 1 and beta 2 synthesis in osteoblasts via divergent signaling pathways. *J Bone Miner Res.* 2000;15:879–884.

174. Sanders JL, Stern PH. Protein kinase C involvement in interleukin-6 production by parathyroid hormone and tumor necrosis factor-alpha in UMR-106 osteoblastic cells. *J Bone Miner Res.* 2000;15:885–893.

175. Takai H, Kanematsu M, Yano K, et al. Transforming growth factor-beta stimulates the production of osteoprotegerin/osteoclastogenesis inhibitory factor by bone marrow stromal cells. *J Biol Chem.* 1998;273:27091–27096.

176. Wrana JL, Overall CM, Sodek J. Regulation of the expression of a secreted acidic protein rich in cysteine (SPARC) in human fibroblasts by transforming growth factor beta. Comparison of transcriptional and post-transcriptional control with fibronectin and type I collagen. *Eur J Biochem.* 1991;197:519–528.

177. Wrana JL, Kubota T, Zhang Q, et al. Regulation of transformation-sensitive secreted phosphoprotein (SPPI/osteopontin) expression by transforming growth factor-beta. Comparisons with expression of SPARC (secreted acidic cysteine-rich protein). *Biochem J.* 1991;273:523–531.

178. Riggs BL. Formation stimulating regimens other than sodium fluoride. *Am J Med.* 1993;95(suppl 5A):62S–68S.

179. Finkelstein JS, Klibanski A, Arnold A, et al. Prevention of estrogen deficiency related bone loss with human PTH: a randomized controlled trial. *JAMA.* 1998;280:1067–1073.

180. Gowen M, Stroup GB, Dodds RA, et al. Antagonizing the parathyroid calcium receptor stimulates parathyroid hormone secretion and bone formation in osteopenic rats. *J Clin Investig.* 2000;105:1595–1604.

181. Ishii H, Wada M, Furuya Y, et al. Daily intermittent decreases in serum levels of parathyroid hormone have an anabolic-like action on the bones of uremic rats with low-turnover bone and osteomalacia. *Bone.* 2000;26:175–182.

182. Slovik DM, Adams JS, Neer RM, et al. Deficient production of 1,25-dihydroxy vitamin D in elderly osteoporotic patients. *N Engl J Med.* 1981;305:372–374.

183. Brandi ML. New treatment strategies: ipriflavone, strontium, vitamin D metabolites and analogs. *Am J Med* 1993;95(suppl 5A):69S–74S.

184. Heikinheimo RJ, Inkovaara JA, Hurju EJ, et al. Annual injection of vitamin D and fractures of aged bones. *Calcif Tissue Int.* 1992;51:105–110.

185. Fisher JE, Rogers MJ, Halasy JM, et al. Alendronate mechanism of action: geranylgeraniol, an intermediate in the mevalonate pathway, prevents inhibition of osteoclast formation, bone resorption, and kinase activation in vitro. *Proc Natl Acad Sci USA.* 1999;96(1):133–138.

186. Mundy G, Garrett R, Harris S, et al. Stimulation of bone formation in vitro and in rodents by statins. *Science.* 1999;286:1946–1949.

187. Chung YS, Lee MD, Lee SK, et al. HMG-CoA Reductase Inhibitors increase BMD in type 2 diabetes mellitus patients. *J Clin Endocrinol Metab.* 2000;85:1137–1142.

188. Wang PS, Solomon DH, Mogun H, Avorn J. HMG-CoA reductase inhibitors and the risk of hip fractures in elderly persons. *JAMA.* 2000;283:3211–3216.

189. Meier CR, Schlienger RG, Kraenzlin ME, et al. HMG-CoA reductase inhibitors and the risk of fractures. *JAMA.* 2000;283:3205–3210.

190. Heath H, Hodgson SF, Kennedy MA. Primary hyperparathyroidism. Incidence, morbidity and potential economic impact in a community. *N Engl J Med.* 1980;302:189–193.

191. Solomon BL, Schaaf M, Smallridge RC. Psychologic symptoms before and after parathyroid surgery. *Am J Med.* 1994;96:101–106.

192. Mallette LE. Primary hyperparathyroidism: clinical and biochemical features. *Medicine.* 1974;53:127–146.

193. Karpati G, Frame B. Neuropsychiatric disorders in primary hyperparathyroidism. *Arch Neurol.* 1964;10:387–397.

194. Clarke OH, Wilkes W, Siperstein AE, et al. Diagnosis and management of asymptomatic hyperparathyroidism: safety, efficacy, and deficiencies in our knowledge. *J Bone Miner Res.* 1991;6:135–142.

195. Consensus Development Conference Panel 1991. Diagnosis and management of asymptomatic primary hyperparathyroidism: consensus development conference statement. *Ann Intern Med.* 1991;114:593–597.

196. Scholz DA, Purnell DC. Asymptomatic primary hyperparathyroidism: 10-year prospective study. *Mayo Clin Proc.* 1981;56:473–478.

197. Silverberg SJ, Shane E, Jacobs TP, et al. A 10-year prospective study of primary hyperparathyroidism with or without parathyroid surgery. *N Engl J Med.* 1999;341:1249–1255.

198. Chen H, Sokoll LJ, Udelsman R. Outpatient minimally invasive parathyroidectomy: combination of sestamibi-SPECT localization, cervical block anesthesia, and intraoperative parathyroid hormone assay. *Surgery.* 1999;126:1016–1021.

199. Lo Gerfo P. Bilateral neck exploration for parathyroidectomy under local anesthesia: a viable technique for patients with coexisting thyroid disease without sestamibi scanning. *Surgery.* 1999;126:1011–1014.

200. McDermott MT, Perloff JJ, Kidd CS. Effect of mild asymptomatic primary hyperparathyroidism on bone mass in women with and without estrogen replacement therapy. *J Bone Miner Res.* 1994;9:509–514.

201. Cosman F, Shen V. Xie F, et al. Estrogen protection against bone resorbing effects of parathyroid hormone infusion. *Ann Intern Med.* 1993;118:337–343.

202. Silverberg SJ, Bone HG III, Marriott TB, et al. Short-term inhibition of parathyroid hormone secretion by a calcium-receptor agonist in patients with primary hyperparathyroidism. *N Engl J Med.* 1997;337:1506–1510.

203. Singer FR, Wallach S. *Paget's Disease of Bone.* New York: Elsevier; 1991.

204. Hosking DJ. Advances in the management of Paget's disease of bone. *Drugs.* 1990;40:829–840.

205. Patel S, Stone MD, Coupland C, et al. Determinants of remission of Paget's disease of bone. *J Bone Miner Res.* 1993;8:1467–1473.

206. Reginster JY, Treves R, Renier JC, et al. Efficacy and tolerability of a new formulation of oral tiludronate in the treatment of Paget's disease of bone. *J Bone Miner Res.* 1994;9:615–619.

207. Singer FR, Fredericks RS, Minkin C. Salmon calcitonin therapy for Paget's disease of bone. The problem of acquired clinical resistance. *Arthritis Rheum.* 1980;23:1143–1154.

44
Orthopedic Problems with Aging

Lawrence A. Pottenger

Musculoskeletal problems are frequently perceived by people as the first concrete signs of aging. The problems tend to be chronic in nature with little or no hope of complete return to the premorbid condition. Although the pains are usually not severe, they make people feel tired, which is interpreted as feeling "old." Increased pain with activity accentuates the feeling of aging by forcing people to accept more sedentary lifestyles. A patient typically complains that she feels like a "45-year-old woman in an 80-year-old body." Depression, which is associated with all forms of chronic pain, can be particularly severe if the patient relates it to fundamental changes such as decreased mobility and growing old.

On the other hand, the presence of musculoskeletal problems can mask heart and lung diseases. Patients may blame their lack of stamina on joint and muscle pains when it is really due to poor oxygenation from heart failure, peripheral vascular disease, or chronic lung disease. It is very important that older patients see a cardiologist or geriatrician before major orthopedic surgery, preferably with a drug-induced stress test, if the patients can barely walk. Their restricted ambulation may be the result of heart disease, and restrictions due to joint pains can reduce patient activities to the point that they do not notice their heart and lung problems.

Osteoarthritis

Age-related changes in joints are different from those of other musculoskeletal tissues. The strength of cartilage does not appear to decrease with age, but cartilage at all ages has very little ability to heal. Injuries to cartilage therefore tend to accumulate with age. Because the function of cartilage is to provide a smooth surface for weight-bearing, disruptions of the surface produce friction that leads to further disruption. Eventually, changes typical of osteoarthritis appear.[1] Although any one particular joint may have escaped injury throughout life, it is virtually

impossible to find people over 65 years of age who do not have at least one osteoarthritic joint somewhere in their bodies. Indeed, anthropologists use evidence of degenerative joint changes in human skeletons to determine the age at time of death.

Any irreversible damage to the cartilaginous surface of a joint will proceed to osteoarthritis if the joint continues to function; this includes damage from trauma, infections, and inflammatory conditions. The rate of progression of osteoarthritis cannot be estimated from a single roentgenograph because it depends upon the degree to which the patient continues to use the joint and the amount of inflammation in the joint.

Roentgenographs of early osteoarthritic joints may show only slight joint space narrowing where some cartilage has been lost. It is therefore very important to take roentgenographs of knees with the patient bearing weight on the affected extremity to detect the narrowing because the articular surfaces of arthritic knees tend to separate when not bearing weight, thus underestimating the severity of the arthritis. As osteoarthritis progresses, the subchondral bone in areas of stress becomes sclerotic with cystlike areas filled with fibrofatty tissue. The edges of the joint develop osteophytes, which are areas of new bone formation with new cartilage on surfaces that face the joint.

Osteophytes are thought, by some people, to make the joints more stable by broadening the surface of weight-bearing. Osteophytes may also stabilize joints by applying lateral pressure on ligaments that have become slack because of loss of cartilage and bone within the joint. Large osteophytes can limit normal motion and cause fixed angular deformities of the joint.[2]

It is generally agreed that the first lesion seen in osteoarthritis is disruption of the articular cartilage in the area of the joint that sustains the greatest loads. In some cases, there is superficial fissuring of the cartilage that propagates down to the subchondral bone. With continued use of the joint, the fissures spread out to form an area of fibrillation, which is a hairlike patch where the cartilage matrix components are lost, leaving only a skeleton of disrupted collagen fibers attached to the bone below. These areas are unable to bear weight because of the loss of proteoglycans from the matrix. The weight then becomes focused upon the intact cartilage surrounding the area of fibrillation, which, in turn, becomes disrupted and fibrillated from the increased stresses. Recent studies indicate that progressive loss of matrix components is related to enzymatic destruction from inflammation.[3]

Sometimes a "blister" lesion forms in an area of normal-looking cartilage. Collagen fibers deep within the cartilage are sheared from their anchorage to the underlying zone of calcified cartilage, whereas the superficial fibers are still intact. Blister lesions eventually break through to the joint, forming a crevice surrounded by undermined flaps of cartilage.

Early cartilage lesions are frequently asymptomatic because cartilage contains no nerves. It is not surprising to see a patient with only a 2-week history of knee pain who has roentgenographic evidence of advanced osteoarthritis. Pain inevitably arrives when cartilage has disappeared from both sides of the joint in an area of weightbearing. Bone contains nerves. Activity-related pain in osteoarthritis is in large part caused by friction from bare bones rubbing together. It responds to analgesics but probably not to anti-inflammatories.

Early cartilage lesions can become painful for several reasons. Large amounts of cartilage debris within the joint cause inflammation of the synovial lining of the joint with swelling and generalized aching in the anterior part of the joint. The inflammation is considered to play a large role in perpetuating the arthritic process. Flaps of undermined cartilage can become painfully caught in the joint and can break off, creating loose bodies that might later become caught in the joint. Osteophytes can also break off the bone to become loose bodies. In the patellofemoral joint, long superficial collagen fibers can partially separate from the cartilage and become caught in the joint even though they are still attached to the bone. If you place your hand on the patella as the knee is bending, you will feel crepitus from catching and giving way of the fibers.

Broken osteophytes that do not separate from the bone can cause pain as the bones rub together at the point of the fracture. Osteophytes can also cause chronic inflammation if they protrude against tendons, ligaments, or joint capsule that move across the joint during motion; this is frequently seen in the knee joint. The quadriceps expansion on both sides of the patella rubs against osteophytes of the anterior femoral condyles as the joint flexes. The synovium under the expansion becomes inflamed because of the increased pressure. The inflamed area becomes fibrotic. The fibrous tissue causes focal eleva-

tions of the synovium, which leads to even greater focal pressures and more inflammation. As the process becomes self-perpetuating, fibrous nodules a centimeter or more in diameter can develop and the pain can become disabling. This condition can easily be diagnosed by placing a hand on the affected knee as it flexes. One feels crepitus on both sides of the patella as the knee is flexed. Patients often get dramatic relief from intra-articular corticosteroid injection, which reduces the inflammation and tends to make the nodules melt away. Large nodules occasionally require excision through an arthroscope.

Chronic entrapment of material within the joint causes a "locked joint." This effect is most often recognized in the knee, although it probably happens in many joints throughout the body. The patient is unable to fully extend the knee. Attempts to forcibly extend the joint cause severe pain in the anterior part of the knee on the side where the material is caught. The patient walks with a painful bent knee. Some knees unlock spontaneously as trapped material escapes from the joint. Others require removal of debris with an arthroscope. A locked knee should be treated with some urgency because material trapped in the knee can cause further cartilage damage during weightbearing. In addition, patients with osteoarthritis who do not fully extend their knee can develop osteophytes on the anterior part of their femoral condyles that permanently prevent the knees from extending. The time required for development of anterior osteophytes varies, but it is probably unwise to leave a knee locked for more than a month.

A torn meniscus in the knee is a frequent cause of locking that may not be associated with osteoarthritis. The menisci are semilunar wedges of fibrocartilage that fit around the outside edge of the medial and lateral compartments of the knee. They function to broadly distribute the weight from the round ends of the femoral condyles onto the flat surface of the tibial plateau. A tear of the meniscus tends to get caught in the part of the joint where the femoral condyle has direct contact with the tibial plateau. In young patients the tears are well defined and are usually the result of a traumatic episode, whereas older patients have "degenerative tears" where the substance of the meniscus has degenerated before the tear. Tears in a front and midportion of the meniscus lead to locking of the knee. Posterior tears cause pain with knee flexion and can actually prevent full flexion. The menisci of obese patients frequently tear at the anterior attachment of the meniscus to the tibial plateau.

There is still much controversy concerning the extent to which tears in the meniscus might initiate cartilage damage, leading to osteoarthritis. Although meniscal degeneration and even total loss of the menisci are frequently seen in knee osteoarthritis, there are also many cases where the femoral and tibial cartilage is severely eroded and the menisci are relatively intact. At arthroscopy, however, focal areas of degenerative loss of femoral cartilage are often seen directly over a torn meniscus, which appears to indicate that the loss of cartilage was caused by abrasion from the piece of torn meniscus trapped in the joint. It is not known if these small areas of cartilage disruption progress to generalized knee osteoarthritis. Doctors frequently mistake the pain of a torn meniscus for "early" arthritis. Meniscus pain is accompanied by focal joint line tenderness where the meniscus is attached to the tibial plateau.

Treatment of Osteoarthritis

In the early stages of osteoarthritis, one can often mitigate the effects of the disease without medications or surgery. The most important way is to reduce the forces transmitted across the affected joints. In the upper extremity, patients find ways to avoid using painful joints by substituting other motions. In the lower extremities where all the joints are used during most activities, the emphasis must be placed on decreasing the forces across the joint by decreasing body weight. For instance, it has been estimated that, during stair climbing, forces of four to six times body weight are placed across the knee joint. Obese patients should at least be encouraged to lose weight because weight loss could have a very beneficial effect on both the symptoms and the progress of the disease.

A cane to help relieve some of the weightbearing on the affected side can also be very beneficial, and is particularly important when medications fall short of relieving the symptoms. Many patients under age 75 refuse to use a cane because they see it as a sign of old age. Some of these patients can be persuaded to use one crutch. The crutch indicates the presence of a physical problem rather than an infirmity of aging.

Exercise can be very beneficial for arthritic patients. Increased activity has both positive and negative influences on the course of arthritic diseases. It causes cartilage wear, but it also keeps muscles and bones strong. With respect to the lower extremities, the best exercises are those that minimize the effects of weightbearing on the joints while promoting muscle strengthening. Swimming, riding a stationary bicycle, and doing low-impact exercises arc generally beneficial in moderation, and they give the patient a feeling of well-being that counteracts some of the chronic pain. Walking, if it is not painful, is also very beneficial. It is a well-known phenomenon that patients with complete loss of cartilage from their joints have less pain if the bone in their joints is very hard, "eburnated," bone with few cysts. It is possible that the nerves in the bone are better protected by the hard bone. These people often have very little inflammation, presumably because there is less wear debris from the harder

bone. They are generally very active people and they appear to be able to tolerate their disease much longer before requiring surgery.

Any exercise that causes joint pain, either at the time of the activity or later, is probably not beneficial. Range of motion exercises in moderation are generally good, but it should be kept in mind that joint contractures in osteoarthritis frequently develop because the muscles have restricted movements that would otherwise be painful. Overcoming that restriction can cause the joint to become more painful.

Braces are generally of little help in lower extremity osteoarthritis. A plastic ankle–foot orthosis that limits ankle motion is sometimes helpful in severe ankle osteoarthritis. Osteoarthritic knee joints tend to collapse toward the most involved side of the knee, so that eventually all the weight is carried by that side. The opposite side of the knee often remains relatively free of arthritis. For a brace to be effective, it would have to apply a great deal of pressure to transfer the weight to the unaffected side; this would be uncomfortable and would rapidly cause skin problems. Small braces around the knee can sometimes be helpful if there is gross instability, but they cannot take the weight off the diseased side of the joint. Many patients get comfort from elastic knee sleeves. Tactile sensations from the sleeve may compete with pain sensations. The sleeves may also enhance proprioception. Braces are of no value in hip arthritis and are generally not useful for upper extremity arthritis.

Medications

Nonsteroidal anti-inflammatory drugs (NSAIDs) can cause dramatic relief of the symptoms of osteoarthritis, but there is little evidence that they slow the progression of the disease, and they may hasten it by allowing the patients to increase their activity levels to the point of causing increased cartilage degeneration. NSAIDs are generally effective in reducing joint inflammation and they have an analgesic effect similar to acetaminophen, but they have no effect upon the frictional pain of bones rubbing together, other than the analgesic effect. Patients frequently report that the drugs lose their effect after about 3 weeks. When one questions them closer, it becomes obvious that they are adjusting their activity by their level of pain and that the NSAIDs have made them more active at the expense of maintaining the same level of pain. It is often necessary to have patients go off the medications, temporarily, so that they can appreciate the benefit they receive from them.

NSAIDs have serious potential side effects including ulcers, gastrointestinal bleeding, renal and liver toxicity, and excessive bleeding secondary to platelet abnormalities. The cyclooxygenase 2 inhibitors have fewer side effects.[4] These drugs should be considered for patients who do not tolerate other NSAIDS, but they are not more clinically effective than other NSAIDS. In the absence of signs of inflammation, NSAIDs should only be employed if they substantially improve the patient's symptoms. Even severely osteoarthritic joints may have only bone pain. Patients often find that one specific NSAID gives them more symptomatic improvement than others they have tried. If one drug is not effective, others should be tried. Alternative oral medications include acetaminophen if the joints are not inflamed.[5] Glucosamine/chondroitin (1500 mg/1200 mg per day) often can relieve arthritic symptoms as effectively as NSAIDs with fewer side effects,[6] but the medication must be taken for several weeks to obtain relief.

Patients frequently show dramatic relief from a corticosteroid injection.[7] Cortisone effectively treats inflammation, but it also has the capacity to inhibit cartilage repair by slowing the metabolism of chondrocytes. Multiple injections at short intervals can damage cartilage. Crystalline corticosteroids that dissolve over several months are probably the most benign. The number of injections into any one joint should be limited unless the joint has degenerated to the point that the only alternative is total joint arthroplasty. Viscosupplementation with intra-articular hyaluronic acid injection can also be effective in eliminating arthritic symptoms.[8] Hyaluronic acid is not as universally effective as corticosteroids, but the effects of one hyaluronic acid injection can last up to 6 months.

Surgery for Osteoarthritis

Current surgical methods cannot restore damaged cartilage or recreate the original anatomy of the joint. Surgery is performed for four reasons: to debride areas of symptomatic cartilage, to redirect the loadbearing to a relatively unaffected part of the joint, to fuse the joint, and to "replace the joint" by attaching artificial surfaces to the ends of the bones comprising the joint.

Arthroscopic Joint Debridement

Flaps of undermined cartilage and frayed cartilage can cause pain and muscle spasm if they become caught in the joint; this is particularly evident in knee arthritis, but can also be present in ankle, hip, and shoulder arthritis. The range of motion of the joint may be limited by reflex muscle spasm or by entrapped cartilage material within the joint. Entrapped meniscal tears are also seen in the older population. Material caught within a joint can cause rapid destruction of the cartilage on both sides of the joint by a process called "three-body wear" that is similar to that seen when a piece of sand is caught in a metal bearing. The treatment for this condition is to remove the symptomatic cartilage by arthroscopy.

Arthroscopic debridement[9] is most effective in early osteoarthritis when the symptoms appear to be much greater than would be predicted by the roentgenographs. The symptoms can be chronic effusions despite NSAIDs or they can be a sudden decrease in range of motion of the joint with pain on attempting to manually increase the motion. Arthroscopic debridement is usually of little benefit in severe osteoarthritis even if a meniscal tear is present. Severely arthritic joints may temporarily benefit from irrigation of the joint, but the effect is usually short lived and in most cases is not justified.[10]

Knee and ankle arthroscopy can usually be performed as an outpatient procedure using only local anesthetic. The risks of complications are small. The possibility of infection is so small that many orthopedists do not use prophylactic antibiotics. The relatively benign effects of arthroscopy make it tempting to expand the indications for its use. This temptation should be resisted because "exploratory arthroscopies" often are not beneficial. Arthroscopy should not be performed for osteoarthritis unless the physical examination and roentgenographs indicate a specific condition, such as a meniscal tear, that is known to benefit from arthroscopic surgery. A preoperative MRI may be needed to have better understanding of the condition of the joint. If there is a question concerning the cause of the arthritis, arthroscopy is a safe way to obtain synovial biopsies for diagnosis.

Realignment Osteotomies

In the early stages of osteoarthritis of the hip and knee, the weightbearing areas of the joint are primarily affected. Osteotomies[11] have been used to redirect body weight to areas of cartilage that have remained relatively intact. Hip osteotomies are rarely performed in the United States because their results are unpredictable, but they continue to be popular in Europe. Knee osteotomies continue to be universally popular, but the effective use of NSAIDs and injections often reduces joint symptoms to the point that surgery is not considered until the joint has degenerated beyond the point that osteotomy would be beneficial. Mild to moderate osteoarthritis of the knee generally affects only the medial or lateral compartments. Knee osteotomy consists of removing a wedge of bone from above or below the knee such that the direction of weightbearing is oriented to the unaffected compartment.

The advantage of osteotomy over total joint replacement is that it does not involve placement of artificial materials within the joint that might wear out or become loose. However, patients with knee osteotomies frequently have return of their symptoms within 5 to 10 years, and some never experience significant relief of pain. In addition, the recovery time following an osteotomy is much longer than for a routine total joint replacement because bone healing is required. Osteotomies should be considered for relatively young patients for whom it is likely that a total joint arthroplasty will fail within the patient's lifetime. Older people who continue to participate in high-impact activities, such as running, should also consider osteotomies as opposed to total joints. Patients over 70 years of age who are not participating in high-impact activities would probably have better results from a total knee arthroplasty.

Joint Fusion

Joint fusion means to remove the joint and hold the bones on either side of the joint together so that they heal to form one longer bone. Joint fusion has always been the most effective way to permanently eliminate the pain of osteoarthritis. In addition, joint fusion is often preferred for manual laborers because it maintains the strength of the extremity better than arthroplasty and it is not as likely to require future surgery. Fusion is the only possible surgical treatment for many of the small joints of the body that become arthritic, including ankles.

Patients are frequently unhappy with fusions. Prolonged postoperative periods of immobilization in a cast are often necessary to obtain a solid fusion, and reoperation may be necessary if the fusion is not successful. In addition, fusion of a large joint such as the hip and knee changes the normal walking pattern, makes it difficult to sit in a chair, and puts additional stress on other joints. Fusions of the hip and knee are generally reserved for young patients with monoarticular disease. Fusions are contraindicated in the lower extremity if more than one joint is arthritic, even if the second joint is only mildly arthritic, because the additional stress can cause rapid degeneration of the second joint. In the geriatric population, the most common indication for a knee fusion is a chronic knee infection from a failed total knee arthroplasty.

Total Joint Arthroplasty

Total joint arthroplasties[12] are procedures that replace the articular surfaces of joints with one or more artificial substances including metal, high-density polyethylene, and ceramic. In most cases, only a small amount of bone is removed to install the joint. Ligaments, joint capsule, and muscles continue to hold the two sides of the joint together. Patients frequently think that a joint arthroplasty involves replacement of a large segment of the extremity and are relieved to find how little bone is actually replaced. Hips and knees are the joints most frequently replaced. Less frequently replaced joints include finger and toe joints, ankles, shoulders, wrists, and elbows.

Arthroplasties of the hip and knee should not be considered unless the joint is irreversibly damaged, with areas of full-thickness loss of cartilage, and the patient's walking capacity is limited to only a few blocks in spite of intensive medical treatment. Roentgenographic indications of the severity of the disease plays little role in the decision to have an arthroplasty except to indicate that the arthritic condition is irreversible because areas of the joint have completely lost their cartilage. Many patients have severe roentgenographic changes with only mild symptoms. Delaying surgery until symptoms become worse rarely makes the surgery more complicated. The best considerations for surgery are the amount of suffering and the degree to which the patients have had to change their lifestyles because of the arthritis.

As with all elective surgeries, the final decision as to whether to have an arthroplasty must be made by an informed patient. The potential benefits of arthroplasty have to be weighed against the risks of surgery. The most common severe complications include infections, pulmonary embolus, cardiac problems, and revision due to mechanical problems such as loosening and malalignment.[13,14] Current hip and knee arthroplasties can be expected to last on average 10 to 15 years. If the patient is active in sports or high-impact physical training, where both feet are off the ground at the same time, alternatives such as fusion or osteotomy must be considered. Arthroplasties are not capable of returning people to high-impact sports and rarely do they make the joint feel completely normal. Patients who can barely function before surgery are usually extremely pleased with their arthroplasty, but those who have an arthroplasty because of mild pain are often unhappy.

Before considering hip or knee arthroplasty, it is necessary to assess all the joints of both lower extremities. Pain from hip arthritis often radiates to the knee. If the ipsilateral hip and knee are both arthritic, sequential intracapsular injections of procaine may be necessary to determine the source of the pain. Osteoarthritis that is well controlled with anti-inflammatory drugs usually hurts only with activity. Pain in a particular joint is often directly related to the amount of activity. An arthritic right knee may not hurt until a patient has walked more than a block. If the left hip hurts after half a block of walking, the patient may not realize that his right knee is severely arthritic until after the left hip has been replaced. Patients become angry and depressed when they realize that they have undergone a major operation with only slight improvement in their ambulatory capacity. This situation is particularly true for patients with rheumatoid arthritis because of the frequent occurrence of arthritis in the joints of the foot and ankle. When a person has extensive arthritic damage in many joints, several arthroplasties as well as other procedures may be necessary to significantly improve the patient's function. Careful preoperative planning and absolute candidness with the patient are very important for a successful outcome.

Operations for hip and knee replacement usually take from 2 to 4 h. The patients are usually out of bed the next day and ambulating in physical therapy on the second postoperative day. The length of stay in the hospital is usually 4 days. Patients are discharged when their wounds are healing well and they can walk independently with crutches or a walker. At home, they do muscle-strengthening exercises and range of motion exercises daily. They continue on protective weightbearing for 1 to 2 months. If a patient has two severely arthritic joints, it is often beneficial to replace both joints during the same hospitalization to reduce the total length of disability and maximize the benefits of postoperative physical therapy. Simultaneous replacement of ipsilateral hips and knees is not recommended because of the high incidence of peroneal nerve problems.

In most cases, two to four units of blood are required for hip replacement and two for knee replacement. Much of the blood loss occurs because patients must receive prophylaxis for deep vein thrombosis before surgery to prevent pulmonary embolism. When medically possible, the patients should be asked to donate their own blood for the operation.

Prophylactic antibiotics are used to reduce the possibility of infection. The antibiotic coverage should include *Staphylococcus aureus* and *Staphylococcus epidermidis*. In uncomplicated cases, the infection rate is less than 2%.[13] Deep wound infections may require removal of the prosthesis. Reimplantation is often possible when the infection is under control. If the infective organism is sensitive to oral antibiotics, older patients are often treated with an irrigation and debridement followed by chronic oral suppression with the prosthesis intact. Patients also need prophylaxis to prevent deep vein thrombosis after surgery.[15]

Most of the newer designs of hip and knee arthroplasties have a coating of porous metal on the side of the prosthesis that faces the bone. The coating is designed to take advantage of the fact that healing bone will grow into porous materials. Loosening of cemented prostheses often occurs at the cement–bone interface with fracture of the cement. A direct bond between the bone and prosthesis eliminates the need for bone cement (methylmethacrylate). Presently, most of the advantages of using cementless prostheses remain theoretical; they have not been implanted long enough to determine if they will last longer than cemented prostheses. If the patient's bones are severely osteoporotic, cement should be used if the replacement is absolutely necessary.

Degenerative Arthritis of the Spine

Degenerative arthritis of the spine is a common problem in older people. Both the intervertebral disks and the posterior facet joints are generally involved. There may be a history of trauma, sports injuries, or occupations that have stressed the neck and back, but many people have no known cause. Intervertebral disk material tends to desiccate and fragment with age. The annulus fibrosus may weaken, allowing disk material to protrude into the spinal canal or laterally into the neural foramina. The arthritic posterior facet joints can develop osteophytes so large that they significantly narrow the foramina.

Pain may be from the arthritic joints or it may be caused by neural impingement. In addition, pain within the spine usually causes reflex spasm of paravertebral muscles, which can also become painful from overwork. Patients with vertebral osteoarthritis tend to restrict their motion to relieve the pain. At first, the loss of disk material may cause painful joint instability. Later, the ligaments tighten with relief of pain, and the joints become nearly fused. Patients with generalized ligament laxity and joint hypermobility tend to have much more back pain because they cannot stabilize their joints to prevent the pain.

Nearly everyone over the age of 60 years has roentgenographic evidence of spinal osteoarthritis. Because of the tendency for ligament tightening to reduce the symptoms of arthritis, there is no correlation between the degree of symptoms and the severity of the arthritis as judged by roentgenographs.[16] Indeed, the worst appearing spines are frequently asymptomatic. Because there are many different causes of back pain, arthritis should be considered as a cause of pain only after other common causes have been ruled out.

Pain from arthritis alone, without nerve compression, can radiate into the shoulder and arm from the neck and into the buttock and thigh from the lumbar spine. The presence or absence of numbness, paresthesias, and specific muscle weakness is very important to differentiate nerve impingement from arthritic pain. Any of these symptoms would suggest nerve root compression. Further workup for nerve root compression can include electromyographic studies to determine which nerve roots are involved and myelographic studies and magnetic resonance imaging to determine the site of compression.

In the neck, the initial treatment of an acute episode of either nerve root compression or arthritis is immobilization with a soft collar. Analgesics and NSAIDS are also helpful. Intermittent cervical traction that can be used in the home can often give dramatic relief of symptoms. Patients with nerve root compression who have persistent symptoms in spite of conservative treatment may require excision of the disk and fusion of the involved vertebrae. Arthritic pain without nerve root involvement usually responds to conservative treatment. Severe unremitting pain can be treated by diskectomy and fusion if it is localized to one level. Fusion of multiple levels is usually unwise because it increases the demand for motion at the remaining levels.

For the lumbar spine, analgesics and anti-inflammatory drugs have been used effectively for acute episodes of both arthritis and radiculopathy secondary to a herniated disk. Treatment beyond medication comes from an understanding of the forces acting upon the vertebrae. The lumbar spine is arched forward (lordotic) to allow upright ambulation. Weight that has been borne primarily through the vertebral bodies in the cervical and thoracic spine is transferred to the facet joints in the lower lumbar spine because of the arch. With good abdominal muscle tone, approximately half the weight of the upper torso is transmitted through the abdomen to the pelvis by hydrolic pressure. With poor abdominal muscle tone, all the weight is transmitted through the spine. Abdominal muscles relax during sitting. Pressures on the spine are therefore greater while sitting than with lying, standing, or walking.

All obese patients with chronic low back pain would benefit from weight reduction to relieve the pressure on the disks and facet joints. Bed rest is frequently advised for patients with disk disease. It has no proven value in treating lumbar arthritis. Bed rest makes all the muscles of the body weak, including the back muscles, which are then less able to stabilize a painful arthritic spine. If patients have acute lumbar arthritis primarily in the area of the vertebrae and disks, a combination of lying with frequent walking and little or no sitting is probably best. Patients with lumbar arthritis primarily in the area of the posterior facet joints have greater pain with standing than with sitting because greater weight is transmitted across the facet joints when the spine is lordotic. They should be allowed to sit. After the arthritic pain has abated, it is important to start an exercise program that strengthens both back and abdominal muscles.

Lumbosacral braces function by increasing intra-abdominal pressure, thus taking the weight off the spine. If the brace is tight, there is some effect even during sitting. The braces also reduce the lumbar lordosis during standing and immobilize the spine to the extent that muscles in spasm may relax. Braces should not be worn constantly because they cause rapid atrophy of back and abdominal muscles. In general, older people do not tolerate lumbosacral braces unless they are accustomed to wearing girdles.

Patients with painful herniated disks that have not responded to conservative therapy may require surgical diskectomy. In cases where nerve roots are compressed by osteophytes of facet joints, resection of the osteophytes with decompression of the nerve roots may be necessary. There is no effective surgery for painful osteoarthritis of the lumbar spine not associated with nerve compression. Lumbar fusions, which have been performed in the past for osteoarthritis, are now indicated only in situations where pain is caused by instability of the joints.

Cervical Spondylotic Myelopathy

In both the cervical and lumbar regions, degenerative arthritis of the spine can cause narrowing of the spinal canal. Cervical myelopathy[17] is the result of bony or soft tissue compression of the spinal cord in the neck that frequently appears in the fifth and sixth decades. Although the signs and symptoms may vary greatly, the sign most frequently found is spasticity of the extremities followed by weakness. Pain is present in less than half of patients. Numbness and painful paresthesias can also be present, as well as fasciculations and sphincter disturbances. Clinical symptoms vary with the part of the cord that is compressed. Patient symptoms can be so vague that their etiology is easily missed if the possibility of myelopathy is not constantly kept in mind. Electromyographic studies are helpful to document the degree of nerve involvement. Magnetic resonance imaging usually can demonstrate the site of compression.

Nonoperative treatment includes use of cervical orthotics, NSAIDs, and isometric neck muscle strengthening. Traction and manipulation of the neck are contraindicated because they may cause further compromise of the spinal cord.

Cervical myelopathy tends to progress to severe disability if left untreated. Surgical decompression of the spinal cord should be considered if progression of the neurologic deficit is observed, or symptoms that have been present for more than 6 months do not improve with conservative treatment or the MRI demonstrates either severe compression of the cord or changes within the substance of the cord.

Lumbar Spinal Stenosis

In the lumbar region, bone hypertrophy from osteoarthritis often narrows both the spinal canal and neural foramina. This condition is called spinal stenosis. Although arthritis of the lumbar spine is frequently seen in the fifth and sixth decade, symptoms of spinal stenosis usually appear in the seventh decade. The first symptoms are vague leg pains, paresthesias and dysesthesias brought on by walking or standing. Patients experience symptoms similar to vascular claudication. After walking a certain distance they find that they have to stop because of increasing leg pain and weakness that abates rapidly if they sit or stand leaning forward. In severe cases, patients walk bent forward at the waist. By bending forward, they are straightening the lordosis in their lumbar spine so that their spinal canal has a maximal diameter. Neurologic deficits are present at rest only in severely affected patients.[18]

The diagnosis of spinal stenosis is made by MRI scan. Most patients with intermittent symptoms respond to rest, anti-inflammatory medications, and back and abdominal strengthening exercises. Severely affected patients may require laminectomy and decompression of neural foramina with approximately an 85% chance of a good result,[19] although stenosis can recur at different lumbar levels.

Pyogenic Osteomyelitis

Bacterial infections in bone can be extremely difficult to eradicate if the circulation to the bone is impaired. Circulation may be disrupted by arterial insufficiency, such as in arterial occlusive disease, by fracture of the bone, or by abscesses caused by the infection itself. Without adequate circulation, antibiotics cannot reach the bacteria. The infection cannot be eliminated unless either circulation is reestablished or the infected bone is removed.[20]

Bacteria reach bone by one of three pathways: hematogenous seeding, direct inoculation, or contiguous spread from a nearby soft tissue infection.

Hematogenous Infection

Hematogenous seeding of the bone by a transient bacteremia is frequently caused by an infection elsewhere in the body, such as pneumonia, cutaneous infection, or urinary tract infection. Bacteremias can also occur during dental and urologic procedures.

Vertebral Osteomyelitis

Vertebral osteomyelitis is the most common type of hematogenous osteomyelitis in adults. Vertebral bodies may be predisposed to hematogenous seeding of bacteria because their marrow is actively producing blood components. The sinusoidal system of the marrow reduces the blood flow greatly and may allow bacteria to move into the tissue. In addition, urologic infections and other pelvic infections can easily spread through Batson's plexus, which is a system of communicating veins that connect the pelvic venous plexus with the venous plexus of the spine.

For many patients, the source of the organism cannot be found. A large majority of the patients have *Staphylococcus aureus* infections. Any vertebra can be involved, but the lower thoracic and lumbar vertebrae have the greatest incidence. All patients have symptoms of back pain that may have been present for as long as several years. A small percentage have symptoms of septicemia such as fevers, night sweats, elevated leukocyte counts, and positive blood cultures. Paraparesis due to neural compression may be present. Surgery is indicated for vertebral osteomyelitis if the spine is unstable, if a large soft tissue abscess is present, or if the infection has not responded to antibiotic therapy.

Direct Inoculation

Infection from direct inoculation of bacteria commonly results from bites and puncture wounds in hands and feet. In older patients. surgery involving bones is also a common cause. The presence of metallic implants or dead bone in the area of the infection can make eradication difficult. Prevention is definitely the best way to treat orthopedic infections. Surgeries should be performed with scrupulous aseptic technique and minimal dissection. Prophylactic antibiotics should be used for all major operations involving implantation of prosthetic materials.

Contiguous Spread of a Soft Tissue Infection

Contiguous spread of soft tissue infection occurs most frequently in areas of poor blood supply, such as decubitus ulcers and ischemia of the lower extremities. Treatment must first be directed toward increasing blood flow to the involved area, which may require arterial bypass procedures or the use of vascularized muscular flaps. Necrotic bone must be completely removed, and intensive soft tissue wound care must be instituted. If amputation is required, it should be performed at a level that is known to have sufficent blood flow to allow healing.

Fractures

Hip Fractures

Fracture of the hip is a frequent occurrence in elderly people and is one the few orthopedic conditions in aged people that is associated with significant mortality. Mortality rates for older patients in the first year following hip fracture have been found to be 14% to 36%.[21] Patients seldom die as a direct result of hip fractures, but hip fractures generally occur in debilitated people. The mortality rate increases in patients with poorly controlled systemic diseases, multiple comorbidities, and dementia.[22] Elderly people tend to think of hip fractures as occurring very close to the end of life because they remember friends and relatives who died shortly after fracturing their hips. If a patient's prognosis for recovery is good, it should be discussed with them because they may hold dark thoughts about their future that would delay recovery and rehabilitation.

Hip fractures are generally the result of trivial trauma. Patients often feel their hips break before they fall. Bedridden patients frequently sustain hip fractures falling out of bed. Inactive elderly patients develop disuse osteoporosis, which, superimposed upon senile osteoporosis, can cause extreme softening of the bone. In addition, poor dietary habits or malabsorption can cause osteomalacia with further softening.

Immediate medical evaluation of patients with hip fractures is very important. Hip fractures can cause rapid loss of several units of blood into the thigh, which can lead to hypotension and possible cardiac ischemia. In addition, patients may have fallen as the result of hypotensive events from cardiac arrthymias. By the time they arrive at the hospital, they may no longer be hypotensive, but they should still be evaluated for the possibility that they might have sustained myocardial damage immediately after the fracture.

People who sustain hip fractures usually require surgery to stabilize the fracture and allow early ambulation. Some types of hip fractures have almost no chance of healing without surgery whereas other types would heal but only after weeks or months of bed rest. The potential morbidity and mortality of bed rest in elderly, debilitated patients is usually greater than the risks of surgery, but bed rest may be the only option for severely ill patients. Each patient must be evaluated with both possibilities in mind.

Hip fractures occur primarily in two areas of the proximal femur, the intratrochanteric region and the femoral neck. Fractures in the intratrochanteric area have a high chance of healing because the fractures have a broad cross-sectional area with good blood supply from both sides. However, if surgery is not performed, several weeks of bed rest are required and the fractures tend to heal in shortened, externally rotated positions. Femoral neck fractures occur between the trochanters and the femoral head. The blood supply to the femoral head comes from the trochanteric region through the femoral neck and vessels surrounding the femoral neck. Displaced femoral neck fractures often totally disrupt the blood supply to the femoral head. If the blood supply is disrupted, the femoral head will become necrotic even if the fracture is surgically stabilized. For these fractures, the femoral head is usually replaced by a prosthesis called a hemiarthroplasty, although in younger patients a trial of internal fixation may be indicated if there is a chance that the blood supply is still intact. If the ends of the fracture have not displaced, the blood supply is usually intact and the fracture can be successfully treated with screws to hold the fracture in place during healing. Very active people with displaced femoral neck fractures should probably have total hip replacements rather than hemiarthroplasties because hemiarthroplasties can be painful in active people.[23] In general, if a patient is community dwelling, ambulatory, and in good health, a total hip replacement should be performed.

Patients occasionally have impacted femoral neck fractures where one side of the fracture becomes stably impacted into the bone of the other side. Patients with these fractures frequently can walk with minimal pain. Sometimes the fractures come apart later, necessitating surgery. If the fracture has impacted in a good position and is relatively painless, it can be treated with protected weightbearing with crutches or a walker.

The goal of surgery for fractured hips is stabilization of the bones of the fracture to the point that the patient can be rapidly mobilized after surgery. Patients are usually allowed to sit up the day after surgery. Physical therapy for ambulation with protected weightbearing is started as soon as medically possible, which is usually the second day after surgery. Prophylaxis to prevent deep vein thrombosis should continue throughout the recovery period.

The possibility of a fractured hip is frequently one of the greatest fears of elderly people who live alone. They have all heard stories of people who have broken their hips and languished for days on the floor of their home unable to get to the telephone. Establishing a system in which they are contacted every day can be very reassuring. Many elderly people carry portable telephones with them while in their home. A home exercise program to strengthen their lower extremities will help prevent falls and alleviate fears of falling.

Vertebral Compression Fractures

Vertebral compression fractures[24] are a major cause of back pain in osteoporotic patients. These fractures are frequently undiagnosed or misdiagnosed as arthritic pain. However, the pain tends to be much more acute and is usually in the middle and upper regions of the back. Some patients give a history of apparently trivial trauma whereas others merely note gradually increasing back pain. The pain can be severe and often radiates in the direction of the dermatome at that level. It is exacerbated by sitting, standing, and mild percussion of the spine at the level of the fracture.

The diagnosis is made with a lateral roentgenograph of the thoracolumbar spine. The silhouettes of the vertebral bodies are normally rectangular. Compression fractures usually cause wedging of the vertebra with loss of anterior height compared to posterior height. In mild cases where the loss of height is minimal, one may see only an increased density of the bone where the collapse has occurred below the endplate of the vertebra. Sometimes, instead of wedging, disk material protrudes through a fracture in the endplate of the vertebra, creating a cystic area within the vertebra called a Schmorl's node.

It is difficult to roentgenographically determine the age of a compression fracture. Previous roentgenographs, if they exist, are often the only way to determine if a fracture is new, because previous compression fractures may have gone undiagnosed and bone scans often show increased activity in the area of a fracture for many years. Mild compression fractures and Schmorl's nodes are frequently missed on the original roentgenographs. Patients with clinical indications of a compression fracture should be treated with the presumptive diagnosis if other causes of the pain have been ruled out.

If there is a history of severe trauma or clinical evidence of a neurologic deficit, computerized tomography or magnetic resonance imaging (MRI) of the spine should be performed to determine if loss of the integrity of the posterior elements of the spine has led to pressure on neural structures. Similar procedures should be performed if there is a significant possibility that the collapse may be due to the presence of tumor.

Osteoporotic compression fractures almost invariably heal because the collapse increases the amount of bone in the area of the fracture. Treatment of the patient is directed toward providing symptomatic relief and preventing possible complications. Originally, the pain may be severe. Patients should be treated with rest in a firm bed until the initial severe pain has abated, which usually takes 3 to 5 days, although some relatively unstable fractures can be painful for as long as 2 months. Strong analgesics may be necessary at first. Patients may have a transient ileus secondary to pain and retroperitoneal hemorrhage. They should not eat if there is abdominal distension or if they are not hungry. Reintroduction of food should be started with a liquid diet. Routine precautions for bedridden patients to prevent thromboembolic disease should be taken. When the patients can sit comfortably, physical therapy for progressive ambulation should be started with a walker or crutches to reduce the weight that is transmitted through the spine.

Soft Tissue Injuries

Chronic soft tissue injuries, also called tendinitis or soft tissue rheumatism, are a common cause of chronic pain in elderly people (Fig. 44.1). There is a tendency for all musculoskeletal tissues to atrophy with age. This atrophy is most apparent with the skin, which slowly becomes thinner and more transparent, and the bones, which show thinning and osteopenia on x-ray, but similar phenomena occur with muscles, tendons, ligaments, and other soft tissues that cannot be as readily assessed. The natural tendency for people to gain weight as they grow older puts increased demands upon weakened tissues. Minor injuries in elderly people heal slowly and have a greater tendency not to heal if there are continued stresses.

Tendons, ligaments, and other tissues that provide tensile strength have very well organized collagen bundles for maximum strength. Chronic stresses on these structures cause fatigue disruption of the collagen that is replaced by relatively weak, poorly organized scar tissue.[26] With rest the patient's symptoms often completely abate but later return after episodes of activity that would not have caused injury to the original tissue but is sufficient to cause injury to the scarred tissue. The result is permanent tissue weakness, frequently accompanied by chronic pain. It is not unusual for a patient to present with a several-year history of intermittent pain in a specific soft tissue structure. They know what makes it worse and what makes it better, and they are not

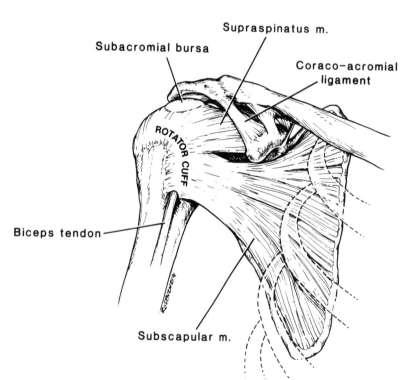

FIGURE 44.1. Rotator cuff and associated structures commonly involved in pain syndromes.

surprised to hear that the pain may never completely disappear.

Commonly affected areas in the upper extremity include the biceps tendon and rotator cuff of the shoulder, the origin of the finger and wrist extensors (tennis elbow), and extensor policis longus and abductor policis brevis tendons (de Quervain's). In the back, the fascial attachment of the erector spinae muscles and the interspinous ligaments are common sites of soft tissue injuries. In the lower extremity, the most commonly affected areas in older people are tendons of gluteus medius at the greater trochanter, the pes anserine (conjoint tendon of the sartorius, gracilis, and semitendinosus) on the medial side of the knee, and the insertion of the plantar fascia of the foot onto the calcaneus (heel spur). In each case, there is an element of overuse. Tendinitis around the hip and knee is frequently associated with intra-articular pathology. Presumably, the tendon damage is caused by increased use of the muscles that protect the knee joints; this is particularly true of the pes anserine, which almost always becomes painful from either a degenerative meniscus tear or osteoarthritis in the medial compartment of the knee.[27] These same conditions cause can cause gluteus medius tendonitis because the gluteus medius stabilized the medial compartment of the knee by abducting the thigh when the knee is planted on the ground.

The subjective nature of the symptoms of chronic soft tissue injuries creates multiple problems for physicians trying to treat the diseases. Roentgenographs and laboratory studies are usually not helpful except to rule out other conditions. The patient is often unable to localize the pain that tends to radiate distally away from its source. The tenderness associated with soft tissue injuries, however, can be well localized to the injured tissue. The diagnosis is made by a physical examination that requires the patient to describe the area of tenderness and the physician to identify the area with regard to underlying anatomic structures.

Treatment of Tendinitis/Bursitis Syndromes

Throughout the body, treatment of tendonitis/bursitis syndromes is similar. It should be kept in mind that these syndromes are primarily caused by overuse of specific muscle groups. The patient history should be carefully examined to determine if they are engaging in activities that might have led to excessive stress of the injured tissues. Obesity is a common contributing cause of lower extremity tendinitis. It may be difficult or impossible to obtain symptomatic relief without weight loss.

Exercise

Patients frequently want to know what exercises might help their tendinitis. Because tendinitis can appear after excessive exercise, it is important to limit exercises that focus on painful muscle groups. Rest, on the other hand, gives rapid relief of symptoms, but also leads to tissue atrophy that renders the tendons more susceptible to future injury when activity is resumed. Gentle muscle-strengthening exercises are probably beneficial. Mild stretching exercises are also important to prevent stiffness and contractures that might render the muscles more susceptible to future injuries. In general, any exercise that does not cause increased pain in the affected tendons is probably beneficial.

NSAIDs

A short trial of oral anti-inflammatory medications may be of benefit. In view of the potential complications, prolonged use of these drugs is probably not warranted except in cases of severe, chronic tendinitis, which have a good response to NSAIDs.

Corticosteroid Injection

There is an acute form of tendinitis that may actually be a different disease in which the patient experiences sharp, incapacitating pain and tenderness without a prior history of pain in the area. Injection of corticosteroids into the affected area frequently provides permanent relief. This acute form is probably an inflammatory condition with little or no damage to the collagen fibers of the tissue. Patients tend to think that all forms of soft tissue pain syndromes can be cured with corticosteroid injections because they know people who have had a good response to the acute form of the disease. Cortisone injections inhibit tissue repair. Repeated injections into chronically weakened tissues are probably detrimental. True bursitis, which is inflammation of a bursa at a bony prominence, is much rarer than tendinitis and can often be cured with cortisone injections.

Palliative Treatments

There are a host of treatments that provide at least temporary relief of the symptoms of soft tissue injuries. These measures include heating pads, liniments, transcutaneous neural stimulation (TENS), acupuncture, aquatic exercising, and ultrasound therapy. These methods are particularly effective if the tendinitis is caused by pain-induced muscle spasms. The treatments relax the muscles, thus reducing the load on the tendons.

Shoulder Pain

Shoulder pain is often very difficult to diagnose because it can have many different causes, including (a) cervical osteoarthritis or a degenerative cervical disk radiating to the shoulder, (b) osteoarthritis of the shoulder or acromioclavicular joint, (c) tendinitis of the long head of the biceps tendon, (d) tears in the rotator cuff, and (e) impingement of soft tissue on the coracoclavicular ligament and anterior border of the acromion (Fig. 44.2). Even carpal tunnel syndrome, which is caused by compression of the median nerve in the carpal canal, can cause pain radiating to the shoulder. In addition, pain from the diaphragm and heart are often felt in the shoulder and arm, and tumors of the periphery of the lung can present as shoulder and arm pain (Pancoast syndrome).

Pain from the shoulder joint and surrounding soft tissues is usually poorly localized and is frequently most severe along the lateral part of the arm just distal to the insertion of the deltoid muscle. Except in cases of severe inflammation, the pain tends to be dull in character. It is often exacerbated by specific shoulder movements.

Primary shoulder pain rarely, if ever, radiates to the neck. If there is a history of neck pain, numbness, paresthesias, or muscle atrophy in the arm, the neck should be considered as a source of the pain. Pain from the neck is usually increased with movement of the neck, and there may be tenderness of the paravertebral muscles and trapezius. Significant limitation of neck motion may also be present. Roentgenographic evidence of cervical arthritis, alone, is insufficient to conclude that the shoulder pain is coming from the neck because even severe cervical arthritis is often asymptomatic.

Osteoarthritis of the shoulder and acromioclavicular joint is easily seen on roentgenographs. Superior displacement of the head of the humerus with respect to the glenoid indicates that the rotator cuff has a significant tear. The area of the lung near the shoulder should always be inspected to rule out Pancoast syndrome.

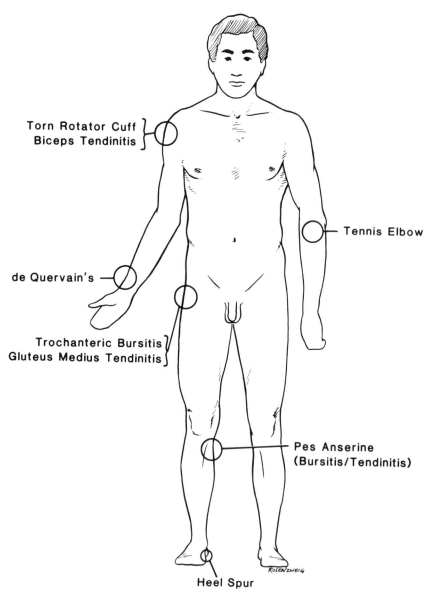

FIGURE 44.2. Common sites of soft tissue pain in the geriatric population.

Rotator Cuff and Bicipital Tendinitis

Tears of the rotator cuff are frequently seen in the older age groups.[28] Patients complain of pain in the shoulder radiating down the lateral part of the arm that is accentuated by abduction or flexion of the shoulder. Combing the hair and putting on a hat can be very painful and sometimes impossible. When much inflammation is present, the pain that normally is present only with movement becomes constant. Normal movements of the shoulder during sleep can wake the patient and exacerbate problems of insomnia frequently seen in older people.

The rotator cuff is formed from the combined tendons of teres minor (from the lateral border of the scapula), infraspinatus (from the dorsal scapular surface below the spine), supraspinatus (from the dorsal scapular surface above the spine), and subscapularus (from the ventral scapular surface). The tendons converge to form the rotator cuff that covers the top and sides of the humeral head superficial to the joint capsule. Laterally, the rotator cuff inserts into the greater tuberosity of the humerus. The tendon of the long head of the biceps courses in the bicipital grove of the humerus anteriorly and then into the shoulder joint under the rotator cuff where it inserts onto the scapula just above the glenoid rim.

Many factors appear to contribute to degeneration of the rotator cuff. The area of the cuff near its insertion on the greater tuberosity has a very limited blood supply, which may at times be insufficient to sustain the cuff.[29] In addition, with flexion of the shoulder the rotator cuff tends to impinge upon the acromiom and coracoacromial ligament, causing local abrasion and thinning. Actual tearing of the cuff may be the result of many years of repetitive movement. The biceps tendon can also be similarly damaged. Tenderness of the tendon is often the first sign of impingement. Crepitus is frequently felt over the anterior part of the shoulder when it is put through a full range of motion, and impingement can be demonstrated by forcibly forward flexing the shoulder when the arm is in neutral rotation.[30]

The muscles of the rotator cuff function to maintain the head of the humerus in the glenoid during arm motion. Tears of the rotator cuff allow the head of the humerus to sublux superiorly during contraction of the deltoid, which would normally cause abduction of the arm. If the tear is large, the superior subluxation of the humeral head can be noted on a roentgenograph of the shoulder. The space between the bottom of the acromion and the top of the head of the humerus is occupied by the joint capsule and rotator cuff. If the space is greatly diminished, the cuff must be torn. Small tears of the rotator cuff often can be demonstrated by MRI.

The treatment of shoulder impingement and rotator cuff tears must be closely tailored to the individual. Patients presenting with shoulder pain who have no loss of motion should be treated with rest, NSAIDs, and gentle range of motion and muscle-strengthening exercises. In particular, strengthening of the posterior shoulder muscles can often pull the femoral head posteriorly with reduction of impingement pain and crepitus. Corticosteroid injections can be tried if NSAIDs are ineffective. Surgical resection of the anterior acromion and coracoacromial ligament, which can be performed arthroscopically, should be considered for those patients with prolonged pain that is not responsive to conservative treatment.

If the patient has recently developed limitation of shoulder motion, an MRI should be performed to determine if the rotator cuff has a complete tear. Large tears should be repaired if the patient's condition permits. Chronic asymptomatic rotator cuff tears in people over 70 years of age are frequently seen on chest roentgenographs as superior subluxation of the humeral head. Although these patients usually have limited shoulder abduction and flexion, the remnants of the rotator cuff are usually so atrophic that surgical reconstruction would be of little benefit.

Frozen Shoulder

The first symptom of frozen shoulder[31] is insidious onset of dull shoulder pain, usually with no prior history of trauma. The pain is worse at night and with activity. Patients often have trouble sleeping and tend to hold their arms tightly against their sides. At first, with some encouragement, the shoulder can be put through a full range of motion. Later, all directions of motion become restricted and the pain subsides so long as the shoulder is not moved.

Frozen shoulder is a diffuse inflammation of the rotator cuff. Frequently there is degeneration of the intra-articular portion of the biceps tendon. Contracture of the subscapularis tendon limits abduction and external rotation of the shoulder. Eventually the shoulder capsule itself becomes contracted. Arthrogram of the shoulder shows decreased potential volume of the joint and obliteration of the normal synovial folds and recesses that allow motion.

Frozen shoulder tends to be a self-limiting disease with spontaneous recovery for most patients within 2 years. Early physical therapy probably reduces the length of disability. Patients are often very reluctant to move the joints. The patient should use a sling to rest the shoulder. Gentle range of motion exercises should be performed in the sling to maintain motion. Pendulum exercises in which the patient bends forward and lets his arms sway in a circular motion like a pendulum are particularly good because they do not require shoulder muscle activity and the natural feeling of the sway tends to relieve the patient's apprehensions about moving their arms.

NSAIDs may help to reduce the pain and stiffness. Occasionally, injections of corticosteroid into the subacromial bursa are helpful. Gentle manipulation of the shoulder under anesthesia may be necessary for patients who are not responding to physical therapy. Patients not responding to manipulation may need arthroscopic debridement of intrascapular adhesions.

Carpal Tunnel Syndrome

Compression of the median nerve at the wrist causes a constellation of signs and symptoms known as carpal tunnel syndrome.[32] The median nerve transverses the carpal canal in conjunction with the long flexor tendons of the fingers. The volume of the carpal canal is limited by the carpal bones dorsally, medially, and laterally, and by the flexor retinaculum ventrally. Swelling of the synovium of the tendons increases the pressure within the canal, which causes nerve compression.

Patients most often complain of painful burning and paresthesias of the first four fingers that is usually most severe at night and often causes insomnia. They report that they have to shake their hands to relieve the tingling. They may say that all their fingers feel numb, but examination demonstrates that numbness, if present, is confined to the first three fingers and the radial side of the fourth. The thenar muscles can be atrophic as a result of compression of the motor branch of the median nerve. Pain will occasionally radiate up the arm to the shoulder.

The most sensitive provocative test for carpal tunnel syndrome is the Phalen test.[33] The patient is asked to completely flex his wrist. Within 1 min, numbness and tingling will be produced, or exaggerated if already present. This test is positive in only 75% of patients. When a Tinel sign (shocklike sensations on percussion of the median nerve at the wrist) is present, the likelihood of carpal tunnel syndrome is great, but absence of a Tinel sign does not preclude the possibility of carpal tunnel syndrome. Electromyography should be performed if the Phalen test is negative in the presence of a high clinical suspicion of carpal tunnel syndrome, or if surgery is being contemplated. Slowing of the nerve conduction velocities is seen when compression of the median nerve is present.

Many diseases are known to cause carpal tunnel syndrome, including all the common chronic inflammatory arthritides, amyloidosis, myxedema, diabetes, and acromegaly. It is frequently seen during pregnancy. An acute form of carpal tunnel syndrome is seen in people who abruptly increase their wrist usage, such as when using crutches. In a large percentage of patients, no etiologic factor can be found. If an etiologic factor is present, therapy should be focused on correcting the problem if possible.

Cock-up splints prevent wrist flexion that causes further compression of the carpal canal. They can be worn at night and also during the day in severe cases. Injection of the carpal canal with corticosteroids often dramatically relieves the symptoms. If the symptoms are not relieved by injection or if they continue to return after multiple injections, surgical release of the flexor retinaculum should be considered. Atrophy of the thenar muscles is an indication for early surgical intervention because patients often have poor return of muscle strength even with surgery.

Foot Problems in the Elderly

Foot problems are often a major source of concern of elderly people. Diseases of aging that affect the musculoskeletal system are frequently first seen in the foot. Osteoarthritis is often first manifested as a bunion of the first metatarsal phalangeal joint. Muscle weakness appears as loss of strength of the interosseous muscles of the foot leading to claw toes. Arterial insufficiency often appears first as pain in the feet. Diabetic vasculopathy and neuropathy often become clinically significant first in the feet.

Shoe Wear

Many of the chronic foot problems seen in older patients are caused by inappropriate footwear. Bunions are not seen in populations that do not wear shoes. High heels can cause contractures of the Achilles tendon and claw toes. Shoes with narrow toes can cause corns as well as bunions. Shoes with hard soles can cause callosities on the bottom of the feet. The time to start wearing appropriate shoes is before the foot deformities appear. After a deformity is present, proper shoes may reduce its effects but cannot correct it.

Fortunately, shoe companies are beginning to make shoes that are both comfortable and acceptable in most social settings. Shoe soles of soft material such as polyurethane have several beneficial effects. They prevent callosities on the bottom of the foot where the soft tissue padding under bony prominences has been lost. Ample arches in the shoes protect the tibialis posterior tendons. They also reduce the amplitude of the forces transmitted from the ground through the foot while walking (ground reactive forces). Reduction of these forces has mitigating effects upon hip and knee osteoarthritis and all types of musculoskeletal low back pain. It may also prevent osteoarthritis in the joints of the foot.

Tarsal Tunnel Syndrome

Compression of the posterior tibial nerve at the ankle causes burning pain on the plantar aspect of the foot known as tarsal tunnel syndrome.[34] The burning is often accompanied by tingling and numbness that is poorly localized. In most patients it is aggravated by activity, but it may also be severe at night. It appears to be analogous to carpal tunnel syndrome in the hand, which is caused by compression of the median nerve in the carpal canal.

Patients usually have a positive Tinel's sign, which is a feeling of electrical shocks when the injured part of the nerve is percussed. The tarsal canal extends around the medial maleolus into the plantar aspect of the foot. The Tinel's sign may be positive anywhere within the tunnel and is sometimes positive along the distal calf, proximal to the medial malleolus. The diagnosis is established by demonstration of decreased nerve conduction velocities of the posterior tibial nerve or one of its branches.

Tarsal tunnel syndrome can often be treated by local injection of steroids or NSAIDs. Occasionally, casting for short periods of time is beneficial. If conservative methods fail, the tarsal tunnel can be surgically released, but the patients should be warned that symptoms often persist after the release.[35]

Hallux Valgus (Bunion)

Bunions[36] are medial protuberances of the first metatarsal phalangeal joints that appear if the first toes deviate laterally. The joints frequently have roentgenographic signs of osteoarthritis. Pressure from shoe wear causes the medial capsule of the joint to become thickened and inflamed, and an exostosis develops on the head of the metatarsal. Superficial nerves that course over the top of bunions often become inflamed, causing feelings of numbness along the medial side of the great toe. In older people, the great toe frequently crosses above or below the second toe, and this can lead to painful sores or areas of maceration. Interposition of a pad between the two toes is frequently helpful.

Although proper footwear helps prevent the appearance of bunions, it cannot correct bunions after they have formed. Abnormal pull of the tendons around the deformed joint with contracture of the joint capsule prevent return of the toe to its correct position. If a bunion is painful and disabling, surgical reconstruction may be necessary. Bunionectomies can usually be performed under local anesthesia, often without hospitalization of the patient. If the bony deformities are mild, removal of the exostosis and soft tissue realignment may be all that is necessary. More complicated bunions require osteotomy of the metatarsal or first phalanx as well.

A "bunionette" or "tailor's bunion" is a prominence along the lateral side of the forefoot resulting from lateral protrusion of the head of the fifth metatarsal bone. At least some prominence of the fifth metatarsal head is a normal finding in most people. The prominence is accentuated by wearing shoes with narrow toes. The fifth toe is pushed medially, and the prominence becomes irritated by direct pressure from the shoe. A callous forms on the skin over the prominence and a bursa often forms between the skin and fifth metatarsal phalangeal joint. In general, bunionettes can be successfully treated by wearing shoes with wide toes and by padding over the painful prominence.

Claw Toes

Claw toes is a common foot deformity that appears to be due to ineffective action of the intrinsic muscles of the foot. Although the leg muscles provide most of the strength of the toes, the lumbricals and interosseous muscles of the foot help to keep the toes elongated during flexion by flexing the metatarsophalangeal joints and extending the interphalangeal joints. Without the intrinsic muscles, flexion of the toes by the leg muscles alone causes hyperextension of the metatarsophalangeal joints and flexion of the interphalangeal joints, which is claw toes. Painful corns develop over the hyperflexed proximal interphalangeal joints, and callosities develop on the tips of the toes that are pushed into the sole of the shoe while walking. Claw toe deformities usually involve all the toes of the foot including the great toe. The deformity of claw toes may be accentuated by wearing high-heeled shoes or shoes that are too narrow and short at the toe.

Conservative treatment for claw toes includes shoes with broad toe width and soft soles to distribute the pressure. In severe cases, surgery to straighten the toes may be necessary.

Heel Spur

Pain in the heel during weightbearing is often caused by inflammation where the plantar aponeurosis attaches to the tuberosity of the calcaneus. As with other forms of tendinitis, the point of attachment to bone appears to be the weakest area and the one most likely to be chronically inflamed, presumably due to microtears. Prolonged inflammation leads to accretion of new bone, called a spur. Tenderness is usually found at the point where the plantar aponeurosis attaches to the calcaneus, which starts in the middle of the bottom of the heel and extends medially.

The distal part of the plantar aponeurosis attaches to the base of the proximal phalanges. Dorsiflexion of the phalanges during normal gait accentuates the arch and therefore shortens the foot. If the heel is everted and the arch is relatively flat, large stresses are put upon the aponeurosis with toe dorsiflexion. The stresses can be relieved by wearing soft-soled shoes with good arch supports. If pain persists, many conservative approaches are possible including foot orthotics to keep the heel inverted, oral anti-inflammatory medications, and local injection of corticosteroid.[37] When pain is unremitting despite conservative measures, surgical excision of the spur is often beneficial.[38]

Diabetic Foot Problems

Foot infection is the most common infection in diabetics that requires hospitalization.[39] Almost all patients with long-standing diabetes have peripheral neuropathies that lead to severe arthropathies (Charcot joints) because the patients are unable to perceive when their joints are being damaged. As the joints are destroyed, the bones around the joints become deformed and often form protuberances below the skin. Foot ulcers appearing over the protuberances inevitably become colonized with bacteria that penetrate the foot because the vascular status of the foot is so poor that it is unable to form a protective barrier against bacterial invasion. Ischemia of the foot appears to be caused by both atherosclerotic narrowing of large arteries and diabetic microangiopathy.

Prevention is the best approach to dealing with diabetic ulcers. Prominences that cause focal pressures with weightbearing should be treated with local padding, soft-soled shoes, and padded stockings. Pressing against the sole of the foot with a nylon fiber can indicate which patients have developed peripheral neuropathy to the point that they no longer have protective sensation.[40] These patients should have frequent inspections for early skin changes.

Treatment of superficial ulcers includes padding to take the weight off the region of the ulcer, intensive wound care, and elevation to reduce swelling. If the arterial blood pressure at the ankle is greater than half the brachial artery pressure, the ulcers have an excellent chance of healing.[41] Treatment of deep infections consists of excision of infected bone, intensive wound care, and intravenous antibiotics.[42] Deep infections can be difficult to diagnose by physical examination alone because of the poor circulation and neuropathy.

References

1. Creamer P, Hochberg M. Osteoarthritis [seminar]. *Lancet.* 1997;350:503–509.
2. Pottenger LA, Phillips FM, Draganich LF. The effect of marginal osteophytes on reduction of varus-valgus instability in osteoarthritic knees. *Arthritis Rheum.* 1990;33:853–858.
3. Goldring MB. The role of inflammatory mediators in osteoarthritis: lessons from animal models. *Connect Tissue Res.* 1999;40:1–11.
4. Silverstein FE, Faich G, Goldstein, et al. Gastrointestinal toxicity with celecoxib vs. nonsteroidal anti-inflammatory drugs for osteoarthritis and rheumatoid arthritis. *JAMA.* 2000;284:1247–1255.
5. Bradley JD, Brandt KD, Katz BP, et al. Comparison of an anti-inflammatory dose of ibuprofen, analgesic dose of ibuprofen and acetaminophen in treatment of patients with osteoarthritis of the knee. *N Engl J Med.* 1991;325:87–91.
6. Deal CL, Moskowitz RW. Nutraceuticals as therapeutic agents in osteoarthritis. The role of glucosamine, chondroitin sulfate, and collagen hydrolysate. *Rheum Dis Clin N Am.* 1999;25:379–395.
7. Rozental TD, Sculco TP. Intra-articular corticosteroids: an updated review. *Am J Orthop.* 2000;29:18–23.
8. Simon LS. Viscosupplementation therapy with intra-articular hyaluronic acid. Fact or fantasy? *Rheum Dis Clin N Am.* 1999;25:345–357.
9. McGinley BJ, Cushner FD, Scott WN. Debridement arthroscopy. A 10-year follow-up. *Clin Orthop.* 1999;367:190–194.
10. Kruger T, Wohlrab D, Birke A, et al. Results of arthroscopic joint debridement in different stages of chondromalacia of the knee joint. *Arch Orthop Trauma Surg.* 2000;120(5–6):338–342.
11. Naudie D, Bourne RB, Rorabeck CH, et al. Survivorship of the high tibial valgus osteotomy. *Clin Orthop.* 1999;367:18–27.
12. Harris WH, Sledge CB. Total hip and total knee replacement. *N Engl J Med.* 1990;323:56–57.
13. Scheller AD, Turner RH, Lowell JD. Complications of arthroplasty and total joint replacement in the hip. In: Epps CH Jr, ed. *Complications in Orthopaedic Surgery, 2nd Ed, vol 2.* Philadelphia: Lippincott; 1986:159–1108.
14. Lonner JH, Lotke PA. Aseptic complications after total knee arthroplasty. *J Am Acad Orthop Surg.* 1999;7:311–324.
15. Kearon C, Hirsh J. Management of anticoagulation before and after elective surgery. *N Engl J Med.* 1997;336:1506–1511.
16. Lawrence JS, Bremner JM, Bier F. Osteoarthritis: prevalence in the population and relationship between symptoms and X-ray changes. *Ann Rheum Dis.* 1966;25:1–24.
17. Dvorak J. Cervical myelopathy: epidemiology, physical examination, and neurodiagnostics. *Spine.* 1998;23:2663–2673.
18. Hilibrand AS, Rand N. Degenerative lumbar stenosis: diagnosis and treatment. *J Am Acad Orthop Surg.* 1999;7:239–249.
19. Hall S, Bartleson JD, Onofrio BM, et al. Lumbar spinal stenosis: clinical features, diagnostic procedures and results of surgical treatment in 68 patients. *Ann Intern Med.* 1985;103:271–275.
20. Lew DP, Waldvogel FA. Current concepts: osteomyelitis. *N Engl J Med.* 1997;336:999–1007.
21. Koval KJ, Zuckerman JD. Functional recovery after fracture of the hip. *J Bone Joint Surg.* 1994;76:751–758.
22. Lyons AR. Clinical outcomes and treatment of hip fractures. *Am J Med.* 1997;103:51S–65S.
23. Gebhard JS, Amstutz HC, Zinar N, et al. A comparison of total hip arthroplasty and hemiarthroplasty for treatment of acute fracture of the hip. *Clin Orthop.* 1992;282:123–131.
24. Rechtine GR. Nonsurgical treatment of thoracic and lumbar fractures. *Instruct Course Lect.* 1999;48:413–416.
25. Holland NW, Gonzalez. Soft tissue problems in older adults. *Clin Geriatr Med.* 1998;14:601–611.

26. Grieco A, Molteni G, De Vito G, et al. Epidemiology of musculoskeletal disorders due to overload. *Ergonomics.* 1998;41:1253–1260.

27. Brookler JA, Mongan ES. Anserina bursitis; a treatable cause of knee pain in patients with degenerative arthritis. *Calif Med.* 193;119:8–10.

28. Jensen KL, Williams GR, Russell IJ, et al. Rotator cuff tear arthropathy. *J Bone Joint Surg. [Am]* 1999;81:1312–1324.

29. Rathbun JB, Macnab I. Vascular anatomy of the rotator cuff of the shoulder. *J Bone Joint Surg [Br].* 1970;52:540–553.

30. Near CS, Welsh RP. The shoulder in sports. *Orthop Clin N Am.* 1977;8:583–591.

31. Goldberg BA, Scarlat MM, Harryman DT II. Management of the stiff shoulder. *J Orthop Sci.* 1999;4:462–471.

32. D'Arcy CA, McGee S. Does this patient have carpal tunnel syndrome? *JAMA.* 2000;283:3110–3117.

33. Gellman H, Gelberman RH, Tan AM, et al. Carpal tunnel syndrome. *J Bone Joint Surg [Am].* 1986;68:735–737.

34. Oh SJ, Meyer RD. Entrapment neuropathies of the tibial (posterior tibial) nerve. *Neurol Clin.* 1999;17:593–615.

35. Pfeiffer WH, Cracchiolo A. Clinical results after tarsal tunnel decompression. *J Bone Joint Surg [Am].* 1994;76: 1222–1230.

36. Scranton PE. Principles of bunion surgery. *J Bone Joint Surg [Am].* 1983;65:1026–1028.

37. Davis PF, Severud E, Baxter DE. Painful heel syndrome: results of nonoperative treatment. *Foot Ankle Int.* 1994;15: 531–535.

38. Baxter DE, Thigpen CM. Heel pain—operative treatment. *Foot Ankle.* 1984;5:16–25.

39. Caputo GM, Cavanagh PR, Ulbrecht JS. Assessment and management of foot disease in patients with diabetes. *N Engl J Med.* 1994;331:854–860.

40. Birke JA, Sims DS. Plantar sensory threshold in ulcerative foot. *Lepr Rev.* 1986;57:261–267.

41. Jacobs RL, Karmondy AM, Wirth C, et al. The team approach in the salvage of the diabetic foot. *Surg Annu.* 1977;9:231–264.

42. Caballero F, Frykberg RG. Diabetic foot infections. *J Foot Ankle Surg.* 1998;37:248–255.

45
Medical Aspects of Hip Fracture Management

R. Sean Morrison and Albert L. Siu

Hip fractures are an important cause of mortality and functional dependence in the United States. Approximately 250,000 hip fractures occur annually in this country, and this number is expected to increase to more than 650,000 by the year 2040.[1,2] For adults over age 65, the annual incidence of hip fracture is 818 per 100,000 persons,[3] and women are two to three times more likely to experience a fracture than men.[4,5] Indeed, it is estimated that a white woman with an average life expectancy of 80 years has a 15% lifetime risk of fracture and that, by age 80, she has a 1% to 2% annual risk.[6] The mortality seen in the Medicare population following fracture is 7% at 1 month, 13% at 3 months, and 24% at 12 months.[7] For those patients who survive to 6 months, 60% will have recovered their prefracture walking ability, 50% will have recovered their prefracture ability to perform their activities of daily living, and about 25% will have recovered their prefracture ability to perform instrumental activities of daily living.[8] However, after 1 year, only 54% of surviving patients are able to walk unaided, and only 40% are able to perform all physical activities of daily living independently.[8] The costs associated with a single hip fracture episode (acute care, rehabilitation, home care services) range between $30,850 and $37,250 in the United States,[9–11] and the annual total costs associated with this disease exceed $5 billion.[12] Furthermore, it is estimated that these total annual costs will increase to $16 billion by the year 2040 as a result of the projected increase in the number of adults over age 65.

Although surgical repair of the fractured extremity is the cornerstone of therapy, available data suggest that the crucial factors that determine optimal functional recovery in hip fracture are independent of the fracture repair but instead are related to prefracture conditions and postfracture complications.[13] Thus, the successful care and outcome of the hip fracture patient require an active partnership between the orthopedic surgeon and medical consultant—the latter's role being to serve as the primary care physician, to medically evaluate and stabilize the patient before surgery, and to prevent and manage post-

operative complications (e.g., delirium). In this chapter, we focus on the medical care processes relevant to the hip fracture patient, with the exception of fall prevention and osteoporosis, which are covered in Chapters 66 and 44, respectively. Readers interested in the surgical management of the hip fracture patient are directed to the article by Zuckerman and Schon.[14]

Diagnosis and Surgical Repair

The majority of hip fractures are easily diagnosed on the basis of history, physical examination, and standard radiographs. Ninety percent of hip fractures result from a simple fall, and the characteristics of the fall (direction, site of impact, and protective response), as well as certain patient characteristics, are recognized as important factors influencing the risk of fracture.[13] A diagnosis of osteoporosis is the leading factor that places patients at increased risk for hip fracture.[13] Other patient characteristics that have been shown to be associated with hip fracture include female sex, white race, maternal history of hip fracture, physical inactivity, low body weight, consumption of alcohol, previous hip fracture, nursing home residence, visual impairment, cognitive impairment, and psychotropic medication use.[13] Patients with hip fracture typically report hip pain on weightbearing following a fall, and on physical exam the involved leg is often foreshortened and externally rotated. Plain radiographs (an anteroposterior view of the pelvis and a lateral view of the femur) of the hip confirm the diagnosis in the majority of circumstances. Occasionally, however, plain films do not reveal evidence of a fracture despite a high clinical suspicion (e.g., pain with weightbearing after a fall). In these cases, an anteroposterior view obtained with the hip internally rotated 15° to 20° may reveal a fracture by providing an optimal view of the femoral neck.[13] In circumstances in which all plain films are negative but clinical suspicion is still high, either a technetium-99m bone scan or an MRI should be undertaken to rule out an occult fracture. The MRI appears to be a more sensitive test to detect early fractures as the bone scan can be normal within the first 72 h following a fracture. If all tests or imaging studies are unrevealing, other diagnoses to consider include fractures of the pubic ramus, acetabulum, or greater trochanter, trochanteric bursitis, or trochanteric contusion.

Hip fractures may be classified as femoral neck (intracapsular), intertrochanteric, or subtrochanteric. Femoral neck fractures occur distal to the femoral head but proximal to the greater and lesser trochanters and are thus located within the capsule of the hip joint. The location of the fracture has important implications for healing and operative repair. Fractures in this region can disrupt the blood supply to the femoral head and can result in complications such as nonunion and avascular necrosis of the femoral head. Thus, although nondisplaced and minimally displaced femoral neck fractures can often be treated by insertion of cannulated screws, displaced femoral neck fractures typically require a hemiarthroplasty procedure to ensure appropriate fracture healing.

Intertrochanteric fractures are located lateral to the femoral neck. These fractures occur in a well-vascularized metaphyseal region between the greater and lesser trochanters, and although intertrochanteric fractures can be associated with considerable blood loss, typically they are not associated with the healing complications associated with femoral neck fractures. Intertrochanteric fracture are typically repaired by open reduction and internal fixation with a compression screw device.

Subtrochanteric fractures occur just below the lesser trochanter and account for only 5% to 10% of hip fractures. These fractures behave clinically like long bone fractures and are repaired either by insertion of an intramedullary device or by placement of a compression screw and long side plate.

Nonoperative management should be considered for nonambulatory patients with advanced dementia. One recent study suggested that mortality following fracture in patients with end-stage dementia exceeds 50% at 6 months.[15] For such patients, aggressive pain management and a return to their previous home environment may be the optimal treatment plan given the burdens associated with routine hospitalization, such as delirium, restraints, and painful therapeutic interventions (phlebotomies, arterial blood gas monitoring, intravenous catheter insertions).[15,16]

Medical Processes of Care

Timing of Surgery

The timing of surgical repair of hip fracture may affect patient outcome in two ways. Delay in surgical repair, and hence delay in return to weightbearing, could affect func-

tional recovery. Conversely, failure to stabilize medical problems before surgery could increase the risk of perioperative complications. Although the scheduling of surgery is set by the orthopedist, the rate-limiting step in this process is often the internist's preoperative medical evaluation.

Ten case series,[17–26] one randomized controlled trial of anesthetic techniques that included surgical delay as an independent variable,[27] and one autopsy series[28] have examined the impact of operative timing on postoperative outcome in hip fracture. The results of these 12 studies suggest that early surgical repair (within 24–48 h) is associated with lower mortality rates at 1 year. However, the majority of these studies did not adjust for the presence and severity of comorbid illness, preoperative functional status, or other physiologic parameters. Additionally, many of the studies excluded patients with complicating medical conditions. Of the 6 studies that did attempt to control for comorbidities,[20,23,25–27] 4 revealed lower mortality rates, 1 revealed shorter length of hospital stay, and 1 reported a lower incidence of confusion and pressure ulcers in patients who underwent surgical repair within 48 h.

In summary, there is evidence from case series that for patients who are medically stable without active comorbid illness (e.g., active heart failure), surgical repair of hip fracture within the first 24 to 48 h of admission is associated with a lower 1-year mortality as compared to patients whose surgery is delayed. Patients who would benefit from delay and further medical evaluation have not been well characterized. Until further data are available, it seems reasonable to attempt surgical repair for the majority of patients with hip fracture within 24 to 48 h of admission to the hospital. Patients with active comorbid medical illness such as congestive heart failure, active infection (e.g., pneumonia), unstable angina, or severe chronic obstructive pulmonary disease probably would benefit from a more extensive preoperative evaluation and medical management of their comorbid condition before repair of their fracture.

Prophylactic Antibiotics

Antibiotic prophylaxis has become the standard of care for major surgical operations to prevent postoperative wound complications. In hip fracture, the timing of administration, the duration of antibiotic therapy, and the effectiveness of antibiotic prophylaxis has been the subject of some debate in the literature.

A recent Cochrane Collaboration Review[29] identified 21 studies that addressed the issue of prophylactic antibiotics in hip fracture. Overall, the quality of the studies was poor to moderate. Although the regimens of antibiotic prophylaxis differed in most of the studies, all reported trials employed agents likely to be widely effective at the time the study was performed against *Staphylococus aureus*, the principal organism implicated in postoperative wound infections. Pooled data from six trials that examined a single preoperative dose of parenteral antibiotics versus placebo or no treatment found reductions in the incidence of deep wound infection (odds ratio, 0.42; 95% CI, 0.26, 0.68), of superficial wound infections (odds ratio, 0.67; 95% CI, 0.47, 0.94), of respiratory infections (odds ratio, 0.42; 95% CI, 0.29, 0.61), and of urinary tract infections (odds ratio, 0.51; 95% CI, 0.39, 0.66). Pooled data from 10 trials that examined the effect of a single preoperative dose and two or more postoperative doses compared to placebo or no treatment revealed similar risk reductions.

Five trials have compared single doses of antibiotics to multiple dose regimens. Pooled data from two trials that compared a single dose of a short-acting parenteral antibiotic with multiple doses of the same antibiotic suggest that a single dose of a short-acting antibiotic is significantly less effective in preventing deep wound, superficial wound, and urinary tract infections as compared to a multiple dose regimen. Three additional trials compared a single dose of a parenteral antibiotic with a long half-life to multiple doses of another agent with a short half-life. Pooled data from these trials revealed no difference in deep wound infections, superficial wound infections, urinary tract infections, or respiratory infections.

The timing of administration of antibiotic prophylaxis has not been well studied. A recent review of the literature[30] found only one study[31] that examined this topic, and this was a cohort study of 2847 elective surgical procedures. In this study, patients administered their first dose of antibiotics less than 2h before surgery had the lowest incidence of postoperative infections as compared to those receiving antibiotics within 3h following surgery (odds ratio, 2.4; 95% CI, 0.9–7.9), 3 to 24h following surgery (odds ratio, 5.8; 95% CI, 2.6–12.3), or more than 2h before surgery (odds ratio, 6.7; 95% CI, 2.9–14.7). These data, in combination with those data described earlier, suggest that the minimum inhibitory concentration of the antibiotic in the tissues must be exceeded for at least the period from incision to wound healing to minimize the risk of postoperative infection.

In summary, the available evidence support the use of a single dose of an intravenous antibiotic with a long half-life to reduce the incidence of deep wound infection, superficial wound infection, urinary tract infections, and respiratory tract infections. Furthermore, economic cost data from two studies[32,33] suggest that antibiotic prophylaxis is cost-effective, with a conservative estimate of cost savings of about $500 per patient given prophylaxis. Given that the major pathogen appears to be *S. aureus*, we recommend administration of a first-generation cephalosporin (e.g., Cefazolin 1–2g intravenously). For patients allergic to penicillins and cephalosporins and for patients admitted to hospitals in which methicillin-resistant *S. aureus* and *Staphylococcus epidermis* are frequent causes of postoperative wound infections, vancomycin is probably the most appropriate prophylactic agent (1g intravenously).[34] Based upon one large cohort study,[31] prophylactic antibiotic therapy should probably be initiated within 2h before surgery and continued for 24h following surgery.

Thromboembolic Prophylaxis

Venous thromboembolism is an important cause of morbidity and mortality in postoperative hip fracture patients. Although thromboembolic prophylaxis is becoming a routine aspect of the care of the patient with hip fracture, a number of questions remain as to the choice of the optimal agent, the timing of prophylaxis, and the duration of prophylaxis after fracture repair. Studies to date have focused on four classes of agents—heparanoids, antiplatelet agents, warfarin sodium, and dextran—and on the use of compression stockings.

Three meta-analyses[35–37] have included hip fracture patients and an additional 11 randomized controlled trials have examined prophylactic antithromboembolic agents in hip fracture.[38–48] There is strong support for the use of prophylactic antithromboembolics based upon the studies reviewed, although the choice of the optimal agent is less clear. Low-dose heparin (5000 international units given subcutaneously twice a day) has been the agent most frequently studied in hip fracture and has been associated with about a 60% reduction in deep venous thromboses by one meta-analysis.[35] Low molecular weight heparin has also been evaluated by meta-analysis and shown to lead to a similar reduction in deep venous thrombosis.[36] This latter meta-analysis also pooled data from four studies that compared low molecular weight heparin to low-dose heparin and found no significant differences between the two agents in the development of deep venous thrombosis. It has been reported recently that low molecular weight heparins, when used concurrently with spinal or epidural anesthesia, may cause bleeding or hematomas within the spinal column.[49] In the trials to date that have involved low molecular weight heparin and hip fracture, there have not been any reported episodes of epidural bleeding. However, these trials were not powered to detect this uncommon complication in the subgroups receiving spinal or epidural anesthesia. Until more data are forthcoming, we believe that the current FDA recommendations, that patients receiving epidural or spinal anesthesia and receiving concurrent low molecular weight heparin be monitored frequently for signs and symptoms of neurologic impairment, are appropriate.[49] It should be noted that this recent FDA report only involved patients receiving low molecular weight heparin and should not deter prophylaxis with low-dose heparin where indicated. Low-dose heparin appears to increase the risk of major bleeding episodes by about 30% to 41% as compared to patients receiving placebo, but the actual percentage increase is small (overall rates, 3.5% in heparin groups as compared to 2.9% in placebo).[35]

The use of aspirin as prophylaxis has been examined in one meta-analysis of 10 orthopedic trauma trials, 9 of which included only hip fracture patients and 1 of which included hip and pelvic fracture patients.[37] Additionally, the efficacy of aspirin has been recently examined in a large randomized controlled trial that enrolled more than 13,000 hip fracture patients.[48] Aspirin has been found to significantly reduce the risk of deep venous thrombosis and pulmonary embolism by about one-third, with much of this benefit appearing to occur after the first postoperative week. Head-to-head comparisons of aspirin to other agents have been limited. In the one study where aspirin was compared to low molecular weight heparin in the prevention of deep venous thrombosis,[47] low molecular weight heparin was found to result in a relative risk reduction of 37% with no significant difference in bleeding complications as compared to aspirin.

A number of other prophylactic agents have been evaluated. Low-dose warfarin (1.5 times control) has been compared to placebo in two studies[38,39] and additionally to low molecular weight heparin[40] and to aspirin.[38] Warfarin significantly reduces the risk of thromboembolic disease as compared to placebo and aspirin, and the magnitude of risk reduction appears to be comparable to that of low-dose unfractionated heparin.[30] When compared directly to low molecular weight heparin, warfarin appears to be less effective (odds ratio, 0.27 for low molecular weight heparin). In summary, low-dose warfarin appears to be an effective agent for thromboembolic prophylaxis. It appears more effective than aspirin but is probably less effective than low molecular weight heparin. The required international normalized ratio (INR) monitoring required for appropriate treatment with warfarin to prevent either over- or underanticoagulation is a potential drawback. Conversely, it might be a better tolerated agent for patients wishing to avoid the discomfort of a twice-daily injection.

Dextran, although not widely employed in the United States, has been perhaps the most extensively studied prophylactic agent after heparin. Five trials have examined the use of dextran, with somewhat conflicting results.[40–44] Dextran clearly appears to be more efficacious than placebo [odds ratio, 0.09 ($p < 0.05$)][41] and appears to be as effective as aspirin [odds ratio, 0.56 ($p > 0.05$)].[41,43] Two studies that compared dextran to low-dose unfractionated heparin observed no significant differences between the two groups in the development of thromboembolic complications.[41,42] However, both these studies were quite small, and it is questionable whether they had

adequate power to detect a true difference. In contrast, two larger studies that compared dextran to low molecular weight heparin observed a significant reduction in thromboembolic events in the heparin groups [odds ratios, 0.25 ($p < 0.001$) and 0.49 ($p < 0.005$)] as compared to the dextran groups.[44,45] In summary, dextran appears to provide protection against the development of thromboembolic events at a level comparable to aspirin. It is probably less efficacious, however, than warfarin or heparin. The potential for dextran administration to cause volume overload resulting in congestive heart failure or renal insufficiency, and the small risk of anaphylaxis associated with this agent argues against its routine use in the geriatric population, particularly given the availability of equally or more efficacious agents. Typically, dextran is administered as a 10% solution in 500 to 1000 mL normal saline per day.

Pneumatic sequential leg compression devices have been shown to decrease the incidence of postoperative deep vein thrombosis in urologic, neurosurgical, and general surgical patients.[50] Compression stockings have also been recently evaluated in patients with hip fracture and have been shown to significantly reduce the incidence of thromboembolic events as compared to no treatment.[46] Given these data, we recommend the routine use of intermittent pneumatic compression devices until the patient is ambulating on a routine basis.

When to begin and how long to continue anticoagulation therapy following fracture is currently not known, and there are no data available with respect to hip fracture that address this issue. Most of the studies have begun anticoagulant therapy on admission, although this has not been studied in a systematic manner. Two autopsy series involving hip fracture patients suggest a role for continuing prophylaxis following hospitalization. In a group of patients who did not receive any form of prophylaxis, the rate of fatal pulmonary embolism declined from 1% at 30 days to 0.4% at 60 days and 0.2% at 90 days.[51] Conversely, in a second autopsy series of patients, all of whom received prophylactic thromboembolic agents, the majority of fatal pulmonary embolisms were observed 30 days or more following fracture repair.[52] The results of these two studies suggest that prolonged prophylaxis might be helpful in some patients, although which patients and for how long need to be empirically studied. At present, it seems reasonable to begin anticoagulation on admission and continue prophylaxis until the patient is fully ambulatory and to extend prophylaxis further in patients in whom the risk of deep venous thrombosis may be increased (patients who experienced prolonged immobility postrepair or patients in whom surgery was delayed).

In summary, there is strong evidence supporting the use of either low-dose heparin or low molecular weight heparin as prophylaxis for deep venous thrombosis. The latter may be slightly more effective but is more expensive and has been associated with bleeding or hemorrhage in the spinal cord following epidural anesthesia in nonhip fracture populations. For these reasons, and until further data are available, low-dose heparin is probably the preferred agent. Aspirin also appears to have some benefit but to a lesser extent and may be considered in patients at high risk for hemorrhagic complications. Several studies support the use of low-dose warfarin; however, the required INR monitoring and risk of over- or underanticoagulation are potential drawbacks. Some patients, however, might strongly prefer weekly INR monitoring to the twice-daily injections required for heparin or low molecular weight heparin. Compression stockings appear to impart benefit with negligible risk and should be utilized. No data are yet available as to the timing of prophylactic thromboembolics and the optimal duration of therapy.

Nutritional Management

Malnutrition has been associated with increased surgical morbidity and mortality,[53,54] increased hospital length of stay,[54] and poorer functional outcomes.[54] It has been reported that as many as 20% of patients experiencing a hip fracture suffer from severe malnutrition.[55] Interventions to improve nutritional status might therefore improve outcomes and decrease complications.

To date, there have been five randomized controlled trials of nutritional supplementation in patients undergoing surgery for hip fracture. Three of the studies examined oral protein supplementation[56–58] and two studies examined supplemental nasogastric tube feeding.[59,60] All the studies suggest that oral protein supplementation can improve outcomes following fracture.

Stableforth[58] compared hip fracture patients randomized to protein supplementation versus usual care and reported significantly improved nitrogen and calorie balance in the supplemented group. Delmi and colleagues[57] and Tkatch and colleagues[56] randomized hip fracture patients to receive either protein supplementation or usual care[57] or placebo.[58] Patients receiving protein supplementation were found to have significantly fewer complications at 6 months, significantly higher albumin levels, and significantly shorter overall lengths of stay than nonsupplemented subjects.

Bastow and colleagues[59] examined the effect of nocturnal nasogastric tube feeding in 122 patients at increased risk for nutritional compromise (arm and trifold skin circumference less than 1 SD below the mean) for home and hospitalized elderly patients.[61] Patients were randomized to usual care or nocturnal tube feedings. There were no significant differences in mortality, although the study lacked statistical power to detect this difference. Very thin patients had a significant reduction in overall length of stay and had significant increases in weight (+4.2 kg;

$p < 0.01$)) as compared to controls. Tube-fed patients achieved independent mobility significantly faster than nontube-fed patients. One-fifth of patients could not tolerate the nocturnal feedings. Hartgrink and colleagues[60] examined the effect of supplemental nocturnal tube feeding on the development of pressure ulcers, serum protein, and serum albumin. No significant differences were found in any of the three outcome measures, although only 26% percent of patients tolerated the tube feedings for the 2-week study period.

Oral protein supplementation appears to be beneficial in reducing minor postoperative complications, preserving body protein stores, and reducing overall length of stay. Patients with evidence of moderate to severe malnutrition may benefit from nocturnal enteral tube feeding if tolerated.

Urinary Tract Management

Urinary retention, incontinence, and urinary tract infections are commonly observed in postoperative hip fracture patients.[62] Because of the frequency of postoperative bladder problems, successful strategies to reduce voiding problems might lead to decreased morbidity. There have been two randomized controlled trials of urinary bladder management in patients undergoing orthopedic surgery.[63,64] One study examined patients with recently sustained hip fracture and the other examined patients undergoing hip or knee replacement.

Michelson and colleagues[64] randomized 100 patients with knee or hip replacement to removal of their indwelling urinary catheter immediately postoperatively or the morning following surgery. The group whose indwelling catheter was removed the morning after surgery had significantly lower rates of urinary retention. Skelly and colleagues[63] randomized 67 hip fracture patients to receive an indwelling catheter for 48h postoperatively, followed by intermittent straight catheterization or intermittent straight catheterization immediately postoperatively. Spontaneous voiding occurred significantly earlier in the intermittent catheterization group. There were no significant differences in the incidence of urinary tract infections in either of the two studies between control and intervention subjects.

Indwelling catheters should probably be removed within 24h of surgery and patients managed by intermittent straight catheterization. Evidence does not exist regarding the management of patients who continue to experience urinary retention following 48h of intermittent catheterization.

Delirium

Delirium, a transient global disorder of cognition and attention characterized by concurrent disorders of attention, perception, thinking, memory, psychomotor behavior, and the sleep–wake cycle,[65,66] may be the most frequent medical complication observed following hip fracture.[67] Delirium occurs in an estimated 11% to 30% of elderly general medical patients[68] and in 13% to 61% of patients with hip fracture.[69] The occurrence of delirium in hospitalized patients has been shown to increase length of stay, risk of complications, mortality, and institutionalization.[70-74] Further, the majority of patients who develop delirium have at least some persistent symptoms as much as 6 months later. In patients with hip fracture, delirium has been associated with poorer functioning in physical, cognitive, and affective domains 6 months postfracture and with slower rates of recovery.[75,76] In this section, we focus specifically on the problem of delirium following hip fracture. A more thorough review of delirium may be found in Chapter 76.

For this discussion, we focused on three types of investigations. First, we identified studies that employed multivariate methods to identify risk factors that, if modified, might prevent delirium; 15 studies met these criteria.[69,74,77-89] Second, because the treatment of the underlying etiology is a cornerstone of the management of delirium, we reviewed studies that systematically described the frequency of different etiologies for this syndrome. We found 4 cohort studies,[79,90,91] 1 of which involved exclusively hip fracture patients. Finally, we identified studies that focused on the prevention and management of delirium in hip fracture patients. We found 2 nonrandomized studies that examined supportive treatment of delirium.[92,93]

The findings with regards to baseline risk factors for delirium appear to be fairly consistent across most studies. Advanced age, history of cognitive impairment, greater illness severity, and history of alcohol use appear to place hospitalized medical and surgical patients at increased risk for the development of confusion. In the two studies of hip fracture patients, only age, dementia, and prefracture functional status predicted the development of delirium.[69,77] Precipitating risk factors have been more difficult to identify and, with few exceptions, a clear understanding of the iatrogenic conditions that place elderly patients at increased risk for delirium has yet to emerge. Although many risk factors have been proposed in the literature (e.g., metabolic disturbances, dehydration, alcohol withdrawal, urinary retention, changes in environment, psychosocial factors, and medications),[94] only a few factors have been consistently identified as precipitating factors in prospective trials, and even these relationships are not consistent across studies. One particularly noteworthy finding, however, has been that two recent studies[88,89] have suggested that untreated or undertreated postoperative pain places patients at increased risk for delirium and that, in this setting, opioid analgesic use does not increase the risk of delirium. No precipitating factors were identified in the two studies of hip fracture patients.[77,93]

Regarding the etiology of delirium, there have been three case series[79,90,91] that examined this issue in medical and surgical patients and one study that examined the etiology of delirium in hip fracture.[95] Delirium in hip fracture appears to result from different etiologies and appears to follow a different clinical course from that observed in the medically ill. Brauer and colleagues[95] found that in more than 60% of observed cases of delirium following hip fracture, the etiology could not be determined. In the majority of cases (74%), the delirium resolved or was nearly resolved at the time of hospital discharge without active intervention. These findings are in contrast to data in the medically ill that suggest that an etiology for delirium can be determined in the majority of circumstances, that delirium tends not to resolve spontaneously but improves only after therapeutic intervention.[72,74]

The management of delirium has been based largely on clinical experience because few systematic and controlled studies have been performed.[94] There have been two nonrandomized studies involving hip fracture patients. Williams and colleagues[92] conducted a time sequence trial using pre- and postoperative nursing interventions (e.g., environmental manipulation, reorientation, reassurance) in hip fracture patients. The incidence of delirium was 44% in the treatment group as compared to 52% in the control ($p < 0.02$). Gustafson and colleagues[93] compared 103 treatment subjects with 111 historical controls admitted 2 to 5 years before the intervention cohort. The intervention in this study consisted of pre- and postoperative geriatric assessments, oxygen therapy for hypoxia, early surgery (performed as soon as patients were medically stable), and aggressive treatment of perioperative blood pressure falls. The incidence of delirium was 61% in the historical controls and 48% in the treatment group ($p < 0.05$). Subjects in the treatment group were less likely to be confused for more than 7 days (9% versus 28%) and had a shorter length of stay (11.6 versus 17.4 days). The individual contributions of each of the various components of the intervention to the reduction in delirium are unknown.

In summary, although many cohort studies have examined the risk factors for developing delirium, most analyses have not specifically focused on hip fracture patients and many studies have lacked adequate statistical power. Nevertheless, the assembled studies indicate a number of recurring potentially modifiable risk factors for developing delirium including electrolyte and metabolic laboratory abnormalities, medications with psychoactive properties, and infection. Environmental manipulation and supportive reorientation appear to reduce the incidence of delirium and benefit the acutely delirious patient, although more research addressing the optimal symptomatic management is needed.

Rehabilitation

Rehabilitative services for hip fracture patients may include limb and joint mobilization and progressive exercises; physical and occupational therapy to regain mobility and independence in activities of daily living; physician oversight of the therapy; psychologic counseling; social work; restorative nursing services; and recreational services. For the purposes of this chapter, we focused on selected aspects of rehabilitation that are particularly salient to the primary care provider (e.g., internist, family practitioner, nurse practitioner), recognizing that rehabilitation is a shared responsibility with the surgeon who, depending on the fracture and type of surgery, may have specific recommendations about mobilization and weightbearing. Specifically, we address the value of (a) early mobilization, (b) intensified interdisciplinary rehabilitation approaches, and (c) intensity and frequency of therapy.

There have been a number of reports of programs that employed early mobilization or early weightbearing policies. From these reports, we excluded studies, primarily from the 1960s through 1970s, that reviewed the experience of "early weightbearing" initiated many days or weeks after the perioperative period and focused only on those studies that reported on early mobilization in the first 24 to 48 h. For this group of interventions, we identified one randomized trial[96] that included early mobilization as part of a larger program of accelerated rehabilitation; we also identified a large number of trials that employed early mobilization policies in the first 24 to 48 h for all subjects.[97–108] In the case of intensified interdisciplinary rehabilitation programs, we identified four randomized trials.[109–112] For the intensity and frequency of physical therapy, we identified two small randomized trials[102,112] and three cohort studies that attempted to control for potential confounding between patient characteristics and receipt of services.[8,26,113]

The one randomized trial that evaluated early mobilization (usually within 24 h of surgery) did so as part of a program that also included early discharge from the hospital and a comprehensive rehabilitation program during and after hospitalization.[96] Although that trial of 252 patients found no differences in physical independence of patients at 4 months, it showed that so-called accelerated rehabilitation could reduce health care costs. Other studies[97–108] have shown that policies on early mobilization from the first postoperative day can be implemented without an increased risk of surgical complications,[97–99] change in discharge destination,[97,101] poorer functional outcomes,[97,100,102] and increased mortality.[99,101]

There have been four, relatively small, randomized trials that evaluated the benefits of geriatric interdisciplinary rehabilitation.[109–112] Two of the studies found no differences in functional outcomes,[112] mortality, or placement.[110] Two studies, however, found positive effects associated with these programs. Kennie and colleagues,[109] in a study of 112 patients, reported improved functional status and found that patients were more likely to be discharged to their own home than to a nursing home following interdisciplinary rehabilitation. Additionally, a randomized trial of geriatric assessment and rehabilitation in which hip fracture was the most common diagnosis (occurring in 18% of the patients) found that geriatric rehabilitation improved the chances of returning to the community.[111]

Two randomized trials have evaluated intensified physical therapy (e.g., therapy sessions twice rather than once a day or supplemental individualized educational sessions).[102,112] Both trials failed to show any benefit in functional outcomes; however, they were both quite small. For that reason, we sought additional evidence of efficacy from cohort studies that attempted to control for potential confounding between patient characteristics and receipt of services. In a cohort study of 162 hospitalized patients, Guccione and colleagues[113] found that more than one physical therapy session per day was associated with improved functional outcome after adjusting for age, prefracture ambulation, and length of stay. In another study of 536 patients, Magaziner and colleagues[8] reported that the number of physical therapy sessions (after adjustment for prefracture and other hospital care variables) was associated with improved physical independence at 1 year but did not affect walking ability or ability to perform instrumental activities of daily living. Finally, in a multisite study involving 284 acute care hospitals in five states, Hoenig and colleagues[26] found that more than five physical therapy/occupational therapy (PT/OT) sessions per week was associated with earlier ambulation [odds ratio (OR), 1.76; 95% confidence limits (CL), 1.50, 2.07), and patients who ambulated earlier had shorter lengths of stay (6.5 fewer days; $p < 0.001$) were more likely to return to the community (OR, 1.45; 95% CL, 1.16, 1.81) and had better than a 6-month survival (OR, 2.8; 95% CL, 2.06, 3.88).

In summary, the available data suggest that early mobilization can be done safely in selected patients, although the potential benefits of early mobilization have not been well studied and quantified. In the case of interdisciplinary rehabilitation featuring geriatric assessment, there is some suggestion from randomized trials that these programs can improve functional outcome and increase the likelihood of patients returning to the community. These trials, however, have been small and limited to programs with personnel with special interests in orthogeriatrics. For physical therapy services, cohort studies that have adjusted for potential confounders suggest that the frequency of physical therapy is likely to have an important impact on outcome and that more than one session per day is probably beneficial.

Falls Assessment

Patients who have fractured a hip have an increased risk of a subsequent fracture.[114] Interventions to reduce the likelihood and number of subsequent falls might therefore have beneficial effects on outcome. A comprehensive review of fall assessment and prevention may be found in Chapter 66.

To date, there have been a number of randomized controlled trials[115-121] and one preplanned meta-analysis[122] of clinical and social interventions to reduce falls. None of the studies were specifically targeted to hip fracture patients. Two of the six studies[116,117] focused on patients at risk for falling on the basis of other factors. Four studies[115,119-121] focused on older persons in the community who were otherwise unscreened for fall risk, and one study focused on frail nursing home residents.[118] The meta-analysis[122] included eight trials, two of which are cited above,[116,118] and examined the impact of exercise and balance on fall prevention.

The five studies[115,118-121] that focused on subjects previously unscreened for fall risk randomly assigned either nursing home residents,[118] senior centers, or households to interventions that included low-intensity exercises, counseling on risk factor reduction, and efforts to identify and correct environmental hazards. Two of the studies[115,119] showed that the intervention slightly reduced the risk of falling (but not that of fractures or falls requiring medical attention). The interventions that targeted older persons at risk of falling were more efficacious. Rubenstein and colleagues[117] randomly assigned ambulatory nursing home residents to either usual care or detailed clinical and environmental assessments within a week of the fall. The intervention did not significantly reduce the risk of subsequent falls, but the intervention group was hospitalized less frequently over the next 2 years. Tinetti and colleagues[116] identified community-dwelling older persons with specific risk factors (e.g., postural hypotension or difficulty in transferring) for falling and randomly assigned them to either social visits or a targeted multifactorial intervention that featured medication adjustment, behavioral instruction, and exercise activities targeted to the patient's risk factors. This intervention reduced the risk of falling (relative risk = 0.69) and the prevalence of targeted risk factors. Province and colleagues[122] performed a meta-analysis of eight trials involving diverse patient populations and several different interventions, all of which, however, included an exercise component. These eight trials demonstrated an adjusted fall incidence rate of 0.90 (95% confidence limits, 0.81–0.99). An adjusted fall incidence rate of 0.83 (95% confidence limits, 0.70–0.98) was observed for treatment groups that included balance training as compared to controls. No specific exercise component was significant for injurious falls, but the studies did not have adequate power to detect this outcome.

These studies suggest that interventions to reduce the incidence of falls are more likely to be beneficial if they focus on persons at risk for falls and if the interventions target specific risk factors or behaviors. Exercise and balance training also appear to be somewhat effective in decreasing fall risk. Because persons who have sustained hip fractures are at higher risk of subsequent falls, these findings may be generalizable to this population.

Conclusion

Hip fracture is a common disorder that results in death or significant loss of function for more than 150,000 Americans annually. Furthermore, the number of hip fractures occurring annually in this country is expected to double by the year 2040.[6,123] Clinical outcomes of hip fracture patients should be improvable by evidence-based medical care. This chapter has identified processes of medical care for which the data are unambiguous (e.g., prophylactic antibiotics and antithrombotics) and others for which the data are less clear and for which more research is needed (e.g., management of delirium, prevention of falls, duration of prophylactic thromboembolics, and cost-effectiveness of low molecular weight heparin as compared to other agents). The recommendations proposed in this chapter should enhance our ability to predict and manage the common complications of hip fracture, improve function and quality of life, and improve the quality of medical care afforded these patients.

References

1. Barrett-Connor E. The economic and human cost of osteoporotic fracture. *Am J Med.* 1995;98:3S–8S.
2. Schneider IL, Guralnik JM. The aging of America: impact on health care costs. *JAMA.* 990;263:2335–2340.
3. *Vital and Health Statistics. Healthy People 2000 Review.* Bethesda: National Center for Health Statistics; 1997.
4. Hedlund R. Lindgren U. Trauma type, age, and gender as determinants of hip fracture. *J Orthop Res.* 1987;5(2):242–246.
5. Gallagher JC, Melton LJ, Riggs BL, Bergstrath E. Epidemiology of fractures of the proximal femur in Rochester, Minnesota. *Clin Orthop.* 1980(150):163–171.
6. Cummings S, Kelsey J, Nevitt M, O'Dowd K. Epidemiology of osteoporosis and osteoporotic fractures. *Epidemiol Rev.* 1985;7:178–208.
7. Lu-Yao G, Baron J, Barrett J, Fischer E. Treatment and survival among elderly Americans with hip fractures: a population-based study. *Am J Public Health.* 1994;84: 1287–1291.
8. Magaziner J, Simonsick E, Kashner M, Hebel J, Kenzora J. Predictors of functional recovery one year following

hospital discharge for hip fracture: a prospective study. *J Gerontol.* 1990;45:M101–M107.

9. Ray NF, Chan JK, Thamer M, Melton LJ III. Medical expenditures for the treatment of osteoporotic fractures in the United States in 1995: report from the National Osteoporosis Foundation. *J Bone Miner Res.* 1997;12(1): 24–35.

10. Brainsky A, Glick H, Lydick F, et al. The economic cost of hip fractures in community-dwelling older adults: a prospective study [see comments]. *J Am Geriatr Soc.* 1997; 45(3):281–287.

11. Office of Technology Assessment. Hip Fracture Outcomes in People Aged 50 and Over: Mortality, Service Use, Expenditures, and Long-Term Functional Impairment. Washington, DC: U.S. Government Printing Office; 1993.

12. Chrischilles E, Shireman T, Wallace R. Costs and health effects of osteoporotic fractures. *Bone.* 1994:15(4):377–386.

13. Zuckerman J. Hip fracture. *N Engl J Med.* 1996;334:1519–1525.

14. Zuckerman JD, Schon LC. Hip fractures. In: Zuckerman JD, ed. *Comprehensive Care of Orthopaedic Injuries in the Elderly.* Baltimore: Urban & Schwarzenberg; 1990. pp. 23–111.

15. Morrison RS, Siu AL. Survival in end-stage dementia following acute illness. *JAMA.* 2000;284(1):47–52.

16. Morrison RS, Siu AL. A comparison of pain and its treatment in advanced dementia and cognitively intact patients with hip fracture. *J Pain Symptom Manag.* 2000;19:240–248.

17. Parker M, Pryor G. The timing of surgery for proximal femoral fractures. *J Bone Joint Surg.* 1992;74B:203–205.

18. Dolk T. Operation in hip fracture patients—analysis of the time factor. *Injury.* 1990;21(6):369–372.

19. Villar R, Allen S, Barnes S. Hip fractures in healthy patients: operative delay versus prognosis. *Br Med J.* 1986;293:1203–1204.

20. Bredhal C, Nyholm B, Hindsholm K, Mortensen J, Olesen A. Mortality after hip fracture: results of operation within 12 hours of admission. *Injury.* 1992;23:83–86.

21. Holmberg S, Kalen R, Thorngren KG. Treatment and outcome of femoral neck fractures. An analysis of 2418 patients admitted from their own homes. *Clin Orthop.* 1987;218:42–52.

22. Kenzora J, McCarthy R, Lowell J, Sledge C. Hip fracture mortality, relation to age, treatment, preoperative illness, time of surgery, and complications. *Clin Orthop Relat Res.* 1984;186:45–46.

23. Rogers F, Shackford S. Keller M. Early fixation reduces morbidity and mortality in elderly patients with hip fractures from low impact falls. *J Trauma Inj Infect Crit Care.* 1995;39:261–265.

24. Todd CJ, Freeman CJ, Camilleri Ferrante C, et al. Differences in mortality after fracture of hip: the east Anglian audit. *Br Med J.* 1995;310(6984):904–908.

25. Zuckerman J, Skovoron M, Koval K, Aharonoff G, Frankel V. Postoperative complications and mortality associated with operative delay in older patients who have a fracture of the hip. *J Bone Joint Surg.* 1995;77A:1551–1556.

26. Hoenig H, Rubenstein L, Sloane R, Horner K, Kahn K. What is the role of timing in the surgical and rehabilitative care of community-dwelling older persons with hip fracture. *Arch Intern Med.* 1997;157:513–520.

27. Davis FM, Woolner DF, Frampton C, et al. Prospective, multi-centre trial of mortality following general or spinal anaesthesia for hip fracture surgery in the elderly. *Br J Anaesth.* 1987;59(9):1080–1088.

28. Perez J, Warwick D, Case C, Bannister G. Death after proximal femoral fracture—an autopsy study. *Injury.* 1995;26:237–240.

29. Handoll HHG, Farrar MJ, McBirnie J, et al. Heparin, low molecular weight heparin and physical methods for preventing deep vein thrombosis and pulmonary embolism following surgery for hip fractures. Cochrane Review. *The Cochrane Library*, 4th Ed. Oxford: Update Software; 2000.

30. Morrison R, Chassin M, Siu A. The medical consultant's role in caring for patients with hip fracture. *Ann Intern Med.* 1998;128:1010–1020.

31. Classen DC, Evans KS, Pestotnik SL, Horn SD, Menlove KL, Burke JP. The timing of prophylactic administration of antibiotics and the risk of surgical-wound infection. *N Engl J Med.* 1992;326(5):281–286.

32. Boxma H, Broekhuizen T, Patka P, Oosting H. Randomised controlled trial of single dose antibiotic prophylaxis in surgical treatment of closed fractures. *Lancet.* 1996;347:1133–1137.

33. Albers B, Patka P, Haarman H, Kostense P. Kosteneffektivat einer antibiotikaprophylaxe bei senkung des infectionsrisikos um 0.25% [Cost effectiveness of antibiotic prophylaxis for closed fractures]. *Unfallchirurg.* 1994;97: 625–628.

34. Abramowicz M, ed. *Handbook of Antimicrobial Therapy.* New Rochelle: Medical Letter; 1998.

35. Collins R, Scrimgeour A, Yusuf S, Peto R. Reduction in fatal pulmonary embolism and venous thrombosis by perioperative administration of subcutaneous heparin. *N Engl J Med.* 1988;318:1162–1173.

36. Lassen M, Borris L, Christiansen H, et al. Clinical trials with low molecular weight heparins in the prevention of postoperative thromboembolic complications: a meta-analysis. *Semin Thromb Hemost.* 1991;17:284–290.

37. Antiplatelet Trialists' Collaboration. Collaborative overview of randomised trials of antiplatelet therapy. III: Reduction in venous thrombosis and pulmonary embolism by antiplatelet prophylaxis among surgical and medical patients. *Br Med J.* 1994;308:235–246.

38. Powers P, Gent M, Jay R, et al. A randomized trial of less intense postoperative warfarin or aspirin therapy in the prevention of venous thromboembolism after surgery for fractured hip. *Arch Intern Med.* 1989;149:771–774.

39. Morris G, Mitchell J. Preventing venous thromboembolism in elderly patients with hip fractures: studies of low-dose heparin, dipyridamole, aspirin, and fluriprofen. *Br Med J.* 1977;1:535–537.

40. Gerhart TN, Yett HS, Robertson LK, Lee MA, Smith M, Salzman EW. Low-molecular-weight heparinoid compared with warfarin for prophylaxis of deep-vein thrombosis in patients who are operated on for fracture of the

hip. A prospective, randomized trial. *J Bone Joint Surg Am.* 1991;73(4):494–502.

41. Bergqvist D, Efsing H, Hallbook T, Hedlund T. Thromboembolism after elective and post-traumatic hip surgery—a controlled prophylactic trial with dextran 70 and low-dose heparin. *Acta Chir Scand.* 1979;145(4):213–218.

42. Pini M, Spadini E, Carluccio L, et al. Dextran/aspirin versus heparin/dihydroergotamine in preventing thrombosis after hip fracture. *J Bone Joint Surg.* 1985;76B:305–309.

43. Feldman D, Zuckerman J, Walters I, Sakales S. Clinical efficacy of aspirin and dextran for thromboprophylaxis in geriatric hip fracture patients. *J Orthop Trauma.* 1993;7:1–5.

44. Bergqvist D, Kettunen R, Fredin H, et al. Thromboprophylaxis in patients with hip fractures: a prospective, randomized, comparative study between Org 10172 and dextran 70. *Surgery.* 1991;109(5):617–622.

45. Oertli D, Hess P. Durig M, et al. Prevention of deep vein thrombosis in patients with hip fractures: LMWH versus dextran. *World J Surg.* 1992;16:980–984.

46. Fisher CG, Blachut PA, Salvian AJ, et al. Effectiveness of pneumatic leg compression devices for the prevention of thromboembolic disease in orthopaedic trauma patients: a prospective, randomized study of compression alone versus no prophylaxis. *J Orthop Trauma.* 1995;9(1):1–7.

47. Gent M, Hirsh J, Ginsberg JS, et al. Low-molecular-weight heparinoid orgaran is more effective than aspirin in the prevention of venous thromboembolism after surgery for hip fracture. *Circulation.* 1996;93(1):80–84.

48. Prevention of pulmonary embolism and deep vein thrombosis with low dose aspirin: Pulmonary Embolism Prevention (PEP) trial. *Lancet.* 2000;355(9212):1295–1302.

49. Nightingale SL. From the Food and Drug Administration. *JAMA.* 1998;279:346.

50. Coe NP, Collins RE, Klein LA, et al. Prevention of deep vein thrombosis in urological patients. A controlled, randomized trial of low-dose heparin and external pneumatic compression boots. *Surgery.* 1978;83:230–234.

51. Schroder HM, Andreassen M. Autopsy-verified major pulmonary embolism after hip fracture. *Clin Orthop.* 1989;293:196–203.

52. Bergqvist D, Fredin H. Pulmonary embolism and mortality in patients with fractured hips—a prospective consecutive series. *Eur J Surg.* 1991;157:571–574.

53. Patterson BM, Cornell CN, Carbone B, Levine B, Chapman D. Protein depletion and metabolic stress in elderly patients who have a fracture of the hip. *J Bone Joint Surg Am.* 1992;74(2):251–260.

54. Koval KJ, Maurer SG, Su ET, Aharonoff GB, Zuckerman JD. The effects of nutritional status on outcome after hip fracture. *J Orthop Trauma.* 1999;13(3):164–169.

55. Bastow M, Rawlings J, Allison S. Undernutrition, hypothermia, and injury in elderly women with fractured femur; an injury response to altered metabolism? *Lancet.* 1983;1983(i):143–146.

56. Tkatch L, Rapin CH, Rizzoli R, et al. Benefits of oral protein supplementation in elderly patients with fracture of the proximal femur. *J Am Coll Nutr.* 1992;11(5):519–525.

57. Delmi M, Rapin CH, Bengoa JM, Delmas PD, Vasey H, Bonjour JP. Dietary supplementation in elderly patients with fractured neck of the femur. *Lancet.* 1990;335(8696):1013–1016.

58. Stableforth PG. Supplement feeds and nitrogen and calorie balance following femoral neck fracture. *Br J Surg.* 1986;73(8):651–655.

59. Bastow MD, Rawlings J, Allison SP. Benefits of supplementary tube feeding after fractured neck of femur: a randomised controlled trial. *Br Med J Clin Res Ed.* 1983;287(6405):1589–1592.

60. Hartgrink HH, Wille J, Konig P, Hermans J, Breslau PJ. Pressure sores and tube feeding in patients with a fracture of the hip: a randomized clinical trial. *Clin Nutr.* 1998;17(6):287–292.

61. Vir S, Love A. Anthropometric measurements in the elderly. *Gerontology.* 1980;26:262–268.

62. Smith NK, Albazzaz MK. A prospective study of urinary retention and risk of death after proximal femoral fracture. *Age Ageing.* 1996;25(2):150–154.

63. Skelly JM, Guyatt GH, Kalbfleisch R, Singer J, Winter L. Management of urinary retention after surgical repair of hip fracture. *Can Med Assoc J.* 1992;146(7):1185–1189.

64. Michelson JD, Lotke PA, Steinberg ME. Urinary-bladder management after total joint-replacement surgery. *N Engl J Med.* 1988;319(6):321–326.

65. Lipowski Z. Delirium in the elderly patient. *N Engl J Med.* 1989;32:278–303.

66. Lipowski Z. Transient cognitive disorders (delirium, acute confusional states in the elderly). *Am J Psychiatry.* 1983;140:1426–1436.

67. Gillick M, Serell N, Gillick L. Adverse consequences of hospitalization in the elderly. *Soc Sci Med.* 1982;16:1033–1038.

68. Rummans T, Evans J, Krahn L, et al. Delirium in elderly patients: evaluation and management. *Mayo Clin Proc.* 1995;70:988–989.

69. Gustafson Y, Berggren D, Brannstrom B, et al. Acute confusional states in elderly patients treated for femoral neck fracture. *J Am Geriatr Soc.* 1988;36(6):525–530.

70. Cole M, Primeau F, McCusker J. Effectiveness of interventions to prevent delirium in hospitalized patients: a systematic review. *Can Med Assoc J.* 1996;155:1263–1268.

71. Francis J, Kapoor WN. Prognosis after hospital discharge of older medical patients with delirium. *J Am Geriatr Soc.* 1992;40(6):601–606.

72. Levkoff S, Evans D, Liptzin B, et al. Delirium: the occurrence and persistence of symptoms among elderly hospitalized patients. *Arch Intern Med.* 1992;152:334–340.

73. Murray AM, Levkoff SE, Wetle TT, et al. Acute delirium and functional decline in the hospitalized elderly patient. *J Gerontol.* 1993;48(5):M181–M186.

74. Rockwood K. Delays in the discharge of elderly patients. *J Clin Epidemiol.* 1990;43:971–975.

75. Dolan MM, Hawkes WG, Zimmerman SI, et al. Delirium on hospital admission in aged hip fracture patients: prediction of mortality and 2-year functional outcomes. *J Gerontol A Biol Sci Med Sci.* 2000;55(9):M527–M534.

76. Marcantonio ER, Flacker JM, Michaels M, Resnick NM. Delirium is independently associated with poor functional

recovery after hip fracture. *J Am Geriatr Soc.* 2000;48(6): 618–624.

77. Williams M, Campbell E, Kaynor W, Musholt M, Mlynarczyk S, Crane L. Predictors of acute confusional states in elderly persons. *Res Nurs Health.* 1985;8:31–40.

78. Foreman M. Confusion in the hospitalized elderly. *Res Nurs Health.* 1989;12:21–29.

79. Francis J, Martin D, Kapoor WN. A prospective study of delirium in hospitalized elderly. *JAMA.* 1990;263(8):1097–1101.

80. Inouye SK, Charpentier PA. Precipitating factors for delirium in hospitalized elderly persons. Predictive model and interrelationship with baseline vulnerability. *JAMA.* 1996; 275(11):852–857.

81. Inouye S, Viscoli C, Horwitz R, Hurst L, Tinetti M. A predictive model for delirium in hospitalized elderly medical patients based on admission characteristics. *Ann Intern Med.* 1993;119:474–481.

82. Jitapunkul S, Pillay I, Ebrahim S. Delirium in newly admitted elderly patients: a prospective study. *Q J Med.* 1992;300:307–314.

83. Marcantonio E, Goldman L, Mangione C, et al. A clinical prediction rule for delirium after elective noncardiac surgery. *JAMA.* 1994;271(2):134–139.

84. Rogers M, Liang M, Daltroy L. Delirium after elective orthopedic surgery: risk factors and natural history. *Int J Psychiatry Med.* 1989;19(2):109–121.

85. Schor JD, Levkoff SE, Lipsitz LA, et al. Risk factors for delirium in hospitalized elderly. *JAMA.* 1992;267(6):827–831.

86. Pompei P, Foreman M, Rudberg M, Inouye S, Braund V, Cassel C. Delirium in hospitalized older persons: outcomes and predictors. *J Am Geriatr Soc.* 1994;42:809–815.

87. Williams Russo P, Urquhart BL, Sharrock NE, Charlson ME. Post-operative delirium: predictors and prognosis in elderly orthopedic patients. *J Am Geriatr Soc.* 1992;40(8): 759–767.

88. Duggleby W, Lander J. Cognitive status and postoperative pain: older adults. *J Pain Symptom Manag.* 1994;9:19–27.

89. Lynch EP, Lazor MA, Gellis JE, Orav J, Goldman L, Marcantonio ER. The impact of postoperative pain on the development of postoperative delirium. *Anesth Analg.* 1998;86:781–785.

90. Moses HD, Kaden I. Neurologic consultations in a general hospital. Spectrum of iatrogenic disease. *Am J Med.* 1986; 81(6):955–958.

91. Purdie FR, Honigman B, Rosen P. Acute organic brain syndrome: a review of 100 cases. *Ann Emerg Med.* 1981; 10(9):455–461.

92. Williams M, Campbell E, Raynor V, Mlynarczyk S, Ward S. Reducing acute confusional states in elderly patients with hip fractures. *Res Nurs Health.* 1985;8:329–337.

93. Gustafson Y, Brannstrom B, Berggren D, et al. A geriatric-anesthesiologic program to reduce acute confusional states in elderly patients treated for femoral neck fractures. *J Am Geriatr Soc.* 1991;39(7):655–662.

94. Francis J. Delirium in older patients. *J Am Geriatr Soc.* 1992;40:829–838.

95. Brauer C, Morrison RS, Silberzweig SB, Siu AL. The cause of delirium in patients with hip fracture. *Arch Intern Med.* 2000;160(12):1856–1860.

96. Cameron ID, Lyle DM, Quine S. Cost-effectiveness of accelerated rehabilitation after proximal femoral fracture. *J Clin Epidemiol.* 1994;47(11):1307–1313.

97. Zuckerman J, Sakales S, Fabian D, Frankel V. Hip fractures in geriatric patients: results of an interdisciplinary hospital care program. *Clin Orthop.* 1992;274:213–225.

98. Stromqvist B, Hansson LI, Nilsson LT, Thorngren KG. Hook-pin fixation in femoral neck fractures. A two-year follow-up study of 300 cases. *Clin Orthop.* 1987;218: 58–62.

99. Arnold WD. The effect of early weight-bearing on the stability of femoral neck fractures treated with Knowles pins. *J Bone Joint Surg Am.* 1984;66(6):847–852.

100. Jarnlo GB. Hip fracture patients. Background factors and function. *Scand J Rehabil Med Suppl.* 1991;24:1–31.

101. Ceder L, Stromqvist B, Hansson LI. Effects of strategy changes in the treatment of femoral neck fractures during a 17-year period. *Clin Orthop.* 1987;218:53–57.

102. Karuumo I. Intensive physical therapy after fractures of the femoral shaft. *Ann Chir Gynaecol.* 1977;66(6):278–283.

103. Skinner P, Riley D, Ellergy J, Beaumont A. Displaced subcapital fractures of the femur: a prospective randomized comparison of internal fixation, hemiarthroplasty and total hip replacement. *Injury.* 1989;20:291–293.

104. Sorenson J, Varmarken J, Bomler J. Internal fixation of femoral neck fractures. Dynamic hip and Gouffon screws compared in 73 patients. *Acta Orthop Scand.* 1992;63:288–292.

105. Elmerson S, Andersson G, Irstam L, et al. Internal fixation of femoral neck fracture. No difference between Rydell four-flanged nail and Gouffon's pin. *Acta Orthop Scand.* 1988;59:372–376.

106. Olerud C, Rehnberg L, Hellquist E. Internal fixation of femoral neck fractures. Two methods compared. *J Bone Joint Surg Br.* 1991;73:16–19.

107. Nungu S, Olerud C, Rehnberg L. Treatment of intertrochanteric fractures: comparison of ender nails and sliding screw plates. *J Orthop Trauma.* 1991;5:452–457.

108. Dalen N, Jacobsson B, Eriksson P. A comparison of nail-plate fixation and enders nailing in pertrochanteric fractures. *J Trauma.* 1988;28:405–406.

109. Kennie D, Reid J, Richardson I, Kiamari A, Kelt C. Effectiveness of geriatric rehabilitative care after fractures of the proximal femur in elderly women: a randomised clinical trial. *Br Med J.* 1988;297:1083–1086.

110. Gilchrist W, Newman R, Hamblen D, Williams B. Prospective randomised study of an orthopaedic geriatric inpatient service. *Br Med J.* 1988;297:1116–1118.

111. Applegate WB, Miller ST, Graney MJ, Elam JT, Burns R, Akins DE. A randomized, controlled trial of a geriatric assessment unit in a community rehabilitation hospital. *N Engl J Med.* 1990;322(22):1572–1578.

112. Jette AM, Harris BA, Cleary PD, Campion EW. Functional recovery after hip fracture. *Arch Phys Med Rehabil.* 1987; 68(10):735–740.

113. Guccione AA, Fagerson TL, Anderson JJ. Regaining functional independence in the acute care setting following hip fracture. *Phys Ther.* 1996;76(8):818–826.

114. Finsen V, Benum P. The second hip fracture: an epidemiologic study. *Acta Orthop Scand.* 1986;57:431–433.

115. Wagner EH, LaCroix AZ, Grothaus L, et al. Preventing disability and falls in older adults: a population-based randomized trial. *Am J Public Health.* 1994;84(11):1800–1816.

116. Tinetti M, Baker D, McAvay G, et al. A multifactorial intervention to reduce the risk of falling among elderly people living in the community. *N Engl J Med.* 1994;331:315–320.

117. Rubenstein L, Robbins A, Josephson K, Schulman B, Osterweil D. The value of assessing falls in an elderly population. *Ann Intern Med.* 1990;113:308–316.

118. Mulrow CD, Gerety MB, Kanten D, et al. A randomized trial of physical rehabilitation for very frail nursing home residents [see comments]. *JAMA.* 1994;271(7):519–524.

119. Hornbrook M, Stevens V, Wingfield D, Hollis J, Greenlick M, Ory M. Preventing falls among community dwelling older persons: results from a randomized trial. *Gerontologist.* 1994;34:16–23.

120. Reinsch S, Macrae P, Lachenbruch P, Tobis J. Attempts to prevent falls and injury: a prospective community study. *Gerontologist.* 1992;32:450–456.

121. Vetter N, Lewis P, Ford D. Can health visitors prevent fractures in elderly people. *Br Med J.* 1992;304:888–890.

122. Province MA, Hadley EC, Hornbrook MC, et al. The effects of exercise on falls in elderly patients. A pre-planned meta-analysis of the FICSIT Trials: Frailty and Injuries: Cooperative Studies of Intervention Techniques. *JAMA.* 1995;273(17):1341–1347.

123. Cummings S, Rubin S, Black D. The future of hip fractures in the United States: number, costs, and potential effects of postmenopausal estrogen. *Clin Orthop.* 1990:252:163–166.

46
Treatment of Diabetes

Kenneth L. Minaker

Sites of Care

Care of the older diabetic patient, similar to the care of other complex geriatric patients, has become a multidisciplinary issue with very high stakes in terms of vascular, renal, and ocular disability. Recent studies have demonstrated the value of careful management on the improvement in patient outcomes, and large-scale studies are under way to deter or prevent the emergence of clinical disease.

Increasingly, the focus of care is planning a comprehensive, multidisciplinary treatment and assessment program designed to prevent end-organ injury and to intervene early in the course of illness. It is an encouraging time to be involved in the treatment of diabetic patients, particularly outpatients treated early in the course of their illness. Improved care of the vascular and renal complications in those with advanced disease has also produced promise for their higher quality of life.

Demographics, Epidemiology, and Risk Factors

Diabetes mellitus prevalence increases with age, and the numbers of older persons with diabetes are expected to grow as the elderly population increases in number[1-3] (Fig. 46.1). The National Health and Nutrition Examination Survey (NHANES III) demonstrated that, in the population over 65 years old, almost 18% to 20% have diabetes. Of great diagnostic and clinical significance is that one-half of those with diabetes mellitus are not aware they have the disease. Other abnormalities in carbohydrate metabolism that have been observed include an additional 20% to 25% older patients meeting the criteria for impaired glucose tolerance. These unknown diabetic individuals and those potentially at risk were uncovered using glucose tolerance tests, which are very sensitive to abnormalities in carbohydrate economy. The incidence of

diabetes mellitus is approximately 2 per 1000 among those older than 45 and increases for those individuals more than 75 years old.[4] Prevalence is much higher in older Hispanics, African Americans, Native Americans (Indians), Scandinavians, Japanese, and Micronesians.

Individuals with diabetes mellitus who are older than 65 usually have noninsulin-dependent diabetes (NIDDM). Insulin-dependent diabetes mellitus (IDDM) accounts for only 5% to 10% newly diagnosed diabetes mellitus in late life.[5] In addition, a small proportion of older individuals who initially have NIDDM appear to become insulin dependent over time. A few clues as to who will require insulin exist. Ketosis at the time of diagnosis suggests that insulin therapy will be necessary. However, some elderly individuals with diabetes and ketosis can subsequently be treated with oral agents. The human leukocyte antigen (HLA)-DR3 serotype is more common in older adults who require insulin treatment. The frequency of antibodies to islet cells in older diabetic patients is not increased.[5]

Specific Clinical Patterns with Aging

A variety of metabolic, sensory, and cardiovascular conditions accompany the widespread prevalence of diabetes in the elderly and contribute to the reduced life expectancy that occurs with diabetes. Life expectancy reductions in diabetic individuals at ages 50 to 59 are 6 to 7 years, at ages 60 to 69 are 4 to 5 years, and at age 70 and above life expectancies are reduced by 3 years. In addition, the longer diabetes has been present, the greater the life expectancy reduction.

Hypertension occurs in 30% to 50% of those with diabetes in 45- to 64-year-olds but is present in 70% of diabetic patients aged 65 to 74. Diabetic ketoacidosis mortality is greater in individuals over age 75 (50 per 100,000 diabetic patients) than age 65 to 74 (20 per 100,000 diabetic patients). Hyperosmolar nonketotic

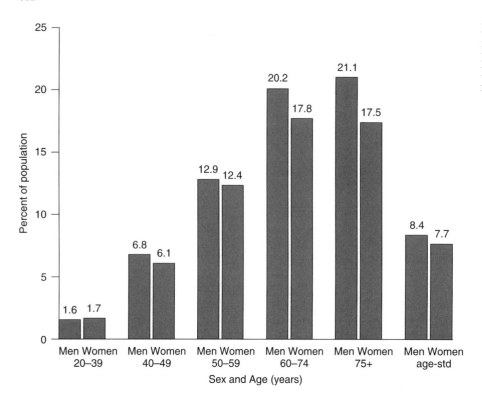

coma is essentially a disorder of the elderly diabetic.[6] Twenty-four percent of all cases of legal blindness occur in diabetic individuals over age 65 years. Peripheral neuropathy, the most common diabetic neuropathy, has a prevalence of 25% to 35% in diabetic patients between 65 and 74 years of age. Absent pulses are twice as frequent in diabetic versus nondiabetic individuals (20% versus 13%) in the age group 55 to 74 years. The risk of leg amputations is 15 to 40 times greater for a person with diabetes. Renal failure requiring dialysis occurs most often from the pool of patients with diabetes mellitus, and recent evidence suggests progression to renal failure is more rapid in older patients.

The incidence of stroke is almost twice as great in diabetic individuals at all ages. Stroke incidence increases with advancing age to incidence rates four times greater: the rate at age 45 to 49 is 30 per 1000 and at age 65 to 69 is 133 per 1000. Between the ages of 45 and 64, 8.4% of diabetic individuals have had a stroke, a prevalence that increases to 12.7% in individuals more than 65 years of age.[7] The incrementally greater impact of the number of risk factors for stroke in the elderly diabetic population has been studied in the Framingham Heart Study. With increasing numbers of risk factors, including hypertension, hypertension treatment, diabetes mellitus, cigarette smoking, preexisting heart disease, atrial fibrillation, and ECG changes compatible with left ventricular hypertrophy, 10-year stroke probability increases geometrically.[8]

Advancing age in diabetic individuals is associated with increasing prevalence of a host of gastrointestinal diseases including hiatus hernia, ulcers, and gallstones, trends that are more apparent in females than males with diabetes mellitus (NHANES II).

Infection rates, particularly urinary tract infections and viral pneumonia, are twice as frequent in diabetic individuals than nondiabetic individuals. Current evidence suggests no age-related increase in infection rates. Periodontal disease shows a linear increase with age in diabetic individuals.[9]

The overall impact of comorbid disease, being more prevalent in older diabetic individuals, is substantial. Although hospital discharges primarily for diabetes mellitus decrease with advancing age, those for associated diseases increase dramatically. Hospitalization rates are 40% to 80% higher in diabetic patients than nondiabetic patients depending on age.[10]

Advancing age is also associated with a progressive increase in length of hospital stay with diabetes mellitus.

Pathogenesis of Age-Associated Glucose Intolerance

Glucose intolerance associated with aging itself may predispose to the development of overt diabetes mellitus. Glucose intolerance is present even in very healthy older individuals. Postprandial blood glucose increases by

5.3 mg/dL per decade after the age of 30[11,12] (Fig. 46.2). Age-related changes in fasting blood glucose levels are 1 to 2 mg/dL (0.05–0.09 mM) per decade after age 30.[13,14]

Several factors appear to contribute to age-associated glucose homeostatic changes. Glucose absorption slows with increasing age, and hepatic glucose production shuts down after food and glucose is delayed, most likely as a result of delayed insulin secretion.[15] Subtle age-related changes in regulation of insulin secretion have been described.[16] The presence of insulin resistance in the elderly has been confirmed in multiple studies.[14,17,18] It is a result of postreceptor events, the specific site(s) of which are not yet understood.[19–21]

Other factors may contribute to glucose intolerance. Both the decline in lean body mass and the increase in body fat that accompany aging may contribute to insulin resistance.[22] Reduced levels of physical activity and altered diet may cause these changes in body composition.[23] Studies of master athletes suggest that some of these changes can be either prevented or modified with exercise.[24] High-carbohydrate, low-fat diets improve insulin sensitivity in older individuals.[25] Drugs commonly used by older individuals, including diuretics, tricyclic antidepressants, estrogen, sympathomimetics, glucocorticoids, niacin, and phenytoin may adversely affect glucose metabolism. Stress states such as myocardial infarction, infection, burns, and surgery may also worsen glucose tolerance.

Impaired glucose tolerance is a risk factor for the development of cardiovascular disease and diabetes mellitus. The Honolulu Heart Study demonstrated that fatal myocardial events among older nondiabetic men were 2.4 times higher in those in the highest quintile for 1 h postchallenge glucose levels than in those in the lowest quintile.[26] The risk of development of diabetes mellitus among those over age 70 who are glucose intolerant is 2% per year, as compared with a risk of 0.04% per year for those with normal glucose tolerance.[27]

The reduction in glucose tolerance associated with aging is correlated with insulin resistance, obesity, hyperlipidemia, and hypertension. The pathogenesis of these associated and interrelated conditions is referred to as the metabolic syndrome or syndrome X. Although the pathogenesis is currently under detailed study, the emergence of insulin resistance as a central feature of diabetes mellitus in the elderly appears secure.

Pathogenesis of Diabetes Mellitus in the Elderly

A strong genetic predisposition to type 2 diabetes in middle-aged and elderly patients exists. The specific genes responsible have not been discovered.[3] Patients with a family history of diabetes are more likely to develop the illness as they age.[4] Elderly patients with peripheral insulin resistance and reduced glucose-induced insulin release are more likely to develop type 2 diabetes than those without.[28] In elderly identical twins discordant for type 2 diabetes, subjects without diabetes have evidence of impaired glucose metabolism.[29] Physiologic and environmental factors compound genetic predisposition. Lower testosterone levels in men[30] and higher testosterone levels in women[31] are risk factors for diabetes development. Elderly individuals who have a high intake of fat and sugar and a low intake of complex carbohydrates are more likely to develop diabetes.[32–35] Physical inactivity and central fat distribution predispose to diabetes in the elderly.[36–46] Unlike younger patients, fasting hepatic glucose production is normal in elderly patients with type 2 diabetes.[47] Elderly type 2 diabetes patients have specific alterations in carbohydrate metabolism. The primary metabolic defect in lean elderly subjects is an impairment in glucose-induced insulin release; the primary abnormality in obese elderly subjects is resistance to insulin-mediated glucose disposal.[47,48]

Glucose uptake occurs by insulin-mediated and noninsulin-mediated mechanisms. Recently, it has been demonstrated that nonmediated glucose uptake (glucose effectiveness) is markedly impaired in elderly patients with type 2 diabetes. The mechanism for this defect is unclear, but impaired glucose effectiveness is a contributing factor to elevated glucose levels in elderly diabetes patients. Given that several interventions, including glucagon-like peptide 1 (GLP-1), have been shown to enhance glucose effectiveness in younger patients, these findings may have important therapeutic relevance for elderly patients with diabetes.[49–51]

Few studies have evaluated molecular biologic abnormalities in elderly patients with diabetes and more are

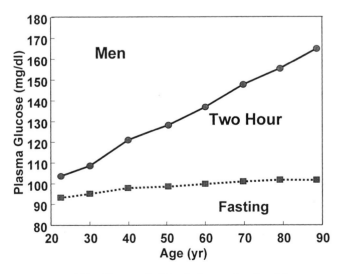

FIGURE 46.2. Changes in blood glucose levels with age.

required. The glucokinase gene is the glucose sensor for the β-cell. Some studies have found that this gene acts as a marker for abnormal glucose tolerance in the elderly, but others have not.[52,53] Insulin receptor number and affinity are normal in elderly patients, but insulin receptor tyrosine kinase activity in skeletal muscle is reduced.[54]

Clinical Presentation

Classic symptoms of polyuria or polydipsia are rarely present. Glucose is not spilled into the urine until the plasma glucose is markedly elevated because the renal threshold for glucose increases with age. Polydipsia is also less common, because thirst is impaired. When symptoms are present, they are generally atypical (falls, failure to thrive, urinary incontinence, or delirium).

Diabetes may present for the first time in elderly individuals as a result of a fasting screening glucose level or be concurrent with the presentation at the time of illness with a complication of illness, such as a myocardial infarction or stroke. Finally, nonketotic hyperosmolar coma may be the first sign of diabetes in older individuals, particularly in older nursing home patients; this results from decreased access to water associated with osmotic diuresis, impaired thirst, and cognitive dysfunction.

Unusual clinical findings also develop in older patients with established diabetes.[55,56] Intradermal bullae of the feet that resolve spontaneously have been described.[57] Painful limitation of the shoulder joints occurs frequently and may be related to nonenzymatic glycation of proteins.[58] Diabetes increases the risk for accidental hypothermia in older individuals.[59] Malignant otitis externa is a necrotizing infection caused by *Pseudomonas*, occurring almost exclusively in elderly patients with diabetes.[56] Renal papillary necrosis can occur in association with urinary tract infections.

Diabetic amyotrophy causes asymmetric and painful weakness of the muscles of the pelvic girdle and thigh, and usually resolves spontaneously in a few months. It is most prevalent in older males.[56] Diabetic neuropathic cachexia occurs in older patients with diabetes, causing weight loss, depression, and painful peripheral neuropathy.[60]

Diagnosis and Differential Diagnosis of Diabetes Mellitus in the Elderly

The diagnosis of diabetes mellitus is made primarily through the findings of elevated glucoses on fasting laboratory samples, random glucoses during outpatient or inpatient care, and, much less commonly now, after formal oral glucose tolerance testing (OGTT). In 1997, the American Diabetes Association (ADA) revised its diagnostic criteria[61] to rely solely on a fasting plasma

glucose value greater than 126 mg/dL (7.0 mmol/L), rather than on a fasting glucose over 140 mg/dL or a 2-h oral glucose tolerance test plasma glucose value over 200 mg/dL, as had been recommended by the 1980–1985 World Health Organization (WHO) diagnostic criteria[62] and the ADA 1979 criteria for diabetes.[63] The new ADA criteria also recommended two other diagnostic classes. Impaired fasting glucose (IFG) is defined as a fasting plasma glucose (FPG) between 110 mg/dL (6.1 mmol/L) and 126 mg/dL (7.0 mmol/L); normal fasting glucose is defined as a fasting plasma glucose less than 110 mg/dL. The OGTT is not recommended for routine diagnosis of glucose intolerance or diabetes. The 1998 preliminary report of WHO essentially endorses the ADA 1997 recommendation, with the exception that they advocate the use of OGTT.[64]

The new ADA 1997 criteria change the incidence of diabetes by age, sex, and ethnicity, resulting in a significant increase in the number of individuals diagnosed with diabetes mellitus while perhaps excluding significant numbers of individuals who would have gained the diagnosis through postchallenge glucose elevations.[61] From all the population data available, the criteria of a 2-h plasma value greater than 200 mg/dL (11.1 mmol/L) would be met by almost all patients who met the older fasting value of 140 mg/dL (7.8 mmol/L). However, it would also be met by many individuals with a lower fasting value.

The new fasting value of 126 mg/dL (7 mmol/L) is reported to be more in agreement with the diagnosis of diabetes by the 2-h post-OGTT plasma glucose value of 200 mg/dL. However, the data suggest this may not be the case. At least 25 studies have examined the impact of the new 1997 ADA criteria with the older 1985 WHO criteria. These reports indicate that 11% to 80% of the individuals diagnosed with diabetes mellitus by the WHO criteria will be missed if the diagnosis is solely based on the lower FPG, which appears to particularly include the elderly. The observations leading to the use of 200 mg/dL level and the difficulties with this level suggest further revisions may be needed. Using data from the NHANES III survey, comparisons of the results of FPG with the 2-h post-OGTT plasma glucose level are more than 50% discrepant.[65] The ADA's 1997 report has stated that the justification for the cut point for the 2-h post-OGTT glucose level of 200 mg/dL is derived, in part, from the evidence that the prevalence of microvascular complications increases dramatically at this point. In addition, the 2-h plasma glucose value following an OGTT from many large populations has a bimodal distribution. The nadir intersection of the two modes is known as the antimode and it shifts to the right with advancing age.[66] The 200 mg/dL level represents the average level of the antimodes from several large population studies (Pima Indians, Naruans, Samoans, Mexican-Americans, and East Indians). However, the antimodes from these populations arc quite variable (range, 143–310 mg/dL) and do not support the average 200 mg/dL level. They do, however, increase with age.

Many of the reported studies show that the 1997 ADA diagnosis standards do not result in equal sensitivity for fasting and 2-h glucose levels, especially in older individuals. Although the use of fasting plasma glucose alone for diabetes diagnosis may simplify testing, the WHO criteria would identify a much greater percentage of elderly subjects with diabetes or impaired glucose testing and move ahead the diagnosis by 5 to 8 years over criteria based on fasting glucose levels. As diabetes prevention efforts increase, a move to a more sensitive bias in diagnosis may be needed. The majority of newly diagnosed diabetic patients (>90%) emerge from the population with impaired glucose tolerance (IGT), no matter how it is defined, and are at higher risk for cardiovascular disorders.[27]

Prognosis and Course of Illness

It had been hoped for many years that intensive treatment of diabetes mellitus would reverse or defer significantly its major complications of microvascular and macrovascular disease, stroke, and heart attack, and be compatible with a healthy lifestyle. While a general impression indicating that intensive and aggressive therapy was potentially a benefit, two major studies have recently provided much greater justification and clarification for control of diabetes mellitus. These two studies, the Diabetes Control Complications Trial research group and the United Kingdom Prospective Diabetes Study Group investigations, are reviewed in detail here to establish more clearly the rationale for close control of diabetes.

Glucose Control

The Diabetes Control and Complications Trial (DCCT)[67] was a randomized, controlled trial of individuals with type 1 diabetes mellitus (aged 13–39 years) comparing the effect of intensive blood glucose management to conventional management on diabetic outcomes over a mean 6.5-year follow-up. Subjects in general were in good health and had diabetes for 1 to 15 years. Patients were stratified by the presence of retinopathy into a primary prevention cohort (no baseline retinopathy) and a secondary prevention cohort (mild retinopathy), and then randomized to either intensive insulin management consisting of three or more insulin doses per day to keep glucose levels as close to normal as possible or to conventional therapy consisting of standard insulin therapy to keep glucoses within accepted guidelines ($A_{1c} < 7.0$).

For primary prevention, the adjusted relative risk of retinopathy was reduced by 76% (95% CI, 62%–85%) in the intensively treated group compared to the conventionally treated group. For secondary prevention, the risk of retinopathy progression was reduced by 54% (CI, 39%–66%) in the intensively treated group. In both cohorts, the reduction in risk increased with time and was not evident until 36 months into the treatment.

When the two cohorts were combined, intensive therapy reduced severe retinopathy and need for laser treatment by 47% and 51%, respectively, clinical neuropathy by 60% (CI, 38%–74%; $p \leq 0.002$), microalbuminuria ($p \leq 0.002$), and albuminuria ($p < 0.04$). Severe hypoglycemia was more common (62 versus 19), as were coma (16 versus 5) and emergency room admission (9 versus 4 cases per 100 patient-years) in the intensively managed group. No significant differences in mortality were observed between the two groups (7 intensive versus 4 conventional).

The DCCT resulted in a number of important recommendations. Intensive therapy with a goal of achieving glucose levels as close to the nondiabetic range as possible should be employed in most IDDM patients. Intensive therapy should be implemented in centers with the requisite nursing, dietary, behavioral, and clinical expertise to ensure safe and effective therapy. Although most diabetes in late life is not of the type 1 variety, this study provided important principles and hopes for improving the long-term prognosis for diabetes patients.

The most comprehensive study of type 2 diabetes to date has been the United Kingdom Prospective Diabetes Study Group.

United Kingdom Prospective Diabetes Study (UKPDS 33)

The UKPDS 33[68] investigated whether tight control of blood glucose in type 2 diabetic patients reduced the risk of microvascular or macrovascular disease. Patients over age 65 were excluded from this multicenter RCT; mean age was 54. Of the 3867 patients, 2729 were randomized to open-label intensive drug therapy with either chlorpropamide, glibenclamide, or insulin, with the goal of lowering FPG to less than 108 mg/dL. The 1138 other patients were randomized to conventional therapy that aimed for the lowest FPG possible with diet alone (although drugs were added if FPG reached as high as 270 mg/dL or in the presence of hyperglycemic symptoms).

Compared to conventional therapy, intensive therapy significantly reduced the risk of microvascular complications, but not macrovascular complications or macrovascular subclinical surrogate endpoints over the 10-year study period. Median hemoglobin A_{1c} levels were significantly lower in the intensive group (7%) than in the conventional group (7.9%). Three grouped endpoints were assessed: all-cause mortality, diabetes-related deaths [myocardial infarction (MI), stroke, peripheral vascular disease, renal disease, hyperglycemia or hypoglycemia, and sudden death], and any diabetes-related endpoint (death from any of the preceding, as well as nonfatal MI, angina, heart failure, stroke, renal failure, amputation, vitreous hemorrhage, retinopathy, blindness, or cataract). Only diabetes-related endpoints were significantly reduced with intensive therapy, with a risk reduction of 12% (95% CI, 1%–21%). Most of this reduction was due to reduction in microvascular outcomes, especially the need for retinal photocoagulation, which was reduced 25% (95% CI, 7%–40%). All three intensive drug regimens reduced microvascular endpoints equally.

Neither all-cause mortality nor diabetes-related deaths differed by intensity of treatment, although a non-significant trend ($p = 0.052$) toward reduction in risk of myocardial infarction was observed in the intensive therapy group, with an RRR of 16% (95% CI, 0–29%). Compared to conventional treatment, intensive therapy was associated with a mean 6.4-pound weight gain (most prominently in the insulin group) and an increased risk of hypoglycemia. Treatment for hypertension was more common with chlorpropamide than with any other regimen, including conventional therapy.

A substudy examined 342 newly diagnosed obese diabetic patients randomized to metformin during UKDPS 33 and compared them to the overweight patients who were included in the UKDPS 33 study already discussed [conventional treatment (411) or intensive treatment (951)]. Based on absolute risk (events per 1000 patient-years) and relative to conventional therapy, metformin treatment reduced risk of any diabetes-related endpoint by 32% (NNT, 10; CI, 6–32), diabetes-related deaths by 42% (NNT, 19; CI, 10–97), and all-cause mortality by 36% (NNT, 15; CI, 8–83). Relative risk of myocardial infarction was also significantly reduced. Metformin was also significantly better than all other drugs used in the intensively treated group in reducing risk of reaching any diabetes-related endpoint, stroke, and all-cause mortality. In these already overweight patients, weight gain was less common with metformin than with other intensive therapies, as were hypoglycemic episodes.[69]

Metformin/Sulfonylurea combined therapy was found to perhaps have less benefit than either drug alone. This observation is important as the popularity of combined drug therapy is increasing.

Blood Pressure Control and Complications in Type 2 Diabetes

UKPDS 38 evaluated the effect of hypertension control on diabetic outcomes. The study involved the randomization of 1148 hypertensive patients (mean age, 56.4 years), to either tight blood pressure control (blood pressures less than 150/85) with either an angiotensin-converting enzyme (ACE) inhibitor (captopril) or a beta-blocker (atenolol), or to less tight control (blood pressures less than 180/105) without these drugs. The actual mean blood pressures obtained were 144/82 in the tight control group and 154/87 in the "less tight."

Endpoints were identical to those in the main study just described. Mean follow-up time was 8.4 years. Tight blood pressure control reduced diabetes-related endpoints by 24% (95% CI, 8%–38%; $p = 0.0046$), diabetes-related deaths by 32% (CI, 6%–51%; $p = 0.019$; NNT = 15), and stroke by 44% (CI, 11%–65%; $p = 0.013$) compared to less tight control. Microvascular endpoints were reduced by 37% (CI, 11%–56%; $p = 0.0092$), with 35% reduction in risk of retinal photocoagulation ($p = 0.023$). There was no difference in all-cause mortality. There were also no differences between captopril or atenolol in terms of treatment benefits.[70]

The DCCT and UKPDS give us important information related to the rationale for treatment of diabetes mellitus in late life. It is clear that microvascular and macrovascular events can be influenced by careful control of diabetes mellitus. As a result, the management of both blood pressure and blood sugar in diabetes mellitus has a sound rationale.

The use of ACE inhibitor therapy in minimizing the development of and the progress of renal damage as measured by micro- and clinical-grade albuminuria has now become an important standard of care in the management of type 2 diabetes. Whether ACE inhibitor itself or blood pressure reduction alone is the factor reducing albuminuria is not fully answered. Additionally, the importance of high lipids as a strong risk factor for future cardiovascular disease in diabetic individuals is gaining attention, and aggressive treatment is becoming the norm.

Treatment and Management of Diabetes Mellitus

The benefits of aggressive treatment in terms of delaying or preventing complications in the elderly diabetic are clear. Life expectancy for the older diabetic person is approximately two-thirds that of a healthy elderly individual. This fact is not an argument against aggressive treatment; in fact, reductions in life expectancy are in large part because most older diabetics have adequate time to develop and suffer from chronic complications of diabetes mellitus. Recent studies confirm that many of the vascular and renal complications of diabetes develop at a relatively similar rate in types 1 and 2 diabetes.[69] Other diabetic complications are aggravated by changes inherent in aging. Creatinine clearance declines with normal aging[71] and may accelerate or enhance risk for diabetic renal failure. Age is also an independent risk factor for the development of peripheral neuropathy, a common condition in diabetes mellitus.[72,73]

The initial approach to the older adult with diabetes mellitus requires assessment of the patient's current medical status and estimated life expectancy. Motivation and commitment of the patient and family also play a large role in determining what level of treatment is appropriate. Support services available in the community and financial status should also be considered.

Following evaluation, one of two levels of care can be recommended: symptom-preventing care or aggressive care. The decision is made jointly by the patient and the primary caregiver. Family members and consultants such as geriatricians, diabetologists, cardiologists, and nephrologists may be helpful. These consultants provide a clearer picture of the current medical condition and estimates of life expectancy.

Symptom-preventing care is indicated for those individuals for whom the primary goal of treatment is avoidance of metabolic complications. The average glucose levels necessary to achieve this goal are approximately 200 mg/dL (11 mM) or the glucose level at which glycosuria is minimal. The elimination of glycosuria removes the risk of volume depletion and the risk of secondary problems related to hypotension and poor tissue perfusion. Hyperglycemic hyperosmolar nonketotic coma due to dehydration and glycosuria is the most dramatic expression of this phenomenon. Glycosuria also is associated with weight loss caused by the loss of calories in the urine. The resultant catabolic state leads to a loss of lean body tissue. The long-term consequences of poor nutrition include increased risk of infections.

Aggressive care has prevention of long-term complications as its goal. Euglycemia is defined as (1) a fasting glucose level lower than 115 mg/dL (6.4 mM), (2) a mean glucose level between 110 and 140 mg/dL (6–8 mM), and (3) normal levels of glycosylated hemoglobin. Prevention of long-term complications in type I patients results from this level of control. These benefits are believed to extrapolate to elderly patients within NIDDM.

Aggressive management programs for older adults with diabetes require high levels of skill, commitment, and diabetes education. Most older individuals are fully able to learn the complicated concepts and tasks required.[74–76] Older adults lead a less hectic, more ordered life than younger adults. Consequently, making the adjustments in lifestyle necessary for adherence to a good diabetes treatment program may at times be easier.

All older adults with diabetes mellitus should receive a standard basic care program regardless of the treatment goal chosen. These standards[77] (Table 46.1) include a complete history and physical examination to detect any complications of diabetes mellitus and any risk factors for

TABLE 46.1. Minimum standards of care for older adults with diabetes mellitus.

Initial evaluation
  Complete history and physical examination
  Geriatric assessment
  Laboratory examination: fasting blood glucose, glycosylated
    hemoglobin, fasting lipid profile, creatinine, urinalysis,
    electrocardiogram
  Ophthalmologic examination
  Dietary assessment
Continuing care
  Use of treatment as needed to meet target glucose levels: diet, oral
    agents, or insulin
  Assessment of blood glucose levels as frequently as needed to
    ensure that treatment goals are being met
  Annual assessment for diabetes complications
  Annual review of geriatric assessment

complications. A geriatric assessment, emphasizing a functional assessment, should be performed at the time of diagnosis. Skills in the basic activities involved in daily life (bathing, grooming, dressing, feeding, toileting, and transferring) and the instrumental activities of daily life (e.g., shopping, telephoning, finances, and housework) should be assessed. Social support systems and financial and insurance status often should also be assessed, by nursing and social work staff. Laboratory evaluation at diagnosis includes determinations of fasting serum glucose level, glycosylated hemoglobin (to assess previous level of control and to be used as a baseline), fasting lipid profile, and serum creatinine; urinalysis with examination for proteinuria; and an electrocardiogram. Ophthalmologic evaluation at the time of diagnosis is recommended by the American Diabetes Association for all patients with NIDDM.[78] This recommendation is particularly relevant for elderly patients who are at high risk for ocular diseases including cataract and glaucoma. Dietary assessment provides an initial dietary therapy for the diabetic patient.

Standard diabetes therapy includes diet, exercise, and if necessary use of oral hypoglycemic agents or administration of insulin.

Oral Hypoglycemic Agents

Increasingly, therapy for type 2 diabetes builds on diet and exercise and has become more mechanistically focused. Single or combination chemotherapy is used. A significant amount of improvement can be expected with improved therapy. Currently, 54% of elderly diabetic patients have hemoglobin A_{1c} levels above normal and 27% of the total had A_{1c} levels greater than 8. Thus, nearly a quarter have "poor" control.[79] Current best practices require a normal hemoglobin A_{1c}, certainly less than 7. For those individuals in whom the demands of therapy are too great, medication side effects are too great, or

TABLE 46.2. Dietary therapy: special considerations for older adults with diabetes.

Financial difficulty
Difficulty with shopping because of transportation or mobility problems
Poor food preparation skills (particularly elderly widowed men)
Ingrained dietary habits
Difficulty following dietary instruction because of impaired cognitive function
Decreased taste
Increased frequency of constipation

access to monitoring is not possible, a reduction in expectations and greater complication rates will be higher. Medications currently available can promote insulin secretion, increase insulin sensitivity, or slow the digestion/processing of complex carbohydrates.

Diet

Diet alone has varying degrees of success. Elderly patients with diabetes are able to improve diabetes control with diet and weight loss.[80] However, they may find it difficult to adhere to a strict dietary regimen and maintain weight loss. Older adults with mobility problems may find exercise to increase caloric expenditure impossible. If dramatic dietary restriction is employed to reduce weight, nutrient and vitamin deficiencies may develop. Aggressive dietary management cannot be recommended under these circumstances. Other considerations specific to older adults may limit the effectiveness of dietary therapy (Table 46.2).[18]

A diabetic diet is relatively high in carbohydrates (50%–60% of total calories), low in fat (<30% of total calories from fat, with 10% saturated fat, 10% polyunsaturated fat, and 10% monosaturated fat), and moderate in protein (~20% of total calories). If malnourished or chronically ill, the elderly patient should increase protein and energy intake. Vitamin and mineral supplements are indicated when caloric intake falls below 1000 kilocalories per day.

Exercise

The role of formalized exercise programs in the management of diabetes mellitus remains controversial. The beneficial effects of exercise on glucose tolerance have been well documented.[81] The effectiveness of exercise in lowering plasma glucose levels is unclear. The effects of exercise on glucose tolerance are disappointingly transient, lessening within days of stopping an exercise program.[82] Exercise for older adults with diabetes may pose additional problems. Perhaps four-fifths of older men with newly diagnosed mild diabetes are unable to participate in a regular training program because of other diseases or treatments.[83] Exercise for control of hyper-

glycemia may thus not be feasible for many older adults. These benefits and the risks of exercise in older adults are outlined in Table 46.3.[77] Because of the prevalence of silent coronary artery disease in this population, older adults with diabetes should be given an exercise tolerance test before they begin any exercise program.

Agents Increasing Insulin Secretion

Sulfonylureas

First-generation agents such as chlorpropamide (Diabinese) are largely of historical interest. Because of chlorpropamide's very long half-life (up to 60h), risk of hypoglycemia, and production of hyponatremia from stimulation of excess antidiuretic hormone, it is rarely used today. Second-generation agents in the sulfonylurea class have largely replaced chlorpropamide. Glipizide (Glucotrol and Glucotrol XL) and Glyburide (Micronase, Glynase, and Diabeta) have been standards for many years. All, however, are associated with weight gain and hypoglycemia and are of less utility the higher the fasting glucose. These drugs rarely produce hyponatremia from central stimulation of antidiuretic hormone. Once fasting glucose levels rise above 200 mg/dL, insulin secretory reserve is very limited and these agents are less likely to be successful. As a general principle, dosing with second-generation agents should be initiated at the lowest end of the dosing range until individual susceptibility to hypoglycemia is known. Dosing is each morning, or twice a day.

Meglitinides

Repaglinide (Prandin) is an agent given before each meal, as it has a short half-life and is a shorter and more rapidly acting agent than classic sulfonylureas. It is therefore most useful when postprandial elevation of glucose dominates the clinical picture. Weight gain and hypoglycemia are shared side effects with sulfonylureas. However, in the treatment design for an individual experiencing between-meal hypoglycemia while taking sulfonylureas, Repaglinide is attractive.

TABLE 46.3. Potential benefits and risks of exercise for older adults with diabetes.

Benefits	Risks
Improved exercise tolerance	Sudden cardiac death
Improved glucose tolerance	Foot and joint injuries
Improved maximal oxygen consumption	Hypoglycemia
Increased muscle strength	
Decreased blood pressure	
Decreased body fat and increased muscle mass	
Improved lipid profile	
Improved sense of well-being	

D-Phenylalanine

Nateglinide (Starlix), which is a chemical derivative of the amino acid phenylalanine, has a similar profile and mode of action as Repaglinide. Because of its very short action, it is most useful in early diabetes when fasting glucoses are only mildly elevated.

Agents Increasing Insulin Action

Because of the recognition of insulin resistance as a fundamental component of noninsulin-dependent diabetes mellitus, agents increasing tissue sensitivity and responsiveness to endogenous insulin have become cornerstones of treatment. A very beneficial treatment side effect is the promotion of weight loss by these agents.

Metformin

Metformin (Glucophage, Glucophage XL) is given once (XL) or twice a day and assists altered diabetes physiology by improving insulin-mediated effects on the liver. The result is improvement in fasting hyperglycemia. On initiating treatment, bloating, cramps, and diarrhea may result. There is still a rare risk of lactic acidosis in individuals with renal, cardiac, or liver failure or in individuals undergoing contrast studies where borderline renal function is already present. Because of this, it is suggested that metformin doses be withheld temporarily in high-risk settings, such as hospitalization, dehydration, or planned radiologic studies. When creatinine clearance is low (when serum creatinine is greater than 1.5 mg/dl), or there is advanced liver, cardiac, or pulmonary disease, this agent should be avoided. Creatinines greater than 1.5 are seen in approximately 5% of all elderly individuals.

Thiazolidinediones

Rosiglitazone (Avandia) and Pioglitazone (Actos), both once or twice per day medicines taken with food that specifically assist in insulin action on muscle and fat, are useful alternatives to metformin. As with metformin, hypoglycemia is rare. However, monthly monitoring of liver function is required as approximately 10% develop hepatic enzyme elevations, and rare fatal hepatitis has occurred. Being new, these drugs are much more expensive than sulfonylureas.

Agents Slowing Carbohydrate Processing in the Gut

The alpha-glucosidase inhibitors Acarbose (Precose) and Miglitol (Glyset) both reduce postprandial increases in blood sugars by inhibiting the breakdown of dietary carbohydrate. These agents are taken with the first food intake of every meal. While they are useful adjunctive therapy for more severe diabetes, Acarbose and Miglitol are helpful in impaired glucose tolerance and mild diabetes as well. High doses of bran have also been associated with improved glucose intolerance and have the additional benefit of lowering cholesterol. The common side effect of all these agents is gas, bloating, and diarrhea.

Combination Therapy

In recent times, the use of drug combinations has increased to avoid or minimize insulin therapy and its inconvenience, hypoglycemia, weight gain, and possible acceleration of other atherogenesis. Several drug combinations have emerged, based on successful experience in combining drugs with complementary mechanisms of action.

Stepwise addition of agents is the practical approach. The most studied combination is sulfonylurea and insulin. Clearly some secretion of endogenous insulin must still be present. In this combination, insulin is given at night and sulfonylurea is given before each meal to produce insulin increments in the postprandial state. Insulin and metformin have been used in combination, with the goal of improving insulin action. Two oral hypoglycemics have been studied in combination, sulfonylurea and metformin; this is an attractive combination as the first produces insulin release, now able to stimulate tissues that have been sensitized by metformin. A three-drug regimen has been described combining NPH insulin at night, preprandial glipizide three times a day, and metformin twice a day. Although this intense regimen will minimize weight gain due to lower overall dosing with insulin, it poses a complexity challenge for elderly individuals.

Combination therapy will be increasingly popular, as combination effects on lipids, hypoglycemic events, and progression of disease is better defined in future years.

Management During Terminal Phases of the Illness: The Elderly Nursing Home Patient

Approximately 3% to 5% of the population over the age of 65 live in nursing homes.[84] One-third of elderly individuals will spend some time in a nursing home.[85,86] Diabetes prevalence in the nursing home population is about twice that in the general population[87] and has progressively increased since 1964.[88,89] The 1987 National Medical Expenditure Survey found that diabetic patients in nursing homes had a high prevalence of diseases associated with diabetes, such as heart disease,[90,91] a high prevalence of amputations and immobility.[90,91] Chronic renal failure, retinopathy, neuropathy, urinary tract infections, and skin infections are also more common among the patients with diabetes than among a similarly aged group of patients without diabetes.[92] In contrast, the prevalence of dementia is low in diabetic nursing home residents.

A significant degree of functional limitation occurs in this population. As life expectancy is markedly reduced for most individuals admitted to nursing homes, the primary goal of therapy is symptom prevention. A recent study of 563 individuals from 24 nursing homes revealed that 75.8% died within 2 years.[93] Poor functional status was a major predictor of mortality.

Control of hyperglycemia in patients in nursing homes is achieved primarily by diet and medication. Exercise does not play a major role. Diet is an important therapeutic option, but weight maintenance may be as important as weight loss for many elderly patients with diabetes in nursing homes. One study found that more than 20% of patients with diabetes in nursing homes were more than 20% underweight.[92] Malnutrition in this population is common. Patients should be weighed monthly, and active dietary adjustments should be made.[94]

The choice of sulfonylureas or insulin therapy should be based on the level of glycemic control desired. Sulfonylureas are preferable both to the patient and to the nursing home staff.[95] Insulin, however, is needed for those patients for whom glycemic goals cannot be achieved with a sulfonylurea. In the nursing home setting, glucose monitoring may be done more frequently, a major asset in the management of diabetes mellitus, resulting in low levels of glycosylated hemoglobin and few episodes of hypoglycemia.[92,96]

Nursing home patients are prone to conditions that may be related to, or are exacerbated by, diabetes mellitus, particularly skin and urinary tract infections. Limiting the use of indwelling bladder catheters and ensuring good urinary output through adequate hydration may reduce urinary tract infections in this population. Skin infections may be prevented by strict pressure ulcer precautions, including frequent turning of immobilized patients, the use of adequate bed and wheelchair cushioning, and the use of heel protectors. The prevalence of all infections is reduced with strict hand-washing regimens. Annual influenza and 5-year pneumococcal vaccination will protect against epidemics of these illnesses in the nursing home. Immunization and PPD (purified protein derivative) status should be verified and documented for all new admissions to the nursing home. Patients with diabetes who have a positive PPD reaction should be considered for prophylaxis with isoniazid if they have not been treated previously for tuberculosis.

Regular ophthalmologic, dental, and foot care services should continue in the nursing home.

Management of the Hospitalized Diabetic Patient

Elderly diabetic individuals are hospitalized about twice as often as elderly people without diabetes. In the NHANES II study, only 16.5% of individuals 65 to 74 years old without diabetes reported having been hospitalized once or more within the previous year, whereas 29.8% of those with known diabetes reported having been hospitalized.[97]

In the hospital, the goal for glycemic management is to minimize the likelihood of insulin deficiency, which can contribute to a catabolic state. Tight control is not necessary to achieve this goal. Reasonable goals would be a mean plasma glucose level of less than 250 mg/dL (14 mM) and minimal glycosuria. Stressful illnesses such as myocardial infarction, pneumonia, influenza, and stroke can exacerbate hyperglycemia and may even precipitate hyperosmolar hyperglycemic nonketotic coma in a patient who is already hospitalized. Fifty percent of all severe episodes of dehydration develop in the hospital.[98] This setting is thus a high-risk environment that could lead to hyperglycemia. Thus, elderly patients usually treated with oral agents may need to be treated temporarily with insulin. Appropriate intravenous fluid therapy to prevent dehydration and worsening of hyperglycemia should be given. Frequent glucose monitoring is recommended to prevent wide variations in glycemia. Sliding scales of regular insulin can be useful for the acutely ill patient or postoperative patient who is unable to eat. However, once oral intake is adequate, split dosing of insulin with adjustments made as needed on the basis of results of frequent glucose monitoring is possible.

Hypoglycemia is a significant problem for all hospitalized patients with diabetes. In general, hypoglycemia in the hospital results from decreased caloric intake or inappropriate changes in insulin dosage.[96] Hypoglycemia may be prevented by frequent glucose monitoring, with adjustments being made in the insulin dose as the patient's medical condition changes.

Prevention of Clinical Diabetes Mellitus

Diabetes mellitus affects more than 100 million individuals worldwide and, because of known risk factors common to many individuals that can be manipulated, the development of type 2 diabetes may potentially be modifiable. A number of clinical trials have addressed this hypothesis through dietary modification, physical activity, and drug treatment. Although some studies indicate protection against diabetes development, conclusions remain limited for reasons of study design problems with randomization, subject selection, or intervention intensity.

Six prospective studies have examined the predictors of progression from impaired glucose tolerance to type 2 diabetes.[99,100] Across the six studies (*n*, 177–693), the incidence rates averaged 57.2 per 1000 patient-years. Incidence rates were sharply higher for those in the top quartile of fasting glucoses, but increased linearly with increasing 2-h postchallenge glucose levels. Native and Hispanic incidence rates were higher than those of Caucasians. Baseline age showed no consistent pattern. Obesity was positively associated with future diabetes mellitus, no matter how body fatness was measured.

One study in the elderly and two in younger patients suggest that diet and exercise may prevent diabetes mellitus in patients with impaired glucose tolerance. In Da Qing, China, a screening program detected 577 individuals (mean age, 45.0) with impaired glucose tolerance (IGT).[101] Following stratification by body weight, patients were assigned to either active treatment (one of three possibilities: diet, exercise, or a combination of both) or to a control group who received brochures on diet, exercise, and IGT. At 6 years, more than two-thirds of the control group (67.7%) developed diabetes, compared to less than half in each of the active treatment groups (43.8% of diet group, 41.1% of exercise group, and 46% in the exercise plus diet group; all *p* < 0.05 compared to control but no significant differences compared to each other). After adjustment for differences in baseline obesity and fasting glucose, reductions in risk of developing diabetes were 31% for diet, 46% for exercise, and 42% for diet plus exercise, each highly significant compared to control.[101]

Another multicenter, partially blind study in Finland identified 522 overweight middle-aged persons with IGT (mean age, 55; persons over age 65 were excluded) who were randomly assigned to usual care or to individualized counseling aimed at reducing weight and total fat intake while increasing fiber intake and exercise.[102] Mean weight loss at 2 years was significantly different between the two groups; 7.7 pounds in the intervention group and 1.8 pounds for the control group. At 2 years, the cumulative incidence of diabetes was 6% in the intervention group versus 14% in controls (at 4 years, 11% and 23%, respectively), a risk reduction of 58% (95% CI, 0.3–0.7; *p* < 0.001).

The largest U.S. study, the Diabetes Prevention Program, recently announced dramatic reductions in the appearance of diabetes in overweight persons with IGT (mean age, 51) through lifestyle modifications.[103] A total of 3234 people were randomized to either metformin (850 mg twice a day), placebo, or 150 min of weekly exercise with a low-fat diet and a goal of 7% weight loss. The incidence of type 2 diabetes over a 3-year period was 4.8% with lifestyle intervention, 7.8% with metformin,

and 11% in the control group. In the subgroup of patients over 60 years of age, reductions in risk of diabetes through lifestyle changes were at least as great as that observed in the overall study population. Thus, substantial reductions in the incidence of diabetes were produced by lifestyle (58%) or metformin (31%). The era of identification of individuals at risk and preventing future disability from targeted practical intervention is well under way.

References

1. Siegel JS. Recent and prospective trends for the elderly population and some implications for health care. In: Haynes S, Feinleib M, eds. *Second Conference on the Epidemiology of Aging.* DHHS (NIH) 80–969. Washington, DC: U.S. Government Printing Office; 1980.
2. Guralnik JM, Fitzsimmons SC. Aging in America: a demographic perspective. *Cardiol Clin.* 1986;4:175–183.
3. Harris MI, Flegal KM, Cowie CC, et al. Prevalence of diabetes, impaired fasting glucose, and impaired glucose tolerance in US adults. *Diabetes Care.* 1998;21:518–524.
4. Harris MI. Undiagnosed NIDDM: clinical and public health issues. *Diabetes Care.* 1993;16:642–652.
5. Kilvert A, Fitzgerald MG, Wright AD, et al. Clinical characteristics and aetiological classification of insulin-dependent diabetes in the elderly. *Q J Med.* 1986;60:865–872.
6. Wachtel TJ, Tetu-Mouradjian LM, Goldman DL, Ellis SE, O'Sullivan PS. Hyperosmolarity and acidosis in diabetes mellitus: a three-year experience in Rhode Island. *J Gen Intern Med.* 1991;6:495–502.
7. Abbott RD, Donahue RP, MacMahon SW, Reed DM, Yano K. Diabetes and the risk of stroke. The Honolulu Heart Program. *JAMA.* 1987;257:949–952.
8. Wolf PA, D'Agostino RB, Belanger AJ, Kannel WB. Probability of stroke: a risk profile from the Framingham Study. *Stroke.* 1991;22:312–318.
9. Shlossman M, Knowler WC, Pettitt DJ, Genco RJ. Type 2 diabetes mellitus and periodontal disease. *J Am Dent Assoc.* 1990;121:532–536.
10. Centers for Disease Control and Prevention. *Diabetes Surveillance, 1993.* Atlanta, GA: U.S. Department of Health and Human Services, Public Health Service; 1993.
11. Elahi D, Muller DC. Carbohydrate metabolism in the elderly. *Eur J Clin Nutr.* 2000;54:S112–S120.
12. Davidson MB. The effect of aging on carbohydrate metabolism: a review of the English literature and a practical approach to the diagnosis of diabetes mellitus in the elderly. *Metabolism.* 1979;28:688–705.
13. Jackson RA, Blix PM, Matthews JA, et al. Influence of aging on glucose homeostasis. *J Clin Endocrinol Metab.* 1982;55:840–848.
14. Minaker KL. What diabetologists should know about elderly patients. *Diabetes Care.* 1990;13(suppl 2):34–46.
15. Jackson RA, Hawa MI, Roshania RD, et al. Influence of aging on hepatic and peripheral glucose metabolism in humans. *Diabetes.* 1988;37:119–129.

16. Chen M, Bergman RN, Pacini G, et al. Pathogenesis of age-related glucose intolerance in man: insulin resistance and decreased beta-cell function. *J Clin Endocrinol Metab.* 1985;60:13–20.

17. DeFronzo RA. Glucose intolerance and aging. *Diabetes Care.* 1981;4:493–501.

18. Lipson LG. Diabetes in the elderly: diagnosis, pathogenesis, and therapy. *Am J Med.* 1986;80(suppl 5A):10–21.

19. Fink RI, Kolterman OG, Kao M, et al. The role of the glucose transport system in the postreceptor defect in insulin action associated with human aging. *J Clin Endocrinol Metab.* 1984;58:721–725.

20. Belfiore F, Vagnoni G, Napoli E, Rabuazzo M. Effect of aging on key enzymes of glucose metabolism in human adipose tissue. *J Mol Med.* 1977;2:89–95.

21. Trischitta V, Reaven GM. Evidence of a defect in insulin-receptor recycling in adipocytes from older rats. *Am J Physiol.* 1988;254:E38–E44.

22. Forbes GB, Reina JC. Adult lean body mass declines with age: some longitudinal observations. *Metabolism.* 1977;19:653–663.

23. Sallis JF, Haskell WL, Wood PD, et al. Physical activity assessment methodology in the Five-City Project. *Am J Epidemiol.* 1985;121:91–106.

24. Seals DR, Hagberg JM, Allen WK, et al. Glucose tolerance in young and older athletes and sedentary men. *J Appl Physiol.* 1984;56:1521–1525.

25. Chen M, Bergman RN, Porte D Jr. Insulin resistance and beta-cell dysfunction in aging: the importance of dietary carbohydrate. *J Clin Endocrinol Metab.* 1988;67:951–957.

26. Donahue RP, Abbott RD, Reed DM, et al. Postchallenge glucose concentration and coronary heart disease in men of Japanese ancestry: Honolulu Heart Program. *Diabetes.* 1987;36:689–692.

27. Agner E, Thorsteinsson B, Eriksen M. Impaired glucose tolerance and diabetes mellitus in elderly subjects. *Diabetes Care.* 1982;5:600–604.

28. Skarfors ET, Selinus KI, Lithell HO. Risk factors for developing noninsulin-dependent diabetes. A 10-year follow-up of men in Uppsala. *Br Med J.* 1991;303:755–760.

29. Vaag A, Henriksen JE, Madsbad S, Holm N, Beck-Nielsen H. Insulin secretion, insulin action, and hepatic glucose production in identical twins discordant for non-insulin-dependent diabetes mellitus. *J Clin Investig.* 1995;95:690–698.

30. Tibblin G, Adlerberth A, Lindstedt GB, Björntorp P. The pituitary-gonadal axis and health in elderly men. *Diabetes.* 1996;45:1605–1609.

31. Goodman-Gruen D, Barrett-Connor E. Sex hormone-binding globulin and glucose tolerance in post-menopausal women. The Rancho Bernardo Study. *Diabetes Care.* 1997;20:645–649.

32. Feskens EJM, Bowles CH, Kromhout D. Carbohydrate intake and body mass index relation to the risk of glucose intolerance in an elderly population. *Am J Clin Nutr.* 1991;54:136–140.

33. Feskens EJM, Virtanen SM, Rasanen L, et al. Dietary factors determining diabetes and impaired glucose tolerance. *Diabetes Care.* 1995;18:1104–1111.

34. Marshall JA, Weiss NS, Hamman RF. The role of dietary fiber in the etiology of non-insulin-dependent diabetes mellitus. The San Luis Valley diabetes study. *Ann Epidemiol.* 1993;3:18–26.

35. Salmeron J, Asherio A, Rimm EB, et al. Dietary fiber, glycemic load, and risk of NIDDM in men. *Diabetes Care.* 1997;20:545–550.

36. Lipton RB, Liao Y, Cao G, Cooper RS, McGee D. Determinants of incident non-insulin-dependent diabetes mellitus among blacks and whites in a national sample. The NHANES I Epidemiologic follow-up study. *Am J Epidemol.* 1993;138:826–964.

37. Cassano PA, Rosner B, Vokonas PS. Obesity and body fat distribution in relation to the incidence of non-insulin-dependent diabetes mellitus. *Am J Epidemiol.* 1992;136:1474–1486.

38. Travia D, Bonora E, Cacciatori V, et al. Study of some putative pathogenic factors of diabetes mellitus in the elderly. *Arch Gerontol Geriatr.* 1991;2(suppl 2):219–222.

39. Morris RD, Rimm AA. Association of waist to hip ratio and family history with the prevalence of NIDDM among 25,272 adult, white females. *Am J Public Health.* 1991;81:507–509.

40. Manson JE, Nathan DM, Krolewski AS, Stampter MJ, Willett HWC, Hennekens CH. A prospective study of exercise and incidence of diabetes among US male physicians. *JAMA.* 1992;268:63–67.

41. Mykkanen L, Kuusisto J, Pyorala K, Laakso M. Cardiovascular disease risk factors as predictors of type 2 (non-insulin-dependent) diabetes mellitus in elderly subjects. *Diabetologia.* 1993;36:553–559.

42. Helmrich SP, Ragland DR, Leung RW, Paffenburger RS. Physical activity and reduced occurrence of non-insulin-dependent diabetes mellitus. *N Engl J Med.* 1991;325:147–195.

43. Edelstein SL, Knowler WC, Bain RP, et al. Predictors of progression from impaired glucose tolerance to NIDDM. *Diabetes.* 1997;46:701–710.

44. Gurwitz J, Field TS, Glynn RJ, et al. Risk factors for NIDDM requiring treatment in the elderly. *J Am Geriatr Soc.* 1994;42:1235–1240.

45. Mooy JM, Grootenhuis PA, de Vries H, et al. Prevalence and determinants of glucose intolerance in a Dutch Caucasian population. *Diabetes Care.* 1995;18:1270–1273.

46. Stolk RP, Pols HA, Lamberts SWJ, de Jong PTVM, Hofman A, Grobbee DE. Diabetes mellitus, impaired glucose tolerance, and hyperinsulinemia in an elderly population. *Am J Epidemiol.* 1997;145:24–32.

47. Meneilly GS, Hards L, Tessier D, Elliott T, Tildesley H. NIDDM in the elderly. *Diabetes Care.* 1996;19:1320–1325.

48. Arner P, Pollare T, Lithell H. Different aetiologies of type 2 (non-insulin-dependent) diabetes mellitus in obese and non-obese subjects. *Diabetologia.* 1991;4:483–487.

49. Best JD, Kahn SE, Ader M, Watanabe RM, Ni TC, Bergman RN. Role of glucose effectiveness in the determination of glucose tolerance. *Diabetes Care.* 1996;19:1019–1030.

50. Forbes A, Elliott T, Tildesley H, Finegood D, Meneilly GS. Alterations in non-insulin-mediated glucose uptake in the elderly patient with diabetes. *Diabetes.* 1998;47:1915–1919.

51. Meneilly GS, Tessier D. Diabetes in the elderly. In: Morley JE, van den Berg L, eds. *Contemporary Endocrinology: Endocrinology of Aging*. Totowa, NJ: Humana Press; 1997: 181–203.

52. McCarthy MI, Hitman GA, Hitchins M, et al. Glucokinase gene polymorphisms: a genetic marker for glucose intolerance in cohort of elderly Finnish men. *Diabet Med*. 1993; 10:198–204.

53. Laakso M, Malkki M, Kekalainen P, Kuusisto J, Mykannen L, Deeb S. Glucokinase gene variants in subjects with late-onset NIDDM and impaired glucose tolerance. *Diabetes Care*. 1995;18:398–400.

54. Obermajer-Kusser B, White MF, Pongratz DE, et al. A defective intramolecular autoactivation cascade may cause the reduced kinase activity of the skeletal muscle insulin receptor from patients with non-insulin-dependent diabetes mellitus. *J Biol Chem*. 1989;264:9497–9504.

55. Morley JE, Kaiser FE. Unique aspects of diabetes mellitus in the elderly. *Clin Geriatr Med*. 1990;6:693–702.

56. Tattersall RB. Diabetes in the elderly—a neglected area. *Diabetologia*. 1984;27:167–173.

57. James WD, Odom RB, Goette DKL. Bullous eruption of diabetes mellitus. *Arch Dermatol*. 1980;116:1191–1192.

58. Friedman NA, LeBan NB. Periarthrosis of the shoulder associated with diabetes mellitus. *Am J Phys Med Rehabil*. 1989;68:12–14.

59. Neil MAW, Dawson JA, Baker JE. Risk of hypothermia in elderly patients with diabetes. *Br Med J*. 1986;293:416–418.

60. Ellenberg M. Diabetic neuropathic cachexia. *Diabetes*. 1974;23:418–423.

61. The Expert Committee on the Diagnosis and Classification of Diabetes Mellitus. Report of the expert committee on the diagnosis and classification of diabetes mellitus. *Diabetes Care*. 1997;20:1183–1197.

62. World Health Organization. *Diabetes Mellitus: Report of a WHO Study Group*. Geneva: WHO; 1985.

63. National Diabetes Data Group. Classification and diagnosis of diabetes mellitus and other categories of glucose intolerance. *Diabetes*. 1979;28:1039–1057.

64. Alberti KGMM, Zimmet PZ. Definition, diagnosis and classification of diabetes mellitus and its complications. Part 1: Diagnosis and classification of diabetes mellitus. Provisional report of a WHO consultation. *Diabet Med*. 1998;15:539–553.

65. Harris M, Flegal K, Cowie C, et al. Prevalence of diabetes, impaired fasting glucose, and impaired glucose tolerance in US adults. The third national health and nutrition examination survey, 1988–1994. *Diabetes Care*. 1998;21: 518–524.

66. Bennett PH, Rushfroth NB, Miller M, Lecompte PM. Epidemiologic studies of diabetes in the Pima Indians. *Recent Prog Horm Res*. 1976;32:333–376.

67. Diabetes Control and Complications Trial Research Group. The effect of intensive treatment of diabetes on the development and progression of long-term complications in insulin-dependent diabetes mellitus. *N Engl J Med*. 1993;329:977–986.

68. UK Prospective Diabetes Study Group. Intensive blood-glucose control with sulphonylureas or insulin compared with conventional treatment and risk of complications in patients with type 2 diabetes (UKPDS 33). *Lancet*. 1998; 352:837–853.

69. UKPDS Group. Effect of intensive blood-glucose control with metformin on complications on overweight patients with type 2 diabetes (UKDPS 34). *Lancet*. 1998;352:854–865.

70. UKPDS Group. Tight blood pressure control and risk of macrovascular and microvascular complications in type 2 diabetes: UKPDS 38. *Br Med J*. 1998;317:703–713.

71. Rowe JW, Andres R, Tobin JD, et al. The effect of age on creatinine clearance in man: a cross-sectional and longitudinal study. *J Gerontol*. 1976;31:513–563.

72. Mackenzie RA, Phillips LH II. Changes in peripheral and central nerve conduction with aging. *Clin Exp Neurol*. 1981;18:109–116.

73. Naliboff BD, Rosenthal M. Effects of age on complications in adult onset diabetes. *J Am Geriatr Soc*. 1989;27:838–842.

74. Albert MS. Cognitive function. In: Albert MS, Moss MB, eds. *Geriatric Neuropsychology*. New York: Guilford; 1988: 33–53.

75. Ciocon JO, Potter JF. Age-related changes in human memory: normal and abnormal. *Geriatrics*. 1988;43(10): 43–48.

76. Einstein GO, McDaniel MA. Normal aging and prospective memory. *J Exp Psychol Learn Mem Cogn*. 1990;16: 717–726.

77. Morrow LA, Halter JB. Treatment of diabetes mellitus in the elderly. In: Weir GC, ed. *Joslin's Diabetes Mellitus*, 13th Ed. Philadelphia: Lea & Febiger; 1993.

78. American Diabetes Association. Standards of medical care for patients with diabetes mellitus. *Diabetes Care*. 1989;12:365–368.

79. Wetzler HP, Synder JW. Linking pharmacy and laboratory data to assess the appropriateness of care in patients with diabetes. *Diabetes Care*. 2000;23:1637–1641.

80. Reaven GM. Beneficial effect of moderate weight loss in older patients with non-insulin-dependent diabetes mellitus poorly controlled with insulin. *J Am Geriatr Soc*. 1985;33:93–95.

81. Holloszy JO, Schultz J, Kursnierkiewicz J, et al. Effects of exercise on glucose tolerance and insulin resistance. Brief review and some preliminary results. *Acta Med Scand Suppl*. 1986;711:55–65.

82. Schneider SH, Amorosa LF, Khachadurian AK, et al. Studies on the mechanism of improved glucose control during regular exercise in type 2 (non-insulin-dependent) diabetes. *Diabetologia*. 1984;26:355–360.

83. Skarfors ET, Wegener TA, Lithell H, et al. Physical training as treatment for type 2 (non-insulin-dependent) diabetes in elderly men. A feasibility study over 2 years. *Diabetologia*. 1987;30:930–933.

84. Ouslander JG, Martin S. Assessment in the nursing home. *Clin Geriatr Med*. 1987;3:155–174.

85. Brock DB, Brody JA. Statistical and epidemiological characteristics. In: Andres R, Bierman EL, Hazzard WR, eds. *Principles of Geriatric Medicine*. New York: McGraw-Hill; 1985;3–71.

86. Kemper P, Murtaugh CM. Lifetime use of nursing home care. *N Engl J Med*. 1991;324:595–600.

87. Tonino RP. Diabetes education. What should health care providers in long-term nursing care facilities know about diabetes? *Diabetes Care.* 1990;13(suppl 2):55.

88. Harris MI, Hadden WC, Knowler WC, Bennett PH. Prevalence of diabetes and impaired glucose tolerance and plasma glucose levels in U.S. population aged 20–74 years. *Diabetes.* 1987;36:523–554.

89. Hing E, Sekscenski E, Strahan G. The national nursing home survey: 1985 summary for the United States. In: *Vital and Health Statistics.* DHHS–PHS 1989;89–1758. Washington, DC: Department of Health and Human Services; 1989.

90. Van Nostrand JF. Nursing home care for diabetics. In: *Diabetes in America: Diabetes Data Compiled in 1984.* DHHS pub 85–1468. Washington, DC: U.S. Government Printing Office; 1985.

91. Edwards WS, Winn DM, Kurlantzick V, Sheridan S, Berk ML, Retchin SC. Evaluation of national health interview survey diagnostic reporting. In: *Vital and Health Statistics, Series 2, No. 120.* DHHS 93–1394. Washington, DC: Department of Health and Human Services; 1994.

92. Mooradian AD, Osterweil D, Petrasek D, et al. Diabetes mellitus in elderly nursing home patients. A survey of clinical characteristics and management. *J Am Geriatr Soc.* 1988;36:391–396.

93. Lewis M, Kane RL, Cretin S, et al. The immediate and subsequent outcomes of nursing home care. *Am J Public Health.* 1985;75:758–762.

94. Tonino RP. What should health-care providers in long-term nursing care facilities know about diabetes. *Diabetes Care.* 1990;13:55–59.

95. Mooradian AD, Osterweil D, Petrasek D, Morley JE. Diabetes mellitus in elderly nursing home patients: a survey of clinical characteristics and management. *J Am Geriatr Soc.* 1988;16:391–396.

96. Fischer KF, Lees JA, Newman JH. Hypoglycemia in hospitalized patients. Cause and outcomes. *N Engl J Med.* 1986;315:1245–1250.

97. Aubert RE, Ballard DJ, Bennett PH, et al. Diabetes in America. In: *National Institutes of Health: National Diabetes and Digestive and Kidney Diseases, 2nd Ed.* NIH 95–1468. Washington, DC: National Institutes of Health; 1995.

98. Snyder NA, Feigal DW, Arieff AI. Hypernatremia in elderly patients. A heterogenous, morbid, and iatrogenic entity. *Ann Intern Med.* 1987;107:309–319.

99. Edelstein SL, Knowler WC, Bain RP, et al. Predictors of progression from impaired glucose tolerance to NIDDM: an analysis of six prospective studies. *Diabetes.* 1997;46(4): 701–710.

100. de Vegt F, Dekker JM, Jager A, et al. Relation of impaired fasting and postload glucose with incident type 2 diabetes in a Dutch population. The Hoorn Study. *JAMA.* 2001; 285(16):2109–2113.

101. Pan XR, Li GW, Hu YH, et al. Effects of diet and exercise in preventing NIDDM in people with impaired glucose tolerance. The Da Qing IGT and Diabetes Study. *Diabetes Care.* 1997;20(4):537–544.

102. Tuomilehto J, Lindstrom J, Eriksson JG, et at. Prevention of type 2 diabetes mellitus by changes in lifestyle among subjects with impaired glucose tolerance. *N Engl J Med.* 2001;344(18):1343–1350.

103. Diabetes Prevention Program Research Group. Reduction in the incidence of type 2 diabetes with lifestyle intervention or metformin. *N Engl J Med.* 2002;346:393–403.

47
Thyroid Disorders

David S. Cooper

Thyroid problems in the elderly are commonly encountered and are challenging to diagnose and treat. In the geriatric population, the prevalence of certain thyroid diseases (e.g., nodules, goiter, hypothyroidism) is high, and some thyroid disorders (e.g., hyperthyroidism) may have subtle or atypical presentations.[1] In older patients with common nonthyroidal illnesses, thyroid function tests may be altered, making their interpretation all the more difficult. Finally, therapy may be more complex than in younger patients because of the presence of underlying chronic illness, especially cardiac disease, and because of altered thyroid hormone metabolism.

Regardless of age, thyroid disorders can be conveniently categorized as functional (hyperthyroidism and hypothyroidism), inflammatory (thyroiditis), or neoplastic (nodules, carcinoma). For unknown reasons, virtually all thyroid problems occur more commonly in women. Before discussing thyroid diseases in depth, however, it is necessary to review normal thyroid function and to emphasize the alterations in thyroid structure and function that occur in the elderly. Fundamental but unanswered questions are whether such changes are part of normal senescence and whether they contribute materially to the aging process itself.

Aging and Thyroid Anatomy and Physiology

Thyroid Anatomy

During normal aging, atrophy and fibrosis of the thyroid occur.[2] There is a corresponding reduction in thyroid weight, making palpation of the normal thyroid more difficult. To an unknown extent, these anatomic and histologic changes reflect autoimmune phenomena,[3] because prevalence of antibodies to thyroglobulin and microsomal antigens approaches 20% in women over age 60 years.[4] In addition, the prevalence of microscopic and macroscopic thyroid nodules rises with age, with a marked increase in clinically palpable disease. However, there does not appear to be a correlation of thyroid weight or histology with thyroid function,[5] at least as assessed by circulating thyroxine concentrations.

Thyroid Physiology
Control of Thyroid Function

The hypothalamic–pituitary–thyroid axis functions as a classic negative feedback system (Fig. 47.1). Thyrotropin-releasing hormone (TRH), a hypothalamic tripeptide, stimulates the thyrotropes in the pituitary to synthesize and release thyroid-stimulating hormone (TSH, thyrotropin). In turn, TSH binds to specific receptors on thyroid follicular cells to stimulate virtually all aspects of thyroid growth and function from the trapping of iodide from the blood to the synthesis and secretion of the thyroid hormones thyroxine (T_4) and triiodothyronine (T_3).

Circulating thyroid hormone exerts negative feedback at the pituitary level, and, as has been recently elucidated, at the hypothalamic level as well. Thus, a rise in thyroid hormone concentrations suppresses TSH and, quite likely, TRH biosynthesis and secretion. On the other hand, a fall in serum thyroid hormone levels stimulates pituitary TSH (and presumably hypothalamic TRH) biosynthesis and secretion. The hypothalamus and pituitary both respond to changes in thyroid hormone concentrations with exquisite sensitivity. Thus, serum TSH levels can fall or rise in response to seemingly minor reciprocal changes in thyroid hormone concentrations, often still within the normal range but not drastic enough to cause clinical evidence of altered thyroid function. For this reason, serum TSH levels are extremely valuable in diagnosing subtle disturbances in thyroid function, which are particularly common in the elderly.

Although the hypothalamic–pituitary unit is of primary importance in the overall control of thyroid function, there is solid evidence that iodide also serves as a regulator of thyroid hormone biosynthesis and secretion. In pharmacologic doses (>30 mg), iodide inhibits thyroid hormone release and blocks thyroidal iodide uptake. Iodide also causes a transient decrease in thyroid hormone biosynthesis, the so-called Wolff–Chaikoff effect. These actions of iodide are probably important in protecting the organism against hyperthyroidism in the event of large iodide loads. Because of its inhibitory effects on thyroid function, iodide occasionally is used to treat hyperthyroidism, but, as is discussed here, it also can cause either hyperthyroidism (the Jod–Basedow phenomenon) or hypothyroidism, given the appropriate clinical substrate.

Thyroid Hormone Synthesis and Transport

Thyroid hormone synthesis is a multistep process that begins with the trapping of iodide by the thyroid follicular cell. Iodine is an essential nutrient and is abundant in the diet of most Western countries. In the United States, the average daily urinary iodine excretion, which reflects dietary iodine intake, has fallen from a mean of 32 μg/dL in 1971 to 1974 to 14.5 μg/dL in 1988 to 1994.[6] Fifteen percent of women over age 60 had low urinary iodine levels (<5 μg/dL), indicative of mild iodine deficiency. The clinical consequences of this nutritional phenomenon, which has also occurred in young individuals, is uncertain.

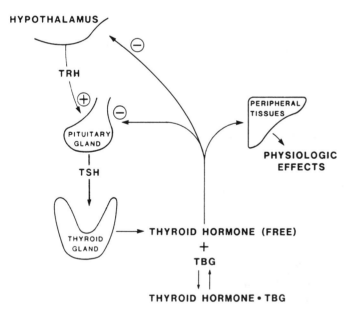

FIGURE 47.1. Regulation of thyroid-stimulating hormone (TSH) and thyroid hormone secretion. The relationship between bound and free thyroid hormones in the serum is depicted, emphasizing the importance of the free thyroid hormone concentration in the feedback control of TSH release and in peripheral tissues.

Trapped iodide is oxidized and bound to tyrosine residues in the large protein thyroglobulin via a process known as organification. The next step is the "coupling" of two iodinated tyrosines to form the *iodothyronines*, T_4 and T_3. Following synthesis, T_4 and T_3 are stored as colloid in the follicular lumen. With TSH stimulation, the colloid (i.e., thyroglobulin) is hydrolyzed inside vacuoles and the free thyroid hormones are released into the bloodstream. The daily T_4 secretion is 10- to 20-fold greater than T_3 secretion (75–100 versus 5–10 μg/day). Once secreted, they are bound (>99.9%) to transport proteins, principally thyroid-binding globulin (TBG), thyroid-binding prealbumin, and albumin. It is believed that only the unbound, or free, hormone is available to enter cells and exert its metabolic effects. Because of the tight binding of thyroid hormones to serum proteins, their clearance is prolonged significantly: the half-life of T_4 is approximately 7 days; because it is less firmly bound, T_3 has a shorter half-life, approximately 1 day.

It is important to emphasize that quantitative and qualitative changes in the binding proteins alter the serum total T_4 and T_3 concentrations but do not affect free thyroid hormone levels. Thus, situations in which thyroid-binding proteins are altered may be confused with true thyroid dysfunction if only total thyroid hormone concentrations are considered.

Thyroid Hormone Metabolism

Although thyroid hormones are metabolized in a variety of ways, the deiodination pathway is the most relevant clinically (Fig. 47.2). Via this route, approximately 50% of the daily T_4 production is converted to T_3 by removal of a single iodine atom from the outer ring of the T_4 molecule. This reaction is catalyzed by a ubiquitous enzyme, 5'- or outer-ring deiodinase, which also degrades the non-biologically active compound, reverse T_3 (rT_3), to another inert product, T_2. About 80% of the daily T_3 production derives from T_4 deiodination in the peripheral tissues. Because T_3 is the more metabolically active hormone and binds to nuclear thyroid hormone receptors with far greater affinity than does T_4, it is likely that T_4 is merely a "pro-hormone" for T_3. In fact, virtually all the biologic effects of thyroid hormone can be accounted for by the actions of T_3 alone.

A variety of clinical states can decrease the conversion of T_4 to T_3 via inhibitory effects on outer-ring deiodinase activity. Starvation, systemic illness, and certain drugs (propranolol, amiodarone, iodinated contrast agents) all cause a fall in serum T_3 concentrations and a reciprocal rise in serum rT_3, resulting from a fall in T_4 to T_3 conversion and in rT_3 degradation. The fall in T_3 concentration reduces protein catabolism and tissue oxygen consumption, which may be beneficial to the organism during periods of illness or decreased caloric intake.

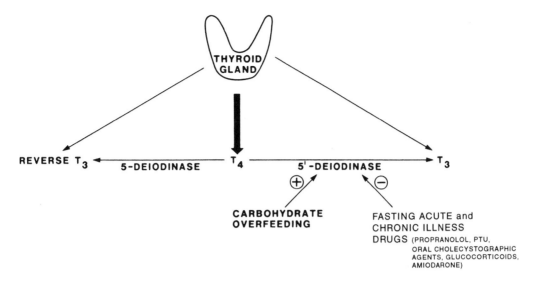

FIGURE 47.2. Peripheral metabolism of T_4 and factors that influence the tissue conversion of T_4 to T_3.

Age-Related Changes in Thyroid Function and Metabolism

A number of studies have examined possible changes in thyroid function with advancing age. Most studies show little, if any, change in circulating T_4 or free T_4 levels in the blood. Plasma iodide levels increase, due to a decrease in thyroidal iodine accumulation. This fall in thyroidal iodine uptake is accompanied by a decrease in T_4 secretion. However, decreased T_4 secretion in the elderly is not necessarily indicative of thyroid failure because it is not accompanied by elevations in serum TSH. Studies of elderly men[7] have also revealed reductions in the T_4 metabolic clearance rate resulting from possible decreases in outer-ring deiodinase activity, lean body mass, or both.[8] Thus, there are two distinct changes in T_4 economy that occur with aging: a decrease in T_4 secretion counterbalanced by a decrease in T_4 degradation, with no net change in T_4 concentrations in the blood.

Possible alterations in serum T_3 concentrations are more controversial. Although several studies have shown age-related reductions in serum T_3 and free T_3 levels, particularly after age 90 years,[9] others have found no significant decline during the fifth through the ninth decade.[10,11] One potential explanation for the discrepancies among the various reports is the inclusion of individuals with subclinical illness in the study populations. Thus, the reported decline in serum T_3 noted by some investigators may be secondary to the presence of subtle or occult infirmities associated with aging, rather than being caused by the aging process itself.

Despite the tentative conclusion drawn by many investigators that serum T_3 levels do not fall with age, it is clear that T_3 levels often are low in randomly selected elderly individuals without obvious illness. Because the major source of daily T_3 production derives from outer-ring deiodination of T_4, one possible explanation for the low T_3 levels in some aged individuals is the well-established decrease in the T_4 secretion rate. Another possible reason is a decline in the T_4 deiodination rate, which is the hallmark of systemic illness or decreased caloric intake. If a fall in deiodination were the explanation, a reciprocal rise in rT_3 would be expected; this has recently been reported in a group of healthy centenarians.[9] Thus, the fall in serum T_3 may be due to the decrease in T_4 production by the thyroid gland or a decrease in peripheral T_4 deiodination or both.

As noted earlier, the decline in thyroidal T_4 secretion is not accompanied by an elevated serum TSH level, which is the most sensitive indicator of thyroid hypofunction. Indeed, some studies using highly sensitive TSH assays have shown a decline in mean TSH levels with age.[10,12] However, other reports suggest that mean TSH levels in the elderly are higher than values observed in younger individuals.[13] Because most studies have shown that elderly women more often have high-normal or frankly elevated TSH levels, and antithyroid antibodies are often (although not always) present in such patients, it is reasonable to conclude that the slight elevation in mean TSH noted in most reports results from the inclusion in the study population of patients with subclinical autoimmune thyroiditis.[2] Thus, the normal range for TSH should not differ between younger and older individuals.

Thyroid Hormone Action

Thyroid hormones enter the cell by diffusion and bind to specific receptors located in the nucleus. The thyroid hormone receptor was recently discovered to be a homologue of the protein product or products of a family of oncogenes (*erb*-A), and shares common structural features with the steroid hormone and retinoic acid receptors.[14] The thyroid hormone receptor protein acts to modify DNA transcription and the synthesis of new proteins by the cell (e.g., angiotensin-converting enzyme, sex hormone-binding globulin, the beta-adrenergic receptor, factor VIII). while it inhibits the transcription and synthesis of other proteins (e.g., TSH and TRH). Future studies of thyroid hormone receptors will undoubtedly enhance our understanding of thyroid hormone action, particularly the reasons why older thyrotoxic individuals have few or no symptoms or signs of thyroid hormone excess (see following).

Virtually all tissues contain thyroid hormone receptors in varying amounts; the degree to which a tissue responds to thyroid hormone is proportional to the thyroid hormone receptor density within that tissue. Clinical observations suggest that elderly persons have decreased responsiveness to thyroid hormones, which is particularly striking in the older patient with thyrotoxicosis, as discussed in the next section. Experimentally, the thyroid hormone response of erythrocyte Ca^{2+}/adenosine triphosphatase (a nonreceptor-mediated activity) falls with age,[15] and in aging rats there is a decrease in hepatic malate dehydrogenase mRNA induction by T_3 compared to young rat.[16] There may also be an age-related decrease in lymphocyte nuclear thyroid hormone receptors.[17] Despite these intriguing data, the decrease in thyroid hormone action that is obvious clinically has yet to be explained at the molecular level.

Thyroid Function Testing

The many recent advances in the laboratory measurement of thyroid function have greatly simplified the evaluation of thyroid dysfunction. Even subtle forms of hypo- and hyperthyroidism can be diagnosed easily, and thyroid hormone therapy can be adjusted with great precision.

Measurement of Thyroid Hormone Concentrations

Radioimmunoassays for T_4 and T_3 are routinely available, with rapid turnaround times. It must be recalled that alterations in TBG affect the total T_4 and T_3 concentrations but not the circulating free thyroid hormone concentrations. Thus, patients with TBG excess or deficiency

TABLE 47.1. Clinical situations associated with abnormal TBG concentrations.

TBG excess	TBG deficiency
Estrogen therapy	Androgen therapy
Acute hepatocellular disease	Chronic liver disease
	Severe catabolic illness
	Congenital X-linked deficiency

TBG, thyroid-binding prealbumin.

TABLE 47.2. Major causes of abnormal serum T_4 concentrations in elderly patients.

Increased T_4	Decreased T_4
Hyperthyroidism	Hypothyroidism
Increased protein binding	TBG deficiency
TBG excess	Serious illness
Anti-T_4 antibodies	Anticonvulsant therapy
Abnormal binding proteins	
Acute illness (transient)	
Decreased T_4 catabolism	
Amiodarone	
High-dose propranolol	

have high or low T_4 and T_3 concentrations, respectively, but are clinically and biochemically euthyroid (Table 47.1). It behooves the clinician to determine the true thyroid status of the patient to avoid erroneous diagnoses and inappropriate therapy. Direct measurement of free T_4 has become more popular due to improved cost-effectiveness; it has rapidly replaced the free thyroxine index (FTI), which is the product of total T_4 and the T_3 resin uptake (T_3RU). The T_3RU is an indirect approximation of TBG binding capacity, and, when used in concert with the total T_4 concentration, it permits distinguishing true thyroid disease from perturbations in TBG concentration. It is important not to confuse the T_3RU, which uses radioactive T_3 in vitro, with the direct assay of serum T_3 (the T_3 radioimmunoassay).

Low Serum Total T_4 Levels

Hypothyroxinemia is characteristic of hypothyroidism, but other conditions also must be considered (Table 47.2). A decrease in serum total T_4 often results from TBG deficiency or inhibition of T_4 binding to TBG by drugs (salsalate, high-dose salicylates) or endogenous factors. A circulating inhibitor of T_4 binding to TBG has been described in nonthyroidal illness and may account for the often extraordinarily low total serum T_4 values (<3 µg/dL) observed in critically ill patients. Unfortunately, most conventional free T_4 assays also yield low results in patients with severe illness that are probably artifactual in nature. Using a technique known as equilibrium dialysis, free T_4 levels are usually found to be normal or even slightly elevated in such circumstances, and most patients are considered to be euthyroid. Low total T_4 and free T_4 levels are also seen in patients taking antiseizure medications because of accelerated hepatic T_4 metabolism and assay artifact, respectively.[18] Because TSH values are normal in this circumstance, these individuals are considered to be euthyroid.

High Serum Total T_4 Levels

Hyperthyroxinemia is seen in most patients with hyperthyroidism. Approximately 10% of patients, however, have T_3 toxicosis, with normal serum T_4 but elevated serum T_3 levels. This circumstance is particularly common in patients with toxic nodules and toxic multinodular goiter. Interestingly, elderly thyrotoxic patients often also develop "T_4 toxicosis," with normal serum T_3 levels, a finding that is rare in younger hyperthyroid patients; this is discussed in more detail in the section on hyperthyroidism.

Euthyroid hyperthyroxinemia (see Table 47.2), that is, a high total T_4 level caused by elevations in TBG or other binding proteins, is commonly confused with biochemical hyperthyroidism. However, use of the free T_4 (fT_4) assay circumvents most problems that arise from alterations in thyroid binding protein levels, and usually permits the correct interpretation of an elevated serum T_4 level and a normal TSH level.

Measurement of TSH

The pituitary gland is exquisitely sensitive to changes in circulating thyroid hormone concentrations. Serum TSH levels therefore are elevated even in mild primary hypothyroidism and, theoretically, TSH levels should be low in virtually all forms of hyperthyroidism. Of course, the serum TSH level will be inappropriately low in hypothyroid patients with pituitary or hypothalamic failure, and, in the rare patient with a TSH-secreting pituitary adenoma causing hyperthyroidism, the TSH level will be inappropriately elevated or normal.

In recent years, TSH assays have been refined, with improvements in their level of sensitivity. Modern techniques can reliably distinguish the low TSH levels in hyperthyroidism from normal TSH levels, which was not possible with older TSH assays. This important modification permits the clinician to diagnose hyperthyroidism (which should yield low or undetectable TSH levels) with greater ease. Most assays in general use are termed sensitive or second-generation assays and typically have a functional detection limit for TSH of approximately 0.1 mU/L. Newer assays, termed ultrasensitive or third generation, are becoming more widespread and have a detection limit in the range of 0.01 to 0.005 mU/L. In both assays, patients with clear-cut hyperthyroidism have undetectable TSH values. Although these new assays have revolutionized the diagnosis of thyroid disease, they have also created difficulties, particularly because a significant fraction of hospitalized patients have TSH values that are subnormal,[19] related to illness or to suppression of serum TSH by high-dose glucocorticoid or dopamine therapy.

A recent metaanalysis of thyroid function screening of geriatric inpatients concluded that there was a high rate of false-positive tests and that the true prevalence of thyroid disease (both hyperthyroidism and hypothyroidism) was similar to that seen in the general population.[20] Screening was not recommended in the absence of symptoms or signs of thyroid disease, but these too lack specificity and sensitivity, it was also pointed out that the likelihood ratio for true thyroid disease was higher (in the range of 7 to 11) with more severely deranged test results (i.e., TSH <0.1 or >20 mU/L).

Recent studies have revealed the existence of a subset of seemingly healthy elderly individuals who have TSH levels that are subnormal and occasionally below the limits of detection in sensitive assays, without evidence of thyroid disease clinically or biochemically.[21] A TSH that is below the detection limit of a third-generation assay (i.e., <0.005 mU/L) is much stronger evidence for true hyperthyroidism than a TSH that is undetectable in a second-generation assay. TSH values will be normal in some patients on repeat testing, but low values will persist in others.[12] Some, perhaps most, of these patients have mild (subclinical) hyperthyroidism, as discussed next, whereas others have no obvious abnormality on long-term follow-up. An isolated subnormal TSH level may be a risk factor for the development of atrial fibrillation,[22] suggesting that seemingly minor changes in T_4 and T_3 levels may be biologically significant.

Radionuclide Evaluation of Thyroid Structure and Function

The thyroid gland traps iodide and other ions, permitting glandular morphology and function to be assessed with isotopes of iodine (^{123}I and ^{131}I) and technetium (^{99m}TcO$_4$). Technetium is used frequently to image the thyroid because it is inexpensive and convenient (imaging after 20 min). However, as it is trapped but not organized (unlike iodide), it cannot provide as much useful information about overall thyroid function as does iodide, with imaging after 6 to 24 h.

Unfortunately, the radioiodine uptake (RAIU) is only occasionally helpful in diagnosing hypo- or hyperthyroidism. The normal 24-h RAIU is between 5% and 25% in most radiology departments, so there is a great deal of overlap between normal and hypothyroid values. Furthermore, many elderly hyperthyroid patients, especially those with toxic nodular goiter, have 24-h RAIU values in the normal range. Additionally, some hypothyroid patients with Hashimoto's thyroiditis can actually have elevated RAIU, whereas patients with hyperthyroidism caused by thyroiditis have low RAIU. Thus, the test is very nonspecific. Stable iodide blocks the uptake of radioactive iodide by the thyroid; therefore, isotopic studies should not be performed within several weeks of receiving iodinated contrast dyes or while patients are taking iodinated drugs such as the antiarrhythmic amiodarone.

Although the 24-h RAIU is of limited usefulness, thyroid scanning is helpful in determining the size and location of thyroid tissue and the functional nature of

TABLE 47.3. Causes of thyrotoxicosis in elderly patients.

Thyroid hormone hypersecretion
  Graves' disease
  Toxic adenoma and toxic nodular goiter
  Iodine-induced hyperthyroidism (rare)
  Metastatic follicular carcinoma (rare)
  Pituitary TSH-secreting tumor (rare)
Follicular disruption
  Subacute thyroiditis
  Painless thyroiditis (rare)
  Radiation thyroiditis, especially after ^{131}I therapy
Exogenous thyroid hormone
  Iatrogenic hyperthyroidism
  Factitious hyperthyroidism

TSH, thyroid-stimulating hormone.

thyroid nodules. Thyroid scanning is also invaluable in the diagnosis of functioning metastases from well-differentiated thyroid cancer.

Other Thyroid-Related Tests

Antithyroid antibodies are important in establishing the diagnosis of autoimmune thyroid disease. Anti-thyroglobulin antibodies are thought to less specific than antithyroid peroxidase (anti-TPO antibodies). Thyrogliobulin is released from the thyroid in a host of thyroid disorders, so it is not useful diagnostically. Its measurement is most crucial in the follow-up of patients with well-differentiated thyroid cancer. Thyroid needle biopsy, thyroid ultrasonography, and neck computed tomography are discussed in the section on thyroid neoplasia and goiter.

Disturbances of Thyroid Function

Thyrotoxicosis

Thyrotoxicosis is being recognized with increasing frequency in the elderly. Although most reports indicate that the peak incidence is in the second and third decades of life, one prospective study found that, of 49 cases of thyrotoxicosis diagnosed over a 3-year period, 28 (57%) were in individuals over the age of 60 years.[23] Graves' disease is the most common cause of thyrotoxicosis in all age groups, but the proportion of patients with toxic multinodular goiter (Plummer's disease) increases with age. Because the prevalence of thyroid nodularity in general is higher in the elderly, some older patients with preexisting nontoxic nodules undoubtedly develop thyrotoxicosis due to Graves' disease, accounting for diagnostic difficulty (Table 47.3). On the other hand, 20% to 50% of elderly thyrotoxic patients have nonpalpable thyroid glands, also making the diagnosis more obscure.[24] In a study of hyperthyroidism in 21 individuals over age 75 years, only 3 had a palpable gland.[25]

Clinical Features

In contrast to the classic symptoms and signs of hyperthyroidism in younger individuals, elderly patients typically display few of the sympathomimetic features that are characteristic of the thyrotoxic state. Thus, the apt term "masked" or "apathetic" thyrotoxicosis has been applied to the elderly thyrotoxic patient who presents with depression, lethargy, weakness, and cachexia. However, most older patients do have symptoms that should bring the diagnosis to mind[26,27] (Table 47.4). Agitation and confusion ("thyrotoxic encephalopathy") can mimic dementia[28] (Table 47.5). Unexplained weight loss, nervousness, palpitations, and tremulousness are present in well over half the patients, with weight loss occurring in up to 80%.[28] In contrast to younger thyrotoxic patients however, elderly patients frequently (but not invariably) have a poor appetite, and constipation is present in a significant minority. The combination of weight loss and diminished appetite often triggers a fruitless evaluation for occult malignancy. Hyperthyroidism causes increased bone turnover, and the presence of what appears to be typical postmenopausal osteoporosis should prompt screening for hyperthyroidism. In a recent prospective study of 9516 white women over age 65 years, a history of hyperthyroidism was an independent risk factor for the development of hip fracture [relative risk (RR), 1.7; 95% CI, 1.2–2.5].[29]

It is well known that the cardiovascular system retains its sensitivity to thyroid hormone action in the elderly. Coupled with a high prevalence of atherosclerotic coro-

TABLE 47.4. Selected symptoms and signs of hyperthyroidism in patients over 70 years of age ($n = 34$) versus patients less than age 50 years ($n = 50$).

Symptom or sign	Percent of elderly+ for finding	Percent of young+ for finding	p value
Fatigue	56	84	0.01
Weight loss	50	51	NS
Tremor	44	84	<0.001
Anorexia	32	4	<0.001
Increased appetite	0	57	<0.001
Nervousness	31	84	<0.001
Heat intolerance	15	92	<0.001
Diarrhea	18	43	0.02
Confusion	16	0	0.01

Source: Data from Ref. 26, with permission.

TABLE 47.5. Most common admission diagnoses in 60 patients with hyperthyroidism over 70 years of age.

Psychiatric disorder	24 (40%)
Hip fracture	11 (18%)
Debility	10 (17%)
Cardiac failure/atrial fibrillation	9 (15%)

Source: Data from Ref. 28, with permission.

nary disease, this probably is the explanation for palpitations, worsening angina, and, more rarely, symptoms of congestive heart failure. Atrial fibrillation, often with a relatively slow ventricular response,[28] is the presenting feature in up to 20% of patients, and the development of atrial fibrillation should always prompt a thorough screen for thyrotoxicosis. One study of nursing home residents over age 65 years found that 11% of men and 31% of women with atrial fibrillation were thyrotoxic.[30] Atrial fibrillation typically develops in patients with dilated left atria, which is apt to be more common in elderly persons.[31]

Despite the fact that Graves' disease is the most common form of thyrotoxicosis in the elderly, infiltrative ophthalmopathy is present less often than in younger of patients,[32] although it may be more severe when it does occur.[33] The reasons for this are unknown.

Laboratory Testing

In contrast to the ease with which the laboratory diagnosis of thyrotoxicosis is made in younger patients, thyroid function test interpretation in the elderly can be a vexing problem. As in younger patients, the serum free T_4 index or free T_4 level, and the T_3 level all are elevated in the average patient. There is controversy, however, regarding the degree of biochemical abnormalities, with one study suggesting that older and younger thyrotoxic patients have similar thyroid function abnormalities[34] and others indicating that the biochemical perturbations are milder in the elderly.[35–38] "T_3 toxicosis" is common in patients with solitary toxic nodules and toxic multinodular goiter. Because these diagnoses occur more frequently in the elderly, the possibility of thyrotoxicosis with normal serum T_4 and free T_4 levels, but an elevated T_3 level, must be kept in mind. Even more problematic is "T_4 toxicosis," which typically occurs in elderly hyperthyroid patients who have concurrent nonthyroidal illness. The decrease in T_4 to T_3 conversion, brought about by the illness, produces normal or even low serum T_3 values. Although the serum T_3 level is virtually always elevated in younger thyrotoxic patients, it is normal in a significant minority of elderly thyrotoxic patients. However, it is of great importance to distinguish T_4 toxicosis from "euthyroid hyperthyroxinemia" because of abnormal protein binding and drugs that inhibit T_4 to T_3 conversion,[39] including amiodarone. It should also be recognized that the serum total T_4 and T_3 levels may actually be normal in debilitated elderly thyrotoxic patients, due to a decrease in serum TBG and a decrease in T_4 to T_3 conversion, respectively. Although the free T_4 index should correct for changes in TBG, it is frequently unreliable in ill patients, and direct measurement of free T_4 is preferable in most cases.

Most truly hyperthyroid individuals have TSH levels that are below the limit of detection in a sensitive or a third-generation assay. Some TSH assays will not distinguish hyperthyroid from normal individuals and yet are called "sensitive" assays.[19] Therefore, a reliable TSH assay is crucial in diagnostic decision making. A low serum TSH is not always the sine qua non of overt hyperthyroidism; some "euthyroid" individuals with nontoxic multinodular goiter may have subclinical hyperthyroidism with normal T_4, free T_4, and T_3 levels, but suppression of the hypothalamic–pituitary axis.[20] One study suggested that measurement of free T_3 could distinguish truly thyrotoxic individuals from those with subclinical hyperthyroidism.[40] TSH levels also may be low in hospitalized patients and may be undetectable even in third-generation TSH assays in critically ill patients.[41] However such patients usually have low rather than high serum T_4 levels, and exclusion of central hypothyroidism is the diagnostic problem, rather than hyperthyroidism.

The 24-h RAIU is normal in up to 30% of elderly patients with Graves' disease and in over two-thirds of elderly individuals with toxic multinodular goiter (Plummer's disease),[34] and is therefore often not helpful in ruling in hyperthyroidism. The measurement of serum T_3 and possibly free T_3 in patients with normal serum T_4 levels and low TSH levels should facilitate the laboratory evaluation and maximize diagnostic accuracy.

Differential Diagnosis

Before initiating a therapy for the thyrotoxic patient, the etiology of hyperthyroidism must be known (see Table 47.3). As stated earlier, Graves' disease is the most frequent cause (in 50%–70% of cases), followed by toxic multinodular goiter. Together, these two account for well over 95% of hyperthyroid patients. Two uncommon forms of thyroiditis cause transient and self-limited hyperthyroidism and are very uncommon in the elderly population. Subacute thyroiditis (De Quervain's) typically presents with severe anterior neck pain, fever, and general malaise and is thought to be viral in origin. Thyroid function test results are elevated due to release of stored hormone into the blood, but the 24-hour RAIU is low, because of damage to the thyroid gland as well as suppression of endogenous TSH by the high thyroid hormone levels. Treatment consists of anti-inflammatory agents (salicylates and other nonsteroidal anti-inflammatory agents, glucocorticoids in severe cases) and beta-adrenergic blocking drugs for symptomatic relief. Painless ("silent") or lymphocytic thyroiditis, rare in the elderly, presents with thyrotoxicosis and small painless goiter.[42] It can be extremely difficult to distinguish from Graves' disease by laboratory testing, except that, as in subacute thyroiditis, the 24-h RAIU is very low. Therapy is limited to the use of beta-adrenergic blockers until the thyrotoxicosis has resolved.

Another diagnosis that should be considered in the elderly patient with thyrotoxicosis is the possibility of a TSH-secreting pituitary tumor. The hallmark is the presence of serum TSH levels that are inappropriate given the elevations in serum T_4 and T_3 levels (i.e., instead of being suppressed, TSH levels are normal or high). A full discussion of inappropriate TSH syndromes is beyond the scope of this chapter but is the subject of a recent review.[43]

Finally, iodine-induced thyrotoxicosis (Jod–Basedow phenomenon) occurs in individuals exposed to iodide or iodide-containing compounds who have an underlying multinodular goiter. The problem has become more common with the recent introduction of the antiarrhythmic amiodarone. There may be two types of amiodarone-induced thyrotoxicosis: one developing in patients with a preexisting multinodular goiter and a second, inflammatory type that resembles painless thyroiditis and may respond to steroid therapy, rather than to antithyroid drugs.[44–46] Although both types of amiodarone-induced thyrotoxicosis are self-limited, they can be very severe, requiring large doses of antithyroid drugs, glucocorticoids, and occasionally even surgery. Although discontinuation of amiodarone would be expected to ameliorate the situation, this is not always possible because of the patient's underlying cardiac disease. Also, the half-life of the drug may be as long as several months, so that stopping it may not afford any immediate benefit.

Treatment

The three treatments for hyperthyroidism are antithyroid drugs, radioactive iodine, and surgery. In elderly patients, surgery is rarely employed because of its attendant morbidity, unless a large toxic multinodular goiter is present and causing local symptoms (dysphagia or dyspnea). Antithyroid drugs (propylthiouracil and methimazole) often are used as primary therapy for Graves' disease in younger patients, for a variety of reasons, including the possibility of spontaneous remission and theoretical but unproved concerns about long-term consequences of radioiodine. In elderly patients, late complications of radioiodine are less relevant and the major goal is definitive therapy with permanent cure. Thus, radioiodine ablation is the treatment of choice for virtually all older thyrotoxic patients.[47]

It must be emphasized, however, that radioiodine therapy cannot be given with impunity to elderly patients. A major concern is possible exacerbation of thyrotoxicosis after radioiodine treatment, due to the release of preformed thyroid hormone into the circulation from radiation-induced thyroiditis. This problem can be life threatening in the elderly thyrotoxic patient, particularly in the presence of underlying cardiac disease. Therefore, many thyroidologists render such patients biochemically

euthyroid with antithyroid drugs before the administration of radioiodine. These drugs impair the biosynthesis of thyroid hormone but not its release. Therefore, at least theoretically, the thyroid is depleted of hormonal stores within 4 to 8 weeks, and radioiodine can be given safely. Traditionally, antithyroid drugs are discontinued for 3 to 5 days before radioiodine administration and are not resumed for 3 to 5 days afterward, so as not to interfere with the intrathyroidal effects of radioiodine. The dosage of the antithyroid drug is tapered over the ensuing months, as the effects of radioiodine are becoming manifest. There is evidence that the use of antithyroid drugs before and after radioiodine therapy results in a higher failure rate of the radioiodine,[48] which can be overcome by using a higher therapy dose of radioiodine.

Antithyroid drugs cause fever, rash, and arthralgias in 1% to 5% of individuals. Agranulocytosis occurs in approximately 1 in 300 to 500 patients (usually in the first 2 months of treatment) and may be more common in elderly patients.[49] Methimazole in low doses (<20 mg/day) may pose less of a risk of agranulocytosis than propylthiouracil, and methimazole has the added advantage of being a once-a-day agent, which improves compliance. Patients beginning antithyroid drug therapy should be warned that if fever or oropharyngitis develops, the medication should be stopped immediately and the physician contacted.

The beta-adrenergic blocking agents are an important adjunct in the management of thyrotoxicosis.[50] Rapid and almost complete resolution of cardiac and neuromuscular symptoms can be accomplished with agents in this class. They do not normalize oxygen consumption or reverse the negative nitrogen balance that typifies the thyrotoxic state, and they should therefore not be used as sole therapy except in those rare patients with self-limited disease due to thyroiditis. These agents are extremely useful before and after antithyroid drug and radioiodine therapy, because euthyroidism generally is not attained for 1 to 2 months after antithyroid drugs are started or for up to 12 months after radioiodine. Propranolol, with its short serum half-life, is not so useful as nadolol or long-acting propranolol. Atenolol and metoprolol, two long-acting cardioselective agents, also are used frequently. The beta-blockers are contraindicated in patients with asthma, and should be used cautiously in patients with congestive heart failure (unless rate related), diabetes treated with oral hypoglycemic agents or insulin, and in patients with Raynaud's phenomenon or intermittent claudication.

Following radioiodine therapy, patients must be followed up expectantly for the development of iatrogenic hypothyroidism. This complication occurs almost inevitably in patients with Graves' disease but is less common in toxic nodular goiter,[51] presumably a result of the failure of radioiodine to be concentrated in suppressed regions of the gland. Posttherapy hypothyroidism develops within 12 months in 40% to 50% of patients with Graves' disease and then occurs at a rate of 2% to 3% per year thereafter. Some patients develop transient hypothyroidism 1 to 6 months after radioiodine therapy, which resolves after a few weeks, then only to be followed by permanent hypothyroidism.[52] The presence of a persistent goiter is a clinical clue that the hypothyroidism is likely to be transient, rather than permanent. Two recent studies suggest that there is an association between radioiodine therapy and subsequent thyroid cancer development, especially in patients with multinodular goiter.[53,54] However, this association may be due to a higher frequency of thyroid cancer in multinodular goiter, rather than a true cause-and-effect relationship.

Atrial fibrillation, especially when present for a relatively short time (less than 6 months), frequently spontaneously converts to normal sinus rhythm with control of thyrotoxicosis. In one study,[55] 62% of patients converted, with 75% converting within 3 weeks of becoming euthyroid; no patient converted after euthyroidism had been established for 4 months. Although age was not predictive of spontaneous conversion in this study, other reports suggest that spontaneous conversion occurs less frequently in elderly patients. Embolic stroke is a recognized complication of atrial fibrillation in thyrotoxicosis. Therefore, routine anticoagulation has been recommended for patients with atrial fibrillation caused by thyrotoxicosis,[56] but therapy must be individualized, and no firm recommendations can be made. If anticoagulation is undertaken, it should be recognized that thyrotoxic patients are *more* sensitive to the effects of coumarin derivatives than are euthyroid patients,[57] and hence require smaller doses to achieve comparable degrees of anticoagulation.

Severe Hyperthyroidism and Thyroid Storm

For those patients who are so severely ill with thyrotoxicosis that hospitalization is required, or if thyrotoxicosis occurs in the setting of severe medical illness (e.g., myocardial infarction), more rapid control of the disease is desirable. Large doses of antithyroid drugs are typically employed (e.g., 200 mg propylthiouracil every 6 h or 40–80 mg methimazole per day as a single dose), which theoretically blocks thyroid hormone production completely. However, because thyroid hormone release is unaffected by antithyroid drugs, other agents must be employed to achieve an expeditious resolution of the thyrotoxic state. Traditionally, potassium iodide (as SSKI, [saturated solution of potassium iodide] containing 35 mg iodide per drop or Lugol's solution, containing 8 mg iodide per drop) has been used for this purpose, because iodine is a potent inhibitor of thyroid hormone release. Doses range form 100 to 500 mg/day in divided doses; iodide should be given only after the patient has been started on antithyroid drugs.

More recently, the iodinated oral cholecystographic contrast agents sodium ipodate (Telepaque) and sodium iopanoate (Oragraffin) have been used in dosages of 1 to 2 g daily in divided doses. These compounds have two beneficial effects. First, they release free iodide into the circulation, which, in turn, inhibits thyroid hormone secretion. Second, these compounds are potent inhibitors of T_4 to T_3 conversion, and they rapidly lower serum T_3 levels toward normal. Thyroxine has a half-life in serum of about 7 days; blocking both synthesis and release does not improve symptoms and signs due to hormone already present in the circulation. By lowering the serum T_3 levels, the iodinated contrast agents should be very useful in this regard. However, it must be acknowledged that there are no clinical trials reporting outcomes with the use of these agents.

The adrenergic blockers also are efficacious in reversing sympathomimetic symptoms and signs caused by circulating thyroid hormone. For life-threatening tachyarrhythmias, 1 mg propranolol hydrochloride can be given slowly intravenously, with the dose repeated every 5 min, or esmolol, a shorter-acting agent, can be employed. For those patients in atrial fibrillation in whom beta-blockers are contraindicated, a calcium channel blocker such as diltiazem can be used.[58]

Thyroid storm is a state of decompensated thyrotoxicosis, defined by severe hypermetabolism, fever, neuropsychiatric changes, and, often, congestive heart failure. Thyroid function test results are no different in patients with thyroid storm than in those with less severe clinical disease. Rather, the ability to deal with the hypermetabolic state is compromised, often by the superimposed stress of acute illness (e.g., infection) or trauma (e.g., surgery). Therapy consists of fluid and electrolyte support, active cooling, and large doses of antithyroid drugs, iodide or iodinated contrast agents, and beta-blockers. Additionally, stress doses of glucocorticoids are usually employed. Because the presentation of hyperthyroidism is relatively more apathetic in elderly patients, they tend to have a better prognosis than younger patients in thyroid storm.[59]

Subclinical Hyperthyroidism

With the development of sensitive TSH assays came the ability to detect a more subtle form of thyroid dysfunction, in which the TSH levels are low or undetectable, but the T_4, free T_4, and T_3 levels are within normal limits. Patients with this constellation of laboratory results generally have few or no symptoms of hyperthyroidism and may or may not have a palpable goiter on physical examination.[60] Subclinical hyperthyroidism has been noted in 1% to 5% of older persons, with a higher frequency if those who are taking excessive quantities of thyroxine are included.[60] Although this syndrome may resolve in

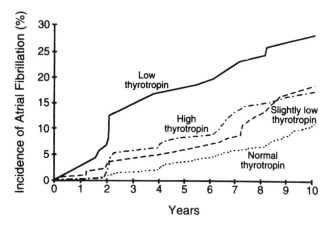

FIGURE 47.3. Incidence of atrial fibrillation in subjects 60 years of age or older, according to serum TSH levels at baseline; 13 of 61 patients developed atrial fibrillation ($p < 0.005$).[22]

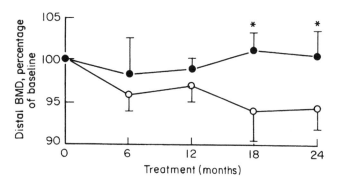

FIGURE 47.4. Mean (±SEM) percentage of baseline bone mineral density in distal forearm in postmenopausal women with subclinical hyperthyroidism randomized to receive methimazole (●, $n = 8$) or no treatment (○, $n = 8$) (*$p < 0.05$).[63]

some patients upon later testing,[12] suggesting that it can be caused by transient intercurrent illness, it usually persists and may evolve into overt hyperthyroidism over time.[59]

One long-term follow-up study found that patients with subclinical hyperthyroidism had a two- to three-fold higher rate of atrial fibrillation than euthyroid controls, suggesting that the low TSH levels have biologic significance[22] (Fig. 47.3). Subclinical hyperthyroidism may[61] or may not[62] be associated with a bone mineral density that is lower than that seen in age-matched controls. However, two recent reports noted an increase in bone mineral density in patients with subclinical hyperthyroidism after either a 2-year course of antithyroid drug therapy[63] (Fig. 47.4) or following radioiodine.[64] Therefore, although treatment of elderly asymptomatic individuals with subclinical hyperthyroidism could be justified to protect the cardiovascular system or the skeleton, it remains controversial.[65] Certainly, if subclinical hyperthyroidism is due to overzealous thyroxine replacement

therapy, the dose of medication should be adjusted until the TSH levels are normal.

Hypothyroidism

Approximately 70% of hypothyroid patients are over age 50 years at the time of diagnosis.[66] The prevalence of hypothyroidism in the population depends on how the condition is defined: if a low serum T_4 or free T_4 level is the criterion, approximately 0.5% of individuals (largely women) over age 65 years will be found to be overtly hypothyroid.[1,2] If the more liberal definition of an elevated serum TSH level with or without a low T_4 level is employed, up to 17.5% of individuals over age 75 years will have mild hypothyroidism.[2,59,67,68] This latter situation may be more appropriately termed subclinical hypothyroidism because serum T_4 and free T_4 levels are still within the broad range of normal.

Etiology

The most common cause of hypothyroidism in the elderly is autoimmune thyroid failure (Hashimoto's thyroiditis, chronic lymphocytic thyroiditis) (Table 47.6). In parallel with the high prevalence of autoimmune thyroiditis in the elderly, the prevalence of antithyroid antibody positivity also rises with age.[69] Over two-thirds of patients with thyroid failure have antithyroid antibodies.[70] Two types of antithyroid antibodies have been described in Hashimoto's thyroiditis: antimicrosomal (now termed antithyroid peroxidase or anti-TPO antibodies) and antithyroglobulin. Antimicrosomal antibodies are highly specific for autoimmune thyroiditis. Antithyroglobulin antibodies, on the other hand, are not as specific for autoimmune thyroid disease, and their presence in the absence of antimicrosomal antibody is not sufficient to establish the diagnosis.

TABLE 47.6. Selected symptoms and signs of hypothyroidism in patients over 70 years of age ($n = 67$) versus patients less than 50 years of age ($n = 54$).

Symptom or sign	Percent of elderly+ for finding	Percent of young+ for finding	p value
Fatigue	68	83	NS
Mental slowness	45	48	NS
Drowsiness	40	43	NS
Dry skin	35	45	NS
Constipation	33	41	NS
Depression	28	52	NS
Cold intolerance	35	65	<0.002
Weight gain	24	59	<0.001
Muscle cramps	20	55	<0.001
Paresthesiae	18	61	<0.001
Slow reflexes	24	31	NS

Source: Data from Ref. 72, with permission.

Iatrogenic hypothyroidism is an additional important, although less frequent, cause of thyroid failure. Radioiodine and surgical therapy for Graves' disease usually lead to permanent hypothyroidism. Additionally, several studies suggest that permanent hypothyroidism is a late phase in the evolution of drug-treated Graves' disease. Not surprisingly, external beam radiotherapy to the head and neck region also can cause late thyroid hypofunction. Lithium- and iodine-containing medications can provoke hypothyroidism; this has become an increasing problem with the antiarrhythmic amiodarone, which used widely in older patients.[71] Finally, many patients with subacute or painless thyroiditis have mild transient hypothyroidism following hyperthyroidism, but this rarely requires therapy. Hypothalamic or pituitary disease are unusual causes of hypothyroidism.

Diagnosis

The diagnosis of hypothyroidism is not difficult in a young patient with typical symptoms of fatigue, weight gain, dry skin, cold intolerance, and constipation. In elderly patients, however, these same complaints are attributed all too often to the aging process itself. The problem is further complicated by the insidious development of symptoms, often over a period of years, and by patients who present in an atypical manner[72] or with no symptoms at all.[73] In a recent study of 67 older hypothyroid patients (mean age, 79 years), they were more likely to present with fatigue and weakness, and less likely to have cold intolerance, weight gain, paresthesiae, and muscle cramps compared to 54 younger hypothyroid patients with a mean age of 41 years.[72] Thus, it behooves the physician to be creative and vigilant and to resist the stereotypical image of the "normal aging process."

Certain findings on physical examination should alert the clinician to the possibility of hypothyroidism. Hypertension, for example, can be a presenting sign, as can bradycardia and, surprisingly, various tachyarrhythmias. Hypothermic patients always should be evaluated for hypothyroidism, hypoglycemia, and sepsis. Although nonpitting edema of the face and limbs is a hallmark of hypothyroidism, pitting edema also is frequently found, possibly due to a lowered glomerular filtration rate and decreased cardiac output. Frank congestive heart failure is unusual in hypothyroidism, and cardiomegaly more often is a result of the presence of pericardial effusion; although the pericardial effusions in hypothyroidism are usually not hemodynamically significant, tamponade has been described. Pleural effusions and ascites also can be seen.

In contrast to younger hypothyroid patients, older individuals rarely have a goiter. Whether this represents the natural history of goitrous autoimmune thyroiditis or a separate, atrophic variant of autoimmune thyroiditis is unclear.[74] Ophthalmopathy also may be present, even in the absence of a history of Graves' disease. Neuropsychiatric signs, including depression, lassitude, impaired cognition, and poor memory, are common; muscle cramps, peripheral neuropathy (carpal tunnel syndrome), and cerebellar ataxia are additional features of hypothyroidism, along with ileus, urinary retention, and sleep apnea. All patients with dementia should be evaluated for possible hypothyroidism.[75] Recent epidemiologic studies suggest an association between Alzheimer's disease and hypothyroidism, but no causal relationship has been proven.[76]

Sometimes hypothyroidism is found serendipitously because of abnormal laboratory data. Elevations in serum cholesterol levels (when previously normal) and high creatine kinase levels are hallmarks of hypothyroidism and are caused by decreased clearance. Hyponatremia commonly is seen in elderly patients and should always prompt an evaluation of thyroid status. Its origin is controversial but probably relates to both decreased glomerular filtration and the inappropriate secretion of vasopressin. A normochromic normocytic anemia, possibly due to decreased erythropoetin secretion, commonly is seen in hypothyroidism, and pernicious anemia occurs frequently in association with autoimmune thyroid disease.

Laboratory Diagnosis

Hypothyroidism is perhaps the simplest thyroid functional abnormality to diagnose. The hallmark of primary hypothyroidism is a low serum free thyroxine index or free T_4, with concomitant elevation of the serum TSH. As previously noted, "subclinical" hypothyroidism is characterized by normal serum T_4 levels with only minimal to modest increases in TSH levels (e.g., 5–20 mU/L, with normal values <5 mU/L). Measurement of T_3 is of little use in the diagnosis of hypothyroidism, because normal serum levels are often maintained until severe hypothyroidism supervenes; this may be related to a shift from T_4 to T_3 secretion by the thyroid gland, under intense stimulation by high levels of TSH.

Several pitfalls in the laboratory diagnosis of hypothyroidism deserve mention. First, some patients with secondary hypothyroidism (i.e., due to hypothalamic or pituitary disease with TSH *deficiency*) have low T_4 values with inappropriately low or normal serum TSH levels. In hypothalamic/pituitary disease, the pituitary may secrete a TSH molecule that is immunologically active in the radioimmunoassay but has lower than normal bioactivity. Thus, if hypothyroidism is suspected clinically and serum T_4 values are low, evaluation of hypothalamic and pituitary anatomy and function is indicated, even if the serum TSH level is "normal." Generally, other hormonal deficits will be present in this clinical circumstance (e.g., adrenal insufficiency, low FSH and LH in a post-menopausal woman, or hypogonadotropic hypogonadism in a man).

A second problem that confounds the diagnosis hypothyroidism is severe illness.[40,77] It may be extremely difficult to distinguish a critically ill patient with low T_4 and normal or low TSH levels from one with secondary hypothyroidism (see previous discussion). To further complicate matters, serum TSH levels occasionally rise during the recovery phase of illness, often to levels consistent with primary hypothyroidism. In this circumstance, repeating the TSH measurement after recovery is complete is the appropriate strategy.

Treatment

Once the diagnosis of primary hypothyroidism is made, therapy with thyroxine should he initiated; patients with chronic fatigue or obesity who are not hypothyroid should never be treated with this drug. Thyroxine is generally well absorbed from the gastrointestinal tract, although the fractional absorption may decline slightly with age.[78] Its long serum half-life produces nonfluctuating serum levels. Cholestyramine, sucralfate, aluminum hydroxide, and possibly ferrous sulfate and calcium supplements interfere with its absorption and should not be taken concurrently. As in healthy untreated individuals, much of the orally administered thyroxine is deiodinated to T_3, at a rate determined by the patient's clinical status (i.e., decreased in illness or starvation). Thyroxine is available in proprietary forms (Synthroid, Levothroid, and Levoxyl) and in generic form. Although most generic brands probably are equivalent to the proprietary preparations in hormonal content, some have been shown to be inferior with respect to hormonal content or bioavailability. And unfortunately, because it is often quite difficult to determine the ultimate manufacturer of a generic product, patients may unknowingly be switched from one generic to another when prescriptions are refilled. Therefore, most endocrinologists prefer the proprietary forms of thyroxine for their proven reliability and consistency.

The dictum "start low, go slow" should be followed in elderly patients when initiating thyroxine therapy, because rapid increases in myocardial oxygen consumption theoretically could trigger or worsen angina. Therefore, it is best to be prudent and initiate treatment with doses of 25 to 50μg/day, with monthly monitoring of thyroid function. The biochemical goal of therapy is the normalization of serum TSH levels in a sensitive TSH assay; the TSH level should not be below the normal range, which would suggest overreplacement. Even seemingly minor changes in dose can cause large changes in serum TSH values.[79] As discussed earlier, the daily thyroxine production rate declines with age, and consequently, as has been noted by most investigators, the daily

thyroxine replacement dose is approximately 10% lower in elderly patients than in young or middle-aged adults.[80] In general, doses of 0.8 to 1.2μg/kg of lean body mass (LBM) are sufficient to normalize serum TSH levels in patients over age 70 years. The thyroxine replacement dose for elderly patients can be predicted by the following formula:[81]

$$T_4(\mu g/day) = 3.6 \times LBM - 30$$
$$LBM(males) = (79.5 - 0.24M - 0.15 \times A) \times M/73.2$$
$$LBM(females) = (69.8 - 0.26M - 0.12 \times A) \times M/73.2$$

where M indicates body weight in kilograms and A indicates age in years. Overreplacement is to be avoided, not only because of untoward cardiac effects[82] but also because of convincing data in postmenopausal women showing that even mild asymptomatic iatrogenic hyperthyroidism can be associated with accelerated bone loss.[83] The dose requirement may be higher in patients with malabsorption or in those taking anticonvulsants or amiodarone.

A large and potentially bewildering number of thyroid hormone preparations are available (Table 47.7). These formulations are traditionally classified as "synthetic" or "biologic." As already described, synthetic thyroxine is the therapy of choice. Another synthetic preparation, liotrix, is a combination of T_4 and T_3 (Thyrolar). This product was developed decades ago, before it was known that T_3 arose from peripheral conversion of T_4, rather than from direct thyroidal secretion. It is now clear that providing T_3 to the patient is unnecessary and theoretically could raise serum T_3 levels to above normal, causing palpitations, anxiety, and other bothersome symptoms. Furthermore, liotrix is more expensive, and its use makes monitoring of therapy more difficult and expensive, because of the necessity of measuring serum T_3 levels as well as T_4 levels. An additional synthetic thyroid hormone, pure L-triiodothyronine (Cytomel), should never be used for long-term replacement therapy. It is often used for short periods in patients with thyroid cancer preparing for radioiodine scanning.

The "biologic" thyroid hormone preparations include desiccated thyroid, derived from the thyroid glands of

TABLE 47.7. Thyroid hormone preparations.

Preparation	Available forms
Synthetic	
Thyroxine (T_4)[a]	Synthoid, Levothyroid, Levoxyl, generics
Triiodothyronine (T_3)	Cytomel, Triostat (i.v.)
Liotrix (T_4 and T_3)	Thyrolar
Biologic	
USP thyroid	Generic, Armour, Thyrar

[a] Drug of choice.

slaughterhouse animals. The generic biologic preparations are notorious for their lack of standardization. The proprietary preparations have better quality control but suffer from the same problem as liotrix and T_3, that is, they contain T_3, which is an undesirable drug for chronic replacement therapy. Most endocrinologists agree that the biologic preparations are of historical interest only; patients who are taking them should be switched to synthetic thyroxine at doses of 0.8 µg/lb body weight per day.

Special Therapeutic Considerations

Hypothyroid Patients with Severe Coronary Artery Disease

Elderly hypothyroid patients not infrequently have concomitant coronary artery disease.[56] Long-standing hypothyroidism, with its attendant hypercholesterolemia, may be an important contributing factor in the development of atherosclerosis. A recent Dutch study found that subclinical hypothyroidism was also an independent risk factor for atherosclerosis (RR, 1.7; 95% CI, 1.1–2.6) and myocardial infarction (RR, 2.3; 95% CI, 1.3–4.0), independent of serum lipid levels.[84] In the setting of overt or silent ischemic heart disease, it may be difficult to replace thyroxine fully without provoking or exacerbating angina. Every effort should be made to maximize the antianginal regimen medically. If that fails, and if the patient remains clinically hypothyroid because of the inability to prescribe an adequate dosage of thyroxine, coronary artery bypass surgery should be considered.[85] Open heart surgery, and, indeed, any surgery, can be performed safely in patients with severe hypothyroidism, so long as scrupulous attention is paid to the patient's pulmonary status and fluid balance in the perioperative period.[86] In the untreated hypothyroid patient with unstable angina, it is probably best to send the patient to surgery or percutaneous transluminal coronary angioplasty (PTCA) rather than risk myocardial infarction by treating the hypothyroidism and delaying surgery.[85]

Subclinical Hypothyroidism

Subclinical hypothyroidism is defined biochemically as normal serum T_4 and free T_4 levels with an elevated serum TSH level. As noted earlier, it is one of the most common thyroid disorders among elderly persons, being present in up to 17.5% of women over age 60 years.[59] Most patients have circulating antithyroid antibodies, suggesting that the condition is autoimmune in nature.[59] Some patients have a history of Graves' disease, while others are taking drugs (lithium- or iodide-containing compounds) that are known to inhibit thyroid function, especially in the presence of underlying autoimmune thyroid disease. Because of the high prevalence of subclinical hypothyroidism in elderly women, routine

screening (every 5 years) of older individuals for hypothyroidism with a serum TSH determination has been recommended by the American Thyroid Association[87] and several other professional organizations, including the American College of Physicians.[88]

A central question is whether patients with subclinical hypothyroidism, who are seemingly asymptomatic and appear to be suffering solely from a biochemical abnormality, should be treated. Although no definite answer can be provided at this time, one study indicated that patients with subclinical hypothyroidism do have subtle symptoms consistent with mild thyroid failure.[89] Furthermore, treatment with small doses of thyroxine (50–100 µg/day) resulted in a statistically significant symptomatic improvement compared with placebo treatment. Improved performance in cognitive function tests[90,91] and serum lipid profiles[92] has been reported, but these findings have not been noted in all studies.[67] In reviewing the results of three randomized trials,[89,90,93] it was concluded that 0 to 28 of 100 symptomatic patients would benefit from thyroxine therapy.[94] However, these authors did not review other studies showing benefit in cognitive function,[91] improvements in intraocular pressure,[95] and possible improvement in coronary angiograms[96] with thyroxine therapy. On the basis of these data, therapy can be justified, if there are no contraindications (e.g., severe angina).

Replacement therapy also can be used as prophylaxis against overt hypothyroidism. Several studies have shown that those patients with subclinical hypothyroidism who also have circulating antithyroid antibodies are likely to develop overt hypothyroidism; in the elderly, the rate may be as high as 20% per year.[97] In a large prospective 20-year follow-up study of 2779 adults, the risk of developing overt hypothyroidism was assessed according to sex, baseline serum TSH level, and antithyroid antibody positivity.[98] In women, the odds ratios (with 95% confidence intervals) for progression to overt hypothyroidism were 8 (3–20) for raised serum TSH alone, 8 (5–15) for positive antithyroid antibodies alone, and 38 (22–65) in women with both elevated serum TSH and antibody positivity. Based on an analysis of the annual incidence data, it was calculated that a woman with a baseline serum TSH of 6 mU/L and positive serum antibodies had a 57% risk of developing overt hypothyroidism over a 20-year period. Helfand and Redfern analyzed these data to examine the implications of therapy in antibody-positive individual.[94] If 1000 people over age 35 are screened, 80 (8%) will be found to be hypothyroid and about half of these will have positive antibodies. By 5 years, very few women will have become hypothyroid (approximately 3 of 40), so the number needed to treat to prevent 1 person from becoming hypothyroid is 13. By 20 years, many more women will have become hypothyroid (roughly 24 of 40), so that 16 of 40 would have taken thyroxine who would not have progressed to overt hypothyroidism. However, such women might have received the benefits alluded to above (improved mild hypothyroid symptoms and cognitive function, etc.). Although definitive data from large randomized trials are lacking, many experts prefer to treat subclinically hypothyroid individuals when they have symptoms consistent with mild hypothyroidism, when antithyroid antibodies are positive, or when there is evidence of an abnormal lipid profile. Hypercholesterolemic patients with serum TSH levels above 10 mU/L are the most likely to benefit from thyroxine therapy, whereas lipid levels are unlikely to change in patients with serum TSH values below 10 mU/L.[99]

If it is elected not to treat a patient with subclinical hypothyroidism, it would be reasonable to test for antithyroid antibodies, because careful monitoring for thyroid failure is necessary if they are present. It should be pointed out, however, that hypothyroidism can develop even in the absence of antithyroid antibodies,[98] so that continuous monitoring of thyroid function is necessary in all untreated patients with subclinical hypothyroidism.

Myxedema Coma

Myxedema coma, as does its hyperthyroid counterpart thyroid storm, results from the physiologic decompensation of a hypothyroid individual.[100,101] Generally, there is a precipitating factor, most often an undiagnosed infection. Patients with myxedema "coma" are not necessarily comatose and can present with stupor, seizures, or psychotic manifestations. Myxedema coma is most often a disease of elderly hypothyroid individuals and generally occurs in the winter months.

The diagnosis of myxedema coma usually is difficult, although it is made easier if there is a history of thyroid disorder or a neck scar or proptosis on physical examination. Hypothermia is a frequent, but not invariable, manifestation; its absence should suggest an occult infection. If the diagnosis is considered, therapy should be initiated, because mortality approaches 50%, even with treatment. Optimal management consists of scrupulous attention to the patient's pulmonary, cardiovascular, gastrointestinal, and renal status. Often intubation and ventilatory assistance are necessary because of carbon dioxide retention. Active warming is contraindicated, because severe hypotension may supervene. A search for infection and prompt treatment is mandatory. Hyponatremia is common, and free water must be administered judiciously. Sedatives and narcotics should be avoided because of the risk of further respiratory depression. Stress doses of glucocorticoids are usually given until adrenal insufficiency has been formally ruled out.

Thyroxine should be administered intravenously because gastrointestinal absorption may be altered because of hypomotility. Initial doses of 0.3 to 0.5 mg have been traditionally recommended to replace the total body thyroid hormone pool, with daily doses of 0.1 mg thereafter. However, lower doses may be more appropriate in older patients (see following). It has been suggested that T_3 therapy might be preferred, because T_3 is the active thyroid hormone and, in the presence of severe illness, insufficient quantities of T_4 might be converted peripherally to T_3. However, it can also be argued that the body's controlled formation of T_3 and T_4 is more desirable than a sudden and dramatic increase in serum T_3. Indeed, a number of deaths have been attributed to T_3-induced cardiac arrhythmias.[100] Therefore, most experts recommend thyroxine rather than T_3 for myxedema coma,[101] although controlled studies are lacking. If the patient fails to respond to T_4 therapy, intravenous T_3 (Triostat) in doses of 10 to 25 μg every 8 to 12 h might be tried.

Because of the rarity of myxedema coma, there are no randomized clinical trials comparing various replacement regimens. In a recent retrospective analysis of 87 cases of myxedema coma, it was observed that higher mortality was associated with greater patient age, cardiac disease, and higher doses of thyroid hormone replacement (T_4 doses >500 μg/day or T_3 doses >75 μg/day), especially when given intravenously.[100] The authors concluded that elderly individuals with myxedema coma should receive lower than conventionally recommended doses of thyroid hormone. Because the study was retrospective, it is possible that sicker patients received the highest doses of thyroid hormone, which might account for the apparent association between higher mortality and thyroid hormone dose. However, the Acute Physiology and Chronic Health Evaluation (APACHE) scores calculated by the authors did not differ between fatal and nonfatal cases. Myxedema coma may be treatable with relatively low doses (e.g., 25 μg) of thyroxine, and very high intravenous doses (>500 μg) may not be suitable for older patients.

Thyroid Neoplasia and Goiter

Thyroid nodularity increases in frequency with age. Autopsy data suggest that 90% of women over age 70 years and 60% of men over age 80 years have one or more thyroid nodules,[1] and ultrasound studies reveal a 40% to 60% prevalence of thyroid nodules in unselected elderly populations.[102] Clinically significant nodules, that is, those that come to medical attention because they are palpable, are also more prevalent in the elderly, with approximately 5% of adults having a palpable nodule in the Framingham study population.[103] As would be expected, palpable nodules are also much more common in women than in men (6% versus 2% in the Framing-

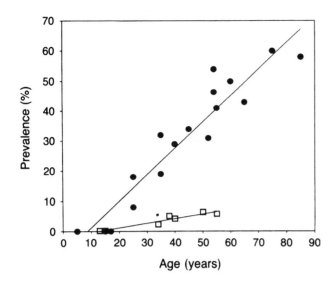

FIGURE 47.5. Prevalence of thyroid nodules detected at autopsy or by ultrasound (●), or by palpation (□) in subjects without a prior history of radiation exposure or known thyroid disease.[105]

ham study)[103] (Fig. 47.5). In the Wickham survey, thyroid nodules were found in about 1% of males and in 9% of women over age 75.[4]

It is clear from surgical or thyroid imaging data that at least one-quarter of nodules that are thought to be solitary on palpation are, in reality, part of a multinodular gland. Nevertheless, it is useful to distinguish clinically solitary nodules and so-called dominant nodules (nodules that are larger than the others that may be palpably present within the gland) because these have a greater likelihood of being malignant. Fortunately, malignancy is present in only about 10% of nodules, a frequency that is no higher and is perhaps lower than in younger patients with thyroid nodules. Given the low likelihood of malignancy, it is a challenge to diagnose and treat those nodules that are cancerous while at the same time avoiding unnecessary surgery in the 90% of patients who have benign disease.

Thyroid Nodules

Clinical Assessment

Although excision of all nodules would be simultaneously diagnostic and curative, surgery, particularly in the elderly, is associated with excess morbidity as well as great potential expense. Although a number of historical features (older-age male,[104] rapid growth, compressive symptoms) and physical findings (firm or rock-hard consistency, fixation to underlying neck structures, and cervical adenopathy) are important clues that suggest malignancy, there is considerable overlap in findings with benign nodules. Indeed, only a distinct minority of malignant nodules have a "classic" clinical presentation.

A history of head, neck, or upper thoracic radiation in childhood or adolescence is important to elicit. From the 1920s through the early 1960s, several million people received external x-irradiation for thymic enlargement, tonsillitis, mastoiditis, acne, and a host of other benign conditions. Many thousands of irradiated patients who are now in the geriatric population are at excess (3- to 10-fold) risk for the development of thyroid cancer, as well as benign nodular disease. In addition, it is becoming clear that radiation for malignancies that included the thyroid gland in the radiation port, for example, the mantle area for Hodgkin's disease, can also be associated with thyroid carcinoma. Thus, a history of radiation exposure warrants a prompt and definitive evaluation.

Differential Diagnosis

Although most thyroid nodules are, in fact, benign tumors, any generalized thyroid disease can present as a thyroid nodule. Thus, the various forms of thyroiditis (subacute, Hashimoto's) are not infrequently asymmetric in their involvement and can mimic a solitary nodule. Other rare causes of an apparent thyroid nodule include congenital hemiagenesis of the opposite lobe of the thyroid, cystic hygromas, and teratomas. Thyroid cysts and neoplasms (benign follicular adenomas, colloid nodules, nodular adenomatous hyperplasia, and carcinomas) comprise the majority of all nodules, however. Although most forms of thyroid cancer (papillary, medullary, anaplastic) are easily diagnosed by means of biopsy, follicular lesions are notoriously difficult to evaluate cytopathologically. The majority of follicular neoplasms are benign, but it can be extremely difficult to distinguish a more atypical benign tumor from a minimally invasive follicular carcinoma. Hürthle cell tumors, a variety of follicular adenoma once thought to always be malignant, are usually benign. Rarely, thyroid nodules are due to metastatic spread of cancer to the thyroid gland.

Laboratory Evaluation

Although a large number of blood tests and radiologic procedures are available to aid in the evaluation of thyroid nodules, most are, unfortunately, of little practical use. Results of routine thyroid function tests are almost always normal, but are worth obtaining to find the rare patient with hyperthyroidism caused by an autonomously functioning nodule and to enable the diagnosis of hypothyroidism, which would suggest Hashimoto's thyroiditis as the underlying disease process.

Other blood tests should be used more selectively. A serum calcitonin determination should be obtained only if there is a family history of medullary thyroid carcinoma or other condition suggestive of multiple endocrine neoplasia syndrome type 2. Antithyroid antibody assays might be performed if the serum TSH level is elevated, suggesting Hashimoto's thyroiditis. Serum thyroglobulin levels are nonspecifically elevated in a host of thyroid diseases, and this determination is used mainly in the follow-up of patients with thyroid cancer.

Traditionally, after routine blood tests, thyroid scanning with radioiodine or technetium has been the next step in the workup of a thyroid nodule. Nodules that concentrate the radionuclide ("hot" nodules) are, for practical purposes, never malignant, and require no further evaluation other than to be sure that hyperthyroidism is not present. On the other hand, hypofunctioning nodules ("cold" nodules) require further evaluation with needle biopsy.

Although categorizing nodules as hot or cold is intellectually satisfying, it is not cost-effective, because at least 90% of all nodules are hypofunctioning. An approach that is gaining wider acceptance is the performance of needle biopsy as the initial diagnostic step.[105,106] The advantage of this scheme is that a scan is avoided in the 90% of patients who would require a biopsy. The disadvantage is that the 10% of patients with hot nodules undergo biopsy needlessly. On the other hand, the fine-needle aspiration biopsy is a relatively painless procedure with virtually no morbidity (see following).

Thyroid ultrasonography, once considered a valuable tool in the evaluation of thyroid nodules, is being used with less frequency nowadays. Although purely cystic lesions are not malignant, pure cysts of the thyroid are rare. In fact, more than 95% of nodules are either solid or complex (having solid and cystic components), the latter having the same clinical implications as a solid lesion. Thus, routine ultrasonography is not a cost-effective initial diagnostic test. It can be a useful technique for monitoring the size of nodules, particularly those that are difficult to palpate.

Incidentalomas of the Thyroid

Studies of normal individuals undergoing thyroid ultrasound have shown a surprisingly high rate of thyroid nodularity, especially in middle-aged and older women. In one report, small, often multiple subcentimeter thyroid nodules were found in 72% of women aged 25 to 75 years, with a nonsignificant trend toward increasing nodule frequency with age.[107] The prevalence of thyroid nodules in similarly aged men was 41%, which was significantly different from that seen in women. When small (<1–1.5 cm), nonpalpable nodules are found serendipitously, most experts recommend monitoring with serial ultrasound examinations, rather than attempting fine-needle aspiration or other diagnostic procedures.[108] If the nodule grows to a size greater than 1.5 cm, needle aspiration using ultrasound guidance would be indicated.

Fine-Needle Aspiration Biopsy of Thyroid Nodules

Thyroid needle biopsy, and more specifically, fine-needle aspiration biopsy, has revolutionized the care of patients with thyroid disease.[105,106] Its diagnostic accuracy depends on the skill of the person performing the procedure, and, even more importantly, on the expertise of the cytopathologist who is interpreting the aspirate. For malignancy, the false-negative rate is low (<1%–5%),[105,106] although the specificity is only about 70% (if suspicious nodules are included). The positive predictive value approaches 99% in most series.[105,106] Most series report that 60% to 70% of lesions are benign and 5% are malignant. About 25% are "indeterminate" or "suspicious," and these include less well differentiated benign follicular adenomas, Hürthle cell neoplasms, and follicular carcinoma. Only 15% of suspicious lesions prove to be malignant at the time of surgery.[109]

Management of Thyroid Nodules

If the nodule is benign, then no further diagnostic evaluation is necessary, although continued follow-up is important. The wisdom of routine suppression therapy with thyroxine has been questioned, especially in the elderly (see following). Malignant nodules, of course, require surgery. If a nodule is suspicious cytologically, the next step would be a thyroid scan, if it had not been performed before the biopsy, because suspicious lesions can be benign functioning (hot) follicular adenomas. If the nodule is hot, then additional laboratory studies should be performed to rule out hyperthyroidism. If the suspicious nodule is cold, then excision is generally recommended. An alternate approach would be a 3- to 6-month trial of suppression therapy with thyroxine. If the nodule fails to decrease in size, then surgery is indicated. If the nodule shrinks, then close follow-up with continued thyroxine therapy is reasonable.

The rationale for thyroxine suppression therapy of suspicious nodules rests with the belief that thyroid growth is dependent upon continued stimulation by TSH. Theoretically, when pituitary TSH secretion is suppressed with exogenous thyroid hormone, both the thyroid and benign nodules should decrease in size. Unfortunately, many benign nodules do not shrink with thyroxine therapy, probably because TSH is not the only factor controlling thyroid growth. Several recent prospective trials comparing thyroxine with placebo have shown little apparent benefit of thyroxine treatment.[110,111] However, decades of clinical experience have shown that some nodules do respond to thyroxine; also, one controlled study indicated that thyroxine is better than placebo in the treatment of multinodular goiter,[112] which might be present in patients with seemingly "solitary" thyroid nodules. Thus, suppression therapy for suspicious thyroid nodules may be an attractive approach in elderly patients in whom coexisting disease makes surgery less appealing.

It should be recognized, however, that suppression therapy is effective in only a minority of patients. In a recent meta-analysis of randomized trials of thyroxine therapy, a decrease in nodule volume of 50% was seen in 17% of patients.[113] Thus, the failure of a nodule to decrease in size with a suppressive dose of thyroxine (1–2 µg/kg of body weight) is not necessarily an indication of malignancy and, in the presence of a benign biopsy, should not be an indication for surgery. If the biopsy is suspicious, however, surgery should be more strongly considered. Continued enlargement despite adequate suppression, even with a benign biopsy specimen, should prompt reevaluation, including repeated biopsy or surgical excision.

Routine suppression therapy in elderly patients with thyroid nodules that are unequivocally benign has been questioned,[114,115] because the benefits of treatment are uncertain, and there are potential risks, especially in elderly patients, because of the intentional production of mild iatrogenic hyperthyroidism. This problem can be compounded if the nodule is part of a multinodular goiter, in which areas of autonomous (i.e., nonsuppressible) function are present. Recent data have documented bone loss in postmenopausal patients undergoing thyroid hormone suppression, with attenuation by concomitant estrogen therapy.[116] Suppression therapy can also cause tachycardia,[81] with the potential for arrhythmias.[22] Therefore, a period of observation without treatment is reasonable, because benign nodules often remain stable or can even resolve spontaneously. If a biopsy-proven benign nodule enlarges, thyroxine therapy might be employed, but care should be taken to employ a dose of thyroxine that will keep the serum TSH level below the lower limit of normal, but above the limit of detection, to avoid skeletal or cardiac complications.[114]

Goiter (Diffuse or Nodular)

Goiter, or a generalized enlargement of the thyroid, is a common problem in the elderly. Indeed, large, nodular, compressive goiters are seen almost exclusively in this age group. Goiters are termed diffuse or nodular, depending on their surface characteristics on physical examination. A significant minority of goiters are caused by Hashimoto's thyroiditis, but most are idiopathic. Pathologically, most idiopathic multinodular goiters consist of areas of nodular adenomatous hyperplasia, interspersed with hemorrhagic cysts, fibrosis, and calcification.

Goiters usually are discovered at physical examination or visualized on routine chest radiographs as a mass in the anterior superior mediastinum. Mild tracheal deviation is frequent and does not necessarily indicate respiratory compromise. Goiter uncommonly causes symptoms by compressing adjacent neck structures (e.g., dysphagia, respiratory difficulty, superior vena cava syndrome). It should be emphasized, however, that such symptoms are most often due to benign disease and not thyroid cancer. A history of rapid growth is worrisome, although benign hemorrhagic cysts frequently present in this manner, often with concomitant pain radiating to the ear. Even recurrent laryngeal nerve paralysis can be caused by benign thyroid enlargement, rather than malignancy.

Aside from the history and physical examination, routine thyroid function tests, including a serum T_3 and/or a high-sensitivity serum TSH determination, should be performed in all patients with goiter because of the possibility of subtle thyrotoxicosis. Antithyroid antibodies (especially antithyroid peroxidase antibodies) are also helpful in diagnosing autoimmune thyroiditis, especially in patients whose goiter is diffuse and firm on palpation. Computed tomography or MRI of the neck and chest can be helpful in delineating the extent of the goiter in the thorax, or the degree of tracheal deviation or compression, but generally these procedures are unnecessary.

The central issues in the patient with a large goiter are (1) whether malignancy is present and (2) whether there is clinically significant compression of adjacent neck structures. Regarding malignancy, if there is any suggestion of a recently enlarging goiter or if there is a dominant nodule within a multinodular goiter, a biopsy should be performed. With respect to esophageal or tracheal compression, a history of dysphagia or dyspnea is usually obtained. It should be emphasized, however, that upper airway compromise may be subtle or asymptomatic or may present as "asthma" or wheezing. Pulmonary function testing, with evaluation of upper airway function by means of flow-volume loops, should be performed in all patients with large goiters who have suggestive respiratory symptoms or evidence of tracheal compression, even in the absence of symptoms.

The indications for surgery in elderly patients with large goiters are more stringent than in younger individuals. Obviously, malignancy or significant esophageal, tracheal, or venacaval compression mandate surgery. Although thyroid surgery is generally well tolerated, even by octogenarians,[117] there is no reason to remove a large asymptomatic goiter simply because "it is there" and may cause trouble "in the future," especially if it is cytologically benign. Suppressive therapy with thyroxine may be helpful[112] but usually is of no benefit in longstanding large goiter and may be potentially hazardous in elderly patients. Recent reports suggest that compressive symptoms can be improved with radioiodine ablation, even in patients who are euthyroid,[118,119] but additional studies are needed before this can be recommended as a routine practice.

As indicated earlier, patients with nontoxic multi-nodular goiter are susceptible to iodine-induced thyrotoxicosis. Iodine-containing compounds, including iodinated contrast media, should be avoided, if possible, in such patients.

Thyroid Cancer

Thyroid cancer in elderly patients shares many features with that seen in younger patients, but there are dramatic differences as well. The histologic types (papillary, follicular, medullary, anaplastic, lymphoma) all occur, but with a shift in histologic type from the more indolent (papillary) to the more aggressive (Hürthle cell, medullary, anaplastic) (Fig. 47.6).[120] Even within a histologic category, advanced age portends a far worse prognosis.[120,121]

Papillary Carcinoma

Papillary carcinoma is the most common kind of thyroid malignancy in the elderly, accounting for approximately 70% of tumors. This tumor often involves ipsilateral cervical lymph nodes, and recent data suggest that nodal involvement confers a higher recurrence rate.[121,122] Although the outlook is generally good, this form of cancer is often aggressive in elderly patients, with local invasion into the trachea or lung metastases. Primary therapy consists of near-total thyroidectomy, whereas in younger patients less extensive surgery is acceptable. Postoperatively, whole-body radioiodine scanning establishes whether residual thyroid tissue or local or distant metastases are present. Radioiodine is administered if the scan reveals remnants or metastatic disease. Follow-up with periodic total body radioiodine scanning, serum thyroglobulin measurements, and other imaging modalities (especially thyroid ultrasound) is important in the detection of recurrent or persistent disease. Patients usually succumb from recurrent local disease, rather than from distant metastases. The recent availability of human recombinant thyrotropin[123] now permits radioiodine scanning and stimulated thyroglobulin measurements without the need for thyroid hormone withdrawal and the unpleasant and occasionally debilitating symptoms of hypothyroidism, which are especially prevalent in older patients.

All patients require lifelong suppressive doses of thyroxine, with doses sufficient to suppress serum TSH to undetectable levels in a sensitive TSH assay. Recently, some have questioned the necessity of maintaining such low TSH levels in elderly postmenopausal women who have been disease free for more than 10 years, given the risk for osteopenia and the low risk of recurrence.[124] Theoretically, patients who have undergone total thyroidectomy and who do not have distant metastases should have undetectable thyroglobulin levels (<2 µg/L). Thyroglobulin levels above 5 ng/dL on thyroxine and above 10 to 20 ng/mL off thyroxine or after human recombinant thyrotropin suggest recurrent or metastatic disease. Details regarding the specifics of management of papillary carcinoma are discussed elsewhere.[125]

Follicular Carcinoma

Follicular carcinoma comprises about 20% of thyroid cancer in the elderly. Tumors tend to spread hematogenously to bone, lungs, and liver. Approximately one-third of patients present with metastases (usually to the bone) as the initial manifestation of disease. The prognosis of follicular cancer is worse in elderly patients, especially in those with metastatic disease.[126] The management is similar to that outlined for papillary cancer. Hürthle cell carcinoma is considered to be a variant of follicular cancer, with a somewhat less favorable prognosis, due to a greater tendency for local and regional metastatic disease, that does not usually concentrate radioiodine.[127]

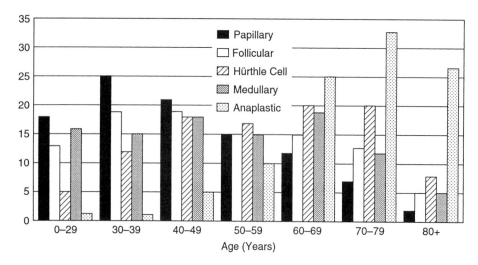

FIGURE 47.6. Age distribution of thyroid cancer by histologic type.[120]

Medullary Cancer

Medullary cancer of the thyroid arises from the calcitonin-producing "C" cells in the thyroid, rather than the follicular cells. This tumor type accounts for 5% to 10% of thyroid cancer in the elderly; it is sporadic in approximately 75% of older patients, with only a minority of tumors being associated with multiple endocrine neoplasia syndrome type 2 (medullary cancer of the thyroid, pheochromocytoma, hyperparathyroidism).[128] Medullary cancer of the thyroid is almost always metastatic to regional cervical nodes at the time of diagnosis, and it frequently metastasizes to the liver and bone. The diagnosis is usually made by means of needle biopsy or after surgical removal of a suspicious nodule. The tumor is frequently bilateral, even in sporadic cases, and total thyroidectomy and central compartment lymph node dissection are recommended because of the high rate of nodal disease. Because it is a neoplasm of calcitonin-producing cells, serum calcitonin can be used as a tumor marker to detect recurrence and to monitor therapy.

Carcinoembryonic antigen is also frequently secreted by medullary cancer of the thyroid and is another useful tumor marker. Because the tumor does not arise from the follicular cells of the thyroid, it does not concentrate radioiodine. Furthermore, suppressive doses of thyroxine are not indicated as the tumor is not dependent upon TSH for growth. Screening of family members for this tumor is indicated because the patient, even if elderly, could be the index case of a kindred with multiple endocrine neoplasia (MEN) syndrome type 2. Family screening involves analysis of germline DNA for mutations in the *ret* proto-oncogene, located on chromosome 10, which have been found in all patients with MEN 2. Screening for these mutations has supplanted the less sensitive screening tests using calcitonin stimulation.

Thyroid Lymphoma

Thyroid lymphoma was once thought to represent a distinct form of "small cell" cancer. It is now known that lymphoma may arise primarily within the thyroid and that it is often, but not always, associated with disseminated extrathyroidal lymphoma.[129] Most thyroid lymphomas are diffuse B-cell lymphomas that arise from mucosa-associated lymphoid tissue (MALT).[130] Typically, thyroid lymphoma presents as a rapidly enlarging neck mass in an elderly woman with a history of Hashimoto's thyroiditis; however, there may be no previous thyroid disease, and antithyroid antibodies are often negative. The diagnosis of thyroid lymphoma is difficult to make with needle biopsy because the cytologic appearance is similar to that of lymphocytic thyroiditis; open biopsy with special immunohistochemical staining for monoclonal B-cell markers often is necessary to establish the diagnosis. Staging for disseminated disease is indicated for all patients. Treatment consists of local radiotherapy and combination chemotherapy, rather than surgery.

Anaplastic Thyroid Cancer

Anaplastic thyroid cancer is one of the most aggressive malignancies of humans.[131] It occurs almost exclusively in elderly persons, often arising in preexisting goiters or in patients who previously have been treated for well-differentiated cancer. Anaplastic cancer presents as a rapidly enlarging mass that quickly produces compressive symptoms. There is no effective treatment. Palliation with radiation therapy and/or chemotherapy to protect the airway should be considered, but surgery is not usually recommended. The median survival is measured in months.

References

1. Mariotti S, Franceschi C, Cossarizza A, Pinchera A. The aging thyroid. *Endocr Rev.* 1995;16:686–715.
2. Irvine RE. Thyroid disease in old age. In: Brocklehurst JC, ed. *Textbook of Geriatric Medicine and Gerontology.* New York: Churchill Livingstone; 1973:435–458.
3. Mariotti S, Chiovata L, Franceschi C, Pinchera A. Thyroid autoimmunity and aging. *Exp Gerontol.* 1998;33:535–541.
4. Tunbridge WMG, Evered DC, Hall R, et al. The spectrum of thyroid disease in a community: the Wickham survey. *Clin Endocrinol.* 1977;7:481–493.
5. Denham MJ, Wills EJ. A clinico-pathological survey of thyroid glands in old age. *Gerontology.* 1980; 26:160–166.
6. Hollowell JG, Staehling NW, Hannon WH, et al. Iodine nutrition in the United States. Trends and public health implications: iodine excretion data from National Health and Nutrition Examination Surveys I and III (1971–1974 and 1988–1994). *J Clin Endocrinol Metab.* 1998;83:3401–3408.
7. Gregerman RI, Gaffney GW, Shock NW, et al. Thyroxine turnover in euthyroid man with special reference to changes with age. *J Clin Investig.* 1962;41:2565–2574.
8. Mokshagundam S, Barzel US. Thyroid disease in the elderly. *J Am Geriatr Soc.* 1993;41:1361–1369.
9. Mariotti S, Barbesino G, Caturegli P, et al. Complex alteration of thyroid function in healthy centenarians. *J Clin Endocrinol Metab.* 1993;77:1130–1134.
10. Kabadi UM, Rosman PM. Thyroid hormone indices in adult healthy subjects: no influence of aging. *J Am Geriatr Soc.* 1988;36:312–316.
11. Hershman JM, Pekary AE, Berg L, Solomon DH, Sawin CT. Serum thyrotropin and thyroid hormone levels in elderly and middle-aged euthyroid persons. *J Am Geriatr Soc.* 1993;41:823–828.
12. Parle JV, Franklyn JA, Cross KW, Jones SC, Sheppard MC. Prevalence and follow-up of abnormal thyrotrophin (TSH) concentrations in the elderly in the United Kingdom. *Clin Endocrinol.* 1991;34:77–83.

13. Lipson A, Nickoloff L, Hsu TH, et al. A study of age-dependent changes in thyroid function tests in adults. *J Nucl Med.* 1979;20:1124–1130.
14. Lazar MA. Thyroid hormone receptors: multiple forms, multiple possibilities. *Endocr Rev.* 1993;14:194–202.
15. Davis PJ, Davis FB, Blas SD, et al. Donor age-dependent decline in response of human RBC Ca^{++}/ATPase activity to thyroid hormone in vitro. *J Clin Endocrinol Metab.* 1987;64:921–925.
16. Mooradian AD. Normal age-related changes in thyroid hormone economy. *Clin Geriatr Med.* 1995;11:159–169.
17. Kvetny J. Nuclear T$_4$ and T$_3$ binding in mononuclear cells in dependence of age. *Horm Metab Res.* 1985;17:35–38.
18. Surks MI, DeFesi CR. Normal serum free thyroid hormone concentrations in patients treated with phenytoin or carbamazepine. *JAMA.* 1996;275:1495–1498.
19. Nicoloff JT, Spencer CA. The use and misuse of the sensitive thyrotropin assays. *J Clin Endocrinol Metab.* 1990;71:553–558.
20. Attia J, Margetts P, Guyatt G. Diagnosis of thyroid disease in hospitalized patients. *Arch Intern Med.* 1999;159:658–665.
21. Sundbeck G, Jagenburg R, Johansson P-M, Eden S, Lindstedt G. Clinical significance of low serum thyrotropin concentration by chemiluminometric assay in 85-year-old women and men. *Arch Intern Med.* 1991;151:549–556.
22. Sawin CT, Geller A, Wolf PA, et al. Low serum thyrotropin concentrations as a risk factor for atrial fibrillation in older persons. *N Engl J Med.* 1994;331:1249–1252.
23. Ronnov-Jessen V, Kirkegaard C. Hyperthyroidism: a disease of old age? *Br Med J.* 1973;1:41–43.
24. Greenwood RM, Daly JG, Himsworth RL. Hyperthyroidism and the impalpable thyroid gland. *Clin Endocrinol.* 1985;22:583–587.
25. Tibaldi JM, Barzel US, Albin J, et al. Thyrotoxicosis in the very old. *Am J Med.* 1986;81:619–622.
26. Trivalle C, Doucet J, Chassagne P, et al. Differences in the signs and symptoms of hyperthyroidism in older and younger patients. *J Am Geriatr Soc.* 1996;44:50–53.
27. Davis PJ, Davis FB. Hyperthyroidism in patients over the age of 60 years: clinical features in 85 patients. *Medicine.* 1974;53:161–181.
28. Martin FIR, Deam DR. Hyperthyroidism in elderly hospitalized patients. *Med J Aust.* 1996;164:200–203.
29. Cummings SR, Nevitt MC, Browner WS, et al. Risk factors for hip fracture in white women. *N Engl J Med.* 1995;332:767–773.
30. Cobler JL, Williams ME, Greenland P. Thyrotoxicosis in institutionalized elderly patients with atrial fibrillation. *Arch Intern Med.* 1984;144:1758–1760.
31. Woeber KA. Thyrotoxicosis and the heart. *N Engl J Med.* 1992;327:94–98.
32. Perros P, Crombie AL, Matthews JNS, Kendall-Taylor P. Age and gender influence the severity of thyroid-associated ophthalmopathy: a study of 101 patients attending a combined thyroid-eye clinic. *Clin Endocrinol.* 1993;38:367–372.
33. Kendler DL, Lippa J, Rootman J. The initial clinical characteristics of Graves' orbitopathy vary with age and sex. *Arch Ophthalmol.* 1993;111:197–200.
34. Caplan RH, Glasser JE, Davis K, et al. Thyroid function tests in elderly hyperthyroid patients. *J Am Geriatr Soc.* 1978;26:116–120.
35. Kawabe T, Komiya I, Endo T, Koizumi Y, Yamada T. Hyperthyroidism in the elderly. *J Am Geriatr Soc.* 1979;27:152–155.
36. Trzepacz PT, Klein I, Roberts M, Greenhouse J, Levey GS. Graves' disease: an analysis of thyroid hormone levels and hyperthyroid signs and symptoms. *Am J Med.* 1989;87:558–561.
37. Aizawa T, Ishihara M, Hashizume K, Takasu N, Yamada T. Age-related changes of thyroid function and immunologic abnormalities in patients with hyperthyroidism due to Graves' disease. *J Am Geriatr Soc.* 1989;37:944–948.
38. Yamada T, Aizawa T, Koizumi Y, Komiya I, Ichikawa K, Hashizume K. Age-related therapeutic response to antithyroid drug in patients with hyperthyroid Graves' disease. *J Am Geriatr Soc.* 1994;42:513–516.
39. Borst GC, Eil C, Burman KD. Euthyroid hyperthyroxinemia. *Ann Intern Med.* 1983;98:366–378.
40. Figge J, Leinung M, Goodman AD, et al. The clinical evaluation of patients with subclinical hyperthyroidism and free triiodothyronine (free T3) toxicosis. *Am J Med.* 1994;96:229–234.
41. Wehmann RE, Gregerman RI, Burns WH, et al. Suppression of thyrotropin in the low-thyroxine state of severe nonthyroidal illness. *N Engl J Med.* 1985;312:546–552.
42. Gordon M, Gryfe CI. Hyperthyroidism with painless subacute thyroiditis in the elderly. *JAMA.* 1981;246:2354–2355.
43. Wynn AG, Gharib H, Scheithauer BW, Davis DH, Freeman SL, Horvath E. Hyperthyroidism due to inappropriate secretion of thyrotropin in 10 patients. *Am J Med.* 1992;92:15–24.
44. Bartalena L, Grasso L, Brogioni S, et al. Serum interleukin-6 in amiodarone-induced thyrotoxicosis. *J Clin Endocrinol Metab.* 1994;78:423–427.
45. Harjai KJ, Licata AA. Effects of amiodarone on thyroid function. *Ann Intern Med.* 1997;126:63–73.
46. Newman CM, Price A, Davies DW, Gray TA, Weetman AP. Amiodarone and the thyroid: a practical guide to the management of thyroid dysfunction induced by amiodarone therapy. *Heart.* 1998;79:121–127.
47. Solomon B, Glinoer D, Lagasse R, Wartofsky L. Current trends in the management of Graves' disease. *J Clin Endocrinol Metab.* 1990;70:1518–1524.
48. Velkeniers B, Cytryn R, Vanhaelst L, Jonckheer MR. Treatment of hyperthyroidism with radioiodine: adjunctive therapy with antithyroid drugs reconsidered. *Lancet.* 1998;1:1127–1129.
49. Cooper DS, Goldminz D, Levin AA, et al. Agranulocytosis associated with antithyroid drugs: effects of patient age and drug dose. *Ann Intern Med.* 1983;98:26–29.
50. Geffner DL, Hershman JM. Beta-adrenergic blockade for the treatment of hyperthyroidism. *Am J Med.* 1992;93:61–68.
51. Erickson D, Gharib H, Li Hongzhe, Van Heerden JA. Treatment of patients with toxic multinodular goiter. *Thyroid.* 1998;8:277–282.

52. Gomez N, Gomez JM, Orti A, et al. Transient hypothyroidism after iodine-131 therapy for Graves' disease. *J Nucl Med.* 1995;36:1539–1542.

53. Ron E, Doody MM, Becker DV, et al. Cancer mortality following treatment for adult hyperthyroidism. *JAMA.* 1998;280:347–355.

54. Franklyn JA, Maisonneuve P, Sheppard M, Betteridge J, Boyle P. Cancer incidence and mortality after radioiodine treatment for hyperthyroidism: a population-based cohort study. *Lancet.* 1999;353:2111–2115.

55. Nakazawa HK, Sakurai K, Ramada N, et al. Management of atrial fibrillation in the postthyrotoxic state. *Am J Med.* 1982;72:903–906.

56. Aronow WS. The heart and thyroid disease. *Clin Geriatr Med.* 1995;11:219–229.

57. Kellett HA, Sawers JSA, Boulton FE, et al. Problems of anticoagulation with warfarin in hyperthyroidism. *Q J Med.* 1986;58:43–51.

58. Roti E, Montermini M, Roti S, et al. The effect of diltiazem, a calcium channel-blocking drug, on cardiac rate and rhythm in hyperthyroid patients. *Arch Intern Med.* 1988;148:1919–1921.

59. Nicoloff JT. Thyroid storm and myxedema coma. *Med Clin N Am.* 1985;69:l005–1117.

60. Samuels MR. Subclinical thyroid disease in the elderly. *Thyroid.* 1998;8:803–813.

61. Faber J, Galloe AM. Changes in bone mass during prolonged subclinical hyperthyroidism due to L-thyroxine treatment: a meta-analysis. *Eur J Endocrinol.* 1994;130:350–356.

62. Bauer DC, Nevitt MC, Ettinger B, Stone K. Low thyrotropin levels are not associated with bone loss in older women: a prospective study. *J Clin Endocrinol Metab.* 1997;82:2931–2936.

63. Mudde AH, Houben AJHM, Nieuwenhuijzen Kruseman AC. Bone metabolism during anti-thyroid drug treatment of endogenous subclinical hyperthyroidism. *Clin Endocrinol.* 1994;41:421–424.

64. Faber J, Jensen IW, Petersen L, et al. Normalization of serum thyrotrophin by means of radioiodine treatment in subclinical hyperthyroidism: effect on bone loss in postmenopausal women. *Clin Endocrinol.* 1998;48:285–290.

65. Utiger R. Subclinical hyperthyroidism—just a low serum thyrotropin concentration, or something more? *N Engl J Med.* 1994;331:1302–1303.

66. Davis PJ, Davis FM. Hypothyroidism in the elderly. *Compr Ther.* 1984;10:17–23.

67. Canaris GJ, Manowitz NR, Mayor G, Ridgway EC. The Colorado thyroid disease prevalence study. *Arch Intern Med.* 2000;160:526–534.

68. Lindeman RD, Schade DS, LaRue A, et al. Subclinical hypothyroidism in a biethnic, urban community. *J Am Geriatr Soc.* 1999;47:703–709.

69. Mariotti S, Sansoni P, Barbesino G, et al. Thyroid and other organ-specific autoantibodies in healthy centenarians. *Lancet.* 1992;339:1506–1508.

70. Sawin CT, Bigos ST, Land S, et al. The aging thyroid: relationship between elevated serum thyrotropin level and thyroid antibodies in elderly patients. *Am J Med.* 1985;79:591–595.

71. Martino E, Safran M, Aghini-Lombardi F, et al. Environmental iodine intake and thyroid dysfunction during chronic amiodarone therapy. *Ann Intern Med.* 1984;101:28–34.

72. Doucet J, Trivalle C, Chassagne P, et al. Does age play a role in clinical presentation of hypothyroidism? *J Am Geriatr Soc.* 1994;42:984–986.

73. Robuschi G, Safran M, Braverman LE, Gnudi A, Roti E. Hypothyroidism in the elderly. *Endocr Rev.* 1987;8:142–152.

74. Dayan CM, Daniels GH. Chronic autoimmune thyroiditis. *N Engl J Med.* 1996;335:99–107.

75. Osterweil D, Syndulko K, Cohen SN, et al. Cognitive function in non-demented older adults and hypothyroidism. *J Am Geriatr Soc.* 1992;40:325–335.

76. Breteler M, Van Duijn C, Chandra V, et al. Medical history and the risk of Alzheimer's disease: a collaborative re-analysis of case-control studies. *Int J Epidemiol.* 1991;20(suppl 2):S36–S42.

77. Docter R, Krenning EP, de Jong M, Hennemann G. The sick euthyroid syndrome: changes in thyroid hormone serum parameters and hormone metabolism. *Clin Endocrinol.* 1993;39:499–518.

78. Hays MT, Nielsen KRK. Human thyroxine absorption: age effects and methodological analyses. *Thyroid.* 1994;4:55–58.

79. Carr D, McLeod DT, Parry G, Thornes HM. Fine adjustment of thyroxine replacement dosage: comparison of the thyrotrophin releasing hormone test using a sensitive thyrotrophin assay with measurement of free thyroid hormones and clinical assessment. *Clin Endocrinol.* 1988;28:325–333.

80. Sawin CT, Herman T, Molitch ME, et al. Aging and the thyroid. Decreased requirement for thyroid hormone in older hypothyroid patients. *Am J Med.* 1983;75:206–209.

81. Cunningham JJ, Barzel US. Lean body mass as a predictor of the daily requirement for thyroid hormone in older men and women. *J Am Geriatr Soc.* 1984;32:204–207.

82. Biondi B, Fazio S, Carella C, et al. Cardiac effects of long term thyrotropin-suppressive therapy with levothyroxine. *J Clin Endocrinol Metab.* 1993;27:334–337.

83. Stall GM, Harris S, Sokoll LJ, Dawson-Hughes B. Accelerated bone loss in hypothyroid patients overtreated with L-thyroxine. *Ann intern Med.* 1990;113:265–269.

84. Hak AE, Pols HAP, Visser TJ, et al. Subclinical hypothyroidism is an independent risk factor for atherosclerosis and myocardial infarction in elderly women: The Rotterdam study. *Ann Intern Med.* 2000;132:270–278.

85. Hay ID, Duick DS, Vlietstra RE, et al. Thyroxine therapy in hypothyroid patients undergoing coronary revascularization: a retrospective analysis. *Ann Intern Med.* 1981;95:456–457.

86. Ladenson PW, Levin AA, Ridgway EC, et al. Complications of surgery in hypothyroid patients. *Am J Med.* 1984;77:261–266.

87. Surks M, Chopra IJ, Mariash CN, Nicoloff JT, Solomon DH. American Thyroid Association guidelines for use of laboratory tests in thyroid disorders. *JAMA.* 1990;263:1529–1532.

88. American College of Physicians. Screening for thyroid disease. *Ann Intern Med.* 1998;129:141–143.

89. Cooper DS, Halpern R, Wood LC, et al. L-thyroxine therapy in subclinical hypothyroidism. A double-blind, placebo-controlled trial. *Ann Intern Med.* 1984;101:18–24.

90. Nystrom E, Caidahl K, Fager G, Wikkelso C, Lundberg P-A, Lindstedt G. A double-blind cross-over 12-month study of L-thyroxine treatment of women with "subclinical" hypothyroidism. *Clin Endocrinol.* 1988;29:63–67.

91. Monzani F, Del Guerra P, Caraccio N, et al. Subclinical hypothyroidism: neurobehavioral features and beneficial effect of L-thyroxine treatment. *Clin Investig.* 1993;71:367–371.

92. Arem R, Patsch W. Lipoprotein and apolipoprotein levels in subclinical hypothyroidism. *Arch Intern Med.* 1990;150:2097–2100.

93. Jaeschke R, Guyatt G, Gerstein H, et al. Does treatment with L-thyroxine influence health status in middle-aged and older adults with subclinical hypothyroidism? *J Gen Intern Med.* 1996;11:744–749.

94. Helfand M, Redfern CC. Screening for thyroid disease: an update. *Ann Intern Med.* 1998;129:144-158.

95. Centanni M, Cesareo R, Verallo O, et al. Reversible increase in intraocular pressure in subclinical hypothyroid patients. *Eur J Endocrinol.* 1997;136:595–598.

96. Perk M, O'Neill BJ. The effect of thyroid hormone therapy on angiographic coronary artery disease progression. *Can J Cardiol.* 1997;13:273–276.

97. Rosenthal MJ, Hunt WC, Garry PJ, et al. Thyroid failure in the elderly: microsomal antibodies as discriminant for therapy. *JAMA.* 1987;258:209–213.

98. Vanderpump MPJ, Tunbridge WMG, French JM, et al. The incidence of thyroid disorders in the community: a twenty-year follow-up of the Wickham survey. *Clin Endocrinol.* 1995;43:55–68.

99. Diekman T, Lansberg PJ, Kastelein JJ, Wiersinga WM. Prevalence and correction of hypothyroidism in a large cohort of patients referred for dyslipidemia. *Arch Intern Med.* 1995;155:1490–1495.

100. Yamamoto T, Fukuyama J, Fujiyoshi A. Factors associated with mortality of myxedema coma: report of eight cases and literature survey. *Thyroid.* 1999;9:1167–1174.

101. Nicoloff JT, LoPresti JS. Myxedema coma: a form of decompensated hypothyroidism. *Endocrinol Metab Clin N Am.* 1993;22:279–290.

102. Brander A, Viikinkoski P, Nickels J, Kivisaari L. Thyroid gland: US screening in a random adult population. *Radiology.* 1991;181:683–687.

103. Vander JB, Gaston EA, Dawber TR. The significance of nontoxic thyroid nodules. *Ann Intern Med.* 1968;69:537–540.

104. Belfiore A, La Rosa GL, La Porta GA, et al. Cancer risk in patients with cold thyroid nodules: relevance of iodine intake, sex, age, and multinodularity. *Am J Med.* 1992;93:363–369.

105. Mazzaferri EL. Management of a solitary thyroid nodule. *N Engl J Med.* 1993;328:553–559.

106. Gharib H, Goellner JR. Fine-needle aspiration biopsy of the thyroid: an appraisal. *Ann Intern Med.* 1993;118:282–289.

107. Ezzat S, Sarti DA, Cain DR, Braunstein GD. Thyroid incidentalomas. Prevalence by palpation and ultrasonography. *Arch Intern Med.* 1994;154(16):1838–1840.

108. Tan GH, Gharib H. Thyroid incidentalomas: management approaches to nonpalpable nodules discovered incidentally on thyroid imaging. *Ann Intern Med.* 1997;126:226–231.

109. Gharib H, Goellner JR, Zinsmeister AR. Fine-needle aspiration biopsy of the thyroid: the problem of suspicious cytologic findings. *Ann Intern Med.* 1984;101:25–28.

110. Gharib H, James EM, Charboneau JW, Naessons JM, Offord KP, Gorman CA. Suppressive therapy with levothyroxine for solitary thyroid nodules. *N Engl J Med.* 1987;317:70–75.

111. Reverter JL, Lucas A, Salinas I, Audi L, Foz M, Sanmarti A. Suppressive therapy with levothyroxine for solitary thyroid nodules. *Clin Endocrinol.* 1992;36:25–28.

112. Berghout A, Wiersinga WM, Drexhage HA, Smits NJ, Touber JL. Comparison of placebo with L-thyroxine alone or with carbimazole for treatment of sporadic non-toxic goitre. *Lancet.* 1990;336:193–197.

113. Zelmanovitz F, Genro S, Gross JL. Suppressive therapy with levothyroxine for solitary thyroid nodules: a double-blind controlled clinical study and cumulative meta-analyses. *J Clin Endocrinol Metab.* 1998;83:3881–3885.

114. Mandel SJ, Brent GA, Larsen PR. Levothyroxine therapy in patients with thyroid diseases. *Ann Intern Med.* 1993;119:492–502.

115. Cooper DS. Thyroxine suppression therapy for benign nodular disease. *J Clin Endocrinol Metab* 1995;80:331–334.

116. Schneider DL, Barrett-Connor EL, Morton DJ. Thyroid hormone use and bone mineral density in elderly women. *JAMA.* 1994;271:1245–1249.

117. Miccoli P, Lacconi P. Cecchini GM, et al. Thyroid surgery in patients aged over 80 years. *Acta Chir Belg.* 1994;94:222–223.

118. Huysmans DAKC, Hermus ARMM, Corstens FHM, Barentsz JO, Kloppenborg PWC. Large, compressive goiters treated with radioiodine. *Ann Intern Med.* 1994;121:757–762.

119. Freitas JE. Radioiodine therapy of non-toxic goiter. *Endocrinologist.* 1999;9:107–112.

120. Hundahl SA, Fleming ID, Fremgen AM, Menck HR. A national cancer data base report on 53,856 cases of thyroid carcinoma treated in the U.S., 1985–1995. *Cancer* 1998;83:2638–2648.

121. Mazzaferri EL, Jhiang SM. Long-term impact of initial surgical and medical therapy on papillary and follicular thyroid cancer. *Am J Med.* 1994;97:418–428.

122. Schlumberger MJ. Papillary and follicular thyroid carcinoma. *N Engl J Med.* 1998;338:297–306.

123. Ladenson PW, Braverman LE, Mazzaferri EL, et al. Comparison of administration of recombinant human thyrotropin with withdrawal of thyroid hormone for radioactive iodine scanning in patients with thyroid carcinoma. *N Engl J Med.* 1997;337:888–896.

124. Cooper DS, Specker B, Ho M, et al. Thyrotropin suppression and disease progression in patients with differentiated thyroid cancer: results from the National Thyroid Cancer Treatment Cooperative Registry. *Thyroid.* 1998;8:737–744.

125. Dulgeroff AJ, Hershman JM. Medical therapy for differentiated thyroid carcinoma. *Endocr Rev.* 1994;15:500–515.

126. McHenry CR, Sandoval BA. Management of follicular and Hurthle cell neoplasms of the thyroid gland. *Surg Oncol Clin N Am.* 1998;7:893–910.

127. Azadian A, Rosen IB, Walfish PG, Asa SL. Management considerations in Hurthle cell carcinoma. *Surgery.* 1995; 118:711–715.

128. Raue F, Frank-Raue K, Grauer A. Multiple endocrine neoplasia type 2: clinical features and screening. *Endocrinol Metab Clin N Am.* 1994;23:137–156.

129. Matsuzuka F, Miyauchi A, Katayama S, et al. Clinical aspects of primary thyroid lymphoma: diagnosis and treatment based on our experience of 199 cases. *Thyroid.* 1993;3:93–99.

130. Kossev P, Livolsi V. Lymphoid lesions of the thyroid: review in light of the revised European-American lymphoma classification and upcoming World Health Organization classification. *Thyroid.* 1999;9:1273–1280.

131. Ain KB. Anaplastic thyroid carcinoma: behavior, biology, and therapeutic approaches. *Thyroid.* 1998;8: 715–726.

48
Changes in Male Sexuality

Thomas Mulligan and Waleed Siddiqi

As men proceed through life, there is a clear change in their sexuality. For example, among men aged 18 to 29 years, 29% report intercourse three or four times per week, whereas only 7% of men aged 60 to 69 years and 2% of men 70 years or older report this same frequency. Years ago, Kinsey et al. first reported that, by age 80 years, the average frequency of intercourse decreases to once every 10 weeks.[1] Pfeiffer et al. corroborated this finding, reporting that 95% of men aged 46 to 50 years had intercourse weekly whereas only 28% of 66 to 71-year-old men reported having intercourse once a week.[2] In healthy Caucasian, upper middle class men aged 80 to 102 years, 26% reported their frequency of sexual intercourse to be several times per month or several times per week. In contrast, among male nursing home residents, 80% no longer engaged in coitus at all despite availability of a sexual partner, moderately strong libido, and preference for vaginal intercourse. Thus, although there is a decline in sexual activity with aging, this decline appears associated with declining health rather than simply advancing age.[3]

Sexual interest seems to decline less than sexual activity. In men 30 to 99 years old, sexual interest decreased with age, but total absence of interest was never reported. In a survey of healthy couples, the desired frequency of sexual contact decreased from a mean score of 6 (based on a scale where 1 = never to 8 = daily) in 45 to 54-year-old men to a mean score of 3 for men aged 65 to 74 years. In another study, of healthy, well-educated men attending a sexuality and aging lecture series (age, 56–85 years), 92% reported that they would like to have sexual activity at least once per week. However, only 33% of this group engaged in sexual activity on a weekly basis.[4] Even in nursing home residents, continued sexual interest, especially among those with partners, has been reported.

The preferred sexual activity remains vaginal intercourse despite aging. With the decline in intercourse, however, some investigators have found a compensatory increase in other forms of sexual contact, such as kissing, caressing, petting, oral sex, or masturbation. Bretschneider and McCoy reported that 83% of their very old subjects engaged in touching or caressing, without sexual intercourse, at least several times per year.[5] Furthermore, 74% expressed moderate to great enjoyment from this activity. Similarly, in the self-selected group of attendees at sex lectures, sexual intercourse and orgasm were the highest rated forms of sexual activity. With aging, however, these forms of sexual expression declined but with an increase in expressions of intimacy without intercourse. Even nursing home residents prefer vaginal intercourse, though 21% prefer hugging or caressing, 5% prefer kissing, and 2% prefer masturbation.[6]

An important factor in sexual behavior during aging is availability of a socially acceptable sexual partner. As one might expect, availability of a marital partner is an important factor, with sexual activity occurring in 74% of older married men and 31% of older unmarried men. Among those with sexual partners, men tended to attribute cessation of sexual intercourse to themselves, which was corroborated by 74% of the women. The main reasons cited were loss of erectile function, decreased libido, and medical illness.[7] In those men who blamed their spouses for stopping, 62% attributed the cause to illness and 37% to loss of interest.

The causes of the age-associated changes in sexual behavior are multifactorial, including organic and social factors. To understand these causes, we review here the anatomy and physiology of male sexual function, then the pathophysiology and treatment of dysfunction.

Physiology of Sexual Function

Libido

In men, libido results from an interplay of psychologic, social, physical, and endocrine factors. Animal research suggests that libido is centered in the medial preoptic area of the hypothalamus.[8] This area of the brain has androgen receptors, and it appears that testosterone (and/or its metabolite dihydrotestosterone) is necessary for normal sexual desire. In data obtained by self-administered questionnaires and serum hormone assays in 102 adolescent boys, serum free testosterone concentration was a strong predictor of sexual motivation and behavior.[9] When the free testosterone index (FTI) was divided into quartiles, 16% of those with the lowest FTI reported having had intercourse, whereas 69% of boys in the highest FTI quartile reported intercourse. Similar findings occurred for noncoital sexual activity and libido. This result suggests that the serum free testosterone concentration affects sexual desire and activity.

In a randomized, double-blind study of healthy, eugonadal men, a gonadotropin-releasing hormone (GnRH) antagonist, Nal-Glu, without testosterone replacement was used to produce acute and profound reversible androgen deficiency. The subjects experienced decreased frequency of sexual desire, fantasies, and intercourse. There was also a decrease in noncoital sexual activity such as kissing, fondling, and masturbation.[10] However, even low-dose testosterone replacement was adequate to maintain normal sexual function and behavior. In eugonadal men complaining of loss of sexual desire, testosterone injection therapy resulted in a modest increase in sexual desire, but no effect on erectile function. Supraphysiologic levels of testosterone increased sexual awareness and arousability but did not modify overt sexual behavior. This finding was in contrast to hypogonadal men, in whom testosterone replacement stimulated both sexual interest and activity. From these and other studies, it appears that the major contribution of testosterone to sexuality is related to libido.[11]

Anatomy

The penis consists of three components, two dorsolateral corpora cavernosa and a ventral corpus spongiosum that surrounds the penile urethra and distally forms the glans penis. A thick fibrous sheath, the tunica albuginea, surrounds each of the corpora cavernosa, and all three corpora are bound together by Buck's fascia. The ischiocavernosus and bulbospongiosus muscles surround the proximal portions of the corpora cavernosa. Each corpus consists of smooth muscle bundles, elastic fibers, collagen, and loose fibrous tissue that forms the trabeculae. In between the trabeculae are blood-filled lacunar spaces that are lined by flat endothelial cells.

The arterial supply to the penis consists of the internal pudendal arteries, which become the penile arteries. Each penile artery terminates in bulbar, urethral, dorsal, and cavernosal arteries. The paired cavernosal arteries penetrate the tunica albuginea and enter the crura of the corpora cavernosa. Each ends in multiple twisted

branches called helicine arterioles that supply the lacunae. There may be two circulatory routes in the human corpora. One route goes from the cavernosal artery to capillary networks underlying the tunica albuginea with the capillaries serving as nutritional vessels. This pathway is the main circulatory route during the flaccid state. The second route is via anastomoses from the cavernosal artery through the helicine arterioles to the cavernosa, which then empties into the postcavernous venules and serves as the main vascular pathway in the mechanism of erection.

Venous return from the penis occurs through the deep and superficial dorsal veins of the penis. Subtunical venules located between the periphery of the erectile tissue and the tunica albuginea drain the lacunar spaces. They coalesce to form emissary veins that penetrate the tunica albuginea and drain into the deep dorsal vein or the circumflex system. Drainage from the proximal crura is mainly through the cavernosal and crural veins. Superficial dorsal veins communicate with the external pudendal vein and/or the saphenous vein to drain the skin and prepuce of the penis.

Mechanism of Erection

Neural Component

Penile erection is a complex event, occurring as a result of the integration of central (cerebral and spinal) and local (smooth muscle and endothelial) factors.[12] It arises in response to sensory stimuli, fantasy, or genital stimulation. Specialized areas in the hypothalamus and thalamus organize the autonomic response to these stimuli.[13]

Sympathetic preganglionic nerve fibers to the penis arise from neurons in the intermediolateral cell columns of Tl2–L2 spinal cord segments, whereas parasympathetic input to the penis arises in the S2–S4 sacral spinal cord segments. Sympathetic impulses travel via the hypogastric nerve, and parasympathetic impulses travel via the pelvic nerve. The pelvic plexus serves as the peripheral integration center for autonomic input to the penis. The pelvic plexus then branches into the cavernous nerves that traverse the posterolateral aspect of the prostate and continue on both sides of the urethra as the cavernosal nerves.[14]

In the flaccid state, tonic contraction of the arterial and corporal smooth muscles is mediated by α-2-adrenergic receptors, which maintains high penile arterial resistance. With erotic stimulation, there is a decrease in sympathetic tone and an increase in parasympathetic activity. Central to erection is a hemodynamic change that decreases penile arterial resistance, with resultant increased penile blood flow.

Parasympathetic stimulation activates cholinergic receptors via acetylcholine, stimulating endothelial cells to produce a nonadrenergic, noncholinergic transmitter nitric oxide (NO). NO relaxes trabecular smooth muscle, and is considered the major neurotransmitter controlling relaxation of penile smooth muscle. NO is formed by conversion of L-arginine into L-citrulline by the enzyme, nitric oxide synthase (NOS). NOS is activated by the influx of calcium ions that occurs with parasympathetic stimulation. The increased oxygen levels derived from the arterialization of cavernosal blood flow further activates NOS and thereby maintains erection.[15]

NO moves from cell to cell through gap junctions and by diffusion into smooth muscle cells, providing the rapidity of the response within the penis. NO activates guanylate cyclase, thereby increasing production of cyclic guanidine monophosphate (cGMP). cGMP depletes intracellular calcium and further induces smooth muscle relaxation with resultant penile vasodilation.[16]

Other chemical entities have been implicated in the control of erection, including prostaglandins E_1 (PGE_1) and E_2 (PGE_2) and vasoactive peptide (VP). PGE_1, PGE_2, and VP stimulate the production of cyclic adenosine monophosphate (cAMP), which decreases intracellular calcium and induces smooth muscle relaxation. VP may also interact with either endothelial or corporal smooth muscle cells to stimulate local formation of NO and thereby sustain penile erection.

Genital stimulation elicits neural impulses that traverse the dorsal nerve of the penis to the pudendal nerve. From the pudendal nerve, the impulses travel to the sacral spinal cord (S2–S4). Efferent impulses travel along the parasympathetic pelvic nerves and produce an erection, as described above.

Vascular Component

Tonic sympathetic stimulation constricts the trabecular smooth muscle and helicine arterioles, keeping the penis flaccid. During flaccidity, blood pressure in the cavernosal lacunae is similar to venous pressure. With sexual stimulation, sympathetic tone decreases and there is parasympathetic-mediated relaxation of arteriolar and trabecular smooth muscle. Penile arterial resistance decreases, resulting in increased blood flow into the corpora cavernosa. The increase in blood volume expands the lacunar spaces and compresses the subtunical venules between the expanding corpora cavernosa and the unyielding tunica albuginea, which results in reduction of venous outflow and trapping of blood within the penis. Penile rigidity develops as intracavernosal pressure rises to mean arterial pressure. Detumescence typically occurs after orgasm. During detumescence, there is a decrease in the arterial flow into the penis, decrease in intracavernosal pressure, increased venous drainage, and restoration of sympathetic nerve impulses, returning the penis to the flaccid state.[17]

Orgasm

Sexual intercourse usually terminates with the motor acts of emission and ejaculation, along with the sensory perception of orgasm. Orgasm occurs in conjunction with the physical events of contraction of smooth muscle of vas deferens, prostate, seminal vesicles, and the buildup of pressure within the proximal urethra. The pleasure of orgasm may derive from the development of this pressure, its release by relaxation of the distal sphincter, and the clonic striated muscle contractions of ejaculation.[18] Electromyography reveals that the onset of the perception of orgasm precedes ejaculation by a few seconds. Also, orgasm may be elicited cerebrally without afferent input from the penis. For example, orgasm has been reported during psychomotor seizures in patients with temporal lobe lesions. Clearly, this area of human sexuality is in need of further research.

Emission and Ejaculation

Emission is the propulsion of semen into the posterior urethra. It is accomplished by peristaltic contractions of the vas deferens, seminal vesicles, and prostatic smooth muscles. Emission is a spinal reflex in response to genital stimulation; but it may be voluntarily stopped, indicating partial cerebral control. It can also be elicited by cerebral erotic stimulation in the absence of afferent genital stimulation.

Expulsion of semen from the urethra marks ejaculation. Intermittent relaxation of the distal sphincter allows semen to enter the bulbous urethra. Contraction of the bulbocavernosus muscle propels the semen through the pendulous urethra. Ejaculation is a reflex reaction in response to semen entrance into the bulbous urethra. Its neural center resides in the spinal cord between Tl2 and L2. The integrity of the vesicle sphincters determines the direction of seminal expulsion. Antegrade ejaculation is achieved by firm closure of the proximal sphincter and a functional distal sphincter. Dripping emission occurs if the distal sphincter is paralyzed, and retrograde ejaculation into the bladder occurs if the proximal sphincter is malfunctioning.

Libido and Aging

Despite the markedly increased prevalence of erectile dysfunction, libido varies much less with advancing age. In an ambulatory geriatric clinic population, 53% of those over the age of 75 years still reported intact libido. When a decline in libido occurs, it is often associated with androgen deficiency.[19] Low sexual interest is typically found in hypogonadal subjects, and testosterone replacement increases libido in a dose-dependent manner. Decreasing serum total and free testosterone concentrations with aging approximate the decline in libido.

Bioavailable testosterone is positively correlated with sexual desire and arousal in the healthy older population.

Erectile Dysfunction and Aging

The National Institutes of Health (NIH) consensus panel suggested that the term erectile dysfunction be used to describe the inability to achieve an erection.[20] It is estimated that 10 to 30 million American men have erectile dysfunction. In a community-based, random sample of men age 40 to 70 years in the Boston area, the overall prevalence of erectile dysfunction was 52%.[21] Kaiser found complete erectile failure in 41% of the men aged 60 to 79 years in a cross-sectional study; none of the men above the age of 70 years was able to achieve a full erection.[7] This high prevalence of sexual dysfunction is important because men with erectile dysfunction report impaired quality of life when compared with unaffected men.

Vascular Disease

The most common etiology of erectile dysfunction in aged men is vascular disease. In a study of 178 men with organic erectile dysfunction, arteriograms revealed lesions in 68%. The investigators also found that the risk of erectile dysfunction increased with the number of vascular risk factors (diabetes mellitus, smoking, hyperlipidemia, and hypertension); 100% of the patients with three or more risk factors had erectile dysfunction.

Vascular disease results in erectile dysfunction by two mechanisms, arterial insufficiency and venous leakage. Obstruction from atherosclerotic arterial occlusive disease of the hypogastric-cavernous arterial bed decreases the perfusion pressure and arterial flow to the lacunar spaces that is necessary to achieve a rigid erection. In an animal model, the hemodynamic alterations created by atherosclerotic occlusive disease of the iliac arteries caused erectile dysfunction. Additionally, atherosclerotic vascular disease may cause ischemia, which results in replacement of smooth muscle by connective tissue. Electron microscopy of cavernosal tissue from men with erectile dysfunction shows marked thickening of the basal lamina, a paucity of contractile filaments, minimal or no glycogen, and fewer vesicles on the cell surface. The degree of smooth muscle cell alterations is correlated with the severity of symptoms. In a rabbit model, the severity of arterial occlusion correlated with the decrease in trabecular smooth muscle content in the corpus cavernosum. This decrease in smooth muscle content impaired cavernosal expandability.[22]

Veno-occlusive dysfunction or venous leakage is characterized by excessive outflow through the subtunical venules, preventing the development of high pressure within the corpora cavernosa and, thereby, interfering with the maintenance of a rigid erection. Venous leakage can result from Peyronie's disease, arteriovenous fistula, or trauma-induced communication between the glans and the corpora.[23] There is an increase in both the size and number of venous outflow channels with advancing age in human cadavers. The structural alteration in the fibroelastic components of the trabeculae causes a loss of compliance and inability to expand the trabeculae against the tunica albuginea, which is necessary to compress the subtunical venules. This decrease in fibroelasticity may result from increased cross-linking of collagen fibers induced by nonenzymatic glycosylation or from hypercholesterolemia associated with altered collagen synthesis. Finally, veno-occlusive dysfunction can occur from insufficient relaxation of trabecular smooth muscle in an anxious patient who has excessive adrenergic-constrictor tone and in patients with injured parasympathetic dilator nerves.

Neurologic Disease

Neurologic disease accounts for the second most common cause of erectile dysfunction in elderly men. Partial or complete erectile dysfunction can result from disorders that affect the parasympathetic sacral spinal cord or the peripheral efferent autonomic fibers to the penis. Such disorders impair penile smooth muscle relaxation and prevent the vasodilation needed for erection. In older men, diabetes mellitus, stroke, and Parkinson's disease can cause autonomic dysfunction, resulting in erectile failure. Additionally, surgical procedures such as radical prostatectomy, cystoprostatectomy, and proctocolectomy frequently disrupt the autonomic nerve supply to the corporal bodies and result in postoperative erectile dysfunction.

Diabetes Mellitus

The prevalence of erectile dysfunction in diabetes mellitus has been reported to be as high as 75%. Greater than 50% of male diabetic patients report erectile dysfunction within 10 years of the diagnosis of diabetes; for some it is the presenting symptom. Although the etiology of diabetic erectile dysfunction is multifactorial, the major cause in older diabetic patients is vascular disease; autonomic neuropathy plays a more important role in younger patients.[24]

The importance of neurologic factors in diabetic erectile dysfunction may be confounded by the fact that many studies fail to categorize diabetic patients into type 1 versus type 2. In a study of type 1 diabetic patients, neuropathy was present in 85% of the impotent diabetic patients. However, 58% of these impotent diabetic patients were still unable to achieve an erection with intracavernosal injection of papaverine, suggesting a vascular component. Nevertheless, the authors concluded that, in type 1 diabetic patients, neurologic factors have a crucial role in the etiology of diabetic erectile dysfunction.[25]

Diabetic men with erectile dysfunction may also have impaired penile cholinergic nerve synthesis and release of acetylcholine, resulting in decreased ability to relax trabecular smooth muscle. In vitro study of human corpus cavernosum tissue from diabetic and nondiabetic patients with erectile dysfunction revealed that impotent diabetic men have impairment in both the autonomic and the endothelium-dependent mechanisms that facilitate relaxation of smooth muscle. Autonomic-mediated contractions were maintained despite impairment in autonomic-mediated relaxation of corporal tissue from diabetic subjects. Thus, there was an imbalance favoring detumescence rather than erection. The decreased response to acetylcholine in tissue from impotent diabetic men is likely caused by decreased synthesis or release of NO, the endothelium-derived relaxing factor.

Another factor contributing to decreased vasodilation in diabetic impotent men may be the inactivation of endothelium-derived NO by basement membrane advanced glycosylation end products (AGE). AGE, which accumulate on tissue proteins such as basement membrane collagen, have been implicated in other long-term complications of diabetes mellitus such as vascular disease.[26]

Testosterone and Erectile Dysfunction

The role of androgens in erection is controversial. Androgen receptors have been demonstrated in sacral parasympathetic nuclei and hypothalamic and limbic system neurons, suggesting potential hormonal regulation of centers involved in erectile function. However, patients with castrate levels of testosterone can attain erections in response to some sexual stimuli. Hypogonadal patients have smaller and slower to develop erections in response to fantasy, and androgen replacement improves erectile response. In hypogonadal men there was also a dose-related response to androgen treatment and the frequency of nocturnal erection and coitus. These findings suggest that erections to certain types of sexual stimuli (i.e., direct penile stimulation) may be androgen independent whereas response to fantasy may be androgen dependent.

Androgen may indirectly affect penile smooth muscle relaxation and resultant rigidity through NOS. Chamness[27] demonstrated decrease in NOS activity and amount of NOS protein in the penis of adult rats after castration. These changes were reversed by testosterone replacement. These investigators also demonstrated a decrease in erectile response with castration and a concomitant decrease in total penile NOS activity.

Drug-Induced Erectile Dysfunction

Many commonly used medications have been associated with erectile dysfunction; there is a reported 25% incidence of drug-induced erectile dysfunction in the medical outpatient clinic population.[28] However, almost all the data available on drug-induced erectile dysfunction are subjective, based on observations, case reports, patient and physician surveys, and pre- and postmarketing drug studies.

The mechanism of drug-mediated erectile dysfunction is often uncertain. Medications such as antidepressants, antipsychotics, and antihistamines have anticholinergic effects that may contribute to erectile dysfunction by blocking parasympathetic-mediated penile artery vasodilation and trabecular smooth muscle relaxation. Antipsychotic medications such as phenothiazines, thioxanthines, and butyrophenones can cause erectile dysfunction through sedation, elevation of the serum prolactin concentration, or anticholinergic or central antidopaminergic effect.

Psychogenic Erectile Dysfunction

Reports on the prevalence of psychogenic erectile dysfunction vary from 10% to 90%. It appears, however, that the likelihood of psychogenic impotence inversely correlates with age. Psychopathology was the cause of erectile dysfunction in only 9% of an aged male veteran population.[29] Psychogenic erectile dysfunction may occur via increased sympathetic stimuli to the sacral cord, inhibiting the parasympathetic dilator nerves to the penis and thereby inhibiting erection. Common causes of psychogenic erectile dysfunction include performance anxiety, conflicts in relationships, sexual inhibition, childhood sexual abuse, and fear of sexually transmitted diseases. A classic psychogenic cause of erectile dysfunction in older men is the "widower's syndrome," where the older man involved in a new relationship feels guilt and develops erectile dysfunction as a defense against perceived unfaithfulness to his dead spouse.

Other Factors in Erectile Dysfunction

In addition to hypogonadism, other endocrine abnormalities have been implicated in the etiology of erectile dysfunction, albeit infrequently.[30] Hyperthyroidism, hypothyroidism, and hyperprolactinemia have been associated with impotence. In hyperprolactinemia, there is an associated decrease in serum testosterone concentration due to inhibition of gonadotropin-releasing hormone secretion. However, normalizing the serum testosterone concentration does not restore erectile function in many patients with hyperprolactinemia, which suggests antagonism by prolactin to the peripheral action of testosterone. Low testosterone secretion and elevated prolactin may also contribute to the erectile dysfunction seen with hypothyroidism. Hyperthyroidism is more often associated with decline in libido rather than with erectile dysfunction.

Chronic alcoholism with associated hypogonadism and peripheral or autonomic neuropathy can also impair erectile function. Hypogonadism in alcoholism occurs through alcohol toxicity at the hypothalamic-pituitary or gonadal levels. Spontaneous reversal of erectile dysfunction occurs with sobriety for at least 1 year, but only if there is no gonadal atrophy or neuropathy. Chronic obstructive lung disease is thought to contribute to erectile dysfunction through hypoxia suppressing the hypothalamic–pituitary–gonadal axis.

Alterations in Emission, Ejaculation, and Orgasm with Aging

In addition to alterations in erectile function, the four stages of sexual response—excitement, plateau, orgasm, and resolution—change with aging.[31,32] During the excitement phase, there is a delay in erection, tensing of the scrotal sac decreases, and testicular elevation may not occur. There is a prolonged duration of the plateau stage and decreased preejaculatory secretion from Cowper's gland. Orgasm is diminished in duration, and there are decreased or spastic prostatic contractions, decreased urethral contractions, and decreased force of emission. Orgasm is less intense, with a smaller quantity of ejaculate being expelled. In the resolution stage, there is rapid detumescence and testicular descent. The refractory period between erections is prolonged with aging. Most young healthy males are capable of achieving an erection, engaging in intercourse, attaining a climax, and repeating this process within minutes. With aging, the rest or refractory period needed before erection and sexual intercourse can be repeated, gradually lengthens. This prolonged refractory period may contribute to the decline in the frequency of sexual intercourse in older men. Older males may experience retrograde ejaculation due to a damaged proximal sphincter following transurethral prostatic resection. Diabetic autonomic dysfunction can also cause retrograde ejaculation and a decline in orgasmic sensation. Last, there is a decrease in penile sensitivity to vibration and light touch with aging. Sexual function and penile sensitivity may be closely related because penile vibrotactile thresholds are higher in subjects with erectile dysfunction than in age-matched control subjects.

Treatment of Erectile Dysfunction

Ideally, treatment of men with erectile dysfunction should be based on the underlying etiology. For example, medications that increase arterial inflow to the penis will not be effective in men with severe arterial occlusive disease. Thus, initial evaluation should include a medical history, focused physical examination, and limited diagnostic tests. The history should include whether the onset of erectile dysfunction was abrupt (suggesting a psychogenic etiology or adverse drug reaction) or gradual (suggesting one of the various organic etiologies). It should also determine which medications (including nonprescription and herbal products) the patient is ingesting, especially whether the patient ingests any nitrates (even illicit use of amyl nitrate). The physical exam should search for gynecomastia, femoral bruits, penile plaques, testicular atrophy, and penile or peripheral neuropathy. There are few laboratory-based tests that are essential, but many authors recommend blood glucose, testosterone, and cholesterol. Also, some investigators recommend a diagnostic penile injection of a vasoactive medication.[33] Based on the history, physical exam, and laboratory assessment, the clinician can then select a treatment strategy that is likely to work and have limited adverse drug reactions.

Sildenafil (Viagra; Pfizer Pharmaceuticals) is the first available orally administered treatment for erectile dysfunction. It is a phosphodiesterase inhibitor that blocks cyclic GMP degradation. Sildenafil has been evaluated in 21 clinical trials with more than 3000 men. In these studies, it was efficacious in approximately 65% of men with organic erectile dysfunction. It has limited effectiveness in men with serious arterial or venous disease. Headache, flushing, and dyspepsia were the most common adverse effects, occurring in 6% to 18% of men. The initial dose should be 50 mg, and should be reduced to 25 mg if side effects occur, or increased to 100 mg if necessary. Each sildenafil dose costs about $9. Importantly, concurrent use of sildenafil and nitrates, in any form, can be fatal. If a man who has taken sildenafil has an ischemic cardiac event, nitrates should not be prescribed within 24 h. A consensus statement from the American College of Cardiology/American Heart Association also urged caution in men with coronary ischemia, congestive heart failure, and low blood pressure as well as those taking a multidrug antihypertensive regimen.[34]

Penile injection therapy with alprostadil (prostaglandin E_1), papaverine, or phentolamine has also been used to induce erection. These drugs, when injected into the corpora cavernosa, induce relaxation of the smooth muscle within the penile erectile bodies. Blood engorges the corpora cavernosa with sufficient pressure to compress the emissary veins that normally drain blood from the penis. The combination of increased arterial inflow and impeded venous outflow creates an erection.

Men can be trained to inject vasoactive medications into one corporal body. Cross-circulation of the penile corpora allows medication to diffuse into the contralateral side. A firm erection can be expected within a few minutes after intrapenile injection.

Three formulations of alprostadil have been used for intracavernous injection: Prostin VR (Pharmacia & Upjohn), Caverject (Pharmacia & Upjohn), and Edex (Schwarz Pharma). The usual dose ranges from 5 to 20 μg. Alprostadil results in erection in more than 70% of patients with organic erectile dysfunction. Depending on which formulation of alprostadil is chosen, the price per dose ranges from $3 to $10.

Papaverine is a nonspecific phosphodiesterase inhibitor that increases cyclic AMP and cyclic GMP concentrations in penile erectile tissue. The usual dose is 15 to 60 mg. It is effective (up to 80%) in men with psychogenic and neurogenic erectile dysfunction, but less effective in men with vasculogenic erectile dysfunction (36%–50%). Its advantages include low cost and stability at room temperature; its major disadvantage is priapism (in up to 35% of cases). The price per dose is approximately $5 (primarily for the syringe, needle, and alcohol pad).

Phentolamine is an alpha-adrenergic receptor antagonist. When used alone, it does not produce rigid erections. Combined with papaverine, success rates range from 63% to 87%. A combination of 30 mg papaverine and 0.5 to 1 mg phentolamine is the usual dose. Side effects include hypotension and reflex tachycardia. The price per dose is approximately $10, primarily because of the compounding fee.

Combinations such as papaverine, phentolamine, and alprostadil (Trimix) are very effective, with response rates as high as 90%. However, this regimen should be reserved for patients who failed to respond to other treatment strategies. The price per dose is approximately $15.

The major side effect of intrapenile alprostadil therapy is penile pain, occurring in about 20% of men. Pain was the side effect most often cited by men who discontinued therapy and is more prominent in men with neuropathy. Priapism, a prolonged erection lasting more than 4 h, is a medical emergency requiring immediate attention. Prolonged erections occur in about 5% of men who use intrapenile alprostadil and 10% of those who use papaverine.

Intraurethral administration of alprostadil (Medicated Urethral System for Erection, MUSE) provides a less invasive alternative to intrapenile injection. The efficacy of intraurethral alprostadil has been evaluated in 1500 men. Two-thirds of these men responded with an erection sufficient for intercourse. Complications such as priapism and penile fibrosis were less common than after penile injection. The cost per dose is approximately $20.

Several mechanical devices have been developed that utilize vacuum pressure to increase arterial inflow and occlusive rings to impede venous outflow from the corpora cavernosae. Mechanical dexterity is required to use these devices. Efficacy is reported to be 67%, and

satisfaction with vacuum-assisted erections has varied from 25% to 49%. The cost per device is $200 to $400.

With the availability of less invasive approaches, enthusiasm for surgical implants has waned. Nevertheless this form of therapy remains a viable option for men who do not respond to sildenafil and find penile injection, urethral, or vacuum therapy unacceptable. Side effects include those related to the anesthesia, local wound infection, and mechanical failure necessitating surgical removal and reimplantation of a new prosthesis. The cost per implant is approximately $5000.

Testosterone supplementation should be discouraged in men in whom erectile dysfunction is not associated with hypogonadism. In men with normal gonadal function, androgen therapy enhances sexual interest without enhancing erectile capacity.

Yohimbine blocks presynaptic alpha-2-adrenergic receptors, and presumably acts in brain centers associated with libido and penile erection. Although folklore has imbued yohimbine with aphrodisiacal properties, it has limited clinical effectiveness. Optimal results are achieved when yohimbine is restricted to men with psychogenic erectile dysfunction.

Summary

Sexuality remains an important issue in the older population. In spite of a decreased ability to achieve an erection, there clearly is continued sexual desire. Many studies suggest that erectile dysfunction in the aged is primarily caused by age-associated chronic disease rather than normal, healthy aging. Therefore, preventive measures aimed at the underlying diseases should be sought. Nevertheless, effective treatment options are now available to successfully regain sexual function and thereby, improve quality of life.

References

1. Kinsey AC, Pomeroy WB, Martin CE. *Sexual Behavior in the Human Male.* Philadelphia: Saunders; 1948.
2. Pfeiffer E, Verwoerdt A, Wang HS. Sexual behavior in aged men and women. *Arch Gen Psychiatry.* 1968;19:753–758.
3. Mulligan T, Retchin SM, Chinchilli VM, et al. The role of aging and chronic disease in sexual dysfunction. *J Am Geriatr Soc.* 1988;36:520–524.
4. Wiley D, Bortz WM. Sexuality and aging—usual and successful. *J Gerontol.* 1996;51A:M142–M146.
5. Bretschneider JG, McCoy N. Sexual interest and behavior in healthy 80-102-year olds. *Arch Sex Behav.* 1988;17:109–129.
6. Mulligan T, Palguta RF. Sexual interest, activity, and satisfaction among male nursing home residents. *Arch Sex Behav.* 1991;20:199–204.

7. Kaiser FE. Sexuality in the elderly. *Urol Clin N Am.* 1996; 23:99–109.

8. Cunningham GR, Hirshkowitz M. Inhibition of steroid 5-alpha-reductase with finasteride: sleep-related erections, potency, and libido in healthy men. *J Clin Endocrinol Metab.* 1995;80:1934–1940.

9. Udry JR, Billy JOG, Morris NM, Groff TR, Raj MH. Serum androgenic hormones motivate sexual behavior in adolescent boys. *Fertil Steril.* 1985;43:90–94.

10. Bagatell CJ, Heiman JR, Rivier JE, et al. Effects of endogenous testosterone and estradiol in sexual behavior in normal young men. *J Clin Endocrinol Metab.* 1994;78:711–716.

11. Mulligan T, Schmitt B. Testosterone for erectile failure. *J Gen Intern Med.* 1993;8:517–521.

12. Lue T. Erectile dysfunction. *N Engl J Med.* 2000;342:1802–1813.

13. Andersson KE, Wagner G. Physiology of penile erection. *Physiol Rev.* 1995;75:191–236.

14. Steers WD. Neural control of penile erection. *Semin Urol.* 1990;8:66–79.

15. Burnett AL. Role of nitric oxide in the physiology of erection. *Biol Reprod.* 1995;52:485–489.

16. Korenman SG. New insights into erectile dysfunction: a practical approach. *Am J Med.* 1998;105:135–144.

17. Wespes E, Schulman C. Venous impotence: pathophysiology, diagnosis, and treatment. *J Urol.* 1993;149:1238–1245.

18. Newman HF, Reiss H, Northup JD. Physical basis of emission, ejaculation, and orgasm in the male. *Urology.* 1982;19:341–350.

19. Vermeulen A. Clinical review 24: androgens in the aging male. *J Clin Endocrinol Metab.* 1991;73:221–224.

20. NIH Consensus Conference. Impotence. *JAMA.* 1993;270:83–90.

21. Feldman HA, Goldstein I, Hatzichristou DG, et al. Impotence and its medical and psychosocial correlates: results of the Massachusetts male aging study. *J Urol.* 1994; 151:54–61.

22. Nehra A, Azadzoi KM, Moreland RB, et al. Cavernosal expandability is an erectile tissue mechanical property which predicts trabecular histology in an animal model of vasculogenic erectile dysfunction. *J Urol.* 1998;59:2229–2236.

23. Azadzoi KM, Siroky MB, Goldstein I. Study of etiologic relationship of arterial atherosclerosis to corporal veno-occlusive dysfunction in the rabbit. *J Urol.* 1996;155:1795–1800.

24. Morley JE, Kaiser FE. Sexual function with advancing age. *Med Clin N Am.* 1989;73:1483–1495.

25. Bemelmans BLH, Meuleman EJH, Doesburg WH, et al. Erectile dysfunction in diabetic men: the neurologic factor revisited. *J Urol.* 1994;151:884–889.

26. Hogan M, Cerami A, Bucala R. Advanced glycosylation endproducts block the antiproliferative effect of nitric oxide. *J Clin Investig.* 1992;90:1110–1115.

27. Chamness SL, Ricker DD, Crone JK, Dembeck CL, Maguire MP, Burnett AL, Chang TS. The effect of androgen on nitric oxide synthase in the male reproductive tract of the rat. *Fertil Steril.* 1995 May; 63(5):1101–1107.

28. Slag ME, Morley JE, Elson MK, et al. Impotence in medical clinic outpatients. *JAMA.* 1983;249:1736–1740.

29. Mulligan T, Katz PG. Why aged men become impotent. *Arch Intern Med.* 1989;149:1365–1366.

30. Johnson AR III, Jarow JP. Is routine endocrine testing of impotent men necessary? *J Urol.* 1992;147:1542–1543.

31. Masters W, Johnson V. *Human Sexual Response.* Boston: Little, Brown; 1970.

32. Rowland DL, Greenleaf WJ, Dorfman LJ, Davidson JM. Aging and sexual function in men. *Arch Sex Behav.* 1993; 22:545–557.

33. Godschalk MF, Sison A, Mulligan T. Management of erectile dysfunction by the geriatrician. *J Am Geriatr Soc.* 1997; 45:1240–1246.

34. Cheitlin MD, Hutter AM Jr, Brindis RG, et al. Use of sildenafil (Viagra) in patients with cardiovascular disease. *Circulation.* 1999;99:168–177 [erratum: *Circulation.* 1999; 100:2389].

49
Sexual Function and the Older Woman

Fran E. Kaiser

Sexual function and dysfunction after menopause and into the later years of a woman's life are poorly defined and even less well studied. However, recognition that sexual function goes well beyond the usual matrix of activity—intercourse—is just beginning to be reconciled to the types of information and data gathered. Sexual function encompasses sense of self, interaction with others, culture, environment, cohort contexts, and myriad levels of affections and expression.[1] It is shaped by these factors, as well as the overlay of physiologic and pathologic and psychologic changes encountered by an individual or her partner. Despite the myths and caricatures created (particularly in females) relating to maintaining sexual interest and performance with aging, the inexorable increase in the population of aging women (and men) and the desire for continued quality of life bring this issue to attention.[1,2] The need for intimacy, touch, and sexual thoughts and fantasies does not end at any age.

More than half a century ago, Kinsey and colleagues noted a general decline in sexual interest and activity that was attributed to age.[3] Subsequent data related to the impact of menopause and the years following have almost invariably reported a decline in both sexual interest and desire.[1] In 1000 consecutive patients who were questioned, patients over age 50 had more sexual complaints than younger individuals.[4] Data from a longitudinal study begun in 1969 with 241 women aged 46 to 71 noted a decline in sexual interest and frequency of intercourse with age.[5,6] Partner issues (death, illness, or performance issues) were noted to be causally linked to women's lack of sexual activity in three-fourths of cases. Postmenopausal status did appear to contribute to diminished sexual interest and frequency but did not appear to mar sexual enjoyment. Some investigators have found an inverse relationship between menopause and sexual interest; however, other data have linked these findings with other life-altering events—partner issues, work or life stressors.[1,7–10] Stress causes a 2.7 times greater

risk of lack of interest in sex; and stress related to diminished arousal has an odds ratio of 4.6 or more.[10] Some studies have shown little or no alternation of sexual desire, response, and satisfaction following menopause.[8,11–13]

In the Massachusetts Women's Health Study II, a longitudinal study of change related to menopausal transition, sexual function data were obtained from 200 women aged 51 to 61 not on hormone replacement.[14] Menopausal status did not relate to sexual satisfaction, frequency of intercourse, orgasmic ability, or dyspareunia. In the Postmenopausal Estrogen/Progesten interventions trial (PEPI), 60% of women 55 to 64 years old were sexually active.[15] Nearly 50% of healthy women over 60 practice masturbation,[1] whereas 25% of women over 70 in nursing homes engage in masturbation.[16]

Menopausal Changes

Hormones, Sexual Responses, and Symptoms of Menopause

The clinical diagnosis and definition of menopause is amenorrhea for 12 months for which there is no other obvious pathologic or physiologic cause. Menopause may occur following irregular menses (perimenopause), which is part of the continuum of change. Perimenopause may be accompanied by symptoms such as hot flashes that predate actual menopause by months or years and are associated with varied hormonal patterns in different women.[17,18] "Natural" menopause (as opposed to surgical menopause) is really only recognized retrospectively a year or more following a final menstrual period and is an event for which a singular biologic marker does not exist. The age at which menopause occurs (mean age, 51) has not substantially changed in the past century, but life span has dramatically altered. Life expectancy was 18 in

1000 B.C., 25 in 100 B.C., and 49 in 1900. Women in 2000 have a life expectancy of 79.7 years (nearly 7 years greater than for men), and nearly two-thirds of women will survive to age 85 or more.[19,20] Thus, women will spend at least one-third or more of their lives postmenopausally. In 2000, there were approximately 41.75 million women in the United States over age 50.

Earlier onset of menopause has been associated with a family history of earlier menopause, and smoking appears to be a dose- and duration-related effect.[17,21–23] The majority of studies indicate that neither age at menarche, number of pregnancies, socioeconomic status, nor race appear to influence the age at which menopause occurs, although increasing parity may be associated with later menopause.

Hormonal Change

Perimenopausally, ovarian follicles decrease, potentially through apoptosis of granulosa cells and oocytes; along with this, ovarian estrogen production diminishes.[24] Serum gonadotropins rise, with follicle-stimulating hormone (FSH) rising to a greater degree than luteinizing hormone (LH).[25] FSH is responsible for follicular maturation and ovulation, while LH provides the stimulation for ovulation and corpus luteum steroid secretion. The etiology of the incremental rise of FSH is not only due to the loss of negative feedback by gonadal steroids but also the cessation of ovarian follicular production of inhibin. In the pituitary, FSH secretion is inhibited by inhibin. In the gonads, gonadotropin-dependent steroidogenesis and cell proliferation are potentiatiated by inhibin. Ovarian production of androgens continues under the elevated LH concentration. Inhibin B appears to fall before Inhibin A.[26] Activin [a member of the transforming growth factor-beta (TGF-β) superfamily] functions as an autocrine/paracrine regulator and plays a role in folliculogenesis and in inducing FSH receptors.[27] Indeed, with postmenopausal estrogen administration, FSH may not be likely to return to premenopausal concentrations. FSH, predominantly under the control of inhibin, which remains low in menopause, will remain somewhat elevated even in the face of estrogen administration, and thus FSH may not be completely reliable as a measure of sufficient or physiologic estrogen administration. Gonadotropins may decline with further aging or with medical comorbidity.[28] During the transition along the way to menopause (perimenopause), both estradiol and estrone concentration fall, although the concentration of estrone is higher than that of estradiol, a reversal of the pattern seen in younger women. In most postmenopausal women the major contribution to circulating estradiol results from peripheral aromatization of androgen (androstenedione) from ovarian and adrenal sources.

Menopause is also associated with decreased ovarian androgen production as well as decreased adrenal androgens, dehydroepiandrostenedione (DHEA) and DHEAS.[29,30] If ovarian stromal hypertrophy or hyperplasia develops because of elevation in LH concentration, this can result in increased testosterone levels. If the ovaries are fibrotic, the adrenal becomes the main androgenic source following menopause. In postmenopausal women, both total testosterone and bioavailable testosterone are reduced in women undergoing TAHBSO (total abdominal hysterectomy with bilateral salpingo-oophorectomy) compared with hysterectomized women who have conservation of one or both ovaries.[31] These data support the importance of the ovary in androgen production. Data related to longitudinal hormonal studies during the menopausal transition reveal declines in both androstenedione and testosterone approximately 3 years before the occurrence of menopause.[32] In postmenopausal women with intact ovaries, low testosterone levels at the time of menopause are found, with a later increment in ovarian synthesis of testosterone, with levels rising to those of premenopausal women. However, because production of androgens is far less altered than estrogen, the estrogen/androgen ratio falls. The hormonal milieu of women also depends to some degree on sex hormone-binding globulin (SHBG). In a recent study of 172 midlife women followed for 7 years, SHBG decreased a mean of 43% from 4 years before the final menstrual period to 4 years after that event.[33] Further, increased levels of estradiol and thyroxine will increase SHBG, whereas testosterone, glucocorticoids, insulin, and obesity decrease SHBG. It seems likely that, in a fashion similar to that of thyroid hormone, it is free bioavailable hormone levels (estradiol and/or estrone, as well as testosterone) rather than total hormone levels that have clinical relevance, but this has not been well studied in women.

Female Sexual Response and Hormonal Change

The complexity of female sexuality comprising libido (desire, drive, interest) and sexual response (biologic, physical ability, view of self, roles, and behavior) has come a long way from the initial physiologic data of Masters and Johnson.[34] In Kaplan's modification of that model[35] in the older woman, desire/libido may show little to mild decrease in both intensity and frequency of desire. The arousal phase is associated with diminished vaginal blood flow and genital engorgement and decreased vaginal lubrication. During the prolonged plateau phase, lessened color change of the labia, indicating lesser blood flow, may occur. Although the multiorgasmic capacity of women is maintained, weaker and less frequent contractions occur. Resolution is associated with a more

TABLE 49.1. Changes with menopause.

Skin, mucous membranes	Atrophy, dryness, hair loss, loss of resilience
Vocal cords	Reduced upper register
Cardiovascular	Atherosclerosis, coronary artery disease (CAD)
Skeleton	Osteoporosis, tooth loss
Breasts	Reduced size, softer consistency
Neuroendocrine	Hot flashes, labile mood
Urogenital atrophy	Dyspareunia, urinary tract infections (UTI)

rapid loss of vasocongestion than in younger years. However, a broadened view of female sexual response that expands to fit different situational roles, those stressing intimacy and relationship with self and others, has been postulated and is likely to be further utilized over time.[36] The loss of estrogen has also been associated with marked diminution of vaginal lubrication, as well as vaginal narrowing and shortening. These changes are less marked in women who have maintained regular sexual activity following menopause. Diminished sensitivity of the clitoris and vulvar area may occur, although whether this is a result of hormonally mediated neuropathy or a direct impairment of vascular flow and ischemic change is unclear.

Androgens and Sexual Function

Although estrogen is a defining hormone for primary and secondary sex characteristics in women, an increasing consensus has developed regarding the role of androgens as a major factor in enhancing libido. In prospective placebo-controlled crossover trials examining androgen administration compared to estrogen, or estrogen plus a progestin (and placebo), androgen or androgen plus estrogen was noted to be more effective in increasing libido, sexual arousal, and the frequency of sexual fantasies in surgically oophorectomized women than the other modalities.[37–39] Low testosterone levels in women have been found to correlate with reduction in the frequency of intercourse and in a study of sexagenarian women, circulating free testosterone positively correlated with sexual desire.[7,13] Testosterone also appears to have benefit in terms of general energy levels and feelings of well-being. Long-term effects of testosterone, especially on cardiovascular risk in women, remain to be determined.

Testosterone administration in women may decrease HDL cholesterol. Methylated testosterone should be avoided as hepatic dysfunction may result. Just as with testosterone replacement in men, only 17β-testosterone should be considered for administration. It is also unclear as to whom and when androgens should be utilized in women. In the absence of depression, low libido is the most compelling reason to consider androgenic therapy. The risk and potential benefits of androgens in women remain to be elucidated. Doses for women must be individualized and the patient carefully monitored for the potential side effects of hirsutism, lipid disorders, hepatic dysfunction, fluid retention, and potential polycythemia. Individual variations in localized production of androgen and estrogens from precursors such as DHEA or DHEAS make clinical application and evaluation of serum concentrations problematic. The roles of hormones on other parameters of sexual stimuli that affect sexual function—touch, vision, hearing, taste, smell—are just beginning to be considered.[40]

Menopausal Symptoms Affecting Sexual Function

Hot Flashes

Hot flashes are one of the characteristic symptoms of menopause, occurring in up to 82% of menopausal women[41] (Tables 49.1, 49.2). Hot flashes may occur for years in the perimenopausal period. About two-thirds of women experience hot flashes for 1 to 5 years, although some (nearly 10%–15%) women experience hot flashes for more than 5 years. There is cultural variability in reports of hot flashes,[42] with reports of fewer hot flashes in women from Indonesia, China, and other cultures. Whether this relates to perceptions of menopause, differences in reporting of symptoms, use of plant/herbal phytoestrogens, genetics, or other factors is unclear. The impact of hot flashes on one's physiology can be extensive. In 506 women with hot flashes, ranging in age from 29 to 82, of those who reported current symptoms 87% had hot flashes daily, 1% reported more than 10 hot flashes per day, lasting 1 to 5 min, but 6% reported flashes that lasted more than 6 min.[43] Described as heat/flushing on the face and/or chest, this can be generalized over the

TABLE 49.2. Menopausal symptoms affecting sexual function.

Hot flashes
  Heat wave
  Flushing, sweating
  Palpitations
  Chills, anxiety
  Sleep disruption
  Mood changes

Vulvovaginal symptoms
  Vaginal dryness
  Vaginal bleeding
  Labial/mons irritation/itching/burning
  Urge incontinence with frequency, dysuria, nocturia
  Dyspareunia
  Urinary tract infections

body (less on lower body), accompanied by sweats, palpitations, chills, shivering, clamminess, and anxiety. Symptoms tend to be reported when the rise in cutaneous temperature exceeds 0.3°C. The rise in cutaneous temperature tends to be inversely proportional to the ambient temperature. Hot flashes can be virtually eliminated with hormonal replacement, but this effect does not occur instantaneously, and up to 12 weeks may be needed for improvement in symptoms to occur. Hot flashes respond to estrogen in a dose–response fashion.[44] Hot flashes can disrupt sleep, work, and social relationships. Body contact may even bring on a hot flash and can clearly be disruptive to intimacy. It is an abrupt drop in estrogen concentration, rather than hypoestrogenemia per se, that appears to be important in the etiology of the hot flash.[45] There are multiple hormonal changes during a hot flash. Although LH pulses are temporally related to the occurrence of a flash, they do not appear to cause the flash. ACTH, cortisol, and neurotensin all increase during a hot flash.[46–48] The central adrenergic system remains an area of active interest. Clonidine, an α_2-adrenergic receptor agonist, has been shown to reduce vascular responsiveness to norepinephrine, epinephrine, and angiotensin.[49] Additionally, it appears to be effective in diminishing hot flashes in women with breast cancer on tamoxifen, whose flashes relate to tamoxifen administration.[50]

Sleep/Depression

Although sleep disruption brought on by hot flashes may produce fatigue and situational loss of coping mechanisms, the majority of studies do not indicate that postmenopausal women have prominent symptoms of depression.[51,52] Clustering of both life events (as well as hormonal change) may appear to link to any temporal peak of depressive symptoms at the time of menopause.

Estrogen replacement appears to enhance mood, although this may relate to improvement in vasomotor symptoms. There are some alterations that may explain estrogenic effects on mood. The association of estrogen with an increase in β-endorphins is one example. In a study of depression that included postmenopausal women (11/18 on estrogen), a serotonin antagonist was administered, and the response of cortisol and prolactin to the anatagonist (1-metachlorophenyl piperazine) was blunted in postmenopausal women compared with younger controls or those on estrogen.[53] This diminished response to serotonin (5-HT) may explain some of the mood-altering effect of estrogen; however, it is not clear that these changes are persistent.[54] The combination of hormone replacement therapy (HRT) plus a selective serotonin reuptake inhibitor (SSRI) may confer benefit in treating depression[55] relative to either estrogen or SSRI alone, and might be considered in postmenopausal

patients who fail an SSRI as monotherapy. The impact of progesterone on mood is also unclear, with studies providing conflicting results, and, as with studies of estrogen, differences in type, dose, and duration of use make cross-comparison of data difficult.[56–58] Lack of compliance with HRT because of effects that are seen as largely progestational—bleeding, mood changes, irritability, cramps, and bloating, to name a few—create a need to advocate the lowest dose that will eliminate endometrial hyperplasia.

Urogenital Atrophy

Vulvovaginal changes are gradual and, unlike vasomotor symptoms that may spontaneously disappear, inexorably worsen if not treated (Tables 49.2, 49.3). Vaginal dryness, soreness, and dyspareunia have been described in 27% of 1761 women.[59] In this same study, 36% complained of micturition symptoms, incontinence, or urinary tract infections. Half of the symptomatic women noted moderate to severe discomfort as a result of these changes. Symptoms can include itching, burning, incontinence, dyspareunia, and other disabling problems.[60] Although the true prevalence of urogenital atrophy is unknown, estimates range from 10% to 40%.[61] About 30% to 65% of women complain of dyspareunia.[62–64] Loss of subcutaneous fat in the labia majora results in shrinkage. The prepuce of the clitoral glans atrophies, and the decrease in lubrication adds to irritation. Loss of vaginal muscularity and the lack of lubrication cause easier trauma to the vagina. Dyspareunia with intercourse and vaginal bleeding may occur.

In the presence of estrogen, vaginal colonization with lactobacilli, which maintain the vaginal pH at 4.5 to 5.0 via lactic acid production, inhibits *Escherichia coli* and other gram-negative organisms that can contribute to urinary tract infections (UTIs). With the loss of estrogen, the rise in vaginal pH results in bacterial population shifts toward coliforms, with staphylococci and streptococci becoming more prominent. Recurrent UTIs are esti-

TABLE 49.3. Specific sexual problems causing dissatisfaction.[a]

	Total number with problem	Number (%) dissatisfied	Odds ratio (95% CI)
Orgasmic dysfunction	160	63 (39.4)	4.1 (3.0–5.6)
Dyspareunia	115	28 (24.3)	5.2 (3.7–7.4)
Vaginal dryness	183	40 (21.9)	1.3 (1.1–1.6)
Arousal problems	101	51 (51)	5.2 (3.7–7.4)
Unpleasurable sex	104	49 (47.1)	4.0 (3.0–5.6)
Any of these	286	77 (26.9)	1.9 (1.5–2.3)

[a] Questionnaire survey of 1768 adults aged 18–75: 290 women (41% reported current sexual problems).
Source: Adapted from Dunn KM, Croft PR, Hackett GI. *J Sex Marital Ther*. 2000;26:141–151.

FIGURE 49.1. Urogenital symptoms in 902 women. (Adapted from Iosif CS, Bekassy Z. Prevalence of genitourinary symptoms in the late menopause. *Acta Obstet Gynecol.* 1984;63:257–260, with permission.)

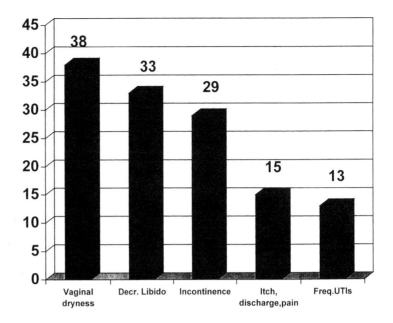

mated to occur in 10% to 15% of women over the age of 60[65] (Fig. 49.1).

With menopause, the cervix atrophies and the transitional zone may be located on the lower endocervix; also, the prevalence of abnormal Pap smears increases with age. Other aspects of urogenital change may include thinning of the urethral epithelium, which reduces the closing pressure for continence. Urethral prolapse may occur, with loss of collagen supporting endopelvic fascia. With menopause and aging, stress as well as urge incontinence may occur. Resultant fears of incontinence may inhibit sexual function. These symptoms are readily reversible with estrogen, and it is important to note that localized application of estrogen may produce a better resolution of urogenital atrophy than is seen with systemic administration. Local absorption is high in the presence of an atrophic vaginal mucosa. Vaginal creams, tablets, or estro-

gen-containing vaginal rings can all provide relief[66,67] (Table 49.4). The tablets and rings appear to have greater acceptance than cream or pessaries. Concern over systemic effects remains even with localized vaginal administration, especially with vaginal cream at a dose the equivalent of 0.625 mg three times a week or more. However, before increasing a systemic dose of hormones to control symptoms, a trial of local administration should be considered.

Urogenital-Vascular Alterations

As part of the urogenital changes seen with menopause, some investigators have postulated a vasculogenic urogenital cause for sexual dysfunction in women,[68,69] similar in nature to the changes that have been described as the primary etiology of sexual dysfunction in aging

TABLE 49.4. Vaginal estrogen preparations.

Generic	Trade name	Content	Administration	Effect beyond local
Estrogen cream	Premarin Cream	0.625 mg conjugated estrogen per gram	Daily for 3 weeks, then 1 week off	Can have systemic effects, elevated E_2, elevated triglycerides
Estriol Cream	Ovestin, Synopause	1 mg/g estriol	0.5 mg estriol twice a week	Low E_1, E_2, elevated E_3, no endometrial hyperplasia noted
Estradiol tablets	Vagifem	25 μg 17β-estradiol	One tablet intravaginally twice a week	Low E_1, E_2, no endometrial hyperplasia
Estradiol ring	Estring	Silicon elastomer ring with 2 mg estradiol releasing 7.5 μg/24 h	Replace every 90 days	Low E_1, E_2, no endometrial hyperplasia

males, that is, atherosclerotic changes. These atherosclerotic changes appear to result in delayed vaginal engorgement, loss of lubrication, diminished vaginal and/or clitoral sensation, and decreased vaginal and/or clitoral orgasm.

Pressure stimulation along the lower third of the vagina increases blood flow and velocity in clitoral arteries.[70] However, it is also clear that sexual function in women goes well beyond any clitoral or vaginal engorgement issues.

Other Factors Affecting Sexual Function in Women

Partner Issues

For women, one of the leading reasons for sexual inactivity is the lack of a partner, even in younger cohorts (under age 70); an assessment of 874 postmenopausal women revealed that although 64% were sexually active, 64% also noted inactivity because of lack of a partner.[71] Erectile dysfunction is a common problem for many older men, so even those women with partners may have some difficulty. A woman may perceive withdrawal of the male, because of libido or erectile difficulties on his part, as loss of interest in her. Depending on the nature of the relationship, a frank discussion of sexual issues and difficulties between the partners may not take place. In the scarce literature on older lesbians, lack of a partner is also cited as the reason for not being sexually active.[72] Few if any recent surveys evaluate masturbation or other activities that can be performed unpartnered.

Medication

The use of medication and its effect on sexual function in women has not received the degree of attention seen in evaluation of drugs that cause erectile dysfunction in men.[73] Although medications can affect libido, arousal, orgasm, or any combination of these, questions related to sexual function are often not assessed in women on medications. Antihypertensive agents can be associated with decreased libido or arousal, whereas antidepressant agents such as SSRIs and tricyclics can decrease libido and inhibit orgasmic function. Depression itself, as well as the therapies directed at its treatment, can be associated with sexual dysfunction. Even over-the-counter agents such as antihistamines may diminish sexual arousal and may often be overlooked in the evaluation of the patient.

Environmental Issues

Women living with their children or in institutional settings such as nursing homes may face environmental barriers to privacy, including the biases and potential disapproval of caregivers or administrators/staff in nursing homes. Maintaining sexual autonomy, avoiding sexual coercion or abuse, and determining capacity for consent in individuals whose cognitive function may not be intact poses another set of issues.[74,75] Neutral or supportive responses by caregivers and recognition that not all touch is sexual and that touching, caressing, and massage are powerful therapies, especially when patients are "touch deprived," are important.

Additional Issues

Surgery: Hysterectomy and Sexual Function

Although the number of women undergoing hysterectomy has decreased from 670,000 in 1985 to 580,000 in 1992, it remains the second most common surgical procedure (following childbirth) in women.[76] Deterioration in sexual function following hysterectomy has been reported in up to 37% of women.[77,78] However, in a 2-year prospective study of 1101 women, dyspareunia, anorgasmia, and rates of low libido all improved following hysterectomy.[79] Shortening of the vaginal vault, loss of uterine contractions, and elimination of cervical movement during orgasm have been cited as contributing to altered sensation during intercourse posthysterectomy but do not appear to produce impaired sexual enjoyment in most women.

Classification of Female Sexual Dysfunction

For the very first time, sexual dysfunction that relates to organic disorders has been classified. Previous definitions of sexual dysfunction noted in the Diagnostic and Statistical Manual of Mental Disorders of the American Psychiatric Society (DSM IV) were not intended to classify organic etiologies of female sexual dysfunction.[80] A recent First Consensus Development Panel on Female Sexual Dysfunction was convened in 1998 and came forward with the following classification[81]:

1. Sexual desire disorders
   A. Hypoactive sexual desire disorder
   B. Sexual aversion disorder
2. Sexual arousal disorder
3. Orgasmic disorder
4. Sexual pain disorders
   A. Dyspareunia
   B. Vaginismus
   C. Other sexual pain disorders

Definitions

Each of the following can be further subdefined as lifelong versus acquired; generalized versus situational; and of etiologic origin (organic, psychogenic, mixed, unknown).

Hypoactive sexual desire disorder is the persistent or recurrent deficiency/absence of sexual fantasies/thoughts and/or desire for, or receptivity to, sexual activity, which causes personal distress.

Sexual arousal disorder is the persistent or recurrent inability to maintain sufficient sexual excitement, causing personal distress, which can be expressed as a lack of subjective excitement or lack of genital (lubrication/swelling) or other somatic responses.

Orgasmic disorder is the persistent or recurrent difficulty, delay, or absence of attaining orgasm following sufficient sexual stimulation and arousal, which causes personal distress.

Sexual pain disorders: dyspareunia is the recurrent or persistent genital pain associated with sexual intercourse. Vaginismus is the recurrent or persistent involuntary spasm of the musculature of the outer third of the vagina that interferes with vaginal penetration, which causes personal distress. Noncoital sexual pain disorder is recurrent persistent genital pain induced by noncoital sexual stimulation.

Evaluating the Patient

Evaluation begins with a careful history. Very few women with sexual problems initiate discussion about them with their physician, but when specifically asked about sexual problems, 19% of women surveyed reported a problem.[82] If the patient is uncomfortable talking about sex, open-ended questions may help create a milieu of a greater level of comfort, such as "Do you have any difficulty with your ability to have sex? Does that refer to intercourse or masturbation or other form of sexual activity?" Nonjudgmental attitudes are paramount in eliciting a sexual history. Specific details on the type of problem, its duration, the rate of progression, and how it has affected sexual function should be obtained. If the patient is not comfortable about providing information that would help define the problem, ask if she would like to speak with someone else, or write out these issues. Libido and orgasmic capacity should be queried as part of both present and past history. Medication, over-the-counter medications, and medical comorbidities and their relation to sexual dysfunction should be explored.

Questions regarding their partner's sexual function and relationship should also be addressed, both as an interview with the patient, regarding their perceptions of the partner issues, and, ideally, with the partner alone. Suggestions for alternatives for those without partners may ease discomfort related to the practice of masturbation. Changes in medication, assessing whether depression is present and addressing that, as well as the recognition of issues such as dyspareunia due to vaginal dryness or vaginitis, may assist in providing appropriate

remedies for these problems. Encouraging frank and open discussion between partners, or, in the nursing home, providing privacy for those whose sexual activity is not coerced, can allow sexual expression and intimacy to continue.

References

1. Roughan P, Kaiser FE, Morley JE. Sexuality and the older woman. *Clin Geriatr Med.* 1993;9:87–106.
2. Kaiser FE. Sexuality in the elderly. *Urol Clin N Am.* 1996;23:99–109.
3. Kinsey AC, Pomeroy WB, Martin CW. *Sexual Behavior in the Human.* Philadelphia: Saunders; 1953.
4. Bachmann GA, Leiblum SR, Grill J. Brief inquiry in gynecologic practice. *Obstet Gynecol.* 1989;73:425–427.
5. Pfeiffer E, VerWoerdt A, Davis GC. Sexual behavior in middle life. *Am J Psychiatry.* 1972;128:1267–1267.
6. Pfeiffer E, Davis GC. Determinants of sexual behavior in middle age, old age. *J Am Geriatr Soc.* 1972;20:151–158.
7. McCoy NL, Davidson JM. A longitudinal study of the effects of menopause on sexuality. *Maturitas.* 1985;7:203–210.
8. Dennerstein L, Smith AMA, Morse CA, Burger HG. Sexuality and the menopause. *J Psychosom Obstet Gynecol.* 1994;15:59–66.
9. Hallstrom T. Sexuality of women in middle age: the Goteburg Study. *J Biosocial Sci (Suppl).* 1979;16:165–175.
10. Laumann EO, Paik A, Rosen RC. Sexual dysfunction in the United States. *JAMA.* 1999;281:537–544.
11. Cawood EH, Bancroft J. Steroid hormones, the menopause: sexuality and well being of women. *Psychol Med.* 1996;26:926–936.
12. Cutler WB, Garcia CR, McCoy N. Perimenopausal sexuality. *Arch Sex Behav.* 1987;16:225–234.
13. Bachmann GA, Leiblum SR. Sexuality in sexagenarian women. *Maturitas.* 1991;13:43–52.
14. Avis NE, Stellato R, Crawford S, Johannes C. How does menopause impact sexual activity? *Menopause.* 1995;2:245.
15. Greendale GA, Hogan P, Shumaker S, for the Postmenopausal Estrogen/Progestin Interventions (PEPI) Trial Investigations. Sexual functioning in postmenopausal women: the Postmenopausal Estrogen/Progestin Interventions (PEPI) Trial. *J Women's Health.* 1996;5:445–456.
16. Kaas MJ. Sexual expression of the elderly in nursing homes. *Gerontologist.* 1978;18:372–378.
17. Cramer DW, Xu H. Predicting age at menopause. *Maturitas.* 1996;23:319–326.
18. Sherman BM, West JH, Korenman SG. The menopausal transition: analysis of LH, FSH, estradiol and progesterone concentrations during menstrual cycles of older women. *J Clin Endocrinol Metab.* 1976;42:629–636.
19. Tauber CM, ed. *Statistical Handbook on Women in America, 2nd Ed.* Phoenix: Oryx Press; 1996:1–5.
20. Olshansky SJ, Carnes BA, Cassel C. In search of Methuselah: estimating the upper limits to human longevity. *Science.* 1990;250:634.

21. Cramer DW, Xu H, Harlow BL. Family history as a predictor for menopause. *Fertil Steril*. 1995;64:740–745.

22. Van Noord PAH, Dubas JS, Dorland N, Boersma H, te Velde E. Age at natural menopause in a population-based screening cohort: the role of menarche, fecundity and lifestyle factors. *Fertil Steril*. 1997;68:95–102.

23. Torgerson DJ, Avenell A, Russell I, Reid DM. Factors associated with onset of menopause in women aged 45–49. *Maturitas*. 1994;19:83.

24. Driancourt MA, Thuel B. Control of oocyte growth and maturation by follicular cells and molecules present in follicular fluid. A review. *Reprod Nutr Dev*. 1998;38:345–362.

25. Santoro N, Adel T, Skurnick J. Decreased inhibin tone and increased activan A secretion characterizes reproductive aging in women. *Fertil Steril*. 1999;71:658–662.

26. Burger HG, Cahir N, Robertson DM, et al. Serum inhibins A and B fall differentially as FSH rises in perimenopausal women. *Clin Endocrinol*. 1998;48:809–813 [erratum 49: 550].

27. Li R, Phillips DM, Mather JP. Activin promotes ovarian follicle development in vitro. *Endocrinology*. 1995;136:849–856.

28. Quint AR, Kaiser FE. Gonadotropin determinations and thyrotropin releasing hormone and luteinizing hormone releasing hormone in critically ill postmenopausal women with hypothyroxinemia. *J Clin Endocrinol Metab*. 1985;60: 464–471.

29. Longcope C. The significance of steroid production by peripheral tissues. In: Scholler R, ed. *Endocrinology of the Ovary*. Paris: SEPE; 1978:23–35.

30. Meldrum DR, Davidson BJ, Tatryn IV, Judd HL. Changes in circulating steroids with aging in postmenopausal women. *Obstet Gynecol*. 1981;57:624.

31. Laughlin GA, Barrett-Connor E, Kritz-Silverstein D, Von Muhlen D. Hysterectomy, oophorectomy and endogenous sex hormone levels in older women: the Rancho Bernardo Study. *J Clin Endocrinol Metab*. 2000;85:645–651.

32. Overlie I, Moen MH, Morkrid L, Skjeraasen JS, Holte A. The endocrine transition around menopause: five years prospective study with profiles of gonadotropines, estrogens, androgens and SHBG among healthy women. *Acta Obstet Gynecol Scand*. 1999;10:642–647.

33. Burger HG, Dudley EC, Cui J, Dennerstein L, Hopper JL. A prospective longitudinal study of serum testosterone, dehydroepiandrosterone sulfate and sex hormone binding globulin levels through the menopause transition. *J Clin Endocrinol Metab*. 2000;85:2832–2838.

34. Masters WH, Johnson VE. *Human Sexual Response*. Boston: Little, Brown; 1966.

35. Kaplan HS. *Disorders of Sexual Desire*. New York: Bronner/Mazel; 1979.

36. Basson R. The female sexual response: a different model. *J Sex Marital Ther*. 2000;26:51–65.

37. Sherwin BB, Gelfand MM, Brender W. Androgen enhances sexual motivation in females: a prospective, crossover study of sex steroid administration in surgical menopause. *Psychosom Med*. 1987;47:339–351.

38. Barrett Connor E, Young R, Notelovitz M, et al. A two-year, double-blind comparison of estrogen-androgen and conjugated estrogens in surgically menopausal women. Effects on bone mineral density, symptoms, and lipid profiles. *J Reprod Med*. 1999;44:1012–1020.

39. Sherwin BB, Gelfand M. Differential symptom response to parenteral estrogen and/or androgen administration in the surgical menopause. *Am J Obstet Gynecol*. 1985;151: 153–160.

40. Graziottin A. Libido: the biologic scenario. *Maturitas*. 2000; 34(suppl 1):S9–S16.

41. Feldman BM, Voda A, Gronseth E. The prevalence of hot flash and associated variables among perimenopausal women. *Res Nurs Health*. 1985;8:261–268.

42. Flint M, Samil RS. Cultural and subcultural meanings of the menopause. *Ann NY Acad Sci*. 1990;592:134–148.

43. Kronenberg F. Hot flashes: epidemiology and physiology. *Ann NY Acad Sci*. 1990;592:52–86.

44. Steingold KA. Treatment of hot flashes with transdermal estradiol administration. *J Clin Endocrinol Metab*. 1985;61: 627–632.

45. Askel S, Schomberg DW, Iyrey L, Hammond CB. Vasomotor symptoms, serum estrogens and gonadotropin levels in surgical menopause. *Am J Obstet Gynecol*. 1996;12:165–169.

46. Lightman SL, Jacobs HS, Maguire AK, McGarrick G, Jeffcoate SL. Climacteric flushing: clinical and endocrine response to infusion of naloxone. *Br J Obstet Gynaecol*. 1981;88:919–924.

47. Kronenberg F, Cote LJ, Linkie DM, Dyrenfurth I, Downey JA. Menopausal hot flashes: thermoregulatory, cardiovascular and circulating catecholamine and LH changes. *Maturitas*. 1984;6:31–43.

48. Freedman RR, Woodward S, Sabharwal SC. Alpha adrenergic mechanism in menopausal hot flushes. *Obstet Gynecol*. 1990;76:573–578.

49. Ginsburg J, O'Reilly B, Swinhoe J. Effects of oral clonidine on human cardiovascular responsiveness: a possible explanation for the therapeutic action of the drug in menopausal flushing and migraine. *Br J Obstet Gynaecol*. 1985;92:1169–1175.

50. Pandya KJ, Raubertas RF, Flynn PJ, et al. Oral clonidine in postmenopausal patients with breast cancer experiencing tamoxifen-induced hot flashes: a University of Rochester cancer center community clinical oncology program study. *Ann Intern Med*. 2000;132:788–793.

51. Kaufert PA, Gilbert P, Tate R. The Manitoba Project: a reexamination of the link between menopause and depression. *Maturitas*. 1992;14:143–155.

52. Matthews KA, Kuller LH, Wing RR, Meilahn EN. Biobehavioral aspects of menopause: lessons from the healthy women study. *Exp Gerontol*. 1994;29:337–342.

53. Halbreich U, Asnis GM, Shindeldecker R, Zumoff B, Nathan RS. Cortisol secretion in endogenous depression. *Arch Gen Psychiatry*. 1985;42:904–908

54. Oppenheim G. A case of rapid mood cycling with estrogen: implications. *J Clin Psychiatry*. 1984;45:34–35.

55. Schneider LS, Small GW, Hamilton SH, Bystritsky A, Nemeroff CB, Meyers BS, and the Fluoxitene Collaborative Study Group. Estrogen replacement and fluoxitene in a multicenter geriatric depression trial. *Am J Geriatr Psychiatry*. 1997;5:97–106.

56. Sherwin BB. The impact of different doses of estrogen and progestin on mood and sexual behavior in postmenopausal women. *J Clin Endocrinol Metab*. 1991;72:336–343.

57. Smith RN, Holland EF, Studd JW. The symptomatology of progestin intolerance. *Maturitas*. 199;18:87–91.

58. Greendale GA, Reboussin BA, Hogan P, et al. Symptom relief and side effects of postmenopausal hormones: results from the Postmenopausal Estrogen/Progestin Interventions Trial. *Obstet Gynecol*. 1998;92:982–988.

59. Van Geelen JM, van de Weijer PH, Arnolds HT. Urogenital symptoms and resulting discomfort in non-institutionalized Dutch women aged 50–75 years. *Int Urogynecol J (Pelvic Floor Dysfunction)*. 2000;11:9–14.

60. Barlow DH, Cardozo LD, Francis RM, et al. Urogenital ageing and its effect on sexual health in older British women. *Br J Obstet Gynaecol*. 1997;104:87–91.

61. Greendale GA, Judd HL. Menopause: health implications and clinical management. *J Am Geriatr Soc*. 1993;41:426–436.

62. Sarrel PM. Sexuality and menopause. *Obstet Gynecol*. 1990;75:26S–30S.

63. Glatt AE, Zinner SH, McCormack WM. The prevalence of dyspareunia. *Obstet Gynecol*. 1990;75:433–436.

64. Bachmann GA, Leiblum SR, Sandler B, et al. Sexual expression and its determination: the postmenopausal woman. *Maturitas*. 1984;6:19–29.

65. Romano JM, Kaye D. UTI in the elderly: common yet atypical. *Geriatrics*. 1981;36:113–115.

66. Keenan JL, Franks AL, Croft JB, Scholes D, Murray ET. Vaginal estrogen creams: use patterns among a cohort of women. *J Am Geriatr Soc*. 1999;47:65–70.

67. Rioux JE, Devlin MC, Gelfand MM, Steinberg WM, Hepburn DS. 17β estradiol vaginal tablet versus conjugated equine estrogen vaginal cream to relieve menopausal atrophic vaginitis. *Menopause*. 2000;7:156–161.

68. Park K, Goldstein I, Andry C, Siroky MB, Krane RJ, Azadzoi KM. Vasculogenic female sexual dysfunction: the hemodynamic basis for vaginal engorgement insufficiency and clitoral erectile insufficiency. *Int J Impot Res*. 1997;9:27–37.

69. Goldstein I, Berman JR. Vasculogenic female sexual dysfunction: vaginal engorgement and clitoral insufficiency syndromes. *Int J Impot Res*. 1998;10(suppl 2):S84–S90.

70. Lavoisier P, Aloui R, Schmidt MH, Watrelot A. Clitoral blood flow increases following vaginal pressure stimulation. *Arch Sex Behav*. 1995;24:37–45.

71. Greendale GA, Hogan P, Schumaker S. Sexual functioning in postmenopausal women. *J Women's Health*. 1996;5:445–448.

72. Kehoe M. *Lesbians over 60 Speak for Themselves*. New York: Harrington Park Press; 1989.

73. Anonymous. Drugs that cause sexual dysfunction: an update. *Med Lett Drugs Ther*. 1992;34:73–78.

74. Kaiser FE, Morley JE. Sexuality and dementia. In: Morris JC, ed. *Handbook of Dementing Illnesses*. New York: Dekker; 1994:539–548.

75. White CB. Sexual interest, attitudes, knowledge and sexual history in relation to sexual behavior in institutionalized elderly. *Arch Sex Behav*. 1992;11:11–21.

76. National Center for Health Statistics. *Health, United States 1993*. Hyattsville, MD: Public Health Service; 1994:188.

77. Goldstein MK, Teng NNH. Gynecological factors in sexual dysfunction of the older women. *Clin Geriatr Med*. 1991;7:41–61.

78. Helstrom L, Lundberg PO, Sorbom D, Backstrom T. Sexuality after hysterectomy: a factor analysis of women's sexual lives before and after subtotal hysterectomy. *Obstet Gynecol*. 1993;81:357–362.

79. Rhodes JC, Kjerulff KH, Langenberg PW, Guzinski GM. Hysterectomy and sexual functioning. *JAMA*. 1999;282:1934–1941.

80. American Psychiatric Association. *DSM-IV: Diagnostic and Statistical Manual of Mental Disorders, 4th Ed*. Washington, DC: American Psychiatric Press; 1994.

81. Basson R, Berman J, Burnett A, et al. Report of the international consensus development conference on female sexual dysfunction: definitions and classifications. *J Urol*. 2000;163:888–893.

82. Utian W, ed. *Menopause Core Curriculum Study Guide*. Cleveland: North American Menopause Society; 2000:326.

50
Gynecologic and Urologic Problems of Older Women

M. Chrystie Timmons

It is well established that the population of the United States and the world is becoming proportionately older.[1] In industrialized countries, there are currently 100 women to 75 men in the 60- to 69-year-old age group but 100 women to only 50 men in the over-80 age group. Women 75 and older continue to be one of the most rapidly growing segments of the population. In response to this demographic change, there is increased interest in treatment of the aging woman. New diagnostic and treatment modalities have been developed for both prevention and treatment of health problems associated with gynecologic aging. All physicians, be they internists, family practitioners, geriatricians, or gynecologists, will need to become adept in evaluation, diagnosis, and management of the common gynecologic and urologic problems of older women.

The concept of geriatric gynecology has evolved since the beginning of the twentieth century because the average life expectancy for women did not reach 50 years until approximately 1900. Now, the life expectancy for a healthy 50-year-old woman is 85 years because, before the past century, women died primarily from infectious diseases and childbirth. Most did not live to suffer conditions associated with aging, such as cardiovascular disease, malignancies, and osteoporosis. Therefore, the challenge to health care providers of the aging woman is to incorporate medical management that includes both prevention and treatment of gynecologic and urologic conditions so that each woman has the optimal chance of health maintenance. Early intervention with consideration of quality of life issues is especially important for this patient group.

The three gynecologic phases of life are prepubertal, reproductive, and peri/postmenopausal. Because of the shorter life expectancy before 1900, women passed through only two gynecologic phases—childhood and reproductive age—before death. The management of conditions in each phase has an impact on a woman's subsequent health in the phases that follow. For example, obstetric management in the reproductive phase may predispose to or help to prevent urogenital prolapse in later years. Healthy lifestyle changes incorporated in the reproductive years can lead to a healthier postmenopausal life. Administration of hormonal replacement therapy in the menopausal years may significantly diminish a woman's risk of developing cardiovascular disease or osteoporosis in the postmenopausal years.

This chapter gives an overview of the effects of aging and hormonal changes on the urogenital system in women, outlines the main features of gynecologic evaluation and diagnosis for these patients, and discusses the common conditions encountered in older women. Practical treatment guidelines are given and the indications for referral are discussed.

Urogenital Changes in Aging Women

Three factors cause urogenital change in the aging woman: the aging process itself, hormonal changes associated with the menopause, or a combination of both. Factors that contribute to the health of the urogenital system include obstetric history and good physical condition and muscle tone with the avoidance of obesity, and heredity. Estrogen deprivation is associated with atrophic changes of the urogenital system. Some of these changes, such as vaginal atrophy, are reversible with the institution of estrogen therapy; others such as prolapse are not. Many of the changes described here are not seen in an older woman who has had hormonal maintenance in the perimenopausal/menopausal years and never experienced any prolonged interval of estrogen deprivation. In this section, the effects of both aging and estrogen deprivation on urogenital anatomy are discussed.

External Genitalia

The vulvar changes seen in the older woman are thinning and graying of the pubic hair, decreased fat content in the labia majora, leading to a shrunken and wrinkled appearance, and dryness and paleness of the labia minora. There may be areas of erythema in the periurethral tissues. The clitoris may appear prominent secondary to relative androgen predominance in a hypoestrogenic woman.

Vagina

Some degree of vaginal atrophy is inevitable in women without estrogen supplementation after menopause. Apical constriction and agglutination leads to vaginal foreshortening, and the caliber of the vagina decreases with age and estrogen deprivation. Women who continue to be coitally active have better preservation of the vagina and a decreased degree of vaginal atrophy.[2] The hypoestrogenic vaginal mucosa has an increased pH, decreased blood flow, and decreased vaginal secretions. These changes can be reversed with estrogen therapy.[3] The appearance of the vaginal mucosa is pale, dry, smooth (denoting decreased rugae and elasticity), mottled, and friable. The associated histologic changes include thinning of the mucosa, loss of squamous cell maturation with basal cell predominance, and a leukocytic inflammatory reaction.

Cervix and Uterus

The cervix undergoes significant change and change in position with aging. The cervical os becomes stenotic and decreases in caliber, often to be virtually unidentifiable in the elderly woman. The cervix itself may become completely flush with the vaginal wall, which has important considerations for potential diagnostic capability for endometrial assessment. The ability to identify or dilate the cervix for endometrial assessment in the office may be limited. The cervix also loses sympathetic and parasympathetic innervation, but this has little clinical significance. In terms of position, the cervix regresses to the top of the vagina. With the decrease in uterine size and volume, the cervix may actually appear elongated when compared with the size of the uterus.

Both the myometrium and the endometrium undergo atrophy with aging. The postmenopausal uterus diminishes in size and weight, with associated decrease in capacity of nuclear binding of estrogen.[4]

Ovaries

The size of the ovary has been noted to decrease beginning at age 35, with a marked decrease after age 45.[5] Histologically, the atrophic ovary has lost primordial follicles, granulosa cells, and theca cells (converted to stromal cells). There are more corpora albicans and stromal cells.

Urethra and Bladder

With aging and progressive hypoestrogenism, the urethral functional length and maximal urethral closure pressure decrease. Because the urethral mucosa and bladder mucosa in the base of the bladder have estrogen receptors, they mimic the changes of the estrogen-deprived vaginal mucosa in undergoing atrophy.

The Gynecologic Examination of the Older Woman

A comprehensive urogynecologic history should be obtained before the urogynecologic examination of the older woman. The important system symptoms to be evaluated are shown in Table 50.1. A review of urogynecologic symptoms is important to anticipate the areas of potentially necessary detailed or procedural evaluation. The elderly patient may tolerate prolonged lithotomy position poorly, so an efficient examination is important. For example, if a patient gives a history of abnormal postmenopausal bleeding, the instruments necessary for

TABLE 50.1. Focused system history for the geriatric woman.

Gynecologic	Urologic

Health maintenance: most recent
   PAP smear
   Mammogram
   Thyroid-stimulating hormone
      (TSH)
	Urethral syndrome/irritative
	   symptoms
	   Dysuria
	   Frequency
	   Urgency
	   Hematuria
	   Nocturia

Menopausal status
   Age at menopause
      Natural or surgical
   Hormone replacement
      Ever or current (regimen)
   Most recent bleeding
	Urinary incontinence
	   Duration, worsening
	   Stress related
	   Urge related

Estrogen deprivation symptoms
   Hot flushes
   Night sweats/sleep disturbance
   Vaginal dryness/dyspareunia
   Vaginal discharge
	Amount of urine lost (spurt,
	   large amount, variable)
	   Fluid intake and pattern
	      Caffeine and alcohol

Prolapse symptoms
   Protrusion
   Pelvic pressure
   Bladder dysfunction:
      Urinary incontinence
      Difficulty voiding
   Bowel dysfunction
      Digital manipulation
      Stool incontinence/soiling
      Constipation
	Voiding dysfunction
	   Difficulty initiating stream
	   Weak stream
	   Prolonged voiding
	   Feeling of being unemptied
	   Postvoid dribbling

endometrial assessment should be available before positioning the patient. Likewise, if a patient describes a vulvar lesion, the local anesthetic and biopsy instrument should be ready before the examination. Because of the changes associated with aging and possible long-term estrogen deprivation, the gynecologic examination of the older woman often requires special techniques and instruments and always requires awareness of the significance of findings compared with those of the examination of a premenopausal patient.

The care in positioning a postmenopausal or elderly woman for gynecologic examination is different from that of a younger woman. The older patient should be allowed to undress and gown privately, if she is able. If not, a nurse or family member should assist. Many gynecologic examining tables still require that the patient step up, turn around on the small step, and sit down. This maneuver should always be done with nursing assistance because of the risk of fall and injury. If the examining table is electronic and lowers to a level comfortable for the patient to sit on without climbing, the patient can do this without assistance. The patient should sit at the end of the table to avoid either having to swing her legs around to the end of the table or to get off the table and go to the end for the gynecologic examination. The initial breast examination should be done with the patient sitting. Any neurologic assessment of the lower extremities, which is important in women complaining of bowel or bladder dysfunction or prolapse, should be done at this time.

The patient should then be placed in the lithotomy position. The patient will be more comfortable if the back of the table can be inclined up for support before her feet are placed in the stirrups. Some offices use birthing chairs, which are easy for the patient to sit in, provide good back and leg support, and can be elevated and tilted for the examination. These chairs are especially useful for evaluating prolapse and bladder function. Special caution is necessary when positioning a patient with severe degenerative disease of the spine and osteoporosis to minimize the stress on spinal deformities. Women with severe osteoarthritis of the hips and knees may not be able to flex these joints for optimal examination. An assistant supporting and gently manipulating the lower extremities can maximize the exposure obtained. If the patient has extreme limitation of motion, she may not be able to be placed in the lithotomy position. Alternative positions include examination with the patient on her back in a modified and supported "frogleg" position or on her side with one leg raised and supported. Once the patient is positioned, the examination should be performed in a thorough, systematic, and expeditious manner. The essential components of the gynecologic and urologic examination are evaluation of the breasts, external genitalia (including Bartholin glands, Skene glands, and urethra), vagina, cervix if present, uterine and vaginal support, uterus, adnexas (ovaries and tubes), and rectum.

Breast Examination

The breast examination of the older woman is not different from that for a younger woman. The patient should initially be sitting to allow the examiner to visually inspect the breasts for asymmetry, dimpling of the skin, and color or contour irregularities. Palpation of the breasts between the examiner's hands may then be performed. After the patient is in the supine position, four-quadrant or concentric circle evaluation may then be performed to detect deep masses in the chest wall. Gentle "milking" from the outer breast toward the nipple should be performed to express any discharge. Finally, all patients should be evaluated for lymphadenopathy, especially of the axillary and parasternal chains. If a patient has had a prior mastectomy, the scar of the chest wall should be palpated for nodules and masses. If a woman has had breast reconstruction, the tissue at the base of the implants should be palpated for nodularity or masses.

The consistency of the breasts of the older woman varies considerably. In many women, particularly those who are older and have not been on estrogen replacement therapy, the dense, firm fibroglandular tissue of the breast has been replaced by fat with resulting breast atrophy. However, fibrocystic breast changes and breast firmness may persist in women who have continued to have estrogen stimulation, either by replacement or their own sex steroid hormone production in peripheral tissues. As with younger women, the geriatric gynecology patient should be instructed in and perform monthly breast self-examinations. For women who are on cyclic progestogens as part of their hormonal replacement regimens, the breast self-examination should be performed the week following the last cyclic dose of the progestogen. The patient should also have annual breast exams by a health care provider.

Despite the importance of breast examinations, one cannot overemphasize the importance of annual mammograms for women over the age of 50. Annual mammograms are recommended by the American Cancer Society and the American College of Obstetricians and Gynecologists. Mammography remains the most sensitive diagnostic screening test available for the detection of breast malignancy. Faulk et al.[6] reported the importance of mammography in women 65 and older, and showed that although women in this age group represented only 34% of women studied (140 women aged 50 or older), they accounted for 45% of all cancers. Medicare coverage for annual mammography should increase compliance in the geriatric age group. However, as discussed in the chapter on breast cancer, some believe that annual mammography is not necessary for older women who have no history of abnormal mammograms or abnormalities on exam. As with younger women, all masses detected in the elderly woman must be evaluated with either ultrasound, aspiration, or biopsy as indicated.

External Genitalia

The external genitalia should be carefully inspected for any evidence of discoloration or mottling, raised or atrophic areas, excoriation or ulceration, or masses. If the patient has given a history of vulvar pruritis, this examination should be geared to identifying infectious, fungal, dystrophic, or malignant etiologies. Swabbings may be used for wet preps to test for fungal dermatoses (with KOH, if needed) and trichomoniasis, but scrapings may be needed to test for parasitic infection (scabies, pediculosis pubis, pediculosis corporis, or pinworms).

Any ulceration or raised lesion should be biopsied. As a general rule, the transition area of a lesion such as the edge of an ulcer rather than the necrotic center and the thickest area of a raised lesion should be sampled. The skin should be anesthetized with a 1% lidocaine with epinephrine subcutaneous injection using a 25 gauge needle. The biopsy itself may be obtained using either a punch biopsy instrument, cervical biopsy forceps, or a scalpel for wider excisions. Topical coagulating preparations such as silver nitrate or Monsel's solution generally will achieve hemostasis. Larger excisions may require interrupted stitches of a fine-gauge, absorbable suture.

Palpation of the Bartholin glands should be performed. Although malignancy of the Bartholin glands is rare, there may be delay in diagnosing it because it is asymptomatic in the early stages. The older patient is less likely to have infectious etiologies for changes in the Bartholin glands. If there is any indication of Bartholin enlargement or mass, aspiration or biopsy should be performed.

The Skene glands, or periurethral glands, are rarely visible or palpable unless there is infection. If this should occur, an area adjacent to the urethra and often proximal to the meatus may be swollen and tender. "Milking" these glands may result in urethral discharge, but this maneuver may be difficult, for the patient may be unlikely to tolerate this maneuver. The urethra in the older woman may be normal in appearance, but it is not uncommon for an older, hypoestrogenic woman to have urethral mucosal prolapse, or caruncle, that appears as fleshy, erythematous tissue extruding from the urethral meatus. This tissue is usually tender and bleeds easily. If these urethral conditions are symptomatic, they often respond to estrogen therapy. If they do not, excision or biopsy under local anesthetic can be performed. Excessive bulging of the anterior vaginal wall below the urethra may indicate either a urethrocele or urethral diverticulum. One should have a higher index of suspicion for a diverticulum in a woman who has frequent urinary tract infections. Again, "milking" the bulge toward the meatus may result in urethral discharge, either urine or purulent.

Vaginal Examination

The purpose of the vaginal examination is to assess estrogenization or atrophy, assess caliber and depth, find any lesions, and assess genitourinary support. If the patient has severe vaginal atrophy with marked reduction in caliber and depth, the remainder of the examination may be extremely difficult. Before doing the speculum examination, it is worthwhile to look at the vaginal introitus. The introitus may be gaping at rest with obvious loss of support of the anterior and posterior vaginal walls to or beyond the introitus, or a woman may have a severe introital stricture as a result of estrogen deprivation and loss of coital function. For these reasons, it is important to have different specula available in the examining room. A Pederson speculum (Fig. 50.1) generally gives adequate exposure of the vagina and cervix. If the cervix has regressed apically, a long Pederson may be required. The advantage of the Pederson is the narrow blades, which are well suited for the narrowed vagina often seen in the older patient.

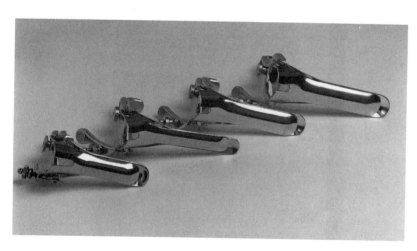

FIGURE 50.1. Pederson and pediatric specula. Note the varying width and length of the blades. The lack of splaying at the end of the blades is an advantage of these specula.

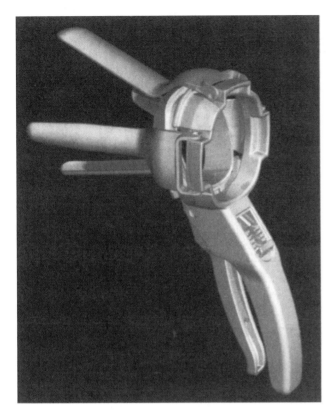

FIGURE 50.2. The Patton speculum allows retraction of the vaginal walls during the examination.

before inserting it will be helpful. The speculum should be inserted to the top of the vagina to visualize the cervix and vaginal cuff (if the patient has had a prior hysterectomy). If there is abnormal vaginal discharge, a swabbing should be taken and placed in a small amount (1 mL or less) of saline for wet prep evaluation after the examination. The speculum is then slowly removed with side-to-side rotation to allow visualization of the anterior, posterior, and lateral vaginal walls. If there is vaginal prolapse, as indicated by relaxation and redundancy of the vaginal mucosa, or frank descent of the pelvic structures (bladder, uterus, vaginal cuff, or rectum), further assessment is needed as described next. Vaginal lesions may be biopsied by cleansing, injecting local anesthetic submucosally, and using cervical biopsy forceps.

Uterus and Cervix

The cervix is assessed visually during the speculum examination. The Pap smear is obtained at that time using some form of notched spatula (many types are marketed) for a circumferential sampling of the ectocervix and a small brush (again, many types are available) for inserting into the cervical canal for endocervical sampling. Both samples should be spread thinly and evenly on slides, using all surfaces of the spatula and brush for

If the patient is severely atrophic, a narrow Pederson, a small pediatric speculum, or nasal speculum may be helpful. If the patient is obese or has vaginal redundancy because of prolapse, a regular or large Graves speculum may be necessary for visualization. If the lateral vaginal walls fold in and prevent cervical or apical visualization, a small examining glove with the fingers cut off can be placed around the blades of the speculum to act as a "dam" laterally, but a new speculum has been developed to enhance the examinations of these patients. It is called the Patton speculum (Fig. 50.2) and has four small blades that fan out to enhance cervical visualization. Finally, to evaluate for prolapse a Sims speculum (Fig. 50.3) is excellent because it is single bladed. However, the bottom half of a jointed speculum with the screw and top blade removed can be very functional when rotated anteriorly and posteriorly to assess prolapse while the patient performs a Valsalva maneuver.

The speculum is inserted into the vagina obliquely to use the length of the vaginal introitus for ease of insertion and to avoid passing the edges of the speculum blades along the urethra. Digital spreading of the posterior vaginal introitus with pressure downward will ease insertion. If a Pap smear is not to be obtained, a water-soluble lubricant should be used before insertion. If a Pap smear is needed, running the speculum under warm water

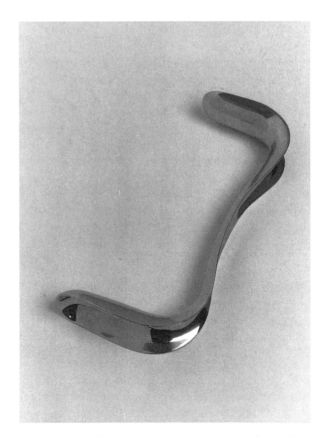

FIGURE 50.3. A Sims speculum is used for assessing prolapse.

adequate specimens. Pap smears, however, may be limited by the presence of atrophic vaginitis, resulting in a report of atypical squamous cells of undermined significance because of marked inflammation. Likewise, endocervical cells may be absent in the Pap smear because of cervical stenosis. In these settings, and if there is availability, the health care provider may choose to use the thin-layer Pap smear technique called AutoCyte PREP (TriPath Imaging, Burlington, NC). With this technique, the cells are obtained with a plastic spatula and transferred directly into a preserving solution. Tench[7] reviewed 10,367 conventional Pap smears and compared them to 2231 thin-layer Pap smears and found a significant reduction in Pap smear reports read as "unsatisfactory" or "unsatisfactory but limited by." There was also an improved rate of detecting squamous intraepithelial lesions.

The uterus is assessed with the bimanual examination. The uterus will not be palpable on the abdominal examination alone unless it is enlarged to at least the size of a 12- to 14-week pregnancy, when it can be palpated just above the pubis. For the bimanual examination, the examiner's two fingers (one, if there is a constricted vagina) are inserted in the vagina and used to elevate the uterus or vaginal cuff. The other hand is used to palpate the uterus, which should be small (approximately 6 cm), firm, and mobile. There may be residua from leiomyomata, which can be palpated as firm (very hard, if calcified), discrete round irregularities. It is helpful if the patient can give a history of having been told that she had fibroids in the past, but if this is a new finding, imaging may be necessary to confirm the appearance of leiomyomata. The uterus of the postmenopausal woman should not be soft or boggy, symmetrically enlarged, or tender. Because these findings are associated with infections, hematometria, pyometria, and malignancies, further evaluation with endometrial and uterine assessment by biopsy or imaging is essential.

Ovaries and Adnexa

The ovaries and adnexa are evaluated with the bimanual examination. For these assessments, the abdominal hand is used to sweep down from the lateral lower abdomen toward the vaginal hand midline to entrap ovaries, tubes, and possible masses between the examiner's two hands for palpation. As reported by Barber and Graber,[8] the postmenopausal ovary should not be palpable, and the ability to palpate it correlates with risk of a neoplastic ovarian process. Miller et al.[9] confirmed this with a neoplasm rate of 60% and a malignancy rate of 15% in 20 postmenopausal women who were asymptomatic with ovaries 5 cm in their greatest diameter. Therefore, palpable ovaries, particularly in geriatric postmenopausal patients, warrant further evaluation with ultrasound and

^{125}Ca. If these are normal, close follow-up and repeat testing should be done to document stability, as needed. Other masses can mimic ovarian neoplasm, such as bowel masses from malignancy or diverticular processes. Likewise, fallopian tube abnormalities such as residual hydrosalpinges or rare fallopian tube neoplasms may appear to be masses of ovarian origin.

Rectovaginal Examination

The rectovaginal examination should be performed after the bimanual examination. If the vaginal examining hand has been contaminated with blood, the glove should be changed, and a lubricant should be applied to the examining fingers. The rectovaginal exam is performed by placing the index finger of the dominant hand in the vagina and the middle finger in the rectum. The rectovaginal septum between the two fingers is palpated to detect masses, induration, fistulas, and tissue thinness on defects. The rectal finger examines the rectum in the usual fashion to assess for masses, hemorrhoids, and stool. The rectal finger is then used to palpate high in the adnexal area bilaterally and posterior to the uterus. Finally, a stool sample is obtained to test for occult blood.

The importance of the rectovaginal exam cannot be overemphasized. It can be especially useful for the assessment of the pelvis in the woman with severe atrophy and a contracted vagina that does not permit vaginal examination. The rectal finger can be used instead of the vaginal finger for bimanual examination, as already described.

Examining the Combative Patient

There will be times when an adequate gynecologic examination cannot be performed. The disoriented, delirious, or demented woman may be combative and not allow examination. When the patient resists the examination, she will be moving, attempting to hold her legs together, and contracting the pelvic muscles, and those actions will preclude examination even with assistants available for patient restraint. Furthermore, attempts by the patient to break away from restraints may cause injury. Establishing eye contact with and gently talking to the patient may allow a partial examination, but once the patient becomes combative, it is better to discontinue. If the examination is unsuccessful, the physician needs to decide what gynecologic information is essential. Abdominal ultrasonography of the pelvis can assess the cervix for masses; the uterus for size and contour; the endometrial cavity for abnormal endometrial thickening, irregularity from polyps or masses, or abnormal fluid collections; the tubes and ovaries for enlargement or masses; and abnormal fluid collection in the pelvis/abdomen. The combative patient may tolerate this imaging, but she may not tolerate any of the preferred vaginal imaging approaches such as transvaginal ultrasonography, saline infusion hysterography, or office hysteroscopy. If the patient has a specific problem that needs gynecologic evaluation such as postmenopausal bleeding, palpable abdominal mass, or abnormal vaginal discharge, referral to a gynecologist is indicated. Complete gynecologic evaluation may require examination under anesthesia with appropriate concomitant testing.

Common Urogynecologic Problems of the Older Woman

This section discusses common urogynecologic presenting symptoms and conditions in geriatric women, office evaluation techniques that can be performed by the primary care provider, diagnostic and therapeutic options, and indications for referral to gynecologists, urogynecologists, or urologists. Gynecologic malignancy, bladder function and urinary incontinence, and hormone replacement therapy are discussed in detail in other chapters in this book. The topics covered in this section are urogenital atrophy, recurrent urinary tract infections, vulvar disorders, postmenopausal bleeding, and pelvic organ prolapse.

Urogenital Atrophy

As discussed previously, estrogen deprivation has a profound effect on the vulva, vagina, cervix, urethra, and bladder. All women who are without estrogen supplementation postmenopausally will have some degree of urogenital atrophy. Endogenous peripheral production of estrogen may provide estrogenization and minimize vaginal and urethral atrophic changes. At least 20% of postmenopausal women with atrophic changes will report significant symptoms of urogenital atrophy, and the actual prevalence of symptomatology is probably higher because of underreporting. The specific presenting symptoms are related to the involved organ.

If significant vaginal atrophy has occurred, the most common presenting symptom is vaginal discharge, which is more irritative than pruritic. It may be malodorous, and there may be vaginal irritation with intercourse. The dyspareunia may be both superficial from the mucosal changes and deep from the changes in vaginal caliber and depth. The superficial dyspareunia is often described as "rawness" and "burning," and the deep dyspareunia is more often described as "tearing," particularly with intromission. Vaginal bleeding may occur in association with physical activity, vaginal manipulation such as douching, or coitus. One must not ascribe postmenopausal bleeding to atrophy, however, unless significant atrophy and vaginal friability are demonstrable on physical exam.

The atrophic vagina appears pale, smooth, dry, and telangectatic. Discharge, if present, is rarely copious, often appears yellowish and slightly purulent, and exhibits white blood cells and bacteria on wet prep. The wet prep should also be assessed for trichomoniasis and candida, although the latter is rare in the atrophic patient without diabetes. Vaginal atrophy responds extremely well to estrogen therapy. Systemic estrogen may be instituted, or administration of vaginal estrogen therapy will give a faster response because of direct effect on the vaginal mucosa. This method is particularly beneficial for the very elderly patient whose symptoms and expected benefits of therapy are related purely to those of urogenital atrophy.

The patient and the health care provider now have different therapeutic options for vaginal estrogen supplementation. In the past, vaginal estrogen cream, either conjugated estrogens or 17β-estradiol, was the only possibility for vaginal treatment of atrophy. The creams tended to be messy and relatively expensive for regular use. The first new product for vaginal estrogenization was the Estring (Pharmacia & Upjohn, Uppsala, Sweden), a small silicone ring impregnated with 2mg 17β-estradiol for slow estrogen release. It is inserted high in the vagina and remains in place for 3 months before replacement. Intercourse is possible without removing the ring. Henriksson et al. reported a 1 year multicenter trial with Estring in 136 women.[10] Only 8 of the patients withdrew from the study because of adverse events such as bleeding not associated with malignancy or endometrial proliferation or vaginal irritation/ulcers. The ring had high patient acceptability, induced a high vaginal maturation index, and corrected vaginal pH to premenopausal levels. Likewise, a 25-μg 17β-estradiol tablet (Vagifem) has been developed for insertion into the vagina once or twice weekly. Rioux et al. compared Vagifem with conjugated estrogen cream in 159 women treated for 24 weeks.[11] At the end of the study, there were fewer systemic effects as evidenced by lowered serum follicle-stimulating hormone (FSH) and increased higher serum estradiol levels, higher patient acceptability, and equal resolution of symptoms of atrophic vaginitis in the vaginal tablet group compared with the cream group.

The atrophic cervix rarely causes symptoms unless it has become very stenotic with resulting fluid collection in the uterus. The fluid collection may be blood in a patient with malignancy or one on hormonal replacement therapy who has stopped having withdrawal bleeding. If ascending infection has occurred, the fluid may represent purulence with associated endometritis. If these situations have occurred, the presenting symptoms include cyclic lower abdominal/pelvic pain in the patient who is on cyclic progestogen and has failed to have withdrawal bleeding, continuous pain in the patient with endometritis and a pyometrium, erratic bleeding sometimes associated with Valsalva maneuvers (i.e., blood is "squeezed" out of the uterus), or purulent discharge. If endometritis is severe, the patient may manifest fever or an elevated white blood cell count, but these symptoms are the exception rather than the expected. On exam, the cervix may appear atrophic but with a normal external os. The internal os, however, may be tightly stenotic. For the primary care physician, obtaining an abdominal or vaginal probe ultrasound to demonstrate endometrial pathology or intrauterine fluid collections may be selected as the first step in evaluation. If pathology is demonstrated, a referral to a gynecologist is indicated. Some primary care physicians, however, are skilled in cervical dilatation and endometrial biopsy and may prefer to attempt these before referral. This procedure should be done with extreme caution, however, because of the risk of cervical or uterine perforation in the presence of malignancy or infection with ensuing potential intraabdominal or vaginal uterine hemorrhage. These procedures should not be done if difficulty is encountered and emergency services including operating room accessibility are not readily available.

If the patient is found to have hematometrium without associated malignancy, the cervix should be dilated on a monthly basis until patency is established and persists. If the patient has a pyometrium (which should be cultured for aerobic and anaerobic bacteria and acid-fast bacteria at the time of endometrial sampling and cervical dilatation) without associated malignancy, she should be treated with antibiotics selected on the basis of the cultured organism's sensitivities, and undergo repeat cervical dilatations as above. If cervical dilatation and patency cannot be accomplished in an office setting, the patient should be referred to a gynecologist for further evaluation and management.

Because the bladder and urethra have estrogen receptive mucosa, atrophic changes affect their function also. The most frequently described symptoms related to this atrophy are those of the urethral syndrome—pain on urination, frequency, and urgency. This syndrome is the classic triad of symptoms of a urinary tract infection. In fact, many postmenopausal women with vaginal atrophy undergo multiple courses of antibiotics for empiric treatment of urinary tract infection. Clean-catch urinalysis will be contaminated with the white and red cells of the vaginal discharge and may give false indices consistent with infection. Urinary tract infection should be documented with culture if antibiotics are to be instituted in the symptomatic patient with urogenital atrophy. Therapy should be based on urinalysis should be from a good catheterized sample with culture submitted.

Another frequently encountered symptom of the urogenital system and atrophy as related to bladder function is urinary incontinence. In past literature such as the report by Faber and Heidenreich[12] and the more recent review by Elia and Bergman,[13] beneficial effects of estrogen on urethral pressure and decrease in stress incontinence have been shown. More recently, other reports such as that of Fantl et al.[14] have indicated no improvement in urethral function or significant decrease in incontinence, but they have shown that patients with estrogen supplementation had a trend to less urinary loss, a significantly decreased rate of nocturia, and a borderline positive effect on maximal bladder capacity. Their findings suggest that hypoestrogenism has its main effect on the bladder/urethral sensory threshold of incontinent postmenopausal women ands leads to the symptomatology described above. Kok et al. confirmed the marked decrease in nocturia with a 65% cure 6 months after beginning a combined estrogen and progestogen regimen (2 mg 17β-estradiol with varying doses of dehydrogesterone). In addition, there was a 23% cure of incontinence.[15] Jackson et al., however, reported the results of a 6-month, double blind, randomized, placebo-controlled trial in 67 women who were treated with either 2 mg estradiol valerate or placebo daily,[16] and found no improvement in postmenopausal stress incontinence. Even more confounding, Grady et al. from the Heart and Estrogen/Progestin Replacement Study reported worsening urinary incontinence in postmenopausal women receiving 0.625 mg conjugated estrogens/2.5 mg medroxyprogesterone acetate for a mean of 4 years when compared to the placebo group.[17] It would appear from the conflicting results of these studies that estrogen treats atrophy of the bladder and urethra and probably does provide some sensory threshold improvement that leads to decreased frequency and nocturia, but it may have little effect on stress incontinence overall.

Recurrent Urinary Tract Infections

The pitfalls of the diagnosis of a bladder infection in the woman with urogenital atrophy have been discussed. In the woman with culture-documented recurrent urinary tract infections, several potential etiologies must be assessed. The symptoms are generally those of urinary tract infection—dysuria, frequency, and urgency. The patient may have fever and persistent lower abdominal or flank pain, but these symptoms are more associated with upper tract infection. Incontinence, both stress and urge, can clearly be caused or worsened by urinary tract infection. The patient may also complain of gross hematuria. Abdominal examination may reveal lower abdominal tenderness, and bimanual examination may reveal focal bladder tenderness.

Hypoestrogenism is an etiologic factor in recurrent urinary tract infections in women. Parsons and Schmidt[18] confirmed prior studies in showing that the atrophic vagina becomes more basic and is colonized by coliform bacteria in postmenopausal women, and they were able to acidify the vagina, revert vaginal flora back to normal, and prevent recurrent urinary tract infections by treating the women with vaginal estradiol. Raz and Stamm confirmed this study in a controlled study also using intravaginal estriol in postmenopausal women with recurrent urinary tract infection.[19] Eriksen added further support that estrogen therapy can prevent recurrent bladder infections in the postmenopausal woman in his multicenter, randomized, parallel group study of 108 postmenopausal women.[20] The Estring treatment group and the placebo group were followed for 36 weeks, and the treatment group had a 45% likelihood of remaining disease free compared to 20% in the placebo group. Therefore, the first line of therapy in the postmenopausal woman with urogenital atrophy and recurrent urinary tract infections is the institution of estrogen replacement therapy, and the vaginal route of administration is effective.

Another important potential contributing factor for recurrent urinary tract infections in the elderly woman is impaired bladder emptying. This problem may occur because of vaginal prolapse with a urethral kinking effect and incomplete emptying, anticholinergic medications, surgical overcorrection of urethral hypermobility or bladder prolapse, and decreased mobility, leading to repetitive overdistension of the bladder and resulting impaired bladder function. The patient may describe difficulty initiating her urinary stream, a vaginal bulge, digital vaginal manipulation necessary for voiding, prolonged voiding, a weak urinary stream, postvoid dribbling, and incontinence (consistent with overflow by history). Examination may reveal significant prolapse or a bladder neck and urethra elevated and fixed retropubically from prior surgery. A useful office test, however, is to have the patient void when she has a full bladder. She should be given a stopwatch (or the nurse or family member may assist) to start at the commencement of voiding and stop when completed. The amount voided should be recorded (the patient may void in a volumetric "hat" placed on the toilet), and then the patient should be immediately catheterized for postvoid residual (this sample should be sent for urinalysis and culture). This simple test will allow the calculation of flow rate (amount voided divided by the number of seconds taken), which should be at least 10 mL/s, and the efficiency of the voiding. The postvoid residual should be less than half the amount voided and, in general, less than 100 mL. If voiding dysfunction is documented, bladder function may be improved by the use of pessaries or surgery to reduce prolapse, and surgery to release prior overcorrection can be performed. If the voiding dysfunction is found to be secondary to medications, these should be changed when possible. Finally, if voiding dysfunction is diagnosed without obvious etiology or means of correction, the patient should have fluid intake monitoring to prevent excessive fluid intake and overdistension of the bladder,

timed voids every 2 h, and consideration for a catheterization regimen (either by the patient herself or nursing staff) with antibiotic suppression.

Perineal hygiene is an important aspect of preventing recurrent urinary tract infections; this is especially pertinent for the elderly patient with arthritic changes, one who has had a stroke with residual impaired movement, the demented patient, or the woman with fecal incontinence for whatever reason. These patients tend to be unable to clean themselves well after defecation. Examination may show fecal soiling of the perianal and perineal areas. Therapy should be aimed at enhancing cleansing, sometimes with the aid of nurses or family members. Another useful technique is to have the patient clean with a squirt bottle, aiming the stream away from the vagina, after defecation. This, however, may not be possible for the impaired patient.

Structural abnormalities of the urinary system should be suspected if there is no obvious cause for recurrent urinary tract infections. Urethral diverticula occur in 1.4% to 4.7% of women. These may be asymptomatic except for recurrent urinary tract infections, urinary incontinence, or dyspareunia. When the diverticulum becomes infected, there is vaginal swelling, erythema, and severe pain. Examination of the noninfected diverticulum may show only a suburethral bulge with egress of urine from the meatus when the diverticulum is "milked." Kidney and bladder stones may serve as a nidus for urinary tract infection. The patient may have the previously described irritative symptoms plus the sensation of passing gravel, colicky pain, and hematuria. Similar symptoms may be produced by bladder or renal malignancy. For this reason, referral to a urologist is indicated for complete evaluation and management.

Vulvar Disorders

The purpose of this section is to discuss conditions affecting the vulva in geriatric patients. Dermatoses such as dermatitis, folliculitis, sebaceous cysts, parasitic infections, and candidiasis are not discussed. Vulvar malignancies are discussed in Chapter 37. Nonneoplastic vulvar disorders (vulvar dystrophies), vulvodynia, abscesses, and cellulitis are presented.

Vulvar dystrophy or nonneoplastic vulvar disorders are general terms to describe a constellation of benign disorders of the vulvae. They are classified into three broad categories; (1) lichen sclerosus; (2) squamous cell hyperplasia not otherwise specified (such as resulting from candidiasis or condylomata); and (3) other dermatoses (e.g., lichen planus, psoriasis, seborrheic dermatitis). Lichen sclerosus and squamous cell hyperplasia may occur together to give a mixed picture of both atrophy and hyperplasia. These conditions affect all age groups and both genders and may affect nongenital skin.

Lichen Sclerosus

The woman with vulvar lichen sclerosus is rarely asymptomatic. Lorenz et al. reported the frequency of presenting symptoms (Table 50.2) of 81 women with biopsy-proven lichen sclerosus.[21] Examination reveals whitened plaques progressing to parchment-like skin, distortion of vulvar architecture (adhesion and obliteration of the labia minora to the labia majora causing obliteration of identifiable labia minora, agglutination of the periclitoral tissues with subsequent burying of the clitoris, and sometimes complete introital contracture), and hematomas and telangestasia with a mottled pattern. Punch biopsy can confirm the diagnosis.

The etiology of lichen sclerosus is unclear. In a study by Scrimin et al., immunologic parameters were evaluated from the serum of 68 women with biopsy-proven lichen sclerosus and compared to serum from 53 matched controls.[22] The changes in the seroimmunologic profiles of the patients showed no evidence of a T-cell-mediated cell response, viral etiology, or autoimmune pathogenesis. Carlson et al.[23] used immunohistochemical techniques to show that activated macrophages and lymphocytes were present, indicating persistent antigen-driven inflammation. Infectious etiologies have been proposed but have not been substantiated.

The goal of therapy is symptom remission and regression of lesions. Historically, testosterone cream or ointment has been used for topical treatment. However, not only has it been proved by Sideri et al.[24] that topical treatment with 2% testosterone in petrolatum is no more effective than treatment with petrolatum alone, but testosterone therapy has also been shown by Joura et al. to result in serum testosterone levels that exceeded the normal range in 8 of 10 women treated with topical testosterone for 4 weeks, that 4 of 10 had clinical symptoms of virilization.[25] In a study by Bracco et al.,[26] only patients treated with clobetasol, a potent topical steroid, had significant improvement in symptoms, gross appearance of lesions, and histology when compared to those treated with testosterone and progesterone creams. In a follow-up study,[27] the same group found clobetasol propionate cream (0.05%) to be effective maintenance therapy for lichen sclerosus when compared to testosterone proprionate (which again was shown to be no more effective than the vehicle alone). Clobetasol propionate cream 0.05% is applied twice a day for 4 weeks, once a day for 2 weeks, and twice a week for 12 weeks. Furthermore, Lewis proposed a maintenance treatment of clobetasol proprionate once a week if symptom free.[28] He showed that 63% were able to use the weekly application for 6 months and remain symptom free. This therapy is begun in conjunction with meticulous perineal hygiene, including blow drying the perineum after bathing and modifications in lifestyle to diminish perineal moisture (cotton underpants, avoidance of slacks and jeans, and allowing free air flow by wearing loose-fitting garments without underpants when at home).

If a patient does not respond to the clobetasol therapy, Virgili et al. reported decreased symptoms and regression of lesions with topical 0.025% tretinoin once a day, 5 days a week, for a year.[29] Likewise, subcutaneous injections of triamcinolone suspension or absolute alcohol (with the patient under general anesthesia) will give relief from intractable pruritus as described by Kaufman.[30] Surgery for treatment of lichen sclerosus should be considered only when all other treatment modalities fail, because of the high rates of recurrence, as high as 50%, as described by Abramov et al.[31]

Because of the association of lichen sclerosus with increased risk of vulvar malignancy (2%–5%), patients with lichen sclerosus must be followed closely with biopsy of suspicious lesions. For cases of severe lichen sclerosus, referral to a gynecologic oncologist for evaluation and management is indicated.

Squamous Cell Hyperplasia

Squamous cell hyperplasia is a disorder characterized by epithelial thickening, as would be expected from the name. The most common presenting symptom is again pruritis. The vulvar and perianal distribution is similar to that seen in lichen sclerosus, but the marked vulvar architectural destruction is rare. The appearance of the skin may range from reddened in early lesions to raised, white plaques in more advanced lesions. As in lichen sclerosus, lichenification, excoriation, and fissures are common in the symptomatic patient. Biopsy is indicated to rule out malignancy. Treatment consists of topical corticosteroid creams, as previously described, and perineal hygiene. Clark et al. reported a study in which patients with lichen sclerosus, squamous cell hyperplasia, and mixed disease were treated twice a day in a 12-week treatment regimen of 4 weeks clobetasol propionate 0.05%, followed by betamethasone valerate 0.1%, and followed by hydro-

TABLE 50.2. Frequency of presenting symptoms of lichen sclerosus.

Symptom	Percent
Itching	98.8
Irritation	60.5
Burning	28.4
Dyspareunia	24.7
Tearing	14.8
Bleeding	9.9
Fissuring	8.8
Discharge	7.4

Source: Lorenz B, Kaufman RH, Ketzner SK. Lichen sclerosus: Therapy with clobetasol propionate. *J Reprod Med.* 1998;43:790–794, with permission.[21]

cortisone 1% with the same regimen.[32] There was a trend for the squamous cell hyperplasia and the mixed disease groups to have a decreased lower cure/improvement rate. Again, severe cases or those not responding to therapy should be referred for evaluation and management to a gynecologic oncologist.

Mixed Vulvar Disorders

The mixed dystrophies are treated and evaluated as the individual components. The important aspect of mixed disorders is their higher rate of associated cellular atypia, reported to be 16% by Fu and Reagan.[33] Therefore, there needs to be increased surveillance for malignant transformation with biopsies of changing lesions.

Vulvodynia

Vulvodynia is a condition characterized by chronic vulvar symptoms of discomfort, burning, itching, and rawness caused by multiple etiologies. Although the symptoms are similar, the etiologies can be infectious (candidiasis, viral with human papilloma virus, etc.), nonneoplastic vulvar disorders as already discussed in detail, dermatoses (lichen planus, psoriasis, dermatitis, etc.), neurologic (postherpetic neuralgia, reflex sympathetic dystrophy, pudendal neuralgia, etc.), and psychologic (a diagnosis of exclusion). There is no mainstay of treatment. The most important aspect in the treatment of this condition is an accurate diagnosis based on detailed history and physical exam to permit the institution of appropriate therapy. Therapies range from antifungals, treatments for vestibular papillomatosis secondary to human papilloma virus (excisional surgery, intralesional interferon injections), low-dose antidepressants (30–50 mg amitriptyline daily), and either topical corticosteroids or discontinuation of these same agents. The primary caregiver needs to be aware that evaluation and treatment of vulvodynia requires time and patience because there are rarely easy diagnoses or rapid cures, as discussed by Jones and Lehr.[34] If the diagnosis is elusive and the therapeutic modalities unsuccessful, gynecologic referral is indicated and would be best if the consultant has a special interest in this complex problem.

Vulvar Cellulitis and Abscesses

These vulvar problems are not common in the elderly woman unless she is diabetic, hypertensive, or has extremely poor hygiene. However, when they do occur they may be life threatening. The patient may present complaining of vulvar pain, swelling, and fever. Examination frequently will reveal vulvar cellulitis with erythema, edema, induration, and tenderness. There may be no fluctuance suggestive of abscess formation. If the patient is diabetic, has symptoms of systemic sepsis (fever, elevated white blood cell count), or has involve-

ment of the Bartholin gland, referral to a gynecologist is indicated for evaluation and probable hospitalization for aggressive parenteral antibiotic therapy and possible surgical incision and drainage. In the absence of such conditions, the physician can mark the borders of the cellulitis with an indelible surgical marking pen, institute broad-spectrum oral antibiotic therapy, and have the patient use sitz baths alternating with warm compresses three to four times per day. CBC should be obtained, and the patient should be reexamined within 24 h. If the induration or borders of the cellulitis are expanding or the patient has developed an abscess or systemic illness, she should be referred to a gynecologist. The reason for this aggressive therapy and vigilance is the potential for the development of necrotizing fasciitis, a polymicrobial synergistic condition characterized by dissolution of the subcutaneous tissues and fascia with resultant severe sepsis and a high mortality. Delay in diagnosis and aggressive therapy, both antibiotic and surgical, increases both morbidity and mortality.

Postmenopausal Bleeding

Postmenopausal bleeding is defined as any bleeding that occurs in a woman with an elevated follicle-stimulating hormone (FSH) after 6 months of amenorrhea. For a postmenopausal woman on hormone replacement therapy, abnormal bleeding is defined by what is expected to occur according to the specific hormonal regimen that she is using. However, abnormal bleeding on hormonal therapy and postmenopausal bleeding are evaluated with the same techniques.

For the postmenopausal, older woman who is not on hormonal replacement therapy, any vaginal bleeding must be evaluated. The patient presents complaining of bleeding, generally painless. It is important to obtain a history of associated activity (physical exercise, coitus, Valsalva maneuvers), any bladder symptomatology, and any bowel symptoms (hemorrhoids, constipation, bloody stools, change in bowel habits, etc.). The importance of the detailed history is to try to differentiate the source of the bleeding. Often, a woman describes blood on the tissue when she wipes herself after urinating or defecating. Likewise, it is important to differentiate between staining, spotting, and actual flow of either blood-tinged discharge, old blood, or bright red blood. The examination should focus on the vagina to detect vulvar lesions (neoplasms, excoriations, or ulcerations), blood in the vagina, a friable atrophic vagina, or evidence of blood in the cervix. The rectal exam should be done with a clean glove to detect gross or occult blood. If genital or rectal blood is not found, a catheterized urine should be obtained to rule out hematuria.

If the bleeding does not appear to be of bowel or bladder source, it must be assumed to be of gynecologic origin. If vulvar lesions are present and are believed to be the source, they should be biopsied. If vaginal bleeding is assumed to be secondary to vaginal mucosal atrophy with demonstrable friability, particularly in a posthysterectomized woman, estrogen therapy should be instituted, and the patient should return for reevaluation in 1 month. Finally, the bleeding may be of uterine or cervical source. The most common cause of postmenopausal uterine bleeding is endometrial polyps, which may be benign, hyperplastic, or malignant. Nonetheless, the patient must have a complete evaluation of the uterus and cervix to rule out malignancy.

Standard evaluation in the past has included Pap smear with colposcopy and directed cervical biopsies if the Pap smear is abnormal. The uterus and endometrium must be assessed. Endometrial assessment has traditionally been achieved with endometrial biopsy or complete fractional dilatation and curettage, and both of these have an 85% correlation with pathology. However, there are now multiple methods to evaluate the uterus and endometrium (Table 50.3). There is a growing trend to do the initial endometrial evaluation with ultrasonographic techniques. Garuti et al. concluded that if the endometrium was less than 4mm thick, further evaluation was unnecessary.[35] However, although transvaginal ultrasonography had a sensitivity of 95.1% and specificity of 54.8%, hysteroscopy had a sensitivity of 96.5% and specificity of 93.6%, making it the more accurate test.

The most exciting new technique for endometrial cavity assessment is the development of saline infusion sonography. This technique involves infusing sterile saline into the uterine cavity to distend it and then passing a small ultrasound probe into the uterus. Laifer-Narin et al. reported 63 patients who underwent saline infusion sonography followed by either endometrial biopsy, hysteroscopy, or hysterectomy.[36] All the polyps and submucosal leiomyomata and endometrial hyperplasia were detected. Of the three endometrial cancers, two had an abnormal endometrial appearance. One could not be assessed because of inability to distend the endometrial canal, common to all three of the studies with malignancy. Hysteroscopy is the test that allows direct visualization of the endometrium and uterine cavity with the capacity for directed biopsies, polypectomies, and resection of submucosal fibroids. Office hysteroscopy was compared to transvaginal ultrasonography by Towbin,[37] who performed office hysteroscopy on 149 patients after transvaginal ultrasonography.

Sixty-five of the patients underwent operative hysteroscopy or hysterectomy after the procedures, and pathology was correlated. Office hysteroscopy had a sensitivity of 79% and specificity of 93% whereas transvaginal ultrasonography had a sensitivity of 54% and specificity of 90%. Although saline infusion sonography is diagnostically more accurate than transvaginal ultrasonography, De Vries et al. recommend that saline infusion sonography be reserved for women who have abnormal bleeding with an endometrial thickness greater than 5mm or endometrial irregularities.[38] If the postmenopausal woman with abnormal bleeding has a normal pelvic examination, endometrial biopsy, and transvaginal ultrasound showing an endometrial thickness less than 5mm and no contour irregularity, the health care provider can be reassured that it is highly unlikely that the patient has a malignancy or serious condition. However, the patient should be followed closely for recurrent abnormal bleeding or change in symptomatology. If this should occur, the patient needs referral for enhanced ultrasonographic evaluation or hysteroscopy.

Pelvic Organ Prolapse

Pelvic organ prolapse is a broad term describing the consequences of relaxation of the supporting structures of the pelvic organs, allowing descent and herniation of these organs. The causes are multiple. DeLancey[39] described the mechanisms of loss of support and possible contributing factors: aging (with decreases in both collagen content and striated muscle function in supporting structures), obesity, and childbirth injury. Other contributing factors are occupational or recreational

TABLE 50.3. Techniques for uterine/endometrial assessment.

Techniques	Advantages	Disadvantages
Endometrial biopsy	Performed in office Histologic diagnosis	Cervical stenosis may preclude
Dilatation and curettage	Histologic diagnosis	Performed in operating room
Hysteroscopy	Performed in some offices Direct visualization Histologic diagnosis	Cervical stenosis may preclude
Transabdominal ultrasonography	Does not require vaginal probe	Limited visualization Difficult with the obese patient Not correlated well with pathology No histologic diagnosis
Transvaginal ultrasonography	Improved urogenital imaging Excellent cervical imaging	No histologic diagnosis Severe vaginal atrophy may preclude
Saline infusion sonography	Best endometrial imaging	No histologic diagnosis Severe vaginal or cervical stenosis may preclude

TABLE 50.4. Compartmental approach to urogenital prolapse.

Compartment	Pathology	Symptoms
Anterior	Cystocele/urethrocele	Urinary incontinence (generally stress)
		Urgency
		Urinary retention if there is urethral kinking
		Pressure/protrusion if large
Middle	Uterine procidentia	Pressure
		Cervical bleeding if protrusion
		Discomfort with activity
	Vaginal vault prolapse	Pressure
	Enterocele (anterior or posterior)	Vaginal irritation
Posterior	Rectocele	Constipation
		Pressure
		Digital manipulation for rectal evacuation
		Stool soiling

lifestyles that lead to increases in intraabdominal pressure, medical conditions (chronic lung disease, lower extremity weakness, etc.) that also increase intraabdominal pressure, and disorders of connective tissue (specifically collagen).

DeLancey[40] further correlated loss of specific support levels with pathology: loss of high support is associated with prolapse of the vaginal apex with uterine descent and/or enterocele formation, middle support with cystourethrocele and rectocele, and lower support with urethrocele or perineal body descent. A simple way to evaluate pelvic organ prolapse is by thinking of the vagina as having three compartments (Table 50.4). In some instances, generally in women who have had previous prolapse or anti-incontinence procedures, enteroceles may occur in either the anterior or posterior compartment instead of the middle compartment. Although a standard prolapse classification system exists, it was developed for use principally by gynecologists, urologists, and urogynecologists. A practical approach for the primary care provider is to think of prolapse as mild (first degree) with the leading edge of the prolapsing organ descending halfway to the vaginal introitus, moderate (second degree) with descent to the introitus, and severe (third degree) with prolapse beyond the introitus. Consistent conditions of grading are important. Most examiners do the grading with the patient in the lithotomy position doing a Valsalva, and although this is the most functional way for the routine office evaluation, it may not detect some prolapse and lead to the underestimation of the degree of prolapse.

Inspection of the introitus at rest may show a gaping introitus with anterior and posterior bulges to or beyond the introitus. The speculum is then inserted to the apex and withdrawn slowly with the patient bearing down so that the examiner can assess apical support and possible descent of the cervix or vaginal vault. The top of the vagina may remain well supported despite significant prolapse at other sites. Half of a speculum or a Sims speculum is then inserted and traction is directed to the floor. Again, the patient is asked to perform a strong Valsalva, and the anterior wall support is assessed. The patient is then asked to cough, and the urethra is observed for loss of urine. The speculum blade is then rotated 180°, and the anterior vaginal wall is retracted upward to allow assessment of the posterior vagina while the patient repeats the bearing down. Bimanual examination is then performed with the patient intermittently bearing down so the examiner can palpate the prolapsing parts and better assess the small bowel prolapse in an enterocele. Rectovaginal examination permits better assessment of rectal bulging and rectovaginal septum thickness as well as a possible high enterocele component to a large rectocele.

There are, however, limitations to this examination. Most women will have their maximal prolapse after physical activity or at the end of the day, but her examination may be in the morning after reduction of the prolapse in the supine position overnight. If the patient gives a history consistent with prolapse, and very little is seen on examination with the patient in the lithotomy position, the patient should be allowed to stand up with one foot on a small stepping stool or the step of the examining table. The examiner should then observe, repeat the observation with the patient performing a Valsalva, and perform a bimanual followed by a rectovaginal examination with and without patient bearing down. A cough stress incontinence test will give a false negative if the patient has an empty bladder. Finally, some patients will have difficulty bearing down because of fear of urinary or fecal incontinence. Reassurance as to the need to assess these dysfunctions and having the patient lift her head off the table and give a strong cough may aid the examiner in eliciting a good patient Valsalva. Complex imaging can be used as a diagnostic tool, although it is rarely necessary. These techniques are not readily available or generally clinically useful for the primary care provider. If a patient's prolapse presents diagnostic difficulty, referral is indicated.

Sagittal sections of the female pelvis and anatomic relationships and prolapses are shown in Figures 50.4 through 50.9. With prolapses beyond the opening of the vagina, the prolapsed parts may ulcerate or incarcerate. It should be noted from the diagram that severe prolapse of the uterus also entails bladder and rectal prolapse. When the patient has a rectocele, it is important to differentiate between true constipation with hard stools versus inability to empty the rectum because of stool impaction in the rectocele. When questioned, the patient

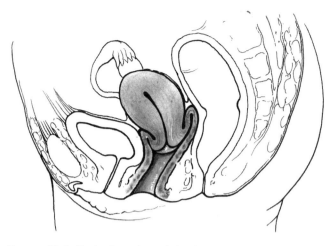

FIGURE 50.4. Sagittal section of the female pelvis with normal anatomic relationships.

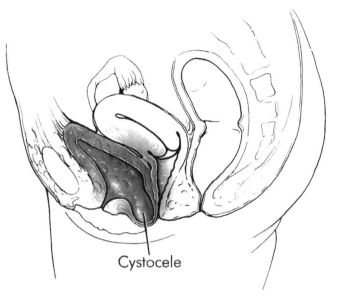

Cystocele

FIGURE 50.5. Second-degree cystocele.

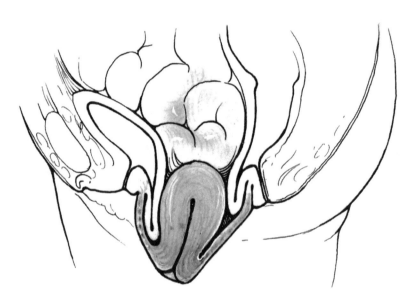

FIGURE 50.6. Total uterine prolapse (procidentia).

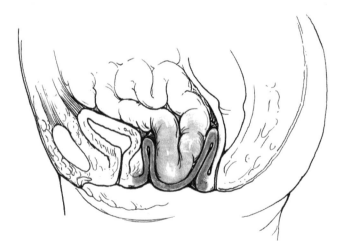

FIGURE 50.7. Second-degree enterocele.

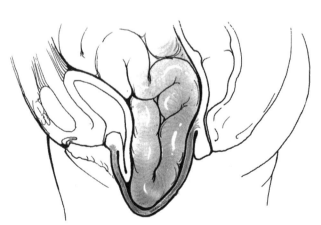

FIGURE 50.8. Total vaginal eversion after hysterectomy.

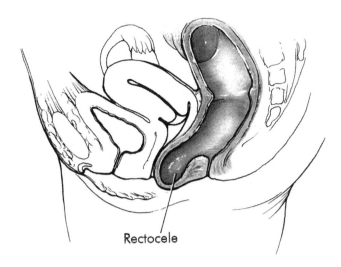

FIGURE 50.9. Second- to third-degree rectocele.

may admit to vaginal, perineal, or rectal digital manipulation for rectal evacuation. Likewise, the stool soiling may not be true stool incontinence of formed stool but rather a leakage of stool slurry from the rectocele.

If the patient has mild to moderate prolapse, therapy is indicated to attempt to prevent progression of prolapse. The patient should be encouraged to modify her lifestyle to avoid causes of stress to the pelvic floor—heavy lifting, high-impact aerobics, repetitive stooping, obesity, chronic coughing. She should also be taught Kegel exercises with both verbal instruction and assessment and written literature. These exercises involve tightening and relaxing the vaginal supporting muscles, particularly the pubococcygeus muscle, and are done both as fast flicks, which are rapid contractions and releases of the muscles, and gradual holds, which are gradual contractions of the muscles with maintaining the contraction for 3s initially with a goal of 10s as the muscles strengthen before gradual relaxation. The patient can tell if she is doing them correctly by starting and stopping her urinary stream with contractions and by feeling a tightening of the vagina when two or three fingers are inserted in the vagina and the exercise performed. The patient should understand that these need to be done twice daily to strengthen and maintain the pelvic supporting muscles, and that the benefits will be lost if she does not continue to do them. Another technique to improve pelvic muscle tone is the use of weighted vaginal cones, which come in a set with progressively increased weight. Starting with the lightest cone, the patient inserts it vaginally and maintains it in the vagina for as long as she can until she can keep it in for 15min several times per day. When she can keep the light cone in, she repeats the process with heavier cones. When the heaviest cone can be retained, the exercises should be continued as with Kegel's.

Patients with problematic urinary incontinence, either stress or urge, and prolapse may benefit from biofeedback or electrostimulation. Biofeedback consists of a computerized program in which a sensor (about the size of a tampon) is inserted in the vagina, the patient does the Kegel exercises, and the ability to sustain contractions of the correct pelvic muscles is shown graphically on a video monitor. The advantage is that the patient learns the correct way to do pelvic floor exercises and can see improvement in strength over the course of therapy. The disadvantages are that the patient must come to the clinic regularly for a variable amount of time, and referral to a urogynecologist or physical therapist for this program is necessary and but may not be widely available in some areas.

Electrostimulation has progressed from requiring clinic equipment to using a small, battery-powered individual unit that a patient can rent or purchase and use at home. The actual stimulator that must be purchased is about the size of a tampon and is inserted into the vagina (the rectum has been used but patients find vaginal insertion preferable). Varying levels and frequency of low-level shock can be set to allow progressively increased muscle stimulation. The advantages are is that this can be used at home. The disadvantages are is that it is expensive (but it is often covered by insurance).

Therapy to reduce prolapse in patients who have any protrusion beyond the vaginal introitus is essential to prevent the complications of severe prolapse—bleeding, ulceration and infection, pain, organ incarceration, and urinary retention with potential urosepsis. In addition, reducing a severe prolapse in a woman improves her quality of life. The options for correction are limited to surgery or pessary use.

Pessaries can be a useful therapy with good patient acceptance, as reported by Sulak et al.[41] They found that 50 of 101 women who were treated with pessaries because they were awaiting surgery, did not want surgery, or were not surgical candidates, were continuing to use them at 2 years. The principal reasons for discontinuation in patients not having surgery were inconvenience/inadequate relief of symptoms (40%), difficulty removing (23%), and discomfort (13%). Only 6% had inability to retain a pessary and 5% could not urinate. This study is important because it shows that pessaries are an acceptable alternative to surgery for some women and are very useful in elderly, infirm women who are not candidates for surgery.

Primary care providers should become familiar with the types, indications for each type, fitting, and management of pessaries if they want to treat third-degree prolapse in geriatric women. Brubaker[42] provided a comprehensive and practical review of pessary use, selection, and management. There are four commonly used pessaries (Fig. 50.10) for reduction of severe uterovaginal

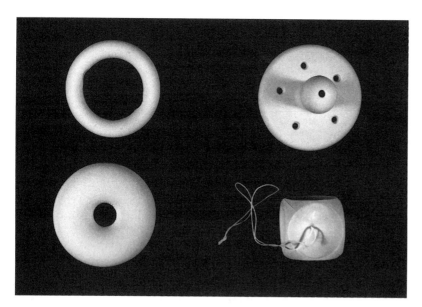

FIGURE 50.10. Commonly used pessaries: dough-nut, ring, Gellhorn, cube.

prolapse. Pessaries are made in silicone material and are more durable, softer, and better quality. There are a wide range of sizes, but the three middle sizes of each pessary type are generally useful for 85% of women with prolapse in a general practice. Women with severe prolapse require the large sizes, and women with introital contracture need the small sizes. The doughnut pessary is the one most familiar to practitioners. It is relatively easy to insert by squeezing the sides, well tolerated, and can often be inserted and removed by the patient. However, it is more often extruded in women who have vaginal vault prolapse without a uterus and who have poor perineal support (gaping introitus and small perineal distance between the anus and the posterior vagina). The ring pessary is excellent for uterine prolapse, easy to insert (the sides are jointed and fold the pessary in half), and is well tolerated. A modification has a fenestrated platform to give additional support.

The Gellhorn pessary has been found to be the most useful in patients with vaginal vault prolapse. These devices maintain support with sidewall apposition and a small amount of central suction due to the concavity of the platform. The flexible pessary is shown, but this type is also made out of rigid acrylic. The insertion is more difficult because the sides do not collapse. Patients can sometimes manage them on their own, but often family or nursing assistance is needed. Finally, the cube pessary is the most effective for reducing severe prolapse in the patient without any significant vaginal support. It works by suction attachment from the concavities of the walls. It is relatively easy to insert because of the softness of the construction material. Unfortunately, this pessary requires medical management because it is associated with vaginal infection, malodorous discharge, and ulceration. The pessary must be removed, cleaned, and

reinserted weekly with accompanying inspection of the vagina. However, it is excellent for short-term use in preparation for surgery.

Before pessary insertion, the patient must empty her bladder. She is placed in the lithotomy position, and the vagina is inspected for ulcerations. Ulcerations per se are not an absolute contraindication to pessary insertion because some will only heal when the prolapse is reduced. However, an actively infected or thin ulcer will require very close medical follow-up until it has healed. Hypoestrogenic patients will be at less risk of pessary complications if aggressive vaginal estrogen cream therapy is instituted for 2 weeks preceding pessary insertion. Vaginal estrogen therapy should always be a component of pessary therapy and should be used at least once a week to lubricate the pessary before reinsertion after cleansing, even in the woman on systemic estrogen replacement. The ability to insert the correct type and size of pessary comes with experience doing it. The patient needs to know that she may need different types or sizes of pessaries before the correct one is found. After the pessary is inserted, the patient should not feel the pessary unless it is too large. The patient should then perform a strong Valsalva. If the pessary is not extruded, the patient may then walk around, and if it continues to be retained and comfortable, she may be allowed to dress. If the patient has the time or she will be returning to a situation without easy access to medical care, she should be allowed to fill her bladder and show that she can void before leaving the clinic. I do not attempt to teach the patient or family member pessary removal, cleansing, or reinsertion at this visit.

Close follow-up is necessary, and the patient should return to the clinic in 1 week at the latest (earlier if the physician is following a preexisting vaginal ulcer). When the patient returns, she is assessed for pessary comfort and retention, vaginal discharge, and bowel and bladder function. The pessary is changed to a different size or type if there are problems with any of these. If the pessary is well tolerated, it is removed, cleansed, and reinserted. At this time outpatient teaching as to pessary management with weekly cleaning, the importance of estrogenization, and the importance of regular follow-up is instituted. If the patient or family member can remove and reinsert the pessary, the patient may return in 1 month for reevaluation, or earlier if she has problems. For the community-dwelling patient or one who cannot manage the pessary, instructions are given to nursing home personnel or home health care nurses are enlisted. Again, the patient needs to return in a month if she does not have reassessment by a health care provider locally. Any retained and neglected pessary can become a nidus for infection, incarcerate, or, even worse, erode into the bladder, rectum, or abdominal cavity. The final issue regarding patient counseling is that the patient may not have any urinary incontinence maintained because of the urethral kinking associated with severe prolapse, and the patient may become incontinent because of underlying stress incontinence (with or without urethral weakness) or detrusor instability when the prolapse is reduced. This occurrence, failure to retain a pessary, or pessary complications are indications for referral to a gynecologist familiar with evaluation and management of pelvic prolapse, bladder function, and reconstructive pelvic surgery.

Surgical correction of pelvic organ prolapse and incontinence is rarely absolutely contraindicated in the elderly patient. Kaminski et al.[43] reported the good outcomes in 24 women with massive vaginal prolapse treated in a rural tertiary care center. Other literature confirms the safety and good results with surgical correction in the older patient. For these reasons and although pessary use is a valid option, referral to a gynecologist or urogynecologist experienced in surgery in the elderly patients with prolapse should always be considered and generally offered to the patient. There are many different surgical approaches including abdominal and vaginal techniques. The specific operation or complex of procedures performed is selected for the individual patient based on her lifestyle, activity level, general health, and desire for preservation of vaginal coital potential.

Conclusion

The gynecologic and urologic evaluation of the older woman is an important part of her medical evaluation. Increased availability of imaging can provide new diagnostic capabilities. Many conditions common in the older woman can be assessed and treated by the primary care provider without referral to specialists. These treatments may successfully improve the quality of life for these women. The primary care provider, however, should have familiarity with these conditions and know the indications for referral.

References

1. United Nations World Assembly on Aging, Vienna. *The Vienna International Plan of Action on Aging; 1983*, paras 9 and 11. [Cf. Swedish Ministry for Foreign Affairs: Forenta Nationeras aldrandekonferens i Wien 26 Juli-6 Augusti 1982.] Stockholm: Norstedt Tryckeri; 1983.
2. Leiblum S, Bachman G, Kemmann E, et al. Vaginal atrophy in the postmenopausal woman: the importance of sexual activity and hormones. *JAMA.* 1983;249:2195–2198.
3. Semmens J, Wagner G. Estrogen deprivation and vaginal function in postmenopausal women. *JAMA.* 1982;248:445–448.
4. Strathy J, Coulam C, Spelsburg T. Comparison of estrogen receptors in human premenopausal and postmenopausal uteri: indication of biologically inactive receptor in postmenopausal uteri. *Am J Obstet Gynecol.* 1982;142:372–382.
5. Tervila L. The weight of the ovaries after stress ending in death. *Ann Chir Gynaecol.* 1982;142:232–244.
6. Faulk R, Sickles E, Sollitto R, et al. Breast screens found useful in elderly women. *Radiology.* 1995;194:193–196.
7. Tench W. Preliminary assessment of the AutoCyte PREP. Direct-to-vial performance. *J Reprod Med.* 2000;45:912–916.
8. Barber H, Graber E. The PMPO syndrome. *Obstet Gynecol.* 1971;38:921.
9. Miller R, Nash J, Weiser E, et al. The postmenopausal palpable ovary syndrome: a retrospective review with histopathologic correlates. *J Reprod Med.* 1991;36:568–571.
10. Henriksson L, Stjernquist M, Boquist L, et al. *Am J Obstet Gynecol.* 1996; 1 74:85–92.
11. Rioux JE, Devlin C, Gelfand MM, Steinberg WM. Hepburn DS. 17beta-estradiol vaginal tablet versus conjugated equine estrogen vaginal cream to relieve menopausal atrophic vaginitis. [Clinical Trial. Journal Article. Multicenter Study. Randomized Controlled Trial] *Menopause.* 2000;7(3):156–161.
12. Faber P, Heidenreich J. Treatment of stress incontinence with estrogen in postmenopausal women. *Urol Int.* 1977;32:221–223.
13. Elia G, Bergman A. Estrogen effects on the urethra: beneficial effect in women with genuine stress incontinence. *Obstet Gynecol Surv.* 1993;48:509–517.
14. Fantl J, Wyman J, Anderson R, et al. Postmenopausal urinary incontinence: comparison between non-estrogen-supplemented and estrogen-supplemented women. *Obstet Gynecol.* 1988;71:823–828.
15. Kok AL, Burger CW, van de Weijer PH, et al. *Maturitas.* 1999;31:143–149.
16. Jackson S, Shepherd A, Brookes S, et al. The effect of oestrogen supplementation on postmenopausal urinary stress incontinence: a double-blind placebo-controlled trial. *Br J Obstet Gynaecol.* 1999;106:711–718.

17. Grady D, Brown JS, Vittinghoff E, et al. *Obstet Gynecol.* 2001;97:116–120.

18. Parsons C, Schmidt J. In vitro bacterial adhesions of vaginal cells of normal and cystitis-prone women. *J Urol.* 1980;126:184–187.

19. Raz R, Stamm W. A controlled trial of intravaginal estriol in postmenopausal women with recurrent urinary tract infections. *N Engl J Med.* 1993;329:753–756.

20. Eriksen B. A randomized, open, parallel-group study on the preventive effect of an estradiol-releasing vaginal ring (Estring) on recurrent urinary tract infections in postmenopausal women. *Am J Obstet Gynecol.* 1999;180:1072–1079.

21. Lorenz B, Kaufman RH, Ketzner SK. Lichen scleroses: therapy with clobetasot propionate. *J Reprod Med.* 1998;43:799–794.

22. Scrimin F, Rustja S, Radillo O, et al. Vulvar lichen sclerosus: an immunologic study. *Obstet Gynecol.* 2000;95:147–150.

23. Carlson JA, Ambrox R, Malfetano J, et al. Vulvar lichen sclerosus and squamous cell carcinoma: a cohort case control, and investigational study with historical perspective; implications for chronic inflammation and sclerosis in the development of neoplasia. *Human Pathology.* 1998;29(9):932–948.

24. Sideri M, Origoni M, Spinaci L, et al. Topical testosterone in the treatment of vulvar lichen scleroses. *Int J Gynaecol Obstet.* 1994;46:53–56.

25. Joura EA, Zeisler H, Bancher-Todesca D, et al. Short-term effects of topical testosterone in vulvar lichen sclerosus. *Obstet Gynecol.* 1997;89:297–299.

26. Bracco CL, Carli P, Sonni L, et al. Clinical and histologic effects of topical treatments of vulval lichen sclerosus: a critical evaluation. *J Reprod Med.* 1993;19:34–36.

27. Cattaneo A, Carli P, DeMaro A, et al. Testosterone maintenance therapy: effects on vulvar lichen scleroses treated with clobetasot propionate. *J Reprod Med.* 1996;41:99–102.

28. Lewis FM. Lichen scleroses: do we need maintenance treatment? *J Reprod Med.* 2000;45:77.

29. Virgili A, Corazza M, Bianchi A, et al. Open study of topical 0.025% tretinoin in the treatment of vulvar lichen sclerosus. One year of therapy. *J Reprod Med.* 1995;40:614–618.

30. Kaufman RH. Optimal management of vulvar lichen sclerosues. *OBG Manag.* 2000;22–28.

31. Abramov Y, Elchalal U, Abramov D, et al. Surgical treatment of vulvar lichen sclerosus: a review. *Obstet Gynecol Surv.* 1996;51:193–199.

32. Clark TJ, Etherington IJ, Luesley DM. Response of vulvar lichen scleroses and squamous cell hyperplasia to graduated topical steroids. *J Reprod Med.* 1999;44:958–962.

33. Fu Y, Reagan J. Pathology of the uterine cervix, vagina, and vulva. In: Bennington JL, ed. *Major Problems in Pathology, vol 21.* Philadelphia: Saunders; 1989.

34. Jones K, Lehr S. Vulvodynia: diagnostic techniques and treatment modalities. *Nurse Pract.* 1994;19:34–36.

35. Garuti G, Sambruni I, Cellani F, et al. Hysteroscopy and transvaginal ultrasonography in postmenopausal bleeding. *Int J Gynaecol Obstet.* 1999;65:25–33.

36. Laifer-Narin S, Ragavendra N, Lu DSK, et al. Transvaginal saline hysterosonography: characteristics distinguishing malignant and various benign conditions. *Am J Radiol.* 1999;172:1513–1520.

37. Towbin NA, Gviazda IM, March CM. Office hysteroscopy vs transvaginal ultrasonography in the evaluation of patients with excessive uterine bleeding. *Am J Obstet Gynecol* 1996;174:1678–1682.

38. DeVries LD, Dijkhuizen FP, Mol BW, et al. Comparison of transvaginal sonography, saline infusion sonography, and hysteroscopy in premenopausal women with abnormal uterine bleeding. *J Clin Ultrasound.* 2000;28:217–223.

39. DeLancey J. Anatomic aspects of vaginal eversion after hysterectomy. *Am J Obstet Gynecol.* 1992;166:1717–1728.

40. DeLancey J. Pelvic floor dysfunction: causes and prevention. *Contemp Obstet Gynecol.* 1993;38:68–79.

41. Sulak P, Kuehl T, Shull B. Vaginal pessaries and their use in pelvic relaxation. *J Reprod Med.* 1994;38:919–924.

42. Brubaker L. The pessary: an important gynecological option. *Menopausal Med.* 1994;2:1–12.

43. Kaminski P, Sorosky J, Pees R, et al. Correction of massive vaginal prolapse in an older population: a four-year experience at a rural tertiary care center. *Obstet Gynecol Surv.* 1993;48:468–470.

51
Benign Prostatic Hyperplasia

Catherine E. DuBeau

The seventh and eighth decades bring many a man to an acute awareness of his prostate and its impact on his quality of life. Lower urinary tract symptoms (LUTS), particularly urgency and nocturia, begin to interrupt his days and, most annoyingly, his nights. After several months he is finally bothered enough to mention his symptoms to his doctor; a rectal exam is done, the news delivered that he has benign prostatic hyperplasia (BPH), and medication is prescribed to shrink his prostate or loosen the grasp of its smooth muscle on his urethra. His brother in a nursing home develops urinary retention; BPH is similarly blamed, but because of his frailty chronic catheterization is deemed the only possible treatment. Yet, although both these men are likely to have age-related proliferation of epithelial and stromal prostate tissue—the hallmark of BPH—it is not necessarily true that BPH is causing their symptoms, or that their prostate is enlarged, or that conventional treatment regimens are their only options.

Although the term BPH often is used synonymously for prostate enlargement, bladder outlet obstruction, and associated urinary tract symptoms, these terms are not equivalent. Histological BPH occurs nearly universally in older men, yet prostate enlargement results in only about half, and symptoms occur in only about half of men with enlargement.[1] Moreover, in older men "prostatism" symptoms often are caused by age-related physiologic lower urinary tract changes, comorbid conditions, or medications independent of any prostate disease[2]; indeed, similar "prostatism" symptoms occur in a significant proportion of older women.[3] Even among symptomatic men with prostate enlargement, bladder outlet obstruction can be demonstrated urodynamically in only two-thirds.[4,5] Thus, the prostate is not inevitably the cause of LUTS in older men, regardless of the presence of prostate enlargement. In this chapter, BPH refers only to the specific histology, as distinct from benign prostate enlargement (BPE) and bladder outlet obstruction (BOO). The term prostatism is abandoned for the more general term BPH-related LUTS.[6]

Epidemiology and Risk Factors

Benign prostatic hyperplasia changes significantly increase with age, occurring in nearly 80% of men by age 80.[7] Population-based data indicate that 28% to 35% of older men without previous prostate surgery have moderate or more severe LUTS.[8,9] Symptoms increase slowly over time, with the greatest rate during the seventh decade,[10] such that nearly one in four men over age 80 receives treatment.[11] Besides advanced age, risk factors for BPH include no alcohol consumption (or, for moderate consumption versus none, 0.59; CI, 0.51–0.70) and smoking 35 or more cigarettes/day (or, compared with nonsmokers, 1.45; CI, 1.07–1.97).[12] LUTS (presumed to be BPH related in older men) also show significant associations with diabetes,[13] cardiovascular disease,[13] diuretics,[13] nocturnal polyuria (excess urine production at night),[14] and an age-related decrease in urine flow rate[15] that is independent of any bladder outlet obstruction.[16]

Natural History of the Aging Prostate

BPH first develops in the third decade, and pathologic and ultrasound studies demonstrate significant increases in the volume of hyperplasia with age.[6,17] In the seventh decade and beyond, however, BPH volume shows an inconsistent or negative relationship with age.[6,17] In cross-sectional studies, the association of BPE with age is strongest in men less than 60 years of age. A small 7-year longitudinal ultrasound study[18] found that prostate volume increased by more than 50% in only 3 of 16 men, with the increase occurring in the seventh decade; in the remaining men, prostate size changed –24% to +22%. In a larger 4-year study using MRI measures, mean prostate volume increased with time, but with wide variability (mean percent change, 14.1 ± 17.5).[19] The strongest predictor of volume increase was not age but baseline prostate-specific antigen (PSA): nearly all men with PSA greater than 2ng/ml had subsequent prostate growth, whereas 33% of men with PSA less than 2ng/ml had prostate shrinkage.

Clinical natural history studies and placebo arms of treatment trials demonstrate that symptomatic progression also is not inevitable, and that associated morbidity occurs only in a minority. Older studies of men on surgical waiting lists for transurethral resection of the prostate (TURP) found that LUTS progressed in only 15% to 20% over 5 years,[20–22] independent of initial symptom severity[22] or radiographic evidence of BOO,[20] when LUTS decreased, symptom remission was durable up to 5 years. Controlled studies of medical therapy consistently show that BPH-related LUTS improve in at least one-third of patients on placebo.[23] In the Veterans Affairs randomized trial of TURP versus watchful waiting for moderately symptomatic BPH-related LUTS with BPE, men with watchful waiting had 38% mean decrease in mean symptom score over 4 years, and 3% developed urinary retention.[24] An observational study of 371 men with BPH-related LUTS surviving 4 years found that symptom progression requiring surgical treatment was related to baseline symptom severity (Table 51.1)[25]; the risk of urinary retention was related to age, symptom severity, and use of anticholinergic drugs, but was low

overall (3% over 3.5 years). Symptom progression may also be related to baseline PSA: men with PSA less than 1.4ng/ml did not have symptom progression over 4 years.[19]

Pathogenesis and Pathophysiology

Hyperplasia occurs when prostate cell proliferation outpaces programmed cell death (apoptosis).[1] BPH may begin with either stimulation of cell growth, inhibition of apoptosis, or both. The mechanisms responsible for BPH are androgen dependent, complex, and incompletely understood. Sex hormones and aging are necessary to develop the characteristic combination of stromal and epithelial hyperplasia. The dominant prostate androgen is dihydrotestosterone, which is produced by 5α-reduction of testosterone within the prostate. The increased incidence of TURP for BPH in men with shorter CAG repeat length in the androgen receptor gene suggests that cellular response to androgens, as well as androgen levels, play an important role.[26]

The observation that castration causes less than complete prostate involution led to the discovery of additional androgen-independent factors supporting prostate

TABLE 51.1. Factors causing lower urinary tract symptoms (LUTS) in older men.

Pathophysiological mechanism	Etiologic factors	
	Outside urinary tract	Within urinary tract

Impaired bladder contractility	Medications:
	  Anticholinergics
	  Calcium channel blockers
	  Narcotics
	Fecal impaction
	Neurologic disease:
	  Lumbosacral spinal disease
	  Neuropathy (alcoholism, diabetes, B_{12} deficiency)
	Pelvic surgery, radiation
		Underactive bladder (idiopathic, age-related)
		Detrusor hyperactivity with impaired contractility (DHIC)

Increased outlet resistance	Medications: α-Adrenergic agonists (OTC "cold" medication)	Urethral obstruction Stricture Bladder sphincter dysynergia

Increased urine volume	Age-related shift to increased nocturnal urine excretion
	  Diuretics: R_x, alcohol, caffeine
	Peripheral edema
	Endocrine:
	  Diabetes
	  Hypercalcemia
	Increased fluid intake
		Urinary retention

Uninhibited contractions	Neurologic:
	  Dementia
	  Cervical spine disease
	Multiple sclerosis
		Detrusor instability
		DHIC

Urethral obstruction		BOO, stricture
Local inflammation		Infection (urine, prostate) Cancer (prostate, bladder) Stone

OTC, over the counter; BOO, bladder outlet obstruction.

TABLE 51.2. Natural history of untreated benign prostatic hyperplasia (BPH)-related LUTS.

| | | Outcomes at 4 years | | | | |
| | | Treatment | | | Symptom severity | |
Baseline symptom severity	n (%)	No treatment (%)	Medical treatment (%)	TURP (%)	Mild–moderate (%)	Severe (±) needed TURP (%)
Mild	60 (16)	63	27	10	83	17
Moderate	245 (66)	45	31	24	59	41
Severe	65 (18)	33	27	39	23	77

TURP, transurethral resection of prostate.
Source: From Barry et al., with permission.[25]

cell growth, including inflammatory infiltrates, autocrine cytokine growth factors, and neuroendocrine cell products.[27,28] Some of these factors, especially stimulatory and inhibitory peptide growth factors, interact with androgens and estrogens to orchestrate some of the stromal–epithelial interactions that regulate prostate cell growth and proliferation.[29] The genetics of BPH are incompletely understood.

The divergence in prevalence between BPH, BPE, and LUTS reflects the variability in the pathophysiologic changes associated with BPH. Histologic diversity exists in the ratio of stromal and epithelial hyperplasia: stromal proliferation predominates in about half of men with BPH, glandular in one-quarter, and mixed in the remainder.[30] Stromal glands tend to be smaller, more symptomatic, and less likely to have good symptomatic response to prostatectomy.[30] BPH nodules occur predominantly in the central transitional and periurethral zones of the lateral prostate lobes, thereby predisposing to mechanical occlusion of the prostatic urethra, yet urethral compression and BOO are not universal with BPH.[4,5] Some men develop significantly enlarged median lobes that compress the bladder base without causing BOO. BPH-related changes in the fibroelastic composition of the prostate capsule may alter prostate compliance and diminish urethral patency in the absence of mechanical blockage.[31] BPH tissue contains an increased number of alpha-adrenergic receptors (primarily of the α_1C class) that mediate prostate smooth muscle contraction.[32] The magnitude of the contractile responsiveness of these receptors is increased in symptomatic men with BPH, especially those with urinary retention.[33]

BPH-related BOO is associated with several changes in bladder detrusor muscle structure and function: increased connective tissue infiltration; smooth muscle hypertrophy and disintegration; and decreased autonomic neuronal number and a conversion from predominantly β-adrenergic (inhibitory) to α-adrenergic (stimulatory) responsiveness.[34,35] BOO also is associated with increased uninhibited contractions [detrusor instability (DI)], but the causality of this relationship is unclear, given that DI occurs in normal asymptomatic elderly men and women.[16] Detrusor instability (DI) disappears in up to two-thirds of men (mean age, 69) following transurethral prostatectomy,[36] yet it tends to persist in very elderly men (mean age, 80).[37]

Clinical Presentation

The most common clinical manifestations of BPH are urgency, frequency, nocturia, hesitancy, weak urine flow, interrupted stream, postvoiding dribbling, and a sense of incomplete emptying. Many men are asymptomatic, even with BPE and BOO. Hematuria (from prostatic varices) and urinary retention can occur, but much less frequently. As noted, the descriptive term prostatism should be avoided, because it falsely implies a single prostatic etiology.[6] LUTS itself is a misnomer, as these symptoms can result from a wide range of age-related physiologic changes, diseases, and medications, as well as lower urinary tract abnormalities other than BPH (Table 51.2; see also Chapter 63 on Urinary Incontinence). Furthermore, the separation of LUTS into "irritative" or "obstructive" groups is a false dichotomy. These groupings do not correlate with symptom bother or severity, urodynamic parameters, or response to medical therapy.[38] Irritative symptoms may result from obstructive pathophysiology (e.g., urinary frequency from severe BOO with overflow) and obstructive symptoms due to irritative pathophysiology (e.g., slowed urine flow rate caused by detrusor hyperactivity with impaired contractility).[39]

BPH, BOO, and LUTS are not equivalent but overlapping concepts (Fig. 51.1).[40] The presence of BPH or BPE does not imply that coexistent LUTS are caused by benign prostate disease. Moreover, even if symptoms are related to BPH, they may not be due to BPE with BOO; up to one-third of symptomatic men with BPH referred to tertiary centers for TURP do not have urodynamic evidence of BOO.[5] Conversely, men with severe BOO and partial or near-complete urinary retention may be entirely asymptomatic. Additionally, some symptomatic men have BOO without BPH (e.g., from urethral stricture) or neither BPH nor BOO.

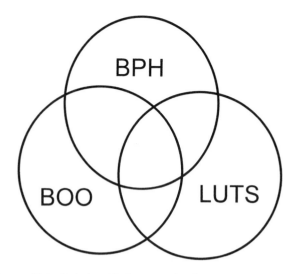

FIGURE 51.1. Relationship between benign prostatic hyperplasia (BPH), bladder outlet obstruction (BOO), and lower urinary tract symptoms (LUTS). (After Hald with permission.[40])

Diagnosis and Differential Diagnosis

Symptoms and Their Impact

LUTS are the usual motivation for men to seek evaluation, especially when symptoms bother, worry, or embarrass them. LUTS are quantified using indices such as the American Urological Association (AUA) symptom score[41] (Table 51.3) or the similar International Prostate Symptom Score (IPSS). Because LUTS are not specific for prostate disease, these indices should never be used for screening or diagnosis of BPH-related LUTS but only

to establish baseline symptom severity and to monitor symptoms over time. Changes in symptom score should be interpreted on the basis of expected intraindividual variation. Data from untreated men with symptomatic BPH who had AUA scores repeated 30 days apart suggest that changes greater than ±4.9 points have at least an 80% probability of indicating a true clinical change.[42] This point should be kept in mind when interpreting treatment studies in which smaller AUA or IPSS changes reach statistical significance because of study size. Any magnitude of change can be due to factors independent of BPH or its progression (see Table 51.2), which should be investigated before attributing symptom variation to prostate disease.

The effect of LUTS on quality of life is central, because for the majority of men the need for treatment depends on symptom bother alone. Bother may reflect interference with daily activities, work, sleep, or sexual function; worry or embarrassment; or physical discomfort.[43,44] The bother from individual symptom(s) may be more important than overall symptom impact. Older men are bothered significantly more by nocturia, frequency, and urgency, independent of overall LUTS severity and the presence of BOO.[45]

The initial step in evaluation always should be a full investigation of potential factors other than benign prostate disease that can cause these symptoms. Indeed, the evaluation of older men with LUTS closely parallels that of any older person with voiding dysfunction. For details of such an evaluation, see Chapter 63 on Urinary Incontinence; the additional points specific to benign prostate disease are emphasized here.

TABLE 51.3. The American Urological Association Symptom Index (score range, 0–35 points)

	Not at all	Less than one time in five	Less than half the time	About half the time	More than half the time	Almost always
1. Over the past month or so, how often have you had a sensation of not emptying your bladder completely after you finished urinating?	0	1	2	3	4	5
2. Over the past month or so, how often have your had to urinate again less than 2 hours after you finished urinating?	0	1	2	3	4	5
3. Over the past month or so, how often have you found you stopped and started again several times when you urinated?	0	1	2	3	4	5
4. Over the past month or so, how often have you found it difficult to postpone urination?	0	1	2	3	4	5
5. Over the past month or so, how often have you had a weak urinary stream?	0	1	2	3	4	5
6. Over the past month or so, how often have you had to push or strain to begin urination?	0	1	2	3	4	5
7. Over the last month, how many times did you most typically get up to urinate from the time you went to bed at night until the time you got up in the morning?[a]	0	1	2	3	4	5

AUA symptom score = sum of questions 1–7.
Mild symptoms: 0–7 points; moderate symptoms: 8–19 points; severe symptoms: 20–35 points.
[a]0, none; 1, one time; 2, two times; 3, three times; 4, four times; 5, five or more times.
Source: Barry et al., with permission.[41]

The medical history and review of systems should inquire about additional urinary symptoms such as hematuria, pelvic pain, and previous episodes of urinary retention; cardiac symptoms (regarding possible congestive heart failure); bowel and sexual function (as clues to potential sacral and pelvic neuropathies); type and amount of fluid intake; and sleep disturbance. All medications (including nonprescription drugs) should be reviewed. In many cases, a 48-h voiding record will provide useful information about the possible role of fluids and urine volume in causing symptoms,[2] especially nocturnal polyuria.[46]

Physical Examination

A complete physical exam is required to exclude nonurologic causes of LUTS, especially congestive heart failure, obstructive sleep apnea, and neurologic disease.

Digital rectal exam (DRE) is done to assess prostate nodularity and rectal tone and to exclude fecal impaction. Prostate sizing by DRE, however, is inaccurate and poorly reproducible, even when performed by specialists.[47] BPH adenomas may occur in the anterior prostate or median lobe, both inaccessible to rectal palpation. Importantly, prostate size or volume, as estimated by DRE, cystoscopy, MRI, or weight of tissue resected at TURP, is not a proxy for BOO.[48,49] Large BPH adenomas may not obstruct the urethra, and small predominantly stromal glands may cause significant obstruction. Prostate size is important for choosing between transurethral and open surgical approaches (see following), but it is not predictive of surgical outcome,[50] with the exception that smaller glands are associated with more postoperative bladder neck contractures.[30]

For men with moderate–severe symptoms, coexistent neurologic disease, or impaired renal function, or those taking bladder suppressant medications, the postvoiding residual volume (PVR) should be checked by urethral catheterization or ultrasound. Radiographic PVR estimates are only qualitative and may be correct only half the time.[51] An elevated PVR may be secondary to detrusor underactivity (due to age, disease, or medication) rather than caused by BOO.[39,52] Inability to pass a urethral catheter also is not diagnostic of BOO, as this is usually due to sphincter spasm from patient discomfort or anxiety.

Testing

Urine flow rates are commonly used to evaluate LUTS in men, yet are frequently misinterpreted. Urine flow rate depends on bladder contractility, outlet patency during voiding, and bladder volume; thus, low flow rates may result from impaired detrusor contractility, BOO, or low bladder volume, alone or in combination. Furthermore,

the prevalence of low flow rate increases with age in men and women independent of BOO.[16,35] Therefore, flow rate is very sensitive for detecting BOO but is not specific. Consequently, a normal flow rate confirms the absence of BOO, but low flow rate is not diagnostic, a point emphasized by the repeated observation that low flow rate does not predict outcome from TURP.[50,53–55] As a general rule, maximum flow rate greater than 12 mL/s for a void of 150 mL or more is normal and excludes BOO.[56]

Maximum flow rate measurement requires an electronic uroflowmeter, whereas average flow rate can be calculated by dividing the volume voided (in milliliters) by the voiding time (in seconds). The dependence of flow on bladder volume can be adjusted for by using one of several nomograms.[56,57] Unfortunately, the derivation populations for these nomograms included few older persons. Care should be taken to note whether the patient strains while voiding, which may falsely elevate the flow.

Voiding cystourethography (VCUG) provides a dynamic evaluation of the urethral outlet during voiding and direct information regarding BOO. The sensitivity and specificity of VCUG for BOO have not been investigated. Radiographic evaluation of bladder morphology and upper urinary tracts are not required routinely in men with LUTS. Although radiographic observation of bladder base indentation or shadowing correlates well with BOO, their detection is inconsistent as a result of contrast dilution by urine, x-ray beam angulation, and prostate morphology.[51] Radiographic evidence of bladder trabeculation correlates poorly with BOO, but more closely with detrusor instability—thus its frequent observation in elderly women.[58,59] Routine screening for hydronephrosis is not necessary because it is uncommon in unselected patients (3%–10%) and mild hydronephrosis is occult in even fewer (1.8%).[60,61] The relationship between elevated PVR and hydronephrosis in individual patients is unclear. Ultrasound is highly sensitive for detecting ureteral obstruction,[62] but intravenous pyleography is necessary for the complete evaluation of upper and lower tracts when hematuria is present.

Cystoscopy is unreliable for assessing BOO because it evaluates the prostate at rest and not during micturition and should not be used diagnostically.[23] In men already selected for surgery, or with hematuria or pelvic pain, cystoscopy provides important information about potential intravesical pathology such as tumors, stones, or marked trabeculation, as well as prostate size, length, and median lobe enlargement.

Urodynamic tests for evaluating LUTS include cystometry (to determine detrusor stability, contractility, and compliance) and pressure–flow studies (to detect BOO and assess detrusor contractility). Voiding profilometry (simultaneous measurement of detrusor and urethral pressures) is comparable to pressure–flow studies in accuracy of BOO diagnosis and may be easier to perform in frail patients.[63] Whether urodynamics are required to confirm BOO in all men with LUTS remains controversial.[6,64] Arguments for their use include these: obstructed men have better symptomatic outcomes from TURP than those without BOO[23]; urodynamics are the most accurate method for diagnosing BOO[6]; and the causes of LUTS in older men are diverse, often multiple, and may not be distinguishable without physiologically based testing. Against routine urodynamic evaluation are the concerns that testing is invasive, expensive, and requires equipment and expertise that are not routinely available even in most urologic practices.[64] Additionally, the marginal difference in TURP outcome for obstructed versus unobstructed men is small in routine cases, making definitive diagnosis of BOO less pressing.[64] The Agency for Health Care Policy and Research (AHCPR)/Agency for Healthcare Research and Quality (AHRQ) Bureau of Primary Health (BPH) guideline designates urodynamics "optional" testing whose performance should be based on the physician's judgment.[23]

For geriatricians, there are two principal issues when considering urodynamic evaluation in older men with LUTS. First, if the man desires and would be a candidate for surgical treatment for BOO, then urodynamics should be strongly considered to exclude other forms of lower urinary tract dysfunction that do not require surgical treatment [e.g., detrusor hyperactivity with impaired contractility (DHIC)]. If he is not suitable for or would refuse surgery, then definitive urodynamic diagnosis is less pressing. Second, urodynamic evaluation should be considered when empiric treatment for BPH-related LUTS has failed, and when there is coexistent neurologic disease (especially spinal cord injury). These guidelines are intended to optimize treatment of older men, while recognizing that the majority of men who today undergo TURP and other invasive treatments for BPH in the United States do not receive preoperative urodynamic evaluation.

Screening for prostate cancer with prostate-specific antigen (PSA) should be considered in the evaluation of older men with LUTS, if the patient would be a candidate for curative treatment of localized cancer with radical prostatectomy or radiation therapy, or if a prostate cancer diagnosis would modify his management. Initial studies suggest that PSA level also may predict the progression of BPH-related LUTS[19] (see earlier). For a full discussion of PSA screening, see Chapter 36.

Treatment

The Decision to Treat

BPH, BPE, and BOO have real but small risks of morbidity and cause variable subjective impact. Moreover, no current treatment prolongs life or abrogates the need for future treatment. Therefore, all treatment decisions should be patient centered,[23] focusing on symptom severity and bother, patient preferences, and potential treatment effects and morbidity. Providers offer critical guidance by exploring these key issues, so that patients do not feel burdened by decision making, but rather supported toward the goal of tailoring treatment to their needs. Importantly, causes of LUTS other than BPH must be evaluated and treated before prostate-specific treatment is initiated. Because many men tolerate mild to moderate symptoms, and only a minority will experience rapid symptom progression or morbidity, care must be taken not to overtreat; many men are best managed with watchful waiting and lifestyle changes.[65]

Symptom bother often drives the decision to initiate therapy. Indices such as the AUA symptom score can be used to quantify voiding symptom severity and overall bother. Asking men specifically which symptom is the most bothersome may be useful in tailoring treatment goals. For example, an older man with slow urinary flow, hesitancy, and nocturia is often most bothered by the latter[45]; nocturia, however, generally responds poorly to BPE/BOO-specific medical and surgical therapies, and may be better addressed by decreasing evening fluid intake and eradicating pedal edema.[46] The specific nature of the bother also is important: for the man most bothered by worry, evaluation and reassurance alone may provide relief, whereas symptom eradication may be most important for the man predominantly bothered by interference with daily activities.

Patient preferences should be elicited regarding the immediacy and permanence of symptom relief, short- and long-term costs and morbidity, and ability to comply with long-term monitoring. As is common in geriatric medicine, decisions must balance individually the probability of desired treatment effect with the need to avoid specific side effects and interactions with comorbid disease. In frail institutionalized men, catheter removal may be the treatment goal, and side effects intolerable in younger men (such as impotence) may be less problematic. Impotence following TURP would not be problematic for an older man with diabetes-related erectile dysfunction, whereas orthostatic hypotension from alpha-blockers could result in a devastating fall for a man with Parkinson's disease.

Time to treatment effect varies significantly among interventions (ranging from days with surgery to months with finasteride), as does duration of symptom relief and need for repeat or further treatment. Symptom palliation alone may or may not be an acceptable outcome short of cure. "Low-cost" medications can result in significant cost burden if treatment is long term, requires frequent monitoring, or results in side effects. The AHCPR Clinical Practice Guideline is a useful source for extensive materials comparing direct and indirect BPH treatment

TABLE 51.4. Probabilities of outcomes from treatment.

Treatment	Symptom improvement		Serious adverse events[a]		Retrograde ejaculation[b]		Five-year retreatment rate	
	Median	90% CI	Median	90% CI	Mean	90% CI	Median	90% CI
Placebo	45%	26%–65%	5%	4%–7%	0%	—	38%	15%–65%
Watchful waiting (WW)	42%	31%–55%	—	—	0%	—	—	—
Alpha-blocker	74%	59%–86%	5%	4%–7%	6%	3.5%–11%	39%	23%–70%
Finasteride	67%	54%–78%	5%	N/A	N/A	—	27%	25%–29%
TUIP	80%	78%–83%	12%	2%–33%	25%	6%–55%	9%[d]	1%–28%
TURP	88%	75%–96%	15%	5%–31%	73%	30%–97%	10%[d]	9%–11%
Open prostatectomy	98%	94%–99.8%	21%	7%–43%	77%	46%–95%	2%[d]	1%–4%

CI, confidence interval; TUIP, transurethral incision of the prostate; TURP, transurethral resection of the prostate; N/A, not available.

[a] Leading to discontinuation of drug treatment or involving immediate postoperative complications.

[b] Probability of retrograde ejaculation.

[c] High estimate based on initial failure rate assumed to be linear up to 5 years. Low estimates, assuming 20% of the initial failure rate over the subsequent period, are for alpha-blockers (13%; 90% CI, 4%–31%) and for finasteride (10%; 90% CI, 9%–12%).

[d] Single point estimates and confidence intervals derived from large clinical series out to and past 5 years.

Source: Modified from AHCPR Clinical Practice Guideline.[23]

outcomes.[23] A selective summary of this information regarding the major forms of treatment is provided in Table 51.4.

Lifestyle Changes

Behavioral approaches such as bladder retraining and unhurried voiding without straining to completely empty the bladder[66] can mitigate LUTS and their impact for some men. Other suggestions are avoidance of diuretic beverages with caffeine or alcohol and, for nocturia, decreasing evening fluid intake or possibly adding an afternoon diuretic for preemptive diuresis in men with a large shift to more nocturnal excretion of their daily fluid load.

Watchful Waiting

The natural history of BPH-related LUTS, along with the repeated observation of marked symptom response without specific therapy and to placebo treatment in trials, established watchful waiting (WW) as sound management. Men most appropriate for WW are those with mild to moderate symptoms who are comfortable with this approach, can be followed reliably, and have no evidence of bladder decompensation (e.g., elevated PVR). Watchful waiting is not, however, the absence of any intervention. Patients must be followed at least yearly to monitor symptoms, renal function, and possibly PVR and PSA level. They should be counseled to avoid medications that may precipitate urinary retention (e.g., over-the-counter "cold" tablets containing alpha-agonists) and monitored carefully if anticholinergic or calcium channel blocking drugs are prescribed.

Watchful waiting may not relieve symptoms, but significant morbidity is uncommon. In a randomized trial of WW versus TURP involving 556 men with moderate symptoms, at 3 years symptom improvement was significantly greater after TURP, although still considerable with WW (mean symptom score decrease, 60% versus 38%).[24] Among WW men, 36% crossed over to TURP, yet the incidence of absolute treatment failures was low (urinary retention, 2.9%; PVR >350 mL, 5.8%; and high symptom score, 4.3%). TURP decreased symptom bother and improved activities of daily living significantly more than WW; there was no difference between treatments, however, regarding sexual performance, general well-being, and social activities. Bother from symptoms improved less in men who were less bothered at baseline, especially following TURP (as in earlier studies[67]).

Medical Therapy

Alpha-Adrenergic Blockers

Smooth muscle contraction in BPH adenomas and the prostatic capsule is mediated by plentiful alpha-1-adrenergic receptors (primarily alpha-1A subtype). Alpha-adrenergic blockers may reduce BPH-related LUTS by decreasing capsule, tissue, and urethral contractility. Most commonly used are alpha-1-selective agents, such as prazosin (1–2 mg twice a day), the longer-acting terazosin (2–10 mg daily), and doxazosin (4–8 mg daily), and the alpha 1A-selective tamulosin (0.4 mg daily). In general, alpha-adrenergic blockers reduce symptoms by 30% to 40% over placebo in 50% to 70% of moderately symptomatic men,[23,68,69] and result in better disease-specific functional outcomes than placebo in men with moderate to severe symptoms.[70] No significant differences have been identified between the different agents.[69] Time to onset of action for alpha-blockers is 2 to 4 weeks, compared with 3 to 6 months for finasteride.[71]

Drug effectiveness appears to be durable, although all long-term (2–4 years) data come from "open label" trials (generally uncontrolled with small numbers of patients self-selected for treatment response).

Side effects of alpha-blockers include asthenia, headache, dizziness, lightheadedness, and orthostatic hypotension; withdrawal rates of 10% to 15% have occurred in published trials and may be higher in practice.[72] The prevalence of dizziness related to terazosin was 19% in one Randomized Clinical Trial (RCT) and was not related to age (less than 65 years of age compared to 65 or older) or changes in blood pressure.[73] Significant blood pressure drops and orthostatic hypotension are more likely in persons with elevated blood pressure (whether treated or not).[74] Alpha-1A-selective agents do not appear to have fewer side effects.[69] Retrograde or delayed ejaculation occurs with tamulosin in 4.5% to 14%.[75] Slow titration from minimal starting doses and nighttime dosing may mitigate first-dose hypotension. Although alpha-blockers may seem a reasonable and concise option in men with BPH-related LUTS and hypertension, alpha-blockers are not recommended as first-line antihypertensive treatment, especially given the increased risk for congestive heart failure observed with doxazosin in men with other cardiac risk factors in the ALLHAT trial.[76]

5α-Reductase Inhibitors

Finasteride causes prostate involution by blocking the 5α-reduction of testosterone to dihydrotesterone, the steroid sustaining prostate growth. Treatment with finasteride 5 mg daily decreases prostate volume by at least one-third in 27% of men by 6 months and in 36% at 12 months; symptom reduction of at least 25% occurs in 54% of men by 6 months and in 58% at 1 year.[77] Significant symptom improvement over placebo did not occur until 10 months.[77] Variability and delay in symptomatic response may reflect heterogeneity of BPH pathology present (with largest responses possibly in men with predominantly glandular rather than stromal tissue) and variable effects on obstructed voiding physiology.[78,79] Combined data from six RCTs[80] and the PLESS trial (Proscar Long-term Efficacy and Safety Study)[81] suggest that IPSS score improvement with finasteride is 55% greater in men with large prostates (>60 versus <20 g) and that prostate size accounts for 80% of the variability in outcome. Finasteride is less effective than terazosin in reducing symptoms[82]; however, finasteride can reduce the risk of urinary retention by 57% and need for TURP by 55%[83] (appropriate trials investigating the effect of alpha-blockers on such BPH complications have not been done). Sustained drug effect requires lifetime use because prostate growth resumes once finasteride is stopped. Cost-effectiveness studies suggest that, in men

with moderate symptoms, finasteride is less expensive and provides more Quality Adjusted Life Years (QALYs) than watchful waiting (for 3 years or less) and TURP (for 14 years or less)[80]; over longer periods, the high cost of the drug is problematic.[84]

Finasteride decreases PSA levels by up to 40% to 60% after 1 year in approximately one-third of men[85]; this heterogeneity in response may make monitoring for prostate cancer difficult.[86] If PSA does not decline in a compliant patient on finasteride, he should be evaluated further with prostate biopsy. Despite maintained or increased testosterone levels, finasteride causes adverse sexual effects, including decreased libido (3%), decreased ejaculate volume (3%), and impotence (3%–4%)[77]; gynecomastia is reported in 0.4% of patients.[83] Preliminary reports suggest that finasteride has little effect on serum lipids or bone density, although adequate long-term studies are lacking.[84]

Phytotherapy

Plant-derived compounds are widely used as over-the-counter treatment for BPH. In general, studies of these agents suffer from short-term treatment (typically 4–24 weeks) and lack of standardized preparations, yet recent meta-analyses suggest these compounds are efficacious. Best studied is *Serenoa repens*, from the dwarf palm tree or saw palmetto. Meta-analyses demonstrate that, compared with placebo, *Serenoa repens* improves urinary symptoms (risk ratio, 1.75; 95% CI, 1.21, 2.54), decreases nocturia (weighted mean difference, −0.76 times a night; 95% CI, −1.22, −0.32), and increases flow rate (weighted mean difference, 1.93 mL/s; 95% CI, 0.72, 3.14 mL/s)[87,88]; in two studies, improvements were similar to those seen with finasteride.[87,88] In a systematic review, beta-sitosterols improved urinary symptoms (IPSS reduction weighted mean difference, −4.9 points; 95% CI, −6.3 to −3.5) and flow rate (weighted mean difference, 3.9 mL/s; 95% CI, 0.91–6.9 mL/s) compared with placebo.[89] Cernilton (pollen from the ryegrass *Secale cereale*) improves symptoms more than placebo (risk ratio, 2.40; 95% CI, 1.21, 4.75) but does not improve flow rate.[90] These agents have few to no reported side effects, but long-term data are lacking.

Antiandrogens

"Medical castration" and resultant prostate involution can be induced through luteinizing hormone-releasing hormone (LHRH) agonists or androgen receptor inhibitors.[91] Small uncontrolled trials suggest that such agents may facilitate the removal of indwelling catheters in frail older men with BOO.[91] A controlled trial of leuprolide demonstrated significant prostate shrinkage over placebo but no significant differences in symptoms until week 48.[92] Similar to finasteride, these agents decrease PSA levels and must be continued indefinitely to maintain prostate reduction. Side effects also include impotence, weight gain, and hot flashes (LHRH agonists and cyproterone acetate) and diarrhea and gynecomastia (flutamide).

Surgery

Transurethral Resection of Prostate (TURP)

Transurethral resection remains the standard against which other BPH treatments are compared because it has the highest rate of symptom improvement, generally 80% to 88%.[23] Despite the advent of alternative surgical treatments for BPH, many urologists continue to employ only TURP: the 1999 Gallup survey of urologists found that only 22% perform laser prostatectomy, 17% microwave thermotherapy, and 7% transurethral needle ablation.[93]

The absolute indications for TURP are severe lower urinary tract obstruction, acute urinary retention, recurrent urinary infections, hydronephrosis, recurrent hematuria, and renal impairment (causes other than BOO excluded).[94] These indications account for nearly one-third of all surgeries; the rate is higher in studies in men over age 80 (48%–61%),[95,96] although causes for retention other than BOO were not excluded. Several studies suggest that men with urodynamically confirmed BOO have better symptomatic outcomes.[64,97]

The efficacy of TURP must be interpreted in light of several considerations. First, quality of life following TURP may be improved only in those with the most severe symptoms.[67] Second, improvement may not be durable: in one trial success rates declined from 87% at 3 months to 75% at 7 years among survivors.[98] Third, success rates tend to be lower in the elderly (less than 80%[96]), often with a concomitant increase in associated morbidity (up to 71%).[94] Fourth, studies of TURP cost-effectiveness in the United States are complicated by marked geographic variability for charges and length of stay.[99] Fifth, although treatment options have expanded widely, there are few trials comparing these to TURP, and no long-term data. Finally, although a subset of men with BOO present initially with retention, bladder decompensation, and renal insufficiency, suggesting that earlier surgery might prevent such outcomes, the time course of decompensation and the true proportion of patients at risk are unknown. These concerns regarding selection for, outcome from, and alternatives to TURP have refocused attention on the indications for surgery in BPH and have fueled the controversy.[6,64,100]

Sexual dysfunction following TURP is a concern for many men. Around 74% of men develop retrograde ejaculation after TURP,[23] which is of concern only if conception is desired. A small but significant proportion of men lose potency after TURP; estimates range as high as 40%, yet the actual rate is closer to 14%, with higher rates in older men.[23,101,102] Urinary incontinence occurs in approximately 5%.[23]

The major complications of TURP are bleeding requiring transfusion, failure to void, and infection; rarer is "TURP syndrome," severe hyponatremia due to systemic absorption of hypotonic bladder irrigation fluid used intraoperatively. Several studies suggest that compared to younger individuals men over age 80 have higher perioperative mortality (2%–3% versus <0.5%) and morbidity (up to 70% versus 18%–30% for major complications)[96,103,104]; these comparisons, however, do not adjust for increased comorbidity in the oldest men. Indeed, in selected robust older men, TURP can be done as an outpatient procedure.[105] In frail patients with small prostates, general or spinal anesthesia can be avoided and TURP performed with sedation and local prostate anesthesia.[106]

Open Prostatectomy

Larger prostates require longer transurethral resection times, with an increased risk of TURP syndrome and analgesia complications. Open prostatectomy by an abdominal or perineal approach generally is recommended for men with marked prostatic hypertrophy (>60 g). In practice, however, open procedures account for 5% or less of prostatectomies, because many surgeons prefer to perform an "incomplete" TURP rather than risk the greater morbidity of open surgery.[100] Retrospective studies suggest that TURP has higher reoperation rate and late mortality compared with open surgery,[107,108] but these did not adequately control for increased age and comorbidity in TURP patients[109] or the secular trend of lower TURP mortality in older men.[110] Unfortunately, a randomized trial under way to address this issue excludes patients with an indwelling catheter, that is, up to 40% of elderly men who undergo prostatectomy.[95,96,104]

Prostate Incision

If the prostate is small (<30 g), prostatotomy or transurethral incision of the prostate (TUIP) may provide similar efficacy to TURP with a technically simpler procedure, shorter operation times, and the potential for using local anesthesia.[111] Randomized studies demonstrate similar symptomatic success rates for TUIP compared with TURP at 1 year; in a select case series with a 2-year mean follow-up, only 8% of patients required later TURP.[112] Additional advantages of TUIP include lower rates of bleeding complications and postoperative retrograde ejaculation. For the higher-risk older man with BOO and a small prostate for whom noninvasive management has failed or is not optimal, TUIP may be a safe and effective alternative to TURP, especially in the hands of a surgeon familiar with the technique.

Laser Prostatectomy

Several different laser systems currently are used to cause prostate vaporization or coagulation necrosis. Randomized trials indicate that at 6 to 7.5 months TURP is superior to noncontact laser for symptom improvement, flow rate, and quality of life, but outcomes equalize at 1 year.[113–115] TURP required longer hospital stay, more transfusions, and resulted in more urethral strictures, while laser therapy had longer catheterization and more infectious complications (including methicillin-resistant *Staphylococcus aureus*, MRSA[116]). The longest study has followed men for only 2 years.[117] Different laser procedures yield results of variable consistency and success.[118] Side effects also vary by method, but include impotence, retrograde ejaculation, increased urgency and frequency for several weeks, incontinence, and bladder neck stricture. Patients may require catheter drainage for several weeks until tissue sloughing is complete. Unlike TURP, laser procedures do not allow tissue examination for occult prostate cancer.

Microwave Hyperthermia

Controlled trials of transurethral microwave thermotherapy (TUMT) have shown variable results regarding symptom improvement, ranging from moderate to no difference from sham,[119,120] and only a modest improvement in peak flow rate (2–4 mL/s).[119] One-third of patients in a 3-year nonrandomized trial required further therapy for their symptoms.[121] Compared with terazosin, TUMT provided less symptom relief at 2 weeks, but was better at 6 months (at least 50% decrease in symptoms; TUMT, 78% versus terazosin, 33%).[122] There are no long-term treatment data.

Other Approaches

One randomized trial found transurethral needle ablation (TUNA) was less efficacious than TURP at 1 year for improving symptoms (decrease in IPSS, 13.6 versus 16 points), although TUNA resulted in no retrograde ejaculation and less bleeding (32% versus 100%).[123] Small, nonrandomized trials indicate that wire urethral stents, placed in the prostatic urethra under endoscopic or radiologic guidance, may restore spontaneous voiding in frail men with acute or chronic retention who are not surgical candidates or for whom indwelling catheters are undesirable. Stents consisting of a wire spiral have been complicated by encrustation, migration of the device, infection, urinary incontinence, and retention. Stents become covered by epithelium in 6 to 8 months, and have fewer infections, but are associated with a high rate of urgency and urge incontinence for up to 2 months.

Summary

BPH is nearly universal among older men, and the associated morbidity from related prostate enlargement, bladder outlet obstruction, and LUTS has a substantial impact on quality of life. The prevalence of BPH ensures a continuing need for geriatricians to be informed regarding issues in evaluation and treatment, while the established role of nonoperative therapy and the recognition of the importance of patient preferences have opened the way for expanded primary care involvement in management. Basic questions regarding the etiology of BPH and LUTS, the role of BOO in predicting treatment outcome, and the measurement of patient-weighted outcomes for invasive and noninvasive treatments await further study. In the interim, geriatricians can significantly help their male patients by understanding the large number of factors that can mimic prostate disease in older men; appreciating the often indolent natural history of BPH and related LUTS; understanding the clinical utility of current evaluation methods; and especially by assisting them in weighing risks and benefits of established and evolving therapies together with their own personal concerns and needs.

References

1. Isaacs JT, Coffey DS. Etiology and disease process of benign prostatic hyperplasia. *Prostate Suppl.* 1989;2:33–50.
2. DuBeau CE, Resnick NM. Controversies in the diagnosis and management of benign prostatic hypertrophy. *Adv Intern Med.* 1992;37:55–83.
3. Lepor H, Machi G. Comparison of the AUA symptom index in unselected males and females between 55 and 79 years of age. *Urology.* 1993;42:36–40.
4. Schäfer W, Rubben H, Noppeney R, Deutz F-J. Obstructed and unobstructed prostatic obstruction: a plea for urodynamic objectivation of bladder outflow obstruction in benign prostatic hyperplasia. *World J Urol.* 1989;6:198–203.
5. Coolsaet BLRA, van Venrooij GEPM, Blok C. Prostatism: rationalization of urodynamic testing. *World J Urol.* 1984;2:216–221.
6. Abrams P. In support of pressure-flow studies for evaluating men with lower urinary tract symptoms. *Urology.* 1994;44:153–155.
7. Berry SJ, Coffey DS, Walsh PC, Ewing LL. The development of human benign prostatic hyperplasia with age. *J Urol.* 1984;132:474–479.
8. Chute CG, Panser LA, Girman CJ, et al. The prevalence of prostatism: a population-based survey of urinary symptoms. *J Urol.* 1993;150:85–89.
9. Diokno AC, Brown MB, Goldstein N, Herzog A. Epidemiology of bladder emptying symptoms in elderly men. *J Urol.* 1992;148:1817–1821.

10. Jacobsen SJ, Girman CJ, Guess HA, Rhodes T, Oesterling JE, Liever MM. Natural history of prostatism: longitudinal changes in voiding symptoms in community dwelling men. *J Urol.* 1966;155:595–600.

11. Jacobsen SJ, Jacobson DJ, Girman CJ, et al. Treatment for benign prostatic hyperplasia among community-dwelling men: the Olmsted County study of urinary symptoms and health status. *J Urol.* 1999;162:1301–1306.

12. Platz EA, Rimm EB, Kawachi I, et al. Alcohol consumption, cigarette smoking and the risk of benign prostatic hyperplasia. *Am J Epidemiol.* 1999;149:106–115.

13. Klein BE, Klein R, Lee KE, Bruskewitz RC. Correlates of urinary symptom scores in men. *Am J Public Health.* 1999;89:1745–1748.

14. Matthiesen TB, Rittig S, Mortensen JT, Djurhuus JC. Nocturia and polyuria in men referred with lower urinary tract symptoms, assessed using a 7-day frequency-voiding chart. *BJU Int.* 1999;83:1017–1022.

15. Jørgensen JB, Jensen KM-E, Mogensen P. Longitudinal observations on normal and abnormal voiding in men over the age of 50 years. *Br J Urol.* 1993;72:413–420.

16. Resnick NM, Elbadawi A. Yalla SV. Age and the lower urinary tract: what is normal? *Neurourol Urodynam.* 1995; 14:557–558.

17. Partin AW, Oesterling JE, Epstein JI, Horton R, Walsh PC. Influence of age and endocrine factors on the volume of benign prostatic hyperplasia. *J Urol.* 1991;145:405–409.

18. Watanabe H. Natural history of benign prostatic hypertrophy. *Ultrasound Med Biol.* 1986;12:567–571.

19. Roehrborn CG, Boyle P, Bergner D, et al. Serum prostate-specific antigen and prostate volume predict long-term changes in symptoms and flow rate: results of a 4-year, randomized trial comparing finasteride versus placebo. *Urology.* 1999;54:662–669.

20. Ball AJ, Feneley RCL, Abrams PH. The natural history of untreated "prostatism." *Br J Urol.* 1981;53:613–616.

21. Birkoff JD, Wiederhorn AR, Hamilton ML, Zinsser HH. Natural history of benign prostatic hypertrophy and acute urinary retention. *Urology.* 1976;6:48–52.

22. Craigen AA, Hickling JB, Saunders CRG, Carpenter RG. Natural history of prostatic obstruction. *J R Coll Gen Pract.* 1969;18:226–232.

23. McConnell JD, Barry MJ, Bruskewitz RC, et al. *Benign Prostatic Hyperplasia: Diagnosis and Treatment. Clinical Practice Guideline, Number 8.* AHCPR Pub 94-0582. Rockville, MD: Agency for Health Care Policy and Research; 1994.

24. Wasson JH, Reda DJ, Bruskewitz RC, Elinson J, Keller AM, Henderson WG. A comparison of transurethral surgery with watchful waiting for moderate symptoms of benign prostatic hyperplasia. *N Engl J Med.* 1995;332:75–79.

25. Barry MJ, Fowler FJ, Bin L, Pitts JC, Harris CJ, Mulley AG. The natural history of patients with BPH as diagnosed by North American urologists. *J Urol.* 1997;157:10–15.

26. Giovannucci E, Stampfer MJ, Chan A, et al. CAG repeat with the androgen receptor gene and incidence of surgery for benign prostatic hyperplasia in U.S. physicians. *Prostate.* 1999;39:130–134.

27. Steiner G, Gessl A, Kramer G, Schöllhammer A, Förster O, Marberger M. Phenotype and function of peripheral and prostatic lymphocytes in patients with benign prostatic hyperplasia. *J Urol.* 1994;151:480–484.

28. Cockett ATK, di Sant'Agnese PA, Gopinath P, Schoen SR, Abrahamsson P-A. Relationship of neuroendocrine cells of prostate and serotonin to benign prostatic hyperplasia. *Urology.* 1993;42:512–519.

29. Steiner MS. Role of peptide growth factors in the prostate: a review. *Urology.* 1993;42:99–110.

30. Dørflinger T, England DM, Madsen PO, Bruskewitz RC. Urodynamic and histological correlates of benign prostatic hyperplasia. *J Urol.* 1988;140:1487–1490.

31. Hinman F Jr. Point of view: capsular influence on benign prostatic hypertrophy. *Urology.* 1986;28:347–350.

32. Chapple CR, Burt RP, Andersson PO, Greengrass P, Wyllie M, Marshall I. Alpha$_1$-adrenoreceptor subtypes in the human prostate. *Br J Urol.* 1994;74:585–589.

33. Lepor H, Shapiro E. Characterization of alpha-1 adrenergic receptors in human benign prostatic hyperplasia. *J Urol.* 1984;132:1226–1229.

34. Chapple CR, Smith D. The pathophysiological changes in the bladder obstructed by benign prostatic hyperplasia. *Br J Urol.* 1994;73:117–123.

35. Elbadawi A, Yalla SV, Resnick NM. Structural basis of geriatric voiding dysfunction. IV. Bladder outlet obstruction. *J Urol.* 1993;150:1681–1695.

36. Abrams PH, Griffiths DJ. The assessment of prostatic obstruction from urodynamic measurements and from residual urine. *Br J Urol.* 1979;51:129–134.

37. Gormley EA, Griffiths DJ, McCracken PN, Harrison GM, McPhee MS. Effect of transurethral resection of the prostate on detrusor instability and urge incontinence in elderly males. *Neurourol Urodynam.* 1993;12:445–453.

38. Barry MJ, Williford WO, Fowler FJ Jr, Jones KM. Lepor H. Filling and voiding symptoms in the American Urological Association symptom index: the value of their distinction in a Veterans Affairs randomized trial of medical therapy in men with a clinical diagnosis of benign prostatic hyperplasia. *J Urol.* 2000;164:1559–1564.

39. Resnick NM, Yalla SV. Detrusor hyperactivity with impaired contractile function: an unrecognized but common cause of incontinence in elderly patients. *JAMA.* 1987;257: 3076–3081.

40. Hald T. Urodynamics in benign prostatic hyperplasia: a survey. *Prostate.* 1989;2(suppl):69–77.

41. Barry MJ, Fowler FJ Jr, O'Leary MP, et al. The American Urological Association symptom index for benign prostatic hyperplasia. *J Urol.* 1992;148:1549–1557.

42. Barry MJ, Girman CJ, O'Leary MP, et al. Using repeated measures of symptom score, uroflowmetry and prostate specific antigen in the clinical management of prostate disease. *J Urol.* 1995;153:99–103.

43. Rhodes PR, Krogh RH, Bruskewitz RC. Impact of drug therapy on benign prostatic hyperplasia—specific quality of life. *Urology.* 1999;53:1090–1098.

44. Garraway WM, Kirby RS. Benign prostatic hyperplasia: effects on quality of life and treatment decisions. *Urology.* 1994;44:629–636.

45. DuBeau CE, Yalla SV, Resnick NM. Implications of the most bothersome prostatism symptom for clinical care and outcomes research. *J Am Geriatr Soc.* 1995;43:985–992.

46. Weiss JP, Blaivas JG. Nocturia. *J Urol.* 2000;163:5–12.

47. Meyhoff HH, Hald T. Are doctors able to assess prostatic size? *Scand J Urol Nephrol.* 1978;12:219–221.

48. Jensen KM-E, Bruskewitz RC, Iversen P. Madsen PO. Significance of prostatic weight in prostatism. *Urol Int.* 1983;38:173–178.

49. Andersen JT, Nordling J, Prostatism, II. The correlation between cystourethroscopic, cystometric, and urodynamic findings. *Scand J Urol Nephrol.* 1980;14:23–27.

50. Bruskewitz RC, Larsen EH, Madsen PO, et al. Three year follow-up of urinary symptoms after transurethral resection of the prostate. *J Urol.* 1986;136:613–615.

51. Andersen JT. Prostatism: clinical, radiological, and urodynamic aspects. *Neurourol Urodynam.* 1982;1:241–293.

52. Coolsaet B, Blok C. Detrusor properties related to prostatism. *Neurourol Urodynam.* 1986;5:435–447.

53. Gerstenberg TC, Andersen JT, Klarskov P, Ramirez D, Hald T. High flow infravesical obstruction in men: symptomatology, urodynamics and the results of surgery. *J Urol.* 1982;127:943–945.

54. Neal DE, Ramsden PD, Sharples L, et al. Outcome of elective prostatectomy. *Br Med J.* 1989;299:762–767.

55. Kadow C, Feneley RCL, Abrams PH. Prostatectomy or conservative management in the treatment of benign prostatic hypertrophy. *Br J Urol.* 1988;61:432–434.

56. Siroky MB, Olsson CA, Krane RJ. The flow rate nomogram: I. Development. *J Urol.* 1979;122:665–668.

57. Haylen BT, Ashby D, Sutherst JR, et al. Maximum and average urine flow rates in normal male and female populations—the Liverpool nomograms. *Br J Urol.* 1989; 64:30–38.

58. Brocklehurst JC, Dillane JB. Studies of the female bladder in old age. I. Cystometrograms in non-incontinent women. *Gerontol Clin.* 1966;8:285–305.

59. Fielding JR, Lee JH, DuBeau CE, Zou KH, Resnick NM. Voiding cystourethrography findings in elderly women with urge incontinence. *J Urol.* 2000;163(4):1216–1218.

60. Mushlin AI, Thornbury JR. Intravenous pyelography: the case against its routine use. *Ann Intern Med.* 1989;111:58–70.

61. Courtney SP, Wightman JAK. The value of ultrasound scanning of the upper urinary tract in patients with bladder outlet obstruction. *Br J Urol.* 1991;68:169–171.

62. Reisman EM, Kennedy TJ, Roehrborn CG, McConnell JD. A prospective study of urologist-performed sonographic evaluation of the urinary tract in patients with prostatism. *J Urol.* 1991;145:1186–1191.

63. DuBeau CE, Sullivan MP, Cravalho E, Resnick NM, Yalla SV. Correlation between micturitional urethral pressure profile and pressure-flow criteria in bladder outlet obstruction. *J Urol.* 1995;154:498–503.

64. McConnell JD. Why pressure-flow studies should be optional and not mandatory studies for evaluating men with benign prostatic hyperplasia. *Urology.* 1994;44:156–158.

65. NHS Centre for Reviews and Dissemination. *Benign Prostatic Hyperplasia. Effective Health Care, vol 2.* York:

66. Root MT. Living with benign prostatic hypertrophy [letter]. *N Engl J Med.* 1979;301:52.

67. Fowler FJ Jr, Wennberg JE, Timothy RP, et al. Symptom status and quality of life following prostatectomy. *JAMA.* 1988;259:3018–3022.

68. Lepor H. Medical therapy for benign prostatic hyperplasia. *Urology.* 1993;42:483–501.

69. Djavan B, Marberger M. A meta-analysis on the efficacy and tolerability of alpha$_1$-adrenoceptor antagonists in patients with lower urinary tract symptoms suggestive of benign prostatic obstruction. *Eur Urol.* 1999;36:1–13.

70. Hillman AL, Schwartz JS, Willian MK, et al. The cost-effectiveness of terazosin and placebo in the treatment of moderate to severe benign prostatic hyperplasia. *Urology.* 1996;47:169–178.

71. Kirby RS, McConnell JD. *Fast Facts: Benign Prostatic Hyperplasia, 2nd Ed.* Oxford: Health Press; 1997:29.

72. Caine M. Reflections on alpha blockade therapy for benign prostatic hyperplasia. *Br J Urol.* 1995;75:265–270.

73. Lepor H, Jones K, Williford W. The mechansim of adverse events associated with terazosin: an analysis of the Veterans Affairs Cooperative Study. *J Urol.* 2000;163: 1134–1137.

74. Guthrie RM, Siegel RL. A multicenter, community-based study of doxazosin in the treatment of concomitant hypertension and symptomatic benign prostatic hyperplasia: the Hypertension and BPH Intervention Trial (HABIT). *Clin Ther.* 1999;21:1732–1748.

75. Lee M. Tamulosin for the treatment of benign prostatic hypertrophy. *Ann Pharmacother.* 2000;34:188–199.

76. ALLHAT Collaborative Research Group. Major cardiovascular events in hypertensive patients randomized to doxazosin vs. chlorthalidone: the antihypertensive and lipid-lowering treatment to prevent heart attack trial (ALLHAT). *JAMA.* 2000;283:1967–1975.

77. Gormley GJ, Stoner E, Bruskewitz RC, et al. The effect of finasteride in men with benign prostatic hyperplasia. *N Engl J Med.* 1992;327:1185–1191.

78. Tammela TLJ, Konturri MJ. Urodynamic effects of finasteride in the treatment of bladder outlet obstruction due to benign prostatic hyperplasia. *J Urol.* 1993;149:342–344.

79. Kirby RS, Bryan J, Eardley I, et al. Finasteride in the treatment of benign prostatic hyperplasia. A urodynamic evaluation. *Br J Urol.* 1992;70:65–72.

80. Wilde MI, Goa KL. Finasteride: an update of its use in the management of symptomatic benign prostatic hyperplasia. *Drugs.* 1999;57:557–581.

81. Boyle P, Gould AL, Roehrborn CG. Prostate volume predicts outcome of treatment of benign prostatic hyperplasia with finasteride: meta-analysis of randomized clinical trials. *Urology.* 1996;48:398–405.

82. Lepor H, Williford WO, Barry MJ, et al. The efficacy of terazosin, finasteride, or both in benign prostatic hyperplasia. Veteran's Afairs cooperative studies benign prostatic hyperplasia study group. *N Engl J Med.* 1996;335:533–539.

83. McConnell JD, Bruskewitz R, Walsh P, et al. The effect of finasteride on the risk of acute urinary retention and the need for surgical treatment among men with benign

NHS Centre for Reviews and Dissemination; 1995:16. [See also Wilde *www.york.ac.uk/inst/crd/.*]

prostatic hyperplasia. Finasteride Long-Term Efficacy and Safety Study Group. *N Engl J Med.* 1998;338:557–563.

84. Rittmaster RS. Finasteride. *N Engl J Med.* 1994;330:120–125.

85. Gormley GJ, Ng J, Cook T, Stoner E, Guess H, Walsh P. Effect of finasteride on prostate-specific antigen density. *Urology.* 1994;43:53–59.

86. Brawer MK, Lin DW, Williford WO, Jones K, Lepor H. Effect of finasteride and/or terazosin on serum PSA: results of VA Cooperative Study #359. *Prostate.* 1999;39: 234–239.

87. Wilt T, Ishani A, Stark G, MacDonald R, Mulrow C, Lau J. Serenoa repens for benign prostatic hyperplasia (Cochrane Review). In: *The Cochrane Library, Issue 3.* Oxford: Update Software; 2000.

88. Boyle P, Robertson C, Lowe F, Roehrborn C. Meta-analysis of clinical trials of permixon in the treatment of symptomatic benign prostatic hyperplasia. *Urology.* 2000; 55:533–539.

89. Wilt TJ, MacDonald R, Ishani A. Beta-sitosterols for the treatment of benign prostatic hyperplasia: a systematic review. *BJU Int.* 1999;83:976–983. [See also: Wilt T, Ishani A, MacDonald R, Stark G, Mulrow C, Lau J. Beta-sitosterols for benign prostatic hyperplasia (Cochrane Review). In: *The Cochrane Library, Issue 3.* Oxford: Update Software; 2000.]

90. MacDonald R, Ishani A, Rutks I, Wilt TJ. A systematic review of Cernilton for the treatment of benign prostatic hyperplasia. *BJU Int.* 2000;85:836–841. [See also: Wilt T, Ishani A, MacDonald R, Ishani A, Rutks I, Stark G. Cernilton for benign prostatic hyperplasia (Cochrane Review). In: *The Cochrane Library, Issue 3.* Oxford: Update Software; 2000.]

91. McConnell JD. Medical management of benign prostatic hyperplasia with androgen suppression. *Prostate Suppl.* 1990;3:49–59.

92. Eri LM, Tveter KJ. A prospective, placebo-controlled study of the luteinizing hormone-releasing hormone agonist leuprolide as treatment for patients with benign prostatic hyperplasia. *J Urol.* 1993;150:359–364.

93. O'Leary MP, Gee WF, Holtgrewe HL, et al. 1999 American Urological Association Gallup survey: changes in physician practice patterns, treatment of incontinence and bladder cancer, and impact of managed care. *J Urol.* 2000;163:1311–1316.

94. Holtgrewe HL, Mebust WK, Dowd JB, et al. Transurethral prostatectomy: practice aspects of the dominant operation in American urology. *J Urol.* 1989;141:248–253.

95. Jenkins BJ, Sharma P, Badenoch DF, Fowler CG, Blandy JP. Ethics, logistics and a trial of transurethral versus open prostatectomy. *Br J Urol.* 1992;69:372–374.

96. Wyatt MG, Stower MJ, Smith PJB, et al. Prostatectomy in the over 80-year-old. *Br J Urol.* 1989;64:417–419.

97. Rodrigues P, Lucon AM, Freire GC, Arap S. Urodynamic pressure flow studies can predict the clinical outcome after transurethral prostatic resection. *J Urol.* 2001;164:499–502.

98. Nielsen KT, Christensen MM, Madsen PO, Bruskewitz RC. Symptom analysis and uroflowmetry 7 years after transurethral resection of the prostate. *J Urol.* 1989;142: 1251–1253.

99. Mushinski M. Prostate surgeries: average charges throughout the United States, 1997. *Stat Bull Metrop Insur Co.* 1999;80:10–18.

100. Neal DE. Prostatectomy: an open or closed case. *Br J Urol.* 1990;66:449–454.

101. Libman E, Fichten CS. Prostatectomy and sexual function. *Urology.* 1987;29:467–478.

102. Tscholl R, Largo M, Poppinghaus E, Recker F, Subotic B. Incidence of erectile impotence secondary to transurethral resection of benign prostatic hyperplasia, assessed by preoperative and postoperative Snap-Gauge tests. *J Urol.* 1995;153:1491–1493.

103. Mebust WK, Holtgrewe HL, Cockett ATK, et al. Transurethral prostatectomy: immediate and postoperative complications. A cooperative study of 13 participating institutions evaluating 3,885 patients. *J Urol.* 1989;141: 243–247.

104. Krogh J, Jensen JS, Iversen H-G, Andersen JT. Age as a prognostic variable in patients undergoing transurethral prostatectomy. *Scand J Urol Nephrol.* 1993;27: 225–229.

105. Klimberg IW, Locke DR, Leonard E, Madore R, Klimberg SR. Outpatient transurethral resection of the prostate at a urological ambulatory surgery center. *J Urol.* 1994;151: 1547–1549.

106. Birch BR, Gelister JS, Parker CJ, Chave H, Miller RA. Transurethral resection of prostate under sedation and local anesthesia (sedoanalgesia). *Urology.* 1991;38:113–118.

107. Roos NP, Wennberg JE, Malenka DJ, et al. Mortality and reoperation after open and transurethral resection of the prostate for benign prostatic hyperplasia. *N Engl J Med.* 1989;320:1120–1124.

108. Roos NP, Ramsey EW. A population-based study of prostatectomy: outcomes associated with differing surgical approaches. *J Urol.* 1987;137:1184–1188.

109. Concato J, Horwitz RI, Feinstein AR, Elmore JG, Schiff SF. Problems of comorbidity in mortality after prostatectomy. *JAMA.* 1992;267:1077–1082.

110. Lu-Yao G, Barry MJ, Chang C-H, Wasson JH, Wennberg JE. Transurethral resection of the prostate among Medicare beneficiaries in the United States: time trends and outcomes. *Urology.* 1994;44:692–699.

111. Orandi A. Transurethral incision of the prostate (TUIP): 646 cases in 15 years—a chronological appraisal. *Br J Urol.* 1985;57:703–707.

112. Riehman M, Bruskewitz R. Transurethral incision of the prostate and bladder neck. *J Androl.* 1991;12:415–422.

113. Donovan JL, Peters TJ, Neal DE, et al. A randomized trial comparing transurethral resection of the prostate, laser therapy and conservative management for lower urinary tract symptoms associated with benign prostatic enlargement: the ClasP study. *J Urol.* 2000;164:65–70.

114. Carter A, Sells H, Speakman M, Ewings P, MacDonagh R, O'Boyle P. A prospective randomized controlled trial of hybrid laser treatment or transurethral section of the prostate, with a 1-year follow-up. *BJU Int.* 1999;83:254–259.

115. Carter A, Sells H, Speakman M, Ewings P, O'Boyle P, MacDonagh R. Quality of life changes following KTP/

Nd:YAG laser treatment of the prostate and TURP. *Eur Urol.* 1999;36:92–98.

116. Jones JW, Carter A, Ewings P, O'Boyle PJ. An MRSA outbreak in a urology ward and its association with Nd:YAG coagulation laser treatment of the prostate. *J Hosp Infect.* 1999;41:39–44.

117. Diana M, Schettini M, Gallucci M. Treatment of benign prostatic hyperplasia with transurethral electrovaporization of the prostate (TUVP) using Vaportrode VE-B. Two years follow-up. *Minerva Urol Nephrol.* 1999;51:191–195.

118. Ogden CW, Reddy P, Johnson H, Ramsay JW, Carter SS. Sham versus transurethral microwave thermotherapy in patients with symptoms of benign prostatic bladder outflow obstruction. *Lancet.* 1993;341:14–17.

119. Bdesha AS, Bunce CJ, Kelleher JP, Snell ME, Vukusic J, Witherow RO. Transurethral microwave treatment for benign prostatic hypertrophy: a randomised controlled clinical trail. *Br Med J.* 1993;306:1293–1296.

120. Brehmer M, Wiskell H, Kinn A. Sham treatment compared with 30 or 60 min of thermotherapy for benign prostatic hyperplasia: a randomized study. *BJU Int.* 1999; 84:292–296.

121. Daehlin L, Frugard J. Three-year follow-up after transurethral microwave thermotherapy for benign prostatic hyperplasia using the PRIMUS U+R device. *Scand J Urol Nephrol.* 1999;33:217–221.

122. Djavan B, Roehrborn CG, Shariat S, Ghawidel K, Marberger M. Prospective randomized comparison of high energy transurethral microwave thermotherapy versus alpha-blocker treatment of patients with benign prostatic hyperplasia. *J Urol.* 1999;161:139–143.

123. Bruskewitz R, Issa M, Roehrborn C, et al. A prospective, randomized 1-year clinical trial comparing transurethral needle ablation to transurethral resection of the prostate for the treatment of symptomatic benign prostatic hyperplasia. *J Urol* 1998;159:1588–1594.

52
Nephrology/Fluid and Electrolyte Disorders

Sharon Anderson

The biologic price of aging includes progressive structural and functional deterioration of the kidney, and the changes in renal function during normal aging are among the most dramatic of any organ system. This chapter considers the functional and structural changes that occur with normal aging; more detailed reviews may be found in several recent publications.[1-6]

Age-Related Changes in Renal Function and Structure

The glomerular filtration rate (GFR) is low at birth, approaches adult levels by the end of the second year of life, and is maintained at approximately 140 mL/min/ 1.73 m² until the fourth decade. Thereafter, GFR declines by about 8 mL/min/1.73 m² per decade.[7,8] Acceleration of age-related loss of renal function has been noted in the setting of systemic hypertension,[9,10] lead exposure,[11] smoking,[12-14] and possibly male gender.[15] Although clinically important in many elderly patients, it should be noted that there is wide variability among individuals in the age-related fall in GFR.[9,16] The age-related reduction in creatinine clearance is accompanied by a reduction in the daily urinary creatinine excretion, due to reduced muscle mass.[8] Accordingly, the relationship between serum creatinine (S_{Cr}) and creatinine clearance changes. The net effect is near-constancy of S_{Cr} while true GFR (and creatinine clearance) decline, and consequently, substantial reductions of GFR despite a relatively normal S_{Cr} level. The creatinine clearance in adult males may be estimated from the S_{Cr} with the following formula:

$$\text{Creatinine clearance} = (140 - \text{age})(\text{weight in kg})/(72 \times S_{Cr})$$

and, in females, by multiplying this value by 0.85.[17]

Similar changes in renal blood flow (RBF) occur, so that RBF is well maintained at about 600 mL/min until approximately the fourth decade, and then declines by about 10% per decade.[18,19] The reduction in RBF is not entirely due to loss of renal mass, as xenon-washout studies demonstrate a progressive reduction in blood flow per unit kidney mass with advancing age.[19] The decrease in RBF is most profound in the renal cortex; redistribution of flow from cortex to medulla may explain the slight increase in filtration fraction seen in the elderly.[18,19]

Studies in laboratory rats, whose age-related renal changes resemble an accelerated version of those in humans, suggest that another functional abnormality in aging is an increase in the glomerular basement membrane (GBM) permeability, leading to an increase in urinary excretion of protein, including both albumin and higher molecular weight proteins.[20] Studies in aging humans demonstrate decreased sulfation of the GBM glycosaminoglycans,[21] which would be expected to render the GBM more permeable to macromolecules. Age-related changes in proteinuria in humans have not been extensively studied, but the incidence of microalbuminuria and proteinuria in the elderly may be slightly elevated.[22-24]

Renal mass increases from about 50 g at birth to more than 400 g during the fourth decade, after which it declines to less than 300 g by the ninth decade. The reduced kidney weight correlates well with the reduction in body surface area.[25-27] Loss of renal mass is primarily cortical, with relative sparing of the medulla.[27,28] Glomerular number decreases, but studies differ on the size of the remaining glomeruli.[26,29,30] Glomerular shape changes as well,[29] with the spherical glomerulus in the fetal kidney developing lobular indentations as it matures. With aging, lobulation tends to diminish, and the length of the glomerular tuft perimeter decreases relative to total area. The GBM undergoes progressive folding and then thickening.[31,32] This stage is accompanied by glomerular simplification, with the formation of free anastomoses between a reduced number of glomerular capillary loops. Frequently, dilatation of the afferent arteriole near the hilum is seen at this stage. Eventually, the folded and thickened GBM condenses into hyaline material with glomerular tuft collapse. Degeneration of cortical glomeruli results in atrophy of both afferent and efferent arterioles, with global sclerosis. In the juxtamedullary glomeruli, glomerular tuft sclerosis is accompanied by the formation of direct channels between the afferent and efferent arterioles, resulting in aglomerular arterioles.[32,33] These aglomerular arterioles, which presumably contribute to maintenance of medullary blood flow, are rarely seen in kidneys from healthy young persons; their frequency increases both in aging kidneys and in the presence of intrinsic renal disease.[33]

The incidence of glomerular sclerosis increases with advancing age. Sclerotic glomeruli comprise fewer than 5% of the total under the age of 40; thereafter, the incidence increases so that sclerosis involves as much as 30% of the glomerular population by the eighth decade.[33–35] Thus, both diminished glomerular lobulation and sclerosis of glomeruli tend to reduce the surface area available for filtration, and therefore contribute to the observed age-related decline in GFP.[29] In addition, age-related changes in cardiovascular hemodynamics, such as reduced cardiac output[36] and systemic hypertension,[9,10] are likely to play a role in the reduced perfusion and filtration of aging.

Age-Related Alterations in Fluid and Electrolyte Homeostasis

Advancing age is not characterized by any specific changes in serum electrolyte or acid–base parameters in healthy subjects. A comprehensive study of serum electrolytes, enzymes, and other parameters in 327 healthy individuals ranging in age from 60 to over 100 years found that healthy aging subjects exhibit no change in serum sodium, potassium, chloride, or CO_2 levels; pH decreases only slightly. Values for blood urea nitrogen (BUN) increase significantly, while serum creatinine does not change.[23] However, the situation changes markedly when hospitalized or ill elderly subjects are considered. Such patients frequently exhibit elevated values for BUN and creatinine (which correlate with the degree of glomerular sclerosis),[37] while alterations in sodium and potassium levels are more prominent, as discussed next. These observations indicate ability of the aging kidney to maintain normal electrolyte homeostasis under steady-state conditions. However, the aging kidney demonstrates impaired ability to respond to perturbations of fluid and electrolyte balance, and therefore a number of these complications are frequently encountered in the presence of intercurrent illness. In concert with the loss of functioning glomeruli, evidence of tubular dysfunction is

found as well, with deterioration of several proximal tubular functions including maximum excretion of para-aminohippurate[38] and diodrast[7] and maximal absorption of glucose.[39] These changes are proportional to changes in GFR, suggesting a constancy of the relationship between GFR and tubular function.[2] However, studies in experimental animals also indicate fewer energy-producing mitochondria,[40] lower enzyme concentrations,[40,41] lower concentrations of total or sodium–potassium-activated adenosine triphosphatase (ATPase),[42] decreased sodium extrusion and oxygen consumption,[43] and decreased brush border sodium–hydrogen exchange and sodium-dependent phosphate transport[44] in old versus younger kidneys. The most prominent abnormalities are found in renal handling of sodium and water, which probably relate to changes in innate tubular transport capacity, as well as to increasingly well-recognized alterations in renal responsiveness to hormonal stimuli.

Disorders of Sodium Balance

In the absence of acquired renal disease, the aging kidney is able to appropriately adjust sodium handling in the face of extracellular sodium deficiency or excess; however, the response time is impaired, and management of these disorders is accordingly complicated.[45–48] The renal response to dietary sodium deprivation in the elderly is blunted. When challenged with an acute reduction in sodium intake (from 100 mEq/day to 10 mEq/day), elderly subjects are able to conserve sodium and achieve sodium balance, but at a slower rate than in younger subjects. An acute study of dietary sodium restriction found that the half-time for reduction in urinary sodium after salt restriction was 17.6 h in young persons but was prolonged to 30.9 h in older subjects.[45] In a more chronic state of sodium deprivation, administration of a 50 mEq/day sodium diet led to urinary sodium conservation and achievement of sodium balance after 5 days in younger subjects, whereas elderly patients did not return to sodium balance after 9 days despite a weight loss of 1.4 kg.[46] Studies in the segmental handling of sodium in elderly patients suggest that sodium handling is fairly normal in the proximal tubule, but that the capacity to reabsorb sodium in the ascending limb of the loop of Henle is markedly impaired.[47] The reduced loop capacity to reabsorb sodium has two important consequences: the amount of sodium delivered to the more distal segments increases, and the capacity to concentrate the medullary interstitium is reduced, therefore also contributing to inability to concentrate the urine.

Age-related abnormalities in several hormonal systems controlling sodium excretion are likely to play a role in this impaired ability to conserve sodium (Table 52.1). Plasma renin levels and blood and urinary aldosterone levels are significantly reduced in the elderly population,

TABLE 52.1. Age-related changes in sodium-modulating factors.

Reduced functioning nephron number
Decreased renin-angiotensin-aldosterone formation and effect
Decreased insulin secretion
Increased atrial natriuretic peptide levels with relatively reduced
    effect
Increased plasma norepinephrine levels
Decreased renal dopamine
Decreased kallikrein-kinin activity

and responses to appropriate stimuli such as sodium restriction are blunted.[48,49] In addition, the tubular response to administration of aldosterone is reduced.[48] The mechanisms for suppression of the renin-angiotensin system are not yet well defined. Hall and coworkers have postulated that these age-related changes result from the loss of nephrons; compensatory hyperfiltration in the remaining nephrons leads to increased sodium chloride delivery to the macula densa, with suppression of renin synthesis and release, and therefore reduced formation of angiotensin II and aldosterone.[50] Studies in aging animals indicate that both renal renin synthesis and renin release in response to volume stimuli are reduced, and that both contribute to the observed fall in plasma renin concentration with aging.[51]

Other mechanisms, although not well studied, could play a role. Theoretically, the observed decrease in insulin secretion with aging[52] could contribute, as insulin is antinatriuretic. In addition, the natriuretic response to head-out water immersion (a physiologic technique used to study redistribution of extracellular fluid) is enhanced in elderly subjects, possibly relating to the greater mean arterial pressure increments.[53] Whatever the mechanisms, the impaired response to sodium deprivation (or relative "salt-wasting") renders the elderly patient more susceptible to developing a cumulative sodium deficit and its attendant systemic complications.

Similarly, the renal response to a sodium load is sluggish in elderly patients.[53,54] In a careful study of renal responses to an acute isotonic sodium load, the amount of sodium excreted acutely did not differ in older individuals. However, these individuals had higher baseline blood pressures, leading to the suggestion that the higher blood pressures in old versus young subjects serves to counteract this potential intrarenal defect.[55] Natriuresis is impaired by both the reduced GFR, leading to a reduced delivery of sodium to the nephron, and by abnormalities in tubular handling of sodium. Studies in aging animals indicate both a greater fall in renal perfusion[56,57] and filtration[57] with angiotensin II administration, as well as impaired natriuresis and augmented kaliuresis with this maneuver.[57] Similarly, animal studies indicate impaired natriuretic responses to increased perfusion pressure, mediated in part by the renal nerves.[58]

Other vasoactive mediators appear to be involved, as well. Plasma levels of norepinephrine increase with age,[59,60] and therefore changes in sympathetic tone could contribute to a tendency to conserve sodium. Both clinical[61–63] and experimental[64] studies indicate that plasma levels of atrial natriuretic peptide (ANP) increase with age. Some investigators have found no differences in natriuretic responses to ANP infusion between young and elderly normal subjects,[65] but changes in fractional excretion of sodium were not measured, and the data indicate the possibility of a lesser augmentation of the fractional excretion of sodium in the older subjects. Most studies have noted similar natriuretic responses to ANP infusion in younger and older subjects,[65–67] but the equivalent responses occur only with much higher increments in plasma ANP levels in older subjects,[66] or the effects in older subjects are more transient than in younger subjects.[67] Other studies have found diminished responses in the elderly.[68] Although indirect, these data are consistent with an altered ANP–sodium dose responsiveness in the older kidney. It has been postulated that several mechanisms underlie the age-related increase in plasma ANP levels: that elevated ANP is secondary to enhanced sensitivity of the atrial afferent system for ANP release, and also that end-organ resistance to ANP actions induces feedback stimulation of ANP release in the elderly.

Less well studied is another vasodilator, kallikrein; it has been reported that there is a negative correlation between age and urinary kallikrein excretion,[69] and that serum kininogen levels decrease with advancing age.[70] Moreover, urinary dopamine excretion declines with advancing age in humans.[71,72] Studies in aging rats have indicated that these changes may be due to a reduction in DA_1 receptor number and subsequent G-protein activation,[73] and that the diminished natriuretic response to dopamine in aging rats is due to an impaired D_1-like receptor signaling pathway.[74] However, the natriuretic response to infusion of dopamine may be preserved in the elderly.[75] Together, altered levels of, or responsiveness to, various natriuretic stimuli most likely contribute to impaired sodium excretion in the elderly (see Table 52.1). Clinical aspects and therapy are discussed next.

Disorders of Water Balance

Renal concentrating and diluting abilities are also impaired in the aging kidney.[76,77] In response to water deprivation, studies in healthy elderly patients indicate that the maximal decrease in urine volume and increase in urine osmolality are both significantly diminished as compared to responses in younger subjects and are not completely explained by the reduced GFR in the elderly.[78]

The mechanisms that underlie the impaired concentrating capacity have been extensively explored. The reduced number of functioning nephrons may contribute to an obligatory solute diuresis in the remaining intact nephrons, as occurs with chronic renal failure. In addition, the effect of age on the renal response to exogenous antidiuretic hormone (ADH) has been studied. Although age-related differences in response to submaximal ADH infusions were not found, such a defect in concentrating ability was found when higher doses of ADH were infused.[79] One explanation for these differences may relate to the relative sparing of medullary blood flow in the aging kidney; this might contribute to a "washout" of the medullary osmotic gradient necessary for urine concentration by the countercurrent multiplier system.

In addition to altered responsiveness to exogenous ADH, the release of endogenous ADH in response to appropriate stimuli is abnormal in elderly subjects. In some cases, there is a diminution in thirst perception to water deprivation[80–83] or saline infusion,[84] so that stimuli such as volume depletion or hyperosmolality are less effective. Some studies have challenged this finding, in adults just over the age of 70.[85] Morphologic studies indicate no evidence of age-related degenerative changes in the supraoptic and paraventricular nuclei, the sites of ADH production.[86] The increase in plasma ADH levels after infusion of hypertonic saline (an osmolar stimulus) is greater in elderly than in younger subjects, indicating enhanced osmoreceptor sensitivity in the elderly.[87] In contrast to the response to an osmolar stimulus, however, the ADH response to volume–pressure stimuli (assumption of upright posture after overnight dehydration) is markedly impaired in some elderly subjects,[88] as is the fall in plasma ADH after drinking water.[82] A portion of the afferent limb of the reflex arc involved in this response is the vasomotor center. In elderly subjects, plasma norepinephrine levels were comparable in those who did and who did not respond appropriately to the pressure–volume stimulus, suggesting that the defect in the afferent limb must exist between the vasomotor center and the hypothalamic area controlling ADH release. This reflex arc is inhibitory to ADH secretion, and a defect in this area would result in a lesser dampening of osmotically stimulated ADH release. These studies suggest that baroreflex input at the hypothalamic level during aging modulates osmotically mediated ADH release, and thus may alter water balance.

Plasma ADH levels under basal conditions do not change with advancing age,[60,87,89] nor are there any differences in ADH pharmacokinetics following ADH administration after adaptation to high or low sodium diets between young and elderly subjects.[90] However, these studies found secondary increases in ADH that were enhanced in magnitude during low sodium intake and absent in elderly subjects. Taken together, these studies indicate that ADH is present in the elderly, and that provocative stimuli can both accentuate its release

and reduce its suppressibility; the mechanisms underlying these observations, as well as the consequences of attenuation of secondary ADH release, remain incompletely defined.

Similarly, the aging kidney demonstrates a modest inability to dilute urine appropriately, as determined by the maximal excretion of free water after water loading.[91,92] This change is most likely due to the reduced GFR and renal perfusion, as well as to functional impairment in the diluting segment of the nephron.[48,91] Recent studies in aging animals indicate that age-related polyuria is associated with downregulation of the aquaporin-2 and -3 receptors in the medullary collecting duct.[93]

Hyponatremia

Serum sodium levels are generally within the normal range in healthy elderly individuals,[23] but the defective sodium and water homeostatic mechanisms render this population markedly susceptible to perturbations. Hyponatremia is the most common electrolyte disorder in the elderly, occurring in as many as one-quarter of all hospitalized or institutionalized elderly patients.[46,94,95] In a survey of hospitalized elderly patients, 3.6% had serum sodium values below 130 mmol/L, even in the absence of drugs known to affect serum sodium.[96] Numerous mechanisms contribute to the susceptibility to hyponatremia and may generally be deduced after clinical evaluation. The most common underlying mechanisms of geriatric hyponatremia are (1) decreased ability to excrete water; (2) water intoxication in the setting of diuretic therapy; and (3) oversecretion of ADH.

As in patients of any age, evaluation of the hyponatremic patient begins with confirmation of true hyponatremia, a hypoosmolar state.[77,97] Pseudohyponatremia may be found in the setting of marked hyperglycemia, hyperlipidemia, and hyperproteinemia. Measurement of plasma osmolality confirms this diagnosis, as plasma osmolality is normal in pseudohyponatremia but reduced in true hyponatremic states. Most clinical laboratories now use specific sodium electrodes, eliminating this form of false positive. Further evaluation requires estimation of extracellular fluid volume status, by physical examination and measurement of urinary sodium concentration. Hyponatremia may be associated with extracellular volume depletion (due to renal or extrarenal losses); with extracellular volume excess (due to cardiac failure, nephrotic syndrome, cirrhosis, or renal failure); or with normal to slightly increased extracellular volume excess in the absence of edema (endocrine disorders, drugs, and excess ADH secretion).

Elderly patients may suffer from any of these disorders, and in fact carry a disproportionate burden of illness associated with extracellular fluid volume deficit and excess.[97] Extracellular volume depletion is quite common, particularly after administration of diuretics; in one series of 77 elderly patients, diuretic therapy accounted for two-thirds of all cases of hyponatremia.[98] In a survey of 631 hospitalized elderly patients, 11.8% of subjects on thiazides were hyponatremic, with the percentage being higher in elderly women.[96] Several age-related abnormalities are likely to contribute to this increased susceptibility: volume depletion, potassium depletion, and inhibition of urinary dilution. As compared to younger subjects, elderly patients challenged with a thiazide diuretic exhibit greater impairment of minimum urine osmolality and clearance of free water, possibly associated with lower prostaglandin production.[92] Diuretic-induced hyponatremia occurs almost exclusively with thiazide diuretics, which interfere with urinary diluting but not concentrating ability and therefore may engender greater defects in free water excretion, particularly in the presence of ADH. Clinically significant hyponatremia tends to occur as early as the first few days of diuretic administration, and the frequency of life-threatening hyponatremia is increased in the elderly population.[99–101] It should also be noted that thiazide diuretics and nonsteroidal anti-inflammatory drugs may have an additive effect in causing hyponatremia in the elderly.[92] Therapy consists of discontinuation of the drug(s) and restriction of water intake. In the setting of severe central nervous system symptomatology, administration of intravenous hypertonic saline is warranted.

Hypervolemic hyponatremia is also common in the elderly, with congestive heart failure being the most common etiology of this disorder. The reduction in renal perfusion, and thus GFR, that accompanies congestive heart failure at any age may be more destructive in the elderly, in whom values for GFR are only half those of younger persons when cardiac function is optimal. Congestive heart failure may be accompanied by increased plasma ADH levels, particularly in elderly patients.[102] Therapy consists of water restriction, and treatment of congestive heart failure with loop diuretics (rather than thiazides) and other usual modalities.

Relatively isovolemic hyponatremia is also prominent in the elderly, who may exhibit elevations in plasma ADH levels in the absence of recognizable stimuli for ADH secretion.[103] The elderly seem to be particularly susceptible to hyponatremia in the setting of the syndrome of inappropriate ADH resulting from pulmonary disease, central nervous system disorders, paraneoplastic syndromes, pain, narcotics, and drugs that cause the syndrome. The presence of excessive levels of ADH, together with impaired ability to excrete free water, render the elderly particularly susceptible to hyponatremia in numerous clinical settings, and particularly in the postoperative setting in the presence of narcotic administration and large amounts of intravenous hypo-

tonic fluids. In one large series of elderly patients, excessive administration of hypotonic intravenous fluids was responsible for 14% of the cases of hyponatremia.[98] More recently, the incidence of hyponatremia due to antidepressant medication has been increasingly realized,[104,105] as has the higher incidence of idiopathic hyponatremia in the elderly.[106,107]

Hypernatremia

Hypernatremia is also particularly prominent in the elderly.[108] The major defense against hypernatremia is thirst, and so the populations at highest risk for hypernatremia are those with impaired access to water. A group at particularly high risk are institutionalized older patients with cognitive impairment, who manifest failure to recognize thirst or physical inability to obtain fluids. Additional evidence, although not entirely unequivocal, suggests that hypodipsia, or failure to recognize thirst despite substantial elevations in serum osmolality, may be more common in elderly patients.[81,84,109] Cerebrovascular disease may also inhibit thirst, as well limiting physical ability to gain access to fluids. These problems, together with the inability of the aging kidney to maximally conserve water, render elderly patients at higher risk for the development of hypernatremia.

Hypernatremia may result from loss of sodium and water with predominant water loss and low total body sodium (renal and extrarenal losses); water losses with normal total body sodium (from nephrogenic and central diabetes insipidus, or inadequate water intake in the presence of normal water losses); and sodium addition with increased total body sodium (endocrine disorders, intravenous or oral sodium administration). Clinical evaluation and measurement of urinary sodium will usually disclose the cause. Therapy consists of administration of hypotonic saline in the setting of low total body sodium; water in the setting of normal total body sodium; and diuretics and water replacement in the setting of high total body sodium.

Alterations in Potassium Balance

Plasma potassium concentrations in the elderly remain within the normal range in the absence of abnormal stresses.[23] However, significant abnormalities in cellular and total body potassium occur with advancing age. Erythrocyte potassium concentration (a reflection of general intracellular potassium content) is decreased, and both total body potassium and total exchangeable body potassium are reduced by about 20% as compared to younger subjects.[46,110–112] Several mechanisms for this reduction in total body potassium concentration have been proposed, including decreased muscle mass, alterations of cell membrane characteristics, nutritional deficiencies, and inability of the kidney to conserve potassium.[46] Renal potassium excretion has been noted to be reduced in elderly subjects, but when corrected for the reduction in GFR, the fractional excretion of potassium may be higher than in younger subjects.[46]

Hypokalemia

Hypokalemia is the most prominent potassium abnormality in the elderly population, and in one series was found in 11% of elderly patients visiting an emergency room, regardless of the reason for the visit.[111] The most prominent etiology of hypokalemia in the elderly population is probably diuretic therapy; aging patients appear to be more susceptible to the hypokalemic effects of these drugs.[98]

Hyperkalemia

Hyperkalemia is relatively uncommon in elderly patients in the absence of renal disease or administration of potassium-sparing diuretics, despite evidence in aging experimental animals of impaired ability to excrete a potassium load.[113] The reduction in total body potassium stores may serve to offset the reduced GFR, thus protecting against significant hyperkalemia. However, the reduced activity of the renin-angiotensin-aldosterone system in the elderly, and the predisposition to the syndrome of hyporeninemic hypoaldosteronism (type IV renal tubular acidosis) may serve to limit potassium excretion, thus enhancing the risk of hyperkalemia in the presence of excessive potassium loads or drugs that predispose to hyperkalemia.[114,115] Elderly patients are less able to mount a sufficient aldosterone defense when faced with hyperkalemia.[116] In fact, hyperkalemia is more prominent in elderly subjects than in younger individuals when administered potassium supplements and other drugs known to increase serum potassium levels, including nonsteroidal anti-inflammatory drugs and trimethoprim-sulfamethoxasole.[117-119] Furthermore, the increasing use of angiotensin-converting enzyme inhibitors and spironolactone for treatment of congestive heart failure is likely to induce further hyperkalemia in elderly patients, in the setting of age-related reductions in renal function.

Disorders of Acid–Base Balance

Abnormalities in both pulmonary and renal acid–base mechanisms may contribute to disorders in elderly patients. Despite evidence for substantial deterioration in lung and kidney function with advancing age, acid–base balance is remarkably well maintained in the elderly, who are generally able to maintain normal values for serum pH, pCO_2, and bicarbonate concentrations.[23,119-122] There

is a modest, significant decrease in bicarbonate levels (within the normal range) in the healthy elderly.[123] Although these systems adequately dispose of the normal daily acid load, studies of ammonium loading in elderly patients indicate a reduced ability to excrete an acute exogenous acid load. However, when corrected for the reduced values for GFR, the response of elderly subjects is similar to that in younger subjects, indicating that nephron loss rather than tubular dysfunction probably accounts for this difference.[122,124] More chronic acid loading, however, may be associated with delayed restoration of normal serum pH and bicarbonate concentrations,[125] and the response to alkali loading may also be delayed in elderly subjects.[126] It seems possible that the numerous etiologies of acidosis and alkalosis (particularly those resulting from drugs) might result in more frequent, profound, and long-lasting acid–base disorders in this population.[120,121] Although relatively few data are available addressing the clinical outcomes of various acid–base disorders in the elderly population, a recent study found that administration of potassium bicarbonate to postmenopausal women resulted in positive calcium and phosphate balance, decreased bone resorption, and increased bone formation.[127]

Calcium/Phosphorus/Magnesium Disorders in Aging

Serum levels of total calcium, ionized calcium, phosphorus, magnesium, and parathyroid hormone (PTH) generally remain within the normal range in the elderly,[23] although some studies have found significant decreases in serum calcium, phosphorus, and vitamin D, and increases in PTH (with values remaining in the normal range), with advancing age.[128] In aging women, there is a sequence of an increase in serum calcium, followed by an increase in calcitriol and PTH.[129] However, calcium metabolism is substantially impaired with aging, due to age-related decreases in intestinal calcium absorption,[130,131] decreased renal 1α-hydroxylase activity and decreased $1,25(OH)_2D3$ activity,[132-136] and decreased intestinal adaptation to dietary calcium restriction.[137] A decrease in vitamin D levels is frequently seen in elderly patients who are in poor health;[138,139] contributing factors may include lack of exposure to sunlight, dietary deficiency, and impaired conversion to $1,25(OH)_2D3$. Other factors, including age-related changes in growth hormone and insulin-like growth factor 1,[140] have also been suggested to influence vitamin D levels in the elderly.[128] However, renal tubular absorption of calcium does not seem to be affected in aging,[129,137] perhaps contributing to the observed constancy of serum calcium levels.

Phosphorus metabolism also changes with aging. The elderly exhibit decreased renal tubular reabsorption of phosphate,[141] and in experimental animals, decreased intestinal phosphate absorption,[130] and impaired renal tubular adaptation to dietary phosphate restriction.[130,142,143] However, as with calcium, these defects do not appear to substantially influence serum levels.

Serum magnesium levels do not change with advancing age.[23] Erythrocyte magnesium content has been shown to increase in elderly women, possibly due to decreased estrogen effect,[144] but no clinical consequences have been identified.

Renal Disease in the Elderly

By itself, age-related loss of functioning nephrons poses little threat to well-being, because even 50% of the normal GFR is ample for sustaining renal excretory function. However, the gradual loss of renal function that accompanies normal aging may be greatly accelerated when surgical loss of renal mass or acquired intrinsic renal disease is superimposed on this process.

The incidence of primary renal disease in the elderly is not significantly different from that in young adults,[1,145–147] although the preponderance of specific forms of glomerular injury varies in different age groups. Several large series of biopsies in elderly patients have indicated the relative incidence of the major forms of glomerular injury. Data from a survey of 12 published series from 1980 through 1993, representing patients with nephrotic syndrome, were recently tabulated by Cameron,[148] and are summarized in Table 52.2. For comparison, results of a large series of patients undergoing biopsy for various reasons, stratified by age, are depicted in Table 52.3.[149] Although differences in reporting classification make exact comparisons difficult, several general trends are apparent from the published studies. In each of these series, approximately two-thirds of the patients were found to have primary glomerular disease, with the remainder exhibiting glomerular disease secondary to systemic disease, or primary tubulointerstitial diseases. Of the primary glomerular diseases, membranous glomerulonephritis was the most frequent etiology,

TABLE 52.2. Etiology of nephrotic syndrome in the elderly.

	n	Percent
Membranous GN	416	37.3
Minimal change disease	140	12.6
Amyloidosis	151	11.8
Other[a]	427	38.3
Total	1114	100.0

[a]Focal sclerosis, membranoproliferative glomerulonephritis (GN), diabetes.
Source: Data are abstracted from 12 published series. Modified from Cameron.[148]

TABLE 52.3. Pathologic diagnoses in patients undergoing biopsies.

	Patient age (years)	
	≥60 (n = 244)	≤60 (n = 875)
Diagnosis		
Nephrosclerosis	13.9	10.7
Membranous GN	11.9	7.5
Crescentic GN	11.1	4.1
Focal glomerular sclerosis	7.8	5.6
Amyloidosis	7.8	2.2
Diabetic nephropathy	7.8	8.1
Chronic GN	4.5	6.4
Acute GN	4.5	3.8
Focal GN	4.1	6.7
Minimal change disease	3.7	8.3
Membranoproliferative GN	2.9	6.3
Vasculitis	2.5	2.1
Systemic lupus erythematosus	2.0	6.6

GN, glomerulonephritis.
Prevalence values are given as percentages.
Source: Adapted from Glickman et al., with permission.[149]

followed in varying degrees by proliferative or rapidly progressive glomerulonephritis, and focal glomerular sclerosis. Of note, most of these series found a substantial proportion of minimal change disease. Although most frequently considered to be a disease of children, in whom it comprises the vast majority of glomerular disorders, this glomerular disease may be found in any age group, including the elderly. Other primary glomerular diseases were found relatively infrequently. Thus, the available data indicated that membranous glomerulonephritis is the most common etiology of nephrotic syndrome in the elderly, whereas rapidly progressive glomerulonephritis is the most common cause of an acute nephritic syndrome in the elderly population.

Although the incidence of primary glomerular diseases is not particularly enhanced in elderly patients, the incidence of renal disease secondary to systemic illness such as atherosclerosis, hypertension, cardiac failure, diabetes, and malignancy clearly increases with advancing age.[145] The etiologies of glomerular diseases secondary to systemic disease are also depicted in Table 52.3. Hypertensive nephrosclerosis, which was not listed as an independent category in all series, may be the most frequent etiology in this category. The next most common causes are vasculitis and amyloidosis, which are relatively infrequent in younger patients. Particularly prominent in the elderly are deposition diseases, including amyloidosis, light chain deposition disease, and fibrillary glomerulonephritis.

Acute Renal Failure in the Elderly

Elderly patients are susceptible to all the causes of acute renal failure seen in the general population, and suscep-

TABLE 52.4. Causes of acute renal failure.

Cause	Young patients ($n = 67$)	Elderly patients ($n = 298$)
Nephrotoxins	6.8	10.8
Volume depletion	15.1	23.4
Septic shock	20.5	25.8
Postsurgery	8.2	5.1
Cardiogenic shock	11.0	5.8
Multifactorial	15.1	11.9
Obstructive	5.5	10.5
Hepatorenal syndrome	4.1	1.0
Glomerular disease	5.5	0.7
Other	8.2	5.8

Data are percent (%).

Source: Adapted from Macias Nuñez and Sanchez Romero, with permission.[150]

tibility to acute renal failure may be enhanced,[1] Presumably, the elderly may be at higher risk for prerenal causes of acute renal failure because of a tendency toward hypodipsia and reduced sodium intake, diuretic administration, and inability to conserve sodium, predisposing to dehydration and sodium depletion. A representative study of the etiology of acute renal failure in 67 young and 298 elderly patients is depicted in Table 52.4,[150] in which volume depletion was deemed primarily responsible in 23.4% of cases in elderly patients. Obviously, preexisting volume depletion would also enhance risk for acute renal failure after administration of contrast agents or nephrotoxic drugs. In addition, advancing age increases risk of acute renal failure associated with surgical complications, aminoglycoside nephrotoxicity, nonsteroidal anti-inflammatory drugs, angiotensin-converting enzyme inhibitor therapy, radiocontrast, and postrenal (obstructive) causes.[1,151] More recently, 4176 consecutive patients admitted to an acute care hospital were evaluated for the incidence and etiology of acute renal failure.[152] Of these, 1.4% developed acute renal failure in the hospital. Contributing factors were nephrotoxic drugs (66%), sepsis and hypoperfusion (45.7% each), contrast media (16.9%), and postoperative acute renal failure (25.4%). Of these, contrast media, surgery, and drugs each predicted acute renal failure on their own. Mortality in the elderly with acute renal failure was significantly higher than in those without acute renal failure (25.4% versus 12.5%; $p = 0.03$). Sepsis (odds ratio, 43), oliguria (odds ratio, 64) and hypotension (odds ratio, 15) were independent predictors of poor patient outcome.[152]

When the cause of acute renal insufficiency is not apparent, a renal biopsy may be required to make the diagnosis. Recently, the pathologic diagnoses in 1065 consecutive patients over the age of 60 who underwent renal biopsy were reviewed.[153] Of these 24.3% had a renal biopsy because of acute renal failure. Results of that survey are depicted in Table 52.5.[153] The most prominent diagnoses, pauci-immune glomerulonephritis and acute

interstitial nephritis, are more frequent in the elderly than in a younger population.

Whether advanced age is an independent risk factor for mortality associated with acute renal failure, dissociable from other systemic illnesses, is not entirely clear.[150] Certain causes of acute renal failure are certainly more frequent in the elderly; these include multiple myeloma; carcinoma leading to obstruction, humoral abnormalities, and risk of nephrotoxicity from chemotherapeutic interventions; polypharmacy with or without inappropriate drug dosing that fails to take into account the marked reduction in GFR in the elderly; obstructive uropathy due to prostatic disease; and atheroembolic renal disease.[150]

End-Stage Renal Disease in the Elderly

The number and relative frequency of elderly patients entering end-stage renal disease (ESRD) programs, and the average age of dialysis patients, is increasing each year in the United States, reflecting the aging of the population in general. The average age of patients starting dialysis for ESRD in the United States is now 62 years. In 1998, the last year for which detailed data are available, there were more than 65,000 patients aged 65 to 74 (up from 13,000 in 1991), and more than 45,000 patients aged 75 or older (up from 8,000 in 1991), in ESRD treatment in the United States.[154] Moreover, the median age of hemodialysis patients is continually rising; some 35% of all ESRD patients are now 65 years of age or older, as are 45% of all hemodialysis patients.

Thus, elderly patients comprise an ever increasing percentage of the patients enrolled in treatment for ESRD. Indeed, while such interventions as improved hypertension control and smoking cessation have dramatically lowered the rates of stroke and fatal myocardial infarction, they have had no discernible impact on the incidence of ESRD. In addition to the direct burden of renal disease, the presence of this condition greatly increases

TABLE 52.5. Pathologic diagnoses in elderly patients with acute renal failure.

Diagnosis	Percent of biopsies
Pauci-immune crescentic GN	31.2
Acute interstitial nephritis	18.6
Acute tubular necrosis with nephrotic syndrome	7.5
Atheroemboli	7.1
Acute tubular necrosis alone	6.7
Light chain cast nephropathy	5.9
Postinfectious GN	5.5
Antiglomerular basement membrane antibody GN	4.0
IgA nephropathy or Henoch–Schonlein nephritis	3.6
Nondiagnostic for acute renal failure	9.9

Source: Adapted from Haas, Spargo, Wit et al., with permission.[153]

cardiovascular risk; ESRD at age 75 confers a relative risk of death of just under 3, as compared with the population without renal disease.[155] All projections indicate that these trends will continue. The direct economic costs ($17 billion in 1998), and the ancillary costs including hospitalization, drugs, disability, and increased cardiovascular risk, together pose a grave challenge for the health care team in the coming years.

Experimental Considerations and Implications for Further Research

The potential mechanisms associated with the normal age-related loss of renal function have been explored in experimental animals, which also exhibit age-related declines in renal blood flow and glomerular filtration rate in association with progressive glomerular sclerosis. The adaptive response to loss of functioning nephrons consists of increases in the glomerular capillary pressures and flows in the remaining functional nephrons, a compensation that serves to preserve total GFR. In the extreme case of extensive surgical removal of renal mass in the rat, the increased filtration in the surviving nephrons is accompanied by systemic hypertension, and progressive azotemia, proteinuria, and glomerular sclerosis. Recent studies using micropuncture techniques have indicated that, at least in some rat strains, development of age-related glomerular injury is associated with glomerular capillary hypertension,[156–158] a hemodynamic abnormality common to many forms of renal disease. As in other diseases, angiotensin-converting enzyme inhibitor delays age-related nephropathy in the rat.[157]

Observations in aging humans and experimental animals are highly reminiscent of changes observed in the setting of acquired renal disease, and lend support to the hypothesis that hemodynamic factors in the aging kidney operate in similar, albeit slower, fashion to injure and ultimately destroy the glomerular population. This formulation suggests that age- or disease-related reduction in functioning renal mass, systemic hypertension, conventionally treated diabetes, and ad libitum protein intake all lead to unrelenting vasodilatation. The resulting long-term elevations in glomerular pressures and flows promote hyperfiltration, impair the permselective properties of the glomerular wall, and injure the component cells of the glomerulus. The resulting glomerular sclerosis exerts a positive feedback stimulus to compensatory hyperfiltration in less affected glomeruli, contributing in turn to their eventual destruction. Numerous dietary, endocrine, and toxic factors that may accelerate nephron loss with normal aging or renal disease have been identified,[1,5,6,159,160] and certain dietary manipulations (particularly dietary protein restriction and total food restriction),[161,162] as well as angiotensin-converting enzyme inhibitors[157] and angiotensin receptor antagonists,[163] have been demonstrated to retard the progression of age-related renal disease in laboratory animals. Given the vulnerability of the aging kidney to acceleration of renal insufficiency after acquired injury, it remains imperative to pay attention to those risk factors (volume depletion, nephrotoxic insults, uncontrolled hypertension, and dietary factors) that may contribute to loss of renal function. Although little information is available specifically addressing these interventions in the elderly population, it seems likely that these hemodynamically protective interventions will prove efficacious in this population as well. With the ever-increasing number of elderly patients entering ESRD programs, clinical studies evaluating these therapeutic interventions in this population at risk are certainly warranted.

References

1. Choudhury D, Raj DSC, Palmer BF, Levi M. Effect of aging on renal function and disease. In: Brenner BM, ed. *The Kidney, 6th Ed*. Philadelphia: Saunders; 2000:2187–2216.
2. Epstein M. Aging and the kidney. *J Am Soc Nephrol*. 1996; 7:1106–1122.
3. Lindeman RD. Overview: renal physiology and pathophysiology of aging. *Am J Kidney Dis*. 1990;16:275–282.
4. Lindeman RD. Renal physiology and pathophysiology of aging. *Contrib Nephrol*. 1993;105:1–12.
5. Baylis C, Schmidt R. The aging glomerulus. *Semin Nephrol*. 1996;16:265–276.
6. Rodrígues-Puyol, D. The aging kidney. *Kidney Int*. 1998; 54:2247–2265.
7. Davies DF, Shock NW. Age changes in glomerular filtration rate, effective renal plasma flow, and tubular excretory capacity in adult males. *J Clin Investig*. 1950;29:496–507.
8. Rowe JW, Andres R, Tobin JD, et al. The effect of age on creatinine clearance in men: a cross-sectional and longitudinal study. *J Gerontol*. 1976;31:155–163.
9. Lindeman RD, Tobin JD, Shock NW. Association between blood pressure and the rate of decline in renal function with age. *Kidney Int*. 1984;27:553–557.
10. De Leeuw P. Renal function in the elderly: results from the European Working Party on High Blood Pressure in the Elderly Trial. *Am J Med*. 1993;90(suppl):40–50.
11. Kim R, Rotnitsky A, Sparrow D, et al. A longitudinal study of low-level lead exposure and impairment of renal function. The Normative Aging Study. *JAMA*. 1996;275:1177–1181.
12. Goetz FC, Jacobs DR Jr, Chavers B, et al. Risk factors for kidney damage in the adult population of Wadena, Minnesota. A prospective study. *Am J Epidemiol*. 1997; 145:91–102.
13. Bleyer AJ, Shemanski LR, Burke GL, et al. Tobacco, hypertension, and vascular disease: risk factors for renal

functional decline in an older population. *Kidney Int.* 2000; 57:2072–2079.

14. Stengel B, Couchoud C, Cenee S, et al. Age, blood pressure and smoking effects on chronic renal failure in primary glomerular nephropathies. *Kidney Int.* 2000;57: 2519–2526.

15. James GD, Sealey JE, Alderman M, et al. A longitudinal study of urinary creatinine and creatinine clearance in normal subjects: race, sex, and age differences. *Am J Hypertens.* 1988;1:124–131.

16. Feinfeld DA, Guzik H, Carvounis CP, et al. Sequential changes in renal function tests in the old old: results from the Bronx longitudinal aging study. *J Am Geriatr Soc.* 1995;43:412–414.

17. Cockcroft DW, Gault MH. Prediction of creatinine clearance from serum creatinine. *Nephron.* 1976;16:31–41.

18. Wesson LG. Renal hemodynamics in physiological states. In: Wesson LG, ed. *Physiology of the Human Kidney.* New York: Grune & Stratton; 1969:96–108.

19. Hollenberg NK, Adams DF, Solomon HS, et al. Senescence and the renal vasculature in normal man. *Circ Res.* 1974;34:309–316.

20. Bolton WK, Benton FR, Maclay JG, et al. Spontaneous glomerular sclerosis in aging Sprague–Dawley rats. *Am J Pathol.* 1976;85:227–302.

21. Cohen MP, Ku L. Age-related changes in sulfation of basement membrane glycosaminoglycans. *Exp Gerontol.* 1976;18:447–450.

22. Jones CA, Francis ME, Eberhardt MS, et al. Microalbuminuria in the US population: Third National Health and Nutrition Examination Survey. *Am J Kidney Dis.* 2002;39: 445–459.

23. Tietz NW, Shuery DF, Wekstein DR. Laboratory values in fit aging individuals—sexagenarians through centenarians. *Clin Chem.* 1992;38:1167–1185.

24. Damsgaard EM, Froland A, Jorgensen OD, et al. Microalbuminuria as predictor of increased mortality in elderly people. *B Med J.* 1990;300:297–300.

25. Kasiske BL, Umen AJ. The influence of age, sex, race, and body habitus on kidney weight in humans. *Arch Pathol Lab Med.* 1986;110:55–60.

26. Nyengaard JR, Bendtsen TF. Glomerular number and size in relation to age, kidney and body surface in normal man. *Anat Rec.* 1992;232:194–201.

27. Emamian SA, Nielsen MB, Pedersen JF, Ytte L. Kidney dimensions at sonography: correlation with age, sex, and habitus in 665 adult volunteers. *Am J Roentgenol.* 1993; 160:83–86.

28. Tauchi H, Tsuboi K, Okutomi J. Age changes in the human kidney of the different races. *Gerontologia.* 1971;17:87–97.

29. McLachlan MSF. The aging kidney. *Lancet.* 1978;ii:143–146.

30. Goyal VK. Changes with age in the human kidney. *Exp Gerontol.* 1982;17:321–331.

31. Ljungqvist A, Lagergren C. Normal intrarenal arterial pattern in adult and aging human kidney. A microangiographical and histological study. *J Anat.* 1962;96:285–300.

32. Takazakura E, Sawabu N, Handa A, et al. Intrarenal vascular changes with age and disease. *Kidney Int.* 1972; 2:224–230.

33. Kaplan C, Pasternack B, Shah H, et al. Age-related incidence of sclerotic glomeruli in human kidneys. *Am J Pathol.* 1974;80:227–234.

34. Kappel B, Olsen S. Cortical interstitial tissue and sclerosed glomeruli in the normal human kidney, related to age and sex. A quantitative study. *Virchows Arch [A].* 1980; 387:271–277.

35. Neugarten J, Gallo G, Silbiger S, et al. Glomerulosclerosis is aging humans is not influenced by gender. *Am J Kidney Dis.* 1999;34:884–888.

36. Wei JY. Age and the cardiovascular system. *N Engl J Med.* 1992;327:1735–1739.

37. Bowker LK, Briggs RSJ, Gallagher PJ, et al. Raised blood urea in the elderly: a clinical and pathological study. *Postgrad Med J.* 1992;68:174–179.

38. Watkin DM, Shock NW. Agewise standard values for C_{In}, C_{PAH} and Tm_{PAH} in adult males. *J Clin Investig.* 1955;34: 969–976.

39. Miller JH, McDonald RK, Shock NW. Age changes in the maximal rate of renal tubular reabsorption of glucose. *J Gerontol.* 1952;7:196–200.

40. Barrows CH Jr, Falzone JA Jr, Shock NW. Age differences in the succinoxidase activity of homogenates and mitochondria from the livers and kidneys of rats. *J Gerontol.* 1960;15:130–133.

41. Burich RJ. Effects of age on renal function and enzyme activity in male C57 BL/6 mice. *J Gerontol.* 1975;30:539–545.

42. Beauchene RE, Fanestil DD, Barrows CH Jr. The effect of age on active transport and sodium-potassium activated ATPase activity in renal tissue of rats. *J Gerontol.* 1965;20: 306–310.

43. Proverbio F, Proverbio T, Marin R. Ion transport and oxygen consumption in kidney cortex slices from young and old rats. *Gerontology.* 1985;31:166–173.

44. Kinsella JL, Sacktor B. Renal brush border Na^+–H^+ exchange activity in the aging rat. *Am J Physiol.* 1987;252: R681–R686.

45. Epstein M, Hollenberg NK. Age as a determinant of renal sodium conservation in normal man. *J Lab Clin Med.* 1976;87:411–417.

46. Macias Nuñez JF, Bondia Roman AB, Rodriguez Commes JL. Physiology and disorders of water balance and electrolytes in the elderly. In: Macias Nuñez JF, Cameron JS, eds. *Renal Function and Disease in the Elderly.* London: Butterworths; 1987:67–93.

47. Mimran A, Ribstein J, Jover B. Aging and sodium homeostasis. *Kidney Int.* 1992;41(suppl 37):S-107–S-113.

48. Macias Nuñez JF, Garcia-Iglesias C, Tabernero-Romo JM, et al. Renal management of sodium under indomethacin and aldosterone in the elderly. *Age Ageing.* 1978;9:165–172.

49. Weidmann P, De Myttanaere-Bursztein S, Maxwell MH, et al. Effect of aging on plasma renin and aldosterone in normal man. *Kidney Int.* 1975;8:325–333.

50. Hall JE, Coleman TG, Guyton AC. The renin-angiotensin system: normal physiology and changes in older hypertensives. *J Am Geriatr Soc.* 1989;37:801–813.

51. Jung FF, Kennefick TM, Ingelfinger JR, et al. Downregulation of the intrarenal renin-angiotensin system in the aging rat. *J Am Soc Nephrol.* 1995;5:1–8.

52. DeFronzo RA. Glucose intolerance and aging. *Diabetes Care.* 1981;4:493–501.

53. Tajima F, Sagawa S, Iwamoto J, et al. Renal and endocrine responses in the elderly during head-out water immersion. *Am J Physiol.* 1988;254:R977–R983.

54. Luft FC, Grim CE, Fineberg N, et al. Effects of volume expansion and contraction in normotensive whites, blacks and subjects of different ages. *Circulation.* 1979;59:643–650.

55. Luft FC, Weinberger MH, Grim CE. Sodium sensitivity and resistance in normotensive humans. *Am J Med.* 1982; 72:726–735.

56. Tank JE, Vora JP, Houghton DC, et al. Altered renal vascular responses in the aging rat kidney. *Am J Physiol.* 1994;266:F942–F948.

57. Baylis C. Renal responses to acute angiotensin II inhibition and administered angiotensin II in the aging, conscious, chronically catheterized rat. *Am J Kidney Dis.* 1993;22:842–850.

58. Masilamani S, Zhang XZ, Baylis C. Blunted pressure natriuretic response in the old rat: participation of the renal nerves. *Am J Kidney Dis.* 1998;32:605–610.

59. Ziegler MJ, Lake CR, Kopin JJ. Plasma noradrenalin increases with age. *Nature.* 1976;261:333–336.

60. Bursztyn M, Bresnahan M, Gavras I, et al. Effect of aging on vasopressin, catecholamines, and alpha₂-adrenergic receptors. *J Am Geriatr Soc.* 1990;38:628–632.

61. Haller BG, Zust H, Shaw S, et al. Effects of posture and aging on circulating atrial natriuretic peptide levels in man. *Hypertension.* 1987;5:551–556.

62. Clark BA, Elahi D, Epstein FH. The influence of gender, age, and the menstrual cycle on plasma atrial natriuretic peptide. *J Clin Endocrinol Metab.* 1990;70:349–352.

63. Ohashi M, Fujio N, Nawata H, et al. High plasma concentrations of human atrial natriuretic polypeptide in aged men. *J Clin Endocrinol Metab.* 1987;64:81–85.

64. Tummala PE, Dananberg J, Grekin RJ. Alterations in the secretion of atrial natriuretic factor in atria from aged rats. *Hypertens.* 1992;20:85–88.

65. Mulkerrin EC, Brain A, Hampton D, et al. Reduced renal hemodynamic response to atrial natriuretic peptide in elderly volunteers. *Am J Kidney Dis.* 1993;22:538–544.

66. Clark BA, Elahi D, Shannon RP, et al. Influence of age and dose on the end-organ responses to atrial natriuretic peptide in humans. *Am J Hypertens.* 1991;4:500–507.

67. Hishida A, Kumagai H, Usozaki T, et al. The role of atrial natriuretic peptide in the natriuretic response to acute saline loading. In: Puschett JB, Greenberg A, eds. *Diuretics IV: Chemistry, Pharmacology and Clinical Applications.* Amsterdam: Elsevier; 1993:669–674.

68. Leosco D, Ferrara N, Landino P, et al. Effects of age on the role of atrial natriuretic factor in renal adaptation to physiologic variations of dietary salt intake. *J Am Soc Nephrol.* 1996;7:1045–1051.

69. Naka T, Ogihara T, Hata T, et al. The effect of aging on urinary kallikrein excretion in normotensive subjects and in patients with essential hypertension. *J Clin Endocrinol Metab.* 1981;52:1023–1026.

70. Pecly IMD, Fagundes VGA, Magalhães SJR, et al. "Normal aging" and renal hemodynamics, kininogen and blood pressure. Effects of protein load. *Am J Hypertens.* 1994;7(4 part 2):132A [abstract].

71. Fukagawa WK, Bandini LG, Rowe JW, et al. Effect of age on renal responses to protein ingestion in man. *Clin Res.* 1989;37:490A [abstract].

72. Kuhlik A, Elahi D, Epstein FH, et al. Urinary dopamine excretion with water diuresis in young and elderly humans. *Clin Res.* 1993;41:190A [abstract].

73. Kansra V, Hussain T, Lokhandwala MF. Alterations in dopamine DA₁ receptor and G proteins in renal proximal tubules of old rats. *Am J Physiol.* 1997;273:F53–F59.

74. Beheray S, Kansra V, Hussain T, et al. Diminished natriuretic response to dopamine in old rats is due to an impaired D₁-like receptor-signaling pathway. *Kidney Int.* 2000;58:712–720.

75. Mulkerrin E, Epstein FH, Clark BA. Reduced renal response to low-dose dopamine infusion in the elderly. *J Gerontol A Biol Sci Med Sci.* 1995;50:M271–M275.

76. Shannon RP, Minaker KL, Rowe JW. Aging and water balance in humans. *Semin Nephrol.* 1984;4:346–353.

77. Sica DA, Harford A. Sodium and water disorders in the elderly. In: Zawada ET Jr, Sica DA, eds. *Geriatric Nephrology and Urology.* Littleton, MA: PSG Publishing; 1985: 127–156.

78. Rowe JW, Shock NW, de Fronzo RA. The influence of age on the renal response to water deprivation in man. *Nephron.* 1976;17:270–278.

79. Lindemann RD, Lee TD, Yiengst MJ, et al. Influence of age, renal disease, hypertension, diuretics and calcium on the antidiuretic responses to suboptimal infusions of vasopressin. *J Lab Clin Med.* 1966;68:206–223.

80. Phillips PA, Rolls BJ, Ledingham JGG, et al. Reduced thirst after water deprivation in healthy elderly men. *N Engl J Med.* 1984;311:753–759.

81. Phillips PA, Bretherton M, Risvanis J, et al. Effects of drinking on thirst and vasopressin in dehydrated elderly men. *Am J Physiol.* 1993;264:R877–R881.

82. Phillips PA, Johnston C, Gray L. Reduced oropharyngeal inhibition of AVP secretion in dehydrated elderly men. *Ann NY Acad Sci.* 1993;689:651–655.

83. McAloon DM, Davis DM, Clark BA, et al. Effects of hypertonicity on water intake in the elderly: an age-related failure. *Geriatr Nephrol Urol.* 1997;7:11–16.

84. Phillips PA, Bretherton M, Johnston CI, et al. Reduced osmotic thirst in healthy elderly men. *Am J Physiol.* 1991; 261:R166–R171.

85. Stachenfeld NS, Mack GW, Takamata A, et al. Thirst and fluid regulatory responses to hypertonicity in older adults. *Am J Physiol.* 1996;271:R757–R765.

86. Frolkis VV, Bezinkov W, Duplinko YK, et al. The hypothalamus in aging. *Exp Gerontol.* 1972;7:169–184.

87. Helderman JH, Vestal RE, Rowe JW, et al. The response of arginine vasopressin to intravenous ethanol and hypertonic saline in man: the impact of aging. *J Gerontol.* 1978; 33:39–47.

88. Rowe JW, Minaker KL, Sparrow D, et al. Age-related failure of volume–pressure-mediated vasopressin release. *J Clin Endocrinol Metab.* 1982;54:661–664.

89. Duggan J, Kilfeather S, Lightman SL, et al. The association of age with plasma arginine vasopressin and plasma osmolality. *Age Ageing*. 1993;222:332–336.

90. Engel PA, Rowe JW, Minaker KL, et al. Stimulation of vasopressin release by exogenous vasopressin: effect of sodium intake and age. *Am J Physiol*. 1984;246:E202–E207.

91. Dontas AS, Karkeros S, Papanayioutou P. Mechanisms of renal tubular defects in old age. *Postgrad Med J*. 1972;48:295–303.

92. Clark BA, Shannon RP, Rosa RM, et al. Increased susceptibility to thiazide-induced hyponatremia in the elderly. *J Am Soc Nephrol*. 1994;5:1106–1111.

93. Preisser L, Teillet L, Aliotti S, et al. Downregulation of aquaporin-2 and -3 in aging kidney is independent of V_2 vasopressin receptor. *Am J Physiol*. 2000;279:F144–F152.

94. Kleinfeld M, Casimir M, Borra A. Hyponatremia as observed in a chronic disease facility. *J Am Geriatr Soc*. 1979;27:156–161.

95. Miller M, Morley JE, Rubenstein LZ, et al. Hyponatremia in a nursing home population. *Gerontologist*. 1985;25:118.

96. Baglin A, Prinseau J, Aegerter P, et al. Electrolytic abnormalities in elderly people. Prevalence and relations with medical treatment: multicentric study of 631 subjects aged 70 years and over. *Presse Méd*. 1992;21:1459–1463.

97. Narins RG, Jones ER, Stom MC, et al. Diagnostic strategies in disorders of fluid, electrolyte, and acid-base homeostasis. *Am J Med*. 1982;72:496–520.

98. Sunderam SG, Mankikar GD. Hyponatremia in the elderly. *Age Ageing*. 1983;12:77–80.

99. Booker JA. Severe symptomatic hyponatremia in elderly outpatients: the role of thiazide therapy and stress. *J Am Geriatr Soc*. 1984;32:108–113.

100. Ashraf N, Locksley R, Arieff A. Thiazide-induced hyponatremia associated with death or neurologic damage in outpatients. *Am J Med*. 1981;70:1163–1168.

101. Fidler HM, Goldman J, Bielawska CA, et al. A study of plasma sodium levels in elderly people taking amiloride or triamterene in combination with hydrochlorothiazide. *Postgrad Med J*. 1993;69:797–799.

102. Rondeau E, de Lima J, Caillens H, et al. High plasma antidiuretic hormone in patients with cardiac failure: influence of age. *Miner Electrolyte Metab*. 1982;8:267–274.

103. Goldstein CS, Braunstein S, Goldfarb S. Idiopathic syndrome of inappropriate antidiuretic hormone secretion possibly due to advanced age. *Ann Intern Med*. 1983;99:185–188.

104. Spigset O, Hedenmalm K. Hyponatremia in relation to treatment with antidepressants: a survey of reports in the World Health Organization data base for spontaneous reporting of adverse drug reactions. *Pharmacotherapy*. 1997;17:348–352.

105. Liu BA, Mittmann N, Knowles SR, Shear NH. Hyponatremia and the syndrome of inappropriate secretion of antidiuretic hormone associated with the use of selective serotonin reuptake inhibitors: a review of spontaneous reports. *Can Med Assoc J*. 1996;155:519–527.

106. Miller M, Hecker MS, Friedlander DA, et al. Apparent idiopathic hyponatremia in an ambulatory geriatric population. *J Am Gerontol Soc*. 1996;44:404–408.

107. Hirschberg B, Ben-Yehuda A. The syndrome of inappropriate antidiuretic hormone secretion in the elderly. *Am J Med*. 1997;103:270–273.

108. Palevsky PM, Bhagrath R, Greenberg A. Hypernatremia in hospitalized patients. *Ann Intern Med*. 1996;124:197–203.

109. Mukherjee AP, Coni NK, Davison W. Osmoreceptor function among the elderly. *Gerontol Clin*. 1973;15:227–233.

110. Lye M. Distribution of body potassium in healthy elderly subjects. *Gerontology*. 1981;27:286–292.

111. McCarthy ST. Body fluid, electrolytes and diuretics. *Curr Med Res Opin*. 1982;7:87–95.

112. Fidler HM, Goldman J, Bielawska CA, Rai GS, Hoffbrand BI. A study of plasma sodium levels in elderly people taking amiloride or triamterene in combination with hydrochlorothiazide. *Postgrad Med J*. 1993;69:797–799.

113. Bengele HH, Mathias R, Perkins JH, et al. Impaired renal and extrarenal adaptation in old rats. *Kidney Int*. 1983;23:684–690.

114. O'Connell JE, Colledge NR. Type IV renal tubular acidosis and spironolactone therapy in the elderly. *Postgrad Med J*. 1993;69:887–889.

115. Billiouw JM, Lornoy W, Becaus I, et al. Severe hyperkalemia in the very old patient. In: Puschett JB, Greenberg A, eds. *Diuretics IV: Chemistry, Pharmacology and Clinical Applications*. Amsterdam: Elsevier; 1993:275–277.

116. Mulkerrin E, Epstein FH, Clark BA. Aldosterone responses to hyperkalemia in healthy elderly humans. *J Am Soc Nephrol*. 1995;6:1459–1462.

117. Perazella MA, Mahnensmith RL. Hyperkalemia in the elderly: drugs exacerbate impaired potassium homeostasis. *J Gen Intern Med*. 1997;12:646–656.

118. Michelis MH. Hyperkalemia in the elderly. *Am J Kidney Dis*. 1990;16:296–299.

119. Marinella MA. Trimethoprim-induced hyperkalemia: an analysis of reported cases. *Gerontology*. 1999;45:209–212.

120. Goodkin DA, Waldman R, Narins RG. Acid-base disorders in the elderly. In: Zawada ET Jr, Sica DA, eds. *Geriatric Nephrology and Urology*. Littleton, MA: PSG Publishing; 1985:157–174.

121. Taberno Romo JM. Proximal tubular function and renal acidification in the aged. In: Macias Nuñez JF, Cameron JS, eds. *Renal Function and Disease in the Elderly*. London: Butterworths; 1987:143–161.

122. Shock NW, Yiengst MJ. Age changes in the acid-base equilibrium of the blood of males. *J Gerontol*. 1950;5:1–4.

123. Frassetto L, Morris RC Jr, Sebastian A. Effect of age on blood acid-base composition in adult humans: role of age-related renal functional decline. *Am J Physiol*. 1996;271:F1114–F1122.

124. Adler S, Lindeman RD, Yiengst MJ, et al. Effect of acute acid loading on urinary acid excretion by the aging human kidney. *J Lab Clin Med*. 1968;72:278–289.

125. Agarwal BN, Cabebe RG. Renal acidification in elderly subjects. *Nephron*. 1980;26:291–295.

126. Hilton JG, Goodbody MF, Kruesi OR. The effect of prolonged administration of ammonium chloride on the blood

acid–base equilibrium of geriatric subjects. *J Am Geriatr Soc.* 1955;3:697–703.

127. Sebastian A, Harris ST, Ottaway JH, et al. Improved mineral balance and skeletal metabolism in post-menopausal women treated with potassium bicarbonate. *N Engl J Med.* 1994;330:1776–1781.

128. Quesada JM, Coopmans W, Ruiz B, Aljama P, Jans I, Bouillon R. Influence of Vitamin D on parathyroid function in the elderly. *J Clin Endocrinol Metab.* 1992;75:494–501.

129. Prine RL, Dick I, Devine A, et al. The effects of menopause and age on calcitropic hormones: a cross-sectional study of 655 healthy women aged 35 to 90. *J Bone Miner Res.* 1995;10:835–842.

130. Armbrecht HJ, Gross CJ, Zenser TV. Effect of dietary calcium and phosphorus restriction on calcium and phosphorus balance in young and old rats. *Arch Biochem Biophys.* 1981;210:179–185.

131. Avioli LV, McDonald JE, Won Lee S. The influence of age on the intestinal absorption of ^{47}Ca in women and its relation to ^{47}Ca absorption in post-menopausal osteoporosis. *J Clin Investig.* 1965;41:1960–1967.

132. Baker MR, Peacock M, Nordin BEC. The decline in vitamin D status with age. *Age Ageing.* 1980;9:249–253.

133. Chapuy M-C, Durr F, Chapuy P. Age-related changes in parathyroid hormone and 25-hydroxycholecalciferol levels. *J Gerontol.* 1983;38:19–22.

134. Gallagher JC, Riggs LB, Eisman J, et al. Intestinal calcium absorption and serum vitamin D metabolites in normal subjects and osteoporotic patients. *J Clin Investig.* 1979;64:729–736.

135. Tsai K-S, Heath H III, Kumar R, et al. Impaired vitamin D metabolism with aging in women: possible role in pathogenesis of senile osteoporosis. *J Clin Investig.* 1984;73:1668–1672.

136. Ambrecht HJ, Zenser RV, Davis BB. Effect of age on the conversion of 25-hydroxy vitamin D_3 to 1,25-dihydroxy vitamin D_3 by kidneys of rats. *J Clin Investig.* 1980;66:1118–1123.

137. Ambrecht HJ, Zenser RV, Gross CJ, Davis BB. Adaptation to dietary calcium and phosphorus restriction changes with age in the rat. *Am J Physiol.* 1980;239:E322–E327.

138. Sakhrani LM, Massry SG. Calcium, phosphorus, and magnesium disorders in the elderly. In: Zawada ET Jr, Sica DA, eds. *Geriatric Nephrology and Urology.* Littleton, MA: PSG Publishing; 1985:175–180.

139. Thomas MK, Lloyd-Jones DM, Thadhani RI, et al. Hypovitaminosis D in medical inpatients. *N Engl J Med.* 1998;338:777–783.

140. Bando H, Zhang C, Takada Y, et al. Impaired secretion of growth hormone-releasing hormone, growth hormone and IGF-1 in elderly men. *Acta Endocrinol (Copenh).* 1991;124:31–36.

141. Insognia KL, Lewis AM, Lipinski BA, et al. Effect of age on serum immunoreactive parathyroid hormone and its biological effects. *J Clin Endocrinol Metab.* 1981;53:1072–1075.

142. Levi M, Jameson DM, Van Der Meer BW. Role of BBM lipid composition and fluidity in impaired renal P_i transport in aged rat. *Am J Physiol.* 1989;256:F85–F90.

143. Sorribas V, Lötscher M, Loffing J, et al. Cellular mechanisms of the age-related decrease in renal phosphate reabsorption. *Kidney Int.* 1996;50:855–863.

144. Henrotte JG, Benech A, Pineau M. Relationship between blood magnesium content and age in a French population. In: Cantin M, Seelig MS, eds. *Magnesium in Health and Disease.* New York: Spectrum; 1980:930–934.

145. Samiy A. Penal disease in the elderly. *Med Clin N Am.* 1983;67:463–480.

146. Murray BM, Raij L. Glomerular disease in the aged. In: Macias Nuñez JF, Cameron JS, eds. *Renal Function and Disease in the Elderly.* London: Butterworths; 1987:298–320.

147. Glassock RJ. Glomerular disease in the elderly population. In: Oreopoulos DG, Hazzard WR, Luke R, eds. *Nephrology and Geriatrics Integrated.* Dordrecht: Kluwer; 2000:57–66.

148. Cameron JS. Nephrotic syndrome in the elderly. *Semin Nephrol.* 1996;16:319–329.

149. Glickman JL, Kaiser DL, Bolton WK. Aetiology and diagnosis of chronic renal insufficiency in the aged: the role of renal biopsy. In: Zawada ET Jr, Sica DA, eds. *Geriatric Nephrology and Urology.* Littleton, MA: PSG Publishing; 1985:485–508.

150. Macias Nuñez JF, Sanchez Tomero JA. Acute renal failure in old people. In: Macias Nuñez JF, Cameron JS, eds. *Renal Function and Disease in the Elderly.* London: Butterworths; 1987:461–484.

151. Mandal AK, Baig M, Koutoubi Z. Management of acute renal failure in the elderly. Treatment options. *Drugs Aging.* 1996;9:226–250.

152. Kohli HS, Bhaskaran MC, Mufhukumar T, et al. Treatment-related acute renal failure in the elderly: a hospital-based prospective study. *Nephrol Dial Transplant.* 2000;15:212–217.

153. Haas M, Spargo BH, Wit E-J C, et al. Etiologies and outcome of acute renal insufficiency in older adults: a renal biopsy study of 259 cases. *Am J Kidney Dis.* 2000;35:433–447.

154. U.S. Renal Data System. Excerpts from the USRDS 2000 Annual Data Report: Atlas of End-Stage Renal Disease in the United States. *Am J Kidney Dis.* 2000(suppl 2):S1–S239.

155. Luke RG, Beck LH. Gerontologizing nephrology. *J Am Soc Nephrol.* 1999;10:1824–1827.

156. Fujihara CK, Limongi DMZP, de Oliveira HCF, et al. Absence of focal glomerular sclerosis in aging analbuminemic rats. *Am J Physiol.* 1992;262:R947–R954.

157. Anderson S, Rennke HG, Zatz R. Glomerular adaptations with normal aging and with long-term converting enzyme inhibition in the rat. *Am J Physiol.* 1994;267:F35–F43.

158. Tolbert EM, Weisstuch J, Feiner HD, et al. Onset of glomerular hypertension with aging precedes injury in the spontaneously hypertensive rat. *Am J Physiol.* 2000;278:F839–F846.

159. Brenner BM. Nephron adaptation to renal injury or ablation. Mechanisms, benefits and risks. *Am J Physiol.* 1985;249:F324–F337.

160. Anderson S. Decline of renal function with age: mechanisms, risk factors and therapeutic implications. In: Oreopoulos DG, ed. *Geriatric Nephrology*. Boston: Nijhoff; 1986:57–71.

161. Saxton JA Jr, Kimball GC. Relation of nephrosis and other diseases of albino rats to age and to modifications of diet. *Arch Pathol*. 1941;32:951–965.

162. Gehrig JJ Jr, Ross J, Jamison RL. Effect of long-term, alternate day feeding on renal function in aging conscious rats. *Kidney Int*. 1988;34:620–630.

163. Ma LJ, Nakamura S, Whitsitt JS, et al. Regression of sclerosis in aging by an angiotensin inhibition-induced decrease in PAI-1. *Kidney Int*. 2000;8:2425–2436.

53
Immunology of Aging

Edith A. Burns and James S. Goodwin

Immunologic function is one of the most intensively studied physiologic processes in gerontology, in part because of the explosive growth in all aspects of immunology research in the past several decades and the ease of obtaining immunocytes (lymphocytes, monocytes, and polymorphonuclear leukocytes) for study. There are more fundamental reasons, however, why the study of immunology is particularly relevant to gerontology. Immunologic function declines and becomes dysregulated with age, as do most physiologic functions. Concomitantly, there is a rise in the incidence of many infections and malignancies with age. There is greater morbidity and mortality associated with infections in adults over 65 years of age. Elderly persons respond less well to protective immunizations against common infections such as influenza and pneumococcal pneumonia. Also intriguing are early observations linking changes in immune function with changes in the life span of various animal species. An understanding of immunologic changes might be important not only in understanding the aging process, but also in developing potential strategies to prevent some of the morbidity and other changes that occur with age.[1,2] This chapter describes changes in the immune system attributed to aging, and tries to give an overall sense of our understanding of aging and immune function at the beginning of the twenty-first century.

Organization of the Immune System

The immune system classically has been divided into the cellular and humoral components, with monocyte and granulocyte function treated separately. The cellular immune response, mediated primarily by T lymphocytes (or thymus-derived lymphocytes), rejects grafts of foreign tissues, kills virus-infected cells, protects against fungi and some intracellular parasites and bacteria, modulates the immune response to prevent autoimmunity, and (possibly) defends against the growth of tumors (Fig. 53.1). The function of the humoral immune system is the production of antibodies (produced by differentiated B cells, or bone marrow-derived lymphocytes), which are the main defense against bacteria and other infectious agents that gain entry into an organism (Fig. 53.2). Cells of the monocyte-macrophage series, in addition to ingesting or killing foreign material that may or may not have been previously opsonized or coated with antibodies, also play an important regulatory role in both humoral and cellular immune responses.

The distinction between cellular and humoral immunity is in some ways artificial, because both B cells (bone marrow derived) and T cells (thymus derived) can participate in each reaction. For example, although T cells are the effectors of cellular immune responses, they are required for the great majority of humoral (antibody) responses. Although B cells evolve into antibody-producing plasma cells, culminating in the humoral response, they can act as antigen-presenting cells in cellular immune responses. Antibodies can be major participants in specific cytotoxic responses. Thus, the high incidence of anergy to delayed-type hypersensitivity skin testing seen in adults over 60 years of age[3–5] could represent problems with antigen recognition, T-cell proliferation, lymphokine production, lymphocyte or monocyte chemotaxis, vascular responses to inflammatory mediators, or a multitude of other steps that are required to produce induration after an intradermal challenge with antigens. As details of age-related changes in immunity grow in quantity and diversity, it may be easier to broadly categorize them as qualitative or quantitative changes in cell populations and production of or response to macromolecules, rather than as changes in cellular versus humoral immunity.

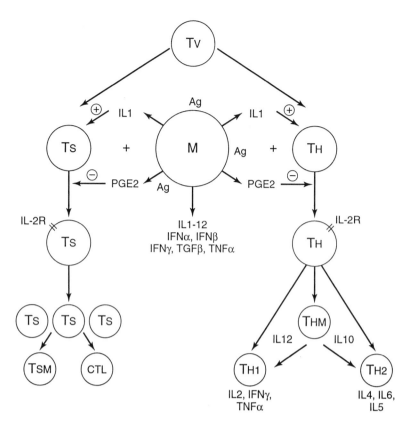

FIGURE 53.1. Model of the cellular immune system. *Ag*, antigen; *CTL*, cytotoxic T lymphocyte; *IFN*, interferon; *IL*, interleukin; *IL-2R*, interleukin-2 receptor; *M*, macrophage/monocyte; *PGE₂*, prostaglandin E₂; *TH*, T-helper (CD4+) lymphocyte; *THM*, T-helper memory lymphocyte; *TS*, T-suppressor (CD8+) lymphocyte; *TSM*, T-suppressor memory lymphocyte; *TV*, virgin T lymphocyte; *TNF*, tumor necrosis factor.

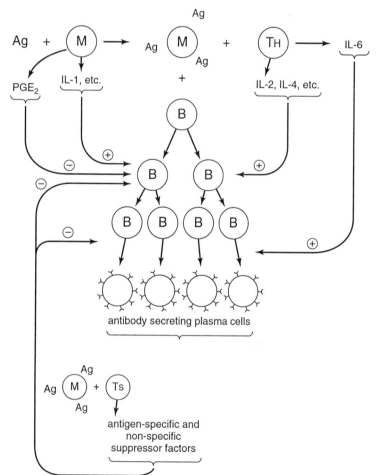

FIGURE 53.2. Model of the humoral immune system. *Ag*, antigen; *B*, B lymphocyte, *BM*, B memory lymphocyte; *IFN*, interferon; *IL*, interleukin; *M*, macrophage/monocyte; *PGE₂*, prostaglandin E₂; *TH*, T-helper (CD4+) lymphocyte; *TS*, T-suppressor (CD8+) lymphocyte; *TSM*, T-suppressor memory lymphocyte.

Changes in Immune Function with Age: Lymphocytes

T Lymphocytes

There are varying reports on quantitative declines in different T-cell populations in aging humans and experimental animals. Studies using monoclonal antibodies to various receptors on T-lymphocyte membranes have shown a consistent decline in "virgin" or reactive T cells and an increase in "memory" or inert T cells in both helper and suppressor cell subpopulations.[2,6–8] Memory T cells from aged individuals produce smaller amounts of interleukin 2 compared to young memory cells, whereas the smaller proportion of virgin T cells produce greater amounts of interleukin 2 than naïve cells from young animals.[9] On a more fundamental level in both animals and humans, there seems to be a loss of stem cell potential to generate T cells.[10,11]

One of the earliest changes reported in qualitative T-lymphocyte function was the decline in proliferative response to mitogens.[3,12,13] In these assays, lymphocytes are isolated from peripheral blood and cultured in media with mitogens, such as phytohemagglutinin (PHA) or pokeweed mitogen, which nonspecifically activate most lymphocytes. The degree of the proliferative response is quantified by adding radiolabeled thymidine to the cultures, harvesting the cells, and measuring the amount of radioactivity incorporated into the lymphocyte DNA. The proliferative response of lymphocytes to specific antigens or nonspecific mitogens is thought to be the in vitro correlate of delayed-type hypersensitivity skin testing. Our study of 300 healthy elderly people showed a substantial decrease in response to phytohemagglutinin (PHA) with age.[4] The mean response of the elderly subjects was significantly less than the mean response of the young control subjects to all mitogen doses. PHA responses were also measured in 24 chronically ill patients over 65 years of age who had a variety of life-threatening medical conditions and who were receiving a number of medications. The responses of this chronically ill group were not different from those of the healthy group. Thus, age per se, and not an accompanying illness, was the major determinant of depressed cellular immunity in this population.

Hyporesponsiveness to mitogens is the sum of several deficiencies.[13] First, the number of mitogen-responsive cells is reduced in lymphocyte preparations from elderly persons. Second, the mitogen-responsive cells from elderly persons do not proliferate as vigorously after exposure to PHA as do lymphocytes from young persons. In old compared to young mice, a smaller percentage of T splenocytes respond to mitogenic stimulation by entering active phases of cell replication.[14] This defect was noted for CD4+ T-helper cells and, to a lesser extent, for CD8+ T-suppressor/cytotoxic cells. The smaller proportion of cells entering active phases of replication is regulated by a balance between genes that stimulate DNA replication and genes which inhibit DNA replication and lead to programmed cell death, or apoptosis.[15,16] Lymphocytes from old donors have a deficit in expression of genes that stimulate DNA synthesis, coupled with decreased proliferative responses.[17,18]

T-helper cells from old mice are less capable of generating cytotoxic effector cells to participate in delayed hypersensitivity reactions.[19] More clinically relevant are studies showing a decreased cytotoxic response to influenza vaccination in old adults, with fewer T-cell subsets able to respond to influenza antigen.[20–22] Old mice are more likely than young mice to develop influenza pneumonia after intranasal inoculation, have impaired cytotoxic T-cell function, and generate ineffective antibody, even in the face of prevaccination.[23] Cytotoxic lymphocytes from aged mice are less able to bind targets, although they appear to be equally effective in destroying their targets.[24]

The role of T-cell lymphocytes in supporting in vitro antibody production appears to change with increasing age. Lymphocytes from older subjects produce greater amounts of IgG and IgM when cultured with pokeweed mitogen than lymphocytes from young control subjects.[25] When lymphocytes are separated into T-cell and B-cell fractions and various combinations of old T cells are cultured with old B cells, old T cells with young B cells, and so on, the old T cells are more capable than the young T cells of supporting immunoglobulin production by either young or old B cells.[26,27] This increased helper activity of the old T cells could result from an actual increase in helper activity or a decrease in suppressor activity. This question was addressed by studying the effects of irradiation of T cells, taking advantage of the fact that suppressor T cells are sensitive to low doses of irradiation whereas helper T cells are relatively radioresistant. Irradiation of T cells from elderly people resulted in smaller increases in immunoglobulin production in subsequent cultures than did irradiation of T cells from young people.[25] This finding suggests that the overall increase in T-cell helper function with age actually was, at least in part, caused by a failure of suppressor cell function.

Failure of tonic inhibition by suppressor T cells is a possible mechanism accounting for the increased incidence of autoimmune antibodies seen in aging. Healthy humans have circulating B cells that are programmed to differentiate into autoantibody-producing plasma cells (producing antinuclear, antithyroid, antimitochondrial, and other antibodies). Suppressor T cells are important in modulating these normal humoral immune responses and preventing the development of autoimmunity. Many investigators have reported an increase in the prevalence of positive tests for various autoantibodies with age (antinuclear antibodies, rheumatoid factors, antithyroid antibodies, antismooth muscle antibodies, and anti-lymphocyte antibodies), with a steep rise in prevalence around 70 years of age.[4,28] The rise in the presence of autoantibodies in elderly persons has been correlated to the decreased ability of T cells to proliferate in response to the mitogen PHA[29] (i.e., the higher the proliferation of T cells to mitogens, the lower was the level of autoantibodies). T-suppressor cells from old adults proliferate less and exert suppressor effects less effectively than those from young adults.[25,30–32] In mice, declines in T-suppressor cell function with age have been associated with the development of oral tolerance.[33] Age-related changes in T lymphocytes are summarized in Table 53.1.

B Lymphocytes

Although the number of circulating B cells does not change appreciably with age,[1] there are alterations in the ratios of surface immunoglobulin and class II molecule expression on the cell surface.[34] Bone marrow precursor cells from old mice are impaired in their ability to generate B cells.[35–37] Similar to studies in T cells, B cells from old individuals proliferate less efficiently, and fewer cells enter active phases of replication.[38,39] Some of the early steps in cell activation are reduced in B cells from old humans[40] (see following).

The functional ability of B cells to mount appropriate antibody responses does change with age.[41] The distinction between antibody responses to T-cell-dependent and T-cell-independent antigens (often made in mice, but less clear in humans) is made on the basis of whether there is an absolute requirement for T-cell help in the antibody response. In experimental animals, the decrease in T-dependent antibody responses is more obvious, with an 80% decrease in antibody-forming cells in older animals.[2,3] The repertoire of B cells appears to change with aging, resulting in an altered ability to recognize

TABLE 53.1. Changes in T lymphocytes with age.

Decreased	Increased
Number of virgin (reactive) T cells	Number of memory (inert) T cells
Number of mitogen-responsive cells	
Stem cell generation of T cells	T-cell help for nonspecific antibody production
Proliferative response	
Expression of early activation genes	
Sensitivity to activating signals	
Cytotoxic cell target binding	
Suppressor cell function	
Help for generation of cytotoxic effector cells	
T-cell help for specific antibody production	

antigens.[32,42] Compared to young animals, old mice develop much larger numbers of immunoglobulin-secreting cells that react with self-antigens after immunization with sheep red blood cells.[43] The accumulation of anti-idiotypes (antibodies directed against other antibodies) with increasing age may also interfere with the production of specific antibody.[44,45]

The ability to respond to a specific antigenic challenge with specific antibody production is decreased in aging.[41,46] Defects in the primary response to flagellin immunization were found in old subjects, who attained similar peak titers of IgG and IgM antibodies but failed to maintain the same levels of IgG antibody over time.[46] We studied a group of 77 healthy older adults not taking any medications who were participating in a larger study of emotions and health behavior. The older adults were less likely to show an in vivo response to immunization with the primary antigen, keyhole limpet hemocyanin, than a group of healthy young control subjects.[47] In contrast, old subjects meeting rigorous health inclusion criteria[48] developed similar numbers of antibody-producing cells after immunization with *Helix pomatia* hemocyanin as did young controls.[49]

Following in vivo immunization, serum antibody levels are significantly lower in old than in young adults.[50–52] The antibody isotypes that are important in the agglutination response against influenza are lower in old adults after immunization.[51] Kishimoto et al.[50] studied specific antitetanus toxoid antibody production and found evidence of declining B-cell function in adults over age 65 years.[50] Purified B cells from elderly or young subjects were cultured with T cells from a young individual who had been immunized with tetanus toxoid a week before. The B cells from the older subjects made significantly less antibody to tetanus toxoid than those from the younger subjects. We also have examined changes in tetanus toxoid-specific antibody production in elderly humans by stimulating lymphocytes from adults of different ages with tetanus toxoid in vitro and measuring the amount of antitetanus toxoid antibody produced.[52] Regardless of the time elapsed since the last booster immunization, the old adults had significantly lower serum levels of antibody to tetanus toxoid. In vitro, old adults had fewer B cells that produced antitetanus toxoid antibody, and each cell produced significantly less antibody than the B cells from young adults. In these studies, the number of antitetanus toxoid precursor cells in the peripheral blood of the older subjects was more than a log magnitude lower than it was in the younger subjects. Thus, the lack of precursor cells with the ability to respond to a specific antigen was primarily responsible for the decreased specific antibody production against tetanus toxoid.[52] Immunizing the subjects with tetanus toxoid led to an increase in the numbers of B cells producing antitetanus toxoid antibody for both age groups. However, the old adults still had sig-

TABLE 53.2. Changes in B cells with age.

Decreased surface MHC class II molecule expression
Decreased proportion of cells capable of clonal expansion
Decreased number of bone marrow precursors
Decreased number of T-cell-dependent antibody-forming cells
Decreased specific antibody production to primary and secondary antigens
Decreased potency
Decreased antigen recognition
Decreased affinity of antibody for targets
Increased anti-idiotypic antibody production

MHC, major histocompatability complex.

nificantly fewer B cells producing specific antibody than did the young adults.[53] Booster immunizations did not alter the mean amount of antibody produced per B cell for either age group.

Although most investigators agree that the observed changes in antibody production are the result of declines in T-lymphocyte function, there is evidence for a decline in intrinsic B-cell function. Findings from our laboratory and others suggest a diminished ability of purified B cells to respond to isolated T-helper cells or to T-cell-derived helper factors.[26,54,55] In old mice, some subsets of B cells function at a much lower level than the same cells from young mice.[56] Compared to young animals, old mice vaccinated with phosphorylcholine generate similar levels of antibody against Streptococcus pneumoniae, but the variable heavy portions of the antibody molecules are different.[57,58] The antibodies produced have lower affinity for the target bacteria and confer less protection.[58,59] Age-related changes in B-cell function are summarized in Table 53.2.

Macrophage Function

Macrophage function in aging has not been as well studied as other lymphocyte subpopulations. Early work suggested that they appear to produce similar levels of cytokines[60,61] and that differences in immune function between age groups may be modulated through changes in T- and B-cell responses to these substances. More recent studies have challenged this concept, showing decreased interleukin 1 secretion with mitogen stimulation.[62] Studies of cutaneous wound healing in old mice also suggest declines in macrophage function with age, as healing took twice as long in old as in young mice.[63] Adding peritoneal macrophages from young and old animals to wounds on old mice sped healing, but macrophages from young mice accelerated the healing process to a greater degree.[63] Studies of the bone marrow in senescence-accelerated mice give some evidence that stem cells are defective in their ability to generate granulocyte-macrophage precursor cells.[64]

There appear to be defects in macrophage–T cell interactions in old animals and humans. Antigenically sensitized macrophages from old mice stimulate significantly lower levels of T-cell proliferation than young macrophages.[65] Dendritic cells (fixed macrophages) from old adults are significantly compromised in their ability to stimulate formation of germinal centers in lymph follicles where B-cell memory develops.[66] By replacing macrophages with other sources of activation, T cells from old adults are able to function at the same level as young T cells, suggesting that the defect may lay in macrophage–T cell communication.[67] Monocytes from old adults display lower cytotoxicity against some tumor cell lines and produce lower levels of reactive oxygen intermediates and lower levels of interleukin 1.[62,68]

Natural Killer Cell Function

Natural killer cells (NK) are cytotoxic cells that are able to lyse targets without the need for antigenic sensitization, differentiating them from cytotoxic T cells. Lymphokine-activated killer cells (LAK cells) are thought to be highly activated NK, and are able to lyse certain cell lines that are resistant to NK. Murine NK show an age-related decline in their ability to lyse spleen cells.[69,70] Most early studies showed little change in NK cytotoxic ability with age,[71] in contrast to more recent work. The actual number of NK cells seems to increase with age, while cytotoxic activity decreases,[72,73] probably due to increased expression of receptors that downregulate activity.[74] There may also be differential requirements for maximal activation of NK by interferon-alpha, with young cells showing maximal responses at lower concentrations of this cytokine.[75] Old adults with a deficiency of growth hormone have less active NK, which can be partially restored in vitro by exposing cells to the hormone's precursor protein.[76] The activity of LAK also may be reduced in aged compared to young humans.[71,75]

Lymphocyte DNA

X chromosomes of T cells from old adults are more fragile than those from young adults,[77] and certain sites on the X chromosome have been shown to be more sensitive to chemical insults. Humans over age 55 exposed to radiation in vivo have lymphocytes that mount poor cellular responses as opposed to humans exposed to radiation when under the age of 15.[78] These results may reflect the increased susceptibility of the aging immune system to radiation. When examining the sensitivity of lymphocyte DNA to irradiation, there were actually fewer breaks in double-stranded DNA in lymphocytes from old adults, but the cells had a significantly reduced ability to repair these breaks compared to lymphocytes from young donors.[79] Other investigators have looked at sister chromatid exchange, a measure of DNA damage, in healthy old individuals and newborns.[80] The basal frequency of sister chromatic exchange was 10 times greater in lymphocytes from the old subjects.

Cell Activation and Membrane Signal Transduction

The proliferative response of T cells to various stimuli results from a complex set of interactions involving T cells and macrophages or other accessory cells. Mitogens such as PHA bind to, cross-link with, and thereby activate the T-cell antigen receptor; this results in activation of phospholipase C, cleavage of membrane phosphatidylinositol phosphates, and liberation of inositol bisphosphate and diacylglycerol. Inositol bisphosphate and its metabolites, inositol triphosphate and tetrakisphosphate, raise intracellular free calcium concentrations by releasing bound calcium from intracellular stores and by opening calcium channels.[81–83] Diacylglycerol binds to and activates protein kinase C, which is further activated by the increased free calcium concentration. At least two families of protein kinases, protein phosphate kinases and protein tyrosine kinases, play a role in cell activation.

Protein kinase activation stimulates transcription and subsequent translation of the gene coding for interleukin 2 (also known as T-cell growth factor) and also of receptors for interleukin 2. Interleukin 2 is thus an autocrine growth factor, produced by the same cells that respond to it. Exposure of interleukin 2 receptor-bearing T cells to interleukin 2 results in proliferation. Monocytes assist T cells in producing and responding to interleukin 2 by presenting antigen that occupies and cross-links T-cell receptors. The antigen-presenting cells secrete a variety of cytokines that provide additional signals necessary for complete T-cell activation. A model of T-cell activation is shown in Figure 53.3.

Several laboratories have investigated whether the decreased proliferative response of lymphocytes from old animals and adults is due to impaired membrane signal transduction in response to various stimuli. Investigations using mouse T cells have found an association between decreased calcium metabolism and defective proliferation in some strains with old age.[6,84] When T cells from old mice are stimulated with mitogens, the rise in intracellular calcium is generally lower than that seen in cells from young mice.[85] Although no change in inositol triphosphate levels was observed in these studies, it was reduced in a different assay system using human peripheral blood neutrophils.[86]

Those T lymphocytes from old mice that retain the ability to proliferate to PHA have normal or enhanced mobilization of calcium compared to cells from young animals.[87] Work with human peripheral blood lymphocytes and isolated T cells has shown contrasting results, indicating that decreased calcium mobilization was a factor in some T-cell subpopulations but not others.[2,33,88]

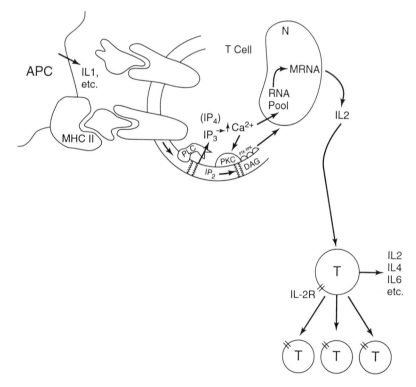

FIGURE 53.3. Model of T-cell activation. *APC*, antigen-presenting cell; *Ca²⁺*, calcium ion; *DAG*, diacylglycerol; *IL*, interleukin; *IL-2R*, interleukin-2 receptor; *IP2*, inositol biphosphate; *IP3*, inositol triphosphate; *MHC II*, major histocompatibility complex molecule; *mRNA*, messenger RNA; *N*, nucleus; *PKC*, protein kinase C; *PLC* phospholipase C; *PPK*, protein phosphate kinase; *PTK*, protein tyrosine kinase.

Compared to young donors, monocyte-depleted lymphocytes from old donors displayed decreased cell–cell binding, a calcium/magnesium-dependent interaction.[89]

Other steps in the signal transduction cascade are altered with aging. Protein kinase activation by mitogens is significantly reduced in cells from old humans.[90] In particular, levels of protein kinase C-alpha are reduced,[91] as well as the level of phosphorylation of the protein phosphokinases[92] and protein tyrosine kinases.[93] The activation of protein kinase C and the protein tyrosine kinases also appears to be reduced in B cells from old humans.[40] The transcription of nuclear factors is also decreased, and correlates with reduced production of interleukin 2.[95]

Production of and Response to Immunoregulatory Factors

Many of the changes in cell function already described may be secondary to age-related changes in sensitivity to a variety of other endogenously produced substances. For example, circulating trough cortisol levels appear to increase with age,[96] resulting in a flattening of the amplitude of diurnal variation of this hormone. Altered sensitivity to glucocorticoids may contribute to poor responses of aged mice to novel immunogens.[97]

Prostaglandins

Arachidonic acid metabolites have been implicated in age-related changes in humoral immunity. Prostaglandin E_2 is a feedback inhibitor of T-cell proliferation in humans,[98] and T cells from adults over 70 years of age are much more sensitive to inhibition by prostaglandin E_2.[99,100] Thus, prostaglandin E_2 may interfere with the expansion of antigen-specific T-cell helper clones. Recent studies have shown not only greater depression of proliferation and interleukin 2 production in T cells from old mice, but also age-related increases in production of prostaglandin E_2 by splenocytes from old mice compared to young mice.[101,102] Old macrophages produce more cyclooxygenase, the enzyme that metabolizes arachidonic acid into prostaglandins.[103]

Increased sensitivity to prostaglandin E_2 was the cause of an impaired primary antibody response of lymphocytes from older adults that were cultured with trinitrophenylated polyacrylamide beads.[60] Removing monocytes (the source of prostaglandin E_2 production) or adding drugs that blocked the production of prostaglandin E_2 partially reversed the depressed response of lymphocytes from older subjects.[60,99] In contrast, other investigators have not found increased prostaglandin production by unstimulated or mitogen-stimulated lymphocytes from old versus young donors,

nor suppression of nonspecific antibody production by prostaglandin.[104]

The increased sensitivity with age to prostaglandin E_2 would not appear to be part of a general increase in sensitivity to all immunomodulators. Lymphocytes from subjects over 70 years of age actually are less sensitive to inhibition by histamine and hydrocortisone than are lymphocytes from young control subjects.[100]

Interleukins

Accessory cells such as monocytes help T cells produce and respond to interleukin 2 by cross-linking T-cell receptors. They secrete interleukin 1 and other monokines that provide additional signals necessary for complete activation of T cells (see Fig. 53.3). The response to interleukin 2 has been extensively studied as one mechanism underlying the age-related defect in cellular immunity. Several laboratories have demonstrated decreased production of interleukin 2 after mitogen stimulation and a decreased density of interleukin 2 receptor expression and decreased proliferation of these cells in response to interleukin 2.[22,105–108] Additional experiments in rodents suggest that the picture might be more complex, with specific defects in production of or sensitivity to interleukin 2, depending on the immunologic stimulus.[109,110] Other investigators have shown that lymphocytes from aged rats are defective in their ability to express messenger RNA for interleukin 2.[111] Some studies have found no differences in T-cell proliferation or interleukin 2 production when stimulating memory T cells from old and young donors.[112] Helper T cells from old mice accumulated similar levels of interleukin 2 transcripts, although they secreted lower levels of interleukin 2.[113] Studies at the molecular level suggest that induction of interleukin 2 involves activation of a complex cascade of cell receptors and gene families.[114] The somewhat conflicting results may be explained by the different systems and substances utilized by different investigators, resulting in differential activation at various steps in the activation pathway.

Interleukins 1 and 2 play a role in activation, recruitment, and proliferation of T lymphocytes. These activated T cells go on to produce a variety of cytokines including B-cell growth and differentiation factors such as interleukin 4, interleukin 6, and gamma-interferon. Experiments with rodents provide evidence that lymphocyte production and response to other cytokines, such as interleukin 1 and tumor necrosis factor, are also defective in aging.[2,115] Monocytes from old adults secrete less interleukin 1 when stimulated with the mitogen lipopolysaccharide, although they produce comparable amounts of interleukin 1 precursor.[68] When lymphocytes from old adults are mixed with cells from other donors, they produce higher levels of interleukin 1, interleukin 2, and tumor necrosis factor-alpha (TNF-α) than cells from young adults.[116] In vivo circulating levels of interleukin 1 may increase with age.[117]

In some studies, lymphocytes from old animals display a lower stimulatory response than when interleukin 4 is added to lymphocytes from young mice,[118] and B-cell proliferation to interleukin 4 and anti-IgM is significantly lower in old mice than in young mice.[119] Memory T cells from old mice produce less interleukin 4 than memory cells from young mice.[120] We have shown that lymphocytes from old adults produce less interleukin 4 when stimulated by specific antigen than lymphocytes from young adults, and are less sensitive to inhibition of specific antibody production when interleukin 4 is added early in the course of stimulation with specific antigen.[121] This finding is similar to findings in murine models.[122] Again, seemingly contradictory findings have been reported in other systems, with either similar or increased production of interleukin 4 by aged cells[117,123] and higher percentages of aged cells participating in production of interleukin 4.[124]

Interferon-gamma (IFN-γ) can have a differential effect on NK activity, depending on the age of the donor.[75] NK cells from old adults secreted less IFN-γ than those from young adults.[125] Lymphocytes from old rats produced smaller amounts of IFN and interleukin 2 when stimulated with concanavalin A.[126] Others found no relationship between the degree of lymphocyte proliferation to mitogen and the production of IFN-γ.[127] In this system, cells from old donors were more sensitive to IFN-γ and interleukin 2. Several other investigators have reported increased IFN-γ mRNA[128] and IFN-γ production by old T cells and lymphocytes.[128–130]

Several investigators have described elevated in vivo blood levels of interleukin 6 in old mice, monkeys, and adults[131–133] whereas some found no differences.[134] In vitro, peritoneal macrophages from old mice stimulated with the mitogen lipopolysaccharide, and human B cells, produce higher levels of interleukin 6 than macrophages from young mice.[135] Interleukin 6 levels are elevated in 24-h, unstimulated culture supernates of lymphocytes from murine spleen and lymph nodes and in peripheral blood mononuclear cells from old humans compared to their young counterparts.[131] Other investigators did not find differences in interleukin 6 production in vitro.[123] Newer investigations utilizing flow cytometry have detected greater intracellular increase in interleukin 6 in T cells from old versus young donors.[117,136,137]

Production of interleukin 8 (neutrophil chemoattractant) by old lymphocytes may be decreased, although this unresponsiveness was observed primarily in cells from male donors.[138] Interleukin 5 has been little studied with aging, but at least one study has reported increased production by lymphocytes from old mice.[139]

The balance between interleukins 10 and 12 is important in determining different patterns of cytokine secretion, with interleukin 10 leading to production of cytokines stimulating B-cell differentiation and antibody production and interleukin 12 leading to production of cytokines stimulating cytotoxic T cells and a cellular immune response (see Fig. 53.3). Cells from old humans have been reported to produce greater levels of interleukin 10 than cells from young humans.[117,140] The increased susceptibility of old mice to infection with *Mycobacterium tuberculosis* is associated with lower levels of interleukin 12 production in the lung.[141] There appears to be a delay in the emergence of IFN-γ-secreting T cells, and these cells are slower in expressing surface adhesion markers that allow migration across endothelial linings to sites of active infection.[142] Other cytokine alterations may contribute to increased spread of the disease in old animals.[143] T cells from young mice are able to protect old mice from infection, suggesting that old macrophages function adequately.[144,145]

At this point, it is unclear which of the age-related changes in cytokine production is the most critical. The defects in interleukin 2 production may well account for some of the fundamental changes in lymphocyte function and have been linked to increased susceptibility to disease. It might be that changes in *patterns* of cytokine production are more important, as these patterns induce commitment to a TH 1 (cellular) response as opposed to a TH 2 (humoral) response. There continue to be conflicting reports as to which pathways are predominant in normal aging.[146,147] Age-related changes in interleukins are summarized in Table 53.3.

Stress, Immunity, and Aging

It has long been known that stress affects the occurrence of disease. Investigators in the field of physiologic psychology have described complex and direct links between the perceptual capabilities of the central nervous system and the immune system. For example, it is possible to elicit specific immune responses in animals with sensory cues. Ader and Cohen have performed a series of elegant taste-aversion learning experiments in rats.[148] In one of these studies, a flavored substance, saccharin water, was administered to the animals along with a dose of cyclophosphamide. Several days later, the animals were injected with sheep red blood cells, with or without readministration of the saccharin solution. Animals given the saccharin had profound suppression of the hemagglutination response to the sheep red blood cells.

The neurohumorally mediated effects of stress on the immune system have been well demonstrated in carefully controlled experiments with animals.[149] In primates, levels of cortisol and complement factors are profoundly affected by a single stressful event.[150] Studies in humans have demonstrated similar effects, although it is impossi-

TABLE 53.3. Changes in interleukins with age.

Decreased	Increased or unchanged
Expression of IL-2 mRNA	In vivo levels of IL-6
Proportion of cells expressing IL-2R	Nonspecific stimulation of T-cell IL-4 and IL-6
High-affinity binding sites for IL-2	Nonspecific stimulation of T-cell IFN-gamma and IFN-gamma mRNA
T-cell production/secretion of IL-2	Memory T-cell production of IL-2
T-cell proliferative response to IL-2	Lymphocyte production of IL-1 in MLC
Memory T-cell production of IL-4	Lymphocyte production of IL-5?
Sensitivity to IL-4	Lymphocyte production of IL-10
B-cell sensitivity to IL-4	
Nonspecific stimulation of lymphocyte-produced IL-8	
Monocyte secretion of IL-1	
IL-2-stimulated NK production of IFN	
IL-12 production in TB-infected mouse lungs	

IL, interleukin; mRNA, messenger RNA; IL-2R, IL-2 receptor; IFN, interferon; MLC, mixed lymphocyte culture; NK, natural killer cells; TB, tuberculosis.

ble to achieve the same degree of control as in the animal studies. Correlational studies have found that clusters of illness (from the common cold to cancer) occur around the time of major life changes.[151] Others have found strong correlations between loneliness and decreased proliferative responses of lymphocytes to mitogens, decreased natural killer cell activity, and impaired DNA splicing and repair in lymphocytes.[151,152] We found that healthy adults over the age of 60 years with a strong social support system (i.e., a close confidant) had significantly lower serum uric acid levels and cholesterol levels, greater total lymphocyte counts, and a stronger immune response (mitogen-induced proliferation of lymphocytes) than those without such a relationship.[153] Indeed, being married has been correlated with lower mortality from any cause, in contrast to being single, widowed, or divorced.[154]

Quasi-experimental or "natural" experiments also have linked stress to depressed immune function and illness. Depressed lymphocyte proliferation in response to mitogens after bereavement has been described.[155] The stress of final examinations has been correlated with the recurrence of herpes simplex type 1 cold sores and rises in serum antibody titers against the virus[156] and with decreased proliferation of memory T cells.[157] Persons experiencing the stress of caring for a spouse with dementia have poorer antibody responses to influenza vaccination than age- and sex-matched controls.[158] Their lymphocytes make less interleukin 1-beta and interleukin 2 when exposed to influenza virus in vitro.[158] The caregivers also showed delayed wound healing after skin punch biopsy compared to controls.[159]

Old age is associated with a greater frequency of major life changes, such as loss of spouse or close friends and changes in lifestyle resulting from retirement. Because of the decreased reserve in immune function with aging, elderly persons may be more sensitive to the effects of such stressful life events.

Immunologic Function, Morbidity, and Mortality

Despite vigorous investigation in the field of immunology, evidence that links depressed or disordered immune function in humans directly to subsequent morbidity or mortality is still scarce. There certainly is evidence that disruption of immune function can result in serious disease, of which the AIDS epidemic is a glaring example. The question of whether decreased immune responses contribute to morbidity and mortality in elderly persons has been addressed by looking for associations between abnormalities in a particular immune response and health status. Several studies have found an association between the response to delayed-type hypersensitivity skin tests and mortality. Elderly subjects who are anergic (responding poorly or not at all to a battery of antigens placed intradermally) have an increased risk of mortality compared to elderly subjects who respond well to one or more of these antigens.[3,160] In our studies of healthy elderly individuals in New Mexico, approximately one-third were anergic at initial testing.[4] The anergic group had about a twofold higher mortality rate and also a twofold higher incidence of pneumonia during 8 years of follow-up.[160]

A similar study examined the in vitro correlate of delayed hypersensitivity skin testing, lymphocyte proliferation in response to mitogens, in a group of 403 adults over the age of 65 years.[12] In this group of community-living adults seen in an outpatient geriatric clinic, 18% had lymphocytes that did not respond to any of three mitogens. A 3-year follow-up found a significantly greater mortality rate among those with no response than among those with a positive response, 26% versus 13%. The increase in overall mortality was not due to an increase in one particular cause of death, such as infection or malignancy, and this increase remained significant after the investigators controlled for medication use, an indirect indicator of health. Clarkson and Alexander demonstrated that vasectomies led to accelerated atherosclerosis in monkeys who were fed a high-fat diet.[174] Monkeys who were vasectomized and maintained on a very low fat, no-cholesterol diet still had an increased incidence of atherosclerosis at autopsy 9 to 14 years later compared with nonvasectomized control monkeys.[174] Thus, a very mild stimulus for autoantibody formation leads to accelerated atherosclerosis even without an atherogenic diet. This evidence provides a strong theoretic basis for proposing that autoantibodies and the resultant circulating immune complexes in humans, by causing a low level of chronic irritation in blood vessels, contribute to the development of atherosclerosis. Indeed, histologic examination of atherosclerotic blood vessels from humans reveals increased lymphocyte and cytokine infiltration in areas of plaque formation.[176]

There are epidemiologic data supporting a link between autoimmunity and atherosclerosis in humans. Mackay and his colleagues found an association between the presence of autoantibodies and the presence of cardiovascular diseases in the adult population of Busselton, Australia.[177] The presence of autoantibodies in the same adults was associated with an increased risk of death due to vascular disease and cancer during 6 years of follow-up.[177]

Reversal of Age-Related Immunodeficiency: Mechanistic Theories

Studies of substances that reverse age-related immunodeficiencies suggest mechanisms that might underlie these changes. One point to keep in mind is that different physiologic systems can display different levels of defect within a single individual and do not appear to be synchronized with each other.[2,45] Immunomodulating substances may affect only some systems and not others. A few more recent studies have added weight to the association between age-related declines in immune measures and mortality.[4,160–163]

As mentioned earlier, one function of the immune system may be to protect against the development of cancer. Early theories of "immune surveillance" proposed that the cellular arm of the immune system was constantly surveying for and eliminating malignancies and that the development of cancer represented a failure of this system.[164–166] If this is indeed the case, elderly persons or those with depressed immune function should have a higher incidence of malignancy. Indeed, advanced age is one of the strongest risk factors for the development of cancer.[167,168] However, the lack of a generalized increase in most malignancies among immunosuppressed

individuals has thrown this theory into relative disrepute.[161] However, there continue to be observations in animal models of cancer that link age-related immune changes to malignant progress, particularly malignant transformation of B cells.[169–171] It is most likely that age-related changes in immune function influence the expression and progression of malignancy, rather than acting as a direct cause of cancer.

Other evidence that links disordered immune function to disease and death concerns the possible role of autoantibodies and circulating immune complexes in the etiology of atherosclerosis. It has been recognized for many years that circulating immune complexes produced by repeated injections of a foreign antigen can cause an acute arteritis. There is also evidence suggesting that the chronic atherosclerosis associated with the acute autoimmune arteritis is exacerbated by an atherogenic diet.[172,173] The links between autoimmunity and atherosclerosis have been demonstrated in primates, as well as in rodents.[174,175] Vasectomy is a mild stimulus for autoantibody and circulating immune complex formation, with antisperm antibodies developing in about 50% of all vasectomized human males and experimental animals.[175] Associated with declines in T-cell function, is the involution of the thymus with subsequent loss of thymic hormone influences.[178] Thymic lymphatic mass, particularly in the cortical area, decreases with age in humans and experimental animals, starting in adolescence. The thymic mass of aging humans and experimental animals is approximately 10% that of a younger thymus.[179] In spite of this involutional process, the remaining thymic tissue from old animals maintains its ability to generate new T cells.[180]

Associated with the loss of thymic mass is a decreased output of thymic hormones, such as thymosin.[179] Exposing lymphocytes of old individuals to thymic hormones either in vivo or in vitro has resulted in at least partial restoration of immunity on a temporary basis.[181–185] Administering thymopentin to aged mice increased their resistance to cutaneous *Leishmania* infection.[186]

Several other hormonal substances whose in vivo production declines with age have been studied for their potential to reverse age-related immune dysfunction. Melatonin, a pineal hormone with free radical-scavenging, antioxidant properties, displays age-related declines in production.[187] Administration of melatonin to old mice increases antibody production, T-helper cell activity and interleukin 2 production.[188] Administering interleukin 2 and melatonin to humans before surgical treatment of gastrointestinal cancer resulted in increased numbers of lymphocytes, T cells, and T-helper cells after surgery.[189] Perhaps more clinically relevant, the combination of interleukin 2 and melatonin appeared to result in at least partial tumor regression and enhanced 1-year survival of patients with some metastatic solid tumors compared to supportive care alone.[190]

Growth hormone and its precursor, insulin-like growth factor 1, have immunoenhancing effects, including stimulation of phagocytes and production of cytokines, which may help protect against bacterial infection.[191] Old patients with growth hormone deficiency have lower NK activity, and this can be partially restored by exposing NK cells to the precursor protein in vitro.[76] By contrast, administering growth hormone to healthy old women for 6 months did not change proliferative responses of lymphocytes or the mean number of virgin T cells compared with untreated controls.[192]

Dehydroepiandrosterone (DHEA), the most abundantly produced adrenal steroid, is another substance whose endogenous levels appear to decline with age. When DHEA is administered in vivo, it augments antibody production by upregulation of T-cell subsets associated with increased antibody production.[193] When aged mice are pretreated with DHEA, they display enhanced responses to vaccination with hepatitis B surface antigen and influenza vaccination, as well as increased resistance to infection with influenza.[194,195] Old humans who received oral DHEA before influenza vaccination displayed a fourfold increase in hemagglutinin inhibition titers compared to untreated elderly individuals.[196]

Often the most intriguing scientific discoveries are those that also are without an obvious practical consequence. An early example was the discovery by McCay and his colleagues in 1935 that caloric restriction of experimental animals markedly prolonged their life span.[197] Restricting total caloric intake to 50% to 60% of that which is required to maintain normal growth in adolescent mice, rats, and guinea pigs resulted in approximately 50% prolongation of the total life span of animals that survived the 6- to 12-month period of restriction. This interesting medical oddity received little attention over the next three decades until other investigators showed that the early starvation of experimental animals resulted in a preservation of normal immune function into old age.[198] Similar effects have been observed with lesser degrees of caloric restriction.[199,200] In contrast to the studies on protein-calorie restriction in animals, nutritional deficiencies in humans are generally associated with poor immune responses.[201] In both nutritionally deficient and healthy elderly adults, caloric supplements and supplementation with vitamins and trace elements have been associated with enhanced immune responses, better responses to vaccines, and fewer days of infectious illness.[202,203] Rasmussen et al. provided "reverse" support for the role of nutrition in immunocompromise by noting significant declines in NK activity in older men ingesting a diet high in polyunsaturated fatty acids.[204]

There has been a tremendous upsurge in interest in antioxidants as potential "antiaging" treatments. Much of this interest is based on solid laboratory-based and epidemiologic and clinical evidence. Some of the most intriguing data involve the effects of vitamin E administration on immune function in old experimental animals and, more recently, in older men and women.[205,206] Supplementation with 400 to 800 U of vitamin E in healthy elderly subjects results in improved immune parameters such as response to delayed-type hypersensitivity skin testing and increased production of interleukin 2 in vitro.[207,208] Vitamin E may cause these effects via inhibition of suppressive factors such as prostaglandin E_2.[205] The most dramatic demonstration of antioxidant effects was in a report by Chandra, who conducted a placebo-controlled, double-blinded trial of supplementation of healthy older men and women with a multiple vitamin containing the recommended daily allowance for most vitamins with the exception of vitamin E and beta carotene, which were at about four times the upper quartile of usual intakes.[203] Supplementation was associated with marked increases in various parameters of immunity. More importantly, the supplemented group had only half the number of days with infection and 60% of days taking antibiotics during the 1-year trial.[203] If these remarkable results can be reproduced in other populations, it will have major implications for recommendations on appropriate intake of the antioxidant vitamins. Although two large studies looking at antioxidant supplementation found a higher incidence of lung cancer in heavy smokers taking beta carotene, vitamin E supplementation was not related to an increased incidence of lung cancer.[209,210]

Another potential means of reversing or improving age-related declines in immunity is by administering drugs that stimulate immune function in one way or another. Prostaglandin synthetase inhibitors, such as the nonsteroidal antiinflammatory drugs (NSAIDs), reduce production of the feedback inhibitor prostaglandin E_2 and stimulate immune responses both in vitro and in vivo.[98] For example, two of our patients with an adult-acquired immunodeficiency who were completely anergic became responsive to delayed-type hypersensitivity skin testing when they were treated with the cyclooxygenase inhibitor indomethacin.[211] Aspirin administration enhanced specific antibody production to A/Beijing after influenza immunization in adults over the age of 75.[212] Such therapeutic strategies might be especially relevant to elderly persons, whose T cells are more sensitive to inhibition by prostaglandin E_2.[99] Other evidence suggests that prostaglandin synthetase inhibitors can also stimulate the primary antibody response to novel antigens[60] and might reduce the increase in autoantibody production that occurs with age.[213]

Investigations studying stress-induced suppression of immune function have explored the effects of psychologic interventions on the same measures of immunity.

Writing about traumatic events, and simple relaxation exercises, have been associated with enhanced immune responses, although the duration of the benefit is unknown.[214,215] The mechanisms underlying such associations are not fully understood.

Another theoretical explanation for age-related immune decline involves the role of cellular oncogenes and antioncogenes in aging. Over long periods of time, the activation of oncogenes, and loss of tumor suppressive genes, have been associated with the progression of malignant lesions.[216] These genes are thus postulated to play a role in the development of malignancies by their regulation of cell growth and differentiation. In vitro experiments in which hybrids are created between senescent cells and immortalized cell lines lead to finite life spans of the hybrids, a property thought to be controlled by antioncogenes.[217] Thus, antioncogenes may play a role in immune senescence by regulating programmed cell death.

The foregoing examples of immunostimulation are representative of the many therapies that have been proposed or tested to reverse age-related immune decline. Although it is difficult to justify medical intervention in a healthy individual with a disordered laboratory parameter (such as chronic nonsteroidal anti-inflammatory use in an individual with low PHA response or skin test anergy), the studies of nutrition and immunity, and stress and immunity, suggest the possibility of more benign interventions that may have a significant impact on the health status of elderly individuals.

References

1. Makinodan T. Biology of aging: retrospect and prospect. In: Makinodan T, Yunis E, eds. *Immunology and Aging.* New York: Plenum Press; 1977:1–8.
2. Miller RA. Aging and immune function. *Int Rev Cytol.* 1991;124:187–215.
3. Roberts-Thompson IC, Whittingham S, Young-Chaiyud U, et al. Aging, immune response and mortality. *Lancet.* 1974; 2:368–370.
4. Goodwin JS, Searles RP, Tung KSK. Immunological responses of a healthy elderly population. *Clin Exp Immunol.* 1982;48:403–410.
5. Hess EV, Knapp D. The immune system and aging: a case of the cart before the horse. *J Chronic Dis.* 1978;31:647–649.
6. Philosophe B, Miller RA. Diminished calcium signal generation in subsets of T lymphocytes that predominate in old mice. *J Gerontol.* 1990;45:B87–B93.
7. Jackola DR, Ruger JK, Miller RA. Age-associated changes in human T cell phenotype and function. *Aging.* 1994; 6:25–34.
8. Miller RA. Age-related changes in T cell surface markers: a longitudinal analysis in genetically heterogeneous mice. *Mech Ageing Dev.* 1997;96:181–196.
9. Dobber R, Tielemans M, Nagelkerken L. Enrichment for Th1 cells in the Mel-14+ CD4+ T cell fraction in aged mice. *Cell Immunol.* 1995;162:321–325.
10. Leclercq G, Plum J, Nandi D, Smedt M, Allison JP. Intrathymic differentiation of V gamma 3 T cells. *J Exp Med.* 1993; 178:309–315.
11. Offner F, Kerre T, De Smedt M, Plum J. Bone marrow CD34+ cells generate fewer T cells in vitro with increasing age and following chemotherapy. *Br J Haematol.* 1999; 104:801–808.
12. Murasko DM, Weiner P, Kaye D. Association of lack of mitogen-induced lymphocyte proliferation with increased mortality in the elderly. *Aging Immunol Infect Dis.* 1988; 1:1–6.
13. Inkeles B, Innes JB, Kuntz MM, et al. Immunological studies of aging. III. Cytokinetic basis for the impaired response of lymphocytes from aged humans to plant lectins. *JP Exp Med.* 1977;145:1176–1187.
14. Ernst DN, Weigle WO, McQuitty DN, Rothermel AL, Hobbs MV. Stimulation of murine T cell subsets with anti-CD3 antibody: age-related defects in the expression of early activation molecules. *J Immunol.* 1989;142:1413–1421.
15. Garkavtsev I, Hull C, Riabowol K. Molecular aspects of the relationship between cancer and aging: tumor suppressor activity during cellular senescence. *Exp Geronol.* 1998;33:81–94.
16. Levine AJ. p53, the cellular gatekeeper for growth and division. *Cell.* 1997;88:323–331.
17. VanAman SE, Whisler RL. Differential expression of p53 tumor suppressor protein and IL-2 in activated T cells from elderly humans. *J Interferon Cytokine Res.* 1998;18: 315–320.
18. Ohkusu-Tsukada K, Tsukada T, Isobe K. Accelerated development and aging of the immune system in p53-deficient mice. *J Immunol.* 1999;163:1966–1972.
19. Vissinga C, Nagelkerken L, Sijlstra J, Hertogh-Huijbregts A, Boersma W, Rozing J. A decreased functional capacity of CD4+ T cells underlies the impaired DTH reactivity in old mice. *Mech Ageing Dev.* 1990;53:127–139.
20. Fagiolo U, Amadori A, Cozzi E, et al. Humoral and cellular immune response to influenza virus vaccination in aged humans. *Aging.* 1993;5:451–458.
21. Swenson CD, Cherniack EP, Russo C, Thorbecke GJ. IgD-receptor up-regulation on human peripheral blood T cells in response to IgD in vitro or antigen in vivo correlates with the antibody response to influenza vaccination. *Eur J Immunol.* 1996;26:340–344.
22. McElhaney JE, Beattie BL, Devine R, et al. Age-related decline in interleukin 2 production in response to influenza vaccine. *J Am Geriatr Soc.* 1990;38:652–658.
23. Ben-Yehuda A, Ehleiter D, Hu AR, Weksler ME. Recombinant vaccinia virus expressing the PR/8 influenza hemagglutinin gene overcomes the impaired immune response and increased susceptibility of old mice to influenza infection. *J Infect Dis.* 1993;168:352–357.
24. Gottesman SRS, Edington J. Proliferative and cytotoxic immune functions in aging mice. V. Deficiency in generation of cytotoxic cells with normal lytic function per cell as demonstrated by the single cell conjugation assay. *Aging Immunol Infect Dis.* 1990;2:19–29.

25. Kishimoto S, Tomino S, Mitsuya H, et al. Age-related changes in suppressor functions of human T cells. *J Immunol.* 1979;123:1586–1592.

26. Rodriguez MA, Cueppens JL, Goodwin JS. Regulation of IgM rheumatoid factor production in lymphocyte cultures from young and old subjects. *J Immunol.* 1989;128:2422–2428.

27. Crawford J, Oates S, Wolfe LA, Cohen HJ. An in vitro analogue of immune dysfunction with altered immunoglobulin production in the aged. *J Am Geriatr Soc.* 1989;37:1141–1146.

28. Delespesse G, Gausset PH, Sarfati M, et al. Circulating immune complexes in old people and in diabetics: correlation with autoantibodies. *Clin Exp Immunol.* 1980;40:96–102.

29. Hallgren H, Buckley C, Gilbertson V, et al. Lymphocyte phytohemagglutinin responsiveness, immunoglobulins, and autoantibodies in aging humans. *J Immunol.* 1973;111:1101–1107.

30. Grossmann A, Ledbetter JA, Rabinovitch PS. Reduced proliferation in T lymphocytes in aged humans is predominantly in the CD8+ subset and is unrelated to defects in transmembrane signaling which are predominantly in the CD4+ subsets. *Exp Cell Res.* 1989;180:367–382.

31. Doria G, Mancini C, Frasca D, Adorini L. Age restriction in antigen-specific immunosuppression. *J Immunol.* 1987;139:1419–1425.

32. Russo C, Cherniak EP, Wali A, Weksler ME. Age-dependent appearance of non-major histocompatibility complex-restricted helper T cells. *Proc Natl Acad Sci USA.* 1993;90:11718–11722.

33. Kawanishi H, Ajitsu S, Mirabella S. Impaired humoral immune responses to mycobacterial antigen in aged murine gut-associated lymphoid tissues. *Mech Ageing Dev.* 1990;54:143–161.

34. Callard R, Basten A, Blanden R. Loss of immune competence with age may be due to a qualitative abnormality in lymphocyte membranes. *Nature.* 1979;281:218–221.

35. Zharhary D. Age-related changes in the capability of the bone marrow to generate B cells. *J Immunol.* 1988;141:1863–1869.

36. Ben-Yehuda A, Szabo P, Dyall R, Weksler ME. Bone marrow declines as a site of B-cell precursor differentiation with age: relationship to thymus involution. *Proc Natl Acad Sci USA.* 1994;91:11988–11992.

37. Viale AC, Chies JA, Huetz F, et al. VH-gene family dominance in aging mice. *Scand J Immunol.* 1994;39:184–188.

38. Hara H, Negoro S, Miyata S, Saiki O, et al. Age-associated changes in proliferative and differentiative response of human B cells and production of T cell-derived factors regulating B cell functions. *Mech Ageing Dev.* 1987;38:245–258.

39. Stephan RP, Lill-Elghanian DA, Witte PL. Development of B cells in aged mice. *J Immunol.* 1997;158:1298–1609.

40. Whisler RL, Grants IS. Age-related alterations in the activation and expression of phosphotyrosine kinases and protein kinase C (PKC) among human B cells. *Mech Ageing Devel* 1993;71:31–46.

41. Delafuente JC. Immunosenescence: clinical and pharmacologic considerations. *Med Clin N Am.* 1985;69:475–486.

42. Schwab R, Russo C, Weksler ME. Altered major histocompatibility complex-restricted antigen recognition by T cells from elderly humans. *Eur J Immunol.* 1992;22:2989–2993.

43. Zhao KS, Wang YF, Gueret R, Weksler ME. Dysregulation of the humoral immune response in old mice. *Int Immunol.* 1995;7:929–934.

44. Arreaza EE, Gibbons JJ Jr, Siskind GW, Weksler ME. Lower antibody response to tetanus toxoid associated with higher auto-anti-idiotypic antibody in old compared with young humans. *Clin Exp Immunol.* 1993;92:169–173.

45. Cinader B, Thorbecke GJ. Aging and the immune system. Report on workshop 94 held during the 7th International Congress of Immunology in Berlin on August 3, 1989. *Aging Immunol Infect Dis.* 1990;2:45–53.

46. Whittingham S, Buckley JD, Mackay IR. Factors influencing the secondary antibody response to flagellin in man. *Clin Exp Immunol.* 1978;34:170–178.

47. Burns EA, l'Hommedieu GD, Patrick-Miller L, et al. Effect of age, sex and depression on response to primary and secondary immunization. *J Am Geriats Soc.* 1993;4:SA41.

48. Ligthart GJ, Corberand JX, Fournier C, et al. Admission criteria for immunogerontological studies in man: the Senieur protocol. *Mech Ageing Dev.* 1984;28:47–55.

49. De Greef GE, Van Staalduinen GJ, Van Doorninck H, Van Rol MJ, Hijmans W. Age-related changes of the antigen-specific antibody formation in vitro and PHA-induced T cell proliferation in individuals who met the Senieur protocol. *Mech Ageing Devel.* 1992;66:1–14.

50. Kishimoto S, Tomino S, Mitsuya H, et al. Age-related decrease in frequencies of B-cell precursors and specific helper T cells involved in the IgG anti-tetanus toxoid antibody production in humans. *Clin Immunol Immunopathol.* 1982;25:1–10.

51. Remarque EJ, van Beek WC, Ligthart GJ, et al. Improvement of the immunoglobulin subclass response to influenza vaccine in elderly nursing home residents by the use of high-dose vaccines. *Vaccine.* 1993;11:649.

52. Burns EA, Lum LG, Giddings BR, Seigneuret MC, Goodwin JS. Decreased specific antibody synthesis by lymphocytes from elderly subjects. *Mech Ageing Devel.* 1990;53:229–241.

53. Burns EA, Lum LG, l'Hommedieu GD, Goodwin JS. Decreased humoral immunity in aging: in vivo and in vitro response to vaccination. *J Gerontol.* 1993;48:B231–B236.

54. Ennist DL, Hones KH, St. Pierre RL, Whisler RL. Functional analysis of the immunosenescence of the human B cell system: dissociation of normal activation and proliferation from impaired terminal differentiation into IgM immunoglobulin-secreting cells. *J Immunol.* 1986;136:99–105.

55. Whisler RL, Williams JW, Newhouse YG. Human B cell proliferative responses during aging. Reduced RNA synthesis and DNA replication after signal transduction by surface immunoglobulins compared to B cell antigenic determinants CD20 and CD40. *Mech Ageing Devel.* 1991;61:209–222.

56. Hu A, Ehleiter D, Ben-Yehuda A, et al. Effect of age on the expressed B cell repertoire: role of B cell subsets. *Int Immunol*. 1993;5:1035–1309.

57. Nicoletti C, Yang X, Cerny J. Repertoire diversity of antibody response to bacterial antigens in aged mice. III. Phosphorylcholine antibody from young and aged mice differ in structure and protective activity against infection with *Streptococcus pneumoniae*. *J Immunol*. 1993;150:543–549.

58. Nicoletti C. Antibody protection in aging: influence of idiotypic repertoire and antibody binding activity to a bacterial antigen. *Exp Mol Pathol*. 1995;62:99–108.

59. Miller C, Kelsoe G. Ig VH hypermutation is absent in the germinal centers of aged mice. *J. Immunol*. 1995;155:3377–3384.

60. Delfraissey J, Galanaud P, Wallon C, et al. Abolished in vitro antibody response in the elderly: exclusive involvement of prostaglandin-induced T suppressor cells. *Clin Immunol Immunopathol*. 1982;24:377–385.

61. Delfraissey JF, Galanaud P, Dormont J, Wallon C. Age-related impairment of the in vitro antibody response in the human. *Clin Exp Immunol*. 1980;39:208–214.

62. McLachlan JA, Serkin CD, Morrey-Clark KM, Bakouche O. Immunological functions of aged monocytes. *Pathobiology*. 1995;63:148–159.

63. Danon D, Kowatch MA, Roth GS. Promotion of wound repair in old mice by local injection of macrophages. *Proc Natl Acad Sci USA*. 1989;86:2018–2020.

64. Izumi-Hisha H, Ito Y, Sugimoto K, Oshima H, Mori KJ. Age-related decrease in the number of hemopoietic stem cells and progenitors in senescence accelerated mice. *Mech Ageing Dev*. 1990;56:89–97.

65. Kirschmann DA, Murasko DM. Splenic and inguinal lymph node T cells of aged mice respond differently to polyclonal and antigen-specific stimuli. *Cell Immunol*. 1992;139:426–437.

66. Szakal AK, Kapasi ZF, Masuda A, Tew JG. Follicular dendritic cells in the alternative antigen transport pathway: microenvironment, cellular events, age and retrovirus related alterations. *Semin Immunol*. 1992;4:257–265.

67. Beckman I, Dimopoulos K, Xaioning X, Bradley J, Henschke P, Ahern M. T cell activation in the elderly: evidence for specific deficiencies in T cell/accessory cell interactions. *Mech Ageing Dev*. 1990;51:265–276.

68. McLachlan JA, Serkin CD, Morrey KM, Bakouche O. Antitumoral properties of aged human monocytes. *J Immunol*. 1995;154:832–843.

69. Itoh H, Abo T, Sugawara S, Kanno A, et al. Age-related variation in the proportion and activity of murine liver natural killer cells and their cytotoxicity against regenerating hepatocytes. *J Immunol*. 1988;141:315–323.

70. Ho S-P, Kramer KE, Ershler WB. Effect of host age upon interleukin-2-mediated anti-tumor responses in a murine fibrosarcoma model. *Cancer Immunol Immunother*. 1990; 31:146–150.

71. Kutza J, Kaye D, Murasko DM. Basal natural killer cell activity of young versus elderly humans. *J Gerontol*. 1995; 50A:B110–B116.

72. Facchini AE, Mariani AR, Mariani S, Papa S, Vitale M, Manzoli FA. Increased number of circulating Leu 11+ (CD16) large granular lymphocytes and decreased NK activity during human aging. *Clin Exp Immunol*. 1987; 68:340.

73. Kutza J, Gross P, Kaye D, Murasko DM. Natural killer cell cytotoxicity in elderly humans after influenza immunization. *Clin Diagn Lab Immunol*. 1996;3:105–108.

74. Dorfman JR, Raulet DH. Acquisition of Ly-49 receptor expression by developing natural killer cells. *J Exp Med*. 1998;187:609.

75. Kutza J, Murasko DM. Effects of aging on natural killer cell activity and activation by interleukin-2 and IFN-alpha. *Cell Immunol*. 1994;155:195–204.

76. Auernhammer CJ, Feldmeier H, Nass R, et al. Insulin-like growth factor I is an independent coregulatory modulator of NK cell activity. *Endocrinology*. 1996;137:5332–5336.

77. Esposito D, Fassina G, Szabo P. et al. Chromosomes of older humans are more prone to aminopterin-induced breakage. *Proc Natl Acad Sci USA*. 1989;86:1302–1306.

78. Akiyama M, Shou O-L, Kusunoki Y, et al. Age- and dose-related alteration of in vitro mixed lymphocyte culture response of blood lymphocytes from A-bomb survivors. *Radiat Res*. 1989;l17:26–34.

79. Mayer PJ, Lange CS, Bradley MO, Nichols WW. Age-dependent decline in rejoining of X-ray-induced DNA double-strand breaks in normal human lymphocytes. *Mutat Res*. 1989;219:95–100.

80. Melaragno MI, De Arruda Cardoso Smith M. Sister chromatid exchange and proliferation pattern in lymphocytes from newborns, elderly subjects and in premature aging syndromes. *Mech Ageing Dev*. 1990;54:43–53.

81. Lewis RS, Cahalan MD. Potassium and calcium channels in lymphocytes. *Annu Rev Immunol*. 1995;13:623–653.

82. Jayaraman T, Ondriasova E, Ondrias K, Harnick, Marks AR. The inositol 1,4,5-trisphosphate receptor is essential for T-cell receptor signaling. *Proc Natl Acad Sci USA*. 1995;92:6007–6011.

83. Zweifach A, Lewis RS. Mitogen-regulated Ca^{2+} current of T lymphocytes is activated by depletion of intracellular Ca^{2+} stores. *Proc Natl Acad Sci USA*. 1993;90:6295–6299.

84. Miller RA, Philosophe B, Ginis I, et al. Defective control of cytoplasmic calcium concentration in T lymphocytes from old mice. *J Cell Physiol*. 1989;128:175–182.

85. Miller RA. Calcium signals in T lymphocytes from old mice. *Life Sci*. 1996;59:469–475.

86. Fultop T Jr, Barabas G, Varga Z, et al. Transmembrane signaling changes with aging. *Ann NY Acad Sci*. 1992;673: 165–171.

87. Philosophe B, Miller RA. Calcium signals in murine T lymphocytes: preservation of response to PHA and to an anti-Ly-6 antibody. *Aging Immunol Infect Dis*. 1990;2:11–18.

88. Lustyik G, O'Leary JJ. Aging and the mobilization of intracellular calcium by phytohemagglutinin in human T cells. *J Gerontol*. 1989;44:B30–B36.

89. Jackola DR, Hallgren HM. Diminished cell-cell binding by lymphocytes from healthy elderly humans: evidence for altered activation of LFA-1 function with age. *J Gerontol*. 1995;50:B368–B377.

90. Whisler RL, Newhouse YG, Bagenstose SE. Age-related reductions in the activation of mitogen-activated protein kinases p44mapk/ERK1 and p42mapk/ERK2 in human T

cells stimulated via ligation of the T cell receptor complex. *Cell Immunol*. 1996;168:201–210.

91. Whisler RL, Newhouse YG, Grants IS, Hackshaw KV. Differential expression of the alpha- and beta-isoforms of protein kinase C in peripheral blood T and B cells from young and elderly adults. *Mech Aging Dev*. 1995;77:197–211.

92. Patel HR, Miller RA. Age-associated changes in mitogen-induced protein phosphorylation in murine T lymphocytes. *Eur J Immunol*. 1992;22:253–260.

93. Shi J, Miller RA. Differential tyrosine-specific protein phosphorylation in mouse T lymphocyte subsets. Effect of age. *J Immunol*. 1993;151:730–739.

94. Whisler RL, Beiqing L, Chen M. Age-related decreases in IL-2 production by human T cells are associated with impaired activation of nuclear transcriptional factors AP-l and NF-AT. *Cell Immunol*. 1996;169:185–195.

95. Whisler RL, Liu B, Wu LC, Chen M. Reduced activation of transcriptional factor AP-l among peripheral blood T cells from elderly humans after PHA stimulation: restorative effect of phorbol diesters. *Cell Immunol*. 1993;152:96–109.

96. Raff H, Raff JL, Duthie EH, et al. Elevated salivary cortisol in the evening in healthy elderly men and women: correlation with bone mineral density. *J Gerontol*. 1999;54:M479–M483.

97. Dozmorov IM, Miller RA. Age-associated decline in response of naïve T cells to in vitro immunization reflects shift in glucocorticoid sensitivity. *Life Sci*. 1999;64:1849–1859.

98. Goodwin JS, Webb DR. Regulation of the immune response by prostaglandins: a critical review. *Clin Immunol Immunopathol*. 1981;15:116–132.

99. Goodwin JS, Messner RP. Sensitivity of lymphocytes to prostaglandin E_2 increases in subjects over age 70. *J Clin Investig*. 1979;64:434–439.

100. Goodwin JS. Changes in lymphocyte sensitivity to prostaglandin E, histamine, hydrocortisone, and X-irradiation with age: studies in a healthy elderly population. *Clin Immunol Immunopathol*. 1982;25:243–251.

101. Hayek MG, Meydani S, Meydani M, et al. Age differences in eicosenoid production of mouse splenocytes: effects on mitogen-induced T cell proliferation. *J Gerontol*. 1994;49:B197–B207.

102. Beharka AA, Wu D, Han SN, Meydani SN. Macrophage prostaglandin production contributes to the age-associated decrease in T cell function which is reversed by the dietary antioxidant vitamin E. *Mech Ageing Dev*. 1997;93:59–77.

103. Hayek MG, Mura C, Wu D, et al. Enhanced expression of inducible cyclooxygenase with age in murine macrophages. *J Immunol*. 1997;159:2445–2451.

104. Yoshikawa T, Suzuki H, Sugiyama E, et al. Effects of prostaglandin E_1 on the production of IgM and IgG class anti-dsDNA antibodies in NZB/W F1 mice. *J Rheumatol*. 1993;20:1701–1706.

105. Negoro S, Hara H, Miyata S, et al. Mechanisms of age-related decline in antigen-specific T cell proliferative response: IL-2 receptor expression and recombinant IL-2 induced proliferative response of purified Tac-positive T cells. *Mech Ageing Dev*. 1986;36:223–241.

106. Vissinga C, Hertogh-Huijbregts, Rozing J, et al. Analysis of the age-related decline in alloreactivity of CD4+ and CD8+ T cells in CBA/RIJ mice. *Mech Ageing Dev*. 1990;51:179–194.

107. Hara H, Tanaka T, Negoro S, et al. Age-related changes of expression of IL-2 receptor subunits and kinetics of IL-2 internalization in T cells after mitogenic stimulation. *Mech Ageing Dev*. 1988;45:167–175.

108. Nagel JE, Chopra RK, Powers DC, Adler WH. Effect of age on the human high affinity interleukin 2 receptor of phytohaemagglutinin stimulated peripheral blood lymphocytes. *Clin Exp Immunol*. 1989;75:286–291.

109. Ajitsu S, Mirabella S, Kawanishi H. In vivo immunologic intervention in age-related T cell defects in murine gut-associated lymphoid tissues by IL-2. *Mech Ageing Dev*. 1990;54:163–183.

110. Ernst DN, Weigle WO, Thoman ML. Retention of IL-2 production and IL-2 receptor expression by Peyer's patch T cells from aged mice. *Aging Immunol Infect Dis*. 1990;2:1–9.

111. Wu W, Pahlavani M, Cheung HT, et al. The effect of aging on the expression of interleukin 2 messenger ribonucleic acid. *Cell Immunol*. 1986;100:224–231.

112. Nijhuis EW, Remarque EJ, Hinloopen B, et al. Age-related increase in the fraction of CD27-CD4+ T cells and IL-4 production as a feature of CD4+ T cell differentiation in vivo. *Clin Exp Immunol*. 1994;96:528–534.

113. Hobbs MV, Ernst DN, Torbett BE, et al. Cell proliferation and cytokine production by CD4+ cells from old mice. *J Cell Biochem*. 1991;46:312–320.

114. Beiqing L, Carle KW, Whisler RL. Reductions in the activation of ERK and JNK are associated with decreased IL-2 production in T cells from elder humans stimulated by the TCR/CD3 complex and costimulatory signals. *Cell Immunol*. 1997;182:79–88.

115. Bradley SF, Vibhagool A, Kunkel SL, Kauffman CA. Monokine secretion in aging and protein malnutrition. *J Leukoc Biol*. 1989;45:510–514.

116. Molteni M, Della Bella S, Mascagni B, et al. Secretion of cytokines upon allogeneir stimulation: effect of aging. *J Biol Regul Homeost* Agents. 1994;8:41–47.

117. Gorczynski RM, Cinader B, Ramakrishna V, Terzioglu E, Waelli TH, Wesphal O. An antibody specific for interleukin-6 reverses age-associated changes in spontaneous and induced cytokine production in mice. *Immunology* 1997;92:20–25.

118. Udhayakumar V, Subbarao B, Seth A, et al. Impaired T cell-induced T cell–T cell interaction in aged mice. *Cell Immunol*. 1988;116:299–307.

119. Thoman ML, Keogh EA, Weigle WO. Aging. *Immunol Infect Dis*. 1988/1989;1:245–253.

120. Li SP, Miller RA. Age-associated decline in Il-4 production by murine T lymphocytes in extended culture. *Cell Immunol*. 1993;151:187–195.

121. Burns EA, l'Hommedieu GD, Cunning J, Goodwin JS. Effects of interleukin 4 on antigen-specific antibody synthesis by lymphocytes from old and young adults. *Lymphokine Cytokine Res*. 1994;13(4):227–231.

122. Dobber R, Tielemans M, Nagelkerken L. The in vivo effects of neutralizing antibodies against IFN-gamma, IL-4, or IL-10 on the humoral immune response in young and aged mice. *Cell Immunol.* 1995;160:185–192.

123. Candore G, Di Lorenzo G, Melluso M, et al. Gamma-interferon, interleukin-4 and interleukin-6 in vitro production in old subjects. *Autoimmunity.* 1993;16:275–280.

124. Mu XY, Thoman ML. The age-dependent cytokine production by murine CD8+ T cells as determined by four-color flow cytometry analysis. *J Gerontol.* 1999;54A:B116–B123.

125. Krishnaraj R, Bhooma T. Cytokine sensitivity of human NK cells during immunosenescence. 2. IL-2-induced interferon gamma secretion. *Immunol Lett.* 1996;50:59–63.

126. Goonewardene IM, Murasko DM. Age associated changes in mitogen induced proliferation and cytokine production by lymphocytes of the long-lived brown Norway rat. *Mech Ageing Dev.* 1993;71:199–212.

127. Faist E, Markewitz A, Fuchs D, et al. Immunomodulatory therapy with thymopentin and indomethacin. Successful restoration of interleukin-2 synthesis in patients undergoing major surgery. *Ann Surg.* 1991;214:264–273.

128. Chopra RK, Holbrook NJ, Powers DC, et al. Interleukin 2, interleukin 2 receptor, and interferon-gamma synthesis and mRNA expression in phorbon myristate acetate and calcium ionophore A23 187-stimulated T cells from elderly humans. *Clin Immunol Immunopathol.* 1989;53:297–308.

129. Nagelkerken L, Hertogh-Huijbregts A, Dobber R, Drager A. Age-related changes in lymphokine production related to a decreased number of CD45RBhi CD4+ T cells. *Eur J Immunol.* l991;21:273–281.

130. Caruso C, Candore G, Cigna D, et al. Cytokine production pathway in the elderly. *Immunol Res.* 1996;15:84–90.

131. Daynes RA, Araneo BA, Ershler WB, et al. Altered regulation of IL-6 production with normal aging. *J Immunol.* 1993;150:5219–5230.

132. Ershler WB. Interleukin-6: a cytokine for gerontologists. *J Am Geriatr Soc.* 1993;41:176–181.

133. Sothern RB, Roitman-Johnson B, Kanabrocki EL, et al. Circadian characteristics of circulating interleukin-6 in men. *J Allergy Clin Immunol.* 1995;95:1029–1035.

134. Liao Z, Caucino JA, Schniffer SM, et al. Increased urinary cytokine levels in the elderly. *Aging Immunol Infect Dis.* 1993;4:139–153.

135. Foster KD, Conn CA, Kluger MJ. Fever, tumor necrosis factor and interleukin-6 in young, mature and aged Fischer 344 rats. *Am J Physiol.* 1992;262:R211–R215.

136. O'Mahony L, Holland J, Jackson J, Feighery C, Hennessy TPJ, Mealy K. Quantitative intracellular cytokine measurement: age-related changes in proinflammatory cytokine production. *Exp Immunol.* 1998;113:213–219.

137. Ye S-M, Johnson RW. Increased interleukin-6 expression by microglia from brain of aged mice. *J Neuroimmunol.* 1999;93:139–148.

138. Clark JA, Peterson TC. Cytokine production and aging: overproduction of IL-8 in elderly males in response to lipopolysaccharide. *Mech Ageing Dev.* 1994;77:127–139.

139. Lio D, D'Anna C, Scola L, et al. Interleukin-5 production by mononuclear cells from aged individuals: implication for autoimmunity. *Mech Ageing Dev.* 1999;106:297–304.

140. Spencer NFL, Norton SD, Harrison LL, Li GZ, Daynes RA. Dysregulation of IL-10 production with aging: possible linkage to the age-associated decline in DHFA and its sulfated derivative. *Exp Gerontol.* 1996;31:3,393–408.

141. Cooper AM, Callahan JE, Griffin JP, et al. Old mice are able to control low-dose aerogenic infections with *Mycobacterium tuberculosis. Infect Immun.* 1995;63:3259–3265.

142. Orme IM, Griffin JP, Roberts AD, Ernst DN. Evidence for a defective accumulation of protective T cells in old mice infected with *Mycobacterium tuberculosis. Cell Immunol.* 1993;147:222–229.

143. Orme IM. Mechanisms underlying the increased susceptibility of aged mice to tuberculosis. *Nutr Rev.* 53:S35–S40.

144. Orme IM. Aging and immunity to tuberculosis: increased susceptibility of old mice reflects a decreased capacity to generate mediator T lymphocytes. *J Immunol.* 1988;140:3589–3593.

145. Orme IM. The response of macrophages from old mice to *Mycobacterium tuberculosis* and its products. *Aging Immunol Infect Dis.* 1993;4:187–195.

146. Sakata-Kaneko S, Wakatsuki Y, Matsunaga Y, Usui T, Kita T. Altered Th1/Th2 commitment in human CD4+ T cells with aging. *Clinical & Experimental Immunology.* 2000;120:267–273.

147. Zhang Y, Acuna CL, Switzer KC, Song L, Sayers R, Mbawuike IN. Corrective effects of interleukin-12 on age-related deficiencies in IFN-gamma production and IL-12R-beta-2 expression in virus-specific CD8+ T cells. *J Interferon Cytokine Res.* 2000;20:235–245.

148. Ader R, Cohen N. Conditioned immunopharmacologic responses. In: Ader R, ed. *Psychoneuroimmunology.* Orlando: Academic Press; 1981:281–317.

149. Borysenko M, Borysenko J. Stress, behavior and immunity: animal models and mediating mechanisms. *Gen Hosp Psychol.* 1982;4:59–67.

150. Rosenberg LT, Coe CL, Levine S. Complement levels in the squirrel monkey. *Lab Anim Sci.* 1982;32:371–372.

151. Minter RE, Patterson-Kimball C. Life events and illness onset: a review. *Psychosomatics.* 1978;19:334–339.

152. Glaser R, Thorn BE, Tarr KL, et al. Effects of stress on methyltransferase synthesis: an important DNA repair enzyme. *Health Psychol.* 1985;4:403–412.

153. Thomas PD, Goodwin JM, Goodwin JS. Effect of social support on stress-related changes in cholesterol level, uric acid level and immune function in an elderly sample. *Am J Psychchol.* 1985;142:735–737.

154. Goodwin JS, Hunt WC, Kay CR, et al. The effect of marital status on treatment and survival of cancer patients. *JAMA.* 1987;255:3125–3130.

155. Schleifer SJ, Keller SE, Camerino M, et al. Suppression of lymphocyte function following bereavement. *JAMA.* 1983;250:374–377.

156. Glaser R, Kiecolt-Glaser JK, Speicher CE, et al. The relationship of stress and loneliness and changes in herpes virus latency. *J Behav Med.* 1985;8:249–260.

157. Glaser R, Pearson GR, Bonneau RH, et al. Stress and the memory T cell response to the Epstein–Barr virus in healthy medical students. *Health Psychol.* 1993;12:435–442.

158. Kiecolt-Glaser JK, Glaser R, Gravenstein S, Malarkey WB, Sheridan J. Chronic stress laters the immune response to influenza virus vaccine in older adults. *Proc Natl Acad Sci USA.* 1996;93:3043–3047.

159. Kiecolt-Glaser JK, Marucha PT, Malarkey WH, et al. Slowing of wound healing by psychological stress. *Lancet.* 1995;346:1194–1196.

160. Wayne S, Rhyne R, Garry P, et al. Cell mediated immunity as a predictor of morbidity and mortality in the aged. *J Gerontol.* 1990;45:45–49.

161. Goodwin JS. Decreased immunity and increased morbidity in the elderly. *Nutr Rev.* 1995;53:S41–S46.

162. Bender BS, Nagel JE, Adler WH, Andres K. Absolute peripheral blood lymphocyte counts and subsequent mortality of elderly men. *J Am Geriatr Soc.* 1986;34:649–654.

163. Ferguson FG, Wikby A, Maxson P, Olsson J, Johansson B. Immune parameters in a longitudinal study of a very old population of Swedish people: a comparison between survivors and nonsurvivors. *J Gerontol.* 1995;50:B378–B382.

164. Burnet FM. The concept of immunological surveillance. *Prog Exp Tumor Res.* 1970;13:1–27.

165. Thomas L. Reactions to homologous tissue antigens in relation to hypersensitivity. In: Lawrence HS, ed. *Cellular and Humoral Aspects of the Hypersensitivity States.* New York: Hoeber-Harper; 1959:529–532.

166. Gatti RA, Good RA. Aging, immunity and malignancy. *Geriatrics.* 1970;25:158–168.

167. Fraumeni JF, Hoover RN, Devesa SS, Kinlen LJ. Epidemiology of cancer. In: DeVita VT Jr, Hellman S, Rosenberg SA, eds. *Cancer. Principles and Practice of Oncology,* 4th Ed. Philadelphia: Lippincott; 1993:150–181.

168. Newell GR, Spitz MR, Sider JG. Cancer and age. *Semin Oncol.* 1989;16:3–9.

169. Phillips J, Mehta K, Fernandez C, Raveche E. The NZB mouse as a model for chronic lymphocytic leukemia. *Cancer Res.* 1997;52:437–443.

170. Shirai T, Okada T, Hirose S. Genetic regulation of CD5+ B cells in autoimmune disease and in chronic lymphocytic leukemia. *Ann NY Acad Sci.* 1992;651:509–526.

171. Davidson WF, Giese T, Fredrickson TN. Spontaneous development of plasmacytoid tumors in mice with defective Fas-Fas ligand interactions. *J Exp Med.* 1998;187:1825–1838.

172. Minick CR, Murphy GE, Campbell WG. Experimental induction of athero-arteriosclerosis by the synergy of allergic injury to arteries and lipid rich diet. *J Exp Med.* 1966;124:635–652.

173. Howard AN, Paterski J, Bowyer DE, et al. Atherosclerosis induced in hypercholesterolemic baboons by immunologic injury. *Atherosclerosis.* 1971;14:17–29.

174. Clarkson RB, Alexander NJ. Long term vasectomy: effects on the occurrence and extent of atherosclerosis in rhesus monkeys. *J Clin Investig.* 1980;65:15–25.

175. Ansbacher R, Keung-Yeung K, Wurster JC. Sperm antibodies in vasectomized men. *Fertil Steril.* 1972;23:640–643.

176. Shimokama T, Haraoka S, Watanabe T. Morphological fate and sequelae of human atherosclerosis: evaluation of immune mechanisms in atherogenesis through immunohistological and ultrastructural analysis. *Pathol Int.* 1995;45:801–814.

177. Mackay IR, Whittingham SF, Mathews JD. The immunoepidemiology of aging. In: Makinodan T, Yunis E, eds. *Immunology and Aging.* New York: Plenum Press; 1977: 35–50.

178. Song L, Kim YH, Chopra RK, Proust JJ, et al. Age-related effects in T cell activation and proliferation. *Exp Gerontol.* 1993;28:313–321.

179. Lewis V, Twomey J, Bealmear P, et al. Age, thymic function and circulating thymic hormone activity. *J Clin Endocrinol Metab.* 1978;47:145–152.

180. Rodewald H. Immunology: the thymus in the age of retirement. *Nature.* 1998;396:630–631.

181. Hirokawa K, Utsuyama M, Kasai M, et al. Aging and immunity. *Acta Pathol Jpn.* 1992;42:537–548.

182. Effros RB, Casillas A, Walford RL. The effect of thymosin-1 immunity to influenza in aged mice. *Aging Immunol Infect Dis.* 1988;1:31–40.

183. Goso C, Frasca D, Doria G. Effect of synthetic thymic humoral factor (THF-gamma 2) on T cell activities in immunodeficient aging mice. *Clin Exp Immunol.* 1992;87: 346–351.

184. Frasca D, Adorini L, Doria G. Enhanced frequency of mitogen-responsive T cell precursors in old mice injected with thymosin alpha 1. *Eur J Immunol.* 1987;17:727–730.

185. Cillari E, Milano S, Perego R, et al. Modulation of IL-2, IFN-gamma, TNF-alpha and IL-4 production in mice of different ages by thymopentin. *Int J Immunopharmacol.* 1991;14:1029–1035.

186. Cillari E, Milano S, Dieli M, et al. Thymopentin reduces the susceptibility of aged mice to cutaneous leishmaniasis by modulating CD4 T-cell subsets. *Immunology.* 1992;76: 362–366.

187. Reiter RJ. Pineal function during aging: attenuation of the melatonin rhythm and its neurobiological consequences. *Acta Neurobiol Exp.* 1994;54:31S–39S.

188. Caroleo MC, Frasca D, Nistico G, Doria G. Melatonin: an immunomodulator in immunodeficient mice. *Immunopharmacology.* 1992;23:81–89.

189. Lissoni P, Brivio O, Fumagalli L, et al. Immune effects of preoperative immunotherapy with high-dose subcutaneous interleukin-2 versus neuroimmunotherapy with low-dose IL-2 plus the neurohormone melatonin in gastrointestinal tract tumor patients. *J Biol Regul Homeost Agents.* 1995;9:31–33.

190. Lissoni P, Barni S, Fossati V, et al. A randomized study of neuroimmunotherapy with low-dose subcutaneous interleukin-2 plus melatonin compared to supportive care alone in patients with untreatable metastatic solid tumour. *Support Care Cancer.* 1995 May;3(3):194–197.

191. Saito H, Inoue T, Fukatsu K, et al. Growth hormone and the immune response to bacterial infection. *Horm Res.* 1996;45:50–54.

192. Bonello RS, Marcus R, Bloch D, Strober S. Effects of growth hormone and estrogen on T lymphocytes in older women. *J Am Geriatr Soc.* 1996;44:1039–1042.

193. Swenson CD, Gottesman SR, Belsito DV, et al. Relationship between humoral immunoaugmenting properties of DHEAS and IgD-receptor expression in young and aged mice. *Ann NY Acad Sci*. 1995;29:249–258.

194. Araneo BA, Woods ML Jr, Daynes RA. Reversal of the immunosenescent phenotype by DHFA: hormone treatment provides an adjuvant effect on the immunization of aged mice with recombinant hepatitis B surface antigen. *J Infect Dis*. 1993;167:830–840.

195. Danenberg HD, Ben-Yehuda A, Zakay-Rones Z, et al. DHEA treatment reverses the impaired immune response of old mice to influenza vaccination and protects from influenza infection. *Vaccine*. 1995;13:1445–1448.

196. Araneo B, Dowell T, Woods ML, et al. DHEA as an effective vaccine adjuvant in elderly humans. Proof-of-principle studies. *Ann NY Acad Sci*. 1995;774:232–248.

197. McCay C, Crowell M, Maynard L. The effects of retarded growth upon the length of life span and upon the ultimate body size. *J Nutr*. 1935;10:63–79.

198. Walford RL, Liu RK, Gerbase-Delima M, Mathies M, Smith GS. Long-term dietary restiction and immune function in mice: response to sheep red blood cells and to mitogenic agents. *Mech Ageing Dev*. 1973;2:447–454.

199. Effros RB, Walford RL, Weindruch R, et al. Influences of dietary restriction on immunity to influenza in aged mice. *J Gerontol*. 46:B142–B147.

200. Ershler WB, Sun WH, Binkley N, et al. Interleukin-6 and aging: blood levels and mononuclear cell production increase with advancing age and in vitro production is modifiable by dietary restriction. *Lymphokine Cytokine Res*. 1993;12:225–230.

201. Chandra RK. Nutrition is an important determinant of immunity in old age. *Prog Clin Biol Res*. 1990;326:321–334.

202. Chandra RK, Puri S. Nutritional support improves antibody response to influenza vaccine in the elderly. *Br Med J*. 1985;291:709.

203. Chandra RK. Effect of vitamin and trace-element supplementation on immune responses and infection in elderly subjects. *Lancet*. 1992;340:1124–1127.

204. Rasmussen LB, Kiens B, Pedersen BK, et al. Effect of diet and plasma fatty acid composition on immune status in elderly men. *Am J Clin Nutr*. 1994;59:572–577.

205. Meydani M. Vitamin E. *Lancet*. 1995;345:170–175.

206. Meydani SN, Hayek M. Vitamin F and immune response. In: Chandra RK, ed. Proceedings of International Conference on Nutrition and Immunity. St. John's, Newfoundland: ARTS Biomedical; 1992:105–128.

207. Meydani SN, Barklund PM, Liu S, et al. Vitamin E supplementation enhances cell-mediated immunity in healthy elderly subjects. *Am J Clin Nutr*. 1990;52:557–563.

208. Meydani SN, Leka L, Loszewski R. Long-term vitamin E supplementation enhances immune response in healthy elderly. *FASEB J*. 1994;8:A274.

209. Omenn GS, Goodman GE, Thornquist MD, et al. Risk factors for lung cancer and for intervention effects in CARET, the Beta Carotene and Retinol efficacy trial. *J Natl Cancer Inst*. 1996;88:1550–1560.

210. Albanes D, Heinonen OP, Taylor PR, et al. Alpha-tocopherol and beta-carotene supplements and lung cancer incidence in the alpha-tocopherol, beta-carotene cancer prevention study: effects of base-line characteristics and study compliance. *J Natl Cancer Inst*. 1996;88:1560–1570.

211. Goodwin JS, Bankhurst A, Murphy S, et al. Partial reversal of the cellular immune defect in common variable immunodeficiency with indomethacin. *J Clin Lab Immunol*. 1978;1:197–199.

212. Hsia J, Tang T, Parrott M, Rogalla K. Augmentation of the immune response to influenza vaccine by acetylsalicylic acid: a clinical trial in a geriatric population. *Methods Find Exp Clin Pharmacol*. 1994;16:677–683.

213. Cueppens J, Rodriguez M, Goodwin JS. Nonsteroidal anti-inflammatory drugs inhibit the production of IgM rheumatoid factor in vitro. *Lancet*. 1982;1:528–531.

214. Pennebaker JW, Kiecolt-Glaser JK, Glaser R. Disclosure of traumas and immune function: health implications for psychotherapy. *J Consult Clin Psychol*. 1988;56:239–245.

215. Kiecolt-Glaser JK, Glaser R, Williger D, et al. Psychosocial enhancement of immunocompetence in a geriatric population. *Health Psychol*. 1985;4:25–41.

216. Ershler WB. The influence of an aging immune system on cancer incidence and progression. *J Gerontol*. 1993;48:B3–B7.

217. Ferluga J. Potential role of anti-oncogenes in aging. *Mech Ageing Dev*. 1990;53:267–275.

54
Infectious Diseases

Thomas T. Yoshikawa

Epidemiology and Risk Factors

Mortality and Morbidity

Today, worldwide, infectious diseases account for one-third of all deaths. It has been estimated by the World Health Organization that approximately 50,000 people die each day throughout the world from an infectious disease.[1] In industrialized countries, such as the United States, infectious diseases were the major causes of death and disabilities until the mid-twentieth century.[2] Advances in sanitation, public health measures, antisepsis, antimicrobial drugs, and immunizations substantially reduced the mortality and morbidity caused by infections in developed nations during the past 50 years. The impact of the reduction in infections can be seen most strikingly in statistics on life expectancy in the United States. The average life expectancy at birth in 1900 in the United States was approximately 47 years (48 years for females and 46 years for males).[3] In contrast, the present life expectancy at birth in the United States is approximately 75 years (80 years for females and 73 years for males).[3] Although persons age 65 years and older constituted only 4% of the entire population in the United States in 1900, they currently represent 1300 of the total number of Americans.[4] Thus the virtual eradication of many death-causing infectious diseases over the past century has resulted in the extraordinary growth in the number of people living to old age. Moreover, it is projected that the very old population (i.e., those persons age 80 years and older) will expand at an even greater rate over the next 50 years.

Unfortunately, the "benefits" of growing older have associated "costs," and one of these is an increased susceptibility and mortality to infections. Although heart disease, cancer, and stroke are now the top three causes of death in the general and geriatric populations, pneumonia/influenza and sepsis are the fourth and ninth leading causes of death, respectively, in the elderly.[5] Dia-betes mellitus, which has a high incidence of infectious complications, is the sixth leading cause of death in those aged 65 years and older.[5] Furthermore, older adults who have infections experience a higher mortality rate than younger adults with the same affliction. Table 54.1 illustrates as a ratio the comparative mortality rates of common infectious diseases in the elderly versus young adults. With the exception of urinary tract infection (UTI), most of the common infections are associated with at least a twofold higher death rate or more in the elderly population.[6-13] Although earlier data suggested that bacteriuria and UTI was associated with a higher mortality rate in the elderly,[14] more recent studies have refuted these findings.[8,15]

In addition to a decreased survival rate, older patients who have infections suffer more complications related to the illness than do younger patients. In Table 54.2, select examples of infectious-related complications are listed along with the relative frequencies of these morbidities in the elderly in comparison with young adults.[16-20] For example, the incidence of bacteremia/sepsis in association with UTI (upper tract; pyelonephritis) was four to five times more common in elderly women than young women.[16] Also, the debilitating complication of postherpetic neuralgia following herpes zoster infection (shingles) is essentially a morbid event confined to persons over the age of 60 years.[20]

The higher rates of complications in the elderly translate into higher rates and longer duration of hospitalization, as well as greater risk for hospital-acquired infections. According to the National Nosocomial Infections Surveillance (NNIS) data between 1986 and 1990, 54% of nosocomial infections occurred in patients age 65 years and older.[21] In another study of 4031 nosocomial infections in 2565 patients, the daily infection rates were 0.59% and 0.40% in patients 60 years and older and under 60 years, respectively.[22] The mean length of hospitalization was 8.1 days for patients age 59 years and younger and 10.4 days for patients 60 years and older.[22]

TABLE 54.1. Comparative mortality rates of infections in elderly and young adults.

Infection	Ratio mortality rates: elderly versus young
Pneumonia[a]	3
Tuberculosis[b]	10
Urinary tract infection[c]	1
Bacteremia/sepsis[d]	3
Cholecystitis	2–8
Appendicitis	15–20
Septic arthritis	2–3
Bacterial meningitis	3
Infective endocarditis[e]	2–3

[a] Community acquired.
[b] From 1979 to 1989.
[c] Bacteremic cases.
[d] With nonfatal and ultimately fatal underlying diseases.
[e] Medically treated cases.
Source: Data from Marston et al.[6]; Centers for Disease Control[7]; Ackermann et al.[8]; McCue[9]; Norman et al.[10]; Norman et al.[11]; Gorse et al.[12]; Werner et al.[13]

Risk Factors and Pathogenesis

The topic of age-associated changes of immune function is discussed in detail in Chapter 53 and thus is mentioned only briefly here. Infection is broadly defined as a host response to the presence of a microbial agent; these responses may include fever, systemic symptoms and signs, markers of inflammation (e.g., presence of neutrophils in tissue or leukocytosis in the blood; production of cytokines), or immune responses. In the elderly, changes in functional status, both physical and cognitive, should also be considered as a host response to microorganisms. In contrast, "colonization" is the presence of microorganisms without an associated host response. An example of colonization is the skin, which normally can be found to have bacteria (e.g., *Staphylococcus epidermidis*) on its surface with no evidence of disease or host reactions in healthy persons. Thus, the skin has a "normal flora."

Whether infection develops or becomes established in a person is dependent on host–microorganism interaction. Three primary factors determine the outcome of a host–microorganism interaction: virulence, inoculum, and host resistance. For an organism to cause infection, it must be pathogenic or virulent to the host, that is, possess inherent properties to (a) gain access to the host (e.g., migrate, attach, and penetrate mucocutaneous surfaces); (b) replicate in the host environment; (c) avoid host defense processes; and (d) induce a host response. Inoculum refers to the number or quantity of microorganisms present at the time of introduction or entry into the host. Although a specific microorganism may have relatively low virulence when the host's defense mechanisms are intact, if an enormous number of these organisms are introduced, the available host resistance processes may

be "overwhelmed" and be unable to mitigate the replication and subsequent tissue and organ injuries of these "pathogens." For example, the large intestine is filled with billions of bacteria that normally cause little damage to or responses from the host (part of the normal bowel flora). However, if in the course of an elective, uncomplicated abdominal surgery, the colon is damaged with subsequent contamination of the peritoneum with normal flora, an infection is immediately established, that is, peritonitis.

The third major factor in the host–microorganism interaction is host resistance. Host resistance or host defenses include the mucocutaneous surfaces, phagocytic cells, complement, humoral immunity, and cellular immunity. Host resistance may also be termed immune responses, which can be divided into two interactive components: innate or natural immunity and acquired or adaptive immunity. Innate immunity is composed of a cellular component, macrophages, polymorphonuclear leukocytes (PMNLs), natural killer (NK) cells, and dendritic cells, and a noncellular component, complement, C-reactive protein, mannose-binding protein, and serum amyloid protein.[23] Compromises in the integrity and function of any or all components of the host's defense mechanisms by age-related changes or underlying diseases or disorders place the elderly at greater risk for contracting an infection as well as experiencing a more severe illness.[24] The relationship of virulence, inoculum, and host resistance can be simply expressed in the following equation:

$$\text{Infection} \cong \frac{\text{virulence} \times \text{inoculum}}{\text{host resistance}}$$

Thus, the risk or severity of infection is directly proportional to the virulence of the microorganism and number of microorganisms and inversely proportional to host

TABLE 54.2. Morbidity from infections in elderly versus young adults.

Infectious complication	Elderly	Young adult
Urinary tract infection and bacteremia (%)[a]	50	11
Pneumococcal pneumonia bacteremia (per 100,000 population)[b]	15–25	1–9
Pneumococcal bacteremia without fever (%)[c]	29	11
Perforation of appendix (%)[d]	32	6
Postherpetic neuralgia (%)[e]	48	4

[a] Less than 65 versus 65 years or older.
[b] 35–59 versus 60 years or older (frequency varies depending on study group and age cohorts (see also Ref. 144).
[c] 20–64 versus 65 years or older.
[d] Less than 60 versus 60 years or older.
[e] Less than 20 versus 70 years or older.
Source: Gleckman et al.[16]; Mufson et al.[17]; Finkelstein et al.[18]; Peltokallio et al.[19]; Demorgas et al.[20]

resistance. Simply stated, susceptibility to infection is greater when the organism is virulent, there are a large number of microorganisms, or there is a reduction in the integrity of the host's defense mechanisms.

Clinical Patterns of Infection

Important Infections

Although there is an apparent increase in susceptibility to infections with aging, there are no data that indicate elderly persons are at greater risk or have a higher mortality rate to all infections. Rather, there is evidence that certain infectious diseases occur with greater incidence, have higher mortality rate, develop more severe complications, or present special or unique diagnostic and management challenges with aging. These important infections in the elderly are summarized in Table 54.3.[25,26]

Intra-abdominal infections, particularly cholecystitis, diverticulitis, perforated appendicitis, and liver abscess, are seen with greater frequency in elderly persons and, as shown earlier (see Table 54.1), may be associated with high mortality.[27,28] Because diabetes mellitus is a major health problem of aging adults, the infections associated with diabetes are a major complication for the elderly. Malignant otitis externa caused by Pseudomonas aeruginosa, and foot infections including osteomyelitis, are especially common in the geriatric diabetic patient and may result in serious complications including death.[29–31] Nearly 50% of the elderly have some form of joint disorder and many have prosthetic joints, which makes them highly vulnerable to septic arthritis. Older adults account for 40% of all nongonococcal joint infections, with most caused by bacteria.[32,33]

TABLE 54.3. Important infections in the elderly.

Pneumonia
Influenza
Tuberculosis
Urinary tract infection
Chronic bacterial prostatitis
Skin and soft tissue infections
Herpes zoster
Cholecystitis
Appendicitis
Diverticulitis
Liver abscess
Infective endocarditis
Malignant otitis externa
Diabetic foot infection/osteomyelitis
Septic arthritis
Meningitis
Tetanus

Source: Yoshikawa et al.[25]; Yoshikawa et al.[26]

Infections by Setting or Environment

Elderly persons can be typically categorized as residing or temporarily staying in three broad types of settings, depending on their overall health status. These three settings include the home or community, acute care facility (hospital), and long-term care facility (e.g., nursing facility). Interactions between the environmental setting, functional status, and underlying disease(s) of the elderly person influence the types of infections often seen in the community, hospital, or long-term care facility.

In the home or community setting, the majority of elderly persons are ambulatory and functionally independent. The most common infections encountered (first diagnosed) under these circumstances include respiratory infections (bronchitis, pneumonia), UTI, gastroenteritis and intra-abdominal infections (cholecystitis, diverticulitis, apendicitis), cellulitis, septic arthritis, herpes zoster, and infective endocarditis.[25] However, depending on the severity of the illness, many of these infections may require hospital management.

If an elderly patient is in the hospital, there is a substantial risk for acquiring a nosocomial infection. These infections typically include UTI (often related to urinary bladder catheterization), aspiration pneumonia (including postendotracheal intubation), skin or soft tissue infections (infected pressure ulcers, wound infection), septic thrombophlebitis (line sepsis from intravenous catheters), gastroenteritis including antibiotic-associated (Clostridium difficile) diarrhea, and bacteremia/sepsis.[21,22,34]

In a long-term care setting, most of the studies on infections have been in nursing facilities (nursing homes). Numerous investigations indicate that pneumonia, urinary tract infection, and skin/soft tissue infections (PUS) account for at least 75% of all infections in nursing facilities.[35] In addition, bacteremia/sepsis, viral respiratory infections, viral hepatitis, and *C. difficile* diarrhea/colitis are being reported with increasing frequency in long-term care facilities.[36–41]

Multidrug-resistant bacteria, that is, penicillin-resistant pneumococci, drug-resistant gram-negative bacilli, methicillin-resistant *Staphylococcus aureus* (MRSA), and vancomycin-resistant enterococci (VRE), are being isolated from residents of long-term care facilities in greater numbers than expected.[42] Approximately 30% of all penicillin-resistant invasive pneumococcal infections occurred in patients aged 65 or older. Strains of pneumococci that have a minimal inhibitory concentration (MIC) greater than $1.0\,\mu g/mL$ are considered resistant. The majority of UTIs in long-term care facilities are caused by gram-negative bacteria. Resistance to a variety of antibiotics is occurring and has been seen for *Escherichia coli*, *Klebsiella*, and *Providencia*.

MRSA was first reported in nursing home residents in 1970, but since then it has appeared in a variety of long-term care settings (LTCF) (community, Veterans Affairs, large, small, adult, pediatric, urban, and rural) throughout the United States. Currently approximately 40% of *Staphylococcus* species are resistant to methicillin. Risk factors for acquiring MRSA are age, Medical Intensive Care Unit (MICU) or prolonged hospital stay, and a history of invasive procedures. Colonization rates with MRSA are approximately 25% with infection rates of approximately 3%. Colonized individuals do not require antimicrobial therapy.

Risk factors for VRE include severe illness, advanced age, prolonged hospitalization, and previous exposure to antibiotics, especially vancomycin. VRE strains are found more frequently in *Enterococcus faecium* than in other species of enterococci. Most older patients with VRE in LTCF are simply colonized, and these patients do not require antibiotic therapy. However, those infected with VRE should receive antimicrobial therapy, preferably in an acute care facility. Therapeutic options are limited, and thus in vitro lab susceptibility testing of VRE as well as in vitro synergy tests of antibiotics should be used to determine appropiate antibiotic therapy. Combinations of penicillin (PCN), vancomycin, and gentamycin have been suggested if the organism is susceptible to gentamycin at an MIC less than $32\,\mu g/mL$, ciprofloxacin with ampicillin, novobiocin, or rifampin if the MIC to ciprofloxacin is less than $8\,\mu g/mL$.

Clinical Manifestations

Fever

The presence of fever has traditionally been viewed as a symptom or sign of an underlying infection, although other noninfectious diseases can cause a febrile response.[43] The pathogenesis of fever is a complex and dynamic process, and a detailed description of this process is beyond the scope of this chapter. It is only mentioned that eliciting an elevation of body temperature from infection involves a cascade of events from exogenous substances (e.g., microorganisms, microbial products), endogenous mediators [cytokines such as interleukin 1 (IL-1), IL-6 tumor necrosis factor, and interferon-gamma], the thermoregulatory center in the anterior hypothalamus, physiologic changes. and behavioral modifications.[43] Alterations along any aspect of this pathway could modify the host's capacity to mount a fever.

There has been accumulating evidence from a variety of human and animal studies that febrile responses may be blunted or abrogated with aging.[44] Approximately 25% of elderly patients who have serious infections, such as bacteremia, pneumonia, infective endocarditis, or meningitis, may not demonstrate a fever on initial pre-

sentation.[45–48] Recent studies in frail nursing facility residents suggest that although febrile responses to infection may be diminished with aging, there are, nevertheless, elderly persons who mount an elevation of core body temperature with an infection but are recorded as being "afebrile." These individuals had low baseline core temperatures but responded with a rise in body temperature of at least 2.4°F (1.3°C) but failed to reach the traditional criterion of fever, that is, 100°F (37.8°C) or 101°F (38.3°C).[49,50] Furthermore, nearly 90% of the nursing facility residents with infection had a temperature of 99°F (37.2°C) or higher. It has been suggested that the criteria for fever in frail elderly persons, especially those in long-term care facilities, be revised to the following: (1) an oral temperature of 99°F (37.2°C) or greater on repeated measurements; (2) a rectal temperature of 99.5°F (37.5°C) on repeated measurements; or (3) a persistent elevation of body temperature of at least 2°F (1.1°C), regardless of technique of measurement.[51]

Conversely, the presence of an elevated body temperature above normal in the elderly is a reliable and specific indicator of an underlying infectious disease process. Elderly patients manifesting robust fevers of at least 101°F (38.3°C) have been shown to be harboring serious bacterial (or viral in some cases) infections.[52–54] Moreover, fever in the presence of leukocytosis and a "left shift" (increased percentage of band neutrophils and metamyelocytes) increases the positive predictive value for diagnosing a bacterial infection.[54] Alternatively, in the absence of any clinical evidence of infection or fever and with a normal leukocyte count and no left shift, the likelihood of a bacterial infection in the elderly is low.

Temperature measurements in incapacitated, debilitated, or cognitively impaired elderly persons may be difficult using oral or axillary thermometry. In addition, rectal temperature measurements may be problematic in persons with fecal incontinence or persistent diarrhea. An alternative approach to measuring body temperature is the use of infrared tympanic membrane thermometry.[55,56] Although studies have been limited in elderly persons, it appears that tympanic thermometry may be a reliable method to measure body temperature and detect fever.[57,58]

Other Symptoms and Signs

Although many older adults with a specific infectious disease manifest symptoms and signs typical for that infection (e.g., cough, fever, and dyspnea for pneumonia; frequency, urgency, and dysuria for UTI), a substantial number of the elderly may only exhibit nonspecific complaints or have confounding findings because of the changes of aging or coexisting chronic diseases.[59] These clinical manifestations may include delirium or other cognitive impairments, lethargy, anorexia, weakness, and fatigue, as well as acute urinary incontinence, falls, and failure to thrive. Furthermore, the presence of an underlying chronic disorder may mask an acute infectious process; for example, a chronic degenerative osteoarthritis of the knee may delay the diagnosis of an active septic arthritis, or an elderly person with underlying Alzheimer's disease may be harboring a tuberculous meningitis but the symptoms are attributed to the dementing process.

Thus, in any elderly person who demonstrates a fever, or experiences a rapid onset of a change in functional capacity—physical or cognitive—or lack of well-being that cannot be explained by other health problems, an infectious disease should be considered as part of the initial differential diagnosis.

Diagnostic Approach and Treatment of Common or Life-Threatening Infections

Once infection is considered as part of the differential diagnosis, the diagnostic approach should be guided by the most likely source(s) or site(s) of infection based on the initial history and physical examination. Furthermore, determining the elderly person's environmental setting, whether community, hospital, or long-term care institution, can provide clues to the most likely primary causes of infection (see earlier discussion). In older patients who are suspected of harboring an infection but in whom no site or focus of infection can be determined on preliminary assessment, it is suggested that the following laboratory and radiologic studies be performed: complete blood count including differential count; urinalysis with urine culture; chest radiograph (posteroanterior and lateral views); renal function tests; and liver function tests. In elderly patients who are ill enough to require hospitalization, blood cultures should also be obtained.

The results of these preliminary studies and continued examination of the patient should allow the clinician to make decisions about additional laboratory, radiologic, or imaging studies. In some instances, older patients may develop prolonged fever and be considered to have a "fever of unknown origin" (FUO).[44] In contrast of younger adults with FUO, the cause can be identified in the majority of older patients with prolonged fever (more than 90% of cases versus 50% cases).[60] Moreover, infections (35%) are the leading cause of FUO in the elderly, followed by multisystem diseases (e.g., polymyalgia rheumatica) (28%).[60]

The following discussions focus on the diagnosis and treatment in different settings of the more common and life-threatening infections encountered in the elderly.

Urinary Tract Infection

Diagnosis

Urinary tract infection (UTI) is the most common bacterial infection in older persons as well as the most frequent cause of bacteremia/sepsis, may be associated with indwelling bladder catheter, and, paradoxically, is most often asymptomatic.[61–63] Chronic bacterial prostatitis may be a contributor to recurrent UTI in elderly men.[64]

In an ambulatory setting, an elderly patient with suspected UTI should have a urinalysis and a confirmatory test for presence of bacteria. A clean-catch midstream urine specimen is the preferred method of urine collection for women; elderly men can provide a reliable specimen by a first-voided urine sample.[65] Besides being a screening test for bacteriuria, a urinalysis provides an estimate of pyuria, which has a high negative predictive value for absence of bacteriuria in the patients with low or absent white blood cells in the urine.[66,67] Alternatively, a dipstick test for leukocyte esterase can be used to determine the presence of neutrophils in the urine.[68] The presence of bacteriuria can be screened by the nitrite (Greiss) test, a dip-strip that becomes positive (pink color) when bacteria convert nitrate to nitrite by the enzyme nitrate reductase.[68] However, the disadvantages of the nitrite test are that it has a sensitivity of only 65%, it fails to detect enterococci, and is best used for the first morning voided specimen (bacteria requires at least 4h incubation in the bladder to convert nitrate to nitrite; thus, random urine samples are less likely to be positive for bacteria). The dip-slide culture is a glass slide coated with nutrient agar on one side and differential agar to isolate gram-negative bacteria on the other side. An estimate of quantity of bacteria is made by comparison of density of bacteria on the slide to a standardized chart.[69] The correlation of the dip-slide culture method to standard culture method is greater than 95%. The dip-slide culture can be sent to a microbiology laboratory for incubation, or a small office incubator can be used. Any growth of organism on the slide can be subcultured for standard microbiologic processing and identification. The leukocyte esterase, nitrite, and dip-slide tests offer convenience, low cost, and a rapid means to screen for bacteriuria in an ambulatory setting.[70] The majority of ambulatory elderly patients with uncomplicated UTI (primarily cystitis; no sepsis, catheterization, underlying genitourinary abnormalities, or recurrence) harbor *Escherichia coli* (60%–70%), with *Proteus* spp. and *Klebsiella* spp. being isolated 20% to 30% of the time. Patients with more complicated infections will be infected with more diverse pathogens (e.g., *Enterobacter* spp., *Pseudomonas aeruginosa*, *Enterococcus* spp.).

For elderly patients who require hospitalization for managing their UTI, in addition to a urinalysis and urine culture, blood cultures should be obtained. Urine should be obtained by standard voided methods as already described; however, in very sick or functionally incapacitated elderly, urinary bladder catheterization may be necessary to obtain a specimen as well as to monitor urine output. Hospitalized patients and those who have complicated infections (upper tract, recurrent, catheter-related) need assessment of renal function (blood urea nitrogen, serum creatinine), as well as evaluation of the genitourinary anatomy (ultrasonography; intravenous pyelography) and bladder function (residual urine volume). Some patients will warrant a cystoscopy, and male patients may require a careful examination of the prostate gland to exclude chronic bacterial prostatitis or prostatic hyperplasia.[71] Uropathogens are similar to those found in ambulatory UTI patients.

In a long-term care setting (e.g., nursing facility), if the resident is clinically stable enough not to require hospitalization, a urinalysis and urine culture are sufficient for the initial evaluation of a UTI. Urine samples from incontinent men in nursing facilities can be collected with excellent accuracy by using an external catheter system.[72] In incontinent women who do not have an indwelling bladder catheter, a straight in-and-out catheterization may be required to obtain an accurate (uncontaminated) urine sample. Residents with long-term bladder catheters should have their catheters changed before obtaining a urine specimen.[73] Catheters remaining in the bladder for prolonged periods become heavily colonized with numerous different species of microorganisms, which may invalidate the isolation of pathogens residing in the bladder. Institutionalized elderly appear to be infected more often with antibiotic-resistant bacteria such as *Citrobacter freundii*, *Pseudomonas aeruginosa*, and *Providencia stuartii*, especially those with chronic urinary catheters.[71] Persons with chronic urinary catheters frequently have polymicrobial bacteriuria, with *Enterococcus* spp. occurring in about 25% of cases.

Treatment

For empiric therapy of elderly ambulatory patients with UTI, the most commonly recommended antimicrobial agent is trimethoprim-sulfamethoxazole.[74,75] Although oral beta lactam agents previously were also prescribed as primary therapy for routine UTI (i.e., ampicillin, amoxicillin-clavulanate, cephalosporins), increasing antimicrobial resistance has reduced their efficacy. Oral fluoroquinolones are now preferred as an alternative to trimethoprim-sulfamethoxazole or as primary treatment in patients who are unable to tolerate trimethoprim or sulfonamides or fail on this regimen.[76,77] Duration of therapy is at least 7 days, with more complicated cases requiring up to 14 days of treatment. Elderly men should generally be prescribed 14 days of antibiotics.

A repeat urine culture should be obtained approximately 7 to 10 days after completion of therapy for evidence of cure.

Older patients requiring hospitalization for UTI should be initially administered antibiotics until there is clinical improvement (afebrile for at least 24h; improvement in other vital signs; able to eat and drink), at which time they may be switched to oral antibiotics based on culture and sensitivity data. Effective parenteral drugs for UTI (pyelonephritis, urosepsis) include fluoroquinolones, extended-spectrum cephalosporins, beta lactam-beta lactamase agents, and aminoglycosides.[76,77] Aminoglycosides should be avoided in the elderly, whenever possible, because of the potential renal and eighth nerve toxicities of these drugs. If *Enterococcus* spp. is isolated or suspected, ampicillin-sulbactam is recommended. Most older patients with UTI in this setting should be treated with 10 to 14 days of antimicrobial therapy. A follow-up urine culture should be obtained 7 to 10 days after completion of treatment.

The management of UTI that requires treatment in the setting of a long-term care facility will be similar to managing UTI in an ambulatory setting. Most residents can be treated with oral antibiotics, that is, trimethoprim-sulfamethoxazole or fluoroquinolones; amoxicillin-clavulanate should be considered for patients with enterococci in the urine. Short-term parenteral therapy can be administered with intramuscular third-generation cephalosporin (e.g., ceftriaxone). Duration of antibiotics is similar to that prescribed for ambulatory UTI patients.

Respiratory Infections

Diagnosis

Pneumonia and influenza are particularly relevant in the elderly because of their associated high mortality rates and the high incidence of pneumonia with aging in both the community and institutional settings.[78–81]

The most important respiratory infection is lower respiratory infection, which includes acute or chronic bronchitis and pneumonia. In the ambulatory setting, acute and chronic bronchitis is the dominant lower respiratory infection managed in an outpatient and home environment. Most acute bronchitis cases are caused by viruses and require no specific diagnostic evaluation. However, if the elderly patient appears to have more severe respiratory symptoms or fever, a chest radiograph may be warranted to exclude possible pneumonia. Chronic bronchitis is especially prevalent in older men, with as many as 40% of cases occurring in men age 65 years and older.[82] Chronic bronchitis is defined as the presence of cough and sputum production on most days for at least 3 months per year for 2 consecutive years.[83] The disease often is a prelude to or is accompanied by airway obstruction, leading to chronic obstructive pulmonary disease (COPD). The most common pathogens found in chronic bronchitis are *Haemophilus influenzae*, *Streptococcus pneumoniae*, and *Moraxella catarrhalis*. However, in more severe lung disease, as determined by the forced expiratory volume in 1 s (FEV$_1$) there appears to be a higher isolation rate of gram-negative bacteria (*Enterobacteriaceae* and *Pseudomonas* species) from sputum in patients with exacerbations of chronic bronchitis. With an FEV$_1$ less than 35%, 40% of chronic bronchitics had gram-negative bacteria isolated from purulent sputum in comparison with only 10% isolation rate for those with FEV$_1$ greater than 50%.[84] The evaluation of an elderly patient with chronic bronchitis should include a chest radiograph to exclude pneumonia or other respiratory complications; collection of expectorated sputum for microbiology is of limited value because of oropharyngeal contamination. Measurement of FEV$_1$ may be considered in those elderly patients with chronic bronchitis who fail to respond to standard therapy (see section on Treatment).

Most elderly patients (nearly two-thirds) with community-acquired pneumonia require hospitalization.[85] In one large study, 18% of outpatient-treated pneumonia cases were in the elderly, but 60% of the hospitalized patients with community-acquired pneumonia were 65 years and older.[86] More recently, the Pneumonia Patient Outcome Research Team (PORT) cohort study established objective criteria to predict prognosis (death) for patients with community-acquired pneumonia within 30 days of presentation.[87] Equally important, this study, by using clinical data and select laboratory/radiologic findings to develop a point scoring system, could infer which patients would most likely benefit from inpatient hospital care for their pneumonia. A total point of 91 or greater (class IV) predicted a poorer prognosis and thus justified hospitalization. With each year of a patient's age counted as 1 point, the elderly patient is more likely to achieve a point score of 91 or greater. Based on the PORT study, in addition to a chest radiograph, the following diagnostic studies are recommended on initial evaluation of an elderly patient with community-acquired pneumonia: arterial blood gas, hematocrit (complete blood count), blood urea nitrogen (BUN), serum sodium (electrolyte panel), and serum glucose. Microbiologic studies include blood cultures, sputum for Gram stain and culture, and tuberculin skin test if tuberculosis is part of the differential diagnosis. The most common reported cause of community-acquired pneumonia in the elderly is *S. pneumoniae* (40%–60%); however, *H. influenzae* (in COPD), gram-negative bacilli, and *Legionella* species may also be isolated.[88] If legionellosis is suspected, appropriate serologic and staining tests should be ordered.

Pneumonia acquired while in the hospital for another medical problem also occurs with greater frequency in elderly patients; the incidence is three times higher in the elderly compared with younger patients.[89] Hospital-acquired pneumonia in the elderly is caused by pathogens similar to those in younger adults, with nearly half of patients having more than one organism isolated; these are gram-negative bacilli (40%–50%), anaerobic bacteria (35%), *Staphylococcus aureus* (31%), and *Streptococcus pneumoniae* (26%).[90] The evaluation of hospital-acquired pneumonia would be similar to that of community-acquired pneumonia (see earlier discussion).

In residents of long-term care facilities who develop pneumonia, most studies are from nursing facilities ("nursing-home" acquired pneumonia).[19] The PORT study predictive index for prognosis and severity of pneumonia has also been successfully applied to nursing facility residents with pneumonia.[91] Whether nursing facility residents with pneumonia require hospitalization or can be treated within the long-term care setting remains unclear and controversial.[92,93] The availability of appropriately trained staff and diagnostic and therapeutic support services in a long-term care facility, as well as the favorable pharmacokinetics of oral antibiotics, facilitate treatment of pneumonia in this setting.[91,94,95] In recently developed practice guidelines endorsed by several geriatric/gerontology and infectious disease professional organizations, the diagnostic evaluation for suspected pneumonia in residents of long-term care facilities should be limited to the following tests: (1) chest radiograph; (2) pulse oximetry to determine oxygen saturation (diagnostic and prognostic value); and (3) respiratory secretions (expectorated sputum or nasopharyngeal aspirate) for assessing purulence (predominance of neutrophils), with subsequent analysis by Gram stain and culture and sensitivity if purulence is present.[96]

Treatment

Acute bronchitis in an ambulatory setting should be managed symptomatically because most cases are caused by viruses. Hydration and nutrition are important in the frail elderly.[74] For severe cough, a mild antitussive agent should be prescribed, but more potent drugs (e.g., codeine) are not recommended for the elderly because of their side effects. If bronchospasm is present, an inhaled bronchodilator will be helpful. When a secondary bacterial infection occurs, empiric antibiotic treatment with such drugs as amoxicillin-clavulanic acid, cefuroxime axetil, azithromycin, clarithromycin, or erythromycin are recommended. Most patients will require only 5 to 7 days of treatment. Acute exacerbation of chronic bronchitis in the elderly generally requires antibiotic therapy.[97] In patients with repeated bouts of cough and purulent sputum, antibiotic therapy may be extended to 7 to 14 days. In elderly patients with FEV_1 less than 35% and failure on standard antibiotic regimens for bronchitis or patients with bronchiectasis, the likelihood of the presence of a gram-negative bacillary organism is high and treatment with an oral fluoroquinolone should be prescribed.[78] Immunization with influenza vaccine should be done on a yearly basis and at least one injection of pneumococcal vaccine should be administered (see section on Immunizations).

Community-acquired pneumonia requiring hospitalization should be managed with intravenous antibiotics until the patient clinically improves and is afebrile for at least 24 to 48h, is able to eat and drink, the respiratory rate is less than 25/min, and pulse rate is less than 100/min.[98] Patients can be discharged if the preceding criteria are present plus the following conditions: (a) negative blood culture(s); (b) oxygen saturation on room air is above 90% (with COPD, arterial oxygen >60mmHg and carbon dioxide <45mmHg, or both values return to baseline); and stable status of underlying diseases.[98] Antibiotic selection depends on severity of disease, suspected pathogens, and drug tolerance. Generally, an extended-spectrum cephalosporin (e.g., third-generation cephalosporin) or beta lactam-beta lactamase inhibitor (e.g., ampicilllin-sulbactam, piperacillin-tazobactam) combined with a macrolide (i.e., azithromycin, clarithromycin, erythromycin) has been commonly recommended as initial empiric therapy until microbiologic data become available.[99] A fluoroquinolone (e.g., levofloxacin, moxifloxacin, gatifloxacin) alone is also acceptable. If aspiration is suspected, clindamycin should be included in the regimen. Patients suspected of harboring *Pseudomonas aeruginosa* should be treated with more than one antipseudomonal agent (e.g., piperacillin or piperacillin-tazobactam plus a fluoroquinolone).[99] Patients allergic to beta-lactam drugs should be treated with a fluoroquinolone plus clindamycin.

Residents who acquire pneumonia in a long-term care facility (e.g., nursing facility) may be treated in this setting or transferred to a hospital.[92–95] The severity of disease, availability of 24-h/7-day per week appropriately trained nursing staff in the facility, physicians willing to follow patients at regular intervals (e.g., daily) in this setting, capacity to provide parenteral therapies and respiratory support treatment, quick and easy access to necessary laboratory and radiologic tests, advance directive or mutually agreed decision between patient/family and physician, and local institutional policies regarding transfer of residents will determine whether treatment occurs in the long-term care facility or hospital. A recent study, using a treatment guideline for nursing facility-acquired pneumonia based on community practices of geriatricians, demonstrated that 72% of residents could be initially treated in the nursing facility with 61% requiring only oral antibiotics.[100] The 30-day mortality rates

between those initially treated in the nursing facility (22%) and those treated in the hospital (31%) was not significant. Additionally, the mortality rates for residents treated in nursing homes with oral agents (21%) versus intramuscularly administered antibiotics (25%) was also similar.[100] A suggested guideline for treating pneumonia in a nursing facility was provided. Residents selected to be managed in the long-term care setting can be treated with a variety of antibiotics, with the route chosen determined by several factors mentioned earlier (i.e., severity of disease including ability to take oral medications, capacity to give intravenous or intramuscular medications, and availability of parenteral antibiotics). Appropriate intravenous antibiotics would be similar to those used to treat hospitalized elderly patients with pneumonia (see earlier discussion). Commonly used intramuscular antibiotics include certain third-generation cephalosporins such as ceftriaxone, cefotaxime, and cefoperazone.[100–103] If oral administration of drugs is feasible,[94,95,102] antibiotics such as amoxicillin-clavulanic acid, second- or third-generation cephalosporins (e.g., cefuroxime axetil, cefixime), or fluoroquinolones (with activity against *S. pneumoniae*, e.g., levofloxacin) would be primary choices. Clindamycin, macrolides (erythromycin, clarithromycin, azithromycin), or trimethoprim-sulfamethoxazole could be prescribed in select circumstances, such as aspiration (clindamycin), beta-lactam allergy (macrolides, clindamycin, trimethoprim-sulfamethoxazole), or possible legionellosis or mycoplasma (macrolides).

Skin and Soft Tissue Infections

Diagnosis

A variety of skin and soft tissue infections afflict older persons, but the most difficult to manage clinically are infected pressure ulcers, which occur most often in frail, debilitated elderly.[104,105]

Cellulitis that is localized and without associated systemic symptoms requires no diagnostic evaluation. Most cellulitis cases are managed in an ambulatory setting. Most cases of cellulitis are caused by either group A streptococci or *Staphylococcus aureus*.[106] In older patients with skin infection associated with diabetes mellitus, the lesions may be ulcerated or at times gangrenous. The microbial agents in diabetic skin lesions are often mixed. In early diabetic cellulitis, the organisms are primarily staphylococci; lesions that are more chronic and ulcerated are generally composed of streptococci, gram-negative bacilli, and anaerobic bacteria.[106] Diabetic skin or soft tissue infections, especially in diabetic foot disease, should have a plain radiograph of the underlying bone to exclude a coexisting osteomyelitis.[107] If plain radiographs are negative and bone infection is still suspected, a bone scan or magnetic resonance imaging (MRI) should be considered.

Another dermal infection occurring primarily in the elderly is herpes zoster (shingles) and its complication, postherpetic neuralgia.[20,108] It is managed primarily in an outpatient setting. This infection is discussed separately in Chapter 71 and is not covered here.

In both hospital and long-term care facility settings, pressure ulcers that become secondarily infected pose major problems for the elderly, especially the frail and debilitated patient or resident. The topic of pressure ulcers is discussed in Chapter 66, and there are numerous excellent reviews on this clinical problem.[109–111] The only comments to emphasize regarding infected pressure ulcers are (a) the microbiota of chronic lesions are generally a mixture of anaerobic and aerobic bacteria; (b) all wounds are always colonized with organisms and thus swab cultures of the surface of ulcers are not clinically useful; and (c) antimicrobial treatment should only be initiated if there are associated signs of purulence, cellulitis, or drainage of the wound or there is evidence of systemic toxicity or osteomyelitis.

Treatment

Cellulitis in ambulatory elderly patients can generally be effectively treated with oral cloxacillin or dicloxacillin for 7 to 10 days. Alternative drugs include oral cephalexin, clindamycin, and amoxicillin-clavulanic acid. Diabetic foot lesions with ulceration or those that are chronic may have anaerobic organisms as part of the flora; treatment with amoxicillin-clavulanic acid or a combination of clindamycin and an oral fluoroquinolone is recommended. If no bone infection is present, diabetic skin infection should be treated for approximately 2 weeks. Wound and foot care are also equally important for these infections.

The treatment of pressure ulcers is discussed in Chapter 66.

Tuberculosis

Diagnosis

Tuberculosis among persons without human immunodeficiency virus (HIV) infection occurs with the highest incidence rate in the geriatric population and poses some diagnostic challenges and a different therapeutic approach.[112–113]

Most cases of tuberculosis in the elderly (or any age group) are diagnosed in an ambulatory setting. The recommended screening test remains the tuberculin skin test, using a purified protein derivative (PPD) antigen in a strength of 5 units and applying the Mantoux technique.[114,115] A two-step procedure for tuberculin test should be implemented in all elderly persons suspected

of tuberculosis because of the "booster effect." In persons over age 55, the booster effect increases; that is, there is previous sensitization to mycobacteria primarily from earlier infection, the initial skin test application is negative, and a repeat test in 1 to 3 weeks becomes positive (10 mm or greater of induration with at least 6 mm increase from the first skin test). If a skin test is positive or if the elderly person has symptoms and signs suggestive of tuberculosis in the absence of a positive skin test, a chest radiograph should be performed.[112] An abnormal chest radiograph with findings consistent with tuberculosis (except old calcified granuloma as the only lesion) warrants sputum collection from the patient for acid-fast bacilli smear and culture for mycobacteria, specifically *Mycobacterium tuberculosis*. Approximately 75% of all tuberculosis in the elderly involves the lung.[112]

Disseminated tuberculosis and tuberculosis involving the pericardium and meninges (pericarditis, meningitis) generally require hospital care initially. The evaluation would be similar as in the ambulatory setting, but additional studies specific to the organ involved would be indicated (e.g., echocardiogram or pericardiocentesis for pericarditis; cerebrospinal fluid examination and imaging of the brain with meningitis).

Tuberculosis in a long-term care setting has been well described.[113,116] The initial evaluation would be the same as described in the ambulatory setting. However, residents identified as having potential tuberculosis disease (active tuberculosis) based on abnormal chest radiograph or positive microbiologic studies require transfer to an acute care facility in which isolation procedures for tuberculosis are available unless (1) chemotherapy is promptly instituted at the time the diagnosis is suspected or confirmed; (2) recent and current contacts are evaluated and placed on appropriate therapy; and (3) new contacts can be prevented for a 1- to 2-week period.[117]

Treatment

The most recent recommendations for chemotherapy for tuberculosis were published in 1994;[118] these are noted in Table 54.4. The recommendations are basically a four-drug regimen at the outset and are based on the assumption that resistance to isoniazid or rifampin may be prevalent.[118] However, if isoniazid resistance is less than 4% in the community, a two- or three-drug regimen is acceptable. Because most elderly patients acquired their tuberculous infection before the usage of isoniazid, most *M. tuberculosis* infections acquired by older adults are drug sensitive to both isoniazid and rifampin.[119] Most elderly patients with pulmonary tuberculosis disease (active infection), whether they are ambulatory, hospitalized, or institutionalized, may be treated with isoniazid and rifampin for 9 months or isoniazid, rifampin, and pyrazinamide for 2 months, followed by isoniazid and rifampin for another 4 months.[119] For

TABLE 54.4. Treatment options for tuberculosis.

Drugs	Frequency
Option 1	
Isoniazid, rifampin, pyrazinamide and ethambutol or streptomycin for 8 weeks[a];	Daily
then isoniazid and rifampin for 16 weeks	Daily or two or three times weekly[b]
Option 2	
Isoniazid, rifampin, pyrazinamide and ethambutol or streptomycin for 2 weeks;	Daily
then same drugs for 6 weeks; then isoniazid and rifampin for 16 weeks	Twice weekly[b]
Option 3	
Isoniazid, rifampin, pyrazinamide and ethambutol or streptomycin for 24 weeks[a]	Three times weekly[b]

[a] If isoniazid resistance is less than 4% in a community, omit fourth drug; streptomycin is not recommended for the elderly because of potential ototoxicity.

[b] Intermittent dosing should be directly observed.

Source: Bass et al.[118]

miliary or disseminated tuberculosis or tuberculous meningitis, osteomyelitis, and pericarditis, therapy should be extended to 12 months.

The indications for chemoprophylaxis (now called treatment of latent tuberculosis infection) for elderly patients or residents with positive tuberculin skin tests are the same as for younger adults.[113,119] Previously, standard chemoprophylaxis was 6 months of isoniazid.[118] More recently, the Centers for Disease Control and Prevention has revised its recommendations for chemoprophylaxis.[120] Isoniazid is now recommended for 9 months; 2 months of rifampin and pyrazinamide is also acceptable. Four months of rifampin alone is an alternative but less acceptable regimen.

Elderly patients may have a higher incidence of isoniazid-associated hepatitis, and thus careful clinical and laboratory monitoring of liver abnormalities is recommended. Baseline and follow-up liver function tests (serum aminotransferase; SGOT) are obtained every 1 to 2 months. Elevation of the SGOT to five times above normal or baseline or clinical signs of liver toxicity is an indication to discontinue isoniazid (and rifampin and pyrazinamide).[113] After resolution of symptoms or abnormal liver function tests, the isoniazid (and other drugs) may be resumed at lower doses with gradual increasing dosages. Recurrence of liver abnormalities requires a trial of an alternative therapeutic regimen.

Infective Endocarditis

Diagnosis

As the American population ages and the incidence of childhood rheumatic heart disease has declined, the incidence of infective endocarditis has risen in the elderly; nearly 50% of all cases of infective endocarditis in the United States occur in persons age 60 years and older.[121,122]

Although the elderly patient with infective endocarditis may be initially seen in an office setting, all patients require diagnostic and therapeutic interventions performed in a hospital. Immediate obtaining of at least three sets of blood cultures at three different points in time and an echocardiogram are the most important tests for the diagnosis of infective endocarditis.[123] More recent criteria for diagnosing infective endocarditis incorporate findings of an echocardiogram.[124] The finding of persistent bacteremia with clinical findings of infective endocarditis (regurgitant murmur, evidence of septic emboli) or evidence of vegetation(s) on echocardiogram is sufficient to make the diagnosis. In general, patients with moderate to severe cardiac failure, prosthetic valve endocarditis, or failure on medical treatment should be evaluated by cardiac surgery (see Treatment section of Infective Endocarditis). The most common organisms causing infective endocarditis in the elderly are streptococci, including viridans group streptococci and occasionally Streptococcus bovis, Enterococcus spp., and Staphylococcus aureus.[125] In patients with prosthetic valve endocarditis, S. aureus and S. epidermidis are the dominant pathogens.

In a long-term care setting, if a resident is suspected of infective endocarditis, he or she should be transferred to an acute care facility for further diagnostic evaluation.

Treatment

Elderly patients with infective endocarditis require hospitalization. Ideally, if the patient is clinically stable, specific antimicrobial therapy should be initiated after identification of the organism from blood cultures. However, most patients with suspected infective endocarditis are empirically treated immediately after blood cultures are obtained, and antibiotics are then adjusted according to the pathogen(s) isolated. Empiric therapy for infective endocarditis in the elderly should be directed toward streptococci, enterococci, and staphylococci. A suggested regimen is intravenous ampicillin, nafcillin (or oxacillin), and an aminoglycoside (e.g., gentamicin) administered in high doses.[126] Patients allergic to beta-lactam antibiotics should be prescribed vancomycin plus an aminoglycoside. Duration of therapy varies depending on severity of illness, sensitivity of the organism(s) to the antibiotics, complications of endocarditis, valve involvement (e.g., aortic valve infection requires longer duration of antibiotics than tricuspid valve endocarditis), and clinical response. Antimicrobial therapy for infective endocarditis generally is for 4 to 6 weeks; prosthetic valve endocarditis requires at least 6 weeks of treatment.

Surgical intervention for infective endocarditis is indicated for the following: (1) refractory congestive heart failure; (2) more than one serious systemic embolic episode; (3) persistent infection despite appropriate antibiotics; (4) significant valve dysfunction as demonstrated by echocardiography; (5) unavailability of effective antimicrobial therapy (e.g., for fungal endocarditis); (6) resection of mycotic aneurysm; (7) antibiotic-resistant organism causing infection; and (8) local valvular or myocardial abscesses.[127] In addition, the American Heart Association has identified the following echocardiographic features as associated with increased potential for surgical intervention: (1) persistent vegetation after a major systemic embolic episode; (2) anterior mitral valve vegetation more than 1 cm in diameter; (3) increase in the size of vegetation after 4 weeks of antimicrobial therapy; (4) acute mitral valve insufficiency; (5) valve perforation or rupture; and (6) periannular extension of infection.[128]

Recent data suggest that with early diagnosis of infective endocarditis using sensitive echocardiographic methods such as transesophageal echocardiography, the clinical outcome of elderly patients with valve infection is similar to that for younger patients.[13] Antimicrobial chemoprophylaxis for preventing infective endocarditis is the same for elderly patients as for the general adult population, as has been published elsewhere.[129]

Meningitis

Diagnosis

As previously mentioned (see Table 54.1), meningitis in the elderly has an especially high mortality rate;[12] in adults, the incidence of bacterial meningitis increases with advancing age.[130,131]

Unless an office setting or outpatient clinic has the capacity for doing spinal punctures and immediate microbiologic studies (e.g., Gram stain), all elderly patients suspected of meningitis should be managed in a hospital. The sine qua non to making a specific diagnosis of meningitis requires examination of the cerebrospinal fluid. Most cases of meningitis in the elderly are caused by bacteria, primarily *Streptococcus pneumoniae*; *Listeria monocytogenes*, *Neisseria meningitidis*, and gram-negative bacilli (*E. coli, Proteus, Klebsiella*) are also important meningopathogens in elderly patients. An immediate Gram stain, immunologic studies for bacterial antigens, and culture of the cerebrospinal fluid are the most important initial tests; the cerebrospinal fluid glucose (with simultaneous serum glucose), white blood cell count with differential, and protein are also useful diagnostically. A low cerebrospinal fluid glucose (below 40 mg/dL or less than 30% of the simultaneously measured serum glucose), high white blood cell count (>500 cells/μL) with a differential of at least 80% neutrophils, and an elevated protein (>100 mg/dL) are consistent with bacterial meningitis.[132] In patients who present with focal neurologic signs, seizures, coma, or suspicion of intracranial hypertension (e.g., papilledema), a brain imaging scan (e.g., computed tomography) should be performed before doing a lumbar spinal tap to exclude a coexisting mass lesion or shifts in brain structures. Under these conditions, the cerebrospinal fluid examination should be postponed to avoid potential herniation of the brain.

Treatment

Because most meningitis cases in the elderly are secondary to a bacterial infection, effective antimicrobial therapy is available for this life-threatening disease. In patients who are clinically stable without evidence of intracranial hypertension or mass lesion in the brain, empiric antimicrobial therapy may be withheld until blood cultures and lumbar spinal puncture are performed. Treatment then can be more specific and directed to a suspected etiologic pathogen based on findings on the initial examination of the cerebrospinal fluid (e.g., Gram stain). However, in elderly patients who are hypotensive, comatose, or having seizures or demonstrating rapid development of focal neurologic deficits (e.g., within 24 h) should receive the initial dose of antibiotics intravenously immediately after blood cultures are obtained and before any other tests are done (e.g., imaging scan of brain).[133] Under these circumstances, studies have shown that delays in antimicrobial therapy seriously affect the clinical outcome.[134] Earlier studies have indicated that prior antimicrobial therapy may affect the yield of organisms on Gram stain and culture, but that the microbiologic data retrieved after a few doses of antibiotics still remain substantial.[135]

Empiric antibiotic treatment in elderly patients suspected of bacterial meningitis should be initiated with a third-generation cephalosporin, that is, cefotaxime or ceftriaxone, that penetrates well into the cerebrospinal fluid and has good antibacterial activity against *S. pneumoniae*, *N. meningitidis*, and gram-negative bacilli. Because *L. monocytogenes* is always a potential meningopathogen in the elderly, either penicillin G or ampicillin should also be added to the empiric therapeutic regimen (cephalosporins are relatively ineffective against this pathogen).[132] In penicillin-allergic patients or if penicillin-resistant *S. pneumoniae* is suspected (e.g., because of a high incidence of this pathogen in the community), vancomycin should be prescribed in place of the cephalosporin for patients with beta-lactam allergy or added to the cephalosporin in penicillin-resistant *S. pneumoniae* cases. In addition, if methicillin-resistant *Staphylococcus aureus* is suspected or isolated, vancomycin would be the drug of choice;

otherwise, nafcillin or oxacillin should be administered for methicillin-sensitive *S. aureus* meningitis. All drugs should be administered intravenously during the entire period of therapy. For *Streptococcus pneumoniae* and *N. meningiditis* meningitis, most elderly patients should be treated for approximately 10 days, assuming there is a good clinical response. Meningitis caused by *L. monocytogenes* and gram-negative bacilli require at least 14 days and as long as 21 days of treatment.

With a good clinical response, repeat lumbar spinal punctures are not necessary at the completion of therapy. Measuring changes in cell counts, glucose, and protein in the cerebrospinal fluid are not better than clinical assessment (symptomatic improvement) in determining when to discontinue antibiotic therapy.[136] Although systemic corticosteroids have been recommended for children with acute bacterial meningitis,[133] data are lacking on their benefits for treatment of routine cases of bacterial meningitis in adults.[137] Nevertheless, in elderly patients with evidence of severely impaired mental status, intracranial hypertension, cranial nerve palsy, or cerebral edema, adjunctive corticosteroid therapy with dexamethasone may be beneficial even though supporting data for this are lacking.[133]

Infectious Diarrhea

Infectious diarrhea has been recognized as a significant cause of morbidity and mortality in older adults in developed countries and is the fourth most common infectious disease in elderly patients confined to chronic care facilities. Acute diarrhea in the elderly is associated with the recovery of a specific diarrhea-inducing microorganism or toxin in the stools of 40% to 50% of patients.

Infectious causes generally result from two main pathophysiologic mechanisms: exudative (inflammatory or invasive) and secretory (noninflammatory or noninvasive). Exudative diarrhea is characterized by inflammation, necrosis, and sloughing of the intestinal mucosa and the presence of fecal leukocytes and occult or gross blood in the stool. Common diarrheal pathogens that operate predominantly by this method include *Salmonella*, *Shigella*, *Campylobacter*, and *Clostridium difficile* (*C. difficile*). Secretory diarrhea involves ion secretions that cause obligatory water loss. This diarrhea is unaffected by fasting and has been associated with viral infections (rotavirus, Norwalk virus), *Giardia lamblia*, and *Vibrio cholerae*.

Clostridium difficile infectious diarrhea following antibiotic use is more protracted and severe in the elderly because of repeated and prolonged use of these agents. It is managed by discontinuation of the offending antibiotic and treatment with oral metronidazole or vancomycin.

Immunizations

Influenza

Epidemics of influenza occur annually during the winter months and account for approximately 20,000 deaths each year in the United States.[138] Although the rates of influenza infection is the highest among children, the rates of serious morbidity and mortality are highest in the population age 65 years and older and in persons of any age with serious underlying medical conditions.[139] Influenza viruses that infect humans are primarily types A and B (there is a type C, but it is not clinically relevant), with influenza type A predominating in most epidemics. During the past three influenza seasons (1997–2000), influenza type A(H3N2) has been the dominant strain.[140]

Vaccination is the primary method for the prevention of influenza and its complications (e.g., death, pneumonia). The primary target groups for immunization against influenza are those with the highest risk of experiencing complications from this infection, that is, all persons age 65 years and older and those persons under 65 years with chronic underlying medical conditions.[81] In addition, individuals who are in contact with the high-risk influenza target groups should also receive immunization to prevent transmission of infection, such as health care personnel, staff of long-term care facilities, employees of assisted living and other residential settings housing high-risk groups, persons providing home to care to high-risk groups, and household members of persons in high-risk groups.[81] Immunization with the influenza vaccine should be administered annually, usually from October through November. The influenza vaccine has a 30% to 40% effectiveness in preventing influenza in residents of long-term care facilities, and perhaps a slightly higher rate of protection in ambulatory elderly.[81] Its greatest benefit is its effectiveness in reducing the severe complications of influenza. It is 50% to 60% effective in preventing hospitalization or pneumonia and 80% effective in preventing death in elderly residents in chronic care institutions.[81]

Use of antiviral agents against influenza is an important adjunct to influenza immunization in the control and prevention of this infection. Presently, amantadine and rimantadine are approved for both treatment and prophylaxis against influenza type A (neither drug is effective against influenza type B). Amantadine and rimantadine must be given within 48 h of onset of illness to be effective in reducing severity and duration of influenza. The standard dosage of 100 mg twice daily of amantadine should be reduced to 100 mg per day in the elderly; rimantadine, similarly, should be prescribed at a dosage of 100 mg/day for those age 65 years and older;[81] further dose reduction is justified with renal impairment.

The drugs are given for 3 to 5 days or discontinued within 24 to 48 h after marked improvement of symptoms. Both drugs can be used as chemoprophylaxis against influenza type A infection during an outbreak but are not a substitute for immunization. It is recommended that chemoprophylaxis be prescribed for high-risk groups who have not been vaccinated, those who cannot be vaccinated (e.g., having allergy to vaccine), or individuals with diseases that are associated with inadequate antibody responses to immunization.[81] In addition, during an outbreak chemoprophylaxis should be considered for all elderly residents in long-term care facilities, even those who have been appropriately vaccinated, because the vaccine has only a 30% to 40% effectiveness in preventing influenza. Duration of prophylaxis is not clear, but most would recommend prescribing the drug until the peak activity of influenza in the community resolves.

Recently, two newer antiviral agents have been approved for treatment of influenza types A and B, the neurominidase inhibitors zanamivir and oseltamivir.[141] The drugs are only recommended for persons with clinical symptoms of influenza for no more than 2 days (efficacy of drug after 48 h of symptoms has not been shown). Data are not available at the time of this writing showing whether either zanamivir or oseltamivir prevents the complications of influenza, but preliminary studies suggest their efficacy in reducing the incidence of influenza in previously vaccinated elderly.[142] Zanamivir is administered via oral inhalation spray and oseltamivir is taken as an oral capsule: both drugs are prescribed for 5 days. Zanamivir and oseltamivir, at present, are not approved for chemoprophylaxis.

Pneumococcal Infection

Invasive *Streptococcus pneumoniae* (pneumococcal) disease in the United States increases with age. In one study, the annual incidence of bacteremia secondary to *S. pneumoniae* in the general population was 15 to 30 cases per 100,000 population; in persons age 65 years and older, the incidence was 50 to 83 cases per 100,000 population.[143] The majority (>60%) of pneumococcal bacteremia in adults is associated with pneumonia.[144] The incidence of pneumococcal meningitis in adults is also the highest in persons age 65 years and older.[145] Pneumococcal infection causes 40,000 deaths annually in the United States, with the case-fatality rates being the highest for bacteremia and meningitis; the highest mortality occurs in the elderly population and patients with serious underlying medical conditions.[145]

Immunization against invasive disease caused by the most common serotypes of *S. pneumoniae* is the most effective means of prevention. In immunocompetent persons aged 65 years and older, the pneumococcal vaccine was shown to have an effectiveness of 75%.[146] A single dose of the pneumococcal vaccine is indicated for all persons aged 65 years and older, including previously unvaccinated persons and persons who have not received the vaccine within 5 years and were less than age 65 years at the time of the vaccination.[145] Persons in whom their vaccination status is unknown should receive the vaccine. A repeat dose is presently not indicated except for immunocompromised persons. In immunocompromised persons (human immunodeficiency virus infection, leukemia, lymphoma, multiple myeloma, generalized malignancy, chronic renal failure or nephritic syndrome, status postorgan transplantation, and receiving immunosuppressive chemotherapy), a single revaccination is recommended after 5 or more years have lapsed since the first dose of pneumococcal vaccine.[145] The pneumococcal vaccine may be administered at the same time the influenza vaccine is given, provided they are injected at opposite sites.

Tetanus

Although the total number of cases of tetanus has continued to decline over the past 50 years, recent reports indicate that 35% of tetanus cases in the United States occurred in persons aged 60 years or older. The case-fatality rate also increased with age.[147]

During 1995 to 1997, the average annual incidence of tetanus among persons age 60 years and older was 0.33 cases per 1 million population, which is a 2-fold increase compared with persons aged 20 to 59 years and a 12-fold increase compared with persons aged 1 to 19 years.[147] The case-fatality ratio was also highest in the older adult age group.[147] The primary explanation for the higher incidence and death rate from tetanus is the lack of adequate immunization.

The Advisory Committee on Immunization Practices (ACIP) recommends that immunization status be reviewed at age 50 and tetanus immunization be administered to all older adults.[148] However, there are no data on the cost-effectiveness of immunizing all persons age 50 and older (or 65 years and older) against tetanus in the United States, given the relatively few number of cases reported annually (average, 25 cases per year). In a Canadian study that examined the cost-effectiveness of implementing a primary tetanus vaccination program among the elderly for family physicians, the conclusion was that there was a questionable value of using health care resources for this program.[149] At that time (1984), in Canadian dollars, the cost of preventing one case of tetanus would be $1.9 million. Some have recommended administering tetanus vaccine to all nursing home residents, which seems premature, given the lack of evidence for cost-effectiveness.[150] Immunization with tetanus vaccine should, perhaps, be considered for older adults who are at risk for wounds or injuries, and for institutionalized elderly who are a significant risk for cutaneous ulcers.

Immunization for tetanus is administered using a combined tetanus-diphtheria toxoid preparation in adults. A primary series of three injections is given, followed by a booster vaccination every 10 years.[147]

References

1. Kupersmith C. *Three Centuries of Infectious Diseases. An Illustrated History of Research and Treatments*. Greenwich, CT: Greenwich Press; 1998.

2. Lyons AS, Petrucelli RJ. *Medicine: An Illustrated History*. New York: Abrams; 1978.

3. National Center for Health Statistics. *Health United States 1985*. DHHS (PHS) 86-1232. Hyattsville, MD: U.S. Department of Health and Human Services, Public Health Service; 1986.

4. U.S. Bureau of Census. *Decennial Censuses of Population, 1900–1980 and Projections of the Population of the United States: 1982–2050 (advance report)*. Current Population Reports Series P-25, No. 922. Washington, DC: U.S. Bureau of Census; 1982.

5. National Center for Health Statistics. *Leading causes of death and number of deaths according to age: United States, 1980 and 1993. Health United States, 1995*. (PHS) 92-1232. Washington, DC: Dept. of Health and Human Services; 1996.

6. Marston BJ, Plouffe JF, File TM, et al. Incidence of community-acquired pneumonia requiring hospitalization. Results of population-based active surveillance study in Ohio. *Arch Intern Med*. 1997;157:1709–1718.

7. Centers for Disease Control. *1989 Tuberculosis Status in the United States*. CDC 91-8322. Atlanta, GA: Dept. of Health and Human Services; 1996.

8. Ackermann RJ, Monroe PW. Bacteremic urinary tract infection in older people. *J Am Geriatr Soc*. 1996;44:927–933.

9. McCue JD. Gram-negative bacillary bacteremia in the elderly: incidence, ecology, etiology and mortality. *J Am Geriatr Soc*. 1987;35:213–218.

10. Norman DC, Yoshikawa TT. Intraabdominal infection: diagnosis and treatment in the elderly. *Gerontology*. 1984; 30:327–338.

11. Norman DC, Yoshikawa TT. Infections of the bone, joint and bursa. *Clin Geriatr Med*. 1994;10:703–718.

12. Gorse GJ, Thrupp LD, Nudleman KL, et al. Bacterial meningitis in the elderly. *Arch Intern Med*. 1984;144:1603–1607.

13. Werner GS, Schulz R, Fuchs JB, et al. Infective endocarditis in the elderly in the era of transesophageal echocardiography: clinical features and prognosis compared with younger patients. *Am J Med*. 1996;100:90–97.

14. Bryan CS, Reynolds KL. Community-acquired bacteremic urinary tract infection: epidemiology and outcome. *J Urol*. 1984;132:490–493.

15. Yoshikawa TT. You are what you urinate: fact or fiction. *J Am Geriatr Soc*. 1998;46:1051–1052.

16. Gleckman RA, Bradley PJ, Roth RM, et al. Bacteremic urosepsis: a phenomenon unique to elderly women. *J Urol*. 1985;133:174–175.

17. Mufson MA, Oley G, Hughey D. Pneumococcal disease in a medium-sized community in the United States. *JAMA*. 1982;248:1486–1489.

18. Finkelstein MS, Petkun WM, Freedman ML, et al. Pneumococcal bacteremia in adults: age-dependent differences in presentation and in outcome. *J Am Geriatr Soc*. 1983;31:19–27.

19. Peltokallio P, Jauhainen K. Acute appendicitis in the aged patient. Study of 300 cases after the age of 60. *Arch Surg*. 1970;100:140–143.

20. Demorgas JM, Kierland RR. The outcome of patients with herpes zoster. *Arch Dermatol*. 1957;75:193–196.

21. Emori TB, Banerjee SN, Culver DH, et al. Nosocomial infections in elderly patients in the United States, 1986–1990. *Am J Med*. 1991;91(suppl 3B):3B-289S–3B-293.

22. Saviteer SM, Samson GP, Rutala WA. Nosocomial infections in the elderly. Increased risk per hospital day. *Am J Med*. 1988;84:661–666.

23. Castle SC. Clinical relevance of age-related immune dysfunction. *Clin Infect Dis*. 2000;31:578–585.

24. Norman DC. Predisposing factors to infection. In: Yoshikawa TT, Norman DC, eds. *Infectious Disease in the Aging: A Clinical Handbook*. Totowa, NJ: Humana Press; 2001:7–12.

25. Yoshikawa TT, Norman DC. *Aging and Clinical Practice: Infectious Diseases. Diagnosis and Treatment*. New York: Igaku-Shoin; 1987.

26. Yoshikawa TT, Norman DC. *Infectious Diseases in the Aging: A Clinical Handbook*. Totowa, NJ: Humana Press; 2001.

27. Hill AB, Meakins JL. Peritonitis. *Clin Geriatr Med*. 1992; 4:869–887.

28. Vo D, Wilson SE. Acute conditions of the abdomen. In: Yoshikawa TT, Norman DC, eds. *Acute Emergencies and Critical Care of the Elderly*. New York: Dekker; 2000:141–164.

29. Yoshikawa TT. Infectious complications of diabetes mellitus in the elderly. *Clin Geriatr*. 1998;6:30–37.

30. Dhawan VK. Osteomyelitis in elderly patients. *Infect Dis Clin Pract*. 1999;8:439–443.

31. Gehanno P. Ciprofloxacin in the treatment of malignant otitis externa. *Chemotherapy*. 1994;1:35–40.

32. Yoshikawa TT. Aging and bacterial arthritis. *Infect Dis Clin Pract*. 1996;5:548–550.

33. Kortekangas P. Bacterial arthritis in the elderly. *Drugs Aging*. 1999;14:165–171.

34. Taylor ME, Oppenheimer BA. Hospital-acquired infection in elderly patients. *J Hosp Infect*. 1998;38:245–260.

35. Yoshikawa TT, Norman DC. Approach to fever and infection in the nursing home. *J Am Geriatr Soc*. 1996;44:74–82.

36. Muder RR, Brennen C, Wagener MM, et al. Bacteremia in a long-term-care facility: a five-year prospective study of 163 consecutive episodes. *Clin Infect Dis*. 1992;14:647–654.

37. Drinka PJ, Gravenstein S, Krause P, et al. Non-influenza respiratory viruses may overlap and obscure influenza activity. *J Am Geriatr Soc*. 1999;47:1087–1093.

38. Simon AE, Gordon M, Bishai FR. Prevalence of hepatitis B surface antigen, hepatitis C antibody, and HIV-1 antibody among residents of long-term-care facility. *J Am Geriatr Soc.* 1992;40:218–220.

39. Chien NT, Dundoo G, Horani MH, et al. Seroprevalence of viral hepatitis in an older nursing home population. *J Am Geriatr Soc.* 1999;47:1110–1113.

40. Thomas DR, Bennett RG, Laughon BE, et al. Postantibiotic colonization with *Clostridium difficile* in nursing home patients. *J Am Geriatr Soc.* 1990;38:415–420.

41. Walker KJ, Gilliland SS, Vance-Ryan K, et al. *Clostridium difficile* colonization in residents of long-term care facilities: prevalence and risk factors. *J Am Geriatr Soc.* 1993;41: 940–946.

42. Yoshikawa TT. VRE, MRSA, PRP, and DRGNB in LTCF: lessons to be learned from this alphabet. *J Am Geriatr Soc.* 1998;46:241–243.

43. Mackowiak PA. *Fever. Basic Mechanisms and Management.* New York: Raven Press; 1991.

44. Norman DC. Fever and fever of unknown origin in the elderly. *Clin Infect Dis.* 2000;31:148–151.

45. Gleckman R, Hibert D. Afebrile bacteremia: a phenomenon in geriatric patients. *JAMA.* 1981;248:1478–1481.

46. Marrie TJ, Haldane EV, Faulkner RS, et al. Community-acquired pneumonia requiring hospitalization. Is it different in the elderly? *J Am Geriatr Soc.* 1985;33:671–680.

47. Terpenning MS, Buggy BO, Kauffman CA. Infective endocarditis: clinical features in young and elderly patients. *Am J Med.* 1987;83:626–634.

48. Norman DC, Yoshikawa TT. Recognizing bacterial meningitis in the elderly. *Geriatr Med Today.* 1984;3:85–88.

49. Castle SC, Norman DC, Yeh M, et al. Fever response in elderly nursing home residents: are the older truly colder? *J Am Geriatr Soc.* 1991;39:853–857.

50. Castle SC, Yeh M, Toledo S, et al. Lowering the temperature criterion improves the detection of infections in nursing home residents. *Aging Immunol Infect Dis.* 1993;4: 76–76.

51. Norman DC, Yoshikawa TT. Fever in the elderly. *Infect Dis Clin N Am.* 1996;10:93–99.

52. Keating MJ III, Klimek JJ, Levine DS, et al. Effect of aging on clinical significance of fever in ambulatory adult patients. *J Am Geriatr Soc.* 1984;32:282–287.

53. Schoeinfeld CN, Hansen KN, Hexter DA, et al. Fever in geriatric emergency patients: clinical features associated with serious illness. *Ann Emerg Med.* 1995;26:18–24.

54. Wasserman M, Levinstein M, Keller E, et al. Utility of fever, white blood cell, and differential count in predicting bacterial infections in the elderly. *J Am Geriatr Soc.* 1989; 37:534–543.

55. Terndrup TE. An appraisal of temperature assessment by infrared emission detection tympanic thermometry. *Ann Emerg Med.* 1992;21:1483–1492.

56. Shinozaki TS, Deane R, Perkins FM. Infrared tympanic thermometer: evaluation of a new clinical thermometer. *Crit Care Med.* 1988;16:148–150.

57. Castle SC, Toledo S, Daskal LS, et al. The equivalency of infrared tympanic membrane thermometry with standard thermometry in nursing home residents. *J Am Geriatr Soc.* 1992;40:1212–1216.

58. Smitz S, Giagoultis T, Dewe W, et al. Comparison of rectal and infrared ear temperatures in older hospital patients. *J Am Geriatr Soc.* 2000;48:63–66.

59. Norman DC. Clinical features of infections. In: *Infectious Diseases in the Aging: A Clinical Handbook.* Totowa, NJ: Humana Press; 2001:13–18.

60. Knockaert DC, Vanneste LJ, Bobbaers HJ. Fever of unknown origin in elderly patients. *J Am Geriatr Soc.* 1993; 41:1187–1192.

61. Raz R, Gennesan Y, Wasser J, et al. Recurrent urinary tract infections in postmenopausal women. *Clin Infect Dis.* 2000;30:152–156.

62. Nicolle LE. Urinary tract infection. In: Yoshikawa TT, Norman DC, eds. *Infectious Disease in the Aging: A Clinical Handbook.* Totowa, NJ: Humana Press; 2001: 99–111.

63. Leibovici L. Bactaeremia in the very old. Features and treatment. *Drugs Aging.* 1995;6:456–464.

64. Pewitt EB, Schaeffer AJ. Urinary tract infection in urology, including acute and chronic prostatitis. *Infect Dis Clin N Am.* 1997;11:623–646.

65. Lipsky BA, Ireton RC, Fihn SD, et al. Diagnosis of bacteriuria in men: specimen collection and culture interpretation. *J Infect Dis.* 1987;155:847–854.

66. Norman DC, Yamamura R, Yoshikawa TT. Pyuria: its predictive value of asymptomatic bacteriuria in ambulatory elderly men. *J Urol.* 1986;135:520–522.

67. Monane M, Gurwitz JH, Lipsitz LA, et al. Epidemiologic and diagnostic aspects of bacteriuria: a longitudinal study in older women. *J Am Geriatr Soc.* 1995;43:618–622.

68. Kunin CM. *Urinary Tract Infection.* Baltimore: Williams & Wilkins; 1997:42–77.

69. Arneil GC, McAllister TA, Kay P. Measurement of bacteriuria by plane dipslide culture. *Lancet.* 1973;1:94–95.

70. Flanagan PG, Davies EA, Rooney PG, et al. Evaluation of four screening tests for bacteriuria in elderly people. *Lancet.* 1989;1:1117–1119.

71. Yoshikawa TT, Nicolle LE, Norman DC. Management of complicated urinary tract infection in older patients. *J Am Geriatr Soc.* 1996;44:1235–1241.

72. Ouslander JG, Greengold BA, Silverblatt FJ, et al. An accurate method to obtain urine for culture in men with external catheters. *Arch Intern Med.* 1987;147:286–288.

73. Grahn D, Norman DC, White ML, et al. Validity of urinary catheter specimen for diagnosis of urinary tract infection in the elderly. *Arch Intern Med.* 1985;145:1535–1537.

74. Yoshikawa TT. Ambulatory management of common infections in elderly patients. *Infect Med.* 1991;8:37–43.

75. Yoshikawa TT. Urinary tract infection. In: Yoshikawa TT, Cobbs EL, Brummel-Smith K, eds. *Practical Ambulatory Geriatrics*, 2nd Ed. St. Louis: Mosby Yearbook; 1998:230–235.

76. Warren JW, Abrutyn E, Hebel JR, et al. Guidelines for antimicrobial treatment of uncomplicated acute bacterial cystitis and acute pyelonephritis in women. *Clin Infect Dis.* 1999; 29:745–758.

77. Stamm WE, Hooton TM. Management of urinary tract infection in adults. *N Engl J Med.* 1993;329:1329–1334.

78. Marrie TJ. Bronchitis and pneumonia. In: Yoshikawa TT, Norman DC, eds. *Infectious Disease in the Aging: A*

Clinical Handbook. Totowa, NJ: Humana Press; 2001:53–65.

79. Medina-Walpole AM, Katz PR. Nursing home-acquired pneumonia. *J Am Geriatr Soc.* 1999;47:1005–1015.

80. Arden NH. Control of influenza in long-term care facility: a review of established approaches and newer options. *Infect Control Hosp Epidemiol.* 2000;21:59–64.

81. Centers for Disease Control and Prevention. Prevention and control of influenza. Recommendations of the Advisory Committee on Immunization Practices (ACIP). *Morb Mortal Wkly Rep (MMWR).* 1999;48(SS-4):1–28.

82. Bulla A, Hitske KL. Acute respiratory infections: a review. *Bull WHO.* 1978;56:481–498.

83. Medical Research Council. Definition and classification of chronic bronchitis for clinical and epidemiological purposes. *Lancet.* 1965;1:775–779.

84. Eller J, Ede A, Schaberg T, et al. Infective exacerbations of chronic bronchitis. Relation between bacterial etiology and lung function. *Chest.* 1998;113:1542–1548.

85. McCue J. Pneumonia in the elderly. Special considerations in a special population. *Postgrad Med.* 1993;94:39–51.

86. Woodhead M. Pneumonia in the elderly. *J Antimicrob Chemother.* 1994;34(suppl A):85–92.

87. Fine MJ, Auble TE, Yealy DM, et al. A prediction rule to identify low-risk patients with community-acquired pneumonia. *N Engl J Med.* 1997;336:243–250.

88. Fein AM, Niederman MS. Severe pneumonia in the elderly. *Clin Geriatr Med.* 1994;10:121–143.

89. Niederman MS. Nosocomial pneumonia in the elderly. In: Niederman MS, ed. *Respiratory Infections in the Elderly.* New York: Raven Press; 1991:207–237.

90. Bartlett JG, O'Keefe P, Tally FP, et al. Bacteriology of hospital-acquired pneumonia. *Arch Intern Med.* 1986;146:868–871.

91. Mylotte JM, Naughton B, Saludades C, et al. Validation and application of pneumonia prognosis index to nursing home residents with pneumonia. *J Am Geriatr Soc.* 1998;46:1538–1544.

92. Fried TR, Gillick MR, Lipsitz LA. Short-term functional outcomes of long-term care residents with pneumonia treated with and without hospital transfer. *J Am Geriatr Soc.* 1997;45:302–306.

93. Mehr DR. Nursing home-acquired pneumonia: how and where to treat? *J Am Board Fam Pract.* 1997;10:168–170.

94. Degalau J, Guay D, Straub K, et al. Effectiveness of oral antibiotic treatment in nursing-home-acquired pneumonia. *J Am Geriatr Soc.* 1995;43:245–251.

95. Peterson PK, Stein D, Guay DRP, et al. Prospective study of lower respiratory tract infections in an extended-care nursing home program: potential role of oral ciprofloxacin. *Am J Med.* 1988;85:164–171.

96. Bentley DW, Bradley S, High K, et al. Practice guidelines for the evaluation of fever and infection in long-term care facilities. *J Am Geriatr Soc.* 2001;49(2):210–22.

97. Marrie TJ. Management of chronic bronchitis in the older patient. *Clin Geriatr.* 1995;11:20–27.

98. Marrie TJ. Clinical strategies for managing pneumonia in the elderly. *Clin Geriatr* (Suppl) 1999:6–10.

99. Bartlett JG, Dowell SF, Mandell LA, et al. Community-acquired pneumonia in adults: guidelines for management. *Clin Infect Dis.* 2000;31(2):347–382.

100. Naughton BJ, Mylotte JM. Treatment guideline for nursing home-acquired pneumonia based on community practice. *J Am Geriatr Soc.* 2000;48:82–88.

101. Yoshikawa TT. Treatment of nursing home-acquired pneumonia. *J Am Geriatr Soc.* 1991;39:1040–1041.

102. Hirata-Dulas CAI, Stein DJ, Guay DRP, et al. A randomized study of ciprofloxacin versus ceftriaxone in the treatment of nursing home-acquired lower respiratory tract infections. *J Am Geriatr Soc.* 1991;39:979–985.

103. Phillips SL, Branaman-Phillips J. The use of intramuscular cefoperazone versus intramuscular ceftriaxone in patients with nursing home-acquired pneumonia. *J Am Geriatr Soc.* 1993;41:1071–1074.

104. Klein NC, Cunha BA. Skin and soft tissue infections. In: Yoshikawa TT, Norman DC, eds. *Infectious Disease in the Aging: A Clinical Handbook.* Totowa, NJ: Humana Press; 2001:139–145.

105. Kertesz D, Chow AW. Infected pressure and diabetic ulcers. *Clin Geriatr Med.* 1992;8:835–852.

106. Cantrell M, Norman DC. Skin and soft-tissue infections in the elderly. In: Bula CJ, Kauffman CA, eds. *Balliere's Clinical Infectious Diseases.* London: Bailliere Tindall; 1998:71–81.

107. Yoshikawa TT. Infectious complications of diabetes mellitus in the elderly. *Clin Geriatr.* 1998;6:30–37.

108. Choo PW, Galil K, Donohue JG, et al. Risk factors for postherpetic neuralgia. *Arch Intern Med.* 1997;157:1217–1224.

109. Allman RM. Pressure ulcers among the elderly. *N Engl J Med.* 1989;320:850–853.

110. Ferrell BA, Osterweil D, Christenson P. A randomized trial of low-air-pressure beds for treatment of pressure ulcers. *JAMA.* 1993;269:494–497.

111. Leigh IH, Bennett G. Pressure ulcers: prevalence, etiology and treatment modalities. A review. *Am J Surg.* 1994;167(1A suppl):25S–30S.

112. Rajagopalan S, Yoshikawa TT. Tuberculosis. In: Hazzard WR, Blass JP, Ettinger WH Jr, et al. eds. *Principles of Geriatric Medicine and Gerontology, 4th Ed.* New York: McGraw-Hill; 1999:737–744.

113. Rajagopalan S. Yoshikawa TT. TB in long-term care facilities. *Infect Control Hosp Epidemiol.* 2000;21(9):611–615.

114. Huebner RE, Schein MF, Bass JB Jr. The tuberculin skin test. *Clin Infect Dis.* 1993;17:968–975.

115. Pouchot J, Grasland A, Collet C, et al. Reliability of tuberculin skin test measurement. *Ann Intern Med.* 1997;126:210-214.

116. Stead W, Lofgren J, Warren E, et al. Tuberculosis as an endemic and nosocomial infection among the elderly in nursing homes. *N Engl J Med.* 1985;312:1483–1487.

117. Centers for Disease Control and Prevention. Prevention and control of tuberculosis in facilities providing long-term care to the elderly. Recommendations of the Advisory Committee for Elimination of Tuberculosis. *Morb Mortal Wkly Rep (MMWR).* 1990;39(RR-10):7–20.

118. Bass JB, Farer S, Hopewell PC, et al. Treatment of tuberculosis and tuberculous infection in adults and children. *Am J Respir Crit Care Med.* 1994;149:1359–1374.

119. Yoshikawa TT. The challenge and unique aspects of tuberculosis in older patients. *Infect Dis Clin Pract.* 1994;3:62–66.

120. Centers for Disease Control and Prevention. Targeted tuberculin testing and treatment of latent tuberculous infection. *Morb Mortal Wkly Rep (MMWR).* 2000;49(RR-6):1–51.

121. Watanakunakorn C, Burkert T. Infective endocarditis at a large community teaching hospital, 1980–1990. A review of 210 episodes. *Medicine.* 1993;72:90–102.

122. Kazanjian PH. Infective endocarditis: review of 60 cases treated in community hospitals. *Infect Dis Clin Pract.* 1993;2:41–46.

123. Fisher EA, Fisher LL, Fuster V, et al. Infective endocarditis: new perspectives in an old disease. *Infect Dis Clin Pract.* 1998;7:12–24.

124. Durack DT, Lukes AS, Bright DK. New criteria for diagnosis of infective endocarditis: utilization of specific echocardiographic findings. *Am J Med.* 1994;96:200–209.

125. Terpenning MS. Infective endocarditis. *Clin Geriatr Med.* 1992;8:903–912.

126. Dhawan V, Yoshikawa TT. Diagnosis and treatment of infective endocarditis in the elderly. In: Vellas B, Albrede JL, Parry PL, eds. *Facts, Research and Intervention in Gerontology.* New York: Springer; 1997:245–259.

127. Bayer AS, Scheld WM. Endocarditis and intravascular infections. In: Mandell GL, Bennett JE, Dolin R, eds. *Principles and Practice of Infectious Diseases, 5th Ed.* Philadelphia: Churchill Livingstone; 2000:857–902.

128. Bayer AS, Bolger AF, Taubert KA, et al. Diagnosis and management of infective endocarditis and its complications. *Circulation.* 1998;98:2936–2948.

129. Dajani AS, Taubert KA, Wilson W, et al. Prevention of bacterial endocarditis. Recommendations by the American Heart Association. *Circulation.* 1997;96:358–366.

130. Wenger JD, Hightower AW, Facklam RR, et al. Bacterial meningitis in the United States, 1986: report of a multistate surveillance study. *J Infect Dis.* 1990;162:1316–1323.

131. Durand ML, Calderwood SB, Weber DJ, et al. Acute bacterial meningitis in adults. A review of 493 episodes. *N Engl J Med.* 1993;328:21–28.

132. Choi C. Bacterial meningitis. In: Yoshikawa TT, Norman DC, eds. *Infectious Disease in the Aging: A Clinical Handbook.* Totowa, NJ: Humana Press; 2001:113–124.

133. Tunkel AR, Scheld WM. Acute meningitis. In: Mandell GL, Bennett JE, Dolin R, eds. *Principles and Practice of Infectious Diseases, 5th Ed.* Philadelphia: Churchill Livingstone; 2000:959–997.

134. Aronin SI, Peduzzi P, Quagliarello VJ. Community-acquired bacterial meningitis: risk stratification for adverse clinical outcome and effect of antibiotic timing. *Ann Intern Med.* 1998;129:862–869.

135. Talan DA, Hoffman JR, Yoshikawa TT, et al. A review of the role of empiric parenteral antibiotics prior to lumbar puncture in suspected bacterial meningitis. *Rev Infect Dis.* 1988;10:365–376.

136. Durack DT, Spanos A. End-of-treatment spinal tap in bacterial meningitis: is it worthwhile? *JAMA.* 1982;248:75–80.

137. McGowan JE Jr, Chesney JP, Crossley KB, et al. Guidelines for the use of systemic glucocorticoids in the management of selected infections. *J Infect Dis.* 1992;165:1–13.

138. Simonsen L, Schoenberger LB, Stroup DF, et al. The impact of influenza on mortality in the USA. In: Brown LE, Hampson AW, Webster RG, eds. *Options for the Control of Influenza.* Amsterdam: Elsevier; 1996:26–33.

139. Glezen WP. Serious morbidity and mortality associated with influenza episodes. *Epidemiol Rev.* 1982;4:25–44.

140. Centers for Disease Control and Prevention. Update: influenza activity—United States, 1999–2000 season. *Morb Mortal Wkly Rep (MMWR).* 2000;49(9):173–177.

141. Centers for Disease Control and Prevention. Neuraminidase inhibitors for treatment of influenza A and B. *Morb Mortal Wkly Rep (MMWR).* 1999;48(RR-14):1–9.

142. Peters PH, Gravenstein S, Norwood P, et al. Long-term use of oseltamivir for prophylaxis of influenza in a vaccinated frail older population. *J Am Geriatr Soc.* 2001;49:1025–1031.

143. Plouffe JF, Breiman RF, Facklam RR, and Franklin County Pneumonia Study Group. Bacteremia with *Streptococcus pneumoniae* in adults—implications for therapy and prevention. *JAMA.* 1996;275:194–198.

144. Afessa B, Greaves WL, Frederick WR. Pneumococcal bacteremia in adults: a 14-year experience in an inner-city university hospital. *Clin Infect Dis.* 1995;21:345–351.

145. Centers for Disease Control and Prevention. Prevention of pneumococcal disease. Recommendations of the Advisory Committee on Immunization Practices (ACIP). *Morb Mortal Wkly Rep (MMWR).* 1997;46(RR-8):1–24.

146. Fine MJ, Smith MP, Carson CA, et al. Efficacy of pneumococcal vaccination in adults: a meta-analysis of randomized controlled trials. *Arch Intern Med.* 1994;154:2666–2677.

147. Centers for Disease Control and Prevention. Tetanus surveillance—United States, 1995–1997. *Morb Mortal Wkly Rep (MMWR).* 1998;47(SS-2):1–13.

148. Centers for Disease Control and Prevention. Assessing adult vaccination status at age 50 years. *Morb Mortal Wkly Rep (MMWR).* 1995;44:561–563.

149. Hutchinson BG, Stoddard GC. Cost-effectiveness of primary tetanus vaccination among elderly Canadians. *Can Med Assoc J.* 1988;139:1143–1149.

150. Richardson JP, Knight AL, Stafford DT. Beliefs and policies of Maryland nursing home medical directors regarding tetanus immunization. *J Am Geriatr Soc.* 1990;38:1316–1318.

55
Hematologic Problems

Gerald Rothstein

The bone marrow and circulating blood cells make up the blood cell system. This system is a dynamic one where, in the nondiseased steady state, production and utilization of blood cells are equal. However, when there is an increased demand for blood cells, such as during anemia or infection, the marrow produces more cells to provide for the increased need. In young and middle-aged adults, the system functions appropriately, responding to physiologic needs and then returning to the steady state ready to respond to new demands. However, as aging proceeds, the response to increased demand for blood cells becomes disordered and a variety of factors combine to increase the prevalence of anemia and hematologic malignancy.

The Bone Marrow During Aging

The bone marrow is the site of production for circulating red blood cells, granulocytes, and platelets. As aging proceeds, the marrow becomes increasingly localized to the axial skeleton. However, in nondiseased elderly persons, the total number of marrow cells in the body is not decreased; it is similar to that of healthy young adults.[1] Consequently, clinical examination of the marrow (the myeloid: erythroid ratio, maturation of cell lines, karyotypic analysis, and presence and distribution of stainable iron) of older persons does not differ from that of normal young adults.

The Blood Cells and Their Laboratory Values During Aging

The concentrations of red cells, platelets, and leukocytes in the blood of healthy older persons do not differ from those of young adults. The normal ranges for hematocrit are expected to increase with altitude and are best interpreted in the context of locally generated means and variances. The prevalence of anemia is increased in populations of community-dwelling, clinic-visiting, and hospitalized elderly. However, anemia is not a consequence of age. Indeed, the distribution of hematocrit values for elderly patients falls roughly into two populations: one that is in the anemic range, and another that overlaps with the distribution for normal young adults.[2] This finding supports the concept that older persons develop anemia because of underlying disease. Indeed, careful diagnostic testing of elderly anemic subjects reveals one or more identifiable causes for the anemia in at least 80% of cases.[2]

Substrates for Blood Cell Production

Critical substrates for blood cell production are iron, vitamin B_{12}, folic acid, dietary calories, and protein. Deficiencies in one or more of these substrates cause anemia, as well as other adverse consequences.

In the elderly, the body's iron is highly conserved. There is no excretory pathway for iron, and aged women are not affected by the iron loss of pregnancy or normal menstruation. Loss of iron from the body is only approximately 1 milligram (mg) per day, occurring as skin and gut cells are shed passively. In contrast to this slight daily insensible loss, total body iron is normally approximately 3 g, distributed roughly equally between red cell hemoglobin and storage iron within reticuloendothelial cells.[3] Consequently, storage iron alone is approximately 1500 times greater than the expected daily insensible loss. This extensive supply of stored iron provides a reserve with which to replace the iron of hemoglobin if blood were lost. Indeed, even if no dietary iron were ingested, more than 4 years would elapse before the iron stores were exhausted by insensible iron loss and anemia began to develop. Therefore, iron deficiency should never be considered to be a consequence of dietary deficiency of iron. *Iron deficiency should always be considered a consequence of blood loss, and should prompt a thorough search for a source of bleeding, such as occult colon carcinoma.* Indeed, in more than 80% of cases of iron deficiency the reason for iron loss is identified, and, at least in a population of variously aged adults, almost always the cause is blood loss.[4]

Folic acid and vitamin B_{12} have a critical role in cellular proliferation. Deficiencies in these vitamins lead to macrocytic anemia with characteristic morphologic alterations (megaloblastic changes) in the precursors of the marrow and circulating neutrophils. Vitamin B_{12} is also important for maintenance of the integrity of the nervous system, and its deficiency leads to subacute combined degeneration of the nervous system with peripheral sensory manifestations and cognitive impairment. The megaloblastic anemia of either vitamin can be corrected by folic acid, so that administration of folic acid can mask the anemic manifestations of vitamin B_{12} deficiency. The neurologic changes of B_{12} deficiency are only inconsistently reversed by replacement therapy and may be irreversible if advanced.[5]

Regulation of Blood Cell Production During Aging

In steady state and during periods of increased demand, blood cell production is regulated by erythropoietin and a variety of cytokine stimulators, as well as being under the influence of endocrine hormones such as thyroxine, and corticosteroids. During aging, steady-state regulation of the marrow appears normal, as evidenced by normal numbers of marrow precursors.[1,6–8] During periods of increased hematopoietic demand, the hematopoietic response of the elderly is dysregulated. For example, phlebotomized aged mice do not repair posthemorrhagic anemia as rapidly as young animals.[6] The cause of this impaired regeneration of red cells is unclear and may be multifactorial. In elderly persons, deficiency of erythropoietin is a frequent contributing or causative factor, and the administration of recombinant erythropoietin is effective in reversing at least some of the anemias in elderly persons due to erythropoietin deficiency.[9] Defects in leukocyte regeneration have also been demonstrated in aged animals, which do not replace utilized neutrophils as briskly as young adults.[7] In fact, in bacterially infected aged mice, there is a *paradoxical reduction* in both the number and proliferative rate of neutrophil precursors.[7] The marrow precursors of elderly persons show a similar defect, with paradoxical reductions in the concentrations of progenitor cells for granulocytes, as well as red cells.

A number of studies have shown that these hematopoietic defects may in part be explained by impaired production of cytokine stimulators such as granulocyte-macrophage colony-stimulating factor (GM-CSF).[10]

However, the disordered production of cytokines is not one of universal impairment; the production of other cytokines, such as interleukin 6 (IL-6) (a promoter of B-lymphocyte survival and growth) appears to be increased in the elderly.[11,12] Consequently, factors that control the production of blood cells appear to be dysregulated during aging, thus impairing the ability of the marrow to appropriately respond to increased demand for blood cells. The age-associated paradoxical reduction in marrow cells during infection and anemia is not yet understood, but it can be speculated that the dysregulated production of cytokines, such as IL-10, which induce programmed cell death (apoptosis), may account for this.[13] It can also be proposed that dysregulated production of cytokines that impair normal marrow growth or promote the growth of neoplastic clones may be factors in the increased prevalence of hematologic malignancies in the elderly. IL-6 is an example of an age-associated increase in cytokine production that can promote the emergence of a specific malignant disease, multiple myeloma. IL-6 is a promoter of the survival and growth of myeloma cells, and IL-6 also impairs the effectiveness of antimyeloma therapy with corticosteroids by blockading their mechanism of action: induction of programmed cell death.[14]

Anemia in the Elderly

Although anemia is more prevalent as aging proceeds, this cannot be assumed to be due to aging alone. In the elderly as in young adults, discrete and identifiable diseases cause anemia. However, elderly persons can be considered to be more susceptible to anemia-inducing events because of an age-associated impairment of the marrow's ability to appropriately increase red cell production.

Prevalence of Anemia in the Elderly

The prevalence of anemia in the elderly is greater than that of young adults, ranging from 5% to 51%, with the lowest prevalence in community-dwelling elderly who consider themselves healthy, intermediate values for prevalence among those enrolled in clinics for health care, and the greatest prevalence among the oldest old who are hospitalized.[2,15–17] This correlation of age-associated anemia and health status supports the concept that anemia is a consequence of disease in the elderly and not due to age alone.

Clinical Presentation of Anemia

The clinical presentation of anemia depends on the degree of anemia, the underlying cause, and the presence of comorbid conditions. Often, anemia in the elderly is

TABLE 55.1. The kinetic categories of anemia: supportive laboratory tests and associated disorders.

Kinetic category of anemia	Laboratory tests	Corresponding disorders
Decreased red cell production	Reticulocyte count[a] (reduced) Marrow cellularity (reduced) Marrow myeloid: erythroid ratio (increased)	Iron deficiency, anemia of chronic disease, megaloblastic anemias, protein/calorie malnutrition, endocrine diseases, erythropoietin deficiency marrow infiltrative diseases, aplastic anemia, anemia secondary to chemotherapy
Increased red cell destruction	Indirect bilirubin[a] (increased) LDH (increased)	Hemolytic anemias, bleeding into closed body spaces, paroxysmal nocturnal hemoglobinuria
Loss of red cells	History of bleeding[a] Stool guaiac (positive)[a]	GI blood loss, surgical blood loss, bleeding diatheses
Ineffective erythropoiesis	Reticulocyte count[a] (reduced) Indirect bilirubin[a] (increased) LDH (increased) Marrow myeloid: erythroid ratio (increased)	Myelodysplastic syndromes, megaloblastic anemia

[a] Tests useful for screening purposes.

associated with such nonspecific symptoms as fatigue, functional decline, and weakess, and is only discovered by laboratory survey. Under these circumstances, the patient's perception of quality of life may be adversely affected, even when hemoglobin levels are as high as 11 g/dL. Importantly, the fatigue and poor quality of life associated with anemia respond to correction of the anemia even when serious underlying conditions such as malignancy are unresponsive to treatment. When anemia is a consequence of malignancy such as myeloma, the dominant presenting symptoms may be those associated with the underlying neoplasm, such as bone pain, symptoms of uremia, or even confusion due to hypercalcemia. When anemia is associated with newly developed postural hypotension, increasing dyspnea, or increasing angina, this may indicate that the anemia has developed acutely, is severe, or is associated with acute bleeding and intravascular volume loss. In such cases, aggressive interventions to restore intravascular volume and red cell mass are indicated.

Determining the Etiology of Anemia

The etiology of anemia should be established to identify the pathologic process responsible for the anemia, to determine the appropriate therapeutic approach for the anemia, and to provide prognostic information. The task of diagnosis is simplified by the consideration that anemia can be categorized kinetically as being due to decreased production of red cells, increased destruction of red cells, loss of red cells (bleeding), or ineffective erythropoiesis. The various laboratory tests that can be used to place anemia in one of these kinetic categories are shown in Table 55.1, as are disorders associated with each kinetic category. It can be seen that the decreased production category is primarily composed of deficiencies of molecular substrates for hematopoiesis, and by infiltrative diseases (e.g., hematopoietic malignancies,

metastases, myelofibrosis). The category of increased destruction is composed of the hemolytic anemias and by bleeding into closed body spaces, such as retroperitoneally. The category blood loss is a simple one, related to mechanical trauma, gastrointestinal lesions, or hemorrhagic diatheses. Ineffective erythropoiesis is associated with clonal hematoproliferative disorders and megaloblastic states.

In addition to the basic tests already listed, the complete blood count (CBC) should include a measure of the mean red cell volume, the MCV. In this way, the anemias may be characterized morphologically as normocytic, microcytic, or macrocytic. The morphologic categories of anemia are shown in Table 55.2, along with diseases associated with them. The need for the tests other than the CBC and MCV varies from example to example, and efficient and effective determination of etiologies is greatly

TABLE 55.2. Morphologic categories of anemia and selected corresponding disorders.

Morphologic category	Disorders
Microcytic	Iron deficiency Anemia of chronic disease Thalassemia, hemoglobin E disease Spherocytic hemolytic anemias
Macrocytic	Megaloblastic anemia (B_{12} and/or folate deficiency, antimetabolites) Liver disease with target cells Greatly increased numbers of reticulocytes
Normocytic	Renal failure Erythropoietin deficiency Endocrine disorders Anemia of chronic disease Protein-calorie malnutrition Infiltrative diseases of the marrow Aplastic anemia Anemia secondary to chemotherapy Polymyalgia rheumatica

enhanced by coupling tests of kinetic parameters with the morphologic information. However, results can sometimes be complex, such as is found in anemia resulting from ineffective erythropoiesis, where the corrected reticulocyte count is low (evidence of decreased production of red blood cells, RBC), the indirect bilirubin is elevated (increased destruction of RBC), and the bone marrow is hypercellular (increased RBC production). Also in hemolytic states, evidence of increased RBC destruction is frequently accompanied by an increased reticulocyte count. Effective use of the morphologic and kinetic information serves the essential process of progressively excluding disorders in the differential diagnosis until the correct cause is identified and confirmed.

Interpretation of Laboratory Tests for Anemia

The utilization of the various laboratory tests for the diagnosis of anemia requires an understanding of the strategies and pitfalls of their interpretation.

Laboratory reports for reticulocyte count are expressed as percent (%), or the number of reticulocytes (young red cells) per 100 red cells in the blood smear preparation. The normal range is from 0.8% to 2.5% in men and 0.8% to 4.1% in women if anemia is not present. However, anemia is expected to stimulate increased production of reticulocytes. In anemic subjects, an adjusted reticulocyte percentage should be calculated by multiplying a patient's raw laboratory reticulocyte percent by the ratio of the patient's hematocrit to an average normal hematocrit value, such as 45%.

Corrected reticulocyte %

$$= \text{uncorrected reticulocyte} \ \% \times \frac{\text{patient hematocrit (\%)}}{45}$$

Measurements of serum folate should be conducted before patients are fed in hospital because single feedings of foods rich in folic acid may raise folate levels into the normal range. Measurements of red cell folate content provide a better estimate of folate status for preceding months. Folic acid deficiency is most frequently caused by decreased dietary intake, although deficiency can also occur because of intestinal malabsorption and because of blockage of absorption by such drugs as anticonvulsants and sulfasalazine.

Serum levels of vitamin B_{12} may also be difficult to interpret. Some reports have suggested that concentrations of less than 100 pg/mL are necessary for establishing the diagnosis of B_{12}-deficient anemia. However, more recent studies suggest that levels greater than 100 pg/mL are found in more than one-third subjects with pernicious anemia.[2] Other investigators suggest that even levels of B_{12} in the low-normal range may be associated with the

central nervous system changes of B_{12} deficiency, so that measurements of methylmalonic acid may be indicated when B_{12} is in the low-normal range (200–300 pg/mL).[2,18,19] Vitamin B_{12} is plentiful in animal products and is stored in considerable quantity, so that strict vegetarian (vegan) diets appear necessary to cause deficiency states based on reduced dietary intake. More frequently, B_{12} deficiency is based on defective absorption, either because of deficiency of gastric-produced intrinsic factor needed for B_{12} absorption, or due to intestinal mucosal atrophy or removal of the jejunum. The Schilling test can be used to assess the mechanism of B_{12} malabsorption but is relatively insensitive as a diagnostic tool for the deficiency state, so that normal Schilling test results do not exclude the diagnosis of B_{12} deficiency.

Measurements of erythropoietin must be interpreted in light of the degree of anemia that is present. In the presence of anemia, erythropoietin production should be increased and circulating levels should rise. Unfortunately, the response of serum erythropoietin to varying degrees of anemia has not been clearly defined and varies among laboratories. However, serum erythropoietin is expected to rise to levels above those described as normal for nonanemic individuals, and many laboratories can supply at least partially complete data for relationship of erythropoietin levels to various degrees of anemia. If such data are not available, a practical approach would be to expect erythropoietin levels in patients with moderate or severe anemia to rise to at least fivefold of the upper limit of the laboratory's normal range.

Evaluation of Renal Function

For the purpose of assessing the role of renal function in anemia, one should use creatinine clearance. The "normal range" reported for serum creatinine by laboratories is derived from studies of young adults and assumptions that depend upon a phenotypically young body composition. During aging, lean body mass comprises a progressively smaller proportion of body weight, so that the source for creatinine diminishes; this change is magnified even further in elderly women. Consequently, reliance on serum creatinine measurements alone results in an overestimate of renal function in the elderly. To correct for the age-related change in body composition, the creatinine clearance can be estimated by the Cockcroft–Gault equation:

Creatinine clearance

$$= 72 \times \frac{140 - \text{age (years)} \times \text{weight (kg)}}{\text{serum creatinine concentration (mg/dL)}}$$

For women, the calculated creatinine clearance from this equation is multiplied by 0.85. Creatinine clearances of 30 mL/min can be expected to be associated with anemia, and when creatinine clearance is 20 mL/min or less, the hematocrit is usually 30% or less.[20] In otherwise unexplained normocytic anemia, measurement of erythropoietin measurement may be useful even if calculated creatinine clearance is more than 40 ml/min because the Cockroft–Gault formula only provides a rough estimate of creatinine clearance, and there may be uncoupling of erythropoietin secretion and renal function.[21]

Serum iron, total iron-binding capacity, transferrin saturation, and ferritin frequently are sufficient to assess iron stores.[22] To avoid artifactual variation related to ingested iron or diurnal variation in iron concentration, the serum iron should be measured fasting and in the morning, and in the absence of medicinal iron supplementation. Normal values among laboratories vary highly and may range from 28 to 122 μmoles/L; consequently, the normal values used should be those established for the laboratory performing the test. The total iron-binding capacity (TIBC) reflects the quantity of iron transport protein, transferrin, and ranges from 250 to 435 μmoles/L. Elevated TIBC values are most often found in iron deficiency; low values are expected in the anemia of chronic disorders and in the presence of protein-calorie malnutrition. The transferrin saturation is calculated by dividing the serum iron × 100 by the TIBC. The transferrin saturation is expected to be reduced to a mean value of 7% in iron deficiency, as compared with a mean of 15% in the anemia of chronic disease, and is between 20% and 45% in normal individuals. Saturations greater than 75% are found in sideroblastic anemia and iron overload conditions. Measurement of serum ferritin is a useful means of indirectly assessing the quantity of stored iron. Values greater than 300 micrograms per liter (μg/L) suggest iron overload, such as can occur with multiple transfusion or hemochromatosis.[21–23] In studies of the elderly, serum ferritin measurements are informative in considering the diagnosis of iron deficiency. Concentrations greater than 100 μg/L are associated with a probability of less than 10% of iron deficiency whereas values less than 18 μg/L indicate a greater than 95% probability of iron deficiency.[24]

Microscopic examination of the blood and marrow is also useful in identifying the etiology of anemia. Examination of the blood smear is highly dependent on the skill of the examiner, and should be carried out when the morphology of circulating RBC and white blood cells is critical to identifying the etiology of anemia. Variations in the size (anisocytosis) and shape (poikilocytosis) of red cells are prominent features of iron deficiency, and also are prominent with certain infiltrative diseases of the marrow, such as myelofibrosis and metatastases to the marrow. Circulating nucleated red cells may also be found in the infiltrative diseases. In iron deficiency, the red cells are microcytic and their hemoglobin concentration (MCHC) is usually reduced (hypochromia) when the hematocrit is as low as 25%. Hypochromia is variably present or absent when the hematocrit is greater than 30%.[25] Young red cells (reticulocytes) can be recognized by their large diameter, a bluish cast to the cytoplasm, and the presence of stippling, which is due to polyribosomes completing the synthesis of hemoglobin. Megaloblastic anemias are characterized by the presence of large, oval-shaped circulating red cells (macrocytes), and further examination usually reveals hypersegmented neutrophils with six or more nuclear lobes. The blood smear in megaloblastic anemia also may disclose a reduction in the numbers of leukocytes and platelets. In addition, examination of the blood smear can reveal leukemic white blood cells, myeloma cells, target cells (large red cells with a target-like distribution of hemoglobin), and a host of other abnormalities. Consequently, examination of the blood may aid substantially in identifying the cause of the anemia.

The marrow can be prepared by smearing cells on a slide, preparing pathologic sections of clotted aspirates, or preparing sections of biopsies obtained by cutting needle or surgical resection. Aspirates may theoretically be obtained from any bone bearing marrow, but most are obtained from the iliac crests. Occasionally, marrow is obtained by aspirate of the sternum, but this procedure is potentially hazardous because of the risk of pericardial or cardiac puncture in all patients; the risk is even greater in elderly persons with osteoporosis. Usually, both aspirated and biopsy specimens are obtained. Aspirated cells examined in smears are useful for morphogic evaluation of cellular maturation, examination for stainable storage iron, and determination of the myeloid: erythroid ratio. Aspirated cells can also be submitted for chromosomal analysis. In cases of megaloblastic anemia, examination of the marrow reveals typical changes characterized by red cell precursors whose nuclei appear younger than expected for the degree of hemoglobin synthesis in the cytoplasm. This "nuclear/cytoplasmic dissociation" is a hallmark of megaloblastic red cell production. Usually, the workup of anemia can be completed without marrow examination, and such examination is only carried out to definitively address issues such as iron status, infiltrative or malignant disease, megaloblastic processes, aplastic anemia, and sideroblastic anemia or myelodysplastic syndromes. The quantitative cellular content (cellularity) of the marrow can be estimated by examination of clot sections of aspirates and biopsies, but not by smears of aspirates.

The Basic Laboratory Approach to Anemia

A practical approach is to begin with the morphologic classification of the anemia and then proceed through additional selected tests to identify the etiology. Note that the values for mean corpuscular volume (MCV) may differ among laboratories, and values specific for each laboratory should be used.

Microcytic Anemias (MCV < 80 fL)

The most common diagnoses are iron deficiency, the anemia of chronic disorders and thalassemia. First, iron status should be defined.

Initial Laboratory Tests

Serum iron
Serum TIBC
% Transferrin saturation
Serum ferritin
Optional: Marrow for stainable iron if the serum tests do not clearly define iron status

Interpretation and Course of Action

This panel of tests defines iron status. Reduced serum iron, increased TIBC and greatly reduced % transferrin saturation establish the diagnosis of iron deficiency. When those results are ambiguous, staining of the marrow for iron represents the "gold standard" for evaluation of iron stores. When iron stores are depleted, stainable marrow iron is absent. The diagnosis of iron deficiency dictates an effort to identify the source of iron loss (bleeding) and to proceed with iron replacement therapy.

Reduced serum iron, decreased or normal TIBC, mildly decreased % transferrin saturation, normal or increased ferritin, the presence of stainable iron in the marrow, and the presence of an active inflammatory disease suggest the anemia of chronic disease. Approximately 30% of patients with the anemia of chronic disease have microcytic red cells, so the absence of microcytosis does not exclude this diagnosis.[25] The anemia of chronic disease may respond partially or completely to effective treatment of the underlying inflammatory condition[26] and, in some cases, erythropoietin administration may be indicated to improve quality of life, even if the underlying condition is not responsive to treatments directed against it.[9,27]

Macrocytic Anemias (MCV > 100 fL)

In general, the diagnoses comprising this category can be divided into those caused by impaired DNA synthesis (megaloblastic anemias), increased reticulocytes, alterations of the RBC membrane due to liver disease, or, more rarely, hemoglobinopathy. The anemias of myelodysplastic disorders usually are also macrocytic. The etiology usually can be identified as follows.

Initial Laboratory Tests

Reticulocyte count
Indirect bilirubin

Interpretation and Course of Action

An increased reticulocyte count signifies increased RBC production in response to either blood loss or hemolytic anemia. In the absence of an elevated bilirubin, blood loss is most likely and the source of blood loss should be identified. If the bilirubin is also elevated, hemolytic anemia should be suspected.

If reticulocyte number is normal or reduced, proceed to examination of blood and bone marrow for megaloblastic changes.

Interpretation and Course of Action

If megaloblastic changes are found in the marrow, this confirms the diagnosis of megaloblastic anemia. Serum vitamin B_{12} and folic acid concentrations should be measured. If a deficient value is found, therapy should be instituted to correct the deficiency. If antimetabolite therapy has been administered, this should be considered the cause of the anemia. If the marrow is not megaloblastic, the blood smear should be examined for the presence of target cells, which may signal the presence of liver disease, hypothyroidism, or, rarely, an inherited hemoglobinopathy such as hemoglobin C disease.

Normocytic Anemias (MCV 81–100 fL)

This morphologic category includes a wide variety of etiologies including posthemorrhagic anemias or hemolytic anemias without extensive reticulocytosis, conditions in which marrow cell production is impaired (e.g., aplastic anemia, infiltrative diseases of the marrow, anemia due to decreased erythropoietin production, the anemia of protein-calorie malnutrition, and most examples of the anemia of chronic disease). A useful initial procedure is to perform a reticulocyte count.

Initial Laboratory Test

Reticulocyte count

Interpretation and Course of Action

An increased reticulocyte count reflects an increase in RBC production and should prompt consideration of the diagnoses of hemolytic anemia or posthemorrhagic anemia. A history of blood loss should be sought, and tests that can reflect increased red cell destruction should be obtained (indirect bilirubin, LDH). If evidence of hemolysis is found, the differential diagnosis should include autoimmune causes with or without underlying malignancy or oxidant sensitivity due to glucose-6-phosphate dehydrogenase deficiency. It should also be noted that bleeding into closed body spaces, such as retroperitoneally, can yield kinetic and morphologic laboratory results that are indistinguishable from those of hemolytic anemia.

A normal or reduced reticulocyte count should prompt the consideration of hepatic or endocrine disorders. If these screening surveys are negative, an additional laboratory test should be preformed.

Microscopic Examination of the Peripheral Blood

Bone marrow aspirate and biopsy
Serum iron, TIBC, transferrin saturation, and ferritin

Interpretation and Course of Action

Examination of the blood and bone marrow is frequently sufficient to establish or exclude the diagnoses of leukemia, myeloma, myelofibrosis, myelodysplasia, or infiltration of the marrow with metastases. Submission of aspirated marrow cells for karyotypic analysis may be useful in differentiating certain of these causes. Iron studies that reveal a reduced serum iron, decreased TIBC, modest decrease in the % transferrin saturation, and normal or elevated ferritin are consistent with the diagnosis of the anemia of chronic disease, in which normocytic RBCs are found in approximately 70% of cases.[26]

Treatment of Anemia

The goal in treating anemia is to increase or completely restore the circulating red cells to normal levels. The appropriate strategies for increasing the red cell mass should be specifically directed by the urgency of the need for treatment and the underlying cause of the anemia. Some remediable causes of anemia and their key laboratory findings and treatment, are displayed in Table 55.3.

Transfusion

Transfusion is associated with significant risks, such as volume overload, immunologic transfusion reactions, and the unintended infusion of infectious agents, such as transfusion-associated hepatitis, Epstein–Barr virus, and human immunodeficiency virus. Consequently, transfusion should not be given simply because a patient's hemoglobin or hematocrit has reached an arbitrary level. Indications for transfusion include acute blood loss with symptoms of hypovolemia, progressive symptoms of decreased oxygen delivery such as angina or increasing confusion, or symptomatic anemia that is refractory to nontransfusion therapy. When transfusion is used to treat refractory anemia without loss of blood volume, concentrated red cells should be used to avoid volume overload. However, even when restoration of blood volume is indicated, blood banks may only supply concentrated red cells rather than whole blood. In such cases, concentrated red cells may be given together with crystalloid or synthetic plasma volume expanders. The infusion of plasma or albumin appears unnecessary except when volume loss has exceeded 50% of total blood volume.[28] When blood transfusion is urgent, it should be given together with measures to ensure restoration of the blood volume.

Correction of Deficiencies of Substrates for Red Blood Cell Production

This strategy represents the ideal for management of anemia. A diagnostic process clearly identifies a deficiency of iron, folic acid, vitamin B_{12}, or protein/calories,

TABLE 55.3. Some remediable causes of anemia, their key laboratory results, and treatment.

Etiology	Laboratory results	Treatment and other interventions/studies
Iron deficiency	Microcytic RBC Reduced serum iron Increased TIBC Reduced Tf saturation Reticulocytes not increased	Identify source of iron loss and correct. Give oral iron 3 months, repeat iron studies. Intravenous iron only if iron cannot be given orally.
Anemia of chronic disease	Normo- or microcytic RBC Reduced serum iron Reduced TIBC Reduced Tf saturation Reticulocytes not increased	Identify underlying inflammatory disease. Apply remedy to underlying disease when available. May be responsive to erythropoietin administration.
B_{12}, folate-deficient anemia	Macrocytic RBC Hypersegmented PMN on blood smear Reduced B_{12} or folic acid Megaloblastic changes on bone marrow exam Reticulocytes not increased	Evaluate diet for sources of B_{12}, folic acid. Rule out malabsorption. Administer B_{12} or folate for replacement. Track response with reticulocyte counts, Hct/Hgb. B_{12} replacement must be for lifetime.
Protein-calorie-deficient anemia	Normocytic RBC Reduced lymphocyte count Reduced serum albunin Reduced serum transferrin	Restoration of protein-calorie nutrition restores the hematocrit to normal.

and administration of the appropriate substrate corrects the anemia. Usually, a response to therapy can be observed within 4 weeks of initiating therapy, and the anemia is repaired in 3 months or less. When iron therapy is needed, oral administration is the preferred route, and the gluconate, sulfate, or fumarate salts of iron are all effective. The iron should be administered with meals to avoid gastrointestinal side effects, and therapy is continued for 3 to 6 months after the anemia is resolved to assure replacement of iron stores.[29] If taken as directed, oral iron therapy is almost always effective in treating iron deficiency, although treatment failures may be encountered because patients may not comply with therapy. Parenteral iron therapy may be necessary in patients who are unable to tolerate oral iron, patients who are noncompliant with oral therapy, situations in which bleeding continues at a rate that exceeds the ability of oral iron to compensate for loss, patients with malabsorption of oral iron, dialysis patients unable to maintain adequate iron by oral intake, and in those who repeatedly and very frequently donate large amounts of blood. Iron-dextran is the preferred preparation for parenteral use and is usually administered intravenously because repeated intramuscular injections are painful and cause staining of the skin at the site of injection. It should be recognized that iron-dextran may cause hypersensitivity reactions.

Vitamin B_{12} can be administered either intramuscularly, monthly at a dose of 1000μg, or orally, in large doses of 1000mg/day, even for treatment of pernicious anemia resulting from intrinsic factor deficiency.[30] Folic acid is also administered orally, and daily doses of 1mg/day provide a generous excess above the minimum daily requirement of 50 to 100μg/day. It should be noted, however, that large doses of folic acid are capable of reversing the anemia of B_{12} deficiency while permitting the neurologic consequences of pernicious anemia to advance. Consequently, therapeutic trials with folic acid are potentially dangerous, and therapy should be directed in a focused manner only after the specific deficiency state has been identified. In some patients, the response to vitamin B_{12} or folate may appear to fail before the anemia is repaired. In such cases, the explanation may be that existing iron stores have been exhausted by utilization for new red cell production. Iron status should therefore be evaluated and, if iron is deficient, its cause should be identified and replacement therapy instituted.

Treatment of Underlying Conditions

Some anemias are partially or completely resolved when therapy is directed toward underlying etiologic conditions. A noteworthy example is the anemia associated with polymyalgia rheumatica (PMR), which resolves when corticosteroid treatment of PMR is successful. Similarly, replacement or thyroid hormone in hypothyroidism induces resolution of the associated anemia, unless it is due to the B_{12} deficiency related to associated gastric autoimmunity.[31] However, the response may be sluggish, requiring 3 to 12 months before the anemia resolves.[32] The anemia associated with myeloma is also resolved by chemotherapeutic measures that induce remission of the malignancy, but may also respond to erythropoietin.

Growth Factors and Erythropoietin

An important characteristic of the hematopoietic progenitors of the elderly is the preservation of their responsiveness to hematopoietic stimulators. With the availability of recombinant growth factors and erythropoietin, an evolving strategy for the treatment of anemia is the use of these agents to directly drive erythropoiesis. For example, it is now clear that in myelodysplastic syndromes (MDS), prolonged administration of a combination of the hematopoietic stimulator, recombinant G-CSF, and erythropoietin can increase the hematocrits of individuals with these disorders.[27]

Alterations of the White Blood Cells

Although the white blood cells (WBC) of the elderly exhibit in vitro changes in their function, the clinically observable function of WBC, laboratory values, and WBC morphology in the elderly are not different from those of young adults. However, some neoplastic disorders of the WBC such as chronic lymphocytic leukemia (CLL), polycythemia vera, atypical chronic myelocytic leukemia, and the myelodysplastic syndromes are particularly prevalent in the elderly.

Aging and Physiologic Function of WBC

The WBC are a system that includes the neutrophils, monocytes, eosinophils, basophils, and lymphocytes. The neutrophils constitute a major physiologic barrier to microbial challenge; their function is based on their ability to migrate toward inflammatory attractants, engulf foreign particles, and kill bacteria via oxidant and enzymic mechanisms. Monocytes also possess migratory and microbial properties and appear particularly important in eradication of microbial organisms that could otherwise survive and proliferate intracellularly. Monocytes also possess the ability to detect and eradicate tumor cells and appear important for eliminating emerging neoplastic clones. Eosinophils participate in resistance to parasitic infections and in hypersensitivity reactions, whereas basophils are thought to serve as sources of histamine. Lymphocytes also participate in hypersensitivity reactions, as well as in antibody synthesis. Both lymphocytes and monocytes synthesize and release a variety of cytokines, which modulate the function of a wide range of cells including blood cell progenitors. Regulation of the production of all the WBC is not completely understood. However, it is clear that neutrophil production can be driven in vitro and in vivo by recombinant growth factors such as G-CSF, and the progenitors of young adults and elderly persons appear to be equally responsive to such stimulation.[33] Proliferation of T lymphocytes is stimulated by interleukin 2, and the production of this cytokine is impaired during aging.[34] However, whether this is the cause of a predominance of naïve T cells that occurs in the elderly is not known.

Specific defects in the function of some types of WBC have been demonstrated in aged animals and man. For example, in in vitro studies, neutrophils from aged individuals do not generate antimicrobial oxidants as vigorously as the neutrophils of young adults.[35] However, this laboratory finding does not correlate with defective function of neutrophils in vivo. Monocytes from aged individuals also generate a reduced flux of antimicrobial oxidants in vitro, and this change may be a contributing factor in the increased susceptibility of aged rodents and man to infection with intracellular microbial agents, such as toxoplasma, legionella, and mycobacteria.[36] Despite observations in animals, which demonstrate impaired production of neutrophils after bacterial challenge,[7] there is no evidence that elderly persons experience impaired neutrophil production during infection. Maldistribution of T cells is observed during aging, with the emergence of a predomination of naïve T cells. This change has been implicated in the reduced and shortened duration of antibody responses to antigen challenge in the elderly.[34]

Laboratory Evaluation of the WBC

WBC are evaluated by numerical counting and morphologic examination. Blood usually is collected in tubes containing calcium chelators to prevent coagulation. The cells are counted electronically as they pass through an aperture and create the electrical resistance characteristic of nucleated cells. Thus, the laboratory "white blood count" is in reality a total nucleated cell count and not specific for WBC. Even so, the white blood count usually accurately reflects the number of leukocytes and not other cells. However, when large numbers of nucleated red cells are present in the circulation, the actual leukocyte count must be calculated by multiplying the WBC by the percentage of leukocytes as determined by differential counting.

Enumeration of the various types of WBC is carried out by performing a differential count, either electronically or by microscopic examination of smeared and stained blood. Laboratories ordinarily perform electronic differ-

TABLE 55.4. Laboratory values for the white blood cell count and absolute counts for specific leukocytes.

Cell type	Mean (10^9/L)	Range (10^9/L)
White cell count	6.6	3.5–9.8
Neutrophils	4.01	1.31–6.71
Lymphocytes	2.1	0.90–3.22
Monocytes	0.37	0.12–0.62
Eosinophils	0.13	0.00–0.30
Basophils	0.0	0.01–0.09

Source: *Wintrobe's Clinical Hematology, 10th Ed*. Philadelphia: Lea & Febiger; 2000, with permission.

ential counts, which do not detect the "band" form, the less mature neutrophils that appear in the blood during infection. Consequently, when WBC are to be evaluated for signs of bacterial infection, microscopically determined differential counts should be ordered. Differential counting adds much to the evaluation of WBC, because this establishes the percentage of the total white blood count for each type of leukocyte. However, differential counting alone is insufficient to quantitatively assess each cell type. To quantify the various types of WBC, absolute cell counts should be calculated by multiplying the percentage for the cell type in question by the white blood count. For example, for a WBC of 8.4×10^3/μL with 33% neutrophils, the absolute neutrophil count is 2.77×10^3/μL (8.4×10^3/μL $\times 0.33$). Values for the WBC and the various types of leukocytes are shown in Table 55.4.

Interpretation of Variations in the Leukocyte Counts

Decreased Leukocyte Counts

A decrease in the WBC (leukopenia) cannot be interpreted without a differential count and calculation of absolute counts.

The significance of neutropenia (neutrophil count $<1.4 \times 10^9$/L) depends on the distribution and kinetics of neutrophils in the blood and their subsequent delivery to sites of infection (Fig. 55.1). Neutrophils are produced in the marrow, and then released into the blood where they have a transit time ($T_{1/2}$) of 4 to 10h.[37] Once they enter the circulation, they may be within a freely circulating pool of cells and available to the phlebotomy needle, or marginated along the walls of vessels where they cannot be obtained in a blood sample and therefore are not counted. Because the circulating and marginated neutrophils freely exchange, together they comprise the total pool of neutrophils available for function. Therefore, the neutrophil count alone does not always reflect the total pool of neutrophils. Indeed, when due to increased margination, even pronounced neutropenia is not associated with an increased risk for infection. The risk for infection

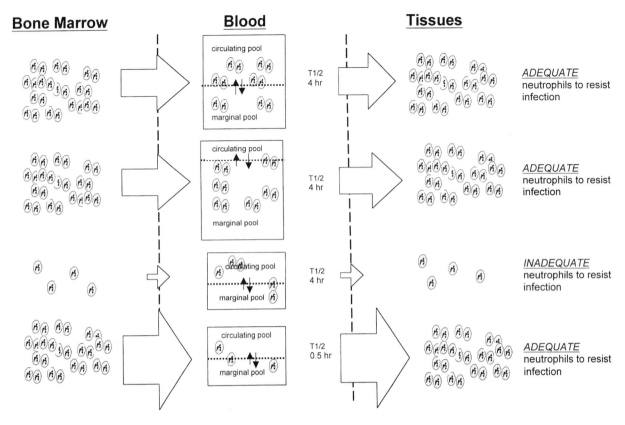

FIGURE 55.1 Distribution and kinetics of neutrophils in blood and tissues.

correlates best with the supply of neutrophils, and neutropenia can exist in circumstances where the total pool of neutrophils is decreased but the rate of production and use of neutrophils is increased, such as in Felty's syndrome. In this latter case, the supply of neutrophils is adequate and the risk for infection is not increased. When neutropenia reflects a reduced total neutrophil pool and production of neutrophils is reduced, the risk of infection increases (see Fig. 55.1). The risk of infection rises significantly with neutrophil counts less than 0.5×10^9/L.[38] Thus, it is neutropenia caused by hypoproduction, which must be differentiated from the neutropenias due to margination or rapid transit of neutrophils through the blood (see Fig. 55.1). The most definitive strategy for estimating the ability of the marrow to produce neutrophils is direct examination of a smear and biopsy of the marrow to determine cellularity, the myeloid : erythroid ratio, and cellular morphology/maturation. The marrow examination is also useful in recognizing the presence of myelodysplastic disorders, in which distinctive morphologic changes, increased numbers of immature blast cells, abnormal iron distribution, and chromosomal abnormalities confirm the diagnosis.

When neutropenia is due to margination or rapid transit of neutrophils in the blood, increased risk of infection is not expected. When neutropenia reflects severely impaired production of neutrophils, fever and symptoms related to the site of infection and infectious organism are prominent. In addition, subjects with neutropenia may experience severe throat or oral pain (agranulocyte angina). Fever or other signs of infection in severely neutropenic patients should be approached as an urgent matter. A thorough workup should be initiated to identify the site and organism responsible for infection, and supportive/antibiotic therapy should either be instituted empirically or as dictated by the site and organisms that are found. In addition, the cause of neutropenia should be identified. Examination of the blood and marrow should be conducted, and a diagnosis of autoimmune disease should be considered. Medications should be reduced to a minimum and an exhaustive search conducted for any medicines that have previously been identified as offending agents.[39]

Lymphopenia (lymphocyte count $<0.9 \times 10^9$/L) can be seen in a variety of conditions, such as following the administration of corticosteroids, in tuberculosis, and during AIDS. Lymphopenia is also a finding in subjects with protein-calorie malnutrition and can be considered as supporting evidence for malnutrition. A reduction in the eosinophil count is observed following corticosteroid administration, during some inflammatory processes, and during bacterial infection.

Increased Leukocyte Counts

The significance of leukocytosis cannot be determined without a differential count and calculation of absolute counts. An increase in the WBC can occur because of large numbers of nucleated red cells in the peripheral blood and may be due to the presence of neoplastic cells, such as leukemia cells. Neutrophilia is defined as a neutrophil count greater than 6.71×10^9/L. Neutrophilia can occur as a consequence of bacterial infection and, under those circumstances, is frequently associated with the appearance of band (nonsegmented) neutrophils in the blood. This appearance of band neutrophils in the blood is referred to as a "left shift." The left shift may also occur after corticosteroid administration. Neutrophilia also occurs as a consequence of movement of neutrophils from the marginal to the circulating pool of cells, without a change in the total circulating neutrophil pool. Neutrophilia due to demargination is not associated with a left shift and can be precipitated by stimuli such as exercise or epinephrine.[37] Lymphocytosis is defined as a lymphocyte count greater than 3.22×10^9/L.

Lymphocytosis occurs in hyperthyroidism, infectious hepatitis, and following blood transfusion when it can signal infection with cytomegalovirus. Unexplained sustained lymphocytosis is usually a reflection of chronic lymphocytic leukemia or, less frequently, lymphoma. Eosinophilia is defined as an eosinophil count greater than 0.7×10^9/L. Eosinophilia is frequently a signal of allergic conditions, such as asthma or allergy to medicines; it also occurs during parasitic infection, and during autoimmune diseases. Monocytosis may be seen in subjects with tuberculosis or during monocytic anemia, but frequently the explanation for it is obscure. Basophilia (basophil counts $>0.09 \times 10^9$/L) may be observed in chronic myelocytic leukemia, polycythemia vera, Hodgkin's disease, and systemic mastocytosis.

Disorders of Hemostasis

Hemostasis is a complex process that depends on vascular factors as well as the formation of an occlusive platelet plug and production of a stable insoluble fibrin clot.

The bleeding history is an indispensable element in evaluating hemostasis. Hemostasis itself is a tightly regulated process with focused hemostatic mechanisms that are intended to restrict the location and duration of the hemostatic process. During aging, chronic solar exposure as well as a reduction in cutaneous collagen and elastin leads to an increased prevalence of ecchymoses, particularly on the extensor surfaces of the forearms and dorsum of the hands. This finding does not signify a systemic disorder of hemostasis. Similar cutaneous ecchymoses are also associated with hyperadrenalcorticism, in which case the clinical findings of Cushing's syndrome may be observed. Numerous unprovoked petechiae are symptoms of decreased platelet function or number, and generalized mucocutaneous bruising should raise the suspicion of a systemic hemostatic defect, particularly that associated with reduced number or function of platelets.

Spontaneous or easily provoked deep bleeding, such as into muscle, retroperitoneally, or into joints, is most likely to reflect a defect in the coagulation process, either due to deficiency of coagulation factors or because of the presence of an endogenously produced or medicinal circulating anticoagulant. The temporal occurrence of bleeding after trauma is also useful in identifying its underlying cause. Defects in platelet function or number are most likely to produce bleeding manifestations that occur within 1 h of procedures such as dental extraction; delay of bleeding until 4 to 6 h is more consistent with a defect in coagulation. Hereditary bleeding disorders are usually recognized and identified before patients reach old age, but a history of lifelong bleeding symptoms my occasionally disclose such disorders, even among the elderly.

Disorders of the restraint of hemostasis also produce distinctive symptoms. For example, unprovoked thrombosis at unusual sites, or even the new and repeated occurrence of deep vein thrombosis in the legs, may reflect a hypercoagulable state. Such events can be caused by deficiency of the naturally occurring endogenous anticoagulants and may be associated with malignancy or antiphospholipid antibody.

Laboratory Evaluation of Hemostasis

The investigation should include a careful history followed by laboratory studies. The basic panel of studies follows.

Initial Studies

Platelet count
Prothrombin time (PT) and international normalized ratio (INR)
Activated thromboplastin time (aPTT)

Interpretation

The platelet count is used to determine whether thrombocytopenia (platelets $<150 \times 10^9$/L) contributes to or causes the bleeding. Thrombocytopenia may be due to decreased production of platelets, increased removal of platates from the circulation, or hemorrhage. A classification of thrombocytopenias is shown in Table 55.5. Bleeding usually is severe when the platelets are below

TABLE 55.5. Classification of the thrombocytopenias.

Decreased platelet production
   Leukemia, other infiltrative diseases of the marrow
   Megakaryocytic hypoplasia
   Hereditary
   Aplastic anemia
   Viral infection
Increased removal of platelets from the circulation
   Heparin-induced thrombocytopenia
   Thrombotic thrombocytopenic purpura (TTP)/hemolytic uremic
     syndrome (HUS)
   Disseminated intravascular coagulation (DIC)
   Immune thrombocytopenic purpura (ITP)
   Microangiopathic processes
Loss of platelets
   Severe hemorrhage, replacement with platelet-poor bank blood
Sequestration of platelets
   Splenic enlargement or infiltrative disease
   Anesthesia coupled with hypothermia

10,000, variably present when platelets are 10,000 to $50,000 \times 10^9$/L, and hemostasis may appear clinically normal in those with counts above $50,000 \times 10^9$/L unless trauma occurs.[40] The thrombocytopenia induced by heparin is due to an IgG antibody toward complexes of heparin and platelet factor 4.[41,42] These antibody–heparin–platelet complexes can cause microvascular occlusive events that result in such consequences as stroke, myocardial infarction, and ischemia of extremities. Thrombotic thrombocytopenic purpura (TTP) is yet another cause of a reduced platelet count and is associated with hemolysis, thrombocytopenia, fever, and mental status changes. TTP represents an urgent condition requiring prompt intervention, such as with corticosteroids and plasma exchange.[43,44]

In some instances, low platelet counts are not associated with clinical signs or symptoms of a bleeding diathesis; this can sometimes be ascribed to pseudo-thrombocytopenia, a laboratory artifact generated by in vitro clumping of platelets, which prevents their accurate electronic counting. Pseudothrombocytopenia can be recognized by examination of blood smears obtained directly from the fingertip and specially anticoagulated specimens.[45]

Several laboratory tests can aid in defining the explanation for thrombocytopenia. The production of platelets is most definitively assessed by examination of a bone marrow biopsy. Assays for antiplatelet antibody may be useful in confirming an antibody-mediated mechanism for thrombocytopenia.[46,47]

The clinical management of thrombocytopenia is dictated by symptoms, urgency of treatment, and etiology. Individuals with active bleeding may require platelet transfusion, although such treatment is not often effective in ITP. When heparin induces slight and asymptomatic reductions in the platelet count, the heparin need

not be discontinued. However pronounced or symptomatic heparin-induced thrombocytopenia should be managed by discontinuing the heparin and active management of the adverse consequences. The diagnosis of ITP dictates the use of steroid therapy or other immunosuppressive interventions. When thrombocytopenia occurs as manifestation of disseminated intravascular coagulation, therapy is directed toward the underlying cause and heparin may be indicated to retard pathologic coagulation, but replacement of platelets and consumed factors is also frequently necessary.

The PT/INR and aPTT are utilized to screen for coagulation disorders. The PT is carried out by activation of the extrinsic pathway of coagulation to generate fibrin (Fig. 55.2) and can only be accurately interpreted by expressing it as an international normalized ratio (INR), which standardizes the test for differing reagents used by various laboratories. The aPTT is performed by activation and fibrin formation via the intrinsic pathway (see Fig. 55.2). Prolongation of either of these tests can be due to (a) a deficiency of one or more coagulation factors or (b) inhibition of the coagulation. Deficiency states can be differentiated from the presence of inhibitors by mixing the patient's plasma with normal plasma, 1:1, and repeating the coagulation assay. In deficiency states, the addition of normal plasma corrects the test; when inhibitors are present, the test is not corrected. Deficiency states are partially clarified by the test that is abnormal: factor VII only functions in the PT, whereas factors VIII, IX, XI, and XII are restricted to the aPTT. Factors, I, II, V, and X function in the common pathway (see Fig. 55.2). Further refinement is obtained by consideration of the vitamin K-dependent factors (II, VII, IX, and X), and those consumed by the coagulation process (I, II, V, and VIII). Factor XIII is consumed with the hemostatic process; proteins S and C are vitamin K dependent, but none of these affect the PT/INR or aPTT.

Inhibitors of coagulation can be considered in two categories: medicinal inhibitors of coagulation, such as heparin, and endogenous inhibitors. Protein S and C, which are present normally, are not potential causes of abnormalities in the PT/INR or aPTT. Heparin preferentially prolongs the aPTT more than the PT, via its acceleration of the anticoagulant activity of antithrombin III. When the coagulation tests are prolonged and not corrected by the addition of normal plasma, the presence of pathologic anticoagulants should be sought. Of these perhaps the most frequently observed is an acquired inhibitor to Factor VIII which, in the elderly, may be found after Factor VIII treatment of classic hemophilics, in the presence of such disorders as rheumatologic disease or cancer, or as an isolated finding.[48] Factor VIII inhibitors are associated with prolongation of the aPTT but not the PT/INR and are usually associated with severe and intractable bleeding.[49] Another cause of prolongation of the aPTT that is uncorrected by normal plasma is the presence of a phospholipid antibody. However, the phospholipid antibody is associated with hypercoagulability, not a hemorrhagic diathesis, and usually presents in subjects less than 60 years of age.[50] Prolongation of both the PT/INR and the aPTT should raise the question of deficiency of vitamin K, or consumption of coagulation factors such as occurs in disseminated intravascular coagulation (DIC). When the PT/INR is prolonged by the induction of vitamin K deficiency with warfarin it is corrected by the addition of normal plasma.

The presence of normal laboratory tests does not rule out a bleeding diathesis. Indeed, even if the complete blood count, PT/INR, and PTT are all normal, diagnoses such as von Willebrand's disease are not ruled out and should be pursued further with tests such as multimeric analysis of von Willebrand's factor (vWF), ristocetin-induced agglutination of platelets, and ristocetin cofactor analysis. In the past, the bleeding time has been con-

sidered as useful for the diagnosis of von Willebrand's disease and as a screening test for preoperative evaluation. However, because of the variability and relatively unreliable nature of the bleeding time, it is no longer recommended.[51] Because of the variability of results for the various tests and their behavior as acute-phase reactants, even repeated sophisticated testing for von Willebrand's disease may be insufficient to definitively rule out this diagnosis.[52]

Estimating the Risk for Bleeding at Surgery

Although routine laboratory tests are frequently ordered with the aim of predicting operative risk, the reliability of such testing is at least suspect, if not misleading, particularly when laboratory tests are normal. However, a history of possible systemic bleeding diathesis (e.g., mucocutaneous bleeding, history of deep hematomata or intra-articular hemorrhage, hemostatic problems with trauma or surgery, or excessive bleeding or rebleeding

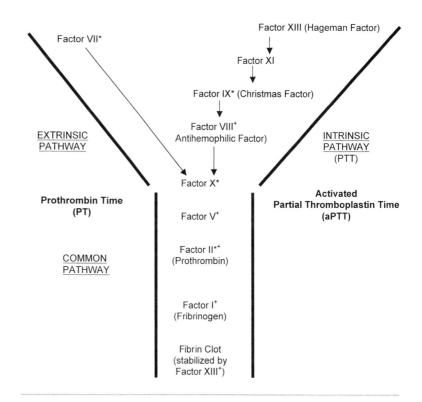

FIGURE 55.2 Pathways of coagulation.

after dental procedures) should prompt a thorough investigation of hemostatic status. In addition, laboratory screening should be performed on patients who are unduly susceptible to the consequences of even minor blood loss or who are to be subjected to surgery that itself carries a particular risk for major blood loss.

Hypercoagulable States

Hypercoagulable states are characterized by a history of excessive or inappropriate (usually venous) thrombotic events. The most common sites of thrombosis are in the lower extremities, although thromboses in unusual sites, such as superficial or deep veins in the arm or shoulder girdle, also occur. The hypercoagulable states may be either hereditary or acquired. Hereditary conditions that cause hypercoagulability usually are manifested in young adulthood, and the history provides the initial and necessary clue to their presence. The hereditary hypercoagulable states include deficiencies of antithrombin III, protein C, or protein S, and specific functional laboratory tests for these proteins are necessary to identify deficiencies of them. Protein S or C are dependent on vitamin K for their synthesis, and their deficiency underlies the phenomenon of warfarin-induced skin necrosis, which is actually a local manifestation of a hypercoagulable state initiated by vitamin K-deficient impairment of physiologic restraints of coagulation. Activated protein C resistance is another inherited cause of hypercoagulability, and is most commonly due to a point mutation in the factor V gene that results in the production of factor V Leiden. This mutation is very common in the Caucasian population (3%–7%) but almost absent among some black or Asian populations. A mutation in the gene for prothrombin (factor II) is also relatively common, and this mutation is found in 6% to 18% of patients with venous thromboembolism. Factor V Leiden and the prothrombin mutation must be diagnosed by specific laboratory testing or by DNA analysis.[53] Acquired hypercoagulable states may be associated with frank malignancy or with such diseases as the myeloproliferative disorders and paroxysmal nocturnal hemoglobinuria. In addition, hypercoagulability may be associated with the antiphospholipid syndrome, although this condition usually presents before age 60.

The management of hypercoagulable states is dictated by management of acute thrombotic events and by preventive therapy with warfarin anticoagulation. Acute thromboses should be treated with either unfractionated or low molecular weight heparin. Patients with two or more spontaneous thromboses, a life-threatening thrombosis, a spontaneous thrombosis at an unusual site, or a thrombosis in the presence of more than one hypercoagulable state should receive anticoaglulation for life.[53]

References

1. Lipschitz CA, Udupa KB, Milton KY, et al. Effect of age on hematopoiesis in man. *Blood*. 1984;63:502–509.
2. Baraldi-Junkins CA, Beck AC, Rothstein G. Hematopoiesis and cytokines. Relevance to cancer and aging. *Hematol Oncol Clin N Am*. 2000;14:45–61.
3. Granick S. Iron metabolism. *Bull NY Acad Med*. 1954;30:81–103.
4. Beveridge BR. Hypochromic anemia. *Q J Med*. 1965;34:135–162.
5. Stabler SP, Allen RH, Savage DG, et al. Clinical spectrum and diagnosis of cobalamin deficiency. *Blood*. 1990;76:871–881.
6. Boggs DR, Patrene K. Hematopoiesis and aging. III: Anemia and a blunted erythropoietic response to hemorrhage in aged mice. *Am J Hematol*. 1985;19:327–338.
7. Rothstein G, Christensen RD, Neilsen GR. Kinetic evaluation of pool sizes and proliferative response in bacterially challenged aged mice. *Blood*. 1987;70:1836—1841.
8. Udupa KB, Lipschitz DA. Erythropoiesis in the aged mouse: I. Response to stimulation in vivo. *J Lab Clin Med*. 1984;103:574–580.
9. Cella D, Bron D. The effect of Epoietin alfa on quality of life in anemic cancer patients. *Cancer Pract*. 1999;7:177–182.
10. Buchanan JJP, Peters CA, Rasmussen C, et al. Impaired expression of hematopoietic growth factors: a candidate mechanism for the hematopoietic defect of aging. *Exp Gerontol*. 1996;31:135–144.
11. Ershler WB, Sun WH, Binkley N, et al. Interleukin-6 and aging: blood levels and mononuclear cell production increase with advancing age and in vitro production is modifiable by dietary restriction. *Lymphokine Cytokine Res*. 1993;4:225–230.
12. Cohen HJ, Pieper CF, Harris T, et al. The association of plasma IL-6 levels with functional disability in the elderly. *J Gerontol A Biol Sci Med Sci*. 1997;52:201–208.
13. Lopatin U, Yao X, Willams RK, et al. Increases in circulating and lymphoid tissue interleukin-10 in autoimmune lymphoproliferative syndrome are associated with disease expression. *Blood*. 2001;97:3161–3170.
14. Frassanito MA, Cusmai A, Iodice G, et al. Autocrine interleukin-6 production and highly malignant multiple myeloma: relation with resistance to drug-induced apoptosis. *Blood*. 2001;97:483–489.
15. Dallman PR, Yip R, Johnson C. Prevalence and causes of anemia in the United States, 1976 to 1980. *Am J Clin Nutr*. 1984;39:437–435.
16. Lipschitz DA, Mitchell CO, Thompson C. The anemia of senescence. *Am J Hematol*. 1981;11:47–54.
17. Timiras ML, Brownstein H. Prevalence of anemia and correlation of hemoglobin with age in a geriatric screening clinic population. *J Am Geriatr Soc*. 1987;35:639–643.
18. Rasmussen K, Vyberg B, Pedersen KO, et al. Methylmalonic acid in renal insufficiency: evidence of accumulation and implications for diagnosis of cobalamin deficiency. *Clin Chem* 1990;36:1523–1524.
19. Allen RH, Stabler SP, Savage DG, et al. Diagnosis of cobalamin deficiency; I. Usefulness of serum methylmalonic acid

and total homocysteine concentrations. *Am J Hematol.* 1990;34:90–98.

20. Radtke HW, Claussner A, Erbes PM, et al. Serum erythropoietin concentration in chronic renal failure: relationship to degree of anemia and excretory function. *Blood.* 1979; 54:877–884.

21. Feinstein S, Becker-Cohen R, Algur N, et al. Erythropoietin deficiency causes anemia in nephrotic children with normal kidney function. *Am J Kidney Dis.* 2001;37:736–742.

22. Jacobs A, Miller F, Worwood M, et al. Ferritin in the serum of normal subjects and patients with iron deficiency and iron overload. *Br Med J.* 1980;4:206–208.

23. Lipschitz DA, Cook JD, Finch CA. A clinical evaluation of serum ferritin as an index of iron stores. *N Engl J Med.* 1974;290:1213–1216.

24. Guyatt GH, Patterson C, Ali M, et al. Diagnosis of iron-deficiency anemia in the elderly. *Am J Med.* 1990;88:205–209.

25. Becutler E, Fairbanks VF. The effects of iron deficiency. In: Jacobs A, ed. *Iron in Biochemistry and Medicine, vol 2.* New York: Worwood Academic; 1980. pp. 394–425.

26. Cartwright GE, Wintrobe MM. The anemia of infection. *Adv Intern Med.* 1952;5:165–226.

27. Mantovani L, Lentini G, Hentschel B, et al. Treatment of anemia in myelodysplastic syndromes with prolonged administration of recombinant human granulocyte colony stimulating factor and erythropoietin. *Br J Haematol.* 2000; 109:367–375.

28. Adamson J, Hillman RS. Blood volume and plasma protein replacement following acute blood loss in normal man. *JAMA.* 1968;205:609–612.

29. Crosby WH. The rationale for treating iron deficiency anemia. *Arch Intern Med.* 1984;144:471–472.

30. Kuzminski AM, Del Giacco EF, Allen RH, et al. Effective treatment of cobalamin deficiency with oral cobalamin. *Blood.* 1998;92:1191–1198.

31. Tudhope GR, Wilson GM. Anaemia in hypothyroidism. *Q J Med.* 1960;29:513–537.

32. Bomford R. Anemia in myxoedema. *Q J Med.* 1938;7:495–536.

33. Shank WA Jr, Balducci L. Recombinant hemopoietic growth factors: comparative hemopoietic response in younger and older subjects. *J Am Geriatr Soc.* 1992;40:151–154.

34. Miller RA. Nathan Shock Memorial Lecture 1992. Aging and immune function: cellular and biochemical analyses. *Exp Gerontol.* 1994;29:21–35.

35. Indelicato SR, Udupa KB, Balazovich KJ, et al. Effect of age on phorbol-ester stimulation of human neutrophils. *J Gerontol.* 1990;45:B75–B80.

36. Gardner ID, Remington JS. Aging and the immune response. I. Antibody formation and chronic infection in *Toxoplasma gondii*-infected mice. *J Immunol.* 1978;120:944–949.

37. Athens JW, Raab SO, Haab OP, et al. Leukokinetic studies. III. The distribution of granulocytes in the blood of normal subjects. *J Clin Investig.* 1961;40:159–164.

38. Walsh SJ, Begg CB, Carbone PP. Cancer chemotherapy in the elderly. *Semin Oncol.* 1989;16:66–75.

39. Kaufman DW. Drugs in the aetiology of agranulocytosis and aplastic anemia. *Eur J Haematol Suppl.* 1996;60:23–30.

40. Lacey JB, Penner JA. Management of idiopathic thrombocytopenic purpura in the adult. *Semin Thromb Hemost.* 1977;3:160–174.

41. Suh JS, Aster RH, Visentin GP. Antibodies from patients with heparin-induced thrombocytopenia/thrombosis recognize different epitopes on heparin platelet factor 4. *Blood.* 1998;91:916–922.

42. Nand S, Wong W, Yuen B, et al. Heparin-induced thrombocytopenia with thrombosis: incidence, analysis of risk factors, and clinical outcomes in 108 consecutive patients treated at a single institution. *Am J Hematol.* 1997;56:12–16.

43. Rock GA, Shumak KH, Buskard NA, et al. Comparison of plasma exchange with plasma infusion in the treatment of thrombotic thrombocytopenic purpura. *N Engl J Med.* 1991;325:393–397.

44. Bell WR, Braine HG, Ness PM, et al. Improved survival in thrombotic thrombocytopenic purpura-hemolytic uremic syndrome. *N Engl J Med.* 1991;325:398–403.

45. Bizzaro N. EDTA-dependent pseudothrombocytopenia; a clinical and epidemiological study of 112 cases, with a 10 year follow-up. *Am J Hematol.* 1995;50:103–109.

46. Berchtold P, Wenger M. Autoantibodies against platelet glycoproteins in autoimmune thrombocytopenic purpura: their clinical significance and response to treatment. *Blood.* 1993;81:1246–1250.

47. Fujisawa K, O'Toole TE, Tani P, et al. Autoantibodies to the presumptive cytoplasmic domain of platelet glycoprotein IIIa in patients with chronic immune thrombocytopenic purpura. *Blood.* 1991;77:2207–2213.

48. White BC. Factor VIII inhibitors: a clinical overview. *Am J Hematol.* 1982;13:335–342.

49. Sahud MA. Factor VIII inhibitors. Laboratory diagnosis of inhibitors. *Semin Thromb Hemost.* 2000;26:195–203.

50. Piette JC, Cacoub P. Antiphospholipid syndrome in the elderly: caution. *Circulation.* 1998;97:295–296.

51. Peterson P, Hayes TE, Arkin CF. et al. The preoperative bleeding time test lacks clinical benefit. College of American Pathologists' and American Society of Clinical Pathologists' position article. *Arch Surg.* 1998;133:134–139.

52. Abilgaard CF, Suzuki A, Harrison J, et al. Serial studies in von Willebrand's disease. Variability versus "variants." *Blood.* 1980;56:712–716.

53. Bauer K. Approach to thrombosis. In: Loscalzo J, Schafer AI, eds. *Thrombosis and Hemorrhage, 2nd Ed.* Baltimore: Williams & Wilkins; 1996. pp 477–490.

56
Gastroenterologic Disorders

Joanne A.P. Wilson

The function of the gastrointestinal tract remains relatively normal during the process of aging,[1–4] probably because of the apparent excess production of hormones and enzymes as well as redundancy in structure of the organ system. In the study of gastrointestinal function in the elderly, most of our studies have attempted to differentiate physiologic changes from pathologic changes that may be associated with systemic disorders. Early studies that did indicate significant physiologic changes appear not to have had essential age-specific controls and frequently represented comparisons of ill hospitalized elderly with younger normal controls. Most recent studies have shown few changes in gastrointestinal function with age.

One important factor in the elderly, however, is the increase in prevalence of certain disorders with age dramatically affecting the differential diagnosis in the elderly patient. For example, the incidence of *Helicobacter pylori* infection in certain populations as well as the incidence of gastric ulcers dramatically increases with age. The effect on the gastrointestinal tract of other disorders such as atherosclerotic vascular disease contributes to ischemic complications. Other vascular abnormalities associated with aging contribute to the development of angiodysplagias and other bleeding lesions within the gastrointestinal tract; these are generally not seen in younger populations. The incidence of other conditions such as cardiovascular dysfunction also contributes to modifications in the management of gastrointestinal problems in elderly patients, particularly with gastrointestinal bleeding and the hemodynamic compromise that may occur. The increased use of medications and the inherent effects of these drugs on the gastrointestinal tract also affect the spectrum of disease seen, which remains an important consideration in the evaluation of the elderly patient. Last, with age, there is an increase in gastrointestinal malignancies. (See Chapter 34, Colon Cancer and Other GI Malignancies.)

Disorders of Swallowing and the Esophagus

Age-related changes in esophageal function are common on careful manometric studies but generally not clinically significant. However, dysphagia and reflux esophagitis are two common problems for elderly patients.

Normal Swallowing

Normal swallowing is accomplished by a series of intricate and interrelated activities. After chewing, the tongue moves the bolus of food to the back of the oropharynx, where voluntary and involuntary muscle movements then occur. The upper esophageal sphincter and the upper third of the esophagus are composed of striated muscle, whereas the lower two-thirds of the esophagus is smooth muscle. Food in the back of the oropharynx initiates reflex progressive muscle contraction in a stripping action known as peristalsis. A voluntary swallow can also initiate peristalsis. As the peristaltic wave reaches the lower esophageal sphincter, reflex relaxation occurs, and food can enter the stomach. Resting pressure in the lower esophageal sphincter then keeps food and acid from refluxing back into the esophagus.

Physiologic Changes with Aging

Healthy older individuals do not have clinically significant evidence of aging when it comes to swallowing or esophageal function. There are, however, histologic and manometric evidence of changes that appear with aging which may predispose the elderly to be less tolerant to other stresses and illnesses. Some illnesses seem more frequently in the elderly may directly affect the ability to swallow.

Oropharyngeal Dysphagia

Age-related changes in the tongue with decrease in the muscle mass may have clinical significant impact on chewing and swallowing in the ill elderly. Age-related olfactory and taste discrimination losses may contribute to anorexia and dietary choices in the elderly as substantial decreases in these functions are noted by age 70 years. Medications may further impair these functions.[4]

Dysphagia

Dysphagia is the sensation that food is sticking or that there is difficulty with swallowing. The feeling of dysphagia is usually associated with the presence of an abnormal movement of food or liquids through the esophagus and should not be considered hysterical.

In general, dysphagia can be due to mechanical abnormalities or to abnormalities of function resulting in motility disturbances. A carefully taken history usually yields a very accurate diagnosis. Symptoms due to mechanical causes of dysphagia are usually consistent in presentation and are most frequently affected by eating solids, especially large solids. Progressive decrease in luminal size, as would be seen with a growing esophageal cancer, may present as progressive loss of ability to swallow meats, then potatoes, and eventually soups. Symptoms associated with motility disorders, on the other hand, are usually intermittent, with liquids playing a major role. Patients can frequently accurately point to the site of the dysphagia. Nonspecific points that represent nerve radiation and are therefore not specific include the sternal notch and the epigastrium. The most common causes of dysphagia can be found in Table 56.1. The reader is referred to a review by Mendez et al.[5] for a more detailed approach to evaluating the patient with dysphagia, or to Sonies for a review of oropharyngeal dysphagia.[6]

Dysphagia is different from odynophagia, or pain on swallowing. Odynophagia usually implies mucosal ulceration, either from irritation (such as one might see from a pill lodged and eroding the mucosa of the esophagus), infection (such as candidial or herpes esophagitis), erosive (such as an esophageal ulcer from reflux esophagitis), or neoplastic.

Most disabling for patients and frustrating for health care practitioners is the problem of oropharyngeal dysphagia, most frequently associated with cricopharyngeal incoordination.[7] Whether due to a large cerebrovascular accident (CVA) or to a point lesion in the swallowing center in the medulla, Parkinson's disease, myasthenia gravis, or myositis, patients with cricopharyngeal incoordination tend to have difficulty initiating swallowing and transferring food from the oropharynx to the upper esophagus and are at high risk of developing aspiration pneumonia. Recurrent coughing or aspiration during eating is the most frequent problem noted. Other symptoms include the sensation of food sticking in the neck or nasal regurgitation. Other evidence of neuromuscular weakness such as dysarthria may also be present. Gag reflex is a poor predictor of intact function.

Treatment usually involves a multidisciplinary approach, including evaluation by a speech therapist and dietary manipulation.[6] In general, semisolids are better tolerated than liquids, as solids will initiate secondary peristalsis whereas liquids may sit in the back of the throat, waiting for the cricopharyngeus to eventually open. If opening does not occur before a breath is taken, then aspiration can occur. Positioning of the head and variation of food consistency may decrease the risk of aspiration. Rehabilitation has had some success after new strokes. For frail patients with recurrent aspiration pneumonia, avoidance of swallowing and tube feeding may be the only alternative.[8] Nasogastric tubes are usually used only as a short-term solution and are not well tolerated by older patients with confusion. Percutaneous endoscopic gastric (PEGs) or duodenal feeding tubes are more permanent solutions.[9]

Some patients with oropharyngeal dysphagia may develop a Zenker's diverticulum, an outpouching through gaps in the muscles of the pharyngeal wall, immediately above the upper esophageal sphincter. These sacs collect food that becomes caught above the uncoordinated sphincter, slowly enlarging over time. They may enlarge enough to become a visible mass in the neck. Patients with Zenker's complain of coughing, gurgling in the neck, postprandial regurgitation, and aspiration. Diverticulectomy will reduce the danger of aspiration. Upper esophageal myotomy is done in some centers to improve the ease of swallowing.

Diabetes mellitus, a common problem in the elderly, can at times be associated with smooth muscle wasting.

TABLE 56.1. Common causes of dysphagia in the elderly.

Motility disorders
  Cricopharyngeal incoordination
  Diabetes mellitus
  Diffuse esophageal spasm
  Presbyesophagus
Mechanical disorders
  Webs or rings
  Carcinoma
  Peptic ulceration or stricture
Extrinsic compression

Intermittent dysphagia to liquids and solids is the major complaint. With involvement of the lower esophageal sphincter, severe reflux esophagitis can also occur. Diagnosis is usually made by manometrically demonstrating loss of primary peristalsis in the body of the esophagus. Little therapeutic progress has been made in this frustrating problem. Having the patient sit upright while swallowing and until food has passed through the stomach may decrease symptoms.

Other problems presenting as motility disorders include scleroderma, especially in patients with Raynaud's phenomena; dermatomyositis; myasthenia gravis; amyotrophic lateral sclerosis; tabes; hyper- and hypothyroidism; and, occasionally, as a finding in patients with a distant carcinoma. The existence of presbyesophagus, the finding of decreased primary peristalsis and the development of spontaneous synchronous nonperistaltic contractions due to aging alone, has been a point of debate. Presbyesophagus, if it does occur, probably does not occur before age 90 unless other neuromuscular problems are present.[10]

Diffuse esophageal spasm (DES) is the development of synchronous, very high amplitude, prolonged nonperistaltic contractions. Known in the past as "nutcracker esophagus," the spasm of DES can produce crushing substernal chest pain that is indistinguishable from cardiac angina in location, character, or radiation. DES represents 10% to 30% of the noncardiac chest pain seen in emergency rooms. Patients with DES sometimes describe onset of pain or dysphagia with ingestion of cold liquids and have intermittent dysphagia for liquids and solids. Diagnosis of DES can be confirmed by barium swallow, where a "corkscrew esophagus" may be seen, or by esophageal manometry, where the multiple concentric nonperistaltic contractions may be shown. As the spasm of DES occurs intermittently, manometry or radiography may be falsely negative if the spasm is not occurring during the testing. Therapy of DES includes treatment of reflux esophagitis if it is present, administration of long-acting nitrates or calcium channel blockers, and occasionally esophageal dilatation or longitudinal myotomy for incapacitating cases with severe dysphagia and weight loss.[7,11]

Achalasia is not frequent in the elderly, but does have a second prevalence peak in old age. Patients complain of a long history, with insidious onset, of intermittent dysphagia to liquids and solids and regurgitation of undigested foods or aspiration. Chest radiographs of patients with achalasia can show a widened mediastinum due to massive dilatation and tortuosity of the esophagus, often with an air–fluid level and evidence of retained secretions. Barium studies show the dilation of the esophagus with "bird beak" narrowing. Esophageal manometry is diagnostic, revealing nonperistaltic contractions, poor relaxation of the lower sphincter, and very high pressure in this sphincter. Neither nitrates nor calcium channel blockers have proven beneficial. Recent studies have shown that botulinum toxin injection into the sphincter muscle is effective for up to 2 years but needs to be repeated.[12] Pneumatic dilatation or surgical myotomy can offer more permanent relief of many of the symptoms for those who can tolerate the procedure. Achalasia-like symptoms of shorter onset can also be seen in patients with carcinoma involving the lower esophageal sphincter. These patients tend to have a more significant weight loss associated with their dysphagia.[13] Endoscopic evaluation is recommended for patients with achalasia.

Mechanical causes of dysphagia in the elderly include problems within the esophagus such as webs, rings, peptic strictures, and carcinoma. A lower esophageal web occurs with some frequency at the junction of the esophagus and the stomach. Known for the radiologist who first reported it, Schatzki rings are the cause of the so-called steakhouse syndrome. Elderly patients who do not chew their food well, especially if they have been drinking, may swallow a piece of steak or other hard food that is larger in diameter than their Schatzki ring. Rings larger than 13 mm in diameter are usually asymptomatic. Blockage of the bolus of food in the distal esophagus can result in significant substernal pressure or pain, and can be mistaken by the patient for cardiac pain. Endoscopic removal, dislodgment, or dissolution of the stuck food can usually be accomplished. A single bougienage with a large-diameter dilator is usually the only treatment that is necessary. Plummer and Vinson reported thin esophageal webs in the upper mid-esophagus in elderly Northern European women with iron deficiency; however, this kind of web is becoming a rare finding in the United States.

Medication-induced esophagitis ("pill esophagitis") and strictures are more likely in the elderly.[14] Recumbency and structural and motility disorders are predisposing factors. Commonly seen medications are potassium chloride, iron compounds, tetracycline, doxycline, and quinidine. Alendronate may cause a severe form of esophagitis. Pills and capsules can lodge in the esophagus near the aortic arch or in the distal esophagus, especially in patients who take their medication while lying in the supine position or patients with decreased primary peristalsis. Prolonged contact of the medication with the esophageal mucosa can result in local inflammation and ulceration. Change to liquid administration, if possible, and acid suppressive therapy is usually satisfactory in reducing the symptomatology if stricture formation has not occurred.

Gastroesophageal Reflux Disease

Gastroesophageal reflux disease (GERD) is a common problem in the elderly, affecting at least 30%, and increasing in prevalence with aging.[15,16] It plays a major role in the annual use of more than $2 billion per year for antacids and other prescription and nonprescription remedies for dyspepsia. Heartburn is most frequent after meals and on reclining in bed; it is typically quickly relieved by ingestion of antacids or milk. Although many elderly present with only occasional mild heartburn, others may have disabling reflux, severe chest pain, bleeding or perforation due to ulceration, laryngeal stridor, asthma, or aspiration pneumonitis because of reflux, or eventually carcinoma if Barrett's esophagus develops. There is no good clinical correlation between the frequency or severity of heartburn and the endoscopic or pathologic evidence of esophagitis. Other symptoms of GERD include water brash, regurgitation, dysphagia, and anginal-like chest pain associated with diffuse spasm. Diagnosis of GERD can frequently be made by history alone. Endoscopy is indicated in patients with chronic reflux (>5 years), late onset, dysphagia, and/or severe pain.

For patients with symptoms that are not quickly responsive or in whom the diagnosis is in doubt, 24-h pH monitoring of the esophagus or barium swallow can demonstrate reflux. Gastroesophageal endoscopy will demonstrate if esophagitis is present and can demonstrate the presence of Barrett's esophagus, ulceration or stricture development, or other intraesophageal pathology.

Barrett's esophagus refers to the finding of one or more islands of gastric columnar epithelium with intestinal metaplasia within the lining of the esophagus, which is usually lined with squamous mucosa. These histologic changes develop after the squamous mucosa has been exposed to acid reflux for years. Barrett's esophagus is a premalignant condition associated with an increased risk of developing adenocarcinoma of the esophagus.[17] The documentation of Barrett's mucosa mandates aggressive acid suppressive therapy with proton pump inhibitors and surveillance endoscopy with biopsy. If dysplasia develops, then ablative or surgical resection is recommended.

Empiric therapy includes elevation of the head of the bed, reduction in nocturnal meal size; avoidance of fat, caffeine, alcohol, and chocolate in the evening; and weight loss if overweight. Mild symptoms may respond to antacids or alginic acid (Gaviscon). Clearly, concerns regarding the administration of aluminum, magnesium, and sodium need to be considered in elderly patients with renal insufficiency or congestive heart failure. H_2 blockers are effective for patients with mild to moderate symptoms; these agents are not effective in patients with severe esophagitis or Barrett's esophagus.

Proton pump inhibitors are the most effective medications in the healing of reflux esophagus.[18] Because reflux esophagitis tends to recur after cessation of therapy, long-term therapy with drugs should probably be considered.[19] Theoretically, metaclopramide tightens the LES, opens the pylorus, and promotes gastric emptying, all of which should decrease reflux; it does not heal esophageal lesions unless taken along with H_2 blockers or other agents that decrease gastric acid production. CNS side effects such as drowsiness, insomnia, agitation, tremor, and dyskinesia may further reduce the usefulness of metaclopramide in the elderly. Elderly patients with significant or recurrent complications of reflux esophagitis should be evaluated for surgical intervention. Criteria for surgical intervention in esophageal disease do not change with age.[20] Laparoscopic Nissen fundoplication is an effective antireflux procedure without significant morbidity and is well tolerated in the elderly.[21]

Disorders of the Stomach and Duodenum

Gastric secretory and motor function has been studied extensively in the elderly during the past several years.[22] Gastric acid secretion, both maximal (stimulated) and basal output, declines with age, probably because of the reduction in parietal cell mass.[23] Grossman et al. demonstrated decreases in basal and stimulated acid output after the age of 50, with the greatest decline in males.[24] Some of these changes were undoubtedly associated with gastric mucosal atrophy.[25] Recent studies have shown many elderly adults have normal gastric acidity.[26] Serum gastrin levels were shown to have increased with age in some studies; this, however, is probably secondary to the acid secretory changes.

Gastric emptying involves a complex interaction of numerous physiologic events. Several early studies have suggested that alterations in gastric emptying with age occur. However, most of these studies did not have adequate controls.[27] It is likely that underlying disease affected some of these findings. Later studies utilizing well-matched controls indicated that liquid emptying was delayed in the elderly whereas solid food emptying appeared to be unaffected.[28] These types of changes in gastric emptying may be an important cause of some age-related variations in drug absorption.[27]

The organism *Helicobacter pylori* (*H. pylori*) has an important impact on gastric function in the elderly.[29–31] This spiral urease-producing organism is seen nestled in the narrow interface between the gastric epithelial cell surface and the overlying mucus layer in the infected patient. The organism has been highly correlated with antral gastritis and with the development of gastric and especially duodenal ulcers. Recent studies indicate that the eradication of the organism effectively eliminates ulcer recurrence.[32] Excellent epidemiologic studies in numerous populations indicate an increased carriage of the organism with age.[33] In the United States, an estimated 50% of adults by age 60 years are seropositive. The organism has been linked to antral gastritis of the type frequently associated with aging. It appears that *H. pylori*-induced gastritis is a pivotal event in development of peptic ulcer disease.

Nonsteroidal anti-inflammatory drugs are one of the most important factors in the development of gastrointestinal damage. This factor is particularly important in the elderly, who are heavy users of these medications.[14] The elderly, especially elderly women, who have increased usage of nonsteroidal medications are at particularly high risk.[34-36] Nonsteroidal use is associated with depletion of mucosal prostaglandins and decreased reparation with an increased risk of gastric and duodenal ulceration and bleeding; this difference may be as great as 50-fold for gastric ulcers and 8-fold for duodenal ulcers, with prevalence of 9% to 31% for gastric ulcers and 0% to 19% for duodenal ulcers. Patients with prior history of peptic ulcer disease and increased age are at particularly high risk.[34,37,38] Newer NSAIDs, the Cox-2 inhibitor, have a significantly lowered risk of ulcerogenesis and although expensive are being used widely in the elderly.

Gastritis and gastric atrophy are two of the most commonly described gastric abnormalities in the elderly. Gastritis is associated with mucosal infiltration of inflammatory cells and with loss of secretory cells, both chief and parietal, from the mucosa. Depending on the type of gastritis, these changes may involve the body and fundus or antrum.[23] Acute forms of gastritis have been associated with alcohol and medication ingestion, in particular, nonsteroidal anti-inflammatory drugs. This type of inflammatory process is highly associated with gastrointestinal bleeding.[36]

Classically, two types of atrophic gastritis have been described. Fundal gastritis (type A) is associated with an absence of fundal glands, which have been replaced by goblet cells, and the appearance of changes suggestive of intestinal metaplasia.[39] The loss of parietal cells is associated with a decrease in acid secretion, and consequently the antrum produces gastrin in response to the decline in acid secretion, resulting in high serum gastrin levels.[40] Antibodies to parietal cells as well as antibody to intrinsic factor are present resulting in vitamin B_{12} malabsorption and the classic picture of pernicious anemia. Other autoantibodies have been described in this clinical situation.

Antral gastritis or type B gastritis is more commonly seen and is probably associated with *H. pylori* infection.[41] This process may be associated with a decrease in serum gastrin levels. Parietal cell antibodies and other serologic abnormalities are not present. Antral mucosa may be variably affected with acute and chronic cellular infiltrates and metaplastic glandular changes. Type B gastritis has been associated with gastric ulcer and gastric cancer.[42,43]

Low-grade and some high-grade gastric lymphomas may be seen in the elderly in association with *H. pylori* infection. These lesions show mucosal infiltration by small lymphocytes and plasma cells, with the appearance of mucosa-associated lymphoid tissue (MALT). These lymphomas have been called B-cell lymphoma of MALT, MALT lymphoma, or MALToma. More than 90% of low-grade MALT lymphomas are positive for *H. pylori* infection. In addition, eradication of *Helicobacter* infection has resulted in resolution of low-grade MALT lymphomas.[41]

Pernicious anemia is an important diagnosis that is usually made secondary to hematologic abnormalities, as GI symptoms are unusual. There is a three- to fivefold increase in the incidence of gastric cancer in patients with pernicious anemia. However, specific screening strategies have not been widely accepted.[44]

Hypertrophic gastropathy (Menetrier's disease) is an uncommon disorder of the stomach presenting with enlarged gastric rugae and is frequently associated with protein loss across the gastric mucosa.[45] Though it is not particularly increased in the elderly, it becomes an important consideration in the differentiation from neoplastic gastric lesions (i.e., lymphoma and carcinoma).

Peptic Ulcer Disease

The clinical picture of the patient with peptic ulcer disease has changed dramatically in the past decade. With the widespread use of nonsteroidal anti-inflammatory drugs (NSAIDs), the incidence of gastric ulcer disease has increased, particularly in the elderly.[38,46] The availability of these drugs as over-the-counter preparations has been associated with markedly increased use. Elderly patients taking these medications frequently present with severe hemorrhage, perforation, and obstruction, often without abdominal pain.[47,48] In addition, the widespread acceptance of *H. pylori* infection as an important factor in the pathogenesis of peptic ulcer disease (especially duodenal ulcer) has significantly changed the therapeutic approach to peptic ulcer disease in all patients.

The incidence of gastric ulcers and gastric erosive disease increases with age, as noted earlier.[37,38,46] This factor is particularly important in those patients using nonsteroidal anti-inflammatory drugs. Gastric ulcers are usually located along the lesser curvature at the junction of body and antral mucosa transition; however, this junction frequently migrates proximally with advancing age.[42] Giant gastric ulcers have been demonstrated frequently in the elderly and are associated with the high rate of complications and mortality.[49] These ulcers are also associated with a greater likelihood of malignancy. Although the incidence of malignancy is low, as many as 6% of apparently benign ulcers may be malignant. It is clinically important to realize that the concurrence of duodenal ulcerations reduces the likelihood of malignancy.[49] Occasionally gastric ulcers, particularly those high in the fundus, may present with atypical symptoms such as chest pain.

Duodenal Ulcers

Duodenal ulcers are likewise common, particularly in elderly men,[38,46] but these do not have as high an association with nonsteroidal anti-inflammatory drug use. The incidence of complications with peptic ulcer disease increases with age. Giant duodenal ulcers are seen more commonly in elderly patients. These ulcers (greater than 2 cm in diameter) may be associated with severe pain and bleeding as well as gastric outlet obstruction.[50] Symptoms and findings on imaging studies (CT scanning) may mimic tumor arising from the pancreas.

The diagnosis of peptic ulcer disease is highly dependent on the use of endoscopic modalities in the elderly. Numerous studies in the elderly have demonstrated excellent tolerance for routine diagnostic endoscopy.[38,51] With monitoring of oxygen saturation and blood pressure as is routinely done for conscious sedation, patients tolerate routine sedation using diazepam and meperidine. The use of midazolam was not recommended for patients over the age of 60 years; however, there are numerous articles discussing its safety for older patients with appropriate titration of the medication.[52] Endoscopy is important in documentation of the presence of active ulceration as well as obtaining tissue biopsy and cytology for histologic examination to determine if malignancy is present.[51] Follow-up endoscopy may be indicated to determine complete healing of gastric ulcers and complicated duodenal ulcers (associated with bleeding or partial obstruction). In patients unable to tolerate endoscopy as a result of severe respiratory compromise or other medical conditions, barium studies may be useful in the diagnosis; however, these cannot determine definitely if malignancy is present.

Once a peptic ulcer is documented, the determination of H. pylori infection is important. A recent NIH consensus panel on H. pylori recommended that if Helicobacter is present in a patient with documented peptic ulcer disease, then the organism should be eradicated by antibiotic therapy.[31] Numerous methods for documentation of H. pylori infection are available. Invasive tests include endoscopy with gastric tissue biopsy and detection of urease activity in the tissue. Histologic evaluation and urea fermentation are more sensitive than culture. Noninvasive tests include breath test of urease activity after oral ingestion of ^{14}C or ^{13}C labeled urea;

these methods have a 90% accuracy.[53] Serologic studies with serology for immunoglobulin G antibodies to H. pylori antigens are most useful in the documentation of prior infection as clearance of the antibody is variable.

Treatment

The treatment of peptic ulcer disease includes the use of antacids, H_2 receptor antagonists, proton pump inhibitors, sucralfate, misoprostol, and antibiotic programs (to eradicate H. pylori).[38,54] Antacids have been used for the treatment of peptic ulcer disease for a number of years; they are most effective in relatively high doses. These doses may be associated with sodium overload, increased magnesium levels (important in patients with a renal dysfunction), and diarrhea or constipation. Antacids may also be associated with altered absorption of certain medications, including antibiotics and quinidine.[54,55]

The H_2 receptor antagonists such as cimetidine, ranitidine, famotidine, and nizatidine remain important drugs in the treatment of peptic ulcer disease. These medications are available over the counter and are widely used. They are generally well tolerated in the elderly, although mental confusion has been described with cimetidine, particularly in high dose and with parenteral use.[54,55] Cimetidine and ranitidine have been associated with altered metabolism of certain medications, such as warfarin, theophylline, and phenytoin. Cimetidine significantly inhibits the cytochrome P-450 system, whereas the other H_2 antagonists have a clinically insignificant effect.

Sucralfate is not absorbed and is effective in healing peptic ulcers. However, it may cause constipation and may bind certain medications.[56,57]

The proton pump inhibitors (PPIs) are an important group of medications, particularly when ulcerogenic medication needs to be continued. These potent inhibitors of the H^+/K^+-ATPase enzyme of the gastric parietal cell result in almost complete suppression of acid secretion, both basal and stimulated. Initially omeprazole was the only available proton pump inhibitor; however, several others are available: lansoprazole, pantoprazole, rabeprazole, and esomeprazole. All appear equally effective. These agents are very effective in treating peptic ulcers, particularly large gastric and duodenal ulcers. PPIs have also been combined with amoxicillin in the treatment of patients with H. pylori-associated ulcers. Recent reports suggest that it is effective in treatment of peptic ulcers where continuation of nonsteroidal medications is necessary.[38,58] PPIs may interact with drugs metabolized by the cytochrome P-450 system. They are associated with hypergastrinemia due to persistent gastric acid suppression; however, long-term treatment has been safe.[38]

Misoprostol, a prostaglandin analogue and cytoprotective agent, has been shown to heal peptic ulcers even when NSAIDs must be continued. This medication has also been used to prevent NSAID-associated ulcers in patients with a history of peptic ulcer disease and is particularly useful in the elderly patient as it has few drug interactions. Diarrhea is its major complication.[57]

Eradication of *Helicobacter pylori* infection results in more rapid healing of ulcers and reduction in recurrence rates.[59,60] Although the organism is sensitive to a number of antibiotics including ampicillin, amoxicillin, metronidazole, cephalosporins, tetracyline quinolones, and macrolides, single-agent treatments have low rates of eradication. The combination therapies including antibiotics and an acid suppressive agent are effective, as sensitivity is dependent on an alkaline environment. Simultaneous administration of bismuth appears to diminish development of resistance in some cases. Triple therapies including PPIs (omeprazole and lansoprazole) and two antibiotics, clarithromycin and amoxicillin or metronidazole, for 1- to 2-week periods are well tolerated and are 80% to 90% effective in eradiacation of the organism. Bismuth salts in combination with metronidazole and amoxicillin or tetracycline are similarly effective. Ranitidine, bismuth citrate in combination with clarithromycin for 2 weeks is likewise effective and well tolerated, although ranitidine must be continued for 4 weeks. After successful eradication, most patients remain free of *Helicobacter* infection and have duodenal ulcer relapse rates of less than 5% per year.[32,38,59,60]

Other Less Common Gastric Lesions

Gastric bezoar and volvulus are two relatively uncommon lesions that may be seen more frequently in the elderly. Bezoars are frequently seen in patients who have a history of vagotomy or subtotal gastrectomy. Metabolic disorders that are associated with decreased gastric emptying may also be associated with bezoars. Patients with diabetes mellitus and autonomic dysfunction are especially at risk.[61,62] Patients generally present with early satiety, weight loss, or unexplained nausea and emesis. Symptoms may mimic those suggestive of gastric neoplasia. Although either barium contrast studies or endoscopy will diagnose the lesion, endoscopy has also been shown to be effective in disruption of the mass of undigested fibrous material by biopsy or jet water spray.[62] Prokinetic agents, such as metoclopramide and cisapride (now withdrawn), are effective in emptying the stomach of residual fragments.[62] Chronic use of enzyme preparations may not be effective because of their low cellulase content.

Volvulus of the stomach may be seen in the elderly and is associated with chronic nausea and emesis or a more acute presentation with abdominal pain and acute abdomen. There are two types of volvulus, the more common being an organoaxial volvulus with rotation of the stomach on its longitudinal axis from cardia to pylorus and, less commonly seen, a mesenteroaxial volvulus with rotation along the vertical axis. Acute volvulus may require emergency surgery for reasons of compromise in blood supply to the stomach. Chronic forms of the former may require no intervention.[61]

Gastrointestinal Bleeding

Gastrointestinal (GI) bleeding is a major problem in the elderly and is associated with high mortality (10%–25%).[63,64] Underlying medical problems such as pulmonary and cardiovascular disease in addition to the use of medications (in particular NSAIDs) may contribute to this increased morbidity and mortality.[65,66] It is important, when treating patients with gastrointestinal bleeding, to determine the initial severity of bleeding and to institute appropriate intervention as early as possible. When one is presented with compromised cardiac and renal reserves, rapid and focused approach to initial intervention is essential. The patient with acute gastrointestinal bleeding may present with hematemesis, melena (dark tarry stools), or hematochezia. Hematochezia is usually associated with lower gastrointestinal bleeding; however, it may occur with massive upper GI hemorrhage with rapid transit of blood through the bowel. The patient with massive gastrointestinal bleeding may present with syncope and/or shock. The elderly person with cardiac disease may present with angina, shortness of breath, or weakness associated with decreased cardiac output and anemia.[66,67]

The initial evaluation and resuscitation of the patient is undertaken in rapid succession. It is important particularly in the elderly to determine whether there is a history of peptic ulcer disease and NSAID or other medication use. The initial clinical evaluation focuses on determination of hemodynamic status with careful monitoring of the blood pressure and pulse. Stigmata of underlying liver disease are important, because management may be altered. Initial laboratory studies should include hematocrit with platelet count, coagulation parameters, blood urea in nitrogen (BUN), and creatinine. It is helpful to compare these to prior studies, noting that hematocrit may not reflect blood loss for 24 to 48 h. In upper gastrointestinal bleeding, the BUN to creatinine ratio may be elevated, reflecting the absorption of blood from the gut; however, this may also occur with hypovolemia. Large-bore intravenous line placement for fluid repletion is imperative. The need to carefully monitor the responses to therapy in the elderly patient with cardiopulmonary compromise may necessitate early central venous pressure measurement. Oxygen support may be necessary in patients with severe anemia, particularly if there is underlying cardiac and pulmonary disease.[67]

Nasogastric lavage is important in the initial evaluation and treatment of bleeding. If the nasogastric lavage is positive for gross blood, this suggests upper GI bleeding, although there is a false-negative rate of approximately 10%.[67–69] Nasogastric lavage with room temperature water may be effective in clearing the stomach of blood, thereby decreasing emesis and facilitating endoscopy.

If an upper GI site is suspected, then upper endoscopy provides important diagnostic and prognostic information as well as therapeutic potential. The elderly patient tolerates endoscopy well, and there is no evidence of increased morbidity. If an active bleeding lesion is seen and treated successfully, studies have demonstrated a decrease in hospital stay and transfusion requirement.[64,66,70] Endoscopy allows the identification of lesions that are associated with poor prognosis and increased incidence of rebleeding: actively bleeding ulcers, the presence of a visible vessel in an active ulcer crater, or stigmata of recent bleeding have up to a 50% chance of rebleeding. Lesions in these patients warrant endoscopic treatment.[70]

Several endoscopic therapeutic modalities are available, including injection with saline and/or epinephrine, thermal coagulation, and laser therapy. The first two are more widely used due to availability and portability and have been shown to be effective.[64,66,71]

Arteriography may be useful as both a diagnostic and a therapeutic modality. The radiologist can examine the celiac and superior mesenteric arteries and selectively embolize arteries with an absorbable gel sponge (gelfoam) or autologous clot. If the initial NG aspirate has been negative and a lower GI source is suspected, angiography can determine a lower GI site with initial examination of the superior mesenteric artery and subsequently the inferior mesenteric artery supply. Infusion of vasopressin is used to control bleeding in lower GI lesions.[63,64,66,72–74]

In patients with suspected small bowel bleeding and colonic bleeding of unclear site, radioactive tagged red blood cell scanning may be effective. Red blood cells are labeled with technetium-99m and injected into the patient. Scanning may occur up to a 30-h period.[75] In cases of lower GI bleeding in which the patient has stopped bleeding or bleeding has slowed, the patient can be prepared for colonoscopy, which can be done in an emergent situation. The preparation with a Golytely purgation may be accomplished in approximately 4h,[76] especially with delivery by nasogastric tube.

Medical Therapy

H_2 antagonists and proton pump inhibitors are commonly given to patients in initial management of their gastrointestinal bleeding. Recent studies have demonstrated a benefit of acid-controlling agents in decreasing recurrent

bleeding; it is certainly associated with the decrease in the incidence of stress ulceration in the intensive care unit setting.[67,77] These agents are typically administered intravenously in bolus or in continuous infusion. Continuous infusion is associated with more consistent lowering of gastric acid. In the United States, proton pump inhibitors have not been available for parenteral use.[78] However, the early use of these agents orally is associated decrease in recurrence of bleeding. Sucralfate has been used as an agent with a lower risk of nosocomial pneumonia than H_2 antagonist therapy in intubated ICU patients.[79]

Peptic ulcers remain the most common causes of upper GI bleeding. In some studies, 33% of the patients presenting with peptic ulcers are over the age of 65; of these, approximately 40% have been reported to have gastrointestinal bleeding.[46,64] Rebleeding rates tend to be higher in the elderly,[64,66,80] which would suggest that elderly patients may frequently need to be monitored for longer periods of time in the hospital than younger patients. Additionally, the mortality rate in gastric ulcers is higher, and these predominate in elderly patients. Giant duodenal and gastric ulcers are also a potential site of bleeding. Dieulafoy's lesion has been reported in the endoscopic literature as a cause of gastric bleeding. This lesion is the result of an arterial bleed from a small mucosal defect that may be difficult to detect unless actively bleeding.[64,76] These lesions respond to endoscopic injection therapy. Vascular ectasia may be noted in the stomach; these are similar to these seen in the distal small bowel and colon.[81]

Surgical Intervention

Surgical intervention may be necessary in patients, especially those requiring massive transfusions (>6 units).[64,70,76] The mortality may be high but depends on underlying medical problems and duration of bleeding. Surgical therapy is mandated when less invasive procedures (therapeutic endoscopy and arteriography) have failed to control hemorrhage. It is important to exercise teamwork in the management of patients with gastrointestinal bleeding, in particular the elderly patient, by combining the primary provider (internist or family practitioner), gastroenterologist, radiologist, and surgeon.[66]

Small Intestine Diseases

Age-related changes in small bowel anatomy and physiology in both animal and human studies have been reported in several studies. Although small intestine motility is maintained throughout the process of aging,[82] studies have demonstrated a decrease in the surface area of villi with shortening and clubbing of villi.[2,83,84] Potential small bowel absorptive deficiency may occur under physiologic stress. Carbohydrate absorption has been demonstrated to be impaired when challenged. More sophisticated studies have demonstrated delayed disaccharidase expression, with a decrease in disaccharidase activities, probably contributing to acquired lactose intolerance.[83,85] In the elderly, calcium absorption is impaired on low-calcium diets. Decreased tissue levels of zinc possibly related to impaired absorption have also been reported. Other investigators have reported vitamin absorption deficiencies. Idiopathic bacterial overgrowth has been demonstrated in some patients and appears to be associated with a decrease in postprandial motility.[1]

Gluten-sensitive enteropathy or celiac sprue has been reported in the elderly, who may represent up to 25% of new cases.[2,83] Patients usually present with classic symptoms of malabsorption, that is, anemia, steatorrhea, and osteomalacia. However, in elderly patients the latter may be confused with osteoporosis. Evidence of folate deficiency may predominate and must be differentiated from primary nutritional deficiency. Management is similar to that in younger patients, with institution of a gluten-free diet and vitamin and mineral supplementation.

Diverticulosis of the small bowel is a common age-associated small bowel lesion. Bacterial overgrowth and malabsorption with diarrhea, abdominal distension, steatorrhea, and weight loss are common presentations. Management includes antibiotic therapy, in conjunction with prokinetic agents such as metoclopramide.

Ischemic Bowel Disease

The superior mesenteric, inferior mesenteric, and hypogastric arteries supply the small bowel and colon. There is extensive collateralization between these arterial supplies, and ischemic disease only occurs when there is significant compromise of two of the three main arterial trunks. This compromise may arise from intrinsic arterial disease or from embolization, both of which are more common in the elderly. Acute occlusion of the superior mesenteric artery with inadequate collateralization may result in infarction of the small bowel[86]; this is frequently a catastrophic event and presents with severe abdominal pain, typically out of proportion to the physical findings.

The patient may initially have an ileus with or without rectal bleeding. Physical findings are associated with transmural infarction and peritoneal irritation. This type of ischemia may frequently go unnoticed in patients in intensive care units with other medical problems.[86,87] One should have a high level of suspicion when caring for the critically ill patient. Diagnostic findings are fairly nonspecific, with elevated white blood cell count and fever. Plain films of the abdomen may show an ileus or thumbprinting in the small bowel and in some instances

portal venous air. When the diagnosis is suspected, angiography is indicated to confirm the diagnosis and to direct surgery.

Chronic occlusion may be associated with "abdominal angina," or abdominal pain worsened by eating. Diarrhea, steatorrhea, and progressive weight loss result. Arteriography followed by revascularization of affected bowel is indicated.[87]

Ischemic colitis is one of the most common causes of lower GI bleeding.[63,64] Patients typically present with rectal bleeding and lower abdominal cramping. Physical examination may be unremarkable if there is no transmural infarction. Ischemia is common in "watershed" areas where two arterial supplies meet, in particular, the sigmoid colon, splenic flexure of the colon, and proximal transverse colon. Less commonly, the ascending colon and cecal areas may also be involved. Plain film of the abdomen may show thumbprinting and narrowing of the affected areas. Initial evaluation is as outlined for the treatment of lower GI bleeding with initial anoscopic and sigmoidoscopic evaluation. Urgent colonoscopy after appropriate bowel cleansing has been very effective in making this diagnosis. Barium enema should be avoided if bleeding has continued and, in particular, if angiographic or endoscopic studies are anticipated. Most patients resolve spontaneously with cessation of bleeding. With deep mucosal injury or transmural injury, resulting strictures may develop. Some patients may present with colonic strictures as a result of ischemic bowel without an acute history.[16,88]

Vascular Ectasias

Vascular ectasias, also called angiodysplagias or arteriovenous malformations, are commonly encountered in the cecum and ascending colon of the elderly. Vascular lesions may also be seen in the small bowel (jejunum, ileum, and duodenum).[81] These lesions are degenerative lesions that form from previously normal vessels. These ectatic, distorted veins and capillaries are thin-walled vessels lined with endothelium. The lesion is characterized in its earliest form by dilated submucosal veins with a progressively enlarged array of dilated and distorted vessels extending into the mucosa.

Boley and colleagues[86] have studied these lesions extensively by angiography and by silicone rubber injection of resected specimens. They have proposed that vascular ectasias develop as a result of intermittent distention of the cecum and right colon with resultant obstruction of venous outflow. According to this hypothesis, cecal location is caused by the large diameter of the cecum and relatively high wall pressures.[56,63,80,89] This theory would not explain small bowel lesions, however.

Vascular ectasias of the colon occur predominantly in the elderly, with two-thirds of the patients over the age of 70 years with equal sex distribution. Bleeding is usually recurrent and subacute, although 15% present with severe hemorrhage. The spectrum of presentation varies between patients and episodes in the same patient. Fifty percent of patients with bleeding have cardiac disease; about one-half of these have been reported to have aortic stenosis. Bleeding can be controlled successfully with endoscopic therapeutic modalities: heater probe, electrocoagulation, laser, or injection. Angiographic infusion of vasopressin is successful in treatment of active bleeding when demonstrated.[64,81,89] If bleeding continues or is recurrent, surgery may be required.

Telangiectasias of the bowel wall may be associated with multiple causes and may be the site of acute and chronic blood loss in elderly patients. Hereditary hemorrhagic telangiectasias (or Osler–Weber–Rendu) may cause bleeding in the elderly. At younger ages, nasal (epistaxis) and oral lesions may be significant. Gastric duodenal and small bowel lesions may be treated endoscopically. Enteroscopy is now available and may diagnose lesions in 15% to 38% of patients studied. Endoscopic therapeutic modalities, as already outlined, can be effective in reduction of bleeding and transfusion requirements.[89]

Hepatobiliary Disorders

The liver changes only slightly with age. Of particular interest is the decrease in the entire weight of the liver and its respective lobules with an overall decrease in the number of hepatocytes. Importantly, the ability of the aged liver to regenerate after injury or resection appears to be somewhat diminished. Liver chemistries and liver function remain normal. However, due to circulatory changes and some metabolic enzyme changes, metabolism of some drugs may be altered and is thus an important concern in the stressed elderly.[90,91]

Cholestatic jaundice occurs more frequently in the elderly in association with an increase in both malignant and benign obstruction (choledocholithiasis). Drug-induced liver disease is an important problem in the elderly, presumably secondary to the increased drug use and drug sensitivity. Jaundice in the elderly may be drug induced in up to 20% of patients.[92,93] The following are some of the commonly used drugs that are offenders: oral hypoglycemics, antibiotics, hormones, nonsteroidals, and anesthetics. Injury may present as primarily hepatocellular, cholestatic, or mixed hepatocellular and cholestatic. The type of injury will determine the pattern of enzyme abnormality in the older patient similar to that seen in younger patients. In most cases, withdrawal of the offending agent will lead to a resolution of biochemical abnormalities. In some cases, however, cholestasis may last for several months, as has been reported with phenothiazines

and imipramine. Several other drugs have been associated with chronic hepatitis.[94]

Alcoholic liver disease may be seen in the elderly, although alcoholic hepatitis is unusual. Patients are more likely to present with cirrhosis in this age group. The anorexia, nausea, abdominal pain, and weight loss seen in alcoholic hepatitis are not dissimilar from viral hepatitis. However, with alcoholic hepatitis, transaminases are typically 300 or less. In severe cases, patients may have fever and leukocytosis. It is important to rule out acetaminophen toxicity as toxicity can occur without overdose and with therapeutic doses of the medication in alcoholic patients.[95,96] Rapid determination of acetaminophen blood levels and therapy with acetylcysteine can be lifesaving.

Acute viral hepatitis is less common in the elderly. The acute course of hepatitis B, in the elderly, is typically very severe secondary due to age-related poor hepatic reserves and regenerative capabilities.[97–99] Hepatitis C, which is frequently transfusion acquired, can be a major problem in the elderly. In particular, about 30% to 50% of patients develop chronic hepatitis after an initial infection, with a rapid progression to cirrhosis. Liver biopsy documentation of progressive liver disease is important in these cases.[100–102]

Ischemic liver injury may occur in patients with circulatory failure, as the result of passive congestion of the liver or decreased blood flow to the liver. Patients with decreased cardiac output may present with a picture similar to acute hepatitis. One may see mild injury or the patient may have dramatically elevated transaminases and LDH.[103]

Congestive failure with severe right heart failure may be associated with jaundice. Typically, patients have an elevation in bilirubin and alkaline phosphatase. In severe cases the liver may be pulsatile. In severe cases, associated passive congestion of the bowel can lead to diarrhea.

Cholelithiasis

Cholelithiasis and choledocholithiasis are common in the elderly. Gallstones may be associated with elevation in cholesterol as well as hemolysis with the formation of pigment stones.[104] When gallstones are asymptomatic, the general approach has been not to recommend surgery, on the basis of studies by Gracie and Ransohoff[105,106] that revealed the probability of developing biliary colic to be 10% after 5 years, 15% after 10 years, and 18% by 15 to 20 years. However, biliary symptomatic cholelithiasis may present itself in the elderly patient as pain and jaundice, pain alone, or jaundice alone. Studies have suggested that the development of choledocholithiasis may be associated with a periampullary duodenal diverticulum. These diverticula increase with age.[107] Choledocholithiasis may be managed nonsurgically with endoscopic sphincterotomy. Elderly patients tolerate endoscopic retrograde pancreatography and endoscopic sphincterotomy well; this may be followed by laparoscopic cholecystectomy, although in some fragile elderly, the gallbladder has been left in situ.[108]

Acute cholecystitis is a serious complication of gallstone disease. Morbidity and mortality associated with acute cholecystitis may be high in the elderly, with one series reporting mortality of 9.8%.[109] With stabilization, some patients may be able to undergo laparoscopic cholecystectomy, which is associated with lower morbidity and mortality.[104]

Pancreatic Disorders

Pancreatic function does not change significantly with age; however, some morphologic changes in the pancreas with age have been noted. The frequency of ductal dilatation of the main pancreatic duct increases by 8% per decade.[110]

Gallstone pancreatitis is a major concern in the elderly. The mortality from acute pancreatitis in the elderly patients has been reportedly as high as 80% as compared to 9% in younger patients.[111,112] Recent studies suggest that early endoscopic retrograde cholangiopancreatography (ERCP) with stone removal may significantly decrease morbidity and possibly mortality.[112,113]

Chronic pancreatitis may manifest in the elderly patient after a long history of alcohol abuse. Pancreatic insufficiency represents one of the major causes of steatorrhea in patients over the age of 65 years. In the setting of weight loss, abdominal pain, and steatorrhea, the differential diagnosis certainly includes pancreatic carcinoma and becomes one of the major diagnoses to be excluded. Pancreatic insufficiency may be difficult to diagnose; 72-h fecal fat collection is imperative to document malabsorption and maldigestion. Pancreatic enzyme replacement effectively treats insufficiency; microencapsulated preparations with high concentrations of pancreatic enzymes are very effective. Use of acid suppressive therapy is not necessary.

Disorders of the Colon

Almost half the gastrointestinal complaints that bring elderly patients to the physician revolve around constipation and irritable bowel syndrome. Other common colonic problems in the elderly include diverticulitis, fecal incontinence, inflammatory bowel disease, ischemic colitis, and appendicitis. Detailed understanding of the relationship between colonic structure, physiology, and clinical symptoms leaves much to be explored.

With aging, some minor changes in the colon do occur that can contribute to some of the problems seen in the elderly. These changes include decreased mucosal secretion, which can decrease the degree of lubrication of the colon; increased connective tissue and atrophy of the muscle layers, which can lead potentially to less effective muscle function; and weakness in the abdominal wall muscles, which can make defecation more difficult.

Studies in healthy active elderly, however, have shown little difference in colonic transit time[114] or in the amplitude or duration of contractions during fasting or after the gastrocolic reflex in the sigmoid, rectosigmoid, or rectum compared to healthy subjects 40 years younger.[115] There is conflicting information on various other measurements of defecation parameters with aging. With disabled elderly who have decreased mobility, transit time may be greatly prolonged.[116]

Constipation

There is a major difference between the medical definition of constipation and a person's perception of their need for laxatives. In general, most authors cite the definition of constipation as having bowel movements of decreased frequency and volume. Normal frequency of bowel movements is between three defecations per day and three per week, regardless of age. Sixty percent to 70% of healthy community-living elderly have a daily bowel movement, yet recurring studies show that 15% to 30% of elderly take laxatives on a regular basis,[117,118] resulting in hundreds of millions of dollars spent yearly on laxatives.

The most frequent reasons for constipation in healthy elderly are chronic suppression of the gastrocolic reflex and poor intake of dietary fiber. Medical conditions that may contribute to constipation in the elderly include immobility, depression, hypothyroidism, and hypercalcemia. Medications that may contribute to constipation are shown in Table 56.3. Chronic use of certain irritant laxatives has been shown to be associated with myoneural degeneration, leading to chronic constipation;[119] however, most cases today are not so associated.

For the patient who is not chronically constipated, many of the over-the-counter preparations, such as saline

TABLE 56.3. Medications that contribute to constipation in the elderly.

Anticholinergics
Opioids and other analgesics
Sedatives and tranquilizers
Antihypertensive ganglionic blockers
Cation-containing agents: iron, calcium
Calcium channel blockers
Anticonvulsants

laxatives and mild stimulants (senna and bisacodyl), will work adequately for the acute incident if obstipation or impaction has not occurred. If impaction is present, then manual disimpaction should occur as soon as the diagnosis is made. Enemas may then be used to evacuate the feces above the rectal vault. Oral laxatives can be used for a time-limited episode of expected constipation, such as the patient acutely immobilized during hospitalization; these agents include milk of magnesia, lactulose, sorbotol, and anthroquinones. The bowel preparation Golytely has also been used in small amounts as an oral laxative in elderly patients.[120] Mineral oil, because it may predispose to aspiration pneumonitis in people with swallowing problems, is usually avoided in the elderly.

Most complaints of constipation can be eliminated or at least reduced by the following: patient education, reduction or elimination of offending medications, addition of fiber through dietary manipulation or supplements, increased physical activity, and bowel stimulation. Dietary fiber in the range of 15 to 20g per day is recommended to increase fecal water content and maintain soft stool of adequate volume. Sources for fiber include whole wheat bread, bran, and shredded wheat cereals; fruit such as apples, bananas, and strawberries; nuts such as peanuts; vegetables such as broccoli, carrots, beans, peas; and bran additives. For patients who cannot or will not increase their dietary bran adequately, fiber supplement with psyllium or methylcellulose supplements are usually more effective than traditional "stool softeners" such as bisacodyl ducosate. Adequate fluid intake needs to be encouraged in patients taking fiber supplements. Addition of dietary fiber has been shown to reduce the need for laxatives even in elderly institutionalized patients.[121] Table 56.4 presents some of the management approaches in the elderly.

Increased water intake has been suggested by some, especially for those elderly with blunted thirst responses and those on diuretics. Increased physical activity has been shown to decrease the need for laxatives in healthy elderly. Even minor increases in physical activity in institutionalized elderly can play a role in decreasing the need for laxatives.

Bowel training is a method of overcoming inhibition of the gastrocolic reflex and includes providing the opportunity to have a bowel movement immediately following the first meal of the day. If a bowel movement does not occur, then a suppository or enema is given to effect the bowel movement. This behavioral training is continued on a daily basis. Usually, by the third to fifth day of reinforcement of the gastrocolic reflex, defecation occurs without the need for a rectal stimulant. Even in institutionalized elderly with neurologic deficits, bowel training has been shown to be effective in more than 85% by day 8.[122]

The complications most frequently associated with constipation include the development of megacolon and

TABLE 56.4. Management of constipation in the elderly.

Chronic therapy
  Education
  Dietary fiber
  Fluid intake
  Bulk laxatives–Fiber supplements
    Psyllium
    Methylcellulose
  Hyperosmolar laxatives
    Sorbitol (cheaper)
    Lactulose
Chronic intermittent therapy
  Stimulant laxatives
    Anthraquinones: senna, cascara, biscodyl
    Diphenylmethanes: phenophthalein (avoid)
    Castor oil (avoid)
  Saline laxative
    Magnesium hydroxide
    Other magnesium salts
  Suppositories/enemas
    Glycerin
    Bisacodyl
  Polyethylene gylcol solutions
Hospitalized patients to decrease straining
  Stool softeners: docusate (ineffective laxative)

overflow fecal incontinence. Fecal incontinence is a frequent reason for institutionalization, accounting in various studies for 10% to 60% of institutionalized elderly, especially female patients; this is a complication of severe constipation in debilitated patients, where it presents as overflow incontinence, and is a major hygienic and health care issue in patients with depressed cerebral function.[123] Treatment is similar to that described for constipation. Make sure that fecal impaction is not present, and then make sure that it does not recur. Bowel training, increased physical activity, biofeedback, and pelvic floor exercises have also been suggested.[124] For patients with neuromuscular causes of fecal incontinence, thickening of stool with bulking agents such as psyllium and cautious use of constipating drugs such as Imodium may be tried.

Irritable bowel syndrome is used to refer to a combination of symptoms including constipation with or without diarrhea, left lower quadrant discomfort, abdominal distension, excessive flatus, and incomplete evacuation. Unlike pathologic conditions that cause constipation, irritable bowel syndrome is never associated with blood in the stool, does not awaken the patient at night, and is not associated with change in appetite or weight loss. Although frequently presenting in middle age, it may not become a significant complaint until the sixth or seventh decade.[125] Treatment is similar to that for constipation and includes increase of fiber content, physical activity, and bowel training. Stress management and behavior modification (biofeedback) have also been successful at times.

Diverticulosis and Diverticulitis

The prevalence of diverticulosis (the presence of numerous colonic diverticula) increases with advancing age and is equally prevalent in men and women. Diverticulosis, which is present in one-third to two-thirds of the American population over the age of 60,[126] represents outpouchings in the colon at sites of insertion of penetrating blood vessels that are most frequently present in the descending colon and sigmoid. Diverticula themselves are usually asymptomatic, unless perforation, infection, or bleeding occurs. Most people who have recurring low-grade discomfort in the left lower quadrant probably have irritable bowel syndrome, even if diverticulosis is present.

Occasionally obstruction of the opening of the diverticulum by a fecalith is associated with microperforation, and diverticulitis occurs. Increased incidence of diverticulitis may also be seen in patients taking nonsteroidal anti-inflammatory drugs.[127] The inflammatory state of acute diverticulitis is classically associated with significant left lower quadrant pain, a left lower quadrant tender inflammatory mass, and fever, with or without chills. Pain increasing with time, anorexia, nausea, and dysuria or abdominal pain aggravated by micturition may also be seen. A left lower quadrant mass with tenderness and local rebound is classically found. In the elderly, many of the classic findings may be diminished, so that pain may be minimal, and tenderness or even the finding of a mass may be absent. Generalized peritoneal findings are unusual. Although fecal occult blood may be found, evidence of gross bleeding is very rare during an attack of acute diverticulitis. Leukocytosis with a shift to the left is classic, but may be blunted in the elderly or in those on steroids. Where there is a suspicion for diverticulitis, absence of a classic finding should not rule out the process. Rather, close observation should be undertaken to ensure that deterioration is not occurring. Evidence of inflammatory cells in the urine may indicate bladder or ureteral involvement. Because presentation of diverticulitis can be so similar to ischemic and inflammatory bowel disease in the elderly, early sigmoidoscopy without bowel preparation is sometimes recommended. Due to risk of perforation, enemas should be avoided if compromise in bowel wall is suspected.

Treatment of suspected acute diverticulitis requires hospitalization for observation, especially for the frail elderly. Bowel rest, fluid replacement, and broad-spectrum antibiotics usually result in defervescence of the inflammatory findings in 3 to 10 days. Radiologic or colonoscopic evaluation of the colon 6 to 8 weeks after an attack is usually recommended to assure that stricture formation has not occurred and that the presenting problem was indeed due to diverticulitis and not to penetrating colon carcinoma.[128]

Decreased recurrence of symptoms and reduced development of additional diverticula has been suggested with the use of a high-fiber diet or bulking agents.[129] Recurrent attacks occur in fewer than 25% of patients.[128]

Acute surgery is necessary in less than 20%, usually in those patients with signs of worsening inflammation or failure to respond despite conservative management. Fistula formation from the perforated diverticulum to urinary bladder, vagina, small bowel, or skin may occur and be another reason to consider surgery.

Diverticula in the right colon are less frequent but, if present, may be a source for major hemorrhage, if erosion of the mucosa underlying the perforating artery occurs. Bleeding from diverticula is said to be the most common cause of major lower intestinal hemorrhage in the elderly, occurring in 10% to 25% of patients with diverticular disease. Diverticular bleeding can be massive, with the patient presenting with mahogany stools or frankly bloody diarrhea. Unlike the pulse and vital sign changes classic for upper gastrointestinal bleeding, older patients with lower gastrointestinal bleeding can experience large volume losses without development of appreciable tachycardia or orthostasis, further complicating diagnosis. Diagnosis can be made by emergency colonoscopy, arteriography, or tagged red cells. Most patients with diverticular bleeding spontaneously resolve bleeding; however, a second bleed is seen in 20%.

Inflammatory Bowel Disease

Both Crohn's disease and ulcerative colitis are now recognized to have a bimodal age presentation, with the second peak between 60 and 75 years of age. Older patients are frequently women and are more likely to have left-sided involvement. Presentation of Crohn's can be very similar to diverticulitis, with acute presentation of left lower quadrant abdominal pain, tender abdominal mass, and fistula development. Ulcerative colitis on the other hand is more likely to present as chronic diarrhea. For more extensive review of the differences and similarities between Crohn's disease and ulcerative colitis, the reader is referred to an excellent review by Lennard-Jones et al.[131–133]

Evaluation includes plain film of the abdomen and examination of the stool for fecal leukocytes, blood, and parasites, as well as flexible sigmoidoscopy to rule out ischemic colitis, pseudomembranous colitis, and neoplasm.

There is growing evidence that presentation in late life is associated with fewer relapses and a milder overall course if the first episode is tolerated.[133] Treatment options for Crohn's colitis and ulcerative colitis include sulfasalazine, 5-aminosalicylic acid agents, and steroids. Systemic steroids are more likely to be necessary in the first attack of late-onset ulcerative colitis than in attacks presenting earlier. Azathioprine and 6-mercaptopurine immunosuppressive agents and infleximab (tumor necrosis factor antibody) are well tolerated in the elderly. Treatment considerations in the elderly include the need to be careful with the use of opiate-containing drugs for diarrhea, with concern for oversedation leading to mental confusion and falls. Loperamide may be better tolerated because of decreased central effects. Anticholinergics should also be used sparingly in the elderly to avoid potential cardiac and neurologic complications.

A severe complication is the development of toxic megacolon, which may be precipitated by anticholinergic drugs and which may progress to colonic perforation. The appearance of acute toxic megacolon is an indication for emergency surgery.

Risk of colon carcinoma is increased with long-standing inflammatory bowel disease, highest in those with active ulcerative colitis for over 10 years.

Pseudomembranous Colitis

Antibiotic-associated colitis, *C. difficile* colitis, is caused by toxins produced by the overgrowth of *Clostridium difficile*. Its name comes from the frequent finding of a necrotic epithelium with an overlying, easily removed yellowish membrane. Alteration of gut flora associated with exposure to broad-spectrum antibiotics and, in some cases, chemotherapy is responsible for colonization and then overgrowth of the pathogenic bacteria.

Person-to-person nosocomial spread has been demonstrated, and several epidemics of pseudomembranous colitis occurring in institutionalized elderly have been reported.[134] Cases occur up to 8 weeks after receiving broad-spectrum antibiotics. Fever, abdominal pain, tenesmus, and blood-streaked diarrhea are common. Diagnosis is confirmed by the isolation of *C. difficile* or its toxin from the stool or characteristic findings on mucosal biopsy.

Withdrawal of the antibiotic and correction of fluid and electrolytes are important. Metronidazole or vancomycin is usually effective in treatment; however, relapses may occur. In the latter case, prolonged treatment course with these agents is indicated. Dehydration and shock may occur. Mortality is high among the elderly so afflicted.

Conclusion

Physiologic changes with aging are usually not clinically significant but predispose the elderly to less ably withstand disease processes. Common problems such as relationship of dysphagia to aspiration, role of NSAIDs and *Helicobacter pylori* in the increased frequency and severity of peptic ulcer disease in the elderly, role of laparascopic treatment of gallstones, approach to GI bleeding, constipation, and diverticulitis are reviewed. Decreases in mortality have come from heightened awareness of presentations in the elderly, early intervention, and development of effective, less invasive treatment approaches.

References

1. Shamburek RD, Farrar J. Disorders of the digestive system in the elderly. *N Engl J Med.* 1990;322:438–443.
2. Holt PR. Gastrointestinal system: changes in morphology and cell proliferation. *Aging.* 1991; 3:392–394.
3. Russell RM. Changes in gastrointestinal function attributed to aging. *Am J Clin Nutr.* 1992;55:1203S–1207S.
4. Blechman MB, Gelb AM. Aging and gastrointestinal physiology. *Clin Geriatr Med.* 1999;15:429–438.
5. Mendez L, Friedman LS, Castell DO. Swallowing disorders in the elderly. *Clin Geriatr Med.* 1991;7:215–7230.
6. Sonies BC. Oropharyngeal dysphagia in the elderly. *Clin Geriatr Med.* 1992;8:569–577.
7. Sallout H, Mayoral W, Benjamin SB. The aging esophagus. *Clin Geriatr Med.* 1999;15:439–456.
8. Ciocon JO. Indications for tube feeding in elderly patients. *Dysphagia.* 1990;5:1–5.
9. O'Gara JA. Dietary adjustments and nutritional therapy during treatment for oral-pharyngeal dysphagia. *Dysphagia.* 1990;4:209–212.
10. Hollis SB, Castell DO. Esophageal function in elderly men: a new look at presbyesophagus. *Ann Intern Med.* 1974;80:371–374.
11. Orlando RC, Borzymski EM. Clinical and manometric effects of nitroglycerin in diffuse esophageal spasm. *N Engl J Med.* 1973;289:23–25.
12. Pasricha PJ, Rai R, Ravich WJ, et al. Botulinum toxin for achalasia: long term outcome and predictors of response. *Gastroenterology.* 1996;110:410–414.
13. Robertson CS, Fellows IW, Mayberry J, et al. Choice of therapy for achalasia in relation to age. *Digestion.* 1988; 40:244–249.
14. Kikendall JW, Friedman AC, Oyewole MA, et al. Pill-induced esophageal injury: case reports and review of the medical literature. *Dig Dis Sci.* 1983;28:174–182.
15. Ellis FH. Current concepts. Esophageal hiatal hernia. *N Engl J Med.* 1972;287:646–669.
16. Spechler SJ. Epidemiology and natural history of gastro-oesophageal reflux disease. *Digestion.* 1992;51(suppl 1): 24–29.
17. Rogers EL, Goldkind S, Goldkind L, et al. Adenocarcinoma of the lower esophagus. *J Clin Gastroenterol.* 1986; 9(6):613–618.
18. Havelund T, Lursen LS, Skoubo-Kristensen E, et al. Omeprazole and ranitidine in treatment of reflux esophagitis: double blind comparative trial. *Br Med J.* 1988; 296:89–92.
19. Sirgo MA, Mills R, Euler AR, Walker S. The safety of ranitidine in elderly versus non-elderly patients. *J Clin Pharm.* 1993;33:79–83.
20. Gorman RC, Morris JB, Kaiser LR. Esophageal disease in the elderly patient. *Surg Clin N Am.* 1994;74:93–112.

21. Bittner HB, Pappas TN. Laparascopic approaches to symptomatic gastroesophageal reflux. *Semin Gastroenterol Dis.* 1994;5(3):113–119.

22. Kekki M, Samloff IM, Ihamake T, et al. Age and sex-related behavior of gastric acid secretion at the population level. *Scand J Gastroenterol.* 1982;17:737–743.

23. Samloff IM, Rotter JI, Siurala M, et al. Aging gastric mucosal histology and gastric secretory function. *Gastroenterology.* 1989;96:297–303.

24. Grossman MI, Kirsner JB, Gillespie IE, et al. Basal and histalog-stimulated gastric secretion in control subjects and in patients with peptic ulcer or gastric ulcer. *Gastroenterology.* 1963;45:14.

25. Steinheber FU. Aging and the stomach. *Clin Gastroenterol.* 1985;14:657–688.

26. Hurwitz, A, Brady DA, Schaal SE, Samloff IM, Dedon J, Ruhl CE. Gastric acidity in older adults. *JAMA.* 1997; 278(8):659–662.

27. Evans MA, Triqqs EJ, Cheung M, et al. Gastric emptying rate in the elderly. Implications for drug therapy. *J Am Geriatr Soc.* 1981;29:201–205.

28. Moore JG, Tweedy C, Christian PE, et al. Effect of age on gastric emptying of liquid-solid meals in man. *Dig Dis Sci.* 1983;28:340–344.

29. Connor BA. Gastrointestinal disorders of the stomach and duodenum in the elderly. In: Gelb AM, ed. *Clinical Gastroenterology.* New York: Dekker; 1996:37–72.

30. DeCross AJ, Marshall BJ. The role of *Helicobacter pylori* in acid-peptic disease. *Am J Med Sci.* 1993;306:381–392.

31. NIH Consensus Development Panel. NIH Consensus Conference on *Helicobacter pylori* in peptic ulcer disease. *JAMA.* 1994;272:65–69.

32. Tytgat GNJ, Noach LA, Rauws EAJ. *Helicobacter* infection and duodenal ulcer disease. *Gastroenterol Clin N Am.* 1993;22:127–139.

33. Perez-Perez GI, Dworkin BM, Chodos JE, et al. *Campylobacter pylori* antibodies in humans. *Ann Intern Med.* 1988; 109:11–17.

34. Allison MC, Torrance CJ, Russell RI. Non-steroidal anti-inflammatory drugs, gastroduodenal ulcers and their complications: prospective controlled autopsy study. *N Engl J Med.* 1992;327:749–754.

35. Skander MP, Ryan FP. Non-steroidal anti-inflammatory drugs and pain-free peptic ulceration in the elderly. *Br Med J.* 1988;297:833–834.

36. Gabriel SE, Jaakkimainendl, Bombardie C. Risk for serious gastrointestinal complications related to use of NSAIDs: a meta-analysis. *Ann Intern Med.* 1991;115: 787–796.

37. Griffin MR, Piper JM, Daughery MS, et al. Nonsteroidal anti-inflammatory drug use and increased risk for peptic ulcer disease in elderly persons. *Ann Intern Med.* 1991;114: 257–263.

38. Borum MA. Peptic-ulcer disease in the elderly. *Clin Geriatric Med.* 1999;15:457–471.

39. Bird T, Hall MRP, Schade ROK, et al. Gastric histology and its relation to anemia in the elderly. *Gerontology.* 1977;23: 309–321.

40. McGuigan JE, Trudeau WL. Serum gastrin concentration in pernicious anemia. *N Engl J Med.* 1970;282:358–361.

41. Leung KM, Hui PK, Chan WY, et al. *Helicobacter pylori*-related gastritis and gastric ulcer: a continuum of progressive epithelial degeneration. *Am J Clin Pathal.* 1992;98:569–574.

42. Parsonnet J. *Helicobacter pylori* and gastric cancer. *Gastroenterol Clin N Am.* 1993;22:89–104.

43. Roggero E, Zucca E, Pinotti G, et al. Eradication of *Helicobacter pylori* infection in primary low-grade gastric lymphoma of mucosa-associated lymphoid tissue. *Ann Intern Med* 1995;122:767–769.

44. Schafer LW, Larson DE, Melton LJ III, et al. Risk of development of gastric carcinoma in patients with pernicious anemia: a population based study in Rochester, Minnesota. *Mayo Clin Proc.* 1985;60;444–448.

45. Cooper BT. Menetrier's disease. *Dig Dis Sci.* 1987;5: 33–40.

46. Kurata JH, Corboy ED. Current peptic ulcer time trends: an epidemiological profile. *J Clin Gastroenterol.* 1988;10: 259–268.

47. Soll AH, Weinstein WM, Karata, et al. Nonsteroidal anti-inflammatory drug and peptic ulcer disase. *Ann Intern Med.* 1991;114:307–319.

48. Fries JF, Miller SR, Spitz PW, et al. Toward an epidemiology of gastropathy associated with nonsteroidal anti-inflammatory drug use. *Gastroenterology.* 1989;96(suppl): 647–655.

49. Tragardh B, Haglund U. Endoscopic diagnosis of gastric ulcer: evaluation of benefits of endoscopic follow-up observation for malignancy. *Acta Chir Scand.* 1985;151:37–41.

50. Klamer TW, Mahr MM. Giant duodenal ulcer: a dangerous variant of a common illness. *Am J Surg.* 1978;135:760–762.

51. Loffeld RJLF, Stobbeningh E, Arends JW. A review of diagnostic techniques for *Helicobacter pylori* infection. *Dig Dis.* 1993;11:173–180.

52. Christe C, Janssens JP, Armenian B, et al. Midazolam sedation for upper gastrointestinal endoscopy in older persons: a randomized, double-blind, placebo-controlled study. *J Am Geriatr Soc.* 2000;48:1398–1403.

53. Rubin W. Medical treatment of peptic ulcer disease. *Med Clin N Am.* 1991;75(4):981–998.

54. Walt RP, Langman MJ. Antacids and ulcer healing. A review of the evidence. *Drugs.* 1991;42(2):205–212.

55. Freston JW. Overview of medical therapy of peptic ulcer disease. *Gastroenterol Clin N Am.* 1990;19(1):121–140.

56. Rees WD. Mechanisms of gastroduodenal protection by sucralfate. *Am J Med.* 1991;91(2A):58S–63S.

57. Scheiman JM. Pathogeneses of gastroduodenal injury due to nonsteroidal anti-inflammatory drugs: implications for prevention and therapy. *Semin Arthritis Rheum.* 1992;21: 201–210.

58. Scheiman JM. NSAID-induced peptic ulcer disease: a critical review of pathogenesis and management. *Dig Dis.* 1994;12:210–222.

59. Marshall BJ. *Helicobacter pylori.* *Am J Gastroenterol.* 1994;89:S116–S128.

60. Tytgat GNJ. Review article: treatments that impact favorably upon the eradication of *Helicobacter pylori* and ulcer recurrence. *Aliment Pharmacol Ther.* 1994;8:359–368.

61. Sandler RS. Miscellaneous diseases of the stomach. In: Yamada T, Alpers DH, Owyang C, et al., eds. *Textbook of Gastroenterology*. Philadelphia: Lippincott; 1991:1398–1408.

62. Delpre G, Kadish V, Glanz I. Metoclopramide in the treatment of gastric bezoars. *Am J Gastroenterol*. 1984; 79:739.

63. Reinus JF, Brandt LJ. Lower intestinal bleeding in the elderly. *Clin Geriatr Med*. 1991;7:301–319.

64. Rosen AM. Gastrointestinal bleeding in the elderly. *Clin Geriatr Med*. 199;15:511–525.

65. Hudson N, Gaulkner G, Smith SJ, et al. Late mortality in elderly patients surviving acute peptic ulcer bleeding. *Gut*. 1995;37:177–181.

66. Farrell JJ, Friedman LS. Gastrointestinal bleeding in the elderly. *Gastroenterol Clin N Am*. 2001;30:377–407.

67. Lieberman D. Gastrointestinal bleeding: initial management. *Gastroenterol Clin N Am*. 1993;22:723–736.

68. Silverstein FE, Gilbert DA, Tedesco FJ, et al. The national ASGE survey on upper gastrointestinal bleeding. *Gastrointest Endosc*. 1981;27:73–79.

69. Silverstein FE, Gilbert DA, Tedesco FJ, et al. The national survey on upper gastrointestinal bleeding. II. Clinical prognostic factors. *Gastrointest Endosc*. 1981;27:80–93.

70. Elta, G. Approach to the patient with gross gastrointestinal bleeding. In: Yamada T, Alpers DH, Owyang C, et al., eds. *Textbook of Gastroenterology*. Philadelphia: Lippincott; 1991:591–616.

71. Lau JYW, Leung JW. Injection therapy for bleeding peptic ulcers. *Gastrointest Endosc Clin N Am*. 1997;7:575–592.

72. Doemeny J, Baum SB. Angiographic diagnosis in acute gastrointestinal hemorrhage. *Semin Interventional Radiol*. 1988;5:1.

73. Fiorito JJ, Brandt LJ, Kozicky O, et al. The diagnostic yield of superior mesenteric angiography: correlation with the pattern of gastrointestinal bleeding. *Am J Gastroenterol*. 1989;84:878.

74. Kovel G, Benner KG, Rosch J, et al. Aggressive angiographic diagnosis in acute lower gastrointestinal hemorrhage. *Dig Dis Sci*. 1987;32:248–253.

75. Bentley DE, Richardson JD. The role of tagged red blood cell imaging in the localization of gastrointestinal bleeding. *Arch Surg* 1991;126:821.

76. Laine L. Acute and chronic gastrointestinal bleeding. In: Feldman M, Scharschmidt BF, Sleisenger MH, eds. *Gastrointestinal and Liver Disease*, *6th Ed*. Philadelphia: Saunders; 1998:198–219.

77. Collins R, Langman M. Treatment of histamine H_2 antagonists in acute upper gastrointestinal hemorrhage: implications of randomized trials. *N Engl J Med*. 1985; 313:660–665.

78. Khuroo MS, Yattoo GN, Khan BA, et al. A comparison of omeprazole and placebo for bleeding peptic ulcer. *N Engl J Med*. 1997;336:1054–1058.

79. Drikes M, Craven D, Celli B, et al. Nosocomial pneumonia in intubated patients given sucralfate as compared with antacids or histamine type 2 blockers: the role of gastric colonization. *N Engl J Med*. 1987;317:1376–1379.

80. Permutt R, Cello J. Duodenal ulcer disease in the hospitalized patient *Dig Dis Sci*. 1982;27:1–6.

81. Reinus JF, Brandt LT. Vascular ectasias and diverticulosis: common causes of lower intestinal bleeding. *Gastroenterol Clin N Am*. 1994;23:7–20.

82. Husebye E, Engedal K. The patterns of motility are maintained in the human small intestine throughout the aging process. *Scand J Gastroenterol*. 1992;27:397–404.

83. Holt PR, Tierney AR, Kotler DP. Delayed enzyme expression: a defect of aging rat gut. *Gastroenterology*. 1985;89: 1026–1034.

84. Holt PR. Gastrointestinal disorders in the elderly: the small intestine. *Clin Gastroenterol*. 1985;14:689–723.

85. Febush JM, Holt PR. Impaired absorptive capacity for carbohydrate in the aging human. *Dig Dis Sci*. 1982;27: 1095–1100.

86. Boley SJ, Brandt LJ, Veith FJ. Ischemic diseases of the intestine. *Curr Probl Surg*. 1978;15:1–21.

87. Williams L. Mesenteric ischemia. *Surg Clin N Am*. 1988; 68:331.

88. Fisher Z, Brandt LJ. Differentiation of ischemic and ulcerative colitis in the elderly. *Gastric Med Today*. 1983; 2:31–49.

89. Foutch PG. Angiodysplasia of the gastrointestinal tract. *Am J Gastroenterol*. 1993;88:807–818.

90. Gilliam JH. Hepatobiliary disorders. In: Hazzard WR, Andres R, Bieoman EL, et al, eds. *Principles of Geriatric Medicine and Gerontology*. New York: McGraw Hill; 1990: 631–640.

91. Wynne HA, Cope LH, Mutch R, et al. The effect of age upon liver volume and apparent liver blood flow in healthy man. *Hepatology*. 1989;9:297–301.

92. Zimmerman HJ. *Hepatoxicity. The Adverse Effects of Drugs and Other Chemicals in the Liver, 2nd Ed*. Philadelphia: Lippincott Williams & Wilkins; 1999.

93. Varanasi RV. Liver diseases. *Clin Geriatr Med*. 1999;15: 559–570.

94. Lewis JH. Drug-induced liver disease. *Med Clin N Am* 2000;84:1275–1311.

95. Saunders JB. Alcoholic liver disease in the 1980's. *Br Med J*. 1983;287:1819.

96. Kaysen GA, Pond SM, Roper MH, et al. Combined hepatic and renal injury in alcoholics during therapeutic use of acetaminophen. *Arch Intern Med*. 1985;145: 2019.

97. Zauli D, Crespi C, Fusconi M, et al. Different course of acute hepatitis B in elderly adults. *J Gerontol*. 1985;40: 415–418.

98. Hoofnagle JH, Carithers RL, Shapiro C, et al. Fulminant hepatic failure. *Hepatology*. 1995;21:240–252.

99. Chien NT, Dundoo G, Horani MH, et al. Seroprevalence or viral hepatitis in an older nursing home population. *J Am Geriatr Soc*. 1999;47:1110–1113.

100. Rubin RA, Falestiny M, Malet PF. Chronic hepatitis C. Advances in diagnostic testing and therapy. *Arch Intern Med*. 1994;154:387–392.

101. Hayashi J. Hepatitis C virus infection in the elderly. Epidemiology prophylaxis and optimal treatment. *Drugs Aging*. 1997;11:296–308.

102. Alter HJ. Descartes before the horse. I clone, therefore I am: the hepatitis C virus in current perspective. *Ann Intern Med*. 1991;115:644–649.

103. Cohen JA, Kaplan MM. Left-sided heart failure presenting as hepatitis. *Gastroenterology.* 1978;74:583.

104. Gollan JL, ed. Proceedings of the NIH Consensus Development Conference on gallstones and laparoscopic cholecystectomy. *Am J Surg.* 1993;165:387–548.

105. Gracie WA, Ransohoff DF. The natural history of silent gallstones: the innocent gallstone is not a myth. *N Engl J Med.* 1982;307:798–800.

106. Ransohoff DF, Gracie WA, Wolfenson LB, Newhauser D. Prophylactic cholecystectomy or expectant management for silent gallstones: a decision analysis to assess survival. *Ann Intern Med.* 1983;99:199.

107. Lotveit T, Osnes M, Larsen S. Recurrent biliary calculi: duodenal diverticula as a predisposing factor. *Ann Surg.* 1982;196:30.

108. Cotton PB. Endoscopic retrograde cholangiopancreatography and laparoscopic cholecystectomy. *Am J Surg.* 1993;165:474–478.

109. Affronti J. Biliary disease in the elderly patient. *Clin Geriatr Med.* 1999;15:571–578.

110. Gullo L, Ventrucci M, Naldoni P, et al. Aging and exocrine pancreatic function. *J Am Geriatr Soc.* 1986;34:790–792.

111. Corfield AP, Cooper MJ, Williamson RC, et al. Prediction of severity in acute pancreatitis: prospective comparison of three prognostic indices. *Lancet.* 1985;2:403–407.

112. Fan ST, Lai ECS, Mok FPT, et al. Early treatment of acute biliary pancreatitis by endoscopic papillotomy. *N Engl J Med.* 1993;328:228–232.

113. Folsch UR, Nitsche R, Ludtke R, et al. Early ERCP and papillotomy compared with conservative treatment for acute biliary pancreatitis: the German study group on acute biliary pancreatitis. *N Engl J Med.* 1997;336:237–241.

114. Read NW, Celik AF, Katsinelos P. Constipation and incontinence in the elderly [review]. *J Clin Gastroenterol.* 1995;20:61–70.

115. Camilleri M, Lee JS, Viramontes B, et al. Constipation, irritable bowel syndrome, and diverticulosis in older people. *J Am Geriatr Soc.* 2000;48:1142–1150.

116. Brocklehurst JC, Kirkland JL, Martin J, Ashford J. Constipation in long stay elderly patients; its treatment and prevention by lactulose, poloxalkol-dihydroxyanthroquinolone and phosphate enemas. *Gerontology.* 1983;29:181–184.

117. Wilson JAP. Constipation in the elderly. *Clin Geriatr Med.* 1999;15:499–510.

118. Whitehead WE, Drinkwater D, Cheskin LJ, et al. Constipation in the elderly living at home—definition, prevalence, and relationship to lifestyle and health status. *J Am Geriatr Soc.* 1989;37:423–429.

119. Smith B. The effect of irritant purgatives on the myenteric plexus in man and mouse. *Gut.* 1968;9:139–143.

120. Andorsky RI, Goldner F. Colonic lavage solution (polyethylene glycol electrolyte lavage solution) as a treatment for chronic constipation: a double blind, placebo-controlled study. *Am J Gastroenterol.* 1990;85:261–265.

121. Sandman RN, Adolfsson R, Hallmans G, et al. Treatment of constipation with high bran bread in long term care of severely demented elderly patients. *J Am Geriatr Soc.* 1983;31:289–293.

122. Munchiando JF, Kendall K. Comparison of the effectiveness of two bowel programs for CVA patients. *Rehabil Nurs.* 1993;18:169–172.

123. Tobin GW, Brocklehurst JC. Faecal incontinence in residential homes for the elderly: prevalence and prognosis. *Age Ageing.* 1986;14:65–70.

124. Whitehead WE, Burgio KL, Engel BT. Biofeedback treatment of fecal incontinence in geriatric patients. *J Am Geriatr Soc.* 1985;33:320–324.

125. O'Keefe E, Talley NJ. Irritable bowel syndrome in the elderly. *Clin Geriatr Med.* 1991;7:2–12.

126. Whiteway J, Morson BC. Pathology of ageing: diverticular disease. *Clin Gastroenterol.* 1985;14:829–835.

127. Campbell K, Steele RJC. Non-steroidal anti-inflammatory drugs and complicated diverticular disease: a case-controlled study. *Br J Surg.* 1991;78:190–193.

128. Farrell RJ, Farrell JJ, Morrin MM. Diverticular disease in the elderly. *Gastroenterol Clin N Am.* 2001;30:475–496.

129. Eastwood MA, Smith AN, Brydon WG, et al. Comparison of bran, ispaghula and lactulose on colon function in diverticular disease. *Gut.* 1978;19:1144–1147.

130. Simmang CL, Shires GT. Diverticular disease of the colon. In: Feldman M, Scharschmidt BF, Sleisenger MH, eds. *Gastrointestinal and Liver Disease, 6th Ed.* Philadelphia: Saunders; 1998:1788–1798.

131. Lennard-Jones JE, Ritchie JK, Zohrab WJ. Proctocolitis and Crohn's disease of the colon: a comparison of the clinical course. *Gut.* 1976;17:477–482.

132. Cooke NT, et al. Crohn's disease: course, treatment, and long-term prognosis. *Q J Med.* 1980;49:363–384.

133. Lindner AE. Inflammatory bowel disease in the elderly. *Clin Geriatr Med.* 1999;15:487–497.

134. Fekety R. Guidelines for the diagnosis and management of *Clostridium difficile*-associated diarrhea and colitis. *Am J Gastroenterol.* 1997;92:739–750.

57
Pulmonary Disease

James R. Webster, Jr.

Evaluation of the Elderly Patient with Pulmonary Disease

In many ways, pulmonary problems in the elderly can be considered classic examples of geriatric medicine. (1) For example, normal lung aging is a benign process with minimal clinical implications.[1] A decline in physiologic reserve is the only truly consistent finding in healthy adults; this results in some mild decrements in vital capacity and peak flow expiratory measurements but does not affect usual activities of daily living and, compared to cardiovascular aging, has only minor effects on exercise capabilities in the elderly. (2) Lifestyle issues, especially relating to cigarette smoking, nutrition, and preventive measures such as immunization, are crucially important in preserving lung health. (3) As usual, in geriatric practice, atypical clinical presentations of pulmonary disease are quite common. (4) Unfortunately, therapeutic nihilism is present with respect to such issues as using bronchodilators in obstructive lung disease, intensive care unit (ICU) admission policies, or recommending pulmonary rehabilitation for older adults.

The effects of repeated environmental exposures, concurrent illness, deconditioning, and especially cigarette abuse can be difficult to assess while evaluating any single individual who presents with dyspnea or other pulmonary symptoms, but these factors are generally more important than any anticipated changes of "normal" aging. Further complicating the issue of normal lung aging is the fact that many studies of lung function in elderly subjects have been cross-sectional and of small size. If a primary lung disease is not present, predictable lung changes due to age in healthy adults below age 85 are relatively mild and should be considered without clinical significance; these include anatomically a decrease in airway size with some qualitative alterations in supporting elastic tissue, gradual increases in chest wall stiffness, and a loss of approximately 20% of intercostal muscle strength beginning after age 50.

As a result of these factors, lung elastic recoil and inspiratory muscle strength (including especially the diaphragm) decrease.[2] With respect to blood gas findings, the arterial–alveolar oxygen gradient widens with a decline in arterial oxygen levels of approximately 1 mmHg per year from ages 60 to 75, after which the levels remain constant in healthy individuals, probably due to cohort survival. There is also a decrease in the sensitivity of the respiratory centers to neurochemical stimuli, in particular hypercapnia. The associated age-related changes in measurable lung functions include increases in residual volume, closing volume, and functional residual capacity. There are also mild decreases in the expiratory flow rate, the total vital capacity, and the 1-s vital capacity (Table 57.1).

Changes occur in the pharyngeal component of swallowing, with slowing of transit times and reduced pharyngeal sensation, which, if neurologic disease supervenes, can set the stage for aspiration. Wide oscillations in upper airway resistance during supine sleep are often present in healthy older persons and may portend problems with sleep disordered breathing. All these changes can combine to contribute to the reduced physiologic reserves and, if an acute insult occurs (for example, an infection or pulmonary embolism), this lack of reserve may be unmasked and both patient and physician may be caught unawares by the steep spiral of disaster that may follow. Finally, the inherited level of lung volume, gender, cigarette smoking, and childhood infections are much more important in determining lung function in older adults than is chronologic age.[3]

It should be noted that pulmonary problems are becoming increasingly recognized as an elderly women's health issue.[4] For example, there is now evidence that women are more susceptible than men to the effects of cigarette smoking, leading to the recently noted disproportionate increase of lung cancer in women (the most common cause of cancer death for women) and the rising incidence of chronic obstructive pulmonary disease

TABLE 57.1. Clinical and functional aspects of age-related lung changes.

Structural	Functional
Increased chest wall stiffness	Increase in elastic work of breathing (+ ? dyspnea)
Muscle loss	Decrease in MVV[a]
Increased anteroposterior diameter	(? increase in dyspnea)
Enlargement of terminal lung units	Decrease in surface area of lung (+ lower PaO₂[b])
Reduced elasticity	Decrease in VC,[c] flow rates
Rearrangement in collagen	Increase in RV[d]
	(? Increase in dyspnea)
Decrease in ciliary function	Decrease in cough effectiveness

[a] MVV, maximum voluntary ventilation; average decrease, 25% between ages 20 and 80.
[b] Arterial pressure of oxygen; average decrease, 1 mmHg/year after age 60.
[c] Vital capacity; average decrease, 18% between ages 20 and 80.
[d] Residual volume.
Source: From Ref. 1, with permission.

(COPD) in women. Currently, the number of women older than 65 years of age who die of COPD is almost the same as men;[5] this is not surprising, given that women have smaller lungs than men and have more hyperresponsive airways and lower elastic recoil at any given lung volume than men.

Atypical presentations of lung disease are not unusual, as with other geriatric situations. Often, this is due to poor patient perception of their symptoms. For example, elderly individuals, even those without lung disease, underestimate dyspnea, presumably because of attenuated upper airway responses, peripheral sensory misinterpretations, and a reduced central nervous system responsiveness to increased mechanical loads.[6] They also have less robust cough responses to irritative stimuli; therefore, they may not appreciate the effects of acute or chronic bronchial obstruction.[7] The use of questionnaires that are specifically designed for elderly patients may provide reliable data.[8] Confusion, especially in cognitively impaired older individuals, may be the ? presenting syndrome for many pulmonary illnesses, making it difficult to obtain an accurate, coherent, or complete history. There are often associated blunted signs as well; for example, a reduced febrile response to infection.

All this makes it a challenge to see such patients but also offers outstanding opportunities to improve their functional status by applying simple medical strategies for acute or chronic pulmonary problems. These measures include exercise programs, bronchodilators, antibiotics, anticoagulants, nutritional interventions, and smoking cessation. In addition, there is the professionally satisfying opportunity to bring all the high-tech wonders of modern medicine to assist in diagnosis and treatment of functionally young older adults. In summary,

the care of these patients is what being a physician is all about.

COPD in the Elderly

Chronic obstructive pulmonary disease (COPD) is a common, underappreciated, underdiagnosed, and therefore undertreated disease that causes significant morbidity and mortality and excess health care utilization in the elderly. It is the most common lung disease causing dyspnea in the older patient.[9] When faced with a patient complaining of shortness of breath, it is of course important that the clinician exclude the myriad nonpulmonary causes of dyspnea, such as anemia, congestive heart failure, and chronic aspiration. With its subcategories of asthma, chronic bronchitis, and emphysema, COPD is the fourth leading cause of death in the elderly in the United States for both men and women.[5] Compared with the general population, patients with COPD are twice as likely to rate their health as fair or poor and to report limitations in ADL and IADL activities. They have a higher incidence of depression than most other chronic diseases, they visit physicians for medical care more frequently than their peers, and they have an increased likelihood of hospitalization and ICU admission. There is virtually a 1:1 male:female prevalence of COPD after age 68. Although men have a slightly higher mortality rate, their rate is stabilizing, while the death rate of women is rising. As discussed in the introduction of this chapter, COPD is becoming a women's health issue.[4] Prognosis of COPD patients is variable; the most important determinants of survival are the presence of comorbidities and the severity and reversibility of the airflow obstruction.

In terms of differentiating the various syndromes of COPD, the diagnosis of "late-onset asthma" in older individuals with its inflammation of conducting airways and its separation from pulmonary emphysema (a disease of inflamed and destroyed alveoli) with a reversible component can be difficult, although from a practical standpoint these two entities can generally be considered to have an anatomic and functional continuum.[10] Classic asthma is a disorder manifested by episodic, reversible airways obstruction, and hyperresponsive airways with a return to normal lung function between attacks. In the elderly asthmatic, however, a complete return to normal baseline is unlikely because most of these patients have a component of permanent lung damage.[11] Usually the symptoms of coughing and wheezing are precipitated or made worse by viral respiratory tract infections, gastroesophageal reflux disease (GERD), or chronic sinus disease, and a history of allergies is often lacking. To further complicate the picture, there may be a remote history of cigarette use. Longitudinal studies of such patients simply are not available at this time, but there is abundant evidence that older patients with asthma are underdiagnosed and undertreated.[12]

In contrast to asthma, classic pulmonary emphysema is manifested anatomically by permanent lung destruction, primarily seen in the terminal lung units, accompanied by irreversible airflow obstruction on testing. It has been described as "a gross exaggeration of what happens to the lung with advancing years."[13] Both chronic bronchitis, with its airways inflammation, mucous production, and peribronchial fibrosis, and asthma, with its bronchospasm, edema and peribronchial fibrosis, and airways remodeling, are susceptible to effective treatment of their somewhat different inflammatory components.

The largest percentage of elderly patients with COPD present with a mixed picture in which maximizing reversibility of airflow obstruction should be a major therapeutic objective. If using the word asthma increases the efforts in this regard, so be it. The American Thoracic Society criteria for reversibility are improvement in forced expiratory volume at 1 s ($FEV_{1.0}$) of at least 15% and an increase of more than 200 mL. Such patients present an outstanding opportunity to improve both functional status and quality of life.

In terms of diagnosis, because the elderly have a decreased perception of dyspnea imposed by mechanical loads or irritative stimuli and the responses to hypoxia and hypercapnea are diminished with age, health professionals need to have a high sensitivity to the possibility of this disease. The diagnosis of COPD can be reliably suggested by the history of smoking and findings on examination of lung hyperinflation with an associated decrease in breath sounds and a prolonged expiratory time, with or without a wheeze, on forced expiration. Cough and breathlessness have a low specificity in older patients with COPD, who often simply complain of fatigue and reduced mobility and ADLs.[8] Recent studies demonstrate that COPD does not impair cognition, although depression is common in these patients, especially in advanced disease when isolation is common.

Confirmation of a diagnosis of COPD can best be made by pulmonary function testing, a simple forced vital capacity (FVC) demonstrating limitation of airflow (less than 70% of predicted $FEV_{1.0}$) being adequate for initial diagnosis and following the effects of therapy.[14] If the results of testing are abnormal, the $FEV_{1.0}$ should be repeated following administration of an inhaled beta-agonist bronchodilator to look for a reversible "hidden asthmatic" component. An arterial blood gas measurement may be obtained, especially in moderate to severe COPD, because the ability of physicians to estimate hypoxia or hypercapnia is notoriously poor. In the patient with unexplained dyspnea, full pulmonary function studies are most often required to help achieve a diagnosis.

There is good evidence that morbidity (i.e., days of illness or hospitalization) can be reduced by treatment of the COPD patient, who will most likely experience a significantly improved quality of life. Therapy of COPD in the elderly should focus on relief of symptoms, reduction of breathlessness, and improvement of functional status. Smoking cessation, specific medications, and adjunctive therapies form the cornerstones of effective management.[14,15]

Smoking cessation is vital to successful management of COPD in any age group, including the elderly. Physicians can play a key role because a direct recommendation to stop can result in a 5% to 10% long-term quit rate. After such advice, a firm quit date should be set. Survey results of older smokers show that they are far less likely than younger persons to believe data about the adverse health effects of smoking and may well view it as a beneficial coping and weight control tactic. Thus clear, specific messages about the risks and the benefits of cessation must be given. "Hard-core" smokers who quit even after the age of 60 have improved pulmonary function, a slower rate of airflow decline, and a decrease in cardiovascular and all-cause mortality compared to those who continue to smoke.[16] Pulmonary benefits include reduction of cough and sputum production, decreased airway irritability, and improved ciliary and macrophage function with subsequent reduction in the frequency and severity of respiratory infections. Ex-smokers have higher levels of physical function, improved appetite and nutrition, and better quality of life than smokers, due in part to fewer cardiovascular problems or strokes.

Management of smoking cessation requires both behavioral and pharmacologic intervention, which include provision of written self-help material, enrollment in formal cessation programs conducted by the Lung and Heart Associations, the use of nicotine gum or patches or bupropion hydrochloride for patients who have significant addiction (smoke one or more packs per day or smoke their first cigarette upon awakening). The use of pharmacologic measures has not been specifically studied in the elderly, but expert opinion recommends their use. Nicotine patch or gum use is contraindicated in patients who have recent myocardial infarction, angina, or serious cardiac arrhythmias. When smokers do quit, the chance of relapse is a strong reality, most occurring within the first 2 to 4 weeks. Follow-up counseling, calls, letters, or visits during this period are important components of success, and patients who relapse should be encouraged to try again with clear discussion of the circumstances of the relapse. Smoking cessation is often an evolving process requiring physician advice and encouragement, patient motivation, and persistence.

Inhaled aerosols are a major component of long-term treatment of COPD. No matter which aerosol is used, metered dose inhaler (MDI) techniques are crucial. In

TABLE 57.2. Proper technique for metered dose inhaler (MDI) use.

Remove the cap. Attach spacer if one is being used.
Shake the canister. Breathe out completely.
Place the mouthpiece fully into your mouth.
Trigger the canister and simultaneously breathe in slowly and deeply.
Hold your breath for as long as you can, at least 10 s.
If more inhalations are prescribed, wait 1 to 5 min and repeat.
When finished, replace the cap on the MDI unit.

terms of outcome, results of using handheld MDIs are equivalent to nebulizer treatments if proper technique is used. Unfortunately, 40% of elderly patients do not use MDIs correctly due to poor hand/breathing coordination or associated illness such as arthritis or cerebral vascular disease.[17] The use of a spacer with the MDI allows for more reliable delivery of medication by slowing the velocity of the aerosol particles, enhancing distal medication deposition in the lungs, and decreasing deposition in the orpharyngeal and laryngeal areas, thus avoiding systemic side affects such as tachycardia or tremors. MDIs that are breath activated have been developed to overcome the hand/breathing coordination problem, but the patient must still develop a rapid inhalation technique. Proper use of a MDI is reviewed in Table 57.2.

Generally, physicians should begin treatment of mild to moderate COPD with inhaled ipratropium, which has been shown to slow the progression of COPD in cohorts of all ages.[18] Cholinergic receptors located in large airways are involved in controlling bronchomotor tone, especially in COPD patients who predominantly have emphysema. The bronchodilatation following inhalation is a local, site-specific effect, not a systemic one. Anticholinergics administered by MDI act locally and therefore do not cause the serious adverse reactions seen if this class of drug is administered to the elderly by oral or parenteral routes; they have a slower onset of action but a longer duration of effect than beta agonists. Tiatroprium is an emerging site-specific agent that only affects the anti-muscarinic M_1 and M_3 receptors. It is still under investigation.

Inhaled selective beta-2 agonists may be short acting for "rescue" (e.g., albuterol) or long acting (e.g., salmeterol) and are particularly useful for symptomatic relief of episodic dyspnea in patients with COPD. These drugs initiate relaxation of bronchial smooth muscle and decrease mucosal edema; they also facilitate mucociliary clearance and decrease goblet cell hypertrophy. They are especially effective in patients with a large component of "asthma"; however, unlike ipratropium, there is no evidence that they slow the progression of disease. There are now combinations of long-acting beta-agonists and ipratrotium that are useful in improving compliance and are especially useful in patients with nocturnal symptoms. Inhaled corticosteroids are sometimes used in patients

with a large reversible "asthmatic" component because they suppress inflammation and reduce airways hyperresponsiveness. They work by interfering with arachnodonic acid metabolism, reducing vascular leaks, and enhancing responsiveness of beta-adrenergic receptors. Patients should follow the package insert recommendations to prevent oral candidiasis. Systemic side effects are negligible although osteoporosis is a long-term concern, particularly at high dose ranges. They have long-term benefits in younger patients with chronic asthma, and their use in the elderly is based on the data generated from these younger populations, with the hypothesis that inflammation of small airways is instrumental in the progression of COPD. Inhaled steroids are most commonly used as an adjunct for patients in whom the disease is difficult to control.

Oral corticosteroids are possibly useful for some moderate to severe COPD exacerbations.[19] An empiric trial of 40 to 60 milligrams (mg) prednisone per day can help return the patient to baseline lung function, shortening the duration of morbidity on average by a few days. Doses are conventionally tapered over 7 to 14 days. The use of oral corticosteroids in the stable phase of COPD is at best very controversial and frequently results in osteoporosis, loss of muscle strength, hyperglycemia, and hypogonadism.

Methyxanthines are considered an archaic third-line agent of treatment. Theophylline preparations can provide consistent but modest bronchodilation and decrease the severity of breathlessness by improving respiratory muscle strength in an occasional patient, but they have a narrow therapeutic window with many side effects (i.e., anorexia, nausea, vomiting, CNS stimulation, and cardiac arrhythmias). The elderly are at greater risk for major toxicity (hypotension, serious arrhythmias, seizures, and death from overmedication) than younger patients.[20] This severely limits their usefulness, and obtaining blood levels is mandatory in patients who are using this group of drugs on a short- or long-term basis. Serum levels of 5 to $10 \mu g/ml$ are appropriate. It should also be noted that adverse drug reactions occur with macrolides and fluoroquinolones. Leukotriene inhibitors have not been systematically studied in the elderly. If they are used, ipratroprium should be discontinued because adverse drug interactions may occur. Patient and physician should also be aware that the international normalized ratio (INR) may be increased by the interaction of leukotriene inhibitors with warfarin.

Oral antibiotics are beneficial in selected COPD patients who have recurrent episodes of bacterial infection.[21] Most commonly these follow a viral upper respiratory illness, and antibiotics can reduce the inflammatory response within the airways. Patients with impaired mucociliary clearance are at risk for a recurrent cycle of infection, tracheobronchial mucosal destruction, and worsening mucociliary clearance. The use of a 2-week course of antibiotics in patients with severe chronic bronchitis and bronchiectasis can break the cycle and provide relief. The most common pathogens associated with such exacerbations are *Haemophilus influenzae*, *Moraxella catarrhalis*, and *Streptococcus pneumoniae*. Ampicillin is frequently used but is ineffective against betalactamase-producing organisms, so that the treating physician must be aware of local sensitivity and resistance patterns. Trimethoprim-sulfamethoxazole, amoxicillin-clavulanate, and third-generation cephalosporins or macrolides may provide broad coverage and can be very effective in treatment of exacerbations. Cost issues are, of course, also a consideration in the choice of antibiotic therapy. The use of long-term antibiotics to prevent exacerbations in patients with COPD is of unproven value, although some interesting new immuno-stimulating vaccines may prove helpful in reducing such events.

Long-term home oxygen therapy (LOT) for 15 to 24 h per day is useful in hypoxemic patients. Raising the arterial oxygen level has been shown to reduce mortality by decreasing pulmonary hypertension in patients with cor pulmonale, as it decreases pulmonary vascular resistance and right ventricular diastolic pressure.[22] In the hypoxemic patient, oxygen therapy also improves neuropsychiatric function, decreases secondary polycythemia, and relieves breathlessness, all of which can improve mobility, functional status, and independence in selected elderly COPD patients. Those patients who are stable on optimal bronchodilator treatment with an arterial oxygen level of less than 55 mmHg (or 55–59 mmHg with concomitant polycythemia, pulmonary hypertension, or right heart failure) are appropriate for treatment and eligible for Medicare reimbursement (Table 57.3). Patients started on oxygen therapy often incorrectly assume that this represents the end of a useful and independent existence. They need to be clearly counseled about benefits of oxygen supplementation and told that therapy will most likely improve overall status and the quality as well as the length of their life.

Oxygen supply systems are of three types: stationary, portable, and ambulatory. Stationary systems refer to any large reservoir of oxygen or oxygen-producing device that cannot easily be moved, including compressed gas cylinders (H or K size), liquid oxygen reservoirs, and oxygen concentrators. Portable oxygen equipment can be moved or transported by the patient. This equipment usually weighs more than 10 lb, involving smaller (E size) compressed oxygen cylinders with a regulator, which is carried on wheels, a cart, or stroller. Ambulatory oxygen can be carried by most adults on their person during activities of daily living; these are small liquid oxygen canisters or lightweight high-pressure cylinders, with a regulator. The liquid oxygen reservoir for home use with an ambulatory liquid system offers an ideal arrangement for the ambulatory patient requiring continuous oxygen rather than the minimum of 15 to 16 h/day. The reservoir will provide a 1-month supply of oxygen and serves as a source to refill the portable ambulatory system, which weighs 5 to 7 lb and provides about 4 h of oxygen. The use of a control valve that delivers oxygen only when the patient inhales can conserve oxygen in patients using ambulatory systems.

The oxygen concentrators that are used for home-bound patients take advantage of a differential separation principle based on the molecular weights of nitrogen and oxygen to concentrate oxygen from room air. Patients using these systems can be active and ambulatory in the home with use of extended tubing. A supply of smaller cylinders is necessary for out-of-home use. These can be pulled on a cart by the patient or carried in a wheelchair but are cumbersome and are a potential cause of falls. Careful evaluation of the patient and knowledge of the patient's activity level and concerns about oxygen therapy will help determine the appropriate system.

As with most older patients (Chapter 21), the perioperative period becomes a time of great hazard for patients with COPD.[23] The frequency of postoperative complications increases with age, particularly if these patients undergo thoracic or upper abdominal procedures. Perioperative evaluation is crucial, with educational interventions stressing the use of effective cough maneuvers, incentive spirometry, and early ambulation. Specific risk factors for an adverse outcome include a $PaCO_2$ level greater than 45 mmHg, poor nutritional status with recent weight loss, current cigarette smoking, and emergency surgery. Careful preoperative evaluation with pulmonary function and arterial blood gas measurements is crucial, and judicious use of analgesics postoperatively to avoid respiratory depression, delirium, and oversedation are important strategies. Recent studies do indicate that elderly postoperative patients in the ICU who need intubation and mechanical ventilation (MV) under any circumstances do as well as younger patients in terms of outcome, although if they have been nutritionally depleted, weaning from MV can be a problem.[24]

TABLE 57.3. Medicare criteria for long-term oxygen therapy indications.

$P_aO_2 \leq 55$ mmHg (on room air)
Oxygen saturation $\leq 88\%$ (on room air)
$P_aO_2 \leq 59$ mm with at least one of these four findings:
   Secondary polycythemia (hematocrit > 55%)
   Clinical cor pulmonale
   Established right ventricular hypertrophy
   Pulmonary hypertension
Optimal medical management established

P_aO_2, partial pressure of arterial oxygen.

Therefore, age alone should never be used to deny older patients either surgery or ICU admission, even though many prognostic rating formulas (e.g., Acute Physiology and Chronic Health Evaluation, APACHE III) list age as an adverse prognostic marker.

Pulmonary rehabilitation can be an important component of successful treatment in patients with moderate to severe COPD.[25] The primary goal is to attain the highest possible functional level using multiple modalities. The rehabilitation model focuses on not only reversing the chronic progressive disease process but on reversing the patient's disability from the disease. Comprehensive patient and family education, breathing retraining, bronchial hygiene, exercise reconditioning, work simplification and energy conservation training, and psychosocial support are all part of pulmonary rehabilitation, which in randomized control trials has been shown to improve functional status and decrease hospitalization rates.[26]

The role of adequate nutrition is also to be stressed, because malnutrition is a common problem among COPD patients. Decreased muscle mass (including muscles of respiration) and impairment of immune function are seen with protein-calorie malnutrition. A body weight of less than 90% of ideal is associated with an increased mortality rate regardless of the severity of COPD. The weight loss may be due to such things as early satiety associated with dyspnea of deglutition or depression, and, according to some recent evidence, tumor necrosis factor (TNF) is increased in these patients.[27] In underweight COPD patients, the increased ventilation requirements during activity require a disproportionately greater increase in energy requirements for respiratory muscle activities compared to well-nourished COPD patients or controls.[28] Malnourished patients also have increased rates of infection, which appear to be partially due to decreased functioning of T cells, complement, and humoral immunity. Treating the malnourished COPD patient requires a comprehensive assessment with an exclusion of treatable causes of weight loss other than pulmonary disease. An assessment (using calorie counts) of the patient's current intake habits and limiting factors (whether physical, environmental, or economic) is important and requires evaluation by dietitians and social workers. Fatigue or dyspnea associated with eating may be reduced by using bronchodilators before meals, assistance with meal preparation, or rests before meal times. Patients can also be encouraged to eat multiple smaller meals and to add liquid protein supplements to their diets. Studies indicated that in severely compromised patients a high percentage of calories from lipids instead of carbohydrates reduces excessive carbon dioxide production and the subsequent increase in minute ventilation at rest.

Immunization against influenza and *S. pneumoniae* plays a significant role in prevention of pneumonia in the elderly COPD patient. Influenza vaccine has been shown to decrease hospitalization, morbidity and mortality, and medical costs and should be given every autumn. In patients who are immunosuppressed or have severely debilitating cardiovascular, pulmonary, renal, or hepatic disease, or diabetes mellitus, the antibody titers from pneumococcal vaccine may not be sustained; therefore, clinicians should consider revaccination after 6 years, although convincing data regarding the effectiveness of such a program in the elderly are currently not available. The pneumococcal vaccine is cost-effective in both community-living and institutionalized older patients.

Because adequate lung or heart/lung donor specimens are very difficult to obtain, most lung transplant programs exclude those applicants over age 60, citing frequent comorbidities (diagnosed or subclinical) as the reason. Some lung transplant programs are still collecting experience as to efficacy for various disease states, but it is not currently an option for the elderly.

In summary, COPD is a common and serious condition often overlooked in the elderly. Clinical suspicion, with confirmative pulmonary function testing, will establish the diagnosis. Successful treatment involves simple, well-established measures that improve functional status and result in significant improvement in the quality of life for these patients.

Pulmonary Embolism in the Elderly

The entities of deep venous thrombosis (DVT) and pulmonary embolism (PE) present a continuum of venous thromboembolic disease (VTE), which is of crucial importance for elderly patients, and offer constant diagnostic and therapeutic challenges to physicians caring for patients of any age. For multiple reasons, the incidence of both DVT and PE increase with age.[29] First, there is often a decrease in the leg muscle mass, setting the stage for stasis. There are increased thrombotic tendencies in the elderly,[30] beginning around age 60, which may involve up to 20% of those over age 85; these include impaired vascular wall fibrinolysis and hypercoagulable states, especially with respect to products of factor X_a activity, Leiden factor V,[31] and likely increased activity of other clotting factors,[32] notably prothrombin. In addition, there may be a decrease in antithrombin III and other antithrombotic components, such as proteins C and S. There is also a dramatic increase in the frequency of triggering risk factors, such as surgery, with its immobility and temporary hypercoagulable state, congestive heart failure, malignancies, lower extremity fractures, and hip and knee joint replacements. This is not only a common problem but a serious one: the in-hospital mortality of elderly patients over the age of 65 with documented pulmonary embolism was 21% in the Prospective Investigation of Pulmonary

Embolism Diagnosis (PIOPED) Study, and the 1-year mortality was 39%.[33] Recent data suggest these numbers may be even higher.[34] Such grim statistics demand optimal vigilance, treatment, and, ideally, prevention.

The diagnosis of VTE in the elderly is difficult, although the presentation is usually quite similar to that seen in younger patient groups. The most common presenting symptom of PE is some complaint of chest discomfort or pain, seen in approximately 35% of patients in most series, usually without hemoptysis. Dyspnea and tachypnea occur frequently. Although circulatory collapse occurs in a relatively small proportion of the elderly, these latter patients are much more likely to have sustained massive pulmonary emboli and often have evidence of neurologic deficits and findings of pulmonary hypertension. Although virtually all younger patients present with one of these syndromes, about 10% of the elderly do not, and in the setting of respiratory distress this minority may show only confusion or atypical new radiographic findings. The major diagnostic strategy[35] required is one of constant suspicion and concern and a consideration that, in any older hospitalized patient who is "failing to thrive," to ask whether this could be due to pulmonary embolism, because both the symptoms and standard laboratory findings are nonspecific and the diagnosis is too often made postmortem. The classic triad of hemoptysis, pleuritic chest pain, and clinically apparent thrombophlebitis is infrequently seen, in less than 10% of elderly patients with VTE.

The first step in making the diagnosis is a careful physical examination to evaluate alternative diagnoses, for example, congestive heart failure, coronary artery disease, malignancy, and infections that are all frequent in the elderly and may on occasion be confused with pulmonary embolism. Studies demonstrate that when clinicians have a high (>90%) certainty of pulmonary embolism, they are most often correct; similarly, when they believe that there is a small (<20%) likelihood, they are also usually correct.[33,35] The problem is the large group of "in-between" patients for whom neither certainty exists.

The most common and serious major error is one of omission, when the diagnosis simply is not considered clinically and is confirmed only at autopsy. The diagnosis should be approached with urgency, once it is considered and diagnostic algorithms are well established.[35] Unfortunately, routine chest roentgenograms are of only limited value at best, to exclude other disorders such as pneumonia or pneumothorax. Most frequently they are unremarkable or demonstrate only scattered areas of atelectasis. Pleural changes and possibly some local asymmetric changes in vascularity may be detected if the film is keenly studied; however, the most common finding is that of an essentially normal chest roentgenogram in a very sick patient. Electrocardiograms are likewise useful in excluding acute myocardial infarction but are not generally helpful in making the diagnosis of PE, because tachycardia and nonspecific ST segment abnormalities are by far the most likely alterations. Recent studies utilizing echocardiography in patients with PE have shown an unexpectedly high incidence of pulmonary hypertension and right ventricular strain.[36] The echocardiogram is, however, not a proven sensitive or specific test for PE. Arterial blood gases generally show mild hyperventilation and hypoxemia (PaO_2 <60mmHg on room air), but again, this is a nonspecific finding.

Ventilation-perfusion lung scans are helpful, particularly when there are segmental mismatches with areas that are well ventilated and not perfused. Lung scans are interpreted as high probability, intermediate probability, low probability, or normal. The PIOPED[33] study demonstrated that combining a high clinical probability and a high-probability lung scan virtually confirmed the diagnosis (>96% certainty). The combination of a low clinical suspicion and low-probability lung scan was associated with low frequency of significant pulmonary embolism (<6%). In patients in whom the lung scan pattern was high probability and clinical suspicion was intermediate, the frequency of pulmonary embolism fell but was still relatively high (86%). The most frequent problem is a high-risk patient with an "intermediate probability" lung scan. Because of the unfortunate lack of specificity of such scans, their utility remains problematic, and with the hazard of "clinical judgment" in such a precarious setting, physicians must often proceed with further studies, either helical computerized tomography (HCT) or pulmonary angiography.

The understanding of the place of HCT in the diagnosis of PE is still an evolving concept. Due to improvements in the technology, and its general availability and safety, the procedure has great appeal. In addition, there is reasonable interobserver reliability in most studies. Unfortunately, it still suffers in published studies from a lack of sensitivity (53%–100%) with specificities of 81% to 100%, and thus is not an ideal test to exclude the diagnosis of PE, especially in the "high clinical suspicion" patient.[37] HCT may be helpful in establishing a diagnosis of pulmonary embolism in selected patients with a nondiagnostic lung scan. It appears to be more accurate in evaluating the central pulmonary arteries (sensitivity, 83%–100%; specificity, 92%–100%) than in the subsegmental vessels (sensitivity, 29%).[38] Future prospective studies of HCT are needed to evaluate its role in the diagnostic algorithm for VTE. These investigations should settle issues of overall specificity, sensitivity, and cost-effectiveness.[39]

Pulmonary angiography is still the gold standard for diagnosis of PE.[40] A positive angiogram requires either a cutoff vessel or clear evidence of an intravascular filling defect, which is typical of a clot. Multiple recent studies indicate that, contrary to some opinions, pulmonary angiography is quite safe in the elderly patient. There is a somewhat increased incidence of postangiogram renal failure in the elderly (1%–2%), but this can be managed quite satisfactorily when identified and is often preventable using hydration and diuretics. One last caveat in the elderly; a small embolus that would not present a serious burden for a younger patient may result in dramatic pulmonary hypertension and significantly impaired cardiovascular status in an elderly patient with underlying heart or lung disease and therefore marginal physiologic reserves. Such patients have been shown to be clinically improved following treatment for PE.

The identification and diagnosis of DVT, the source of PE, may also be difficult. It is well demonstrated that for this entity, clinical signs are notoriously unreliable. Virchow's triad (stasis, hypercoagulability, and vessel wall injury) is still the physiologic basis of DVT, which forms the continuum with PE. Elderly patients who have "idiopathic" thrombophlebitis most likely have an acquired hypercoagulable state, most commonly due to Leiden factor V or a prothrombin mutation. In the absence of an obvious precipitating cause or clotting problem, a clinically focused search for a malignancy is appropriate based on a history and physical exam with routine screening studies. One review[41] reported a standardized incidence ratio of 1.5 for malignancies in such patients. Recent data suggest that cancers diagnosed concurrently with or within a year of an episode of VTE are associated with an advanced stage and have a poor prognosis.[42] Tumors of pancreas, lung, ovary, and brain were the most common sites.

Noninvasive studies of veins in the lower extremities (the site of more than 95% of emboli) are now widely available and have been demonstrated to have good specificity and sensitivity. B-mode ultrasonography with flow Doppler is the most commonly used diagnostic method because it avoids some of the confounding false positives of the impedance plethysmography methods [e.g., congestive heart failure (CHF), extrinsic obstruction]. Contrast venography is the gold standard for the diagnosis, but it is usually reserved for extremely serious and equivocal situations. Approximately 70% of patients with demonstrated PE have positive noninvasive lower extremity studies. Presumptive explanations for the "30%" are either that the clot has migrated, leaving no demonstrable residue, or possibly that clots were coming from elsewhere in the venous system, particularly the pelvic veins or the right ventricle. This finding means that although a positive study is a call to therapy, a single negative study does not completely exclude the diagnosis; serial investigations are appropriate[43] if suspicion is high and a decision is made not to begin anticoagulant therapy.

The use of D-dimers as a secondary strategy to exclude the diagnosis of VTE has been recommended because the test has a high sensitivity, although a low specificity. False positives may occur in patients with recent trauma or surgery, malignancy, pregnancy, severe infections, and liver disease. It is somewhat dependent on the specific methods used, and most series show that a normal plasma level (e.g., <500 μg/ml by immunosorbent assay) is useful in conjunction with other strategies to exclude the diagnosis of VTE, although false negatives up to 3%–5% are reported.[44]

The treatment of VTE has been revolutionized by the emergence of low molecular weight heparins (LMWH), which have been demonstrated to be effective for both DVT and PE.[45] They are given on a weight-adjusted schedule, often only once a day, and the treating physician should be familiar with the specifics of the preparation being used. They are easier to use than older treatment protocols because they do not require frequent partial thromboplastin time testing to adjust dose schedules, as is required for the intravenous unfractionated heparins.

The thrombocytopenias that were occasionally (3%–6%) a problem with the unfractionated preparations are seen in less than 1% of patients treated with LMWH. Studies indicate that they are safe in terms of bleeding complications and can even be given on an outpatient basis to compliant patients with uncomplicated DVT. It is usually recommended that warfarin be started concurrently and, after a 4- to 7-day crossover, that the warfarin be continued, maintaining an international normalized ratio (INR) of approximately 2:3. Bleeding complications of warfarin therapy are more frequent in the elderly, particularly in older women, and increase with duration of therapy; however, with careful clinical and laboratory monitoring in formalized programs, bleeding should not become a major problem in most cases.

The question of how long to continue warfarin therapy is always a difficult clinical judgment. In general, it is recommended that therapy be sustained for 3 to 4 months in patients for whom the initial risk factor can be controlled or eliminated. Patients may need long-term therapy if they are considered to remain at high risk, and recent studies show that recurrences can be cut to 6% by maintaining anticoagulation for 1 year. Current recommendations for "idiopathic" VTE are for up to 2 years of therapy for the first episode and that a second episode requires lifelong anticoagulation, possibly with INRs of 3 to 3.5.[46] Thrombolytic therapy, particularly tissue plasminogen activator (TPA), is occasionally used in the elderly patient with massive PE and circulatory collapse but is generally not required.[47]

Although the experience is relatively small, there seems to be an increased incidence of bleeding in the elderly, especially intracranial hemorrhages, with even a single administration. Supportive therapy, such as oxygen, fluids, and vasopressors for hypotension and

TABLE 57.4. Prevention of venous thromboembolism (VTE)

Risk	Recommended R$_x$
High	
Bed confined with:	Low molecular weight heparin (LMWH)
Congestive heart failure	? Intermittent pneumatic compression
Active malignancy	
Postoperative: lower extremity, orthopedic, extensive abdominal, or pelvic surgery	
Previous diagnosis of DVT or PE	
Moderate	LMWH or warfarin
Medical illness with:	
Immobilization, e.g., stroke, COPD	
Less extensive surgery, of shorter duration	

For patients who cannot be anticoagulated (e.g., postoperative neurologic surgery), pneumatic compression boots or graduated pressure stockings provide some proven effectiveness.
Source: From Ref. 49, with permission.

hypovolemia, and pain control, are of course standard treatments that must be used in the critically ill patient. Vena caval interruption, for example, use of the Greenfield filter, may be needed in patients with PE who cannot immediately be anticoagulated. Chronic venous complications are common with use of these devices, and such patients, if possible, should have lifelong anticoagulation as studies show that they are at risk of proximal clot formation above the filter.[48] Pulmonary embolectomy is not recommended in the elderly because it has a very low success rate and medical therapy is generally quite effective.

Preventive guidelines are fairly straightforward at this time. Patients who are at risk due to bed rest, postoperative status, congestive heart failure, or malignancies are best treated according to the measures listed in Table 57.4. Intermittent pneumatic compression boots have been demonstrated to be useful for prophylaxis in patients who are at high risk of critical local wound hemorrhage (for example, following neurosurgical procedures) but who cannot be immediately anticoagulated. Graded compression antiembolic stockings also have some limited effectiveness in prevention. Low-dose warfarin with an INR adjusted to 1.5 to 2 units, or subcutaneous LWMH, appear to be the preventive treatments of choice. Studies demonstrate that, for unknown reasons, such preventive strategies are not used on a regular basis by physicians, probably because of the mistaken opinions that pulmonary embolism is not a common or serious problem, that preventive strategies do not work, or that such anticoagulation protocols are actually dangerous. None of these beliefs is true. Particularly in the elderly, for whom an ounce of prevention is worth more than a pound of cure, these procedures should regularly be found in the armamentarium of geriatricians.[49]

In conclusion, the continuum of DVT and PE in the elderly is quite similar to that of the younger patient. Constant consideration of the diagnosis and application of standard diagnostic and therapeutic strategies will benefit patients and also enhance the mental equanimity and professional satisfaction of physicians caring for the elderly.

Interstitial Lung Disease

The term interstitial lung disease covers a heterogeneous group of disorders that are lumped together as a result of common radiographic and clinical findings which are nonspecific and not related to etiology (Table 57.5).[50] The conventional wisdom on the pathogenesis of interstitial lung disease postulates an etiologic insult resulting in alveolitis, followed by an abnormal, hyperexuberant repair process that causes excess connective tissue generation, fibrosis, and ultimately a "honeycomb" appearance of a scarred, destroyed lung, both on biopsy and radiographically. The presentation is usually one of cough, dyspnea, and frequent associated systemic symptoms such as fatigue and arthralgias. The astute geriatrician will focus on the clinical history, seeking drug exposures, disorders of swallowing leading to chronic

TABLE 57.5. Disorders associated with interstitial lung disease in the elderly.

Common
  Recurrent gastric aspiration
  Drugs
  Infection
    Acute: viral, bacterial
    Chronic: granulomatosis, especially TB
  Atypical congestive heart failure
  Environmental/occupational exposures
  Lymphangitic spread of malignancies
  Idiopathic
Less common
  Sarcoidosis
  Eosinophilic and lymphocytic infiltrative disorders
  Collagen vascular disease

Source: From Ref. 50, with permission.

aspiration with lower lobe infiltrates, often without classic symptoms of gastroesophageal reflux,[51] classic rheumatologic symptoms (which would suggest rheumatoid arthritis or vasculitis), and environmental exposures during previous employment or at home (e.g., to humidifiers, hobbies, or pets) as possible etiologic clues. There are few data on the incidence or outcomes of these diseases in elderly patients.

The laboratory findings are often nonspecific, but useful findings may occasionally be elicited. For example, abnormal liver function tests suggest the possibility of metastatic malignancy, and hematuria or impaired renal function suggests Wegner's granulomatosis or Goodpasture's syndrome. The chest radiograph usually shows an increase in interstitial markings and on serial films an associated progressive decrease in lung volume. Diagnostic inferences may be made by correlating pleural changes or adenopathy. The various specific syndromes relating to radiographic findings are beyond the scope of this text; contemporary review articles are available.[50] High-resolution computerized tomography (CT) of the lung is of considerable value in determining the extent and severity of these interstitial disorders, although, like roentgenograms, it does not give an etiologic diagnosis—that is the job of the clinician. Gallium scans are nonspecific, have serious problems of interobserver variability, and are totally useless in evaluating these entities. Pulmonary function studies, on the other hand, may be clinically helpful in diagnosis and for following the results of therapy, demonstrating classic restrictive changes, that is, a decrease in lung volumes, diffusing capacity, compliance, and, frequently, a low PaO_2.

If diagnosis cannot be achieved on the basis of a careful history, physical examination, and consideration of the patient's overall medical diagnoses, and if it appears that lung biopsy will likely be useful in terms of management, this invasive intervention can be performed. Transbronchial biopsy with a fiberoptic bronchoscope (FOB) may be helpful and is safe in older patients, although the tissue sample size is usually quite limited and the ability to achieve a firm diagnosis is disappointingly small in most series. Open lung biopsy with sampling of several sites gives a higher probability of a definitive diagnosis, although it carries a small (approximately 1%) risk of mortality and a 5% to 10% incidence of complications. In more than 50% of patients, the diagnosis is idiopathic pulmonary fibrosis (IPF), leaving both the patient and physician unsatisfied. Prognosis is related to the specific etiology. IPF, which occurs on average at age 61, has an especially poor prognosis, with a 50% mortality in 2 years.

Therapy is often difficult, disappointing, and limited to supportive measures. Corticosteroids or cytotoxic agent treatments have significant side effects, and if they are used, short therapeutic trials of 3 to 4 months with objective PFT and CT measurements for follow-up and prog-

nosis should be the strategy utilized. Colchicine has been recommended and is safer than steroids or immunosuppression, but long-term results show no difference from untreated patients. Recent data suggest that interferon gamma-1b may provide a better outcome than steroids in patients with IPF.[52] Advanced patient age, even with a diagnosis of IPF, should not deter physicians from offering nondrug treatments that may improve physical and social functional status and even survival (e.g., pulmonary rehabilitation). Portable oxygen can improve exercise capacity and quality of life in these patients.

Sleep Disordered Breathing

Sleep complaints increase in the elderly, partly because of changes in central nervous system control of breathing during sleep. The sensitivity of brainstem receptors to carbon dioxide and oxygen levels decreases with aging to as much as one-half of the awake response. The resultant reduction in ventilation can combine with an increase in upper airway resistance and lead to rises in the blood levels of carbon dioxide ($PaCO_2$) and decreases in oxygen (PaO_2) during sleep. These changes all help to explain the increase in sleep disordered breathing that occurs with aging, with increasingly frequent apneic or hypopneic events being more common in older men than women.[53] (See Chapter 70 for details.)

Perioperative Care of the Elderly

Pulmonary complications in the postoperative period occur with increased frequency in older as compared to younger patients, especially in those undergoing thoracic or upper abdominal procedures.[23,54] Proper preoperative evaluation, patient education, and postoperative management will decrease the risk of pulmonary complications such as atelectasis, impaired gas exchange, and infection. The elderly are at higher risk of complications, not because of age, but as a result of decreased pulmonary and cardiovascular reserves associated with aging and an increased number of accompanying comorbidities. Congestive atelectasis is the predominant pulmonary complication seen in the immediate postoperative period. Following thoracic or upper abdominal procedures, it may take to 2 to 3 weeks for pulmonary function capability to return to a baseline. These procedures cause impaired diaphragmatic and intercostal muscle function, and this impairment results in a decreased functional residual capacity (FRC) with an associated increase in residual volume (RV) and a closing capacity (CC), which rises into the tidal volume (TV). This change means that some alveoli remain unventilated throughout the entire respiratory cycle, primarily because of an increase in lung recoil and decrease in chest wall compliance. In recumbency, the decrease in FRG is approximately 500 mL, or 20% of the awake value, so that bed rest exacerbates this problem.

Postoperative patients generally show a significant restrictive pattern of breathing, with a decrease in forced vital capacity (FVC), TV, FRC, and peak expiratory flow rate. They demonstrate a shallow breathing pattern without the deep breaths that are needed to replete surfactant and prevent atelectasis. The work of breathing is also increased, and cough effectiveness is reduced.[23] Patients with underlying pulmonary disorders and minimal pulmonary reserve due to cigarettes are at particularly high risk of postoperative atelectasis. Thorough preoperative evaluation and patient education will identify these patients and guide postoperative management to reduce complications. A careful history and physical examination with special focus on cardiopulmonary symptoms and findings, smoking history, and functional status is at the center of this endeavor. The use of additional testing is often necessary to clarify the evaluation of pulmonary function and to guide pre- and postoperative treatment.

The routine use of preoperative pulmonary function testing is controversial because many of the frequently cited studies in this area were conducted 20 to 30 years ago when different surgical, anesthetic, and perioperative management practices prevailed. However, patients who are to have abdominal or thoracic surgery, and who have a history of smoking or signs or symptoms of pulmonary disease identified preoperatively, will benefit from spirometry measurements before and after bronchodilators.[55] The pulmonary function testing assists in making a specific pulmonary diagnosis, assessing the degree of impairment and risk, and identifying appropriate maximal pre- and postoperative therapy. An increase in perioperative complications and mortality is seen in patients with an elevated $PaCO_2$ (>45), which makes the arterial blood gas measurement an important component of a complete preoperative evaluation of the high-risk patient.[54] High-risk warning signs include emergency surgery, poor nutritional status, and continued cigarette use.[23,54] The use of pancuronium during surgery has been associated with a 3.2 increase in relative risk of postoperative pulmonary complications.[23]

Preoperative patient education is essential to reduce the risk of postoperative pulmonary complications. The use of incentive spirometry has been shown to decrease atelectasis and other postoperative pulmonary complications and is equivalent to chest physiotherapy.[56] The use of intermittent positive pressure breathing (IPPB) is much more expensive, has more complications, and offers no advantage over incentive spirometry. The objective of incentive spirometry is to increase the low postoperative FRC. The teaching and implementation of incentive spirometry preoperatively has been shown to improve its effective use after surgery. Patients should use the device for at least 5 min every waking hour. The preoperative teaching of the effective cough at the end of a deep inspiration is also an important strategy. The high alveolar and airway pressures obtained during the periods of glottic closure are beneficial in clearing secretions and expanding atelectatic portions of the lung. The patient should hold a pillow or other "splint" over the incisional area, take a breath to total lung capacity, hold for 4 to 6 s, then cough repeatedly throughout exhalation, and finish by expectorating the mobilized secretions.

Counseling patients preoperatively to cease smoking is essential. The benefit of stopping smoking can be dramatic in improving overall prognosis. Cigarette smoking is associated with a fourfold increase in postoperative pulmonary complications. Smoking cessation 4 to 8 weeks before surgery is accompanied by a demonstrated decrease in postoperative pulmonary complications, predominantly due to improved tracheobronchial clearance, with a decrease in cough and sputum and an increase in vital capacity and PaO_2.[23] Smoking cessation even the day before surgery theoretically can be beneficial due to a decrease in carboxyhemoglobin concentration (CO-HgB). The half-life of CO-HgB is 6 h, and a decreased level of CO-HgB will improve oxygen delivery to tissues. The patient should be counseled to continue smoking abstinence in the postoperative period and beyond.

Pain control measures in the postoperative period can both cause or prevent postoperative complications. Elderly patients are at very high risk for oversedation and postoperative delirium from narcotic pain medications. The education in and use of patient-controlled analgesia (PCA) is often the best option for pain relief.[57] When compared with intermittent intramuscular opiate injections in a population of frail elderly in the postoperative period, PCA is easier to use, provides better analgesia, is associated with less frequent pulmonary complications or postoperative confusion, and shows less variability in serum morphine levels.[57] Avoiding oversedation is critical in preventing a complicated prolonged postoperative course. In the patient with a thoracic or abdominal procedure, proper pain control improves cough effectiveness. The use of epidural anesthesia or intercostal nerve block also can be used to provide effective pain control in the postoperative period.[23]

In conclusion, there is a rationale for the routine use of pulmonary function tests and arterial blood gas measurements in the perioperative assessment of elderly patients with a history of smoking or previous pulmonary disease. It is especially crucial in those patients undergoing thoracic or upper abdominal operations. Comprehensive education regarding incentive spirometry, effective coughing, and smoking cessation is critical to prevent postoperative pulmonary complications. The judicious use of analgesia is likewise of benefit. Recent studies have demonstrated that even the oldest-old (those over 85 years of age) can safely undergo operations.[58] Thus, age alone should never be a criteria for denying a patient the benefits of surgery.

Critical Care Issues

Elderly persons are more frequently admitted to ICUs than are those in younger cohorts and currently represent 25% to 45% of days of ICU occupancy.[59] This rate no doubt reflects the generally high rate of hospitalization of elderly and their multiple interacting acute and chronic diseases. Age, per se, is not a reason for exclusion from ICUs, as functional status and comorbidities have been shown to be much more important initial prognostic factors than chronologic age, both for survival and for return to a meaningful life following an ICU stay.[24] However, critically ill elderly patients are more likely to develop respiratory failure requiring mechanical ventilation (MV) than are younger individuals; this is due to their decrease in pulmonary reserve, with declines in $FEV_{1.0}$, and PaO_2, blunted respiratory responses to stimuli such as hypercapnia and hypoxemia, decreased muscle strength and endurance with reduced ability to generate inspiratory and expiratory pressures, a reduced cardiac reserve, and, finally, an increased likelihood of sepsis. Specific management of the elderly while on MV and strategies for "weaning" from support are not covered here, although they are of crucial importance in day-to-day management and have been the focus of several recent reviews.[60] Specific adverse prognostic factors for recovery and survival in the elderly, some of which are apparent at time of admission for an acute illness, are the following:

- A diagnosis of pneumonia
- A diagnosis of COPD
- Poor prior functional status
- Severity of illness (APACHE III score >30)
- Difficulty maintaining oxygenation (e.g., $PaO_2 < 55$ mmHg, $FIO_2 > 60\%$)
- Advanced age (greater than 90 years old) plus 24 or more h of ventilation
- Prolonged mechanical ventilation requirements (more than 3 days)

The issue of ICU costs (totaling more than $60 billion per year in the United States), which are proportionally higher for the elderly, and the relation of these costs to outcomes is a topic under intense study at this time by health economists and physicians.[61] Firm conclusions are hampered by the fact that, although mortality is an easy endpoint to evaluate, quality of life following survival is crucial and much more difficult to evaluate.

Terminal Care: Palliative Care Issues

An especially vexing problem is that of the patient dying of respiratory failure who seemingly cannot be effectively treated, with dyspnea as a devastating symptom. This range includes both patients on mechanical ventilation (MV) in a hospital setting and those patients cared for outside the hospital who are dying of respiratory insufficiency, most often with severe COPD. In counseling such patients and their families, a strategy of open communication is essential, so that after exploration of the patient's life values advance directives can be implemented. This plan is enhanced if there has been a prior physician–patient relationship and is an area where the primary care physician (geriatrician) can provide a crucial service as he or she takes over management from the intensivist staff.

Palliative care of patients who are clearly dying in the end stages of respiratory insufficiency and who have no reversible aspects is a difficult but extremely important undertaking; this can be a gratifying professional experience and of true value for patient, family, and the care team. First, it is important to share the knowledge that death, although unpredictable (due to well-documented physician inability to render accurate prognosis in this situation), is coming soon and that in the absence of a clear acute reversible complication, MV or CPR with prolongation of dying would not be in the best interests of the patient.[62] Data show that survival, much less a return to a meaningful quality of life, in such situations is nil. At this time, previous advance directives should be reviewed. Most often patients are well aware of their status and are relieved by the knowledge that such frank discussions can be held and that their physician will not abandon them at this time. Palliative care interventions and what to expect and how they will die can then be discussed with emphasis on effective control of dyspnea, cough, mental or physical suffering, and pain. This discussion should focus on support of activities of daily living, symptomatic treatment of infection, and the aggressive use of medical measures for comfort (as in the previous discussion of COPD) to reduce symptoms. These support measures can be arranged at home, as well as in the inpatient hospice setting.

Special attention must be given to help with emotional needs. Depression and panic are common problems at this time, and, in addition to sensitive communication and counseling interventions, patients may respond to seritonin reuptake inhibitors, benzodiazapines, or even low-dose opiates, which can reduce dyspnea without significantly altering respiratory rate or oxygenation. The provision of sleep and a dignified transition should be assured. A détente with death can usually be achieved with supportive discussions and judicious pharmacologic interventions, with the focus concentrated on comfort and symptom control. Frequently, with CO_2 retention, supplemental oxygen is all that is required for tranquility in the patient who is within hours of dying with severe COPD. Sedation can be achieved with diazepam, lorazepam, or most effectively with an intravenous morphine sulfate drip that can be titrated to control terminal restlessness, *not* for euthanasia, but as an excellent way to provide continuous relief of dyspnea. Intravenous haloperidol is also useful with a rapid onset of action in the dyspneic agitated patient, and it does not suppress respiratory drive. The use of alcohol, or sedatives, if previously utilized by the patient, is appropriate, even if by secondary effect they hasten the moment of death. Cutaneous scopolamine patches may be used to control troublesome secretions.

Management of withdrawal of MV must be done using "best practices" to avoid excess suffering, and guidelines are available.[63,64] Discontinuation of MV in the ICU in the comatose patient is relatively straightforward. The ventilator is disconnected, 100% oxygen at atmospheric pressure is maintained, and a quiet and peaceful death occurs. The endotracheal tube can be left in place to prevent disturbing upper airway obstructive phenomena ("gurgling," etc.). Sedatives and anticholenergics for control of secretions can be utilized as needed. In the patient in whom ventilatory support is to be terminated and where mental status is perhaps more a stupor than coma, once all good-byes have been said and the course has been set (most easily done when explicit discussions and advance directives have been previously completed), adequate sedation must be assured. Intravenous opiates with or without an optional benzodiazapine should be instituted until the patient is comfortable and has spontaneous respirations but is clearly fully sedated and comfortable. Muscle relaxants should never be used to give an appearance of comfort. Then and only then should the ventilator be disconnected and 100% oxygen at atmospheric pressure be given. With an endotracheal tube in place, no "struggle" should occur.

The staff should be aware that as many as 10% of patients may survive for up to a day or longer following withdrawal of MV. Frequently it is beneficial for the family to be present at the bedside at this time so that they can be part of the process, which should be similar to a tranquil sleep leading to apnea and death. Colleagues involved in palliative care hospice and critical care programs and hospital ethics committees are useful consultants in all these difficult situations.[63]

References

1. Rossi A, Genassini A, Tantucci C, Grassi V. Aging and the respiratory system. *Aging.* 1996;8:143–161.
2. Pitcher WA, Cunningham HS. The oxygen cost of increased tidal volume and diaphragm flattening in obstructive lung disease. *J Appl Physiol.* 1993;74:2750–2756.
3. Petty TL. It's never too late to stop smoking, but how old are your lungs? *JAMA.* 1993;269:2785.
4. Petty TL. The rising epidemic of COPD in women. *Women's Health Primary Care.* 1999;2(12):942–953.
5. Peters KD, Kochanek KD, Murphy SE. Deaths: final data for 1996. National Center for Health Statistics. *Natl Vital Stat Rep.* 1998;47(9).
6. Connolly MJ, Crowley JJ, Charan NB, et al. Reduced subjective awareness of bronchoconstriction provoked by methacholine in elderly asthmatic and normal subjects as measured on a simple awareness scale. *Thorax.* 1992;47: 410–413.
7. Newnham DM, Hamilton SJ. Sensitivity of the cough reflex in young & elderly subjects. *Age Aging.* 1997;26:185–188.
8. Yohannes AM, Roam J, Winn S, Connolly MJ. The Manchester respiratory activities of daily living questionnaire: development, reliability, validity and responsiveness to pulmonary rehabilitation. *J Am Geriatrics Soc.* 2000;48: 1496–1500.
9. Enright PL, Kronmal RA, Higgins MW, et al. Prevalence and correlates of respiratory symptoms and disease in the elderly. *Chest.* 1994;106:827–834.
10. Mannino DM, Gagnon RC, Petty TL, Lydicke E. Obstructive lung disease and low lung function in adults in the United States. *Arch Intern Med.* 2000;160:1683–1689.
11. Reed CE. The natural history of asthma in adults: the problem of irreversibility. *J Allergy Clin Immunol.* 1999;103: 539–547.
12. Enright P, McClelland RL, Newman AB, et al. Underdiagnosis and undertreatment of asthma in the elderly. *Chest.* 1999;116:603–613.
13. Bates DV, Chistie RV. Effects of aging on respiratory function in man. In: Wolstenholme EV, Cameron MF, eds. *Ciba Foundation Colloquia on Aging: General Aspects.* Boston: Little, Brown; 1955:58.
14. BTS guidelines for the management of chronic obstructive pulmonary disease. *Thorax.* 1997;52(suppl 5):510–528.
15. Chan ED, Welsh CH. Geriatric respiratory medicine. *Chest.* 1998;114:1707–1733.
16. Scanlon PD, Cannett JE, Waller LA, et al. Smoking cessation and lung function in mild-to-moderate chronic obstructive pulmonary disease. *Am J Respir Crit Care Med.* 2000; 161:381–390.
17. Allen SC, Prior A. What determines whether an elderly patient can use a metered dose inhaler correctly? *Br J Dis Chest.* 1986;80:45–49.
18. Rennard SI, Serby CW, Ghafouni M, et al. Extended therapy with ipratropium is associated with improved lung function in patients with COPD: a retrospective analysis of data from seven clinical trials. *Chest.* 1996;110:62–70.
19. Niewoehner DE, Erbland MC, Devpree RH, et al. Effect of systemic glucocorticoids on exacerbations of chronic obstructive pulmonary disease. *N Engl J Med.* 1999;340: 1941–1947.
20. Shannon M. Predictors of major toxicity after the theophyllin overdose. *Ann Intern Med.* 1993;119:1161–1167.
21. Sethi S. Infectious exacerbations of chronic bronchitis: diagnosis and management. *J Antimicrob Chemother* 1999; 43(suppl A):97–105.
22. Nocturnal Oxygen Therapy Trial Group. Continuous or nocturnal oxygen therapy and hypoxemic chronic obstruc-

tive lung disease: a clincal trial. *Ann Intern Med.* 1980;93: 391–398.

23. Smetana GW. Preoperative pulmonary evaluation. *N Engl J Med.* 1999;340:937–944.

24. Ely EW, Evanst GW, Haponik EF. Mechanical ventilation in a cohort of elderly patients admitted to an intensive care unit. *Ann Intern Med.* 1999;131:96–104.

25. Roomi J, Johnson MM, Waters K, et al. Respiratory rehabilitation, exercise capacity and quality of life in chronic airways disease in old age. *Age Aging.* 1996;25:12–16.

26. Ries AL, Kaplan RM, Limberg TM, Prewitt LM. Effects of pulmonary rehabilitation on physiologic and psychosocial outcomes in patients with chronic obstruction pulmonary disease. *Ann Intern Med.* 1995;122:832–832.

27. Di Francia M, Barbier D, Mege JL, Onhek J. Tumor necrosis factor levels and weight loss in chronic obstructive pulmonary disease. *Am J Respir Crit Care Med.* 1994;150: 1453–1455.

28. Mannix ET, Manfredi F, Faber MD. Elevated O_2 cost of ventilation contributes to tissue wasting in chronic obstructive pulmonary disease. *Chest.* 1999;115:708–713.

29. Hanson PO, Tibblin G, Eriksson H. Deep vein thrombosis and pulmonary embolism in the general population: the study of men born in 1913. *Arch Intern Med.* 1997;157:1665–1670.

30. Ibbotson SH, Tate GH, Davies JA. Thrombin activity by intrinsic activation of plasma in vitro acceleration with increasing age of the donor. *Thromb Haemostasis.* 1992;67: 377–380.

31. Price DT, Ridken PM. Factor V Leiden mutation and the risks for thromboembolic disease: a clinical perspective. *Ann Intern Med.* 1997;127:895–903.

32. Lindmarker P, Schulman S, Stern-Lindesz S, et al. The risk of recurrent venous thromboembolism in carriers and noncarriers of G1691A allele in the prothrombin gene DURAG trial study group (Duration of Anticoagulation). *Thromb Haemostasis.* 1999;81:684–689

33. PIOPED Investigators. Valve of the ventilation/perfusion scan in acute pulmonary embolism: results of the prospective investigation of pulmonary embolism diagnosis (PIOPED). *JAMA.* 1990;263:2753–2759.

34. Heit JA, Silverstein MD, Mohr DN, et al. Predictors of survival after deep vein thrombosis and pulmonary embolism: a population-based cohort study. *Arch Intern Med.* 1999; 159:445–456.

35. Wells PS, Ginsberg JS, Andersen DR, et al. Use of a clinical model for safe management of patients with pulmonary embolism. *Ann Intern Med.* 1998;129:997–1005.

36. Goldhaber SZ. Medical progress: pulmonary embolism. *N Engl J Med.* 1998;339:93–104.

37. Rathburn SW, Raskob GE, Whitsett JL. Sensitivity and specificity of helical computed tomography in the diagnosis of pulmonary embolism: a systematic review. *Ann Intern Med.* 2000;132:227–232.

38. Mullins MD, Becker DM, Hagspiel KD, Philbrick JT. The role of spiral volumetric computed tomography in the diagnosis of pulmonary emboilsm. *Arch Intern Med.* 2000;160.293–298.

39. Hull RD, Felstein W, Stein PD, et al. Cost effectiveness of pulmonary embolism diagnosis. *Arch Intern Med.* 1996;156: 68–72.

40. Stein PD, Anthansoulis C, Alavi A, et al. Complications and validity of pulmonary angiography in acute pulmonary embolism. *Circulation.* 1992;85:462–469.

41. Sorensen HT, Mellemkjaer L, Steffensen FH, et al. The risk of cancer after primary deep venous thrombosis or pulmonary embolism. *N Engl J Med.* 1998;338:1169–1173.

42. Sorensen HT, Mellemks L, Olsen JH, Baron JA. Prognosis of cancers associated with venous thromboembolism. *N Engl J Med.* 2000;343:1846–1850.

43. Kearon C, Julian JA, Newman JE, et al. Noninvasive diagnosis of deep venous thrombosis. *Ann Intern Med.* 1998;128: 663–677.

44. Quinn DA, Fogel RB, Smith CD, et al. D-Dimers in the diagnosis of pulmonary embolism. *Am J Respir Crit Care Med.* 1999;159:1445–1449.

45. Dolovich LR, Ginsberg JS, Douhetis JD, et al. A meta-analysis comparing low molecular weight heparin with unfractionated heparin in the treatment of venous thromboembolism. *Arch Intern Med.* 2000;160:181–188.

46. Kearon C, Gent D, Hirsh J, et al. A comparison of three months of anticoagulation with extended anticoagulation for a first episode of idiopathic venous thromboembolism. *N Engl J Med.* 1999;340:901–907.

47. Goldhaber SZ, Kessler CM, Heit J, et al. Randomized controlled trial of recombinant tissue plasminogen activator versus urokinase in the treatment of acute pulmonary embolism. *Lancet.* 1988;2:293–298.

48. Haine WD. Vena caval filters for the prevention of pulmonary embolism. *N Engl J Med.* 1998;338:463–468.

49. Clagett GB, Anderson FN, Gerts W, et al. Preventing venous thromboembolism. *Chest.* 1998;114:531–560.

50. American Thoracic Society. Idiopathic pulmonary fibrosis: diagnosis and therapy. *Am J Respir Crit Care Med.* 2000;161: 640–664.

51. Tobin RW, Pope CE II, Pellegrini CA, et al. Increased prevalence of gastroesophageal reflux in patients with idiopathic pulmonary fibrosis. *Am J Respir Crit Care Med.* 1998;158:1804–1808.

52. Ziesche R, Hofbauer F, Wittmann K, et al. A preliminary study of long-term treatment with interferon gamma-1b and low dose prednisone in patients with idiopathic pulmonary fibrosis. *N Engl J Med.* 1999;341:1264–1269.

53. Bixler EO, Vgontzas AN, Have TT, et al. Effects of age on sleep apnea in men: prevalence and severity. *Am J Respir Crit Care Med.* 1998;l57:144–148.

54. Dales RE, Dionne G, Leech JA, Lunau M, Schweitzer I. Preoperative prediction of pulmonary complications following thoracic surgery. *Chest.* 1993;104:155–159.

55. Zibrak JD, O'Donnell CR. Indications for preoperative pulmonary function testing. *Clin Chest Med.* 1993;14(2):227–236.

56. Hall JC, Tarala R, Harris J, Tapper J, Christiansen K. Incentive spirometry versus routine chest physiotherapy for prevention of pulmonary complications after abdominal surgery. *Lancet.* 1991;337:953–956.

57. Egbert AM, Parks LH, Short LM, et al. Randomized trial of postoperative patient-controlled analgesia versus intramuscular narcotics in frail elderly men. *Arch Intern Med.* 1990;150:1897–1903.

58. Thomas DR, Ritche CS. Perioperative assessment of older adults. *J Am Geriatr Soc.* 1995;43:811–821.

59. Heuser MD, Case LD, Ettinger WH. Mortality in intensive care patients with respiratory disease, is age important? *Arch Intern Med.* 1992;152:1683–1688.

60. Krieger BP. Respiratory failure in the elderly. *Clin Geriatr Med.* 1994;10:103–119.

61. Cohen IL, Lombrinos J, Fein A. Mechanical ventilation for the elderly patient in intensive care: incremental charges and benefits. *JAMA.* 1993;269:1025–1029.

62. Sullivan KE, Hebart PC, Logan J, et al. What do physicians tell patients with end stage COPD about intubation and mechanical ventilation? *Chest.* 1996;109:258–264.

63. Faber-Longeduen K, Lanken PN. Dying patients in the intensive care unit: foregoing treatment, maintaining care. *Ann Intern Med.* 2000;133:886–893

64. Brody H, Campbell ME, Faber-Langen Coen K, Ogle KS. Withdrawing intensive life-sustaining treatment—recommendation for compassionate clinical management. *N Engl J Med.* 1997;336:652–657.

58
Dermatologic Diseases and Problems

Amy Krupnick Freeman and Marsha Gordon

Structure and Physiology of Aging Skin

Epidermis

Overall, the epidermis thins with advancing age. The stratum corneum loses its basket-weave pattern and becomes thin and compact, providing a less effective barrier. Keratinocytes exhibit some nuclear irregularity, especially in sun-exposed areas. Melanocyte density decreases by 10% to 20% each decade, but the exact decrease varies according to anatomic site. There is loss of cellular immunity with aging, as demonstrated by a nearly 50% decrease in the bone marrow-derived dendritic Langerhans' cells.[1]

Dermis

With aging, the dermis loses roughly 20% of its thickness secondary to the loss of proteoglycan as well as collagen. Collagen fibers become more cross-linked. Elastic fibers decrease and fragment, particularly in sun-exposed skin. In addition to decreased cellularity, the dermis becomes less vascular, as demonstrated by the loss of capillary loops. These vascular alterations may lead to pallor and contribute to decreased inflammation, a decreased rate of healing after injury, and delayed clearance of foreign materials.[2]

Subcutaneous Fat

The underlying subcutaneous fat also undergoes atrophy with age. These changes predispose the elderly to the effects of trauma and cold. The loss of subcutaneous fat in the face contributes to what we interpret as an aged appearance.[1]

Appendages

Age-related changes of the hair include most notably loss and graying of the hair. The loss of hair is determined by both androgenetic and involutional alopecia. The former begins before age 40 and is dependent upon male sex hormones and genetics. It is marked by bitemporal recession and hair loss on the vertex and frontal areas of the scalp in men, and by hair loss just posterior to the frontal rim in women, as the hair changes from thick to fine vellus-like hairs. Involutional alopecia, seen after the age of 40, is a process where there is a decrease in the hair shaft diameter and a decrease in the number of hair units, resulting in diffuse hair thinning. This phenomenon poses a cosmetic issue for some people. Therapy is available for androgenetic alopecia. Topical minoxidil, 2% solution 1.0 mL twice daily, has been shown to significantly increase hair counts. Oral finasteride at a dose of 1 mg daily has also been proven to increase hair counts and improve scalp coverage in men. There is also the option of scalp reduction and hair transplants to restore hair.[3]

Hair graying, often synonymous with aging, is a hereditary loss of functional melanocytes in the hair bulb. By age 50, roughly half of all body hairs become gray.[4]

Nail plate thickness and linear growth rate also decrease with age. Nails become thinner, more brittle, and may develop longitudinal ridges. This fragility may be improved with the application of lactic acid 12% lotion or a creamy moisturizer massaged daily into unpolished nails.

Sebaceous glands undergo hypertrophy with age, although sebum production decreases with age, partly due to a decline in androgen levels.[5] Apocrine and eccrine sweat glands decrease in density as they accumulate lipofuscin, an aging pigment of unknown significance. These glandular changes contribute to decreased thermoregulatory abilities, making the elderly person more susceptible to hyperthermia.[1]

Changes in Aging Skin from Physical Elements

In addition to the intrinsic process of senescence, there is the extrinsic component of skin aging that results from photodamage, smoking, and diet. The cutaneous changes of chronic ultraviolet (UV) damage manifest as wrinkling, solar lentigines ("liver spots"), telangiectasias, mottled pigmentation, and, most significantly, premalignant and malignant neoplasms.[5] Therefore, it is very important to take appropriate measures to protect the skin from these environmental effects.

Sun Exposure

Dermatoheliosis

The sun is the most damaging physical element to the skin. The cumulative effects of chronic sun damage on the skin is called dermatoheliosis. Appropriate lifelong use of sunscreens, protective clothing (hats and long-sleeved shirts), and avoiding sunlight between 10 A.M. and 3 P.M. may significantly reduce the cutaneous effects of photoaging. It is now known that both ultraviolet A (320–400 nm) and ultraviolet B (290–320 nm) light are responsible for chronic damage from the sun.[6] Therefore, the ideal photoprotectant agent shields against both UVB and UVA radiation and has a sun protection factor rating of 15 or more.

The epidermal changes that occur with chronic sun exposure range from benign hyperplasia to epidermal dysplasia and neoplasia. There is thinning of the epidermis with a predominance of atypical keratinocytes. Melanocyte hyperplasia and uneven melanin distribution lead to the blotchy pigmentation characteristic of photodamage. With solar damage, there is deposition of abnormal clumps of elastin within the dermis, called elastosis.[2] Actinically damaged skin, which is thicker than intrinsically aged skin, has smaller and fewer collagen fibers. Clinically, elastosis leads to wrinkling. Wrinkling is determined by solar damage as well as genetics. Facial movements play a role in those wrinkles formed at the nasolabial fold, forehead, and periorbital areas. Cosmetic treatment of aging skin is discussed in detail at the end of this chapter.

The American Academy of Dermatology consensus conference estimated that most of the UV-induced photoaging occurs within the first 20 years of life.[2] Thus, early preventive measures play a key role in the defense against solar radiation. By age 70, the number of melanocytes per unit area decreases by 40%. Fair-skinned persons inherently have less photoprotectant melanin pigment, so they are far more susceptible to sun damage than others with greater pigmentation.

Cutis Rhomboidalis Nuchae

This condition is characterized by thickened, furrowed skin that forms a rhomboid pattern at the back of the neck.[7] It is most often seen in men. Treatment is not necessary, unless it poses an aesthetic problem for the patient.

Nodular Elastoidosis with Cysts and Comedones (Favre–Racouchot Syndrome)

Cysts and comedones develop most commonly at the temporal and periorbital areas in patients with advanced actinic damage. Clinically, they appear as either a blackhead (filled with a greasy blue-black plug) or a whitehead with no apparent opening (milium).[7] Like cutis rhomboidalis nuchae, this condition does not require medical intervention, unless it is cosmetically bothersome to the patient.

Colloid Milium

Clinically, colloid milium is an entity in which numerous, translucent papules, approximately 2 mm in diameter, form on the dorsal hands and face. Histologically, the dermis is expanded by discrete lobules of homogeneous, eosinophilic material called colloid, formed after years of overexposure to sunlight.[7]

Senile/Solar Purpura (Bateman's Purpura)

This term refers to the transient red-purple patches on the forearms and dorsal hands in older persons (Fig. 58.1).[8] The elastotic dermis does not provide adequate structural support for the blood vessels. Therefore, even minor trauma to the aging skin can cause small vessels to rupture and form purpuric lesions.

Stellate Pseudoscars

These white, atrophic, irregularly shaped scars form after minor trauma.[8] They are commonly found on the fore-

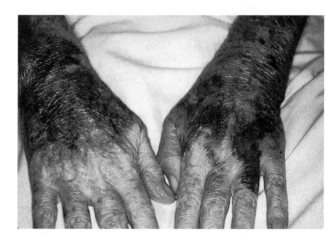

FIGURE 58.1. Senile purpura on the dorsal hands. (See color plate)

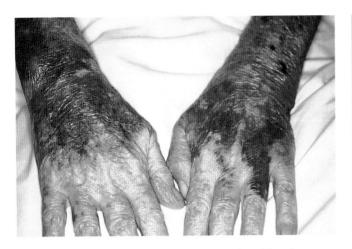

FIGURE 58.1. Senile purpura on the dorsal hands.

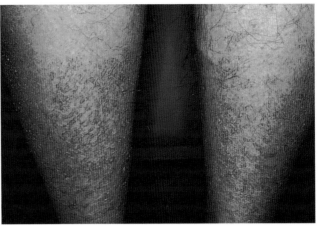

FIGURE 58.2. Eczema craquele', characterized by fissured and inflamed skin, located on bilateral lower extremities.

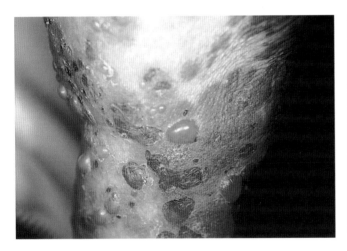

FIGURE 58.3. Bullous pemphigoid on the upper aspect of the arm.

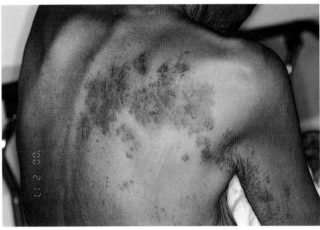

FIGURE 58.4. Herpes zoster of the back, with grouped vesicles in a dermatomal distribution.

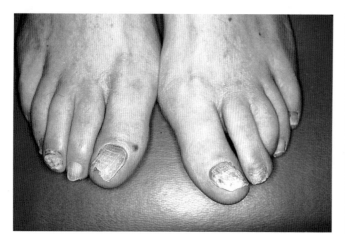

FIGURE 58.5. Onychomycosis of toenails with distal subungual hyperkeratosis and onycholysis.

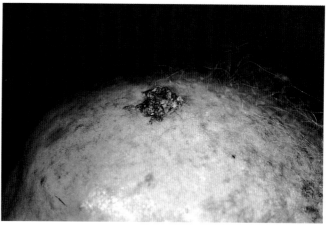

FIGURE 58.6. Squamous cell carcinoma of the scalp with thick keratotic scale.

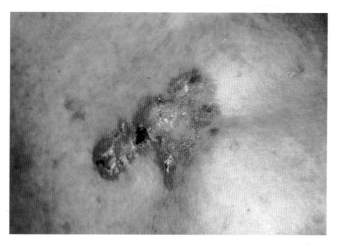

FIGURE 58.7. Basal cell carcinoma, appearing as a nodule with irregular borders and a scarlike quality.

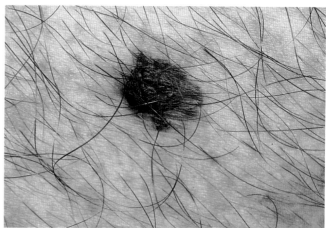

FIGURE 58.8. Malignant melanoma with characteristic features.

arms. Chronic sun exposure leading to solar purpura and atrophy with subsequent shearing from minor trauma and poor reparative abilities may be responsible for this clinical entity.

Heat

Erythema Ab Igne

Erythema ab igne is a condition caused by chronic exposure to heat.[9] This problem often occurs in elderly people who warm themselves by a fire, or a space heater, or with a heating blanket. They develop a reticulated brown pigmentation in the heat-exposed areas that may become keratotic and rarely develops into squamous cell carcinoma.

Cold

Cold is also poorly tolerated by older adults. Winter weather causes the aging skin, with less eccrine and sebaceous gland function, to become dry and pruritic. The loss of subcutaneous fat and reduced vascularity makes aging skin more susceptible to frostbite. Thus, extreme weather conditions can be damaging to the elderly.

Inflammatory Dermatoses in Aging Skin

Xerosis and Asteatotic Eczema

Xerosis or dryness is frequently seen in the elderly, particularly during the wintertime with the low humidity of heated rooms.[10] The decrease in eccrine and sebaceous gland function as well as an increase in transepidermal water loss due to impaired barrier function of the stratum corneum all likely play an etiologic role. Xerosis, seen most commonly on the extremities and trunk, is dry, scaly, and oftentimes pruritic. It may progress to asteatotic eczema, which in turn may progress to fissured, cracked, inflamed skin called eczema craquelé (Fig. 58.2).

During the winter months, xerosis can be reduced by limiting the amount of bathing and avoiding hot bath water and soap. The daily use of a topical emollient, preferably an ointment, can further prevent drying of the skin. It may be necessary to use a daily topical application of an alpha-hydroxy acid, such as lactic acid 12% lotion. For inflammatory changes, a low-dose topical corticosteroid ointment, such as 1% to 2.5% hydrocortisone, may be used twice daily, but with caution in thin, aging skin. To control pruritus, a low-dose systemic antihistamine at bedtime may be useful.[11]

Nummular Eczema

This eczema is characterized by scattered oval patches with scaly erythema and sometimes crusted papulovesi-

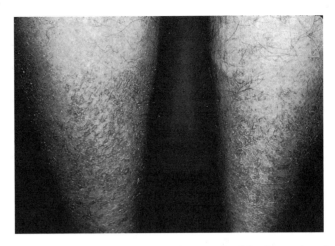

FIGURE 58.2. Eczema craquelé, characterized by fissured and inflamed skin, located on bilateral lower extremities. (See color plate)

cles on the trunk and extremities of people with dry skin. Nummular eczema may be treated with emollients and low-dose topical corticosteroids.

Lichen Simplex Chronicus

This is an eczematous eruption that results from chronic scratching or rubbing.[12] Pruritus precedes the scratching, which causes lichenification and further itching, resulting in a perpetual cycle. The lesion is usually a thick plaque with enhanced skin markings, and perhaps erythema and excoriations. It commonly involves the dorsum of the feet and ankles, the back of the neck, and the wrists. Potent topical corticosteroids, menthol-containing preparations, or topical doxepin may be helpful. Lichen simplex chronicus resolves when scratching or rubbing ceases.

Pruritus

Pruritus is a common complaint in the geriatric population, yet remains a challenge for physicians. It may be caused by a primary skin disease, or by an underlying systemic disease, or be idiopathic. First, the clinician should look for a skin condition, such as xerosis, scabies, urticaria, contact dermatitis, dermatitis herpetiformis, or eczema. If a skin disease is not evident, a systemic cause may be present. Systemic disorders include renal failure, liver disease, cancer (especially myeloproliferative disorders), thyrotoxicosis, diabetes, and psychiatric and neurologic disorders. Treatment is aimed at the underlying disease. Oftentimes, there is no apparent etiology for the pruritus and the patient must be treated symptomatically. Emollients and topical antipruritic agents with 0.5% menthol may be helpful. The use of low-dose oral antihistamines and topical corticosteroids can also be useful. Doxepin 5% cream applied every 3 to 4 h has proven to be successful, but should be limited to 8 days of use and to no more than 10% of the body surface.[11]

Angular Cheilitis

This inflammatory condition is characterized by erythema and fissuring at the corners of the mouth.[13] It is frequently seen in elderly people who do not have teeth. In this situation, the cheek loses support and the angles of the mouth overlap trapping saliva. As a result, maceration and sometimes secondary *Candida* infections develop. Properly fit dentures and nightly application of petrolatum are measures that can prevent this condition. Topical antifungals can treat the secondary candidal infection and low-dose topical corticosteroids can minimize the inflammation.

Seborrheic Dermatitis

This is an extremely common chronic eczematous condition affecting more than 20% of the geriatric population. It affects the hairy regions of the body, where there is an abundance of sebaceous glands, such as the scalp, eyebrows, nasolabial creases, ears, chest, and intertriginous areas. Clinically, it appears as erythematous patches and plaques with yellowish, greasy scale. The etiology is unclear but is thought to be, in part, caused by an inflammatory reaction against the resident skin yeast, *Pityrosporum ovale*. In light of this, therapy can include a topical antifungal agent, such as ketoconazole 2% cream or shampoo applied to nonhair-bearing areas or the scalp, respectively. There is only symptomatic treatment for this chronic condition. For the scalp, one can use either selenium sulfide, tar-based, or as mentioned before, ketoconazole shampoo, applied twice weekly. In addition to ketoconazole cream, a low-dose topical corticosteroid may be helpful. Seborrheic dermatitis has a wide differential diagnosis that includes atopic dermatitis, candidiasis, dermatophytosis, histiocytosis X, psoriasis vulgaris, rosacea, systemic lupus erythematosus, tinea capitas, tinea versicolor, and vitamin deficiency.[14]

Rosacea

Rosacea, also known as "adult acne," tends to occur on the face of those with fair hair and skin. Facial flushing is thought to be one of the causative factors in rosacea, eventually leading to persistent erythema and telangiectasias, which then progress to inflammatory papules, pustules, and nodules. In a minority with long-standing rosacea, the sebaceous glands and connective and vascular tissue of the nose proliferate, causing a bulbous hypertrophy of the nose, called rhinophyma. Rosacea may cause ocular problems such as blepharitis and conjunctivitis. Avoidance of factors that trigger flushing is central to the management of rosacea. These provocative factors include exposure to extreme temperature changes (especially heat), consumption of hot or spicy foods, alcohol (especially red wine), sunlight, and stress. The mainstay of treatment has been topical metronidazole 0.75% gel twice daily with or without an oral antibiotic, such as erythromycin or a tetracycline. For the rare patient with resistant disease, systemic isotretinoin may be necessary, but its use is limited by side effects. Therapy for telangiectasias and rhinophyma is surgical. New approaches include use of a tunable dye laser for vascular lesions and dermabrasion, excision and skin grafting, scalpel shaving, cryosurgery, electrosurgery, or laser for cases of rhinophyma.[15]

Grover's Disease

Grover's disease, also known as transient acantholytic dermatosis, is a self-limited, pruritic, papulovesicular eruption primarily on the central trunk. Its classic presentation is an erythematous, scaling, papular eruption after an extreme environmental stress such as heavy exercise/sweating, excessive sun exposure, or high fever in a middle-aged male, although there are many cases reported in female patients. The characteristic histologic finding is acantholysis, or separation of epidermal cells and formation of an intraepidermal vesicle. Treatment may prove frustrating. However, the disease may resolve spontaneously or with topical corticosteroids. Treatment should also be aimed at avoiding the precipitating factors, such as excessive heat or exercise or extreme environmental stresses such as dryness. Soothing baths, emollients, or topical antipruritics may relieve the pruritus. If the eruption is severely pruritic, persistent, or extensive, systemic therapy may be necessary.[16]

Psoriasis

Psoriasis is a condition that most often appears in young adulthood, but increases in prevalence with age.[17] Therefore, it affects a significant proportion of the geriatric population. Psoriasis is an inflammatory rash with increased epidermal proliferation of unclear etiology. Its characteristic lesions are sharply demarcated, oval or round erythematous plaques surmounted by silvery scales, typically located on the scalp and extensor aspects of the elbows and knees. There are four main clinical forms of psoriasis, plaque type being the most common, which include guttate (eruptive), inverse (flexural), erythrodermic, and pustular. Inverse psoriasis is mainly observed in the elderly population. Approximately 7% of psoriatic patients, usually those with severe disease or with nail involvement, develop arthritis. Because there is no cure for psoriasis, the goal of treatment is remission and prevention of recurrence. Topical therapies include coal tar preparations, dithranol, topical corticosteroids, tazarotene, calcipotriol (a vitamin D_3 analogue), and ultraviolet light. Systemic treatment is indicated in those with severe disease or in patients who are resistant to topical agents. The elderly person may be at particular risk for the adverse side effects of systemic therapy, and therefore it is important to carefully evaluate the risks and benefits in this age group. The various systemic agents are psoralen with long-wave ultraviolet light (PUVA), methotrexate, and etretinate (an oral retinoid), recently replaced by its metabolite acitretin. Cyclosporin is effective, but its use in the elderly is limited by the adverse effects of nephrotoxicity and hypertension. The major concerns with methotrexate are liver toxicity and myelosuppression. The retinoids have numerous side effects, but myalgias, arthralgias, xerosis, and headache are particularly common in older people.

Contact Dermatitis

Contact dermatitis is an inflammatory reaction to either an irritant or allergen. The typical acute lesions are erythematous macules, papules, and vesicles with exudation and crusting. Elderly people may present with milder clinical disease because of depressed inflammatory responses. Instead, older individuals may present with severe itching, associated with mild erythema, scaling, or early hyperpigmentation, and lichenification rather than vesiculation and inflammation.[10] Therefore, contact dermatitis can be a difficult diagnosis. Common causative agents in older persons include neomycin, parabens (a common preservative in medications), lanolin, ethylenediamines, nitrofurazone, and acrylate adhesives in transdermal medications. Plants, nickel, and rubber compounds commonly cause allergic contact dermatitis. The key to treatment is removal of the offending agent. Topical corticosteroids of moderate to high potency and antihistamines are also mainstays of therapy.

Drug Eruptions

Elderly patients are particularly susceptible to drug eruptions because of their numerous comorbidities and the increased likelihood of polypharmacy in this age group. Approximately 2% of medical inpatients have cutaneous drug reactions, and this rate is significantly higher in those receiving eight or more medications.[18] There are myriad clinical presentations including erythematous, lichenoid, eczematous, acneiform, urticarial, bullous, fixed drug, exfoliative, nodular, photosensitive, and purpuric. However, morbilliform (erythematous macules and papules) represents nearly 75% of the eruptions. The penicillins, cephalosporins, and sulfonamides have high reaction rates. Once the offending agent is discontinued, the rash clears within 1 to 2 weeks.

Bullous Pemphigoid

This is the most common blistering disorder in older persons, occurring in the sixth, seventh, and eighth

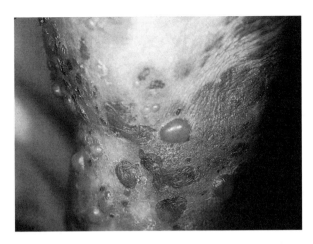

FIGURE 58.3. Bullous pemphigoid on the upper aspect of the arm. (See color plate)

decades.[10] The bullae are large, tense, and nonscarring and may contain clear or hemorrhagic fluid (Fig. 58.3). They occur on normal or urticarial skin over flexural surfaces of the extremities and abdomen. Approximately one-third of patients may have oral involvement. Diagnosis is made by skin biopsy. The bullae are subepidermal according to light microscopy. Immunofluorescence reveals linear deposits of immunoglobulin G and C3 along the basement membrane.[19] Typically, the disease subsides after months to years, but relapses do occur. Debilitated patients with widespread blistering have died of this condition. Initial therapy is prednisone (0.5–1 mg/kg/day) to suppress blister formation. Steroids should be tapered as soon as clinically feasible. Azathioprine, gold, methotrexate, or cyclophosphamide may be used for their steroid-sparing effects. When prescribing a systemic corticosteroid in an older person, it is important to also start vitamin D and calcium to counteract the adverse side effects of osteoporosis. For mild disease, dapsone or treatment with tetracycline with or without niacinamide may be used. Local care with compresses, topical corticosteroids, and, sometimes, topical antibiotics is helpful.

Pemphigus vulgaris is a blistering disease predominant in middle-aged people. The bullae are flaccid, fragile, and intraepidermal. Therapy consists of systemic corticosteroids and immunosuppressive agents. Untreated pemphigus is fatal.

Anogenital Disease in Aging Skin

Pruritus Ani

This is a common frustrating problem in the elderly population. Fecal soiling and moisture accumulation in the anal region cause irritation, which starts the vicious cycle of itching, rubbing with subsequent development of lichenification, and further pruritus.[20] Major causative factors may be incomplete cleansing after defecation and fecal incontinence. Or, there may be a primary condition as the etiology, such as hemorrhoids, candidiasis, and psoriasis. Treatment always includes education on proper hygiene (cleansing, baths) and, in cases of incontinence, application of barrier preparations. Hydrocortisone cream may allieviate the pruritus.

Senile Vulvar Atrophy

Postmenopausal women frequently experience vulvar atrophy.[8] Specifically, there is atrophy of the labia majora, labia minora, and clitoris and the vaginal mucosa becomes dry. This condition may be pruritic. A topical emollient or topical estrogen preparation may be very helpful.

Lichen Sclerosus et Atrophicus, Balanitis Xerotica Obliterans

Lichen sclerosus et atrophicus commonly occurs in menopausal women, but can also affect children. Clinically, it appears as ivory-white, well-defined atrophic plaques that often form a "figure-of-eight" arrangement on the vulva and anus.[20] Patients may experience pruritus, dyspareunia, or discomfort. There is a waxing and waning course, with roughly 50% of people developing leukoplakia. Squamous cell carcinoma rarely develops, but surveillance for it necessitates follow-up every 12 months. Treatment options include the application of bland emollients and topical corticosteroids for pruritus and inflammation. Topical testosterone, once the mainstay of therapy, has fallen out of favor because of minimal results and masculinizing side effects.

Balanitis xerotica obliterans is the male equivalent.[20] The white atrophic lesions occur on the glans and prepuce. Urethral stricture and phimosis may occur.

Angiokeratomas of Fordyce

This entity is characterized by dilated venules that appear as dark red to purple lesions with minimal hyperkeratosis.[21] These benign lesions are located on the scrotum and are asymptomatic, making removal unnecessary.

Infections in Aging Skin

Herpes Zoster

Herpes zoster (shingles) is a vesicular dermatomal disease caused by the varicella virus (chicken pox).[22] (See Chapter 72 for a detailed discussion on herpes zoster.) It can be severe and debilitating in the elderly. After the primary infection, the varicella-zoster virus remains dormant in the dorsal root ganglion. Herpes zoster develops after reactivation of the latent virus, perhaps precipitated by trauma, radiotherapy, immunosuppression, or stress. People with neoplastic disease and those on immunosuppresive therapy are also at increased risk.

A prodrome of pain and paresthesia precedes the eruption of unilaterally grouped vesicles on an erythematous base (Fig. 58.4). The lesions are situated in a dermatomal distribution. Any dermatome may be involved, but the thoracic and trigeminal nerves are the most common. Disseminated disease is more common in patients with lymphoreticular disease or in immunosuppressed individuals; this can be life threatening. Postherpetic neuralgia is a complication that increases in incidence with age. Elderly people also have increased recurrence of herpes zoster infection.

Diagnosis can quickly be made by demonstration of multinucleated giant cells on Tzanck smear. Analgesics and topical compresses to dry the vesicles are helpful. Secondary infection may be controlled with oral antibiotics that provide staphylococcal and streptococcal coverage.

Ongoing pain after the acute infection has subsided is called postherpetic neuralgia and can be a debilitating condition.[22] Topical capsaicin or various oral psychoactive medications for pain have been useful for this condition.

Dermatophytes and Candida

Dermatophyte infection of the toenail plate, called tinea unguium or onychomycosis, is a common disorder, especially in elderly people.[23] The involved nail becomes thick and yellow, with subungual accumulation of debris (Fig. 58.5). Often the nail changes cannot clinically be distinguished from nail dystrophy of aging, psoriasis, or trauma. Onychomycosis is usually associated with tinea pedis and can be diagnosed by demonstration of hyphae on KOH

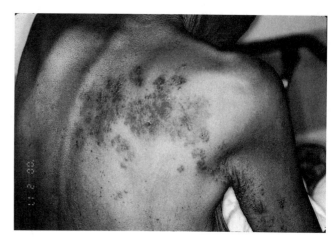

FIGURE 58.4. Herpes zoster of the back, with grouped vesicles in a dermatomal distribution. (See color plate)

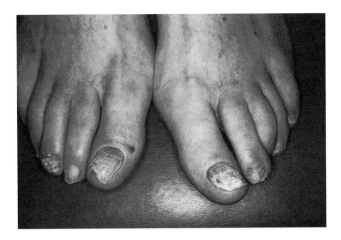

FIGURE 58.5. Onychomycosis of toenails with distal subungual hyperkeratosis and onycholysis. (See color plate)

preparation, histologic preparation of a nail clipping, or fungal culture.[24] Oral antifungals are considerably more effective than topical preparations. In the past, a 1- to 2-year course of griseofulvin with monitoring of renal, hepatic, and hematopoietic functions was the treatment of choice. Newer antifungals, including terbinafine or itraconazole, require only 3 months of treatment.[25] However, close monitoring of hepatic function and blood counts is still necessary. After successful treatment of onychomycosis, interdigital application of a topical antifungal preparation may be necessary to prevent the recurrence of tinea pedis, from which a future case of onychomycosis may develop. Additionally, it is important to be aware that the interdigital scale of tinea pedis can act as the portal of entry for bacteria, which may lead to cellulitis of the lower extremity.

Older people, particularly those who are obese or bedridden, can develop candidiasis in the moist areas of the groin, axilla, and submammary region. This infection appears as a "beefy-red" rash with satellite papules and pustules. Drying moist areas thoroughly and frequent turning of bedridden patients are important preventive measures. Candidiasis may be treated with topical antifungal agents such as nystatin or ketoconazole cream applied twice a day.

Benign and Malignant Skin Tumors in Aging Skin

Elderly patients frequently develop various benign, premalignant, or malignant skin tumors, which can be of epidermal, melanocytic, or dermal origin.

Seborrheic Keratosis

This extremely common benign epidermal growth may occur anywhere on the body. The keratoses are crusty, greasy appearing, "pasted-on" papules or plaques that are sharply marginated. The color ranges from tan to black, and the occasional dark lesion may require biopsy to distinguish from malignant melanoma. The elderly may develop stucco keratosis, a variant form marked by white, keratotic papules on the extremities. Treatment is not necessary for these benign lesions unless they are cosmetically unacceptable, inflamed, or atypical in appearance.[26] Curettage and liquid nitrogen cryosurgery are two simple treatment options. Of note is the rare paraneoplastic sign of Leser–Trelat, which is the rapid increase in size and number of these lesions.[27] This development signifies an internal malignancy, usually adenocarcinoma of the gastrointestinal tract.

Skin Tags (Acrochordons)

These are benign, fleshy, pedunculated papules that are frequently acquired in adult life.[20] The lesions have a predilection for the axilla, neck, eyelids, and flexural areas. Removal is not necessary but can easily be performed by scissor excision or light electrodesiccation.

Sebaceous Hyperplasia

This benign clinical entity often occurs on the face in the elderly patient.[28] It appears as one or multiple, yellowish dome-shaped papules with central umbilication. The lesions range in size from 1 to 3 mm in diameter and may be mistaken for a basal cell carcinoma. Therefore, a biopsy is sometimes necessary. Lesions can be removed with light electrodesiccation.

Cherry Angiomas

These extremely common benign lesions appear as bright-red, dome-shaped vascular lesions. They are principally found on the trunk. They first appear at about age 30 then tend to become more numerous and larger with age. If cosmetically problematic, then electrodesiccation or excision for larger lesions can be used.

Venous Lakes

Venous lakes are dilated venules characterized by a blue to black soft papule. They occur on the face, lips, and ears of people over the age of 50 years. The etiology is unknown but may be secondary to solar exposure. The differential diagnosis includes malignant melanoma and blue nevus. Treatment is cosmetic and can be performed with electrodesiccation or excision.

Spider Veins

This common complaint in older women is often a frustrating cosmetic problem. Spider veins are dilated purple veins, approximately 1 to 2mm in diameter, on the lower extremities that result from elevated venous pressure over time. Treatment, called sclerotherapy, involves injection of 23.4% hypertonic saline or an alternative sclerosing agent into the vessel lumen.[29]

Solar Lentigos (Senile Lentigos)

Solar lentigines, also called "liver spots" or "age spots," are commonly seen on sun-exposed areas in Caucasians over 60 years of age.[6] They appear as uniformly colored tan to dark brown macules that vary in size. Biopsy may be required to distinguish the lesion from lentigo maligna. Treatment is not necessary for these benign lesions, but can be accomplished with liquid nitrogen cryotherapy, trichloroacetic acid, or laser modalities. Additionally, tretinoin cream with 4% hydroquinone cream applied twice daily for 6 to 8 weeks can fade solar lentigines.

Actinic Keratosis

Actinic, or solar, keratosis is a premalignant lesion caused by exposure to ultraviolet light.[30] Therefore, actinic keratoses are most commonly found on sun-exposed areas, such as the face and dorsal hands, in fair-skinned, middle-aged to elderly people. Clinically, the lesions are pink macules or papules with dry adherent scale. They are often more easily felt than seen secondary to their rough nature.

A small percentage of actinic keratoses develop into squamous cell carcinoma, necessitating removal of these lesions.[31] With fewer lesions, options of removal are cryosurgery, curettage, or application of 30% to 50% trichloroacetic acid. Topical 5-fluorouracil cream (efudex) applied twice daily for 3 to 6 weeks is an effective means of treating multiple lesions. This antimetabolite selectively destroys the pathologic cell, leaving normal skin relatively unharmed, but may cause much discomfort and inflammation. Once therapy is stopped, the inflamed skin resolves. In cases where large areas are involved, dermabrasion or chemical peeling may be useful.[32] Prevention by avoidance of excessive sun exposure is the best approach.

Bowen's Disease

Bowen's disease, or squamous cell carcinoma in situ, is an intraepidermal tumor.[6] It is differentiated from actinic keratoses in that it is not found on sun-exposed skin.[33] The lesion of Bowen's disease is a slowly enlarging, sharply defined erythematous plaque with scale, which may be clinically confused with psoriasis or eczema. Biopsy will differentiate these entities. Electrodesiccation and curettage, cryosurgery, excision, ionizing radiation, and Mohs' surgery can all be used to remove the lesion. Close follow-up is essential.

When this lesion occurs on the glans penis in uncircumcised men, it appears as a red, moist, or velvety, well-circumscribed oval to round patch and is known as erythroplasia of Queyrat.[20] This entity is histologically identical to Bowen's disease, but metastasizes more frequently. Therefore, it is important to identify these lesions immediately so treatment can be initiated.

Squamous Cell Carcinoma

Squamous cell carcinoma often appears on sun-exposed areas in fair-skinned patients.[34] It may arise from an actinic keratosis or de novo. Clinically, the lesion is an erythematous, scaly nodule that may become ulcerated, crusted, or verrucous as it enlarges (Fig. 58.6). Squamous cell carcinoma arising in sun-damaged skin rarely metastasizes and is typically only locally destructive. Lesions arising on mucous membranes, however, such as the lip, vulva, or penis, or lesions arising from a chronic skin ulcer, all have a greater tendency to metastasize. Complete eradication of the lesion can be accomplished with excision or Mohs' surgery. Other treatment modalities are curettage and electrodesiccation, useful in early lesions, and ionizing radiation, useful in older people.

Keratoacanthoma

Keratoacanthoma is a rapidly growing, benign tumor that clinically and histologically resembles squamous cell carcinoma.[35] It commonly occurs in older light-skinned individuals on sun-exposed, hair-bearing sites. Clinically, the lesion is a solitary, firm, dome-shaped nodule with a central keratinous plug. It may suddenly grow over 4 to 6 weeks, stabilize, and then regress, leaving a scar. Surgical excision or curettage with electrodesiccation are the

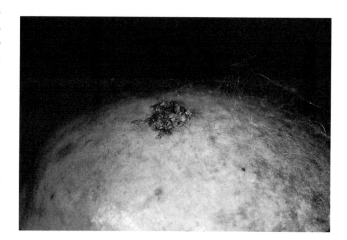

FIGURE 58.6. Squamous cell carcinoma of the scalp with thick keratotic scale. (See color plate)

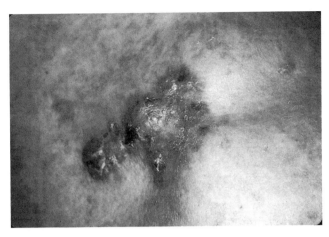

FIGURE 58.7. Basal cell carcinoma, appearing as a nodule with irregular borders and a scarlike quality. (See color plate)

best treatment modalities, as they allow for histologic confirmation of diagnosis.

Basal Cell Carcinoma

Basal cell carcinoma is the most common malignant tumor.[36] Chronic exposure to UV light is strongly associated with these slow-growing lesions on sun-exposed areas of older, fair-skinned individuals. Metastasis is extremely rare, but basal cell cancers may become very large and be locally destructive.

There are several clinical presentations of basal cell carcinoma ranging from nodular to flat in nature. The most common is the nodular ulcerative type, characterized by a pearly, translucent papule or nodule with a central depression, rolled borders, and telangiectasias. These lesions may ulcerate, become crusted, or bleed (Fig. 58.7). Superficial basal cell carcinoma usually appears on the trunk and is characterized by a slowly growing, erythematous slightly scaling plaque. It may be clinically similar to a patch of eczema. Sclerosing basal cell carcinoma has a flat scarlike quality and often has a poorly defined border. Pigmented basal cell carcinomas contain brown pigment and may be clinically indistinguishable from melanomas. In all types, histologic examination confirms the diagnosis.

Treatment options include curettage and electrodesiccation (usually reserved for small lesions and nonsclerosing basal cell carcinomas) or excision with a possible skin graft or flap in large lesions. Ionizing radiation may be used in elderly patients. However, in middle-aged or younger patients, concerns about future radiation dermatites severely limits its use. Mohs' surgery, a microscopically controlled technique in which a lesion's perimeter is histologically examined to ensure tumor-free margins, has the highest cure rate.[37] It is employed when treating lesions that abut a functional structure such as the eye, or in lesions from areas with high risk of recur-

rence, such as the nasolabial fold near the nose. It is also the treatment of choice for recurrent basal cell carcinoma and for very large lesions. Evolving therapies include intralesional injection of interferon and prophylactic oral retinoid therapy. Long-term follow-up is necessary because of the possibility of recurrence and the high risk for developing new lesions.[38]

Lentigo Maligna and Lentigo Maligna Melanoma

Lentigo maligna is a slowly enlarging pigmented macular lesion found on sun-exposed skin in older people.[39] It can reach a size of several centimeters. There is often variation in color within the same lesion. Lentigo maligna is a form of melanoma in situ. It may have a horizontal growth phase of many years before dermal invasion, at which time it is called lentigo maligna melanoma. In fact, many elderly patients succumb to other conditions before lentigo maligna transforms into lentigo maligna melanoma. However, because of the concern of invasion, treatment is complete surgical excision.

The A, B, C, D, Es of melanoma recognition are valuable for clinicians and for patient education: Asymmetry, Border irregularities, Color variegation, Diameter greater than 6 mm, Enlargement (Fig. 58.8). Excisional biopsy is the diagnostic procedure of choice for clinically suspicious lesions. It is important to completely excise the lesion, providing a full-thickness specimen extending to the subcutaneous fat, as tumor thickness, measured from the granular layer of the epidermis to the deepest area of involvement, determines prognosis of the disease.[40,41] Accurate staging involves complete examination of the skin, lymph nodes, liver, and spleen, along with a review of systems. Surgical excision is the treatment of choice for melanoma. Current recommendations are based on the histologic depth of the melanoma and no longer rely on the principle of "deep and wide" excisions that predominated in previous years. For

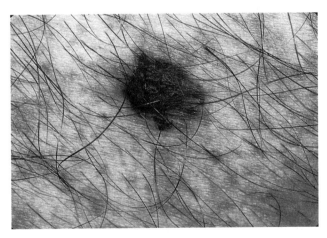

FIGURE 58.8. Malignant melanoma with characteristic features. (See color plate)

in situ melanomas, a margin of 0.5 cm of normal skin is recommended and, for melanomas less than 1 mm thick, a margin of 1 cm is accepted. The benefit of lymph node dissection remains controversial.[42] Patients with lesions greater than 4 mm thick are at high risk for metastatic disease. Interferon alpha-2b has been approved for the treatment of metastatic melanoma.[43] Chemotherapy and radiation therapy are, unfortunately, of minimal help in most cases of melanoma, as most melanomas are relatively resistant to these modalities. Vaccines and gene therapies are experimental treatment options.[44,45] Of course, reducing risk by using a broad-spectrum sunscreen with both UVA and UVB coverage of at least spf 15, wearing sun-protecting clothing, and avoiding midday sun is strongly recommended.

Paget's Disease

Paget's disease is an intraepidermal carcinoma of glandular origin with two forms, mammary[46] and extra-mammary.[47] In mammary Paget's disease, the carcinoma involves the nipple and areola, stimulating a sharply marginated, eczematous plaque. It is associated with underlying intraductal carcinoma of the breast. Management consists of surgery, radiotherapy, or chemotherapy. Extramammary Paget's disease, clinically and histologically similar to Paget's disease of the breast, involves the anogenital and axillary skin. It is often associated with an underlying adenocarcinoma of the secretory glands, lower gastrointestinal, urinary, or female genital tracts. Treatment involves surgical excision and examination for a possible underlying malignancy. Paget's disease clinically resembles eczema, so any treatment-resistant dermatitis should be biopsied.

Kaposi's Sarcoma

Kaposi's sarcoma (KS) is a malignant, vascular tumor characterized by purple macules, papules, or nodule, usually on the lower legs.[48] This malignancy is typically seen in three settings. Classic Kaposi's occurs in elderly men of Eastern European or Jewish descent and progresses very slowly; or, it is an endemic disease in Africa, presenting as an aggressive lymphadenopathic tumor that is often fatal; and last, Kaposi's sarcoma is found in association with the acquired immunodeficiency syndrome (AIDS), particularly in homosexual patients. It is more extensive and has a poorer prognosis in these individuals than in the elderly. Approximately 95% of KS lesions have been found to be infected with Kaposi's sarcoma-associated herpesvirus (also known as human herpesvirus 8). Therapy often depends on the extent and form of the disease. Kaposi's sarcoma may respond to radiotherapy or chemotherapy, such as vinblastine. Palliative destruction of individual lesions by cryosurgery or excision may also be helpful.

Angiosarcoma

Angiosarcoma is a rare, aggressive vascular tumor that occurs typically on the head of the elderly. It appears as reddish-purple nodules or plaques that are asymptomatic. Because the lesions often metastasize early, treatment is usually unsuccessful.

Cutaneous Metastases

Metastatic cancer to the skin is characterized by solitary or multiple hard nodules, often intradermal.[20] Approximately 4% of internal malignancies eventually spread to the skin by hematogenous, lymphatic, or direct extension. The most common sites of primary tumor are breast, lung, gastrointestinal tract, and kidney. The average survival after detection of cutaneous metastases is only 3 months, with the exception of breast cancer. The lesions may be treated with excision or systemic therapy.

Ulcerations in Aging Skin

Further discussion of these conditions can be found in Chapter 66.

Stasis Dermatitis and Venous Ulceration

Stasis dermatitis is caused by elevated venous pressures secondary to either valvular incompetence or obstruction.[10] It is an eczematous eruption of the lower extremities with brown hemosiderin-derived pigmentation and, sometimes, petechiae, often preceded by edema and swelling. The predominant site of involvement is the medial malleolus. Predisposing factors include a history of thrombophlebitis, a positive family history, obesity, or multiple pregnancies. Low-dose topical corticosteroids and reduction of edema, by such measures as leg elevation and compression stockings, are the mainstays of treatment.[49]

The most common cause of ulcerations in older people is venous ulcers, which may arise spontaneously or from a superficial injury in the setting of chronic venous insufficiency. The ulcer is usually surrounded by brown-red pigmentation, located at the medial malleolus, and has irregular borders. There may be surrounding edema and pigmentation. Cellulitis may complicate venous ulcers. Ulcerations often recur unless the underlying risk factors are corrected. Leg elevation and use of elastic support stockings can alleviate the venous hypertension.[50,51] Dressings can facilitate healing by maintaining a moist environment that promotes reepithelialization.[52] Options include wet or dry nonadherent dressings, occlusive dressings (such as OpSite and DuoDerm), or zinc paste-impregnated bandages (known as the Unna boot). An associated eczematous dermatitis can be treated with moist compresses, if needed, and corticosteroid ointment. If a secondary bacterial infection develops, a systemic antibiotic may be used.

Arterial Ulceration

Arterial ulcers are caused by artherosclerosis-induced ischemia of the skin.[53] Arterial ulcers are clinically different from venous ulcers. These lesions are gray-black, sharply demarcated ulcers, located at the pretibial area or on the toes. The ulcer is often painful and is associated with other ischemic findings, such as loss of hair and cold, atrophic skin. Pulses may be diminished or absent. Control or elimination of risk factors, such as smoking, hypertension, diabetes, obesity, and high cholesterol, are important in management. Local therapy includes moist saline dressings, changed frequently, although healing is slow. Analgesics for pain may be necessary.

Diabetic Ulceration

Leg ulcers in diabetics are multifactorial, resulting from complications of small and large vessel disease and neuropathy.[49] Diabetes mellitus causes proliferation of endothelial cells and thickening of the basement membrane in small vessels, which leads to decreased blood flow through the vessel lumen. Furthermore, patients with diabetes are at increased risk for artherosclerosis of medium- and large-sized vessels. Therefore, arterial ulcerations commonly develop in these patients.

Long-standing diabetes can also cause peripheral and autonomic neuropathy. Patients eventually lose sensation in their feet and, as a result, cannot perceive trauma, pressure, or chronic friction. Mal perforans refers to the neurotrophic ulcer that develops in these patients. The diabetic foot is typically numb, warm, and dry. The ulcer is gray to black, surrounded by hyperkeratotic skin, and located at points of pressure or trauma, such as the heel, sole, metatarsal head, and great toe. These ulcers may evolve into cellulitis, osteomyelitis, or gangrene, which requires amputation. This diabetic complication can be prevented by daily inspection of the feet for early signs of trauma, properly fitted shoes, and avoidance of trauma and going barefoot. Surrounding callus may need debridement, and associated infections may require antibiotic therapy. Also see Chapter 66 for further detail on this condition.

Nutritional Deficiencies and Aging Skin

Many elderly people, particularly those who live alone, have a fixed income, or suffer from chronic disease, suffer from malnutrition.[54] The skin is a rapidly dividing tissue and, therefore, is particularly sensitive to nutritional deficiencies. Skin desquamation and alopecia often result from malnutrition. Certain vitamin deficiencies are marked by specific cutaneous changes. Vitamin A deficiency leads to generalized scaling with hyperkeratosis and dry eyes. Pellagra (vitamin B complex deficiency) causes cheilitis and dermatitis. Patients who lack vitamin C suffer from perifollicular hemorrhage with coiled hairs, impaired wound healing, and swollen, bleeding gums (scurvy).

Cosmetic Treatment of Aging Skin

With society's emphasis on physical appearance, elderly people are becoming increasingly interested in cosmetic options to improve aging skin. When elderly patients feel physically attractive, their mental well-being also improves. Therefore, it is important to provide options for these patients seeking advice on the use of cosmetics for wrinkling, mottled pigmentation, or rough skin.

Tretinoin (all-*trans* retinoic acid) is a topical cream effective in improving fine wrinkling, rough skin, hyperpigmentation, and lentigines, when used daily.[55] A pea-sized drop should be applied nightly to clean, dry skin approximately 20 to 30 min after washing the face. In the morning, the face should be washed and a broad-spectrum sunscreen (blocking UVA and UVB) should be applied, as well as a moisturizer, if needed. Side effects include redness, scaling, burning, and irritation; these often improve with time or with a reduction in dosing strength or frequency. The alpha-hydroxy acids, especially glycolic acid, have recently been used to improve sun-damaged skin and wrinkling.[56] Lower concentrations in a cream or lotion formulation (5%–10%) can be used twice daily at home, alternating with use of higher concentrations applied as a peel. The latter is typically used at the physician's office, or now in beauty salons, at a concentration up to 70% for 2 to 6 min every 1 to 6 weeks. Each of the topical approaches exfoliates the skin and, therefore, may cause irritation in sensitive individuals. With patience, however, a regimen can be found for nearly everyone.

In cases of more severe sun damage, other procedures have been used. Injections of augmenting agents into the nasolabial fold, perioral, chin areas, and, less often, the forehead, may improve wrinkles. Several materials such as collagen, hyaluronic acid, and silicone have been used, but at the present time, collagen is a popular choice. These injections, which place collagen into the dermis underneath a wrinkle, plump up the depressed furrow of the wrinkle and therefore smooth the appearance of the skin. Several products and formulations are available. The choice of material used is dictated by the location and depth of the wrinkle, as well as by the experience of the physician. The effects are temporary, and patients often require touch-up injections every 3 to 6 months. Chemical peels, using either trichloroacetic acid or phenol, dermabrasion, and laser resurfacing have been used to treat wrinkles and lentigines. In experienced hands, trichloroacetic acid is a safe way to induce a medium-depth peel that may decrease the appearance of some wrinkles and even out skin tone. It is important to note that even a relatively safe peeling material such as 30% trichloroacetic acid may cause scarring as well as other complications. Therefore, it should be used only by experienced physicians. Phenol penetrates deeper, but it can cause hypopigmentation and cardiac arrhythmias, necessitating cardiac monitoring. An infrequent side effect of dermabrasion may be hypertrophic scarring. Laser may leave persistent erythema and, rarely, scarring. Botilinum A exotoxin has also been used to minimize those lines and wrinkles caused by muscular movement (i.e., "kinetic" wrinkles).[57] It is safest and most effective on crow's feet and glabellar and forehead lines. The toxin produces reversible paralysis of striated muscle. A facelift and eye surgery are other options for improving wrinkles and sagging skin.

References

1. Newcomer VD, Young EM Jr. *Geriatric Dermatology: Clinical Diagnosis and Practical Therapy.* New York: Igaku Shoin; 1989.
2. Leyden JJ. Clinical features of ageing skin. *Br J Dermatol.* 1990;122:1–3.
3. Price VH. Treatment of hair loss. *N Engl J Med.* 1999;341:964–973.
4. Rook A, Dawber R. *Diseases of the Hair and Scalp.* Boston: Blackwell; 1982.
5. Bolognia JL. Aging skin. *Am J Med.* 1995;98(1A):99S–103S.
6. Beacham BE. Solar-induced epidermal tumors in the elderly. *Am Fam Physician.* 1990;42:153–160.
7. Calderone DC, Fenske NA. The clinical spectrum of actinic elastosis. *J Am Acad Dermatol.* 1995;32:1016–1024.
8. Ogawa CM. Degenerative skin disorders: toll of age and sun. *Geriatrics.* 1975;30:65–69.
9. Shahrad P, Marks R. The wages of warmth: changes in erythema ab igne. *Br J Dermatol.* 1977;97:179–186.
10. Beacham BE. Common dermatoses in the elderly. *Am Fam Physician.* 1993;47:1445–1450.
11. Fleischer AB Jr. Pruritus in the elderly: management by senior dermatologists. *J Am Acad Dermatol.* 1993;28:603–609.
12. Lookingbill DP, Marks JG Jr. *Principles of Dermatology, 2nd Ed.* Philadelphia: Saunders; 1993.
13. Schoenfeld RJ, Schoenfeld FL. Angular cheilitis. *Cutis.* 1977;19:213–216.
14. Janniger CK, Schwartz RA. Seborrheic dermatitis. *Am Fam Physician.* 1995;52:149–155.
15. Thiboutot DM. Acne rosacea. *Am Fam Physican.* 1994;50:1691–1697.
16. Parsons JM. Transient acantholytic dermatosis (Grover's disease): a global perspective. *J Am Acad Dermatol.* 1996;35:653–666.
17. Bonifati C, Carducci M, Mussi A, et al. Recognition and treatment of psoriasis: special considerations in elderly patients. *Drugs Aging.* 1998;12:177–190.
18. Roujeau JC, Stern RS. Severe adverse cutaneous reactions to drugs. *N Engl J Med.* 1994;331:1272–1285.
19. Nousari HC, Anhalt GJ. Pemphigus and bullous pemphigoid. *Lancet.* 1999;354:667–672.
20. Fitzpatrick TB, Eisen AZ, Wolff K, et al. *Dermatology in General Medicine, 4th Ed.* New York: McGraw-Hill; 1993.
21. Imperial R, Helwig EB. Angiokeratoma of the scrotum (Fordyce type). *J Urol.* 1967;98:379–387.
22. Cohen JI, Brunell PA, Straus SE, et al. Recent advances in varicella-zoster virus infection. *Ann Intern Med.* 1999;130:922–932.
23. Ellis DH. Diagnosis of onychomycosis made simple. *J Am Acad Dermatol.* 1990;40:S3–S8.
24. Elewski BE. Diagnostic techniques for confirming onychomycosis. *J Am Acad Dermatol.* 1996;35:S6–S9.
25. Scher RK. Onychomycosis: therapeutic update. *J Am Acad Dermatol.* 1999;40:S21–S26.
26. Beacham BE. Common skin tumors in the elderly. *Am Fam Physician.* 1992;46:163–168.
27. Burg G. *Atlas of Cancer of the Skin.* Philadelphia: Churchill Livingstone; 2000.
28. Mehregan AH, Rahbari H. Benign epithelial tumors of the skin. II: Benign sebaceous tumors. *Cutis.* 1977;19:317–320.
29. Bodian EL. Techniques of sclerotherapy for sunburst venous blemishes. *J Dermatol Surg Oncol.* 1985;11:696–704.
30. Schwartz RA. Premalignant keratinocytic neoplasms. *J Am Acad Dermatol.* 1996;35:223–242.
31. Marks R, Rennie G, Selwood TS. Malignant transformation of solar keratoses to squamous cell carcinoma. *Lancet.* 1988;1:795–797.
32. Coleman WP III, Yarborough JM, Mandy SH. Dermabrasion for prophylaxis and treatment of actinic keratoses. *Dermatol Surg.* 1996;22:17–21.
33. Miller DL, Weinstock MA. Nonmelanoma skin cancer in the United States: incidence. *J Am Acad Dermatol.* 1994;30:774–778.
34. Kuflik AS, Schwartz RA. Actinic keratosis and squamous cell carcinoma. *Am Fam Physician.* 1994;49:817–820.
35. Schwartz RA. Keratoacanthoma. *J Am Acad Dermatol.* 1994;30:1–19.
36. Kuflik AS, Janniger CK. Basal cell carcinoma. *Am Fam Physician.* 1993;48:1273–1276.
37. Drake LA, Ceilley RI, Cornelison RL, et al. Guidelines of care for basal cell carcinoma. *J Am Acad Dermatol.* 1992;26:117–119.
38. Karagas MR, Stukel TA, Greenberg ER, et al. Risk of subsequent basal cell carcinoma and squamous cell carcinoma of the skin among patients with prior skin cancer. Skin

Cancer Prevention Study Group. *JAMA.* 1992;267:3305–3310.

39. Cohen LM. Lentigo maligna and lentigo maligna melanoma. *J Am Acad Dermatol.* 1995;33:923–936.

40. Johnson TM, Smith JW, Nelson BR, et al. Current therapy for cutaneous melanoma. *J Am Acad Dermatol.* 1995;32:689–707.

41. Schucter L, Schultz DJ, Synnestvedt M, et al. A prognostic model for predicting 10-year survival in patients with primary melanoma. *Ann Intern Med.* 1996;125:369–375.

42. Piepkorn M, Weinstock MA, Barnhill RL. Theoretical and empirical arguments in relation to elective lymph node dissection for melanoma. *Arch Dermatol.* 1997;133:995–1002.

43. Cole BF, Belber RD, Kirkwood JM, et al. Quality-of-life adjusted survival analysis of interferon alpha-2b adjuvant treatment of high-risk resected cutaneous melanoma: an Eastern Cooperative Oncology Group study. *J Clin Oncol.* 1996;14:2666–2673.

44. Bystryn JC, Shapiro RL, Harris M, et al. Use of vaccines in treatment of malignant melanoma. *Clin Dermatol.* 1996;14:337–341.

45. Bonnekoh B, Bickenbach JR, Roop DR. Immunological gene therapy approaches for malignant melanoma. *Skin Pharmacol.* 1997;10:105–125.

46. Ashikari R, Park K, Huvos AG, et al. Paget's disease of the breast. *Cancer.* 1970;26:680–685.

47. Lee SC, Roth LM, Ehrlich C, et al. Extramammary Paget's disease of the vulva: a clinicopathologic study of 13 cases. *Cancer.* 1977;39:2540–2549.

48. Antman K, Chang Y. Kaposi's sarcoma. *N Engl J Med.* 2000;342:1027–1038.

49. Goodfield M. Optimal management of chronic leg ulcers in the elderly. *Drugs Aging.* 1997;10:341–348.

50. Douglas WS, Simpson NB. Guidelines for the management of chronic venous leg ulceration. Report of a multidisciplinary workshop. *Br J Dermatol.* 1995;132:446–452.

51. Partsch H. Compression therapy of the legs. *J Dermatol Surg Oncol.* 1991;17:799–805.

52. Ryan TJ. Wound dressing. *Dermatol Clin.* 1993;11:207–213.

53. Leu HJ. Differential diagnosis of chronic leg ulcers. *Angiology.* 1963;14:288–296.

54. Gambert SR, Gaunsing AR. Protein-calorie malnutrition in the elderly. *J Am Geriatr Soc.* 1980;28:272–275.

55. Weiss JS, Ellis CN, Headington JT, et al. Topical tretinoin improves photoaged skin: a double-blind, vehicle-controlled study. *JAMA* 1988;259:527–532.

56. Van Scott EJ, Yu RJ. Alpha-hydroxy acids: procedures for use in clinical practice. *Cutis.* 1989;43:222–227.

57. Carruthers A, Kiene K, Carruthers J. Botulinum A exotoxin use in clinical dermatology. *J Am Acad Dermatol.* 1996;34:788–797.

59
Changes and Diseases of the Aging Eye

Bruce P. Rosenthal

The eye is a complex dynamic structure that undergoes physiologic and functional changes as well as significant pathological changes with age. In addition, vision may be affected by systemic conditions that are more prevalent after the age of 50, such as hypertension and diabetes. Visual performance, however, is not limited only to changes in the eye itself but may also be affected by changes to the surrounding structures, such as the eyelids, orbit, and internal and external muscles, as well as the visual pathways.[1-6]

There are other common functional as well as physiologic changes that take place in the aging visual system, including a decrease in visual acuity, accommodation, visual field, contrast sensitivity function, color vision, and recovery from a glare source. Bullimore et al.[7] found that the functional losses may ultimately affect the most basic of activities of daily living, including reading, and driving performance, as well as the ability to recognize faces.

Ginsberg[8] and Ginsberg et al.[9] found that contrast sensitivity function (CSF) is one of the most important measures of functional visual performance. Rubin et al.[10] found that contrast sensitivity function decreases from the early sixties to the nineties. It is especially important in the detection of changes of aging and ocular pathology in the visual system. Contrast sensitivity function is the eye's ability to detect the whiteness to the blackness of a target or the blackness to the whiteness of a target. Contrast sensitivity testing gives some indication of how a person sees under nonideal conditions and may give a more realistic indication of how a person sees. Rubin[11] also found that glare sensitivity and recovery from a bright light source are changes that may take place in the visual system with age. Glare recovery is a measure of the speed with which the visual system regains function following exposure to bright light.

Prevalence Studies

The Lighthouse National Survey on Vision Loss[12] revealed that the prevalence of vision impairment substantially increases with age. In fact, 15% of Americans aged 45 to 64 years (representing 7.2 million persons) self-report some form of vision impairment. This number increases to 17% of Americans aged 65 to 74 years and older (representing 3.1 million persons) and to 26% of Americans (3.5 million persons) aged 75 years and older.

Moderate and significant vision impairment can result in an inability to continue to perform activities of daily living (ADLs), such as reading, driving, watching television, or writing a check.[13,14] Horowitz and Reinhardt[15] and Kleinschmidt et al.[16] found that this could result in a loss of independence and social integration, as well as depression.

Demographics, Epidemiology, and Risk Factors

Definitions related to vision loss are important in a discussion on the demographics and epidemiology of the aging eye. Colenbrander[17] and Bailey[18] have categorized vision impairment as a condition that encompasses the continuum from near-normal vision with a slight deficit in the visual acuity or visual field to low vision with significantly reduced vision to profound vision loss and blindness (no light perception). About 7 million, or 21% of persons age 65 and over, report some form of visual impairment. This number will dramatically increase to 8.3 million in the year 2010, 11.2 million in 2020, and 15 million in 2030.[19] Blindness is defined as no usable vision with the exception of light perception. It is estimated by the American Foundation for the Blind that there are about 220,000 persons nationally in this category.[20] Only 1% of the functionally blind population at Lighthouse International are from the 45 to 64 age group; 5% are from the 65 to 84 age group and 0.6% are from the 85-plus age group.[21]

Legal blindness is another term that is important to define in determining disability, state, and social security benefits. Legal blindness is defined as a visual acuity of 20/200 or less in the better eye or a visual field of 20° or less in the better eye in the widest meridian.[22] Approximately 1.1 million Americans were in this category in 1992.[23]

Ocular Anatomy and Surrounding Structures

The eye and its surrounding structures are unique, often dependent structures that work in concert for optimum visual performance. The major anatomic ocular structures include (anterior to posterior in the eye) the eyelids, eyelashes, the cornea and its overriding tear film, conjunctiva, sclera, aqueous fluid, the canal of Schlemm and the trabecular meshwork (the aqueous fluid drainage complex), pupil, the lens and the zonules of Zinn (supporting "wires" for the lens), ciliary body, vitreous, retina, choroid, and optic nerve.[24]

The photons of light energy entering the eye are converted into chemical energy when the image falls on the retina. This image is then transferred via the optic nerve of the right and the left eye to the brain. Some of the fibers from the optic nerve of the right and the left eye cross over to the other side of the brain at the optic chiasm while some fibers remain uncrossed. Some of the visual information from the right nasal visual field is transmitted to the left visual cortex and some left nasal visual field information is transmitted to the right visual cortex. The visual information is processed and integrated in the brain with sensations such as form, texture, size, and taste. A cerebral vascular accident, however, may disrupt transmission and result in the loss of vision on one side (hemianopia) as well as visual neglect contralateral to the involved side.

In addition, two internal muscles and six external muscles are associated with each eye. The internal muscles, known as the dilator and constrictor, control the pupil's ability to constrict or dilate in response to ambient light. The six external muscles associated with each eye include the superior, inferior, internal, and external recti as well as the superior and inferior obliques. These muscles enable the eyes to work as a yoked "binocular" team for horizontal, vertical, and oblique movements as well as enable the eyes to converge to a point focus when reading.[25]

Sites of Care

Eyelids

The lids, which are not only protective in nature but also help to spread the tear film and prevent desiccation of the cornea, are predisposed to aging changes. They thin out with age, while the dermis[26] becomes dehydrated and loses its vascularity. The loss in tonicity is often associated with a condition such as myasthenia gravis[27] and results in a lid droop (ptosis) that may obscure the pupil. Non-surgical prosthesis, such as the ptosis crutch, which holds up the drooping lid, as well as surgical techniques may be indicated if the pupillary aperture is either partially or fully obscured.[28,29]

Dermatochalasis is another condition that may occur normally with aging. This condition is characterized by thin, loose redundant skin of the eyelids that may be severe enough to restrict peripheral vision.[30]

Another normal consequence of aging is ectropian or eversion of the lower lid. The eyelids lose tonicity and droop, which may result in exposure of the protective inner lining of the eyelids, the conjunctiva. Ectropian results not only in chronic conjunctival inflammation but in a thickening of the lid margins, excess tearing (epiphora), exposure keratitis (inflammation of the cornea),[31] and chronic dry eye. The latter is caused by the inability of the tears to reach the drainage canal of the lid (puncta).

Entropian, which is an involution of the eyelid (it may also be cicatricial or paralytic, i.e., cranial nerve VII palsy),[32] may result in the eyelashes rubbing up against and scratching the delicate epidermis of the cornea. Epilation (removal of the eyelashes) or surgical intervention may be required if the condition persists.

The eyelids may also be the sites of neoplasms, such as the most common malignant eyelid tumor, basal cell carcinoma, as well as squamous cell carcinoma.[33]

Tear Layer

The layer of tears produced by the lacrimal glands protects the cornea, as well as the inner surface of the lids, to keep them from drying out. DeRoetth,[34] Paschides et al.,[35] and others found that tear production begins to decrease markedly after age 40. By age 50, an individual produces half the tears produced at age 20 and by age 80 this is reduced to one-quarter in males and females. This decreased supply of tears may cause erosion of the cornea, dry spots, neovascularization, and scarring. Tear production is also decreased in the meibomian and goblet cells (contributors to the makeup of the tears); this may result in a thinning of the tear film that, in turn, reduces the stability of the tear layer.[36]

Talal[37] and Preston and Buchanan[38] have also found that systemic conditions, such as rheumatoid arthritis and

FIGURE 59.1. Cross section of the eye. (Courtesy of the National Eye Institute.)

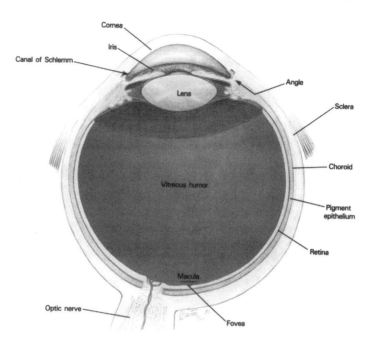

Sjögren's syndrome (over 90% are women, with the age of onset between 40 and 60) may also affect the supply of the tears to the eyes.

Conjunctiva

The conjunctiva is a transparent mucous membrane that overlies the sclera and lines the inside of the eyelids. It protects the eye from infection and injury. The conjunctiva is subject to infectious, allergic, metabolic, degenerative, vascular, and neoplastic changes in the elderly.

Cornea

The cornea is a multilayered transparent window of the eye that is composed of five distinct layers. It is one of the two major refracting structures of the eye (the other being the lens) that enable light to reach the retina. It is affected by pathologic and degenerative changes, becomes yellower with age, loses some of its transparency, and becomes more astigmatic in shape[39] (Fig. 59.1).

Corneal disease, in the elderly, may be the result of infections, metabolic changes, viruses, fungi, a decrease in the tear film, trigeminal nerve involvement, degenerations, and neoplasms.

Fuch's dystrophy is one of the common corneal conditions associated with aging and is found after the fifth decade. Kachmer et al.[40] have described it as an autosomal dominant disease that is 2.5 times more prevalent in women.[41] The condition, which may result in severe pain as well as a loss in transparency of the cornea, may be medically managed. However, transplantation of the cornea may be necessary to restore vision as well as to relieve pain.

Dry eye may also contribute to the changes in the integrity of the corneal structure. If left untreated, dry eye can result in severe visual disability. Remedies include insertion of small plugs (inserted into the drainage canal on the lid, the puncta) to increase tear supply, as well as supplementation with artificial tears.

Aqueous Fluid, Canal of Schlemm, and Glaucoma

The aqueous fluid, which is produced by the ciliary body, helps to maintain the intraocular pressure of the eye and is eventually drained through a structure known as Schlemm's canal and into the venous system.

Any change in the outflow of aqueous through Schlemm's canal can result in an elevation of the intraocular eye pressure. This elevation in pressure, known as glaucoma, in turn can result in damage to the optic nerve as well as the retina.

Glaucoma

Glaucoma is a group of diseases rather than a simple disease. It is generally classified into open- and closed-angle types. It is estimated that between 2 and 4 million people 40 and older have glaucoma.[42,43] The Baltimore Eye Study and the Barbados Eye study revealed an incidence of glaucoma of 6% in the African-American population and persons of West African ancestry in the Caribbean region.[44,45] Kahn and Milton[46] found a prevalence of glaucoma in 1.2% to 2% of the Caucasian population in the Framingham Eye Study.

Quigley and Vitale[47,48] estimated, from glaucoma prevalence studies, that there would be 2.43 million cases of open-angle glaucoma in the year 2000 in the United States and 67 million cases worldwide. There are no comparable statistics for closed angle.

There is no agreement that changes in the anterior chamber structures of the aging eye, including the trabecular meshwork and Schlemm's canal, are associated with glaucoma.[49] Grierson and Calthorpe,[50] however, believe that a change in resistance to outflow appears to be a primary causative agent in glaucoma that is associated with the normal aging changes. The aging changes include a loss of cells, increase in pigment in the endothelial cells of the trabecular meshwork, increase in thickening of the meshwork, and deposition of plaque in key areas[51] (Fig. 59.2).

The diagnosis of glaucoma[52] is generally made on the basis of elevated intraocular pressure, changes in the visual field, changes in the appearance of the optic nerve and optic disk, changes in the nerve fiber layer, and family history.

The symptoms of glaucoma, may include halos around lights, difficulty with mobility, difficulty in seeing under low levels of illumination, and difficulty with contrast. Glaucoma, if left untreated, will result in significant changes in the ganglion cell layer of the retina, optic nerve, and visual field.

Tonometry, the measurement of eye pressure, has traditionally been one of the tests to diagnose as well as manage glaucoma. However, damage may take place in the optic nerve even with "normal" eye pressures for that individual. Visual field testing (perimetry) is another measure used to determine the extent of vision loss in glaucoma. The newer types of automated perimeters help to precisely measure the damage of the visual field in decibels and are very analogous to a hearing test; this technique will enable the examiner to measure the effect of the various treatments used to preserve the remaining visual field.

The diagnosis and evaluation of the optic nerve head has changed dramatically with the introduction of retinal color photography, automated stereoscopic evaluation, digital optic nerve head analysis, scanning laser ophthalmoscopes, and nerve fiber layer analyzers.

Traditional treatment for glaucoma has included the instillation of eyedrops as well as surgery. However, there are numerous new medications that work on different mechanisms in the eye to reduce the eye pressure. Some beta-blockers are used to inhibit production by blocking beta receptors in the ciliary body. There are also carbonic anhydrase inhibitors that similarly reduce the production of aqueous, whereas epinephrine reduces aqueous production and to a less extent increases outflow of the fluid. In addition, there are adrenergic agonists, pilocarpine, and prostaglandin analogues that also increase aqueous outflow. Unfortunately, laser surgery or other filtering procedures may be indicated if damage continues.

Pupil

The pupil is basically an opening in the iris through which the aqueous fluid flows. Its size may vary in response to light, medication, emotional states, disease, or trauma as well as surgical procedures. The pupil functions in much the same manner as a diaphragm in a camera. It dilates under conditions of dim illumination and constricts when the illumination is increased.

Lowenfeld[53] found that the pupillary aperture decreases by about 2.5 mm between the age of 20 and 80 due to the loss in muscle tonus. This resultant decrease in the ambient light reaching the photosensitive layer, the retina, in turn may affect mobility as well as reading performance.[54]

Morgan[55] found that the pupillary response to ambient light diminishes with age and results in a smaller pupillary diameter. He found that the pupillary diameter diminishes from about 6 to 7 mm in the 20-year-old to 4 mm and less in the 75-year-old person.

Lens: Normal Aging Changes

The lens is commonly known as the crystalline lens, because of its impressive regularity, precise organization, and clarity in the early years of life.[56] It is avascular (no blood vessels) and is biconvex in shape. Positioned just behind the pupillary aperture, the lens is supported in place by tiny "guy wires" known as the zonules of Zinn.

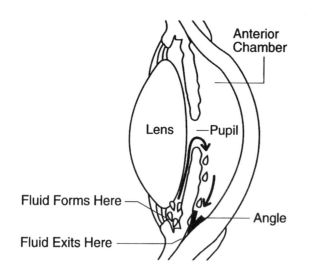

FIGURE 59.2. Aqueous outflow. (Courtesy of the National Eye Institute.)

Its construction is very similar to that of an onion or peach pit, having a cortex, nucleus, and capsule.

Weale[57] found that aging changes affect the transmission of light through the lens in the visible and the ultraviolet regions of the spectrum. In addition, there is a yellowing of the crystalline lens due to the slow growth of the lens throughout life. These factors result in a significant decrease of light reaching the retina with advancing age. In fact, Weale[58] found that only one-third of the amount of light reaches the retina of a 60-year-old compared to the retina of a 20-year-old.

Lens: Presbyopia

The most common of these "normal" aging changes, known as presbyopia, begins in the fourth decade. Beers and van der Hiejde,[59] Hamasaki et al.,[60] Ramsdale and Charman,[61] and Wagstaff[62] defined presbyopia as a natural age-related condition that is the result of a gradual decrease in accommodative amplitude, from about 15 diopters (D) in early childhood to 1 D before the age of 60 years.

Presbyopia is basically the inability to focus clearly on close objects or to see print clearly. The lens, which is a flexible structure that can change its shape into a more or less convex structure, begins to lose its elasticity in the third and fourth decade. Reading is not generally affected, however, until the early or mid-forties.

Pointer,[63] Patorgis,[64] and Jain et al.[65] found that the major risk factors for presbyopia are age, short stature, the occurrence of certain systemic diseases such as diabetes and cardiovascular disease, medications, trauma, hyperopia (farsightedness), and side effects of drugs. However, there are still major unanswered questions on the influence of genetics, caloric intake, hypertension, ethnic and racial factors, and environmental influences.

There has been a paradigm shift in the treatment for most eye conditions. Presbyopia was traditionally treated with reading lenses, contact lenses, bifocals, or trifocals. The latest optical designs include bifocal contact lenses as well as optical systems that allow the viewer to see simultaneously at distance and near. One of the more recent changes in the treatment of presbyopia, known as monovision, involves correction of the dominant eye for distance vision. Patients may either wear a contact lens or, more recently, have corrective surgery on the cornea to correct for near vision, which is done by inserting an intraocular lens (lens placed in the eye) to correct for close vision. One of the newest surgical advances includes a foldable silicone multifocal intraocular lens that allows the viewer to see more clearly at different distances.

The future will see intraocular lenses that will eventually be able to focus and reproduce the same effect as the normal lens does before the age of 40, as well as surgical procedures to reverse the effect of presbyopia.[66]

Lens: Cataracts

Leske, in The National Health and Nutritional Examination Survey (NHANES),[67] Taylor et al. in the Waterman Eye Study,[68] and Klein et al. in the Framingham Study[69] showed that there is also a significant increase in the prevalence of cataract with age. Podgor et al. showed, in The Framingham Eye Study,[70] that the prevalence of cataract was 5% in the 52 to 64 age group, 18% in the 65 to 74 group, and 46% of persons aged 75 to 85 years.

There is a steady increase in cataracts with age according to Kahn et al.[71]: 45.5% in individuals 52 to 64 years of age; 18.0% in individuals 65 to 74 years of age, and 45.9% in individuals 75 to 85 years of age. The Framingham Eye, NHANES, Punjab, and the Tibet Eye studies also showed a higher prevalence in females.[72]

Some of the risk factors for cataract development include excessive exposure to sunlight (UVB), age (as already noted), cigarette smoking,[73] high cholesterol and triglycerides, diabetes mellitus, cortisone medication, and eye injury.[74]

Surgical procedures have dramatically shifted to a procedure known as extracapsular cataract extraction.[75] Ophthalmic treatment for cataract has also evolved rapidly over the past 25 years from the prescription of thick heavy glass and plastic lenses to contact lenses to the posterior chamber-placed intraocular implant (IOL).[76] The IOL is the treatment of choice for more than 95% of persons undergoing cataract surgery in the Western world.

Vitreous

The vitreous is an avascular and acellular transparent jelly-like substance that occupies the central cavity of the eye and helps to maintain its shape. The vitreous is generally transparent throughout life but may contract, liquefy, shrink, and possibly detach in the aging eyes.

Vitreous hemorrhage, often a complication of proliferative diabetic retinopathy, results in a clouding of the vitreous. Charles[77] and Machemer[78] were instrumental in developing a procedure to remove the vitreous, known as a vitrectomy. The vitreous is often removed and replaced when delicate surgery is performed on the retina and the macular region.

Retina

The posterior lining of the eye, the retina, is a multilayered structure that contains the light-sensitive photoreceptors known as the rods and cones (Fig. 59.3). The cones, which respond to color, are tightly packed into the central area of the eye, known as the macula. The rods, which occupy the majority of the peripheral retina, respond to black and white and to low levels of illumi-

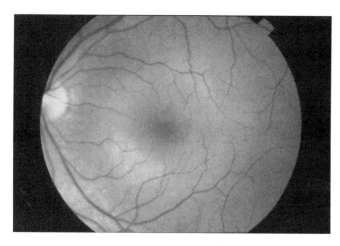

FIGURE 59.3. Normal retina: macula is pigmented area at the center. (Courtesy of the National Eye Institute.)

nation and are important in mobility. The central as well as the peripheral retina may be significantly affected by pathologic changes later in life from conditions such as macular degeneration, diabetic retinopathy, retinal detachment, central and branch artery and vein occlusions, and hemorrhagic disease.

The value of the macula far outweighs its size in relation to the rest of the retina, It is the area that contains the sharpest vision. Everyday tasks such as reading print and seeing facial features, television, and street signs are dependent upon an intact macula.

The choroid is the pigmented, heavy vascular layer lying between the retina and the sclera. It is a layer that is prone to the growth of new fragile leaky blood vessels in the "wet" form of macular degeneration.

Macular Degeneration

More than 13.2 million Americans (15%) have signs of age-related macular degeneration. That number climbs to 1 in 3 over the age of 75.[79] It is estimated that as the population ages, more people will become legally blind from macular degeneration than from glaucoma and diabetic retinopathy combined.[80]

Age-related macular degeneration, formerly known as senile macular degeneration, is primarily found in the Caucasian population. Known risk factors include smoking, light-colored irises, women over 60, familial history, and postmenopausal women who have not undergone hormonal replacement therapy, individuals taking antihypertensive drug therapy, and those having a high serum cholesterol level.[81]

Visual function may be dramatically affected in macular degeneration. Age-related macular degeneration might also be manifested by blurred vision, with difficulty

in seeing words, letters, faces, or street signs, as well as difficulty in differentiating colors.

There are primarily two types of age-related macular degeneration (AMD). The dry (atrophic) type, for which there is no treatment at this time, accounts for 90% of the new cases diagnosed. The wet type, also known as choroidal neovascularization or exudative maculopathy, accounts for the remaining 10% of the cases. The wet AMD is generally characterized by a more profound loss of visual function. However, despite the profound vision loss, there is usually enough peripheral vision to be able to function and travel safely.

Remediation includes traditional "thermal" laser as well as nonthermal photodynamic therapy for the wet AMD. The latter treatment may arrest the progressive loss of vision but never results in complete restoration of visual function. Additional research on AMD is being done with low-dose radiation, submacular surgery, cell transplantation, macular translocation, blood filtration, and vasogenic factors that stimulate the growth of new blood vessels.

Diabetic Retinopathy

Diabetic retinopathy is a microvascular complication of chronic diabetes mellitus.[82] Forty percent or 4.8 million of the estimated 12.7 million people over the age of 40 have diabetic retinopathy,[83] the majority having the more common background diabetic retinopathy. However, there are 700,000 people who have the proliferative, more destructive type of the disease. It is also estimated that 12,000 to 24,000 persons lose their sight from diabetic retinopathy.[84]

In addition to ongoing medical care, the diabetic may need laser photocoagulation and cataract extraction as the disease progresses. Vision rehabilitation is often indicated for the diabetic, especially those with advanced vision loss.

Optic Nerve

The optic nerve contains the retinal nerve fibers and consists of ganglion cell axons. It transmits the images falling on the retina to the visual pathway and eventually to the visual cortex. The optic nerve is also synonymous with the blind spot of the eye and contains no light-sensitive receptors where it exits the eye. The optic nerve may be affected by a number of disease processes including glaucoma, multiple sclerosis, and brain tumors.

Visual Field Loss

The etiology of visual field loss is generally glaucoma, stroke, or brain tumor. The vast majority (92%) of all strokes occur in patients aged 50 and older.[85] The incidence doubles with each successive decade.[86] The ocular consequences of stroke are often serious and may include transient vision loss as well as the loss of the right or the left side of vision (hemianopia) in both eyes or partial field loss. Hemianopia can also be the result of brain tumors that affect the older individual between 50 and 70 years.[87] Depending upon the location of the visual field loss, reading, as well as mobility, may be affected.

Individuals with hemianopia often read the entire eyechart to the 20/20 line because of macular sparing. However, there may still be an absolute or relative loss in the visual field. Many people are unaware that the vision is actually lost and can injure themselves unless instructed on the management of using the residual vision.

Stroke rehabilitation often requires a team approach and usually includes a variety of professionals for re-education in the areas of vision, mobility, speech, and cognitive functioning. The low-vision specialist may recommend techniques, and optical and nonoptical devices, as well as special lens systems to enhance visual performance.

Low Vision and Vision Rehabilitation

Vision rehabilitation may be an essential component in the management of the person with a visual impairment from macular degeneration, inoperable cataracts, glaucoma, diabetic retinopathy, or visual field loss from a stroke or tumor. Vision rehabilitation may involve many other professionals, including the eyecare professionals specializing in low vision, the optometrist (O.D.) or ophthalmologist (M.D.), as well as vision rehabilitation teachers, an orientation and mobility instructor, social workers, and an occupational therapist. The low-vision specialist will prescribe specialized optical, nonoptical, and electronic low-vision devices for distance and near tasks. A rehabilitation teacher may be called upon to teach how to safely manage one's kitchen and personal affairs, and an orientation or mobility instructor may be involved to teach safe independent cane travel.

Low-Vision Evaluation and Low-Vision Devices

A low-vision evaluation is an eye examination that may be ordered when the vision is not corrected with ordinary glasses, contact lenses, or medical treatment including surgery. The examiner will use specialized eyecharts to test visual acuity function at distance and near to determine the visual potential. Various researchers[88–91] have outlined specialized tests of visual function, including a contrast sensitivity test, evaluation of the macular function with the Amsler grid, visual field tests, color vision analysis, and photostress tests, that may be indicated.

Rosenthal and Williams[92] have demonstrated the value of the prescription of specialized low-vision devices for persons with a visual impairment ranging from mild to profound. These low-vision devices would be especially valuable with persons having a visual acuity ranging from 20/40 to 20/800, as well as for individuals with visual field and loss in contrast sensitivity function.

These specialized low-vision devices include high-powered reading lenses (microscopic lenses), hand and stand magnifiers, handheld and head-borne telescopic systems, absorptive and tinted lenses, closed-circuit television, and systems for persons with visual field defects. In addition, there are numerous nonoptical devices including lighting and illumination systems, reading stands, and talking devices, as well as high-contrast devices, that will help to improve visual performance.

References

1. Dutton JJ. Gliomas of the anterior visual pathway. *Surv Ophthalmol.* 1992;38:427–452.
2. Sadun AA, Rubin R. Sensory neuro-ophthalmology and vision impairment. In: Silverstone B, Lang MA, Rosenthal BP, Faye EE, eds. *The Lighthouse Handbook on Vision Impairment and Vision Rehabilitation.* New York: Oxford University Press; 2000.
3. Arnold AC, Hepler RS. Natural history of nonarteritic anterior ischemic optic neuropathy. *J Neuro-Ophthalmol.* 1994; 14:66–69.
4. Gentile M. *Functional Visual Behavior: A Therapist's Guide to Evaluation and Treatment Options.* Bethesda MD: The American Occupational Therapy Association; 1997.
5. Beard C. *Ptosis.* St. Louis: Mosby; 1976.
6. Mahoney BP. Sjogren syndrome. In: Mark ES, et al., eds. *Primary Eyecare in Systemic Disease.* Norwalk: Appleton and Lange; 1995.
7. Bullimore MA, Bailey IL, Wacker RT. Face recognition in age-related maculopathy. *Investig Ophthalmol Vis Sci.* 1991; 1:776–783.
8. Ginsburg AP. A new contrast sensitivity vision test chart. *Am J Optom Physiol Opthalmol.* 1984; 61:403–407.
9. Ginsburg AP, Rosenthal BP, Cohen JM. The evaluation of the reading capability of low vision patients using the Vision Contrast Test System (VCTS). In: Woo CG, ed. *Low Vision: Principles and Applications.* New York: Springer-Verlag; 1987:17–28.
10. Rubin GS, Bandeen-Roche K, Prasada-Rao P, Fried LP. Visual impairment and disability in older adults. *Optom Vision Sci.* 1994;71:750–760.
11. Rubin GS. Perceptual correlates of optical disorders of middle and later life. In: Silverstone B, Lang MA, Rosenthal BP, Faye EE, eds. *The Lighthouse Handbook on Vision Impairment and Vision Rehabilitation,* New York: Oxford University Press; 2000.

12. The Lighthouse Inc. *The Lighthouse National Survey on Vision Loss: The Experience, Attitudes, and Knowledge of Middle-Aged and Older Americans.* New York: The Lighthouse; 1995.

13. Kircher C. Economic aspects of blindness and low vision: a new perspective. *J Visual Impairment Blindness.* 1995;89: 506–513.

14. Horowitz A. Vision impairment and functional disability among nursing home residents. *Gerontologist.* 1994;34(3): 316–323.

15. Horowitz A, Reinhardt JP. Mental health issues in vision impairment. In: *The Lighthouse Handbook on Vision Impairment and Vision Rehabilitation.* New York: Oxford University Press; 2000.

16. Kleinschmidt JJ, Trunnell EP, Reading JC, White GL, Richardson GE, Edwards ME. The role of control in depression, anxiety, and life satisfaction among the visually impaired older adult. *J Health Educ.* 1995;26:26–36.

17. Colenbrander A. Dimensions of visual performance. *Trans Am Acad Ophthalmol Otolaryngol.* 1977;83:322.

18. Bailey IL. Measurement of visual acuity: towards standardization. In: *Vision Science Symposium.* Bloomington: Indiana University; 1988:215–230.

19. The Lighthouse Inc. *The Lighthouse National Survey on Vision Loss: The Experience, Attitudes, and Knowledge of Middle-Aged and Older Americans.* New York: The Lighthouse; 1995.

20. American Foundation for the Blind. Prevalence Estimates of Blindness and Low Vision in the United States: Late 1980's. New York: American Foundation for the Blind; 1989.

21. Annual Statistical Report of New York Lighthouse Vision Rehabilitation Services, Fiscal Year 2000.

22. Silverstone B, Lang MA, Rosenthal BP, Faye EE. *The Lighthouse Handbook on Vision Impairment and Vision Rehabilitation,* vol. 1. *Vision Impairment.* New York: Oxford University Press; 2000:xvii.

23. Chiang YP, Bassi LJ, Javitt JC. Federal budgetary costs of blindness. *Milbank Q.* 1992;70(2):319–340.

24. Spalton DJ, Hitching RA, Hunter PA. *Atlas of Clinical Ophthalmology.* Philadelphia: Lippincott; 1984.

25. London R. Versions and ductions. In: Eskridge JB, Amos JF, Barlett JD, eds. *Clinical Procedures in Optometry.* Philadelphia: Lippincott, 1991:61–71.

26. Michael D. Ocular disease in the elderly. In *Vision and Aging,* 2nd ed., Boston: Butterworth-Heinemann; 1992: 112–113.

27. Oosterhuis HJGH. The ocular signs and symptoms of myasthenia gravis. *Doc Ophthalmol.* 1982;52:363.

28. Innes AL. Prescribing conventional lenses for the low vision patient. In: Cole RG, Rosenthal BP, eds. *Remediation and Management of Low Vision.* St. Louis: Mosby-Year Book; 1996:194.

29. Steinbery I, Levine MR. Cysts, tumors, and abnormal positions of the eyelids in the elderly. In: Kwitko ML, Weinstock FJ, eds. *Geriatric Ophthalmology.* Orlando: Grune & Stratton; 1985:165–168.

30. Collins J. *Your Eyes: An Owners Guide.* Englewood Cliffs: Prentice Hall; 1995:158.

31. Michael DD. Ocular disease in the elderly. In: Rosenbloom AA, Morgan MW, eds. *Vision and Aging.* Boston: Butterworth-Heinemann; 1993:124–125.

32. Harkins T. Geriatric ocular disease. In: Aston SJ, Maino JH, eds. *Clinical Geriatric Eyecare.* Boston: Butterworth-Heinemann; 1993:66–67.

33. Katowitz JA. *Orbit, Eyelids and Lacrimal System.* San Francisco: American Academy of Ophthalmology; 1990.

34. De Roetth A. Lacrimation in normal eyes. *Arch Ophthalmol.* 1953;49:185–189.

35. Paschides CA, Petroutsos G, Psilas K. Correlation of conjunctival impression cytology with lacrimal function and age. *Acta Ophthalmol (Copen).* 1991;69(4):422–425.

36. Patel S, Farrell JC. Age-related changes in precorneal tear film stability. *Optom Vis Sci.* 1989;66:175.

37. Talal N. Sjogrens syndrome and connective tissue disease with other immunologic disorders. In: McCarty DJ, ed. *Arthritis and Allied Conditions.* Philadelphia: Lea & Febiger; 1989:810.

38. Preston SJ, Buchanan WW. Rheumatic manifestions of immune deficiency. *Clin Exp Rheumat.* 1989;7:547.

39. Rubin GS. Perceptual correlates of optical disorders of middle and later life. In: Silverstone B, Lang MA, Rosenthal BP, Faye EE. *The Lighthouse Handbook on Vision Impairment and Vision Rehabilitation,* vol. 1. *Vision Impairment.* New York: Oxford University Press; 2000.

40. Krachmer JH, Purcell JJ, Young CW, Bucher KD. Corneal endothelial dystrophy. *Arch Ophthalmol.* 1978;96:2035–2039.

41. Doughman DJ. Corneal disorders. In: Silverstone B, Lang MA, Rosenthal BP, Faye EE, eds. *The Lighthouse Handbook on Vision Impairment and Vision Rehabilitation.* New York: Oxford University Press; 2000:135–136.

42. Prevent Blindness America. *Vision Problems in the U.S.* 1994.

43. Glaucoma Foundation, Inc. [Online] http://www.glaucomafoundation.org. 2000.

44. Tielsch JM, Sommer A, Katz J, et al. Racial variations in the prevalence of primary open angle glaucoma: the Baltimore Eye Survey. *JAMA.* 1991;266:369–374.

45. Leske MC, Connell AMS, Schachat AP, Hyman L. The Barbados Eye Study: prevalence of open angle glaucoma. *Arch Ophthalmol.* 1994;112:821–829.

46. Kahn HA, Milton RC. Revised Framingham Eye Study: prevalence of glaucoma and diabetic retinopathy. *Am J Epidemiol.* 1980;111:769–776.

47. Quigley HA, Vitale S. Models of open-angle glaucoma prevalence and incidence in the United States. *Investig Ophthalmol Vis Sci.* 1997;38:83–91.

48. Quigley HA. Number of people with glaucoma worldwide. *Br J Ophthalmol.* 1996;80:389–393.

49. Chapman SA, Bonshek RE, Stoddart RW, O'Donoghue E, Gooda II K, McLeod D. Glycans of trabecular meshwork in primary open angle glaucoma. *Br J Ophthalmol.* 1996;80: 435–444.

50. Grierson I, Calthorpe CM. Characteristics of meshwork cells and age changes in the outflow system of the eye: their relevance to primary open-angle glaucoma. In: Mills KB, ed. *Glaucoma: Proceedings of the Fourth International Symposium of the Northern Eye Institute.* Manchester, UK: Pergamon Press; 1988:12–31.

51. Lewis T, Fingeret M. *Primary Care of the Glaucomas.* New York: McGraw-Hill; 2000.
52. Yablonski ME, Zimmerman TJ, Kass MA, Becker B. Prognostic significance of optic disc cupping in ocular hypertensive patients. *Am J Ophthalmol.* 1980;89:585–590.
53. Lowenfeld IE. Pupillary changes related to age. In: Thompson HS, Daroff R, Frisen L, et al., eds. *Topics in Neuro-Ophthalmology.* Baltimore: Williams & Wilkins; 1979:124–150.
54. Chylack LT. Age-related cataract. In: *The Lighthouse Handbook on Vision Impairment and Vision Rehabilitation.* New York: Oxford University Press; 2000.
55. Morgan MW. Changes in visual function in the aging eye. In: Rosenbloom AA, Morgan MW, eds. *Vision and Aging.* New York: Fairchild Publications; 1986:121–134.
56. Chylack LT. Age-related cataract. In: Silverstone B, Lang MA, Rosenthal BP, Faye EE, eds. *The Lighthouse Handbook on Vision Impairment and Vision Rehabilitation*, vol. 1, *Vision Impairment.* New York: Oxford University Press; 2000:35.
57. Weale RA. Age and the transmittance of the human crystalline lens. *J Physiol.* 1988;395:577–587.
58. Weale RA. Spatial and temporal resolution. In: *The Aging Eye.* New York: Harper & Row; 1963:144–153.
59. Beers APA, van der Hiejde GI. Age-related changes in the accommodative mechanism. *Optom Vis Sci.* 1996;73:235–242.
60. Hamasaki D, Ong J, Marg E. The amplitude of accommodation in presbyopia. *Am J Optom.* 1956;33:3–14.
61. Ramsdale C, Charman WN. A longitudinal study of the changes in the state accommodative response. *Opthalmol Physiol Optom.* 1989;9:255–263.
62. Wagstaff DF. The objective measurement of the amplitude of accommodation. Part VII. *Optician.* 1966;151:431–436.
63. Pointer JS. Broken down by age and sex. The optical correction of presbyopia revisited. *Ophthalmol Physiol Optom.* 1995;15(5):439–443.
64. Patorgis CJ. Presbyopia. In: Amos JF, ed. *Diagnosis and Management in Vision care.* Boston: Butterworths; 1987:203–238.
65. Jain IS, Ram J, Bupta A. Early onset of presbyopia. *Am J Optom Physiol Ophthalmol.* 1982;59:1002–1004.
66. Eye TECH update. July/August 2000.
67. Leske MC, Sperduto RD. The epidemiology of senile cataract: a review. *Am J Epidemiol.* 1983;118(2):152–165.
68. Taylor HR, West SK, Rosenthal FS, et al. Effect of ultraviolet radiation on cataract formation. *N Engl J Med.* 1988;319(22):1429–1433.
69. Klein BEK, Klein RK, Linton KLP. Prevalence of age-related lens opacities in a population. The Beaver Dam Eye Study. *Ophthalmology.* 1992;99:546–552.
70. Podgor MJ, Leske MC, Ederer F. Incidence estimates for lens changes, macular changes, open angle glaucoma and diabetic retinopathy. *Am J Epidemiol.* 1983;118(2):206–212.
71. Kahn HA, Leibowitz HM, Ganley JP, et al. The Framingham Eye Study: I. Outline and major prevalence findings. *Am J Epidemiol.* 1977;106:17–32.
72. *Clinical Practice Guideline* Number 4: *Cataract in Adults: Management of Functional Impairment.* Cataract Management Guideline Panel, U.S. Dept of Health and Human Services, Public Health Service, Agency for Health Care Policy and Research, Rockville, MD, AHCPR Publication No. 93-0542, Feb 1993, 13–15.
73. Rouhiainen P, Rouhiainen H, Salonen JT. Association between low plasma vitamin E concentration and progression of early cortical lens opacities. *Am J Epidemiol.* 1996;144:496–500.
74. Faye EE, Rosenthal BP, Sussman-Skalka CJ. Cataract and the aging eye. New York: Lighthouse International, Center for Vision and Aging; 1995.
75. Jaffe NS, Jaffe MS, Jaffe GF. *Cataract Surgery and Its Complications, 5th Ed.* St. Louis: Mosby-Yearbook; 1990:34.
76. Lindquist TD, Lindstrom RL. Ophthalmic surgery: loose-leaf and update service. St. Louis: Mosby-Yearbook; 1994:1-F-1.
77. Charles S. *Vitreous Microsurgery.* Baltimore: Williams & Wilkins; 1981.
78. Machemer R. *Vitrectomy: A Pars Plana Approach.* New York: Grune & Stratton; 1975.
79. Prevent Blindness America. *Vision Problems in the U.S.* 1994.
80. National Advisory Eye Council. *Vision Research—A National Plan: 1994–1998.* (NIH 95-3186.) Bethesda, MD: National Institutes of Health; 1993.
81. Rosenthal BP. *Living Well with Macular Degeneration.* New York: NAL Penguin/Putnam; 2001.
82. Leonard B, Charles S. Diabetic retinopathy. In: Silverstone B, Lang MA, Rosenthal BP, Faye EF, eds. *The Lighthouse Handbook on Vision Impairment and Vision Rehabilitation.* New York: Oxford University Press; 2000:106–111.
83. Prevent Blindness America. *Vision Problems in the U.S.* 1994.
84. Will JC, Geiss LS, Wetterhall SF. Diabetic retinopathy [letter to the editor]. *N Engl J Med.* 1990;323:613.
85. Cockburn DM. Ocular implications of systemic disease in the elderly. In: Rosenbloom A, Morgan M, eds. *Vision and Aging.* Boston: Butterworth-Heinemann; 1993.
86. Blaustein BH. Cerebrovascular disease. In: Marks ES, Adamczyk DT, Thomann KH, eds. *Primary Eyecare in Systemic Disease.* Norwalk, CT: Appleton & Lange; 1995:55.
87. Messner LV. Primary intracanial tumors. In: Marks ES, Adamczyk DT, Thomann KH, eds. *Primary Eyecare in Systemic Disease.* Norwalk, CT: Appleton & Lange; 1995:67.
88. Rosenthal BP, Fischer ML. Optometric asessment of low vision. In: Gentile M, ed. *Functional Visual Behavior: A Therapist's Guide to Evaluation and Treatment Options.* Bethesda, MD: American Occupational Therapy Association; 1997:345–373.
89. Cole RG, Rosenthal BP. *Remediation and Management of Low Vision.* St. Louis: Mosby; 1997.
90. Rosenthal BP, Cole RG. *Functional Assessment of Low Vision.* St. Louis; Mosby; 1996.
91. Faye EE. *Clinical Low Vision, 2nd ed.* Boston: Little, Brown; 1984.
92. Rosenthal BP, Williams DR. Devices primarily for people with low vision. In: Silverstone B, Lang MA, Rosenthal BP, Faye EE, eds. *The Lighthouse Handbook on Vision Impairment and Vision Rehabilitation,* vol. 1. *Vision Impairment.* New York: Oxford University Press; 2000.

60
Otologic Changes and Disorders

George A. Gates and Thomas S. Rees

Age-related hearing loss is one of the most frequent health problems encountered in geriatric medicine. It is the third most prevalent major chronic disability in the over-65-year-old age group. Unfortunately, hearing loss is a disorder that is frequently unrecognized, frequently misunderstood, and all too frequently neglected, both by the affected themselves as well as by health care providers.

Presbycusis, literally meaning "elder hearing," is the generic term applied to age-related hearing loss and is used to signify the sum of all the processes that affect hearing with the passage of time. The prevalence of self-reported hearing problems among the elderly is 30%.[1] The prevalence increases substantially with age, with a 10-dB reduction in hearing sensitivity per decade of life after age 60. Although only slightly more than 1% of people under the age of 17 have hearing loss, the prevalence rises to 12% between the ages of 45 and 64, to 24% between the ages of 65 and 74, and up to 39% for those over 75 years. In the Framingham Heart Study Cohort (ages 63–95), the prevalence of hearing loss for the speech frequencies was 42%.[2] It is predicted that, by the year 2030, older adults will comprise 32% of the population, and as many as 60% to 75% of the elderly will suffer hearing loss, approximately 21 million persons.

Hearing loss impairs communication, subtly at first, and increasingly so as the magnitude of the hearing loss increases. Impairment in the ability to hear and understand speech leads older adults to withdraw from life's activities, resulting in social isolation and depression.[3,4] Significant social, emotional, and communication difficulties have been associated with hearing loss in the elderly. Social and emotional handicaps are present even in those with only mild to moderate hearing loss. Bess and associates analyzed the impact of hearing impairment in elderly patients by using the Sickness Impact Profile (SIP) to measure functional and psychosocial impairment.[3] Poor hearing was associated with higher SIP scores (greater impairment) and increased dysfunc-

tion. Even mild amounts of hearing loss were related to poorer function. Hearing loss has also been implicated as a cofactor in senile dementia.[5] Although measures for hearing loss identification and remediation are widely available, they are frequently underutilized.

Symptoms of Presbycusis

Age-related hearing loss is manifested by deterioration in each of the two critical dimensions of hearing: reduction in threshold sensitivity and reduction in the ability to understand speech. The loss in threshold sensitivity is insidious in onset, beginning in the highest frequencies (8000 Hz) and slowly progressing to involve those frequencies important in speech understanding (1000–3000 Hz range). The most common complaint of presbycusic patients is not that "I can't hear"; rather, it is "I can't understand." The high frequency hearing impairment causes the voiceless consonants (t, p, k, f, s, and ch) to be rendered unintelligible. For example, people confuse "mash, math, map, and mat," or "Sunday" with "someday." Seniors often complain that others "mumble" and they cannot participate in conversations because bits and pieces of speech are missing. As the hearing loss worsens to affect the lower frequencies with advancing years, the older person requires greater volume for speech detection and often needs repetition or confuses what is said. Everyday sounds, such as beepers, turn signals, and escaping steam are not heard, which places the hearing-impaired at greater risk of injury and makes them more isolated from the everyday world.

Whenever the speech message is degraded, the older listener's understanding difficulties increase dramatically. Rapid speech, foreign accents, and speech through poor transmitting equipment (i.e., airport intercoms) are often not understood. In addition, speech understanding in poor acoustic environments, such as noisy restaurants and large reverberant rooms, presents substantial difficulties for the hearing-impaired senior. Older adults typically have greater difficulties in speech understanding and processing than do younger persons with comparable hearing loss.[6] It has been postulated that some of these difficulties are due to a central integrative and synthesizing hearing disability that reflects a progressive deterioration within the central auditory pathways.[7]

Pathogenesis of Presbycusis

The major components of presbycusis are noise toxicity and aging.[8] Other factors are genetic susceptibility, age-related diseases, and ototoxic medications. Damage to the hearing is cumulative from the effects of these various factors. Much of our knowledge about presbycusis comes from cross-sectional studies of large cohorts. While it is generally possible to sort out the components of presbycusis in individuals, it is difficult to do so with group data. Therefore, presbycusis is best used as an inclusive term to signify all the processes that affect hearing with the passage of time, rather than limiting its meaning to aging per se.

The aging process has three distinct components: physiologic degeneration, extrinsic insults, and intrinsic insults. These factors are superimposed on a genetic substrate and possibly overshadowed by age-related susceptibility to disease. In the auditory system, the extrinsic component (nosocusis) includes hearing loss due to otologic disease, hazardous noise exposure, acoustic trauma, and ototoxic agents. The intrinsic component (sociocusis) indicates the wear-and-tear effects of exposure to the everyday sounds of normal living.[9] People who live in nonindustrialized regions avoid both nosocusis and sociocusis and demonstrate excellent hearing into old age.[10]

Although hearing steadily worsens with age, the rate of change is not linear, is highly variable, and is only weakly associated with chronologic age. For example, in comparing the change in hearing thresholds of the Framingham subjects over the 6-year interval between examinations 15 and 18, less than 10% of the variance is accounted for solely by age.[11] This finding suggests that other factors affect hearing more than age alone. In our industrialized society, it is difficult to escape from noise pollution. It is likely that much of the variance in levels of presbycusis is due to unmeasured effects of noise damage, which is the most common form of ototoxicity. The effects of systemic disease on hearing are still incompletely understood but may contribute as well. For example, older people with prior cardiovascular disease (CVD) events have poorer hearing than do those without CVD.[12]

Four types of presbycusis have been described, based on audiograms and postmortem histopathologic findings.[13] Sensory presbycusis involves loss of cochlear hair cells in the basal end of the cochlea and secondary degeneration of associated neurons. It usually begins in middle age and is characterized by steeply sloping high-frequency hearing loss and proportional reduction in word recognition. Neural presbycusis involves primary degeneration of cochlear neurons and central auditory pathways. The most significant clinical finding is disproportionately severe loss of word recognition ability, much poorer than would be expected from pure tone findings. Metabolic presbycusis is characterized by a flat pure tone audiogram with excellent word recognition and is due to atrophy of the stria vascularis in the cochlea. Mechanical (cochlear conductive) presbycusis is thought to result from stiffening of the basilar membrane and is reflected by a gradually sloping audiogram and word recognition that is correspondingly affected to a greater degree. In clinical practice, the majority of cases of age-related hearing loss appear as a mixture of types. The data of the Framingham Cohort showed most patients fell into the sensory category, and pure neural types were infrequent.[14]

Hearing Loss Types

Hearing loss is traditionally classified as conductive, sensorineural, and central. These types are based on the site of structural damage or blockage in the auditory system. Conductive hearing loss arises from obstruction of sound transfer through the external or middle ear space or both. Cerumen impaction represents the most common external ear cause of conductive hearing loss and is a frequently overlooked problem in elderly people whose ear canals often "collapse" with age. Cerumen impaction is commonly the result of misguided attempts by people to clean their ear canals with Q-tips. Other types of conductive loss, such as otitis media and otosclerosis, seldom arise primarily in the senior years. Unilateral middle ear effusion can be a sign of nasopharyngeal cancer but is more commonly the result of an ear infection.

A sensorineural hearing loss involves damage to the cochlea or fibers of the eighth cranial nerve. "Nerve deafness" and "perceptive deafness" are obsolete terms for sensorineural hearing loss that are occasionally encountered. Sensorineural hearing loss may be sensory only (cochlear hair cell loss), may involve the auditory nerve or brainstem (neural), or both. Newer diagnostic methods permit finer distinctions between sensory and neural losses. Now, by measuring otoacoustic emissions (OAEs) the status of the outer hair cells in the cochlea can be determined quickly and objectively. OAEs are very soft sounds produced by the contraction of the outer hair cells either spontaneously or in response to sound input into the ear. Sensorineural hearing loss due to presbycusis affects both ears equally and generally begins in the higher frequencies. Unilateral sensorineural hearing loss may be caused by a neoplasm (acoustic neuroma), acoustic trauma (blast injury), or a viral infection or vascular event (sudden sensorineural hearing loss). Sudden sensorineural hearing loss may be accompanied by vestibular symptoms of vertigo, dizziness, and nystagmus. Idiopathic sudden sensorineural hearing loss often recovers with prompt corticosteroid therapy. Therefore, immediate otologic referral is indicated for evaluation and treatment. Metabolic causes of hearing impairment are seen in endocrine diseases—thyroid, pancreatic, and adrenal, and in renal disease, diabetes mellitus, and hypertension.

Central auditory dysfunction is far less common and is seen in conditions such as stroke and Alzheimer's disease, neoplasm, multiple sclerosis, and degenerative disorders.[15]

Clinical Evaluation of Hearing Loss

The History and Physical Examination

The otologic examination is preceded by a carefully taken patient history. In the case of hearing loss, the time of onset, whether the loss was gradual or sudden, and the presence or absence of associated symptoms, especially vertigo, tinnitus, discharge, or pain, should be noted. Family history, noise exposure history, previous ear or head trauma, and use of ototoxic drugs should also be included. People with substantial exposure to workplace noise, recreational noise, and firearm use are more likely to have irreversible high-frequency hearing loss. Medication history should be explored to determine possible ototoxicity. Aminoglycoside antimicrobials, *cis*-platinum, loop diuretics, and anti-inflammatory agents may contribute to hearing loss. Metabolic evaluation is indicated if the patient has not had a recent health examination. Diabetes, hypertension, and hyperlipidemia should be excluded as cofactors. Patients receiving renal dialysis often have poorer hearing than would be expected from age alone. Hearing loss does cluster in families, particularly the strial form of presbycusis.

The physical examination of the ear canal and tympanic membrane is typically normal in most seniors, with the exception of cerumen accumulation in some. Cerumen removal with either ear canal irrigation, often preceded by use of cerumen-dissolving drops (10% sodium bicarbonate is the most effective), or manual (instrumental) removal is necessary. Although the removal of occluding cerumen can result in hearing improvement for some individuals, most often the locus of the hearing loss is in the sensorineural system. Itching and dryness of the external canal is a common complaint among seniors. The itching is often temporarily relieved

TABLE 60.1. Medical referral guidelines.

Visible congenital or traumatic deformity of the ear, including perforation of the eardrum
History of, or active, drainage from the ear within the previous 90 days
History of sudden or rapidly progressive hearing loss within the previous 90 days
Acute or chronic dizziness
Any unilateral hearing loss
Visible evidence of significant cerumen accumulation or foreign body in the ear canal
Pain or discomfort in the ear

by their Q-tip use, but this habit inevitably worsens the dryness and itching due to trauma of the canal. Aging causes atrophy of the canal epithelium and underlying sebaceous and cerumen glands, which results in decreased hydration of the canal skin and increased susceptibility to Q-tip abrasion. Patients should avoid putting anything in their canals. Canal itching can be controlled with steroid-based creams as needed.

Examination of the tympanic membrane should be accompanied by pneumatic otoscopy to assess tympanic membrane mobility. In people with middle ear effusion, the drum does not move or moves very little. Relying on the "color" of the tympanic membrane to diagnose effusion may be misleading. Commonly seen is opacification of the normally translucent tympanic membrane (tympanosclerosis); this has no effect on conduction of sound energy into the inner ear and is simply a manifestation of age.

Imaging studies are not indicated except where the loss is unilateral or significantly asymmetric, or where tinnitus is unexplained by the audiogram. Screening MRI examinations using the T_2 fast spin echo technique provide superb visualization of the eighth nerve and brainstem and can detect tumors in the millimeter range, even before hearing is affected.[16] Table 60.1 lists several "warning signs" associated with the history and physical examination that should prompt referral to an otolaryngologist for complete evaluation and treatment.

Screening Audiometry

Although it would seem prudent for health care providers to screen for one of the most prevalent chronic conditions affecting the elderly, this is unfortunately not the practice with hearing loss identification.[4] Moreover, even when elderly patients have discussed their hearing difficulties with their primary care providers, they are often told that their hearing loss is minor or that it cannot be improved with a hearing aid.[17] When one considers the adverse effects of hearing loss on quality of life and that such effects are reversible with hearing aids, it is surprising that in-office hearing loss screening is not common practice.

TABLE 60.2. Audiometric screening chart.

Intensity	Frequency		
	1000 Hz	2000 Hz	3000 Hz
25 dB (normal)			
40 dB (borderline)			
60 dB (fail)			

25 dB, normal hearing; 40 dB, borderline (referral dependent upon patient's self-perceived handicap); 60 dB, fail; 0, right ear; X, left ear.

Tuning forks, whispered/spoken voice, or finger friction test, which are used by many practitioners, are not effective and reliable approaches to hearing loss identification. The use of screening audiometry is the tool of choice in the identification of hearing loss. Screening audiometry can be quickly and easily administered by a trained office nurse or medical assistant. The equipment needed for screening audiometry is lightweight and low cost. There are portable, battery-operated audiometers and even specially developed otoscopes with audiometric capabilities available for the practitioner.[18] A portable audiometer can be used to screen hearing at 1000, 2000, and 3000 Hz at intensity levels of 25 dB (normal), 40 dB (borderline), and 60 dB HL. Failure at any one frequency at 25 dB for younger adults or 40 dB for older adults suggests the need for referral for a complete audiologic evaluation.[19] A sample form for recording audiometric screening results is shown in Table 60.2.

Self-Assessment

The simplest self-assessment screening method is to ask patients if they think they have a hearing problem. This single question is more sensitive than multi-item questionnaires, which are more specific. A number of self-assessment inventories have been developed as a means of evaluating hearing handicap. These scales quantify hearing handicap by including questions about the self-perceived situational and psychosocial effects of decreased hearing on various aspects of daily function. One of these scales, the Hearing Handicap Inventory for the Elderly–Screening Version (HHIE-S), is specifically designed for use with noninstitutionalized elderly (Table 60.3).[20] It has been shown to be a reliable and valid method for delineating handicapping hearing impairment among aging persons and is a good screening tool for primary care practices.[21] The HHIE-S can be completed by patients in about 10 min while they are waiting for their appointment or may be verbally administered by the practitioner or assistant. The inventory consists of 10 questions about circumstances related to hearing. Patients simply circle whether or not they have a problem in that situation. A "yes" response scores 4 points, a "sometimes" scores 2 points, and a "no" scores 0. Total scores range from 0 to 40, with a score of 40 representing the maximum self-perceived hearing handicap. Scores of 0 to 10 are unlikely to occur in people with significant hearing loss; scores of 26 to 40 should prompt referral for otologic/audiologic evaluation. Intermediate scores are ambiguous. The person with a score of 12 to 24 who notes having a hearing problem should be referred for testing, but a similar score in one who denies having a problem should not be a cause for action.

Patients who fail audiometric screening tests, or have a high self-perceived hearing handicap, should be referred for formal audiologic and otologic assessment. This evaluation will delineate the pattern and degree of loss, indicate the likely site of loss, and predict the suitability of otologic treatment or amplification for rehabilitation. Central auditory tests are widely available and should be considered when the possibility of early dementia exists. People with clinical Alzheimer's disease have poor central auditory function. We have recently shown that poor performance on a standard central auditory test (Synthetic Sentence Identification with

TABLE 60.3. Hearing Handicap Inventory for the Elderly—Screening Version (HHIE-S).

Please answer the following questions by circling the appropriate letter: **Y** = yes, **N** = no, **S** = sometimes.

	Y	N	S
1. Does a hearing problem cause you to feel embarrassed when meeting new people?	Y	N	S
2. Does a hearing problem cause you to feel frustrated when talking to members of your family?	Y	N	S
3. Do you have difficulty hearing when someone speaks in a whisper?	Y	N	S
4. Do you feel handicapped by a hearing problem?	Y	N	S
5. Does a hearing problem cause you difficulty when visiting friends, relatives, or neighbors?	Y	N	S
6. Does a hearing problem cause you to attend religious services less often than you would like?	Y	N	S
7. Does a hearing problem cause you to have arguments with family members?	Y	N	S
8. Does a hearing problem cause you difficulty when listening to TV or radio?	Y	N	S
9. Do you feel that any difficulty with your hearing limits or hampers your personal or social life?	Y	N	S
10. Does a hearing problem cause you difficulty when in a restaurant with relatives and friends?	Y	N	S

"Yes" = 4 points; "Sometimes" = 2 points; "No" = 0 points; total possible = 40.

Contralateral Competing Message) precedes the clinical onset of dementia by many years.[22] With the possibility of treatments to forestall the progression of Alzheimer's disease, early identification may be of great importance.

Hearing Loss Rehabilitation

Medical–Surgical Treatment

Hearing loss caused by conductive deficits (e.g., otosclerosis, otitis media, eardrum perforations, etc.) can most often be successfully treated with medical or surgical intervention by an otolaryngologist. Eardrum perforations can be surgically repaired (myringoplasty), middle ear fluid can be removed and the middle ear aerated (myringotomy with placement of a pressure equalization tube), a nonmobile stapes can be removed and replaced with a prosthesis (stapedectomy), and an absent or disarticulated ossicle can be replaced with a prosthesis (ossicular chain reconstruction). These procedures generally can eliminate the conductive hearing loss and return hearing to normal or near-normal levels.

Once thought to be untreatable, some cochlear lesions are now responding to medical therapy. About one-third of people with sudden hearing loss recover hearing. For example, the majority of people with autoimmune hearing loss recover substantial amounts of hearing with corticosteroid and other anti-immune treatment, such as methotrexate and plasmapheresis. However, for the vast majority of people with presbycusis, definitive treatment must await the results of our ongoing research programs in hair cell regeneration. This section will undoubtedly be expanded in the next decade or two.

Hearing Aid Amplification

The most common site of age-related hearing loss is dysfunction in the cochlea or associated neural structures. Of all patients with sensorineural hearing loss, less than 5% can be helped medically. Consequently, hearing aid amplification is the principal resource for improving communication and reducing hearing handicaps in persons with sensorineural hearing loss. Unfortunately, only 10% of people who might benefit from an aid actually own one, which indicates a substantial underservice. Current hearing aids include devices that fit behind the ear, in the canal, and, most recently, completely in the canal. Those seniors with dexterity problems or vision impairments are often unable to insert and adjust the smaller aids properly and are better served with larger hearing aids. The audiologist reviews such issues with the hearing-impaired individual during the prefitting session.

Today's hearing aids have evolved from simple devices to remarkably sophisticated technologically advanced instruments. In just the past few years, more advances in hearing aid technology have been made than throughout history. Hearing aids no longer merely provide linear amplification but may include compression circuitry to reduce the amplification for loud sounds. There are also hearing aids that include several programs for use at the listener's discretion, because a single amplification paradigm may not be of benefit for all listening situations. One may choose a wide frequency band amplification for quiet environments, another program that reduces low frequencies for noisier situations, and a program specifically suited for telephone use. These hearing aids are digitally programmed by an external programmer or computer through a microchip within the hearing aid itself. Customized programming of the hearing aid enables the dispenser to make significant electroacoustic modifications to an individual's needs and to change the hearing aid parameters if the hearing loss should change in future years.

Conventional hearing aids typically use omnidirectional microphones, which pick up sounds from all directions. These microphones are helpful in quiet situations, but persons often complain of amplification of background noise in restaurants and groups. Directional and dual microphones are now available in hearing aids that attenuate sounds from the back or side and focus on sounds from the front of the listener. The hearing aid user can choose either the directional microphone or omnidirectional microphone to suit the listening situation.

The most recent introduction in hearing aid technology is the fully digital instrument. These aids offer complex sound processing, fitting flexibility, precision in signal manipulation, multiple memories, multiple channels, and automatic feedback reduction capabilities, which are not available in conventional devices. Although digital aids are considerably more expensive than conventional aids, the benefits may by justified by many hearing-impaired persons. One must consider the acoustic and communicative needs of an individual patient and determine the appropriate level of hearing aid technology. If the patient does not participate in social activities and has few demands placed on their hearing, a digital hearing aid is inappropriate. If, on the other hand, the patient is socially active and encounters a variety of listening environments and high hearing demands, digital hearing aids with multiple memories and dual microphone technology are highly beneficial and worth the added cost.

The choice of hearing aid depends on the type of hearing loss, cosmetic concerns, and manual ability to insert/remove and care for the device. A telephone coil (T coil) should be available to optimize telephone use. Dispensing audiologists provide sophisticated evaluations to select and program the optimal device, and also provide training and long-term rehabilitative services.

These audiologists may practice in an otology office, a speech and hearing clinic, or independently. Some hearing aid dealers are relatively skilled in the fitting of hearing aids, but others possess only minimal training or are more oriented to sales. Many states, in fact, require that a hearing aid dealer meet only the minimum requirements of being 18 years old and passing a state licensing examination; there are typically no educational requirements. The clinical audiologist, on the other hand, holds at least a master's degree in the evaluation and rehabilitation of hearing loss. The audiologist is uniquely qualified to provide a full range of auditory assessment and rehabilitative services to elderly persons.

The industry standard of practice is to provide the user with at least a 30-day trial period with amplification and to refund the cost of the hearing aid if it is returned. The new amplification systems are considerably more expensive than conventional hearing aids. Currently, digital in-the-canal aids cost approximately $2500 per aid, and binaural aids are typically most beneficial. Neither Medicare nor most insurance carriers provide financial coverage for hearing aids. The specific hearing needs, lifestyle, and adaptability of the hearing aid wearer must be taken into account during the prefitting process.

Assistive Listening Devices

Although substantial improvements have been achieved in hearing aid design and application, few of the hearing-impaired can ever come close to achieving "normal" auditory function with the use of hearing aids alone. The inherent physiologic restrictions imposed by age-related hearing loss, coupled with the electronic constraints of hearing aids, render "normal hearing" impossible, especially considering the levels of noise and background interference found in most public places. The amplification of unwanted sounds (e.g., multiple speakers in groups, background noise, ventilation) by hearing aids often causes the desired message to be rendered unintelligible.

Assistive listening devices (ALDs) constitute a growing number of situation-specific amplification systems designed for use in difficult listening environments. ALDs commonly use a microphone placed close to the desired sound source (e.g., a television, theater stage, or speaker's lectern), and sound is directly transmitted to the listener. Several transmission methods include infrared, audio loop, FM radio, or direct audio input. Desired sounds are enhanced while competing extraneous noises are decreased, thus permitting improved understanding. These ALDs are becoming more available in churches, theaters, and classrooms, enabling hearing-impaired seniors to avoid the isolation imposed by the inability to hear a sermon, play, or public address.

Other assistive listening devices, such as small portable pocket amplifiers, are very helpful in medical situations.

These amplifiers are particularly well suited for health care professionals' communication with the hearing-impaired elderly. Often it is in the setting of acute health care delivery that older patients have misplaced or forgotten their own hearing aids. Portable amplifiers can save the voice and patience of the health care provider and allow respectful and private interactions to take place. Amplified telephones, low-frequency doorbells, amplified ringers, and closed-captioned TV decoders are just a few examples of the number of devices currently available for the hearing-impaired for everyday use. Flashing alarm clocks, alarm bed vibrators, and flashing smoke detectors provide valuable help for severely hearing-impaired individuals. Audiologists can provide such devices for their patients.

Implantable Hearing Aids

Surgically implantable hearing systems are in field testing in the United States and Europe. These systems avoid the discomfort many people experience with ear molds and they eliminate the telltale "squeal" or acoustic feedback that is so common when the ear mold does not fit tightly. It is likely that some of these systems will be available commercially in the very near future.

Cochlear Implants

Cochlear implants are used frequently for older deafened adults with excellent results. The cochlear implant is a neural stimulator with an electrode array that is surgically placed inside the cochlea. Speech sounds are extracted and encoded via an external speech processor, and transmitted to the electrodes through a transcutaneous radio coil. For patients whose hearing loss is so severe that amplification is of little or no benefit, the cochlear implant is a standard, safe, and effective method of auditory rehabilitation. Most insurance plans now include cochlear implantation as a benefit. There are approximately 25,000 implantees in the United States and 35,000 worldwide.

Audiologic Rehabilitation

While the hearing aid serves as the nucleus of audiologic rehabilitation, other avenues of hearing loss management are becoming increasingly more important. Audiologic rehabilitation can include speech reading (lipreading) training, auditory training, and hearing loss counseling. Speech reading training teaches the use of visual cues to help in understanding speech. Cues include the use of lip movement, facial expression, body gestures, and context. Auditory training teaches strategies to improve listening skills and encourages the acceptance of amplified sound. Informational counseling sessions address numerous issues including implications of hearing loss on everyday life, coping mechanisms, speech conservation, and other specific concerns of the patient. Patients can find support through self-help groups and hearing loss informational materials, such as those offered by SHHH (Self Help for Hard of Hearing People, Inc.). SHHH has local chapters throughout the country and provides a valuable resource for hearing-impaired seniors.

Effective Communication with the Hearing-Impaired

Communication with the hearing-impaired adult can be frustrating at times, both for the affected individual and for those who communicate with them. The hearing-impaired person may confuse words, give inappropriate answers, ask for repetition, or just not hear and respond to questions or comments. These difficulties are even greater in background noise or group environments. Some persons unfortunately avoid communicating with a hearing-impaired person or show displeasure or irritation when asked for repetition. Others talk around the person by talking with their spouse or companion and ignoring the hearing-impaired person. Health care practitioners may at times talk with the spouse or caregiver about the patient's symptoms or medical treatment options while treating the hearing-impaired patient as if their cognitive abilities were affected. This obviously causes much frustration and isolation to the patient.

The practitioner should be aware of the communicative difficulties associated with hearing loss and use techniques to enhance communication. A quiet office environment without distracting noises is an ideal setting for the hearing-impaired patient. The examination door should be closed to reduce the noise from other rooms, and there should not be competing music or equipment noise. The patient should be spoken to face to face in a slower than usual voice. Table 60.4 lists several ways to enhance communication with hearing-impaired persons. These "guidelines" can be very helpful for improved communication in the practitioner–patient relationship.

TABLE 60.4. Guidelines for communicating with the hearing-impaired.

1. Get listener's attention before speaking.
2. Face listener directly to give visual cues.
3. Do not cover mouth while talking or turn away.
4. Try to reduce background noise: turn down TV, radio, etc.
5. Use facial expressions and gestures.
6. Speak slowly and clearly with more pauses than usual.
7. Speak only slightly louder than normal: do not shout.
8. Rephrase if listener does not understand rather than repeating word for word.
9. Alert listener to changes in topic before proceeding.
10. Do not turn and walk away while talking.
11. Use written notes if necessary.

Hearing-impaired persons most often remove their hearing aids when sleeping, so it is important that their aids are in place before talking with them; this is especially true with nursing home patients or those in health care facilities. Once the hearing aids are inserted, a simple question such as "Can you hear me now?" is helpful before conversing with the patient. Patients with hearing loss will appreciate such efforts in establishing effective communication with the health care provider.

Quality of Life and Amplification

The "treatment" of hearing impairments with hearing aid amplification, assistive listening devices, or aural rehabilitation therapy does not "cure" the impairment or restore hearing and communicative efficiency to normal, but such approaches do represent the best treatments to date. They will improve the ability of most older persons to communicate and reduce the handicapping consequences of hearing loss.

Numerous studies have shown that hearing aids do improve the quality of life for older persons with hearing loss. Successful hearing aid users have been found to show an advantage in self-perceived communication effectiveness, assertiveness in managing difficult listening situations, and an increased ability to accept their hearing loss as opposed to nonhearing aid users. Malinoff and Weinstein reported dramatic reductions in hearing handicap following only 3 weeks of hearing aid use that was sustainable after 1 year of use.[23] Mulrow and colleagues reported statistically significant improvements in cognitive and mental status scores and on a geriatric depression scale for hearing aid users compared to a nonhearing aid user control group.[24]

There is mounting evidence to suggest that the psychosocial implications of hearing handicap can be reduced with hearing aids and that these positive outcomes can be sustained over time. Studies using self-report methods to assess hearing aid benefit are providing overwhelming evidence of the efficacy of hearing aids. Unfortunately, only 10% of the people who might benefit from amplification actually have hearing aids.

Tinnitus Management

Tinnitus is a common consequence of presbycusis, noise-induced hearing loss, and, indeed, of most types of hearing loss. Tinnitus sensations are probably generated central to the cochlea; tinnitus has been noted to worsen in some cases after section of the cochlear nerve (e.g., as with tumor surgery). Given that spontaneous neural activity is typical of normal auditory nerve fibers, the absence of such activity may be a code for silence and may trigger the central generation of tinnitus sensations. However, the exact mechanism for tinnitus remains poorly defined.

Most patients with tinnitus adapt to the new sensation without difficulty and accept it as part of their existence. A small percentage, 5% or less, are unduly bothered by the unwanted sound. High proportions of these tinnitus sufferers are clinically depressed. Many are also bothered by loud sounds (hyperacusis). It is important to recognize that the characteristics of the tinnitus (as determined psychoacoustically) are no different in sufferers and nonsufferers. Rather, it is the psychologic status of the sufferer that is the focal point.

Management of the tinnitus sufferer may require amplification (which masks much of the unwanted sound) and antidepressive therapy, in addition to education about the nature of tinnitus. Cognitive psychotherapy may be useful in difficult cases. Drug therapy of the tirnnitus, per se, is futile.

Summary

Hearing loss is a normal accompaniment of old age. Many specific steps can be taken to overcome the potentially devastating effects on the individual. The geriatrician should be alert to the signs of hearing impairment and assist the patient in obtaining and using appropriate rehabilitation.

References

1. Lavizzo-Mourey RJ, Siegler EL. Hearing impairment in the elderly. *J Gen Intern Med.* 1992;7:191–198.
2. Gates GA, Cooper JC, Kannel WB, et al. Hearing in the elderly: the Framingham Cohort, 1983–1985. *Ear Hear.* 1990; 4:247–256.
3. Bess FH, Lichtenstein MJ, Logan SA, et al. Comparing criteria of hearing impairment in the elderly: a functional approach. *J Speech Hear Res.* 1989;32:795–802.
4. Mulrow CD, Aguilar C, Endicott JE, et al. Quality-of-life changes and hearing impairment: a randomized trial. *Ann Intern Med.* 1990;113(3):188–194.
5. Uhlmann RF, Larson EB, Koepsell TD. Hearing impairment and cognitive decline in senile dementia of the Alzheimer type. *J Am Geriatr Soc.* 1986;34:207–210.
6. Jerger J, Jerger S, Oliver T, et al. Speech understanding in the elderly. *Ear Hear.* 1989;10:79–89.
7. Welsh LW, Welsh JJ, Healy MP. Central presbycusis. *Laryngoscope.* 1985;95:128–136.
8. Working Group on Speech Understanding and Aging. Speech understanding and aging. *J Acoust Soc Am.* 1988; 3:859–895.
9. Kryter KD. Addendum and erratum: presbycusis, sociocusis, and nosocusis. *J Acoust Soc Am.* 1983;73:1897–1919.
10. Goycoolea MV, Goycoolea HG, Farfan CR, et al. Effect of life in industrialized societies on hearing in natives of Easter Island. *Laryngoscope.* 1986;90:1391–1396.
11. Gates GA, Cooper JC. Incidence of hearing decline in the elderly. *Acta Otolaryngol* 1991;111:240–248.
12. Gates GA, Cobb JL, D'Agostino RB, et al. The relation of hearing in the elderly to the presence of cardiovascular disease and cardiovascular risk factors. *Arch Otol Head Neck Surg.* 1993;119:156–161.
13. Schuknecht HF. Further observations on the pathology of presbycusis. *Arch Otolaryngol.* 1964;80:369–382.
14. Gates GA, Popelka GR. Neural presbycusis: a diagnostic dilemma. *Am J Otol.* 1992;13:313–317.
15. Sinha UK, Hollen KM, Rodriguez R, et al. Auditory system degeneration in Alzheimer's disease. *Neurology.* 1993;43: 779–785.
16. Shelton C, Harnsberger HR, Allen R, et al. Fast spin echo magnetic resonance imaging: clinical application in screening for acoustic neuroma. *Otolaryngol Head Neck Surg.* 1996; 114:71–76.
17. Logan SA, Hedley A. The elderly and hearing loss. *Semin Hear.* 1988;9:325–330.
18. Frank T, Petersen DR. Accuracy of a 40 dB HL audioscope and audiometer screening for adults. *Ear Hear.* 1987;8:180–183.
19. ASHA Ad Hoc Committee on Hearing Screening in Adults. Considerations in screening adults/older persons for handicapping hearing impairments. ASHA. *J Am Speech Hear Assoc.* 1992;8:81–87.
20. Ventry IM, Weinstein BE. The Hearing Handicap Inventory for the Elderly: a new tool. *Ear Hear.* 1982;3:128–134.
21. Weinstein BE. Age-related hearing loss: how to screen for it, and when to intervene. *Geriatrics.* 1994;49:40–45.
22. Gates GA, Karzon RK, Garcia P, et al. Auditory dysfunction in aging and senile dementia of the Alzheimer's type. *Arch Neurol.* 1995;52:626–634.
23. Malinoff RL, Weinstein BE. Changes in self-assessment of hearing handicap over the first year of hearing aid use by older adults. *J Am Acad Rehabil Audiol.* 1989;22:54–60.
24. Mulrow CD, Aguilar C, Endicott JE, et al. Association between hearing impairment and quality of life of elderly individuals. *J Am Geriatr Soc.* 1990;38(1):45–50.

61
Aging and the Oral Cavity

Gretchen Gibson and Linda C. Niessen

Many myths surround aging and the oral cavity. The stereotype of your grandmother going to bed with her teeth in a cup on the nightstand will fade rapidly as the baby boomers, those Americans born between 1946 and 1964, reach older adulthood in the twenty-first century.

The key roles of the oral cavity include initiation of alimentation and production of speech. Any discussion of the age-related and disease-related changes that occur in the oral cavity must address the effect of the changes on these functions. The oral cavity has developed specialized tissues to speak and to process food. The teeth and their supporting structures, called the periodontium, and the muscles of mastication, including the tongue, participate in preparing food for swallowing. The secretions of the salivary glands participate in digestion but also lubricate and protect the oral tissues.

The goal of this chapter is to provide clinicians with a better understanding of the effects of aging on the oral cavity in the hope of preventing as many disease-related changes as possible.

Oral Changes Associated with Aging

Tooth loss is the most common oral change associated with aging. However, no one ever lost a tooth because they celebrated a 75th birthday. Adults lose teeth because of disease, primarily dental caries or periodontal disease.

Although tooth loss does increase with age in cross-sectional and longitudinal studies, the percent of adults who have lost all their teeth (i.e., are completely edentulous) has decreased from the 1960s through the 1990s.[1-4] Figure 61.1 shows the percent of edentulous adults aged 65 to 74 years for 1960 to 1962, 1971 to 1974, 1985 to 1986, and 1993. The trend is a quite dramatic decrease in the rate of edentulousness from the high in the 1960s of 49.4% to the current low in the 1990s of 25% for this age group.

The tooth consists of enamel and cementum, which cover the outer surfaces of the crown and root, respectively (Fig. 61.2). Enamel is the hardest substance in the body, composed of more than 90% mineralized tissue. Dentin is the layer beneath both the enamel and cementum. Both dentin and cementum are softer than enamel, consisting of only 50% mineralized tissue. Dental caries (tooth decay) can affect enamel, dentin, or cementum surfaces. The dental pulp in the center of the tooth is composed of soft tissue where the nerve, blood, and lymphatic supply are located.

The supporting structures of the teeth (i.e., the periodontium) are those tissues that support the teeth in the jawbones. The periodontium consists of soft tissues [the gingiva (gums) and periodontal ligament (a ligament that attaches cementum to alveolar bone)] and mineralized tissues (cementum and bone support). Gingivitis occurs when the gingival tissues are inflamed. Periodontal disease or chronic periodontitis occurs when inflammation of the attachment tissues results in loss of bony support for the teeth.

Changes in the teeth do occur with aging. Teeth appear to darken with age. It is not clear what accounts for this change. It is hypothesized that wearing away of the enamel layers allows for the yellow dentin color to become more predominant. Clinically, some of the age-related oral changes have led to an increased interest in esthetic or cosmetic dentistry among senior patients. The ability to smile confidently and improve self-esteem is fueling the esthetic dentistry movement among older adults. Affluent older adults who are contemplating plastic surgery are also exploring a smile makeover, such as tooth whitening to eliminate darkened teeth and crowns or veneers to correct shortened, elongated, or even crooked teeth.

The dental pulp decreases in size as a result of aging. The clinical implications of a decreased dental pulp are not clear. Enamel and cementum surfaces continue to absorb fluoride, thus promoting remineralization of early

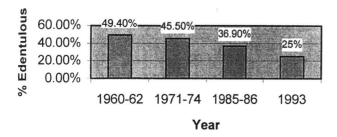

FIGURE 61.1. Edentulous rates for seniors, age 65–74 years. (From References 1–4, with permission.)

carious lesions, which contributes significantly to the theoretical basis for fluoride use in adults to prevent dental caries.

At one time, salivary flow was thought to decrease with aging. However, much of the research conducted on aging and salivary flow often compared healthy young adults with medically compromised older adults. Failure to draw appropriate samples and characterize the sample populations according to medical conditions and medication use resulted in the erroneous conclusion that salivary flow decreased as a result of aging.

More recent studies have shown that, in healthy adults, decreased salivary flow is not a normal consequence of aging.[5,6] Although histologic changes in salivary glands are noted with aging, it is thought that the glands contain

sufficient reserve capacity to offset these morphologic changes. Thus, a patient's complaint of oral dryness should not be attributed to aging. The differential diagnosis for salivary dysfunction is discussed later in this chapter.

Disease-Related Changes of the Mouth

Disease-related changes of the mouth appear to play a larger role in poor oral health than the currently known age-related changes. Most diseases of the oral cavity are either treatable or, more importantly, preventable.

Infectious Diseases of the Oral Cavity

The oral cavity, as a part of the gastrointestinal complex, is not only accessible to bacterial colonization from the environment but is a natural host to many species. Both dental caries and periodontal disease, the two most common diseases of the dentition, are the results of chronic bacterial infections.

Caries and periodontal disease occur when there is a shift in the oral environment and normal bacterial balance. This shift allows pathogenic organisms to flourish. The *Candida* species of fungus is also found in the oral cavity and other parts of the body of most healthy adults.

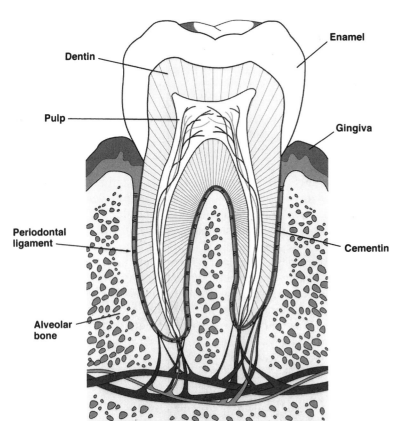

FIGURE 61.2. Anatomy of tooth and supporting structures.

Patients with dental caries or periodontal disease may or may not experience pain. Patients with root surface caries may be unaware of its presence until the caries has progressed circumferentially around the tooth and broken off the crown of the tooth. Patients may be unaware of the presence of periodontal disease until they wake up one morning and notice that their teeth are loose. Periodontal disease, like dental caries, requires dental intervention to stop disease progression.

Factors that affect the body's immune potential, or the natural colonization of the oral cavity, can lead to opportunistic infection of yeast, such as an overgrowth of *Candida albicans*.[7] Oropharyngeal colonization of gram-negative bacteria is the most common route of acquiring gram-negative pneumonia.[8,9] It has been hypothesized that bacterial infections, such as those found in periodontal disease, may play a role in aspiration pneumonia.[10] For these reasons, it is important to maintain good oral hygiene, even for nonresponsive patients who are parenterally fed.

Dental Caries

Dental caries is often thought of as a disease of childhood. Currently, an increasing number of older adults are afflicted with this infectious condition. In fact, caries has been shown to be a major cause of tooth loss in adults.[11] With the rate of edentulism continuing to decline, there will be an increase in the number of people with natural teeth who are at risk for caries.[12] Thus, the preventive dental methods that have contributed to declining tooth decay rates in children will need to be applied to a growing older population.

Caries is identified by the surface of the tooth on which the lesion is found. Caries attacking enamel surface is classified as coronal (the crown portion of the tooth). Caries attacking cementum, which covers the tooth root, is classified as root surface caries. Most current epidemiologic studies report coronal and root caries as two separate diseases.

The etiology of caries is threefold. It requires (1) a predominance of cariogenic bacteria; (2) a food source for the bacteria, such as fermentable carbohydrates; and (3) an acidic environment for continued bacterial growth. Because caries can be site specific in the oral cavity, the bacterial environment can vary from tooth to tooth within the same mouth and surface to surface on the same tooth. The bacteria most commonly associated with both coronal and root caries are *Streptococcus mutans*, a gram-positive coccus, and to a lesser degree, *Lactobacillus*, a gram-positive rod, and *Actinomycetes*.[13–15]

Risk factors for caries among older adults are similar to those for all adults. Unfortunately, these risk factors are often enhanced by local and systemic diseases that are more prevalent in old age. Poor oral hygiene allows both an acidic environment and prolonged access to food sources for bacterial proliferation. Poor oral hygiene can be exacerbated by decreased dexterity, as occurs in arthritic or stroke victims. As a general rule, persons who have difficulty with their activities of daily living, particularly feeding, will have difficulty with daily oral care and are at greater risk for dental caries.

Dietary choices made by older adults can greatly affect their caries activity. A decreased ability to chew and poor economic status among older adults have been shown to contribute to a diet that is higher in fermentable carbohydrates, softer, and therefore more cariogenic.[16,17]

Periodontal disease also acts as a risk factor specific for root caries. Chronic periodontal disease often leads to recession of gingival tissue with resulting tooth root exposure. Once the root surface or cementum of a tooth is exposed to the oral environment, it can be quickly demineralized when exposed to the acidic by-products of bacteria.

Decreases in salivary flow contribute significantly to increased caries activity. Patients who have a significantly decreased flow rate secondary to radiation therapy to the head or neck, which affects the salivary glands, have demonstrated a significant increase in caries activity.[18] Medication use and primary salivary gland disease can also cause low salivary flow, as is discussed later in this chapter.

Periodontal Diseases

The periodontal diseases consist of various disease processes, including gingivitis and periodontitis. Gingivitis is an inflammatory response of the gingival tissue to the metabolic products of bacteria found in oral plaque. Plaque-associated gingivitis most commonly presents as erythematous, edematous tissue that halos the teeth (Fig. 61.3). The gingiva bleed easily on tissue manipulation, such as during an examination or routine tooth brushing.

The primary risk factor for gingivitis is poor oral hygiene. Removal of the plaque eliminates the inflammatory response and, in most cases, the gingivitis will heal. Some research has shown that although gingivitis forms more quickly in older adults, healing is not impaired.[19]

Medications can also alter the gingival tissue. Steroid-induced gingivitis has been associated with postmenopausal women receiving hormone replacement therapy.[20] Gingival overgrowth can be induced by certain medications, such as cyclosporins, nifedipine, and phenytoin. Poor oral hygiene increases the risk of gingival hyperplasia when taking any of these medications.[21,22] This overgrowth further decreases a person's ability to maintain good oral hygiene. To eliminate the overgrowth, oral hygiene must be improved and any plaque or calculus removed from beneath the gingival tissue. If the tissue does not satisfactorily resolve after a dental scaling

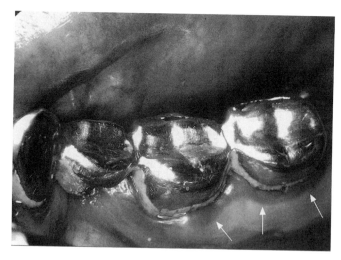

FIGURE 61.3. Gingivitis. Dark halo (indicated by *arrows*) on gingival tissue surrounds gold crowns, which are covered with plaque.

(cleaning), the overgrown tissue can be surgically removed.

Periodontitis is the destruction of the supporting structure of the tooth. If a sufficiently large amount of supporting bone is lost, clinically a patient may present with a chief complaint of tooth migration or movement, loose teeth, and tooth loss.

Periodontal disease in older adults is commonly referred to as chronic periodontitis (Fig. 61.4). Chronic periodontitis (referred to as periodontitis in this discussion) is now believed to be composed of short bursts of disease activity or destruction and longer periods of quiescence.[23,24] Because periodontitis is a chronic disease, much of the ravages of the disease we see in older adults results from an accumulation of the disease over time. Research has shown that the advanced stages of periodontitis are less prevalent than the moderate stages in the elderly population.[3,25] It is theorized that many of the sites of advanced periodontal disease have resulted in tooth loss earlier in life, suggesting that older age is not a risk factor for periodontal disease.[20]

As with caries, bacteria-containing plaque is the primary risk factor for periodontal disease. An altered immune response can exacerbate the inflammatory reaction in periodontal disease. Certain nutritional deficiencies, such as vitamin C, calcium, and zinc, may all play a role in the susceptibility and progression of periodontitis.[26,27] People who smoke are at greater risk for periodontal disease.[28] Smoking has been shown to be as important as bacterial destruction in the formation of this oral disease.[29,30]

Recently, strong evidence has begun to suggest a link between periodontal disease and the severity and progression of diabetes. Diabetic patients are at risk for a more severe form of periodontal disease, when compared

to healthy adults. More recently, preliminary data have suggested that controlling the gram-negative chronic infection of periodontal disease can have a positive impact on the control of diabetes.[31]

The evidence for the relationship between periodontal disease and coronary atherosclerosis is still somewhat controversial. Multiple studies have shown periodontal disease to have an independent association with coronary artherosclerosis, even after adjustment for other obvious and known risk factors, whereas others show no evidence of causal association between periodontal disease and coronary heart disease.[32,33] Theoretical causes include similar inflammatory mediators for both periodontitis and atherosclerosis,[32] increased platelet aggregation, and possible formation of an embolus due to an oral plaque organism.[34] Finally, there is recent evidence from a national prospective study that found periodontal disease to be a risk factor for nonhemorrhagic stroke.[35]

Yeast

As part of the gastrointestinal tract, the oral cavity is a natural host to many species of microorganisms. Yeast is one of these microorganisms. Most healthy adults who are cultured may at various times have a low yeast count. *Candida albicans* is the primary cause of pathogenic yeast infection in the oral cavity. Overproliferation of the organism and infiltration into the mucosal layers result in a pathogenic infection. The causes can be both local and systemic, and the infection is collectively termed candidiasis. The various types of candidiasis are classified by their onset and appearance.

Oral candidiasis can be classified as acute or chronic. The acute form can present as pseudomembranous or

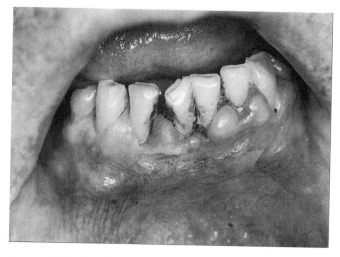

FIGURE 61.4. Periodontal disease. Note the bone loss and the elongated appearance of the lower teeth, as well as puffy or inflamed gums. Also note verrucous appearance of tissue below the gums due to smokeless tobacco.

atrophic. Chronic candidiasis can present as atrophic or hyperplastic. In older adults, the two most common types of candidiasis are acute pseudomembranous (traditionally called thrush) and chronic atrophic.

Thrush is characterized by white plaques described as having a curdlike appearance. Patients with *Candida* often complain of a burning mouth. Thrush can be found on any soft tissue in the oral cavity and pharynx, including the tongue. For diagnostic purposes, the white lesions can be wiped away with gauze, leaving an erythematous area under the white lesion. For clinical laboratory verification, a smear of the white lesion can be placed on a slide with 20% potassium hydroxide and viewed for hyphae. The presence of budding yeast and hyphae will confirm the presence of *Candida*.

Any condition compromising a patient's immune system or altering normal flora can be considered a risk factor for candidiasis. Oral candidiasis can occur with long-term use of medications such as antibiotics, steroid therapies, or chemotherapy. Diabetes mellitus, human immunodeficiency virus (HIV) disease, and head and neck radiation are risk factors for thrush.

Candidiasis located under a denture can be either atrophic or hyperplastic. It occurs as an erythematous area under a maxillary denture that vividly outlines the tissue covered by the prosthesis (Fig. 61.5). An ill-fitting upper denture is the most commonly cited risk factor. There is a decrease in the pH of the salivary film between denture and oral tissue from breakdown of carbohydrates (food debris) under a poorly fitting denture. This acidic atmosphere may be part of the etiology of the candidal overgrowth.[36] In patients without a prosthesis, chronic atrophic candidiasis may present as a generalized redness or even generalized burning of the mouth.

Because of the difficulty of identifying an area of tissue to scrape for a smear in this type of candidiasis, the

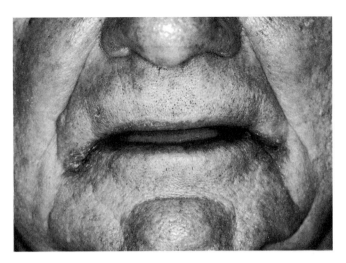

FIGURE 61.6. Angular cheilitis caused by *Candida albicans* in the commissures of the mouth.

patient may also swish with sterile saline for 1 min. The saline is subsequently cultured for the *Candida* species and read as the number of microorganisms per milliliter.[37] Patients showing more than 75 to 100 organisms per milliliter should be considered for treatment.

Chronic atrophic candidiasis associated with denture use is usually accompanied by poor oral hygiene of both the oral tissue and the prosthesis. Many patients wear their prosthesis 24 h per day and therefore do not allow the tissue to heal from the fungal infection. Xerostomia, or dry mouth, can also predispose a patient to this type of *Candida* infection, which causes a burning sensation in the oral cavity.

When chronic atrophic candidiasis manifests itself in the creases or commissures of the lips, it is called angular chelitis (Fig. 61.6); this occurs when a patient has a tendency to pool saliva around the corners of the mouth or, in some cases, constantly lick the lips. It presents as a reddened or raw area in the commissures on either one or both sides.

Treatment for Oral Candidiasis

The treatment for all types of candidiasis includes an antifungal medication. Topical (nystatin, chlortrimazole troches) or systemic (ketoconazole, fluconazole) medications are available. Topical medications should be used for at least 14 days to assure total eradication of the fungus. If the infection is more widespread than just the oral cavity or does not subside within 3 to 6 weeks of topical treatment, then systemic medication may be necessary. Fluconazole is a good drug of choice because of its once-daily dosing regimen and minimal drug interactions compared with other systemic antifungals, but is also costly in comparison. Table 61.1 lists the various medications that are indicated for treating candidiasis, as well as prescription information and comments.

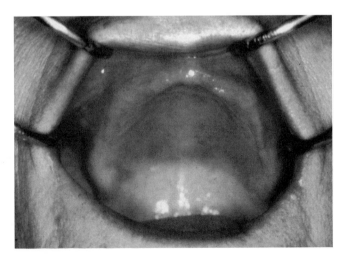

FIGURE 61.5. Chronic atrophic candidiasis. Note the dark outline of maxillary (*top*) denture on the palate.

Table 61.1. Medications for treatment of oral candidiasis.

Medication	Prescription	Comments and cautions
Nystatin oral suspension 100,000 U/ml	Disp: 240 ml Sig: Rinse w/5 ml and expectorate qid × 14 days	*50% sucrose, which can be highly cariogenic in patients with natural teeth *Patient may swallow if candidiasis extends in GI tract beyond oral cavity
Nystatin powder	Disp: 1 billion units Sig: Mix 1/8 t to 1/2 cup water, swish for 1 min and expectorate qid × 14 days	*Can be mixed with sugar-free, noncarbonated drink *Sugar substitute may be added to water to improve taste *May be difficult to find in pharmacy
Nystatin ointment 100,000 U/g	Disp: 15 g Sig: Apply thin coat to inner surface of denture qid OR apply to corners of mouth qid × 14 days	*Used for denture stomatitis or angular chelitis
Nystatin pastille	Disp: 28 pastilles Sig: Dissolve in mouth qid × 14 days	*Denture must be out when using pastilles or troches for medication to reach areas affected by denture stomatitis *May be hard to dissolve if patient has xerostomia
Chlortimazole troches	Disp: 50 tabs Sig: Dissolve one tab in mouth 5 ×/day for 10–14 days	*Can also use OTC vaginal chlortrimazole troches: dissolve 1/2 troche in mouth bid × 14 days
0.12% Chlorhexidine gluconate	Disp: 1 bottle Sig: Swish with 1 capful for 1 min and expectorate bid × 14 days	*Can also be swabbed on affected areas *Can cause taste alterations and staining *Contains 12% alcohol, which may cause discomfort in xerostomic patients
Ketoconazole 100 mg	Disp: 14 tabs Sig: Take 1 tab/day × 14 days	Multiple drug interactions that must be assessed before prescribing
Fluconazole 100 mg	Disp: 15 tabs Sig: Take 2 tabs on day 1, and 1 tab each day for 13 days	Medication is expensive compared to other treatments mentioned
Soaking solutions for infected dentures	*1 teaspoon sodium hypochlorite to 1 C water *1/2 capful 0.12% chlorhexidine gluconate added to soaking liquid *Full solution mouthrinse containing cetylpyridinium chloride (Cepacol or Gum)	*Dentures must be soaked every night while treating oral cavity for denture stomatitis *Solution must be changed each evening before soaking

Both nystatin and 0.12% chlorhexidine gluconate are effective antifungal agents. However, if both are prescribed, they must be taken at different times of the day because, when taken together, the overall efficacy is decreased. The decreased efficacy may be the result of a precipitation reaction that renders both medications much less effective when used together.[38]

Salivary Gland Pathology

Saliva has numerous functions in the maintenance of overall health and oral health. Saliva starts the digestive process by mediating taste acuity and combining food for further digestion. Saliva also lubricates and repairs the oral tissues to allow comfortable oral function and speech. It aids in maintaining the oral pH balance by buffering acids produced by oral bacteria, contains minerals that remineralize teeth, and provides mechanical cleansing and antimicrobial and antifungal activities.

For various reasons, salivary flow may be reduced. The subjective feeling of dry mouth is termed xerostomia. Table 61.2 provides a differential diagnosis for oral dryness. Xerostomia may be reversible or irreversible. Some xerostomic patients have salivary flow when stimulated (i.e., during eating), whereas others with glandular damage, such as Sjögren's syndrome, have a greatly

Table 61.2. Diseases or conditions that can cause oral dryness: differential diagnosis for xerostomia.

Alcoholism
Autoimmune disorders
Dehydration
Diabetes
Glandular blockage
Habitual oral breathing
Medication use
Parkinson's disease
Psychologic disorders
Radiation of salivary glands
Surgery affecting salivary glands

reduced flow, even when stimulated. It is imperative to diagnose the cause of the oral dryness to appropriately select treatment.

Oral dryness can adversely affect oral tissues, both mineralized and soft tissues. Oral dryness can cause an increase in caries activity, alterations in taste and smell, or a decrease in the ability to comfortably speak, chew, or swallow. Patients with dry mouth are at increased risk for oral *Candida* infections. If the patient wears a removable prosthesis, lack of adequate saliva for lubrication can make the denture uncomfortable or sometimes impossible to wear without damaging the underlying soft tissue.

Medication Use and Xerostomia

Medication use is the most common cause of oral dryness. More than 400 medications currently prescribed have xerostomia as an adverse drug effect. The actual mechanism of xerostomia resulting from medication use is varied and often is not completely understood. Some, such as anticholinergics, have been linked to actual salivary reduction. Others may dehydrate the tissue, causing the feeling of oral dryness. It is important to note that, in most cases of drug-induced xerostomia, stimulation of the glands does produce adequate salivary flow, which is an important distinction between drug-induced xerostomia and xerostomia attributed to gland destruction caused by disease or radiation.

The effects of drug-induced xerostomia are also reversible. If the patient discontinues the medication or if their dosage is altered, salivary flow returns to the previous normal rates.[39] Methods to stimulate the salivary flow will help ease the patient's symptoms.

Treatment of oral dryness is dependent on the cause. In the case of medication-induced xerostomia, an evaluation of the causative drugs and possible dose or medication changes should be considered. Also, consider the dosing schedule so that the primary time of dryness is at night, during sleep, or close to mealtime when the patient will have more salivary stimulation to overcome the dryness.

Because medication-induced oral dryness is not the result of a destructive process within the gland, treatment directed at salivary stimulation will be helpful, including the use of sugarless chewing gums, sugarless candies, and flavored drinks that do not contain sugar or caffeine. Patients must also be advised to drink adequate amounts of water daily to avoid dehydration and to provide the major component of saliva, that is, water.

Salivary substitutes serve as a palliative measure. Most of these products do not stimulate salivary flow but do provide relief from the discomforts of xerostomia. An oral gel, such as Oralbalance (Laclede, Gardena, CA, USA), will help coat and protect the oral tissues, especially during the night. A gel can also be used daily under dentures to provide moisture and reduce friction.

Alcohol-free mouthwashes should be recommended for xerostomic patients to avoid oral tissue irritation. Caffeine and alcohol are both known to increase oral dryness and should be avoided by xerostomic patients. Because dry oral tissue may be both more sensitive and more fragile, a toothpaste with mild flavoring agents (avoid a strong peppermint or cinnamon flavoring) may provide relief from burning. A children's toothpaste may contain less of the flavorings associated with burning.

Most toothpastes contain fluoride (1100 ppm F^-). For the patient with severe oral dryness and natural teeth, an additional at-home fluoride gel (5000 pmm F^-) or high-fluoride toothpaste (5000 ppm F^-) should be prescribed to prevent the severe tooth decay seen in these patients. Proper oral hygiene care is also essential to avoid the rapid carious breakdown that can occur without the adequate antibacterial protection of saliva.

Sjögren's Syndrome

Sjögren's syndrome is an autoimmune disorder characterized by an immune infiltrate of the exocrine glands, such as the salivary and lacrimal glands, that occurs primarily in middle-aged and older women. Individuals with the disease complain of both dry mouth and dry eyes. A diagnosis of Sjögren's syndrome with only dry eyes and dry mouth as symptoms is termed primary. If, however, there is an associated connective tissue disorder with these symptoms, such as systemic lupus erythematosus or scleroderma, it is termed secondary Sjögren's syndrome.[40]

The inflammatory damage of this disease on salivary glands is irreversible. Many patients, however, do have some remaining residual gland function. For this reason, treatment for these patients should focus both on ways to stimulate their remaining gland function and on palliative measures to increase their comfort. Treatment options for stimulation and palliative relief already mentioned are also applicable for Sjögren's syndrome patients. Five milligrams of oral pilocarpine given four times daily has shown positive results in increasing salivary flow and decreasing xerostomic symptoms in Sjögren's syndrome patients.[41] Contraindications for this medication include narrow-angle glaucoma and patients who suffer from respiratory problems. Because 5% to 10% of Sjögren's patients will progress to a systemic lymphoproliferation that may become malignant,[42] it is important to monitor these patients for any suspicious changes. At increased risk of rampant caries, these patients should be seen regularly by a dental professional and encouraged to practice good daily oral hygiene care.

Bacterial Infection of Salivary Glands

Reduced salivary flow can sometimes lead to a bacterial infiltrate and subsequent infection within the salivary

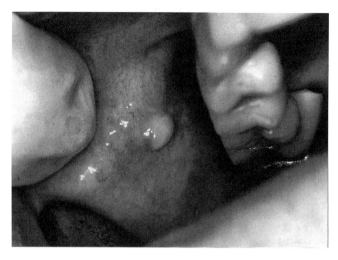

FIGURE 61.7. Exudate caused by a bacterial infection expressed from the parotid gland duct.

gland and duct. Patients may present with pain within the gland, swelling of the gland, possible headache and fever, or a purulent exudate upon milking the salivary gland. The patient will complain of the pain worsening during mealtime (Fig. 61.7).

If not in the acute phase, this problem can be diagnosed using a sialogram. Infection is noted by the classic dilated duct with segmental strictures within the gland.[43] Bacterial infections are seen primarily within the parotid glands. If the gland is still functional, antibiotics may also be utilized in treatment. However, often antibiotics may not reach the duct where the bacteria are residing, and hydration and salivary stimulation are the only means of treatment to help flush the duct as much as possible.

Sialolith

Sialoliths are radiopaque stones seen primarily within the submandibular glands and are composed mostly of calcium salts that can form anywhere within the gland. Symptoms include swelling or pain in the gland. The swelling is often associated with salivary stimulation occurring at mealtime and during eating. Sialoliths may cause glandular blockage, which may require surgical removal of either the sialolith or the gland itself. Soft tissue radiographs in the area of glandular blockage may aid in diagnosing the sialolith.

Salivary Gland Tumors

Tumors can occur in salivary glands as in other parts of the oral cavity. The percentage of malignant salivary tumors varies according to the type of salivary gland; 90% of parotid tumors and 50% of submandibular tumors are benign, whereas only 10% of sublingual tumors are benign.[44,45]

As with most oral cancers, pain is usually not present with salivary gland tumors. Indications of a salivary tumor include nerve damage and paresthesia, rapid growth, fixation of the gland, and telangiectatic vessels over the tumor site.[46]

Early diagnosis is an important factor in treatment outcomes. Most tumors of the salivary glands require excision of the gland with or without radiation therapy.

Mucocele

A mucocele is a surface swelling of the salivary gland due to trauma, a severed duct, or ductal blockage. These lesions occur primarily in the lower lip but may be seen wherever minor salivary glands are located, such as the palate, floor of the mouth, and tongue. They appear as a bluish or translucent swelling in the affected area. Deeper mucoceles may appear as nondescript swellings of normal color. These lesions may appear when the salivary gland is stimulated and not recede until the mucinous saliva is absorbed. Because the lesion often is traumatized before it has receded, causing the patient discomfort, the minor salivary gland is often removed to prevent further trauma in the area.

Radiation-Induced Xerostomia

If salivary glands are included in the radiation field for head and neck cancer, the result is most often destruction of much of the salivary gland, leading to radiation-induced xerostomia. Whole saliva (saliva collected from the oral cavity, which includes flow from all major and minor salivary glands) is usually measurably reduced at 2000 cGy of radiation.[47] Along with all the negative sequelae of xerostomia described earlier, the altered oral environment can lead to rampant caries and loss of teeth.

Loss of glandular function from radiation is irreversible. The patient must learn to function with whatever salivary flow is remaining after therapy. Current research includes investigating materials that will block the radiation in the specific areas of the salivary glands, leaving some function intact.

Oral pilocarpine has been recommended both during and following radiation treatment, which includes that of the salivary glands. Research found that patients who received a 5-mg dose of pilocarpine three times per day had the best outcomes in terms of increased salivary production and relief of symptoms with minimal adverse reactions.[48] Another study proposed the use of 5 mg pilocarpine four times daily during and for a time following radiation treatment to decrease the damage and flow loss of salivary glands.[49]

Disease Processes of the Temporomandibular Joint

The temporomandibular joint (TMJ) is a ball-and-socket joint with a cartilaginous disk between the skull and mandible to aid in movement within the joint. Although complications with the TMJ decrease with increasing age, they are still present within the older population.[50] Many older adults exhibit sounds described as clicking, popping, or crepitus on joint manipulation. However, treatment is usually not initiated unless discomfort or pain is involved.

Symptoms of temporomandibular disorder (TMD) include pain in the area of the joint and inability to fully open the mouth. Symptoms range from vague or non-specific, such as diffuse pain of the head and neck, to vertigo, tinnitus, paresthesia, visual, and hearing disturbances.[51]

Loss of occlusal function may predispose a person to TMD pain. It has been shown that persons with missing teeth are more likely to have pain and clicking on the side with the missing teeth.[52] Persons wearing dentures are also susceptible to TMD and should be evaluated if symptoms of the disorder are reported by the patient; however, edentulous patients without prostheses rarely report temporomandibular joint pain.[53]

Acute and life-threatening causes of temporomandibular pain, such as malignancies or infectious processes, should always be considered in the initial differential diagnosis. Malignancies in this area are rare. The clinical signs would be similar to those listed for a parotid gland tumor. Infections of the TMJ are also rare and include pain and swelling in the area that has been distinguished from a parotid swelling, which is much more common as the result of Sjögren's syndrome or parotid gland infection. Due to the threat of intracranial spreading, aggressive treatment is advised for this type of infection.

Both osteoarthritis and rheumatoid arthritis affect the TMJ. Although osteoarthritis is the most common type noted in the TMJ, many patients do not exhibit pain or symptoms with this type of arthritis. Rheumatoid arthritis of the TMJ is seen primarily in younger women and usually occurs in conjunction with inflammatory responses in other joints. Common complaints with this type of TMD include stiffness, crepitus, tenderness, swelling, masticatory pain, hypomobility of the mandible, and, in severe cases, mandibular fixation.[51] One study linked severe degradation of the TMJ from rheumatoid arthritis to upper airway obstruction in 70% of the cases with severe rheumatoid arthritis[54]; this was hypothesized to result from an induced micrognathia-causing tongue retrusion that blocks the airway. During acute exacerbation of rheumatoid arthritis, the patient may benefit from decreased mandibular movement and a soft diet, along with pharmacologic therapy for rheumatoid arthritis.

Oral Cancer

Oral cancer refers to lesions of the lips, tongue, pharynx, and all other hard and soft tissue within the oral cavity.

Oral cancer accounts for 3% of all diagnosed cancers. The average age of diagnosis of oral cancer is 60 to 63 years. Men account for the majority of oral cancers, with 20,200 cases estimated in the year 2000, and 10,000 new cases estimated in women in the same year. Oral cavity and pharyngeal cancer are among the 10 leading sites for men, but not for women.[55] Although oral cancer has traditionally been considered a disease of older men, recent data have shown an increase in oral cancer rates in women, with the gender ratio of 6:1 (male to female) in 1950 changing to 2:1 (male to female) in 1980.[56]

Unlike many other cancers, there has been little improvement in the mortality rate of oral cancer through the years. Even if mortality is avoided, the morbidity of this disease and the treatment can be very disfiguring.[57] Many patients suffer from decreased self-esteem due to altered appearance from radical surgery, a decrease in the ability to speak and masticate, and a severe decrease in saliva secondary to surgery or radiation therapy or both.

Use of alcohol and of tobacco are the primary risk factors for oral cancer. Sunlight is a risk factor for lip cancer. The combination of alcohol and tobacco use has been shown to have a multiplicative effect on the incidence of oral cancer, accounting for 75% of all oral cancers in the United States.[58]

Oral cancer is primarily squamous cell carcinoma. (For the purpose of this discussion, oral cancer and squamous cell carcinoma are used synonymously.) The most common sites in men are the floor of the mouth (under the tongue) and the retromolar area (just behind the last molar teeth in the mandible). For women, the most common area is the gingiva. Other common sites include the lateral borders of the tongue and the soft palate area.[59]

Oral cancer can present as a red or white lesion that does not heal. When performing an oral examination, the health professional should note anything that appears unusual. Oral cancer is rarely associated with pain. When a patient does present with pain or paresthesia associated with a cancerous lesion, it usually suggests invasive disease.

Although white lesions, or leukoplakia, are common in older adults, their cause should always be diagnosed. If there is no obvious cause for the leukoplakia, such as friction or trauma, then the lesion should be biopsied if it has not resolved within 1 to 2 weeks.

Red lesions (erythroplakia), red and white mixed lesions, and ulcerations without pain should be held as highly suspicious. Again, if resolution of the lesion is not noted within 1 to 2 weeks, a biopsy should be performed to confirm or rule out oral cancer.

Oral Examination

Currently, early detection is the most effective way to reduce the mortality and morbidity associated with oral cancer. Because the mouth is easily accessible, physicians and nurses should include a routine oral cancer screening as part of the physical examination for all older adults.

To efficiently perform an oral examination, a focused source of light, a tongue blade, and gauze are all that are required. These instruments are readily available in most examination rooms. The examiner should always wear gloves when conducting an oral examination.

As any other part of the physical examination, an oral examination should proceed in a systematic and consistent manner. Emphasis should be placed on the areas where oral cancer most often occurs, which are the areas where saliva would pool. These areas include the floor of the mouth, lateral borders of the tongue, retromolar area (area behind the last molar tooth on the bottom arch), and soft palate. The examiner should first examine the buccal mucosa for red, white, and ulcerative lesions or any swellings that cannot be readily explained. From the buccal mucosa, the examiner should proceed to the hard and soft palate. The tongue blade should be used to manipulate the tissue, as well as to hold the tongue to adequately view the soft palate. The examiner should be sure to fully visualize the soft palate and oropharynx by asking the patient to stick out the tongue and say "ah," while depressing the tongue with the tongue blade. The examiner should also view the floor of the mouth, retromolar area, and lateral borders of the tongue. The lateral borders of the tongue can be best seen by asking the patient to stick out the tongue. The examiner then holds the tongue with a gauze and moves the tongue from side to side so that the most posterior lateral borders can be visualized (Fig. 61.8).

Just as patient self-examination has become an important part of other cancer prevention campaigns, oral cancer prevention may also benefit from teaching

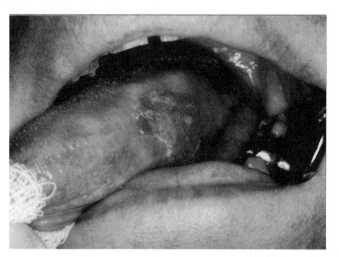

FIGURE 61.8. Correct retraction of tongue to assure complete observation of posterior lateral tongue reveals an oral cancer lesion.

patients the warning signs of oral cancer and how to examine their mouth during daily oral hygiene care.

Soft Tissue Lesions Common in Older Adults

Soft tissue lesions are common in older adults, most with identifiable causative factors. The most common lesions noted in older adults are ulcerations, white or leukoplakic areas, and maculopapular lesions (to be discussed with ill-fitting prostheses).[60]

Oral Ulcerations

Ulcerations are most often associated with trauma, and patients usually present with a complaint of pain. The most common sites for oral ulcerations include the tongue, lips, buccal mucosa, and gingiva.[60] Many ulcerative lesions in older adults are associated with an ill-fitting or broken prosthesis (denture). Risk factors that make a patient more susceptible to ulcerations under a prosthesis include diabetes, xerostomia, and a compromised immune complex. Patients who have received radiation therapy encompassing either the mandible or maxilla are at high risk for oral ulcerations that may lead to osteoradionecrosis. For this reason, a dentist may choose to wait up to 1 year after radiation therapy before making removable prostheses. Fractured teeth may also cause ulcerations, and patients should be referred to a dentist for treatment.

As stated earlier, an ulceration that is painless or does not heal within 1 to 2 weeks should be biopsied to rule out cancer. Painful lesions will usually cease being painful in 3 to 4 days and completely heal within 7 to 10 days following removal of the source of irritation. Any treatment is usually palliative, consisting of an emollient with a topical anesthetic.

If no source of trauma is noted and the lesion is located on unattached tissue (tissue not directly attached to bone), the diagnosis may be recurrent aphthous ulcerations. Patients will give a history of recurrence of these lesions. The exact etiology is unknown, but stress plays an important factor in reoccurrence. The lesions are small and self-limiting, healing in 7 to 10 days. Treatment, if necessary, is usually palliative. On rare occasions these ulcerations may become quite large (major aphthous ulcerations) and require systemic steroids or surgery for proper healing.

Lichen planus is a chronic inflammatory mucocutaneous disease that has been suggested to be an autoimmune disorder. It may be initiated by stress, drug hypersensitivity, bacterial or viral infection, or a genetic predisposition.[61] Biopsy of a lesion is required for definitive diagnosis of the disease. The lesions often appear as eroded or ulcerative areas surrounded by white lines radiating from the ulcerations in a lacelike pattern. These

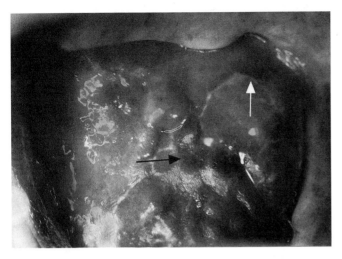

FIGURE 61.9. Lichen planus. *White arrow* indicates white stria (Wickham's stria), which radiate from a red central lesion (*black arrow*) in a lacelike pattern on the buccal mucosa.

white lines, called Wickham's striae, are characteristic of this disorder (Fig. 61.9).

Lesions are seen primarily in the buccal mucosa, gingiva, and tongue and less frequently on the lips and hard and soft palate. Erosive painful lesions are noted during exacerbations of the disease, often from a source of local or systemic stress. Secondary *Candida* infection may occur during exacerbations.

Treatment during exacerbations is a topical steroid applied to the lesions after they have been gently dried. Three topical medications of choice include fluocononide gel 0.05%, triamcinolon acetonide in gel base 0.1%, and clobetasol propionate ointment 0.05%. All these should be applied three times daily and at bedtime. Various topical antihistamines and topical anesthetics have also been suggested to help ease the symptoms. If the symptoms worsen, or are not responding to topical treatment, systemic steroids may be used.[62] Diagnosis and treatment of oral candidal infections should be done regularly for patients suffering with lichen planus.

Leukoplakia

Leukoplakia, a white plaque on the oral tissue, is most often attributable to chronic friction resulting in a hyperkeratotic lesion. It is often seen under a denture or on the lateral borders of the tongue. Again, oral cancer should be ruled out. If the cause of the lesion is known, treatment of the lesion consists of removing the source of trauma or friction. If the lesion is raised and causing discomfort for the patient, its excision may be necessary.

Burning Mouth

Burning mouth or burning tongue is primarily seen in middle-aged and older women. The exact etiology is unknown and may be varied or multifactorial. The primary symptom, as the name describes, is a burning sensation in the oral cavity. It may manifest as a diffuse burning within the mouth or a localized burning, often specific to the tongue.

The most common cause of a burning mouth is an oral *Candida* infection. Oral *Candida* should be ruled out before considering other causes. Burning mouth has also been associated with chronic or severe xerostomia, vitamin B deficiency, diabetes mellitus, hematologic deficiencies such as iron, nonfunctional oral habits, allergies, and peri- and postmenopause.[63]

Treatment is based primarily on proper evaluation of etiology. Treatments include antifungal medications, vitamin or iron supplements, and improved oral hygiene of both natural and prosthetic dentition. Treatment for the xerostomia, which is described elsewhere in this chapter, may help decrease the burning or discomfort. A dentist should be consulted.

Treatment as simple as smoothing roughened tooth surfaces or fabricating a splint to protect the tongue from rubbing on the teeth, may help ease the discomfort. A patient's oral hygiene regimen should always be evaluated to look for products to which the patient may be sensitive. Possibilities include products with cinnamon, tartar control toothpaste, or even strong flavorings. It is sometimes helpful to have the patient switch to a milder flavored children's toothpaste that still contains fluoride. Some postmenopausal women suffering from burning mouth and with no other noted etiology have found relief after implementation of estrogen replacement therapy.[64]

Oral Lesions Associated with Prostheses (Dentures)

For this discussion, prostheses refers to removable dentures, either full or partial, made to replace natural teeth and enhance oral function. A full or complete denture replaces all the teeth in an arch. A partial denture replaces some teeth, and the remaining teeth help to retain the partial denture.

Most oral problems attributed to prostheses are due to an ill-fitting prosthesis. Natural teeth serve as the main stabilizing factor in maintaining mandibular and maxillary osseous ridges. When teeth are removed, most persons lose some alveolar bone when functional stress is placed on the ridge. This loss of bony support is a primary factor for an ill-fitting prosthesis. Other factors that may cause oral lesions include need for adjustment after placing a new prosthesis and poor oral hygiene causing a *Candida* infection.

Ulcerative lesions caused by trauma from ill-fitting prostheses and their treatment were discussed earlier in this chapter. (See Ulcerative Lesions.) When a prosthesis does not fit in the border areas (the edge of the denture), fibrous connective tissue can form to protect the area from chronic trauma. This overgrowth of tissue is termed epulis fissuratum or chronic fibrous hyperplasia. It usually appears as an overgrowth of tissue where the denture fits in the mouth. There may or may not be an associated ulcer, depending on the duration of the lesion. The lesion may shrink with removal of the overextended border of the denture, but it usually does not completely resolve. Before a new denture is made, this lesion should be removed to ensure a properly fitting prosthesis.

Papillary hyperplasia is a lesion described as multiple papillary nodules primarily covering the palate vault. It is usually erythematous or red in color, painless, and not associated with dysplasia. It is a reactive lesion caused by an ill-fitting prosthesis and is sometimes linked to candidiasis. Treatment includes having the patient remove the prosthesis for at least 6h each day or night, proper hygiene of the prosthesis and underlying soft tissue, and treatment of candidiasis, if present. The patient should be counseled on the need for a new prosthesis.

Oral Manifestations of Systemic Disease

In addition to the previously described primary oral diseases, many systemic disease can present oral manifestations.

Arthritis

Arthritis is currently the most prevalent chronic condition in older adults in the United States. Arthritis can have temporomandibular manifestations, as described earlier in this chapter. A more common oral problem is decreased oral hygiene abilities. Patients with hands deformed from rheumatoid arthritis may be unable to grip or maneuver a toothbrush or floss. For patients with such problems, devices are available to assist with brushing and flossing. Referrals or consultations with dental professionals will assist physicians and nurses in preventing the patient's arthritis from causing additional oral disease.

Stroke

Stroke is the third leading cause of death in the United States.[4] Paralysis of extremities and speech impairments, two of the residual effects of strokes, are among the most common chronic impairments of the older adult population. Both dentate and edentulous persons are at risk for oral sequela of stroke. These risks include swallowing disorders, a decrease in oral motor function, decreased oral hygiene abilities, oral numbness or sensitivity, an alteration in the ability to wear a prosthesis, and altered bite or occlusion.

Decreased swallowing ability can lead to aspiration and the possibility of an aspiration-type pneumonia.

Eighty-five percent of patients surviving a stroke have been found to have swallowing abnormalities of either the oral or pharyngeal stage.[65] Dental professionals should be advised of a patient's swallowing disorder to avoid the risk of aspiration of fluids during dental treatment.

The residual hemiparesis associated with a stroke can result in decreased oral hygiene abilities. The guiding principle in dentistry is if a patient can be taught to feed themselves then the patient can be retaught oral hygiene skills. A patient may need some assistance from a caregiver during the rehabilitation period. The patient should be evaluated for competence in providing oral hygiene and be referred to a dental professional, if necessary.

Poststroke patients will sometimes present with very poor oral hygiene or food packing on the affected side. Although patients may report brushing or caring for their mouth, they seem unaware of this food buildup. Loss of sensation on the affected side may account for this condition (Fig. 61.10). Oral hygiene should be monitored after a stroke and the patient informed if this problem is noted. The patient or a caregiver may need to visually check this area after the patient brushes or eats to ensure that the food has been removed. Because poststroke patients may also have increased pain sensitivity or numbness in the oral cavity, it is important to have periodic oral examinations to rule out infections or oral lesions.

Current recommendations suggest delaying elective dental treatment for 6 months poststroke. The time varies according to an individual's rehabilitation progress. It is optimal for the patient to have regained the maximum amount of oral motor function before denture fabrication to achieve a properly fitting prosthesis.

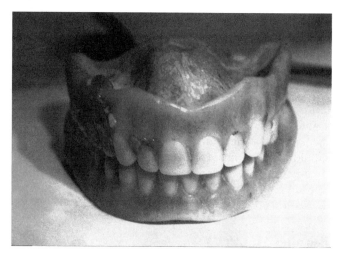

FIGURE 61.10. Denture with one-half covered with food debris on the affected side in a poststroke patient.

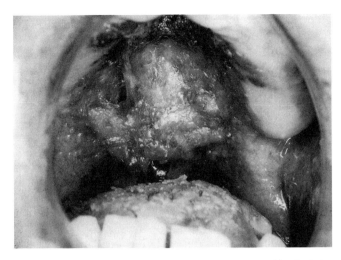

FIGURE 61.11. Dried oral secretions in the palate (roof of the mouth) of a patient who breathes through his mouth and is fed parenterally.

Often after a stroke, an edentulous patient with full removable prostheses will complain that the prosthesis no longer fits. The patient may have lost weight during an extended hospital stay, causing a decrease in the adipose pads of the maxilla, leading to a loose maxillary prosthesis. More often, however, the muscles that once accommodated a slightly ill fitting prosthesis before the stroke are no longer compensating for the poor fit after the stroke. The treatment in either case requires the dentist to temporarily reline the denture by adding a soft material to the tissue side of the denture until the patient is able to undergo more definitive treatment.

Good oral care should be maintained as well for patients who are nonresponsive or using parenteral nutrition. Because many are at high risk for aspiration of secretions, the oral flora should be reduced as much as possible. If a patient is unable to brush their teeth, the caregiver may swab an antimicrobial in the oral cavity daily to reduce the aspiration risk.

Another oral problem occurring in patients with difficulty swallowing and who are mouth breathers is drying oral tissues and secretions (Fig. 61.11). Dried oral secretions should be removed at least two times per day with a wet gauze. After the secretions are removed, the caregiver may swab the tissues with a small amount of a lubricating gel or a water-soluble lubricant.

Dementia

Oral health should not decline simultaneously with cognitive function.[66] Unfortunately, a large percentage of patients suffering with dementia also suffer from various oral diseases. Because of the increasing cognitive decline expected as the disease progresses, physicians and nurses must assist caregivers in reminding them to provide daily oral care as part of their 36-h day. This plan may begin

with a referral to the dentist to obtain needed dental care early in the course of the disease. The caregiver can provide daily reminders to the patient to perform daily oral hygiene. During the latter stages of the disease, the caregiver must provide total oral care for the patient.

Food packing in the buccal pouches of the maxilla often occurs in dementia patients, causing an increase in caries and an increase in the susceptibility to oral infections. Research suggests that dementia patients may have an increased craving for sweets, also increasing their risk for dental caries.[67] The increase in caries risk, coupled with decreased oral hygiene abilities, suggests the need for an aggressive preventive dental plan.[66] This plan can include daily oral hygiene care and use of a prescribed at-home fluoride gel or high-fluoride toothpaste and chlorhexidine mouth rinse.

Many patients with later stages of dementia may not communicate pain effectively to caregivers and subtle signs must be investigated. For all these reasons, scheduled oral exams should be performed for these patients, at a minimum of once per year.

Because of the progressive nature of this disease, early intervention and planning are key to maintaining oral health. Dental treatment in the early stages should be aggressive, knowing that treatment may not be possible in the later stages. If removable prostheses are made, two sets may be fabricated in case of loss in later stages of the disease. Prostheses should be labeled with the patient's name in case the patient misplaces the dentures. In the later stages of dementia, it may be necessary to remove the prosthesis if the patient no longer tolerates it. A removable partial denture may become a danger to the oral cavity if the patient can no longer place it in their mouth properly as it may puncture the lip or other soft tissue with the metal projections or clasps. Some patients, however, feel comfortable wearing their prosthesis until very late in the disease; this should always be evaluated on an individual basis. Often it is difficult for family members to see the patient without the prosthesis.

Nutritional Deficiencies and Oral Health

Nutritional deficiencies can cause oral symptoms, and poor oral health can lead to decreased nutritional intake.[16] For example, malnutrition and zinc deficiency may result in increasing susceptibility to periodontal disease. Poor food choices, such as softer foods that may be easier to chew with compromised dentition, may also be more cariogenic.

Changes in the tongue, such as reddening, balding, and burning are associated with deficiencies in B_{12} and iron. Mucosal pallor may be due to anemia. Hyperkeratosis of soft tissue may be seen with a deficiency of vitamin A, and gingival inflammation, such as acute gingivitis, may be associated with vitamin C deficiency.

Systemic Sequelae Requiring Antibiotic Prophylaxis

The American Heart Association (AHA) periodically reviews and publishes standardized guidelines for antibiotic prophylaxis for the prevention of bacterial endocarditis.[68] These guidelines speak specifically about dental procedures and prophylaxis needs. Table 61.3 lists specifics of the latest recommendations.

Although a 91% efficacy has been shown for endocarditis prophylaxis in patients with prosthetic heart valves,[69] the AHA guidelines are not always followed. Researchers from one study found that only 22% of the cases identified as needing antibiotic premedication before invasive procedures were premedicated according to the guidelines.[70] This issue is still somewhat controversial. Strom et al., in 1998, through a population-based, case-control study, concluded that even with 100% effectiveness of antibiotic prophylaxis preceding invasive dental care, few cases of infective endocarditis would be prevented.[71] However, at this time the standard of care is still the AHA recommendations (see Table 61.3).

Of even greater controversy is the issue of antibiotic premedication before dental care for patients with prosthetic joints. The evidence that links dental procedures with the failure of prosthetic joints is highly debatable. Most infections around a joint prosthesis are staphylococcal organisms, yet most transient bacteremias secondary to dental manipulation are streptococcal in nature. Even the choice of antibiotic is questioned, because although a penicillin would be the choice for a dentally induced bacteremia, a first-generation cephalosporin is the choice of most physicians.

In 1997 the American Dental Association and the American Academy of Orthopedic Surgeons produced an advisory statement that was published in the *Journal of the American Dental Association*.[72] Both organizations recognized the fact that not all patients with a prosthetic joint share the same high risk for failure. The joint statement recognized that patients with such systemic complications as immunosuppression, poorly controlled diabetes, history of previous joint failure, malnourishment, hemophilia, and a joint placed as recently as 2 years earlier all increase the possibility of joint failure. Their recommendation for a drug regimen is the same as the AHA guidelines for premedication for bacterial endocarditis because of the nature of the bacteremias most often seen from a dental procedure.

Oral Problems Resulting from Medical Treatment

Oral Adverse Drug Reactions

With the increase in the number of older adults with chronic diseases in the United States, medication use by older adults will continue to increase. As a result, adverse drug reactions or oral complications of medication use may also increase. An assessment of the top 22 medications in the United States shows that 79% have oral adverse drug reactions listed. The three most common

TABLE 61.3. Antibiotic prophylaxis (AP) for prevention of infective endocarditis (IE): conditions and regimens.

	AP recommended	AP *not* recommended
Cardiac conditions	• Prosthetic cardiac valves • Previous IE • Most congenital cardiac malformations • Surgically constructed systemic pulmonary shunts and conduits • Acquired valvular dysfunction (ex. rheumatic heart dx) • Hypertrophic cardiomyopathy • Mitral valve prolapse with valve; regurgitation or thickened leaflets	• Isolated secundum atrial septal defect • Surgical repair of atrial septal or ventricular septal defects or patent ductal arteriosus • Previous coronary artery bypass graft surgery • Mitral valve prolapse without valvular regurgitation • Physiologic, functional or innocent murmurs • Previous Kawasaki dx without valvular dysfunction • Previous rheumatic heart dx without valvular dysfunction • Cardiac pacemaker and defibrillators
Dental procedures	• Tooth extraction • Periodontal procedures • Dental implant placement • Root canal • Intraligamentary local anesthetic injections • Dental prophylaxis	• Fillings not near the gingival • All other local anesthesia injections • Suture removal • Prosthesis fabrication steps • Fluoride treatment • Taking radiographs

Recommended oral regimens: Amoxicillin, adult dose 2.0 g 1 h before dental procedure; for patients allergic to penicillin, clindamycin, adult dose 600 mg 1 h before dental procedure; cephalixin, adult dose 2.0 g 1 h before dental procedure; azithromycin or clarithromycin, adult dose 500 mg 1 h before dental procedure.
Source: Adapted from Dajani AS, Taubert KA, Wilson W, et al. Prevention of bacterial endocarditis. Recommendations by the American Heart Association. *JAMA*. 1997;277:1794–1801, with permission.[68]

oral side effects are xerostomia, taste alteration, and stomatitis.[73]

Tardive dyskinesia, an oral movement disorder, results from neuroleptics, lithium, antipsychotics, and antiparkinson agents. Tardive dyskinesia, unlike most oral adverse drug reactions, is usually irreversible. Gingival overgrowth can result from the use of calcium channel blockers, phenytoin, and cyclosporins. For these patients, good oral hygiene is imperative to reduce the risk of severe periodontal disease and caries.

Patients on anticoagulation therapy may be at risk for excessive bleeding during surgical dental procedures. If the patient's international normalized ratio (INR) is below 3.0 and the surgery is limited to a single tooth extraction or deep scaling or cleaning of only one-quarter or one-half of the mouth, the treatment is most likely feasible without alteration of the anticoagulation therapy. If however, the oral surgery consists of more than one tooth extraction, periodontal surgery, or implant surgery or the patient has further risk factors for excessive bleeding, cessation of the anticoagulation therapy for at least 3 days may be required. If the patient is unstable and stopping anticoagulation is not feasible, consideration should be given to hospitalizing the patient to switch therapy to heparin, which has a shorter half-life and can be stopped for the minimal amount of time during the dental procedure and immediately postoperatively. Over-the-counter medications, such as aspirin and nonsteroidal anti-inflammatories, can also cause an increased bleeding time that can pose problems during dental treatment.

The systemic effects of chemotherapy for malignant lesions include oral manifestations due to the myelosuppressive and cytotoxic effects, which include mucositis, or inflamed and tender oral tissues, primarily resulting from the high mitotic rate of the oral epithelium and its sensitivity to the chemotherapy. Oral infections, including fungal infections, and bleeding are increased because of bone marrow suppression and overall immunosuppression. Fifty percent of patients undergoing chemotherapy for leukemia experience oral complications, and the percentage for patients undergoing chemotherapy for lymphomas and carcinomas is 33% and 12%, respectively.[74,75]

Good oral health before the chemotherapy begins will help prevent many oral infections. If dental treatment is required during chemotherapy, it is essential to treat either immediately before or after an episode of chemotherapy, when the immunosuppression effect is at its lowest.

Research has shown that placing patients on a 0.12% chlorhexidine gluconate rinse during chemotherapy can both reduce the severity of the mucositis and help resolve the mucositis more rapidly.[76] Palliative treatment for stomatitis include rinses such as 1/2 t salt, 1/2 t soda, and 1 quart of water; a 50:50 mixture of diphenhydramine and kaolin-pectate; and for existing ulcerative lesions, sucralfate suspension. If oral hemorrhagic oozing occurs easily, the patient may be required to use a very soft toothbrush or to swab the teeth with chlorhexidine to avoid bleeding from brushing but still remove oral bacteria.

Oral adverse effects from head and neck radiation include osteoradionecrosis of osseous tissue, xerostomia, rampant caries, mucositis, trismus, altered taste, and an increased susceptibility to oral infections. Osteoradionecrosis, the sloughing of injured or dying bone, can affect large areas of the jaw due to suppressed osteoblastic activity and a decrease in the bony vascularity caused by hyalinization of the vessels and endarteritis. The mandible is the most susceptible oral osseous structure because of its density. Risks for osteoradionecrosis include extractions, trauma, or even ulcerations from wearing a prosthesis. Signs and symptoms include pain, exposure sloughing, and suppuration of the osseous tissue.

Before initiating radiation therapy to the head and neck, a thorough dental evaluation is essential. All sources of oral infection should be treated aggressively. Xerostomia and mucositis may be treated as listed in other sections of this chapter, although the therapeutic benefit of 0.12% chlorhexidine to prevent mucositis from radiation therapy has been questioned.[76] Patients who have had teeth removed before head and neck radiation therapy are usually required to wait 1 year after therapy to help decrease the risk of severe bone destruction due to osteoradionecrosis from ulcerations that often occur while wearing a new prosthesis. Good oral hygiene must be a lifetime commitment for the postradiation patient with remaining teeth to avoid the rampant tooth decay and risk of osteoradionecrosis that will always be present.

With the addition of the baby boomer seniors, who are retaining their natural teeth longer, there will most likely come an increase in the prevalence of oral disease and infection seen in geriatric patients. It is imperative that all health care providers understand the symbiotic nature of good oral health and good systemic health. The good news is that, unlike many of the chronic conditions faced in later years, oral disease is preventable and in most cases curable.

References

1. Johnson ES, Kelly JE, VanKirk LE. Selected findings in adults by age, race and sex. United States, 1960–62. Washington, DC: U.S. Government Printing Office; 1965.
2. Kelly JE, Harvey CR. Basic data on dental examination findings in persons 1–74 years, United States, 1971–74. Washington, DC: U.S. Government Printing Office; 1979.
3. National Institute of Dental Research. *Oral Health of United States Adults: The National Survey on Oral Health in*

U.S. Employed Adults and Seniors: 1985–86: National Findings. NIH 87-2868. Hyattsville, MD: National Institutes of Health; 1987.

4. Kramarow E, Lentzner H, Rooks R, et al. *Health and Aging Chartbook. Health, United States, 1999.* Hyattsville, MD: National Center for Health Statistics; 1999.

5. Baum BJ. Evaluation of stimulated parotid saliva flow rate in different age groups. *J Dent Res.* 1981;60(7):1292–1296.

6. Chauncey HH, et al. Parotid fluid composition in healthy aging males. *Adv Physiol Sci.* 1981;28:323.

7. Levy B. Disease-related changes in older adults. In: Papas A, Niessen L, Chauncey H, eds. *Geriatric Dentistry: Aging and Oral Health.* St. Louis: Mosby Year Book; 1991:83–102.

8. Levinson M, Daye D. Pneumonia caused by gram-negative bacilli: an overview. *Rev Infect Dis.* 1985;7(suppl 4):S656–S665.

9. Berk S, Verghese A. Emerging pathogens in nosocomial pneumonia. *Eur J Clin Microbiol Infect Dis.* 1989;8:11–14.

10. Ship J. Oral sequelae of common geriatric diseases, disorders, and impairments. *Clin Geriatr Med.* 1992;8(3):483–497.

11. Chauncey HH, Glass RL, Alman JE. Dental caries: principal cause of tooth extraction in a sample of US male adults. *Caries Res.* 1989;23(3):200–205.

12. Niessen LC, Jones JA. Facing the challenge: The Graying of America. In: Papas AS, Niessen LC, Chauncey HH, eds. *Geriatric Dentistry. Aging and Oral Health.* St. Louis: Mosby Yearbook; 1991:3–13.

13. Fitzgerald FJ, Deyes PH. Demonstration of the etiologic role of streptococci in experimental caries in the hamster. *J Am Dent Assoc.* 1960;61:9–19.

14. Houte JV. Bacterial specificity in the etiology of dental caries. *Int Dent J.* 1980;30:305–326.

15. Bowden GHW. Microbiology of root surface caries in humans. *J Dent Res.* 1990;69:1205–1208.

16. Chauncey HH, Meunch ME, Kapur KK, et al. The effect of the loss of teeth on diet and nutrition. *Int Dent J.* 1984;34:98–104.

17. Gordon SR, Kelley SL, Sybyl JR, et al. Relationship in very elderly veterans of nutritional status, self-perceived chewing ability, dental status and social isolation. *J Am Geriatr Soc.* 1985;33:334–339.

18. Brown LR, Dreizen S, Daly TE, et al. Interrelations of oral microorganisms, immunoglubulins, and dental caries following radiotherapy. *J Dent Res.* 1978;57(9–10):882–893.

19. Holm-Pederson P, Agerbaek N, Theilade E. Experimental gingivitis in young and elderly individuals. *J Clin Periodontol.* 1975;2:14–24.

20. Suzuki J, Niessen L, Fedele D. Periodontal diseases in the older adult. In: Papas A, Niessen L, Chauncey H, eds. *Geriatric Dentistry: Aging and Oral Health.* St. Louis: Mosby Yearbook; 1991:189–201.

21. Addy V, McElnay JC, Eyre DG, et al. Risk factors in phenytoin-induced gingival hyperplasia. *J Periodontol.* 1983;54:373–377.

22. Wynn RL. Calcium channel blockers and gingival hyperplasia. *Ger Dent.* 1991;39:270–243.

23. Socransky S, Haffajee A, Goodson J, et al. New concepts of destructive periodontal disease. *J Clin Periodontol.* 1984;11:21–32.

24. Haffajee A, Goodson J, Socransky S. Periodontal disease activity. *J Periodont Res.* 1982;17:521–522.

25. Hunt R, Levy S, Beck J. The prevalence of periodontal attachment loss in an Iowa population aged 70 and older. *J Public Health Dent.* 1990;50(4):251–260.

26. Palmer C. Nutrition and oral health in the elderly. In: Papas A, Niessen L, Chauncey H, eds. *Geriatric Dentistry: Aging and Oral Health.* St. Louis: Mosby Yearbook; 1991:83–102.

27. Albanese A, Edelson A, Lorenze E, et al. Problems of bone health in elderly. Ten year study. *NY State J Med.* 1975; 75(3):326–336.

28. Feldman RS, Bravocos JS, Rose C. Association between smoking different tobacco products and periodontal disease indexes. *J Periodont Res.* 1983;54:481–485.

29. Grossi SA, Zambon JJ, Ho AW, et al. Assessment of risk for periodontal disease. 1. Risk indicators for attachment loss. *J Periodontol.* 1994;65:260–267.

30. Page RC. The pathobiology of periodontal disease may affect systemic diseases: inversion of a paradigm. *Ann Periodontol.* 1998;3(1):108–120.

31. Grossi SC, Genco RJ. Periodontal disease and diabetes mellitus: a two-way relationship. *Ann Periodontol.* 1998; 3(1):51–61.

32. Beck JD, Offenbacher S, Williams R, et al. Periodontitis: a risk factor for coronary heart disease? *Ann Periodontol.* 1998;3(1):127–141.

33. Hujoel PP, Drangsholt M, Spiekerman C, DeRouen TA. Periodontal disease and coronary heart disease risk. *JAMA.* 2000;284(11):1406–1410.

34. Herzberg MC, MacFarlane GD, Gong K. The platelet interactivity phenotype of *Streptococcus sanguis* influences the course of experimental endocarditis. *Infect Immun.* 1992;60:4809–4818.

35. Wu T, Trevisan M, Genco RJ, et al. Periodontal disease and risk of cerebrovascular disease. *Arch Intern Med.* 2000;160:2749–2755.

36. Rao M, Bhargava K. Oral lesions in relation to prosthetics. A review. *Indian J Dent Res.* 1994;5:39–46.

37. Samaranayake LP, McFarlane TW, Lamey PJ, et al. A comparison of oral rinse and imprint sampling techniques for the detection of yeast, coliform and *Staphylococcus aureus* carriage in the oral cavity. *J Oral Pathol.* 1986;15:386–388.

38. Barkvoll P, Attramedal A. Effect of nystatin and chlorhexidine gluconate on *Candida albicans. Oral Surg Oral Med Oral Pathol* 1989;67:279–281.

39. Bertram U, Dragh-Sorensen P, Rafelsen O, et al. Salivary secretion following long-term antidepressant treatment with nortriptyline controlled by plasma levels. *Scand J Dent Res.* 1979;87(1):58–64.

40. Moutsopuolos HM, Chused TM, Mann DL, et al. Sjögren's syndrome (sicca syndrome): current issues. *Ann Intern Med.* 1980;92:212–226.

41. Vivino FB, Al-Hashimi I, Khan Z, et al. Pilocarpine tablets for the treatment of dry mouth and dry eye symptoms in patients with Sjogren's syndrome: a randomized, placebo-controlled, fixed-dose, multicenter trial. P92-01 Study Group. *Arch Intern Med.* 1999;159(2):174–181.

42. Talal N. Sjogren's syndrome: historical overview and clinical spectrum of the disease. *Rheum Dis Clin N Am.* 1992;18(3):507–515.

43. Rankow RN, Polayes IM. Diseases of the salivary glands. Philadelphia: Saunders; 1975:180–185.

44. Batsakis JG. *Tumors of the Head and Neck: Clinical and Pathologic Considerations*. Baltimore, MD: Williams & Wilkins; 1979:161–164.

45. Foote EW, Frazell EL. Tumors of the major salivary glands. *Ca.* 1953;6(1):65–133.

46. Langlais RP, Benson BW, Barnett DA. Salivary gland dysfunction: infections, sialoliths and tumors. *Ear Nose Throat J.* 1989;68:758–770.

47. Valdez IH. Radiation-induced salivary dysfunction: clinical course and significance. *Spec Care Dent.* 1991;11(6):252–255.

48. Johnson JT, Ferretti GA, Dethery WJ, et al. Oral pilocarpine for post-irradiation xerostomia in patients with head and neck cancer. *N Engl J Med.* 1993;329:390–395.

49. Zimmerman RP, Mark RJ, Juillard GF. Concomitant pilocarpine during head and neck irradiation is associated with decreased posttreatment xerostomia. *Int J Radiat Oncol Biol Phys.* 1997;37(3):571–575.

50. Reider C, Martinoff ZJ, Wilcox S. The prevalence of mandibular dysfunction: sex and age distributions of related signs and symptoms. *J Prosth Dent.* 1983;50:81–88.

51. Iacopino AN, Wathen WF. Craniomandibular disorders in the geriatric patient. *J Orofac Pain.* 1993;7(1):38–53.

52. Harriman LP, Snowden DA, Soberay AH. Temporomandibular joint dysfunction and selected health parameters in the elderly. *Oral Surg Oral Med Oral Pathol.* 1990;70:406–413.

53. Wilding RJ, Owen CP. prevalence of temporomandibular joint disease in edentulous non-denture wearing individuals. *J Oral Rehabil.* 1987;14:175–182.

54. Redlund-Johnell I. Upper airway obstruction in patients with rheumatoid arthritis and temporomandibular joint destruction. *Scand J Rheumatol.* 1988;17:273–239.

55. Greenlee RT, Murray T, Bolden S, Wingo PA. Cancer Statistics, 2000. *CA Cancer J Clin.* 2000;50:7–33.

56. Center for Disease Control. *Cancers of the Oral Cavity and Pharynx: A Statistics Review and Monograph, 1973–1987.* Bethesda: National Institutes of Health, U.S. Dept. of Health and Human Services, 1991.

57. Fedele DI, Jones JA, Niessen, LC. Oral cancer screening in the elderly. *J Am Geriatr Soc.* 1991;39:920–925.

58. Blot WJ, McLaughlin JK, Winn DM, et al. Smoking and drinking in relation to oral and pharyngeal cancer. *Cancer Res.* 1988;48:3282–3287.

59. National Cancer Institute. *Oral Cancer Research Report.* NIH 88-2876. Bethesda, MD: USDHHS; 1988.

60. Greer RO. A problem oriented approach to evaluation of common mucosal lesions in the geriatric patient. *Gerodontics.* 1985;1:68–74.

61. Bottomly WK, Rosenberg SW. *Clinical Guide to Treatment of Common Oral Conditions.* American Academy of Oral Medicine; 1987:14.

62. Ship JA, Lin BP. Oral medical problems in older persons. Part II. *Clin Geriatr.* 1996;4(9):39–58.

63. Lamey PH, Lamb AB. Prospective study of etiological factors in burning mouth syndrome. *Br Med J Clin Res.* 1988;296(6631):1243–1260.

64. Wardrop RW, Hailes J, Burger H, et al. Oral discomfort at menopause. *Oral Surg Oral Med Oral Pathol.* 1989;67(5):535–540.

65. Chen MY, Ott DJ, Peele VN, et al. Oropharynx in patients with cerebrovascular disease: evaluation with videofluoroscopy. *Radiology.* 1990;176(3):641–643.

66. Niessen LC, Jones JA. Alzheimer's disease: a guide for dental professionals. *Spec Care Dent.* 1986;6(1):6–12.

67. Mungas D, Cooper JK, Wieler PG, et al. Dietary preference for sweet foods in patients with dementia. *J Am Geriatric Soc.* 1990;38:999–1007.

68. Dajani AS, Taubert KA, Wilson W, et al. Prevention of bacterial endocarditis: recommendations by the American Heart Association. *JAMA.* 1997;277(22):1794–1801.

69. Imperiale TF, Horwitz RJ. Does prophylaxis prevent post-dental endocarditis? A controlled evaluation of protective efficacy. *Am J Med* 1990;88:131–136.

70. Sagert G, Austin TW, Bombassaro AM, Parbtani A. Conformity with guidelines for antimicrobial prophylaxis against bacterial endocarditis. *Am J Hosp Pharm.* 1994;51:2403–2408.

71. Strom BL, Abrutyn E, Berlin JA, et al. Dental and cardiac risk factors for infective endocarditis. A population-based, case-control study. *Ann Intern Med.* 1998;129:761–769.

72. American Dental Association, American Academy of Orthopedic Surgeons. Advisory statement. Antibiotic prophylaxis for dental patients with total joint replacements. *J Am Dent Assoc.* 1997;128:1004–1007.

73. Smith RG, Burtner AB. Oral side effects of the most frequently prescribed drugs. *Spec Care Dent.* 1994;14(3):96–102.

74. Dreizen S, McCredie KB, Bodey GP, et al. Quantitative analysis of the oral complications of anti-leukemia chemotherapy. *Oral Surg Oral Med Oral Pathol.* 1986;62:650–653.

75. Sonis ST, Sonis AL, Lieberman A. Oral complications in patients receiving treatment for malignancies other than the head and neck. *J Am Dent Assoc.* 1978;97:468–472.

76. Ferretti GA, Raybould TP, Brown AT, et al. Chlorhexidine prophylaxis for chemotherapy and radiotherapy induced stomatitis: randomized double-blind trial. *Oral Surg Oral Med Oral Pathol.* 1990;69:331–338.

Part V
Medical Care

Section C
Common Problems in Older Adults

62
Dietary Supplements for Geriatric Patients

Cynthia X. Pan and Charles Mobbs

Information about the safety and efficacy of nutritional supplements is increasingly important to the geriatrician because these supplements are widely used by elderly patients, often without the knowledge of their physicians, yet the use of such supplements can have deleterious effects, including interference with prescribed drugs. Recent studies indicate that adults are increasingly using nutritional supplements such as herbal therapy[1] and other forms of complementary/alternative medicine (CAM) in the United States.[2-4] Several epidemiologic studies spanning different nations suggest that older individuals of both sexes use such therapies.[2,5-7] In a study of more than 1000 patients who complained of "arthritis," one-third had received treatment from a nonorthodox medical practitioner.[8] Risberg et al. noted that 20% of a population of hospitalized cancer patients used alternative medicine.[9] A 1995 study of 101 primary caregivers of dementia patients found that 55% of caregivers attending support groups had tried at least one type of alternative therapy in an attempt to improve the memory of the demented individual for whom they were caring.[10] A Canadian telephone survey of 115 caregivers and patients (with dementia) found that 9.6% of the patients were using complementary medicine as a treatment to help with their memory or thinking problems.[11]

More recent data reveal CAM use patterns in older adults. In a cross-sectional survey examining patterns of complementary therapy use in urban multiethnic populations, 421 older participants were interviewed at two sites: an academic geriatrics primary care practice and a veterans medical clinic.[12] Fifty-eight percent (58%) of all subjects surveyed used some form of CAM, almost 75% at the academic practice alone. In a national survey of Californians enrolled in a Medicare risk product that offers coverage for acupuncture and chiropractic care, surveys were sent to 1597 members and responses received from 728 (51% response rate). Forty-one percent of seniors reported use of CAM. Herbs (24%), chiropractic (20%), massage (15%), and acupuncture (14%) were the most frequently cited therapies. Respondents also expressed considerable interest in receiving third-party coverage for CAM. Although 80% reported that they had received substantial benefit from their use of CAM, the majority (58%) did not discuss the use of these therapies with their medical doctor.[13]

The widespread use of nutritional supplements in elderly patients was corroborated by a study of one of the authors (Pan), who conducted a multisite survey of 503 patients aged 65 and older.[14] This survey included a diverse population whose mean age was 77 years; 50% were white, 34% African-American, and 13% Hispanic-American. Approximately 57% of respondents used some form of complementary therapy within 12 months of being surveyed, of which 35% consisted of dietary supplements and another 35% was herbal supplements. The most common herbal supplements used were garlic, gingko, fish oils, ginger, and ginseng, and the most common vitamin supplements used were vitamin E, vitamin C, the B vitamins, and carotenes/vitamin A. Physicians increasingly may be called upon by patients to advise them about the use of nutritional supplements. Physicians also need to be aware of potentially hazardous interactions between supplements and drugs and when appropriate should ask patients specifically about the use of such supplements. Nevertheless, despite the widespread use of herbal treatments, a recent survey indicated that only about half of responding physicians reported discussing complementary, including herbal, therapies with their patients.[15] Another study compared results of a convenience sample survey of older adults with documentation in medical charts.[16] Authors measured the proportion of CAM supplements and herbs (CAMsh) reported by patients *also* documented in patients' charts: only 35% of all self-reported supplements were documented in the charts. Of 182 patients, 46% reported taking CAM with anticoagulant properties: of these, 52% took a prescribed anticoagulant (per chart). This lack of knowledge of patient use of herbal and dietary sup-

TABLE 62.1. Internet (Google) searches: January 2001.

	Health	Cholesterol	Cancer	Memory	Fatigue
Garlic	181,000	91,000	60,800	45,000	28,200
Gingko biloba	12,600	2,900	4,600	3,000	2,490
Fish oils	99,100	17,000	29,000	7,000	10,000
Ginseng	102,000	32,000	39,700	33,000	35,000
Zingiber (ginger)	5,000	2,000	2,000	1,500	1,400
Vitamins	500,000	157,000	212,000	88,000	89,000
Wine	800,000	60,000	189,000	283,000	33,000
St. John's wort	67,800	22,000[a]	39,700	33,000	35,000
Glucosamine	70,400				
Chondroitin	34,000				
DHEA (dehydroepi-androsterone)	59,400	22,000	24,700	12,200	28,700

[a] Many discussed how St. John's wort can interfere with cholesterol-lowering drugs.

plements can have potentially serious and lethal consequences.

Garlic (*Allium sativum*)

Garlic (*Allium sativum*) is a common folk remedy for many conditions, as well as a ubiquitous component in food preparation. One index of popular interest of supplements is a simple search on the Internet of the supplement combined with various health concerns such as "health," "cholesterol," "cancer," "memory," and "fatigue" (Table 62.1). Of the supplements we searched, garlic was one of the most popular, particularly in connection with cholesterol.

Although garlic has been reported to improve certain cardiovascular risk factors, especially cholesterol, there is currently no evidence that these effects translate into reduction of morbidity or mortality. A recent meta-analysis concluded that garlic preparations may reduce plasma cholesterol, a finding not seen in some small well-designed studies. Therefore, the cholesterol-lowering effect of garlic is likely to be weak and requires a highly powered study to demonstrate a significantly positive effect.[17] Conversely, another report indicated that although the trial failed to demonstrate an effect of garlic powder on plasma cholesterol levels,[18] meta-analysis of previous data supported that garlic probably can have a beneficial effect. Another well-designed double-blind placebo study did find a significant effect of a garlic preparation on reducing total serum cholesterol as well as low-density lipoprotein and blood pressure.[19] Similarly, an uncontrolled study indicated that daily consumption of a fresh garlic clove for 16 weeks reduced serum cholesterol

by 20%, but also reduced serum thromboxane a remarkable 80%.[20]

Earlier meta-analyses had reported that garlic reduced cholesterol by about 12%[21] or 9%.[22] However, observing effects on potential risk factors may not predict clinical outcomes [such as coronary artery disease (CAD), myocardial infarction (MI), and mortality]. For example, a meta-analysis in the Cochrane review series has concluded that the use of garlic has no significant effect on at least one cardiovascular outcome, peripheral occlusive arterial disease.[23] In terms of garlic for cancer, a recent meta-analysis of epidemiologic evidence concluded that the evidence supports that high intake of both raw and cooked garlic may protect against stomach and colorectal cancer.[24] However, there have been no clinical trials to study this conclusion. All these data should be framed in the context of a 1998 ruling[25] that the U.S. Food and Drug Administration (FDA) issued prohibiting the use on foods of a claim relating to the relationship between garlic, decreased serum cholesterol, and the risk in adults of cardiovascular disease.

The use of garlic provides a good example of the issues faced by practitioners on the subject of nutritional supplements. First, garlic represents the most commonly used nutritional supplement, probably because it is a common component of cooking. For this reason, garlic is perceived as safer than most herbal nutritional supplements. Second, there is a literature substantiating that the use of garlic as a nutritional supplement (specifically entailing the consumption of fresh garlic or garlic powder at levels far exceeding levels normally consumed in food) produces clinically desirable effects, especially on plasma cholesterol, although similar controlled trials on cancer prevention have not yet been undertaken. Thus, when a patient asks about the advisability of consuming garlic, the answer is not clear-cut. In general, relatively high-level consumption of garlic is unlikely to cause harm and may marginally reduce plasma cholesterol. In patients with clinically significant hypercholesterolemia, numerous treatments, including weight loss and pharmacologic intervention with statins, are far more likely to produce clinically significant effects. The main concern of the clinician is that the use of garlic as a nutritional supplement may produce a false sense of security in some patients and undermine their compliance with clinically more efficacious treatments. Clinicians also need to advise patients about garlic halitosis, expense issues, and potential drug–herb interactions, such as with warfarin.[26]

Ginkgo biloba

Extracts from the leaves of the ginkgo biloba tree have been used in traditional Chinese medicine to treat a variety of ailments associated with "cerebral insufficiency." In comparison with most of the other supplements reviewed here, which average around 100,000 hits when searched with the word "health," ginkgo appears to be of much less popular interest, at least as reflected in Web pages. Ginkgo use does hold a special place in geriatric medicine, however, because of its positive effects in treating cognitive impairment associated with dementia.

For more than a decade the effectiveness of ginkgo extracts to improve cognitive function in dementia has been extensively studied, and such extracts have even been approved for the treatment of dementia in Germany.[27] A meta-analysis of these studies concluded that ginkgo extracts do improve cognitive symptoms in dementia, although the effects are modest.[28] Consistent with that analysis, a later study also concluded that ginkgo in the form of the EGB761 extract produces effects in patients with Alzheimer's disease, as measured by the Alzheimer's Disease Assessment Scale–Cognitive subscale (ADAS-Cog) scale, that are comparable to those produced by cholinesterase inhibitors including tacrine;[29] furthermore, EGB761 use resulted in a lower dropout rate than tacrine.[29] A recent large trial reached a similar conclusion.[30] This trial was a double-blind, placebo-controlled, parallel group, and multicenter study on mildly to severely demented patients with either Alzheimer's disease or vascular dementia. The patients' mean age was 69 years, and their Mini-Mental Status score ranged from 9 to 26. The extract EGB761 was used at 120 mg/day in three divided doses and given for 26 weeks. The extract stabilized and modestly improved patients' cognitive performance and social functioning. The findings were documented objectively by ADAS-Cog and noticed by caregivers. The study's conclusions are valid mostly for Alzheimer's disease patients with mild to moderate cognitive impairment. However, another study found no effect of treatment with higher doses of the same extract given for 12 weeks.[31] Thus, one may need to take ginkgo for a long period of time (e.g., 26 weeks) to observe an effect. In terms of ginkgo extracts for fatigue, no randomized, placebo-controlled double-blind trials exist to date.

In conclusion, the EGB761 preparation of ginkgo produces real but modest improvements in cognitive function in individuals with mild moderate cognitive impairment, probably comparable to that produced by tacrine or other cholinesterase inhibitors. Ginkgo extracts may be better tolerated by some patients than cholinesterase inhibitors, so in those patients it may be the treatment of choice. It is essential to emphasize, however, that no current treatment, including Aricept and other prescription drugs, produces more than a slight delay in the deterioration of cognitive function in Alzheimer's disease or other dementias.

Fish Oils (3-Omega Fatty Acids)

Interest in fish oils, especially omega-3 fatty acids (including eicosapentaenoic acid and docosahexaenoic acid), was stimulated by epidemiologic findings that indigenous Inuit people in Greenland were often obese but suffered lower than expected levels of cardiovascular complications, apparently due to a diet consisting mainly of fish.[32,33] The highest ranked of our Internet searches reviewed published data reporting beneficial effects of omega-3 fatty acids on a rather large variety of clinical conditions, especially related to cardiovascular function and cancer. It is interesting that although the Web pages exhibit greater popular interest in the use of fish oils to prevent or reduce cancer, there are far more scientific data to support a role in cardiovascular disease risk reduction.

Recent meta-analyses of controlled clinical trials confirm that use of omega-3 fatty acids up to 3 g/day for 3 to 24 weeks produced clinically significant reductions in blood pressure.[34,35] Similarly, a recent meta-analysis concluded that consumption of omega-3 fatty acids, especially eicosapentaenoic acid and docosahexaenoic acid, produced clinically significant reduction of triglycerides in diabetic patients.[36,37] Despite these data, the position of the FDA, as of 1998, was typically cautious, and prohibited a claim by commercial vendors that consumption of omega-3 fatty acids would produce cardiovascular benefits.[38] Nevertheless, while the literature supports that consumption of omega-3 fatty acids up to 3 g/day leads to reduction of some risk factors for cardiovascular disease, there has not yet been definitive proof that reduction in these risk factors will lead to reduction in actual cardiovascular events.

Ginseng (from Root of *Panax ginseng*)

Ginseng is one of the most popular herbal and nutritional supplements and is a major mainstay of the traditional Chinese medicine pharmacopeia. In contrast to the substantial data supporting statistically significant, if modest, effects of other nutritional supplements including garlic, ginkgo, and St. John's wort, there is relatively little objective evidence that ginseng produces significant clinical effects. For example, an extensive systematic review[39] searched the computerized literature for double-blind, randomized, placebo-controlled trials of ginseng root extract for any indication. Sixteen trials met the inclusion criteria and were reviewed. These trials looked at physical performance, psychomotor performance and cognitive function, immunomodulation, diabetes mellitus, and herpes simplex type 2 infections. The authors concluded that efficacy of ginseng was not firmly established for any of those indications. There are several reports in the literature, however, that ginseng may produce subjective improvements that many patients may consider valuable. For example, in a randomized, double-blind placebo-controlled study of symptomatic perimenopausal women,[40] ginseng was found to produce significant improvements in self-rated assessments of depression, well-being, and health. Similarly, a randomized, double-blind study assessed effects of a ginseng plus vitamin preparation on responses to a quality of life questionnaire in 625 patients, compared to a vitamin regimen.[41] The ginseng preparation did not produce a significant improvement in every item assessed, whereas the vitamin preparation was reported not to produce an improvement in any item. Although subjective outcomes are difficult to measure and more subject to bias, they are patient centered and should not be dismissed. Also, ginseng may have pharmacologic activity for which we have not yet found the appropriate objective measures.

Ginger (*Zingiber officinale*)

The main interest in ginger appears to be its effects on nausea: a search on "zingiber" and "nausea" produced 2900 hits. Indeed, this indication of ginger is the only one for which clinical trials exist. A recent meta-analysis of randomized clinical trials concluded that the six trials that met the criterion of the analysis suggested that ginger reduces nausea more than placebo and may in fact be as effective as metoclopramide for postoperative nausea.[42] As with garlic, the use of ginger may be effective, and is probably not as likely to produce iatrogenic effects as some pharmaceuticals.

Vitamins

There is tremendous interest in vitamin supplements, which are widely used. A search on the Internet (Google) on "vitamin" and "health" in January 2001 resulted in almost 500,000 hits. There is however surprisingly little support for a clinically significant effect of vitamin supplementation, at least in well-nourished Western populations. Two recent meta-analyses concluded that although epidemiologic evidence clearly suggests that higher intake of antioxidant vitamins C and E are protective against cardiovascular disease, controlled clinical trials, examining high doses up to 400 IU per day, have not convincingly demonstrated this effect.[43-45] While current studies are continuing to assess this question in more detail, it is instructive that vitamin supplementation is far more common than other supplements described in the review, but there is actually less evidence supporting the

value of their use than there is for most of the other supplements. However, they are also not likely to be harmful.

Wine

The observation that incidence of coronary heart disease is relatively low in France, despite high levels of dietary fat, led to the hypothesis that the relatively high levels of wine consumed in France may produce a protective effect against heart disease.[46-48] Like garlic, drinking wine is a common component of dining habits in many societies, and there is intense popular interest in the health consequences of drinking wine. A search on the Internet (Google) on "wine" and "health" in January 2001 resulted in almost 800,000 hits, "wine" and "cholesterol" generated about 60,000 hits, "wine" and "cancer" generated about 189,000 hits, "wine" and "memory" generated about 283,000 hits, and "wine" and "fatigue" generated about 33,000 hits.

Extensive epidemiologic data have demonstrated a J-shaped relationship between consumption of alcohol, especially red wine, and reduction of mortality resulting from cardiovascular disease.[49-52] However, such data do not address the effects of alcohol consumption specifically in the elderly. Furthermore, clinical trials to assess the effects of alcohol consumption on any health parameter have not actually been undertaken, and as with vitamins, it remains possible that the epidemiologic data may be misleading. It is plausible that consumption of wine reduces the development of cardiovascular impairments but does not reverse them. For both pharmacokinetic and pharmacodynamic reasons, older adults have a greater response to the same amount of wine they were able to tolerate when younger. Considering the increased risk of falls and other potential major injuries that might be exacerbated by alcohol in the elderly, it may be that the optimal use of alcohol is to consume it during the middle-age years and abstain during older adulthood. Currently, these precise relationships remain unclear. Therefore, the current thinking is that if moderate drinking of wine has been part of the normal lifestyle of an elderly individual, there is no reason to recommend a marked change in habit, but the evidence also does not support a recommendation to begin consumption of wine in elderly individuals who would otherwise abstain.

St. John's Wort (*Hypericum perforatum*): Potential for Lethal Drug Interactions

There is much evidence supporting extracts of St. John's wort, or *Hypericum perforatum*, as an effective treatment for depression. A search on the Internet (Google) on "St. John's wort" and "health" in January 2001 resulted in about 67,800 hits, while "St. John's wort" and "cholesterol" generated about 22,000 hits (many of which discussed how St. John's wort can interfere with cholesterol-lowering drugs). Recent studies have demonstrated an unexpected danger in the use of these extracts, however, especially in elderly patients who are more likely to be under treatment with several medications simultaneously.

Hypericum extracts are now commonly used by patients to treat depressive symptoms, often without consultation with medical professionals;[53] a high percentage of such patients report positive effects of the treatment, although some patients cease using the extracts because of side effects, including symptoms of serotonin syndrome.[53] Several meta-studies have concluded that hypericum extracts are more effective than placebo to reduce depressive symptoms[54-56] and may be as effective as prescription pharmacologic treatments of depression[57] although a recent large study failed to show a benefit.[57a] Hypericum extracts have been reported to be as effective as imipramine in reducing depressive symptoms, with fewer iatrogenic effects than imipramine.[58] Similarly, hypericum extracts were reported to be as effective as sertraline[59] and fluoxetine[60,61] in reducing symptoms of mild depression. Hypericum extracts were also found to reduce obsessive-compulsive symptoms.[62] At least one report specifically suggests that hypericum extracts may be a particularly useful treatment for even severe depression in the elderly, because these extracts are both efficacious and may be better tolerated than tricyclic antidepressants.[63]

Hypericum extracts appear to exert their antidepressant activity by enhancing serotonin tone, as is the case with many antidepressants, but the mechanism by which this occurs may be different from the mechanisms engaged by classic serotonin uptake inhibitors,[64] including an effect to stimulate dopamine release,[65] inhibit norepinephrine synthesis,[66] and reduce reuptake of glutamate and GABA.[67] Interestingly, some compounds extracted from hypericum may interact directly with receptors for corticotropin-releasing factor,[68] a system known to influence anxiety. As is typically the case with herbal extracts, the specific chemical constituents that mediate the antidepressant effects of hypericum extracts remain to be determined. In the case of hypericum extract, the main candidates are hypericin and hypaphorine, but the role of these and other constituents are unclear.[69]

As with any drug, hypericum extracts can have iatrogenic effects, including inducing reversible mania in some patients.[70,71] On the whole, such iatrogenic effects are thought to be less problematic for hypericum extracts than for prescription drugs. Several recent reports have indicated that hypericum extracts can dramatically reduce the bioavailability of cyclosporin A in liver trans-plant patients, leading to almost fatal rejection of the transplanted liver.[72] After cessation of ingestion of hypericum, cyclosporin A levels returned to normal, as did liver function.[72] Similar observations were made in patients with kidney transplantations[73,74] and with heart transplantations.[75] Part of the mechanism by which hypericum extracts reduce drug bioavailability is through the activation of the pregnane X orphan steroid receptor,[76,77] which in turn activates the hepatocyte cytochrome P-450 A34 (CYPA34) enzyme that is involved in the oxidative inactivation of more than 50% of all drugs.[77,78] Because activation of CYPA34 may enhance inactivation of many drugs, the effect of hypericum extracts to activate CYPA34 may be particularly dangerous in elderly patients who are more likely to be treated with several drugs simultaneously. Thus, the wide use of hypericum extracts constitutes a particularly clear example of the need for physicians to obtain a complete appraisal of the use of nutritional supplements that their patients are consuming, as well as a renewed effort to monitor medications that are metabolized by the P-450 cytochrome system.

Glucosamine and Chondroitin

Glucosamine and chondroitin sulfate have become increasingly popular nutritional supplements to treat symptoms of osteoarthritis.[79] A search on the Internet (Google) on "glucosamine" and "arthritis" generated about 46,000 hits, and "chondroitin" and "arthritis" generated about 20,000 hits. In a recent meta-analysis[79] assessing the efficacy of glucosamine in treating symptoms of osteoarthritis, 13 randomized clinical trials compared glucosamine to placebo; glucosamine was found to be superior in all except 1, using a variety of outcomes including patient reports of pain and mobility. In the four randomized clinical trials in which glucosamine was compared to a nonsteroid anti-inflammatory drug, glucosamine was superior in two, and equivalent in two, again using the same outcomes. However, the present data are considered preliminary by the American College of Rheumatology because of the small number of patients examined so far. A large NIH-sponsored trial is under way to more definitively assess the efficacy of glucosamine and chondroitin in osteoarthritis and to include some objective outcomes in addition to patients' subjective reports.[80]

DHEA (Dehydroepiandrosterone)

Plasma levels of dehydroepiandrosterone (DHEA) and its more abundant sulfated form, DHEA-S, decrease more markedly during aging (maximum levels observed in the early twenties) than levels of any other hormone in humans, with the exception of the decrease of estradiol in postmenopausal women.[81,82] The most recent meta-analysis of trials assessing effects of DHEA concluded that DHEA replacement produced no significant objective benefit, although it may produce subjective benefit.[83] To date the most complete study published that addresses the effects of DHEA supplementation in aging humans has been by Morales et al.[84] This randomized, double-blind, placebo-controlled crossover trial involved nightly oral DHEA administration (producing pharmacologic levels of the hormone) or placebo over 6 months in a group of healthy men and women 40 to 70 years of age, a regimen that restored plasma DHEA and DHEA-S to youthful levels. This study examined a wide variety of outcomes, including concentration of androgens, lipids, apolipoproteins, insulin-like growth factor 1 (IGF-1), IGF-binding protein 1 (IGFB-1), IGFB-3, insulin sensitivity, percent body fat, libido, and sense of well-being. In a subgroup, blood was taken every 20 min over 24 h for measurement of growth hormone. Of all these parameters, the only objective measurements that were significantly influenced by DHEA replacement were an increase in IGF-1 (20% in men and 12% in women) and a decrease in IGFB-1 (29% in men, 23% in women). The significance of these isolated effects remains unclear.

Despite the rather impressive lack of effect of DHEA supplementation in the study by Morales et al.[84] on objective parameters, the increase in perceived physical and psychologic well-being was dramatic. Although fewer than 10% of the subjects on placebo reported an improvement in sense of well-being, 82% of women and 67% of men given the DHEA replacement reported an improvement in sense of well-being. Specific statements included improved quality of sleep, increased sense of relaxation, and increased sense of energy. Furthermore, several subjects given DHEA self-reported marked improvements of preexisting joint pains and mobility. Because this study was double blinded, these subjective improvements were impressive despite the paucity of objective measurements that showed any improvement. It is plausible that DHEA replacement may produce physiologic effects, which we have not yet been able to measure, that lead to improvements in the sense of well-being. Nevertheless, as with any steroid hormone, the use of DHEA can be potentially dangerous (high levels are associated with increased risk of some cancers and reduced HDL levels[85]), and there is currently little basis to recommend the use of DHEA.

Growth Hormone

Similar to that of DHEA, growth hormone secretion decreases during aging.[86] Growth hormone (GH) is not a nutritional supplement; it is available only by injection.

Reports by Rudman et al.[87,88] that treatment of elderly hyposomatotropic men with growth hormone significantly increased muscle mass and partially reversed other age-related impairments greatly stimulated interest in this treatment during aging. Replacement of growth hormone has even been touted as an antiaging regimen.[89] However, this possibility must be approached with considerable caution, because acromegalic humans with elevated growth hormone secretion exhibit shortened life span.[90] Similarly, it was observed that transgenic mice expressing elevated levels of growth hormone, like acromegalic humans, actually exhibit a reduced life span compared with wild-type mice.[91,92] Even more surprisingly, it has recently been observed that mice with growth hormone secretion or receptors genetically ablated actually live longer than wild-type controls.[93,94] Thus the concept of using growth hormone replacement as an antiaging regimen must be considered to be highly suspect.

Discussion

The nutritional supplements and "antiaging" medicines discussed in this review are available commercially (except for GH) and are widely popularized on the Internet and other sources. Several studies document that older adults use these supplements, often without the knowledge of the health care provider. Because nutritional supplements are increasingly popular, the clinician is increasingly called upon to address the use of these supplements in several capacities: to recommend whether or not the patient should begin or continue using a supplement, to compare a supplement with a medication to decide which one to try first, and to advise about potential drug–herb interactions. When advising patients about nutritional supplements, we must consider the following. First, many people seek nutritional/dietary supplements because they think they are "natural" and therefore safe. We must advise our patients that natural does not automatically mean safe, especially because supplements are not regulated by the FDA, are not required to follow strict manufacturing standards, and can potentially contain contaminants such as lead or other compounds. Second, when recommending the use of a supplement that has been tested in a clinical trial, it is probably safest to recommend that the patient buy the brand that was used in that trial, thus ensuring the patient receives as standardized a dose as possible. Third, evidence for efficacy of supplements is derived from different sources: anecotal evidence, epidemiologic evidence, uncontrolled studies, and controlled clinical trials. Thus, all supplements are not created equal. Although clinical trial evidence would support using glucosamine for osteoarthritis, it would not support using GH to reverse the aging process. Finally, we should educate patients about dosing their supplements. The maxim, "The difference between a drug and poison is dose" may be helpful for some patients to understand why in vitro effects may not predict therapeutic value.

References

1. Bauer BA. Herbal therapy: what a clinician needs to know to counsel patients effectively. *Mayo Clin Proc.* 2000;75(8): 835–841.

2. Eisenberg DM, Kessler RC, Foster C, et al. Unconventional medicine in the United States. Prevalence, costs, and patterns of use. *N Engl J Med.* 1993;328(4):246–252.

3. Eisenberg DM, Davis RB, Ettner SL, et al. Trends in alternative medicine use in the United States, 1990–1997: results of a follow-up national survey. *JAMA.* 1998;280(18):1569–1575.

4. Paramore LC. Use of alternative therapies: estimates from the 1994 Robert Wood Johnson Foundation National Access to Care Survey. *J Pain Symptom Manage.* 1997; 13(2):83–89.

5. Thomas KJ, Carr J, Westlake L, et al. Use of non-orthodox and conventional health care in Great Britain. *Br Med J.* 1991;302(6770):207–210.

6. MacLennan AH, Wilson DH, Taylor AW. Prevalence and cost of alternative medicine in Australia. *Lancet.* 1996; 347(9001):569–573.

7. Furnham A, Kirkcaldy B. The health beliefs and behaviors of orthodox and complementary medicine clients. *Br J Clin Psychol.* 1996;35(pt 1):49–61.

8. Resch KL, Hill S, Ernst E. Use of complementary therapies by individuals with "arthritis." *Clin Rheumatol.* 1997;16(4):391–395.

9. Risberg T, Kaasa S, Wist E, et al. Why are cancer patients using non-proven complementary therapies? A cross-sectional multicentre study in Norway. *Eur J Cancer.* 1997; 33(4):575–580.

10. Coleman LM, Fowler LL, Williams ME. Use of unproven therapies by people with Alzheimer's disease. *J Am Geriatr Soc.* 1995;43(7):747–750.

11. Hogan DB, Ebly EM. Complementary medicine use in a dementia clinic population. *Alzheimer Dis Assoc Disord.* 1996;10(2):63–67.

12. Cherniack EP, Senzel RS, Pan CX. Correlates of use of alternative medicine by the elderly in an urban population. *J Altern Complement Med.* 2001;7(3):277–280.

13. Astin JA, Pelletier KR, Marie A, Haskell WL. Complementary and alternative medicine use among elderly persons: one-year analysis of a Blue Shield Medicare supplement. *J Gerontol A Biol Sci Med Sci.* 2000;55(1):M4–M9.

14. Pan CX, Cherniack EP, Ness J, et al. Complementary medicine use in older adults. Presented at the Gerontological Society of America Annual Meeting, San Francisco, Nov 20, 1999 [abstract].

15. Einarson A, Lawrimore T, Brand P, et at. Attitudes and practices of physicians and naturopaths toward herbal products, including use during pregnancy and lactation. *Can J Clin Pharmacol.* 2000;7(1):45–49.

16. Cohen R, Ek K, Pan CX. Complementary and alternative medicine (CAM) use by older adults: a comparison of self-report and physician chart documentation. The Journals of Gerontology Series A: Biological and Medical Sciences 2002:57:M223–227.

17. Stevinson C, Pittler MH, Ernst E. Garlic for treating hypercholesterolemia. A meta-analysis of randomized clinical trials. *Ann Intern Med.* 2000;133(6):420–429.

18. Neil HA, Silagy CA, Lancaster T, et al. Garlic powder in the treatment of moderate hyperlipidaemia: a controlled trial and meta-analysis. *J R Coll Physicians Lond.* 1996;30(4):329–334.

19. Steiner M, Khan AH, Holbert D, et al. A double-blind crossover study in moderately hypercholesterolemic men that compared the effect of aged garlic extract and placebo administration on blood lipids. *Am J Clin Nutr.* 1996; 64(6):866–870.

20. Ali M, Thomson M. Consumption of a garlic clove a day could be beneficial in preventing thrombosis. *Prostaglandins Leukot Essent Fatty Acids.* 1995;53(3):211–212.

21. Silagy C, Neil A. Garlic as a lipid lowering agent—a meta-analysis. *J R Coll Physicians Lond.* 1994;28(1):39–45.

22. Warshafsky S, Kamer RS, Sivak SL. Effect of garlic on total serum cholesterol. A meta-analysis. *Ann Intern Med.* 1993;119(7 pt 1):599–605.

23. Jepson RG, Kleijnen J, Leng GC. Garlic for peripheral arterial occlusive disease. In: Review TC, ed. *The Cochrane Library.* Oxford: Oxford; 2001.

24. Fleischauer AT, Poole C, Arab L. Garlic consumption and cancer prevention: meta-analyses of colorectal and stomach cancers. *Am J Clin Nutr.* 2000;72(4):1047–1052.

25. FDA. Food labeling: health claims; garlic, reduction of serum cholesterol, and the risk of cardiovascular disease in adults. Interim final rule. *Fed Reg.* 1998;63(119): 34110–34112.

26. Fugh-Berman A. Herb–drug interactions. *Lancet.* 2000; 355(9198):134–138.

27. Forstl H. Clinical issues in current drug therapy for dementia. *Alzheimer Dis Assoc Disord.* 2000;14(suppl 1): S103–S108.

28. Oken BS, Storzbach DM, Kaye JA. The efficacy of *Ginkgo biloba* on cognitive function in Alzheimer disease. *Arch Neurol.* 1998;55(11):1409–1415.

29. Wettstein A. Cholinesterase inhibitors and *Gingko* extracts—are they comparable in the treatment of dementia? Comparison of published placebo-controlled efficacy studies of at least six months' duration. *Phytomedicine.* 2000;6(6):393–401.

30. Le Bars PL, Kieser M, Itil KZ. A 26-week analysis of a double-blind, placebo-controlled trial of the *Ginkgo biloba* extract EGb 761 in dementia. *Dernent Geriatr Cogn Disord.* 2000;11(4):230–237.

31. van Dongen MC, van Rossum E, Kessels AG, et al. The efficacy of ginkgo for elderly people with dementia and age-associated memory impairment: new results of a randomized clinical trial. *J Am Geriatr Soc.* 2000;48(10): 1183–1194.

32. O'Keefe JH Jr, Harris WS. From Inuit to implementation: omega-3 fatty acids come of age. *Mayo Clin Proc.* 2000; 75(6):607–614.

33. Burr ML. Lessons from the story of *n*-3 fatty acids. *Am J Clin Nutr.* 2000;71(suppl 1):397S–398S.

34. Appel LJ, Miller ERD, Seidler AJ, et al. Does supplementation of diet with "fish oil" reduce blood pressure? A meta-analysis of controlled clinical trials. *Arch Intern Med.* 1993;153(12):1429–1438.

35. Morris MC, Sacks F, Rosner B. Does fish oil lower blood pressure? A meta-analysis of controlled trials. *Circulation.* 1993;88(2):523–533.

36. Friedberg CE, Janssen MJ, Heine RJ, et al. Fish oil and glycemic control in diabetes. A meta-analysis. *Diabetes Care.* 1998;21(4):494–500.

37. Farmer A, Montori V, Dinneen S, et al. Fish oil in people with type 2 diabetes mellitus. In: Review TC, ed. *The Cochrane Library.* Oxford: Oxford; 2001.

38. FDA. Food labeling: health claims; omega-3 fatty acids and the risk in adults of cardiovascular disease. Interim final rule. *Fed Reg.* 1998;63(119):34107–34110.

39. Vogler BK, Pittler MH, Ernst E. The efficacy of ginseng. A systematic review of randomised clinical trials. *Eur J Clin Pharmacol.* 1999;55(8):567–575.

40. Wiklund IK, Mattsson LA, Lindgren R, et al. Effects of a standardized ginseng extract on quality of life and physiological parameters in symptomatic postmenopausal women: a double-blind, placebo-controlled trial. Swedish Alternative Medicine Group. *Int J Clin Pharmacol Res.* 1999;19(3):89–99.

41. Caso Marasco A, Vargas Ruiz R, Salas Villagomez A, et al. Double-blind study of a multivitamin complex supplemented with ginseng extract. *Drugs Exp Clin Res.* 1996;22(6):323–329.

42. Ernst E, Pittler MH. Efficacy of ginger for nausea and vomiting: a systematic review of randomized clinical trials. *Br J Anaesth.* 2000;84(3):367–371.

43. Dagenais GR, Marchioli R, Yusuf S, et al. Beta-carotene, vitamin C, and vitamin E and cardiovascular diseases. *Curr Cardiol Rep.* 2000;2(4):293–299.

44. Yusuf S, Dagenais C, Pogue J, et al. Vitamin E supplementation and cardiovascular events in high-risk patients. The Heart Outcomes Prevention Evaluation Study Investigators. *N Engl J Med.* 2000;342(3):154–160.

45. Lonn EM, Yusuf S. Is there a role for antioxidant vitamins in the prevention of cardiovascular diseases? An update on epidemiological and clinical trials data. *Can J Cardiol.* 1997;13(10):957–965.

46. Constant J. Alcohol, ischemic heart disease, and the French paradox. *Clin Cardiol.* 1997;20(5):420–424.

47. Burr ML. Explaining the French paradox. *J R Soc Health.* 1995;115(4):217–219.

48. Renaud S, de Lorgeril M. Wine, alcohol, platelets, and the French paradox for coronary heart disease. *Lancet.* 1992; 339(8808):1523–1526.

49. Poikolainen K. Alcohol and mortality: a review. *J Clin Epidemiol.* 1995;48(4):455–465.

50. Cleophas TJ. Wine, beer and spirits and the risk of myocardial infarction: a systematic review. *Biomed Pharmacother.* 1999;53(9):417–423.

51. Deev A, Shestov D, Abernathy J, et al. Association of alcohol consumption to mortality in middle-aged U.S. and Russian men and women. *Ann Epidemiol.* 1998;8(3): 147–153.

52. Kannel WB, Ellison RC. Alcohol and coronary heart disease: the evidence for a protective effect. *Clin Chim Acta.* 1996;246(1–2):59–76.

53. Beckman SE, Sommi RW, Switzer J. Consumer use of St. John's wort: a survey on effectiveness, safety, and tolerability. *Pharmacotherapy.* 2000;20(5):568–574.

54. Stevinson C, Ernst E. Hypericum for depression. An update of the clinical evidence. *Eur Neuropsychopharmacol.* 1999;9(6):501–505.

55. Linde K, Mulrow CD. St. John's wort for depression. *Cochrane Database Syst Rev.* 2000;2.

56. Gaster B, Holroyd J. St. John's wort for depression: a systematic review. *Arch Intern Med.* 2000;160(2):152–156.

57. Williams JW Jr, Mulrow CD, Chiquette E, et al. A systematic review of newer pharmacotherapies for depression in adults: evidence report summary. *Ann Intern Med.* 2000;132(9):743–756.

57a. Shelton RC, Keller MB, Gelenberg A, et al. Effectiveness of St. John's wort in major depression: a randomized controlled trial. *JAMA.* 2001;285(15):1978–1986.

58. Woelk H. Comparison of St. John's wort and imipramine for treating depression: randomised controlled trial. *Br Med J.* 2000;321(7260):536–539.

59. Brenner R, Azbel V, Madhusoodanan S, et al. Comparison of an extract of hypericum (LI 160) and sertraline in the treatment of depression: a double-blind, randomized pilot study. *Clin Ther.* 2000;22(4):411–419.

60. Volz HP, Laux P. Potential treatment for subthreshold and mild depression: a comparison of St. John's wort extracts and fluoxetine. *Compr Psychiatry.* 2000;41(2 suppl 1): 133–137.

61. Schrader E. Equivalence of St. John's wort extract (Ze 117) and fluoxetine: a randomized, controlled study in mildmoderate depression. *Int Clin Psychopharmacol.* 2000;15(2):61–68.

62. Taylor LH, Kobak KA. An open-label trial of St. John's Wort (*Hypericum perforatum*) in obsessive-compulsive disorder. *J Clin Psychiatry.* 2000;61(8):575–578.

63. Vorbach EU, Arnoldt KH, Wolpert E. St. John's wort: a potential therapy for elderly depressed patients? *Drugs Aging.* 2000;16(3):189–197.

64. Yu PH. Effect of the *Hvpericum perforatum* extract on serotonin turnover in the mouse brain. *Pharmacopsychiatry.* 2000;33(2):60–65.

65. Di Matteo V, Di Giovanni G, Di Mascio M, et al. Effect of acute administration of hypericum perforatum-CO_2 extract on dopamine and serotonin release in the rat central nervous system. *Pharmacopsychiatry.* 2000;33(1): 14–18.

66. Denke A, Schempp H, Weiser D, et al. Biochemical activities of extracts from *Hypericum perforatum* L., 5th communication: dopamine-beta-hydroxylase-product quantification by HPLC and inhibition by hypericins and flavonoids. *Arzneim-forsch.* 2000;50(5):415–419.

67. Wonnemann M, Singer A, Muller WE. Inhibition of synaptosomal uptake of 3H-*L*-glutamate and 3H-GABA by hyperforin, a major constituent of St. John's wort: the role of amiloride sensitive sodium conductive pathways. *Neuropsychopharmacology.* 2000;23(2):188–197.

68. Wirz A, Simmen U, Heilmann J, et al. Bisanthraquinone glycosides of *Hypericum perforatum* with binding inhibi-

tion to CRH-1 receptors. *Phytochemistry.* 2000;55(8):941–947.

69. Daudt R, von Poser GL, Neves G, et al. Screening for the antidepressant activity of some species of hypericum from south Brazil. *Phytother Res.* 2000;14(5):344–346; 2000; 14(8):661.

70. Moses EL, Mallinger AG. St. John's wort: three cases of possible mania induction. *J Clin Psychopharmacol.* 2000; 20(1):115–117.

71. Barbenel DM, Yusufi B, O'Shea D, et al. Mania in a patient receiving testosterone replacement postorchidectomy taking St. John's wort and sertraline. *J Psychopharmacol.* 2000;14(1):84–86.

72. Karliova M, Treichel U, Malago M, et al. Interaction of *Hypericum perforatum* (St. John's wort) with cyclosporin A metabolism in a patient after liver transplantation. *J Hepatol.* 2000;33(5):853–855.

73. Mai I, Kruger H, Budde K, et al. Hazardous pharmacokinetic interaction of Saint John's wort (*Hypericum perforatum*) with the immunosuppressant cyclosporin. *Int J Clin Pharmacol Ther.* 2000;38(10):500–502.

74. Breidenbach T, Kliem V, Burg M, et al. Profound drop of cyclosporin A whole blood trough levels caused by St. John's wort (*Hypericum perforatum*). *Transplantation.* 2000;69(10):2229–2230.

75. Ruschitzka F, Meier PJ, Turina M, et al. Acute heart transplant rejection due to Saint John's wort. *Lancet.* 2000;355(9203):548–549.

76. Wentworth JM, Agostini M, Love J, et al. St John's wort, a herbal antidepressant, activates the steroid X receptor, *J Endocrinol.* 2000;166(3):R11–R16.

77. Moore LB, Goodwin B, Jones SA, et al. St. John's wort induces hepatic drug metabolism through activation of the pregnane X receptor. *Proc Natl Acad Sd U S A.* 2000; 97(13):7500–7502.

78. Roby CA, Anderson GD, Kantor E, et al. St John's Wort: effect on CYP3A4 activity. *Clin Pharmacol Ther.* 2000; 67(5):451–457.

79. Towheed TE, Anastassiades TP, Shea B, et al. Glucosamine therapy for treating osteoarthritis (Cochrane Review). *Cochrane Database Syst Rev.* 2001;1.

80. O'Rourke M. Determining the efficacy of glucosamine and chondroitin for osteoarthritis. *Nurse Pract.* 2001;26(6): 44–46, 49–52.

81. Orentreich N, Brind JL, Rizer RL, et al. Age changes and sex differences in serum dehydroepiandrosterone sulfate

concentrations throughout adulthood. *J Clin Endocrinol Metab.* 1984;59(3):551–555.

82. Orentreich N, Brind JL, Vogelman JH, et al. Long-term longitudinal measurements of plasma dehydroepiandrosterone sulfate in normal men. *J Clin Endocrinol Metab.* 1992;75(4):1002–1004.

83. Huppert FA, Van Niekerk J, Herbert J. Dehydroepiandrosterone (DHEA) supplementation for cognition and well-being. *Cochrane Database Syst Rev.* 2000;2.

84. Morales AJ, Nolan JJ, Nelson JC, et al. Effects of replacement dose of dehydroepiandrosterone in men and women of advancing age [published erratum appears in *J Clin Endocrinol Metab.* 1995;80(9):2799]. *J Clin Endocrinol Metab.* 1994;78(6):1360–1367.

85. Sirrs SM, Bebb RA. DHEA: panacea or snake oil? *Can Fam Physician.* 1999;45:1723–1728.

86. Xu X, Sonntag WE. Growth hormone and the biology of aging. In: Mobbs CV, Hof P, eds. *Functional Endocrinology of Aging.* Basel: Karger; 1998:67–88.

87. Rudman G, Feller AG, Cohn L, et al. Effects of human growth hormone on body composition in elderly men. *Horm Res.* 1991:1:73–81.

88. Rudman D, Feller AG, Nagraj HS, et al. Effects of human growth hormone in men over 60 years old. *N Engl J Med.* 1990;323(1):1–6.

89. Shomali ME. The use of anti-aging hormones. Melatonin, growth hormone, testosterone, and dehydroepiandrosterone: consumer enthusiasm for unproven therapies. *Md Med J.* 1997;46(4):181–186.

90. Hennessey JV, Jackson IM. Clinical features and differential diagnosis of pituitary tumours with emphasis on acromegaly. *Baillieres Clin Endocrinol Metab.* 1995;9(2):271–314.

91. Brem G, Wanke R, Wolf E, et al. Multiple consequences of human growth hormone expression in transgenic mice. *Mol Biol Med.* 1989;6(6): 531–547.

92. Miller DB, Bartke A, O'Callaghan JP. Increased glial fibrillary acidic protein (GFAP) levels in the brains of transgenic mice expressing the bovine growth hormone (bGH) gene. *Exp Gerontol.* 1995;30(3–4):383–400.

93. Brown-Borg HM, Borg KE, Meliska CJ, et al. Dwarf mice and the ageing process. *Nature.* 1996;384(6604):33.

94. Coschigano KT, Clemmons D, Bellush LL, et al. Assessment of growth parameters and life span of GHR/BP gene-disrupted mice. *Endocrinology.* 2000;141(7):2608–2613.

63
Urinary Incontinence

Neil M. Resnick

Urinary incontinence poses a major problem for the elderly. Afflicting 15% to 30% of older people living at home, one-third of those in acute care settings, and at least half of those in nursing homes,[1] it predisposes to rashes, pressure ulcers, urinary tract infections, urosepsis, falls, and fractures.[1-3] It is also associated with embarrassment, stigmatization, isolation, depression, and risk of institutionalization,[1] as well as caregiver burden and depression.[4] Finally, it cost more than $26 billion to manage in America in 1995,[5] exceeding the amount devoted to dialysis and coronary artery bypass surgery combined.

Although both providers and older patients often neglect incontinence or dismiss it as a normal part of growing older,[6,7] it is abnormal at any age.[1,8] Although its prevalence increases with age, at no age does incontinence affect the majority of individuals, even above age 85.[9] Moreover, the reason for its increased prevalence in the elderly is likely the diseases and functional impairments that become more common with age rather than age itself.[8-10] Regardless, incontinence is usually treatable and often curable at all ages, even in frail elderly,[11-14] but the approach must differ significantly from that used in younger patients.

Lower Urinary Tract Anatomy and Physiology

Details of the anatomy and physiology of normal micturition remain controversial. For present purposes, however, both can be simplified. The lower urinary tract includes the bladder (detrusor), the urethra, and two urethral sphincters. The internal sphincter lies in the proximal urethra, at the bladder neck and is composed predominantly of smooth muscle. The external sphincter lies distally, at the level of the urogenital diaphragm, and is composed of striated muscle.

Innervation of the lower urinary tract is derived from the parasympathetic (S2–S4), sympathetic (T10–L2), and somatic (voluntary) nervous systems (S2–S4). The parasympathetic nervous system innervates the detrusor; increased cholinergic activity increases the force and frequency of detrusor contraction, while reduced activity has the opposite effect. The sympathetic nervous system innervates both the bladder and the urethra, with its effect determined by local receptors. Adrenergic receptors are sparse in the bladder body, but those normally present are beta receptors; their stimulation relaxes the bladder. Receptors in the bladder base and proximal urethra are alpha receptors; their stimulation contracts the internal sphincter. Thus, activation of the sympathetic nervous system facilitates storage of urine in a coordinated manner. The somatic nervous system is the primary source of innervation for the urogenital diaphragm and the external sphincter. The central nervous system integrates control of the urinary tract; the pontine micturition center mediates synchronous detrusor contraction and sphincter relaxation, while higher centers in the frontal lobe, basal ganglia, and cerebellum (among others) exert inhibitory and facilitatory effects.

Storage of urine is mediated by detrusor relaxation and closure of the sphincters. Detrusor relaxation is accomplished by central nervous system inhibition of parasympathetic tone, while sphincter closure is mediated by a reflex increase in the activity of the alpha-adrenergic and somatic nervous systems. Voiding occurs when detrusor contraction, stimulated by the parasympathetic nervous system, is coordinated with sphincter relaxation.

The Impact of Age on Incontinence

At any age, continence depends on not only the integrity of urinary tract function and innervation, but also the presence of adequate mentation, mobility, motivation, and manual dexterity. Although incontinence in younger patients is rarely associated with deficits outside the urinary tract, such deficits are found commonly in older patients. It is crucial to detect them, both because they exacerbate and occasionally even cause incontinence in the elderly and because design of an efficacious intervention requires that they be addressed.

In addition, the lower urinary tract changes with age, even in the absence of disease. Data from continent elderly are sparse, and longitudinal data virtually non-existent, but bladder contractility and capacity, as well as the ability to postpone voiding, appear to decline in both sexes. Urethral length and closure pressure, as well as striated sphincter muscle cells, probably decline with age in women.[15–18] The prostate enlarges in most men and appears to cause urodynamic obstruction in half.[17] In both sexes, the prevalence of involuntary detrusor contractions increases while the postvoiding residual volume (PVR) probably increases, but to no more than 50 to 100 mL.[15–17] In addition, the elderly often excrete most of their fluid intake at night, even in the absence of venous insufficiency, renal disease, heart failure, or prostatism.[19,20] This fact, coupled with the age-associated increase in sleep disorders, leads to one to two episodes of nocturia in the majority of healthy elderly.[19,20] Finally, at the cellular level, detrusor smooth muscle develops a "dense band pattern" characterized by dense sarcolemmal bands with depleted caveolae.[21,22] This depletion may mediate the age-related decline in bladder contractility. In addition, an "incomplete dysjunction pattern" develops, characterized by scattered protrusion junctions, albeit not in chains; these changes likely underlie the high prevalence of involuntary detrusor contractions.[17,23]

None of these age-related changes causes incontinence, but they do predispose to it. This predisposition, coupled with the increased likelihood that an older person will encounter an additional pathologic, physiologic, or pharmacologic insult, explains why the elderly are so likely to become incontinent. The implications are equally important. The onset or exacerbation of incontinence in an older person is likely to be caused by precipitant(s) *outside* the lower urinary tract that are amenable to medical intervention. Furthermore, *treatment of the precipitant(s) alone may be sufficient to restore continence, even if there is coexistent urinary tract dysfunction.* For instance, flare of hip arthritis in a woman with age-related detrusor overactivity may be sufficient to convert her urinary urgency into incontinence. Treatment of the arthritis—rather than the involuntary detrusor contractions—will not only restore continence but also lessen pain and improve mobility. These principles, depicted in Figures 63.1 and 63.2, provide the rationale in the older patient for adding, to the established lower urinary tract causes of incontinence, a set of transient causes. Because of their frequency, ready reversibil-

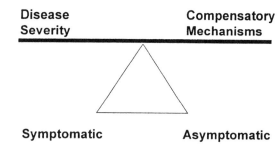

FIGURE 63.1. Incontinence results when the ability to compensate for bladder dysfunction is inadequate. For instance, in the intact older person, detrusor overactivity or sphincter weakness may not cause leakage if the patient is more attuned to bladder fullness, drinks less, voids more often, eliminates precipitants such as coughing, and stays close to a toilet. This behavior explains how older patients may remain continent despite such abnormalities and also suggests alternate therapeutic approaches independent of the urinary tract. (Modified from Resnick NM. *JAMA.* 1996;276:1832–1840, with permission.)

ity, and association with morbidity beyond incontinence, the transient causes are discussed first.

Causes of Transient Incontinence

Incontinence is transient in up to one-third of community-dwelling elderly and up to half of acutely hospitalized patients.[8,15] Although most of the transient causes of incontinence in the elderly lie outside the lower urinary tract, three points are worth emphasizing. First, the risk of incontinence developing from a transient cause is increased if, in addition to physiologic changes of the lower urinary tract, the older person also suffers from pathologic changes. Anticholinergic agents are more likely to cause overflow incontinence in individuals with a weak or obstructed bladder, whereas excess urine output is more likely to cause urge incontinence in people with detrusor overactivity and/or impaired mobility.[24,25] Second, although termed "transient," these causes of incontinence may persist if left untreated and cannot be dismissed merely because incontinence is long-standing. Third, similar to the situation for established causes (see following), identification of "the most common cause" is of little value. The likelihood of each cause depends on the individual, the clinical setting (community, acute hospital, nursing home), and the referral pattern. Moreover, geriatric incontinence is rarely the result of a single etiology.

The causes of transient incontinence can be recalled easily using the mnemonic "DIAPERS" (Table 63.1). In the setting of *delirium*, incontinence is merely an associated symptom that abates once the underlying cause of confusion is identified and treated. The patient needs medical rather than bladder management.[15]

Symptomatic urinary tract *infection* (UTI) causes transient incontinence when dysuria and urgency are so prominent that the older person is unable to reach the toilet before voiding. Asymptomatic bacteriuria, which is much more common in the elderly, does not cause incontinence.[15,26–28] Because illness can present atypically in older patients, however, incontinence is occasionally the only atypical symptom of a UTI. Thus, if otherwise asymptomatic bacteriuria is found on the initial evaluation, it should be treated and the result recorded in the patient's record to prevent future futile therapy.

Atrophic urethritis/vaginitis frequently causes lower urinary tract symptoms, including incontinence. As many as 80% of elderly women attending an incontinence clinic have atrophic vaginitis, characterized by vaginal mucosal atrophy, friability, erosions, and punctate hemorrhages.[29] Incontinence associated with this entity usually is associated with urgency and occasionally a sense of "scalding" dysuria, mimicking a urinary tract infection, but both symptoms may be unimpressive. In demented individuals, atrophic vaginitis may present as agitation. Atrophic vaginitis also can exacerbate or even cause stress incontinence.

Atrophic vaginitis is important to recognize because it responds to low-dose estrogen (e.g., 0.3–0.6 mg con-

TABLE 63.1. Causes of transient incontinence.

D	elirium/confusional state
I	nfection—urinary (only symptomatic)
A	trophic urethritis/vaginitis
P	harmaceuticals
E	xcess urine output (e.g., CHF, hyperglycemia)
R	estricted mobility
S	tool impaction

Source: Adapted from Resnick NM. Urinary incontinence in the elderly. *Medical Grand Rounds*. 1984;3:281–290, with permission.

jugated estrogen/day, orally or vaginally).[1] Moreover, as for the other causes of transient incontinence, treatment has other benefits; in this case, treatment ameliorates dyspareunia and reduces the frequency of recurrent cystitis[15,30,31] Recently, estrogen has been given transcutaneously, but studies of its impact on atrophic vaginitis are not yet available. The transcutaneous route seems promising, however, because it requires application only twice weekly and preliminary data suggest that it may have beneficial effects on lipids without adverse hepatic effects. Whichever route is chosen, symptoms remit in a few days to several weeks, but the intracellular response takes longer.[32]

The duration of therapy has not been well established.[33] One approach is to administer a low dose of estrogen daily for 1 to 2 months and then taper it. Most patients probably can be weaned to a dose given as infrequently as two to four times per month. After 6 months, it can be discontinued entirely in some patients, but recrudescence is common. Because the estrogen dose is low and given briefly, its carcinogenic effect is likely slight, if any. However, if long-term treatment is required, a progestin probably should be added if the patient has a uterus. Hormone treatment is contraindicated for women with a history of breast cancer. For those without such a history, mammography should be performed before initiating therapy. There may be a small increased risk of breast cancer among women using estrogen daily for more than 5 years, but fortunately, such high-dose, frequent, and long-term therapy is rarely required. Of note, the estrogen dose for atrophic vaginitis is lower than the more typically used daily dose of 0.625 mg.

Pharmaceuticals are one of the most common causes of geriatric incontinence, and they precipitate leakage by a variety of mechanisms (Table 63.2). Experts often cite dosages and serum levels below which side effects are uncommon. Unfortunately, such rules are of limited use in the elderly because they are generally derived from studies of younger people who have no other diseases and take no other medications. Of note, many of these agents also are used in the treatment of incontinence, underscoring the fact that most medications are "double-edged swords" for the elderly.

Incontinence: Young vs Old

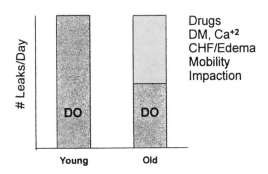

FIGURE 63.2. This cartoon shows why treatment of urinary incontinence (UI) in older adults has to differ and is often easier to treat than in younger adults. Both these patients with detrusor overactivity (DO) have the same frequency of leakage. However, in the younger patient with intact compensatory mechanisms, such leakage reflects solely the contribution of the DO. In the older adult, other comorbid conditions make it more difficult to appreciate bladder fullness, adjust fluid output, and reach the bathroom. Such conditions magnify the impact of DO and will be unaffected by bladder relaxant therapy. However, addressing them will result in a marked improvement in the UI even without treatment of the DO and will make bladder relaxant therapy, if still required, more effective. (Modified from Resnick NM, Marcantonio ER. *Lancet*. 1997;350:1157–1158, with permission.)

TABLE 63.2. Commonly used medications that may affect continence.

Type of medication	Examples	Potential effects on continence
Sedatives/hypnotics	Long-acting benzodiazepines (e.g., diazepam, flurazepam)	Sedation, delirium, immobility
Alcohol		Polyuria, frequency, urgency, sedation, delirium, immobility
Anticholinergics	Dicyclomine, disopyramide, antihistamines (sedating)	Urinary retention, overflow incontinence, delirium, impaction
Antipsychotics	Thioridazine, haloperidol	Anticholinergic actions, sedation, rigidity, immobility
Antidepressants (tricyclics)	Amitriptyline, desipramine	Anticholinergic actions, sedation
Anti-Parkinsonians	Trihexyphenidyl, benztropine	Anticholinergic actions, sedation
Narcotic analgesics	Opiates	Urinary retention, fecal impaction, sedation, delirium
α-Adrenergic antagonists	Prazosin, terazosin, doxazosin	Urethral relaxation may precipitate stress incontinence in women
α-Adrenergic agonists	Nasal decongestants	Urinary retention in men
Calcium channel blockers	All dihydropyridines[a]	Urinary retention; nocturnal diuresis due to fluid retention
Potent diuretics	Furosemide, bumetanide	Polyuria, frequency, urgency
Angiotensin-converting enzyme (ACE) inhibitors	Captopril, enalapril, lisinopril	Drug-induced cough can precipitate stress incontinence in women and in some men with prior prostatectomy
Vincristine		Urinary retention caused by neuropathy

[a] Examples include nifedipine, nicardipine, isradipine, felodipine, nimodipine.
Source: Adapted from Resnick NM. Geriatric medicine. In: Isselbacher KJ, Braunwald E, Wilson JD, Martin JB, Fauci AS, Kasper DJ, eds. *Harrison's Principles of Internal Medicine*. New York: McGraw-Hill; 1994:34, with permission.

Anticholinergic agents are used often by older people, even when not prescribed (e.g., sedating antihistamines used for allergies, coryza, and insomnia). These substances are particularly important to ask about because they cause or contribute to incontinence in several ways. In addition to provoking overt urinary retention, they often induce subclinical retention. The resultant decrease in functional bladder capacity allows bladder capacity to be reached more quickly, exacerbating incontinence from detrusor overactivity as well as that caused by functional impairment. By increasing residual volume, anticholinergic agents also can aggravate leakage due to stress incontinence. Additionally, many of these drugs decrease mobility (e.g., antipsychotics that induce extrapyramidal stiffness) and precipitate confusion. Finally, several agents intensify the dry mouth that is already so common in the elderly; the resultant increased fluid intake contributes to incontinence. Attempts should be made to discontinue anticholinergic agents, or to substitute those with less anticholinergic effect. Bethanechol may be useful for nonobstructed patients whose urinary retention is associated with use of an anticholinergic that cannot be discontinued.[34]

Because the proximal urethra, prostate, and prostatic capsule all contain alpha-adrenergic receptors, urethral tone can be increased by alpha-adrenergic agonists and decreased by alpha antagonists. In men with otherwise asymptomatic prostatic obstruction, alpha-adrenergic agonists can provoke acute retention. Particularly problematic are nonprescription decongestants, because they also often contain an (anticholinergic) anti-histamine and are taken with a nonprescription (sedating antihistamine) hypnotic as well. In other words, both agents can come together (e.g., Contac) or separately (e.g., Sudafed, Benadryl). Because older individuals often fail to mention nonprescription agents to a physician, urinary retention due to use of a decongestant, nose drops, and a hypnotic may result in premature or even unnecessary prostatectomy. In older women, in whom urethral length and sphincter strength decline with age, alpha-adrenergic antagonists (many antihypertensives) may induce stress incontinence by blocking receptors at the bladder neck.[35] Before considering other interventions, one should substitute an alternative agent and reevaluate.

Calcium channel blockers also can cause incontinence. As smooth muscle relaxants, they may increase residual volume and occasionally even provoke overflow incontinence, particularly in obstructed men with coexisting detrusor weakness. The dihydropyridine class of these agents (e.g., nifedipine, nicardipine, isradipine, nimodipine) also can cause peripheral edema, which may exacerbate nocturia and nocturnal incontinence.

Angiotensin-converting enzyme inhibitors (ACEI) can induce a chronic cough. Because the risk of this side effect increases with age, these agents may exacerbate what otherwise would be minimal stress incontinence in older women.

Excess urine output commonly contributes to or even causes geriatric incontinence. Causes include excessive fluid intake, diuretics, metabolic abnormalities, and disorders associated with fluid retention. Excess output is a likely contributor when incontinence is associated with nocturia (Table 63.3).

Restricted mobility commonly contributes to geriatric incontinence. It can result from numerous treatable conditions including arthritis, hip deformity, deconditioning, postural or postprandial hypotension, claudication, spinal stenosis, heart failure, poor eyesight, fear of falling, stroke, foot problems, drug-induced disequilibrium or confusion, or being restrained in a bed or chair.[36] A careful search will often identify these or other correctable causes. If not, a urinal or bedside commode may still improve or resolve the incontinence.

Finally, *stool impaction* is implicated as a cause of urinary incontinence in up to 10% of older patients admitted to acute care hospitals or referred to incontinence clinics[15]; the mechanism may involve stimulation of opioid receptors.[37] Patients usually present with either urge or overflow incontinence and typically have associated fecal incontinence as well. Disimpaction restores continence.

These seven reversible causes of incontinence should be assiduously sought in every older patient. In one series of hospitalized elderly, when these causes were identified, continence was regained by most of those who became incontinent in the context of acute illness.[15] Regardless of their frequency, however, their identification is important in all settings because they are easily treatable and contribute to morbidity beyond incontinence.

TABLE 63.3. Causes of nocturia.

I. *Volume related*
   Age related
   Excess intake/alcohol
   Diuretic, caffeine, theophylline
   Endocrine/metabolic
      Diabetes mellitus/insipidus
      Hypercalcemia
   Peripheral edema
      Congestive heart failure
      Low albumin states
      Peripheral vascular disease
      Drugs (e.g., lithium, NSAIDs, nifedipine)
II. *Sleep related*
   Insomnia
   Pain
   Dyspnea
   Depression
   Drugs
III. *Lower urinary tract related*
   Small bladder capacity
   Detrusor hyperactivity
   Prostate related
   Overflow incontinence
   Decreased bladder compliance
   Sensory urgency

Source: Adapted from Resnick NM. Noninvasive diagnosis of the patient with complex incontinence. *Gerontology.* 1990;36(suppl 2):8–18, with permission.

Established Incontinence

Causes Unrelated to the Lower Urinary Tract ("Functional" Incontinence)

In contrast with transient causes, the established causes of geriatric incontinence generally lie *within* the urinary tract. The exception is "functional incontinence," a type of incontinence attributed to deficits of cognition and mobility. However, this concept is problematic for several reasons.[38] First, "functional incontinence" implies that urinary tract function is normal, but studies of both institutionalized and ambulatory elderly reveal that normal urinary tract function is the exception even in continent subjects and is rarely observed in incontinent elderly patients.[15,17,39,40] Second, incontinence is not inevitable with either dementia or immobility. For instance, we found that 17% of the most severely demented institutionalized residents (mean age, 89) were continent; more impressive, if they could merely transfer from a bed to a chair, nearly *half* were *continent*.[10] Third, because functionally impaired individuals are the most likely to suffer from factors causing transient incontinence,[10,41–43] a diagnosis of functional incontinence may result in failure to detect reversible causes of incontinence. Finally, functionally impaired individuals may still have obstruction or stress incontinence and benefit from targeted therapy.[15,40,41]

Nonetheless, the importance of functional impairment as a factor *contributing* to incontinence should not be underestimated, because incontinence is also affected by environmental demands, mentation, mobility, manual dexterity, medical factors, and motivation. Although lower urinary tract function is rarely normal in such individuals, these factors are important to keep in mind because small improvements in each may markedly ameliorate both incontinence and functional status. In fact, once one has excluded causes of transient incontinence and serious underlying lesions, dealing with functional impairment often obviates the need for further investigation.

Lower Urinary Tract Causes

If incontinence persists after transient and functional causes have been addressed, the urinary tract causes of incontinence should be considered. The lower urinary tract can malfunction in only four ways. Two involve the bladder and two involve the outlet: the bladder either contracts when it should not (detrusor overactivity) or fails to contract when or as well as it should (detrusor underactivity); alternatively, outlet resistance is high when it should be low (obstruction) or low when it should be high (outlet incompetence). Because incontinence in

TABLE 63.4. Lower urinary tract causes of established incontinence in the elderly.

Urodynamic diagnosis	Some neurogenic causes	Some nonneurogenic causes
Detrusor overactivity	Multiple sclerosis Stroke Parkinson's disease Alzheimer's disease	Urethral obstruction/incompetence Cystitis Bladder carcinoma Bladder stone
Detrusor underactivity	Cauda equina disc compression Plexopathy Surgical damage (e.g., abdominoperineal resection) Autonomic neuropathy (e.g., diabetes mellitus, alcoholism, B_{12} deficiency)	Idiopathic (common in women) Chronic outlet obstruction
Outlet incompetence	Surgical lesion (rare) Lower motor neuron lesion (rare)	Urethral hypermobility (type 1 and 2 SUI) Intrinsic sphincter deficiency (type 3 SUI) Postprostatectomy
Outlet obstruction	Spinal cord lesion with detrusor-sphincter dyssynergia (rare)	Prostatic enlargement Prostate carcinoma Prolapsing cystourethrocele Following bladder neck suspension

SUI, stress urinary incontinence.
Source: Adapted from Resnick NM. Voiding dysfunction and urinary incontinence. In: Beck JC, ed. *Geriatric Review Syllabus*. New York: American Geriatrics Society; 1991:141–154, with permission.

older individuals is frequently due to a cause other than the classic types of "neurogenic bladder," it is better to think of the causes of incontinence in terms of these four pathophysiologic mechanisms and to realize that each mechanism can be caused by "neurogenic" as well as "nonneurogenic" conditions (Table 63.4). This section provides an overview of the four basic mechanisms and their causes; a later section provides treatment strategies for each.

Detrusor overactivity (DO), characterized by involuntary bladder contractions, is the most common form of urinary tract dysfunction in incontinent elderly of either sex.[15,40] DO is associated with increased spontaneous activity of detrusor smooth muscle. Recently, we found that it is also associated with unique changes at the cellular level. Termed the "complete dysjunction pattern," these changes include widening of the intercellular space and replacement of normal (intermediate) muscle cell junctions by novel "protrusion" junctions and ultraclose abutments connecting cells together in chains. These junctions and abutments may mediate a change in cell coupling from a mechanical to an electrical mechanism, which could facilitate propagation of heightened smooth muscle activity and provide the "final common pathway" by which such spontaneous cellular contractions result in involuntary contraction of the entire bladder.[23,44–46]

A distinction is generally made between detrusor overactivity that is associated with a CNS lesion (detrusor hyperreflexia) and that which is not (detrusor instability). In the latter situation, the etiology of the DO may be in the urinary tract itself, where a source of irritation—such as cystitis (interstitial, or radiation- or chemotherapy-

induced), bladder tumor, or stone—overwhelms the brain's ability to inhibit bladder contraction. Two other important local causes are prostate obstruction and stress incontinence, each of which may lead to secondary detrusor overactivity. However, in older patients the distinction is often unclear because many of these causes may be present concomitantly, even in a patient with Alzheimer's disease. Unfortunately, there is still no reliable way to determine the source of such contractions, which obviously complicates treatment decisions. It also suggests that DO coexisting with urethral obstruction or stress incontinence may be less likely to resolve postoperatively than in younger individuals without other reasons for detrusor overactivity.[15,47]

Traditionally, detrusor overactivity has been thought to be the primary urinary tract cause of incontinence in demented patients. While this is true, it is also the most common cause in nondemented patients, and the three studies that have examined it failed to find an association between cognitive status and DO.[40,48,49] This lack of association likely reflects the fact that in the elderly there are multiple causes of DO unrelated to dementia, including cervical disk disease or spondylosis, Parkinson's disease, stroke, subclinical urethral obstruction or sphincter incompetence, and age itself. Moreover, demented patients also may be incontinent due to the transient or functional causes already discussed. Thus, it is not tenable to ascribe incontinence in demented individuals a priori to detrusor overactivity.

Detrusor overactivity in the elderly exists as two physiologic subsets, one in which contractile function is preserved and one in which it is impaired.[50] The latter condition is called detrusor hyperactivity with impaired contractility (DHIC), and it has proved to be the most common form of DO found in the elderly.[40,44] Evidence suggests that DHIC may represent the coexistence of DO and bladder weakness, rather than a separate physiologic entity.[44] Nonetheless, DHIC has several implications. First, because the bladder is weak, urinary retention develops commonly in these patients, and DHIC must be added to outlet obstruction and detrusor underactivity as a cause of retention. Second, even in the absence of retention, DHIC mimics virtually every other lower urinary tract cause of incontinence. For instance, if the involuntary detrusor contraction is triggered by or occurs coincident with a stress maneuver and the weak contraction (often only 2–6 cmH$_2$O) is not detected, DHIC will be misdiagnosed as stress incontinence or urethral instability.[51] Alternatively, because DHIC is associated with urinary urgency, frequency, weak flow rate, elevated residual urine, and bladder trabeculation, in men it may mimic urethral obstruction.[52] Third, bladder weakness often frustrates anticholinergic therapy of DHIC because urinary retention is induced so easily. Thus, alternative therapeutic approaches are often required (see Therapy, following).

Regardless of etiology or bladder strength, DO is characterized by frequent and precipitant voiding. Leakage is usually moderate to large, nocturnal frequency and incontinence are common, sacral sensation and reflexes are preserved, voluntary control of the anal sphincter is intact, and postvoiding residual volume is generally low. A residual volume in excess of 50 mL in a patient with detrusor overactivity suggests outlet obstruction (although there may be no residual in early obstruction), DHIC, or pooling of urine in a woman with a cystocele. It is also found in patients with Parkinson's disease or spinal cord injury.

Stress incontinence is the second most common cause of incontinence in older women. As in younger women, it is usually a result of pelvic muscle laxity; this results in "urethral hypermobility," which allows the proximal urethra and bladder neck to "herniate" through the urogenital diaphragm when abdominal pressure increases. Such herniation may result in unequal transmission of abdominal pressure to the bladder and urethra and consequent stress incontinence (Fig. 63.3). The defect is thus one of urethral support, rather than sphincter strength. Leakage due to urethral hypermobility is characterized by daytime loss of small to moderate amounts of urine, infrequent nocturnal incontinence, and low postvoiding residual volume (in the absence of urine pooling in a large cystocele). The hallmark of the diagnosis is leakage that, in the absence of bladder distension, occurs *coincident* with the stress maneuver.

A much less common cause of stress incontinence is intrinsic sphincter deficiency (ISD) or "type 3 stress incontinence,"[53,54] in which the sphincter is intrinsically weak. Afflicted women usually leak with even trivial stress maneuvers (e.g., walking) and may even note continuous seepage when standing quietly. The prevalence of ISD may be lower than thought, however, because the diagnosis is often based solely on documenting a very low urethral "leak point" or "closure pressure" during

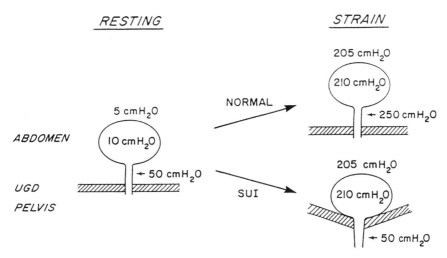

FIGURE 63.3. Pathophysiology of stress incontinence (SUI) caused by urethral hypermobility. Normally, resting urethral pressure is greater than bladder pressure. With a stress maneuver (such as coughing, straining, laughing, or bending over), the increase in abdominal pressure is transmitted equally to the bladder and the outlet, and the individual remains dry. In a woman with urethral hypermobility, however, the proximal urethra "herniates" through the urogenital diaphragm (UGD) into the pelvis with a stress maneuver. Because abdominal pressure is no longer transmitted equally, instantaneous leakage occurs but stops coincident with the drop in intra-abdominal pressure. (From Resnick NM. Urinary incontinence—a treatable disorder. In: Rowe JW, Besdine RW, eds. *Geriatric Medicine*, 2nd Ed. Boston: Little, Brown; 1988, with permission.)

urodynamic testing. Because pressure declines with age and low pressures are seen commonly in older women without stress incontinence, this finding does not establish the presence of ISD. Moreover, because urethral pressure falls reflexly with detrusor contraction, leakage coinciding with low urethral pressure can be seen in patients with DHIC in whom the low-pressure contraction is missed.

When it occurs, ISD is usually due to operative trauma. However, a milder form also occurs in older women, resulting only from urethral atrophy superimposed on the age-related decline in urethral pressure. Instead of leaking with any bladder volume, such women often leak only at higher amounts (e.g., >200 ml); many become dry if bladder volume is kept below this level.

A rare cause of stress incontinence in older women is urethral instability, in which the sphincter paradoxically relaxes in the absence of apparent detrusor contraction.[55] However, most older women thought to have this condition actually have DHIC.[51]

In men, stress incontinence is uncommon and usually caused by sphincter damage following prostatectomy. In both sexes, stress-associated leakage also can occur in association with urinary retention, but in this situation leakage is not due to outlet incompetence.

Outlet obstruction is the second most common cause of incontinence in older men, although most obstructed men are not incontinent. If caused by neurologic disease, obstruction is invariably associated with a spinal cord lesion. In this situation, pathways are interrupted to the pontine micturition center, where outlet relaxation is coordinated with bladder contraction. Rather than relaxing when the bladder contracts, the outlet contracts simultaneously, leading to severe outlet obstruction, a "Christmas tree bladder," hydronephrosis, and renal failure—a condition termed detrusor-sphincter dyssynergia.

Much more commonly, obstruction results from prostatic enlargement, prostate carcinoma, or urethral stricture. Such men present with postvoid dribbling, urge incontinence (because detrusor overactivity coexists in two-thirds of cases), or, less commonly, overflow incontinence due to urinary retention. Because symptoms, ease of catheterization, and palpated prostate size correlate poorly with obstruction, and PVR is insufficiently specific, obstruction is difficult to exclude without further testing.[56]

Anatomic obstruction is rare in women. With age, urethral elasticity decreases in most women. In a small proportion of them, in whom it may be compounded by fibrotic changes associated with atrophic vaginitis, moderate urethral stenosis may occur. Frank outlet obstruction, however, is usually caused not by stricture but by kinking associated with a large cystocele or obstruction following bladder neck suspension. Rarely, bladder neck obstruction or a bladder calculus is the cause.

Detrusor underactivity, which causes 5% to 10% of incontinence in older persons, may be caused by mechanical injury to the nerves supplying the bladder (e.g., disk compression or tumor involvement) or by the autonomic neuropathy of diabetes, B_{12} deficiency, Parkinson's disease, alcoholism, vincristine therapy, or tabes dorsalis. Alternatively, the detrusor may be replaced by fibrosis and connective tissue, as occurs in men with chronic outlet obstruction, so that even when the obstruction is removed, the bladder fails to empty normally. Detrusor weakness in women is generally idiopathic; instead of fibrosis, the detrusor displays degeneration of both muscle cells and axons, without accompanying regeneration.[22]

A mild degree of bladder weakness occurs commonly in older individuals. Although insufficient to cause incontinence, it can complicate treatment of other causes (see Therapy). However, when severe enough to cause leakage, detrusor underactivity is associated with overflow incontinence.[15,16,40] Leakage of small amounts occurs frequently throughout the day and night. The patient also may notice hesitancy, diminished and interrupted flow, incomplete emptying, and a need to strain to void. If the problem is neurologically mediated, perineal sensation, sacral reflexes, and anal sphincter control are frequently impaired.

Diagnostic Approach

Evaluation

The evaluation should identify transient and established causes of incontinence, assess the patient's environment and available support, and detect uncommon but serious conditions that may underlie incontinence, including lesions of the brain and spinal cord, carcinoma of the bladder or prostate, hydronephrosis, bladder calculi, detrusor-sphincter dyssynergia, and decreased bladder compliance. Assessment must be tailored to the individual's clinical status and goals and be tempered by the realization that not all detected conditions can be cured, that simple interventions may be effective even in the absence of a diagnosis, and that for many elderly persons, diagnostic tests are themselves often interventions. Because the evaluation generally requires a comprehensive approach, it should be conducted over several visits to ease the burden and to obviate further testing in those who respond to simple measures.

History

After assessing functional status, one elicits a detailed description of the incontinence, focusing on its onset, frequency, severity, pattern, precipitants, palliating features,

TABLE 63.5. Evaluation of the incontinent elderly patient.

History
  Type (urge, reflex, stress, overflow, or mixed)
  Frequency, severity, duration
  Pattern (diurnal, nocturnal, or both; also after taking medications, for example)
  Associated symptoms (straining to void, incomplete emptying, dysuria, hematuria, suprapubic/perineal discomfort)
  Alteration in bowel habit/sexual function
  Other relevant factors (cancer, diabetes, acute illness, neurologic disease, urinary tract infections, and pelvic or lower urinary tract surgery or
    radiation therapy)
  Medications, including nonprescription agents
  Functional assessment (mobility, manual dexterity, mentation, motivation)

Physical examination
  Identify other medical conditions (e.g., orthostatic hypotension, CHF, peripheral edema)
  Test for stress-induced leakage when bladder is full, but not during abrupt urgency
  Observe/listen to void for force, continuity, straining
  Palpate for bladder distension after voiding
  Pelvic examination (atrophic vaginitis or urethritis; pelvic muscle laxity; pelvic mass)
  Rectal examination (skin irritation; resting tone and voluntary control of anal sphincter; prostate nodules; fecal impaction. *Note*: ease of
    catheterization and prostate size correlate poorly with presence or absence of urethral obstruction)
  Neurologic examination (mental status and affect, mobility, and elemental examination, including sacral reflexes and perineal sensation)

Laboratory investigation
  Voiding record (incontinence chart)
  Metabolic survey (measurement of electrolytes, calcium, glucose, and urea nitrogen)[a]
  Measurement of postvoiding residual volume (PVR) by catheterization or portable ultrasound

Urinalysis and culture
  Renal ultrasound for men whose residual urine exceeds 100–200 ml[a]
  Urine cytology for patients with sterile hematuria, suprapubic/perineal pain, or unexplained new onset or worsening of incontinence[a]
  Uroflowmetry for men in whom urethral obstruction is suspected[a]
  Cystoscopy for patients with hematuria, suspected lower urinary tract pathology (e.g., bladder fistula, stone, or tumor; urethral diverticulum),
    or need for surgery
  Urodynamic evaluation when the risk of empiric therapy exceeds the benefit, when empiric therapy has failed or might be improved by more
    precise assessment, or when surgery would be clinically appropriate if a correctable condition were found[a]

[a] Tests indicated only for selected individuals, as described.
Source: Adapted from Resnick NM, Yalla SV. Management of urinary incontinence in the elderly. *N Engl J Med*. 1985;313:800–805, wtih permission.

and associated symptoms and conditions (Table 63.5). It is also helpful to know if the patient leaks at night. Generally, individuals with detrusor overactivity gush intermittently both day and night, whereas those with pure stress incontinence are usually dry at night because they are in the supine position and not straining. However, individuals with intrinsic sphincter deficiency, especially those who also have a poorly compliant bladder, may leak only at night if they allow their bladder to fill to a volume greater than their weakened outlet can withstand. Such individuals also have the almost continuous seepage mentioned earlier.

Although the clinical type of incontinence most often associated with detrusor overactivity (DO) is urge incontinence, "urge" is neither a sensitive nor specific symptom; it is absent in 20% of older patients with detrusor overactivity, and the figure is higher in demented patients.[40] "Urge" is also reported commonly by patients with stress incontinence, outlet obstruction, and overflow incontinence.

A more useful term for the symptom associated with DO is "precipitancy," which can be defined in two ways. For patients with no warning of imminent urination

("reflex" or "unconscious" incontinence), the abrupt gush of urine in the absence of a stress maneuver can be termed precipitant leakage, and it is almost invariably due to DO. For those who do sense a warning, it is of less value to focus on the leakage, because the presence and volume of leakage in this situation depend on bladder volume, amount of warning, toilet accessibility, the patient's mobility, and whether the individual can overcome the relative sphincter relaxation that normally accompanies detrusor contraction.[57] Instead, precipitancy should be defined as the *abrupt sensation* that urination is imminent, *whatever the interval or amount of leakage that follows*; defined in these two ways, precipitancy is both a sensitive and specific symptom.[58]

Similar to the situation for urgency, other symptoms ascribed to DO also can be misleading unless explored carefully. Urinary frequency (more than seven diurnal voids) is common,[15,26,59] and may result from voiding habit, preemptive urination to avoid leakage, overflow incontinence, sensory urgency, a stable but poorly compliant bladder, excessive urine production, depression, anxiety, or social reasons.[58] Conversely, incontinent individuals may severely restrict their fluid intake so that

Date	Time	Volume voided (mL)	Are you wet or dry?	Approximate volume of incontinence	Comments
4/5	3:50 pm	240	Wet	Slightly	
	6:05 pm	210	Dry		
	8:15 pm	150	Dry		
	10:20 pm	150	Wet	15 mL	Running water
	10:30 pm	30	Dry		Bowel movement
4/6	3:15 am	270	Dry		
	6:05 am	300	Dry		
	7:40 am	200	Dry		
	9:50 am	?	Dry		
	11:20 am	200	Dry		
	12:50 pm	180	Dry		
	1:40 pm	240	Dry		
	3:35 pm	160	Wet	Slightly	
	6:00 pm	170	Wet	Slightly	Running water
	8:20 pm	215	Wet	Slightly	
	10:25 pm	130	Dry		

FIGURE 63.4. Sample voiding record. Voiding diary of an in-continent 75-year-old man. Urodynamic evaluation excluded urethral obstruction and confirmed a diagnosis of detrusor hyperactivity with impaired contractility (DHIC). However, note the 24-h urine output of nearly 3 L due to the belief that drinking 10 glasses of fluid/day was "good for my health." (Patient did not mention this until queried about the voiding record.) Given the typical voided volume of 150–250 mL and a measured postvoiding residual (PVR) of 150 mL, excess fluid intake was overwhelming his usual bladder capacity of 400 ml (150 + 250 ml). Although uninhibited bladder contractions were present, the easily reversible volume component of the problem—coupled with the risk of precipitating urinary retention with an anticholinergic agent—prompted treatment with volume restriction alone. After daily urinary output dropped to 1500 mL, frequency abated and incontinence resolved. (Adapted from DuBeau CE, Resnick NM. Evaluation of the causes and severity of geriatric incontinence: a critical appraisal. *Urol Clin North Am.* 1991;18:243–256, with permission.)

even in the presence of DO they do not void frequently. Thus, the significance of urinary frequency—or its absence—can be determined only in the context of more information.

Nocturia also can be misleading unless it is first defined (e.g., two episodes may be normal for the individual who sleeps 10 h but not for one who sleeps 4 h) and then approached systematically (see Table 63.3). There are three general reasons for nocturia: excessive urine output, sleep-related difficulties, and urinary tract dysfunction. These causes can be differentiated by careful questioning and examination of a voiding diary that includes voided volumes (Fig. 63.4). One inspects the record of voided volumes to determine the functional bladder capacity (the largest single voided volume) and compares the capacity to the volume of each nighttime void. For instance, if the functional bladder capacity is 400 mL and each of three nightly voids is approximately 400 mL, the nocturia is due to excessive production of urine at night. If the volume of most nightly voids is much smaller than bladder capacity, nocturia is due to either (1) a sleep-related problem (the patient voids because she is awake anyway) or (2) a problem with the lower urinary tract. Like excess urine output, sleep-related nocturia may also be due to treatable causes, including age-related sleep disorders, pain (e.g., bursitis, arthritis), dyspnea, depression, caffeine, or a short-acting hypnotic (e.g., triazolam). Bladder-related causes of nocturia are displayed in Table 63.3. Whatever the cause, the nocturnal component of incontinence is generally remediable.

Prostatism is another symptom complex that warrants comment. Regardless of whether the patient has "irritative" or "obstructive" symptoms, the physician can be easily misled. Most investigators have found that one-third of middle-aged patients referred for prostatectomy are not obstructed. Usually, the problem is an overactive detrusor, which, if unaccompanied by outlet obstruction, may be exacerbated by operative intervention. In older men, the specificity of "prostatism" for obstruction is even lower, owing to the high prevalence of medication use, altered fluid excretion,[60] constipation, and DHIC, as well as the impairment of bladder contractility that accompanies aging. Thus, symptoms of prostatism are a clue to the diagnosis but are alone insufficiently specific to confirm it.[61]

When asking women about leakage with stress maneuvers, it is important to ensure that the absence of such leakage is not due simply to the lack of coughing or sneezing. For those without such precipitants, it is useful to inquire about leakage that occurs instantaneously with lifting or bending over to put on a shoe or stockings.

Finally, patients or their caregivers should be asked which voiding symptom is most bothersome. For example, although a woman may have both stress and urge incontinence, the urge component may be her worst problem and should become the focus of evaluation and treatment. A man with "prostatism" may be most bothered by nocturia,[62] which may be remedied without any consideration of his prostate (see Fig. 63.4). Failure to address symptom bother can lead to frustration for patient and provider alike.

Voiding Record

One of the most helpful components of the history is the voiding diary. Kept by the patient or caregiver for 48 to 72 h, the diary records the time of each void and incontinent episode. No attempt is made to alter voiding pattern or fluid intake. Many formats have been proposed; a sample is shown in Figure 63.4.

To record voided volumes at home, individuals use a measuring cup, coffee can, pickle jar, or other large-mouth container. Information regarding the volume voided provides an index of functional bladder capacity and, together with the pattern of voiding and leakage, can suggest the cause of leakage. For example, incontinence occurring only between 8 A.M. and noon may be caused by a morning diuretic. Incontinence that occurs at night in a demented man with congestive heart failure, but not during a 4-h nap in his wheelchair, is likely due to neither dementia nor prostatic obstruction but to postural diuresis associated with his heart failure. A woman with volume-dependent stress incontinence may leak only on the way to void after a full night's sleep, when her bladder contains more than 400 mL, more than it ever does during her continent waking hours. A patient may also void frequently because of polyuria.

The voiding record should also guide therapy. For instance, in a patient with DO or prostatic obstruction, excess nocturnal fluid excretion may result in nocturnal incontinence that is more severe and troublesome than daytime leakage; successful therapy must address the excess excretion. In contrast, another patient with the same urinary dysfunction and excretion, but able to hold more urine when asleep, might be bothered more by daytime leakage. Shifting his excess nocturnal excretion to the daytime will *exacerbate* the problem.

The information gathered from the history and voiding record permits symptomatic characterization of the incontinence as *urge*, in which precipitant leakage of a large volume is preceded by a brief warning of seconds to minutes; *reflex*, in which precipitant leakage is not preceded by a warning; *stress*, in which leakage occurs coincident with, and only in association with, increases in abdominal pressure; *overflow*, in which continual drib-

bling occurs; and *mixed*, which is usually a combination of urge and stress. Each of these types correlates fairly well with the pathophysiologic mechanisms already mentioned: urge and reflex with detrusor overactivity; stress with urethral incompetence (owing to either urethral hypermobility or ISD); overflow with urethral obstruction or detrusor underactivity; and mixed with both an overactive detrusor and an incompetent outlet.

Targeted Physical Examination

Similar to the history, the physical examination is essential to detect transient causes, comorbid disease, and functional impairment. One should check for signs of neurologic disease, such as delirium, dementia, stroke, Parkinson's disease, cord compression, and neuropathy (autonomic or peripheral), as well as for atrophic vaginitis and general medical illnesses such as heart failure and peripheral edema. One also should check for bladder distension and for spinal column deformities suggestive of vertebral anomalies that may impinge on the spinal cord.

The rectal exam checks for fecal impaction, masses, and prostate nodularity and consistency. Prostate size is less important to assess because, as determined by palpation, it correlates poorly with the presence or absence of outlet obstruction.[56] The remainder of the rectal exam is actually a detailed neurourologic examination because the same sacral roots (S2–S4) innervate both the external urethral and the anal sphincters. Gluteal fold symmetry should be assessed. Then, with the finger in the rectum, one assesses motor innervation by asking the patient to volitionally contract and relax the anal sphincter. Because abdominal straining may mimic sphincter contraction, it is useful to place one's other hand on the patient's abdomen to check for this. Many neurologically unimpaired elderly patients are unable to volitionally contract their sphincter, but if they can, it is evidence against a cord lesion. When the perineum is relaxed, one can assess motor innervation further by testing the anal wink (S4–S5) and bulbocavernosus reflexes (S2–S4). In an older person, however, the absence of these reflexes is not necessarily pathologic, nor does their presence exclude an underactive detrusor (due to a diabetic neuropathy, for example). Finally, afferent supply is assessed by testing perineal sensation.

In women, one can check for pelvic muscle laxity (cystocele, rectocele, enterocele, uterine prolapse). After removing one blade of the vaginal speculum (or using a "tongue blade"), one sequentially places the remaining blade on the anterior and posterior vaginal walls and asks the patient to cough. If bulging of the anterior wall is detected when the posterior wall is stabilized, a cystocele is present; conversely, if bulging of the posterior wall is detected, a rectocele or enterocele is present. While the extent of pelvic muscle laxity may be underestimated if one checks in only the supine position, the presence of laxity can usually be determined in any position. It is important to realize, however, that the presence or absence of pelvic muscle laxity reveals little about the cause of an individual's leakage. Detrusor overactivity may exist in addition to a cystocele, and stress incontinence may exist in the absence of a cystocele. Thus, knowledge of pelvic muscle laxity is useful primarily in informing the surgeon's choice of operation. The one exception occurs in the woman with a large cystocele: descent of the cystocele may kink the urethra and cause obstruction.

Stress Testing and PVR Measurement

Stress testing is important for incontinent women. Optimally, it is performed when the bladder is full and she is relaxed (check gluteal folds to corroborate) and in as close to the upright position as possible. The cough or strain should be vigorous and *single*, so that one can determine whether leakage coincides with the increase in abdominal pressure or follows it. Stress-related leakage can be missed if any of these conditions is not met. Delayed leakage, typical of stress-induced DO, should be differentiated from leakage typical of stress incontinence, which is instantaneous and ceases as abdominal pressure declines. *To be useful diagnostically, leakage must replicate the symptom for which help is sought*, because many older women have incidental but not bothersome leakage of a few drops. The test should not be performed if the patient has an abrupt urge to void, because this is usually due to an involuntary detrusor contraction that will lead to a falsely positive stress test. Falsely negative tests occur when the patient fails to cough vigorously or fails to relax the perineal muscles, the bladder is not full, or the test is performed in the upright position in a woman with a large cystocele (which kinks the urethra). If performed correctly, the stress test is reasonably sensitive and quite specific (>90%).[63–65]

Following the stress test, the patient is asked to void into a receptacle and the PVR is measured. If the stress test was negative but the history suggests stress incontinence *and* the combined volume of the void and PVR is less than 200 mL, the bladder should be filled with sterile fluid so that the stress test can be repeated at an adequate volume. There is no need to repeat a well-performed positive stress test or to repeat it in a woman whose history is negative for stress-related leakage; the sensitivity of the history for stress incontinence, unlike its specificity, exceeds 90%,[66,67] making the likelihood of stress incontinence remote in this situation.

Optimally, the PVR is measured within 5 min of voiding. Measuring it after an intentional void is better than after an incontinent episode, because many patients are able to partially suppress the involuntary contraction during the episode and more than the true PVR remains. In cognitively impaired patients this may not be possible; however, as the resulting artifact will lead to a falsely elevated PVR, a low value is still useful. The PVR will also be spuriously high if measurement is delayed (especially if the patient's fluid intake was high or included caffeine), the patient was inhibited during voiding, or there is discomfort due to urethral inflammation or infection. It will be spuriously low if the patient augmented voiding by straining (most important in women), if the catheter is withdrawn too quickly, and if the woman has a cystocele that allows urine to "puddle" beneath the catheter's reach. Of note, relying on the ease of catheterization to establish the presence of obstruction can be misleading, because difficult catheter passage may be caused by urethral tortuosity, a "false passage," or catheter-induced spasm of the distal sphincter, whereas catheter passage may be easy in even obstructed men.[68]

Two other tests should be mentioned. Because pelvic muscle laxity may be present regardless of the cause of incontinence in an older woman, the "Q-tip test" used to detect such laxity is of little value.[61] The Bonney (or Marshall) test assesses whether leakage that coincides with increased abdominal pressure can be prevented by stabilizing (not occluding) the bladder base and thereby preventing its herniation through the urogenital diaphragm. The test is performed by placing a finger in each lateral vaginal fornix and asking the patient to cough again. Stress incontinence owing to urethral hypermobility is considered present if leakage is prevented. The value of this test is limited in elderly women because vaginal stenosis is common and may lead to a false-positive result by precluding accurate finger placement; if one's fingers are not placed far enough laterally, they may occlude the bladder outlet rather than stabilizing it and prevent leakage even in a patient with detrusor instability. Furthermore, even if the test is performed correctly, a false-positive result may occur if the first episode of leakage was due to a cough-induced detrusor contraction, which, having emptied the bladder, does not recur during bladder base elevation.

Laboratory Investigation

One should check the blood urea nitrogen (BUN), creatinine, urinalysis, and PVR in all patients.[1,61,69,70] Urine culture should be obtained in those with dysuria or an abnormal urinalysis. Serum sodium, glucose, and calcium should be measured in patients with confusion. If the voiding record suggests polyuria, serum glucose and calcium should be determined. Sterile hematuria suggests partially or recently treated bacteriuria, malignancy, calculus, or tuberculosis.

Empiric Diagnostic Categorization

After transient and serious causes have been addressed, the optimal diagnostic strategy for persistent incontinence is unknown.[1,70,71] "Bedside" cystometry has been proposed, but its utility is limited because it misses low-pressure contractions of DHIC; its feasibility and accuracy are low in frail elderly[72]; and detected DO may be either incidental and unrelated to leakage or due to urethral obstruction or incompetence and warrant different therapy. The following approach,[11] although still unproved, is relatively noninvasive, accurate, cost-effective, and easily tolerated. A similar approach forms the basis for the AHCPR Clinical Practice Guideline,[1] as well as the Minimum Data Set/Resident Assessment Instrument that we designed and validated for use in all American nursing homes.[73]

The first step is to identify the 5% to 10% of individuals with overflow incontinence (e.g., PVR > 450 mL). Because its causes (obstruction and underactive detrusor) cannot be differentiated clinically,[73–75] further assessment is warranted for those in whom it would affect therapy, and catheterization should be used for the rest.

For the remaining patients, the next step depends on their sex. In women, obstruction is rare. Thus, in the absence of previous bladder neck suspension or prolapsing cystocele, the differential diagnosis is generally between stress incontinence and DO. If the contemplated intervention is nonoperative, this distinction usually can be made on clinical grounds alone, informed by the caveats mentioned earlier.

In men, stress incontinence is uncommon and presents with a characteristic drip (similar to a "leaky faucet") that is exacerbated by standing or straining. Thus, the usual problem in men is differentiating DO from obstruction. Figure 63.5 summarizes the approach. Uroflowmetry is helpful, but only if peak flow is normal (e.g., >12 mL/s for voided volume of 200 mL); the age-related decrease in bladder contractility means that a normal unstrained flow rate, together with PVR less than 100 mL, effectively excludes clinically significant obstruction in an older man.[74] The next step is to search for hydronephrosis in men whose PVR exceeds 200 mL and to decompress those in whom it is found.[56] Further evaluation is also reasonable for men without hydronephrosis who would be amenable to surgery if obstructed. For the rest, it seems

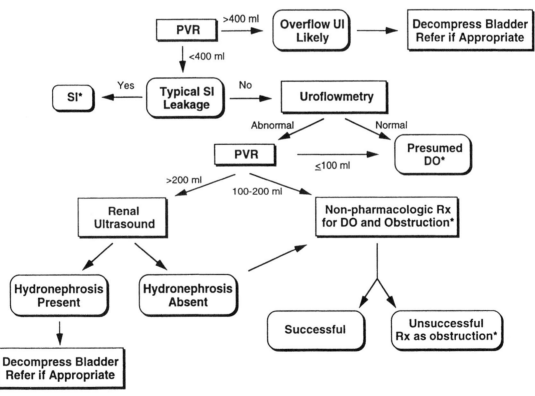

FIGURE 63.5. Stepwise evaluation of incontinent men. Assumes transient (DIAPERS) causes have been excluded. Cutoffs for postvoiding residual urine volumes are intended as guidelines rather than absolute values, which are not available; see text for further details and caveats. *Rectangles*, denote tests/actions; *rounded boxes*, findings/diagnoses; *UI*, urinary incontinence; *PVR*, postvoiding residual volume; *SI*, stress incontinence; *DO*, detrusor overactivity. (See Table 63.6 for management suggestions.)

sensible to treat those with urge incontinence for presumed DO, provided they are compliant and can be taught signs of incipient urinary retention; bladder relaxants should be avoided in those with significantly elevated PVR (e.g., >150 mL). A similar approach is advocated for cognitively impaired men who can be closely observed (e.g., institutionalized residents).[73,76] Men without urge incontinence, those who fail empiric therapy, and those who are cognitively impaired and less supervised should be evaluated further if findings would affect therapy.

Urodynamic Testing

Although its precise role in the elderly is unclear, multi-channel urodynamic evaluation is probably warranted when diagnostic uncertainty may affect therapy and when empiric therapy has failed and other approaches would be tried. Because conditions that closely mimic obstruction and stress incontinence are so common in the elderly—including altered fluid excretion,[60] medication use, Detrusor Hyperactivity (DH), and DHIC[51,52]—urodynamic corroboration of the diagnosis is strongly recommended if surgery will be performed.[1,51,73,76] Whatever its role, however, urodynamic evaluation of elderly patients is reproducible, safe, and feasible to perform, even in frail and debilitated individuals.[40,77]

Urodynamic evaluation consists of a battery of tests that characterize bladder and urethral function during both the filling and voiding phases of the micturition cycle. Optimally, bladder, urethral, and rectal pressures are measured simultaneously and during both phases of the cycle. Concurrent fluoroscopic monitoring is extremely helpful for the elderly patient, because pressure monitoring alone may miss involuntary contractions, obstruction, and stress incontinence. Some of the more commonly used tests are described next.

Cystometry

Cystometry (CMG) assesses only the bladder, not the outlet, and only during filling, not voiding. Therefore, it yields only part of the information needed to establish a diagnosis. It is performed by inserting a catheter into the bladder, filling it with gas or fluid, and observing the bladder's pressure response to increasing volume. In addition to providing information about bladder proprioception (sensation), compliance, and capacity, cystometry detects involuntary detrusor contractions (detrusor overactivity), which generally appear as phasic increases in bladder pressure. However, if the contraction amplitude is low (as in DHIC) or if the patient talks, coughs, or moves during the contraction, these contractions may be missed.[51,52] Furthermore, artifacts are common, especially when investigating the elderly. These artifacts can be minimized by having the test performed by a knowledgeable physician (not a technician), by infusing fluid rather than gas, by using moderate infusion rates (<100 mL/min) rather than rapid ones, by using fluoroscopy, and—most importantly—by measuring abdominal and bladder pressures simultaneously to differentiate rises in bladder pressure from rises in abdominal pressure.

Finally, because involuntary contractions may occur in the elderly as an incidental finding rather than as the cause of incontinence or since they may be merely secondary to primary urethral pathology (e.g., stress incontinence or obstruction), their significance is difficult to discern without further testing. Such differentiation is important to avoid misdirected therapy; for instance, anticholinergic therapy of DO in a man in whom the DO is incidental to obstruction could precipitate painful urinary retention.

Urethral Profilometry (During Filling and Voiding)

There are two types of profilometry, depending on whether urethral pressure is measured when the bladder is at rest or contracting. The first is called urethral closure pressure profilometry (UCPP) and the second micturitional urethral pressure profilometry (MUPP). UCPP is performed by inserting a catheter into the bladder, slowly withdrawing it through the urethra, and plotting urethral pressure at each point. The diagnostic value of UCPP is limited. In women with known stress incontinence, however, very low urethral pressures suggest that leakage may reflect intrinsic sphincter deficiency (ISD) rather than urethral hypermobility; in the former, urethral pressure is consistently low (e.g., <10 cmH$_2$O), while in the latter it is normal. Determining "leak point pressure," the pressure at which the sphincter becomes incompetent during coughing or straining, is another way to identify ISD. Urethral profilometry is also used to exclude detrusor-sphincter dyssynergia. Generally, only evaluation of the distal urethral sphincter is required; this sphincter should relax just before, or coincident with, detrusor contraction.

MUPP is useful for evaluating men.[78] It is performed by simultaneously measuring pressure in the bladder and along the urethra as the patient voids. With urethral obstruction, the pressure distal to the obstruction is lower than bladder pressure. If obstruction is detected, fluoroscopy can localize the site. MUPP is more accurate than cystoscopy for determining the presence of an obstruction and judging its severity.[56]

Uroflowmetry

Uroflowmetry is often used to screen men for urethral obstructions.[74] The flow rate depends not only upon the presence of obstruction, however, but also upon the strength of detrusor contraction. To interpret the test, one must know the voided volume, residual volume, whether the void was augmented by abdominal straining, the peak and mean flow rates, and the configuration of the accompanying trace. Interrupted and oscillatory patterns are suggestive of abdominal straining, bladder weakness, or outlet obstruction. Although age-related norms have been devised to facilitate interpretation of the test, the studies on which they are based are flawed and included few patients over age 70. Moreover, although the sensitivity of the test likely increases with age, its specificity almost certainly declines.[74] Thus, the utility of isolated uroflowmetry in elderly males remains undefined. One can, however, derive some information from it. In the older man with symptoms of prostatism, a normal flow rate and PVR less than 100 mL exclude clinically significant obstruction.

Electromyography

Electromyography (EMG) evaluates the distal urethral sphincter by determining the integrity of its innervation, testing its response to reflex stimuli [such as bladder filling (guarding reflex) and bulbocavernosus stimulation], and characterizing its behavior during voiding. Several techniques are available for EMG, depending on whether one employs surface or needle electrodes, records the response of single or multiple nerve fibers, and evaluates the nerve supply to the urethral sphincter or the pelvic floor musculature (through vaginal, anal, or perineal probes). The most accurate technique is to insert a needle electrode directly into the distal urethral sphincter. Although most elderly patients can tolerate this, the results can be difficult to interpret, the equipment is expensive, and, if urodynamic testing is performed as already detailed, EMG adds little. If fluoroscopically monitored multichannel urodynamic capability is not available, however, EMG is useful. Unfortunately, in these situations, only surface or anal EMG is usually performed. As these techniques are fraught with artifact, they should be interpreted with caution.

Radiographic Evaluation

Optimally, the radiographic and urodynamic evaluations are performed simultaneously, allowing correlation of visual and manometric information. If this is not feasible, substantial information can still be gleaned from cystography. A full evaluation includes posteroanterior and oblique (or lateral) views of the bladder, at rest and during straining and voiding. These films check for bladder trabeculation, diverticula, masses, bladder neck competence, and ureteral reflux. Although the urethrovesical angle and axis are also often measured, their reliability and relevance are limited. The *voiding* films

allow one to check for outlet obstruction. Postvoiding residual volume also can be assessed radiographically, but there are pitfalls. Elderly patients are frequently rushed through busy radiography departments and may feel too inhibited to void to completion; the radiologist, who may have been absent during the exam, may then erroneously conclude that the residual volume is elevated. Conversely, a low volume does not exclude a weak bladder if the patient augmented voiding by straining or by multiple voids before the film was obtained. Therefore, the radiographer should be viewed as a partner in the evaluation, rather than being asked to read films blindly after the examination is completed.

Therapy

Like the diagnostic approach, treatment must be individualized because factors outside the lower urinary tract so often affect feasibility and efficacy. For instance, although both may have detrusor overactivity that can be managed successfully, a patient with impaired cognition and mobility must be treated differently from one who is ambulatory and cognitively intact. This section and Table 63.6 outline several treatments for each condition and provide guidance for their use. It is assumed that serious underlying conditions, transient causes of incontinence, and functional impairments have already been addressed. It cannot be overemphasized that successful treatment of established incontinence, especially in the elderly, is usually multifactorial and requires addressing factors beyond the urinary tract, as well.

Detrusor Overactivity

The initial approach to detrusor overactivity is to identify and treat its reversible causes. Unfortunately, many of its causes are not amenable to specific therapy or a cause may not be found, so treatment usually must be symptomatic. Simple measures, such as adjusting the timing or amount of fluid excretion (see Fig. 63.4) or providing a bedside commode or urinal are often successful. If not, the cornerstone of treatment is behavioral therapy. If the patient can cooperate, bladder training regimens will extend the voiding interval.[79–82] For instance, if the voiding record documents incontinence when the interval exceeds 3 h, the patient is instructed to void every 2 h and to suppress urgency in between. Once dry, the patient can extend the interval by half an hour and repeat the process until a satisfactory result or continence is achieved. Patients need not follow this regimen at night, because nighttime improvement parallels daytime success. Biofeedback may be added,[80,81,83,84] but its marginal benefit is unclear[82,85]

TABLE 63.6. Stepwise approach to treatment.[a]

Condition	Clinical type of incontinence[b]	Treatment
Detrusor overactivity with normal contractility (DO)	Urge	1. Bladder retraining or prompted voiding regimens 2. ±Bladder relaxant medication (anticholinergic, smooth muscle relaxant, calcium channel blocker), if needed and not contraindicated 3. Indwelling catheterization alone is often unhelpful because detrusor "spasms" often increase, leading to leakage around the catheter 4. In selected cases, induce urinary retention pharmacologically and add intermittent or indwelling catheterization[f]
Detrusor hyperactivity with impaired contractility (DHIC)	Urge[c]	1. If bladder empties adequately with straining, behavioral methods (as above) ±bladder relaxant medication (low doses; especially feasible if sphincter incompetence coexists) 2. If residual urine >150ml, augmented voiding techniques[d] or intermittent catheterization (±bladder relaxant medication); if neither feasible, undergarment or indwelling catheter
Stress incontinence	Stress	1. Conservative methods [weight loss if obese; treatment of cough or atrophic vaginitis; physical maneuvers to prevent leakage (e.g., tighten pelvic muscles, cross legs); occasionally, use of tampon or pessary is useful] 2. If leakage threshold ≥150ml identified, adjust fluid excretion and voiding intervals 3. Pelvic muscle exercises ±biofeedback/weighted intravaginal "cones" 4. Imipramine (or doxepin) or alpha-adrenergic agonists, ±estrogen, if not contraindicated 5. Surgery [urethral suspension, or compression ("sling"), periurethral bulking injections, artificial sphincter]
Urethral obstruction	Urge/overflow[e]	1. Conservative methods (including adjustment of fluid excretion, bladder retraining/prompted voiding) if hydronephrosis, elevated residual urine, recurrent symptomatic UTI, and gross hematuria have been excluded 2. Bladder relaxants if DO coexists, PVR is small, and surgery is not desired or feasible 3. Alpha-adrenergic antagonists, finasteride, antiandrogens, and/or LHRH analogues if not contraindicated and the patient either prefers them or is not a surgical candidate 4. Surgery (incision, prostatectomy)
Underactive detrusor	Overflow	1. If duration unknown, decompress for several weeks and perform a voiding trial 2. If cannot void, PVR remains large, or retention is chronic, try augmented voiding techniques[d] ±alpha-adrenergic antagonist, but only if some voiding possible; bethanechol rarely useful unless bladder weakness due to an anticholinergic agent that cannot be discontinued 3. If fails, or voiding is not possible, intermittent or indwelling catheterization[f]

UTI, urinary tract infection; PVR, postvoiding residual volume.

[a] These treatments should be initiated only after adequate toilet access has been ensured, contributing conditions have been treated (e.g., atrophic vaginitis, heart failure), fluid management has been optimized, and unnecessary or exacerbating medications have been stopped. For additional details, recommendations, and drug doses, see text.

[b] *Urge*: Leakage in the absence of stress maneuvers and urinary retention, usually preceded by *abrupt* onset of need to void.
Stress: Leakage that coincides *instantaneously* with stress maneuvers, in the absence of urinary retention or detrusor contraction.
Overflow: Frequent leakage of small amounts associated with urinary retention.

[c] May also mimic stress or overflow incontinence.

[d] Augmented voiding techniques include Crede (application of suprapubic pressure) and Valsalva (straining) maneuvers, and "double" voiding. They should be performed only *after* voiding has begun.

[e] Also can cause postvoid "dribbling" alone, which is treated conservatively (e.g., by sitting to void and allowing more time, "double voiding," and by gently "milking" the urethra after voiding).

[f] UTI prophylaxis can be used for recurrent symptomatic UTIs, but only if catheter is not indwelling.

Source: Adapted from Resnick NM. Voiding dysfunction and urinary incontinence. In: Beck JC, ed. *Geriatric Review Syllabus*. New York: American Geriatrics Society; 1991:141–154, with permission.

For cognitively impaired patients, "prompted voiding" is used.[12,86] Asked every 2 h whether they need to void, patients are escorted to the toilet if the response is affirmative. Positive verbal reinforcement is employed and negative comments are avoided. Prompted voiding reduces incontinence frequency in nursing homes by roughly 50%, and leakage can be virtually eliminated during daytime hours in one-third of residents.[87–89] The latter group can be identified within 3 days. When prompted *hourly* to void during the daytime, they urinate into a toilet or commode more than two-thirds of the time that they indicate the need to do so, or they become continent on more than 80% of checks. Response is maintained when the prompting interval is increased to 2 h. Half the remaining patients also improve with prompting, but they remain wet more than once during the daytime. For the quarter of patients who do not respond to prompting at baseline, little benefit is obtained by further prompting. Importantly, response does not correlate with the degree of dementia. In addition, these results were obtained without drugs, and urodynamic evaluations were not performed.[89,90] Tailoring the regimen to the cause and pattern of incontinence should further improve outcome.

The voiding record also can be helpful if it reveals that nocturnal incontinence correlates with nocturnal diuresis. If caused by systolic congestive heart failure, it should improve with diuretic therapy. If due to peripheral edema in the absence of heart failure and hypoalbuminemia (i.e., venous insufficiency), it should respond to pressure gradient stockings. If it is not associated with peripheral edema, it may respond to alteration of the pattern of fluid intake or administration of a rapidly acting diuretic in the early evening.[60,91] For patients with DHIC whose voiding record and PVR suggest that involuntary detrusor contractions are provoked only at high bladder volumes, catheterization at bedtime will remove the residual urine, thereby increasing functional bladder capacity and restoring both continence and sleep.

Drugs augment behavioral intervention but do not supplant it because they generally do not abolish involuntary contractions, Timed toileting or bladder retraining, in conjunction with a bladder relaxant, is thus especially useful for older adults who have little warning before detrusor contraction.[13] Table 63.7 provides information on drugs used to treat DO. There are few data on comparative efficacy or toxicity of standard drugs in the elderly, but available studies show similar efficacy for most agents, except flavoxate, which fares poorly in controlled trials[1]; no controlled data are available for hyoscyamine in the elderly.

Both oxybutynin and tolterodine have proved effective in well-conducted trials that included older adults,[13,92,93] and healthy elderly participants appeared to respond as well as younger patients. Fewer data are available for extended-release oxybutynin in the elderly,[1,13,94] but our randomized and controlled data, in which low-dose immediate-release oxybutynin was given three or four times daily, suggest that the more constant serum concentrations achieved with extended release oxybutynin should yield similar results to the immediate-release form given frequently. For instance, in our trial of community-dwelling patients, two-thirds of patients (mean age, 73 years) became continent, including 71% whose bladder had normal contractility and 47% of those with DHIC, as compared with 17% on placebo.[95] Immediate-release oxybutynin, which has a short half-life, can be employed prophylactically if incontinence occurs at predictable times. Intravesical instillation of several agents is also effective in younger patients,[92] but the need for self-catheterization makes this strategy less useful in the elderly.

Unlike tolterodine or extended-release oxybutynin, immediate-release oral oxybutynin has been assessed in

TABLE 63.7. Bladder relaxant medications used to treat urge incontinence.[a]

Medication class, name, and dosage	Comments
Smooth muscle relaxant Flavoxate 300–800 mg daily (100–200 mg po tid-qid)[b]	Has not proved effective in placebo-controlled trials

Calcium channel blocker
  Diltiazem 90–270 mg daily (30–90 mg po qd-tid)
  Nifedipine 30–90 mg daily (10–30 mg po qd-tid)
	No controlled trial data; most useful for the patient with another indication for the drug (e.g., hypertension, angina pectoris, or abnormalities of cardiac diastolic relaxation)

Combination smooth muscle relaxant and anticholinergic
  Oxybutynin IR 7.5–20 mg daily (2.5–5 mg po tid-qid)[c]
  Oxybutynin XL 5–30 mg daily (given once daily)
  Tolterodine 2 mg twice daily
  Dicyclomine 30–90 mg daily (10–30 mg po tid)
	Both oxybutynin and tolterodine have proved effective in rigorous controlled trials when used continuously; fewer controlled data are available for dicyclomine but efficacy appears to be similar; because immediate release oxybutynin and dicyclomine have a rapid onset of action, they can be tried prophylactically if incontinence occurs at predictable times

Tricyclic antidepressants[d]
  Doxepin 25–75 mg daily (10–25 mg po qd-tid)
  Imipramine 25–100 mg daily (10–25 mg po qd-qid)
	May be particularly helpful in women with coexistent stress incontinence; orthostatic hypotension often precludes their use, but a tricyclic antidepressant may be preferred for a depressed incontinent patient without orthostatic hypotension

IR, immediate release; XL, extended release.
[a] All drugs should be started at the lowest dose and increased slowly until encountering maximum benefit or intolerable side effects. All are given in divided doses, except the antidepressants and long-acting forms of oxybutynin and tolterodine, which may be given as a single daily dose.
[b] Some uncontrolled reports suggest that doses up to 1200 mg/day may be effective with tolerable side effects; efficacy has not been supported by randomized controlled trials at any dose.
[c] May also be applied intravesically in patients who can use intermittent catheterization.
[d] May give as single daily dose of 25–100 mg after determining the optimal dose.
Source: Adapted from Resnick NM. Urinary incontinence. *Lancet*. 1995;346:94–99, with permission.

nursing home patients. In a randomized controlled trial, 2.5 mg qid proved well tolerated and effective, albeit less so than in more independent people. On this dose, 10% of these frail patients (mean age, 89 years) became completely continent, and incontinence frequency decreased by at least half in 27% and by at least one-third in 54% (Resnick et al., unpublished data).

For depressed patients, imipramine may be tried,[1] but only if the depression has not already remitted and there is no evidence of orthostatic hypotension. Other tricyclic agents should work similarly, but efficacy data are available only for imipramine and doxepin.[92]

Regardless of which bladder relaxant is used, urinary retention may develop. PVR and urine output should be monitored, especially in DHIC in which the detrusor is already weak. Subclinical urinary retention also may develop, reducing functional bladder capacity and attenuating or even reversing the drug's benefit. Thus, if incontinence worsens as the dose is increased, PVR should be remeasured. Another reason for drug failure is excess fluid ingestion engendered by anticholinergic-induced xerostomia. For patients whose incontinence defies other remedies (such as those with DHIC), inducing urinary retention and using intermittent catheterization may be viable if catheterization is feasible. Other remedies for urge incontinence, including electrical stimulation[96–98] and selective nerve blocks,[99] are successful in selected situations but have not been studied adequately in the elderly.

Vasopressin has little efficacy for geriatric incontinence,[100–102] and the high prevalence of contraindications to its use [e.g., renal insufficiency, heart failure (even subclinical)], the risk of inducing serious hyponatremia and fluid retention,[102] and the considerable expense suggest that use of desmopressin acetate (DDAVP) in the elderly should await results of further studies. These caveats are underscored by recent data that suggest that nocturnal polyuria may reflect more of a disordered release of atrial natriuretic hormone (ANH) than of vasopressin.[103] If corroborated, such increased ANH release could result in a natriuresis that would underlie the older patient's predisposition to hyponatremia when treated with vasopressin.

Adjunctive measures, such as pads and special undergarments, are invaluable if incontinence proves refractory. Many types are now available, allowing the recommendation to be tailored to the individual's problem.[104–107] [Most are included in an illustrated catalog (NAFC, P.O. Box 8310, Spartanburg, SC 29305; *www.nafc.org*)]. For bedridden individuals, a launderable bedpad may be preferable, whereas for those with a stroke, a diaper or pant that can be opened using the good hand may be preferred. For ambulatory patients with large gushes of incontinence, wood pulp-containing products are usually superior to those containing polymer gel because the gel generally cannot absorb the large amount and rapid flow, whereas the wood pulp product can easily be doubled up if necessary. Optimal products for men and women differ because of the location of the "target zone" of the urinary loss. Finally, the choice will be influenced by the presence of fecal incontinence.

Condom catheters are helpful for men, but they are associated with skin breakdown, bacteriuria, and decreased motivation to become dry[12,86,108,109]; these also are not feasible for the older man with a small or retracted penis. External collecting devices have been devised for institutionalized women[110]; whether they will adhere adequately in more active women remains to be determined. Indwelling urethral catheters are not recommended for detrusor overactivity because they usually exacerbate it. If they must be used (e.g., to allow healing of a pressure sore), a small catheter with a small balloon is preferable to avoid leakage around the catheter; such leakage almost invariably results from bladder contractions rather than a catheter that is too small. Increasing catheter and balloon size only aggravates the problem and may result in urethral erosion and sphincter incompetence. If spasms persist, drugs such as oxybutynin can be tried. More potent anticholinergic agents, such as belladonna suppositories, should be avoided in the elderly.

Stress Incontinence

Urethral hypermobility, the most common cause of stress incontinence in older women, may be improved by weight loss if the patient is obese, by postural maneuvers,[111] by therapy of precipitating conditions such as atrophic vaginitis or cough (e.g., due to an angiotensin-converting enzyme inhibitor), and (rarely) by insertion of a pessary.[112,113] If the voiding diary reveals that leakage is volume dependent, it may be improved by adjusting fluid excretion and voiding intervals to keep bladder volume below this threshold. However, if the threshold is less than 150 to 200 ml, this strategy generally is not alone sufficient.

Pelvic muscle (Kegel) exercises can decrease incontinence substantially, especially if the patient also contracts her pelvic muscles at the time of stress. The exercises are performed by "drawing in" the perianal and perivaginal muscles while relaxing the abdominal, gluteal, and thigh muscles. The patient should place her hand on her abdomen to ensure that it remains relaxed. Another method is to interrupt voiding midstream by contracting the sphincter, again ensuring that nearby muscles remain relaxed. The exercise can be taught during the examination; for patients who need more help, an inexpensive audiotape is available from NAFC (National Association for Continenc, at the above address). Once she identifies the correct muscles, the patient should try to increase the number and duration of contractions, exercising at any time and during any activity. The optimal regimen remains to be determined, but proven regimens involve 30 to 200 contractions/day for up to 10s at a time.[1,114-117] Unfortunately, these exercises must be pursued indefinitely, efficacy is limited for severe incontinence, only 10% to 25% of women become fully continent, and many older women are unable or unmotivated to follow such regimens. Adding vaginal cones, biofeedback, or electrical stimulation likely enhances efficacy, but their marginal benefit is unclear.[1,115,117,118] Urethral plugs are still under development.

If not contraindicated by other conditions, treatment with an alpha-adrenergic agonist, such as phenylpropanolamine (PPA) or pseudoephedrine, may be added and is often beneficial for women, especially when administered with estrogen.[1,92,116] Pseudoephedrine and estrogen may also work for women with sphincter deficiency. Unfortunately, PPA, the agent for which most data are available, was recently withdrawn from the American market, owing to reports of a very small risk of stroke.[119] Pseudoephedrine remains available, inexpensive, and obtainable without a prescription. As it is also contained in nonprescribed remedies for coryza and allergy, however, the physician should prescribe the dose and guide the choice of preparation, because some capsules also contain agents such as chlorpheniramine in doses that can be troublesome for elderly patients. The physician should also closely supervise its use in patients with hypertension, if it is used at all. Imipramine, with beneficial effects on the bladder and the outlet, is a reasonable alternative for patients with evidence of both stress and urge incontinence, but it should be used only if symptoms as well as signs of postural hypotension have been excluded.

If these methods fail or are unacceptable, further evaluation of the urinary tract may be warranted. If urethral hypermobility is confirmed, surgical correction is successful in the majority of selected elderly patients.[15,120-122] If sphincter incompetence is diagnosed instead, it can be corrected with a different procedure (pubovaginal sling),[123] but the morbidity is higher and precipitation of chronic retention is more likely than with correction of urethral hypermobility. The influence of coincident DO on outcome in older women has been inadequately investigated for either type of stress incontinence. Other treatments for sphincter incompetence include periurethral bulking injections (e.g., bovine collagen) and insertion of an artificial sphincter.[124] Each is effective in selected cases, but reported experience with these approaches in individuals over age 75 is still limited, and so is long-term follow-up.[125] Many devices other than pessaries have been developed to contain the leakage. Most are applied as a "cap" over the urethral meatus. Unfortunately, most are available for only a brief period, and few objective data have yet been accrued on any, especially in older women for whom atrophic mucosa makes application of such devices more problematic.

For men in whom these interventions fail, prostheses such as condom catheters or penile clamps may be useful, but most require substantial cognitive capacity and manual dexterity and are often poorly tolerated. Penile sheaths (e.g., McGuire prosthesis or adhesive underwear liners) are an alternative. As already discussed, pads and undergarments are used as adjunctive measures. However, in these cases, polymer gel pads are frequently successful because the gel can more readily absorb the smaller amount of leakage. Some products can be flushed down the toilet, a convenient feature for ambulatory individuals.

Outlet Obstruction

For older men, conservative management often suffices. In the absence of urinary retention, modification of fluid excretion and voiding habits may be effective. If not, alpha-adrenergic antagonists are useful and generally well tolerated, except for men with diastolic dysfunction or significant aortic stenosis, in whom these agents should be used with more caution. Tamsulosin may be better tolerated than less specific alpha-blocking agents, but definitive clinical data are still not available.[26] Finasteride, a 5α-reductase inhibitor, is another alternative, but fewer men appear to benefit, the effect is more modest, and the benefit is more delayed.[127] Devices and surgical approaches are discussed elsewhere. Of note, DO probably resolves less often following removal of obstruction in older persons than in younger ones; however, incontinence may still improve, even in cognitively impaired individuals.[47,128] In addition, less extensive resection often suffices for frail elderly men, in whom recurrence of symptoms with adenoma regrowth years later is often not an issue. This fact, coupled with surgical techniques that now permit resection under local anesthesia, has made surgery increasingly feasible for this population. More detailed discussion of these and other options is provided in Chapter 52.

In women, if a large cystocele is the problem, surgical correction is usually required and should include bladder neck suspension if urethral hypermobility is also present. Prior urodynamic evaluation is helpful as well: if intrinsic sphincter deficiency is identified, a different surgical approach is required to avoid converting incontinence due to obstruction into incontinence due to sphincter incompetence. Bladder neck obstruction is also corrected easily, in even the frailest patient. Distal urethral stenosis can be dilated and treated with estrogen. If meatal stenosis is present, more extensive intervention may be necessary; alternatively, dilation can be repeated at fairly frequent intervals. It should be noted that most women who undergo dilation do not have urethral stenosis but rather an underactive detrusor; for these women, dilation is usually unhelpful and may be harmful.

Underactive Detrusor

Management of detrusor underactivity is directed at reducing the residual volume, eliminating hydronephrosis (if present), and preventing urosepsis. The first step is to use indwelling or intermittent catheterization to decompress the bladder for up to a month (at least 7–14 days), while reversing potential contributors to impaired detrusor function (fecal impaction and medications). If an indwelling catheter has been inserted, it then should be withdrawn (Table 63.8). If decompression does not fully restore bladder function, augmented voiding techniques [such as double voiding and implementation of the Credé (application of suprapubic pressure during voiding) or Valsalva maneuver] may help if the patient is able to initiate a detrusor contraction or if there is coexistent stress incontinence, especially in a woman. Bethanechol (40–200 mg/day in divided doses) is occasionally useful in a patient whose bladder contracts poorly because of treatment with anticholinergic agents that cannot be discontinued (e.g., tricyclic antidepressant).[34] In other patients, bethanechol may decrease the PVR if sphincter function and local innervation are normal, but evidence for its efficacy is equivocal at best, and residual volume should be monitored to assess its effect.[129,130]

On the other hand, if after decompression the detrusor is acontractile, these interventions are apt to be fruitless,

and the patient should be started on intermittent or indwelling catheterization; a condom catheter is contraindicated in the setting of retention. For individuals at home, intermittent self-catheterization is preferable and requires only clean, rather than sterile, catheter insertion. The patient can purchase two or three of these catheters inexpensively. One or two are used during the day and another is kept at home. Men can carry their catheter in a coat pocket, and women can carry theirs in a purse (the catheter used for females is only a few inches long). Catheters are cleaned daily, allowed to air dry at night, sterilized periodically, and may be reused repeatedly. Antibiotic or methenamine prophylaxis against urinary tract infection is probably warranted if the individual gets more than an occasional symptomatic infection or has an abnormal heart valve.[131,132] Intermittent catheterization in this setting is generally painless, safe, inexpensive, and effective, and allows individuals to carry on with their usual daily activities. For debilitated patients, however, intermittent catheterization is usually less feasible, although sometimes possible.[107,133] If used in an institutional setting, sterile rather than clean technique should be employed until studies document the safety of the latter.

Unfortunately, despite the benefits and proven feasibility of intermittent catheterization,[134,135] most elderly individuals choose indwelling catheterization instead.

TABLE 63.8. Removing an indwelling urethral catheter.

Ensure that bladder has been decompressed for at least several days, and 7–21 days if possible; the higher the residual volume, the longer the bladder should be decompressed.

Correct reversible causes of urinary retention: fecal impaction; pelvic/perineal pain; and use of anticholinergic, alpha-adrenergic agonist, or calcium channel blocker medications. If an anticholinergic antidepressant/antipsychotic agent cannot be stopped, consider switching to one with fewer or no anticholinergic side effects, or consider adding bethanechol. Addition of an alpha-adrenoceptor antagonist may be helpful, but is unproven in women.

Treat delirium, depression, atrophic vaginitis, or urinary tract infection, if present.

Record urinary output at intervals of 6–8 h for 2 days to establish a pattern of baseline urine excretion.

Remove the catheter at a time that permits accurate recording of urine output and allows for postvoiding recatheterization; clamping the catheter before removal is not necessary and can be dangerous.

Reinsert the catheter *only*:

- After the patient voids, to determine PVR volume; or
- After the expected bladder *volume* (based on records of urine output)—not the time since the catheter was removed—exceeds a preset limit (e.g., 600–800 ml); or
- If the patient is uncomfortable and unable to void despite ensured privacy and maneuvers performed to encourage voiding (e.g., running water, tapping suprapubic area, or stroking inner thigh).

If the patient voids and the PVR volume is:

- Greater than 400 ml—reinsert the catheter and evaluate further, if appropriate.[a]
- 100–400 ml—watch for delayed retention and evaluate further, if appropriate.[a]
- Less than 100 ml—watch for delayed retention.

If the patient is unable to void, evaluate further if appropriate. If not, resident requires permanent catheterization.[a]

PVR, postvoiding residual.

[a] Further evaluation is appropriate when the patient and physician feel that if a surgically correctable condition were found (e.g., urethral obstruction), an operation would be preferable to chronic catheterization or the other options described in the text.

Source: Modified from Resnick NM. Incontinence. In: Beck JC, ed. *Geriatric Review Syllabus*. New York: American Geriatrics Society; 1991:141–154, with permission.

TABLE 63.9. Principles of indwelling catheter care.

Maintain sterile, closed-gravity drainage system:

- Secure the catheter to upper thigh or abdomen to avoid urethral irritation and contamination. Rotate the site of attachment every few days.
- Empty the bag every 8h.
- Do not routinely irrigate the catheter.
- Do not clamp or kink the drainage tubing, and keep the collection bag below bladder level at all times.
- Avoid frequent cleaning of the urethral meatus; washing with soap and water once daily is sufficient; periurethral application of antimicrobial creams is ineffective.

If "bypassing" occurs in the absence of obstruction, it is likely caused by a bladder spasm, which can be minimized by using the smallest balloon that will keep the catheter in place and by treating with a bladder relaxant medication if necessary.

Infection prophylaxis, as well as treatment of asymptomatic bacteriuria, is fruitless and usually leads to the emergence of resistant organisms. Surveillance cultures are unnecessary and potentially misleading because bacteriuria is universal, frequently changing, and often polymicrobial.

If symptomatic urinary tract infection (UTI) develops, change the catheter before obtaining a culture specimen, because cultures obtained through the old catheter may reflect organisms colonizing encrustations rather than the infecting organism. Pending culture results, antibiotic treatment should include coverage of common uropathogens, as well as uncommon ones such as *Providencia stuartii* and *Morganella morganii*.

If catheter obstruction occurs frequently, and urine cultures reveal *Providencia stuartii* or *Proteus mirabilis*, antibiotic treatment may reduce the frequency of obstruction but induces emergence of resistant organisms. In the absence of urea-splitting organisms, consider urine acidification if urine output is normal (at low output, acidification may increase blockage due to uric acid crystals). If frequent blockage persists, consider using a silicon catheter.

In the absence of obstruction and symptomatic UTI, there is no consensus on the best time to change the catheter. Some persons form material that frequently clogs the lumen; their catheter probably should be changed often enough to reduce such obstruction. Other individuals can use the same catheter for years, but it is customary to change it every 1–2 months. For patients who are difficult to catheterize, the catheter can be changed less frequently if it remains patent and complication free.

Source: Adapted from: Resnick NM. Voiding dysfunciton and urinary incontinence. In: Beck JC, ed. *Geriatric Review Syllabus*. New York: American Geriatrics Society; 1991;141–154, with permission.

As in younger individuals, complications of chronic indwelling catheterization include renal inflammation and chronic pyelonephritis,[136] bladder and urethral erosions, bladder stones and cancer, as well as urosepsis.[132] Principles of catheter care are summarized in Table 63.9.

When indicated, indwelling catheters can be extremely effective, but their use should be restricted. They are indicated in the acutely ill patient to monitor fluid balance, in the patient with a nonhealing pressure ulcer, for temporary bladder decompression in patients with acute urinary retention, and in the patient with overflow incontinence refractory to other measures. Even in long-term care facilities, they are probably indicated for only 1% to 2% of patients. However, patient preference and values are also important. Thus, an indwelling catheter may also be justified for a cognitively intact patient who is willing to accept the risk in return for the security and convenience the catheter can provide.

Summary

Regardless of age, mobility, mentation, or institutionalization, incontinence is never normal. By attenuating physiologic reserve, aging increases the likelihood of becoming incontinent in the setting of additional physiologic, pharmacologic, or pathologic insults. Because many of these problems lie outside the urinary tract, so too must the diagnostic and therapeutic focus. However, such a strategy—coupled with a multifactorial, creative, persistent, and optimistic approach—will increase the chances of a successful outcome and generally reward patient and physician alike.

References

1. Fantl JA, Newman DK, Colling J. *Urinary Incontinence in Adults: Acute and Chronic Management. Clinical Practice Guideline, No. 2, 1996 Update.* AHCPR Pub 96-0682. Rockville, MD: U.S. Department of Health and Human Services, Public Health Service, Agency for Health Care Policy and Research; 1996.
2. Tromp AM, Smit JH, Deeg DJH, Bouter LM, Lips P. Predictors for falls and fractures in the Longitudinal Aging Study Amsterdam. *J Bone Miner Res*. 1998;13:1932–1939.
3. Brown JS, Vittinghoff E, Wyman JF, et al. Urinary incontinence: does it increase risk for falls and fractures? *J Am Geriatr Soc*. 2000;48:721–725.
4. Flaherty JH, Miller DK, Coe RM. Impact on caregivers of supporting urinary function in non-institutionalized, chronically ill seniors. *Gerontologist*. 1992;32:541–545.
5. Wagner TH, Hu T-W. Economic costs of urinary incontinence. *Urology*. 1998;51:355–361.
6. Branch LG, Walker LA, Wetle TT, DuBeau CE, Resnick NM. Urinary incontinence knowledge among community-dwelling people 65 years of age and older. *J Am Geriatr Soc*. 1994;42:1257–1262.

7. Cohen SJ, Robinson D, Dugan E, et al. Communication between older adults and their physicians about urinary incontinence. *J Gerontol.* 1999;54A:M34–M37.

8. Herzog AR, Fultz NH. Prevalence and incidence of urinary incontinence in community-dwelling populations. *J Am Geriatr Soc.* 1990;38:273–28l.

9. Wetle TT, Scherr PA, Branch LG, et al. Difficulty with holding urine among older persons in a geographically-defined community: prevalence and correlates. *J Am Geriatr Soc.* 1995;43:349–355.

10. Resnick NM, Baumann MM, Scott M, Laurino E, Yalla SV. Risk factors for incontinence in the nursing home: a multivariate study. *Neurourol Urodyn.* 1988;7:274–276.

11. Resnick NM. Urinary incontinence. *Lancet.* 1995;346:94-99.

12. Ouslander JG, Schnelle JF. Incontinence in the nursing home. *Ann Intern Med.* 1995;122:438–449.

13. Wagg A, Malone-Lee J. The management of urinary incontinence in the elderly. *Br J Urol.* 1998;82(suppl 1):11–17.

14. Weinberger MW, Goodman BM, Carnes M. Long-term efficacy of nonsurgical urinary incontinence treatment in elderly women. *J Gerontol.* 1999;54A:M117–M121.

15. Resnick NM. Voiding dysfunction in the elderly. In: Yalla SV, McGuire EJ, Elbadawi A, Blaivas JG, eds. *Neurourology and Urodynamics: Principles and Practice.* New York: Macmillan; 1988:303–330.

16. Diokno AC, Brown MB, Brock BM, Herzog AR, Normolle DP. Clinical and cystometric characteristics of continent and incontinent noninstitutionalized elderly. *J Urol.* 1988;140:567–571.

17. Resnick NM, Elbadawi A, Yalla SV. Age and the lower urinary tract: what is normal? *Neurourol Urodyn.* 1995;15:577–579.

18. Strasser H, Tiefenthaler M, Steinlechner M, Bartsch G, Konwalinka G. Urinary incontinence in the elderly and age-dependent apoptosis of rhabdosphincter cells. *Lancet.* 1999;354:918–919.

19. Miller M. Nocturnal polyuria in older people: pathophysiology and clinical implications. *J Am Geriatr Soc.* 2000;48:1321–1329.

20. Morgan K, Bergmann M, DuBeau CE, Resnick NM. The voiding pattern of normal elders. *J Am Geriatr Soc.* 2000;48:S6[abstract].

21. Elbadawi A, Yalla SV, Resnick NM. Structural basis of geriatric voiding dysfunction. I. Methods of a correlative study, and overview of the findings. *J Urol.* 1993;150:1650–1656.

22. Elbadawi A, Yalla SV, Resnick NM. Structural basis of geriatric voiding dysfunction. II. Aging detrusor: normal vs. impaired contractility. *J Urol.* 993;150:1657–1667.

23. Hailemariam S, Elbadawi A, Yalla SV, Resnick NM. Structural basis of geriatric voiding dysfunction. V. Standardized protocols for routine ultrastructural study and diagnosis of endoscopic biopsies. *J Urol.* 1997;157:1783–1801.

24. Fantl JA, Wyman JF, Wilson M, Elswick RK, Bump RC, Wein AJ. Diuretics and urinary incontinence in community-dwelling women. *Neurourol Urodyn.* 1990;9:25–34.

25. Diokno AC, Brown MB, Herzog AR. Relationship between use of diuretics and continence status in the elderly. *Urology.* 1991;38:39–42.

26. Brocklehurst JC, Dillane JB, Griffiths L, Fry J. The prevalence and symptomatology of urinary infection in an aged population. *Gerontol Clin.* 1968;10:242–253.

27. Baldassare JS, Kaye D. Special problems in urinary tract infection in the elderly. *Med Clin North Am.* 1991;75:375–390.

28. Ouslander JG, Schapira M, Schnelle JF, et al. Does eradicating bacteriuria affect the severity of chronic urinary incontinence in nursing home residents? *Ann Intern Med.* 1995;122:749–754.

29. Robinson JM. Evaluation of methods for assessment of bladder and urethral function. In: Brocklehurst JC, ed. *Urology in the Elderly.* New York: Churchill Livingstone; 1984:19–54.

30. Raz R, Stamm WE. A controlled trial of intravaginal estriol in postmenopausal women with recurrent urinary tract infections. *N Engl J Med.* 1993;329:753–756.

31. Cardozo L, Bachmann G, McClish DK, Fonda D, Birgerson L. Meta-analysis of estrogen therapy in the management of urogenital atrophy in postmenopausal women: second report of the Hormones and Urogenital Therapy Committee. *Obstet Gynecol.* 1998;92:722–727.

32. Semmens JP, Tsai CC, Semmens EC, Loadholt CB. Effects of estrogen therapy on vaginal physiology during menopause. *Obstet Gynecol.* 1985;66:15–18.

33. Pandit L, Ouslander JG. Postmenopausal vaginal atrophy and atrophic vaginitis. *Am J Med Sci.* 1997;314:228–231.

34. Everett HC. The use of bethanechol chloride with tricyclic antidepressants. *Am J Psychiatry.* 1975;132:1202–1204.

35. Marshall HJ, Beevers DG. α-Adrenoceptor blocking drugs and female urinary incontinence: prevalence and reversibility. *Br J Clin Pharmacol.* 1996;42:507–509.

36. Resnick NM. Geriatric medicine. In: Braunwald E, Isselbacher K, Wilson JD, Martin JB, Fauci A, Kasper D, eds. *Harrison's Principles of Internal Medicine.* 15th edition. New York: McGraw-Hill; 2001:36–46.

37. Hellstrom PM, Sjoqvist A. Involvement of opioid and nicotinic receptors in rectal and anal reflex inhibition of urinary bladder motility in cats. *Acta Physiol Scand.* 1988;133:559–562.

38. Resnick NM, Marcantonio ER. How should clinical care of the aged differ? *Lancet.* 1997;350:1157–1158.

39. Ouslander JG, Hepps K, Raz S, Su H-L. Genitourinary dysfunction in a geriatric outpatient population. *J Am Geriatr Soc.* 1986;34:507–514.

40. Resnick NM, Yalla SV, Laurino E. The pathophysiology and clinical correlates of established urinary incontinence in frail elderly. *N Engl J Med.* 1989;320:1–7.

41. DuBeau CE, Resnick NM. Urinary incontinence and dementia: the perils of guilt by association. *J Am Geriatr Soc.* 1995;43:310–311.

42. Skelly J, Flint AJ. Urinary incontinence associated with dementia. *J Am Geriatr Soc.* 1995;43:286–294.

43. Brandeis GH, Baumann MM, Hossain M, Morris JN, Resnick NM. The prevalence of potentially remediable urinary incontinence in frail older people: a study using the Minimum Data Set. *J Am Geriatr Soc.* 1997;45:179–184.

44. Elbadawi A, Yalla SV, Resnick NM. Structural basis of geriatric voiding dysfunction. III. Detrusor overactivity. *J Urol.* 1993;150:1668–1680.

45. Elbadawi A, Hailemariam S, Yalla SV, Resnick NM. Structural basis of geriatric voiding dysfunction. VI. Validation and update of diagnostic criteria in 71 detrusor biopsies. *J Urol.* 1997;157:1802–1813.

46. Tse V, Wills E, Szonyi G, Khadra MH. The application of ultrastructural studies in the diagnosis of bladder dysfunction in a clinical setting. *J Urol.* 2000;163:535–539.

47. Gormley EA, Griffiths DJ, McCracken PN, Harrison GM, McPhee MS. Effect of transurethral resection of the prostate on detrusor instability and urge incontinence in elderly males. *Neurourol Urodyn.* 1993;12:445–453.

48. Castleden CM, Duffin HM, Asher MJ. Clinical and urodynamic studies in 100 elderly incontinent patients. *Br Med J.* 1981;282:1103–1105.

49. Dennis PJ, Rohner TJ, Hu TW, Igou JF, Yu LC, Kaltreider DJ. Simple urodynamic evaluation of incontinent elderly female nursing home patients. A descriptive analysis. *Urology.* 1991;37:173–179.

50. Resnick NM, Yalla SV. Detrusor hyperactivity with impaired contractile function. An unrecognized but common cause of incontinence in elderly patients. *JAMA.* 1987;257:3076–3081.

51. Resnick NM, Brandeis GH, Baumann MM, DuBeau CE, Yalla SV. Misdiagnosis of urinary incontinence in nursing home women: prevalence and a proposed solution. *Neurourol Urodyn.* 1996;15:599–618.

52. Brandeis GH, Yalla SV, Resnick NM. Detrusor hyperactivity with impaired contractility (DHIC): the great mimic. *J Urol.* 1990;143:223A.

53. McGuire EJ. *Urinary Incontinence.* New York: Grune & Stratton; 1981.

54. Blaivas JG, Olsson CA. Stress incontinence: classification and surgical approach. *J Urol.* 1988;139:727–731.

55. McGuire EJ. Reflex urethral instability. *Br J Urol.* 1978;50: 200–204.

56. DuBeau CE, Resnick NM. Controversies in the diagnosis and management of benign prostatic hypertrophy. *Adv Intern Med.* 1992;37:55–83.

57. Dyro FM, Yalla SV. Refractoriness of urethral striated sphincter during voiding: studies with afferent pudendal reflex arc stimulation in male subjects. *J Urol.* 1986;135: 732–736.

58. Resnick NM. Noninvasive diagnosis of the patient with complex incontinence. *Gerontology.* 1990;36(suppl 2): 8–18.

59. Diokno AC, Brock BM, Brown M, Herzog AR. Prevalence of urinary incontinence and other urological symptoms in the non-institutionalized elderly. *J Urol.* 1986;136:1022–1025.

60. Reynard JM, Cannon A, Yang Q, Abrams P. A novel therapy for nocturnal polyuria: a double-blind randomized trial of frusemide against placebo. *BJU Int.* 1998;81:215–218.

61. DuBeau CE, Resnick NM. Evaluation of the causes and severity of geriatric incontinence: a critical appraisal. *Urol Clin North Am.* 1991;18:243–256.

62. DuBeau CE, Yalla SV, Resnick NM. Most bothersome symptom in men presenting with prostatism: implications for outcomes research. *J Am Geriatr Soc.* 1995;43:985–993.

63. Hilton P, Stanton SL. Algorithmic method for assessing urinary incontinence in elderly women. *Br Med J.* 1981; 282:940–942.

64. Diokno AC. Diagnostic categories of incontinence and the role of urodynamic testing. *J Am Geriatr Soc.* 1990;38:300–305.

65. Kong TK, Morris JA, Robinson JM, Brocklehurst JC. Predicting urodynamic dysfunction from clinical features in incontinent elderly women. *Age Ageing.* 1990;19:257–263.

66. Jensen JK, Nielsen FR Jr, Ostergard DR. The role of patient history in the diagnosis of urinary incontinence. *Obstet Gynecol.* 1994;83:904–910.

67. Diokno AC, Wells TJ, Brink CA. Urinary incontinence in elderly women: urodynamic evaluation. *J Am Geriatr Soc.* 1987;35:940–946.

68. Klarskov P, Andersen JT, Asmussen CF, et al. Symptoms and signs predictive of the voiding pattern after acute urinary retention in men. *Scand J Urol Nephrol.* 1987;21: 23–28.

69. Resnick NM. Initial evaluation of the incontinent patient. *J Am Geriatr Soc.* 1990;38:311–316.

70. Resnick NM, Ouslander JG, eds. National Institutes of Health consensus development conference on urinary incontinence. *J Am Geriatr Soc.* 1990;38:263–386.

71. Scientific Committee of the First International Consultation on Incontinence. Assessment and treatment of urinary incontinence. *Lancet.* 2000;355:2153–2158.

72. Ouslander JG, Colling J, and the PURT study group. Use of simple urodynamic tests in nursing homes. *Neurourol Urodyn.* 1992;11:159–160.

73. Resnick NM, Brandeis GH, Baumann MM, Morris JN. Evaluating a national assessment strategy for urinary incontinence in nursing home residents: reliability of the Minimum Data Set and validity of the Resident Assessment Protocol. *Neurourol Urodyn.* 1996;15:583–598.

74. DuBeau CE, Yalla SV, Resnick NM. Primary care screening for outlet obstruction in men with voiding symptoms. *J Am Geriatr Soc.* 1998;46:1118–1124.

75. Sonke GS, Heskes T, Verbeek ALM, De La Rosette JJMCH, Kiemeney LALM. Prediction of bladder outlet obstruction in men with lower urinary tract symptoms using artificial neural networks. *J Urol.* 2000;163:300–305.

76. Resnick NM, Baumann MM. Urinary incontinence. In: Morris JN, Lipsitz LA, eds. *Quality Care for the Nursing Home Resident.* St. Louis: Mosby 1996;376–406.

77. Resnick NM, Yalla SV, Laurino E. Feasibility, safety and reproducibility of urodynamics in the elderly. *J Urol.* 1987;137:189A.

78. Yalla SV, Resnick NM. Vesicourethral static pressure profile during voiding: methodology and clinical utility. *World J Urol.* 1984;2:196–202.

79. Fantl JA, Wyman JF, McClish DK. Efficacy of bladder training in older women with urinary incontinence. *JAMA.* 1991;265:609–613.

80. Burgio KL, Locher JL, Goode PS, et al. Behavioral vs. drug treatment for urge urinary incontinence in older women: a randomized controlled trial. *JAMA.* 1998;280:1995–2000.

81. Berghmans LCM, Hendriks HJM, DeBie RA, et al. Conservative treatment of urge urinary incontinence in women: a systematic review of randomized clinical trials. *BJU Int.* 2000;85:254–263.

82. Payne CK. Behavioral therapy for overactive bladder. *Urology.* 2000;55(5A):3–6.

83. Baigis-Smith J, Jakovac Smith DA, Rose M, Newman DK. Managing urinary incontinence in community-residing elderly persons. *Gerontologist.* 1989;29:229–233.

84. Cardozo L. Biofeedback in overactive bladder. *Urology.* 2000;55(5A):24–28.

85. Resnick NM. Improving treatment of urinary incontinence. *JAMA.* 1998;280:2034–2035.

86. Ouslander JG. Intractable incontinence in the elderly. *BJU Int.* 2000;85(suppl 3):72–78.

87. Hu TW, Igou JF, Kaltreider DL. A clinical trial of a behavioral therapy to reduce urinary incontinence in nursing homes. *JAMA.* 1989;261:2656–2662.

88. Engel BT, Burgio LD, McCormick KA. Behavioral treatment of incontinence in the long-term care setting. *J Am Geriatr Soc.* 1990;38:361–363.

89. Schnelle JF. Treatment of urinary incontinence in nursing home patients by prompted voiding. *J Am Geriatr Soc.* 1990;38:356–360.

90. Ouslander JG, Schnelle JF, Uman G, et al. Predictors of successful prompted voiding among incontinent nursing home residents. *JAMA.* 1995;273:1366–1370.

91. Pedersen PA, Johansen PB. Prophylactic treatment of adult nocturia with bumetanide. *Br J Urol.* 1988;62:145–147.

92. Andersson K-E, Appell R, Cardozo LD, et al. The pharmacological treatment of urinary incontinence. *BJU Int.* 1999;84:923–947.

93. Chapple CR. Muscarinic receptor antagonists in the treatment of overactive bladder. *Urology.* 2000;55(5A):33–46.

94. Bemelmans BLH, Kiemeney LALM, Debruyne FMJ. Low-dose oxybutynin for the treatment of urge incontinence: good efficacy and few side effects. *Fur Urol.* 2000; 37:709–713.

95. Miller KL, DuBeau CE, Bergmann M, Resnick NM. Dose titration key to oxybutynin efficacy for geriatric incontinence, even for DHIC. *Neurourol Urodyn.* 2000;19: 538–539 [abstract].

96. Brubaker L. Electrical stimulation in overactive bladder. *Urology.* 2000;55(5A):17–23.

97. Yamanishi T, Yasuda K, Sakakibara R, Hattori T, Suda S. Randomized, double-blind study of electrical stimulation for urinary incontinence due to detrusor overactivity. *Urology.* 2000;55:353–357.

98. Galloway NTM, El-Galley RES, Sand PK, Appell RA, Russell HW, Carlin SJ. Update on extracorporeal magnetic innervation (ExMI) therapy for stress urinary incontinence. *Urology.* 2000;56(suppl 6A):82–86.

99. Bosch JLHR, Groen J. Sacral nerve neuromodulation in the treatment of patients with refractory motor urge incontinence: long-term results of a prospective longitudinal study. *J Urol.* 2000;163:1219–1222.

100. Asplund R, Åberg H. Desmopressin in elderly subjects with increased nocturnal diuresis. A two-month treatment study. *Scand J Urol Nephrol.* 1993;27:77–82.

101. Dequecker J. Drug treatment of urinary incontinence in the elderly. *Gerontol Clin.* 1965;7:311–317.

102. Cannon A, Carter PG, McConnell AA, Abrams P. Desmopressin in the treatment of nocturnal polyuria in the male. *BJU Int.* 1999;84:20–24.

103. Carter PG, Cannon A, McConnell AA, Abrams P. Role of atrial natriuretic peptide in nocturnal polyuria in elderly males. *Eur Urol.* 1999;36:213–220.

104. Brink CA, Wells TJ. Environmental support for incontinence: toilets, toilet supplements, and external equipment. *Clin Geriatr Med.* 1986;2:829–840.

105. Brink CA. Absorbent pads, garments, and management strategies. *J Am Geriatr Soc.* 1990;38:368–373.

106. Snow TL. Equipment for prevention, treatment, and management of urinary incontinence. *Top Geriatr Rehabil.* 1988;3:58–77.

107. Fonda D, Benvenuti F, Castleden M, et al. Management of incontinence in older people. In: Abrams P, Khoury JM, Wein AJ, eds. *Incontinence. From the 1st International Consultation on Incontinence. Co-Sponsored by the WHO.* Monaco: Health Publication; 1999:731–773.

108. Johnson ET. The condom catheter: urinary tract infection and other complications. *South Med J.* 1983;76:579–582.

109. Jayachandran S, Moopan UMM, Kim H. Complications from external (condom) urinary drainage devices. *Urology.* 1985;25:31–34.

110. Johnson DE, Muncie HL, O'Reilly JL, Warren JW. An external urine collection device for incontinent women. *J Am Geriatr Soc.* 1990;38:1016–1022.

111. Norton PA, Baker JE. Postural changes can reduce leakage in women with stress urinary incontinence. *Obstet Gynecol* 1994;84:770–774.

112. Suarez GM, Baum NH, Jacobs J. Use of standard contraceptive diaphragm in management of stress urinary incontinence. *Urology* 1991;37:119–122.

113. Zeitlin MP, Lebherz TB. Pessaries in the geriatric patient. *J Am Geriatr Soc.* 1992;40:635–639.

114. Wells TJ. Pelvic (floor) muscle exercises. *J Am Geriatr Soc.* 1990;38:333–337.

115. Burns PA, Pranikoff K, Nochajski TH, Hadley EC, Levy KJ, Ory MG. A comparison of effectiveness of biofeedback and pelvic muscle exercise treatment of stress incontinence in older community-dwelling women. *J Gerontol.* 1993;48:M167–M174.

116. Wells TJ, Brink CA, Diokno AC, Wolfe Robert, Gillis GL. Pelvic muscle exercise for stress urinary incontinence in elderly women. *J Am Geriatr Soc.* 1991;39:785–791.

117. Berghmans LCM, Hendriks HJM, Bo K, Hay-Smith EJ, DeBie RA, Van Doom ES. Conservative treatment of stress urinary incontinence in women: a systematic review of randomized clinical trials. *Br J Urol.* 1998;82:181–191.

118. Burgio KL, Engel BT. Biofeedback-assisted behavioral training for elderly men and women. *J Am Geriatr Soc.* 1990;38:338–340.

119. Haller CA, Benowitz NL. Adverse cardiovascular and central nervous system events associated with dietary supplements containing ephedra alkaloids. *N Engl J Med.* 2000;343:1833–1838.

120. Eriksen BC, Hagen B, Eik-Nes SH. Long-term effectiveness of the Burch colposuspension in female urinary stress incontinence. *Acta Obstet Gynecol Scand.* 1990;69:45–50.

121. Griffith-Jones MD, Abrams PH. The Stamey cndoscopic bladder neck suspension in the elderly. *Br J Urol.* 1990;65:170–172.

122. Nitti VW, Bregg KJ, Sussman EM, Raz S. The Raz bladder neck suspension in patients 65 years old and older. *J Urol.* 1993;149:802–807.

123. Blaivas JG, Jacobs BZ. Pubovaginal fascial sling for the treatment of complicated stress urinary incontinence. *J Urol.* 1991;145:12l4–l218.

124. Chaliha C, Williams G. Periurethral injection therapy for the treatment of urinary incontinence. *Br J Urol.* 1995;76:151–155.

125. Winters JC, Chiverton A, Scarpero HM, Prats LJ. Collagen injection therapy in elderly women: long-term results and patient satisfaction. *Urology.* 2000;55:856–861.

126. Mann RD, Biswas P, Freemantle S, Pearce G, Wilton L. The pharmacovigilance of tamsulosin: event data on 12,484 patients. *BJU Int.* 2000;85:446–450.

127. Gormley GJ, Stoner E, Bruskewitz RC, et al. The effect of finasteride in men with benign prostatic hyperplasia. *N Engl J Med.* 1992;327:1185–l191.

128. Eastwood HD, Smart CJ. Urinary incontinence in the disabled elderly male. *Age Ageing.* 1985;14:235–239.

129. Downie JW. Bethanechol chloride in urology—a discussion of issues. *Neurourol Urodyn.* 1984;3:211–222.

130. Finkbeiner A. Is bethanechol chloride clinically effective in promoting bladder emptying? A literature review. *J Urol.* 1985;134:443–449.

131. Chawla JC, Clayton CL, Stickler DJ. Antiseptics in the long-term urological management of patients by intermittent catheterization. *Br J Urol.* 1988;62:289–294.

132. Warren JW. Urine collection devices for use in adults with urinary incontinence. *J Am Geriatr Soc.* 1990;38:364–367.

133. Hunt GM, Whitaker RH. A new device for self-catheterization in wheelchair-bound women. *Br J Urol.* 1990;66:162–163.

134. Bennett CJ, Diokno AC. Clean intermittent self-catheterization in the elderly. *Urology.* 1984;24:43–45.

135. Bakke A, Brun OH, Hoisæter PÅ. Clinical background of patients treated with clean intermittent catheterization in Norway. *Scand J Urol Nephrol.* 1992;26:211–217.

136. Warren JW, Muncie HL, Hebel JR, Hall-Craggs M. Long-term urethral catheterization increases risk of chronic pyelonephritis and renal inflammation. *J Am Geriatr Soc.* 1994;42:1286–1290.

64
Syncope in the Elderly

Wishwa N. Kapoor

Syncope is defined as a sudden transient loss of consciousness associated with loss of postural tone from which the patient recovers spontaneously. Syncope has a large differential diagnosis, ranging from common benign problems to severe life-threatening disorders. As a result, the approach to this symptom frequently results in hospital admission and performance of many diagnostic tests. Although evaluation is often focused on explaining the symptom by a single disease process, this approach may not apply to the elderly because multiple physiologic processes and age-related changes may contribute to syncope. This chapter briefly reviews the pathophysiology and etiologies of syncope and provides a practical and directed evaluation of syncope in the elderly.

Pathophysiology

Syncope is caused by a sudden decrease in cerebral blood flow to those areas of the brain that are responsible for consciousness (reticular activating system and both hemispheres). Elderly patients often have multiple comorbid conditions that interact with age-related physiologic derangement, leading to a reduction in cerebral blood flow when even mild acute processes are superimposed. Elderly patients with hypertension and atherosclerotic vascular disease have baseline decreased cerebral blood flow, which may be further reduced by multiple comorbid conditions. Additionally, elderly patients are often taking multiple medications, which may further reduce cerebral blood flow by altering vascular tone or volume.

Physiologic changes related to aging may diminish the ability to adapt to a sudden drop in blood pressure.[1] These changes include the following events.

Age-Related Cardiovascular Changes

Baroreflex sensitivity diminishes with aging, manifesting as a reduction in vascular response to hypotensive stimuli; this may be due to a blunting of beta-adrenergic-mediated vasodilation. Additionally, there is an increase in plasma norepinephrine and a greater norepinephrine response to acute hypotension in the elderly, suggesting impaired end-organ responsiveness to adrenergic stimulation with normal central and afferent components of the baroreflex circuit. As a result of decreased baroreceptor reflex sensitivity, elderly persons may not be able to maintain cerebral blood flow by increasing heart rate and vascular tone in the setting of hypotension. Thus, the elderly are more sensitive to the effects of vasodilators and other hypotensive drugs and are more likely to have exaggerated hypotension from volume loss, hemorrhage, and upright posture.

Systolic hypertension, prevalent in more than 30% of persons over age 75, also leads to diminished baroreflex sensitivity and decreased vascular and ventricular compliance. Hypertension may also increase the threshold for cerebral autoregulation, which can lead to a decrease in cerebral blood flow with modest acute decreases in blood pressure to levels within the normotensive ranges.[1] Thus, the age-related physiologic changes just described may be worsened by the presence of systolic hypertension.

Decreased Ability to Maintain Extracellular Volume

With aging, kidneys develop impairment of sodium conservation when salt intake is restricted. Basal plasma levels of renin and aldosterone are also decreased. These changes may increase the susceptibility of the elderly to orthostatic hypotension and syncope. As a result, the effects of diuretics, salt restriction, and upright posture may be more pronounced in the elderly.

Clinical Classification

Although syncope has a large differential diagnosis, the etiologies can be classified into four major categories (Table 64.1).

TABLE 64.1. Etiologies of syncope.

Neurally mediated syndromes
  Vasovagal
  Situational
    Micturition
    Cough
    Swallow
    Defecation
  Carotid sinus syncope
  Neuralgias
  High altitude
  Psychiatric disorders
  Others (exercise, selected drugs)
Orthostatic hypotension
  Neurologic diseases
    Migraines
    TIAs
    Seizures
Decreased cardiac output
  Obstruction to flow
    Obstruction to LV outflow or inflow
      Aortic stenosis, IHSS
      Mitral stenosis, myxoma
    Obstruction to RV outflow or inflow
      Pulmonic stenosis
      PE, pulmonary hypertension
      Myxoma
  Other heart disease
    Pump failure
      MI, CAD, coronary spasm
    Tamponade, aortic dissection
  Arrhythmias
    Bradyarrhythmias
      Sinus node disease
      Second- and third-degree
        atrioventricular block
      Pacemaker malfunction
      Drug-induced bradyarrhythmias
    Tachyarrhythmias
      Ventricular tachycardia
      Torsades de pointes (e.g., associated with congenital long QT
        syndromes or acquired QT prolongation)
      Supraventricular tachycardia

TIA, transient ischemic attack; LV, left ventricular; IHSS, idiopathic hypertrophic subaortic stenosis; RV, right ventricular; PE, pulmonary embolism; MI, myocardial infarction; CAD, coronary artery disease.

Neurally Mediated Syndromes

Neurally mediated or neurocardiogenic syncope are terms used synonymously that refer to syncope resulting from reflex mechanisms associated with inappropriate vasodilatation and/or bradycardia.[2,3] These terms encompass more specific syndromes such as vasovagal, vasodepressor, situational, or carotid sinus syncope.

The mechanism of neurally mediated syncope is poorly understood, but receptors that respond to pain, mechanical stimuli, and temperature are widely believed to be important in the pathophysiology of these spells. These receptors appear to serve as the origins of the afferent signals triggering the various neurally mediated syncopal syndromes.[2,3] For example, in carotid sinus hypersensitivity, carotid artery baroreceptors, and vasovagal syncope, left ventricular baroreceptors (mechanoreceptors) serve as triggers. Similar receptors in the aortic arch, carotid arteries, atrial and ventricular myocardium, respiratory tree, bladder, and the gastrointestinal tract may trigger various other neurally mediated syndromes.[2] The afferent pathway consists of neural fibers that transmit signals to the central nervous system sites (in the medulla, particularly the nucleus tractus solitarius). The efferent outflow results in vasodilatation and bradycardia. The effect of higher CNS centers is not fully understood.

Vasovagal syncope is a common etiology of syncope in the elderly. Vasovagal syncope is commonly associated with pallor, nausea, vomiting, and sweating but may occur without associated symptoms. It is often a response to fear or injury. Examples of precipitating factors include fatigue, prolonged standing, venipuncture, blood donation, heat, dental surgery, and eye surgery.

Syncope in the elderly may be associated with a wide variety of daily situations (termed situational syncope). In a study of institutionalized elderly, syncope in association with micturition, defecation, postural change, and meals was found in 20% of patients.[4] Other situations include coughing, laughing, and swallowing. Mechanisms of syncope in these circumstances may be similar to vasovagal syncope with activation of inhibitory reflexes mediated by these activities. In the elderly, impaired homeostasis and orthostatic hypotension may facilitate situational syncope.

Postprandial hypotension can be associated with syncope during or after a meal. In a nursing home elderly population, up to 36% may have a systolic blood pressure decline of more than 20 mmHg after a meal (generally at 45–60 min).[5] However, acute symptoms are rare. In institutionalized elderly patients with syncope, 8% of patients had postprandial syncope.[4] The mechanism of postprandial hypotension is not well understood. Impaired compensation for the pooling of blood in the splanchnic blood vessels, insufficient increase in cardiac output, impaired baroreflex function, poor peripheral vasoconstriction, and other factors may contribute to postprandial hypotension.[6]

Carotid sinus hypersensitivity results from the stimulation of baroreceptors located just above the bifurcation of the common carotid artery. Carotid sinus hypersensitivity may be cardioinhibitory (asystole ≥3 s), vasodepressor (a systolic blood pressure decline ≥50 mmHg in the absence of significant bradycardia), or mixed (combination of cardioinhibitory and vasodepressor response). Spontaneous loss of consciousness, termed carotid sinus syncope, is reported in 5% to 20% of individuals with carotid sinus hypersensitivity. Attacks may be precipitated by a tight collar, shaving, or sudden turning. This disorder occurs primarily in the elderly, and the majority of patients have coronary artery disease and hypertension. Other factors leading to carotid sinus hypersensitivity include neck pathology such as enlarged lymph nodes, tissue scars, carotid body tumors, parotid, thyroid, head, and neck tumors, and drugs such as digitalis, alpha-methyldopa, and propranolol.

Stress and psychiatric illnesses such as generalized anxiety disorder, panic disorder, and major depression probably cause syncope by precipitating vasovagal reactions. A neurally mediated mechanism is also implicated for syncope in association with exercise, especially immediately postexercise in individuals without structural heart disease, where mild volume depletion and shifts of blood flow to dissipate heat may precipitate neurally mediated syncope. Neurally mediated syncope may also occur with drugs that decrease venous return to the heart in an upright position, such as nitroglycerine. Syncope with aortic stenosis, hypertrophic cardiomyopathy, supraventricular tachycardias, paroxysmal atrial fibrillation, and related to pacemakers (i.e., pacemaker syndrome) appear to be consistent with neurally mediated syndrome.

Orthostatic Hypotension

Blood pressure is maintained by homeostatic adjustments in the brain and reflexes in the systemic circulation. Upon standing, pooling of blood in the lower extremities and the splanchnic circulation results in reduced venous return to the heart and a decrease in cardiac output, leading to stimulation of aortic, carotid, and cardiopulmonary baroreceptors. An increase in sympathetic outflow and a decrease in parasympathetic activity result, leading to an increase in heart rate and vascular resistance to maintain systemic blood pressure. A number of pathophysiologic processes, disease states, and medications may alter blood pressure homeostasis, leading to orthostatic hypotension (Table 64.2).

Age-related physiologic changes and systolic hypertension contribute significantly to the development of orthostatic hypotension in the elderly. Volume depletion is another major cause of orthostatic hypotension because salt and water homeostasis is impaired in the elderly. Thus, the elderly can readily develop volume depletion with the use of even low-dose mild diuretics or during acute illnesses that increase insensible water losses. This state is further exacerbated because the elderly experience less thirst than younger people in the setting of hyperosmolality. Medications are also a common cause of orthostatic hypotension in the elderly and often in the usual therapeutic doses rather than in toxic amounts (see Table 64.2).

TABLE 64.2. Causes of orthostatic hypotension.

Primary
  Autonomic failure with multiple system atrophy (Shy–Drager syndrome)
Secondary
  General medical disorders: diabetes; amyloid; alcoholism
  Autoimmune disease: Guillain–Barré syndrome; mixed connective tissue disease; rheumatoid arthritis; Eaton–Lambert syndrome; systemic lupus erythematosus
  Metabolic disease: vitamin B_{12} deficiency; porphyria; Fabry's disease; Tangier disease
  Hereditary sensory neuropathies, dominant or recessive
  Central brain lesions: vascular lesion or tumors involving the hypothalamus and midbrain, for example, craniopharyngioma; multiple sclerosis; Wernicke's encephalopathy
  Spinal cord lesions
  Familial dysautonomia
  Aging
Drugs
  Tranquilizers: phenothiazines; barbiturates
  Antidepressants: tricyclics; monoamine oxidase inhibitors
  Vasodilators: prazosin; hydralazine; calcium channel blockers
  Centrally acting hypotensive drugs: methyldopa; clonidine
  Adrenergic neuron-blocking drugs: guanethidine
  α-Adrenergic blocking drugs: phenoxybenzamine; labetalol
  Ganglion-blocking drugs: hexamethonium; mecamylamine
  Angiotensin-converting enzyme inhibitors: captopril; enlapril; lisinopril

Source: Adapted from Bannister SR, ed. Autonomic Failure, 4th Ed. New York: Oxford University Press, 1999, with permission.

A wide variety of diseases affecting the autonomic nervous system may cause chronic orthostatic hypotension (Table 64.2). Idiopathic orthostatic hypotension is a rare illness that affects men five times more than women. Its manifestations may include sphincter disturbances, impotence, impaired erection and ejaculation, and impaired sweating. Supine basal plasma norepinephrine levels are markedly low and remain unchanged on standing, suggesting a peripheral dysfunction with depletion of norepinephrine from sympathetic nerve endings. Shy–Drager syndrome consists of autonomic failure and involvement of the corticospinal, extrapyramidal, and cerebellar tracts, including a Parkinson-like syndrome. Basal norepinephrine levels are normal at rest but do not increase substantially on standing, suggesting an inability to stimulate normally functioning peripheral neurons.

Neurologic Diseases

Neurologic disorders are infrequent causes of syncope. Approximately 6% of persons with ischemic stroke or transient cerebral ischemia have associated syncope. In 483 syncope patients seen in an emergency room, 7.7% had transient ischemic attacks.[7] All patients had concurrent neurologic symptoms, most frequently vertigo, ataxia, and paraesthesia. Almost all patients had vertebrobasilar transient ischemic attacks (TIAs).[7] Migraines may lead to a vasovagal reaction secondary to pain, although they are unusual in the elderly.

Less than 2% of patients presenting with syncope are diagnosed as having a seizure disorder as a cause of their loss of consciousness.[8] These events may include atonic seizures and sudden falls associated with temporal lobe epilepsy (termed temporal lobe syncope). Unwitnessed grand mal seizures may also be mistaken as syncope if the patient cannot provide detailed information.

Cardiac Syncope

Obstruction to Flow

Obstruction to outflow may result from structural lesions of either the left or right side of the heart (see Table 64.1). Exertional syncope is a common manifestation of all types of heart disease in which cardiac output is fixed and does not rise with exercise. The most likely mechanism of exertional syncope is ventricular baroreceptor-mediated hypotension and bradycardia. Exercise leads to a marked increase in left ventricular systolic pressure, which may result in excessive stimulation of left ventricular mechanoreceptors that leads to inhibition of sympathetic and activation of parasympathetic tone through cardiac vagal afferent fibers. Syncope in hypertrophic cardiomyopathy may also be due to neurally mediated syndrome or ventricular tachycardia, which is commonly found in these patients.

Syncope, which may occasionally occur with exertion, is reported in 10% to 15% of patients with pulmonary embolism and is more likely with massive embolism. The mechanism may be acute right ventricular failure with decreased cardiac output and hypotension or activation of cardiopulmonary mechanoreceptors leading to neurally mediated syncope.

Other Organic Heart Disease

Syncope may be the presenting symptom in 5% to 12% of elderly patients with acute myocardial infarction because of (1) sudden pump failure producing a decrease in perfusion pressure of the brain, (2) rhythm disturbance that may include ventricular tachycardia or bradyarrhythmias, and (3) vasovagal reactions resulting from stimulation of left ventricular baroreceptors during acute inferior infarction or ischemia involving the right coronary artery.

Arrhythmias

Bradyarrhythmias and tachyarrhythmias may cause a sudden decrease in cardiac output and syncope. The elderly are less able to compensate for sudden decrease in cardiac output caused by arrhythmias. Physiologic impairments with aging and the effects of multiple medications and comorbidity may predispose elderly to syncope in the setting of brief arrhythmias whereas such arrhythmias may not lead to symptoms in the young.

Sick sinus syndrome and ventricular tachycardia were the most common arrhythmic causes of syncope in the elderly, occurring in 22% of this group. Syncope is a central manifestation of sick sinus syndrome, reported in 25% to 70% of these patients. Electrocardiographic findings include sinus bradycardia, pauses, arrest, or exit block. These bradyarrhythmias may be associated with supraventricular tachycardia or atrial fibrillation (tachycardia-bradycardia syndrome).

Ventricular tachycardia commonly occurs in the setting of known organic heart disease. Torsades de pointes and syncope in the elderly occur in the setting of acquired long QT syndromes associated with drugs, electrolyte abnormalities, and central nervous system disorders. Antiarrhythmic drugs such as quinidine (quinidine syncope), procainamide, disopyramide, flecainide, and encainide are the most common causes of torsades de pointes.

Multiple Abnormalities

The evaluation of the elderly should initially focus on a single disease as explaining the loss of consciousness. If a single disease is found (such as severe aortic stenosis, symptomatic bradycardia, or symptomatic orthostatic hypotension), treatment of that disease can be planned. However, a single disease as the cause of syncope is often not apparent. In these patients, inability to compensate for common situational stresses in the setting of multiple medical problems, medications, and physiologic impairments may be responsible for the loss of consciousness. Once these potential processes are identified, treatment should be directed to correcting these factors. As an example, consider an elderly patient presenting with syncope, who has taken enalapril 10mg/day, has anemia (hemoglobin 9.0), mild orthostatic hypotension, and a recent upper respiratory tract infection. In this patient, if no other etiology of syncope is apparent based on clinical findings and selective use of laboratory tests, volume repletion, treatment of anemia, and adjustment or change of antihypertensive medication may help prevent further episodes of syncope.

Diagnostic Evaluation

The most important elements in the evaluation of syncope in the elderly are (1) determining whether the patient had syncope; (2) risk stratification; and (3) selective use of diagnostic tests to define the etiology of loss of consciousness.

Determining Whether the Patient Had Syncope

A history from the patient and the witness, if present, is needed to separate syncope from other entities such as dizziness, vertigo, drop attacks, coma, and seizure. A particularly important issue is the distinction between syncope and seizure, as videometric analysis of syncope has shown myoclonic activity in 90%, predominantly consisting of multifocal arrhythmic jerks in both proximal and distal muscles.[9] Historical features are often sufficient to distinguish syncope from seizures. Seizures are associated with blue face (or not pale), frothing at the mouth, tongue biting, disorientation, aching muscles, sleepiness after the event, and duration of unconsciousness of more than 5 min. On the other hand, symptoms associated with syncope are sweating or nausea before the event and being oriented after the event. The best discriminatory symptom is disorientation after the episode, which often signifies a seizure.[10]

Risk Stratification

Risk stratification is important for initial management decisions such as admission to the hospital and the use of invasive testing such as electrophysiologic studies. The issues include prediction of risk of sudden death and likelihood of cardiac syncope. In the assessment of risk, the cause of syncope, presence of underlying cardiac disease, and abnormalities on ECG are important.[11–13]

Previous studies have consistently shown increased mortality and sudden death rates in patients with cardiac causes of syncope, thus identifying patients with cardiac causes as a high-risk subset.[8,14] Examples include aortic stenosis, pulmonary hypertension, and arrhythmic syncope. Arrhythmias are primarily of concern in patients with heart disease or abnormal ECG. Thus, the presence of heart disease and certain abnormalities on ECG help stratify patients into low- and high-risk groups.[11] Congestive heart failure, valvular heart disease, hypertrophic cardiomyopathy and other types of organic heart disease constitute a high risk group. AV block, old myocardial infarction, and Wolf–Parkinson–White syndrome (WPW) are examples of high-risk findings on ECG. If the presence or absence of heart disease cannot be determined clinically, specific tests such as echocardiogram, stress test, and ventricular function studies may be needed for risk stratification.

Selective Use of Diagnostic Tests

The evaluation of syncope is best approached by using the history and physical examination, ECG, and risk stratification to guide further diagnostic tests.

History, Physical Examination, and Baseline Laboratory Tests

A detailed account of syncope, the events leading to loss of consciousness, and symptoms following the episode are crucial to diagnosing specific entities. Table 64.3 shows

TABLE 64.3. Clinical features suggestive of specific causes.

Symptom of finding	Diagnostic consideration
After sudden unexpected pain, fear, unpleasant sight, sound, or smell	Vasovagal
Prolonged standing at attention	Vasovagal
Well-trained athlete after exertion (without heart disease)	Vasovagal
During or immediately after micturition, cough, swallow, or defecation	Situational syncope
Syncope with throat or facial pain (glossopharyngeal or trigeminal neuralgia)	Neurally mediated syncope with neuralgia
With head rotation, pressure on carotid sinus (as in tumors, shaving, tight collars)	Carotid sinus syncope
Immediately upon standing	Orthostatic hypotension
Medications that may lead to long QT or orthostasis/bradycardia	Drug induced
Associated with headaches	Migraines, seizures
Associated with vertigo, dysarthria, diplopia	TIA, subclavian steal, basilar migraine
With arm exercise	Subclavian steal
Confusion after spell or loss of consciousness more than 5 min	Seizure
Differences in BP or pulse in two arms	Subclavian steal or aortic dissection
Syncope and murmur with changing position (from sitting to lying, bending, turning over in bed)	Atrial myxoma or thrombus
Syncope with exertion	Aortic stenosis, pulmonary hypertension mitral stenosis, hypertrophic cardiomyopathy, coronary artery disease
Family history of sudden death	Long QT syndrome, Brugada syndrome
Brief loss of consciousness, no prodrome, with heart disease	Arrhythmias
Frequent syncope, somatic complaints, no heart disease	Psychiatric illness

Source: Reproduced with permission from Kapoor WN. Syncope. N Engl J Med. 2000;343:1856–1862, with permission.

clinical presentations that may suggest specific entities. Physical examination is used to diagnose specific entities and exclude others. Orthostatic hypotension, cardiovascular findings, and neurologic examination are critical in this regard.

Orthostatic hypotension is generally defined as a decline of 20 mmHg or more in systolic pressure on assuming an upright position. However, this finding is reported in up to 24% of the elderly and is frequently not associated with symptoms. Thus, the clinical diagnosis of orthostatic hypotension should incorporate the presence of symptoms (e.g., dizziness and syncope) in association with a decrease in systolic blood pressure.

In detection of orthostatic hypotension, supine blood pressure and heart rate should be measured after the patient has been lying down for at least 5 min. Standing measurements should be obtained immediately and for at least 3 min. Sitting blood pressures are not reliable for detection of orthostatic hypotension.

Several cardiovascular findings are crucial diagnostically. Differences in the pulse intensity and blood pressure (generally >20 mmHg) in the two arms are suggestive of aortic dissection or subclavian steal syndrome. Special focus on cardiovascular examination for aortic stenosis, idiopathic hypertrophic subaortic stenosis, pulmonary hypertension, myxomas, and aortic dissection may uncover clues to these entities.

In a study of syncope in the elderly, a history and physical examination led to 40% of the diagnoses that could be assigned.[14] Furthermore, in an additional 15%, a diagnosis was suggested by history and physical examination and confirmed by specific tests (e.g., echocardiogram or catheterization for aortic stenosis).[14] In comparing elderly to young, arrhythmias are more often diagnosed as the etiology in the elderly, and several entities were primarily found in the elderly including aortic stenosis, TIAs, and carotid sinus syncope.[14]

Initial laboratory blood tests rarely yield diagnostically helpful information. Hypoglycemia, hyponatremia, hypocalcemia, or renal failure are found in 2% to 3% of patients, but most of these conditions appear to result in seizures rather than syncope.[15,16] These tests are often confirmatory of clinical suspicion of these laboratory abnormalities. In the elderly patients in whom a cause of syncope is not established by the initial history and physical examination, further evaluation should focus on the following issues: (1) arrhythmia detection, (2) tilt testing, and (3) multiple abnormalities causing symptoms.

Arrhythmia Detection

In diagnosing arrhythmias, every attempt should be made to attain symptomatic correlation. When this is not possible, uncertainty may remain regarding the cause of syncope because at the current time there are no vali-dated criteria for attributing syncope to most arrhythmias by the use of electrocardiographic or electrophysiologic abnormalities during asymptomatic periods.

Arrhythmias are evaluated by prolonged electrocardiographic monitoring or electrophysiologic studies, although rarely (in 2%–9%) the initial electrocardiogram or a rhythm strip may show an arrhythmia.[8,14,15,16] In one study of the elderly, ECG led to a diagnosis in 9% of patients as compared to 4% of the young group.[14] Exercise ECG can be used to evaluate syncope with exercise for the diagnosis of ischemia, exercise-induced tachyarrhythmias or bradyarrhythmias after abrupt termination of exercise. However, the yield of this test for arrhythmias is very low.

Prolonged Electrocardiographic Monitoring

One method of assessing the impact of ambulatory monitoring in syncope is to determine the presence or absence of arrhythmias in patients who develop symptoms during monitoring. In studies that evaluated syncope or presyncope with monitoring and reported on symptoms, only 4% of patients had symptomatic correlation with arrhythmias.[17] In approximately 17% of patients, symptoms were not associated with arrhythmias, thus potentially excluding rhythm disturbance as an etiology for syncope.[17] In approximately 80% of patients, no symptoms occurred but arrhythmias were often found. The causal relation between these arrhythmias and syncope therefore is uncertain. Furthermore, finding brief or no arrhythmias (without symptoms) on monitoring does not exclude arrhythmic syncope because of the episodic nature of arrhythmias. In patients with high pretest likelihood of arrhythmias, further evaluation for arrhythmias needs to be pursued by event monitoring or electrophysiologic studies. Extending the duration of monitoring to 72 h may increase the yield of arrhythmias detected but not the yield for arrhythmias associated with symptoms.[18]

Long-term monitoring (weeks to months) is possible with patient-activated intermittent external loop recorders that can capture the rhythm during syncope after the patient has regained consciousness because several minutes of retrograde electrocardiographic recording can be obtained. Loop monitoring is most useful in patients with a history of recurrent unexplained syncope because their probability of recurrence is higher, making it more likely for arrhythmias to be captured during an event. Recently, long-term monitoring (up to 24 months) has become possible with subcutaneously inserted loop monitors. This device, roughly the size of a pacemaker, is usually inserted in the left pectoral or inframammary region, and can record an episode from 6 to 40 min before activation and 1 to 2 min afterward. Although this is an invasive test, it may be useful in patients with brief episodic arrhythmias not captured by other means who have infrequent episodes. In one study of 85 patients with recurrent syncope, a positive yield of 27% was found that included tachycardias and bradycardias (5 of 18 patients with bradycardias were considered to have neurally mediated syncope).[19]

Electrophysiologic Studies

Electrophysiologic studies are more likely to be "positive" in patients with known heart disease, abnormal ventricular function, or abnormalities on electrocardiogram or ambulatory monitoring. Predictors of ventricular tachycardia by electrophysiologic studies include organic heart disease, premature ventricular contractions (PVCs) by ECG, and nonsustained ventricular tachycardia by Holter monitoring. Sinus bradycardia, first-degree AV block, and bundle branch block by ECG predict bradyarrhythmic outcome.

Predictors of a negative electrophysiologic study in patients with syncope include the absence of heart disease; an ejection fraction greater than 40%; normal electrocardiogram and Holter monitoring; absence of injury during syncope; and multiple or prolonged (>5 min) episodes of syncope.

Electrophysiologic studies are abnormal in approximately 50% of patients undergoing this test. The most common finding is inducible ventricular tachycardia. In the elderly, a study of 75 patients who were 75 years old or older showed electrophysiologic testing to be abnormal in 68%.[20] The abnormalities were mostly conduction disturbances, such as sinus node disease in 55% and His bundle conduction abnormalities in 39%. Inducible ventricular tachycardia was found in 14% of the patients.[20]

The limitations of electrophysiologic testing for syncope are similar to the problems with prolonged monitoring. Symptomatic correlation is often not possible, and the criteria for significant abnormalities are controversial. For example, criteria for significantly abnormal HV interval have ranged from greater than 55 ms to greater than 100 ms. Furthermore, some of the abnormalities such as polymorphic ventricular tachycardia have poor specificity.

Electrophysiologic studies identify a group of patients who are at high risk of mortality. Mortality rates as high as 61% and sudden death rates of 48% have been reported at 3 years in patients with abnormal studies as compared to 15% and 9% in the negative group.[21] These differences are probably largely due to the higher prevalence of cardiac comorbidity in patients with positive findings. A low rate of mortality and sudden death in patients with negative studies can also be reassuring because this defines a low-risk group of syncope patients.

Patients with abnormal electrophysiologic studies generally have lower rates of recurrence of syncope in follow-up as compared to patients with normal findings. At a mean of 26 months, recurrence of syncope in the elderly with positive electrophysiologic studies was 16% as compared to 25% in the negative group.[21] These studies have been observational and not controlled. Because of differences in the prevalence of heart disease in patients with normal and abnormal electrophysiologic testing, it is difficult to be sure that the outcome differences are a result of this procedure.

Tilt Testing

The pathophysiologic mechanism of inducing syncope by upright tilt testing is poorly understood. One postulated mechanism centers around the stimulation of cardiac mechanoreceptors. Upright posture leads to pooling of blood in the lower limbs, resulting in decreased venous return. Normal compensatory response to standing upright is reflex tachycardia, more forceful contraction of the ventricles, and vasoconstriction. However, in individuals susceptible to vasovagal syncope, this forceful ventricular contraction in the setting of a relatively empty ventricle may excessively stimulate the cardiac sensory nerves (mechanoreceptors). Afferent impulses are relayed to the medulla, resulting in a decrease in sympathetic and increase in parasympathetic tone. Catecholamine release (as may occur with anxiety, fear, and panic), by increasing ventricular contraction, may also activate the nerve endings responsible for triggering this reflex. The role of higher cortical centers is controversial.

The American College of Cardiology Expert Consensus has recommended tilt testing methods and indications.[22] Tilt testing methods generally involve the use of provocative agents such as isoproterenol or nitroglycerine because rates of positive responses without chemical stimulation appear to be low.[22–24] In patients with unexplained syncope, positive responses occur in approximately 66% with isoproterenol protocols.[24,25] The results with the use of nitroglycerine appear to be similar.[26,27] The specificity of most currently used tilt testing approaches 90% with chemical stimulation.[24,25]

Studies of upright tilt testing in syncope of unknown origin in the elderly (studies of patients with a mean age of 60 years or older or specified as elderly) mostly have used passive protocols. The overall percent positive response is 54% (range, 26%–90%).[24,25] The rate of positive response in elderly control subjects without syncope is approximately 11% with a range of 0% to 100%.[24] Isoproterenol should be avoided in the elderly whenever possible. Protocols with the use of nitroglycerine may be more suitable for testing in the elderly.

Other Tests

Skull films, lumbar puncture, radionuclide brain scan, and cerebral angiography have not yielded diagnostic information for a cause of syncope in the absence of clinical findings suggestive of a specific neurologic process.[8] EEG shows an epileptiform abnormality in 1%, but almost all these are suspected clinically. Head CT scans are needed if subdural bleed due to head injury is suspected or in patients suspected to have a seizure as a cause of loss of consciousness, but the yield is low when used in a nondirected fashion.[8]

Approach to Evaluation

The majority of the causes of syncope are identified by a careful history and physical examination. Additionally, history and physical examination may suggest specific entities as possible causes (e.g., findings of aortic stenosis or neurologic signs and symptoms suggestive of a seizure disorder). These entities can then be approached in a directed fashion by performing further noninvasive or invasive tests for establishing a diagnosis and initiating treatment. An electrocardiogram is generally needed for the initial evaluation of patients with syncope. Although the diagnostic yield of electrocardiogram for arrhythmias or suspicion of myocardial infarction is low, abnormalities can be acted upon quickly if found.

In patients with a negative history, physical examination, and ECG, further testing can be approached by stratifying patients into those with and without heart disease.

Patients with heart disease (e.g., coronary artery disease, congestive heart failure, valvular heart disease, obstructive cardiomyopathy, and ECG abnormalities such as bundle branch block) have a higher likelihood of arrhythmic syncope. In elderly patients without clinical heart disease and unexplained syncope, cardiac assessment with stress testing or echocardiogram may be needed to define the presence of occult heart disease. Prolonged electrocardiographic monitoring provides an initial step in the evaluation of patients with syncope and heart disease or when arrhythmias are suspected based on clinical presentation. If prolonged monitoring is nondiagnostic, these patients may be candidates for electrophysiologic studies. Because in the elderly, diseases may present in an atypical fashion or multiple abnormalities may be important in causing syncope, the clinical assessment should be particularly focused on these issues. If multiple abnormalities are found that could have led to loss of consciousness, a trial of empiric treatment of those factors is warranted before considering an invasive workup with electrophysiologic tests. Carotid sinus syncope is a disorder of the older individuals. Carotid sinus massage is recommended in all elderly patients.

The prognosis of patients with negative electrophysiologic studies is favorable. Upright tilt testing may define a potential etiology in these patients, but therapy is only recommended for patients with recurrent or disabling symptoms as the effectiveness of therapy has not been established, especially in patients with single or rare episodes. In the elderly patients without heart disease and with a normal electrocardiogram, the likelihood of arrhythmias is low. A large proportion of these patients may also have vasovagal syncope. If there is a clinical suspicion of arrhythmias, ambulatory monitoring or loop monitoring (when there is recurrent syncope) may help define an etiology. Because the yield of electrophysiologic studies is low in this group, these studies should generally be avoided in these patients.

Management Issues in the Elderly

Management issues include hospitalization decision, treatment selection, and patient instructions and education.

Hospital Admission

There are no studies evaluating the need for hospital admission in syncope. Table 64.4 lists reasons for admis-

TABLE 64.4. Reasons for hospital admission.

Admission for diagnostic evaluation:
  Structural heart disease
    Known coronary artery disease
    Congestive heart failure
    Valvular or congenital heart disease
    History of ventricular arrhythmias
    Physical findings of heart disease (e.g., findings of aortic stenosis)
  Symptoms suggestive of arrhythmias or ischemia
    Associated with palpitations
    Chest pain suggestive of coronary disease
    Exertional syncope
  Electrocardiographic abnormalities
    Ischemia
    Conduction system disease (e.g., bundle branch block, first-degree atrioventricular block)
    Unsustained ventricular or supraventricular tachycardia
    Prolonged QT
    Accessory pathway
    Right bundle branch block with ST elevation in V1–V3
    Pacemaker malfunction
  Neurologic disease
    New stroke or focal neurologic findings
Admission for treatments:
  Structural heart disease
    Acute myocardial infarction, pulmonary embolism, other cardiac diseases diagnosed as causing syncope
  Orthostatic hypotension
    Acute severe volume loss (e.g., dehydration, gastrointestinal bleeding)
    Moderate to severe chronic orthostatic hypotension
  Treatment of multiple coexisting abnormalities
  Discontinuation or dose modification of offending drug
    Drugs causing torsades de pointes and long QT
    Drug reaction such as anaphylaxis, orthostasis, bradyarrhythmias

sion. Generally patients are admitted if a rapid diagnostic evaluation is needed because of concerns about serious arrhythmias, sudden death, newly diagnosed serious cardiac disease (e.g., aortic stenosis, myocardial infarction), and new onset of seizure or stroke. Admission may also be needed for treatment when etiology is clear (e.g., management of dehydration). In the large group of patients with unexplained syncope after initial history, physical examination, and ECG, risk stratification for arrhythmias and sudden death should guide the admission decision.

Treatment Selection

Because the treatment largely depends on the cause of syncope, a discussion of the treatment of all the causes is beyond the scope of this review. General management issues and treatments of neurally mediated syncope that have recently received considerable attention are reviewed here.

Neurally Mediated Syncope

Because of potential side effects, treatment should be reserved for elderly patients with frequent or disabling symptoms. As psychiatric illnesses (especially depression and anxiety) probably lead to vasovagal reactions, screening for the psychiatric illnesses noted here should be performed. Treatment of the psychiatric illness often results in resolution of recurrent syncope.

Various drugs and pacemakers have been tried for patients with vasovagal syncope, and a decrease in recurrence of syncope or resolution of symptoms have been reported in almost every uncontrolled study. There are very few controlled studies of drug therapy for neurally mediated syncope. The drugs most commonly used are beta-blockers[28] (e.g., metoprolol 50–200mg/day, atenolol 25–200mg/day, propranolol 40–160mg/day), which may inhibit the activation of cardiac mechanoreceptors by decreasing cardiac contractility. Other drugs include anticholinergic drugs, such as transdermal scopolamine (one patch every 2–3 days), disopyramide (200–600mg/day), paroxetine (20–40mg/day),[29] or theophylline (6–12mg/kg/day), and measures to expand volume (increased salt intake, custom-fitted counterpressure support garments from ankle to waist, and fludrocortisone acetate at 0.1–1 mg per day). Dual-chamber atrioventricular pacing with rate drop response has been reported to decrease recurrence in patients with frequent recurrent neurally mediated syncope associated with bradycardia and can be considered when medications are ineffective.[30,31]

Orthostatic Hypotension

The initial approach to treatment of orthostatic hypotension is to ensure adequate salt and volume intake and to discontinue drugs that cause orthostatic hypotension. Patients with orthostatic hypotension should be advised to raise the head of the bed at night, to rise from bed or chair slowly, and to avoid prolonged standing. Compression stockings applied up to thigh level may help decrease venous pooling. Frequent small feedings may be helpful in patients with marked postprandial hypotension.

Pharmacologic agents of potential benefit include fludrocortisone (0.1–1 mg/day), in conjunction with increased salt intake. Various agents have been used including midodrine, ephedrine, and phenylephrine.

Patient Instruction and Education

Issues in patient education include instruction in prevention of syncope, nonpharmacologic treatment, and restriction of activities. Many patients with vasovagal syncope have precipitating factors or situations that should be identified and the patient instructed to avoid these situations. Common triggers include prolonged standing, venipuncture, large meals, and heat (such as hot baths or sunbathing). Additionally, fasting, lack of sleep, and alcohol intake may predispose to vasovagal syncope and should be avoided. Postexercise vasovagal syncope may occasionally be related to chronic inadequate salt and fluid replacement. Syncope may be prevented with the use of electrolyte-containing solutions and water in such instances. In other patients, exercise may have to be curtailed.

Although 84% of states in the United States have specific regulations for driving restriction for seizures, only 26 states (52%) have regulations that limit driving after an episode of loss of consciousness other than seizure[32] (e.g., vasovagal syncope, arrhythmias, diabetic coma). In nonseizure loss of consciousness, the average mandated duration of driving restriction is 4.3 months. In addition to adhering to state regulations on driving, the likelihood of recurrent episodes and the probability of treatment efficacy should be considered in restricting driving.[32]

References

1. Lipsitz LA. Altered blood pressure homeostasis in advanced age: clinical and research implications. *J Gerontol.* 1989;44(6):M179–M183.
2. Benditt DG, Remole S, Bailin S, et al. Tilt table testing for evaluation of neurally-mediated (cardioneurogenic) syncope: rationale and proposed protocols. *PACE.* 1991;14:1528–1537.
3. Abboud FM. Neurocardiogenic syncope. *N Engl J Med.* 1993;15:1117–1120.
4. Lipsitz LA, Wei JY, Rowe JW. Syncope in an elderly, institutionalized population: prevalence, incidence, and associated risk. *Q J Med.* 1985;55:45–55.

5. Vaitkevicius PV, Esserwein DM, Maynard AK, et al. Frequency and importance of postprandial blood pressure reduction in elderly nursing-home patients. *Ann Intern Med.* 1991;115:865–870.

6. Jansen RW, Lipsitz LA. Postprandial hypotension: epidemiology, pathophysiology, and clinical management. *Ann Intern Med.* 1995;122(4):286–295.

7. Davidson E, Rotenbeg Z, Fuchs J, et al. Transient ischemic attack-related syncope. *Clin Cardiol.* 1991;14:141–144.

8. Kapoor W. Evaluation and outcome of patients with syncope. *Medicine.* 1990;69:160–175.

9. Lempert T, Bauer M, Schmidt D. Syncope: a video metric analysis of 56 episodes of transient cerebral hypoxia. *Ann Neurol.* 1994;36:233–237.

10. Hoefnagels WAJ, Padberg GW, Overweg J, et al. Syncope or seizure? The diagnostic value of the EEG and hyperventilation test in transient loss of consciousness. *J Neurol.* 1991;54:953–956.

11. Martin TP, Hanusa BH, Kapoor WN. Risk stratification of patients with syncope. *Ann Emerg Med.* 1977;29(4):495–466.

12. Kapoor WN, Hanusa B. Is syncope a risk factor for poor outcomes? Comparison of patients with and without syncope. *Am J Med.* 1996;100(6):646–655.

13. Oh JH, Hanusa BH, Kapoor WN. Do symptoms predict cardiac arrhythmias and mortality in patients with syncope? *Arch Intern Med.* 1999;159(4):375–380.

14. Kapoor W, Snustad D, Peterson J, et al. Syncope in the elderly. *Am J Med.* 1986;80:419–428.

15. Linzer M, Yang EH, Estes NA, Wang P, Vorperian V, Kapoor WN. Diagnosing syncope. Part 1: Value of history, physical examination, and electrocardiography. The clinical efficacy assessment project of the American College of Physicians. *Ann Intern Med.* 1997;126:989–996.

16. Linzer M, Yang EH, Estes NA, Wang P, Vorperian V, Kapoor WN. Diagnosing syncope. Part 2: Unexplained syncope. The clinical efficacy assessment project of the American College of Physicians. *Ann Intern Med.* 1997;126:989–996.

17. DiMarco JP, Philbrick JT. Use of ambulatory electrocardiographic (Holter) monitoring. *Ann Intern Med.* 1990;113:53–68.

18. Bass EB, Curtiss EI, Arena VC, et al. The duration of Holter monitoring in patients with syncope: is 24 hours enough? *Arch Intern Med.* 1990;150:1073–1078.

19. Krahn AD, Klein GJ, Yee R. Use of extended monitoring strategy in patients with problematic syncope. *Circulation.* 1999;99(3):406–410.

20. Sugrue DD, Holmes DR, Gersh BJ, et al. Impact of intracardiac electrophysiologic testing on the management of elderly patients with recurrent or near syncope. *J Am Geriatr Soc.* 1987;35:1079–1083.

21. Bass EB, Elson JJ, Fogoros RN, et al. Long-term prognosis of patients undergoing electrophysiologic studies for syncope of unknown origin. *Am J Cardiol.* 1988;62:1186–1191.

22. Benditt DG, Ferguson DW, Grubb BP, et al. Tilt table testing for assessing syncope. *J Am Coll Cardiol.* 1996;28:263–275.

23. Grubb BP, Kosinski D. Current trends in the etiology, diagnosis and management of neurocardiogenic syncope. *Curr Opin Cardiol.* 1996;11:32–41.

24. Kapoor WN. Using a tilt table to evaluate syncope. *Am J Med Sci.* 1999;317(2):110–116.

25. Kapoor WN, Smith M, Miller NL. Upright tilt testing in evaluating syncope: a comprehensive literature review. *Am J Med.* 1994;97:78–88.

26. Raviele A, Menozzi C, Brignole M, et al. Value of head-up tilt testing potentiated with sublingual nitroglycerin to assess the origin of unexplained syncope. *Am J Cardiol.* 1995;76:267–272.

27. Raviele A, Giada F, Brignole M, et al. Diagnostic accuracy of sublingual nitroglycerin test and low-dose isoproterenol test in patients with unexplained syncope. A comparative study. *Am J Cardiol.* 2000;85:1194–1198.

28. Mahanonda N, Bhuripanyo K, Kangkagate C, et al. Randomized double-blind, placebo-controlled trial of oral atenolol in patients with unexplained syncope and positive upright tilt table test results. *Am Heart J.* 1995;130:1250–1253.

29. Di Girolamo E, Di Iorio C, Sabatini P, Leonzio L, Barbone C, Barsotti A. Effects of paroxetine hydrochloride, a selective serotonin reuptake inhibitor, on refractory vasovagal syncope: a randomized, double-blind, placebo-controlled study. *J Am Coll Cardiol.* 1999;33(5):1227–1230.

30. Connolly SJ, Sheldon R, Roberts RS, Gent M. The North American Vasovagal Pacemaker Study (VPS). A randomized trial of permanent cardiac pacing for the prevention of vasovagal syncope. *Am J Coll Cardiol.* 1999;33(1):21–23.

31. Sutton R, Brignole M, Menozzi C, et al. Dual-chamber pacing in treatment of neurally-mediated tilt-positive cardioinhibitory syncope. Pacemaker versus no therapy: a multicentre randomized study. *Circulation.* 2000;102:294–299.

32. Strickberger SA, Cantillon CO, Friedman PL. When should patients with lethal ventricular arrhythmia resume driving? An analysis of state regulations and physician practices. *Ann Intern Med.* 1991;115:560–563.

65
Management of Chronic Wounds

David R. Thomas

Sites of Care

Chronic wounds, including pressure ulcers, diabetic ulcers, and venous stasis ulcers, occur across the spectrum of care. In 1997, among 265 acute care hospitals the overall prevalence of pressure ulcers was 10.1% (range, 1.4%–36.4%), with the sacrum and heels the most common sites. Seventy-four percent of pressure ulcers were superficial (i.e., stages I and II).[1] A 1995 analysis of the Minimum Data Set data for 2011 nursing home residents aged 60 or older who lived in 270 facilities from 10 states found a prevalence of 11.2% for stage II through IV lesions and a 6-month incidence of 6.2%. Logistic regression analysis determined that dependence in transfer or mobility, being bedfast, having diabetes mellitus, and having had a pressure ulcer in the past were significantly associated with a stage II through IV pressure ulcer.[2] Among persons with diabetes, 15% develop a foot ulcer, and 14% to 24% of these will require amputation.[3] Venous stasis ulcers affect 0.2% to 1.3% of the adult population.[4]

Diagnosis and Differential Diagnosis

The differential diagnosis of chronic ulcers is imperative because the management of each wound type differs substantially. Pressure ulcers are the visible evidence of pathologic changes in dermal blood flow caused by pressure. The most common sites of occurrence are found on the sacrum, posterior heels, and trochanteric areas. Diabetic ulcers are often caused by recurrent pressure in neuropathic extremities and may be complicated by diminished blood flow in small and larger vessels. These ulcers frequently occur at sites on the foot subjected to pressure, especially over the plantar aspect of the foot and metatarsal heads. Diabetic ulcers often coexist with arterial ischemic ulcers due to macrovascular and microvascular complications of the diabetic state. Arterial ischemic ulcers usually occur in areas not necessarily subjected to pressure and result from decreased blood flow to that area.

Most often the diagnosis of ulcer type is made by wound location, wound appearance, and the presence of pain. Ischemic ulcers typically occur distally to the impaired blood supply and frequently are painful, particularly with leg elevation. Microemboli from infection or cholesterol plaques can cause the sudden onset of pain and discoloration in the distal extremity.[5,6] Venous stasis ulcers develop in the lower extremities as a result of incompetent valves in the veins. Edema may or may not be present, but hyperpigmentation changes are usually present when the condition is chronic. Typically, venous stasis ulcers occur on the lateral aspect of the calf. The sites of occurrence among these various wounds overlap, but careful history and physical examination usually establishes the correct etiology. Adequate tissue perfusion with blood is important for healing of all types of wounds, particularly on the extremities. Examination of pulses and an ankle–brachial blood pressure index can assess healing adequacy. An ankle–brachial index below 0.7 is abnormal, and an index below 0.4 is associated with a poor likelihood of healing.

Course of Illness

Chronic wounds fail to proceed through an orderly and timely process to produce anatomic or functional integrity.[7] Normally, fibroblasts and epithelial cells grow rapidly in skin tissue cultures, covering 80% of in vitro surfaces within the first 3 days. In contrast, biopsy specimens from pressure ulcers usually do not grow until much later, covering only 70% of surfaces by 14 days.[8] The lack of hemorrhage in chronic wounds interferes with bringing wound-healing factors into contact with tissue. Platelet release and fibrinolytic activity are diminished.

Finally, these wounds contain complex polymicrobial colonizations that are poorly understood.[9]

The result is slow healing. Eight weeks were required to heal 75% of stage II pressure ulcers while only 17% of stage III or IV pressure ulcers healed in that time.[10] In a similar study, 23% of stage II pressure ulcers and 48% of stage IV pressure ulcers remained unhealed at 1 year. At 2 years, 8% of stage II pressure ulcers, 29% of stage III, and 38% of stage IV remained unhealed.[11] An estimated 76% of diabetic wounds remain unhealed at 12 weeks of follow-up and 69% remain unhealed at 20 weeks.[12] Thus, treatment of these chronic wounds extends over months to years.

Pressure ulcers have been associated with more than a fourfold increase in mortality rates in both acute and long-term care settings. Death has been reported to occur during acute hospitalization in 67% of patients who develop a pressure ulcer compared to 15% of at-risk patients without pressure ulcers.[13] Patients who develop a new pressure ulcer within 6 weeks after hospitalization are three times as likely to die as patients not developing a pressure ulcer.[14] In long-term care settings, development of a pressure ulcer within 3 months among newly admitted patients was associated with a 92% mortality rate, compared to a mortality rate of 4% among residents who did not subsequently develop a pressure ulcer.[15] Residents in a skilled nursing facility who had pressure ulcers experienced a 6-month mortality rate of 77.3% whereas patients without pressure ulcers had a mortality rate of 18.3%.[11] Interestingly, patients whose pressure ulcers healed within 6 months had a significantly lower mortality rate (11% versus 64%) than patients whose pressure ulcers did not heal.[16]

Despite this association with death rates, it is not clear if pressure ulcers contribute to increased mortality or are mainly a marker for increased frailty. The severity of the pressure ulcer has not correlated with an increased mortality risk. Patients with stage II pressure ulcers have been equally as likely to die as patients with stage IV pressure ulcers.[14] In the absence of complications, it is difficult to imagine how stage I or II pressure ulcers contribute to death. Evidence suggesting that the association with mortality may result from their occurrence in otherwise frail, sick patients comes from a prospective study of residents of 51 nursing homes, where pressure ulcers were associated with an increased rate of mortality but not with the rate of acute hospitalization.[14] Additionally, a correction for the presence and severity of coexistent conditions can eliminate the association of pressure ulcers with death. In a prospective study of high-risk patients in an acute hospital setting, the development of a new pressure ulcer predicted death within 1 year. Independent risk factors for mortality in this study included weight loss reported in the 6 months before admission relative risk (RR 2.4), the admitting physician's estimate of life expectancy of less than 5 years (RR 2.1), and the Co-morbidity Damage Index score (RR 1.1). When adjusted for measures of disease severity, comorbidity, and a history of weight loss, the development of a pressure ulcer was no longer a predictor of mortality at 1 year.[17]

The incidence of bacteremia from pressure ulcers is about 1.7 per 10,000 hospital discharges.[18] However, sepsis is a serious complication of pressure ulcers and a frequent cause of death. In a study of 21 patients with sepsis syndrome attributed to pressure ulcers, 76% had bacteremia that originated from the pressure ulcer. Overall, mortality was 48% and all patients over age 60 died despite empiric antibiotic treatment. In 5 patients, bacteremia persisted despite antibiotic treatment and resolved only after local debridement.[19] The bacteremia occurring with pressure ulcers is likely to be polymicrobial.[18]

Osteomyelitis is a frequent complication of pressure ulcers and diabetic ulcers, reported in 38% of patients who have infected pressure ulcers[20] and in 59 of 96 (61%) of foot infections in diabetic patients.[21] Diagnosis of contiguous osteomyelitis in pressure ulcers is difficult. Plain radiographs are unable to differentiate true osteomyelitis from pressure changes to bone.[22] Radionuclide studies, including technetium-99m and gallium-67, are sensitive but have a false-positive rate of 41%.[20] Computed tomography may be more useful, with a specificity of 90%, although the sensitivity is only 10%.[23] A needle biopsy of bone is the most useful single test, with a sensitivity of 73% and a specificity of 96%,[24] and should be used whenever osteomyelitis must be excluded.

Infection occurs in up to 25% of diabetic foot ulcers.[25,26] Similar problems with the diagnosis of osteomyelitis occur in diabetic ulcers. Gentle probing of the wound with a steel probe to detect palpable bone demonstrated a 66% sensitivity and specificity of 89% with a positive predictive value of 89% and negative predictive value of 56%. Thus, a positive probe test was accurate in detecting osteomyelitis, but a negative probe does not exclude osteomyelitis.[27]

An estimated 8000 foot amputations are performed annually on patients with diabetes in the United States.[28] More than 70% of these amputations are due to complicated foot ulcers.[29] The higher risk factors for lower extremity amputation include a transcutaneous oxygen of 50 mmHg or less, insensitivity to monofilament testing, and a lower extremity ulcer.[30] Peripheral vascular disease is the major cause of morbidity associated with diabetic foot ulcers in older patients. Peripheral vascular disease and peripheral neuropathy, occurring in 11% and 42% of diabetic patients respectively,[31] may further predispose patients with diabetes to develop foot ulcers. The presence of peripheral vascular disease results in delaying ulcer healing and has been shown to associate significantly with the incidence of amputation.[32]

Treatment and Management

Pain Management

A primary goal of wound assessment should be to relieve pain. Except in neurologically impaired patients, chronic ulcers may be painful. Relief of pressure results in pain relief. Unfortunately, persons who develop pressure ulcers often are unable to report pain due to cognitive deficits and persons with diabetic neuropathy often cannot feel pain due to neuropathies. A decrease in wound pain with occlusive dressings has been noted in donor sites and venous stasis ulcers,[33,34] but studies in pressure ulcers have been limited. Analgesics should be used when pain assessment reveals discomfort. Principles of pain therapy are discussed in Chapter 28 and elsewhere[35] and should be incorporated into management of chronic wounds.

Nutrition

One of the most important reversible host factors contributing to wound healing is nutritional status. Several studies suggest that dietary intake, especially of protein, is important in healing pressure ulcers. Greater healing of pressure ulcers has been reported with a higher protein intake irrespective of positive nitrogen balance.[36] Breslow et al. evaluated 48 patients with stage II through IV pressure ulcers in a dietary intervention trial. Malnutrition was defined as a serum albumin below 3.5 mg/dL or body weight more than 10% below the midpoint of the age-specific weight range. The results suggested that patients fed a 24% protein diet healed their pressure ulcers at a greater rate than those fed a 14% protein standard diet. However, changes in body weight or in biochemical parameters of nutritional status did not occur between groups. The study was limited by a small sample size (only 28 patients completed the study), nonrandom assignment to treatment groups, confounding effects of air-fluidized beds, and the use of two different feeding routes.[37] Chernoff et al. randomized 12 enterally fed patients to formulas containing 17% versus 25% of calories as protein. The group that received 1.8 g/kg of protein had a 73% improvement in pressure ulcer surface area compared to a 42% improvement in surface area in the group receiving 1.2 g/kg of protein, despite the fact that the group that received the higher protein level began the study with larger surface area pressure ulcers (22.6 cm^2 versus 9.1 cm^2). Serum albumin did not appear to be a predictor of the development of pressure ulcers or their healing rate, although values were not given.[36]

An optimum dietary protein intake in patients with pressure ulcers is unknown, but may be much higher than current adult recommendations of 0.8 g/kg/day. Half of chronically ill elderly persons are unable to maintain nitrogen balance at this level.[38] Increasing protein intake beyond 1.5 g/kg/day may not increase protein synthesis and may cause dehydration.[39] A reasonable protein requirement is therefore between 1.2 and 1.5 g/kg/day.

The deficiency of several vitamins and minerals has significant effects on wound healing. However, supplementation to accelerate wound healing is controversial. High doses of vitamin C have not been shown to accelerate wound healing.[40] In a 12-week study of 88 patients who received either 10 or 500 mg of ascorbic acid twice daily, the healing rate and the healing velocity of their pressure ulcers were not different in the higher-dose group.[41] No evidence of benefit from topical or oral zinc sulfate in patients with chronic leg ulcers has been shown. Oral zinc sulfate may be beneficial in the treatment of patients with leg ulcers who have a low serum zinc level, but evidence of benefit is lacking in patients who are not zinc deficient.[42,43] High serum zinc levels interfere with healing, and supplementation above 150 mg/day may interfere with copper metabolism.[44,45]

Nutritional therapy in diabetic ulcers is aimed at control of hyperglycemia and hyperlipidemia. The risk for a lower extremity amputation increases 25% with each 1% rise in glycolsylated hemoglobin above normal.[46] Whether tight diabetic control can reduce this risk is not known. Proper glycemic control is also essential for ulcer healing.[47] Hyperglycemia interferes with immune function.[48,49] Glucose levels greater than 216 mg/dl are associated with a lower phagocytosis index of leukocytes.[50] Correction of hyperglycemia has been shown to normalize leukocyte function.

Local wound treatment is directed to providing an optimum wound environment and improving host factors.

Dressings

Moist wound healing allows experimentally induced wounds to resurface up to 40% faster than air-exposed wounds.[51–53] The concept of a moist wound environment led to development of occlusive dressings. The term "occlusive" describes the lessened ability of a dressing to transmit moisture vapor from a wound to the external atmosphere. The degree to which dressings dry the wound can be measured by the moisture vapor transmission rate (MVTR). An MVTR of less than 35 g of water vapor per square meter per hour is required to maintain a moist wound environment. Woven gauze has an MVTR of 68 g/m^2/h and impregnated gauze has an MVTR of 57 g/m^2/h. In comparison, hydrocolloid dressings have an MVTR of 8 g/m^2/h.[54] In chronic wounds, occlusion has been shown to reduce wound pain,[55,56] enhance autolytic debridement,[57,58] and prevent bacterial contamination.[59,60]

TABLE 65.1. Agents that promote epidermal resurfacing.

Dressing	Relative rate of healing (%)
DuoDerm	+36
Blisterfilm	+33
Benzoyl peroxide (20%)	+33
Bacitracin zinc	+30
Silvadene	+28
Neosporin	+28
Polysporin	+25
J&J First Aid Cream	+20
Bioclusive	+20
Op-Site	+18

Source: Alvarez O. Moist environment: matching the dressing to the wound. *Ostomy/Wound Manage*. 1988;12:64–83,[68] with permission.

Wound exudate in chronic ulcers has been found to be an excellent medium for fibroblast stimulation.[61] Removal of this medium by aggressive scrubbing or drying has been shown to be detrimental. Wound fluid is thought to contain a variety of growth factors such as interleukin-1, epidermal growth factor, and platelet-derived growth factor-beta, which may enhance healing.[62] A moist environment may maintain a normal electrical voltage gradient across the wound necessary for epithelial migration.[63] Wound fluid under occlusive dressings may also increase bacterial overgrowth, stimulating epidermal migration.[50]

Because of the appreciation of the importance of wound fluid, dressings that preserve this environment have become important. Any therapy that dehydrates the wound, such as dry gauze, heat lamps, air exposure, or liquid antacids, is detrimental to chronic wound healing.[64–67] Several types of topical wound treatments can promote more rapid epidermal resurfacing. Results of controlled trials for several agents are shown in Table 65.1.[68] The range of acceleration in healing varies from 18% to 36%. Note that most of these agents, or their vehicles, are occlusive. Whether the benefit is independent of the occlusive vehicle is not known. Certain antiseptic agents are cytotoxic to human fibroblasts, including povidone iodine (Betadine), Hibicles, pHisohex, benzalkonium chloride, and Granulex.[69–72] In animal models, povidone-iodine 1%, acetic acid 3%, and sodium hypochlorite 0.5% adversely affected wound healing.[73] In human pressure ulcers, Dakins solution 0.05% was clearly inferior to a hydrocolloid dressing[60] (Table 65.2).

Hydrocolloid dressings under a compression system have been shown to heal 62% to 82% of venous stasis ulcers at 12 weeks[74,75] and to be superior to an Unna's boot alone.[76] Topical cadexomer iodine produced a mean reduction in venous ulcer size of 62% versus 41% and 24% for hydrocolloid and paraffin gauze (ns).[77] Use of pentoxifylline and compression produces a 30% increase in complete healing compared to compression alone.[78]

Occlusive dressings can be divided into broad categories of polymer films, polymer foams, hydrogels, hydrocolloids, alginates, and biomembranes. Each has several advantages and disadvantages; no single agent is perfect. The choice of a particular agent depends on the clinical circumstances. The available agents differ in their properties of permeability to water vapor and wound protection. Understanding these differences is the key to planning for wound management in a particular patient.

Comparative qualities among available agents are shown in Table 65.3.[79,80] All the occlusive dressings offer pain relief. Only absorbing granules or polymers fail to reduce pain. Polymer films are impermeable to liquid but permeable to both gas and moisture vapor. Because of low permeability to water vapor, these dressings are not dehydrating to the wound. Nonpermeable polymers such as polyvinylidine and polyethylene can be macerating to normal skin. Polymer films are not absorptive and may leak, particularly when the wound is highly exudative. Most films have an adhesive backing that may remove epithelial cells when the dressing is changed. Polymer films do not eliminate deadspace and do not absorb exudate.

Hydrogels are three-layer hydrophilic polymers that are insoluble in water but absorb aqueous solutions. They are poor bacterial barriers and are nonadherent to the wound. Because of their high specific heat, these dressings are cooling to the skin, aiding in pain control and reducing inflammation. Most of these dressings require a secondary dressing to secure them to the wound.

Hydrocolloid dressings are complex dressings similar to ostomy barrier products. They are impermeable to moisture vapor and gases and are highly adherent to the skin. Their adhesiveness to surrounding skin is higher than that of some surgical tapes, but they are nonadherent to wound tissue and do not damage epithelialization of the wound. The adhesive barrier is frequently overcome in highly exudative wounds. Hydrocolloid dressings

TABLE 65.2. Agents that delay epidermal resurfacing.

Dressing	Relative rate of healing (%)
Neomycin sulfate	−5
Dakins Solution (1%)	−6
Hebiclens	−7
Hydrogen peroxide (3%)	−8
Povidone iodine solution	−10
Wet to dry gauze	−15
Liquid detergent	−28
Furacin	−30
Triamcinalone acetonide (0.1%)	−34

Source: Alvarez O. Moist environment: matching the dressing to the wound. *Ostomy/Wound Manage*. 1988;12:64–83,[68] with permission.

TABLE 65.3. Comparison of occlusive wound dressings.

	Moist saline gauze	Polymer films	Polymer foams	Hydrogels	Hydro-colloids	Alginate granules	Biomembranes
Pain relief	+	+	+	+	+	±	+
Maceration of surrounding skin	±	±	−	−	−	−	−
O_2 permeable	+	+	+	+	−	+	+
H_2O permeable	+	+	+	+	−	+	+
Absorbent	+	−	+	+	±	+	−
Damage to epithelial cells	±	+	−	−	−	−	−
Transparent	−	+	−	−	−	−	−
Resistant to bacteria	−	−	−	−	+	−	+
Ease of application	+	−	+	+	+	+	−

Source: Adapted from Helfman T, Ovington L, Falanga V. Occlusive dressings and wound healing. *Clin Dermatol.* 1994;12:121–127.[79] Witkowski JA, Parish LC. Cutaneous ulcer therapy. *Int J Dermatol.* 1986;25:420–426,[80] with permission.

cannot be used over tendons or on wounds with eschar formation. Several of these dressings include a foam padding layer that may reduce pressure to the wound.

Alginates are complex polysaccharide dressings that are highly absorbent in exudative wounds. This high absorbency is particularly suited to exudative wounds. Alginates are nonadherent to the wound, but if the wound is allowed to dry, damage to the epithelial tissue may occur with removal.

Only the hydrocolloid and biomembranes offer bacterial resistance. The biomembranes are very expensive and not readily available. Hydrocolloid dressings theoretically have a disadvantage because of impermeability to oxygen. These dressings could be problematic in wounds contaminated by anaerobes, but this effect has not been demonstrated clinically.

The agents differ in the ease of application. This difference is important in pressure ulcers in unusual locations, or when considering for home care. Dressings should be left in place until wound fluid is leaking from the sides, a period ranging from days to 3 weeks.

Saline-soaked gauze that is not allowed to dry is an effective wound dressing. When moist saline gauze has been compared to occlusive-type dressings, healing of pressure ulcers has been similar with both dressings.[81–83] The use of occlusive-type dressings has been shown to be more cost-effective than traditional dressings, primarily due to decrease in nursing time required for dressing changes.[82,83]

The optimal dressing choice for diabetic wounds remains controversial.[86] No differences in healing were seen comparing cadexomer iodine, vaseline gauze, gentamicin solution, or streptodornase/stretokinase treatments in 25 diabetic patients over a 12-week period.[87] Moist saline gauze remains the standard dressing for diabetic ulcers. Use of cultured human dermis tissue weekly for 8 weeks demonstrated a higher healed rate compared to standard treatment (50% versus 8%).[88]

Partial-thickness skin grafts for venous stasis ulcers have resulted in healing rates of 52% to 70%, with recurrence rates of 22% to 30%.[89,90] Bioengineered skin tissue grafting resulted in healing of 61% of venous ulcers compared to 44% of control ulcers.[91] Complete wound healing occurred by 12 weeks in 60% of diabetic wounds treated with a culture human dermis compared to 8% of controls.[88]

Debridement

Necrotic debris increases the possibility of bacterial infection and delays wound healing.[92] The preferred method of debriding the pressure ulcers remains controversial. Options include mechanical debridement with gauze dressings, sharp surgical debridement, autolytic debridement with occlusive dressings, or application of exogenous enzymes. Surgical sharp debridement produces the most rapid removal of necrotic debris and is indicated in the presence of clinical wound infection. Mechanical debridement can be easily accomplished by letting the saline gauze dressing dry before removal. Remoistening of gauze dressings in an attempt to reduce pain can defeat the debridement effect. Aggressive surgical or mechanical debridement can damage healthy tissue or fail to completely clean the wound.

Thin portions of eschar can be removed by occlusion under a semipermeable dressing. Both autolytic and enzymatic debridement requires periods of several days to several weeks to achieve results. Enzymatic debridement can dissolve necrotic debris, but whether it harms healthy tissue is debated. Penetration of enzymatic agents is limited in eschar and requires either softening by autolysis or cross-hatching by sharp incision before application.

Enzymatic debridement evaluated in pressure ulcer trials include streptokinase/streptodornase (SK/SD)\ combination, collagenase, trypsin, and papain. Debridement with SK/SD combination was equivalent to zinc oxide/gauze at 8 weeks,[93] and worse than dextranomer granules at 7 days.[94] Collagenase reduced necrosis, pus, and odor, compared to inactivated control ointment,[95] and produced debridement in 82% of pressure ulcers at 4 weeks compared to petrolatum.[96] Papain produced measurable debridement in 4 days compared to the control vehicle ointment.[97] Trypsin in balsam of Peru and castor oil was not better than mechanical gauze debridement.[98] Three enzyme preparations are currently marketed in the United States for debridement: collagenase, papain/urea, and a papain/urea–chlorophyll combination. A trial in 21 patients with pressure ulcers found a greater reduction in necrotic tissue using papain/urea (95.4%) compared to collagenase (35.8%) at 4 weeks, but the rate of complete healing was not different between groups.[99]

Diabetic ulcers require extensive debridement to remove callous formation and nonviable tissue. Removal of necrotic debris has been reported to be the chief factor associated with healing in diabetic ulcers.[100] Frequent sharp debridement has been shown to heal diabetic neuropathic wounds more rapidly.

Growth Factors

Acute wound healing proceeds in a carefully regulated fashion that is reproducible from wound to wound. A number of growth factors have been demonstrated to mediate the healing process. The factors described include transforming growth factor-alpha and -beta, epidermal growth factor, platelet-derived growth factor, fibroblast growth factor, interleukin-1 and -2, and tumor necrosis factor-alpha. Accelerating healing in chronic wounds by using these acute wound factors is attractive. The development of wound healing factors is still in infancy but shows great promise. Several of these factors have been favorable in animal models; however, they have not been as successful in human trials.

In pressure ulcers, recombinant human platelet-derived growth factor (rhPDGF-BB) failed to improve the rate of complete healing,[101] although a 15% difference in percentage of initial volume of ulcers was shown with PDGF-BB in another study.[102] Another report showed that more subjects had greater than 70% wound closure with basic fibroblast growth factor at 100 μg/mL ($p = 0.05$).[103]

The topical use of rhPDGF-BB has been shown to accelerate wound healing in diabetic ulcers. In ulcers present for at least 8 weeks, the addition of 30 μg rhPDGF-BB to moist saline dressings resulted in complete closure of 48% of ulcers compared to 25% of ulcers treated with placebo gel. However, in another trial, 10 μg rhPDGF-BB was superior to 30 μg and placebo (complete closure 50% versus 36% versus 35%, respectively). Using 10 μg rhPDGF-BB, placebo gel, and moist saline gauze alone, the rate of complete closure at 20 weeks was 44% versus 36% versus 22%, respectively. Finally, in another trial of 10 μg rhPDGF-BB compared to moist saline alone, there was no difference in rate of closure at 20 weeks (36% versus 32%; $n = 250$).[104]

A small study of basic fibroblast growth factor (bFGF) in diabetic neurotrophic foot ulcers showed 63% of ulcers completely healed at 12 weeks in the placebo group compared to 33% using bFGF,[105] suggesting a detrimental effect on healing.

Infection

Quantitative microbiology alone is a poor predictor of clinical infection in chronic wounds.[106] Although normal skin flora in numbers greater than 10^5 organisms/mL produce local disease in intact skin[107] and skin grafts and flaps show poor healing when greater than 10^5 organisms of certain species of bacteria are present,[108] chronic wounds do not appear to follow these rules. Greater than 10^5 organisms may persist for months or years in chronic wounds without apparent clinical effect. Colonization with bacteria is common and unavoidable. All chronic wounds become colonized, initially with skin organisms, followed in 48 h by gram-negative bacteria.

The diagnosis of infection in chronic wounds must be based on clinical signs—erythema, edema, odor, fever, or purulent exudate. A foul odor is a particularly important clinical sign, usually signifying anaerobic organisms.[84] However, wounds with a reported foul odor are not always infected. When there is evidence of clinical infection, topical or systemic antimicrobials or antibiotics are required. Reduction of colony-forming units (CFUs) has been used as the endpoint in evaluating antimicrobial efficacy in acute wounds. Several antimicrobial or antibiotic agents reduce CFUs without damaging the wound, including silver sulfadiazine 1% cream, combination antibiotic ointments, and propylene glycol.[85] Topical gentamicin and silver sulfadiazine have been shown to improve clinical appearance of infected wounds and may improve healing.[109,110] Iodine and thimerosal have been noted to increase pain and delay healing.[111] Infections with anaerobes may respond to topical metronidazole.[112] Systemic antibiotics are indicated when the clinical condition suggests spread of the infection to bone or to the bloodstream.

In worsening pressure ulcers, *Pseudomonas aeruginosa* and *Providencia* species were found in 88% and 34% of ulcers, compared to 0% of stationary wounds and 7% of rapidly healing ulcers. Peptococci, *Bacteroides* species, or *Clostridia* were found in more than half of worsening or stationary ulcers but were absent in healing pressure ulcers. Staphylococci and enterococci were frequently isolated from rapidly healing ulcers.[113,114] Based on these findings, *Pseudomonas aeruginosa* and *Providencia* species should not be regarded as simple colonization.

Similar principles apply to diabetic ulcers. Systemic antimicrobial therapy is clearly indicated in the presence of systemic signs of infection or underlying osteomyelitis. Mild to moderate infections without systemic signs may respond to oral agents.[115] Topical antiseptics may have a role in this setting.

Despite an increase in numbers of bacteria, occlusive dressings used to treat chronic wounds very rarely cause a clinical infection. Hutchinson and McGuckin reviewed 36 studies comparing infection rates under occlusive dressings to gauze or impregnated gauze. Infection rates were 2.6% for occlusive dressings and 7.1% for nonocclusive gauze.[116]

Pressure-Relieving Devices

Pressure-relieving devices have a therapeutic role in treating pressure ulcers. This therapy is successful in the acute hospital and in some nursing home studies but is very expensive. When patients with pressure ulcers in an acute hospital setting were randomized to air-fluidized therapy or a vinyl alternating air mattress, patients treated on air-fluidized beds had a decrease in ulcer size over a mean of 15 days. However, there was no difference in the number of ulcers showing a size reduction of at least 50%. The cost was estimated at an additional $80 per day.[117]

In 95 nursing home patients with severe pressure ulcers treated on air-fluidized beds, 14% of pressure ulcers healed in a mean of 79 days; 44% of patients had greater than 50% reduction in surface area of the index ulcer. Very few patients had a reduction in ulcer surface area after 1 month of treatment on the specialized bed. The median length of time to healing was 119 days and of time to improvement was 127 days. The additional cost for the bed was $50 to $100 per day.[118] Low-air-loss beds have produced substantial improvement in ulcer size (9.0 versus 2.5 mm^2 per day) compared to a 10-cm convoluted foam mattress in nursing home patients.[10]

Repetitive mechanical trauma is the most common cause of foot ulcers in diabetic individuals.[119] Mechanical trauma resulting in foot ulceration may be the result of abnormal foot mechanics, abnormal foot structure, or ill-fitting shoes or socks.[120] Chronic sensorimotor neuropathy may contribute to the development of foot deformity that results from the denervation of foot muscles.[121] Accompanying autonomic neuropathy may also result in dry skin as well as cutaneous arteriovenous shunting that further predisposes the skin to damage.[122]

In the presence of diabetic sensory neuropathy, trauma to soft tissue from foot deformity (e.g., hammertoes, or bunions) or ill-fitting footwear may remain undetected and result in foot ulceration. Removal of recurrent pressure, particularly in the presence of bony deformity, is critical to prevent recurrence.[123] When therapeutic shoes were prescribed, the recurrence rate has been reduced to 17% compared to an 83% recurrence rate in regular shoes.[124]

Although pressure relief is required for pressure ulcers and diabetic ulcers, the critical component of healing of venous stasis ulcers is compression therapy.[125] Compression can be achieved with a rigid boot or external multi-layered elastic compression.[126]

Surgical Management

Pressure Ulcers

Nowhere does the difference in pressure ulcers among younger spinal cord injury patients and elderly patients become so pronounced as in discussing surgical management. Surgical closure of pressure ulcers results in a more rapid resolution of the wound. The chief problems are the frequent recurrence of ulcers and the inability of the frail patient to tolerate the procedure.

The efficacy of surgical repair of pressure ulcers is high in the short term. The efficacy for long-term management has been questioned, even in younger patients.[127] In a series of 40 patients selected for surgical closure of pressure ulcers, patients were divided into three subgroups. In nontraumatic, nonparaplegic elderly patients with a mean age of 73, 84% of surgically treated pressure ulcers were healed at discharge. Twelve percent of surgically treated patients had another pressure ulcer at discharge. Within 7.7 months, 40% of surgically treated pressure ulcers recurred and 69% of the patients had a pressure ulcer at a different site. In patients with traumatic paraplegia, 74% of operated pressure ulcers were healed at discharge and 76% of patients were free of pressure ulcers. Within 10.9 months, 79% of operated ulcers recurred, and 79% of patients had additional pressure ulcers. Only 21% of traumatic paraplegics and 31% of nontraumatic nonparaplegic elderly patients remained healed after muscle-flap coverage for pressure ulcers.[128] After 10 years of follow-up in 16 surgically treated patients, only 1 patient remained alive and free of pressure ulcers.[129]

A decision analysis demonstrated that myocutaneous flap procedures for stage III pressure ulcers was favorable unless the success rate for surgery was less than 30% or the healing rate with medical therapy was less than 40%. The added cost for the procedure was estimated at $17,000 per treatment episode compared to medical therapy.[130]

Diabetic Ulcers

Indications for revascularization in diabetic ischemic ulcers include rest pain, impending gangrene, and failure to progress toward healing. An ankle–brachial pressure index (determined by dividing the systolic pressure in the foot arteries by that of the brachial artery) value greater than 0.45 has been shown to predict healing in diabetic foot ulcers (10).[131] Distal arterial reconstruction can result in lower rates of amputation in diabetic patients.[132]

Venous Stasis Ulcers

Surgical graft techniques have been used for venous stasis ulcers. In 51 venous ulcers in older patients who had not responded to conservative treatment, split skin grafts resulted in an 88% healing rate after a mean of 15 days. However, 49% of the healed venous ulcers recurred after a mean of 4 months. After a mean of 4 years, 18 of the patients were dead and 10 had had the leg in question amputated. Of the 34 patients still alive who had not had amputations, 7 patients had open leg ulcers. The mean cost for treating one leg ulcer by skin grafting was estimated at $11,125.[133] Pinch grafting demonstrated a healing rate after 12 weeks for venous ulcers of 45%.[134]

Summary

Chronic wounds represent complex clinical problems for which no gold standard for prevention or treatment has yet been established. In practice guidelines for the treatment of pressure ulcers published by the Agency for Health Care Policy and Research, approximately 85 specific recommendations were made based on a careful literature review.[135] Only four level A recommendations and 10 level B recommendations were made. The remaining recommendations were made using expert opinion. In those areas where supporting data are insufficient, local and national consensus determines management.

References

1. Barczak CA, Barnett RI, Childs EJ, Bosley LM. Fourth national pressure ulcer prevalence survey. *Adv Wound Care.* 1997;10(4):18–26.
2. Brandeis GH, Berlowitz DR, Hossain M, Morris JN. Pressure ulcers: the Minimum Data Set and the Resident Assessment Protocol. *Adv Wound Care.* 1995;8(6):18–25.
3. Consensus Development Conference of Diabetic Foot Wound Care. *Diabetes Care.* 1999;22:1354–1360.
4. Lyon RT, Veith FJ, Bolton L, Machado F. Clinical benchmark for healing of chronic venous ulcers. *Am J Surg.* 1998;176:172–175.
5. Coffman JD. Atheromatous embolism. *Vasc Med.* 1996;1:267–273.
6. O'Keefe ST, Woods BB, Reslin DJ. Blue toe syndrome: causes and management. *Arch Intern Med.* 1992;152:2197–2202.
7. Lazarus GS, Cooper DM, Knighton DR, et al. Definitions and guidelines for assessment of wounds and evaluation of healing. *Arch Dermatol.* 1994;130:489–493.
8. Seiler WO, Stahelin HB, Zolliker R, et al. Impaired migration of epidermal cells from decubitus ulcers in cell culture: a cause of protracted wound healing? *Am J Clin Pathol.* 1989;92:430–434.
9. Baxter CR. Immunologic reactions in chronic wounds. *Am J Surg.* 1994;167:12S–14S.
10. Ferrell BA, Osterweil D, Christenson P. A randomized trial of low-air-loss beds for treatment of pressure ulcers. *JAMA.* 1993;269:494–497.
11. Brandeis GH, Morris SN, Nash DJ, et al. The epidemiology and natural history of pressure ulcers in elderly nursing home residents. *JAMA.* 1990;264:2905–2909.
12. Margolis DJ, Kantor J, Berlin JA. Healing of diabetic neuropathic foot ulcers receiving standard treatment. *Diabetes Care.* 1999;22:692–695.
13. Allman RM, Laprade CA, Noel LB, et al. Pressure sores among hospitalized patients. *Ann Intern Med.* 1986;105:337–342.
14. Berlowitz DR, Wilking SVB. The short-term outcome of pressure sores. *J Am Geriatr Soc.* 1990;38:748–752.
15. Bergstrom N, Braden B. A prospective study of pressure sore risk among institutionalized elderly. *J Am Geriatr Soc.* 1992;40:747–758.
16. Reed JW. Pressure ulcers in the elderly: prevention and treatment utilizing the team approach. *Md State Med J.* 1981;30:45–50.
17. Thomas DR, Goode PS, Tarquin PH, et al. Pressure ulcers and risk of death. *J Am Geriatr Soc.* 1996;44:1435–1440.
18. Byran CS, Dew CE, Reynolds KL. Bacteremia associated with decubitus ulcers. *Arch Intern Med.* 1983;143:2093–2095.
19. Galpin JE, Chow AW, Bayer AS. Sepsis associated with decubitus ulcers. *Am J Med.* 1976;61:346.
20. Sugarman B, Hawes S, Musher DM, et al. Osteomyelitis beneath pressure sores. *Arch Intern Med.* 1983;143:683–688.
21. Grayson MI, Gibbons GW, Habershaw GM, et al. Use of ampicillin/sulbactam versus imipenem/cilastine in the treatment of limb-threatening foot infections in diabetic patients. *Chin Infect Dis.* 1994;18:683–693.
22. Thornhill-Joyness M, Gonzales G, Stewart CA, et al. Osteomyelitis associated with pressure ulcers. *Arch Phys Med Rehabil.* 1986;67:314–318.
23. Firooznia H, Rafii M, Golimbu C, et al. Computed tomography of pressure ulcers, pelvic abscess, and osteomyelitis in patients with spinal cord injury. *Arch Phys Med Rehabil.* 1982;63:545–548.
24. Lewis VL, Bailey MH, Pulawski G, et al. The diagnosis of osteomyelitis in patients with pressure sores. *Plast Reconstr Surg.* 1988;81:229–323.
25. Lipsky BA, Pecoraro RE, Wheat IJ. The diabetic foot: soft tissue and bone infection. *Infect Dis Chin North Am.* 1990;4:409–432.

26. Most RS, Sinnock P. The epidemiology of lower extremity amputation in diabetic individuals. *Diabetes Care.* 1983;6: 87–91.

27. Grayson MI, Lindsay M, Gibbons GW, et al. Probing to bone in infected pedal ulcers: a clinical sign of underlying osteomyelitis in diabetic patients. *JAMA.* 1995;27:721–723.

28. Landsman A, Sage R. Off-loading neuropathic wounds associated with diabetes using an ankle-foot orthosis. *J Am Podiatr Med Assoc.* 1997;87:349–357.

29. Reiber GE. The epidemiology of diabetic foot problems. *Diabet Med.* 1996;13:S6–S11.

30. Adler AI, Boyko EJ, Ahroni JH, et al. Lower-extremity amputation in diabetes. The independent effects of peripheral vascular disease, sensory neuropathy, and foot ulcers. *Diabetes Care.* 1999;22:1029–1035.

31. Kumar S, Ashe HA, Parnell LN, et al. The prevalence of foot ulceration and its correlates in type 2 diabetic patients: a population-based study. *Diabet Med.* 1994; 11(5):480–484.

32. Weiman TJ, Griffiths GD, Polk HC Jr. Management of diabetic midfoot ulcers. *Ann Surg.* 1992;215(6):627–630.

33. Handfield-Jones SE, Grattan CEH, Simpson RA, et al. Comparison of hydrocolloid dressing and paraffin gauze in the treatment of venous ulcers. *Br J Dermatol.* 1988;118: 425–427.

34. Nemeth AJ, Eaglstein WH, Taylor JR, et al. Faster healing and less pain in skin biopsy sites treated with an occlusive dressing. *Arch Dermatol.* 1991;127:1679–1683.

35. Acute Pain Management Guideline Panel. *Clinical Practice Guideline.* AHCPR pub 92-0032. Rockville, MD: Agency for Health Care Policy and Research, Public Health Service, U.S. Department of Health and Home Services; 1992.

36. Chernoff RS, Milton KY, Lipschitz DA. The effect of very high-protein liquid formula (Replete) on decubitus ulcer healing in long-term tube-fed institutionalized patients. Investigators Final Report 1990. *J Am Diet Assoc.* 1990; 90(9):A–130.

37. Breslow RA, Hallfrisch J, Guy DG, et al. The importance of dietary protein in healing pressure ulcers. *J Am Geriatr Soc.* 1993;41:357–362.

38. Gersovitz M, Motil K, Munro HN, et al. Human protein requirements: assessment of the adequacy of the current Recommended Dietary Allowance for dietary protein in elderly men and women. *Am J Clin Nutr.* 1982;35:6–14.

39. Long CL, Nelson KM, Akin JM Jr, et al. A physiologic basis for the provision of fuel mixtures in normal and stressed patients. *J Trauma.* 1990;30:1077–1086.

40. Vilter RW. Nutritional aspects of ascorbic acid: uses and abuses. *West J Med.* 1980;133:485.

41. ter Riet G, Kessels AG, Knipschild PG. Randomized clinical trial of ascorbic acid in the treatment of pressure ulcers. *J Clin Epidemiol.* 1995;48:1453–1460.

42. Wilkinson EA, Hawke CI. Does oral zinc aid the healing of chronic leg ulcers? A systematic literature review. *Arch Dermatol.* 1998;134:1556–1560.

43. Sandstead HH, Henriksen LK, Greger JL, et al. Zinc nutriture in the elderly in relation to taste acuity, immune response, and wound healing. *Am J Clin Nutr.* 1982; 36(suppl):1046–1059.

44. Thomas DR. Specific nutritional factors affecting wound healing. *Adv Wound Care.* 1997;10:40–43.

45. Prasad AS. Discovery of human zinc deficiency and studies in an experimental human model. *Am J Clin Nutr.* 1991;53:403–412.

46. Moss SE, Klein R, Klein BE. The 14-year incidence of lower-extremity amputations in a diabetic population. *Diabetes Care.* 1999;22:951–959.

47. Romani A, Nayak SS, Gopalakrishna K, et al. Glycemic control and its relationship to diabetic foot ulcers. *Indian J Pathol Microbiol.* 1991;34(3):161–165.

48. Rayfield EJ, Ault MJ, Keusch GT, et al. Infection and diabetes: the case for glucose control. *Am J Med.* 1982;72: 439–450.

49. Sabioncello A, Rabatic S, Kadrnka-Lovrencie M, et al. Decreased phagocytosis and antibody-dependent cellular cytotoxicity (ADCC) in type-1 diabetes. *Biomedicine.* 1981;35:227–229.

50. Jakelic J, Kokic 5, Hozo I, et al. Nonspecific immunity in diabetes: hyperglycemia decreases phagocytic activity of leukocytes in diabetic patients. *Med Arh.* 1995;49:9–12.

51. Eaglstein WH, Mertz PM. New method for assessing epidermal wound healing. The effects of triamcinolone acetonide and polyethylene film occlusion. *J Invest Dermatol.* 1978;71:382–384.

52. Odland G. The fine structure of the interrelationship of cells in the human epidermis. *J Biophys Biochem Cytol.* l958;4:529–535.

53. Winter GD. Formation of scab and the rate of epithelialization of superficial wounds in the skin of the young domestic pig. *Nature.* l962;193:293–294.

54. Bolton L, Johnson C, van Rijswijk L. Occlusive dressings: therapeutic agents and effects on drug delivery. *Clin Dermatol.* 1992;9:573–583.

55. Eaglstein WH. Experiences with biosynthetic dressings. *J Am Acad Dermatol.* 1985;12:434–440.

56. May SR. Physiology, immunology and clinical efficacy of an adherent polyurethane wound dressing Op-Site. In: Wise DL, ed. *Burn Wound Coverings, vol II.* Boca Raton: CRC Press; 1984:53–78.

57. Freidman S, Su DWP. Hydrocolloid occlusive dressing management of leg ulcers. *Arch Dermatol.* 1984;120:1329–1336.

58. Kaufman C, Hirshowitz B. Treatment of chronic leg ulcers with Op-Site. *Chir Plast.* 1983;7:211–215.

59. Buchan IA. Clinical and laboratory investigation of the compositions and properties of human skin wound exudate under semi-permeable dressings. *Burns.* 1981;7: 326–334.

60. Mertz RM, Marshall DA, Eaglstein WH. Occlusive wound dressings to prevent bacterial invasion and wound infection. *J Am Acad Dermatol.* 1985;12:662–668.

61. Sporr M, Roberts A. Peptide growth factors and inflammation, tissue repair and cancer. *J Clin Investig.* 1986;78: 329–332.

62. Lawrence WT, Diegelmann RF. Growth factors in wound healing. *Clin Dermatol.* 1994;12:157–169.

63. Falanga V. Occlusive wound dressings: why, when, which? *Arch Dermatol.* 1988; 124;872–877.

64. Fowler E, Goupil D. Comparison of the wet-to-dry dressing and a copolymer starch in the management of derided pressure sores. *J Enterostomal Ther.* 1984;11:22–25.

65. Gorse GJ, Messner RL. Improved pressure sore healing with hydrocolloid dressings. *Arch Dermatol.* 1987;123:766–771.

66. Kurzuk-Howard G, Simpson L, Palmieri A. Decubitus ulcer care: a comparative study. *West J Nurs Res.* 1985;7:58–79.

67. Sebern MD. Pressure ulcer management in home health care: efficacy and cost effectiveness of moisture vapor permeable dressing. *Arch Phys Med Rehabil.* 1986;67:726–729.

68. Alvarez O. Moist environment: matching the dressing to the wound. *Ostomy/Wound Manage.* 1988;12:64–83.

69. Custer J, Edlich RF, Prusak M, et al. Studies in the management of the contaminated wound. V. An assessment of the effectiveness of pHisohex and Betadine surgical scrub solutions. *Am J Surg.* 1971;121:572–575.

70. Johnson AR, White AC, McAnalley B. Comparison of common topical agents for wound treatment: cytotoxicity for human fibroblasts in culture. *Wounds.* 1989;1:186–192.

71. Rodeheaver GT, Kurtz L, Kircher BJ, et al. Pluronic F-68: a promising new skin wound cleanser. *Ann Emer Med.* 1980;9:572—576.

72. Rydberg B, Zederfeldt B. Influence of cationic detergents on tensile strength of healing skin wounds in the rat. *Acta Chir Scand.* 1968;134:317–320.

73. Lineaweaver W, Howard R, Soucy D, et al. Topical antimicrobial toxicity. *Arch Surg.* 1985;120:267–270.

74. Van Rijswijk L, Brown D, Friedman S, et al. Multicenter clinical evaluation of a hydrocolloid dressing for leg ulcers. *Cutis.* 1985;35:173.

75. Friedman SJ, Su WP. Management of leg ulcers with hydrocolloid occlusive dressing. *Arch Dermatol.* 1984;120:1329–1336.

76. Cordts PR et al. A prospective, randomized trial of Unna's boot vs. DuoDerm hydroactive dressing plus compression in the management of venous leg ulcers. *J Vasc Surg.* 1992;15:480.

77. Hansson C. The effects of cadexomer iodine paste in the treatment of venous leg ulcers compared with hydrocolloid dressing and paraffin gauze dressing. Cadexomer Iodine Study Group. *Int J Dermatol.* 1998;37:390–396.

78. Weitgasser H. The use of pentoxifylline in the treatment of leg ulcers: results of a double-blind trial. *Pharmatherapeutica.* 1983;2S:143–151.

79. Helfman T, Ovington L, Falanga V. Occlusive dressings and wound healing. *Clin Dermatol.* 1994;12:121–127.

80. Witkowski JA, Parish LC. Cutaneous ulcer therapy. *Int J Dermatol.* 1986;25:420–426.

81. Alm A, Hornmark AM, Fall PA, et al. Care of pressure sores: a controlled study of the use of a hydrocolloid dressing compared with wet saline gauze compresses. *Acta Dermato-Venereol.* 1989;149(suppl):142–148.

82. Colwell JC, Foreman MD, Trotter JP. A comparison of the efficacy and cost-effectiveness of two methods of managing pressure ulcers. *Decubitus.* 1992;6:28–36.

83. Xakellis GC, Chrischilles EA. Hydrocolloid versus saline gauze dressings in treating pressure ulcers: a cost-effective analysis. *Arch Phys Med Rehabil.* 1992;73:463–469.

84. Sapico FL, Ginunas VJ, Thornhill-Joynes M, et al. Quantitative microbiology of pressure sores in different stages of healing. *Diagn Microbiol Infect Dis.* 1986;5:31–38.

85. Bolton L, Oleniacz W, Constantine B. Repair and antibacterial effects of topical antiseptic agents in vivo. *Models Dermatol.* 1985;2:145–158.

86. Hanft JR, Fish SE, Frykbery R, et al. Wound management in the diabetic foot. *J Foot Ankle Surg.* 1997;36:240–254.

87. Apelqvist J, Ranarson TG. Cavity foot ulcers in diabetic patients: a comparative study of cadexomer iodine ointment and standard treatment. *Acta Dermato-Venereol.* 1996;76:231–235.

88. Gentzkow GD, Iwasaki SD, Herson KS, et al. Use of Dermagraft, a cultured human dermis, to treat diabetic foot ulcers. *Diabetes Care.* 1996;19:350–354.

89. Lofgren KA, Laustad WA, Bonnemaison MF. Surgical treatment of large stasis ulcers: review of 129 cases. *Mayo Clin Proc.* 1965;40:560–563.

90. Kirsner RS, Mata SM, Falanga V, Kerdel FA. Split-thickness skin grafting of leg ulcers. *Dermatol Surg.* 1995;21:701–703.

91. Sabolinski ML, Rovee DT, Parenteau NL, et al. The efficacy and safety of Graftskin for the treatment of chronic venous ulcers. *J Wound Repair Regen.* 1995;3:78.

92. Constantine BE, Bolton LL. A wound model for ischemic ulcers in the guinea pig. *Arch Dermatol Res.* 1986;278:429–431.

93. Agren MS, Stromberg HS. Topical treatment of pressure ulcers. A randomized comparative trial of Varidase and zinc oxide. *Scand J Plast Reconstr Surg.* 1985;19:97–100.

94. Hulkko A, Holopainen YV, Orava S, et al. Comparison of dextranomer and streptokinase-streptodornase in the treatment of venous leg ulcers and other infected wounds. *Ann Chir Gynecol.* 198;1;70:65–70.

95. Varma AO, Bugatch E, German F. Debridement of dermal ulcers with collagenase. *Surg Gynecol Obstet.* 1973;136:281–282.

96. Lee LK, Ambrus JL. Collagenase therapy for decubitus ulcers. *Geriatrics.* 1975;30:91–98.

97. Piana M. An economical enzymatic debriding agent for chronic skin ulcers. *Psychiatr Q.* 1968;42:98–101.

98. Yucil VE, Basmajian JV. Decubitus ulcers: healing effect of an enzymatic spray. *Arch Phys Med Rehabil.* 1974;55:517–519.

99. Alvarez OM, Fenandez-Obregon A, Rogers RS, Bergamo L, Masso J, Black M. Chemical debridement of pressure ulcers: a prospective, randomized, comparative trial of collagenase and papain/urea formulations. *Wounds.* 2000;12:15—25.

100. Steed D, Donohoe D, Webster M, et al. Effect of extensive debridement and treatment on the healing of diabetic foot ulcers. *J Am Coll Surg.* 1996;183:61.

101. Robson MC, Phillips LG, Thomason A, et al. Recombinant human derived growth factor-BB for the treatment of chronic pressure ulcers. *Ann Plast Surg.* 1992;29:193–201.

102. Robson MC, Phillips LG, Thomason A, et al. Platelet-derived growth factor BB for the treatment of chronic pressure ulcers. *Lancet.* 1992;339:23–25.

103. Robson MC, Phillips LG, Lawrence WT, et al. The safety and effect of topically applied recombinant basic fibroblast growth factor on the healing of chronic pressure sores. *Ann Surg.* 1992;216:401–408.

104. Federal Drug Administration. *Prescribing Information.* Ortho-McNeil Pharmaceuticals; revised February 1998.

105. Richard J-L, Purer-Richard C, Daures JP, et al. Effect of topical basic fibroblast growth factor on the healing of chronic diabetic neuropathic ulcer of the foot. *Diabetes Care.* 1995;18:64–69.

106. Thomson PD, Smith DJ Jr. What is infection? *Am J Surg.* 1994;167(suppl):7–11.

107. Eleck SD. Experimental staphylococcal infections in the skin of man. *Ann NY Acad Sci.* 1956;65:85–90.

108. Krizek TJ, Robson MD, Kho E. Bacterial growth and skin graft survival. *Surg Forum.* 1967;18:518.

109. Bendy RH Jr, Nuccio PA, Wolfe E. Relationship of quantitative wound bacterial counts to healing of decubiti: effect of topical gentamicin. *Antimicrob Agents Chemother.* 1964;4:147–155.

110. Kucan JO, Robson MC, Heggers JP, et al. Comparison of silver sulfadiazine, povidone-iodine and physiologic saline in the treatment of chronic pressure ulcers. *J Am Geriatr Soc.* 1981;29:232–235.

111. Leyden JL, Bartelt NM. Comparison of topical antibiotic ointments, a wound protectant, and antiseptics for the treatment of human blister wounds contaminated with *Staphylococcus aureus. J Fam Pract.* 1987;6:601–604.

112. Gomolin IH. Pressure sore in the elderly: topical metronidazole therapy for anaerobically infected pressure sores. *Geriatr Med Today.* 1988;3:93–99.

113. Daltrey DC, Rhodes B, Chattwood JG. Investigation into the microbial flora of healing and non-healing decubitus ulcers. *J Clin Pathol.* 1981;34:701–705.

114. Seiler WO, Stahelin HB, Sonnabend W. Effect of aerobic and anaerobic germs on the healing of decubitus ulcers. *Schweiz Med Wochenschr.* 1979;109:1594–1599.

115. Lipsky BA, Pecoraro RE, Larson SA, et al. Outpatient management of uncomplicated lower-extremity infections in diabetic patients. *Arch Intern Med.* 1990;150:790–797.

116. Hutchinson JJ, McGuckin M. Occlusive dressings: a microbiological and clinical review. *Am J Infect Control.* 1990;18:257–268.

117. Allman RM, Walker JM, Hart MK, et al. Air-fluidized beds or conventional therapy for pressure sores: a randomized trial. *Ann Intern Med.* 1987;107:641–648.

118. Bennett RG, Bellantoni MF, Ouslander JG. Air-fluidized bed treatment of nursing home patients with pressure sores. *J Am Geriatr Soc.* 1989;37:235–242.

119. Hong TF, Brodsky J. Surgical treatment of neuropathic ulcerations under the first metatarsal head. *Foot Ankle Clin.* 1997;2:57–75.

120. Jacobs AM, Appleman KK. Foot-ulcer prevention in the elderly diabetic patient. *Clin Geriatr Med.* 1999;15(2):351–369.

121. Lippman H. Must loss of limb be a consequence of diabetes mellitus? *Diabetes Care.* 1979;2:432.

122. Boulton AJM. Peripheral neuropathy and the diabetic foot. *Foot.* 1992;2:67–72.

123. Armstrong DG, Lavery LA. Evidence-based options for off-loading diabetic wounds. *Clin Podiatr Med Surg.* 1998;15:95–104.

124. Edmonds ME, Blundell MP, Morris ME, et al. Improved survival of the diabetic foot: The role of a specialized foot clinic. *Q J Med.* 1986;60:763–771.

125. Fletcher A, Cullum N, Sheldon TA. A systematic review of compression treatment for venous leg ulcers. *Br Med J.* 1997;315:576–580.

126. Eagle M. Compression bandaging. *Nurs Standard.* 199;13:49–54.

127. Evans GRD, Dufresne CR, Manson PN. Surgical correction of pressure ulcers in an urban center: is it efficacious? *Adv Wound Care.* 1994;7:40–46.

128. Disa JJ, Carlton JM, Goldberg NH. Efficacy of operative cure in pressure sore patients. *Plast Reconstr Surg.* 1992;89:272–278.

129. Goldberg NH. Outcomes in surgical intervention. *Adv Wound Care.* 1995;8:69–70.

130. Siegler EL, Lavizzo-Mourey R. Management of stage III pressure ulcers in moderately demented nursing home residents. *J Gen Intern Med.* 1991;6:507–513.

131. Jacobs AM, Appleman KK. Foot-ulcer prevention in the elderly diabetic patient. *Clin Geriatr Med.* 1999;15(2):351–369.

132. LoGerto FW, Gibbons GW, Pomposelli FB Jr. Trends in the care of the diabetic foot: expanded role of arterial reconstruction. *Arch Surg.* 1992;127:617–621.

133. Turczynski R, Tarpila E. Treatment of leg ulcers with split skin grafts: early and late results. *Scand J Plastic Reconstr Surg Hand Surg.* 1999;33:301–305.

134. Oien RF, Hansen BU, Hakansson A. Pinch grafting of leg ulcers in primary care. *Acta Dermato-Venereol.* 1998;78:438–439.

135. Bergstrom N, Bennett MA, Carlson CE, et al. *Treatment of Pressure Ulcers. Clinical Practice Guideline No. 15.* AHCPR Pub 95-0652. Rockville, MD: U.S. Dept of Health and Human Services, Public Health Service, Agency for Health Care Policy and Research; 1994.

66
Falls

David C. Thomas, Helen K. Edelberg, and Mary E. Tinetti

Until the 1940s, falls and fall-related injuries were considered accidents, that is, "acts of God," random or chance events without observable or understandable explanations.[1] Since the early studies by Droller,[2] Sheldon,[3] and Fine,[4] falls have gained appreciation, first as predictable, then as preventable health problems worthy of careful evaluation and preventive efforts. Up through the early 1990s, risk factors were identified in various settings, that is, community and nursing home. Simultaneously, the notion of falls as multifactorial events was established as the norm. Over the past decade, studies have focused more on the prevention and treatment of falls as well as on identifying subgroups of patients who would benefit most from preventive interventions.

Falling is an important clinical marker of frailty, as evidenced by its association with other functional problems, such as incontinence, and with a high mortality rate that is not directly attributable to fall-related injuries.[5] As a consequence of its associated morbidity, falling is also an important health problem in its own right among frail as well as healthier older persons.

As discussed here, although some falls have a single intrinsic (disease- or impairment-related) or extrinsic (environmental) cause, many falls by elderly persons are multifactorial in origin, resulting from an interaction between stability-impairing characteristics of the individual and the hazards and demands of the environment. As recent evidence indicates that individual interventions may play a key role in fall prevention and treatment, these are also presented. We address nonsyncopal rather than syncopal falls, that is, those events that are not associated with a loss of consciousness, stroke, or epileptic seizure nor related to sustaining a violent blow.[6]

Prevalence and Morbidity

Community

Each year, approximately one-third of community-living adults over age 65 years and 50% of persons over age 80 years sustain a fall.[7-9] Half of these individuals experience multiple falls. Among individuals under age 75, women fall more frequently than men do. This gender difference in prevalence lessens, however, among adults over age 75.[10]

Unintentional injury is the sixth leading cause of death in persons over the age of 65 years; the majority of these deaths are attributed to falls and their complications, especially among persons 85 years of age and older.[11] Although women are about twice as likely to suffer a serious injury during a fall,[12,13] the rates for fall-related deaths are consistently higher among men, who are 22% more likely than women to sustain a fatal fall.[14]

About 7% of persons over 75 years visit emergency rooms for a fall injury event each year; more than 40% of these visits result in hospitalizations.[15] As many as 10% of falls in this age group are complicated by serious injury, such as a fracture, joint dislocation, or severe head trauma.[16] An estimated 5% of falls by community-living elderly persons result in a fracture, fewer than 1% in a hip fracture.[15] In persons over age 75, fractures of the lower extremity are about twice as common as fractures of the upper extremity. An additional 5% of falls result in serious soft tissue injuries requiring medical attention.[9,11] These injuries include hemarthroses, joint dislocations, sprains, and hematomas. Subdural hematomas and cervical fractures are devastating, but rare. About 30% to 50% of falls by elderly persons result in minor injuries such as bruises, lacerations, and abrasions.

Being unable to get up after a fall is a potentially hazardous consequence of falling that can occur with or without serious injury. Community-based studies have reported that 50% of older fallers are unable to get up without help after at least one fall.[10,13] Factors associated with the inability to get up without assistance include age over 80 years, decreased upper and lower extremity strength, poor balance, arthritis, and greater dependency in activities of daily living (ADL).[10,13] Older individuals who are unable to get up after a fall are at risk for complications such as dehydration, pressure sores, rhabdomyolysis, and pneumonia.

Fear of falling is common among community-living older adults, particularly among older women. Many older women express concern over the loss of independence and quality of life resulting from a fall and hip fracture.[17] One in four fallers reports that they avoid acivities because of fear of falling.[9,18] As a result of this fear, patients report a poorer quality of life with a loss of function and independence.[19] Fear of falling has been independently associated with requiring assistance to climb stairs, poor vision, restriction in instrumental activities of daily living (IADL), poor self-related health, and poor performance on tests of balance.[20,21] The concept of self-efficacy or confidence in the ability to perform specific activities in specific situations has been applied to fear of falling to understand the relationship between fear and function.[6] Self-efficacy shows a stronger association with functioning in basic and instrumental activities of daily living and higher-level physical and social activities than does self-reported fear of falling.[22]

Limitation of functioning and activity, whether because of physical impairment from injury or fear of future falls, is a common adverse consequence of falling. In a national survey, falls and their sequelae accounted for 18% of restricted activity days among elderly persons, the highest proportion for any health condition.[23] In a prospective study, more than 40% of fallers restricted their activities at least temporarily after a fall.[24] Pain or limitation of activity after a fall was present 8 weeks later in 40% of fallers treated in an emergency room; almost half these persons had not yet fully recovered by 8 months.[24]

Falling has been associated with an increased likelihood of hospitalization, nursing home placement, and death.[25–27] Much of this relationship, however, may be accounted for by older age, chronic conditions, and ADL disabilities.[27] Noninjurious as well as injurious falls have been found to be independent predictors of nursing home placement, after adjusting for other known risk factors, and falls with serious injury were twice as likely as noninjurious falls to result in nursing home placement.[28]

Nursing Home

More than half of ambulatory nursing home residents fall each year.[29] The annual incidence of falling among nursing home residents is 1.5 falls per bed per year. About 4% of falls within nursing homes result in fractures and 11% in other serious injuries such as head trauma, soft tissue injuries, and severe lacerations. Each year, about 1800 fatal falls occur in nursing homes. Among persons 85 years and older, 1 of 5 fatal falls occurs in a nursing home. The contribution of falls to fear and functioning has been less studied among nursing home than among community, residents.

The use of physical restraints in nursing homes to prevent high-risk persons from falling has been associated with an increased frequency of serious injury, as well as increased agitation, depression, and immobility.[30] Immobilization by physical restraint may result in vasomotor instability and decreased muscle mass, strength, and joint flexibility, all of which can contribute to falls and injuries.[31] Although some restraint reduction programs have resulted in an increase in falls and minor injuries, the discontinuation of physical restraints has not led to an increase in serious fall injuries.[32,33]

Pathogenesis

Community

Nonsyncopal falls occur when environmental hazards or demands exceed the individual's ability to maintain postural stability. Specific diseases such as Parkinson's syndrome, normal pressure hydrocephalus, white matter disease, and high cervical myelopathy may result in severe postural instability. Some authors also describe a gait disturbance of unknown central nervous system etiology, referred to as senile or essential gait disorder. Overall, these central nervous system diseases account for a relatively small percentage of falls by older persons.

Immediate Causes

Investigators have attempted, through a careful review of fall circumstances, to identify the most likely immediate cause of falls. Summarizing the results of several studies, Rubenstein et al. reported that an environmentally related factor was the most likely cause of 41% (range, 23%–53%) of falls, gait or balance disturbance or weakness of 13% (2%–29%), drop attack of 13% (0%–25%), dizziness or vertigo of 8% (0%–19%), confusion of 2% (0%–7%), and postural hypotension of 1% (0%–6%), while visual disorder, syncope, acute illness, drugs, and other factors accounted for an additional 17% of falls.[29] The cause was unknown for 6% (0%–16%) of falls. The relative frequency of the various causes varied widely among the studies.

Classification Schemes

Several classification schemes have been developed to explain the pathogenesis of falls. One approach has been to classify balance and gait dysfunctions based on anatomy and physiology. One such scheme, described by Nutt et al.,[34] proposed four categories of balance and gait disorders: (1) lower-level disorders, due to problems with sensory systems (proprioceptive, vestibular, or visual) or strength; (2) middle-level disorders, involving the spinal cord or brainstem; (3) higher-level disorders, concerning the cerebellum, basal ganglia, or corticospinal tracts; and (4) highest-level gait disorders, relating to the frontal cortex.[34] Although this classification system has helped advance research into postural instability and falls, many older persons with the presumed anatomic or physiologic lesions do not fall and many fallers do not possess a readily identifiable single lesion within the sensory or neuromuscular systems. Another classification system, used in a large prospective community study, divided falls into four broad categories: (1) falls related to extrinsic factors, slips, trips, or displaced center of gravity (55%); (2) falls related to intrinsic factors, such as poor mobility, balance, cognitive, or sensory impairments (39%); (3) falls from a nonbipedal stance, such as falling out of bed or while using an assistive device (8%); and (4) unclassified falls (7%).[35] Although investigators have used such classification schemes to identify differences in types of falls by age, gender, and other factors, these schemes fail to account for the multifactorial etiology of most falls.

Multifactorial Etiology

The epidemiologic model of host, activity, and environmental factors addresses the multifactorial etiology of most falls. Under this model, there is a reciprocal relationship among host, activity, and environmental factors. The importance of these three categories of factors varies with individual falls. Host factors contributing to falls can best be understood by considering that postural stability requires input from sensory, central integrative, and effector neuromuscular components in a highly integrated manner.[36] These components are overlapping and compensatory. Cardiac, circulatory, respiratory, metabolic, and other conditions may further influence the functioning of these three primary components. Postural instability and predisposition to falling may not be evident until several contributing components are impaired.

A related and clinically useful method for explaining fall etiology is to consider both predisposing as well as situational factors. Predisposing risk factors are those intrinsic characteristics of the individual that chronically impair stability and render the individual vulnerable to new insults. Situational factors are those host, activity, and environmental factors that are present at the time of the fall (Tables 66.1 and 66.2).

Predisposing Risk Factors

As noted, stability depends on the intricate functioning of sensory, central integrative, and musculoskeletal effec-

TABLE 66.1. Results of univariate analysis of most common risk factors for falls identified in 16 studies that examined risk factors.[a]

Risk factor	Significant/total[b]	RR-OR[c]	Range
Muscle weakness	10/11	4.4	1.5–10.3
History of falls	12/13	3.0	1.7–7.0
Gait deficit	10/12	2.9	1.3–5.6
Balance deficit	8/11	2.9	1.6–5.4
Use assistive device	8/8	2.6	1.2–4.6
Visual deficit	6/12	2.5	1.6–3.5
Arthritis	3/7	2.4	1.9–2.9
Impaired ADL	8/9	2.3	1.5–3.1
Depression	3/6	2.2	1.7–2.5
Cognitive impairment	4/11	1.8	1.0–2.3
Age >80 years	5/8	1.7	1.1–2.5

[a] References: 9, 18, 51, 57, 58, 68–71, 74, 80, 87, 107–109.
[b] Number of studies with significant odds ratio or relative risk ratio in univariate analysis/total number of studies that included each factor.
[c] Relative risk ratios (RR) calculated for prospective studies–odds ratios (OR) calculated for retrospective studies.
Source: Modified and used with permission: *J Am Geriatr Soc.* 49(5): 665.

TABLE 66.2. The relationship between falls and medication use.

Medication class[a]	Number of studies	Pooled OR	95% CI
Psychotropics	20	1.73	1.52–1.97
Neuroleptics	23	1.5	1.25–1.79
Sedative/hypnotics	23	1.54	1.40–1.70
Any antidepressant	28	1.66	1.4–1.95
Tricyclic antidepressants	13	1.51	1.14–2.00
Benzodiazepines	14	1.48	1.23–1.77
Diuretics	27	1.08	1.02–1.16
Digoxin	18	1.22	1.05–1.42
Class IA antiarrhythmics	11	1.59	1.02–2.48
Three or more medications	11	—[b]	—[b]
Four or more medications	9	—[b]	—[b]

[a] References: 48, 50.
[b] Pooled odds ratio and 95% confidence interval not calculated due to heterogeneity in the definition of medication, however or significantly increased in recurrent fallers.

tor components. Accumulated impairments and diseases affecting these components, superimposed on age-related physiologic changes or lifestyle factors (e.g., past physical activity), result in a predisposition to falling.[37]

The major sensory modalities responsible for orienting the individual in space and identifying hazards include the visual, auditory, vestibular, and proprioceptive systems. These modalities have multiple interconnections with one another. Age-related visual changes include decreased visual acuity, contrast sensitivity, dark adaptation, and accommodation. In addition, ocular diseases that are common in older persons, such as macular degeneration, glaucoma, and cataracts, may adversely affect visual functioning. Visual acuity, contrast sensitivity, and depth perception, a visual function involved in spatial orientation, have been shown to be especially relevant to postural stability and falling.[38-40]

An age-related decline in vestibular function has been suggested as an explanation for increased postural sway as well as dizziness and perhaps falling in elderly persons.[41] The vestibular system contributes to spatial orientation at rest as well as during acceleration and is responsible for visual fixation during head and body movements. An age-related decline in vestibular function has been attributed to changes in the otoconia. Predisposing factors include past aminoglycoside use as well as present use of aspirin, furosemide, quinine, quinidine, and perhaps tobacco and alcohol. Head trauma, mastoid or ear surgery, and middle ear infections are other possible predisposing factors. Elderly persons with vestibular problems complain of worsening stability in the dark because of increased reliance on visual input.

Hearing contributes directly to stability through the detection and interpretation of auditory stimuli, which help localize and orient the individual in space, particularly when other sensory modalities are impaired. More than 50% of elderly persons have some hearing loss.[42]

The proprioceptive system provides spatial orientation during position changes, while walking on uneven ground, or when other modalities are impaired.[36] The proprioceptive system includes peripheral nerves, apophyseal joint mechanoreceptors, and the posterior columns, as well as multiple central nervous system connections. It is unclear whether age-related changes occur in peripheral nerves. Nevertheless, peripheral neuropathy from a variety of different causes is common among elderly persons. The contribution of cervical mechanoreceptors to proprioception is not well appreciated.[43] Predisposing factors for cervical disorders include whiplash injuries and cervical degenerative diseases such as rheumatoid arthritis or spondylosis. Older adults with proprioceptive problems complain of worsening difficulties in the dark or on uneven ground. They may complain of true vertigo. Gait often improves in these individuals with even minimal support.

The central nervous system channels inputs from the sensory modalities to the appropriate efferent components of the musculoskeletal system. Given the multiple connections and their complexity, virtually any central nervous system disorder can contribute to instability and falling. Specific diseases such as Parkinson's disease, normal pressure hydrocephalus, and stroke are associated with an increased risk of falling. Central nervous system processes that adversely affect cognition further impede stability because problem solving and judgment are needed to interpret and respond appropriately to environmental stimuli. Individuals with impaired mental status or dementia have consistently been found to have an increased incidence of falling, even in the absence of

a clinical gait disorder. Additional studies have demonstrated the relationship between white matter disease, even in the absence of cognitive impairment, and gait disorders.[44]

Any impairment within the musculoskeletal system, including joints, muscles, and bones, will decrease stability and increase fall risk. Arthritis, myopathies, and hemiparesis are all associated with falling. Arthritis likely increases the risk of falling through several mechanisms including pain, periarticular muscle weakness, and compromised proprioception due to deterioration of joint mechanoreceptors. Hip, knee, and ankle weakness have all been found to significantly increase risk of falling.[45] Reciprocal flexion and extension of lower extremity muscles appears essential to postural stability. Ankle dorsiflexion weakness may explain the tendency of some elderly persons to fall backward with even minimal displacement. Alternatively, the predisposition to falling backward may result from a smaller posterior than anterior base of support. Foot abnormalities such as calluses, bunions, and deformed toes and nail abnormalities may provide incorrect proprioceptive information and adversely affect gait patterns.

Systemic diseases may contribute to instability by impairing sensory, neurologic, or musculoskeletal functioning or by causing a reduction in cerebral oxygenation or perfusion, fatigue, or confusion. Common examples include anemia, electrolyte disturbances, hypoglycemia or hyperglycemia, acid–base disturbances, or hypothyroidism.

Postural hypotension may result in instability by compromising cerebral blood flow.[46] The prevalence of postural hypotension ranges from 10% to 30% in community-dwelling persons over 65 years of age. As is falling, postural hypotension is frequently multifactorial. Contributing factors include age-related autonomic changes, decreased baroreceptor sensitivity, decreased renin-angiotensin response to upright position, decreased venous and lymphatic return, and salt and water depletion. The effects of diseases such as diabetes or Parkinson's disease and of medications such as antidepressants, neuroleptics, antihypertensives, nitrates, and diuretics are further contributing factors. Postural hypotension should be considered if the fall occurred while moving from a lying or sitting to a standing position, after prolonged standing, or during exertion. Another abnormality in blood pressure homeostasis is postprandial hypotension.[46] The mechanisms and mediators of postprandial hypotension remain unknown, although inability to compensate for splanchnic blood pooling after the meal has been postulated as a possible etiology.

Medications may contribute to gait instability through a variety of mechanisms, including impairment of cognitive functioning, postural hypotension, dehydration, impaired balance, fatigue, or electrolyte disturbance.

(Table 66.2) Centrally acting medications, including sedative-hypnotics, tranquilizers, antidepressants, and neuroleptics have repeatedly been associated with an increased risk of falls and injuries.[47,48] Both selective serotonin reuptake inhibitors (SSRIs) and tricyclic antidepressants have been implicated in falls and hip fractures.[49] Other classes of medications associated with falls in older adults include diuretics, type 1A antiarrhythmics, and digoxin.[50] In addition to specific medications, recent changes in dose and the total number of medications have been associated with an increased risk of falling.[51] Conversely, evidence suggests that postural instability, as manifested by impaired balance, dizziness, and falling, is one of the most frequent presentations of adverse drug effect in an older population.[52,53]

Situational Factors

Falling is well recognized as a nonspecific presentation of acute illness in older adults. Acute febrile illnesses (e.g., pneumonia or urinary tract infections) and chronic disease exacerbations (e.g., congestive heart failure or diabetes mellitus) likely precipitate falls by temporarily impairing stability.[9] Some cardiac dysrhythmias cause a decrease in cerebral blood flow and loss of consciousness, resulting in a fall.[53] Carotid baroreceptor hypersensitivity may contribute to syncopal, as well as nonsyncopal, falls.

One type of fall, mentioned most frequently in the British literature, is the drop attack.[3] This term refers to a sudden loss of postural tone without loss of consciousness. Drop attacks may occur while walking, while turning the neck, while looking up, or without an obvious precipitating movement. Some individuals note that their knees buckled or "just gave out." It is likely that at least some of those who report their knees buckling have impaired mechanoreceptors secondary to arthritic joint changes. Difficulty getting up is often reported. The etiology and frequency of drop attacks are unknown. Although reported in up to 25% of falls in the earlier literature,[3] more recently "just going down" without any obvious intrinsic or environmental cause is reported in less than 5% of falls.[9,29]

The majority of falls by community-living elderly persons occur during the course of usual, relatively nonhazardous activities such as walking, changing position, or performing basic activities of daily living. Only a small percentage of falls occur during clearly hazardous activities such as climbing on chairs or ladders or participating in sports activities.[9]

Although major environmental hazards account for few falls, environmental factors probably contribute to the majority of falls by community-dwelling older adults. The precise role of environmental factors is difficult to ascertain because studies lack control data on nonfallers or fallers at times other than their fall. Over 70% of falls by community-dwelling older adults occur at home. About 10% of falls occur on stairs, well out of proportion to time spent on them, with descending being more hazardous than ascending.[9,54] The most commonly mentioned environmental hazards include carrying heavy or bulky objects, and negotiating obstacles that can be tripped over, slippery floors, and poor lighting.[55] Slippery or improperly fitting shoes are another potential hazard. Finally, patterns on floors or walls, depending on their quality, may either distort or improve visual perception.[56]

Nursing Homes

Immediate Causes and Predisposing Factors

As in community-based studies, investigators have attempted to identify the "most likely cause" of individual falls by nursing home residents.[57] Studies of nursing home residents have found a higher incidence of falls caused by gait, balance, or strength disorders (25%; range, 20%–39%), by dizziness (25%; range, 0%–30%) and by confusion (10%; range, 0%–14%).[29] Only 16% (range, 6%–27%) of falls are primarily attributed to an environmental factor.[29] Visual disorders (4%; range, 0%–5%), postural hypotension (2%; range, 0%–16%), and drop attacks (0.3%; range, 0%–3%) are other less frequently cited causes. Other causes such as acute illness, drugs, and pain were believed to account for 12% of falls among nursing home residents. Although investigators have attempted to identify the "most likely cause of individual falls," falling among nursing home residents, as among community-living residents, most often results from the accumulated effect of multiple specific impairments and diseases.[51,58] The predisposing impairments are the same as those cited for community-dwelling older adults. The prevalence of the impairments is higher among nursing home than among community residents, which may partially explain the higher frequency of falling.[29] Similar to community studies, studies of nursing home residents have identified an increased risk of falling with an increased number of impairments and diseases possessed.[51,58]

Situational Factors

Host factors such as acute illness, postural hypotension, dizziness, or medications have been described. Environmental factors are thought to be less important among institutionalized than community-dwelling older adults. The greater frailty and larger number of impairments predispose institutionalized elderly persons to fall in situations where healthier persons would not. Also, by and large, institutions are safer environments than the community because many potential hazards have been removed. Further, institutionalized elderly persons have fewer opportunities to engage in such hazardous activities as climbing stairs, walking on ice, or climbing on ladders. Even so, environmental factors do contribute to falls among institutionalized older adults.[29] Examples include ill-fitting shoes, untied shoelaces, long pants, or slippery floors.[59] Furniture may be hazardous; beds that are either too high or too low, bed rails that can be climbed over, and chairs that are too low or soft may also be dangerous. Walking aids are an unappreciated fall hazard. Canes and footrests can be tripped over, and the added weight of a walker may displace an individual backward. Many residents are able to remove their restraints. In addition, restrained persons may take their wheelchairs or chairs over with them in a fall. As one study points out, falls are a possible, but not inevitable, outcome in the nursing home setting. Through the implementation of a standardized and structured safety program, the impact of these falls can be minimized.[60]

Risk Factors for Serious Fall Injury

Recent interest has focused on factors that increase the risk of serious injury, particularly fractures, during a fall. The likelihood of suffering a serious injury during a fall has been postulated to depend on factors such as the velocity of the fall, the energy-absorbing capacity of the surface landed on, the protective responses of the faller, the injury threshold of the tissue, and the direction and location of impact.[61,62] Characteristics of fallers shown to be independently associated with serious injury include older age, female gender, white race, decreased bone mineral density, decreased body mass index, cognitive impairment, the use of certain medications, abnormal neuromuscular findings such as decreased reaction time and balance disturbance, poor visual acuity, history of previous falls and fall injuries, and the presence of specific chronic diseases, such as diabetes, and stroke.[12,18,63–74] Increased physical activity level has been associated with both an increased and a decreased risk of suffering a serious fall injury event.[12,72] Circumstances of the fall that increase likelihood of serious injuries such as fractures include the direction and impact of the fall, the height of the fall, and the hardness of the landing surface, as well as low body mass index (BMI).[73–75] A discussion of the risk factors and medical aspects of hip fracture management are covered in Chapter 45.

Evaluation and Management

The goal of a fall evaluation and prevention strategy is to minimize the risk of falling without compromising mobil-

ity or functional independence. Given the inherent trade-offs between safety and independence, this goal may be difficult to achieve in some individuals. Perhaps a better goal, rather than to prevent all falls, would be to prevent relevant fall-related morbidities such as serious injury, fear, and the inability to get up. As the ability to identify the subset of fallers at risk for these fall sequelae improves, evaluative and preventive efforts can be better targeted. A recent report by an expert panel provides an evidence-based approach to the management and prevention of falls: The Quality Indicators for Assessing Care of the Elderly (ACOVE) project.[75–77]

As already described, the etiology and risk factors for falls are similar in nursing home and community residents, but the relative frequency and modifiability of contributing risk factors may differ in these two populations. Therefore, the recommended evaluation and preventive strategies are discussed separately for community and nursing home residents. The American Geriatrics Society and British Geriatrics Society Panel on Falls in Older Persons has published the most up-to-date guidelines for the prevention of falls in older persons, and the reader is referred there for a discussion of these guidelines.[78]

Community

The first step in evaluating individuals who have experienced a fall or who are at risk for falling is to identify possible contributing factors.[79,80] The following components of the evaluation provide complementary information: (1) a thorough assessment of predisposing risk factors and diseases; (2) a balance and gait assessment; and (3) a review of previous fall situations.

Predisposing Risk Factor Assessment
History and Examination

The risk assessment begins with a careful history and physical examination aimed at identifying all predisposing risk factors. It is important to bear in mind that the multiple diseases and disabilities suffered by many older individuals may render the signs and symptoms of specific conditions obscure, vague, or nonspecific. For example, nonvestibular disorders may present with vertigo, whereas individuals with vestibular dysfunction may complain only of vague dizziness or unsteadiness. Therefore, a thorough systematic assessment of all possible contributing factors is essential. The governing concept in fall assessment is that it may be possible to decrease fall risk by ameliorating as many contributing factors as possible.

The neurologic diseases that predispose to falls can be diagnosed from a thorough neurologic history and examination. Although most neurologic diseases associated with falling result in postural instability and pathologic gait patterns, these findings are not disease specific. Common features of gait seen in persons with central neurologic diseases include flexed posture, step-to-step variability, path deviation, decreased step height that results in shuffling if severe, instability on turning, and easy displacement backward.[36,81] Many of these findings, however, can also be seen in individuals with sensory abnormalities and may represent compensatory, rather than primary, changes. Thus, in diagnosing neurologic diseases, gait findings must be considered in association with findings from other components of the neurologic examination including cranial nerve findings, sensation, tone, muscle strength, and coordination. The neurologic examination is helpful not only in diagnosing specific diseases but also in identifying other contributing factors to fall risk such as decreased sensation or muscle weakness.

Other important components of the risk assessment are included in Table 66.3. Simple screening tests such as the Snellen chart can be used to measure near and distant visual acuity. If there are any questions concerning visual function, the individual should be referred to an ophthalmologist or optometrist for a full evaluation. Portable audiometry or the Whisper Test[82] can be used to screen for hearing problems. Although vestibular dysfunction is difficult to diagnose from simple clinical tests, a vestibular contribution to instability should be suspected if the individual complains of vertigo, worsening stability in the dark or with specific head positions, or provides a history of predisposing factors including past aminoglycoside use, use of aspirin, furosemide, quinine, or quinidine, or has a past history of head trauma, mastoid or ear surgery, or middle ear infections. If vestibular problems are suspected, attempts should be made to provoke vertigo with the Dix–Hillpike maneuver (see Chapter 67). Selected patients should be referred to audiology for a complete hearing evaluation or to otolaryngology for full vestibular testing.

Individuals with proprioceptive impairments complain of worsening stability in the dark, on uneven ground, on inclines, or on thick rugs. Decreased position and vibration sense are noted on examination. During gait testing, individuals with decreased proprioception may markedly improve their gait pattern simply by holding on to the examiner's finger or using a straight cane. If a cervical disorder is the cause of the proprioceptive problem, the complaints will be similar to those for peripheral neuropathy, but the individual will also complain of worsening symptoms with head turning or true vertigo. In some cases, the examination may reveal signs of radiculopathy or myelopathy; there may be clumsiness with fine motor tasks and even mild spastic quadriparesis. Many elderly individuals will, on examination of neck range of motion while standing, exhibit decreased neck range of motion

and complaints ranging from vague dizziness to marked instability. It may be difficult to determine whether these individuals suffer from a mechanoreceptor-related cervical disorder or whether the decreased neck range of motion is secondary to vestibular dysfunction and inadvertent avoidance of neck movements that precipitate the symptoms. It is important to distinguish between the two because a decrease in neck movements will exacerbate the underlying vestibular disorder by impeding compensation by the central nervous system. The musculoskeletal examination may reveal various patterns of muscle weakness.

As noted earlier, all of hip, knee, and ankle strength and range of motion are essential to postural stability and the response to perturbations. Thus, any arthritic or musculoskeletal process may contribute to fall risk. Individuals with knee arthritis may complain of falls because their "knee gave out." Individuals with proximal muscle weakness may report difficulty getting in and out of chairs, in and out of the bathtub, and climbing stairs, whereas individuals with distal weakness will complain of frequent tripping. The contribution of upper extremity arm movements to postural stability and response to perturbation is unappreciated and needs to be considered. Foot problems, including bunions, calluses, and deformity, can affect gait patterns and decrease proprioception and thus should be identified.

Although postural hypotension has not been identified as a frequent risk factor for falls among community-dwelling elderly persons, this is likely because it is not feasible to assess blood pressure change at the time of a fall. Blood pressure change with position change should be part of the risk factor assessment. Individuals may complain of lightheadedness or other vague sensations on position change, prolonged standing, or walking, although many individuals with significant postural hypotension may be asymptomatic and thus unaware of the blood pressure drop. Many, but not all, of these individuals may have concomitant diseases such as Parkinson's syndrome or diabetes. In addition, as noted next, many medications can contribute to the risk of falling by causing postural hypotension. Particularly important medications to ask about include nitrates, antihypertensives, and antidepressants.

The screen for depressive symptoms may reveal vegetative complaints, poor concentration, or apathy. Finally, a careful medication review is an essential component of a fall risk assessment. The assessment should involve the direct recording of all prescription medications from the original containers and verification of the dose and timing of each medication. Over-the-counter medications, particularly sedative-hypnotics, cold preparations, and nonsteroidal anti-inflammatory agents, must be ascertained as well. In addition, possible medication side effects including confusion, lightheadedness, fatigue,

TABLE 66.3. Predisposing and situational factors associated with risk of falling.

Predisposing factors with contribution to falling	Possible interventions
Sensory	
Vision: acuity, perception	Medical: refraction; cataract extraction
Impaired hazard recognition; distorted environmental signals; spatial disorientation	Rehabilitative: balance and gait training
	Environmental: good lighting; home safety assessment; architectural design that minimizes distortions and illusions
Hearing	Medical: cerumen removal; audiologic evaluation with hearing aid if appropriate
Spatial disorientation; balance impairment; distorted environmental signals (auditory)	Rehabilitative: training in hearing aid use
	Environmental: decrease background noise
Vestibular dysfunction	Medical: avoid vestibulotoxic drugs; surgical ablation
Spatial disorientation at rest; impaired visual fixation; balance impairment especially with head or body turning	Rehabilitative: habituation exercises
	Environmental: good lighting (increased reliance on visual input); architectural design that minimizes distortions and illusions
Proprioceptive: cervical disorders; peripheral neuropathy	Medical: diagnose and treat specific disease (e.g., spondylosis, B_{12} deficiency)
Spatial disorientation during position changes or while walking on uneven surfaces or in dark	Rehabilitative: balance exercises; correct walking aid
	Environmental: good lighting (increased reliance on visual input); appropriate footwear; home safety assessment
Central neurologic	
Central nervous system diseases	Medical: diagnose and treat specific diseases (e.g. Parkinson's syndrome, Normal Pressure hydrocephalus)
Impaired problem solving, strength, sensation, balance, gait, tone, or coordination	Rehabilitative: physical therapy; balance and gait training; correct walking aid
	Environmental: home safety assessment; appropriate adaptations (e.g. high, firm chairs, raised toilet seats, grab bars in bathroom)
Dementia/cognitive impairment	Medical: minimize sedating or centrally acting drugs
Impaired problem solving, impaired gait	Rehabilitative: supervised exercise and ambulation
	Environmental: safe, structure, supervised environment
Musculoskeletal	
Muscle weakness: upper and lower extremity,	Medical: diagnose and treat specific diseases
Impaired postural stability	Rehabilitative: balance and gait training; Tai Chi, muscle-strengthening exercises; back exercises; correct walking aid; correct footwear; good foot care (nails, bunions)
Arthritides	
Impaired postural stability	
Feet	
Impaired proprioception; impaired postural instability; altered gait pattern	Environmental: home safety assessment; appropriate adaptations
Back	
Impaired ability to regain stability	
Other	
Postural hypotension	Medical: diagnose and treat specific disease; avoid offending drugs; rehydrate; replenish salt
Impaired cerebral blood flow leading to fatigue, weakness, postural instability; syncope if severe	Rehabilitative: tilt table if severe; reconditioning if component of deconditioning; graded pressure stockings; dorsiflexion and hand flexion exercises before arising
	Environmental: elevate head of bed
Depression	Medical: ?antidepressants associated with increased risk of falling; ? select least anticholinergic
? accident-proneness; ? poor concentration	
Medications: especially sedatives, phenothiazines, antidepressants; total number and dose of medications	Medical: lowest effective dose of essential medications; readjust or discontinue when possible
Impaired alertness; postural hypotension; postural instability; fatigue	

Situational factors	Possible interventions
Acute host factors	
Acute illness; new or increased medications	Medical: diagnose and treat specific diseases; start medications low and increase slowly
Transiently impaired alertness; postural hypotension; fatigue	Environmental: increase supervision during illnesses or with new medication
Displacing activity	Rehabilitative: recommend avoiding only clearly hazardous and unnecessary activities (e.g., climbing on chairs); balance and gait training
Increased opportunity to fall	
Environmental hazards	Environmental: home safety assessment with appropriate adaptive or structural changes (see Ref. 7)
Slipping or tripping hazards (e.g., loose rugs, wet floors, ice, small objects) stairs, lighting, and furniture	
Nursing home: movable tables; inappropriate bed or chair height; ill-fitting shoes or pants; restraints	

weakness, or postural hypotension should be elicited from the patient.

Carotid hypersensitivity should be suspected if the individual gives a history of "just going down" or falling with head turning or with looking up. Carotid sinus massage should be performed if carotid sinus syndrome is suspected, if there is no evidence of cerebrovascular disease or cardiac conduction abnormality, and if the procedure is judged safe in the individual patient. The carotid sinus syndrome is defined as greater than a 3-s sinus pause or more than a 5 mmHg drop in systolic blood pressure.

Laboratory Evaluation

All elderly persons who have experienced falls should undergo routine laboratory screening including a complete blood count, thyroid function tests, electrolytes, including blood urea nitrogen (BUN) and creatinine, and serum glucose, as well as a determination of vitamin B_{12} levels. These tests are warranted to screen for anemia, thyroid dysfunction, electrolyte abnormalities, dehydration, hyperglycemia or hypoglycemia, and B_{12} deficiency because of the prevalence, nonspecific presentation, and potential for modification of underlying diseases by these diagnoses. Drug levels, for example, should be measured in individuals taking anticonvulsants, tricyclic antidepressants, antiarrhythmics, and high-dose aspirin. History and examination should guide other laboratory investigations.

As already noted, in approximately 10% of cases falls by community-dwelling older adults are a nonspecific manifestation of an acute illness. In these situations the laboratory and diagnostic evaluation in these situations should be dictated by the suspected etiology. Examples of potentially useful tests include the electrocardiogram, cardiac enzymes, chest x-ray, urine analysis and culture, and blood cultures.

Brain imaging with computed tomography or magnetic resonance imaging is indicated only when focal abnormalities are noted on the neurologic examination. Cervical spine films may be helpful in individuals with impaired gait, lower extremity spasticity, and hyperreflexia suggestive of cervical spondylosis. A lateral dimension of the spinal canal of less than 12 mm is suggestive of a significant encroachment on the cervical cord. Magnetic resonance imaging should be pursued to confirm this finding only if the individual is deemed a candidate for neurosurgery.

A 24 h ambulatory cardiac monitor (Holter) is not warranted for the routine evaluation of nonsyncopal falls. The yield of ambulatory electrocardiographic monitoring is very low in these individuals. In addition, the results may be difficult to interpret because of the high prevalence of asymptomatic arrhythmias in older adults.

Balance and Gait Evaluation

Balance and gait represent end products of the accumulated effects of disease, age-related and lifestyle changes, and impairments in sensory, neurologic, and musculoskeletal functioning. Therefore, a careful assessment of balance and gait is an essential component of the fall evaluation. There is strong epidemiologic evidence to support balance and gait assessment as the single best means of identifying individuals at increased risk of falling.[9,10,13,18,83,84] Simple but reliable methods for observing an individual's balance and gait performance are available for use in clinical practice.[58,85]

Tests of balance and gait typically reproduce the position changes, postural responses, and gait maneuvers used during daily activities. The "Get Up and Go" test and the Performance-oriented Assessment of Mobility are two examples of clinical observation tests of balance and gait that have been used extensively in clinical practice.[58,85] Both assessments involve observing the individual perform various combinations of maneuvers such as getting up from a chair, reaching up, turning, bending over, assuming various narrowed stances, walking at a usual and rapid pace, and sitting in a chair. The examiner watches for instability or difficulty with performing each maneuver. Components of a simple balance and gait assessment are included in Table 66.4. The assessment may help to identify not only individuals at risk for falling but the circumstances in which falls are most likely to occur. As discussed next, combinations of medical, rehabilitative, and environmental interventions can be recommended based on the simple observations of balance and gait.

The role of computerized posturography in the clinical evaluation and treatment of balance and falling disorders remains to be determined. Posturography may be helpful in determining the relative contribution of visual, vestibular, and proprioceptive abnormalities to postural instability.[83] Posturography may further reveal the method by which the individual responds to postural perturbations. Although still under investigation, preliminary studies suggest that these findings may help in the development of effective rehabilitative interventions.[86]

Review of Fall Situations

The fourth component of the fall evaluation is a careful review of recent fall situations. In determining the contribution of possible intrinsic factors, the clinician should obtain information on premonitions; feelings of lightheadedness, vertigo, or unsteadiness; recent medications, particularly focusing on recent changes; preceding alcohol consumption; or symptoms of acute illness, postural hypotension, or dysrhythmias. A precise description of activity at the time of the fall is important as well.[87] Was the individual standing still, performing a simple

TABLE 66.4. Position changes, balance maneuvers, and gait components included in performance-oriented mobility assessment.

Position change or balance maneuver	Observation: fall risk if
Getting up from chair[a]	Does not get up with single movement; pushes up with arms or moves forward in chair first; unsteady on first standing
Sitting down in chair	Plops in chair; does not land in center
Withstanding nudge on sternum or pull at waist	Moves feet; begins to fall backward; grabs object for support; feet not touching side by side
Side by side standing with eyes open and shut	Same as above; eyes closed tests patient's reliance on visual input for balance
Neck turning	Moves feet; grabs object for support; feet not touching side by side; complains of vertigo, dizziness, or unsteadiness
Bending over	Unable to bend over to pick up small object (e.g., pen) from floor; grabs object to pull up on; requires multiple attempts to arise

Gait component or maneuver	Observation: fall risk if
Initiation[b]	Hesitates; stumbles; grabs object for support
Step height (raising feet with stepping)	Does not clear floor consistently (scrapes or shuffles); raises foot too high (more than 2 in.)
Step continuity	After first few steps, does not consistently begin raising one foot as other foot touches floor
Step symmetry	Step length not equal (pathologic side usually has longer step length; problem may be in hip, knee, ankle, or surrounding muscles)
Path deviation	Does not walk in straight line; weaves side to side
Turning	Stops before initiating turn, staggers; sways; grabs object for support

[a] Use hard, armless chair. Other more difficult balance maneuvers include tandem, semitandem, and one-leg standing.
[b] Patient walks down hallway at "usual pace," turns and comes back using usual walking aid. Repeat at "rapid pace." Examiner observes single component of gait at a time (analogous to heart examination). Other gait observations include heel–toe sequencing; armswing; trunk sway; stepping over objects.
Source: Modified with permission from *JAMA*. 1988; 259: 1191. "Copyright 1988, American Medical Association."

activity of daily living such as getting dressed, or walking? If walking, on what type of surface? Was the individual getting up or sitting down, arising from a lying position, going up or down stairs or curbs? If the fall occurred during routine and relatively nonhazardous activities, the goal of intervention will be to improve the safety and effectiveness of the maneuver during which the fall occurred. If, on the other hand, the fall occurred while performing more hazardous activities such as climbing on chairs or ladders, substitution of safer activities or avoidance should be recommended.

Environmental details that should be ascertained include obstacles in the immediate area of the fall; the volume and intensity of lighting; the floor or ground surface; objects being carried; footwear, including the fit, heel height, and type of sole; and walking aids used at the time of the fall. A home safety evaluation as well as careful review of specific fall situations may reveal remedial environmental hazards. While common sense dictates eliminating obvious hazards such as throw rugs and obstacles, these have not been shown to be independent risk factors. Still, a recent Cochrane review supports interventions to reduce home hazards, particularly by a trained professional for patients in the immediate posthospitalization period.[88,90]

Prevention and Therapy

The appropriate intervention strategy depends on the health status and fall history of the individual. For healthy individuals who have not suffered falls, the treatment goal is to maintain or improve balance, gait, flexibility, and endurance to decrease the risk of falls and to maintain mobility and functional independence. Recent clinical trials suggest that strength and balance training are effective in increasing lower extremity strength in healthier, more vigorous elderly persons.[91] In a case-control study, older persons who perform vigorous physical activity at least three times per week and have no limitations in their ADLs may be at a lower risk for fall-related fractures.[92] Recent evidence suggests that older adults who participate in a program of resistance exercise training once or twice weekly demonstrate improved neuromuscular performance and achieve muscle strength gains similar to those training 3 days per week.[93]

Further studies are needed to define the long-term effectiveness, optimal combination of exercise components, and minimal intensity required. In a recent randomized controlled trial, a low-cost multifactorial intervention based at a community organization was shown to be effective in reducing slips by 61%, trips by 56%, and falls by 29% in a group of healthy older adults during 1 year.[94] Evidence is emerging that among "healthier," less-impaired persons, exercise seems to have as strong an effect on falls as does the multifactorial approach in the less healthy.[95] The aim of treatment in older individuals who have already experienced falls or who suffer from chronic diseases and impairments is to reduce the rate of subsequent falls and decrease the incidence of fall-related morbidity such as injury, fear, inability to get up, functional decline, and immobility. The treatment strategy should be guided by the results of the assessment.[96–98] The governing concept should be that it is possible to reduce the risk of falls and fall sequelae by eliminating or modifying as many contributing factors as possible. Because of the overlapping, compensatory nature of the systems affecting stability as described earlier, simple interventions may result in major improvements, even if the interventions are not targeted at the systems believed to be most impaired.

As most of the factors contributing to fall risk are chronic diseases or impairments that may be modifiable, but only rarely curable, the treatment strategy should combine appropriate combinations of medical, surgical, rehabilitative, and environmental interventions. These interventions are summarized in Table 66.3. Similarly, the balance and gait assessment is useful not only for identifying individuals at risk for falling and the situations under which falls are likely to occur but can also be used to determine rehabilitative and environmental interventions that may decrease risk. Examples of using the results of balance and gait examination to guide treatment are outlined in Table 66.4. Rather than targeting one area of risk, an individualized, interdisciplinary, multifactorial approach to modifying all risk factors was shown to be most beneficial in reducing falls in older adults.[90] The withdrawal of psychotropic medications in association with a home-based exercise program had a relative hazard for falls of 0.34 (95% CI, 0.16–0.74) compared with maintaining the psychoactive medications and the exercise program.[99]

As can be seen from reviewing Tables 66.3 and 66.4, physical therapy is an integral part of any fall assessment and treatment program.[97] A home safety evaluation with recommendations for modification and adaptation, prescription of and training in the appropriate use of assistive devices, transfer and gait training, and instruction in muscle-strengthening and balance exercises are examples of fall preventive interventions carried out by a trained physical therapist.[97] The physical therapist may also help in treating the consequences of falls by teaching strategies for how to fall, or for getting up from the floor after a fall, and by encouraging confidence in performance of activities of daily living without falling. Recent evidence suggests that a home exercise program may reduce falls, but further evidence is needed to determine the long-term effects of this intervention.[100]

A randomized controlled trial of thrice-weekly progressive resistance exercises, walking, and balance training in a group of high-risk community-dwelling male fallers resulted in improved endurance and lower extremity strength and decreased fall rates.[101] A pre-planned meta-analysis of the seven federally funded Frailty and Injuries: Cooperative Studies of Intervention Techniques (FICSIT) Trials showed a 10% reduction in the adjusted fall incidence ratio for studies that included endurance, resistance, and flexibility exercise programs and a 17% reduction for those that only used balance.[102] After adjusting for fall risk factors, a moderate Tai Chi training program was found to reduce the risk of multiple falls by 48%.[103]

Promising treatment modalities for the prevention of fall-related fractures include treatment of osteoporosis, discussed in Chapter 43. Additionally, an assessment of falls is recommended for those patients who have already sustained a hip fracture.[104] Providing extra padding, through the use of various types of hip protectors, appears to be a promising approach for the prevention of hip fractures, one of the most serious consequences of falls among elderly persons.[105] These devices were recently shown to improve self-efficacy in high-risk community-dwelling older adults and to reduce the risk of hip fracture in a group of frail ambulatory elderly.[106]

Nursing Home

The first step to developing and implementing a fall evaluation and prevention program for institutionalized older adults is to establish appropriate goals. Not only are institutionalized older adults more likely than their community-dwelling counterparts to be frail, they are also more likely to have readily available alternatives to walking as a means of mobility. It is important to carefully assess the trade-offs of safety versus functional independence and mobility in institutionalized older adults, as an increase in physical activity may increase the risk of injury. Although the components of a fall evaluation are the same in nursing home and community-dwelling older adults, the relative contribution of chronic or situational risk factors may differ.

Predisposing Risk Factor Assessment

A thorough clinical evaluation aimed at identifying all contributing risk factors is the cornerstone of the evaluation among nursing home residents.[107] As with community-living elderly persons, the risk of falling increases with the number of impairments, suggesting again that ameliorating or eliminating as many risk factors as possible may decrease risk.[51,58,108] A careful examination of the risk factors noted in Table 66.3 is essential as the number and severity of impairments and diseases is greater among nursing home than community residents, and nonspecific and vague presentations, particularly among the large number of nursing home residents with cognitive impairment, render the clinical history less reliable.[109]

Laboratory Evaluation

As among community-living elderly persons, routine laboratory testing should be targeted toward conditions that are common and treatable. Additional testing should be considered on an individual resident basis, guided by the history and examination. There is no role for routine ambulatory cardiac monitoring for nonsyncopal falls among nursing home residents.

Balance and Gait Evaluation

Balance and gait assessment plays the same role in nursing home as in community residents. Reliable and validated assessments have been developed specifically for use among frail nursing home residents and hospital patients.[110]

Review of Fall Situations

Although many falls among nursing home residents are unwitnessed, there is greater opportunity to identify acute intrinsic and environmental contributors to falling among nursing home residents compared with community residents.[29,57] Symptoms experienced near the time of the fall such as dizziness may suggest postural hypotension, hypoglycemia, dysrhythmia, or a medication side effect. Chest pain may suggest angina or myocardial infarction. The immediate postfall physical examination should include a careful evaluation of postural blood pressure and pulse changes at both 1 and 3 min, focal neurologic signs, and signs of any acute illnesses that may present as a fall.

Environmental factors that are particularly relevant to nursing home residents include the presence of side rails, inappropriate use of walking aids such as walkers or wheelchairs, and the presence and application of vest, belt, or other restraints. Among nonambulatory nursing home residents, injurious falls are more likely to occur while seated or during transfers from the chair or bed level and to involve ill-fitting or poorly maintained equipment such as wheelchairs, shower chairs, or commodes.[111]

Prevention and Therapy

Although earlier studies demonstrated that careful assessment and intervention among nursing home residents who fall reduces the risk of hospitalization, there was little evidence that it prevents subsequent falls.[112] A recent randomized controlled trial of a nursing home consultation service demonstrated a reduction in the proportion of nursing home residents who were recurrent fallers, especially among those who adhered to the recommendations. These interventions included targeting environmental and personal safety issues, wheelchair use, transferring, and ambulation, along with psychotropic drug use.[60] The specific role of physical therapy in fall prevention among nursing home residents remains to be determined. Although on the one hand studies have not found physical therapy interventions to be effective,

other studies have shown that intense strength training results in increased strength, balance, and gait in even very frail elderly nursing home residents.[113,114] These seemingly conflicting results suggest that the optimal cost-effective strategy is to identify and treat those elderly persons most likely to benefit from a multifactorial intervention to prevent falls. At the very least, a physical therapy evaluation is warranted to prescribe and ensure the correct use of assistive devices, including walkers, canes, crutches, orthotics, and shoe modification.

Although researchers have failed to establish a causal link between medications and falls by nursing home residents, the strong association between medications and falling and the contribution of polypharmacy to other adverse events warrants frequent medication review and adjustment. The goal should be to reduce the total number and dosage of medications taken by nursing home residents. On the strength of the current evidence it is suggested that efforts to prevent falls in nursing homes should focus on decreasing the use of psychoactive medications, training staff members to perform safe transfers, and repairing broken equipment such as wheelchairs.

Environmental Assessment

In addition to assessing the environment at the time of a fall, ongoing environmental assessment aimed at removing potential hazards and modifying the environment to improve mobility and safety should be an ongoing practice in nursing homes. The provision of adequate lighting without glare; dry, nonslippery floors that are free of obstacles; high, firm chairs with arms; beds at appropriate heights for individual residents (feet should touch the floor with the knees bent at 90°); beds without upper side rails; and raised toilet seats with arms are preventive measures that should be implemented for all nursing home residents. Movable bed trays, which are often used by residents for support, should be considered a serious fall hazard. Footwear should be scrutinized; shoes that are ill fitting, have worn soles or heels, or are left untied are unsafe for nursing home residents. Slippers without backs, with soles that are either too slippery or have too high friction, or which provide little foot and ankle support are particularly hazardous, as is wearing stockings without shoes.

Restraints

Recent efforts, guided by federal regulations as well as by the results of several studies, have aimed at reducing the use of physical restraints. Although controlled studies are lacking, observational evidence suggests that physical restraints may contribute to falls, injuries, and death through strangulation as well as to other adverse outcomes such as withdrawal and depression.[30,115,116] One prospective study showed a 25% to 40% reduction in restraint use in a nursing home with restraint education with consultation compared to restraint education or control alone.[117] Increasingly, nursing homes are implementing alternative measures such as increased nurse-to-resident ratio, alternative seating, lowered side rails and bed heights for residents who climb out of bed, and alarms that are activated when residents try to get out of bed or move unassisted.[29] Although the effectiveness of these various techniques and devices remains to be determined, restraint reduction does appear to decrease the injury rate in those who fall.[33]

As noted for community-living elderly persons, injury prevention alternatives such as hip protectors are currently being tested.[105,118] It has been proven that hip protectors can be particularly effective in preventing hip fractures. At this point, however, patients complain about the discomfort and practicality of the device, thereby resulting in only a small percentage of at-risk patients wearing them. As a result, nursing home patients should be encouraged to use hip protectors to prevent injury from falls.[119]

Summary

Falling is a common event among community and nursing home residents. These falls may result in considerable morbidity, ranging from self-imposed activity restriction to serious injury and death. Until methods are available for accurately identifying those falls or fallers at risk for serious morbidity, all fallers should be assumed to be at risk. A small percent of falls result from a single, overwhelming intrinsic event such as a stroke, from the effects of a single disease process such as Parkinson's disease, or from overwhelming environmental hazards. The majority of falls are multifactorial, resulting from various combinations of intrinsic, activity-related, and environmental factors. Recent studies suggest that careful assessment and interventions aimed at identified risk factors and well-designed exercise programs may decrease the risk of falling. Most often, the goal of fall prevention programs should be to minimize the risk of falls and injuries without compromising function or mobility. As with all older individuals, however, the goals and priorities may be different for individual persons.

References

1. Hogue CC. Epidemiology of injury in older age. In: *Second Conference on the Epidemiology of Aging*. Bethesda: National Institutes of Health; 1980:127–138.
2. Droller H. Falls among elderly people living at home. *Geriatrics*. 1955:293–344.
3. Sheldon JH. On the natural history of falls in old age. *Br Med J*. 1960;2:1685–1690.
4. Fine W. An analysis of 277 falls in hospital. *Gerontol Clin*. 1959;1:292–300.
5. Tinetti ME, Inouye SK, Gill TM, Doucette JT. Shared risk factors for falls, incontinence, and functional dependence. Unifying the approach to geriatric syndromes. *JAMA*. 1995;273:1348–1353.
6. Kennedy TE, Coppard LC. The prevention of falls in later life: a report of the Kellogg International Group on Prevention of Falls in the Elderly. *Dan Med Bull*. 1987; 34:1–24.
7. Campbell AJ, Reinken J, Allan BC, Martinez GS. Falls in old age: a study of frequency and related clinical factors. *Age Ageing*. 1981;10(4):264–270.
8. Prudham D, Evans JG. Factors associated with falls in the elderly: a community study. *Age Ageing*. 1981;10(3): 141–146.
9. Tinetti ME, Speechley M, Ginter SF. Risk factors for falls among elderly persons living in the community. *N Engl J Med*. 1988;36:1701–1707.
10. Tinetti, ME, Liu WL, Claus EB. Predictors and prognosis of inability to get up after falls among elderly persons. *JAMA*. 1993;269:65–70.
11. Sattin RW. Falls among older persons: a public health perspective. *Annu Rev Public Health*. 1992;13(7):489–508.
12. O'Loughlin JL, Robitaille Y, Boivin JF, Suissa S. Incidence of and risk factors for falls and injurious falls among the community-dwelling elderly. *Am J Epidemiol*. 1993; 137(3):342–354.
13. Nevitt MC, Cummings SR, Hudes ES. Risk factors for injurious falls: a prospective study. *J Gerontol*. 1991;46(5): M164–M170.
14. Stevens JA, Hasbrouck LM, Durant TM, Dellinger AM, et al. Surveillance for injuries and violence among older adults. *MMWR CDC Surveill Summ*. 1999;48(8):27–50.
15. Sattin RW, Lambert Huber DA, DeVito CA, Rodriguez JG, et al. The incidence of fall injury events among the elderly in a defined population. *Am J Epidemiol*. 1990;131:1028–1037.
16. Tinetti ME, Doucette J, Claus E, Marottoli R. Risk factors for serious injury during falls by older persons in the community. *J Am Geriatr Soc*. 1995;43(11):1214–1221.
17. Salkeld G, Cameron ID, Cumming RG, Easter S, et al. Quality of life related to fear of falling and hip fracture in older women: a time trade off study [see comments]. *Br Med J*. 2000;320(7231):341–346.
18. Nevitt MC, Cummings SR, Kidd S, Black D. Risk factors for recurrent nonsyncopal falls. A prospective study. *JAMA*. 1989;261(18):2663–2668.
19 Cumming RG, Salkeld G, Thomas M, Szonyi G. Prospective study of the impact of fear of falling on activities of daily living, SF-36 scores, and nursing home admission. *J Gerontol A Biol Sci Med Sci*. 2000;55(5):M299–M305.
20. Maki BE, Holliday PJ, Topper AK. Fear of falling and postural performance in the elderly. *J Gerontol*. 1991; 46(4):M123–M131.
21. Arfken CL, Lach HW, Birge SJ, Miller JP. The prevalence and correlates of fear of falling in elderly persons living in the community. *Am J Public Health*. 1994;84(4):565–570.

22. Tinetti ME, Mendes de Leon CF, Doucette JT, Baker DI. Fear of falling and fall-related efficacy in relationship to functioning among community-living elders. *J Gerontol.* 1994;49(3):M140–M147.

23. Kosorok MR, Omenn GS, Diehr P, Koepsell TD, Patrick DL. Restricted activity days among older adults. *Am J Public Health.* 1992;82(9):1263–1267.

24. Grisso JA, Schwarz DF, Wolfson V, Polansky M, LaPann K. The impact of falls in an inner-city elderly African-American population. *J Am Geriatr Soc.* 1992; 40(7):673–678.

25. Wolinsky FD, Johnson RJ, Fitzgerald JF. Falling, health status, and the use of health services by older adults. A prospective study. *Med Care.* 1992;30(7):587–597.

26. Kiel DP, O'Sullivan P, Teno JM, Mor V. Health care utilization and functional status in the aged following a fall. *Med Care.* 1991;29:221–228.

27. Dunn JE, Rudberg MA, Furner SE, Cassel CK. Mortality, disability, and falls in older persons: the role of underlying disease and disability. *Am J Public Health.* 1992;82(3): 395–400.

28. Tinetti ME, Williams CS. Falls, injuries due to falls, and the risk of admission to a nursing home. *N Engl J Med.* 1997; 337(18):1279–1284.

29. Rubenstein LZ, Josephson KR, Robbins AS. Falls in the nursing home. *Ann Intern Med.* 1994;121:442–451.

30. Tinetti ME, Liu WL, Ginter SF. Mechanical restraint use and fall-related injuries among residents of skilled nursing facilities. *Ann Intern Med.* 1992;116(5):369–374.

31. Capezuti E, Strumpf NE, Evans LK, Grisso JA, Maislin G. The relationship between physical restraint removal and falls and injuries among nursing home residents. *J Gerontol A Biol Sci Med Sci.* 1998;53(1):M47–M52.

32. Capezuti E, Evans L, Strumpf N, Maislin G. Physical restraint use and falls in nursing home residents. *J Am Geriatr Soc.* 1996;44(6):627–633.

33. Neufeld RR, Libow LS, Foley WJ, Dunbar JM, Cohen C, Breuer B. Restraint reduction reduces serious injuries among nursing home residents. *J Am Geriatr Soc.* 1999; 47(10):1202–1207.

34. Nutt JG, Marsden CD, Thompson PD. Human walking and higher-level gait disorders, particularly in the elderly. *Neurology.* 1993;43(2):268–279.

35. Lach HW, Reed AT, Arfken CL, Miller JP, Paige GD, et al. Falls in the elderly: reliability of a classification system. *J Am Geriatr Soc.* 1991;39(2):197–202.

36. Tinetti ME. Instability and falling in elderly patients. *Semin Neurol.* 1989;9(1):39–45.

37. Wolfson LI, Whipple R, Amerman P, Kaplam J, Kleinberg A. Gait and balance in the elderly. Two functional capacities that link sensory and motor ability to falls. *Clin Geriatr Med.* 1985;1(3):649–659.

38. Lord SR, Ward JA, Williams P, Anstey KJ. Physiological factors associated with falls in older community-dwelling women. *J Am Geriatr Soc.* 1994;42(10):1110–1117.

39. Glynn RJ, Seddon JM, Krug JH, Sahagian CR, et al. Falls in elderly patients with glaucoma. *Arch Ophthalmol.* 1991; 109(2):205–210.

40. Tobis JS, Reinsch S, Swanson JM, Bryd M, Scharf T. Visual perception dominance of fallers among community-

dwelling older adults. *J Am Geriatr Soc.* 1985;33(5): 330–333.

41. Hazell JW. Vestibular problems of balance. *Age Ageing.* 1979;8(4):258–260.

42. Woolf SH, Kamerow DB, Lawrence RS, Medalie JH, Estes EH. The periodic health examination of older adults: the recommendations of the U.S. Preventive Services Task Force. Part II. Screening tests. *J Am Geriatr Soc.* 1990; 38(8):933–942.

43. Wyke B. Cervical articular contribution to posture and gait: their relation to senile disequilibrium. *Age Ageing.* 1979;8(4):251–258.

44. Masdeu JC, Wolfson L, Lantos G, Tobin JN, Grober E, et al. Brain white-matter changes in the elderly prone to falling. *Arch Neurol.* 1989;46(12):1291–1296.

45. Whipple RH, Wolfson LI, Amerman PM. The relationship of knee and ankle weakness to falls in nursing home residents: an isokinetic study. *J Am Geriatr Soc.* 1987;35(1): 13–20.

46. Lipsitz LA. Orthostatic hypotension in the elderly. *N Engl J Med.* 1989;321:952–957.

47. Ray WA, Griffin MR. Prescribed medications, and the risk of falling. *Top Geriatr Rehabil.* 1990;5:12–20.

48. Leipzig RM, Cumming RG, Tinetti ME. Drugs and falls in older people: a systematic review and meta-analysis: I. Psychotropic drugs. *J Am Geriatr Soc.* 1999;47(1):30–39.

49. Liu B, Anderson G, Mittmann N, To T, Axcell T, et al. Use of selective serotonin-reuptake inhibitors of tricyclic antidepressants and risk of hip fractures in elderly people. *Lancet.* 1998;351(9112):1303–1307.

50. Leipzig RM, Cumming RG, Tinetti ME. Drugs and falls in older people: a systematic review and meta-analysis: II. Cardiac and analgesic drugs. *J Am Geriatr Soc.* 1999;47(1): 40–50.

51. Robbins AS, Rubenstein LZ, Josephson KR, Schulman BL, et al. Predictors of falls among elderly people. Results of two population-based studies. *Arch Intern Med.* 1989; 149(7):1628–1633.

52. Gray SL, Mahoney JE, Blough DK. Adverse drug events in elderly patients receiving home health services following hospital discharge. *Ann Pharmacother.* 1999;33(11): 1147–1153.

53. Kapoor WN. Syncope in older persons. *J Am Geriatr Soc.* 1994;42(4):426–436.

54. Startzell JK, Owens DA, Mulfinger LM, et al. Stair negotiation in older people: a review. *J Am Geriatr Soc.* 2000;48(5):567–580.

55. Stevens M, Holman CDJ, Bennett N. Preventing falls in older people: impact of an intervention to reduce environmental hazards in the home. *J Am Geriatr Soc.* 2001;49:1442–1447.

56. Owen DH. Maintaining posture and avoiding tripping. Optical information for detecting and controlling orientation and locomotion. *Clin Geriatr Med.* 1985;1(3):581–599.

57. Lipsitz LA, Jonsson PV, Kelley MM, et al. Causes and correlates of recurrent falls in ambulatory frail elderly. *J Gerontol.* 1991;46:M114–M122.

58. Tinetti ME, Williams TF, Mayewski R. Fall risk index for elderly patients based on number of chronic disabilities. *Am J Med.* 1986;80(3):429–434.

59. Donald IP, Pitt K, Armstrong E, et al. Preventing falls on an elderly care rehabilitation ward. *Clin Rehabil.* 2000; 14(2):178–185.

60. Ray WA, Taylor JA, Meador KG, et al. A randomized trial of a consultation service to reduce falls in nursing homes. *JAMA.* 1997;278(7):557–562.

61. Melton LJ, Riggs BL. Risk factors for injury after a fall. *Clin Geriatr Med.* 1985;1(3):525–539.

62. Cummings SR, Nevitt MC. A hypothesis: the causes of hip fractures. *J Gerontol.* 1989;44(4):M107–M111.

63. Lord SR, McLean D, Stathers G. Physiological factors associated with injurious falls in older people living in the community. *Gerontology.* 1992;38(6):338–346.

64. Kelsey JL, Browner WS, Seeley DG, et al. Risk factors for fractures of the distal forearm and proximal humerus. The Study of Osteoporotic Fractures Research Group. *Am J Epidemiol.* 1992;135(5):477–489.

65. Ryynanen OP, Kivela SL, Honkanen R, et al. Recurrent elderly fallers. *Scand J Prim Health Care.* 1992;10(4): 277–283.

66. Greenspan SL, Myers ER, Maitland LA, et al. Fall severity and bone mineral density as risk factors for hip fracture in ambulatory elderly. *JAMA.* 1994;271(2):128–133.

67. Grisso J. Risk factors for falls as a cause of hip fracture in women. *N Engl J Med.* 1991;324(19):1326–1331

68. Myers AH, Baker SP, VanNatta ML, et al. Risk factors associated with falls and injuries among elderly institutionalized persons. *Am J Epidemiol.* 1991;133(11): 1179–1190.

69. Campbell AJ, Borrie MJ, Spears GF. Risk factors for falls in a community-based prospective study of people 70 years and older. *J Gerontol.* 1989;44(4):M112–M117.

70. Mahoney J, Sager M, Dunham NC, et al. Risk of falls after hospital discharge. *J Am Geriatr Soc.* 1994;42(3):269–274.

71. Oliver D, Britton M, Seed P, et al. Development and evaluation of evidence based risk assessment tool (STRATIFY) to predict which elderly inpatients will fall: case-control and cohort studies [see comments]. *Br Med J.* 1997;315(7115):1049–1053.

72. Sorock GS, Bush TL, Golden AL, et al. Physical activity and fracture risk in a free-living elderly cohort. *J Gerontol.* 1988;43(5):M134–M139.

73. Schwartz AV, Kelsey JL, Sidney S, et al. Characteristics of falls and risk of hip fracture in elderly men. *Osteoporos Int.* 1998;8(3):240–246.

74. Davis JW, Ross PD, Nevitt MC, et al. Risk factors for falls and for serious injuries on falling among older Japanese women in Hawaii. *J Am Geriatr Soc.* 1999;47(7):792–798.

75. Wenger NS, Shekelle PG. Assessing care of vulnerable elders: ACOVE project overview. *Ann Intern Med.* 2001;135(8 pt 2):642–646.

76. Shekelle PG, MacLean CH, Morton SC, et al. ACOVE quality indicators. *Ann Intern Med.* 2001;135(8 pt 2): 653–667.

77. Rubenstein LZ, Powers CM, MacLean CH. Quality indicators for the management and prevention of falls and mobility problems in vulnerable elders. *Ann Intern Med.* 2001;135(8 pt 2):686–693.

78. Guideline for the prevention of falls in older persons. American Geriatrics Society, British Geriatrics Society, and American Academy of Orthopaedic Surgeons Panel on Falls Prevention. *J Am Geriatr Soc.* 2001;49(5):664–672.

79. Tinetti ME, Speechley M. Prevention of falls among the elderly. *N Engl J Med.* 1989;320:1055–1059.

80. Vellas BJ, Wayne SJ, Garry PJ, et al. A two-year longitudinal study of falls in 482 community-dwelling elderly adults. *J Gerontol A Biol Sci Med Sci.* 1998;53:M264–M274.

81. Sudarsky L. Geriatrics: gait disorders in the elderly. *N Engl J Med.* 1990;322(20):1441–1446.

82. MacPhee GJ, Crowther JA, McAlpine CH. A simple screening test for hearing impairment in elderly patients. *Age Ageing.* 1988;17(5):347–351.

83. Maki BE, Holliday PJ, Topper AK. A prospective study of postural balance and risk of falling in an ambulatory and independent elderly population. *J Gerontol.* 1994; 49(2):M72–M84.

84. Hausdorff JM, Rios DA, Edelberg HK. Gait variability and fall risk in community-living older adults: a 1-year prospective study. *Arch Phys Med Rehabil.* 2001;82(8): 1050–1056.

85. Mathias S, Nayak US, Isaacs B. Balance in elderly patients: the "Get-up and Go" test. *Arch Phys Med Rehabil.* 1986; 67(6):387–389.

86. Rose DJ, Clark S. Can the control of bodily orientation be significantly improved in a group of older adults with a history of falls? *J Am Geriatr Soc.* 2000;48(3):275–282.

87. Berg WP, Alessio HM, Mills EM, et al. Circumstances and consequences of falls in independent community-dwelling older adults. *Age Ageing.* 1997;26(4):261–268.

88. Carter SE, Campbell EM, Sanson-Fisher RW et al. Environmental hazards in the homes of older people. *Age Ageing.* 1997;26(3):195–202.

89. Cumming RG, Thomas M, Szonyi G, et al. Home visits by an occupational therapist for assessment and modification of environmental hazards: a randomized trial of falls prevention. *J Am Geriatr Soc.* 1999;47(12):1397–1402.

90. Gillespie LD, Gillespie WJ, Cumming R, et al. Interventions for preventing falls in the elderly. *Cochrane Database Syst Rev.* 2000;5(2)CD000340.

91. Judge JO, Whipple RH, Wolfson LI. Effects of resistive and balance exercises on isokinetic strength in older persons. *J Am Geriatr Soc.* 1994;42(9):937–946.

92. Stevens JA, Powell KE, Smith SM, et al. Physical activity, functional limitations, and the risk of fall-related fractures in community-dwelling elderly. *Ann Epidemiol.* 1997;7(1): 54–61.

93. Taaffe DR, Duret C, Wheeler S, et al. Once-weekly resistance exercise improves muscle strength and neuromuscular performance in older adults. *J Am Geriatr Soc.* 1999;47(10):1208–1214.

94. Steinberg M, Cartwright C, Peel N, et al. A sustainable programme to prevent falls and near falls in community dwelling older people: results of a randomised trial. *J Epidemiol Commun Health.* 2000;54(3):227–232.

95. Buchner DM, Cress ME, de Lateur BJ, et al. The effect of strength and endurance training on gait, balance, fall risk, and health services use in community-living older adults. *J Gerontol A Biol Sci Med Sci.* 1997;52(4):M218–M224.

96. Tinetti MA, Baker DI, McAvay G, et al. A multifactorial intervention to reduce the risk of falling among elderly

people living in the community. *N Engl J Med.* 1994; 331(13):821–827.

97. Koch M, Gottschalk M, Baker DI, et al. An impairment and disability assessment and treatment protocol for community-living elderly persons. *Phys Ther.* 1994;74(4): 286–294; discussion 295–298.

98. Lipsitz LA. An 85-year old woman with a history of falls. *JAMA.* 1996;276(1):447–454.

99. Campbell AJ, Robertson MC, Gardner MM, et al. Psychotropic medication withdrawal and a home-based exercise program to prevent falls: a randomized, controlled trial. *J Am Geriatr Soc.* 1999;47(7):850–853.

100. Lord SR, Ward JA, Williams P, et al. The effect of a 12-month exercise trial on balance, strength, and falls in older women: a randomized controlled trial. *J Am Geriatr Soc.* 1995;43(11):1198–1206.

101. Rubenstein LZ, Josephson KR, Trueblood PR, et al. Effects of a group exercise program on strength, mobility, and falls among fall-prone elderly men. *J Gerontol A Biol Sci Med Sci.* 2000;55(6):M317–M321.

102. Province MA, Hadley EC, Hornbrook MC, et al. The effects of exercise on falls in elderly patients. A pre-planned meta-analysis of the FICSIT Trials. Frailty and Injuries: Cooperative Studies of Intervention Techniques [see comments]. *JAMA.* 1995;273(17):1341–1347.

103. Wolf SL, Barnhart HX, Kutner NG, et al. Reducing frailty and falls in older persons: an investigation of Tai Chi and computerized balance training. Atlanta FICSIT Group. Frailty and Injuries: Cooperative Studies of Intervention Techniques [see comments]. *J Am Geriatr Soc.* 1996;44(5): 489–497.

104. Morrison RS, Chassin MR, Siu AL. The medical consultant's role in caring for patients with hip fracture. *Ann Intern Med.* 1998;128(12 pt 1):1010–1020.

105. Lauritzen JB, Petersen MM, Lund B. Effect of external hip protectors on hip fractures. *Lancet.* 1993;341(8836):11–13.

106. Kannus P, Parkkari J, Niemi S, et al. Prevention of hip fracture in elderly people with use of a hip protector. *N Engl J Med.* 2000;343(21):1506–1513.

107. Kiely DK, Kiel DP, Burrows AB, et al. Identifying nursing home residents at risk for falling. *J Am Geriatr Soc.* 1998: 46(5):551–555.

108. Thapa PB, Gideon P, Fought RL, et al. Psychotropic drugs and risk of recurrent falls in ambulatory nursing home residents. *Am J Epidemiol.* 1995;142(2):202–211.

109. Luukinen H, Koski K, Laippala P, et al. Risk factors for recurrent falls in the elderly in long-term institutional care. *Public Health.* 1995;109(1)57–65.

110. Winograd CH, Lemsky CM, Nevitt MC, et al. Development of a physical performance and mobility examination. *J Am Geriatr Soc.* 1994;42(7):743–749.

111. Thapa PB, Brockman KG, Gideon P, et al. Injurious falls in nonambulatory nursing home residents: a comparative study of circumstances, incidence, and risk factors. *J Am Geriatr Soc.* 1996;44(3):273–278.

112. Rubenstein LZ, Robbins AS, Josephson KR, et al. The value of assessing falls in an elderly population. *Ann Intern Med.* 1990;113(4):308-316.

113. Mulrow CD, Gerety MB, Kanten D, et al. A randomized trial of physical rehabilitation for very frail nursing home residents. *JAMA.* 1994;271(7):519–524.

114. Fiatarone MA, O'Neill EF, Ryan ND, et al. Exercise training and nutritional supplementation for physical frailty in very elderly people. *N Engl J Med.* 1994:330(25): 1769–1775.

115. Miles SH, Irvine P. Deaths caused by physical restraints. *Gerontologist.* 1992;32(6):762–766.

116. Evans LK, Strumpf NE. Tying down the elderly. A review of the literature on physical restraint. *J Am Geriatr Soc.* 1989;7(1):65–74.

117. Evans LK, Strumpf NE, Allen-Taylor SL, et al. A clinical trial to reduce restraints in nursing homes. *J Am Geriatr Soc.* 1997;45(6):675–681.

118. Kannus P, Parkkari J, Poutala J. Comparison of force attenuation properties of four different hip protectors under simulated falling conditions in the elderly: an in vitro biomechanical study. *Bone.* 1999;25(2):229–235.

119. Parker MJ, Gillespie LD, Gillespie WJ. Hip protectors for preventing hip fractures in the elderly. *Cochrane Database Syst Rev.* 2000;5(2):CD001255.

67
Chronic Dizziness and Vertigo

Aman Nanda and Mary E. Tinetti

Dizziness is a subjective sensation of postural instability or of illusory motion. It is a nonspecific term that includes vertigo, disequilibrium, lightheadedness, spinning, giddiness, faintness, floating, feeling woozy, and many other sensations. As the etiologies differ, dizziness is often classified on the basis of duration as acute (present for less than 1–2 months) or chronic (present for more than 1–2 months). Because the causes of acute dizziness are usually identical for patients of all ages, this chapter is therefore limited to a discussion of chronic dizziness.

Prevalence and Morbidity

Dizziness is one of the most common presenting complaints in primary care practice for persons aged 65 years and older.[1] The prevalence of dizziness ranges from 4% to 30% in this age group.[2-4] Dizziness increases with age, with a 10% increase every 5 years. After adjusting for age, women are 30% more likely than men to report dizziness.[3]

Chronic dizziness has been associated with an increased risk of falls, syncope, functional disability, and, in some studies, strokes and death.[4-12] It is strongly associated with fear of falling and reduced confidence in performing daily activities.[13] In one study, 47% of patients with dizziness expressed a fear of falling compared to only 3% of the controls.[14] It has also been associated with worsening of depressive symptoms, self-rated health, and participation in social activities.[15]

Types of Dizziness

There is no universally accepted classification of dizziness. Dizziness has been categorized by either duration (acute/chronic) or types of sensations. Drachman and Hart[16] categorized dizziness into four subtypes based on sensations: vertigo, presyncope, disequilibrium, and other.

Vertigo is a spinning or rotational sensation, either of the patient with respect to the environment (subjective vertigo) or of the environment with respect to the patient (objective vertigo). The key element is the perception of motion. Vertigo often begins instantaneously, is episodic, and when severe may be associated with nausea, vomiting, and a staggering gait. Vertigo is considered to result from a disturbance within the vestibular system or its connections. However, the lack of a spinning sensation may not be used to exclude vestibular diseases, as patients with vestibular problems can describe dizziness as an imbalance, disequilibrium, or other sensation. Also, etiologies outside the vestibular system (e.g., cervical causes of dizziness) may result in vertigo.

Presyncope is a feeling of lightheadedness or impending faintness or a feeling that one is about to pass out. It is usually considered to result from a hypoperfusion of the brain. A number of cardiovascular conditions may cause presyncope and syncope.

Disequilibrium is a feeling of imbalance or unsteadiness usually not associated with any abnormal head sensations. The patient feels as if he or she is going to fall. Disequilibrium usually results from abnormalities in the proprioceptive system.

The category "other" is defined as a vague feeling other than vertigo, presyncope, or disequilibrium. The patient may describe "floating," "wooziness," "spaciness," "whirling," and other nonspecific sensations.

A person may have a combination of two or more of these four types of dizziness; this is the most common type of dizziness reported by older persons[17,18] and is believed to result from systemic disorders such as anemia, electrolyte imbalances, diabetes, and hypothyroidism, or from the presence of combinations of diseases affecting the vestibular, central nervous, visual, or proprioceptive system.

These sensations as noted here have diagnostic specificity among persons of all ages with acute dizziness and among younger persons with chronic dizziness. Among older persons with chronic dizziness, however, there is a less consistent correlation between the type of sensation and specific organ systems.

Mechanisms of Equilibrium

Given that dizziness is a sensation of postural instability, a review of the mechanisms determining balance and equilibrium may help in understanding the pathophysiology of dizziness. Maintenance of balance and equilibrium results from a complex integration of sensory information obtained from the visual, auditory, vestibular, and proprioceptive systems by the cerebral cortex and cerebellum and the use of this information for the appropriate motor response.

The visual system helps in maintaining balance by providing signals from the retina to the occipital cortex, necessary for providing a stable retinal image during head movement. The vestibulo-ocular reflex (VOR) controls the position of the eyes, enabling maintenance of a stable visual image during head movement. The VOR depends on the information relayed by the vestibular nucleus to the sixth (abducens) cranial nerve nucleus in the pons and, via the medial longitudinal fasciculus, to the third (oculomotor) and fourth (trochlear) cranial nerve nuclei in the midbrain. Binocular vision and depth perception also are important visual signals for spatial orientation.

Hearing assists in stability by detecting and interpreting auditory stimuli, which enables one to localize and be oriented in space. Hearing is particularly helpful when other sensory modalities are impaired. Hearing impairment, common in older persons, may be secondary to aging, to disease processes, or to the presence of excess cerumen. Although impaired hearing may be a marker of vestibular dysfunction as both sensory modalities operate through the eighth cranial nerve, studies have reported an independent association between decreased hearing and dizziness.[4,18]

The vestibular system contributes to spatial orientation at rest, as well as during acceleration, and is responsible for visual fixation during head and body movements. The vestibular system includes the semicircular canals, utricle, saccule, vestibular nerve, and vestibular nucleus in the brainstem. The semicircular canals respond to changes in angular acceleration, and the utricle and saccule respond to linear acceleration. The sensory epithelium of the semicircular canals, utricle, and saccule consists of hair cells. The afferents from these hair cells relay information to the vestibular nuclei in the brainstem. The vestibular nuclei relay this information to the nuclei of the third, fourth, and sixth cranial nerves, spinal cord (vestibulospinal tract), and cerebellum (vestibulocerebellar pathway).

The proprioceptive system provides information about changes in position and movements and helps maintain equilibrium during changes in position. The components of the proprioceptive system are mechanoreceptors in the joints, peripheral nerves, posterior columns in the spinal cord, and multiple central nervous system connections. The afferent impulses relay information to the cerebral cortex via the thalamus and to the cerebellum via the spinocerebellar tract.

The cerebral cortex, cerebellum, and brainstem integrate information received from the visual, auditory, vestibular, and proprioceptive systems and direct the musculoskeletal system via efferent pathways toward the response appropriate for maintaining balance and equilibrium. Lesions in the brain may cause disordered integration of information from these systems, resulting in imbalance/dysequilibrium.

Effects of Aging on Sensory Systems

Evidence suggests that age-related changes occur in each of the vestibular, visual, auditory, and proprioceptive systems. Although these age-related changes do not likely cause clinical disease, they may predispose older persons to the occurrence of dizziness by making them more vulnerable to the effects of superimposed impairments and diseases. Degenerative changes and reductions in the number of sensory cells (hair cells) in the semicircular canals, saccule, and utricle have been reported with aging.[19,20] Richter noted a significant decrease in the number of cells in Scarpa's ganglion.[21] Bergstrom found a 37% reduction in the number of nerve fibers in the vestibular nerves of five people over age 75.[22] Age-related visual changes include a decrease in visual acuity, dark adaptation, contrast sensitivity, and accommodation.[23,24] Age-related decline in proprioception has not been extensively studied. Skinner et al. reported a significant deterioration in joint-position sense in older individuals, but Kokemen et al. concluded that there is no major decline in joint-position sensation with aging.[25,26]

Causes of Chronic Dizziness

Dizziness results from either discrete or combined effects of disorders or impairments in the multiple systems responsible for maintaining equilibrium. Acute and, to a lesser extent, chronic dizziness result when a disorder in one of these systems causes abnormal or decreased sensory input, resulting in a mismatch of information about the movements of the head or body. Discrete causes of chronic dizziness can be divided into central nervous system disorders, vestibular disorders, psychogenic causes, systemic causes, medications, and miscellaneous. The relative frequency of these causes is unclear, as there has been a wide variability in their reported prevalences.[9,10,16–18,27–31]

Discrete Diseases Causing Dizziness

Central Nervous System Causes

Cerebrovascular diseases have been identified as a primary or contributing cause of dizziness in 4% to 70% of older patients.[9,10,16–18,28–32] Vertebrobasilar ischemia results from an obstruction of the blood flow in the vertebrobasilar arteries, most commonly caused by arteriosclerosis leading to either transient ischemic attacks (TIA) or infarction. Because the basilar artery is responsible for the blood supply to the eighth nerve and vestibular nuclei, dizziness is one of the cardinal signs of basilar artery insufficiency. Apart from acute dizziness, which is usually in the form of prodromal symptoms in patients with vertebrobasilar TIA, patients may complain of chronic dizziness following a brainstem infarct. Dizziness may also result from anterior or posterior inferior cerebellar artery ischemia but is uncommon with internal carotid cerebral artery disease.[32]

Other central nervous system disorders such as parkinsonism, acoustic neuroma, and basilar artery migraine (rare in older persons) may also cause dizziness.[33–35]

Vestibular Causes

Vestibular diseases have been identified as a primary or contributing cause in 4% to 71% of cases of dizziness.[9,16,17,27,28,30,31] Common vestibular diseases causing chronic dizziness in older persons include benign paroxysmal positional vertigo, Meniere's disease, recurrent vestibulopathy, and acoustic neuroma. Ototoxic medications may also lead to complaints of dizziness.

Benign paroxysmal positional vertigo (BPPV), reportedly responsible for between 4% and 34% of cases of recurrent episodes of dizziness,[9,16,17,27,28,30] is characterized by brief bouts (seconds) vertigo of sudden onset that is provoked by certain changes in the head position (e.g., rolling over in bed into a lateral position, gazing upward, or leaning forward). Another characteristic feature of BPPV is an accompanying rotational nystagmus. The vertigo is often associated with nausea or vomiting. Patients typically experience recurrent bouts of positional vertigo over days to months, with quiescent periods between episodes.

Most BPPV cases have no identifiable cause. The most common known causes are a history of head trauma and viral neurolabyrinthitis.[36] The currently accepted pathophysiologic mechanism of BPPV is the presence of free-floating particulate matter, most likely dislodged otoconia (tiny calciferous granules that form part of the

receptor mechanism in the otolith apparatus) in the endolymph of the posterior semicircular canal. The exact mechanism by which free-floating particulate matter causes paroxysmal vertigo and nystagmus is unknown, but presumably it is the result of the movement of the debris causing alterations in endolymphatic pressure.[37–39] The otoconia have been shown to undergo degenerative changes with aging, which might also be responsible for their dislodgment from the utriculus.[40] A definitive diagnosis of benign paroxysmal positional vertigo can be made by the Dix–Hallpike test (discussed here).[41]

Meniere's disease is an idiopathic inner ear disorder characterized by episodic vertigo, tinnitus, fluctuating hearing loss, and a sensation of fullness in the inner ear. The frequency of this disease has been reported to be 2% to 8% in dizziness cases.[9,16,17,27,28,30] Males and females are affected equally, with onset usually occurring during the fifth decade of life. The main pathologic finding in patients with Meniere's disease is an excess of endolymph within the cochlea and vestibular labyrinth. The patient develops a varying degree of sensations of fullness or pressure, along with hearing loss, and tinnitus in the affected ear. Vertiginous episodes usually last from 1 to 24 h. The patient may complain of a sense of unsteadiness after the acute episode. In the early stages, the hearing loss is completely reversible, but in later stages, partial or complete hearing loss occurs in about 90% of the patients.[42] The hearing loss has a sensorineural pattern, with hearing at the lower frequencies tending to be worse.

Recurrent vestibulopathy was first described by LeLeiver and Barber in 1981.[43] This clinical entity is characterized by recurrent episodes of vertigo, usually lasting from 5 min to 24 h, without auditory or neurologic signs or symptoms. The exact cause is not known.[44] The absence of auditory symptoms differentiates it from Meniere's disease. Spontaneous recovery has been reported in 62% of patients over an 8.5-year follow-up.[45]

An acoustic neuroma is a benign tumor of the eighth cranial nerve, characterized by tinnitus and progressive unilateral sensorineural hearing loss that is greater for higher frequencies. This tumor has been reported in 2% to 3% of older persons with dizziness.[17,28] Vertigo is a complaint of 19% of patients, whereas 48% complain of imbalance or disequilibrium.[46] As the tumor grows, patients may complain of parasthesias or pain in the trigeminal nerve distribution. A large tumor can cause cerebellar ataxia.

Postural Hypotension

In various studies, postural hypotension has been identified as a primary or contributing cause in 2% to 15% of dizziness cases.[18,27–29] Postural hypotension has commonly been defined as a drop in systolic arterial blood pressure of at least 20 mmHg or a fall in diastolic blood pressure of 10 mmHg after standing up from a supine position. However, there are no uniform criteria for postural hypotension in older persons, and at least 15 different definitions exist for postural hypotension.[47,48] Blood pressure is commonly measured at 1 and 3 min after standing, but in some older persons a significant orthostatic drop occurs only after 10 to 30 min (delayed orthostatic hypotension).[49] Some older persons complain of dizziness on standing, but their blood pressure changes do not meet the criteria of postural hypotension. In one study of 9672 elderly women, postural hypotension was reported in 14% of the participants, but only 3% of these patients complained of dizziness, whereas 16% of the subjects reported dizziness on standing without any postural blood pressure changes.[6] In another study, 9% of patients with postural blood pressure changes complained of dizziness, while 31% complained of dizziness on standing with no postural blood pressure changes.[29] These results suggest that a postural drop in blood pressure is not always symptomatic and that, conversely, not all dizziness with postural changes is the result of orthostatic blood pressure changes.

Postprandial hypotension, usually defined as a decrease in systolic blood pressure of 20 mmHg or more in a sitting or standing posture within 1 to 2 h of eating a meal, may also cause dizziness.[50,51] A recent study showed that the effects of postprandial hypotension and orthostatic hypotension are additive but not synergistic, suggesting that the two entities have different pathophysiologic mechanisms.[52] Postprandial reductions in blood pressure may result in falls, syncope, weakness, or dizziness.

Systemic Causes

Systemic disorders may contribute to instability or dizziness by affecting the sensory, central, or effector components. In addition, systemic disorders may result in decreased cerebral perfusion or oxygen delivery, fatigue, or confusion, many of which in turn may result in instability or dizziness. Common examples include anemia, hypothyroidism, congestive heart failure, and diabetes mellitus with anatomic dysfunction. Carotid sinus hypersensitivity or carotid sinus syndrome can also cause dizziness, falls, or syncopal episodes. Wearing tight collars can precipitate dizziness, syncopal episodes, or falls upon sudden head turning or looking up. Carotid sinus syndrome is defined as a sinus pause of more than 3 s or a drop in systolic blood pressure of more than 50 mmHg following carotid sinus massage for 5 s. In one study, carotid sinus syndrome was reported in 45% of patients with dizziness, falls, and syncope.[53] However, this high percentage is likely because the study population was a select group referred to a syncope clinic.

The prevalence of dizziness in patients with systemic disorders is not known, but studies have found a significant association between dizziness and a history of angina, myocardial infarction, hypertension, or diabetes mellitus and with the total number of chronic conditions.[4,17,18,54]

Psychogenic Causes

Psychogenic causes of dizziness have been reported in the range of 0% to 57% in older persons with dizziness.[9,16–18,29–31,54,55] The most common conditions in older persons are depressive and anxiety disorders, either the primary cause or a contributing factor. Patients usually present with a vague sensation of dizziness, along with other somatic complaints and with symptoms of psychologic disorders. Studies have reported an independent association between dizziness and depression or anxiety.[3,4,17,54]

Cervical Causes

The reported frequency of dizziness caused by cervical spine disorders ranges from 0% to 65%.[16,27,29,30] Disorders of the cervical spine should be suspected when dizziness worsens with head turning or walking on uneven surfaces. Both proprioceptive and vascular mechanisms have been postulated.[56,57] *Proprioceptive* deficits in the cervical spine can cause dizziness secondary to the impaired information from proprioceptive receptors present in the facet joints of the cervical spine. In older persons, cervical osteoarthritis most likely causes dizziness via this mechanism. The patient usually complains of pain in the neck on movement, along with a worsening of dizziness. There is often a history of arthritis or whiplash injury. Further examination may reveal a decreased range of motion of the neck or signs of radiculopathy or myelopathy or spastic gait.

A *vascular mechanism* causing cervical dizziness is thought to result from an obstruction to the vertebral arteries. One theory is that when there is an extensive blockage of one vertebral artery, rotation of the head can sufficiently obstruct the other vertebral artery to cause brainstem ischemia.[56] Another theory is that when a person turns their head or neck, an osteoarthritic spur may press upon the nearby vertebral artery, causing a transient disruption of the blood flow.[57]

Medications

Medications have frequently been reported to cause or contribute to chronic dizziness.[17,18,28] Several classes of medications, such as anxiolytic drugs, antidepressants, antihypertensive drugs, aminoglycosides, chemotherapeutic agents, and nonsteroidal anti-inflammatory drugs, are known to produce dizziness as a side effect.[58]

Medications may cause dizziness through various mechanisms. Antihistamines and tricyclic antidepressants trigger dizziness through their anticholinergic side effects. Aminoglycosides have direct ototoxic effects when used in high dosages or for longer durations, especially when renal function is impaired. Other ototoxic agents include nonsteroidal anti-inflammatory agents such as aspirin, quinine, loop diuretics, and erythromycin and vancomycin analogues.[59] Meclizine, often prescribed for dizziness, has anticholinergic properties and may even exacerbate the dizziness caused by nonlabyrinthine disease.[57] When taking a medication history, one should also inquire about over-the-counter drugs such as cold preparations, which are prone to cause dizziness. In addition to specific medications, an independent association between the use of multiple medications and dizziness has been reported.[18,54]

Diseases Causing Impairment of Vision

Diseases such as cataracts, glaucoma, and macular degeneration, which are common in older persons, may cause dizziness by impairing the visual functions. Davis, in his study of 117 patients with complaints of dizziness, reported that 26% suffered from disorders of the visual system, but he concluded that it was the major cause of dizziness in only 1% of the cases.[28] In this study, 13% of the patients had cataracts. Other studies have also reported an association between poor vision or cataracts and dizziness.[4,54]

Chronic Dizziness as a Geriatric Syndrome

In the previous section, dizziness in older persons was considered a symptom of one or more discrete diseases. The results of recent studies, however, suggest the possibility of a multifactorial etiology of dizziness.[3,4,18,30] In these studies, chronic dizziness has been associated with risk factors such as angina, myocardial infarction, stroke, arthritis, diabetes, syncope, anxiety, depressive symptoms, impaired hearing, alcohol consumption, smoking, nervousness, and the use of several classes of medications. In a recent cohort study of a large community sample, the authors found an association between factors in multiple domains and the occurrence of chronic dizziness. The factors that were independently associated with chronic dizziness included anxiety, depressive symptoms, decreased hearing, postural hypotension, impaired balance and gait, the use of five or more medications, and a past history of myocardial infarction. A person with more than five of the risk factors was five times more likely to report chronic dizziness than a person with fewer than two factors.[18] These findings were validated in a cohort of patients seen in a geriatric assessment center.[54]

An association among the characteristics in multiple domains and dizziness suggests that dizziness may be considered as a geriatric syndrome, similar to delirium and falls.[18] Geriatric syndromes are health conditions experienced more frequently by older than by younger persons and result from the accumulated effect of impairments and diseases involving multiple systems. The importance of considering chronic dizziness a geriatric syndrome is that a multifactorial assessment and intervention strategy, as described in the following section, may be more effective at alleviating the symptom than the standard disease-oriented approach.

The concept of a geriatric syndrome does not preclude the possibility that a single disease may be primarily responsible for impairment in a subset of persons. Rather, it acknowledges that many symptoms such as dizziness in older persons cannot be explained adequately on the basis of a single disease.

Evaluation

Dizziness is a challenging problem for physicians who take care of older persons. The differential diagnosis as presented in the previous section is broad. The potential workup is extensive and expensive. The goal should be to eliminate the cause of the dizziness, if possible. If not, the goal should then be to alleviate the dizziness to the extent possible and to avoid the adverse consequences such as falls, functional disability, and increased depressive symptoms. Based on these goals and on the available evidence, a stepwise approach to the evaluation of chronic dizziness seems warranted. The existence of discrete diseases is usually suggested by the results of the history, physical examination, and routine laboratory evaluation. Only in the subset of patients in whom discrete diagnosis is suggested by their routine evaluation should a targeted battery of expensive tests be pursued, and only if the results of these tests are likely to influence treatment or prognosis. For the majority of older persons in whom a routine evaluation does not suggest a single discrete cause, the clinician should identify the various factors contributing to dizziness, some of which may be amenable to treatment. This approach is based on the fact that identifying and ameliorating one or more of these contributors might help alleviate the dizziness and its adverse consequences. Table 67.1 lists the possible causes of chronic dizziness, the salient history and examination findings, relevant investigations, and treatment.

An evaluation of dizziness begins with the clinical history. The patient should be asked to be as precise as possible about the sensations of dizziness, an often difficult task because patients may experience more than one

TABLE 67.1. Evaluation and treatment of chronic dizziness

Possible causes	History	Examination	Investigations	Treatment
Central nervous system				
Brainstem (vertebrobasilar) and/or cerebellar infarcts/ hemorrhages	History of dizziness (e.g., vertigo, near fainting, wooziness) usually associated with slurred speech; visual changes; one-sided weakness and/or gait ataxia; truncal ataxia	Detailed neurologic examination, localizing the lesion	CT or MRI scan; MRI is preferred	Low-dose aspirin or ticlopidine or clopidigel if infarct; rehabilitation therapy
Cerebellopontine angle tumor: acoustic neuroma, schwanomma, etc.	History of vertigo or dysequilibrium; unilateral hearing loss; tinnitus	Detailed neurologic examination	Audiometry reveals asymmetric hearing loss; which may be further evaluated by MRI	Surgical excision
Parkinson's disease	Dysequilibrium; imbalance; slow motor activities; slow walking, etc.	Increased muscular rigidity; bradykinesia; tremor; orthostatic hypotension	Diagnosis is made by history and examination	Antiparkinson treatment
Vestibulocochlear system				
Benign paroxysmal positional vertigo	Sudden and fleeting episodes of intense vertigo with specific head position (e.g., rolling over in bed into lateral position; looking upward; bending forward); episodes last days to months and are often recurrent	History of episodic vertigo; nystagmus; confirmed by Dix–Hallpike maneuver; along with absence of signs suggesting other pathology, especially central involvement	None	Epley maneuver is helpful in treatment provided the side of the vertigo is known; vestibular rehabilitation and sometimes a short course of vestibular suppressants
Meniere's disease	Episodic vertigo for a few hours; there are no symptoms between episodes; tinnitus; fluctuating hearing loss; sensation of fullness in ears	If unilateral, then bedside vestibulo-ocular reflex test will be abnormal	An audiogram revealing a sensorineural hearing loss (low more than high frequencies) is confirmatory; MRI scan to rule out retrocochlear lesions	Salt restriction and diuretics are the mainstay; during acute attacks vestibular suppressants may be helpful to relieve vertigo; surgical interventions, including endolymphatic decompression, gentamicin perfusion, vestibular nerve section, and labyrinthectomy should be considered only in severe cases
Peripheral nerves				
Diabetes; vitamin B_{12} deficiency; hypothyroidism; syphilis; idiopathic	Disequilibrium; worse in dark or on uneven surfaces	Decreased vibration or position sense; steppage gait	Serum glucose; B_{12} levels; thyroid function test; VDRL	Treatment of the underlying disease; good lighting; appropriate walking aid and footwear; gait and balance training exercises
Cervical spine				
Degenerative or inflammatory arthritis, spondylosis, whiplash injury	Neck pain, usually episodic dizziness secondary to change in position of the neck; history of trauma or arthritis	Decreased neck range of motion; decreased vibratory or joint position sense; signs of radiculopathy or myelopathy or vertebrobasilar ischemia	Cervical spine series	Treatment of underlying disease; cervical or balance exercises; cervical collar; consider surgery
Vision				
Presbyopia, cataract; glaucoma; macular degeneration	Difficulty in vision; use of bifocals or trifocals	Abnormalities in near/distant acuity	Vision testing; referral to ophthalmologist	Good lighting without glare; appropriate refraction; consider avoiding bifocals or trifocals; drugs for glaucoma; surgery

Cause	History/Symptoms	Examination	Investigations	Management
Hearing Cerumen; presbycusis; otosclerosis	Difficulty in hearing in social situations; unilateral or bilateral deafness	Otoscopy: cerumen; abnormal findings with whisper test, Rinne's test, Weber's test	Audioscopic examination; audiometry	Cerumen removal; ear wax drops; hearing aid; surgery (for otosclerosis); hearing rehabilitation; listening devices
Hypotension Orthostatic volume/salt depletion; drugs; vasovagal attack; autonomic dysfunction; diabetes; parkinsonism; deconditioning	Near fainting; worse when getting up, walking, exercising; may be asymptomatic; complaints consistent with predisposing diseases; medication history	Blood pressure and heart rate; signs of predisposing diseases	Investigations relevant to predisposing diseases	Salt and water repletion; dosage adjustment or removal of the offending drugs; treatment of relevant diseases; ankle pumps; slow rising; elevate head of bed; graduated stockings; reconditioning exercises; drug therapy, fludrocortisone, midodrine, if needed
Postprandial	Same as orthostatic hypotension except the onset is within 1h of eating	Postprandial blood pressure and heart rate measurement	None	Frequent small meals; avoid exertion after meals; have caffeine with meals; slow rising; avoid antihypertensive drugs with or near meal time
Systemic diseases Cardiac/metabolic/respiratory: e.g., cardiac arrhythmias, valvular lesions, coronary artery disease, cardiomyopathy; heart failure; COPD; diabetes; thyroid disorders; renal disorders; anemia	Symptoms of the underlying diseases	Signs of the underlying diseases	Relevant investigations	Variable, depending on the underlying disease
Psychiatric disorders Anxiety, depression	Usually continuous nonspecific dizziness; fatigue; poor appetite; sleep problems; somatic complaints; poor concentration	Positive results on anxiety or depression screening		Psychotherapy; antidepressant therapy after considering risks and benefits
Medications Ototoxic: aminoglycosides, diuretics, nonsteroidal anti-inflammatory drugs, vestibular suppressants	Vestibulocochlear symptoms (as discussed above)	Presence of nystagmus, bedside vestibular function test can be abnormal, abnormal caloric test		Eliminate, substitute, or reduce specific offending medication if possible; reduce the drugs to lowest possible dose
Others: antihypertensives, antianxiety drugs, anticholinergics, antidepressants, anticonvulsants, antipsychotics	H/o fatigue; confusion; dizziness often vague, can be continuous, dizziness can be postural	May have postural hypotension		

manifestation or a vague sensation. The frequency and duration of dizziness, as well as any associated symptoms such as hearing loss, ear fullness, tinnitus, diplopia, dysarthria, and syncopal episodes, are all important. Recurrent episodes of dizziness lasting less than 1 min are seen in BPPV, whereas recurrent episodes of dizziness associated with fluctuating hearing loss or tinnitus and ear fullness are suggestive of Meniere's disease. The clinician should ask the patient whether the dizziness is episodic or continuous. For example, in BPPV, Meniere's disease, or CNS disorders, the dizziness is episodic whereas psychogenic dizziness is usually continuous. The patient should also be asked about any precipitating or provoking factors, such as standing from a supine or sitting position, rolling over in bed, or changing the position of the head or neck (i.e., looking up or from side to side). One should inquire as to whether dizziness occurs after eating meals, which can be caused by postprandial hypotension. The physician should also ask about comorbid conditions, such as cardiac diseases, diabetes, renal disorders, anxiety, or depression, which can predispose or exacerbate dizziness. A careful review of all medications, including over-the-counter drugs, is also important. All patients with complaints of dizziness should be evaluated for depressive symptoms or anxiety disorders.

The physical examination should include measurements of orthostatic changes in blood pressure. Blood pressure and heart rate measurements should be taken after at least 5 min of quiet lying and then at 1 to 2 min after standing. The patient's ears should be examined for excessive wax or structural abnormalities in the external ears. Hearing should be tested by either a whisper test or an audioscope. Near and distant vision should also be tested.

The examiner should look for spontaneous nystagmus. The nystagmus in peripheral vestibular lesions is usually horizontal or rotatory and is suppressed by visual fixation, whereas that in central lesions is vertical and is not suppressed by visual fixation. Frenzel glasses (high-diopter lenses in a frame with a light source) should be used, if available. These lenses eliminate visual fixation and magnify nystagmus. Another possible method of detecting vestibular dysfunction is to do a one-leg or tandem stand on thick foam with the eyes closed, which eliminates visual and proprioceptive input to maintain balance. However, the sensitivity and specificity of this method have not been determined.

In the examination of cranial nerves, diplopia, dysarthria, dysphagia, or facial weakness are suggestive of vertebrobasilar involvement. One should look for cerebellar signs, such as gait ataxia, truncal ataxia, or dysmetria, which suggest etiologies such as a cerebellar stroke or cerebellopontine angle tumors. In the latter,

patients may present with unilateral hearing loss, tinnitus, absence of corneal reflex, and facial parasthesias and ataxia as well as dizziness. Gait and balance examinations should be performed. A poorer performance with eyes closed rather than open suggests a vestibular or proprioceptive etiology. A steppage gait suggests a proprioceptive etiology, as does an improvement in gait when the patient places a fingertip on the examiner's fingertip. Vibration sense testing is a more sensitive test of proprioception than is testing for joint position sense.

Range of neck motion, preferably in a standing position, should be assessed. A decrease in the range of motion, with or without symptoms of dizziness, may be due to a cervical process or, secondarily, to vestibular dysfunction. (The sensation of dizziness on head turning leads to a voluntary restriction in head turning, which, in turn, may lead to a decreased range of neck motion.) Because decreased head turning can interfere with central compensation, recognizing it in patients with vestibular dysfunction is important because vestibular rehabilitation is helpful.

A detailed history and physical examination should help the physician in identifying one or more causes responsible for dizziness. Apart from the history and physical examination, certain provocative tests can be done at bedside to evaluate the vestibular system.

Provocative Tests

1. To see if the vestibulo-ocular reflex (VOR), which helps to maintain visual stability during head movement, is intact, the following three tests can be done. The sensitivities, specificities and predictive values of these tests for vestibular lesions in older persons have not been established.

a. In the head-thrust test, the patient is asked to fixate on the examiner's nose, and the head is moved rapidly by the examiner about $10°$ to the left or right. In a normally functioning VOR, the eyes will be fixed on the target. In patients with a vestibular deficit, the eyes are carried away from the target along with the head, followed by a corrective saccade back to the target. For example, in a patient with a right-sided vestibular lesion, head thrusts to the right will produce a slipping away of the pupils from the target, followed by a corrective movement back to the target, whereas head thrusts to the left will produce a normal response of the eyes.[60,61]

b. In the postheadshake test, with fixation eliminated by Frenzel lenses, the head is rotated either passively by the examiner or actively by the subject at a frequency of about 2 Hz in the horizontal plane for about 10 s, and then the examiner looks for nystagmus when the head is stopped. In unilateral peripheral vestibular lesions, there is a horizontal nystagmus with the fast phase usually beating toward the stronger ear, whereas in central lesions the nystagmus may be vertical.[60,62]

2. Dynamic visual acuity testing is done by asking the patient to read a fixed eye chart while the examiner moves the head horizontally at a frequency of 1 to 2 Hz. A drop in acuity of two rows or more from the baseline is suggestive of an abnormal vestibulo-ocular reflex.[63] This test is sometimes difficult to perform because patients may be able to read at times when the head is not in motion (i.e., at turnaround points or by resisting movements).[60]

These tests are more helpful in detecting unilateral than bilateral vestibular dysfunction. It is important to remember that compensatory mechanisms may mask a vestibular deficit when these maneuvers are used in patients with long-standing vestibular loss.[60] If the findings of these tests are abnormal, then the patient can be referred for more sophisticated vestibular testing, such as electronystagmography and rotational testing.

3. The Stepping Test, originally described by Unterberger[64] and later modified by Fukuda,[65] is positive when there is a lesion in the vestibulospinal system. The patient is asked to stand at the center of a circle drawn on the floor. The circle is divided into sections by lines passing at 30° angles. The patient is blindfolded and is asked to outstretch both arms at 90° to the body. The patient is then asked to flex and raise high first one knee and then the other and to continue stepping forward at a normal walking speed for a total of 50 or 100 steps. The examiner notes body sway while the patient marches in place with the eyes closed. In a unilateral vestibular lesion or in acoustic neuroma, there will be a gradual rotation of the body (more than 30°) toward the affected side.[60,65,66]

4. The Dix–Hallpike Maneuver[41] can definitively establish a diagnosis of BPPV.[37] The patient is seated on an examination table with the head rotated 30° to 45° to one side. The patient is asked to fix his vision on the examiner's forehead. The examiner holds the patient's head firmly in the same position and moves the patient from a seated to a supine position with the head hanging below the edge of the table and the chin pointing slightly upward. The examiner should note for the direction, latency, and duration of the nystagmus and the latency and duration of vertigo, if present. The diagnostic criteria for BPPV are (1) vertigo associated with a rotatory nystagmus; (2) a latency (typically of 1–2 s) between the completion of the maneuver and the onset of vertigo and nystagmus; (3) a paroxysmal nature of the vertigo and nystagmus (lasting for 10–20 s); and (4) fatigability (decrease in the intensity of the vertigo and nystagmus with repeated testing).[37]

Routine Laboratory Evaluation

A small battery of laboratory tests should be performed on all patients with chronic dizziness because the prevalence of undetected abnormalities is high and because results often lead to effective treatment. Hematocrit, glucose, blood urea nitrogen, electrolytes, thyroid function tests, and vitamin B_{12} levels should be ordered in all patients complaining of dizziness. If a cardiovascular etiology is suspected, an ECG to evaluate for the presence of cardiac arrhythmia is indicated. Holter monitoring and tilt table testing are indicated only if there is a strong suspicion of transient/intermittent cardiac arrhythmia or unexplained syncope. Audiometry, which includes pure tone assessment, speech discrimination, impedance measurement, and evoked responses, is recommended for evaluating dizzy patients with hearing loss. Gradual hearing loss is characteristic of acoustic neuroma, while Meniere's disease typically presents with fluctuating hearing loss. Also, in acoustic neuroma an audiogram reveals a sensorineural hearing loss, which is more for higher than for lower frequencies, whereas in Meniere's disease sensorineural hearing loss is more for lower frequencies.

Specialized Testing

Vestibular Function Tests

Several tests for vestibular function that might be considered in patients with a history and physical examination finding suggestive of vestibular disease include electronystagmography, rotational testing, and computerized posturography.

Electronystagmography is the most established and widely used test. Eye movements are recorded with electrodes that record changes in scalp potential produced by the corneal–retinal potential. The procedure consists of a battery of tests designed to record eye movements in response to visual and vestibular stimuli, including oculomotor evaluation, positional testing, and caloric testing.[67] The oculomotor evaluation involves saccade testing, pursuit testing, optokinetic nystagmus, and spontaneous and gaze-evoked nystagmus. The positional testing is designed to detect nystagmus evoked when the head is held in different positions. The *caloric testing* assesses the symmetry of vestibular functions. This test can indicate the side of involvement in unilateral vestibular lesions. Each ear is stimulated first with warm (44°C) and then cool water (30°C), each instilled over 30 s. The temperature change stimulates or suppresses the respective horizontal semicircular canals, resulting in nystagmus.[68] A decreased response will occur on the ipsilateral side in peripheral vestibular disorder. Patients with suspected bilateral vestibular loss should undergo rotational chair testing to confirm the finding.[67] Aging minimally affects responses to the caloric test.[69]

The *rotational chair test* uses a series of well-controlled rotational stimuli to provoke nystagmus. The patient is seated on a chair in a dark, soundproof room. The patient is asked to fixate on an imaginary visual target while the chair is oscillated at different frequencies and the eye movements are recorded. This test reflects the function of the vestibulo-ocular system. Findings can reveal the degree of peripheral or central vestibular dysfunction; serial measurements can be used to detect improvement or worsening of the dysfunction. The effects of aging on the rotational chair test are not well documented because inconclusive results have been produced by too few studies that lack standardization.[69]

Computerized posturography provides information related to functional ability of the patient to maintain balance. It quantifies the functions of the vestibulospinal system. The patient stands on a platform that is embedded with four sensors to monitor sway. This test has two components, a sensory organization test (SOT) and a motor control test (MCT). The SOT measures the ability of the patient to maintain her balance when visual and somatosensory inputs are systematically disrupted, whereas in the MCT the patient experiences abrupt changes in the center of gravity produced by horizontal movements and rotations of the platform.[67] Rather than providing localizing information, this test provides information regarding which types of stimuli (visual, vestibular, and proprioceptive) the patient can or cannot use to maintain balance.[67] This test is useful in providing additional information when peripheral vestibular pathology is suggested by the vestibular function test, but the results are inconclusive.[70] Effects of aging on posturography have been documented and consist of an inability to perform well with reduced visual or somatosensory information and a general reliance on a hip strategy to maintain balance.[71]

Neuroimaging

Not all patients with dizziness need neuroimaging. Magnetic resonance imaging scans should be done if the history or physical examination is suggestive of a stroke or cerebellopontine angle tumor.

Treatment

Treatment is ideally directed toward a specific cause. However, investigators have acknowledged the limitations of a diagnosis-oriented approach for the evaluation and management of chronic dizziness.[18,72] Also, the presentation sometimes does not permit identification of a specific cause. Therefore, if the history, examination, and routine laboratory testing do not suggest a discrete cause, therapeutic trials are often the best way to determine significant contributors. Older persons often have multiple comorbid diseases and impairments that contribute to dizziness. The most effective treatment, therefore, may be to ameliorate one or more potential etiologic factors.[73]

Medical Therapy

Medical therapy for individual diseases is discussed in Table 67.1. Patients should be treated for anxiety or depression. If there is impairment of vision or hearing, it should be corrected. Medication-associated dizziness responds to dosage adjustment or to medication withdrawal. One should try to reduce all drugs to the lowest possible dosages.

Vestibular suppressants, including antihistamines (e.g., meclizine) and anticholinergic agents (scopolamine), are commonly used for symptomatic relief. These agents are effective for acute dizziness but play little role in managing chronic dizziness. Meclizine is a weak antihistaminic agent usually taken orally in doses of 12.5 to 25 mg three times a day, as needed. Vestibular suppressants should not be used long term because of their CNS side effects and because they suppress central and vestibular adaptation and thus may worsen or exacerbate dizziness.[74] Benzodiazepines (e.g., diazepam) may be beneficial to patients with severe unilateral peripheral vestibular dysfunction. Scopolamine should not be used in older persons due to its anticholinergic side effects such as urinary retention and deficits in cognition.

Rehabilitation

Vestibular rehabilitation therapy is an important and effective management strategy for patients with peripheral and central vestibular causes of dizziness. Studies have shown a reduction in symptoms and disability following rehabilitation therapy.[75–78] Vestibular rehabilitation includes combinations of exercises involving head and eye movements (while sitting and standing) designed to provoke vertigo and unsteadiness. It also involves various dynamic balance exercises and exercises to improve gait stability during head movement, visual and vestibular interactions, and vestibular spinal responses. The movements are repeated until they can no longer be tolerated, and the number of repetitions are gradually increased over a period of 6 to 8 weeks.[79] Initially, the exercises may worsen the dizziness, but over time (weeks to months) movement-related dizziness improves, likely because of central adaptation. Generally, a good functional recovery can be achieved by patients with peripheral vestibular disorders, but rarely does complete recovery occur in patients with central vestibular dysfunction, although they can experience considerable functional improvement.[80] Vestibular rehabilitation can be administered in a classroom setting or one-to-one with a physical therapist. Also, patients can perform exercises independently at home after being instructed by a physical therapist. This therapy also has been shown to alleviate dizziness in patients who have anxiety, probably by educating them about their dizziness and by encouraging them to cope actively with their problem.[81]

The *canalith repositioning procedure*, introduced by Epley,[82] is a currently recommended treatment for benign positional vertigo.[37] The purpose of this bedside maneuver is to move free-floating debris by the effects of gravity from the posterior semicircular canal into the utriculus of the vestibular labyrinth, where it will no longer affect the dynamics of the semicircular canals.[82] In this procedure, a Dix–Hallpike maneuver is performed with the patient's head rotated 45° toward the affected ear and hanging below the edge of the table, and a vibrator is applied to the ipsilateral mastoid process. After the cessation of the provoked vertigo and nystagmus, the head, which is hanging below the edge of the table, is rotated 45° to the opposite side. This maneuver may induce a brief episode of vertigo. The examiner should hold the head in this position and wait for about 10 to 15 s or until the vertigo ceases. Then the head and body are further rotated until the head is in a facedown position. This maneuver may again induce a brief vertigo. The patient should be kept in the final facedown position for about 10 to 15 s or until the vertigo ceases.

Then, with the head kept in the same position, the patient is brought to a seated position. Once the patient is upright, the head is turned forward with the chin tilted slightly downward. The patient should be instructed not to lie flat and to keep the head relatively upright for the next 24 to 48 h. Another option would be to instruct the patient to wear a cervical collar and neither to lie supine nor to tilt the head upward, downward, or to the right or left more than 30°.[83] These strategies are to prevent the loose debris from gravitating back to the posterior semicircular canal. There are no data available to support these recommendations. Investigators have tried gentle manual vibration of the head instead of using a vibrator during the treatment and have found it effective; 60% of the patients reported improvement with this procedure without using a vibrator and 92% reported improvement with the use of the vibrator.[83]

In patients who cannot keep their head in a relatively upright position for 1 to 2 days, a different maneuver described by Brandt and Daroff[84] can be used.[85] The patient is asked to sit on a table sideways with eyes closed and to rotate the head horizontally about 45°. Then the patient should rapidly lie on their side in the opposite direction and should wait in the same position until the vertigo has resolved or for 30 s. The patient should then sit up rapidly and wait for another 30 s. The movement is then repeated in the opposite direction.[85] This maneuver can be repeated every 3 h while awake and can be terminated if the patient is symptom free for 2 consecutive days.[84] The patient can perform these exercises at home. It usually takes 1 to 2 weeks for the symptoms to be resolved. These exercises likely work either by habituation or by dislodging debris from the posterior semicircular canals.[85]

Physiotherapy in the form of cervical exercises and relaxation techniques has been found to be effective for patients with cervical dizziness.[86] Progressive, competency-based balance exercises have proved effective in enhancing a sense of stability and may be useful for patients with dizziness related to sensory or motor deficits.

Surgery

Surgical therapy is needed in a small group of dizzy patients. Surgical excision is the treatment of choice for cerebellopontine angle tumors. Surgery is reserved for disabling unilateral peripheral disease unresponsive to medical therapy. Surgical procedures can be ablative or nonablative. Ablative procedures include transmastoid labyrinthectomy and partial vestibular neurectomy. The primary indication for either procedure is uncontrolled Meniere's disease or peripheral vestibulopathy.[87] Nonablative procedures include endolymphatic sac decompression and posterior canal occlusion. Endolymphatic sac decompression is confined to cases of Meniere's disease but its role is controversial.[87,88] Surgery is indicated for only those disabled patients of BPPV who are refractory to the canalith repositioning procedure despite multiple attempts. The two procedures used to disable the posterior semicircular canal include singular neurectomy or occlusion of the posterior semicircular canal.[87,89,90]

Patient Education

Patients should be given basic education concerning the functioning of the balance system and the pathophysiology of dizziness. This knowledge enables patients to understand the body movements responsible for these symptoms and also alleviates their anxiety about this problem.[81] They should be instructed on modifying their activities; for example, if orthostatic hypotension is detected, patients should be instructed to rise slowly from sitting or supine positions. Movements such as looking up, reaching up, or bending down are to be avoided, in part by storing items at home strategically. However, patients should be cautioned not to habitually avoid other movements such as head turning because doing so may compromise central adaptation, thereby exacerbating dizziness. Patients should be instructed to avoid walking in the dark. They should be reminded to avoid over-the-counter drugs that may exacerbate dizziness.

References

1. Sloane PD. Dizziness in primary care. Results from the national ambulatory medical care survey. *J Fam Pract.* 1989: 29:33–38.
2. Hale WE, Perkins LL, May FE, Marks RG, Stewart RB. Symptom prevalence in the elderly. An evaluation of age, sex, disease, and medication use. *J Am Geriatr Soc.* 1986:34: 333–340.
3. Colledge NR, Wilson JA, Macintyre CCA, MacLennan WJ. The prevalence and characteristics of dizziness in an elderly community. *Age Ageing.* 1994:23:117–120.
4. Sloane P, Blazer D, George LK. Dizziness in a community elderly population. *J Am Geriatr Soc.* 1989:37:101–108.
5. Tilvis RS, Hakala S-M, Valvanne J, Erkinjuntii T. Postural hypotension and dizziness in a general aged population: a four-year follow-up of the Helsinki Aging Study. *J Am Geriatr Soc.* 1996:44:809–814.
6. Ensrud KE, Nevitt MC, Yunis C, Hulley SB, Grimm RH, Cummings SR. Postural hypotension and postural dizziness in elderly women. *Arch Intern Med.* 1992:152: 1058–1064.
7. Boult C, Murphy J, Sloane P, Mor V, Drone C. The relation of dizziness to functional decline. *J Am Geriatr Soc.* 1991:39: 858–861.
8. Sixt E, Landahl S. Postural disturbances in a 75 year old population: prevalence and functional consequences. *Age Ageing.* 1987:16:393–398.
9. Kroenke K, Lucas CA, Rosenberg ML, et al. Causes of persistent dizziness: a prospective study of 100 patients in ambulatory care. *Ann Intern Med.* 1992:117:898–904.
10. Grimby A, Rosenhall U. Health related quality of life and dizziness in old age. *Gerontology.* 1995:41:286–298.
11. O'Loughlin JL, Robitaille Y, Boivin JF, Suissa S. Incidence of and risk factors for falls and injurious falls among the community-dwelling elderly. *Am J Epidemiol.* 1993:137: 342–354.
12. Tinetti ME, Doucette J, Claus E, Marottoli R. Risk factors for serious injury during falls by older persons in the community. *J Am Geriatr Soc.* 1995:43:1214–1221.
13. Tinetti ME, Mendes de Leon CF, Doucette JT, Baker DI. Fear of falling and fall-related efficacy in relationship to functioning among community-living elders. *J Gerontol.* 1994:49:M140–M147.
14. Burker EJ, Wong H, Sloane PD, Mattingly D, Preisser J, Mitchell CM. Predictors of fear of falling in dizzy and non dizzy elderly. *Psychol Aging.* 1995:10:104–110.
15. Tinetti ME, Williams CS, Gill TM. Health, functional and psychological outcomes among older persons with chronic dizziness. *J Am Geriatr Soc.* 2000:48:417–421.
16. Drachman DA, Hart CW. An approach to the dizzy patient. *Neurology.* 1972:22:323–334.
17. Sloane PD, Baloh RW. Persistent dizziness in geriatric patients. *J Am Geriatr Soc.* 1989:37:1031–1038.
18. Tinetti ME, Williams CS, Gill TM. Dizziness among older adults: a possible geriatric syndrome. *Ann Intern Med.* 2000: 132:337–344.
19. Johnson LG. Degenerative changes and anomalies of the vestibular system in man. *Laryngoscope.* 1971:81: 1682–1694.
20. Rosenhall U. Degenerative patterns in the aging human vestibular neuro-epithelia. *Acta Otolaryngol.* 1973:76: 208–220.
21. Richter E. Quantitative study of human Scarp's ganglion and vestibular sensory epithelium. *Acta Otolaryngol.* 1980:90:199–208.
22. Bergstrom B. Morphology of the vestibular nerve. The number of myleinated vestibular nerve fibers in man at various ages. *Acta Otolaryngol.* 1973:76:173–179.
23. Sekuler R, Hutman LP. Spatial vision and aging. 1: Contrast sensitivity. *J Gerontol.* 1980:35:692–699.
24. Hutman LP, Sekuler R. Spatial vision and aging. 2: Criterion effects. *J Gerontol.* 1980:35:700–706.
25. Skinner HB, Barrack RL, Cook SD. Age-related decline in proprioception. *Clin Orthop Relat Res.* 1984:184:208–211.
26. Kokmen E, Bossemeyer RW, Williams WJ. Quantitative evaluation of joint motion sensation in an aging population. *J Gerontol.* 1978:33:62–67.
27. Lawson J, Fitzgerald J, Birchall J, Aldren CP, Kenny RA. Diagnosis of geriatric patients with severe dizziness. *J Am Geriatr Soc.* 1999:47:12–17.
28. Davis LE. Dizziness in elderly men. *J Am Geriatr Soc.* 1994: 42:1184–1188.
29. Colledge NR, Barr-Hamilton RM, Lewis SJ, Sellar RJ, Wilson JA. Evaluation of investigations to diagnose the cause of dizziness in elderly people: a community-based controlled study. *Br Med J.* 1996:313:788–792.
30. Katsarkas A. Dizziness in aging. A retrospective study of 1194 cases. *Otolaryngol Head Neck Surg.* 1994:110:296–301.
31. Hoffman RM, Einstadter D, Kroenke K. Evaluating dizziness. *Am J Med.* 1999:107:468–478.
32. Fisher CM. Vertigo in cerebrovascular disease. *Arch Otolaryngol.* 1967:85:529–534.
33. Harker LA, Rassekh CH. Episodic vertigo in basilar artery migraine. *Otolaryngol Head Neck Surg.* 1987:96:239–250.
34. Reichert WH, Doolittle J, McDowell FH. Vestibular dysfunction in Parkinson disease. *Neurology.* 1982:32:1133–1138.
35. Hitselberger WE. Tumors of the cerebellopontine angle in relation to vertigo. *Arch Otolaryngol.* 1967:85:539–541.
36. Baloh RW, Honrubia V, Jacobson K. Benign positional vertigo: clinical and oculographic features in 240 cases. *Neurology.* 1987:37:371–378.
37. Furman JM, Cass SP. Benign paroxysmal positional vertigo [review article]. *N Engl J Med.* 1999:341:1590–1596.
38. Welling DB, Parnes LS, O'Brien B, Bakaletz LO, Brackmann DE, Hinojosa R. Particulate matter in the posterior semicircular canal. *Laryngoscope.* 1997:107:90–94.
39. Parnes LS, McClure JA. Free-floating endolymph particles: a new operative finding during posterior semicircular canal occlusion. *Laryngoscope.* 1992:102:988–992.
40. Ross MD, Peacor D, Johnson LG, et al. Observations on normal and degenerating human otoconia. *Ann Otol Rhinol Laryngol.* 1976:85:310–326.

41. Dix MR, Hallpike CS. The pathology, symptomatology and diagnosis of certain common disorders of the vestibular system. *Proc R Soc Med.* 1952:45:341–354.

42. Green DJ, Blum DJ, Harner SG. Longitudinal follow-up of patients with Meniere's disease. *Otolaryngol Head Neck Surg.* 1991:104:783–788.

43. LeLiever WC, Barber HO. Recurrent vestibulopathy. *Laryngoscope.* 1981:91:1–6.

44. Wallace IR, Barber HO. Recurrent vestibulopathy. *J Otolaryngol.* 1983:12:61–63.

45. Rutka JA, Barber HO. Recurrent vestibulopathy: third review. *J Otolaryngol.* 1986:15:105–107.

46. Selesnick SH, Jackler RK, Pitts LW. The changing clinical presentation of acoustic tumors in the MRI era. *Laryngoscope.* 1993:103:431–436.

47. Ooi WL, Barrett S, Hossain M, Kelly-Gagnon M, Lipsitz LA. Patterns of orthostatic blood pressure change and their clinical correlates in a frail, elderly population. *JAMA.* 1997: 277:1299–1304.

48. Mader SL. Aging and postural hypotension. An update. *J Am Geriatr Soc.* 1989:37:129–137.

49. Sloane PD. Dizziness. In: Cobbs EL, Duthie EH, Murphy JB, eds. *Geriatric Review Syllabus: A Core Curriculum in Geriatric Medicine, 4th Ed.* Iowa: Kendall/Hunt, for the American Geriatric Society; 1990:149–151.

50. Jansen RWMM, Lipsitz LA. Postprandial hypotension: epidemiology, pathophysiology, and clinical management. *Ann Intern Med.* 1995:122:286–295.

51. Lipsitz LA, Fullerton KJ. Postprandial blood pressure reduction in healthy elderly. *J Am Geriatr Soc.* 1986:34: 267–270.

52. Maurer MS, Karmally W, Rivdeneira H, Parides MK, Bloomfield DM. Upright posture and postprandial hypotension in elderly persons. *Ann Intern Med.* 2000:133: 533–536.

53. Mcintosh S, Costa DD, Kenny RA. Outcome of an integrated approach to the investigations of dizziness, falls and syncope in elderly patients referred to a syncope clinic. *Age Ageing.* 1993:22:53–58.

54. Kao A, Nanda A, Williams CS, Tinetti ME. Validation of dizziness as a possible geriatric syndrome. *J Am Geriatr Soc.* 2001:49:72–75.

55. Sloane PD, Hartman M, Mitchell CM. Psychological factors associated with chronic dizziness in patients aged 60 and older. *J Am Geriatr Soc.* 1994:42:847–852.

56. McClure JA. Vertigo and imbalance in the elderly. *J Otolaryngol.* 1986:15:248–252.

57. Sloane PD. Evaluation and management of dizziness in the older patient. *Clin Geriatric Med.* 1996;12:(4):785–801.

58. Kerstin W, Carsten W. Drug-related dizziness. *Acta Otolaryngol Suppl.* 1998:455:11–13.

59. Rybak LP. Ototoxicity. *Otolaryngol Clin North Am.* 1993:26:705–845.

60. Walker MF. Zee DS. Bedside vestibular examination. *Otolaryngol Clin North Am.* 2000;33(3):495–506.

61. Halmagyi GM, Curthoys IS. A clinical sign of canal paresis. *Arch Neurol.* 1988:45:737–739.

62. Takahashi S, Fetter M, Koenig E, Dichgans J. The clinical significance of head-shaking nystagmus in the dizzy patient. *Acta Otolaryngol (Stockh).* 1990:109:8–14.

63. Longridge NS, Mallinson AI. The dynamic illegible E-test. A technique for assessing the vestibulo-ocular reflex. *Acta Otolaryngol (Stockh).* 1987:103:273–279.

64. Unterberger S. Neue objective registrierbare vestibularis-drehrealktion, erhalten durch treten auf der stelle. Der "Tretversuch." *Arch Ohren Nasen Kehlopfheilkd.* 1938:145: 478–492.

65. Fukuda T. The stepping test. *Acta Otolaryngol (Stockh).* 1958:50:95–108.

66. Moffat DA, Harries MLL, Baguley DM, Hardy DG. Unterberger's stepping test in acoustic neuroma. *J Laryngol Otol.* 1989:103:839–841.

67. Ruckenstein MJ, Shepard NT. Balance function testing. A rational approach. *Otolaryngol Clin North Am.* 2000:33: 507–517.

68. Hart CW. Caloric tests. *Otolaryngol Head Neck Surg.* 1984: 92:662–670.

69. Sloane PD, Baloh RW, Honrubia V. The vestibular system in the elderly: clinical implications. *Am J Otolaryngol.* 1989: 10:422–429.

70. Rubin W. How do we use state of the art vestibular testing to diagnose and treat the dizzy patient? An overview of vestibular testing and balance system integration. *Neurol Clin.* 1990;8(2):225–234.

71. Manchester D, Woollacott M, Zederbauer-Hylton N, Marin O. Visual, vestibular and somatosensory contributions to balance control in the older adult. *J Gerontol.* 1989:44: M118–M127.

72. Sloane PD, Dallara J. Clinical research and geriatric research: the blind men and the elephant [editorial]. *J Am Geriatr Soc.* 1999:47:113–114.

73. Tinetti ME. Chronic dizziness and postural instability. In: Beers MH, Berkow R, eds. *The Merck Manual of Geriatrics, 3rd Ed.* Whitehouse Station: Merck Research Laboratories; 2000:181–194.

74. Zee DS. Perspective on the pharmacotherapy of vertigo. *Arch Otolaryngol.* 1985:11:609–612.

75. Shepard NT, Smith-Wheelock M, Telian SA, Raj A. Vestibular and balance rehabilitation therapy. *Ann Otol Rhinol Laryngol.* 1993:102:198–205.

76. Cowand JL, Wrisley DM, Walker M, Strasnick B, Jacobson JT. Efficacy of vestibular rehabilitation. *Otolaryngol Head Neck Surg.* 1998:118:49–54.

77. Norre ME, Beckers A. Benign paroxysmal positional vertigo in the elderly. Treatment by habituation exercises. *J Am Geriatr Soc.* 1988:36:425–429.

78. Yardley L, Beech S, Zander L, et al. A randomized controlled trial of exercise therapy for dizziness and vertigo in primary care. *Br J Gen Practice.* 1998:48: 1136–1140.

79. Isaacson JE, Rubin AM. Otolaryngologic management of dizziness in the older patient. *Clinics in Geriatric Medicine.* 1999:15:179–191.

80. Whitney SL, Rossi MM. Efficacy of vestibular rehabilitation. *Otolaryngol Clin North Am.* 2000:33:659–672.

81. Yardley L, Luxon L. Treating dizziness with vestibular rehabilitation (editorial). *BMJ.* 1994:308:1252–1253.

82. Epley JM. The canalith repositioning procedure: for treatment of benign paroxysmal positional vertigo. *Otolaryngol Head Neck Surg.* 1992:107:399–404.

83. Li JC. Mastoid oscillation: A critical factor for success in the canalith repositioning procedure. *Otolaryngol Head Neck Surg.* 1995:112:670–675.

84. Brandt T, Daroff RB. Physical therapy for benign paroxysmal positional vertigo. *Arch Otolaryngol.* 1980:106:484–485.

85. Tusa RJ. Episodic vertigo. In: Conn HF, et al, eds. *Conn's Current Therapy*, 2000 Ed. Philadelphia: Saunders; 2000: 884–892.

86. Karlberg M, Magnusson M, Malmstrom EM, Melander A, Mortiz U. Postural and symptomatic improvement after physiotherapy in patients with dizziness of suspected cervical origin. *Arch Phys Med Rehabil.* 1996:77:874–882.

87. Goebel JA. Management options for acute versus chronic vertigo. *Otolaryngol Clin North Am.* 2000:33:483–493.

88. Ruckenstein MJ, Rutka JA, Hawke M. The treatment of Meniere's disease: Torok revisited. *Laryngoscope.* 1991:101: 211–218.

89. Parnes LS, McClure JA. Posterior semicircular canal occlusion for intractable benign paroxysmal positional vertigo. *Ann Otol Rhinol Laryngol.* 1990:99:330–334.

90. Gacek RR. Technique and results of singular neurectomy for the management of benign paroxysmal positional vertigo. *Acta Otolaryngol (Stockh).* 1995:115:154–157.

68
Nutrition

David A. Lipschitz

Human aging may be defined as a complex interaction between an individual and the environment over time. In relation to external variables that affect aging, perhaps none is more important than nutrition. Evidence obtained from animal studies has shown that life expectancy can be significantly extended by restricting food intake. Nutritional factors have been shown to contribute substantively to many diseases that occur in late life. With advancing age, the risk of developing serious nutritional deficiencies also increases because of age-related reductions in total food intakes combined with the presence of debilitating disease. The presence of malnutrition increases functional dependency, morbidity, mortality, and use of health care resources. This chapter discusses the relevance of these findings and describes rational approaches to the diagnosis and management of nutritional problems in the elderly.

The Role of Caloric Restriction in Aging

Many animal studies have shown that nutritional deprivation delays maturation and significantly prolongs life expectancy.[1] These investigations have shown that caloric restriction causes delays in virtually every biomarker of aging. Classic studies have shown delays in the appearance of the well-described age-related declines in cell-mediated and humoral immunity. This effect has been suggested as the mechanism by which dietary restriction results in the later appearance of neoplasms. Food restriction also leads to a marked reduction in the generation of free radicals postulated to result in many declines in cellular function that occur with age. The mechanism by which food restriction results in prolongation of life span is still not clear. It appears that total calorie intake is a more important variable than are either total protein or fat intakes. Caloric restriction results in the presence of leaner and more active animals who utilize energy very efficiently. Overall metabolic requirements are markedly reduced. This lifelong diminution in metabolic activity has recently been suggested as an important factor in prolonging life.

The importance of these observations in relation to humans remains unclear. Affluent societies who frequently consume high-caloric, high-fat diets usually demonstrate the longest life expectancy. It must be emphasized, however, that the shorter life span noted in the less affluent can be ascribed to pathologic malnutrition, diminished sanitation, and the increased prevalence of communicable diseases. In industrialized societies, high-fat, high-calorie diets are associated with high prevalence rates of age-related diseases, such as atherosclerosis, hypertension, and colon and breast cancer. For these reasons, recent dietary recommendations have focused on the need for a prudent diet that not only restricts total and saturated dietary fats but also avoids excessive calorie intake. These recommendations may be important in the minimization of the role of nutrition in the common cancers that occur in the Western world.

Energy Requirements

Aging results in a significant decrease in energy needs.[2] The major mechanism is a decrease in resting energy expenditure as a consequence of declines in muscle mass. Reduced thyroid function does not appear to contribute to the reduced energy needs of the elderly. Diminished energy needs also result from age-related declines in physical activity, which has been demonstrated longitudinally in men and confirmed in women. Decreased activity is the result primarily of coexisting diseases, such as bone and joint disorders, loss of postural stability, and chronic diseases that may limit activity, such as angina pectoris and intermittent claudication. However, reduced strength as a consequence of declines in muscle mass does contribute to reductions in mobility.

Total caloric (food) intake is determined primarily by energy needs. Thus, a 30% reduction in energy need will be accompanied by a 30% reduction of food intake. This reduced caloric intake has been confirmed in both cross-sectional and longitudinal studies. As compared with younger subjects, individuals over the age of 70 consume a third fewer calories. The importance of this effect relates to the fact that the average intake of all nutrients is reduced in parallel. Yet the requirements for virtually every other nutrient, with the exception of carbohydrates, do not decline significantly with age (see following). As a consequence, epidemiologic studies of dietary intakes of healthy elderly individuals reveal deficient intakes. In contrast, biochemical assessments of nutritional status indicate that significant deficiencies of both macro- and micronutrients (vitamins and minerals) are quite rare in ambulatory healthy elderly. This is explained by the fact that inadequate dietary intake of a nutrient is determined by the comparison of the actual intake with the recommended dietary allowance (RDA) for that nutrient. The RDA is generally much higher than an intake that would result in a nutritional deficiency. Nevertheless, decreased intake results in reduced reserve capacity. In the presence of disease with increased nutritional requirements or because of declining intake caused by anorexia, severe nutritional deficiencies are very common in hospitalized or institutionalized elderly individuals with acute or chronic diseases.

Protein Requirements

On first principles it seems likely that, because of declines in muscle mass, aging should result in decreased protein needs. At the current time, the RDA for protein for younger subjects is 0.8 g/kg body weight. Studies in the elderly have shown that, even in healthy elderly subjects, the requirements for protein are modestly increased.[3] At the current time a protein intake of 1 g/kg body weight is recommended in healthy elderly. Most importantly, the presence of acute or chronic diseases further increases protein requirements. In this circumstance, protein intake in the older patient is frequently grossly inadequate. This is particularly important in wound healing and in decubitus ulcer, where inadequate protein intake adversely affects outcome.

Although aging results in significant declines in muscle mass, protein synthetic and degradation rates are only minimally compromised. Visceral protein stores and turnover are generally unchanged with aging so that no significant reductions are noted in serum albumin, retinol binding protein, or prealbumin, which reflect visceral protein stores.

Fat Requirements

Aging does not alter any of the specific requirements for any of the essential lipids. Advancing age is generally associated with an increase in the proportion of body weight as fat, which is the result of decreases in muscle mass accompanied by an increase in fat mass. Body fat stores increase until the seventh decade, after which reductions in total weight and fat stores are frequently noted. Although obesity is not as common a problem in the elderly as it is in younger individuals, approximately 20% of subjects over the age of 65 are significantly overweight. Studies have shown that even in the very old obesity is associated with increased mortality. Furthermore, there is evidence that the risks of atherosclerotic heart disease and stroke in the elderly can be reduced by consuming a diet low in saturated fats and cholesterol. These facts make dietary recommendations in the elderly difficult. For older individuals, a palatable acceptable diet is very important. Recommending drastic changes in dietary intake should therefore be undertaken with caution and with careful clinical judgment. For individuals in their late sixties and early seventies who are very healthy and ambulatory but significantly overweight, hypercholesterolemic, and perhaps hypertensive, an effort to reduce calories, fat, and sodium intake is warranted. In many circumstances, drastic reductions in diet may not be beneficial; this particularly applies to institutionalized elderly where medically prescribed diets are frequently not palatable, are not adequately consumed, and may result in weight loss. It must be noted that the value of serum or high-density lipoprotein (HDL) cholesterol in the prediction of coronary artery disease is less for the elderly than it is for younger subjects.[3] For this reason, the efficacy of aggressive dietary or pharmacologic attempts to lower cholesterol in subjects over the age of 70 is far from clear.

Water Requirements

In the elderly, fluid balance is extremely important because of the propensity of the elderly to develop dehydration and the ease at which overhydration can occur in elderly individuals with compromised renal function or other disorders associated with fluid retention. As a general rule, water intake should be 1 mL/kcal or 30 mL/kg body weight. Dehydration is extremely prevalent in hospitalized elderly and is the single most common cause of an acute confusional state in the elderly; this is primarily related to the well-described age-related decline in thirst drive. Studies have demonstrated a decreased ability of the elderly to respond to fluid deprivation, which becomes a particularly serious problem in frail elderly who develop a minor pathologic insult, such as a respiratory or urinary tract infection, resulting in fever, increased metabolism, and fluid loss. If fluid intake does not readily replace fluid lost, dehydration rapidly develops. This leads to confusion, worsening dehydration, and the rapid development of a serious disease that may be life threatening, warrant hospitalization, and necessitate a prolonged period of recuperation.

For these, aggressive attempts at assuring adequate hydration are essential in the elderly. Furthermore, this must commence soon after the development of a minor or major pathologic stress. Patients and their families must be educated to emphasize the importance of maintaining adequate fluid intake at all times and to carefully monitor intake if a minor illness develops or if fluid requirements are increased, as occurs during heat waves. In the hospitalized older patient, the possibility that confusion or delirium is caused by dehydration should be high on the differential diagnosis list. Physicians must assure that their patients have adequate access to water. Furthermore, total fluid intake should be carefully monitored by frequent weight and intake and output measurements.

Mineral Requirements

Numerous studies indicate that, for a wide variety of minerals and vitamins, intake is significantly lower than the RDA for a large proportion of ambulatory elderly.[4]

Calcium

Of most importance is the evidence that lifelong inadequate intakes of calcium contribute to the high prevalence of osteoporosis in the elderly. It is generally recommended that calcium intake in the elderly be between 1.0 and 1.5 g/day.

Zinc

The prevalence of zinc deficiency is important because of the role that this mineral plays in food intake and in wound healing. In elderly subjects with chronic debilitating diseases, modest zinc deficiency may contribute to anorexia. Although not clinically proven, there is also evidence that zinc supplementation aids in wound healing in general and in the healing of pressure ulcers in particular.[5] Zinc supplementation has also been shown to improve immune function and impede the rate of development of macular degeneration in the elderly.

Iron

In younger patients, iron deficiency is the most common cause of anemia and the most common global deficiency leading to widespread morbidity and decreased work performance. Aging is associated with a gradual increase in iron stores in both men and women. As a consequence, iron deficiency is rare in the elderly and invariably is caused by pathologic blood loss. It is important to emphasize that the anemia of chronic disease, which is associated with iron-deficient erythropoiesis, including a low serum iron concentration and a reduced transferrin saturation, is frequently misdiagnosed as iron-deficiency anemia in the elderly. This error results in the inappropriate administration of oral iron therapy and unnecessary invasive investigative procedures to identify the source of iron loss. The anemia of chronic disease is associated with an impaired ability of the reticuloendothelial system to recirculate iron obtained from the breakdown of phagocytosed senescent red cells. Thus, in the anemia of chronic disease, iron stores are normal or increased, whereas in iron deficiency iron stores are absent.

Recent studies indicate a correlation between increased iron stores and risks of neoplasia and coronary artery disease. Because aging is associated with increasing iron stores, supplementation with oral iron may not be desirable in older persons. Consuming a multivitamin with minerals containing the RDA for iron, combined with adequate intake from the diet, may result in inappropriately high intakes. If current evidence confirms adverse effects of iron stores, the use of iron-containing supplements in the elderly may well be unwise.

Selenium

There is suggestive evidence that selenium deficiency may contribute to age-related declines in cellular function. The mineral may be involved in minimizing free radical accumulation, as it is essential for the normal function of glutathione peroxidase. Significant selenium deficiency has been reported frequently in the elderly, although syndromes associated with selenium deficiency are very rare (cardiomyopathy, nail abnormalities, and myopathies). There is some evidence that selenium deficiency may contribute to a greater neoplastic risk and declines in immune function.

Copper

Aging generally is associated with increases in serum copper concentrations, although the significance of this increase is unknown. Copper deficiency is very rare and has been reported only in total parenteral nutrition.

Chromium

Recent evidence has suggested an important role for chromium in carbohydrate metabolism. Studies have shown age-related declines in tissue chromium levels. It is possible that chromium deficiency may contribute to glucose intolerance in the elderly, although the therapeutic efficacy of chromium replacement is controversial.

Vitamin Requirements

Studies have shown that dietary intake of many vitamins is inadequate in the elderly, including an intake of 50% or less for folic acid, thiamine, vitamin D, and vitamin E. In other studies intakes were shown to be less than 66%

of the RDA for most vitamins. It must be emphasized again that deficiencies identified on the basis of inadequate intake are invariably significantly higher than the prevalence of biochemical deficiency of most vitamins.

Water-Soluble Vitamins

Vitamin C

Studies have indicated inadequate dietary intake of vitamin C in the elderly. Others have shown a high prevalence of vitamin C supplementation in the elderly. There is no evidence, however, that vitamin C deficiency is of any clinical relevance in healthy elderly or that replacement with megadoses of vitamin C is of any clinical value. In elderly subjects with chronic debilitating diseases, there is some evidence that vitamin C supplementation improves the rate of wound and pressure ulcer healing. There is little evidence that megadoses of vitamin C have any relevant side effects, although falsely negative occult bloods have been reported, as have inaccuracies in serum and urine glucose determinations.

Thiamine

Clinically relevant deficiencies of the B vitamins are very rare in the elderly. Thiamine deficiency, however, is common in elderly alcoholics and can be an important contributing factor in the development of disordered cognition, neuropathies, and perhaps cardiomyopathies. Relevant deficiencies of this vitamin are relatively common in institutionalized elderly.

Folate Acid

Like thiamine, folate deficiency in the elderly is predominantly found in alcoholics. It is also common in elderly subjects who are taking drugs that interfere with folate metabolism (trimethoprim, methotrexate, and Dilantin) or in disorders associated with increased folate needs (hemolytic anemia and ineffective erythropoiesis). Folate deficiency may result in cognitive loss or significant depression and should always be evaluated in the workup of elderly subjects with a memory disorder.

Vitamin B$_{12}$

Low serum vitamin B$_{12}$ concentrations have been shown to occur in as many as 10% of otherwise healthy elderly subjects. Many comprehensive workups indicate early pernicious anemia, the commonest cause of vitamin B$_{12}$ deficiency, whereas in others no obvious cause can be identified. B$_{12}$ deficiency classically causes a severe megaloblastic anemia. Not uncommonly, the nonhematologic manifestations of B$_{12}$ deficiency can occur in the absence of anemia; these include gait disorders, sensory and motor neurologic deficits, and highly significant memory loss. This vitamin should be measured routinely in the

workup of any elderly patient with disordered cognition or depression, and replacement therapy should be given to any patients in whom low serum levels are found. The lower limit of normal varies in different laboratories, but a value below 150 pg/mL is highly suspect and should always result in the commencement of replacement therapy.

Fat-Soluble Vitamins

Recent evidence has suggested that vitamin A is one of the only nutrients in which requirements decrease with advancing age. Studies have shown that aging is associated with an increase in absorption of vitamin A from the gastrointestinal tract, accompanied by a reduction of hepatic uptake. These effects make the elderly susceptible to toxicity if excessive amounts of the vitamin are consumed as a supplement. Side effects of daily intakes in excess of 50,000 IU include headaches, lassitude, reduction in white cell counts, impaired hepatic function, and bone pain. The vitamin plays an important role in visual acuity. However, there is no evidence that vitamin A supplements improve age-related declines in eyesight. Vitamin A and its precursor beta-carotene have been suggested as exerting a protective effect against an array of neoplasms. Recent large-scale controlled trials have, however, failed to definitively prove a beneficial effect of beta-carotene in the development of skin cancers.

Vitamin D

Recent studies suggest that vitamin D deficiency may be a serious concern in the elderly. In addition to the vitamin's known role in bone metabolism, it also affects macrophage function in general and pulmonary macrophages in particular. Vitamin D deficiency increases susceptibility to the development of pulmonary tuberculosis by compromising macrophage function. This has been suggested as contributing to the high prevalence of tuberculosis in nursing home patients in whom deficiencies are common and aggravated by diminished exposure to sunlight. In any patient with severe osteoporosis, fracture, or bone pain, vitamin D-induced osteomalacia must be excluded.

Vitamin E

Vitamin E (alpha-tocopherol) is abundant in the diet and deficiencies of the vitamin virtually never occur. It is involved in the function of the enzyme glutathione peroxidase, which is involved in free radical generation. The vitamin also affects the biophysical properties of the cell membrane, reducing the age-related increase in membrane microviscosity. It also influences immune function, and recent evidence indicates that administration of the vitamin enhances immune function in the elderly and may minimize infectious risk. Despite these effects, which may be of benefit in improving age-related declines in cellular function, no good evidence exists indicating a beneficial effect of vitamin E supplementation in subjects of any age.

Vitamin K

Vitamin K is essential for the production of a number of factors involved in both the intrinsic and extrinsic clotting cascade. There is evidence that vitamin K administration is beneficial in elderly people who have an unexplained prolongation of their prothrombin time. Although dietary intake is adequate, deficiencies can result from the administration of drugs that interfere with the vitamin's absorption or interfere with bacterial flora.

A Practical Approach to Nutritional Assessment

General Considerations on History and Physical Examination

A high index of suspicion of nutritional problems is very important in patients who have a primary diagnosis associated with malnutrition, such as chronic alcoholism, disorders of cognition, chronic myocardial, renal, or pulmonary insufficiency, malabsorption syndromes, and multiple medication use.[6] In addition, particular attention should focus in the history on evidence of anorexia, early satiety, nausea, change in bowel habits, fatigue, apathy, or memory loss. Physical findings that may also provide clues to the presence of nutritional deficits include poor dentition, cheilosis, angular stomatitis, and glossitis, which is common in a number of vitamin deficiencies. Pressure ulcers or poorly healing wounds, edema, dehydration, and poor dental status are common physical findings in severely malnourished patients.

Clinically, a number of important questions must be addressed in the nutritional assessment. Increased risk of malnutrition can usually be identified from the history and physical examination. Commonly recognized risk factors are listed in Table 68.1. Generally, factors leading to malnutrition can be categorized into disorders resulting in anorexia, inadequate or inappropriate nutrient intake, and social or economic isolation.

Has the Patient Lost Weight?

Weight loss is perhaps the most important finding indicating the presence of malnutrition. Recent studies have clearly indicated that this finding in patients with serious disease is a very poor prognostic sign and is associated with increased morbidity and mortality.[7] To be significant, weight loss must be involuntary. It has often been said

TABLE 68.1. Causes of weight loss in the elderly.

Anorexia
  Depression
  Medications
    Digoxin
    Serotonin reuptake inhibitors
  Diseases
    Cancer
    Chronic organ failure (cardiac, renal, pulmonary)
  Chronic infections
    Tuberculosis
  Polymyalgia rheumatica and other collagen vascular diseases
  Single nutrient deficiencies that affect taste and appetite
    Vitamin A
    Zinc

Malabsorption
  Intestinal ischemia
  Celiac disease

Swallowing disorders
  Neurologic
  Esophageal candidiasis
  Web stricture
  Dental disease

Metabolic
  Thyroid disease
  Diabetes
  Liver disease

Social
  Isolation
  Poverty
  Caregiver fatigue
  Neglect
  Abuse
    Physical
    Alcohol
  Food preference not met
  Inappropriate food choices

Physical
  Inability to purchase or cook food
  Decreased activity

No cause identified

that to be significant, weight loss must have exceeded 10% or more of body weight in 6 months, 7.5% or more in 3 months, or 5% or more in 1 month. In older persons, any weight loss that clearly cannot be ascribed to alterations in fluid balance (common in older persons receiving diuretic therapy) should be taken seriously. It must be emphasized that significant malnutrition can be present in individuals who are not underweight. Any significant weight loss that is involuntary indicates that nutritional intake is inadequate and that the patient's needs are not being met.

Is the Patient Underweight?

To determine if the patient is underweight or has lost weight requires an evaluation of body composition.[8] In this regard, virtually every anthropometric measure of body composition employs height as the reference point. In both males and females, height decreases by approximately 1 cm per decade after the age of 20. This is caused by vertebral bony loss, increased laxity of vertebral supportive ligaments, reductions in disk spaces, and alterations in posture. Historical estimations of height are also frequently inaccurate in the elderly, and its measurement is difficult in bedridden patients or in those with significant postural abnormalities. For this reason, it has been suggested that alternatives to height should be used in the development of standards for body composition for the elderly. Options suggested include arm length and knee-height measurements.

In general, a gradual increase in weight occurs with advancing age, peaking in the early forties in males and a decade later in females. After age 70, reductions in weight are not uncommon. Lean body mass decreases by approximately 6.0% per decade after the age of 25. By the age of 70, lean body mass has decreased an average of 5 kg for females and 12 kg for males. Thus, in the elderly, fat constitutes a far greater percentage of total weight than it does in subjects of younger ages. Fat distribution also alters with aging. Truncal and intrabdominal fat content increase while limb fat diminishes. Skinfold measurements are often employed to estimate fat and muscle stores. Although the triceps skinfold thickness is the most frequently obtained, multiple skin folds are much more reliable than single measurements. In the elderly, subscapular and suprailiac skinfolds are the best predictors of fat stores in males, while the triceps skinfold and thigh measurements are of greater value in females. Total body water is also decreased in parallel to declines in lean body mass. Evaluating ideal body weight for height can be employed to determine if a patient is underweight. Tables are available for older persons that provide a guide to their ideal body weight. These are based upon an assessment of height, weight, and body frame. On the basis of these tables, being significantly underweight is defined as being 15% below the ideal weight for that individual patient. Unfortunately, current tables are based upon relatively small samples and often are not representative of the individual being evaluated.

A more accurate assessment is the determination of the body mass index (BMI), which is the ratio of weight to height squared. This obviates the need to create gender tables, although the confounding effect of age remains to be determined and the problems with assessing height persist. A standard nomogram is available from which BMI can be calculated from height and weight. It is generally recommended that persons over the age of 65 have a BMI between 24 and 29. As a general rule, a BMI below 22 is a cause for concern and indicates that the patient is significantly underweight, while a value above 29 indicates obesity.

Does the Patient Have Protein-Energy Malnutrition?

This condition is best described as a metabolic response to stress that is associated with increased requirement for energy and protein. The pathophysiologic events leading to this disorder are illustrated in Figure 68.1. The metabolic response to a stress such as injury or infection is characterized by hormonal changes and the release of cytokines that lead to the development of anorexia, despite the presence of increased nutrient needs. In older persons, the negative sequelae of this response can develop quickly. Protein-energy malnutrition (PEM) is associated with marked depletion of visceral protein stores characterized by the presence of hypoalbuminemia. Inadequate supply of protein leads to liver dysfunction, which contributes to the low serum albumin. Decreased clearance of drugs and toxins also occurs, increasing the risk of toxicities and adverse drug reactions. Inadequate supply of protein primarily affects organ systems with the highest turnover of cells, which are the skin, immunohematopoietic system, and gastrointestinal tract. Thus, PEM is characterized by a dry skin and "flaky paint" dermatitis. Impaired immune responses lead to compromised host defenses, increasing the risk of life-threatening infections. Malabsorption also develops as a result of impaired jejunal and ileal mucosal cell proliferation, creating a vicious cycle of malnutrition causing malabsorption and worsening malnutrition. As a result of disease and deficiencies of taste-related nutrients, anorexia is usually present. The disorder is also referred to as hypoalbuminemia malnutrition and is usually diagnosed by the presence of a serum albumin level of less than 3.0 g/dL.

In the elderly, relatively minor stress of short duration can result in PEM. Thus, PEM is common in elderly patients who develop minor pulmonary and urinary infections and is often found soon after an elective surgical procedure. The problem of PEM in the elderly is compounded by the ease at which these patients develop severe dehydration as a consequence of an age-related decline in thirst drive.[9] This leads to the development of confusion, hypotension, and a vicious cycle in which the patient's overall condition can deteriorate very rapidly. Furthermore, in contrast to younger people, the positive benefits of this disorder in the elderly are limited to a very short period. If nutritional needs are not met within 2 to 3 days of the onset of the acute illness, the declines in immune, hepatic, and gastrointestinal function appear to contribute significantly to increased morbidity, mortality, and prolonged hospital stays.

In the nursing home, PEM should be suspected in any patient who develops an acute medical problem. It is also frequently seen in patients with chronic infections and in those with decubitus ulcers. Any patient presenting with

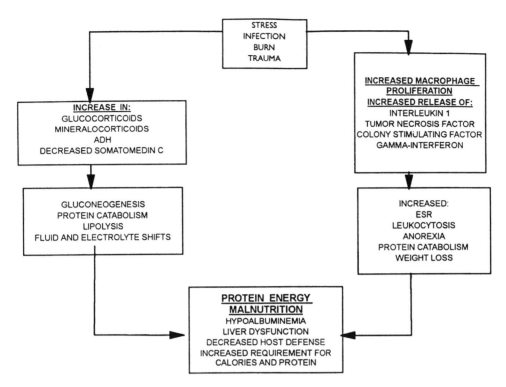

FIGURE 68.1. Pathophysiology of protein-energy malnutrition. ADH, antidiuretic hormone; ESR, erythrocyte sedimentation rate.

confusion, lassitude, anorexia, decreased activity, or greater functional dependence may have developed an acute medical problem such as an infection, which, if not treated, will result in the development of significant PEM.

Does the Patient Have Isolated Nutrient Deficiencies?

These are quite rare in older persons but should be considered in special circumstances. Zinc deficiency has been reported to be increased in patients with pressure ulcers and may contribute to decreased rates of healing. For this reason, zinc supplementation is frequently prescribed in patients with pressure ulcers. Vitamin D deficiency is relatively common in homebound and institutionalized older persons and may contribute to declines in host defense mechanisms in the elderly. Frank osteomalacia has also been reported. Folate deficiency is limited to patients with malabsorption and to older alcoholics (not uncommon). Vitamin B_{12} deficiency has been reported to be frequent in older persons. Its level should be measured in any patient being evaluated for memory loss. Low levels warrant replacement. Whether this affects memory is not clear.

Significance of Malnutrition in Older Persons

There is compelling evidence indicating that malnutrition is highly significant in older persons. Being underweight or losing weight is associated with increased morbidity and mortality in older persons. There is even suggestive evidence that voluntary weight loss may be associated with an increased adverse outcome in older persons. In the acute care hospital setting, the presence of protein-energy malnutrition has been shown to be an independent predictor of increased morbidity and mortality in older persons. This information is important, as studies have shown that the nutritional status of hospitalized patients is often ignored and that nutritional therapy is inadequate with a high complication rate.

Management of Nutritional Problems in Older Persons

Weight Loss and Being Underweight

As indicated, a major predictor of increased morbidity and mortality makes being underweight or losing a significant amount of weight highly relevant clinically. While no study has shown that correcting the decline in weight improves survival in this patient population, it is obvious that every attempt must be made to identify and treat the cause.

The initial approach to management should be a careful attempt to identify the cause of the weight loss and, if found, to aggressively attempt correction. Table 68.1 lists the common causes of weight loss in older persons, highlighting potentially correctable causes. Figure 68.2 lists an approach to treatment of weight loss

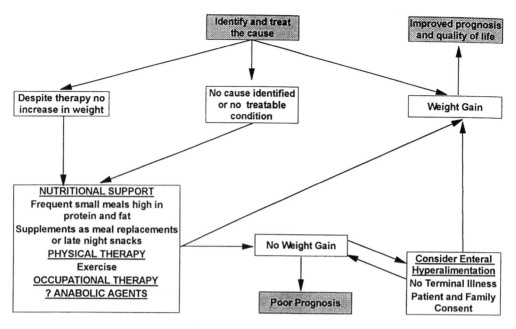

FIGURE 68.2. A rational approach to the treatment of weight loss in the elderly.

in the elderly. Identifying a potentially treatable cause such as drug use (digoxin, fluoxytene), thyrotoxicosis, and depression can usually result in weight gain if the underlying condition is corrected with appropriate medical interventions. Other conditions that may well contribute to weight loss that are potentially improvable include social or economic isolation, difficulties with cooking or feeding as a consequence of physical disability, dental or swallowing problems, and not providing palatable or preferred foods. Failure to identify a cause for weight loss is generally accompanied by a poor prognosis despite aggressive medical and nutritional interventions.

Older persons who have experienced weight loss are consuming inadequate calories to meet their needs. Thus nutritionally the aim must be to increase caloric intake. This can be achieved by assuring the use of palatable meals, often recommending diets high in both protein and fats. All too frequently the underweight older person may, for apparent health reasons, be consuming a low-fat, low-protein diet that may well contribute to or minimize the chances of weight gain. In these patients, risks of hypercholesterolemia are small compared with those from losing weight. For this reason, in underweight older persons we often recommend high-fat diets, including red meats, pork, full cream milk, and ice cream, all of which are dense in both calories and proteins. Frequent small meals should be recommended, using nutritional supplements that are calorie dense and high in protein as meal

replacements or late night snacks. Providing supplements with meals is not recommended, as total caloric intake will not be improved. The importance of a comprehensive rehabilitation program cannot be overemphasized. Recent evidence has shown that increased caloric intake can only be achieved when nutritional supplementation is accompanied by an aggressive and proactive program of exercise and physical therapy (Fig. 68.3).[10] Patients who fail to respond to treatment of their underlying medical condition and fail to gain weight despite nutritional and physical rehabilitation carry a very poor prognosis.

Management of Nutritional Problems in the Acute Care Setting

Protein Energy Malnutrition

Figure 68.4 summarizes a rational approach to the management of nutritional problems in the acute care setting. Once a diagnosis of PEM has been made, clinical judgment is extremely important in deciding the appropriate time to commence nutritional support. In the acutely ill patient, attention should first be directed at correcting the major medical abnormalities. Thus, management of infections, control of blood pressure, and the restoration of metabolic, electrolyte, and fluid homeostasis must assume priority. During this period, fluid and nutrient intake should be recorded so that an assessment of future needs can be made. Once the acute process has stabilized, daily calorie counts should be performed and the patients should be encouraged by the staff to voluntarily consume as much of their food as possible. If fluid overload is not a major concern, the use of polymeric dietary supplements between meals and in the late evening should be considered. The aim is to obtain a caloric intake of approximately 35 kcal/kg, based upon an ideal rather than the actual body weight.

It is our experience that by encouragement alone only 10% of elderly subjects with PEM can consume sufficient food voluntarily to correct their nutritional deficiency. Thus, most subjects require a more aggressive form of nutritional intervention. As a general rule, more aggressive attempts to assure adequate nutrient intake must commence within 48 h of admission. The approach taken depends upon the clinical presentation of the patient and whether or not short-term or more long-term nutritional support is required. For those patients requiring short-term support (fewer than 10 days), peripheral hyperalimentation is the method of choice. Using this approach it is possible, through a peripheral vein, to provide adequate calories and protein to meet the patient's needs using amino acid solutions, 10% dextrose, and intralipid.

Nasogastric feeding should be avoided in any confused older patient because of the risk of aspiration and the need for restraints to prevent the patient from pulling out the uncomfortable and irritating tubes. For those who are not confused and who have a normal gastrointestinal tract, enteral hyperalimentation through a small-bore nasogastric polyethylene catheter should be considered. These tubes are nonirritating and do not interfere with patient mobility or the ability to swallow food. It is extremely important that after the tube is passed, placement in the stomach be confirmed before commencing nutritional feedings. For patients likely to require nutritional support for periods of 6 weeks or longer, a feeding gastrostomy or jejunostomy is recommended. For both nasogastric feeding gastrostomies, infusions should begin with an undiluted, commercially available polymeric dietary supplement at a continuous rate of 25 mL/h. The supplement should contain no more than 1 kcal/mL, as caloric-dense fluids are too viscous to pass through the tube with ease. The rate can gradually be increased so that after 48 h the total daily protein and calorie requirements of the patient are met by this route.

Enteral hyperalimentation has major side effects of which the attending physician must be aware. One of the most commonly encountered side effects is excessive fluid retention. When nutritional support begins, weight gain is invariably noted within the first 2 to 3 days. This almost certainly reflects fluid retention, as the weight gain is associated with significant reductions in the serum albumin and hemoglobin levels. The average increase in weight during this time in our patients is 1.3 kg, while the level of the serum albumin falls from a mean of 2.8 g/dL in patients before nutritional support to a value of 2.3 g/dL at day 3. Occasionally, and particularly in elderly

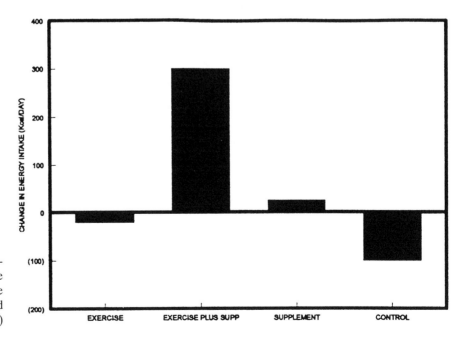

FIGURE 68.3. Effect of nutritional supplementation with and without exercise on daily increase in energy (food) intake in underweight older persons. (Adapted from Fiatarone et al., with permission.[10])

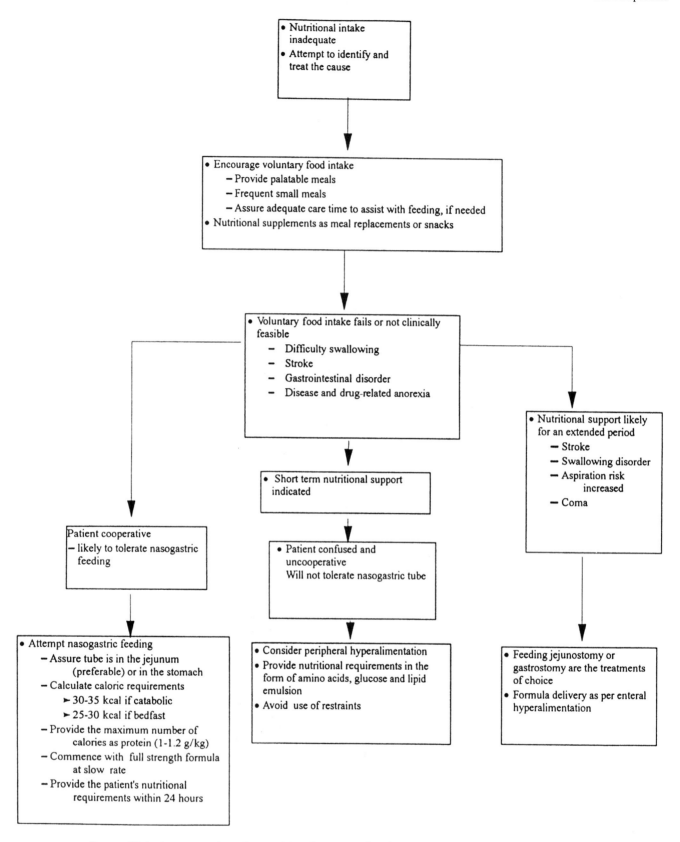

FIGURE 68.4. An approach to the nutritional support of malnourished hospitalized elderly patients.

subjects with inadequate renal function, excessive retention of fluid can result in peripheral edema or even heart failure. When this occurs, diuretic therapy can correct the underlying problem or the use of calorie-dense supplements should be considered. Major alterations in circulating electrolytes have also been described. Hyponatremia and hypocalcemia occur frequently. In addition, hypophosphatemia and decreased magnesium levels can occur, resulting in worsening confusion and delirium. Hyperglycemia and glycosuria are occasionally noted, and frank diabetic coma can develop. An additional problem seen occasionally is severe diarrhea. The risk of diarrhea can be minimized if supplements are given by slow infusion. Bolus administration of dietary supplements through a nasogastric tube increases the risk of diarrhea and, particularly in the elderly, enhances the possibility of vomiting and aspiration pneumonia. Nutritional management requires a great deal of clinical skill, particularly when frail aged subjects are being supported. With suitable training and monitoring, the side effects of enteral hyperalimentation can be minimized and, when they occur, easily corrected.

Although anecdotal evidence has demonstrated that aggressive nutritional intervention can result in weight gain (Fig. 68.5), improved immune and hematologic functions, as well as the return of serum albumin, transferrin, and other parameters of visceral protein stores to the normal range, increases in muscle mass, as measured by anthropometric measurements, usually do not occur.[11] Because a major goal of any geriatric rehabilitation is to improve functional independence and improve strength, strategies aimed at improving muscle mass are particularly important. For this reason, the recent observation that administration of recombinant growth hormone can improve muscle mass and performance in frail elderly is particularly significant. It may well be that this will become a useful tool as an adjunct to nutritional support in older patients receiving rehabilitation. A similar beneficial effect of appropriate exercise has also been recently reported. These studies emphasize the need for a comprehensive approach to the management of elderly malnourished patients. Aggressive nutritional intervention is only a part of a complete strategy aimed at restoring, in the appropriate patient, functional independence.

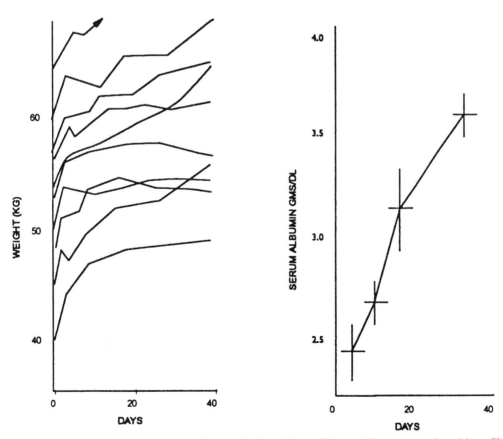

FIGURE 68.5. Response to enteral hyperalimentation in 10 elderly patients with protein-energy malnutrition. Changes in weight and serum albumin are shown.

Nutritional Support of Patients with Pressure Ulcers

Debility, immobility, and prolonged pressure are well-known contributors to the development of pressure ulcers.[5] There is also good evidence that treatment and prevention of nutritional deficiencies can decrease the risk of developing pressure ulcers and aid in the rate of healing. There is some evidence to suggest that the rate of pressure ulcer healing can be improved by administration of relatively large doses of zinc and vitamin C. In addition, total protein intake has been shown to affect the rate of pressure ulcer healing. In a recent study, we examined the effects of dietary protein intake on pressure ulcer healing in a group of geriatric patients receiving enteral hyperalimentation. A significant increase in pressure ulcer healing rates was found in subjects fed a very high protein formula containing 25% of calories as protein as compared with a group receiving 16% of calories as protein. The percent improvement averaged 76% in the very high protein formula as compared with 36% in the group fed 16% protein diet. This finding was also observed in a recent report that demonstrated a correlation between dietary protein intake and pressure ulcer healing.

Nutritional Support of Long-Term Tube Feeders

Most long-term care facilities have a number of bed-bound older patients who are receiving long-term nutritional support either via a nasogastric tube, or more common at the current time, via feeding gastrostomies or jejunostomies. In bedbound patients, energy requirements are determined exclusively via resting metabolic rate and, as such, are generally lower than ambulatory older persons.

In our experience, weight gain can be maintained when as little as 25 kcal/kg body weight is provided on a daily basis.[12] This amount will increase if an active disease process is present, such as an infection or a pressure ulcer. As a general rule, supplements with the highest protein content are favored. This is based on studies in which we have demonstrated that nitrogen balance is only maintained when more than 20% of total calories are provided in the form of protein. It is important to assure that the water needs of patients receiving enteral hyperalimentation are being met. Water needs average 35 mL/kg, even in the bedbound patient. Thus in patients receiving supplements containing 1 or more cal/mL, fluid needs may not be met without the provision of free water, in addition to the dietary supplement.

Paying attention to fluid status is critically important because of the well-known negative sequelae of dehydration in older persons.

Summary

Management of nutritional problems in the elderly constitutes an important challenge. Few health care professionals pay much attention to the nutritional status of their patients, which may have adverse effects on morbidity, mortality, and quality of life. While overnutrition is a common problem in younger persons, aging is associated with increases in the incidence of weight loss, being underweight, and having protein-energy malnutrition. Identifying and appropriately treating the underlying cause is a critical component of nutritional rehabilitation. However, it is important to simultaneously assure that the patient's energy and protein needs are met, which can be done by dietary manipulation and by the use of dietary supplements. In the hospitalized setting, the presence of anorexia and inadequate voluntary food intake may necessitate the need for nutritional hyperalimentation. Peripheral hyperalimentation is recommended for the older confused patient requiring short-term nutritional support and who is unlikely to tolerate nasogastric feeding. For long-term nutritional support, feed via nasogastric tube or percutaneous endoscopic gastrostomy (PEG) placement should be considered. It is important to emphasize that nutritional care is a critical component of comprehensive rehabilitation program that must include physical and occupational therapy if overall improvement of the patient and functional independence are to be achieved.

References

1. McCarter RJM. Role of caloric restriction in prolongation of life. *Clin Geriatr Med*. 1995;11:553–565.
2. Shock NW, Gruelich RC, Andres R, et al, eds. *Normal Human Aging: The Longitudinal Study of Aging*. NIH Pub 84-2450. Washington, DC: National Institutes of Health; 1984.
3. Gersovitz M, Motil K, Munro H, et al. Human protein requirements: assessment of the adequacy of the current recommended dietary allowance for dietary protein in elderly men and women. *Am J Clin Nutr*. 1982;35:6–14.
4. Chernoff R. Effects of age on nutrient requirements. *Clin Geriatr Med*. 1995;11(4):641–651.
5. Allman R. Pressure sores among the elderly. *N Engl J Med*. 1989;320:850–853.
6. Ham RJ. The signs and symptoms of poor nutritional status. *Prim Care*. 1994;21:33–67.

7. Sullivan DH, Walls RC. Impact of nutritional status on morbidity in a population of geriatric rehabilitation patients. *J Am Geriatr Soc.* 1994;42:471–477.

8. The Nutrition Screening Initiative. *Incorporating Nutrition Screening and Interventions into Medical Practice: A Monograph for Physicians.* Washington, DC: The Nutrition Screening Initiative; 1994.

9. Silver AJ, Morley JE. Role of the opioid system in the hypodypsia associated with aging. *J Am Geriatr Soc.* 1992;40:556–560.

10. Fiatarone MA, O'Neill EF, Ryan ND, et al. Exercise training and nutritional supplements for physical frailty in very elderly people. *N Engl J Med.* 1994;330:1769–1775.

11. Lipschitz DA, Mitchell CO. The correctability of the nutritional, immune and hematopoietic manifestations of protein calorie malnutrition in the elderly. *J Am Coll Nutr.* 1982;1:17–25.

12. Lipschitz DA. Approaches to the nutritional support of older patients. *Clin Geriatr Med.* 1995;11:715–724.

69
Exercise

Eric B. Larson and Robert A. Bruce

Introduction

The health benefits of exercise, *particularly for a sedentary society*, have gained an increasingly compelling evidence base in the past decade. For earlier generations of seniors, exercise was a regular feature of everyday life. Beginning sometime after the industrial revolution and culminating in today's most advanced societies, there is a seemingly inevitable tendency leading to everyday lives that require progressively less energy expenditure through exercise.

Exercise in the last half of the twentieth century was viewed primarily as recreation, and especially recreation for younger people. The therapeutic benefits of exercise were initially explored for younger people—in whom the principal benefits are for cardiovascular risk reduction.

We believe that the health benefits of exercise may be even greater in older persons. Younger adults have considerably more physiologic reserve, both muscular strength and cardiovascular capacity. Older individuals, by contrast, experience a progressive decline in many physiologic functions, including muscular strength and cardiovascular capacity.[1,2] Habitual exercise, by improving strength and maximum aerobic capacity ($\dot{V}O_2$ max) as a result of conditioning effects, can provide added physiologic reserve as well as enhance well-being by reducing effort and fatigue associated with activities of daily living.[3] Most importantly, habitual exercise in moderation can slow development of disability and thereby prolong active life expectancy.[4,5]

In addition to habitual exercise for conditioning, there is increasing evidence that *resistance exercise to improve muscle strength* along with more tailored exercise therapies, including those designed to improve balance, and rehabilitate persons with various chronic disease and acute ailments, may be of particular value for older patients.[6–8] Thus, exercise should be considered an important part of general care of so-called healthy agers as well as for persons with age-related illnesses.[9]

Society should focus health promotion on the elderly as well as the young. Life expectancy at age 65 averages at least 15 years for men and 19 years for women,[10] long periods during which risk reduction and health promotion can provide beneficial effects.

Most older people in advanced countries have grown older during an era when advancing technology at home and in the workplace has promoted a lifestyle characterized by progressively less habitual physical activity. A physically active lifestyle (before today's ongoing exercise craze) was usually associated with lower socioeconomic manual labor or the considerable activity provided by raising children. As people aged, they typically became progressively more sedentary. Leisure time was for resting, and heavy physical activity was not viewed as desirable. Thus, it may come as a surprise to many older patients when a physician recommends habitual exercise as a "treatment" or when tailored exercise programs are prescribed as part of a care plan for managing ongoing chronic diseases. There is now a growing evidence base that exercise programs offer measurable health benefits, ranging from increased life expectancy to mitigation of adverse sequelae of aging and of many chronic diseases. Nowadays, the greatest challenge with regard to achieving the health benefits of exercise is caused by limited access to effective programs and poor compliance.[11]

Exercise and Aging

Dynamic aerobic exercise is commonly defined as the rhythmical alternating flexion and extension of large muscle masses for pleasure or improved fitness and stamina.[3] Aerobic metabolism of muscle increases in proportion to the mass of muscles involved and the intensity of exertion. The functional limits are determined by the body's ability to circulate oxygen and substrates and remove CO_2, metabolites, and heat from the muscles, which is determined by cardiac output and arterial-mixed venous oxygen (a-v O_2) differences at symptom-limited maximal exercise.[12] Beyond these limits, additional energy for a short interval is achieved by anaerobic metabolism with release of lactate.

A variety of acute changes occur during dynamic aerobic exercise. Knowledge of the physiology of exercise was originally derived from studies of young, typically athletic male volunteers; however, subsequent work has been directed to other adults, including the elderly.[13] The circulatory response to dynamic exercise is most prominent in the exercising muscle. Blood flow increases from 4 to 7 mL/100 g/min up to 50 to 70 mL/100 g/min due to decreased vascular resistance and opening of capillary beds in working muscles.[14] The muscle itself generates adenosine triphosphate (ATP), increases oxygen consumption, and consumes more substrates, especially free fatty acids. Oxygen extraction at the tissue level increases from 5 to 15 mL/100 mL of nutrient flow.[15] Overall, total oxygen uptake increases 10- to 20-fold in well-trained athletes.

Cardiac output increases linearly with oxygen uptake, and heart rate increases linearly with cardiac output.[15] Stroke volume increases to a lesser extent as a result of enhanced systolic emptying. The increase in cardiac output, however, is not sufficient to account for all the increase in oxygen uptake. Increased extraction of oxygen at the tissue level occurs also.

There is a prominent rise in systolic blood pressure as well as a modest increase in mean arterial pressure. Diastolic blood pressure usually is unchanged or decreases. Arterial vasoconstriction during exercise restricts regional blood flow to the hepatosplanchnic and renal circulations to transfer more blood flow to working skeletal muscle groups and to a lesser extent the coronary circulation.

In the working muscle, heat is generated up to 41°C at maximal effort. A maximum of about 25% of the chemical energy produced is turned into work; 75% is given off as heat and must be dissipated. The most important mechanism for handling excess heat is circulatory; adequate blood flow is required to allow heat to flow from the contracting muscle to the surface for dissipation through the skin. In the lungs, the minute ventilation increases in proportion to the generation of carbon dioxide[14] and aids in heat dissipation.

Most people perform dynamic aerobic exercise repeatedly for a training or conditioning effect. The training effect consists of an increase in the capacity for maximal effort and decrease in circulatory and relative metabolic changes at any given level of submaximal effort. The increase in maximum aerobic capacity ($\dot{V}O_2$ max) that occurs is related to the person's baseline, limitations imposed by the presence of any disease, and the intensity and consistency of duration and frequency of training.[14] Physical training increases $\dot{V}O_2$ max, and because capac-

ity is greater, the effort required for any given level of submaximal exertion as a percent of $\dot{V}O_2$ max, cardiac output, and heart rate is reduced. Approximately half the increase occurs as a result of peripheral changes, that is, an increase in the capacity of aerobic metabolism and extraction of substrate and oxygen at the tissue level. These peripheral changes include an increased density of mitochondria in the muscle, increased amount of mitochondrial enzymes, and therefore an increased capacity to oxidize fat, carbohydrate substrates, and ketones; the amount of myoglobin is increased as is the ability to generate ATP. The net result is an increased capacity for oxygen extraction and a decrease in lactate production during submaximal exercise.[16] The other half of the training effect occurs primarily in the cardiovascular system.[15,17] Thus, skeletal muscles are more efficient and myocardial oxygen requirements are actually less due to the reduction in afterload.

Dynamic exercise may be sustained for hours without fatigue if activity is below 50% of the individual's maximum oxygen consumption ($\dot{V}O_2$ max).[18] To obtain physiologic adaptation, training should begin at lower levels, gradually increasing to 58% to 78% of $\dot{V}O_2$ max or to 70% to 85% of the individual's maximal heart rate.[18,19] Exertion at this level, 20 to 40 min three times per week, for several weeks is required for physical conditioning to occur. If not maintained, deconditioning occurs. Thus, *an active life is necessary to maintain the benefits of such training.* Strenuous exertion or training activities sustained above 85% of maximal heart rate can trigger adverse effects such as heart attacks, especially in sedentary persons with coronary heart disease.[20,21]

Aging alters structures and reduces functions of cells and tissues of all organ systems. $\dot{V}O_2$ max defines the functional limits of aerobic metabolism and the cardiovascular system that occur with aging.[1,18] In the absence of bronchopulmonary disease or anemia, neither ventilation nor arterial oxygen content limits $\dot{V}O_2$ max before the cardiovascular limits are obtained.

Much research has focused on the relationship of $\dot{V}O_2$ max and age. The general results are that $\dot{V}O_2$ max increases with age during growth and in childhood development, reaches a peak with adolescence, and then declines with advancing age.[1,22] $\dot{V}O_2$ max is higher in men than women in proportion to differences in amount of skeletal muscle mass. For both men and women, higher values are found in physically active persons compared to those who are sedentary. After adjusting $\dot{V}O_2$ max for weight, the highest value for aerobic capacity is observed during the first decade of life, and a roughly linear decline then follows throughout life. The relationship follows the declining maximal heart rate with age.[23]

The rate of decline in $\dot{V}O_2$ max with aging is lower, based on cross-sectional selective sampling of healthy individuals of different ages, compared to the rate of decline found in longitudinal studies of the same persons over time. In cross-sectional studies, the coefficient for this rate of change averages $-0.4\,ml\,min^{-1}\,kg^{-1}\,yr^{-1}$ compared to $-0.9\,ml\,min^{-1}\,kg^{-1}\,yr^{-1}$ observed in longitudinal studies.[23] Extrapolations based on cross-sectional data result in implausibly long-lived preservation of aerobic capacity due to selective survival effects whereas, using longitudinal data, the age at which basal or minimal oxygen uptake is intersected (minimal aerobic requirement for survival) corresponds to observed survival of healthy persons.[18,23] Longitudinal measurements are needed to describe the effects of aging on $\dot{V}O_2$ max; such data are difficult to obtain.

The critical observation with regard to exercise and aging is that the rate of decline in weight-adjusted $\dot{V}O_2$ max with aging is not identical in habitually active compared to sedentary men who remain healthy. Regression lines computed for aerobic capacity and age from longitudinal reports of aerobic capacity and aging show separation for active and sedentary men. The slopes were remarkably similar for the same categories of men, even though data[24–26] were derived from different population samples over different durations between measurements. The slopes of the regression lines calculated were $-0.54 \pm 1.5\,mL\,min^{-1}\,kg^{-1}\,yr^{-1}$ for physically active men compared to $-1.32 \pm 0.85\,ml\,min^{-1}\,kg^{-1}\,yr^{-1}$ for sedentary mean[23]; thus, there is a twofold difference in the rate of decline in $\dot{V}O_2$ max based on habitual activity levels. For men in the 50- to 59-year-old range, this is equivalent to a 10-year difference in the intersection of the extrap-

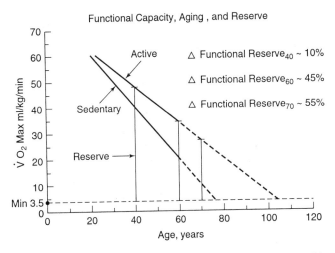

FIGURE 69.2. The relationship between functional aerobic capacity, aging, and functional reserve. Δ functional reserve is the difference between functional reserve for active and sedentary persons at ages 40, 60, and 70, respectively.

olated regression lines with the $\dot{V}O_2$ min necessary to maintain life (Figure 69.1).[3,18]

The consequences of a difference in the rate of declining aerobic capacity are obviously important for aging persons. One important consequence is expressed by the concept of functional reserve.[27,28] Functional aerobic reserve can be defined as the amount of reserve between maximum aerobic capacity ($\dot{V}O_2$ max) and the weight-adjusted resting oxygen requirement of about 3.5 ml/kg/min, which is the minimal aerobic requirement for survival. Figure 69.2 shows that at age 40 the difference in rates of $\dot{V}O_2$ max and minimal functional capacity associated with survival (or the functional aerobic reserve) is considerable.[27] Furthermore, the relative difference between conditioned and unconditioned persons is small. As the two curves diverge and one approaches age 60, there still is considerable functional aerobic reserve but the difference between active and sedentary persons' functional reserve is greater. By the time a person reaches age 70, the functional reserve in the sedentary group becomes much less as aerobic capacity approaches the minimum aerobic requirements for survival, and thus there is more likely to be a clinically significant difference in functional aerobic reserve. The clinical importance of the difference between sedentary and active groups may be manifest as improved ability to withstand the stress of illness, more rapid recovery from illness or injury, and greater likelihood to have the ability to perform activities of daily living during the course of an acute illness or during exacerbations of chronic illnesses.[3,27] These data form the theoretical basis for postulating that aerobic exercise and conditioning may not only prolong life but, more importantly, prolong *active* life expectancy,[3,5] the health benefit most desired by patients.

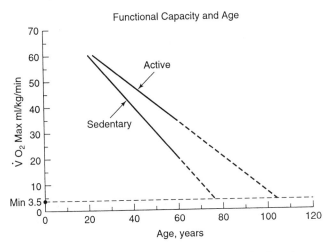

FIGURE 69.1. Age-related decline in physiologic function, as measured by maximum oxygen consumption ($\dot{V}O_2$ max). *Solid lines* represent regression lines based on longitudinal studies of $\dot{V}O_2$ max; *dotted segments* are extrapolations based on regression line (decline) observed. Extrapolation of this decline in persons who have been followed longitudinally and classified as habitually active or sedentary suggests that minimum $\dot{V}O_2$ min (3.5 ml/kg/min) occurs at a later age in the habitually active group.

Exercise Programs for Older Persons

It is tempting (and probably justified) to simply prescribe exercise as a general tonic for all older persons. However, there are special benefits for older persons with chronic disease and disabilities for whom more focused prescriptions should be considered. Current evidence supports exercise programs for persons with ischemic heart disease, including those with congestive heart failure, osteoporosis, osteoarthritis, spinal stenosis, degenerative central nervous system diseases such as Parkinson's disease, diabetes, hypertension, peripheral vascular disease, and possibly psychiatric illnesses, such as depression and anxiety disorders.[8,9,29,30–35] In general, current evidence indicates that older adults with chronic diseases enjoy benefits from exercise. If anything, we believe exercise offers relatively more benefits to older adults in whom the baseline level of risk is higher, and thus the opportunity to reduce risk is greater. We now know that the underlying plasticity of the muscles, autonomic nervous system, bones, and joints exists in both young and old persons and is amenable to the effects of conditioning and therapeutic exercise.[6,36–39]

Habitual exercise in older adults has been shown to produce as much conditioning effect as in younger persons.[13,40] The most important concern with regard to the overall health benefits of exercise in older persons is the risk of exercise.[41] Except for the risks, exercise is essentially a "low-cost" intervention and may require relatively little in the way of health care resources. If the individual has time that is not encumbered with other activities (work, raising a family, etc.), the marginal cost to the individual of time spent exercising is low. Thus, the key element to the question of efficacy in older persons is risk and injuries.[41]

The hazards of exercise are related to extremes of intensity and duration. When exercise is excessively intense and/or prolonged, extreme fatigue, exhaustion, or delayed recovery is experienced. In addition, more prolonged or intense exercise is associated with increased risk of injury.[42] Injuries and sudden death are the most important complication for elderly persons.[3]

The risk of injury has been documented in numerous studies to be directly related to the intensity of training.[3,41,43] For example, for participants in the Peach Tree Road Race in Atlanta, Georgia, there was a nearly linear relationship between miles run per week and likelihood of suffering an injury in the previous year. At the highest level of training, more than 70% of participants had at least one injury the preceding year.[42] On the other hand, studies of a "runners' club" from Stanford demonstrate that habitual exercise need not be associated with increased overall utilization of health service.[43] In this group of patients with mean age of 58.6 years who ran approximately 27 miles per week, visits to physicians, dis-

ability days, and disability levels were more favorable in the running group compared to a group of community controls. Nonetheless, 35% of the visits to physicians in the runners' club were for running-related injuries.[43]

The risk of sudden death and nonfatal myocardial infarction is quite small, but detectable, during unsupervised activity.[44] Risk factors for sudden death among those participating in exercise programs include attaining a heart rate in excess of 85% of that individual's maximum; marked ST depression with exercise despite the absence of chest pain; poor adherence to limiting heart rate; and attainment of above-average $\dot{V}O_2$ max for gender and age due to peripheral mechanisms.[20] Overall, however, the risk of primary cardiac arrest in more active individuals is less.[44] The incidence of primary cardiac arrest attributable to lack of exercise was greatest in older, hypertensive, or obese males.[45] Bouts of heavy exertion in sedentary people appear to pose a threat.[21]

Thus, any general exercise program should be moderate in intensity and duration and should minimize risk of injury, cardiac arrest, and nonfatal myocardial infarction, as well as excessive fatigue. It may also be important to maintain adequate hydration to counteract fluid losses of sweating.

Four goals should be a part of an exercise program established for older individuals.[27] First, the program should increase conditioning, especially endurance. Second, the intervention should improve muscle strength, especially lower extremity strength, given the importance of walking to independent functioning. Both these goals are likely to improve a person's ability to perform activities of daily living, decrease fatigue associated with the day's activity, improve a sense of well-being, and perhaps forestall such adverse events as falls by improving muscle strength. The third goal of an exercise program should be to minimize risk of injury due to the program, and a fourth goal should be to promote enjoyment without causing excessive fatigue.

The components of the exercise program include two essentials: the first is dynamic aerobic exercise[3,19] in the form of walking, swimming, cycling, jogging, and so forth; the second is a program that promotes lower extremity strengthening. Also desirable are a period to warm up and cool down and muscle and tendon stretching.

The exercise program should be tailored, especially so for older individuals. The program should take account of an individual's physical capacities and coexistent disabilities as well as mitigating social, psychologic, and economic factors.[19] Among all forms of exercise available to the elderly, brisk walking is one of the most ideal and has, in fact, been recommended by a number of groups.[46–48] Brisk walking does produce a training response in many older individuals. More vigorous exercise may be required for persons to obtain a conditioning effect if they start from higher baseline fitness levels. Physicians and other health professionals should be prepared to give appropriate guidelines for exercise.[19] In particular, habitually sedentary persons may need to be advised of the normal responses to exercise, which include increased heart rate and breathing; mild perspiration; an increased awareness of one's heartbeat; and, at least initially, mild muscle aches. Such responses are normal and do not indicate that a person should stop exercising.[27] The warning signs of *excessive* exercise include severe dyspnea, wheezing, coughing; any form of chest discomfort; excessive perspiration; syncope or near syncope; prolonged fatigue and exhaustion lasting at least half an hour after exercise; and local muscle or joint discomfort. Heart rate guidelines are most appropriate for persons with coexistent cardiac disease. An exercise tolerance test will allow one to calculate the desired heart rate based on the observed or extrapolated maximal heart rate. The typical target heart rate for achieving a conditioning effect is 70% to 80% of maximal heart rate.[2] There also are tables listing average exercise heart rates for various age groups; however, such tables may be less useful given the wide variation in baseline and maximal aerobic capacity seen in the elderly.

In our own experience, it is perhaps more useful to teach individual guidelines for pacing. One guideline is the so-called talk test in which persons know they are not exercising excessively when they can carry on a normal conversation while exercising. For many elderly persons, a reliable heart rate guide is to aim for an exercise heart rate 15 to 20 beats per minute over their resting heart rate.[48] Most persons who have not exercised excessively will also find that their pulse returns to resting levels or nearly so within 20 min after stopping exercise. Finally, it is important to emphasize that exercise for conditioning is not "competition." Many people associate exercise with competition and thus need to be counseled to avoid external comparisons. Competitive urges can be focused on the goal of making progress or minimizing decline over time.

Perhaps the most important pacing guide is to emphasize starting a program slowly and increasing activity by small increments. Many older persons abandon exercise programs because they expect too much too fast, become discouraged, and thereby give up their programs before benefits are achieved (Table 69.1).

The duration to be prescribed is driven by the amount of time required to produce the conditioning effect. In general, a minimum of 20 to 30 min of aerobic exercise three times per week at 70% to 80% of maximum heart rate is required to achieve a conditioning effect, which will begin approximately 2 weeks after commencing an exercise program. Moderate exercise (such as brisk walking) is more likely to produce a conditioning effect at levels of 30 to 40 min for 5 days per week, which is the level recommended by the U.S. Prevention Services Task

Force. Deconditioning begins as soon as a program is abandoned. Deconditioning is dramatic and malignant when persons "take to bed."[49]

Table 69.1 demonstrates two programs recommended by advisory groups for elderly individuals.[48] Both plans begin at extremely modest levels (5 min of walking three times per week or 1/4 mile walking three times per week) and eventually proceed to a brisk walking pace lasting 30 to 60 min.

Compliance, along with low levels of physician counseling, is the major barrier to successful exercise programs in the elderly.[11,50] This is a common issue for many health promotion activities. More research is required to define strategies for improving compliance with habitual exercise recommendations. A related issue is the relative lack of social and community resources for habitual activity. Much of our advancing technology consists of "labor-saving" devices. In our large northern cities, especially, there may be few opportunities and almost no facilities for older persons to get habitual exercise. During the prolonged cold or wet winters, the opportunity for outside activity is particularly restricted. The social issues involved in creating facilities that provide a range of exercises at reasonable costs have yet to be solved. Walking in shopping malls is a solution that works in some communities. Older adult living communities are beginning to "invest" in exercise facilities containing a treadmill, bicycling, and cross-country skiing and other exercise machines.

Recent work on the feasibility of high-intensity resistance exercise training has demonstrated that rather vigorous, supervised progressive resistance training exercise designed to improve strength is both feasible and effective.[6,37,38,39,51] Muscle dysfunction is an important factor in the development of falls, fractures, dependence in activities of daily living, and need for institutionalization.[52,53] The feasibility and effectiveness of strength training represents an important advance, which could lead to effec-

TABLE 69.1. Two examples of brisk walking programs.

Week	Program 1: miles of walking[46]	Program 2: minutes of walking[47]
1	1/4 [a]	5
2	1/4	7
3	1/2	9
4	1/4	11 (approx. 1/2 mile)
5	1	13
6	1	15
7	1 (20 min)	18
8	1 1/2 (30 min)	20 (approx. 1 mile)
9	2 (40 min)	23
10	2 (20 min)	26
11	2 1/2 (50 min)	28
12	3 (60 min)	30 (approx. 1 1/2 mile)

[a] Three times weekly.
Source: From Ref. 46, with permission.

tive programs to reverse frailty. The results also demonstrate that aged, wasted, and unused muscles retain their plasticity at virtually any age.

What emerges as this chapter goes to press is that habitual exercise and tailored exercise programs are important components in the therapeutic armamentarium of geriatric medicine. Habitual moderate intensity exercise is a proven way to reduce risk of death from heart disease[53] and will also improve bone density, strength, stamina, and balance, which reduces risk of falling and injury, hypertension, glucose control, sleep, depression, constipation, and other common maladies.[3,27] Age-related decline in exercise capacity and functional reserve is attenuated by habitual exercise.

The development of specifically tailored programs is likely best accomplished with the assistance of specially trained physical therapists or in group programs often found in senior centers, through voluntary groups such as YMCAs in some residential facilities or in some medical centers. We recently established a program at the University of Washington Medical Center (*Strong and Steady*), whose purpose is to provide seniors with the tools to maintain or increase their level of independent physical function and enhance their health through exercise. The *Strong and Steady Program* uses a combination of exercise and education to accomplish these goals. The services provided through the *Strong and Steady Program* include individual therapy sessions, group classes, and individualized fitness programs. Education focuses on the importance of exercise to health maintenance and measures that can be taken to maintain safe mobility function.

The program includes a comprehensive evaluation and the development of an individualized exercise program. The evaluation performed by a physical therapist focuses on assessment of balance, mobility and fall risk, and components of function such as strength, range of motion, and coordination. The tools of the program include strengthening exercises, balance retraining, aerobic conditioning, flexibility exercises, and gait retraining. More information on the Strong and Steady Program can be found on the University of Washington Medical Center Web site, http://www.washington.edu/medical/uwmc/uwmc_clinicals/bonejo/strong.html.

We believe that programs like Strong and Steady should help address the challenge of providing access to facilities, therapeutic expertise, and programs for older adults—both those with good health and those with chronic disease. The need for such services likely exceeds supply in most communities. Geographic access is often a problem for many patients. Financial viability of the programs themselves is a critical issue. The Strong and Steady Program was started with a small grant from the UWMC Service League to cover modest startup costs. The Program receives most of its revenue from billed charges and is expected to cover operational costs in 2 to 3 years, when it reaches its expected clinical capacity. The services are charged as physical therapy evaluation, therapeutic exercise, balance training, and gait training. Most charges are to Medicare, with supplemental or private pay covering the other 20%. Group classes are all private pay. We believe evidence strongly supports such efforts by clinicians, provider institutions, geriatric self-help activist groups, and older persons in general to promote exercise—both habitual and tailored programs—for long periods of time to maintain strength, fitness, health, and function.

References

1. Astrand PO. Physical performance as a function of age. *JAMA*. 1968;205:729–733.
2. Larson EB, Bruce RA. Exercise and aging. *Ann Intern Med*. 1986;105:793–785.
3. Larson EB, Bruce RA. Health benefits of exercise in an aging society. *Arch Intern Med*. 1987;147:353–356.
4. Fries JF, Singh G, Morfeld D, Hubert HB, Lane WE, Brown BW. Running and the development of disability with age. *Ann Intern Med*. 1994;121:502–509.
5. Katz S, Branch LG, Branson MH, Papsidero JA, Beck JC, Greer DS. Active life expectancy. *N Engl J Med*. 1983;309:1218–1224.
6. Fiatarone MA, Marks EC, Ryan ND, et al. High intensity strength training in nonagenarians. *JAMA*. 1990;263:3029–3034.
7. Buchner DM, Cress ME, de Lateur BJ, et al. The effect of strength and endurance training on gait, balance, fall risk and health services use in community-living older adults. *J Gerontol Med Sci*. 1997;52A:M218–24.
8. Wolff J, van Croonenborg JJ, Kemper HC, Kostense PJ, Twisk JW. The effect of exercise training on bone mass: a meta-analysis of published clinical trials in pre- and post-menopausal women. *Osteoporos Int*. 1999;9:1–12.
9. Girolami B, Bernardi F, Prinz MH, et al. Treatment of intermittent claudication with physical training, snacking cessation, pentoxifylline, or nafronyl: a meta-analysis. *Arch Intern Med*. 1999;159:337–345.
10. Van Nostrand JF, Furner SE, Suzman R, eds. *Health Data on Older Americans: United States, 1992*. Vital Health Statistics, Series 3. US Department of Health and Human Services, Hyattsville, MD; 1993.
11. Elward K, Larson EB, Wagner EH. Factors associated with regular aerobic exercise in an elderly population. *J Am Board Fam Pract*. 1992;5:467–474.
12. Mitchell JN, Sproule BJ, Chapman CV. The physiological meaning of the maximal oxygen intake tests. *J Clin Investig*. 1958;37:538–547.
13. Posner JD, Gorman KM, Windsor-Landsberg L, et al. Low to moderate intensity endurance training in healthy older adults: physiological responses after four months. *J Am Geriatr Soc*. 1992;40:1–7.
14. Clausen JP. Circulatory adjustments to dynamic exercise and effect of physical training in normal subjects and

patients with coronary artery disease. *Prog Cardiovascular Dis.* 1976;18:459–495.

15. Wallace AG. Cardiovascular adaptations to exercise. In: Smith LH, Their SO, eds. *Pathophysiology: The Biological Principles of Disease.* Philadelphia: Saunders; 1981;1136–1142.

16. Holloszy JO. Adaptations of muscular tissue to training. *Prog Cardiovasc Dis.* 1976;18:445–458.

17. Detry JR, Russeau M, Vanderbrouche G, Kasumi F, Brasseur LA, Bruce RA. Increased arteriovenous oxygen differences after physical training in coronary heart disease. *Circulation.* 1974;44:109–118.

18. Bruce RA. Exercise, functional aerobic capacity and aging—another viewpoint. *Med Sci Sports Exerc.* 1984;16:8–13.

19. Goldberg L, Eliot EL. Prescribing exercise. *West J Med.* 1984;141:383–836.

20. Hossack KF, Hartwig R. Cardiac arrest associated with supervised cardiac rehabilitation. *J Cardiac Rehabil.* 1982;2:402–408.

21. Curfman GD. Is exercise beneficial or hazardous to your heart? *N Engl J Med.* 1993;329:1720–1731.

22. Robinson S. Experimental studies of physical fitness in relationship to age. *Arbeitsphysiologie.* 1938;10:251–323.

23. Dehn MM, Bruce RA. Longitudinal variations in maximal oxygen intake with age and activity. *J Appl Physiol.* 1972;33:805–807.

24. Dill DB, Robinson S, Ross JC. A longitudinal study of 16 champion runners. *J Sports Med.* 1967;7:4–32.

25. Hollman W. *Korperliches Training als Pravention von Herz Kreislauf-Krankheiten.* Stuttgart: Kippokrates-Verlag; 1965.

26. Irving JB, Kusumi F, Bruce RA. Longitudinal variations in maximal oxygen consumption in healthy men. *Clin Cardiol.* 1980;3:134–136.

27. Larson EB. A general approach to health promotion and disease prevention in the older adult. *Geriatrics* 1988;43:31–39.

28. Williams MA. Clinical implications of aging physiology. *Am J Med.* 1984;76:1049–1054.

29. Arroll B, Baeglehole R. Exercise for hypertension. *Lancet.* 1993;34:1248–1249.

30. Hambrecht R, Wolf A, Grelen S, et al. Effect of exercise on coronary endothelial function in patients with coronary artery disease. *N Engl J Med.* 2000;342:454–460.

31. Kasch FW, Boyer JL, Schmidt DK, et al. Aging of the cardiovascular system during 33 years of aerobic exercise. *Aging* 1999;28:531–536.

32. Paluska SA, Schwenk TL. Physical activity and mental health: current concepts. *Sports Med.* 2000;29:167–180.

33. Singh NA, Clements KM, Fiatarone MA. A randomized trial of progressive resistance training in depressed elders. *J Gerontol A Biol Sci Med.* 1997;52:27–35.

34. Wei M, Gibbons LW, Kampert JB, Nichamon MZ, Blair SW. Low cardiorespiratory fitness and physical inactivity as predictors of mortality in men with type 2 diabetes. *Ann Intern Med.* 2000;132:605–611.

35. Walker RD, Nawaz S, Wilkinson CH, Saxton JM, Pockley AG, Wood RF. Influence of upper- and lower-limb exercise program on cardiovascular function and walking distances

in patients with intermittent claudication. *J Vasc Surg.* 2000;31:662–669.

36. Beere PA, Russell SD, Morey MC, Kitzman DW, Higginbotham MB. Aerobic exercise training can reverse age-related peripheral circulation changes in healthy older men. *Circulation.* 1999;100:1085–1094.

37. Pyka G, Lindenberger E, Charette S, Marcus R. Muscle strength and fiber adaptations to a yearlong resistance training program in elderly men and women. *J Gerontol.* 1994;49:M22–M27.

38. Fiatarone MA, Evans WJ. The etiology and reversibility of muscle dysfunction in the aged. *J Gerontol.* 1993;48:77–83.

39. Fiatarone MA, O'Neill EF, Ryan ND, et al. Exercise training and nutritional supplementation for physical frailty in very elderly people. *N Engl J Med.* 1994;330:1769–1775.

40. De Vries HA. Physiological effects of an exercise training regimen upon men aged 52 to 88. *J Gerontol.* 1970;25:325–336.

41. Koplan JP, Siscovick DS, Goldbaum GM. Risks of exercise: public health view of injuries and hazards. *Public Health Rep.* 1985;100:189–194.

42. Koplan JP, Powell KE, Sikes RK, Shirley RW, Campbell OC. An epidemiologic study of the benefits and risks of running. *JAMA.* 1982;248:3118–3121.

43. Lane NE, Bloch DA, Woud PD, Fries JF. Aging, long-distance running and the development of musculoskeletal disability. *Am J Med.* 1987;82:772–780.

44. Siscovick DS, Weiss NS, Fletcher RH, et al. The incidence of primary cardiac arrest during vigorous exercise. *N Engl J Med.* 1984;311:874–877.

45. Siscovick DS, Weiss NS, Fletcher RH, Schoenbach VJ, Wagner EH. Habitual vigorous exercise and primary cardiac arrest: effect of other risk factors on the relationship. *J Chron Dis.* 1984;37:625–631.

46. President's Council on Physical Fitness and Sports. *Pep Up Your Life—A Fitness Book for Seniors.* Washington, DC: American Association for Retired Persons.

47. *Exercise and Your Heart.* Bethesda, MD: U.S. Dept. of Health and Human Services, Public Health Services, National Institutes of Health; 1981.

48. Mielchen SD, Larson EB, Wagner E, et al. Getting started: a guide to physical activity for seniors. Seattle: Center for Health Promotion, Group Health Cooperative; 1987.

49. Clark LP, Dion DM, Barker WH. Taking to bed: rapid functional decline in an independently mobile older population. *J Am Geriatr Soc.* 1990;38:967–972.

50. Wee CC, McCarthy EP, Davis RB, Phillips RS. Physician counseling about exercise. *JAMA.* 1999;282:1583–1588.

51. Mulrow CD, Gerety MD, Kanton D, et al. A randomized trial of physical rehabilitation for very frail nursing home residents. *JAMA.* 1994;271:519–524.

52. Tinetti ME, Baker DI, McAvay MS, et al. A multifactorial intervention to reduce the risk of falling among elderly people living in the community. *N Engl J Med.* 1994;331:821–827.

53. Paffenbarger RS Jr, Hyde RT, Wing AL, Lee IM, Jung DL, Kampert JB. The association of changes in physical activity level and other lifestyle characteristics with mortality among men. *N Engl J Med.* 1993;328:538–545.

70
Sleep and Sleep Disorders

Tamar Shochat and Sonia Ancoli-Israel

The prevalence of sleep complaints increases dramatically with age and is estimated to be about 40% in the elderly population.[1] These complaints include difficulty falling asleep, waking up at night, waking up too early in the morning, not feeling well rested, and needing to nap during the day. In an epidemiologic study of more than 9000 participants aged 65 and over, more than half reported at least one sleep complaint occurring most of the time.[2] Women were more likely to report nighttime complaints but were less likely to nap during the day compared to men. The most common complaint was waking up at night (30%), followed by daytime naps (25%) and difficulty falling asleep (19%). Less than 20% reported rarely or never having any sleep complaint. Sleep complaints were associated with coexisting health disorders, including poor self-perceived health, depressive symptoms, respiratory symptoms, physical disabilities, chronic medical conditions, and medication use. However, of the healthy minority in this study, over one-fourth reported at least one chronic sleep complaint.

Although age-related changes do occur in normal sleep, sleep problems in the elderly are not a consequence of the aging process per se but are strongly related to medical and psychiatric comorbidity as well as psychosocial changes in later life. Furthermore, some specific sleep disorders such as sleep disordered breathing, periodic limb movements in sleep, and REM sleep behavior disorder are more prevalent with age, although not exclusive to this age group.

Physiologic Sleep and Its Measurement

In the 1950s, scientists discovered that sleep is an active process, not, as formerly believed, a passive state not worthy of scientific investigation. By recording brainwave activity (the electroencephalogram, EEG), eye movements, and muscle tension, it was determined that sleep is broken down into two major states, rapid eye movement (REM) and nonrapid eye movement (NREM). NREM sleep is further subdivided into sleep stages 1 through 4, which represent a continuum from light sleep (stage 1) to deep sleep (stages 3 and 4). REM sleep is characterized by rapid eye movements similar to those seen in the waking state, as well as muscle atonia.

Healthy human individuals show stable and distinct patterns of sleep architecture, that is, the cyclic alternations of the different sleep stages. Sleep is entered through the transitional stage 1, and followed by stages 2, 3, and 4, respectively. After about 90 min, through stage 2 sleep, REM sleep begins. The first appearance of REM sleep during the night is termed REM latency. This 90- to 100-min cycle repeats itself typically four to five times during the night. However, the internal temporal structure changes, so that at the beginning of the night stages 3 and 4 are long while REM sleep is short, and as the night progresses, the amount of stages 3 and 4 decreases, while the amount of REM sleep increases.

Both REM sleep and non-REM sleep stages 3 and 4 are homeostatically driven; that is, selective deprivation of each of these states subsequently causes a rebound in their appearance once the person is allowed to sleep. This finding leads to the ubiquitous assumption that both are essential in the sleep process and its many functions.[3] REM sleep may also be driven by a circadian oscillator, as studies have shown that REM is temporally coupled with the circadian rhythm of temperature.[4]

Specific Clinical Patterns in Aging

Because the prevalence of several medical and psychiatric conditions that affect sleep, as well as the prevalence of specific sleep disorders, is high in the elderly population, it is extremely difficult to portray the picture of the "normal" elderly sleeper. Nevertheless, studies of age-related changes in sleep architecture have found some common characteristics. Sleep efficiency, defined as the amount of time asleep relative to the amount of time in bed, is decreased to 70% to 80%,[5] compared to 90% or more in younger adults. Total sleep time is reduced, particularly in the later part of the sleep episode.[6] The amount of stage 1 sleep, which is the transitional state between wake and sleep, is increased, while the amount of stages 3 and 4 (also termed slow-wave sleep or delta sleep) is much decreased.[4,7] Specifically, the amplitude of slow-wave activity is significantly reduced.[8] Therefore, older people spend more of the night in light sleep and are more likely to arouse (awaken) in response to external stimuli during the night.

Changes in the amount of REM sleep and latency of REM (time from sleep onset to the first REM sleep period) in the elderly are controversial.[5] While some studies report a reduction in the percentage of REM,[4] others report few or no changes in REM with aging.[9] Feinberg[7] reported a shorter REM latency and longer duration of REM sleep in the first sleep cycle. Reynolds et al.[10] reported a "flat" temporal distribution of REM, with no changes in the percentages of REM sleep throughout the night, unlike the increase in REM sleep in the second half of the night typically seen in young adults. Some studies have shown shorter REM latencies in the elderly; however, this may be due to the decrease in the amount of non-REM sleep in stages 3 and 4. Alternatively, as REM sleep is coupled to the circadian rhythm of core body temperature, which has been found to be phase advanced in the elderly population, it is possible that changes in circadian timing account for the reduced REM latency compared to young adults.[4]

Studies looking at gender differences have shown that despite the tendency for women to complain about their sleep more often than men, older women sleep somewhat better than older men.[11] This conclusion is consistent with polysomnographic findings showing that slow-wave sleep is more preserved in older women than it is in older men.[10,12] Sleep maintenance, particularly in the last part of the night, was also reported to be poorer in older men than women.[10] Although sleep disruption in elderly women may be milder compared to elderly men, women tend to report their sleep problems and seek help more often than their male counterparts.

Sleep Disordered Breathing

Definition and Prevalence

Sleep disordered breathing (SDB) or sleep apnea is characterized by complete or partial cessation of breathing, lasting at least 10s, that occurs repeatedly throughout the night. The respiratory disturbance index (RDI) represents the number of complete pauses (apnea) and partial pauses (hypopnea) in respiration per hour of sleep.

There are two types of apnea: obstructive and central. Obstructive apneas are caused by an anatomic obstruction of the airway during sleep. Patients attempt to breathe and may appear to be choking or gasping for breath; however, despite their respiratory effort the airway is shut down. The obstruction may be located in different areas, but most often it is in the lower pharynx, between the base of the tongue and the larynx. Many patients with obstructive sleep apnea are heavy, loud snorers, as snoring in itself is also a result of a partial obstruction of airflow. In mild to moderate cases, obstructive apnea may be related to body position.[13] Sleeping in a supine position may increase the frequency and severity of the apnea, as the tongue falls back to the anterior neck and oropharynx. Respiratory events may occur in all sleep stages; however, in some patients the length and severity of the events increases during REM sleep.[14]

Central apneas are caused by failure of the central nervous system respiratory centers. Respiratory neurons fail to stimulate the motor neurons that activate the respiration process, resulting in an absence of respiratory effort. Central apnea is common in patients with heart failure or stroke. Many patients have mixed apneas, with both central and obstructive components.

Ancoli-Israel et al.[15] have reported the prevalence of SDB with RDI greater than 10 in 70% of elderly men and 56% of elderly women, respectively, compared to only 15% and 5% of younger men and women, respectively.[16]

Consequences of the Disorder

Patients with SDB stop breathing in their sleep. To start breathing again, they must awaken. Often these awakenings are so brief that they are not recalled the next morning. However, these short repetitive arousals may cause sleep fragmentation, which in turn may lead to excessive sleepiness during the day. The respiratory events may cause oxyhemoglobin desaturation, which may cause morning headaches and decreased cognitive functioning.

SDB is also an independent risk factor for hypertension[17] and is associated with obesity and cardiac arrhythmias.[18,19] In severe cases, SDB has been linked to increased mortality.[20,21] However, in a review of the literature, Wright et al.[22] claimed that evidence for an association between SDB and morbidity and mortality was not sound, and other confounding factors such as age, body mass index, smoking, and alcohol use were often not properly considered.

Epidemiologic studies have linked SDB in the elderly with cognitive impairment and dementia.[23,24] Ancoli-Israel et al. found significant associations between SDB and cognitive functioning in community-dwelling elderly,[25] as well as in the nursing home, where severe apnea was significantly correlated with severe dementia.[26]

Clinical Presentation

The two chief complaints of the apnea patient are loud snoring (usually the spouse suffers from this and is motivated to seek help) and excessive daytime sleepiness. Patients usually do not complain of sleep disruption, as they do not remember the nighttime arousals. However, the daytime sleepiness may have extreme consequences, as some patients may fall asleep at work or while driving. Morning headaches, confusion, and cognitive impairment are also common, particularly in the elderly. Some studies have linked these disturbances to the hypoxemia or to the excessive sleepiness.[27,28]

Risk Factors

Patients with SDB are often obese, although this is less true in the elderly. Smoking has been implicated as a risk factor.[29]

Diagnosis

Sleep disordered breathing (SDB) must be evaluated by an all-night sleep recording. Traditionally, this is done in a sleep laboratory, with a full EEG montage, including a nasal thermistor that records airflow and chest and abdomen movements, and oximetry, to determine oxyhemoglobin level. Portable equipment that can be set up in the patient's home is also available. This alternative is particularly appropriate for elderly individuals who may become confused or disoriented or simply uncomfortable while sleeping away from home. Based on the sleep recording, the RDI is computed and treatment options are evaluated. SDB is diagnosed slightly differently in the various sleep clinics, but generally the cutoff point is an RDI greater than 10 to 15.

Treatment and Management

Weight loss in obese patients with SDB can significantly reduce or eliminate the respiratory events.[30] For positional apnea, sewing a pocket to the back of a nightshirt and placing a tennis ball inside the pocket is a simple, noninvasive method to avoid lying in a supine position.[31] Alcohol and sedating medications should be avoided, as these may exacerbate the severity of the apnea.[32,33] Smoking cessation may help.[29]

The treatment of choice for obstructive sleep apnea is continuous positive airway pressure (CPAP).[34] This machine is connected by a hose to a face mask worn over the patient's nose. Positive pressure is administered continuously at an appropriately titrated level, acting as a splint to keep the airway from collapsing during sleep. When used appropriately, CPAP is extremely effective in eliminating the respiratory events, the oxygen desaturations, the snoring, and the excessive daytime sleepiness. CPAP has also been found to improve measures such as mood, general health, fatigue, and functional status even in mild cases of SDB.[35] However, CPAP does not cure SDB, and it must be worn every night unless another solution, such as weight loss or surgery (see following), is achieved. Compliance is therefore an important issue, and initial acceptance rate has been found to be 70% to 80%. Long-term compliance has been found to be 80% to 90%.[36,37]

Surgical procedures for the correction of anatomic abnormalities of the airway have been developed for the treatment of obstructive sleep apnea. Obstructions are most often found in three major regions, including the nose, the soft palate, and the base of the tongue. Usually patients have multiple obstructions. The goal of surgery is to cure the apnea or to obtain results comparable to those observed with CPAP treatment.[38]

Nasal reconstruction is used for the correction of obstruction in the nasal airway. Pharyngeal reconstruction, or uvulopalatopharyngoplasty (UPPP), is indicated for the correction of excess tissue in the soft palate, a large uvula, and enlarged tonsillar adenoidal tissue. Unfortunately, UPPP is only effective in about 50% of the cases.[39] Laser-assisted uvulopalatoplasty (LAUP) is a similar procedure mostly used for the treatment of snoring. Its success rate for obstructive sleep apnea is lower than that of UPPP.[39,40] Genioglossus advancement is used for obstruction at the base of the tongue, with the tongue being moved forward to enlarge the airway. UPPP combined with genioglossus advancement has a success rate of 61%.[41] Maxillomandibular advancement is indicated for patients who do not respond to other forms of surgery. It is relatively contraindicated in the elderly population as they tend to have more risk factors such as heart disease, for example, atherosclerosis, placing them at risk for complications from this invasive surgical procedure. Tracheostomy was one of the first procedures for obstructive sleep apnea. Today it is used only for severe cases, when all else has failed, or in conjunction with UPPP.

Drug treatments for SDB have generally been only marginally successful. For central sleep apnea, respiratory stimulants such as progesterone and acetazolamide may be appropriate. For SDB associated with REM sleep, tricyclic antidepressants may be indicated, as they reduce the amount of REM, thus indirectly reducing the number of respiratory events.

Oral appliances have been developed for both obstructive sleep apnea and snoring, including the tongue-retaining device and the mandibular advancement device. Both devices are designed to enlarge the airway at the base of the tongue by advancing the tongue or the mandible forward. Although compliance rates are estimated to range between 50% and 100%, success rates (i.e., achieving a RDI < 10) are only about 50%.[42] Thus, oral appliances are indicated for patients who do not respond to behavioral treatment such as weight loss or body position, who are intolerant to CPAP, or who are not candidates for surgery.[43] Treatment options are based on the severity of the apnea, the patient's medical status, the level of urgency in treating the apnea, and the patient's own preference.

Periodic Limb Movements in Sleep

Definition and Prevalence

Periodic limb movements in sleep (PLMS) is a disorder of unknown etiology, in which patients involuntarily kick their limbs (most often it is their legs) in short, clustered episodes lasting between 0.5 and 5 s and occurring about every 20 to 40 s. The kicks are often accompanied by arousals. These episodes occur repeatedly throughout the night. The myoclonus index (MI) represents the number of kicks with arousals per hour of sleep.

The prevalence of PLMS seems to increase with age. Ancoli-Israel et al.[44] reported that 45% of randomly selected elderly adults aged 65 years and older had PLMS, compared to 5% to 6% of the younger adult population.[45]

Consequences of the Disorder

As with SDB, the nighttime arousals are often too short to be recalled. However, patients with PLMS may complain of insomnia, as they may have difficulty falling asleep as well as settling back to sleep following these episodes. PLMS occur most often in the first half of the night, during sleep stages 1 and 2. Sleep is fragmented, with reduced amounts of stages 3 and 4 and REM.

Clinical Presentation

In addition to complaining of difficulty falling asleep, patients may also complain of excessive daytime sleepiness, as they suffer from sleep fragmentation throughout the night. They may also note that the bedding is disorganized or jumbled when they wake up in the morning. Bed partners often complain of the leg kicks disturbing their sleep as well, and often it is important to obtain information from the bed partner in diagnosing and assessing the disorder.

Risk Factors

A related disorder that occurs during the relaxed, awake state often just before sleep onset is restless leg syndrome (RLS). Patients report unpleasant sensations in their legs and irresistible movement of the legs. The disagreeable, sometimes painful leg sensations are alleviated by rubbing or squeezing the legs or simply by walking. The prevalence of RLS is not well defined. Most patients with RLS also suffer from PLMS, suggesting that these disorders may be related. Furthermore, many patients with PLMS also suffer from other sleep disorders, including SDB and REM sleep behavior disorder.[46,47]

Diagnosis and Differential Diagnosis

PLMS is diagnosed in a full night sleep recording in the sleep clinic, which includes the recording of the anterior tibialis muscles to establish the MI. The muscular jerks are often accompanied by EEG signs of arousal, which may appear following the leg jerks. As with SDB, ambulatory equipment is available to record sleep in the comfort of one's own home. PLMS is diagnosed with a MI greater than 5.

PLMS and RLS may be associated with some medical conditions, including uremia, anemia, chronic lung disease, myelopathies, and peripheral neuropathies. Use of medications, such as tricyclic antidepressants and lithium carbonate, and withdrawal from benzodiazepines and anticonvulsants may all induce these disorders. Other movement disorders that should be differentiated from PLMS include the hypnic myoclonus, nocturnal leg cramps, and jerks associated with long-term use of L-dopa.[48]

Treatment and Management

PLMS is treated by medications aimed at reducing or eliminating the leg jerks or the arousals. Dopaminergic agents such as carbidopa/levodopa, pergolide,[49] and a newer drug, pramipexol, are the treatment of choice for PLMS, as they decrease or eliminate both the leg jerks and the arousals. These medications are also successful for the treatment of RLS.[49] In one study, carbidopa/levodopa was superior to propoxyphene in decreasing the number of leg kicks and the number of arousals per hour of sleep.[50] However, carbidopa/levodopa and, to a lesser extent, pergolide may shift the leg movements from the nighttime to the daytime.[49]

Benzodiazepines, such as clonazepam and temazepam, are sometimes used to treat PLMS. These drugs do not eliminate the limb movements but do decrease the arousals, so that the patient sleeps more continuously throughout the night.[51] Triazolam has been shown to be effective in older patients,[52] although because of age-related changes in pharmacokinetics and the need to avoid daytime sedation, it is recommended that low doses of triazolam be prescribed in this population.[53] Furthermore, caution should be used in prescribing a sedative hypnotic to elderly patients who might have SDB, because sedatives exacerbate the severity of the respiratory events. Some of the longer-acting medications, particularly clonazepam, may not be eliminated by morning, particularly in older adults, causing daytime sedation. Opiates such as propoxyphene or Tylenol with codeine are effective in decreasing the leg kicks; however, the arousals may continue to occur.[54]

REM Sleep Behavior Disorder

Definition and Prevalence

REM sleep behavior disorder (RBD) is a disorder in which the muscle atonia typical of the REM state is absent, causing motor disinhibition presenting as vigorous movements that may be violent or aggressive toward the patient or the bed partner. Vivid dreams are often remembered on awakening and are consistent with the observed behavior. Most often the patients report not being the aggressors in the dream, but being the defenders of themselves or their family members. The harmful behavior is uncharacteristic of the waking individual.

RBD is considered a neuropathologic disorder, although most often it is idiopathic. It has been associated with neurodegenerative impairments such as dementia, parkinsonism, Guillain–Barre syndrome, olivo-ponto-cerebellar degeneration, and subarachnoid hemorrhage.[55] Some patients exhibit other sleep disorders, including narcolepsy and PLMS. It is also associated with psychiatric disorders such as depression and drug and alcohol abuse and withdrawal.

The prevalence of REM behavior disorder (RBD) in the population has not been estimated; however, those diagnosed with the disorder are predominantly older men.[56]

Consequences

The majority of the patients report injuries to themselves and to their spouses, including ecchymoses, lacerations, and fractures.[56]

Clinical Presentation

Episodes usually begin during the second half of the night when REM is most abundant, but usually no earlier than 60 to 90 min after sleep onset, which is when the first REM period is expected to occur.

RBD may become more frequent over time. Patients may experience an episode once every 2 to 3 weeks, or as many as four episodes a night for several nights in a row. Some experience a nightly episode. There have been no reports of spontaneous remission.

One-fourth of the patients report a prodrome in their history, which involved behavioral disinhibition of dreams, or other parasomnias, including sleeptalking, yelling, and limb jerks. Sleep recordings show elevated percentages of REM sleep, as well as a shortened REM latency.

Diagnosis and Differential Diagnosis

A detailed history of the sleep disorder, from both the patient and the bed partner, should include the timing and frequency of the episodes and the type of the behavioral disturbance. Mahowald and Schenck[57] have suggested minimal criteria for diagnosing RBD, including a history or videotape recording of abnormal sleep behavior, with an EMG recording showing elevated muscle tone and/or phasic limb twitching.

Differential diagnoses include night terrors and sleepwalking, which are also disruptive behavioral enactments during sleep; however, unlike RBD, these are parasomnias that occur during non-REM sleep, often in the early part of the night.

Another differential diagnosis is parkinsonism, as 30% of patients with this disease who are treated with L-dopa may exhibit similar sleep disturbance.[58] In a longitudinal follow-up study of 29 male patients initially diagnosed with idiopathic RBD, 38% were subsequently diagnosed with a parkinsonian disorder.[59] Compared with the idiopathic RBD group, those who developed parkinsonism had significantly elevated PLMS in non-REM sleep, as well as elevated REM sleep percentage. The authors implicate the pathology of the pedunculopontine nucleus in these combined disorders.

Treatment and Management

Clonazepam is remarkably efficient in the treatment of both the vivid dreams and the disruptive behaviors in RBD. It can be taken at low doses for extended periods of time with minimal side effects.[56] Alprazolam may be used when clonazepam is not well tolerated.[58] However, benzodiazepines may be contraindicated in cases of SDB or excessive daytime sleepiness. Other treatment options include tricyclic antidepressants such as desipramine[55,60] and carbamazepine.[61]

Insomnia

Definition and Prevalence

Unlike SDB, PLMS, or RBD, insomnia is not considered a sleep disorder in itself, but rather a complaint of insufficient and nonrestorative sleep. There are several possible causes for the insomnia complaint, including medical, psychiatric, drug and medication use, changes in circadian rhythms, and psychophysiologic issues.

Insomnia may be short or transient, lasting only a few days to a few weeks. Most often, transient insomnia may be related to a specific event, such as taking an exam, moving to a new house, starting a new job, divorce, or loss of a loved one. The anxiety associated with the stressful event may interfere with sleep and, if not resolved effectively, poor sleep habits may turn into long-term psychophysiologic insomnia.

The prevalence of insomnia increases with age.[62] In a survey of more than 9000 elderly adults 65 years and older, 28% complained of difficulty initiating sleep, and 42% reported difficulty in both initiating and maintaining sleep.[2] In a study done in the general practice, more than 50% of elderly patients reported insomnia, with 80% of those reporting that the insomnia was a chronic condition.[63] Insomnia was associated with poor sleep hygiene and with depression. Women complained of insomnia more than men.[64,65] The annual incidence rate of insomnia in the elderly was found to be 5% and was associated with depressed mood, respiratory symptoms, poor perceived health, physical disabilities, widowhood, and use of sedatives.[66] Remission was estimated as 15% annually and was associated with improved self-perceived health, no new medical conditions such as heart disease and stroke, and improved physical functioning.[66] African-American women were found to have a higher incidence of insomnia than either African-American men or Caucasian men and women.[67]

Clinical Presentation

Insomnia may present as a difficulty in falling asleep, which is referred to as sleep onset insomnia, or as a difficulty in maintaining sleep throughout the night, which is called sleep maintenance insomnia. In sleep onset insomnia, the patient may lie in bed without falling asleep from 30 min to a few hours. With sleep maintenance insomnia, falling asleep is achieved easily, but the patient awakens one to several times during the night and has difficulty falling back to sleep. Some patients have both sleep onset and sleep maintenance insomnia. In the elderly, waking up too early in the morning and having difficulty getting back to sleep is particularly prevalent, often secondary to advanced sleep phase syndrome (ASPS). ASPS is a common circadian rhythm sleep disorder in the elderly, in which the timing of the sleep period is advanced to an earlier hour and wake-up time is correspondingly advanced as well.

Risk Factors

Long-term or chronic insomnia may be caused by chronic medical conditions, such as cerebrovascular disease, arthritis, chronic obstructive pulmonary disease, and neurologic disorders.[68] The pain and discomfort associated with these disorders may interfere with sleep. Psychiatric disorders are strongly related to the insomnia complaint.[69] Depression is one of the most common causes of insomnia, and depressive symptoms are very common in the elderly population[70] (see Chapter 79). Alerting or stimulating medications may cause insomnia, such as CNS stimulants, decongestants, beta-blockers, calcium channel blockers, corticosteroids, bronchodilators, and stimulating antidepressants.[31] Substances such as alcohol, caffeine, and nicotine can all cause insomnia. Sedating medications may cause daytime drowsiness, which may lead to daytime napping, which subsequently may also lead to insomnia at night. Circadian rhythm changes with age may also present as an insomnia complaint.

Diagnosis and Differential Diagnosis

Unlike the specific sleep disorders already discussed, a sleep recording in the sleep clinic is usually not warranted for complaints of insomnia because insomnia may not occur every night and often patients experience insomnia in their own bed but not in new environments.

As multiple factors may contribute to the insomnia complaint, a comprehensive history should be taken with the patient and, when possible, with the bed partner. This information should include medical and psychiatric history and current medication use, including dosage and time of administration. Possible sleep disorders may present as insomnia, including PLMS and SDB. Identification of the underlying problem causing the insomnia is the key to successful treatment.

A history should also include sleep-related habits such as napping, sleep–wake patterns on weekends versus weekdays, exercise regimens, timing and duration of bright light exposure, and caffeine or alcohol intake. Much of the sleep patterns and habits information can easily be obtained by asking the patient to fill out a sleep log for 1 or 2 weeks. An example of a typical sleep log can be seen in Table 70.1.

Some sleep clinics also use a wrist activity monitor, called an actigraph, which reliably distinguishes sleep from waking based on level of activity,[71,72] to diagnose insomnia. Patients wear this watchlike device and fill out a sleep log for about a week. Contrasting the objective actigraphic-based information with the subjective reports may reveal some misperceptions of the patient regarding their sleep. For example, insomnia patients may overestimate their sleep latency, that is, the amount of time that

TABLE 70.1. Sleep diary.

Day: __ Date: __ Patient ID:
Complete before bedtime:
1. Time actigraph removed for bathing: __ : __ am/pm
   Time put back on: __ : __ am/pm
2. How many naps did you take today?
   Times: From: __ : __ am/pm To: __ : __ am/pm
          From: __ : __ am/pm To: __ : __ am/pm
3. How many cups of coffee or other beverages with caffeine did you drink?
   Times: __ : __ am/pm
          __ : __ am/pm
4. How many alcoholic beverages did you drink?
   Time: __ : __ am/pm
         __ : __ am/pm
Complete in the morning:
1. What time did you go to bed? __ : __ am/pm
2. What time did you turn out the lights and go to sleep?
   __ : __ am/pm
3. How long did it take you to fall asleep? __ hours and __ minutes
4. How many awakenings did you have during the night?
5. What time did you wake up in the morning? __ : __ am/pm
6. What time did you get out of bed? __ : __ am/pm
7. Did you feel refreshed when you got up? yes/no

it takes them to fall asleep[73,74] and underestimate their sleep efficiency.[74]

Abnormal sleep–wake patterns may indicate a circadian rhythm sleep disorder. These disorders occur when the physiologic propensity for sleep is misaligned with the environmental light–dark cycle. Thus, although sleep may not be disrupted, its timing is inappropriate with respect to the normal environment. Elderly patients often complain of early morning awakenings, which may be caused by advanced sleep phase, that is, they are tired early in the day and they wake up early in the morning, due to an advancement of their sleep–wake cycle. Duffy et al.[6] have suggested that older individuals have a narrow window of time in which sleep is efficiently maintained, and this window is at an advanced clock time relative to younger adults. It is important to stress that although advanced sleep phase may present as insomnia, there is no sleep disruption associated with it, and only the timing of sleep is inappropriate or inconvenient. The differential diagnosis is important in terms of modes of treatment.

Treatment and Management

As many factors may contribute to the insomnia complaint, identifying and treating the underlying cause is the key for a successful outcome. If insomnia is caused by a painful medical problem, successful treatment of the medical disorder will improve the insomnia as well. If depression is causing the insomnia, treatment of the depression will help resolve the insomnia.

Changing the timing of medication administration may be important for resolving the insomnia. Ideally, stimulating medications should be taken early in the day, while sedating medications should be taken near bedtime.

Some behavioral modification techniques have proven successful for the alleviation of psychophysiologic or primary insomnia. In a recent review by Morin et al.,[75] 70% to 80% of patients with primary chronic insomnia benefited from nonpharmacologic treatments.

Sleep hygiene[76] is a set of guidelines aimed at maintaining healthy sleep habits. Commonsense rules include avoiding or limiting naps, particularly late in the day, as daytime napping may interfere with nighttime sleep; avoiding substances that interfere with sleep, such as alcohol, caffeine, and nicotine; maintaining a stable sleep–wake pattern throughout the week; and exercising regularly, but not late in the day (physical or mental stimulation at night may interfere with sleep). For a summary of sleep hygiene rules for the elderly, see Table 70.2.[77]

Stimulus control therapy[78] is another behavioral technique designed to remove all negative associations from the bedroom environment. The patient is instructed to go to bed only when sleepy. If unable to fall asleep in 15 to 20 min, the patient must leave the bedroom and engage in a relaxing activity, such as reading a magazine or writing a letter. Only when patients feel sleepy again can they return to bed. This procedure should be repeated as needed, until sleep is achieved in less than 15 min. For a summary of stimulus control therapy, see Table 70.3. Stimulus control therapy is appropriate for patients who feel stress, tension, or anxiety that are conditioned to the bedroom or the bed. They are caught in a vicious cycle, in which negative thoughts and feelings disrupt their ability to fall asleep, leading to more intensified adverse thoughts and feelings associated with the bedroom. Learning to associate the bedroom with relaxing feelings of sleepiness breaks the cycle and allows the patient to regain control over their sleep.

Sleep restriction therapy[79] is based on reducing time in bed to improve sleep efficiency. Many insomniacs try to

TABLE 70.2. Rules of sleep hygiene in the elderly.

1. Maintain a regular sleep/wake schedule.
2. Take no more than one nap per day.
3. Limit nap time to less than 60 min early in the day.
4. Exercise regularly.
5. Spend time in bright outdoor light.
6. Avoid caffeine, especially after lunch.
7. Avoid alcohol and nicotine.
8. Check the effects of medications on sleep.
9. Limit liquid intake in the evening.

Source: From Martin J, Shochat T, Ancoli-Israel S. Assessment and treatment of sleep disturbances in older adults. *Clin Psychol Rev.* 2000;20:783–805, with permission.

TABLE 70.3. Instructions for stimulus control therapy.

1. Patient goes to bed only when sleepy.
2. If not asleep within about 20 min, patient gets out of bed and engages in relaxing activity.
3. Patient returns to bed only when sleepy.
4. If patient again does not fall asleep within 20 min, repeat as necessary.
5. Wake-up time remains the same every day (regardless of number of hours asleep).
6. Daytime naps must be avoided.
7. Bed is used only for sleeping (not for reading, paying bills, or watching television).

Source: From Bootzin RR, Nicassio PM. Behavioral treatments for insomnia. In: Hersen M, Eisler RM, Miller PM, eds. *Progress in Behavior Modification, vol 6.* New York: Academic Press; 1978:1–45,[78] with permission.

get more sleep by going to bed early and spending more time in bed, when in fact this only worsens the problem. Thus, patients are instructed to stay in bed only for the amount of time that they actually sleep, plus 15 min. Actual sleep time is assessed by a subjective sleep log or an actigraph.[80,81] When sleep efficiency reaches 85% or above, time in bed may be increased by 15 min. The procedure is repeated until the desired amount of time in bed is reached.

Sleep restriction therapy was found to be superior to relaxation techniques[80] and comparable to sleep hygiene therapy[81] for the treatment of insomnia in community-residing elderly after a 3-month follow-up.

Bright light therapy is an effective treatment for circadian rhythm sleep disorders. The light–dark cycle is the most important synchronizer of our internal biologic clock, and changes in the timing of bright light exposure effectively shift altered circadian rhythms to a more appropriate phase.

In the elderly, who most commonly have advanced sleep phase syndrome, exposure to bright light in the evening hours on a daily basis delays the sleep episode to a later phase, so that they no longer experience the early morning awakenings that often present as an insomnia complaint. Avoidance of bright light in the early morning hours is also important, as light exposure early in the day causes an advancement of the sleep episode.

There is growing evidence that institutionalized elderly patients receive disturbingly low levels of illumination during the day, and this has been associated with poor sleep at night.[82–84]

Pharmacologic Treatment

The use of sedative-hypnotics in the elderly population must be approached with caution. Because of changes in metabolic and elimination rates, the lowest effective dose must be used. The specific type of sleep disturbance should be determined to establish the appropriate type of sedative; that is, a short-acting, fast-absorbing hypnotic would be appropriate for sleep-onset insomnia (e.g., zolpidem or zaleplon), whereas a medium-acting hypnotic should be used for sleep maintenance insomnia (e.g., temazepam). Long-acting hypnotics are usually contraindicated, as they are bound to create excessive daytime sleepiness and diminished performance the following day, and may increase the risk of car accidents.[85] Ultra-short-acting hypnotics, such as zaleplon, may be used both at the beginning of the night and again, if needed, in the middle of the night, without residual sedation in the morning.[86,87]

Pharmacologic treatment should be used in combination with behavioral therapy. In a small trial, Morin et al.[88] compared the effectiveness of behavioral, pharmacologic, and combined behavioral and pharmacologic treatment for insomnia in the elderly. All three modes of treatment were effective compared to placebo in the short term, and the combined approach was slightly better than the behavioral or pharmacologic approaches alone. However, long-term follow-up revealed that those who received pharmacologic treatment alone showed a worsening of their sleep, whereas those who received behavioral treatment alone maintained their gains from posttreatment. For the combined approach group, follow-up results were more variable, that is, some patients maintained their gains in the long run while some did not.

The use of melatonin for the alleviation of insomnia in the elderly has received much attention both in the scientific community and in the general media. Melatonin is a natural hormone that is secreted during the nighttime and is associated with sleep promotion and circadian rhythm regulation. The amount of melatonin secreted at night has been found to drop in the elderly, and this has been associated with the decline in sleep quality in older adults.[89] Melatonin replacement in elderly insomniacs has been found to improve sleep efficiency.[90] In a recent study, insomnia patients were able to discontinue benzodiazepine treatment and maintain good sleep quality with melatonin substitution.[91]

However, melatonin may be effective only in those insomnia patients whose melatonin levels are particularly low or depleted. Furthermore, caution should be used, as there is still much debate regarding the correct dosage and timing of administration. Finally, melatonin is currently sold as a food supplement and lacks proper quality control.

Sleep Disorders in Dementia

Definition and Prevalence

Dementia is highly associated with sleep disruption. Sleep–wake patterns in dementia are often polyphasic, with frequent nighttime awakenings and redistribution of sleep episodes throughout the day.[92] Ancoli-Israel and colleagues have reported that many institutionalized demented patients were neither awake nor asleep for a full hour in the day or night,[93] and that while the mildly to moderately demented patients had extremely fragmented sleep at night, the severely demented patients were extremely sleepy during the day and night.[94]

Clinical Presentation

Sleep structure is also altered in demented patients compared to healthy elderly individuals, with significantly lower amounts of stages 3 and 4 and REM sleep and significantly more awakenings, as well as more time spent awake during the night.[92] Increased stage 1 sleep and decreased sleep efficiency have also been reported.[95] REM latency has been found to increase in dementia patients, possibly due to the general reduction in the amount of REM found in these patients.[96]

The neuronal degeneration seen in Alzheimer's disease is most likely the cause of these sleep changes. Neuronal structures that are damaged in this population and are implicated in sleep regulation include the basal forebrain and the reticular formation of the brainstem.[96] As sleep changes are already evident in the early, mild stages of dementia, they may serve as markers of early dementia in clinical assessment.

Nocturnal awakenings, often accompanied by agitation, confusion, and wandering, are typical in demented patients. These events are often referred to as "sundowning" behaviors, and as they typically occur at the same time of day, it has been suggested that they are related to a circadian rhythm disorder.[97]

Support for this hypothesis has come from studies using bright light treatment for circadian rhythm disorders. Satlin et al.[98] used bright light therapy in the evening to improve sleep and behavioral disturbances in Alzheimer's disease patients. Mishima et al. found similar results using morning bright light therapy.[99] Lovell et al.[100] reported that bright light therapy in the morning hours decreased agitated behaviors in the late afternoon in a group of institutionalized demented patients.

In a recent study, Martin et al.[101] challenged the idea of sundowning by showing that peak levels of agitation occur during various times of the day, but more often in the afternoon, rather than in the evening or night. However, they did find associations between circadian rhythms of activity, agitation, and light exposure, indicating that sleep disruption in demented individuals may be amenable to treatment using bright light exposure.

Risk Factors

Ancoli-Israel et al.[26] have reported a strong relationship between demented patients and sleep apnea, with the most severe apnea in the most severely demented group of patients. This positive association has been confirmed by several research studies, as summarized by Ancoli-Israel and Coy.[102] In a review of the literature, the prevalence of SDB in demented patients ranged between 33% and 70%.[103] In a recent study of institutionalized Alzheimer's disease patients, the prevalence of SDB was 80% with RDI of 10 or more and 48% with an RDI of 20 or more.[104]

Cognitive impairment is a common symptom in both dementia and SDB patients. In SDB, cognitive impairment is associated with the nocturnal hypoxemia, as well as the sleep fragmentation.[27,28] In an epidemiologic study, Dealberto et al. (24) found a strong relationship between symptoms of SDB and cognitive impairment. Bliwise has suggested that SDB may contribute to cognitive decline in demented elderly, together with cerebrovascular disease and hypertension.[5,105] Furthermore, he suggests that treatment of SDB may reverse the cognitive decline in demented patients or at least slow the dementia process. In a pilot study, Shochat et al.[106] examined the possibility of treating demented patients with SDB using CPAP. They concluded that CPAP may be tolerated and may partially reverse cognitive decline (e.g., global mental functioning and memory) in some mildly demented patients.

In summary, severe sleep disturbance is commonly found in the demented elderly population, which may be the result of neurodegenerative processes in areas in the brain that regulate sleep/wake and possibly circadian rhythm mechanisms. The high presence of SDB in this population may indicate that neuronal damage is also contributing to the respiratory difficulties during sleep, and these respiratory disturbances may be contributing to the cognitive impairment associated with the dementia.

References

1. Vitiello MV. Sleep disorders and aging: understanding the causes. *J Gerontol.* 1997;52A:M189–M191.
2. Foley DJ, Monjan AA, Brown SL, Simonsick EM, Wallace RB, Blazer DG. Sleep complaints among elderly persons: an epidemiologic study of three communities. *Sleep.* 1995; 18:425–432.
3. Rechtschaffen A. Current perspectives on the function of sleep. *Perspect Biol Med.* 2000;41:359–390.
4. Weitzman ED, Moline ML, Czeisler CA, Zimmerman JC. Chronobiology of aging: temperature, sleep-wake rhythms and entrainment. *Neurobiol Aging.* 1982;3:299–309.
5. Bliwise DL. Review: sleep in normal aging and dementia. *Sleep.* 1993;16:40–81.
6. Duffy JF, Dijk DJ, Klerman EB, Czeisler CA. Later endogenous circadian temperature nadir relative to an earlier wake time in older people. *Am J Physiol.* 1998;275: R1478–R1487.

7. Feinberg I. Changes in sleep cycle patterns with age. *J Psychiatr Res.* 1974;10:283–306.

8. Zepelin H. Normal age related changes in sleep. In: Chase M, Weitzman ED, eds. *Sleep Disorders: Basic and Clinical Research.* New York: SP Medical; 1983:431–434.

9. Brezinova V. The number and duration of the episodes of the various EEG stages of sleep in young and older people. *Electroencephalogr Clin Neurophysiol.* 1975;39:273–278.

10. Reynolds CFI, Kupfer DJ, Taska LS, Hoch CC, Sewitch DE, Spiker DG. Sleep of healthy seniors: a revisit. *Sleep.* 1985; 8:20–29.

11. Rediehs MH, Reis JS, Creason NS. Sleep in old age: focus on gender differences. *Sleep.* 1990;13(5):410–424.

12. Reynolds CFI, Monk TH, Hoch CC, et al. Electroencephalographic sleep in the healthy "old old": a comparison with the "young old" in visually scored and automated measures. *J Gerontol.* 1991;46(2):M39–M46.

13. Cartwright R. Effect of sleep position on sleep apnea severity. *Sleep.* 1984;7:110–114.

14. Findley LJ, Wilhoit SC, Suratt PM. Apnea duration and hypoxemia during REM sleep in patients with obstructive sleep apnea. *Chest.* 1985;87:432–436.

15. Ancoli-Israel S, Kripke DF, Klauber MR, Mason WJ, Fell R, Kaplan O. Sleep disordered breathing in community-dwelling elderly. *Sleep.* 1991;14(6):486–495.

16. Young T, Palta M, Dempsey J, Skatrud J, Weber S, Badr S. The occurrence of sleep disordered breathing among middle-aged adults. *N Engl J Med.* 1993;328:1230–1235.

17. Lavie P, Herer P, Hoffstein V. Obstructive sleep apnea syndrome as a risk factor for hypertension: population study. *Br Med J (Clin Res Ed).* 2000;320:479–482.

18. Wittels EH. Obesity and hormonal factors in sleep and sleep apnea. *Med Clin North Am.* 1985;69:1265-1280.

19. Guilleminault C. Natural history, cardiac impact and long-term follow-up of sleep apnea syndrome. In: Guilleminault C, Lugaresi E, eds. *Sleep/Wake Disorders: Natural History, Epidemiology, and Long-term Evolution.* New York: Raven Press; 1983:107–124.

20. Lavie P, Herer P, Peled R, et al. Mortality in sleep apnea patients: a multivariate analysis of risk factors. *Sleep.* 1995; 18:149–157.

21. Ancoli-Israel S, Kripke DF, Klauber MR, et al. Morbidity, mortality and sleep disordered breathing in community dwelling elderly. *Sleep.* 1996;19:277–282.

22. Wright J, Johns R, Watt I, Melville A, Sheldon T. Health effects of obstructive sleep apnea and the effectiveness of continuous airway pressure: a systematic reveiw of the research evidence. *Br Med J.* 1997;314:851–860.

23. Foley DJ, Monjan AA, Masaki KH, Enright PL, Quan SF, White LR. Associations of symptoms of sleep apnea with cardiovacular disease, cognitive impairment and mortality among older Japanese-American men. *J Am Geriatr Soc.* 1999;47:524–528.

24. Dealberto MJ, Pajot N, Courbon D, Alperovitch A. Breathing disorders during sleep and cognitive performance in an older community sample: the EVA study. *J Am Geriatr Soc.* 1996;44:1287–1294.

25. Kullen AS, Stepnowsky C, Parker L, Ancoli-Israel S. Cognitive impairment and sleep disordered breathing. *Sleep Res.* 1993;22:224.

26. Ancoli-Israel S, Klauber MR, Butters N, Parker L, Kripke DF. Dementia in institutionalized elderly: relation to sleep apnea. *J Am Geriatr Soc.* 1991;39(3):258–263.

27. Valencia-Flores M, Bliwise DL, Guilleminault C, Cilveti R, Clerk A. Cognitive function in patients with sleep apnea after acute nocturnal nasal continuous positive airway pressure (CPAP) treatment: sleepiness and hypoxemia effects. *J Clin Exp Neuropsychol.* 1996;18:197–210.

28. Findley LJ, Barth JT, Powers DC, Wilhoit SC, Boyd DG, Suratt PM. Cognitive impairment in patients with obstructive sleep apnea and associated hypoxemia. *Chest.* 1986;90: 686–690.

29. Wetter DW, Young TB, Bidwell TR, Badr MS, Palta M. Smoking as a risk factor for sleep-disordered breathing. *Arch Intern Med.* 1994;154:2219–2224.

30. Loube DI, Loube AA, Mitler MM. Weight loss for obstructive sleep apnea: the optimal therapy for obese patients. *J Am Diet Assoc.* 1994;94:1291–1295.

31. Ancoli-Israel S. Sleep problems in older adults: putting myths to bed. *Geriatrics.* 1997;52:20–30.

32. Guilleminault C, Silvestri R, Mondini S, Coburn S. Aging and sleep apnea: action of benzodiazepine, acetazolamide, alcohol, and sleep deprivation in a healthy elderly group. *J Gerontol.* 1984;39:655–661.

33. Block AJ, Hellard DW, Slayton PC. Effect of alcohol ingestion on breathing and oxygenation during sleep. Analysis of the influence of age and sex. *Am J Med.* 1986;80:595–600.

34. American Thoracic Society. Indications and standards for use of nasal continuous positive airway pressure (CPAP) in sleep apnea syndromes. *Am J Respir Crit Care Med.* 1994;150:1738–1745.

35. Redline S, Adams N, Strauss ME, Roebuck T, Winters M, Rosenberg C. Improvement of mild sleep disordered breathing with CPAP compared with conservative therapy. *Am I Res Crit Care Med.* 1998;157:858–865.

36. Fleury B, Rakotonanahary D, Tehindrazanarivelo AD, Hausser-Hauw C, Lebeau B. Sleep and breathing: long term compliance to continuous positive airway pressure therapy (nCPAP) setup during a split-night polysomnography. *Sleep.* 1994;17:512–515.

37. Collard P, Pieters T, Aubert P, Delguste P, Rodenstein DO. Compliance with nasal CPAP in obstructive sleep apnea. *Sleep Med Rev.* 1997;1:33–44.

38. Powell NB, Guilleminault C, Riley RW. Surgical therapy for obstructive sleep apnea. In: Kryger MH, Roth T, Dement WC, eds. *Principles and Practice of Sleep Medicine, 2nd Ed.* Philadelphia: Saunders; 1994:706–721.

39. Walker RP, Grigg-Damberger M, Gopalsami C. Uvulopalatopharyngoplasty versus laser-assisted uvulopalatoplasty for the treatment of obstructive sleep apnea. *Laryngoscope.* 1997;107:76–82.

40. Walker RP, Grigg-Damberger M, Gopalsami C. Laser-assisted uvulopalatoplasty for the treatment of mild, moderate and severe obstructive sleep apnea. *Laryngoscope.* 1999; 109:79–85.

41. Riley RW, Powell NB, Guilleminault C. Obstructive sleep apnea syndrome: a review of 306 consecutively treated surgical patients. *Otolaryngol Head Neck Surg.* 1993;108: 117–125.

42. Schmidt-Nowara WW, Lowe A, Wiegand L, Cartwright R, Perez-Guerra F, Menn S. Oral appliances for the treatment of snoring and obstructive sleep apnea: a review. *Sleep*. 1995;18:501–510.

43. An American Sleep Disorders Associations Report. Practice parameters for the treatment of snoring and obstructive sleep apnea with oral appliances. *Sleep*. 1995; 18:511–513.

44. Ancoli-Israel S, Kripke DF, Klauber MR, Mason WJ, Fell R, Kaplan O. Periodic limb movements in sleep in community-dwelling elderly. *Sleep*, 1991;14(6):496–500.

45. Bixler EO, Kales A, Vela-Bueno A, Jacoby JA, Scarone S, Soldatos CR. Nocturnal myoclonus and nocturnal myoclonic activity in a normal population. *Res Commun Chem Pathol Pharmacol*. 1982;36:129–140.

46. Guilleminault C, Crowe C, Quera-Salva MA, Miles L, Partinen M. Periodic leg movement, sleep fragmentation and central sleep apnoea in two cases: reduction with Clonazepam. *Eur Respir J*. 1988;1(8):762–765.

47. Mahowald MW, Schenck CH. REM sleep behavior disorder. In: Thorpy MJ, ed. *Handbook of Sleep Disorders*. New York: Dekker; 1990:567–593.

48. Montplaisir J, Godbout R, Pelletier G, Warnes H. Restless leg syndrome and periodic limb movements during sleep. In: Kryger MH, Roth T, Dement WC, eds. *Principles and Practice of Sleep Medicine, 2nd Ed*. Philadelphia: Saunders; 1994:589–597.

49. Earley CJ, Allen RP. Pergolide and carbidopa/levodopa treatment of the restless legs syndrome and periodic leg movements in sleep in a consecutive series of patients. *Sleep*. 1996;19:801–810.

50. Kaplan PW, Allen RP, Buchholz DW, Walters JK. A double-blind, placebo-controlled study of the treatment of periodic limb movements in sleep using carbidopa/levidopa and propoxyphene. *Sleep*. 1993;16(8):717–723.

51. Mitler MM, Browman CP, Menn SJ, Gujavarty K, Timms RM. Nocturnal myoclonus: treatment efficacy of clonazepam and temazepam. *Sleep*. 1986;9:385–392.

52. Bonnet MH, Arand DL. The use of triazolam in older patients with periodic leg movements, fragmented sleep, and daytime sleepiness. *J Gerontol*. 1990;45(4):M139–M144.

53. Greenblatt DJ, Harmatz JS, Shapiro L, Engelhardt N, Gouthro TA, Shader RI. Sensitivity to triazolam in the elderly. *N Engl J Med*. 1991;13:1691–1698.

54. Kavey N, Walters AS, Hening W, Gidro-Frank S. Opioid treatment of periodic movements in sleep in patients without restless legs. *Neuropeptides*. 1988;11(4):181–184.

55. Schenck CH, Bundlie SR, Ettinger M, Mahowald MW. Chronic behavioral disorders of human REM sleep: a new category of parasomnia. *Sleep*. 1986;9:293–308.

56. Schenck CH, Mahowald MW. Polysomnographic, neurologic, psychiatric, and clinical outcome report on 70 consecutive cases with the REM sleep behavior disorder (RBD): sustained clonazepam efficacy in 89.5% of 57 treated patients. *Clevel Clin J Med*. 1990;57:S10–S24.

57. Mahowald MW, Schenck CH. REM sleep behavior disorder. In: Kryger MH, Roth T, Dement WC, eds. *Principles and Practice of Sleep Medicine, 2nd Ed*. Philadelphia: Saunders; 1994:574–588.

58. Sforza E, Krieger J, Petiau C. REM sleep behavior: clinical and physiopathological findings. *Sleep Med Rev*. 1997; 1:57–69.

59. Schenck CH, Bundlie SR, Mahowald MW. Delayed emergence of a parkinsonian disorder in 38% of 29 older men initially diagnosed with idiopathic rapid eye movement sleep behavior disorder. *Neurology*. 1996;46:388–393.

60. Schenck CH, Bundlie SR, Patterson AL, Mahowald MW. Rapid eye movement sleep behavior disorder. A treatable parasomnia affecting older adults. *JAMA*. 1987;257:1786–1789.

61. Bamford CR. Carbamazepine in REM sleep behavior disorder. *Sleep*. 1993;16:33–34.

62. Mellinger GD, Balter MB, Uhlenhuth EH. Insomnia and its treatment. Prevalence and correlates. *Arch Gen Psychiatry*. 1985;42:225–232.

63. Hohagen F, Kappler C, Schramm E, et al. Prevalence of insomnia in elderly general practice attenders and the current treatment modalities. *Acta Psychiatr Scand*. 1994; 90:102–108.

64. Morgan K, Dallosso H, Ebrahim S, Arie T, Fentem PH. Characteristics of subjective insomnia in the elderly living at home. *Age Ageing*. 1988;17:1–7.

65. Chui HFK, Leung T, Lam LCW, et al. Sleep problems in Chinese elderly in Hong Kong. *Sleep*. 1999;22:717–726.

66. Foley DJ, Monjan A, Simonsick EM, Wallace RB, Blazer DG. Incidence and remission of insomnia among elderly adults: an epidemiologic study of 6800 persons over three years. *Sleep*. 1999;22:S366–S372.

67. Foley DJ, Monjan A, Izmirlian G, Hays JC, Blazer DG. Incidence and remission of insomnia among elderly adults in a biracial cohort. *Sleep*. 1999;22:S373–S378.

68. Wooten V. Medical causes of insomnia. In: Kryger MH, Roth T, Dement WC, eds. *Principles and Practice of Sleep Medicine*. Philadelphia: Saunders; 1994:456–475.

69. Ford DE, Kamerow DB. Epidemiologic study of sleep disturbances and psychiatric disorders: an opportunity for prevention? *JAMA*. 1989;262(11):1479–1484.

70. Blazer D, Burchett B, Service C, George LK. The association of age and depression among the elderly: an epidemiologic exploration. *J Gerontol*. 1991;46(6): M210–M215.

71. Hauri PJ, Wisbey J. Wrist actigraphy in insomnia. *Sleep*. 1992;15(4):293–301.

72. Sadeh A, Sharkey KM, Carskadon MA. Activity-based sleep-wake identification: an empirical test of methodological issues. *Sleep*. 1994;17:201–207.

73. Bootzin RR, Wyatt JK, Valdiserri M, Ludwig C. Assessment of insomnia at home with wrist actigraphy and sleep diaries. *Sleep Res*. 1993;22:355.

74. Brooks JO III, Friedman L, Bliwise DL, Yesavage JA. Use of the wrist actigraph to study insomnia in older adults. *Sleep*. 1992;16(2):151–155.

75. Morin CM, Hauri PJ, Espie CA, Spielman AJ, Buysse DJ, Bootzin RR. Nonpharmacologic treatment of chronic insomnia. An American Academy of Sleep Medicine review. *Sleep*. 1999;22:1134–1156.

76. Hauri P, Linde S. *No More Sleepless Nights*. New York: Wiley; 1990:1–262.

77. Hauri P. *Case Studies in Insomnia.* New York: Plenum; 1991: 1–268.

78. Bootzin RR, Nicassio PM. Behavioral treatments for insomnia. In: Hersen M, Eisler RM, Miller PM, eds. *Progress in Behavior Modification, vol 6.* New York: Academic Press; 1978:1–45.

79. Glovinsky PB, Spielman AJ. Sleep restriction therapy. In: Hauri PJ, ed. *Case Studies in Insomnia.* New York: Plenum; 1991:49–63.

80. Friedman L, Bliwise DL, Yesavage JA, Salom SR. A preliminary study comparing sleep restriction and relaxation treatments for insomnia in older adults. *J Gerontol.* 1991; 46(1):P1–P8.

81. Friedman L, Benson K, Noda A, et al. An actigraphic comparison of sleep restriction and sleep hygiene treatments for insomnia in older adults. *J Geriatr Psychiatry Neurol.* 2000;13:17–27.

82. Ancoli-Israel S, Klauber MR, Jones DW, et al. Variations in circadian rhythms of activity, sleep and light exposure related to dementia in nursing home patients. *Sleep.* 1997; 20:18–23.

83. Martin J, Shochat T, Marler M, Ancoli-Israel S. Circadian activity rhythms, sleep/wake and light exposure in nursing patients. *Sleep.* 2000;23:A216.

84. Martin J, Shochat T, Gehrman P, et al. Light, sleep and agitation in Alzheimer's disease patients. *Soc Light Treat Bio-Rhythms.* 2000;12:13.

85. Hemmelgarn B, Suissa S, Huang A, Boivin JF, Pinard G. Benzodiazepine use and the risk of motor vehicle crash in the elderly. *JAMA.* 1997;2:27–31.

86. Walsh JK, Pollack CP, Scharf MB, Schweitzer PK, Vogel GW. Lack of residual sedation following middle-of-the-night zaleplon administration in sleep maintenance insomnia. *Clin Neuropharmacol.* 2000;23:17–21.

87. Ancoli-Israel S, Walsh JK, Mangano RM, Fujimori M, Zaleplon Clinical Study Group. Zaleplon, a novel non-benzodiazepine hypnotic, effectively treats insomnia in elderly patients without causing rebound effects. *Prim Care Comp J Clin Psychiatry.* 1999;1:114–120.

88. Morin CM, Colecchi C, Stone J, Sood R, Brink D. Behavioral and pharmacological therapies for late life insomnia. *JAMA.* 1999;281:991–999.

89. Haimov I, Laudon M, Zisapel N, et al. Sleep disorders and melatonin rhythms in elderly people. *Br Med J.* 1994;309: 167.

90. Haimov I, Lavie P, Laudon M, Herer P, Vigder C, Zisapel N. Melatonin replacement therapy of elderly insomniacs. *Sleep.* 1995;18(7):598–603.

91. Garfinkel D, Zisapel N, Wainstein J, Laudon M. Facilitation of benzodiazepine discontinuation by melatonin: a

new clinical approach. *Arch Intern Med.* 1999;159:2456–2460.

92. Prinz PN, Peskind ER, Vitaliano PP, et al. Changes in the sleep and waking EEGs of nondemented and demented elderly subjects. *J Am Geriatr Soc.* 1982;30:86–92.

93. Jacobs D, Ancoli-Israel S, Parker L, Kripke DF. Twenty-four hour sleep-wake patterns in a nursing home population. *Psychol Aging.* 1989;4(3):352–356.

94. Pat-Horenczyk R, Klauber MR, Shochat T, Ancoli-Israel S. Hourly profiles of sleep and wakefulness in severely versus mild-moderately demented nursing home patients. *Aging Clin Exp Res.* 1998;10:308–315.

95. Bliwise DL. Sleep in dementing illness. *Annu Rev Psychiatry.* 1994;13:757–777.

96. Prinz PN, Vitaliano PP, Vitiello MV, et al. Sleep, EEG and mental function changes in senile dementia of the Alzheimer's type. *Neurobiol Aging.* 1982;3:361–370.

97. Bliwise DL, Carroll JS, Lee KA, Nekich JC, Dement WC. Sleep and sundowning in nursing home patients with dementia. *Psychiatry Res.* 1993;48:277–292.

98. Satlin A, Volicer L, Ross V, Herz L, Campbell SS. Bright light treatment of behavioral and sleep disturbances in patients with Alzheimer's disease. *Am J Psychiatry.* 1992; 149:1028–1032.

99. Mishima K, Okawa M, Hishikawa Y, Hozumi S, Hori H, Takahashi K. Morning bright light therapy for sleep and behavior disorders in elderly patients with dementia. *Acta Psychiatr Scand.* 1994;89:1–7.

100. Lovell BJ, Ancoli-Israel S, Gevirtz R. The effect of bright light treatment on agitated behavior in institutionalized elderly. *Psychiatry Res.* 1995;57:7–12.

101. Martin J, Marler MR, Shochat T, Ancoli-Israel S. Circadian rhythms of agitation in institutionalized Alzheimer's disease patients. *Chronobiol Int.* 2000;17:405–418.

102. Ancoli-Israel S, Coy T. Are breathing disturbances in elderly equivalent to sleep apnea syndrome? *Sleep.* 1994; 17:77–83.

103. Ancoli-Israel S. Epidemiology of sleep disorders. In: Roth T, Roehrs TA, eds. *Clinics in Geriatric Medicine.* Philadelphia: Saunders; 1989:347–362.

104. Ancoli-Israel S, Poceta JS, Stepnowsky C, Martin J, Gehrman P. Identification and treatment of sleep problems in the elderly. *Sleep Med Rev.* 1997;1:3–17.

105. Bliwise DL. Is sleep apnea a cause of reversible dementia in old age? *J Am Geriatr Soc.* 1996;44:1407–1409.

106. Shochat T, Cohen-Zion M, Ancoli-Israel S. The effects of CPAP treatment on cognitive function in dementia: a pilot study. *Sleep.* 2000;23:A21.

71
Herpes Zoster

Kenneth Schmader

Herpes zoster is a neurocutaneous disease caused by the reactivation of varicella-zoster virus (VZV) from a clinically latent state in dorsal sensory or cranial ganglia. VZV reactivation preferentially affects elderly persons and usually results in dermatomal pain and a vesicular skin eruption. Zoster has been recognized since ancient times, but only recently have large numbers of persons experienced the disease, owing to population aging and increasing numbers of immunosuppressed hosts. Although a scourge for the patient, zoster is a remarkable phenomenon for clinical observers. Dr. Hope-Simpson said it best when lecturing the Royal College of Physicians in England: "Herpes zoster is fascinating because it arrives unpredictably, is readily diagnosed—a rare pleasure for most of us—and difficult to explain."[1]

Epidemiology

Risk Factors

Aging

The cardinal epidemiologic feature of herpes zoster is its striking relationship to aging. Primary VZV infection usually occurs during childhood and adolescence in temperate zones (childhood to young adulthood in tropical zones), and VZV establishes a latent infection in more than 95% of the adult population (Fig. 71.1).[2] However, the likelihood of symptomatic VZV reactivation increases sharply with aging.[1-5] For example, Hope-Simpson's study of zoster cases in England showed an incidence of 0.74 per 1000 per year in children under 10 years old, 2.5 per 1000 per year in adults aged 20 to 50 years, and 7.5 per 1000 per year in those older than 60 years old.[1] Ragozzino et al. found a similar dramatic increase with aging in Minnesota, where the incidence of zoster was less than 1 per 1000 per year under 44 years old but peaked at 4 to 4.5 per 1000 per year at ages

greater than 75 years.[3] Donahue et al. confirmed this relationship in Boston where they reported an incidence of 1.9, 2.3, 3.1, 5.7, and 11.8 per 1000 person-years for the age groups 25 to 34, 35 to 44, 45 to 54, 55 to 64, and 65 to 75+ years, respectively.[5]

Cellular Immunity

The other strong risk factor for zoster is cellular immune dysfunction. In vitro lymphoproliferative responsiveness to VZV antigens is significantly diminished in immunosuppressed patients and in the elderly. In vivo, zoster is more frequent and severe in patients with hematologic malignancies, organ transplants, HIV infection, immunomediated diseases, and immunosuppressive therapies.[6-10] Patients with solid tumors are at lesser risk for zoster, but in one large series treated patients of any age with lung, breast, or gynecologic cancers were more likely to have zoster than those with other solid tumors.[6] Conversely, zoster is not a risk factor for cancer, so the presence of zoster in an elderly patient should not trigger a diagnostic search for a presumed underlying malignancy.[10]

Other Factors

Other potentially important but less well-established risk factors include physical trauma, radiation therapy, psychologic stress, and white race. In a case-control study of stressful life events and zoster in the elderly, cases experienced negative life events significantly more often than controls at 2 months before zoster onset [odds ratio (OR) 2.64, 95% confidence interval (CI) 1.13, 6.27] and 3 months before onset (OR 2.64, 95% CI 1.20, 6.04).[11] In the Duke Established Populations for the Epidemiological Studies of the Elderly (EPESE), stressful life events increased the risk of zoster but the result was borderline for statistical significance [adjusted relative risk (RR) = 1.38, 95% CI 0.96–1.97, p = 0.078], and methodologic limitations precluded definitive conclusions about these results.[12] Regarding race, in the Duke EPESE, blacks

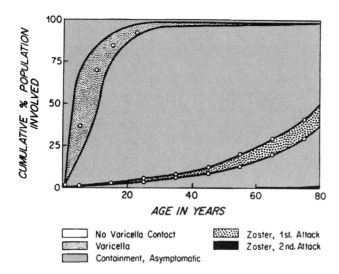

FIGURE 71.1. Age-related activity of varicella-zoster virus in a population in a temperate region. (Reprinted by permission of the *New England Journal of Medicine* 1983;309:1366.[2])

were four times less likely than whites to develop zoster over their lifetimes, after adjusting for age, cancer, sex, and education (adjusted OR 0.25, 95% CI 0.18–0.35).[13] In a follow-up prospective study of the incidence of zoster in blacks and whites in the Duke EPESE, blacks were significantly less likely than whites to develop zoster (adjusted risk ratio 0.35, 95% CI 0.24–0.51).[12] Gender, education, residence, season, and exposure to zoster or to chickenpox do not predict zoster.[1,3,13,14]

Incidence

The incidence of herpes zoster in Western populations of all ages is estimated to be between 1.3 and 3.4 per 1000 person-years.[1,3,5,15] Estimates of the incidence of zoster in the elderly vary from 3.9 to 11.8 cases per 1000 person-years.[1,3,5,13,15] The incidence of zoster in populations limited to immunosuppressed patients is substantially higher. For example, the incidence of zoster in HIV-infected individuals ranges from 29 to 51 per 1000 person-years.[8,16,17] Investigators have used these data to calculate an overall lifetime incidence of zoster of 10% to 20% and to estimate the total number of cases in the United States each year to be at least 600,000.[18] Elderly patients usually experience zoster only once, but second attacks occur in 1% to 5% of zoster victims. With population aging, the total number of zoster cases worldwide will increase significantly in the future.

Transmission

The potential infectivity of the elderly zoster patient is an important component of the disease. Viable, cell-free, infectious VZV is present in vesicular lesions. Although less infectious than varicella patients, an elderly zoster patient can transmit varicella to an uninfected susceptible host. There is no evidence that the elderly zoster patient transmits varicella or herpes zoster to latently infected individuals.[14] Regarding infection control, susceptible, seronegative persons should avoid contact with the zoster patient until the rash has crusted over. To protect susceptible staff and patients, the Centers for Disease Control recommends a private room and standard precautions for immunocompetent hospital patients with localized zoster. For immunocompromised patients in hospital with localized zoster or any patient with disseminated zoster, the recommendations are a private room with special ventilation and airborne and contact precautions. The risk of VZV transmission is thought to be higher in these patients.[19] Similar measures are advocated for zoster patients in long-term care facilities but modified for the special problems and limited resources of these facilities.[20] For example, private rooms may be available only for the patient with disseminated zoster. These precautions no longer apply when the rash has crusted over because VZV is very difficult to recover and the patient is no longer contagious.

Pathogenesis

Varicella-Zoster Virus

The causative agent is a double-stranded DNA virus of the herpesvirus family. The VZV genome contains approximately 125,000 nucleotide base pairs and encodes about 70 gene products.[21,22] These products include glycoproteins located in the viral envelope that bind to host cell receptors, initiate cellular infection, and stimulate the host immune response. Other protein products include the enzymes thymidine kinase and viral DNA polymerase. Viral thymidine kinase catalyzes the transformation of nucleoside analogues such as acyclovir to the triphosphate form that inhibits VZV DNA polymerase and viral replication.

Primary and Latent Infection

VZV causes primary infection when it invades the respiratory tract of a VZV-naive individual. From the respiratory tract, VZV disseminates in the blood and infects the skin, causing the rash of chickenpox. During this time, VZV also infects dorsal sensory and cranial nerve ganglia where it establishes a latent, lifelong infection. The persistence of VZV in asymptomatic adults has been confirmed by the detection of VZV DNA and RNA in spinal and trigeminal ganglia by in situ hybridization and by amplification of VZV DNA using the polymerase chain reaction (PCR).[23,24] The virus is present in both neurons and satellite cells during latency.[22] VZV appears to evade the immune system during latency by limiting expression of viral proteins and downregulating the expression of MCH class I antigens.

Reactivation

The molecular mechanisms responsible for VZV reactivation are poorly understood. Available evidence suggests that VZV sporadically replicates throughout life but the host immune response prevents clinical manifestations. As host immunity wanes, the likelihood of reactivated VZV causing zoster increases.[25] As with other herpesviruses, cell-mediated immunity is much more important than humoral immunity in defending VZV reactivation. For example, patients with agammaglobulinemia do not have an increased risk for zoster whereas diseases and therapies that affect T cells (hematologic malignancies, AIDS, cancer chemotherapy) markedly increase the incidence and severity of zoster.

Age-related decline in the number and function of T-cell responders to VZV plays a role in the development of zoster in old age. Studying lymphocytes from young ($n = 14$) and old ($n = 15$) subjects, Miller first demonstrated that the proliferative response of these cells to VZV antigen in vitro was significantly less in the elderly.[26] Berger et al. confirmed age-related differences in VZV antigen-dependent lymphocyte proliferation by demonstrating a low or absent stimulation index in lymphocytes from 33 of 100 (33%) healthy elderly and 0 of 43 (0%) persons aged 20 to 40 years.[27] Burke et al. studied lymphocyte proliferation and skin test reactivity to VZV antigen in 157 healthy, latently infected subjects of all ages.[28] Mean stimulation indices declined steadily by decade from a peak mean of 6.28 in 1- to 10-year-olds ($n = 24$) to 2.10 in 60- to 70-year-olds ($n = 12$), 1.56 in 70- to 80-year-olds ($n = 12$), and 1.39 in 90- to 100-year-olds ($n = 13$). In addition, the percent of positive skin test responses to VZV progressively decreased with aging, starting at 89% in 30- to 40-year-olds to 18% in 60- to 70-year-olds, 8% in 70- to 80-year-olds, and 0% in 80- to 100-year-olds. Finally, Hayward et al. used lymphoproliferative responses to VZV antigens to estimate the frequency of VZV-responsive lymphocytes in blood from healthy old ($n = 6$) and young ($n = 6$) subjects.[29] Mean responder cell frequency was $1:14,300 \pm 2000$ (one VZV-responsive lymphocyte per 14,300 lymphocytes) in young volunteers and $1:78,000 \pm 6600$ in elderly subjects ($p = 0.002$). Further studies by Hayward et al. have confirmed these findings in larger numbers of subjects.[30] Although these studies were limited by cross-sectional design and small sample size, they demonstrated consistent results using similar methodologies. Whether the age-related decline in tests of in vitro VZV cellular immunity and the age-related increase in herpes zoster are coincidence or cause and effect is unknown.

Clinical Features

Acute Herpes Zoster

Prodrome

As VZV spreads in the dorsal ganglion and afferent nerve, the patient usually experiences a prodrome of pain, discomfort, or paresthesias in the affected dermatome. This distressing prelude bewilders patients, caregivers, and physicians because the cause is not readily apparent and it masquerades as many other conditions in the elderly, such as biliary colic, appendicitis, kidney stones, pleuritis, myocardial infarction, acute musculoskeletal pain, trigeminal neuralgia, and migraine headaches. One potentially useful clue to the diagnosis is tender or hyperesthetic skin in the affected dermatome during this prodrome. The experienced clinician should keep herpes zoster in the differential diagnosis of any acute, unilateral, localized pain syndrome in the elderly, particularly if unexplained after the history and examination.

Rash

After a few days of the prodrome, the rash erupts and the diagnosis of zoster becomes apparent (see Fig. 59.4). The rash begins as an erythematous maculopapular eruption that is unilateral and dermatomal. Within a day or two, vesicles form on this erythematous base. The exanthem may be confluent or scattered about the dermatome and a few satellite lesions may be found in adjoining dermatomes. It appears most frequently on the areas of the trunk innervated by T3 to L3 and on the areas of the face innervated by the ophthalmic division of the trigeminal nerve.[1,3,31] Typically, the vesicles crust over in 7 to 10 days (2–3 weeks in immunocompromised individuals) and the crusts persist for 2 to 3 weeks. The impact of the rash ranges from an uncomfortable nuisance to serious problem in the elderly, including dissemination to other areas of skin, secondary bacterial infection, scarring, embarrassment and social withdrawal when on the face, and inaccessibility for proper care when on the back.

Pain

The acute neuritis produces significant pain in most elderly patients but the pain experience is remarkably variable, reflecting the variability of many conditions in geriatrics. A small percentage (~10%) of elderly zoster patients undergo little or no pain.[32] For those with pain or discomfort, the severity ranges from mild to severe; the quality includes terms like burning, deep aching, tingling, itching, and stabbing; and the temporal aspects vary from constant to intermittent. The acute zoster pain experience can have a tremendous effect on the patient's quality of life and functional status by interfering with personal care, mobility, sleep, energy, mood, and socialization.

Atypical Presentations

Zoster is no different from other conditions in geriatrics in its ability to present atypically. The rash may be small and inconspicuous or it may be disseminated over several dermatomes. In AIDS patients, chronic, indolent VZV replication can generate a hyperkeratotic, verrucous rash.[33] In other clinical scenarios, the rash may not be present as a diagnostic guide. For example, investigators have described prodromal pain for a month or more before the appearance of the rash, so-called preherpetic neuralgia.[34] Typical unilateral, dermatomal, neuralgic pain due to zoster can occur without a rash, an event entitled zoster sine herpete.[35] Besides dermatomal pain, acute facial palsy, hearing loss, vertigo, and/or dysgeusia (cranial polyneuritis); blurred vision and a painful eye (acute retinal necrosis); fever, delirium, and meningismus (meningoencephalitis); back pain, leg paraparesis and ascending paresthesias (myelitis); and hepatitis may be the first manifestations of zoster without a rash.[36–39]

Postherpetic Neuralgia

Postherpetic neuralgia (PHN) is the most debilitating and feared feature of zoster in the elderly. A common definition of PHN is pain 1 month after the onset of the rash, although alternative definitions include pain after the rash has healed or pain 3 months after rash onset.[40,41] Like zoster, the overriding epidemiologic feature of PHN is its striking relationship to aging. For example, deMoragas and Kirkland reported pain greater than 1 month in 10% of zoster patients less than 40 years old, 42.3% of those 40- to 59 years old, and 68% of those greater than 60 years old.[32] Other risk factors include greater severity of the acute pain, greater rash severity, the degree of sensory impairment in the affected dermatome, and a painful prodrome.[42–44] In the placebo group of a large acyclovir trial in zoster patients over 60 years old, 61% of patients had pain 1 month after rash onset.[45]

PHN victims describe their suffering with words like burning, throbbing, stabbing, shooting, sharp, aching, gnawing, tiring, and tender.[46] These descriptors and clinical studies have revealed that PHN pain is spontaneous and/or stimulus evoked.[47] The spontaneous pain usually involves constant pain and/or brief, intermittent shock-like pain. Patients may also note distracting tingling or itching. Stimulus-evoked pain consists of allodynia or hyperpathia. Allodynia is pain elicited by an innocuous stimulus, but that definition does not convey how terrible this can be for the elderly patient. The touch of bedsheets or clothing may be so unbearable that patients remain partially naked, effectively trapped in their home. Hyperpathia is an exaggerated pain after a mildly painful stimulus. For example, a minor bump of the affected dermatome against an object can send the patient to bed with severe pain that lasts for hours. Cutaneous scarring and disordered sensation is not uncommon in the affected dermatome. Careful sensory testing often reveals a discrete area of tenderness in the affected dermatome but absent or diminished thermal, touch, vibration, or pinprick sensation.[48] These findings are curious because PHN is a "positive" neurologic phenomenon (pain) but the exam shows "negative" findings (decreased or absent sensation).

PHN profoundly affects the elderly patient's quality of life and functional status. Patients can suffer from a variety of constitutional symptoms including chronic fatigue, anorexia, weight loss, and insomnia. PHN is a well-known cause of depression in the elderly. The social activities of many patients and their spouses are often curtailed by the illness, and the patient's social role may change from a vital member of the community to an inactive individual in a household. Furthermore, PHN can interfere with dressing, bathing, grooming, eating, and mobility. For example, the patient with allodynic skin may be forced to avoid bathing or clothing around the affected area. Instrumental ADLs commonly affected include traveling, shopping, cooking, and housework.

Other Complications

Ocular

VZV reactivates in the ophthalmic division of the trigeminal nerve in 10% to 15% of zoster patients.[3,40] The appearance and location of the facial rash do not necessarily predict the location and extent of eye involvement. Rash on the tip of the nose, indicating involvement of the nasociliary branch, appears to increase the likelihood of inflammation of the eye. The uvea and the cornea are the most common sites of inflammation, but any part of the eye is vulnerable.[49,50] VZV-induced damage to these structures can result in glaucoma, optic neuritis, optic atrophy, corneal anesthesia and ulceration, cataract, eyelid scarring and retraction, compromised vision, and blindness.[51] In one study of the natural history of ophthalmic zoster in untreated patients, 50% of patients developed ocular complications and 28% had active ocular disease 6 months or more after rash onset.[49]

VZV can also cause acute retinal necrosis, which is characterized by destructive retinal inflammation and affects adults of any age.[51–53] Patients do not exhibit facial rash; instead, they present with blurred vision and a painful eye. The fundus shows peripheral yellow-white patches indicative of retinal inflammation. These changes are not specific for VZV but VZV is frequently found in the lesions. The inflammation usually persists for 4 to 5 weeks and is followed by retinal scarring and detachment. Years later, the unaffected eye can develop the same pathology.

Neurologic

Considering the focus and spread of VZV within the peripheral and central nervous system, it is not surprising that zoster is associated with several neurologic complications along with PHN.[54] Up to 5% of zoster patients develop focal motor pareses involving muscle groups innervated by ventral horn neurons in proximity to dorsal horn neurons of the affected dermatome. The most commonly affected muscles are those of the extremities with zoster of the accompanying dermatome and the face with zoster of the seventh cranial nerve. Oculomotor weakness (cranial neuritis), unilateral diaphragmatic paralysis (cervical zoster), bladder and anorectal dysfunction (sacral zoster), and intercostal muscle weakness (thoracic zoster) have also been reported. These deficits usually occur at the time of or within a few weeks after the onset of the rash. Full or partial recovery of motor function occurs in 65% to 85% of patients within months of the onset of weakness, but VZV-induced facial palsy has a much lower rate of recovery (30%–40%).[55,56]

Other important neurologic complications include cranial neuropathy, meningoencephalitis, transverse myelitis, and cerebral stroke. Zoster-induced cranial nerve symptoms include facial weakness with involvement of cranial nerve (CN) V or VII; hearing loss, imbalance, hyperacusis, and tinnitus with CN VIII; dysgeusia and mouth lesions with CN V, mandibular branch, and CN IX; and pharyngitis and laryngitis with CN IX, X.[54,57] The patient may have multiple symptoms because more than one cranial nerve can be involved in an attack. Cephalic herpes zoster (Ramsay Hunt syndrome) refers to VZV-induced facial palsy and otic vesicles, often in association with CN VIII and/or other cranial nerve symptoms.[54]

Clinically overt meningoencephalitis rarely occurs in the elderly. The clinical manifestations of fever, delirium, headache, and meningismus may occur days or weeks before, during, or up to 2 months after the rash.[58] Most patients survive and regain premorbid cognitive functioning. Cerebral stroke or transient ischemic attacks are a recognized complication of ophthalmic zoster in older patients.[59,60] VZV appears to infect cerebral arteries adjacent to the ophthalmic division of the trigeminal nerve and cause granulomatous angiitis with resultant thrombosis. Weeks to months after zoster, patients present with fixed or transient motor deficits contralateral to the zoster-affected side. The delayed manifestation may preclude the clinician from making the link between the stroke and the prior occurrence of ophthalmic zoster. These patients show segmental narrowing or occlusion of cerebral arteries next to the affected ophthalmic division on a cerebral arteriogram.

Visceral

Under conditions of severe immunosuppression, reactivated VZV can cause pneumonitis, hepatitis, esophagitis, gastritis, cystitis, and arthritis.[25] These complications are unusual in the typical elderly zoster patient.

Diagnosis

Clinical

The clinical diagnosis of herpes zoster in the elderly is ordinarily unmistakable and sufficient. Burns and contact dermatitis may infrequently resemble zoster, but the history and clinical course will lead to the diagnosis. The principal condition in the differential diagnosis is zosteriform herpes simplex. The differentiation is most challenging in the elderly when the herpes simplex virus (HSV) reactivates in sacral and trigeminal dermatomes and produces lesions on the buttocks or face that are indistinguishable from zoster. HSV commonly produces a short, mild prodrome; generates smaller, closely grouped vesicles; recurs many times; affects younger adults; and very rarely causes postherpetic neuralgia.[25] However, the appearance of the rash and the clinical situation may make it impossible to distinguish the two conditions and lead to misdiagnosis.[61,62]

Laboratory

Diagnostic testing is useful for differentiating herpes zoster from herpes simplex, for suspected organ involvement, and for atypical presentations. Available tests can provide a definitive diagnosis of herpes zoster by detecting (1) VZV antigens using immunofluorescent antibody (IFA) techniques, (2) VZV replication in culture, (3) VZV antibody by serology, or (4) VZV DNA by the polymerase chain reaction (PCR) in the target specimen (vesicle fluid/scrapings, involved tissue, CSF, or blood) (Table 71.1). Of these options, IFA is the most expedient and useful test because it is rapid, specific, and sensitive.[63] A rash specimen is easily prepared by scraping or swabbing the base of an unroofed vesicle, placing the material on a slide, and fixing it by air-drying or acetone. The slide

TABLE 71.1. Laboratory diagnostic tests for herpes zoster.

Test	Sensitivity	Specificity	Turnaround	Comment
IFA	Very high	High	Hours	Preferred test in most patients
Culture	Low	High	Days	Positive test needs confirmatory test
Serology	Moderate	Moderate	Weeks	Retrospective diagnosis
PCR	Very high	High	Hours	Limited availability, expensive

IFA, immunofluorescent antibody (direct or indirect); PCR, polymerase chain reaction.

is stained with an anti-VZV monoclonal antibody that is tagged with an immunofluorescent label. The microscopic detection of fluorescence indicates the presence of VZV antigen and confirms the diagnosis.

Cell culture of infected specimens can isolate VZV. A positive culture shows the typical cytopathic effects (CPE) of in vitro herpes virus infection—distinct foci of enlarged, fused cells that appear multinucleated and contain intranuclear inclusions. However, VZV culture is limited by the slow time for a result (usually several days but as little as 1–2 days with the shell vial technique), the nonspecific nature of CPE (a positive culture requires immunologic confirmation), and significant insensitivity (VZV is very labile).[64]

Serologic tests can provide a retrospective diagnosis if acute and convalescent sera are obtainable and show a fourfold or greater increase in VZV IgG titers. The most sensitive and specific tests are fluorescent antimembrane antibody (FAMA), enzyme-linked immunofluorescent antibody (ELISA), latex agglutination, and radioimmunoassays (RIA).[25] Although not useful for acute infection, serologic tests are occasionally helpful for atypical syndromes such as zoster sine herpete. The PCR detects VZV DNA by repeated amplification of target segments of the VZV genome. The PCR is a powerful, extremely sensitive, specific technique that can produce results in a day. Researchers have used the PCR to detect VZV DNA in the rash, conjunctiva, synovial fluid, cerebrospinal fluid, a variety of tissues, and in the air surrounding patients with chickenpox and zoster and in mononuclear cells of asymptomatic elderly persons.[65–69] The principal disadvantage of the PCR is its extreme sensitivity and potential for false positives.

Prognosis

The prognosis of herpes zoster is related to the duration and severity of pain. The duration and severity of zoster pain is significantly greater in older patients than younger patients. In general, the number of elderly zoster patients with pain declines over weeks to months from rash onset. Specific data on pain duration in elderly zoster patients is limited by the lack of population-based studies of this phenomenon. Nonetheless, data from patient groups and recent clinical trials provide some useful information.

Studies of predominantly older adults in the preantiviral era found that the percentage of patients with any pain 6 months after rash onset was 41% to 46% and one year after rash onset was 28% to 41%.[1,32] The upper figures in these ranges are partly elevated by referral bias. In a meta-analysis of acyclovir trials, the percent of patients 50 years of age or older with any pain in the placebo group was 54% at 3 months and 35% at 6 months after rash onset (12-month data not available).[70] These data indicate that a substantial subset of elderly zoster patients have a poor prognosis with respect to pain. Many of these patients are refractory to all treatments, and some may actually get worse over time.[71] Furthermore, some patients have pain-free intervals of weeks or even months only to note the return of their pain. Nonetheless, the geriatrician can offer hope to the acute zoster pain sufferer because the majority of elderly zoster patients note the loss of pain in the weeks or months after rash onset. Furthermore, some patients with long-lasting pain eventually have a good outcome. In a study of 88 patients with PHN of 1 year or more, 31 (35%) had mild pain and no disability after an average of 2 years of follow-up.[71]

Treatment

Acute Herpes Zoster

Rash

Recommended treatments for the rash are empirical because there are no clinical trials of topical therapy. The stage of the rash determines the choice of therapy. For an uncomplicated rash, soap and tap water are sufficient to keep the wound clean and provide some comfort. For the patient with multiple, oozing vesicles, wet dressings with aluminum acetate (Burow's solution), acetic acid, or zinc sulfate dry lesions and prevent secondary infection. Calamine lotion, cornstarch, or baking soda are said to be useful by some patients in this phase. The typical rash heals in 3 to 4 weeks. Oral antiviral therapy reduces the time of rash healing by a mean of 1 to 2 days.[45]

Pain

The principal goal of the treatment of herpes zoster in the elderly is the reduction or elimination of pain. Antiviral therapy, anti-inflammatory drugs, and analgesics are three strategies to achieve that goal.

Antiviral Therapy (Table 71.2)

Available anti-VZV drugs are nucleoside analogues that are converted first by VZV thymidine kinase and then cellular kinases to the nucleoside triphosphate form. This compound stops VZV from replicating by inhibiting VZV DNA polymerase and by incorporation into the VZV DNA chain. In general, these drugs are safe and well tolerated in the elderly. The most common side effects are nausea and/or vomiting, diarrhea, and headache in about 8% to 17% of patients.[45,72,73] To be effective, the drugs must be used early during zoster. The beneficial effects occur most when the drugs are begun within 48 to 72h of rash onset. They are all renally excreted.

Acyclovir

When used early, oral acyclovir can reduce acute zoster pain.[74] The effect of acyclovir on chronic pain is less apparent because clinical trial data conflict. It is difficult to combine data from available studies because of differences in study methods and definitions of postherpetic neuralgia. Nonetheless, a recent meta-analysis combined the results of five randomized, placebo-controlled trials of oral acyclovir and used any pain at 6 months as the outcome.[75] None of these studies reported significant differences in the proportion of treated or placebo patients with pain at 6 months, but there was a trend favoring acyclovir in four of the studies. When the data were combined, the summary odds ratio for the incidence of any pain at 6 months for patients treated with acyclovir was 0.54 (95% CI, 0.36–0.81).

Acyclovir is useful for ophthalmic zoster, visceral, and central nervous system infections, and for the immunosuppressed host. Oral acyclovir reduced keratitis, uveitis, and ocular complications significantly in placebo-controlled trials of older patients with ophthalmic zoster.[76] Depending on the nature of the pathology, some ophthalmologists employ topical corticosteroids to reduce severe inflammation and mydriatics to reduce pupillary sphincter and ciliary body muscle spasm and prevent anterior lens and pupil synechiae.[77] Intravenous (i.v.) acyclovir, at doses of 10mg/kg every 8h for 7 to 10 days, is recommended in severely immunosuppressed patients

with localized zoster and for any patient who develops serious VZV-induced disease such as meningoencephalitis, pneumonitis, acute retinal necrosis, generalized dissemination, or other organ system complications.[78] Acyclovir i.v. does not appear to affect PHN but it does reduce the likelihood of cutaneous, visceral, or central nervous system complications in the immunosuppressed host.[79] Oral acyclovir is sufficient for localized zoster in mildly immunosuppressed patients. Acyclovir-resistant VZV, mediated by the lack of thymidine kinase, has been reported only in AIDS and transplant patients on prolonged acyclovir therapy and not in elderly patients.[80,81]

Famciclovir

Famciclovir is a prodrug that is well absorbed in the gastrointestinal tract and metabolized in the liver to penciclovir. Penciclovir has a chemical structure very similar to that of acyclovir. A placebo-controlled trial of famciclovir in immunocompetent zoster patients more than 18 years old (mean, 51 years old) demonstrated a significantly shorter overall duration of zoster pain in the treated group.[73] The proportion of patients with pain at rash healing (the study definition of PHN) was the same in both groups. Of the patients with pain at rash healing (about 54% of the total group), the median duration of PHN was significantly less in the treated group (median time to loss of pain, 60–63 days with famciclovir and 120 days with placebo group, 500-mg dose versus placebo, $p = 0.02$). Similar results were reported in a subgroup analysis of patients over 50 years old. In another trial of immunocompetent zoster patients greater than 18 years old, famciclovir (at doses of 250mg, 500mg, or 750mg three times daily for 7 days) was compared to standard doses of acyclovir.[82] Famciclovir and acyclovir were equally effective in reducing acute pain and the duration of zoster-associated pain. The efficacy of famciclovir in ophthalmic zoster and the immunosuppressed host is unknown. Famciclovir dosage must be decreased when the creatinine clearance falls below 60ml/min.

Valacyclovir

Valacyclovir is well absorbed in the gastrointestinal tract and metabolized in the liver to acyclovir, thereby bypassing the poor absorption of acyclovir. Valacyclovir, at 1g for 7 days ($n = 384$) or 14 days ($n = 381$) was compared to acyclovir in standard doses ($n = 376$) in immuno-

TABLE 71.2. Oral anti-varicella-zoster virus medications.

Name	Active agent	Reduce zoster pain?	Oral dose	Form
Acyclovir	Acyclovir	Yes	800mg five times daily	Tablet, liquid
Famciclovir	Penciclovir	Yes	500mg three times daily	Tablet
Valacyclovir	Acyclovir	Yes	1g three times daily	Tablet

competent zoster patients over 50 years old (mean, 68 years old).[72] Median days to pain cessation for 7-day valacyclovir was 38 days; for 14-day valacyclovir, 44 days; and for acyclovir, 51 days. The recommended dose is 1 g three times a day, with downward adjustments for renal insufficiency when the creatinine clearance falls below 50 ml/mm. A thrombotic thrombocytopenic purpura/hemolytic-uremic syndrome has been reported in severely immunosuppressed patients while taking valacyclovir.[83]

In summary, antiviral therapy appears to reduce acute pain and the duration of pain in elderly zoster patients who are treated within 72 h of rash onset. The longer the patient presents after 72 h of rash onset, the less sense it makes to prescribe antiviral therapy, unless the patient continues to form new vesicles or has ocular involvement. Acyclovir reduces ocular complications in ophthalmic zoster and organ system complications in the severely immunosuppressed host. The disadvantages of antiviral therapy are marginal or no effect on PHN in some patients, gastrointestinal side effects, and cost. The very early use of antiviral therapy is paramount because days of VZV replication, neuronal destruction, and inflammation have occurred by the time the patient reaches the doctor. Currently available data suggest that acyclovir, famciclovir, or valacyclovir are acceptable agents with factors other than efficacy determining the choice.

Anti-inflammatory Agents

Several well-designed clinical trials of corticosteroids compared to placebo or acyclovir in zoster have shown no significant effect on chronic zoster pain and argue against routine treatment of elderly zoster patients for preventing PHN.[84,85] The most common adverse effects were gastrointestinal symptoms (dyspepsia, nausea, vomiting), edema, and granulocytosis. Interestingly, corticosteroids reduced acute zoster pain from 2 to 8 weeks after rash onset in most of these trials, although that beneficial effect was not sustained. In the most recent trial, Whitley et al. studied acyclovir plus prednisone ($n = 51$), acyclovir plus prednisone placebo ($n = 48$), prednisone plus acyclovir placebo ($n = 50$), and placebos for acyclovir and prednisone ($n = 52$) in immunocompetent zoster patients of median age 60 to 63 years.[86] Standard doses of acyclovir were given for 21 days and prednisone was given as 60 mg/day for the first week and tapered over the next 2 weeks. There were no significant differences between the four groups or between prednisone versus no-prednisone groups (hazard ratio, 1.26; 95% confidence interval, 0.91–1.75) in time to cessation of zoster-associated pain. However, time to uninterrupted sleep, return to daily activity, and cessation of analgesic therapy was significantly accelerated in the prednisone versus no-

prednisone groups in this relatively healthy group of 60-year-olds. Therefore, oral corticosteroids may be considered for otherwise healthy older adults with moderate to severe pain and no contraindications to corticosteroids. Some clinicians use corticosteroids for VZV-induced facial paralysis and cranial polyneuritis to improve motor outcomes and pain.

Analgesics

Clinicians should employ analgesics to reduce acute zoster pain regardless of effects on chronic zoster pain. The choice of nonopiate or opiate analgesics depends on the patient's pain severity, underlying conditions, and response to the drug. The principles of excellent pain management, such as scheduled analgesia, use of standardized pain measures, and close follow-up, should be applied to acute zoster pain management as with any other painful condition. If pain control from antiviral agents and analgesics is inadequate, then regional or local anesthetic nerve blocks should be considered. Although there are no randomized controlled trials of this approach for the treatment of acute pain or the prevention of PHN, several published case series have consistently reported acute pain relief from a variety of anesthetic techniques.[87,88]

The effectiveness of well-managed opiates, regional anesthetic nerve blocks, anticonvulsants, and tricyclic antidepressants in reducing chronic zoster pain is not known but needs to be tested in rigorous clinical trials. In one randomized double-blind study of amitriptyline or placebo during acute zoster in 72 elderly patients, the percentage of patients who were pain-free at 1 and 3 months after rash onset was not significantly different. However, at 6 months after rash onset, 32 (84%) patients in the amitriptyline group were pain-free compared to 22 (65%) patients in the placebo group ($p = 0.05$).[89] This study was small, the use of acyclovir was unbalanced between the groups, and amitriptyline is a hazardous drug in the elderly. These points argue against using amitriptyline acutely in elderly zoster patients, but the result is interesting and deserves better study with less toxic alternatives.

Nonpharmacologic approaches to zoster pain are also important. Elderly zoster victims need education and reassurance because shingles myths and fears are commonplace. Social support, mental and physical activity, adequate nutrition, and a caring attitude go a long way toward coping with this illness.

Postherpetic Neuralgia

No one treatment is uniformly effective in all elderly PHN patients. Clinicians have employed many treatments for

PHN, but few of these treatments have been evaluated in randomized, double-blind, placebo-controlled trials. However, recent clinical trials indicate that topical lidocaine, gabapentin, opiates, and tricyclic antidepressants can significantly reduce pain in PHN patients.

Topical Therapies

Topical therapies are low-risk interventions that include topical lidocaine, capsaicin, and nonsteroidal anti-inflammatory (NSAID) drugs. The topical lidocaine patch and the topical anesthetic cream EMLA (eutectic mixture of lidocaine and prilocaine) have produced significant pain relief in PHN patients in uncontrolled and controlled clinical trials.[90–93] Galer et al. enrolled PHN patients who were successfully treated with topical lidocaine patches and randomized them to continue the topical patch or receive a vehicle patch for 2 weeks and then cross over to the opposite treatment for 2 weeks.[94] Patients were allowed to exit either treatment period if their pain relief scores decreased by 2 or more on a 6-item pain relief scale for 2 consecutive days. The lidocaine patch exit time was 14 days and the vehicle patch exit time was 3.8 days ($p < 0.001$), indicating that vehicle-treated patients wanted the active ingredient after a few days. At study completion, 25 of 32 (78.1%) of subjects preferred the lidocaine patch compared to 3 of 32 (9.4%) of vehicle patch recipients. Hence, the topical lidocaine patch provided significantly more pain relief than a placebo patch. The 10 by 14 cm patch contains 5% lidocaine base and other ingredients on a polyester backing. One or more patches are applied over the affected area for 12 h/day. It may take up to 2 weeks to determine whether it is effective. Systemic lidocaine toxicity has not been reported with topical lidocaine preparations. The disadvantages of the patch are application site reactions such as skin redness or rash and substantial cost.

Capsaicin (0.025% or 0.075%), the active principle in hot peppers, has had divergent results in controlled clinical trials and in systematic reviews.[95–97] It is difficult to blind patients and investigators because of the burning associated with the treatment. An adequate trial requires 6 weeks of therapy of either the 0.025% or 0.075% concentration applied to the affected area three to four times per day. The utility of the drug is limited by intense burning that becomes tolerable for some patients and unbearable for many others. NSAID creams and aspirin or indomethacin in solution [chloroform, ether, dimethylsulfoxide (DMSO)] are reported to reduce pain in limited studies.[98–101] The extent of clinical benefit from these treatments is uncertain, but these agents deserve further study in large, controlled clinical trials. All topical therapies may be impractical when the involved area of skin is too large or difficult to reach.

Anticonvulsants

Clinicians have used phenytoin and carbamazepine for PHN, but there is little evidence for their effectiveness and they can have significant adverse effects in the elderly. However, there is evidence that gabapentin is effective in reducing the severity of PHN. Rowbotham et al. conducted a randomized, placebo-controlled trial of gabapentin in 229 patients with PHN over an 8-week period.[102] Study participants received an initial dose of 300 mg, and the dose was titrated over a 4-week period to 300 mg tid, 600 mg tid, 900 mg tid, and 1200 mg tid or until intolerable adverse effects. On an 11-point pain scale (0–10), the average daily pain score of treated patients declined from 6.3 to 4.2 compared with a decline from 6.5 to 6.0 in the placebo group ($p < 0.001$). Forty-three percent of the treated group rated their pain as moderately or much improved compared to 12% of the placebo group. On average, treated patients experienced significant improvement in health-related quality of life, sleep, and mood compared to placebo recipients. The adverse effects of gabapentin included somnolence (27%), dizziness (24%), and ataxia (7%). These adverse effects will limit the use of gabapentin in the frail elderly and elderly patients with falls and gait disturbance.

Tricyclic Antidepressants (TCAs)

Five randomized controlled clinical trials of amitriptyline, one trial of desipramine, and one trial of nortriptyline have demonstrated moderate to good pain relief in 44% to 67% of elderly PHN patients.[103–108] Nortriptyline and desipramine are preferred alternatives to amitriptyline because they cause less sedation, cognitive impairment, orthostatic hypotension and constipation in the elderly. Given the adverse effects of amitriptyline in the elderly and the data supporting its use, Watson et al. compared amitriptyline and nortriptyline in PHN patients using a double-blind crossover design.[108] The two agents reduced pain in roughly 55% of patients but nortriptyline was better tolerated. A conservative dosing regimen of nortriptyline begins with 10 mg at night and increases the dose every 4 to 7 days by the same amount until reduction in pain or intolerable side effects. At least 4 weeks of therapy is required (4–8 weeks recommended) and therapy should be continued for 3 to 6 months if adequate pain reduction.

Opiates

There is increasing evidence that a subset of PHN patients respond to chronic opioid therapy. Small studies of intravenous morphine and oral opioids have reported significant pain relief in PHN.[109–112] Watson and Babul conducted a randomized, placebo-controlled, double-blind, crossover trial of sustained release oxycodone in 38 PHN patients over an 8-week period.[113] The initial dose of controlled-release oxycodone was 10 mg every 12 h. The dose was increased weekly to 20 mg every 12 h and to a possible maximum of 30 mg every 12 h. The results showed significant pain relief in constant, intermittent, and allodynic pain as measured by visual analogue scale and a numerical-verbal 6-point pain scale. Sixty-seven percent of patients expressed marked preference for oxycodone compared to 11% for placebo. The most frequently reported adverse effects were constipation, nausea, and sedation.

Other Modalities

Transcutaneous electrical nerve stimulation (TENS) may be beneficial in some patients and it has little risk.[114] The ideal candidate for a TENS trial has truncal or extremity PHN and adequate cognition, vision, and manual dexterity. Some patients derive short-term relief from the application of cold to the affected area. Acupuncture has been used in PHN, but there is little evidence to support its efficacy.[115,116] Ablative surgical procedures are usually considered for the desperately ill PHN patient who has failed all attempts at medical management. The literature is restricted to case reports or series of limited quality.[117] In general, the likelihood of success from surgical procedures appears to be very small whereas the risks are significant. Chronic pain coping strategies, social support, physical activity as tolerated, and a supportive doctor–patient relationship are beneficial for elderly PHN patients.

In summary, available evidence indicates that the lidocaine patch, gabapentin, tricyclic antidepressants (preferably nortriptyline or desipramine), and opiates (e.g., oxycodone) are effective in providing pain relief in a significant number of elderly patients with PHN. The choice for initial treatment depends on patient comorbidity, the drug's adverse event profile, patient preference, and cost. If an adequate trial of the first choice is not effective, then the other agents may be employed. Whether combinations of these agents are superior to single drug therapy is unknown. The chances of pain reduction are likely to be increased if nonpharmacologic principles of chronic pain management are employed. In particular, the value of regular follow-up and a supportive relationship cannot be overstated. If these widely available therapies show no pain reduction after adequate trials, then more specialized treatments are available. Those treatments include regional neural blockade (best if tried <3–6 months of rash onset), spinal cord stimulators, higher-potency opiates (e.g., morphine), and psychologic strategies such as relaxation therapy or cognitive-behavioral therapy. The frontline approaches are in the province of geriatricians but the specialized treatments are probably best managed in a multidisciplinary pain clinic. These therapies represent a reasonable approach based on available research, clinical experience, and the opinions of PHN experts. This summary does not cover all possible treatments of PHN (there are hundreds), nor will it satisfy every clinician or patient who has their own favorite nostrum.

Prevention

Takahashi et al. developed a live, attenuated varicella vaccine in 1974 by isolating VZV from a child with chickenpox and passing the isolate in human embryonic lung fibroblasts and guinea pig embryo cells.[118] The vaccine has been studied carefully for its ability to prevent chickenpox in uninfected children and adults. The vaccine induces protective antibodies and cellular immunity for many years in these individuals. About 85% to 90% of healthy and immunocompromised children and 70% of healthy adults experience long-lasting protection against chickenpox after vaccination.[119–122] In addition, "breakthrough" chickenpox in vaccinees is mild. The vaccine is safe and causes mild, transient side effects of a vaccine-induced rash, sore arm, fever, or fatigue in a minority of vaccinees.

Given that cellular immunity to VZV declines with age, might vaccination of latently infected elderly persons with the varicella-zoster vaccine prevent zoster or postherpetic neuralgia?[123] The vaccine induces significant increases in mean anti-VZV antibody levels, interferon-gamma production, T-cell proliferation indices, cytokine secretion, and VZV-specific T-cell responder frequency in the elderly.[124–126] Levin et al. reported that, 6 years after vaccination, VZV responder cell frequency was still significantly improved over baseline in 130 individuals aged 55 to 87 years at the time of vaccination.[127] In this study, 10 herpes zoster-like clinical events were recorded but the patients had little acute pain and no postherpetic neuralgia. Furthermore, the vaccine has been well tolerated, with minor, transient injection site reactions being the most common adverse event. A randomized, double-blind, placebo-controlled Veterans Affairs Cooperative Studies trial is in progress in the United States to evaluate the effects of a more potent formulation of the vaccine on zoster and postherpetic neuralgia in the elderly.

References

1. Hope-Simpson RE. The nature of herpes zoster: a long-term study and new hypothesis. *Proc R Soc Med (Lond)*. 1965;58:9–20.
2. Weller TH. Varicella and herpes zoster. Changing concepts of the natural history, control, and importance of a not-

so-benign virus. *N Engl J Med.* 1983;309:1362–1368, 1434–1440.

3. Ragozzino MW, Melton LF, Kurland LT. Population-based study of herpes zoster and its sequelae. *Medicine.* 1982; 61:310–316.

4. Glynn C, Crockford G, Gavaghan D, et al. Epidemiology of shingles. *J R Soc Med.* 1990;83:617–619.

5. Donahue JG, Choo PW, Manson JE, et al. The incidence of herpes zoster. *Arch Intern Med.* 1995;155:1605–1609.

6. Rusthoven JJ, Ahlgren P, Elhakim T, et al. Varicella-zoster infection in adult cancer patients. *Arch Intern Med.* 1988;148:1561–1566.

7. Locksley RM, Flournoy N, Sullivan KM, et al. Infection with varicella-zoster virus after marrow transplantation. *J Infect Dis.* 1985;152:1172–1181.

8. Buchbinder SP, Katz MH, Hessol NA, et al. Herpes zoster and human immunodeficiency virus infection. *J Infect Dis.* 1992;166:1153–1156.

9. Manzi S, Kuller LH, Kutzer J, et al. Herpes zoster in systemic lupus erythematosus. *J Rheumatol.* 1995;22:1254–1258.

10. Ragozzino MW, Melton LJ, Kurland LT, et al. Risk of cancer after herpes zoster: a population-based study. *N Engl J Med.* 1982;307:393–397.

11. Schmader KE, Studenski S, MacMillan J, et al. Are stressful life events risk factors for herpes zoster? *J Am Geriatr Soc.* 1990;38:1188–1195.

12. Schmader KE, George LK, Burchett BM, et al. Race and stress in the incidence of herpes zoster in the elderly. *J Am Geriatr Soc.* 1998;46:973–977.

13. Schmader KE, George LK, Hamilton JD. Racial differences in the occurrence of herpes zoster. *J Infect Dis.* 1995; 171:701–705.

14. Weller TH. Varicella-herpes zoster virus. In: Evans AS, Kaslow RA, eds. *Viral Infections of Humans. Epidemiology and Control.* New York: Plenum; 1997:870–878.

15. Helgason S, Sigurdsson JA, Gudmundsson S. The clinical course of herpes zoster: a prospective study in primary care. *Eur J Gen Pract.* 1996;2:12–16.

16. Veenstra J, Krol A, van Praag RM, et al. Herpes zoster, immunological deterioration and disease progression in HIV-1 infection. *AIDS.* 1995;9:1153–1158.

17. Schmader KE. Herpes zoster epidemiology. In: Arvin A, Gershon A, eds. *Varicella-Zoster Virus.* Cambridge: Cambridge University Press; 2000:220–245.

18. Straus SE. Shingles: sorrows, salves, and solutions. *JAMA.* 1993;269:1836–1839.

19. Garner JS. Guideline for isolation precautions in hospitals. The Hospital Infection Control Practices Advisory Committee. *Infect Cont Hosp Epidemiol.* 1996;17:53–80.

20. Pritchard VG. Infection control measures to block transmission: isolation and beyond. In: Smith PW, ed. *Infection Control in Long-Term Care Facilities, 2nd Ed.* Albany: Delmar; 1994:227–251.

21. Davison AJ, Scott JE. The complete DNA sequence of varicella-zoster virus. *J Gen Virol.* 1986;67:1759–1816.

22. Cohen JI, Brunell PA, Straus SE, et al. Recent advances in varicella-zoster virus infection. *Ann Intern Med.* 1999; 130:922–932.

23. Mahalingham R, Wellish M, William W, et al. Latent varicella-zoster viral DNA in human trigeminal and throracic ganglia. *N Engl J Med.* 1990;323:627–631.

24. Hyman RW, Ecker JR, Tenser RB. Varicella-zoster virus RNA in human trigeminal ganglia. *Lancet* 1983;2:814–816.

25. Straus SE, Oxman MN. Varicella and herpes zoster. In: Freedberg IM, Eisen AZ, Wolff K, et al. eds. *Fitzpatrick's Dermatology in General Medicine.* New York: McGraw-Hill; 2000:2427–2448.

26. Miller AE. Selective decline in cellular immune response to varicella-zoster in the elderly. *Neurology.* 1980; 30:582–587.

27. Berger R, Forest G, Just M. Decrease of the lymphoproliferative response to varicella-zoster antigen in the aged. *Infect Immun.* 1981;32:24–27.

28. Burke BL, Steele RW, Beard OW, et al. Immune responses to varicella-zoster in the aged. *Arch Intern Med.* 1982; 142:291–293.

29. Hayward AR, Herberger M. Lymphocyte responses to varicella-zoster virus in the elderly. *J Clin Immunol.* 1987;7:174–178.

30. Hayward AR, Levin M, Wolf W, et al. Varicella-zoster virus-specific immunity after herpes zoster. *J Infect Dis.* 1991;163:873–875.

31. Rogers RS, Tindall JP. Geriatric herpes zoster. *J Am Geriatr Soc.* 1971;19:495–504.

32. deMorgas JM, Kierland RR. The outcome of patients with herpes zoster. *Arch Dermatol.* 1957;75:193–196.

33. Hoppenjans WB, Bibler MR, Orme RL, et al. Prolonged cutaneous herpes zoster in acquired immunodeficiency syndrome. *Arch Dermatol.* 1990;126:1048–1051.

34. Gilden DH, Dueland AN, Cohrs R, et al. Preherpetic neuralgia. *Neurology.* 1991;41:1215–1218.

35. Easton HG. Zoster sine herpete causing trigeminal neuralgia. *Lancet.* 1970;2:1065–1066.

36. Gilden DH, Dueland AN, Devlin ME. Varicella-zoster virus reactivation without rash. *J Infect Dis.* 1992; 166(suppl 1):230–234.

37. Mayo DR, Booss J. Varicella-zoster associated neurologic disease without skin lesions. *Arch Neurol.* 1989;46:313–315.

38. Dueland AN, Devlin M, Martin JR, et al. Fatal varicella-zoster virus meningoradiculitis without skin involvement. *Ann Neurol.* 1991;29:569–572.

39. Heller HM, Carnevale NT, Steigbigel RT. Varicella zoster virus transverse myelitis without cutaneous rash. *Am J Med.* 1990;68:550–551.

40. Hope-Simpson RE. Postherpetic neuralgia. *J R Coll Gen Pract.* 1975;25:571–575.

41. Dworkin RH, Portenoy RK. Proposed classification of herpes zoster pain [letter]. *Lancet.* 1994;343;1648.

42. Dworkin RH, Portenoy RK. Pain and its persistence in herpes zoster. *Pain.* 1996;67:241–251.

43. Choo PW, Galil K, Donahue JG, et al. Risk factors for postherpetic neuralgia. *Arch Intern Med.* 1997;157:1217–1224.

44. Dworkin RH, Boon RJ, Griffin DRG, et al. Postherpetic neuralgia: impact of famciclovir, age, rash severity, and acute pain in herpes zoster patients. *J Infect Dis.* 1998; 178(suppl 1):S76–S80.

45. Wood MJ, Ogan PK, McKendrick MW, et al. Efficacy of oral acyclovir treatment of acute herpes zoster. *Am J Med.* 1988;85(suppl 2A):79–83.

46. Bhala BB, Ramamoorthy C, Bowsher D, et al. Shingles and post-herpetic neuralgia. *Clin J Pain.* 1988;4:169–174.

47. Rowbotham MC, Fields HL. Post-herpetic neuralgia: the relation of pain complaint, sensory disturbance, and skin temperature. *Pain.* 1989;39:129–144.

48. Nurmikko T, Bowsher D. Somatosensory findings in postherpetic neuralgia. *J Neurol Neurosurg Psychiatry.* 1990;53:135–141.

49. Harding, SP, Lipton JR, Wells JCD. Natural history of herpes zoster ophthalmicus, predictors of postherpetic neuralgia and ocular involvement. *Br J Ophthalmol.* 1986; 71:353–358.

50. Galil K, Choo PW, Donahue JG, et al. The sequelae of herpes zoster. *Arch Intern Med.* 1997;157:1209–1213.

51. Liesgang TJ. Diagnosis and therapy of herpes zoster ophthalmicus. *Ophthalmology.* 1991;98:1216–1229.

52. Culbertson WW, Blumenkranz MS, Pepose JS, et al. Varicella zoster virus is a cause of the acute retinal necrosis syndrome. *Ophthalmology.* 1986;93:559–569.

53. Soushi S, Ozawa H, Matsuhashi M, et al. Demonstration of varicella zoster virus antigens in the vitreous aspirates of patients with acute retinal necrosis syndrome. *Ophthalmology.* 1988;95:1394–1398.

54. Gilden DH, Kleinschmidt-DeMasters BK, LaGuardia JJ, et al. Neurologic complications of the reactivation of varicella-zoster virus. *N Engl J Med.* 2000;342:635–645.

55. Adour KK. Diagnosis and management of facial paralysis. *N Engl J Med.* 1982;307:348–351.

56. Gupta SK, Helal BH, Keily P. The prognosis in zoster paralysis. *J Bone Joint Surg B.* 1969;51:593–603.

57. Adour KK. Otological complications of herpes zoster. *Ann Neurol.* 1994;35(suppl):S62–S65.

58. Jemsek J, Greenberg L, Taber D, et al. Herpes zoster-associated enchephalitis: Clinicopathologic report of 12 cases and review of the literature. *Medicine.* 1983;62:81–97.

59. Bourdette DN, Rosenberg NL, Yatsu FM. Herpes zoster ophthalmicus and delayed ipsilateral cerebral infarction. *Neurology.* 1983;33:1428–1432.

60. Eidelberg D, Sotrel A, Horoupian DS, et al. Thrombotic cerebral vasculopathy associated with herpes zoster. *Ann Neurol.* 1986;19:7–14.

61. Kalman CM, Laskin OL. Herpes zoster and zosteriform herpes simplex virus infections in immunocompetent adults. *Am J Med.* 1986;81:775–778.

62. Rubben A, Baron JM, Grussendorf-Conen EI. Routine detection of herpes simplex virus and varicella-zoster virus by polymerase chain reaction reveals that initial herpes zoster is frequently misdiagnosed as herpes simplex. *Br J Dermatol.* 1997;137:259–261.

63. Rawlinson WD, Dwyer DI, Gibbons VL, et al. Rapid diagnosis of varicella-zoster virus infection with a monoclonal antibody based direct immunoflourescence technique. *J Virol Methods.* 1989;23:13–18.

64. Schirm J, Meulenberg JJ, Pastoor GW, et al. Rapid detection of varicella-zoster virus in clinical specimens using monoclonal antibodies on shell vials and smears. *J Med Virol.* 1989;28:1–6.

65. Nahass GT, Goldstein BA, Shu WY, et al. Comparison of Tzanck smear, viral culture, and DNA diagnostic methods in detection of herpes simplex and varicella-zoster infection. *JAMA.* 1992;268:2541–2544.

66. Sawyer MH, Chamberlin CJ, Wu YN, et al. Detection of varicella-zoster virus DNA in air samples from hospital rooms. *J Infect Dis.* 1994;169:91–94.

67. Devlin ME, Gilden DH, Mahalingam R, et al. Peripheral blood mononuclear cells of the elderly contain varicella-zoster virus DNA. *J Infect Dis.* 1992;165:619–622.

68. Puchhammer-Stockl E, Popow-Kraupp T, Heinz FX, et al. Detection of varicella-zoster virus DNA by polymerase chain reaction in the cerebrospinal fluid of patients suffering from neurological complications associated with chicken pox or herpes zoster. *J Clin Microbiol.* 1991; 29:1513–1516.

69. Tamura T, Yoshida M, Tezuka T. Detection of varicella-zoster virus DNA in conjunctivas of patients with herpes zoster. *Ophthalmologica.* 1994;208:41–43.

70. Wood MJ, Kay R, Dworkin RH, et al. Oral acyclovir therapy accelerates pain resolution in patients with herpes zoster: a meta-analysis of placebo-controlled trials. *Clin Infect Dis.* 1996;22:341–347.

71. Watson CPN, Watt VR, Chipman M, et al. The prognosis with postherpetic neuralgia. *Pain.* 1991;46:195–199.

72. Beutner KR, Friedman DJ, Forszpaniak C, et al. Valaciclovir compared with acyclovir for improved therapy for herpes zoster in immunocompetent adults. *Antimicrob Agents Chemother.* 1995;39:1546–1553.

73. Tyring S, Barbarash RA, Nahlik JE, et al. Famciclovir for the treatment of acute herpes zoster: effects on acute disease and postherpetic neuralgia. *Ann Intern Med.* 1995;123: 89–96.

74. McKendrick MW, McGill JI, White JE, et al. Oral acyclovir in acute herpes zoster. *Br Med J.* 1986;293:1529–1532.

75. Jackson JL, Gibbons R, Meyer G, et al. The effect of treating herpes zoster with oral acyclovir in preventing postherpetic neuralgia: a meta-analysis. *Arch Intern Med.* 1997;157:909–912.

76. Cobo LM, Foulks GN, Liesgang T, et al. Oral acyclovir in the treatment of acute herpes zoster ophthalmicus. *Ophthalmology.* 1986;93:763–770.

77. Harding SP. Management of ophthalmic zoster. *J Med Virol.* 1993;40(suppl 1):97–101.

78. Whitley RJ, Gnann JW. Acyclovir: a decade later. *N Engl J Med.* 1992;327:782–789.

79. Balfour HH, Bean B, Laskin OL, et al. Acyclovir halts progression of herpes zoster in immunocompromised patients. *N Engl J Med.* 1983;308:1448–1453.

80. Safrin S, Berger TG, Gilson I, et al. Foscarnet therapy in five patients with AIDS and acyclovir-resistant varicella zoster virus infection. *Ann Intern Med.* 1991;115:19–25.

81. Jacobson MA, Berger TG, Fikrig S, et al. Acyclovir re-sistant varicella-zoster virus infection after chronic oral acyclovir therapy in patients with the acquired immunodeficiency syndrome (AIDS). *Ann Intern Med.* 1990;112:187–191.

82. DeGreef H and the Famciclovir Herpes Zoster Clinical Study Group. Famciclovir, a new oral antiherpes drug: results of the first controlled clinical study demonstrating its efficacy and safety in the treatment of uncomplicated

herpes zoster in immunocompetent patients. *Int J Antimicrob Agents.* 1994;4:241–246.

83. Anonymous. Valacyclovir. *Med Lett Drugs Ther.* 1996;38: 3–4.

84. Wood MJ, Johnson RW, McKendrick MW, et al. A randomized trial of acyclovir for 7 days or 21 days with and without prednisolone for treatment of acute herpes zoster. *N Engl J Med.* 1994;330:896–900.

85. Kost RG, Straus SS. Postherpetic neuralgia—pathogenesis, treatment, and prevention. *N Engl J Med.* 1996;335:32–42.

86. Whitley RJ, Weiss H, Gnann JW, et al. Acyclovir with and without prednisone for the treatment of herpes zoster: a randomized, placebo-controlled trial. *Ann Intern Med.* 1996;125;376–383.

87. Fine PG. Nerve blocks, herpes zoster and postherpetic neuralgia. In: Watson CPN, ed. *Herpes Zoster and Postherpetic Neuralgia.* Amsterdam: Elsevier; 1993:173–182.

88. Riopelle J, Lopez-Anaya A, Cork RC, et al. Treatment of the cutaneous pain of acute herpes zoster with 9% lidocaine (base) in petrolatum/paraffin ointment. *J Am Acad Dermatol.* 1994;30:757–767.

89. Bowsher D. The effects of pre-emptive treatment of postherpetic neuralgia with amitriptyline: a randomized, double-blind, placebo-controlled trial. *J Pain Symptom Manage.* 1997;13;327–331.

90. Stow PJ, Glynn CJ, Minor B. EMLA cream in the treatment of post-herpetic neuralgia. Efficacy and pharmacokinetic profile. *Pain.* 1989;39:301–305.

91. Collins PD. EMLA cream and herpetic neuralgia. *Med J Aust.* 1991;155:206–207.

92. Rowbotham MC, Davies PS, Fields HL. Topical lidocaine gel relieves post-herpetic neuralgia. *Ann Neurol.* 1995; 37:246–253.

93. Rowbotham MC, Davies PS, Verkempinck C, et al. Lidocaine patch: double-blind controlled study of a new treatment method for post-herpetic neuralgia. *Pain.* 1996;65:39–44.

94. Galer BS, Rowbotham MC, Perander J, et al. Topical lidocaine patch relieves postherpetic neuralgia more effectively than a vehicle topical patch: results of an enriched enrollment study. *Pain.* 1999;80:533–538.

95. Bernstein JE, Korman NJ, Bickers DR, et al. Topical capsaicin treatment of chronic postherpetic neuralgia. *J Am Acad Dermatol.* 1989;21;265–270.

96. Watson CP, Tyler KL, Bickers DR. A randomized vehicle-controlled trial of topical capsaicin in the treatment of postherpetic neuralgia. *Clin Ther.* 1993;15:510–526.

97. Volmink J, Lancaster T, Gray S, et al. Treatments for post-herpetic neuralgia—a systematic review of randomized controlled trials. *Fam Pract.* 1996; 13:84–91.

98. King RB. Topical aspirin in chloroform and the relief of pain due to herpes zoster and postherpetic neuralgia. *Arch Neurol.* 1993;50:1046–1053.

99. McQuay HJ, Carroll D, Moxon A, et al. Benzydamine cream for the treatment of post-herpetic neuralgia: minimum duration of treatment periods in a cross-over trial. *Pain.* 1990;40:131–135.

100. Bowsher D, Gill H. Aspirin-in-choloroform for the topical treatment of postherpetic neuralgia. *J Pain Soc Great Br Ireland.* 1991;9:16–17.

101. DeBenedittis G, Besana F, Lorenzetti A. A new topical treatment of acute herpetic neuralgia and postherpetic neuralgia: the aspirin/diethyl ether mixture: an open label study plus a double-blind, controlled clinical trial. *Pain.* 1992;48:383–390.

102. Rowbotham M, Harden N, Stacey B, et al. Gabapentin for the treatment of postherpetic neuralgia: a randomized controlled trial. *JAMA.* 1998;280:1837–1842.

103. Watson CPN, Evans RJ, Reed K, et al. Amitriptyline versus placebo in postherpetic neuralgia. *Neurology.* 1982;32: 671–673.

104. Max MB, Schafer SC, Culnane M, et al. Amitriptyline, but not lorazepam, relieves postherpetic neuralgia. *Neurology.* 1988;38:1427–1432.

105. Kishore-Kumar R, Max MB, Schafer SC, et al. Desipramine relieves postherpetic neuralgia. *Clin Pharm Ther.* 1990;47:305–312.

106. Watson CPN, Evans RJ. A comparative trial of amitriptyline and zimeldine in post-herpetic neuralgia. *Pain.* 1985; 23:387–394.

107. Watson CPN, Chipman M, Reed K, et al. Amitriptyline versus maprotiline in postherpetic neuralgia: a randomized, double-blind, crossover trial. *Pain.* 1992;48:29–36.

108. Watson CPN, Vernich L, Chipman M, Reed K. Nortriptyline versus amitriptyline in postherpetic neuralgia: a randomized trial. *Neurology.* 1998;51:1166–1171.

109. Rowbotham MC. Managing post-herpetic neuralgia with opioids and local anesthetics. *Ann Neurol.* 1993; 35(suppl):S46–S49.

110. Watson CPN, Evans RJ, Watt VR, et al. Postherpetic neuralgia: 208 cases. *Pain.* 1988;35:289–297.

111. Rowbotham MC, Reisner LA, Fields HL. Both intravenous lidocaine and morphine reduce the pain of post-herpetic neuralgia. *Neurology.* 1991;41:1024–1028.

112. Pappagallo M, Campbell JN. Chronic opioid therapy as alternative treatment for post-herpetic neuralgia. *Ann Neurol.* 1994;35(suppl):S54–S56.

113. Watson CPN, Babul N. Efficacy of oxycodone in neuropathic pain: a randomized trial in postherpetic neuralgia. *Neurology.* 1998;50:1837–1841.

114. Nathan PW, Wall PD. Treatment of post-herpetic neuralgia by prolonged electric stimulation. *Br Med J.* 1974; 3:645–647.

115. Lewith GT, Field F, Machin D. Acupuncture versus placebo in postherpetic pain. *Pain.* 1983;17:361–368.

116. Dung HC. Acupuncture for the treatment of post-herpetic neuralgia. *Am J Acupunct.* 1987;15:5–14.

117. Loeser J. Surgery for postherpetic neuralgia. In: Watson CPN, ed. *Herpes Zoster and Postherpetic Neuralgia.* Amsterdam: Elsevier; 1993:221–237.

118. Takahashi M, Otsuke T, Okuno Y, et al. Live vaccine used to prevent the spread of varicella in children in hospital. *Lancet.* 1974;2:1288–1290.

119. Gershon AA, Steinberg S, Gelb L, NIAID Collaborative Varicella Vaccine Study Group. Live attenuated varicella vaccine: efficacy for children with leukemia in remission. *JAMA.* 1984;252:355–362.

120. Gershon AA, Steinberg S, LaRussa P, NIAID Collaborative Varicella Vaccine Study Group. Immunization of

healthy adults with live attenuated varicella vaccine. *J Infect Dis.* 1988;158:132–137.

121. Weibel R, Neff BJ, Kuter BJ, et al. Live attenuated varicella virus vaccine: efficacy trial in healthy children. *N Engl J Med.* 1984;310:1409–1415.

122. White CJ. Varicella-zoster virus vaccine. *Clin Infect Dis.* 1997;24:753–761.

123. Schmader KE. Postherpetic neuralgia in immunocompetent elderly people. *Vaccine.* 1998;16:1768–1770.

124. Takahashi M, Iketani T, Sasada K, et al. Immunization of the elderly and patients with collagen vascular diseases with live varicella vaccine and use of varicella skin antigen. *J Infect Dis.* 1992;166(suppl 1):S58–S62.

125. Levin MJ, Murray M, Rotbart HA, et al. Immune response of elderly individuals to a live attenuated varicella vaccine. *J Infect Dis.* 1992;166:253–259.

126. Trannoy E, Berger R, Hollander G, et al. Vaccination of elderly immunocompetent elderly subjects with a live attenuated Oka strain of varicella-zoster virus: a randomized, controlled dose response trial. *Vaccine.* 2000; 18:1700–1706.

127. Levin MJ, Barber D, Goldblatt E, et al. Use of a live attenuated varicella vaccine to boost varicella-specific immune responses in seropositive people 55 years of age and older: duration of booster effect. *J Infect Dis.* 1998;178(suppl 1): S109–S112.

72
Elder Mistreatment

Terry Fulmer and Maria Hernandez

Elder mistreatment (EM) is a complex syndrome including such actions as abuse, neglect, exploitation, and abandonment of an older person. Such phenomena can be overlooked by clinicians who are not careful to elicit a detailed history and physical to determine the nature of common signs and symptoms, which can be ascribed to aging or disease in old age. In every setting (hospitals, nursing homes, clinics), there is an opportunity to screen, diagnose, and treat cases of elder mistreatment. In this chapter, the authors present an overview of the problem, provide specific screening approaches for different patterns of mistreatment, and discuss intervention protocols for care.

Overview

Elder mistreatment is a form of family violence that takes place in the homes and lives of people every day. Domestic violence is noted to be a major issue in the United States. The goals of Healthy People 2010, the national health promotion and disease prevention initiative, is to increase the quality and years of healthy life and eliminate health disparities.[1] Within that document, domestic violence is addressed within the sections pertaining to age groups (e.g., "infant mortality," "elder abuse"). There is no overall estimate of prevalence for domestic violence across the lifespan, but instead estimates of different subtypes within age groups.

Family violence encompasses much of what can go wrong among and between individuals in a family or familiar relationship. Physical abuse, financial exploitation, neglect, and abandonment of older adults take place every day.

Elder mistreatment represents an array of interactions between older adults and their caregivers ranging from physical abuse to fatal neglect. It is a part of the constellation of domestic violence that can affect individuals at any point in the lifespan, and it is particularly difficult to assess in older adults who are likely to have other geriatric syndromes, which may mask or mimic mistreatment. Over the past two decades, mandatory state reporting laws and a heightened sensitivity to the problem have helped clinicians define and channel cases of mistreatment.

Within the broad category of elder mistreatment, four patterns are generally discussed in the literature,[2] including physical abuse, psychologic abuse, financial abuse, and neglect. Conceptual definitions appear to be consistent but the operational definitions categorize abuse in different ways. For example, Pillemer and Wolf[3] note the behavioral category, "withholding of personal care," is defined in different studies as psychologic neglect, physical abuse, or active neglect. Social scientists have typically used a broader framework than clinicians.

The mistreatment literature is quite compartmentalized. Literature searches on the topic of domestic violence reflect research on mistreatment of women, while child abuse and elder abuse searches come under different terms and, therefore, do not overlap across age groups. Discussion of child abuse and elder abuse take place in specialty journals with little synthesis across the lifespan. This challenge needs to be addressed. Some investigators have begun by looking at widely held beliefs and examining the literature for evidence. In one study, the belief that individuals who are abused as children are more likely to abuse their own children are examined. Studies published between 1965 and 2000 were reviewed. In 10 studies, the relative risk (RR) of maltreatment in children was significantly increased (RR 4.75–37.8), whereas in 3 others the relative risk was less than 2 and not significant. A number of methodologic flaws were discerned across the studies, and none examined mistreatment across the lifespan within families, which needs to be done.[4] Currently, however, it appears from the evidence that a relationship exists between child abuse and abusing one's own child. Lifespan studies will help place knowledge of elder mistreatment in a context and framework that can help create more appropriate treatment plans.

Sites of Care

Most older adults live independently or at home with care supports from family or social services. Fewer than 2 million older adults reside in nursing homes, and most do so when they are infirm or at a very advanced age. The discussion of elder mistreatment, therefore, is a discussion, in most cases, of mistreatment in the home setting. Cases come to the attention of authorities and agencies when these older adults come to a point of contact such as the office, the clinic, or the hospital emergency room.

Community Settings

According to Tatara,[5] abuse in domestic settings is widespread and affects thousands of vulnerable elderly people across the country. Pillemer and Finkelhor[6] estimated that only 1 of about 14 domestic elder abuse cases comes to the attention of authorities. Data from the National Elder Abuse Incidence Study (NEAIS)[7] reported approximately 450,000 new cases of abuse and neglect in adults over age 60 in 1996,[8] all community-dwelling elders. This study used a sentinel approach with a random sample of counties across the nation to detect new cases. Prevalence data for EM came from a random sample survey conducted in the metropolitan Boston area in 1986. In that survey, Pillemer and Finkelhor surveyed more than 2000 older persons and reported 700,000 to 1.2 million annually.[6]

Primary care of the elderly takes place in private offices and clinics. Elder mistreatment screening is thought to take place here, but there are few data-based studies to support this. In health department prenatal clinics, incorporation of an abuse assessment protocol into the routine procedures increased the assessment, identification, and documentation of and referral for abuse among pregnant women. Evaluation was conducted at three matched prenatal clinics; two clinics used the abuse protocol and one did not. An audit was performed at the clinics on a randomly selected sample of 540 maternity patient charts for the 15 months before the protocol was initiated and the 540 records for the 15 months after the protocol was introduced. At the clinics using the protocol, abuse assessment increased from 0% to 88%. Detection of abuse increased from 0.8% to 7%. There were no changes at the comparison clinic. The authors suggested that an abuse protocol should be a routine part of maternity care. The obvious parallels and opportunities for elder abuse screening and detection are apparent.

Emergency departments (EDs) have been noted to be key clinical settings for screening for elder mistreatment.[4,9–13] Older adults may wait until they are extremely overwhelmed or debilitated before coming forth and seeking the help of EDs at that time. Emergency departments are often the first point of contact for elder neglect victims. The prevalence is not clear; however, in one study,[14] 3153 consecutive visits to the ED over a 6-month period were retrospectively reviewed for abuse and neglect. The records for every person 70 years or older were reviewed daily to detect any suspicion for abuse or neglect as noted by the ED nurses who were specifically trained in elder mistreatment detection. The 3153 visits were made by 2175 people. Of these, there were 127 cases of elder mistreatment (4%). Delirium and dementia were found to be risk factors for EM. In another study, of 182 elder victims of physical abuse who were identified over a 7-year period, 114 (62.6%) were seen in an ED at least once during a 5-year window surrounding the initial identification of abuse. These 114 persons accounted for 628 visits (median, 3; range, 1–46) and 30.6% of the visits resulted in hospital admission. Clearly, EDs are extremely important for the initial screen for EM.

Elder neglect protocols appear to be feasible in busy emergency departments, and neglect can be accurately detected by nurses when screening procedures are in place. In an ED pilot study which focused on neglect, ED nurses received special training and their ability to conduct accurate screening protocols for elder neglect in the context of their busy practice was measured. During a 3-week period, 180 patients older than 70 years of age (90% of all possible elderly patients during the screening hours) were screened to determine if they met the study criteria and could be enrolled into the protocol. Thirty-six patients met the eligibility criteria to enroll in the study, and 7 patients screened positive for neglect by a home caregiver. The nurses were able to screen and detect elder neglect with more than 70% accuracy according to the "gold standard" of the Neglect Assessment Team. Sensitivity was 71%, and specificity was 93%.

Nursing Home Mistreatment

Nursing homes demonstrate different types of mistreatment. There may be abuse or neglect by staff or by other patients. The Omnibus Budget Reconciliation Act (OBRA) of 1987[15] clearly states that abuse in nursing homes will not be tolerated. Since this act, cases on abuse in nursing homes have gone to trial and have been won. National standards for care in nursing homes are based on public policy set forth in the Nursing Home Reform Act of 1987 (Public Law 100–203; Social Security Act, Title C). This law, as part of OBRA, became effective October 1990. The intent of the law and its regulation is to promote high-quality care and to prevent substandard care, abuse, and neglect. Nurses and other health care providers, including M.D.s, are identified by many states as the professionals who must report suspected abuse and neglect to state officials. Failure to report is usually a misdemeanor and may be punishable by a fine or penalty, although it is clear that punishment alone will not improve reporting. It is when clinicians believe that reports make a difference in care going forward that they readily comply with mandated reporting.[16]

Pillemer and Bachman-Prehn,[17] through a literature review of characteristics that predict abuse in nursing homes, found that (1) quality of care increases with the number of beds in a nursing home; (2) nonprofit homes are superior to proprietary homes for medical and personal care; (3) nursing home costs and better service were positively related; (4) nurses and nursing aides with lower levels of education tend to be more abusive than those with higher levels of education; (5) younger staff held more negative attitudes toward older people; (6) nurses were more empathetic toward the residents than nursing aides (or assistants); and (7) staff who work for a long time with older people have fewer negative attitudes toward the elderly. The nursing staff, especially nurses' aides, may have little training in dealing with the problems of institutionalized elderly persons. Sometimes there are ethnic, cultural, or linguistic barriers to good care. The high turnover rate of nurse's aides reflects the high stress of the job, the low pay, and low morale. Prevention of staff burnout lessens the likelihood of institutional elder abuse. Sometimes there is a fine line between protective restraint and abusive or unnecessary restraint. Providing education for employees and a means for ventilating pent-up frustrations reduces elder abuse and minimizes staff turnover in nursing homes.[18]

A random sample survey of 577 nurses and nursing aides working in long-term care facilities sought to determine the extent of abuse by nursing home staff. Data suggested that abuse by nursing aides was a prevalent phenomenon within the facilities selected. Of the sample surveyed, at least 23% had observed abuse by a staff member. In addition, 10% of the respondents had self-reported that they committed at least one physically abusive act, and 40% self-reported that they committed at least one psychologically abusive act over the past year.[19] Patient-to-patient abuse can also take place, especially in the context of dementia and mental illness.

Risk Factors

Risk factors can be divided into characteristics of the victim, the abuser, and the situation in which both find themselves.

Victims

Particular groups of elderly people have been identified as having a greater risk for abuse than the general public. Studies have described the demographic, physical, and mental characteristics of older adults who are at risk.[3,6,20] It appears that those more likely to be EM victims are very old, female, and in poor physical and mental health. Situational factors that increase the risks of victimization include poor social support, low income, and dependency.

Longitudinal risk factors for abuse and neglect in community-dwelling older adults were examined by linking an established cohort of community-dwelling older adults ($n = 2812$) to the elderly protective service database over a 9-year follow-up period.[21] Protective services saw 184 (6.5%) individuals in the cohort for any indication of mistreatment and 47 for abuse and neglect, for a sampling prevalence of 1.6% (95% CI 1%, 2.1%). In a pooled logistic regression, age, race, poverty, functional disability, and cognitive impairment were identified as risk factors for reported elder mistreatment. However, the authors carefully noted that because of the mechanism for case finding (a social welfare system), the race and poverty risk factors were likely overestimates due to a reporting bias.

Another study examined the characteristics of abused or neglected patients to compare the prevalence of depression and dementia in neglected patients with that of patients referred for other reasons. Using a case-control approach in a large academic hospital-based geriatric clinic, 47 older persons were referred for neglect and 97 were referred for other reasons. Comprehensive geriatric assessment with standard geriatric assessment tools was used in this study. There was a statistically significant higher prevalence of depression (62% versus 12%) and dementia (51% versus 30%) in victims of self-neglect compared to patients referred for other reasons. No overall prevalence of mistreatment was given for the clinic. The authors concluded that geriatric clinicians should consider elder neglect or abuse in their depressed or demented patients.[11]

Abusers

Abusers are most often care custodians, employees of the facilities, or children of the abused.[6,19,22–24] These are the individuals with greatest contact with the abused. Theories for why EM might occur have provided some guidance to clinicians in terms of anticipating when these relationships may result in EM. They are briefly reviewed here.

The social learning or transgenerational violence theory contends that violence is learned. Espoused by child abuse experts, this theory contends that abused children grow up to abuse their own children; extended to elder abuse, it further espouses that abused children grow up to abuse their parents as well. As noted earlier, there are no data to support this theory; only anecdotal case evidence exists. The stressed caregiver theory contends that elder abuse and neglect occur when stresses in the caregiver's life become overwhelming (either from caregiving or external sources) and cause the caregiver to act in abusive or neglectful ways toward the older adult. The isolation theory asserts that a shrinking social network is the major risk factor for elder abuse and neglect, in that no one is able to evaluate the well-being of the older person on a regular basis until it might be too late. The dependency theory holds that functional frailty and medical illness set the stage for EM, because care demands will eventually exceed care resources and set the stage for inadequate care. Finally, the psychopathology of the abuser theory focuses on caregivers who have mental health impairment, such as substance abuse, mental retardation, or some other psychiatric diagnosis. These individuals may not be able to provide appropriate care.[25] All these theories are in need of research to determine which aspects, if any, are supported by data.

Situations

According to Fulmer and O'Malley,[26] some of the high-risk situations, as experienced from clinical practice, that result in EM are these:

1. Persons with chronic progressive, disabling illnesses that impair function and create care needs that exceed or will exceed their caretaker's ability to meet them, such as dementia, parkinsonism, severe arthritis, severe cardiac disease, severe chronic obstructive pulmonary disease (COPD), severe adult onset diabetes mellitus (AODM) and recurrent strokes.

2. Persons with progressive impairments who are without informal supports from family or neighbors, or whose caretakers manifest signs of "burnout."

3. Persons with a personal history of substance abuse or violent behavior or a family member or caretaker with the same problem.

4. Persons who live with a family in which there is a history of child or spouse abuse.

5. Persons with family members who are financially dependent on them.

6. Persons residing in institutions that have a history of providing substandard care.

7. Persons whose caretakers are under sudden increased stress, caused by, for example, loss of job, health, or spouse.

Diagnosis and Differential

Symptoms of elder mistreatment may result from physical, psychologic, financial, or material abuse or neglect, or any combination of these.

The natural history of chronic and acute illness in the elderly may mask the presence of abuse or neglect because it is difficult to determine whether the elderly person's worsening physical condition is due to the natural progression of illness or to omissions or active interventions on the part of a caretaker.[26] The interdisciplinary team approach is the most thorough way to avoid overlooking a case of elder mistreatment. One assessment instrument can be found in the appendix, the Fulmer Elder Assessment Instrument.[27] This valid and reliable instrument is used to screen individuals who are suspect for EM.[26,26]

The following observations should raise the index of suspicion that elder abuse has occurred. The caregiver may (1) show a loss of control or fear losing control, (2) present a contradictory history or one that does not or cannot explain the injury, (3) project the cause of injury onto a third party, (4) delay bringing in the elderly person for care, (5) overreact or underreact to the seriousness of the situation, (6) complain continuously about problems that are unrelated to the injury, and (7) refuse consent for further diagnostic studies and remove the patient from the facility. Because some frail elderly persons are prone to underlying conditions (instability of gait, poor vision, and frequent falls) that give rise to trauma, it may be difficult to differentiate accidental from willful injuries. The simultaneous presence of fresh and healing injuries suggests ongoing episodes of trauma, and elder abuse should be considered in the differential diagnosis.

Clinical assessment of EM is made complex by the variations across cultures and groups regarding what constitutes acceptable behavior. Differences in the way people define quality of life, survival needs, and well-being are widespread. Difficult ethical issues are frequently inherent in describing elder neglect and abuse. What if the older person asks the clinician to keep the abusive situation confidential? What if the choice is to return to a dangerous situation? What if there is beginning cognitive impairment, which is not yet impairing function, yet presents issues for decision making? All these complex and disturbing questions are best answered within a team approach where interdisciplinary members can come together with the patient, either in person or telecommunication, to review and evaluate strategies that can improve the situation. Each case is highly individual. Safety and security measures for one person may be perceived as threatening or restrictive to another person. The elderly person's perception of a situation as abuse, abusive, or nonabusive may further influence their perception of whether or where they would seek help in that situation. In one study, Caucasian, African-American, and Korean women were surveyed using case studies as to what they thought constituted abuse. Korean women were least likely to perceive abuse while African-American women were most likely to perceive abuse.[28] Given that it is unlikely that there will be

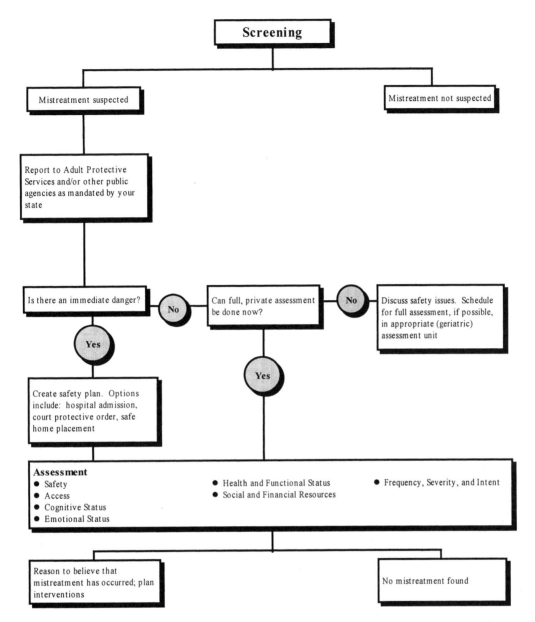

FIGURE 72.1. **Intervention and case management: part 1.** Screening and assessment for elder mistreatment should follow a routine pattern. Assessment of each case should include the following. (Reprinted with permission of the American Medical Association. *Diagnostic and Treatment Guidelines on Elder Abuse and Neglect*, 1992:1.)

a universal definition that is accepted by all cultures, it is essential that clinicians be aware of the values and cultural beliefs of those for whom they care. Clinicians must also be prepared to use principles of ethical decision making as guidelines for screening and intervention.

Intervention and Treatment

Clinicians have relied on their professional associations to help guide practice protocols. The American Medical Association[29] guidelines summarize the clinical approach

to screening and assessment of EM and have developed particularly useful algorithms to help clinicians decide how to develop care plans for those who might be mistreated (Figs. 72.1, 72.2). It is important to note that algorithm 1 indicates screening approaches whereas algorithm 2 indicates intervention approaches.

The focus of intervention and treatment is on maintaining the independence and functional capabilities of both the abused elderly person and their family or support system. Interdisciplinary teams ensure a variety of perspectives from which to consider potential problems and solutions.[30] Institutionalization may be the

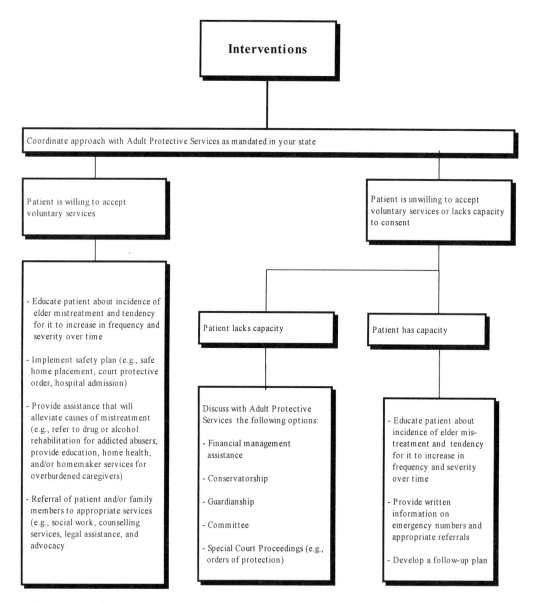

FIGURE 72.2. **Intervention and case management: part 2.** Case management should be guided by choosing the alternatives that least restrict the patient's independence and decision-making responsibilities and fulfill state mandated reporting requirements. Intervention will depend on the patient cognitive status and decision-making capability and on whether the mistreatment is intentional or unintentional. (Reprinted with permission of the American Medical Association. *Diagnostic and Treatment Guidelines on Elder Abuse and Neglect*, 1992:14.)

solution to the problem in cases where abuse is a reflection of a need for care that outstrips the caregiver's ability to provide it. Great care should be taken before this action, however, as the tensions that potentiate elder abuse may be ameliorated through improved in-home services such as the visiting nurse service, social services agencies, or Meals on Wheels. Sending services into the home also provides trained outsiders who watch and are able to offer informal counseling and support.

Most states have legislation that addresses elder mistreatment; such statutes are usually contained in adult protective service or domestic violence legislation. Protective services laws with provisions for reporting EM are in place in all 50 states and the District of Columbia.[31]

Summary

Elder mistreatment is a significant clinical problem, and clinicians have an important role in assessing, detecting, referring, and care planning for these victims. The medicalization of the elder mistreatment research portends very favorably in increasing the number of providers available to intervene in a rapid fashion. Research needs to be conducted in the sensitivity and specificity of EM questions in the clinical setting. In the meantime, clinicians who ask, "Is there any abuse in your home?" will help address this serious issue. Vigilance in assessment and avoidance of labeling signs and symptoms as sequelae of aging are essential.

References

1. U.S. Department of Health and Human Services PHS. *Healthy People 2010*. Washington, DC: Government Printing Office; 2000.
2. Fulmer T, Ashley J. Clinical indicators of elderly neglect. *Appl Nurs Res*. 1989;2(4):161–167.
3. Pillemer KA, Wolf RS. *Elder Abuse: Conflict in the Family*. Dover: Auburn House; 1986.
4. Ertem IO, Leventhal JM, Dobbs S. Intergenerational continuity of child physical abuse: how good is the evidence? *Lancet*. 2000;356:814–819.
5. Tatara T. Understanding the nature and scope of domestic elder abuse with the use of state aggregate data: summaries of key findings of a national survey of state APS and aging agencies. *J Elder Abuse Neglect*. 1993;5:35–57.
6. Pillemer KA, Finkelhor D. Prevalence of elder abuse: a random sample survey. *Gerontologist*. 1988;28:51–57.
7. The National Center on Elder Abuse at The American Public Human Services Association (formerly the American Public Welfare Association) in collaboration with Westat, Inc. *The National Elder Abuse Incidence Study: Final Report*. Washington, DC: National Aging Information Center; 1998.
8. Tatara T. Personal communication with T. Fulmer, 1996.
9. Fulmer T, Paveza G, Abraham I, Fairchild S. Elder neglect assessment in the emergency department. *J Emerg Nurs*. 2000;26:436–443.
10. Wiist WH, McFarlane J. The effectiveness of an abuse assessment protocol in public health prenatal clinics. *Am J Public Health*. 1999;89:1217–1221.
11. Dyer CB, Pavlik VN, Murphy KP, Hyman DJ. The high prevalence of depression and dementia in elder abuse or neglect. *J Am Geriatr Soc*. 2000;48:205–208.
12. Rosenblatt DE, Cho KH, Durance PW. Reporting mistreatment of older adults: the role of physicians. *J Am Geriatr Soc*. 1996;44:65–70.
13. Lachs MS, Williams CS, O'Brien S, et al. ED use by older victims of family violence. *Ann Emerg Med*. 1997;30:448–454.
14. Fulmer T, McMahon DJ, Baer-Hines M, Forget B. Abuse, neglect, abandonment, violence, and exploitation: an analysis of all elderly patients seen in one emergency department during a six-month period. *J Emerg Nurs*. 1992; 18:505–510.
15. Omnibus Budget Reconciliation Act of 1987. *Public Law 100–203. Subtitle C: Nursing Home Reform*. Department of Health and Human Services, Washington, DC. *Fed Reg*. 1987;52:38582, 38584.
16. Greenberg S, Ramsey G, Mitty E, Fulmer T. Elder mistreatment: case law and ethical issues in assessment, reporting and management. *J Nurs Law*. 1999;6(3):7–20.
17. Pillemer KA, Bachman-Prehn R. Helping and hurting: predictors of maltreatment of patients in nursing homes. *Res Aging*. 1991;13:74–95.
18. Pillemer KA, Hudson B. A model abuse prevention program for nursing assistants. *Gerontologist*. 1993;33: 128–131.
19. Pillemer KA, Moore DW. Abuse of patients in nursing homes: findings from a survey of staff. *Gerontologist*. 1989; 29:314–320.
20. Blakely BE. 1990–91 Assessment of adult protective services in Indiana. In: Tatara T, Rittman MM, eds. *Findings of Five Elder Abuse Studies from the NARCEA Research Grants Program*. Washington, DC: National Aging Resource Center on Elder Abuse; 1991:81–133.
21. Lachs MS, Williams C, O'Brien S, Hurst L, Horwitz RI. Risk factors for reported elder abuse and neglect: a nine-year observational cohort study. *Gerontologist*. 1997;37: 469–474.
22. Watson M, Cesario T, Ziemba S, McGovern P. Elder abuse in long-term care environments: a pilot study using information from long-term care Ombudsman reports in one California county. *J Elder Abuse Neglect*. 1993;5(4):95–111.
23. Pillemer KA. Maltreatment of patients in nursing homes: overview and research agenda. *J Health Soc Behav*. 1988; 29:227–238.
24. Tellis-Nayak V, Tellis-Nayak M. Quality of care and the burden of two cultures: when the world of the nurse's aide enters the world of the nursing home [see comments]. *Gerontologist*. 1989;29:307–313.
25. Lachs MS, Fulmer T. Recognizing elder abuse and neglect. *Clin Geriatr Med*. 1993;9(3):665–681.
26. Fulmer T, O'Malley T. *Inadequate Care of the Elderly: A Health Care Perspective on Abuse and Neglect*. New York: Springer; 1987.
27. Fulmer T, Street S, Carr K. Abuse of the elderly: screening and detection. *J Emerg Nurs* 1984;10:131–140.
28. Moon A, Williams O. Perceptions of elder abuse and help-seeking patterns among African-American, Caucasian American, and Korean-American elderly women. *Gerontologist*. 1993;33:386–395.
29. Aravanis SC, Adelman RD, Breckman R, et al. *Diagnostic and Treatment Guidelines on Elder Abuse and Neglect*. Chicago: American Medical Association; 1992.
30. Carr K, Dix G, Fulmer T, et al. An elder abuse assessment team in an acute hospital setting. The Beth Israel Hospital Elder Assessment Team. *Gerontologist*. 1986;26:115–8(2): 115–118A.
31. Capezuti E, Brush BL, Lawson WT. Reporting elder mistreatment. *J Gerontol Nurs*. 1997;23:24–32.

Appendix. Fulmer Elder Assessment Instrument

General Assessment

	Very Good	Good	Poor	Very Poor	Unable to Assess
1. Clothing	1	2	3	4	9999
2. Hygiene	1	2	3	4	9999
3. Nutrition	1	2	3	4	9999
4. Skin Integrity	1	2	3	4	9999

Neglect Assessment

	No Evidence	Probably No Evidence	Probably Evidence	Evidence	Unable to Assess
5. Bruising	1	2	3	4	9999
6. Contractures	1	2	3	4	9999
7. Decubiti	1	2	3	4	9999
8. Dehydration	1	2	3	4	9999
9. Diarrhea	1	2	3	4	9999
10. Impaction	1	2	3	4	9999
11. Lacerations	1	2	3	4	9999
12. Malnutrition	1	2	3	4	9999
13. Urine burns/excoriations	1	2	3	4	9999

Usual Lifestyle

	Totally Independent	Mostly Independent	Mostly Dependent	Totally Dependent	Unable to Assess
14. Administration of meds	1	2	3	4	9999
15. Ambulation	1	2	3	4	9999
16. Continence	1	2	3	4	9999
17. Feedings	1	2	3	4	9999
18. Maintenance of hygiene	1	2	3	4	9999
19. Management of finances	1	2	3	4	9999
20. Family support	1	2	3	4	9999

Social Assessment

	Very Good Quality	Good Quality	Poor Quality	Very Poor Quality	Unable to Assess
21. Financial situation	1	2	3	4	9999
22. Interaction with family	1	2	3	4	9999
23. Interaction with friends	1	2	3	4	9999
24. Interaction with nursing home personnel	1	2	3	4	9999
25. Living arrangement	1	2	3	4	9999
26. Observed relationship with care provider	1	2	3	4	9999
27. Participation in daily social activities	1	2	3	4	9999
28. Support systems	1	2	3	4	9999
29. Ability to express needs	1	2	3	4	9999

Medical Assessment

	No Evidence	Probably No Evidence	Probably Evidence	Evidence	Unable to Assess
30. Duplication of similar medications (e.g., multiple laxatives, sedatives)	1	2	3	4	9999
31. Unusual doses of medication	1	2	3	4	9999
32. Alcohol/substance abuse	1	2	3	4	9999
33. Greater than 15% dehydration	1	2	3	4	9999
34. Bruises and/or trauma beyond what is compatible with alleged trauma	1	2	3	4	9999
35. Failure to respond to warning of obvious disease	1	2	3	4	9999
36. Repetitive admissions due to probable failure of health care surveillance	1	2	3	4	9999

Emotional/Psychological Neglect	No Evidence	Probably No Evidence	Probably Evidence	Evidence	Unable to Assess
37. Elder states being left alone for long periods of time	1	2	3	4	9999
38. Elder states being ignored or given the "silent treatment"	1	2	3	4	9999
39. Elder states failure to receive companionship, news, changes in routine, information	1	2	3	4	9999
40. Subjective complaint of neglect	1	2	3	4	9999

Summary Assessments	No Evidence	Probably No Evidence	Probably Evidence	Evidence	Unable to Assess
41. Evidence of neglect	1	2	3	4	9999
42. Evidence of physical abuse	1	2	3	4	9999
43. Evidence of psychological abuse	1	2	3	4	9999
44. Evidence of financial abuse	1	2	3	4	9999

Disposition	Yes	No
45. Referral to social service	1	0
46. Referral to other? If yes, please specify	1	0

73
Frailty

Linda P. Fried, Jonathan Darer, and Jeremy Walston

Clinical Import and Definition of Frailty

Older patients who are frail have been described as the central focus of the practice of geriatric medicine, as they are thought to be the subset at highest risk for adverse outcomes. These outcomes range from falls to dependency, hospitalization, and mortality. Frail patients are the target group for a number of geriatric health care delivery systems, including geriatric assessment. Effective delivery of care to frail older adults has been described as the major challenge to medicine in the twenty-first century.[1]

Remarkably, given the centrality of frailty to the practice of geriatric medicine, a standardized definition has been challenging to achieve. Practitioners and researchers have historically assigned a broad range of meanings to "frailty," from referring to the very old (80 or 85 and older), to those with comorbid diseases, or to the presence of disability and dependency as frailty. Frequently, frailty has been used interchangeably with disability. However, recent work suggests that frailty is likely etiologically related to each of these states but is not identical to them.

The Clinical Syndrome of Frailty

Growing evidence suggests that frailty is a biologic syndrome of decreased reserves in multiple systems that results from dysregulation that can occur with aging and is initiated by physiologic changes of aging, disease, and/or lack of activity or inadequate nutritional intake. It is thought that these changes are manifested in loss of skeletal muscle mass and bone, and in abnormal function in inflammatory, immune, and neuroendocrine systems, as well as in energy regulation; this results in homeostenosis, or a decreased range of physiologic responses available to maintain homeostasis. It is hypothesized that the underlying system dysregulation might be latent in a non-stressed state, becoming clinically apparent when the system is stressed, for example, by extremes of temperature, infection, or injury. These hypotheses as to the physiology of frailty could explain the clinical picture of frail older adults being vulnerable to stressors, whether endogenous or exogenous, and, through this vulnerability, to the outcomes described above that are clinically associated with frailty.

Although these physiologic alterations may be the underpinnings of frailty (described further below), the clinical presentation, or phenotype, of frailty before the development of adverse outcomes appears centered around weight loss or sarcopenia (loss of muscle mass with aging), resulting weakness, low exercise tolerance or endurance, slowed task performance (such as walking speed), and low activity levels.[2-4] More end-stage frailty is thought to also include biochemical abnormalities consistent with a wasting syndrome, including hypoalbuminemia and hypocholesterolemia.[5] In a survey of U.S. geriatricians, 97% indicated that clinically apparent frailty involves more than one characteristic being present,[6] consistent with the definition of a syndrome. The consensus, in this survey and the geriatrics literature, is that this syndrome presents clinically with at least several of the manifestations described here, not including the biochemical abnormalities, in most frail, community-dwelling older adults. There is strong evidence in the literature for pairwise associations between most of these symptoms and signs, suggesting that they may be related in a cycle of frailty (Fig. 73.1).[4,7] This cycle of physiologic decline is hypothesized to be the basis for the phenotype of frailty in older adults. Clinically, such a cycle appears self-perpetuating once initiated, ultimately leading to a spiral of decline and death.

The components of the cycle of frailty are laid out in Figure 73.1—undernutrition, sarcopenia and weight loss, weakness, lower exercise tolerance, slowed motor performance, and low activity levels. These factors may com-

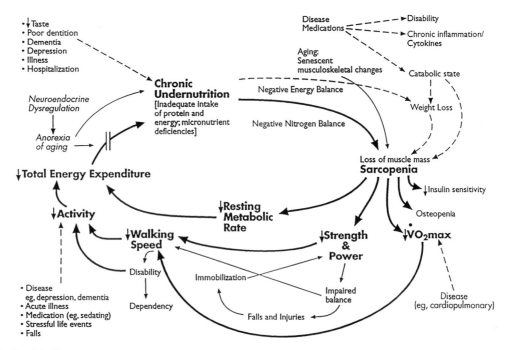

FIGURE 73.1. Cycle of frailty, integrating known pairwise causal relationships between symptoms and signs. Factors central to the cycle are indicated in *bold*. Potential etiologic causes and outcomes are also indicated. (From Ref. 3, with permission)

prise a clinical phenotype of the geriatric syndrome of frailty. A study was conducted to validate whether these components were found in community-dwelling older adults, and whether they, together, predicted a group at high risk of adverse outcomes that geriatricians clinically associate with being frail. To this end, community-dwelling adults 65 years and older in four U.S. communities who were participating in the Cardiovascular Health Study (CHS) were assessed for each of the characteristics described here.[4] Using the criteria of having three or more of five criteria being present to constitute frailty (Fig. 73.1, Appendix), 6.9% were found to be frail; the 3-year incidence of frailty was 7%. Frailty increased dramatically with age, being present in 3% of those 65 to 70 years of age and increasing to 26% of those 85 to 89. Frailty was more prevalent in women (7%) than men (5%) in the predominantly Caucasian cohort, whereas in a second, smaller group of African-Americans, frailty was twice as frequent as in the first group, found in 14% of the women and 7% of the men. The higher rates of frailty in women are thought to be because women have a lower lean body mass initially, suggesting that loss of muscle mass with aging would lead them to cross a threshold associated with increased vulnerability more rapidly than would men.[8] Those who were frail in this cohort were at high risk of mortality, falls, hospitalization, and incident or worsening disability, compared to those with none of the frailty manifestations. As seen in Table 73.1, there was a 1.3- to 2.2-fold increased risk of each of these outcomes, after 3 years, for those who were frail at the initial eval-

uation, adjusting for a number of other diseases and health conditions. Thus, this clinical presentation or phenotype of frailty identifies a high risk group of older adults. The screening criteria for frailty based on this phenotype are provided in the Appendix. Future work will offer alternative approaches to identifying those who are frail, with the approach that is ultimately most useful being the one that detects those at highest risk.

Association of Disability and Comorbidity with Frailty

As stated initially, frailty has often been used in the literature as synonymous with disability and comorbidity. Increasing evidence suggests, rather, that these conditions are etiologically related, with frailty being a cause of disability, whereas both comorbidity and disability may exacerbate frailty itself. Support for distinguishing frailty from disability comes, in part, from a survey at six U.S. medical schools which found that 98% of geriatricians thought that frailty was different from disability, with 40% supporting the idea that frailty was usually or always a cause of disability and 13% indicating that they thought disability would also cause frailty.[6] Additionally, the individual components of the frailty phenotype (see Fig. 73.1) are each, separately, known to predict the development of disability in mobility and activities of daily living (ADLs); this further suggests that the aggregate syndrome of frailty might, itself, be a powerful predictor of

TABLE 73.1. The phenotype of the syndrome of frailty identifies older adults at high risk of adverse geriatric outcomes: Hazard ratios (HR) estimated over 3 years for frail versus nonfrail[a]

Outcome	Frail (vs. nonfrail)[a]
Incident fall	
Unadjusted	HR = 2.06
	CI = (1.64–2.59)
	$p < 0.0001$
Covariate adjusted	HR = 1.29
	CI = (1.00–1.68)
	$p = 0.054$
Worsening mobility	
Unadjusted	HR = 2.68
	CI = (2.26–3.28)
	$p < 0.0001$
Covariate adjusted	HR = 1.50
	CI = (1.23–1.82)
	$p < 0.0001$
Worsening ADL (= disability)	
Unadjusted	HR = 5.61
	CI = (4.50–7.00)
	$p < 0.0001$
Covariate adjusted	HR = 1.98
	CI = (1.54–2.55)
	$p < 0.0001$
First hospitalization	
Unadjusted	HR = 2.25
	CI = (1.94–2.62)
	$p < 0.0001$
Covariate adjusted	HR = 1.29
	CI = (1.09–1.54)
	$p < 0.004$
Death	
Unadjusted	HR = 6.47
	CI = (1.09–1.54)
	$p < 0.004$
Covariate adjusted	HR = 2.24
	CI = (1.51–3.33)
	$p < 0.0001$

Note: Covariate adjustment includes age, gender, indicator for minority cohort, income, smoking status, brachial and tibial blood pressure, fasting glucose, albumin, creatinine, carotid stenosis, history of CHF, cognitive function, major ECG abnormality, use of diuretics, problem with IADLs, self-report health measure, CES-D modified depression measure.
[a] Frail is defined as three or more of the following factors being present: weight loss, weakness, exhaustion, slow walking speed, and low physical activity (see Appendix for definitions).
Source: From Ref. 4, with permission of the authors.

developing disability in tasks requiring strength, mobility, or exercise tolerance. This expectation is supported by the findings in Table 73.1, after adjusting for the major diseases present (both clinical and subclinical), age, gender, baseline disability level, health habits, and depressive symptoms. Thus, it appears that disability may result from frailty. These different clinical states are etiologically related, but distinct.

Regarding the role of comorbidity in frailty, it has been hypothesized that frailty is a wasting syndrome that *can*

occur as the end stage of a number of chronic diseases (e.g., congestive heart failure, certain cancers), as well as the consequence of cumulative physiologic changes of aging; this would constitute secondary frailty. This biologic hypothesis differs from other contentions that frailty and comorbidity are the same. As with disability, this was assessed in the CHS study already mentioned, where it was found that those who were older and had more comorbid disease had higher rates of frailty, although 7% of those who were frail had no major diseases and about 25% had only one. The latter group may well represent primary frailty. Additionally, the presence of frailty was associated with higher rates of depressive symptoms and with lower Mini-Mental scores (between 18 and 23), providing some insight into other possible causes.[4] In a work by Newman et al.[9] evaluating this same cohort, subclinical and clinical cardiovascular diseases, including infarct-like lesions on brain MRI scan, were associated with the phenotype of frailty. This finding suggests that the extent of atherosclerosis may be a precipitant of frailty, or that the decreased physiologic reserve caused by cardiovascular disease, or other related mechanisms such as inflammation, may be intermediary causes of frailty. Thus, older age and chronic diseases may be etiologic risk factors for frailty, whereas frailty itself may lead to disability in mobility and exercise tolerance-demanding tasks.

The Physiology, Natural History, and Continuum of Frailty

It is likely that frailty includes a range of severity—and reversibility—of physiologic changes. Hypothetically, there is progressive dysregulation of physiologic systems with aging, including sarcopenia or loss of lean body mass, chronic inflammation, immune system compromise, and altered function of the neuroendocrine axis (Table 73.2). These changes may be etiologically interrelated, themselves (Fig. 73.2).[7] To date, no study has evaluated all these potential etiologies together in a frail population. However, several systems have been individually studied in older, compared to younger, persons, and provide supportive evidence that age-related changes in both the neuroendocrine and the immune systems may influence the development of frailty. For example, there

TABLE 73.2. Age-related alterations in neuroendocrine and immune system markers that may influence the development of frailty.

↓ testosterone	↓ growth hormone	↑ cortisol	↑ IL-6
↓ estrogen	↓ DHEA-S	↑ SNS activity	

SNS, sympathetic nervous system.
Source: From Ref. 7, with permission of the authors.

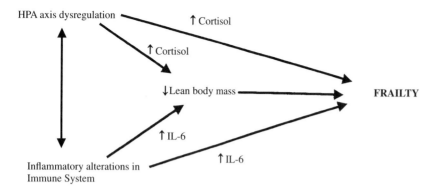

FIGURE 73.2. Hypothetical physiologic causal pathway that influences the development of frailty.

is a clear, age-related decline in growth hormone, its major messenger molecule IGF-1, and dehydroxy-epiandrosterone (DHEA-S),[10] and these declines are related to loss of muscle mass and strength. In addition, the sex steroids estrogen and testosterone clearly affect muscle mass maintenance, and the age-related decline in these hormones correlate with strength loss. Age-related alterations in the hypothalamic–pituitary–adrenal (HPA) axis, along with related increased inflammation, have also been hypothesized to contribute to the development of frailty.[11] Cortisol secretion appears to be moderately increased in older, compared to younger, adults, and there is some evidence that HPA reactivity to stress is increased in older adults.[10] Long-term elevations in cortisol levels have been associated with increased insulin resistance, increased rates of osteoporosis and hip fracture, and memory decline. These elevations may contribute to inflammation, which itself may contribute to frailty. High levels of IL-6 downregulate genes important in muscle mass maintenance and act to amplify production of nor-epinephrine and cortisol via increased HPA axis activity. Based on etiologies of altered body composition in individuals with rheumatoid arthritis, Roubenoff and Rall proposed that age-related losses of lean body mass and strength are influenced by inflammatory cytokines.[12] Frailty appears to present a similar picture. Several recent population studies have also suggested that elevations in the inflammatory cytokine IL-6 predicts functional decline and early morbidity and mortality.[13,14] These relationships likely contribute to the development of frailty.

More inclusively, Lipsitz et al. posited that there is a decrease with aging, in a number of systems, in the range of responses that are available physiologically to respond to stressors; one example is the decreased complexity of heart rate response with aging.[15] Lipsitz suggests that the aggregate alterations across systems may underlie the clinical vulnerability of frail older adults. Changes at the molecular level may also contribute to the decreased reserve of those who are frail. Even more theoretically, Bortz has proposed a "physics of frailty," postulating a loss of functional competence at a cellular level, with

thermodynamic decline and a loss of cellular energy stores predisposing to generalized physiologic decline.[16] There is some early evidence that such subclinical changes may not be apparent in the static state, but may be manifested under stress; this has been observed for cortisol responses to a stressor, as already mentioned.[17] However, this has not yet been demonstrated in frail older adults. Buchner and Wagner suggested that a reduced physiologic reserve plus decreased neurologic control and lower energy metabolism, in the presence of a specific physiologic trigger (see following), leads to frailty.[18] Such aggregate declines in reserve across multiple physiologic systems could lead to a subclinical stage of frailty manifesting as decreased ability to maintain homeostasis in the face of stressors such as acute infection. This change would confer greater vulnerability to poor outcomes for patients with such physiologic alterations.

A cycle of frailty, suggested in Figure 73.1, could potentially be initiated at any of multiple points, thus precipitating the transition from a preclinical toward a clinically apparent state. There is evidence from the study performed to validate the frailty phenotype described here[4] that the presence of only one or two of the major components of the phenotype of frailty does predict development of the full syndrome (with three or more components present) over 3-year follow-up, and also carries an increased risk of the same adverse outcomes listed in Table 73.1, but with weaker associations than the full frailty syndrome. This evidence suggests that there is a prefrail stage that is associated with some risk, even though not yet clinically apparent as frailty. It is possible that this stage is the most remediable.

On the extreme end of the continuum of frailty, an end-stage presentation has been termed "failure to thrive." This stage has been described as including unexplained weight loss, wasting, dependency, and possibly cognitive impairment.[5] Signs include hypocholesterolemia and hypoalbuminemia, both known predictors of mortality.[5,19] Studies of hospitalized patients with these characteristics indicate that this is frequently a nonreversible stage that presages death and identifies patients often not able to participate in therapy, such as rehabilitation.[20] Therapeutic interventions appear unlikely to reverse this presentation or the outcomes, and the goals of treatment are generally stabilization and comfort care.

Acute Precipitants of Frailty

Although the biologic basis of frailty may develop slowly and progressively, Buchner and Wagner[18] suggested that it may develop clinically in a stepwise process, with increments of decline precipitated by acute events, such as an infection or injury. Acute illness is often associated with a period of bed rest and undernutrition, with resulting loss of muscle mass, strength, and conditioning. According to Buchner's proposal, incomplete recovery from an illness, perhaps through inadequate rehabilitation or another acute illness before the period of recovery is complete, puts the individual at risk for still more decline with another insult. This scenario has clinical face validity and is consistent with the evidence for a prefrail stage, as mentioned. If correct, it suggests that it is critical to maximize recovery of strength and function after an acute illness.

Some diseases may contribute to frailty through direct biologic pathways, such as a potential role of atherosclerosis or inflammation. Other diseases could potentially trigger the onset of the cycle of frailty (see Fig. 73.1) by affecting the key components of the phenotype itself: nutritional status, muscle wasting, exercise tolerance, or activity level. For example, depression or congestive heart failure could each lead to both decreased dietary intake and low physical activity. Additionally, it is possible that medications could worsen frailty status, for example, through appetite suppression, increasing inflammation affecting muscle wasting, or lassitude affecting activity levels.

Diagnostic Approaches to Frailty

To decrease the high levels of morbidity and mortality observed in frail older adults, a more consistent diagnostic approach to the identification and management of the frail older adult needs to be developed and put into clinical practice. A diagnostic approach based on signs and symptoms of frailty, rather than either targeting just comorbidity or disability or awaiting the outcomes of frailty, has emerged in the past few years. Chin et al. identified weight loss and inactivity as important criteria in the identification of frail, older adults and provided validation by demonstrating higher levels of mortality and functional decline in that same study.[2] Fried et al. have validated a more specific phenotype of frailty described previously, which is diagnosed by three or more of five criteria: weight loss, low grip strength, low levels of phys-

ical activity, subjective exhaustion, and slow walking speed[4] (see Appendix). Whatever approach is used, a screening phenotype will only identify clinically manifest frailty. The subclinical or prefrail stages described here may mark a less-advanced but still vulnerable group, wherein early identification of declines in weight, strength, dietary intake, walking speed, *or* activity could make a difference in outcomes.

Differential Diagnosis of Frailty

When considering the prevention and treatment plan for clinical care for the frail older adult, it is important to keep in mind the numerous medical illnesses with a cachectic component that may either mimic or trigger frailty.[21] Frailty is, in part, a wasting syndrome of complex etiology, one that can coexist with acute and chronic disease. It is therefore frequently challenging to differentiate the wasting caused by a specific disease state from the wasting of frailty. Because signs and symptoms of all wasting syndromes often include weight loss, declines in strength and physical activity, and physical exhaustion, it is important that a full differential diagnosis of wasting syndromes that may mimic frailty be considered (Table 73.3). Severe congestive heart failure or cardiac cachexia has a well-described wasting syndrome associated with it. Cachexia related to occult malignancies is also common in older adults. Many connective tissue or collagen vascular diseases can be accompanied by a wasting syndrome, including rheumatoid arthritis and polymyalgia rheumatica. Chronic infections can also lead to wasting. Major depression can also present with several of the classic signs and symptoms of frailty. All these disorders are potentially treatable and must be ruled out in any older adult who presents with wasting symptoms. Because many of these disorders may well trigger the apparently independent and self-perpetuating syndrome of frailty as well as wasting syndromes in their own right, aggressive management of these disorders may slow the corresponding functional and medical declines that lead into the cycle of frailty (see Fig. 73.1).

TABLE 73.3. Differential diagnosis of common chronic diseases of older adults that have wasting features that can mimic or trigger frailty.

Congestive heart failure
Occult malignancy
Chronic infection
Rheumatoid arthritis
Polymyalgia rheumatica
Major depression
Parkinson's disease

Treatment of Frailty

The physiologic and functional vulnerability of frail, older adults should be used to guide their clinical management. Most frail older adults have numerous medical problems, many of which present atypically. The diagnosis and management of these medical problems must be addressed, selecting treatment in context with the overall physiologic and functional tolerance for their treatments, including special attention to altered pharmacokinetics and higher risk for complications in this population. In addition, numerous social, psychologic, and functional issues profoundly affect the health status of frail older adults and need to be included in any comprehensive treatment plan.

Independent of treatment for the numerous medical illnesses that can coexist with frailty, several groups of investigators have evaluated exercise and nutrition as potential treatments for frailty. Most studies have clearly shown a benefit of strength training exercise in improving strength and functionality in frail, older adults.[22,23] Evans has reported that high-intensity strength training has highly anabolic effects in older adults. He reported a 10% to 15% decrease in nitrogen excretion after initiation of such training, which persisted for the 12-week duration of training.[24] In other words, progressive resistance exercise improved nitrogen balance. As a result, older patients performing resistance training had a lower mean protein intake requirement than did sedentary subjects. Tai Chi has also proven beneficial in the prevention of falls and injuries in older adults who practice it on a regular basis, perhaps having similar effects.[25] Nutritional interventions are less clearly indicated in frail older adults, at least when they are the only intervention.[26] Poehlman et al. have shown that older men and women must increase energy expenditure by 1000 kcal per week to obtain compensatory increases in energy (food) intake and increases in resting metabolic rate.[27] Indeed, there appears to be minimal physiologic response to increased protein calorie nutrition in frail persons unless it is done in conjunction with an exercise program.[23,26,27] A benefit to functional outcomes was suggested in a cohort of very old, frail adults through combining strength training exercises and increased nutrition.[23]

The endocrine system has long been proposed to play a role in the development of frailty, and there have been a number of endocrinologic intervention trials seeking to improve muscle mass or strength in older adults. In part, such trials have been based on observations of age-related declines in hormone levels, such as declines in testosterone levels identified in older men. However, no direct relationship of *age-related* decline in testosterone levels to strength has ever been demonstrated. While the replacement of testosterone in *hypogonadal* younger and older men has proven effective in increasing muscle mass and strength, no study has clearly demonstrated a benefit of testosterone for the treatment of frail, older men with normal, age-related declines in testosterone. Growth hormone and its major messenger molecule IGF-1 have also been extensively studied in older adults, and a number of interventions have been tested to improve muscle mass or strength. Although there is a clear indication for growth hormone (GH) replacement in adults who have pituitary deficiency, no study has yet demonstrated that interventions with growth hormone or GH-releasing factor benefit normal adults or frail older adults.[28]

Organizational Approaches Effective for Frail Older Adults

Frail older adults, in addition to being clinically vulnerable, have the added difficulty of often being financially and socially vulnerable. They may also have diminished capacity to access appropriate health care services, navigate multiple providers, and obtain supplies and medications. Devising viable and effective systems to coordinate the complexities of frailty care within the increasingly cost-conscious health care environment is a major challenge for providers taking care of frail adults. During the past 30 years, geriatricians have developed and tested numerous models for care of the frail elderly. From this experience a series of best practices is emerging.

To determine the appropriate delivery systems for frail patients, we consider the following questions.

- What are the principles of high-quality care for frail older adults?
- What are the best strategies for delivering care to frail older adults?

Principles of High-Quality Care for Frail Older Adults

Frail older adults are complex, fragile, and often chronically ill patients, and as such require a more intensive approach to the delivery of care than healthy geriatric patients. Traditional medical care, generally designed to treat acute illnesses in patients actively seeking care, tends to employ episodic interactions where physicians perform medical diagnosis and offer treatment options. These traditional models of care often do not provide for the ongoing management of chronic conditions and prevention that frail patients require. They also are not geared to care for patients who require coordination of care or are unable to seek the care they need (Fig. 73.3).

Effective interventions for care of frail older adults incorporate a number of activities that can be distilled into a series of five steps.

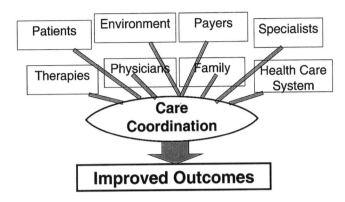

FIGURE 73.3. Coordination of care.

1. <u>Targeting</u>: Successful interventions focus their efforts on high-risk patients with reversible problems or who would benefit from stabilization.

2. <u>Assessment</u>: Having the appropriate expertise available to comprehensively identify medical and nonmedical needs is central to implementing effective interventions. Conversely, lack of expertise may lead to missed care needs or failed interventions, Assessing these needs often requires the skills of a multidisciplinary team.

3. <u>Intervention</u>: Knowing and using the up-to-date evidence-based interventions that make a difference is vital to improving outcomes.

4. <u>Implementation</u>: Patient adherence to treatment regimens is highly variable, requiring time to follow up on patient tolerance of a new treatment plan. There are, however, implementation strategies that physicians and health care teams can perform to improve adherence to treatment plans.

5. <u>Evaluation</u>: Assessing the processes and outcomes of care delivery enables providers to modify their approach to be more responsive to the needs of patients or more effective in care. Integrating performance improvement into the design of care facilitates the implementation of real improvements over time.

Successful Care Strategies for Frail Older Adults

Although these five steps are common approaches to management of complex medical issues, with modifications they provide an important framework for the care of frail older adults. Successful care models tend to perform these steps, and many of them have been able to demonstrate improved outcomes such as reduced mortality, reduced hospitalizations, and improved function. Conceptually, the type of care shown to improved outcomes varies by health and severity of frailty status (Fig. 73.4). We briefly describe some of the different care models that have been developed to treat patients across the frailty spectrum, from the prefrail older adult to the acutely ill, hospitalized frail patient, and the frail, dependent individual.

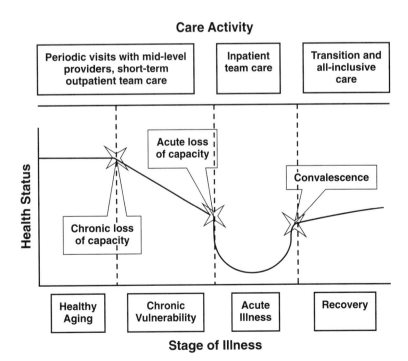

FIGURE 73.4. Geriatric care across settings.

Periodic Visits with Midlevel Providers

Successful models designed to prevent community-dwelling seniors from becoming frail include the use of periodic visits with midlevel providers. Stuck et al. were able to improve function and reduce nursing home days in community-dwelling seniors through a series of home visits by a geriatric nurse practitioner designed to identify unmet needs, facilitate access to appropriate services, and provide limited care recommendations with the support of a geriatrician.[29] In an analogous delivery model using geriatric nurse practitioner visits at a local senior center, designed to link seniors to existing community resources, provide chronic disease management and exercise classes, and increase social contact with other elders, Leveille et al. reduced hospital days and improved physical function in community-dwelling chronically ill patients aged 70 and over.[30]

Short-Term Outpatient Team Care

The use of outpatient multidisciplinary care teams on a short-term basis to perform comprehensive assessments and manage unmet needs can be effective in prefrail and frail patients as well. Hospital days and costs were reduced over a 1-year period through outpatient, multidisciplinary team assessment and short-term intervention in frail older adults with changing medical needs.[31] Fall prevention in older patients has been achieved using comprehensive assessment by nurse practitioners and physical therapists, coupled with a 3-month intervention in seniors aged 70 and older at risk for falls.[32] One-time multidisciplinary geriatric consultation can reduce functional decline in the outpatient setting in elderly patients with urinary incontinence, depression, falls, or functional impairment, when combined with aggressive adherence-improving strategies including phone calls to patients and primary care physicians.[33] Comprehensive assessment followed by interdisciplinary primary care of a population-based sample of community-dwelling Medicare beneficiaries ages 70 and older who were at high risk of hospital admission led to less functional decline and less use of home health care than controls.[34] One-time multidisciplinary consultations in isolation appear to be substantially less effective than those utilizing such implementation strategies.[35]

Inpatient Team Care

Inpatient multidisciplinary teams led by geriatricians can improve clinical and cost outcomes for hospitalized seniors.[36,37] In addition to geriatrically trained nurses and team care, modifying the hospital environment, for example, through the use of rails and carpets, can help reduce the complications of hospitalization and reduce length of hospital stay. Multidisciplinary team care can also be effective in an inpatient rehabilitation setting for older patients with reversible functional impairments.[38] In contrast, studies evaluating the effectiveness of inpatient geriatric consultation alone have failed to demonstrate an improvement in clinical outcomes for geriatric patients. Further work may need to be performed to clarify the obstacles to finding an effect; in some cases, this may have been due to the methods used for identifying those to receive the care being tested.

Transitional Care

Providing rehabilitation and aggressive clinical follow-up for patients after acute illness can be effective in improving outcomes for elderly patients with acute exacerbations of chronic illnesses or undergoing major surgery and potentially in preventing frailty. Naylor et al. showed that nurses working with specific transitional care protocols, following patients from hospital to home, were able to significantly reduce readmissions and costs.[39]

All-Inclusive Care

The Program for All-Inclusive Care for the Elderly (PACE), a Health Care Financing Administration (HCFA) demonstration project based upon the On Lok model in San Francisco, has been the most comprehensive care delivery system designed to address the needs of community-dwelling disabled and often frail seniors. In this capitated program, nursing home-eligible patients over the age of 55 are cared for by interdisciplinary teams, primarily in a day hospital setting. Focus is placed upon preventive, rehabilitative, and end-of-life care; short-term hospital and nursing home care are provided as necessary. This all-inclusive model has been successful at reducing hospitalizations by approximately 25%, when compared to the experience of similarly functionally impaired non-PACE seniors.[40]

In summary, a spectrum of geriatric care models can be matched to the stage of frailty in older patients (see Fig. 73.4) and effectively improve outcomes for each stage.

References

1. Report of the Council on Scientific Affairs. American Medical Association White Paper on Elderly Health. *Arch Intern Med.* 1990;150:2459.
2. Chin APM, Dekker JM, Feskens EJ, Schouten EG, Kromhout D. How to select a frail elderly population? A comparison of three working definitions. *J Clin Epidemiol.* 1999;52(11):1015–1021.
3. Dayhoff NE, Suhrheinrich J, Wigglesworth J, Topp R, Moore S. Balance and muscle strength as predictors of frailty among older adults. *J Gerontol Nurs.* 1998;24(7):18–27.

4. Fried LP, Tangen C, Walston J, et al. Frailty in older adults: evidence for a phenotype. *J Gerontol Med Sci.* 2001;56A: M146–M156.

5. Verdery RB. Failure to thrive in the elderly [review]. *Clin Geriatr Med.* 1995;11(4):653–659.

6. Williamson JD, Fried LP. Characteristics of frail older adults (unpublished data).

7. Fried LP, Walston J. Frailty and failure to thrive. In: Hazzard WR, Blass JP, Ettinger WH Jr, Halter JB, Ouslander J, eds. *Principles of Geriatric Medicine and Gerontology*, 4th Ed. New York: McGraw-Hill; 1998:1387–1402.

8. Walston J, Fried LP. Frailty and the older man. *Med Clin North Am.* 1999;83(5):1173–1194.

9. Newman AB, Gottdiener JS, McBurnie MA, et al. Associations of subclinical cardiovascular disease with frailty. *J Gerontol Med Sci.* 2001;56A:M158–M166.

10. Lamberts SW, van den Beld AW, van der Lely AJ. The endocrinology of aging. *Science.* 1997;278(5337):419–424.

11. Stouthard JM, Romijn JA, Van der PT, et al. Endocrinologic and metabolic effects of interleukin-6 in humans. *Am J Physiol* 1995;268(5 pt 1):E813–E819.

12. Roubenoff R, Rall LC. Humoral mediation of changing body composition during aging and chronic inflammation. *Nutr Rev.* 1993;51(1):1–11.

13. Cohen HJ, Pieper CF, Harris T, Rao KM, Currie MS. The association of plasma IL-6 with functional disability in community-dwelling elderly. *J Gerontol Med Sci.* 1997;52: M201–M208.

14. Ferrucci L, Harris TB, Guralnik JM, et al. Serum IL-6 level and the development of disability in older persons. *J Am Geriatr Soc.* 1999;47:639–646.

15. Lipsitz LA, Goldberger AL. Loss of "complexity" and aging. Potential applications of fractals and chaos theory to senescnce. *JAMA.* 1992;267(13):1806–1809.

16. Bortz WM. The physics of frailty. *J Am Geriatr Soc.* 1993; 41(9):1004–1008.

17. McEwen BS. Protective and damaging effects of stress mediators. Seminars in Medicine of the Beth Israel Deaconess Medical Center. *N Engl J Med.* 1998;338:171–179.

18. Buchner DM, Wagner EH. Preventing frail health. *Clin Geriatr Med.* 1992;8(1):1–17.

19. Corti MC, Guralnik JM, Salive ME, Sorkin JD. Serum albumin level and physical disability as predictors of mortality in older persons. *JAMA.* 1994;272(13):1036–1042.

20. Berkman B, Foster LWS, Campion E. Failure to thrive: paradigm for the frail elder. *Gerontologist.* 1989;29(5)654–659.

21. Kotler DP. Cachexia. *Ann Intern Med.* 2000;133(8):622–634.

22. Brown M, Sinacore DR, Ehsani AA, Binder EF, Holloszy JO, Kohrt WM. Low-intensity exercise as a modifier of physical frailty in older adults. *Arch Phys Med Rehabil.* 2000;81(7):960–965.

23. Fiatarone MA, O'Neill EF, Ryan ND, et al. Exercise training and nutritional supplementation for physical frailty in very elderly people. *N Engl J Med.* 1994;330(25):1769–1775.

24. Evans WJ. Effects of exercise on body composition and functional capacity of the elderly [review]. *J Gerontol A Biol Sci Med Sci.* 1995;50(spec no):147–150.

25. Wolf SL, Barnhart HX, Kutner NG, McNeely E, Coogler C, Xu T. Reducing frailty and falls in older persons: an investigation of Tai Chi and computerized balance training. Atlanta FICSIT Group. Frailty and Injuries: Cooperative Studies of Intervention Techniques. *J Am Geriatr Soc.* 1996; 44(5):489–497.

26. Hogarth MB, Marshall P, Lovat LB, et al. Nutritional supplementation in elderly medical in-patients: a double-blind placebo-controlled trial. *Age Ageing.* 1996;25(6):453–457.

27. Poehlman ET, Toth MJ, Fishman PS, et al. Sarcopenia in aging humans: the impact of menopause and disease [review]. *J Gerontol A Biol Sci Med Sci.* 1995;50(spec no): 73–77.

28. Lamberts SW. The somatopause: to treat or not to treat? *Horm Res* 2000;53(suppl 3):42–43.

29. Stuck AE, Aronow HU, Steiner A, et al. A trial of annual in-home comprehensive geriatric assessments for elderly people living in the community [see comments]. *N Engl J Med.* 1995;333(18):1184–1189.

30. Leveille SG, Wagner EH, Davis C, et al. Preventing disability and managing chronic illness in frail older adults: a randomized trial of a community-based partnership with primary care [see comments]. *J Am Geriatr Soc.* 1998; 46(10):1191–1198.

31. Williams ME, Williams TF, Zimmer JG, Hall WJ, Podgorski CA. How does the team approach to outpatient geriatric evaluation compare with traditional care: a report of a randomized controlled trial. *J Am Geriatr Soc.* 1987;35(12): 1071–1078.

32. Tinetti ME, Baker DI, McAvay G, et al. A multifactorial intervention to reduce the risk of falling among elderly people living in the community. *N Engl J Med.* 1994;331(13): 821–827.

33. Reuben DB, Frank JC, Hirsch SH, McGuigan KA, Maly RC. A randomized clinical trial of outpatient comprehensive geriatric assessment coupled with an intervention to increase adherence to recommendations. *J Am Geriatr Soc.* 1999;47(3):269–276.

34. Boult C, Boult LB, Morishita L, Dowd B, Kane RL, Urdangarin CF. A randomized clinical trial of outpatient geriatric evaluation and management. *J Am Geriatr Soc.* 2001;49:351–359.

35. Epstein AM, Hall JA, Fretwell M, et al. Consultative geriatric assessment for ambulatory patients. A randomized trial in a health maintenance organization. *JAMA.* 1990; 263(4):538–544.

36. Landefeld CS, Palmer RM, Kresevic DM, Fortinsky RH, Kowal J. A randomized trial of care in a hospital medical unit especially designed to improve the functional outcomes of acutely ill older patients. *N Engl J Med.* 1995; 332(20):1338–1344.

37. Rubenstein LZ, Josephson KR, Wieland GD, English PA, Sayre JA, Kane RL. Effectiveness of a geriatic evaluation unit. A randomized clinical trial. *N Engl J Med.* 1984; 311(26):1664–1670.

38. Applegate WB, Miller ST, Graney MJ, Elam JT, Burns R, Akins DE. A randomized, controlled trial of a geriatric assessment unit in a community rehabilitation hospital. *N Engl J Med.* 1990;322(22):1572–1578.

39. Naylor MD, Brooten D, Campbell R, et al. Comprehensive discharge planning and home follow-up of hospitalized

elders: a randomized clinical trial [see comments]. *JAMA.* 1999;281(7):613–620.

40. Wieland D, Lamb VL, Sutton SR, et al. Hospitalization in the Program of All-Inclusive Care for the Elderly (PACE): rates, concomitants, and predictors. *J Am Geriatr Soc.* 2000; 48(11):1373–1380.

Appendix. Cutoffs Used to Define Frailty

- Weight loss: In the past year, have you lost more than 10 lb unintentionally (i.e., not due to dieting or exercise)? If yes, then frail for weight loss criterion.
  At follow-up, weight loss was calculated as: (weight in previous year – current measured weight)/(weight in previous year) = K. If K ≥ 0.05 and the subject does not report that he/she was trying to lose weight (i.e., unintentional weight loss of at least 5% of previous year's body weight), then frail for weight loss = Yes.

- Exhaustion: Using the CES-D Depression Scale, the following two statements are read. (a) I felt that everything I did was an effort; (b) I could not get going. The question is asked: How often in the last week did you feel this way? 0 = rarely or none of the time (<1 day), 1 = some or a little of the time (1–2 days), 2 = a moderate amount of time (3–4 days), or 3 = most of the time. Subjects answering "2" or "3" to either of these questions is categorized as frail by the exhaustion criterion.

- Physical Activity: Based on the short version of the Minnesota Leisure Time Activity questionnaire, asking about walking, chores (moderately strenuous), mowing the lawn, raking, gardening, hiking, jogging, biking, exercise cycling, dancing, aerobics, bowling. golf, singles tennis, doubles tennis, racquetball, calisthenics, swimming. Kilocalories per week expended are calculated using standardized algorithm. This variable is stratified by gender.

  Males: Those with Kcal of physical activity per week <383 are frail.
  Females: Those with Kcal per week <270 are frail.

- Walk time, stratified by gender and height (gender-specific cutoff at median height):

Male	*Cutoff for time to walk 15 feet criterion for frailty:*
Height ≤173 cm	≥7 s
Height >173 cm	≥6 s
Female	
Height ≤159 cm	≥7 s
Height >159 cm	≥6 s

- Grip strength, stratified by gender and body mass index (BMI) quartiles:

Males	*Cutoff for grip strength (kg) criterion for frailty:*
BMI ≤24	≤29
BMI 24.1–26	≤30
BMI 26.1–28	≤30
BMI >28	≤32
Females	
BMI ≤23	≤17
BMI 23.1–26	≤17.3
BMI 26.1–29	≤18
BMI >29	≤21

Summary for frailty: a subject is frail if he/she has 3, 4, or 5 components identified as frail. Intermediate subjects have 1 or 2 components, and subjects with 0 positive frailty factors are considered not frail.

Source: From Ref. 4, with permission of the authors.

Part VI
Neurologic and Psychiatric Disorders

74
Dementia

Gary J. Kennedy

Dementia is a syndrome of progressive, global decline in cognition that is severe enough to degrade the individual's well-being and social function. Persons with dementia have learning and memory problems, plus at least one of the following: impairments in communication (aphasia), reasoning, and planning (executive function); recognition and manipulation of objects in space (agnosia, apraxia); orientation; and the regulation of emotion and aggression. Dementia is the most common cause of disability among older Americans.[1] With the number of dementia cases projected to double over the next 40 years,[2] even modestly effective interventions will have substantial benefits if achieved in the population at large. However, rates of underrecognition and undertreatment are considerable.[3] A comprehensive approach combining proven interventions can have a major impact on the patient and family's well-being and on the costs of long-term care.

Epidemiology and Costs

There were 360,000 new cases of Alzheimer's dementia diagnosed in 1997, with prevalent cases from all forms of dementia approaching 4 million Americans.[4] Costs of dementia care provided by professionals, institutions, and agencies total $100 billion a year. Yet, most persons with dementia are cared for in the community rather than institutions. The expense to the family members providing community-based care is estimated to be an additional $100 billion. Alzheimer's disease alone affects 8% to 15% of persons 65 and older. The prevalence of dementia increases exponentially, doubling every 5 years at least to age 85, at which point the incidence may decline.[5] Among individuals 85 and older with a demented first-degree relative, however, the prevalence approaches 50%.[6] And, despite improved survival rates associated with cardiovascular disease, an increase in vascular dementia may be expected.[7] Pathogenesis of

primary neuronal degeneration and genetic and other risk factors are discussed in the next chapter. What follows here is a commonsense, evidence-based approach to treatment.

Differential Diagnosis

Table 74.1 characterizes the various cognitive disorders, as well as the specific dementias. The diagnosis is challenging in the early stage because there are no definitive biologic markers, the onset is often insidious, and other reversible causes of cognitive impairment either resemble or accompany dementia. Clinical history from patient and family, physical examination, mental status assessment, and laboratory procedures are carried out to detect reversible or partially reversible disease. Although few dementias are reversible, most have elements that will partially remit.[8]

Delirium (see Chapter 76) is perhaps the most common cognitive disorder and often complicates dementia. The hallmarks are fluctuating level of awareness, impaired attention, disorganized thinking, and demonstrable physiologic disturbance. Symptoms should remit once the disturbance is reversed, but recovery may be delayed in older persons. Delirium can also be chronic and difficult to distinguish from dementia.[9] Cognitive impairment due to depressive disorders is distinguished by the patient's prominent complaints of difficulty with memory and concentration. Apathy, irritability, and reluctance to complete cognitive testing are apparent. Aphasia is usually absent.[10] However, there is a growing body of evidence that late-life depression accompanied by cognitive impairment often heralds the onset of dementia, even when the initial impairment remits with antidepressant therapy.[11]

Age-associated memory impairment (AAMI) is characterized by memory complaints in persons age 50 or older whose performance falls 1 SD below the mean on

TABLE 74.1. Differential diagnosis of cognitive impairment in adults.

Condition	Distinguishing features
Dementia	Progressive decline, global cognitive impairment with learning and memory deficits (recent > remote), aphasia, apraxia, agnosia, executive dysfunction; patients tend to minimize deficits
Developmental disorder	Childhood onset without progressive decline; history of diminished educational and work attainment; attention unimpaired
Delirium	Sudden onset and fluctuating course with inattention, disorganized thinking, and altered level of awareness; impairment reversible but recovery may be prolonged by advanced age
Major depressive disorder with cognitive impairment	Memory and concentration complaints prominent; aphasia absent, apathy or irritability present; cooperation with testing difficult, risk of subsequent dementia elevated
Age associated	Age >50, memory complaints prominent; performance below 1 SD from the mean on tests normed with young adults, information retrieval slowed; learning, orientation, communication intact; functional independence preserved
Mild cognitive impairment	Age >50, memory complaints prominent; performance below 1.5 SD from the mean on tests compared to age mates, information retrieval slowed; learning, orientation, communication intact; functional independence preserved
Alzheimer's disease	Insidious onset with smooth, inexorable decline, cortical atrophy; apolipoprotein E, ε4 allele, and cardiovascular disease elevate risk; more rapid decline in middle-stage onset; mood disturbance early, psychosis and behavioral disturbance later in the course
Vascular dementia	Sudden onset, fluctuating course with temporary improvements or prolonged plateau; multiple infarcts, diffuse white matter lesions, diabetes, cardiovascular disease present; focal neurologic exam
Huntington's disease	Autosomal dominant but incomplete penetrance inheritance pattern; atrophic caudate nuclei; premorbid DNA testing quantifies risk, age of onset, severity
Parkinson's disease	Characteristic tremor with unilateral onset, bradykinesia, bradyphrenia, cognition may be spared
Acute cognitive impairment due to stroke, traumatic brain injury	Focal neurologic exam; circumscribed rather than global cognitive deficits may improve significantly over 6 months
Frontal lobe degeneration, Pick's disease	Personality, sociability, executive function prominently impaired; disinhibition, impaired judgment, and social indifference significant; aphasia, apraxia, amnesia, loss of calculation less notable
Lewy body dementia	Sudden onset, fluctuating level of awareness, psychosis (visual and auditory hallucinations more often than delusions) prominent, parkinsonian signs and falls; adverse response to typical antipsychotic
Corticonuclear degeneration	Marked visuospatial impairment, substantial apraxia, memory behavior disturbance less prominent
Creutzfeldt–Jakob disease	Rapid progression, death in 6–12 months, characteristic EEG, myoclonic jerks
Alcohol-related dementia	Massive, prolonged abuse; may remit with abstinence
Normal pressure hydrocephalus	Gait disturbance ("magnetic gait"), incontinence, ventricular enlargement disproportionate to cortical atrophy
AIDS dementia	HIV positive, may present with behavioral disturbance, parkinsonian features

Source: Used with permission from Kennedy GJ. *Geriatric Mental Health Care: A Treatment Guide for Health Professionals*. New York: Guilford; 2000:48.

tests normed for younger adults. Although lower memory scores are predictive of dementia, only 1% to 3% of these individuals will experience global cognitive decline in the ensuing 12 to 24 months.[12] In contrast, 5% to 15% of persons with mild cognitive impairment (MCI) will develop dementia within the year. MCI is characterized by performance between 1 and 1.5 SD below the mean on tests of memory. As with AAMI, persons with MCI have memory complaints but do not meet diagnostic criteria for dementia; they exhibit slowed information retrieval, but orientation and communication are usually intact.[13]

Although a histologic examination of brain tissues sets the criteria for "definite" Alzheimer's disease, the diagnosis of "probable" Alzheimer's dementia can be accurately made in 90% of cases by history from the patient and family and clinical examination.[1] "Possible" cases may have atypical features but no identifiable alternative

diagnosis. Alzheimer's disease is the most frequent dementia. The onset is insidious; the decline is smooth, but more rapid in the middle stage in which behavioral disturbances emerge. Individuals with Alzheimer's disease often minimize their deficits, unlike persons with MCI or depression. Alzheimer's and Pick's disease represent cortical dementias in which there is primary neuronal degeneration.[14] Huntington's and Parkinson's disease represent the subcortical dementias. Dementia associated with Lewy bodies overlaps with both Parkinson's and Alzheimer's disease in presentation and distribution of pathology.

The secondary neuronal degeneration of the vascular dementias is caused by angiopathic disorders, most commonly ischemic heart disease and arrhythmias, hypertension, and diabetes. Hemiparesis, gait disorder, and other signs of past stroke also suggest vascular dementia. However, the pathology of vascular dementia is frequently of a mixed type (cortical and subcortical) with diverse presentations in which the loss of brain volume, ventricular dilatation, bradykinesia, and the cognitive deficits are difficult to distinguish from Alzheimer's disease.

Although perceptual distortions are common in dementia, when visual or auditory hallucinations are prominent, signs of Parkinson's disease are evident, the onset was abrupt, and the course characterized by lucid moments alternating with confusion, Lewy body disease may be diagnosed.[15] Paranoid delusions, falls, and depression are also characteristic of diffuse Lewy body dementia. More importantly, patients with diffuse Lewy body disease experience marked disruptions in dopaminergic systems, accounting for their exquisite sensitivity to antipsychotic medications.[16]

Alzheimer's, vascular, and Lewy body disease make up the majority of dementia diagnoses. Table 74.2 offers a simplified algorithm that will capture 95% of the dementias encountered by the average practitioner. The rare dementias would be easy to overlook were it not for their distinctive features. Marked deficits in visual perception and praxis out of proportion to memory impairment suggest corticonuclear degeneration. Changes in affect, typically depression but also hypomania and irritability preceding signs of dementia, suggest a non-Alzheimer's diagnosis.[17] Early deterioration in personality, loss of social inhibitions, and frontal lobe atrophy indicate Pick's dementia.[18] Physical signs such as the tremor and bradykinesia of Parkinson's disease, the choreoathetoid movements of Huntington's disease, the myoclonic twitching of Creutzfeldt–Jakob disease, or the pseudo-bulbar palsy of vascular dementia may not present before intellectual deterioration is observed. Huntington's disease is typical of the subcortical dementias in that various cortical functions, including communication,

praxis, and visual perception, are generally spared. Emotional disturbances and personality change are regular features of Huntington's disease and are frequently the first signs of the illness.[19] Normal pressure hydrocephalus is characterized by incontinence, abnormal ("magnetic") gait, and ventricular atrophy out of proportion to cortical loss.

Dementia may also be secondary to infectious systemic disease such as syphilis or acquired immunodeficiency syndrome.[20] Transmissible disorders of the prion type (Creuztfeldt–Jakob disease) may also cause dementia through exposure to infected foodstuffs or transplanted tissues or extracts.[21]

Diagnostic Procedures

Routine diagnostic laboratory procedures include complete blood count, blood chemistries, liver function studies, serologic test for syphilis, thyroid-stimulating hormone and vitamin B_{12} and folate levels, and cardiogram. In less than 1% of patients will these procedures detect a reversible cause of dementia. However, the identification of comorbid conditions whose less than optimal treatment compounds the disability or worsens the prognosis of the dementia will be more substantial. Chest x-ray, human immunodeficiency virus (HIV) test, and test of Lyme disease may also be included, based on physical examination and history. For patients with syncope or suspected seizures, an electroencephalogram may be ordered. A review of prescribed and over-the-counter medications and intake of alcohol and tobacco products is mandatory. Medications may be the most common cause of reversible dementia.

Imaging studies are used to confirm the diagnosis when clinical findings are equivocal, to distinguish one demen-

TABLE 74.2. Simplified algorithm for the differential diagnosis of dementia.

Insidious onset with smooth decline and motor function minimally impaired?		
	Abrupt onset or fluctuating course, little if any psychosis?	
YES NO →		
↓		
Alzheimer's dementia		
	History of stroke or significant ischemic brain injury on CAT scan or MRI?	
		Marked fluctuation in cognitive impairment, hallucinations prominent, signs of Parkinson's syndrome evident, falls
	YES NO →	
	↓	YES
	vascular dementia	↓
		Lewy body disease

Source: Used with permission from Kennedy GJ. Geriatric Mental Health Care: A Treatment Guide for Health Professionals. New York: Guilford; 2000:51.

tia from another, and to detect reversible causes. Because the incidence of irreversible dementia is age related, the detection rate for reversible causes with imaging declines with advancing age. Computerized tomography of the brain, without contrast, should be performed when focal neurologic signs are present, when change in mental status is sudden, or when trauma or mass effects are suspected. Magnetic resonance imaging may be indicated when vascular dementia is suspected. However, the white matter changes seen on T_2-weighted images are not necessarily indicative of dementia.[1] Functional imaging studies with positron emission tomography or single photon emission computerized tomography may detect the temporoparietal metabolic deficits of Alzheimer's disease or the diffuse irregular deficits of vascular dementia when objective signs of memory impairment are equivocal.[22] Functional imaging is far from being a routine clinical procedure. As treatments become available for early intervention, however, the desire for early detection may yet bring functional imaging into everyday practice.

Cognitive Assessment

Cognitive assessment should be conducted without family present to avoid distractions and any potential embarrassment over failed items. Because the patient is asked to actively demonstrate errors, considerable care is required to place the person at ease and accurately administer the exam. It is useful to discuss findings and recommendations in the individual interview and then gain the patient's permission to share the information with family. A premium is placed on openness and disclosure. However, certain individuals will be too anxious or suspicious to be examined alone or to accept a discussion of findings and recommendations in their presence. In such cases, tact and ingenuity are required to obtain consent for disclosure to the family. The use of a cognitive screening instrument allows the clinician to demonstrate the presence and, with longitudinal administrations, the course of deficits objectively.

A number of factors may influence cognitive performance yet not be indicative of dementia. These aspects include inefficient learning strategies, slowed processing capacity, reduced attention, sensory deficits, and age-associated memory impairment.[23] Age, education, and other demographic factors also alter performance.[24] Language, visuospatial ability, and abstract reasoning are less affected by age than memory and learning. Long-term and procedural memories are relatively preserved, whereas recent and episodic recall decline.[25] For example, the older musician may perform pieces from early life with both facility and feeling but not recall what was played the next day. New music will be impossible to master, despite good command of the instrument.

The Mini-Mental State Examination (MMSE) is the most widely used screening exam for impaired cognition in the United States and has been translated to a number of languages and normed for age and education. Molloy and Standish[26] have standardized the administration procedures for the MMSE to reduce test time and uncertainty about scoring (Table 74.3). Their techniques also reduce test anxiety. A perfect score is 30, with mild to moderate impairment falling between 18 and 24. For persons with fewer than 9 grades of education, a score of 17 or less is evidence of at least mild impairment. The average decline in MMSE scores among Alzheimer's patients is 2 to 4 points per year. In the study by Kelman et al. of 1855 older community residents, an impaired MMSE score whether mild, moderate, or severe was a stronger predictor of mortality than physical disability, number of conditions, or age.[27]

MMSE scores of 19 and above, memory loss and disorientation, repetitiousness, loss of interests, and change in personality characterize mild Alzheimer's dementia.[28] Although depression may appear early, delusions, agitation, sleep disturbance, and wandering are more characteristic of moderate dementia. Persons with moderately advanced dementia have MMSE scores ranging between 10 and 19. They require supervision to complete tasks of daily living, such as dressing, and to be safe from dangerous wandering. Severe dementia is evidenced by marked aphasia, loss of capacity to recognize family, incontinence, and dependency in all aspects of daily living.

Of the widely used screens for cognitive impairment, the Clock Drawing Test is the briefest, requiring less than 5 min to complete. The patient is asked to draw a clock face with all the numbers and hands and then to state the time as drawn. The number 12 must appear on top (3 points), there must be 12 numbers present (1 point), there must be two distinguishable hands (1 point), and the time must be identified correctly (1 point) for full credit. A score less than 4 is considered impaired.[29] The Free and Cued Selective Reminding may be useful to distinguish age-associated memory impairment from dementia. The Free and Cued Selective Reminding test reduces the age-related decrements in learning and processing to elicit genuine deficits in recall, which are characteristic of dementia. The measures may also be less sensitive to educational attainment.[23] For intellectually gifted persons, those with higher educational attainment, and when decline is subtle, referral to a neuropsychologist is warranted. For annual screening of seniors in primary care without signs or symptoms of dementia, the MMSE combined with the Clock Drawing Test provides adequate sensitivity and specificity.[29] Serial assessments at 6-month intervals are helpful when the diagnosis remains suspect. However, like imaging studies, none of the cognitive screening or neuropsychologic batteries can be considered diagnostic.

TABLE 74.3. Standardized Mini-Mental State Examination.

Preparations
    Ensure that the patient is willing and that vision and hearing aids if needed are in place. Ask *"Would it be all right to ask you some questions about your memory"?* Ask each question a maximum of 3 times. If the patient does not respond score the item as 0. If the answer is incorrect, score 0. Do not hint, prompt, or ask the question again once an answer has been given. If the patient answers, "What did you say?" do not explain or engage in conversation—merely repeat the same directions up to a maximum of 3 times. If the patient interrupts or wanders from the task, redirect the person by saying *"I will explain in a few minutes when we are finished. Now if we could just proceed please . . . we are almost finished."*

Begin by saying I am going to ask you some questions and give you some problems to solve.

	Max Score
1. (Allow no more than 10 seconds for each reply)	
a) *"What year is this?"* (Accept exact answer only)	1
b) *"What season is this?"* (In the last week of the old season or first of the new, accept either)	1
c) *"What month of the year is this?"* (On the first day of the new month or last day of the previous, accept either month)	1
d) *"What is today's date?"* (The day before of after is acceptable, e.g., on the 7th accept the 6th or 8th)	1
e) *"What day of the week is this?"* (Exact day only)	1
2. (Allow no more than 10 seconds for each reply)	
a) *"What county/borough are we in?"*	1
b) *"What province/state/country are we in?"*	1
c) *"What city/town are we in?"*	1
d) If in the clinic, *"What is the name of this hospital/building?"* (Exact name of hospital/institution/building only)	1
If in the patient's home *"What is the street address of this house?"* (Street name and house number or equivalent in rural areas)	
e) If in the clinic *"What floor of the building are we on?"* (Exact answer only)	1
If in the home *"What room are we in?"* (Exact only)	
3. *"I am going to name 3 objects. After I have said all 3, I want you to repeat them. Remember what they are because I am going to ask you to name then again in a few minutes."* (Say the objects slowly at 1-second intervals)	3
"BALL (1 second) *CAR* (1 second) *MAN. Please repeat the 3 items for me."*	
(Score 1 point for each reply on the first attempt. Allow 20 seconds for the reply, if the patient cannot repeat all 3 on the first attempt, repeat until they are learned but no more than 5 times)	
4. *"Now please subtract 7 from 100 and keep subtracting 7 from what's left until I tell you to stop."* (May repeat 3 times if the patient pauses—allow 1 minute for answer. Once the patient starts do not interrupt until 5 subtractions have been completed. If the patient stops, repeat "keep subtracting 7 from what's left" for a maximum of 3 times. See scoring examples below)	5
5. *"Now what were the 3 objects that I asked you to remember?"* (Score 1 point each regardless of the order; allow 10 seconds)	3

BALL CAR MAN

	Max Score
6. Show the patient a wristwatch and ask; *"What is this called?"* (Accept "wristwatch or "watch" but not "clock" or "time")	1
7. Show a pencil and ask; *"What is this called?"* (Do not accept "pen")	1
8. *I'd like you to repeat a phrase for me: say "no if's, and's, or but's."* (Exact reply only)	1
9. *"Read the words on the page and then do what it says."* (Hand the patient the sheet with CLOSE YOUR EYES on it. Instructions may be repeated 3 times but patient must close eyes for correct score)	1
10. Ask if the patient is right or left handed. The paper is held in front of the patient and should be taken with the nondominant hand.	3
"Take this paper in your right/left hand, fold it in half, and place it on the floor."	
Takes paper with nondominant hand = 1	
Folds it in half = 1	
Places it on the floor = 1	
11. Give the patient a pencil and paper and say *"Write any complete sentence on this piece of paper."* (Allow no more than 30 seconds. Sentence should make sense. Ignore spelling.)	1
12. Place intersecting pentagons design, pencil, and paper in front of the patient. Say: *"Please copy this design."* Allow multiple attempts up to 1 minute. To be correct the patient's copy must show a 4-sided drawing within two 5-sided figures. Ignore rotation and distortions.)	1

Scoring serial sevens:

93, 86, 79, 72, 65	5 points
93, 88, 81, 74, 67	4 points
92, 85, 78, 71, 64	4 points
93, 87, 80, 73, 64	3 points

Scource: Adapted with permission from the author, Dr. D.W. Molloy, McMaster University. Also see Molloy DW, Alemayehu E, Roberts R. (1991) A standardized Mini-Mental State Examination (SMMSE): its reliability compared to the traditional Mini-Mental Sate Examination (MMSE). *American Journal of Psychiatry.* 148:102–105.

TABLE 74.4. Evolution of Alzheimer's disease (AD) as measured with the Functional Assessment Staging/Global Deterioration Scale (FAST/GDS), Clinical Dementia Rating (CDR) Scale, and Mini-Mental State Examination (MMSE).

FAST/GDS stage	CDR stage	MMSE score	Diagnosis	Elapsed Time	Progression of Disability
1	0	29	Normal	0	No difficulties either subjectively or objectively
2	0.5		Age-associated memory impairment		Complaints of forgetting location of object, subjective work difficulties
3	0.5	25	Mild cognitive impairment		Decreased job functioning evident to co-workers; difficulty in traveling to new locations
4	0.5	19	Mild AD	7 years	Decreased ability to perform instrument ADL's
5	1	14	Moderate AD	9 years	Requires assistance in choosing proper clothing
6a	2	5	Moderately severe AD	10.5 years	Difficulty putting clothing on properly
6b	2				Unable to bathe properly; may develop fear of bathing
6c	3				Inability to handle mechanics of toileting
6d	3				Urinary incontinence
6e	3				Fecal incontinence
7a	3	0	Severe AD	13 years	Ability to speak limited (1 to 5 words a day)
7b	3				All intelligible vocabulary lost
7c	3				Nonambulatory
7d	3				Unable to sit up independently
7e	3				Unable to smile
7f	3				Unable to hold head up

Source: Adapted from Reisberg B. Alzheimer's disease. In: Sadavoy J, Lazarus LW, Jarvik LF, Grossberg GT, eds. *Comprehensive Review of Geriatric Psychiatry—II, 2nd Ed.* Washington, DC: American Psychiatric Press; 1996:401–458, with permission.

Assessment of Functional Impairment

Although the examination of cognition occurs between patient and practitioner, functional impairment is more reliably assessed with collateral informants, most often family.[30] An assessment of activities of daily living not only covers the maintenance of physical hygiene and grooming, but also the more instrumental tasks such as management of finances, property, and household chores. Patients may appear in immaculate condition as a result of attentive caregivers, yet not be able to shop, cook, bathe, dress, or pay the bills without total assistance. The Global Deterioration Scale and Functional Assessment Staging (Table 74.4) is a widely used measure of dementia-related dependency.[31]

Treatment

The comprehensive approach to dementia care seeks to preserve the patient's independence by delaying disability to the end of the natural life span. There are five elements to the comprehensive approach. First is accurate diagnosis of the specific dementia and recognition of other conditions that contribute excess disability. Second is caregiver education, counseling, and support. The third element is the pharmacologic palliation of cognitive impairment. Fourth are interventions, both pharmacologic and environmental, to lessen behavioral and psychologic disturbances. Fifth is early advance care planning in anticipation of late-stage and end-of-life care issues.

Reduction of Excess Disability

Beyond recognition of the specific dementia, the optimal treatment of associated conditions is critical. One-half of persons with dementia have a concurrent physical or mental illness that contributes to their functional impairments. Half that number will experience at least temporary benefits from treatment of the comorbid condition. And, in half that group, the benefits will last a year or more.[32] Weight control, exercise, elimination of tobacco use, and minimizing alcohol intake represent good preventive health at any age, perhaps more so for individuals with dementia. However, some persons would rather not forgo real pleasures in the present for the promise of potential benefits in the uncertain future. For patients with suspected vascular dementia, the use of 325 mg aspirin daily should be recommended.[33]

Counseling and Coaching the Caregiver

The cornerstones of caregiver counseling are education, emotional support, and telephone availability. When combined with support groups, these techniques delayed nursing home admission an average of 9 months without increasing the caregiver's burden.[34] The majority of dementia care is provided by female family members who vary widely in their capacity to adapt to the burdens of the illness.[35] Rehabilitation of the patient should always include consultation with the family, and failure of the family to appear should alert the clinician to future problems. Most families are remarkably creative in providing care. Others seem enmeshed, trapped in maintaining conflict rather than resolving it.[36] Clinical depression is a problem for 20% to 60% of the primary family caregivers.[37,38] The focus of care in these instances shifts to the family member and includes supportive psychotherapy or antidepressant medication. In rare instances, elder abuse, most often in the form of neglect, will require involvement of community agencies.

Caregivers should be instructed to modify the physical environment to be safe and predictable. A regular schedule of activities including rising, meals, medications, and exercise lessens the burden on memory. Unfamiliar people, places, and events require accommodation for which the patient is poorly equipped. Travel that disrupts the person's routine will be disorienting. Cherished holidays are better celebrated in the patient's home. The withdrawal of firearms, opportunities to cook or smoke unsupervised, and automobile driving requires compassion and at times imagination.

Psychotic and affective disturbances occur in as many of 80% of patients and account for much of the needed caregiver counseling. Behavioral disturbances are more distressing than forgetfulness or incontinence. Aggression, assault, accusations, nighttime wandering, and loss of capacity to recognize the caregiver predict nursing home admission.[39,40] Pharmacologic improvement of cognition will help, but behavioral and other measures often need to be instituted, as discussed in subsequent sections.

Pharmacologic Palliation of Impaired Cognition

Brietner predicts that medications emerging in the next two decades will significantly reduce the morbidity of Alzheimer's disease.[41] Simply delaying the onset of dementia by 5 years would reduce the prevalence by one-third.[42] Until those agents have been administered to a generation at risk, however, the pharmacologic alternative will continue to be drugs that may palliate but cannot prevent the disability of dementia (Table 74.5). Because the common dementias overlap diagnostically, every patient with the diagnosis of dementia should be offered a trial of a cholinesterase inhibitor.[43] In mild to moderately impaired persons, cholinesterase inhibitors may improve cognition, delay decline, lessen the disability in activities of daily living,[44] improve psychologic and behavioral disturbances including psychosis,[45,46] and forestall nursing home admission.[47]

Using randomized controlled trials of cholinesterase inhibitors, Livingston and Katona[48] performed a number needed to treat analysis to calculate the number of patients receiving active treatment needed to demonstrate a beneficial effect compared to placebo. For example, 29 patients with atrial fibrillation would need to be treated with coumadin to prevent stroke in 1. In contrast, with 10 mg donepezil, 6 (95% confidence interval, 4–12) Alzheimer's patients need to be treated to stabilize

TABLE 74.5. Agents used to palliate the cognitive impairment of dementia.

Generic name	Trade name	Initial dose	Final dose	Arrhythmia potential	Hypotensive potential	Sedative potential	Precautions	Advantages
Anticholinesterases								
Donepezil	Aricept	5 mg qd	10 mg qd	Bradycardia	Low	Low	Transient, initial GI upset, abrupt withdrawal leads to abrupt decline, may interact with paroxitine	Once a day dosing, safety
Rivastigmine	Exelon	1.5 mg bid	6 mg bid	Low	Low	Low	Transient, initial GI upset, titrated up at 2-week intervals, abrupt withdrawal leads to abrupt decline, bid dosing	Wider dose range, no drug interactions
Galantamine	Reminyl	4 mg bid	16 mg bid	Bradycardia	Low	Low	Transient, initial GI upset, titrated up at 4-week intervals, abrupt withdrawal leads to abrupt decline, bid dosing	Wider dose range, nicotinic receptor modulation
Antioxidants								
Selegiline	Eldepryl	5 mg qd	5 mg bid	Low	Moderate	Low	Potentially life-threatening diet and drug interactions are rare at recommended doses	Available as a transdermal patch
Alpha-tocopherol	Vitamin E	30 IU qd	1000 IU bid	NA	NA	NA	Liver toxicity, coagulopathy	Low toxicity, OTC
Others								
Extract of *Ginkgo biloba*	Ginkgold Tebonin forte	60 qd	60 qid	Low	Low	Low	qid dosing, an "herbal" not subject to FDA quality controls, few data available at max dose	Low toxicity, OTC

T½, half life; OTC, over the counter; FDA, U.S. Food and Drug Administration; NA, not applicable; AD, Alzheimer's disease; VaD, vascular dementia.
Source: Used with permission from Kennedy GJ. *Geriatric Mental Health Care: A Treatment Guide for Health Professionals*. New York: Guilford; 2000:58.

or reverse cognitive decline by 1 year in 1 person; with 12 mg rivastigmine, 5 (95% confidence interval, 4–7) patients need to be treated.

On average, cholinesterase inhibitors restore the person to a level of impairment seen 6 months previously. Although the effect is palliative, the less impaired time and delay in nursing home admission may be precious, particularly for patients whose improvement is marked. The side effects of cholinergic enhancement are nausea, diarrhea, sweating, bradycardia, and insomnia; these are most often are transient, occurring in 10% to one-third of patients at the initiation of treatment depending on the agent. To lessen adverse reactions, the cholinesterase inhibitors should be taken with meals and not at bedtime. Promethazine may be administered to counter nausea and vomiting but should not be required beyond the initial phase. The medication should be titrated up at 2- to 4-week intervals to the maximum recommended or tolerated dose. Phasing in the increase on an every other day schedule may enhance tolerability. Roughly one patient in four will experience improvement readily noticeable to family and practitioner within weeks of beginning the drug. That number increases to one in three by the third month of treatment.[49]

However, the majority of those who are not obviously better will experience less decline in the coming months with medication than without. As a result, the identification of genuine nonresponders who might be offered an alternative cholinesterase inhibitor is a real dilemma. Also, there is as yet no evidence for or against switching from one cholinesterase inhibitor to another. In theory, use of serial MMSE assessments might demonstrate a stabilizing effect of the medication. In practice, patients and families who find the benefits trivial compared to the burden of side effects, cost, and pill taking will opt to withdraw from treatment. However, cholinesterase inhibitors should not be withdrawn simply because the patient has been admitted to a nursing home. When withdrawn, the cognitive impairment of genuine responders will fall to that of patients treated with placebo. However, once the patient is bedbound, free of behavioral disturbances, and no longer recognizes family or caregivers, the benefits of the drug are questionable.

Two cholinesterase inhibitors are approved and a third is under consideration (galantamine) by the FDA for mild to moderate Alzheimer's disease. Donepezil possesses a prolonged action and specificity for brain tissue. The starting dose is 5 mg once daily and should be increased to 10 mg. Although it is metabolized by the cytochrome P-450 system, drug interactions are rare. Many practitioners find it has an alerting effect in late-stage patients.[43] Rivastigmine (Exelon) is a brain-specific cholinesterase inhibitor administered twice daily. The dose ranges from 1.5 to 6 mg bid.[50] Patients able to tolerate the gastrointestinal difficulties of higher doses may

benefit more. It is not metabolized by the cytochrome P-450 system, and drug interactions are thought to be rare.

Rivastigmine also inhibits butylcholinesterase, which may be more active in the latter stages of dementia, but the clinical significance of this property is uncertain.[51] The acetylcholinesterase inhibitor galantamine (Reminyl) is a plant-derived alkaloid with nicotinic receptor-modulating activities. Its capacity to allosterically modulate nicotinic receptors avoids the undesirable cardiovascular effects of direct nicotinic stimulation.[52] However, the clinical significance of this property is uncertain. Galantamine is taken twice daily at doses ranging from 4 to 16 mg. Because multiple enzymes of the cytochrome P-450 system metabolize galantamine, drug interactions should be rare.[53]

Although the cholinesterase inhibitors should not be prescribed together, many practitioners combine them with vitamins C (500 mg) and E (400–1000 IU bid). Both are antioxidants and appealing in theory, but evidence of benefit in dementia exists only for vitamin E. The author generally discourages patients from adding extract of Ginkgo biloba to the foregoing regimen for reasons of minimal benefit, cost, and possible coagulopathy, particularly in the presence of high-dose vitamin E. Selegiline, a selective monoamine oxidase-B inhibitor, and vitamin E (α-tocopherol) reduce the rate of functional decline and delay nursing home placement in moderately impaired persons with dementia. However, cognitive performance is not enhanced, and the combination of the two agents is no more beneficial than vitamin E alone.[54] Estrogen is associated with lesser prevalence of dementia among more highly educated women in epidemiologic studies. It also has a trophic effect on cultured neurons. However, the use of estrogen to treat established cases of or prevent Alzheimer's disease has not yet been convincingly demonstrated.[55]

Management of Behavioral and Psychologic Symptoms

Mental and behavioral disturbances are prevalent, occurring in more than half of community-residing elders who meet diagnostic criteria for dementia.[56] Their relative prevalence is displayed in Table 74.6 with significant differences between vascular dementia and Alzheimer's disease noted. The causes of behavioral symptoms are usually multiple, including the caregiving context, the caregiver's capacities and tolerance, as well as the patient's disease. Intervention to make the disturbed behavior less disruptive is a more realistic goal than outright elimination. A wait-and-see attitude may be reasonable when transient depression occurs, but agitation and psychosis are more likely to be persistent and disruptive.[28] The key to behavioral intervention is improved communication and patient perception. Adequate time

TABLE 74.6. Prevalence of specific[a] behavioral or psychologic symptoms among community-residing persons with dementia.

Apathy	25%
Depression (Vascular > Alzheimer's)	24%
Agitation/Aggression	24%
Irritability	20%
Delusions (Alzheimer's > vascular)	18%
Anxiety	17%
Hallucinations	14%
Pacing, wandering	14%

[a] More than half of diagnosed persons exhibited one or more symptoms.
Source: Data from Lyketsos et al. Am J Psychiatry. 2000;157:708–714, with permission.

must be allowed to communicate. Visual cues and verbal suggestions should be coupled. Caregivers should stay at eye level with the patient, avoid provocative stances or gestures, speak softly and slowly, use "sound bite"-size statements or instructions, check that the patient understands and is ready, eliminate visual distractions, reduce ambient noise, and attend to one thing at a time. Glasses and hearing aids should be available, and they will need to be replaced when lost.

Characterization of the three-point sequence or ABC's of problematic behavior is central to the task of management.[57] First, the caregiver is asked (A) to identify the "Antecedents" or triggering events such as changes in daily routine, interpersonal conflict, emotional or physical stressors. The antecedents can then be removed or minimized as a preventive measure. (B) The caregiver should describe the "Behavior" in detail, how often it occurs, when and where it is most likely to happen, and how long it lasts. Caregivers may need to step back and observe or take note to provide sufficient detail and to set the baseline for objective measurement of improvement. This observation period also refines recognition of antecedents and how the problem behavior fits into other aspects of the patient's life. (C) The caregiver identifies the "Consequences" of the behavior, how the caregiver or others react to reinforce or deter the activity, and what happens when the activity ceases.

Roca[58] advocates a different three-part approach to behavioral disturbances of encompassing empathic, behavioral, and medical perspectives. The patient's point of view, the environmental precipitants, and the extent to which unrecognized or undertreated diagnoses contribute to the disturbances are each assessed to arrive at effective interventions. The male resident of the facility who is occasionally combative and wanders out of the home provides an example of each perspective. The man may have been a boxer early in life who is now protecting himself from the intrusion of unfamiliar nursing staff. Staff should be alerted to his characteristic defense. He may have a bed near the entrance to the facility and simply be following others out as a result of echopraxia. Or, he may have a past history of bipolar illness with untreated mania as the explanation for his behavior. The intervention should be tailored to the individual characteristics of each patient.

Agitation

Behavioral disturbances naturally cluster into predominantly psychotic or affective groups, with agitation occurring in both.[59] Agitation is a common, persistent problem, and the etiology varies. Delirium may be the most frequent acute cause. However, environmental stressors such as sleep deprivation and unfamiliar or chaotic surroundings can induce confusion indistinguishable from toxic delirium. Patients may be "talked down" and reoriented, but attempts to flee or remove intravenous lines or life supports as a result of delirium require medication, most often an antipsychotic agent such as haloperidol. Depression, psychosis, anxiety, boredom, and pain also contribute to agitation.[60] Mania in dementia may also cause agitation, particularly when elevated mood, irritability, and hyperactivity appear. Frontal lobe degeneration impairs the person's judgment and capacity to sequence steps to gain attention or comfort. Patients whose needs cannot be accurately expressed because of aphasia may also become agitated. Their inability to comprehend spoken cues may compromise staff efforts to reassure them. Recognizing the impediments to communication will lessen the caregiver's frustration and justify the time and patience required to reduce, if not prevent, agitation. Impairments in hearing and vision add to the problem.

Psychotic Symptoms: Delusions, Hallucinations, Paranoia, Suspicions

It is important to distinguish persistent false beliefs or perceptions from transitory illusions that result from impairments in vision, hearing, and cortical deficits.[61] Similarly, if antecedents can be identified, they may be manipulated to reduce the problem to manageable proportions. Change in routine and caregiving personnel should be minimized. Better lighting to reduce shadows, correct sensory deficits, a modulated level of activity, and attention may also be effective. The suspicious person may be set at ease by reassurance or redirection to a less threatening theme or activity. Distraction, physical activity, or gentle touch (the elbow is neutral territory) may also restore trust. Attention provided when suspicions are silenced will lay a foundation for trust and reassurance at more problematic times.

However, when patients act on their delusions through reclusiveness, threats, accusations, or assault, antipsychotic medication is necessary. Suspicious patients may retain enough regard for an empathic physician that they will consent to medication to restore sleep, alleviate stress, or help control their temper. Patients can be informed that family or nursing staff will place liquid medication in their juice or cereal each morning if they agree. Consent need not be renewed with each dose.

Affective Symptoms: Apathy, Depression, Anxiety, Sleep Disturbance

Loss of interest, initiative, and responsiveness are seen in at least one-quarter of persons with dementia.[56] For patients who sleep too much, exercise, coffee, or tea may be useful. Other patients who are apathetic or nap too frequently may benefit from low-dose methylphenidate (5–15 mg after breakfast and lunch). Transient depressive symptoms are not uncommon in dementia, but persistent depressed mood and suicidal behaviors are less frequent. Depressed expressions may be evoked when the patient is reminded of sad events, when frustration overwhelms, or when the person feels neglected or alone. To lessen depressive expressions as well as apathy, caregivers should focus on pleasant memories, avoid or minimize frustrating, unpleasant circumstances, and increase pleasurable activities and social interaction. Teri et al.[62] found that combined behavioral and psychoeducational approaches significantly improved depressive symptoms in the majority of dementia patients and their caregivers. However, when there is a prior history of major depressive episodes, an antidepressant may be indicated.

Sleep disturbance is common in dementia and disrupts both the patient's and the caregiver's rest. A brief assessment of the sleep pattern, time spent in bed, and daytime activities can identify the need for changing the sleep schedule, adding exercise, or prescribing medication. If physical discomfort awakens the patient, an analgesic at bedtime may help. Holding fluids after 6:00 P.M. may reduce the frequency of nighttime urination. Sedation will solve the problem, but predisposes the patient to falling and increased daytime confusion.

Verbally Disruptive Behaviors

Verbally disruptive behaviors include screaming, abusive language, and repetitive verbalizations. These behaviors disturb others and may signal the person's unmet needs. In theory, screaming may result from cortical disinhibition or be reinforced by attention. However, it more often results from undiagnosed and untreated pain, physical discomfort, sensory deprivation, or social isolation. Often the behavior can be reduced in frequency and volume without resorting to sedation. Individual social interaction is most effective. Examples include simple conversation, range of motion exercises, and sensory stimulation with photos, fabrics, fragrances, and occupational therapy games.[63]

Family and staff generally prefer a little unpleasant vocalization to a patient made inaccessible with psychotropics. However, risk to the patient and risk to others must be parceled out. The concept of negotiated autonomy helps to avoid futile power struggles over patient rights. Negotiated autonomy means that once the patient is dependent on others, the autonomy of those others becomes a shared concern. Behavior that is disagreeable to others with whom the patient resides or on whom the patient depends is a justified focus of intervention. Thus, accommodation rather than autonomy is the issue.

Sundowning

Increased confusion at evening time can usually be managed by recognizing that change in the environmental routine triggers the problem. Patients who become troubled at change of shift in the nursing home or hospital may be responding to the increase in stimulation. Others may be bothered by the reduction in stimulation as daylight fades. In either situation, providing the optimum of stimulation is preferable to medication. Food, brief personal contact, music, or improved hearing or vision are only some of the alterations in the care routine that reduce sundowning.[63]

Indiscreet or Unwelcome Sexual Behavior

Demented persons seeking sexual gratification should not be labeled pathologic even though they may disturb caregivers and facility staff. However, when sexual advances are unwelcome or when self-stimulation is not managed discreetly, more may be required than directing the patient to a private area. The problem should be discussed directly with the patient at the time of the behavior and disapproval indicated for the circumstances surrounding the act, not the impulse. A matter-of-fact approach with family and staff also helps alleviate their reluctance to discuss the issue. Pathologic sexuality in dementia is more often seen with frontal lobe disease and represents disinhibition rather than willfulness. Staff and family will be less morally outraged once the neurologic basis of the behavior is explained.

Difficulties Accepting Personal Care

Efforts to assist with feeding, bathing, or transfer from bed to chair or toilet are sometimes met with assaultive behavior, particularly when the caregiver is not familiar with the patient. Assaultiveness results from protective reflexes and disinhibition directly related to the dementia. Apraxia, aphasia, and agnosia, made worse by impairment in vision and hearing, reduce the patient's ability to complete or comprehend simple tasks or to recognize the caregiver. It is helpful to educate staff that the objectionable behavior is the result of neurologic deficits and protective responses rather than malice. With time, staff become accustomed to the patient's needs and, through perseverance and intuition, develop an effective routine of care. Two persons may be required for bathing to prevent assault. The time saved by team approach to "problem bathers" more than compensates for the added personnel. Nonetheless, for some patients, a low dose of risperidone, olanzapine, or the short-lived benzodiazepine lorazepam is necessary to counter combativeness.

Willful Behavior and Personality Disorders

Despite accusations that objectionable behavior is "done on purpose," most often staff and family are mistaken in attributing willfulness to the demented person's behavior. However, individuals with personality disorders may also become demented. Problematic interpersonal relations across adult life are the key indicator that psychotropic medications may not be beneficial. Limit setting and confrontation are more effective. Because the behavior is part of an established pattern, staff should adjust their expectations accordingly.

Falls, Wandering, Pacing

Gait disturbance due to apraxia, quadriceps weakness, rigidity, sedatives, and poor vision predispose the patient to falls, soft tissue injury, and fractures. Physical therapy, if the patient will actively engage and sustain the benefits, may reduce the risk but not eliminate it. A change in medications may help, but environmental modifications are more likely needed. Restraints are usually employed to reduce the risk of falls. However, they degrade the patient's quality of life, cause soft tissue injury, and have led to documented cases of strangulation. As a result, there has been a national effort to reduce if not eliminate restraints in long-term care.[64] The dilemma of balancing safety and freedom should be shared with staff and family to reach a consensus. The substituted judgment of family in an informed or negotiated model of consent is most helpful.[65] Faced with the progressive decline in a loved relative, the family may choose near-term freedom from restraints and sedation rather than long-term freedom from injury.

The patient who walks about the backyard or enclosed garden of a nursing home presents no problem. However, when someone with dementia becomes lost in the neighborhood or wanders into traffic, safety becomes the issue. In the acute care setting, where wandering poses a more imminent risk, placing the patient under close observation may be necessary. In nursing facilities, an ankle bracelet set to electronically trip an exit alarm can help staff to redirect the patient to a safe destination. A family member may volunteer to provide supervised walking. Alternatively, physical therapy or other forms of low-risk exercise may be substituted. Exercise for the demented person is an underutilized modality to remedy behavioral disturbance. Caregivers should seek to determine whether there is a temporal or event-related pattern to the wandering. Do reminders of leaving (hat, coat) need to be removed? Pictures of family prominently displayed in the patient's room may assist when helping the patient to "go home." Pacing or wandering may also signal unmet needs or discomfort. Staff may need to experiment with toileting, snacks, or analgesics to find the right solution.

Catastrophic Reactions

Persons with dementia can be transiently overwhelmed, displaying anxious confusion, unwarranted suspicions, or tearful self-reproach. This catastrophic response follows overstimulation and a sense of failure or threat. An overbearing attitude, rapid questions, excessive commands, or too much noise or activity can provoke the response. Criticism, whether real or implied, such as intrusive efforts to correct or reorient the person, may also contribute. Patient fatigue or conflict with certain individuals may also be to blame. To counter a catastrophic reaction, it is helpful to change the subject or defer the task to a less distressing time. A soothing tone, with empathic comments spoken slowly with eye contact, may abort the response. At times it will be necessary to create a distraction or to remove the patient from the source of conflict or supply a pleasurable alternative.

Medications for Behavioral and Psychologic Disturbances

"Start low, go slow" is the catchphrase of prescribing for older adults. However, the most common error when using medication to control behavioral disturbance is failure to follow through, to monitor the effects, and to adjust doses accordingly. A short-acting benzodiazepine (lorazepam 0.5mg oral or intramuscular) can help the patient through procedures such as a CAT scan or MRI. For sleep disturbance, however, low doses of the sedating antidepressant trazodone (25–50mg) may be effective. Hypotension may ensue as the dose is increased.[66]

Antipsychotics

Haloperidol (0.5mg), and risperidone (0.5mg) are available in liquid form, which allows the dose to be given in food or a beverage for patients who have difficulty swallowing or accepting pills. Haloperidol, because of its lengthy track record, lack of cardiovascular effects, and availability of an intramuscular injection, may be preferable for short-term use in acute care settings. Although more expensive, the atypical antipsychotics are preferable for longer-term treatment. Risperidone, a mildly sedative atypical antipsychotic, does not induce movement disorders or hypotension at low doses (1–2 mg daily). Katz et al.[67] found it superior to placebo for the treatment of suspiciousness and aggressive behavior in dementia; however, at 2 mg, extrapyramidal signs began to appear. Olanzapine (2.5–10 mg) is less likely to induce extrapyramidal effects than resperidone but may cause somnolence, gait disorder, and elevated fasting blood glucose. It rarely lowers blood pressure, and the weight gain associated with its use may be desirable for some individuals. It also reduces agitation, aggression, and other manifestations of psychosis, as well as reducing their impact on caregivers.[68] Quetiapine (Seroquel) is more sedative than olanzapine but less likely to cause extrapyramidal effects. It is also relatively free of interactions with other drugs. At a mean dose of 100 mg (25 mg initially then up to 50 mg bid), it reduces behavioral disturbances, most notably hostility.[69]

In summary, both the typical and atypical antipsychotic medications are modestly effective for psychosis in dementia. They exhibit a therapeutic window in which low doses are ineffective and high doses are either ineffective or induce intolerable side effects. Based on the controlled trials, ease of administration, and duration in clinical practice, risperidone is the initial choice, followed by olanzapine then quetiapine. If these agents fail, either a typical antipsychotic or clozapine would be next in line. If extrapyramidal side effects appear with risperidone, another atypical antipsychotic should be substituted. Although antipsychotics have been the main treatment of aggression, valproate (125 mg twice daily to start) has gained increasing recognition as an antiaggression agent, as well as a mood stabilizer. It is relatively safe, and not amnestic, arrhythmogenic, or hypotensive, but should be monitored with the same therapeutic levels used for anticonvulsant therapy.[70]

Antidepressants

For the agitated or sleep-deprived depressed patient, trazodone is an effective antidepressant but is hypotensive and very sedative (25 mg initial dose). Nefazadone (50 mg twice daily to begin) is virtually free of amnestic and arrhythmic effects and is less sedative than trazodone. Sertraline (25 mg to begin) is not sedative and improves the signs of depression among nursing home residents in the late stages of dementia.[71] Citalopram (20–40 mg), which is FDA approved for recurrent depression, is somewhat longer acting than sertraline. Paroxetine (10–20 mg daily) is a more calming selective serotonergic reuptake inhibitor. Like sertraline and citalopram, it is free of cardiovascular and amnestic risk but may cause

nausea and jitteriness in a minority of persons. For the frail patient in whom no risk of side effects can be tolerated, buproprion (75–150 mg twice daily), which is selectively noradrenergic, is reasonable.

In similar instances, methylphenidate (5–15 mg after breakfast and lunch) may be prescribed and has the advantage of rapid onset of therapeutic response for the apathetic or somnolent patient.[72] Venlafaxine (25–100 mg twice daily) has the advantage of lacking sedative and hypotensive properties but may impair appetite.[73] In contrast, mirtazapine (7.5–30 mg) will improve sleep and appetite.[74] Antidepressants are frequently effective in combating anxiety. Sertraline, venlafaxine, and paroxetine are each FDA approved for one or more of the anxiety disorders and are less sedating than the benzodiazepines. Some practitioners also use nefazadone for this purpose.

Preparations for Late-Stage and End-of-Life Care

In the early stage of the disease, when incapacity is minimal, the practitioner should anticipate the need for supportive services and urge referral before the need becomes acute. Arrangements for home health aides, day treatment, respite care, and residence in nursing facilities can be patched together with a good deal of continuity. However, providing these arrangements exceeds the capacity of any one individual and is best coordinated by a social worker or other professional functioning as a case manager. Legal advice for the management of financial assets is another important area of consideration for the family. Nursing home placement will devastate even substantial estates, and prolonged care at home is also expensive.[75] Durable power of attorney assigned to a family member while the patient is still capable of exercising the necessary judgment will ensure adequate access to resources once the person is no longer able to manage financial decisions.

Cost considerations aside, patients and families need assistance throughout the treatment process to confront end-of-life care issues early, while the patient can still participate in appointing a surrogate decision maker and expressing preferences about future care. The appointment of a durable power of attorney for health care decisions (health care proxy) is the first step. A backup proxy may also be appointed. Some ethicists prefer the appointment of a health care proxy over the designation of advance directives. The proxy is empowered to act across an array of contingencies, which may be difficult to anticipate. However, the use of "feeding tubes" (gastrostomy or nasogastric tube), "breathing machines" (respirators), and "artificial kidney" (hemodialysis) for reasons beyond treatment of acute illness will be rejected by most older patients under circumstances of irreversible loss of mental ability. Late-stage dementia patients become so impaired that they are unable to allow others to feed them or to swallow without aspiration. Difficulty with feeding may signal terminal decline. Artificial nutrition and hydration through a gastrostomy tube has not been demonstrated to reduce suffering or prolong life in advanced dementia.[76] Further, feeding tubes are associated with aspiration pneumonia, fecal and urinary incontinence, cellulitus at the tube site, and other morbidities. Placement of a feeding tube also signals loss of the human contact gained through spoon-feeding.

Given the real risks and scant benefits of feeding tubes, their use is considered an option rather than an imperative. When those who care for the person are at odds about placing a feeding tube it is helpful to determine by consensus the specific goal to be achieved by the treatment. Typical examples include decubitus healing or a return to oral feeding. The involved parties can then agree to a time limited trial of tube feeding and, if the desired goal is not met the tube can be removed once proven to be ineffective.[77] (Also see Chapter 29.)

Cardiac resuscitation should also be carefully discussed before the indication arises. Late in the stage of dementia, when the patient has lost awareness of caregivers and surroundings, the use of antibiotics or hospitalization for acute illness has not been shown to prolong life and is associated with significant distress and agitation. These are difficult decisions, but they are more easily approached when the practitioner anticipates the need and is experienced in the discussion.[77]

Medical Legal Issues

Physicians are increasingly being called upon to provide affidavits and expert testimony regarding the capacity of an older individuals to manage assets and property and to make essential life decisions. A credible evaluation should include a diagnostic assessment that emphasizes the evaluation of functional capacity and is substantiated by validated measures of cognitive impairment and functional deterioration. Ideally, the evaluation should include a visit to the allegedly incapacitated person's home where the ability to manage personal documents, mail, medications, financial transactions, and telephone can be directly observed. A history of functional decline from collateral informants and a review of medical assessments to ensure that reversible causes of mental impairment have not been neglected are mandatory. The report should delineate life skills that are preserved, as well as those that are deficient. For example, an individual may take pride in keeping house and preparing meals but not be able to balance the checkbook or make change in the market. A court-ordered financial guardian and assistance with shopping are required, but a housekeeper is not. (See also Chapter 84.)

Summary

A comprehensive approach based on evidence from the scientific literature promises to reduce the disability of dementia substantially in the near future. However, the use of medications and modifications in staff or family's approach to the patient still requires ingenuity and perseverance. Even modest individual benefits, when spread over the large numbers of older Americans who will become demented, means sizable reductions in projected costs of care.

How to Contact Community-Based Services

National Association of State Units on Ageing: 202-898-2578

Alzheimer's Association: 800-621-0379, *www.alz.org*

National Association of Home Care: 202-547-7424, *www.nahc.org*

ABA Commission on Legal Problems of the Elderly: 202-662-8690, *www.abanet.org*

Assisted Living Federation of America: 703-691-8100, *www.alfalorg*

National Academy of Elder Law Attorneys: 520-881-4005, *www.naela.org*

Eldercare Locator: 800-677-1116, *www.aqeinfo.org/elderloc*

References

1. Small GW, Rabins PV, Barry PP, et al. Diagnosis and treatment of Alzheimer disease and related disorders. *JAMA*. 1997;278:1363–1371.
2. Ernst RL, Hay JW. The US economic and social costs of Alzheimer's disease revisited. *Am J Public Health*. 1994;84:1261–1264.
3. Ross GW, Abbot RD, Petrovich H, et al. Frequency and characteristics of silent dementia among elderly Japanese-American men: the Honolulu-Asia Aging Study. *JAMA*. 1997:277:80–85.
4. Brookmeyer R, Gray S, Kawas C. Projections of Alzheimer's disease in the United States and the public health impact of delaying disease onset. *Am J Public Health*. 1998;88:1337–1342.
5. Ritchie K, Kildea D. Is senile dementia "age-related" or "ageing related"?—evidence from meta-analysis of dementia prevalence in the oldest old. *Lancet*. 1995;346:931–934.
6. Mohs RC, Breitner JCS, Silverman JM, Davis KL. Alzheimer's disease; morbid risk among first-degree relatives approximates 50% by 90 years of age. *Arch Gen Psychiatry*. 1987;44:405–408.
7. Kennedy G, Hofer M, Cohen D, Schindledecker R, Fisher J. Significance of depression and cognitive impairment

in patients undergoing programmed electrical stimulation of cardiac arrhythmias. *Psychosom Med.* 1987;49:410–421.

8. Katzman R. Alzheimer's disease. *N Engl J Med.* 1986;314: 964–973.

9. Inouye SK, Bogardus ST, Charpentier PA, et al. A clinical trial of a multicomponent intervention to prevent delirium in hospitalized older patients. *N Engl J Med.* 1999,340:669–676.

10. Reifler BV. Mixed cognitive-affective disturbances in the elderly: a new classification. *J Clin Psychiatry.* 1986;47:354–356.

11. Jost BC, Grossberg GT. Evolution of psychiatric symptoms in Alzheimer's disease: a natural history study. *J Am Geriatr Soc.* 1996;44:1078–1081.

12. Richards M, Touchon J, Ledesert B, Richie K. Cognitive decline in ageing: are AAMI and AACD distinct entities? *Int J Geriatr Psychiatry.* 1999;14:534–540.

13. Peterson R, Smith G, Waring S, et al. Mild cognitive impairment; clinical characterization and outcome. *Arch Neurol.* 1999;56:303–308.

14. Huber SJ, Paulson GW. The concept of subcortical dementia. *Am J Psychiatry.* 1985;142:1313–1317.

15. McKieth LG, Galasko D, Kosaka K, et al. Consensus guidelines for the clinical and pathologic diagnosis of dementia with Lewy bodies (DLB): report of the consortium on DLB international workshop. *Neurology.* 1996; 47:1113–1124.

16. Luis CA, Barker WW, Gajaraj K, et al. Sensitivity and specificity of three clinical criteria for dementia with Lewy bodies in an autopsy-verified sample. *Int J Geriatr Psychiatry.* 1999;14:526–533.

17. Mahendra B. Depression and dementia: the multi-faceted relationship. *Psychol Med.* 1985;15:227–236.

18. Heston LL, White JA, Mastri AR. Pick's disease; clinical genetics and natural history. *Arch Gen Psychiatry.* 1987;44: 409–411.

19. Folstein SE, Folstein MF. Psychiatric features of Huntington's disease. *Psychiatr Dev.* 1983;2:193–206.

20. Koenig S, Gendelman HE, Orenstein JM, et al. Detection of AIDS virus in macrophages in brain tissues from AIDS patients with encephalopathy. *Science.* 1986;233:1089–1093.

21. Harrington MG, Merril CR, Asher DM, Gajdusek DC. Abnormal proteins in the cerebrospinal fluid of patients with Creutzfeldt–Jakob disease. *N Engl J Med.* 1986;315: 279–283.

22. Cutler NR, Haxby JV, Duara R, et al. Brain metabolism as measured with serial assessment in a patient with familial Alzheimer's disease. *Neurology.* 1985;35:184.

23. Grober E, Lipton RB, Hall C, et al. Memory impairment on free and cued selective reminding predicts dementia. *Neurology.* 2000;54:827–832.

24. Folstein M, Anthony JC, Parhad I, Duffy B, Gruenberg EM. The meaning of cognitive impairment in the elderly. *J Am Geriatr Soc.* 1985;33:228–235.

25. Sherwin BB. Mild cognitive impairment: potential pharmacological treatment options. *J Am Geriatr Soc.* 2000;48:431–441.

26. Molloy DW, Standish TIM. A guide to the standardized Mini-Mental State Examination. *Int Psychcogeriatr.* 1997;9: 87–94.

27. Kelman HR, Thomas C, Kennedy GJ, Chen J. Cognitive impairment and mortality among older community residents. *J Am Public Health.* 1994;84:1255–1260.

28. Devanand DP, Jacobs DM, Tang M-X, et al. The course of psychopathology in mild to moderate Alzheimer's disease. *Arch Gen Psychiatry.* 1997;66:205–210.

29. Stahelin HB, Monsch AU, Spiegel R. Early diagnosis of dementia via a two-step screening and diagnostic procedure. *Int Psychogeriatr.* 1997;9:123–130.

30. Kasper JD. Cognitive impairment among functionally limited elderly people in the community: future considerations for long-term care policy. *Milbank Q.* 1990;68: 81–109.

31. Auer S, Reisberg B. The GDS/FAST system. *Int Psychogeriatr.* 1997;9:167–171.

32. Reifler BV, Larson E. Excess disability in demented elderly outpatients: the rule of halves. *J Am Geriatr Soc.* 1988;36: 82–83.

33. Nyenhuis DL, Gorelick PB. Vascular dementia: a contemporary review of epidemiology, diagnosis, prevention, and treatment. *J Am Geriatr Soc.* 1998;46:1437–1448.

34. Mittelman MS, Ferris SH, Shulman E, Steinberg G. The effects of a multicomponent program on spouse-caregivers of Alzheimer's disease patients: results of a treatment/control study. In: Heston LL, ed. *Progress in Alzheimer's Disease and Similar Conditions.* Washington, DC: American Psychiatric Association Press; 1995:259–270.

35. Butler RN. Sounding board; on behalf of older women. *N Engl J Med.* 1996;334:794–796.

36. Boss P, Caron W, Horbal J, Mortimer J. Predictors of depression in caregivers of dementia patients: boundary ambiguity and mastery. *Fam Process.* 1990;29:245–254.

37. Cohen D, Eisdorfer C. Depression in family members caring for a relative with Alzheimer's disease. *J Am Geriatr Soc.* 1988;36:885–889.

38. Gallagher D, Rose J, Rivera P, et al. Prevalence of depression in family caregivers. *Gerontologist.* 1989;29:449–456.

39. Coleridge PT, George LK. Predictors of institutionalization among caregivers of patients with Alzheimer's disease. *J Am Geriatr Soc.* 1986;34:493–498.

40. Gwyther LP. *Care of Alzheimer's Patients: A Manual for Nursing Home Staff.* Washington, DC: American Health Care Association and the Alzheimer's and Related Disorders Association; 1988.

41. Breitner JCS. The end of Alzheimer's disease? *Int J Geriatr Psychiatry.* 1999;14:577–586.

42. Rosenberg RN. The molecular and genetic basis of AD: the end of the beginning. The 2000 Wartenberg lecture. *Neurology.* 2000;54:2045–2054.

43. Cummings JL. Cholinesterase inhibitors: a new class of psychotropic compounds. *Am J Psychiatry.* 2000;157:4–15.

44. Rogers SE, Friedhof LT, Apter JT, et al. The efficacy and safety of donepezil in patients with Alzheimer's disease: results of a US multi-center, randomized, double-blind, placebo controlled trial. *Dementia.* 1996;7:293-303.

45. Kaufer DI, Cummings JL, Christine D. Effect of tacrine on behavioral symptoms in Alzheimer's disease: an open label study. *J Geriatr Psychiatry Neurol.* 1996;9:1–6.

46. Becker RE, Colliver JA, Markwell SJ, et al. Effects of metrifonate on cognitive decline in Alzheimer's disease: a

double-blind, placebo-controlled, 6-month study. *Alzheimer Dis Relat Disord.* 1998;12:54–67.

47. Knopman D, Schneider LS, Davis K, et al. Long term tacrine (Cognex) treatment effects on nursing home placement and mortality: the Tacrine Study Group. *Neurology.* 1996;47:166–177.

48. Livingston G, Katona C. How useful are cholinesterase inhibitors in the treatment of Alzheimer's disease? A number needed to treat analysis. *Int J Geriatr Psychiatry.* 2000;15:203–207.

49. Cameron I, Curran S, Newton P, et al. Use of donepesil for the treatment of mild-moderate Alzheimer's disease: an audit of the assessment and treatment of patients in routine clinical practice. *Int J Geriatr Psychiatry.* 2000;15:887–891.

50. Vellas B, Inglis F, Potkin S, et al. Interim results from an international clinical trial with rivastigmine evaluating a 2-week titration rate in mild to severe Alzheimer's disease patients. *Int J Geriatr Psychopharm.* 1998;1:140–144.

51. Röseler M, Anand R, Cicin-Sain A, et al. Efficacy and safety of rivastigmine in patients with Alzheimer's disease: international randomized controlled trial. *Br Med J.* 1999;318:633–638.

52. Maelicke A. Allosterric modulation of nicotinic acetylcholine receptors as a treatment strategy for Alzheimer's disease. *Dement Geriatr Cogn Disord.* 2000;11(suppl 1):11–18.

53. Krall WJ, Srmek JJ, Cutler NR. Cholinesterase inhibitors: a therapeutic strategy for Alzheimer's disease. *Ann Pharmacother.* 1999;33:441–450.

54. Sano M, Ernesto C, Thomas RG, et al. A controlled trial of selegiline, alpha-tocopherol, or both as treatment for Alzheimer's disease. *N Engl J Med.* 1997;336:1216–1222.

55. Marden K, Sano M. Estrogen to treat Alzheimer's disease: too little, too late? So what's a woman to do? *Neurology.* 2000;54:2035–2036.

56. Lyketsos CG, Steinberg M, Tschanz JT, et al. Mental and behavioral disturbances in dementia: findings for the Cache County Study on Memory and Aging. *Am J Psychiatry.* 2000;157:708–714.

57. Teri L, Rabins P, Whitehouse P, et al. Management of behavior disturbance in Alzheimer disease: current knowledge and future directions. *Alzheimer Dis Assoc Disord.* 1992;6:77–88.

58. Roca RP. Managing the behavioral complications of dementia. In: Cobbs EL, Duthie EH, Murphy JB, eds. *Geriatric Review Syllabus: A Core Curriculum in Geriatric Medicine,* 4th Ed., Iowa: Kendall/Hunt; 1999:183–186.

59. Lyketsos CG. Remarks before the FDA Psychopharmacological Drugs Advisory Committee, March 18, 2000.

60. Greenwald BS, Kramer-Ginsberg E, Mann DB, et al. Dementia with coexistent major depression. *Am J Psychiatry.* 1989;146:1472–1478.

61. Wragg RE, Jeste VD. Overview of depression and psychosis in Alzheimer's disease. *Am J Psychiatry.* 1989;146:577–587.

62. Teri L, Logsdon R, Uomoto J, et al. Behavioral treatment of depression in dementia: a controlled trial. *J Gerontol.* 1997;32B:P159–P166.

63. Cohen-Mansfield J, Werner P. Management of verbally disruptive behaviors in nursing home residents. *J Gerontol Med Sci.* 1996;52:M369–M377.

64. Swauger KC, Tomlin C. Moving toward restraint-free patient care. *J Nurs Admin.* 2000;30:325–329.

65. Moody HR. From informed consent to negotiated consent. *Gerontologist.* 1988;28:64–70.

66. Houlihan DJ, Mulsant BH, Sweet RA, et al. A naturalistic study of trazodone in the treatment of behavioral complications of dementia. *Am J Geriatr Psychiatry.* 1994;2:78–85.

67. Katz IR, Jeste VD, Mintzer JE, et al. Comparison of resperidone and placebo for psychosis and behavioral disturbances associated with dementia: a randomized, double-blind trial. *J Clin Psychiatry.* 1999;60:107–115.

68. Street JS, Clark WS, Gannon KS, et al. Olanzapine treatment of psychotic and behavioral symptoms in patients with Alzheimer's disease in nursing care facilities: a double-blind, randomized, placebo-controlled trial. The HGEU Study Group. *Arch Gen Psychiatry.* 2000;57:968–976.

69. McManus DQ, Arvantis LA, Kowalcyk BB. Quetiapine, a novel antipsychotic: experience in elderly patients with psychotic disorders. Seroquel Trial 48 Study Group. *J Clin Psychiatry.* 1999;60(5):292–298.

70. Maletta GJ. Treatment of behavioral symptomatology of Alzheimer's disease, with emphasis on aggression: current clinical approaches. *Int Psychogeriatr.* 1992;4:117–130.

71. Magai C, Cohen C, Kennedy GJ, Gomberg D. A controlled clinical trial of sertraline in the treatment of depression in nursing home residents. *Am J Geriatr Psychiatry.* 2000;8:66–75.

72. Salzman C. Practical considerations for the treatment of depression in elderly and very elderly long-term care patients. *J Clin Psychiatry.* 1999;60(suppl 20):30–33.

73. Clerc GE, Ruimy P, Verdeau-Palles J. A double blind comparison of venlafaxiine and fluoxitine in patients hospitalized for major depression and melancholia. *Int Clin Psychopharmacol.* 1994;9:139–143.

74. Burrows G, Kremer C. Mirtazapine: clinical advantages in the treatment of depression. *Psychopharmacology.* 1997;17(suppl 1):34S–39S.

75. Overman W, Stoudemire A. Guidelines for legal and financial counseling of Alzheimer's disease patients and their families. *Am J Psychiatry.* 1988;145:1495–1500.

76. Gillick MR. Rethinking the role of tube feeding in patients with advanced dementia. *N Engl J Med.* 2000;342:206–210.

77. Karlawish JH, Quill T, Meier DE. A consensus-based approach to providing palliative care to patients who lack decision-making capacity. ACP-ASIM End-of-Life Care Consensus Panel. American College of Physicians—American Society of Internal Medicine. *Ann Intern Med.* 1999;130:835–840.

75
Neurobiologic Basis of Age-Related Dementing Disorders

Patrick R. Hof, Thierry Bussière, Joseph D. Buxbaum, and John H. Morrison

Over the past decade, we have witnessed a remarkable increase in our knowledge of the structural, molecular, and biochemical determinants of Alzheimer's disease (AD). Alzheimer's disease is the most common form of dementia, as it affects approximately 11% of the population over age 65, and up to 50% of individuals over 85 can be diagnosed as having "probable AD."[1] The exact pathogenetic events that lead to dementia are not yet known, although numerous hypotheses regarding the formation of the typical lesions of AD have been proposed and many risk factors have been identified. The current knowledge of the pathologic changes that occur in AD suggests that structurally and functionally AD is predominantly a disease of the cerebral cortex. However, it is not a generalized loss of cortical function: it involves only certain populations of neurons that share specific regional and laminar distribution and connectivity patterns, whereas other neuron types are spared.[2] Thus, different degrees of neuronal vulnerability exist in AD that can be related to the morphologic and biochemical characteristics of select neuronal populations and connections.

In this context, neuroanatomic analyses of nonhuman primate brain have considerably expanded our knowledge of the organization of the major afferent and efferent systems of the cerebral cortex, as well as its intrinsic organization. These analyses have fostered the development of an organizational scheme for the cerebral cortex that relates various molecules of interest to specific groups of neurons or circuits and have been particularly illuminating in regard to the organization of neocortical connectivity and interactions between the neocortex and the hippocampus. Furthermore, specific histochemical techniques have made it possible to investigate issues such as neuronal typology, connectivity, and localization within the context of their neurochemical identity. Certain neuron types within the cerebral cortex and some of the major cortical afferent systems have now been characterized as to the presence of structural proteins and neurotransmitters, and the extension of these studies to the human cerebral cortex is currently on its way. There are obvious limitations as to the application of such experimental paradigms to the study of the human brain, and it should be kept in mind that the human brain has become the object of intensive analyses with chemically specific techniques only relatively recently. However, many of the histochemical procedures work very reliably in the postmortem human brain, and to some extent it is possible to draw certain correlations across species that have allowed for the application to the human brain of organization principles described in several species of nonhuman primates. Such correlations have been particularly useful in regard to issues pertaining to the neuropathology of AD, as well as to the normal functional anatomy of the human cerebral cortex, although caution must be used when transposing information extracted from analyses of the monkey to the human brain.

Overview of Neuronal Vulnerability in Dementia

It is instructive to consider briefly the links between the distribution of pathologic changes in AD and related dementing conditions and the localization of specific elements of the cortical circuitry that are affected by these alterations. The current state of knowledge on the molecular components of the principal neuropathologic lesions observed in AD can be considered in the context of observations that relate the neurochemical phenotype of a given neuron to its relative vulnerability or resistance to the degenerative process. Selective neuronal vulnerability has been particularly well studied in AD but is a cardinal feature of all the major age-related neurodegenerative disorders.[2] The notion of differential vulnerability can be best understood in the context of an inclusive and integrative definition of neuronal typology that includes single cell morphology, regional and laminar location, connectivity, and neurochemical phenotype. This approach is useful

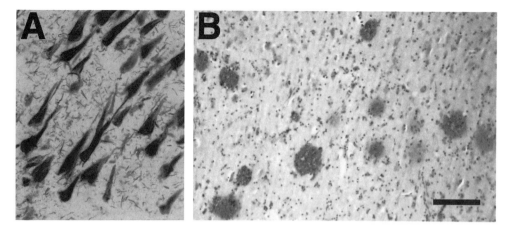

Figure 75.1. Examples of neurofibrillary tangles (NFT) (A) and senile plaques (SP) (B) from the hippocampus of a severe Alzheimer's disease (AD) case. Note the flameshape morphol-ogy of NFT and the more variable features of SP. In (B), several SP stained with an antiamyloid protein antibody are visible. *Bar* (on B) 100 μm (A); 200 μm (B).

to explore the cellular organization of the neocortex, as well as the cellular pathologic changes in diseases such as AD, as it considers the complex relationships among these morphologic and functional parameters.

In a very general sense, the most vulnerable group of cortical neurons includes large pyramidal cells, and more specifically those providing long corticocortical projections between association neocortical areas and hippocampal projections. These systems utilize the excitatory amino acid neurotransmitter glutamate and are driven by glutamatergic input. The occurrence of modifications in the expression during aging or dementia of some of the various subunit proteins that constitute the glutamate receptors, in particular those subunits regulating calcium permeability through the receptor channels, may determine susceptibility to calcium-mediated toxicity, which may play an important role in the degenerative processes leading to neuronal death in dementing illnesses. For example, neurons that express high cytoplasmic levels of certain calcium-binding proteins may have an increased calcium-buffering capacity and are likely to resist the toxic effects of abnormal intracellular calcium concentrations. Other neurons, in particular, pyramidal cells, are not equipped with such molecular mechanisms and demonstrate enhanced vulnerability to a variety of noxious stimuli that may lead to the formation of the neurofibrillary tangles (NFT), one of the cardinal pathologic changes of AD. It appears, therefore, that specific neurochemical and morphologic characteristics of certain pyramidal neurons may predispose them to degeneration, as well as NFT formation. Because only certain neuronal circuits are affected in AD, the relevance and impact of pathologic alterations in AD are best understood within the context of the organized systems that underlie neocortical function. For example, integrated processing in a given sensory modality such as vision involves the simultaneous activity of numerous distinct

cortical domains that have extensive, ordered interconnections establishing a distributed, hierarchical system and subserving the proper integration of the visual information. Similarly, cognition and language, not modality-specific functions, presumably rely on more complex networks. Such corticocortical circuits are provided by the particular neurons that degenerate in AD, leading in turn to a global neocortical disconnection syndrome that presents clinically as dementia.[2,3]

Lesion Types and Distribution in Alzheimer's Disease

Alzheimer's disease is a neurodegenerative disorder classically characterized by the presence of two major types of histopathologic lesions, neurofibrillary tangles (NFT) and senile plaques (SP), in the cerebral cortex (Fig. 75.1). The distribution and density of NFT and SP have been analyzed in great detail and constitute the basis of the neuropathologic diagnosis of AD.[4] NFT are characterized by the accumulation of abnormal components of the neuronal cytoskeleton that form paired helical filaments, whereas SP are composed of dystrophic neurites and glial elements with or without a central amyloid core.[3,5,6] These lesions are consistently observed throughout the brain but predominate in the cerebral cortex, where NFT are located in the soma of large pyramidal neurons, and SP are distributed throughout the cortical regions but are particularly numerous in association areas.[7] Tangles are also found in a number of subcortical structures connected with the cerebral cortex, such as the amygdala and the thalamus, as well as cholinergic and aminergic nuclei in the basal forebrain and brainstem. Variable densities of SP are also observed in other subcortical structures, such as the cerebellum and basal ganglia. Other pathologic alterations commonly seen in the brain of AD patients include neurophil threads, which also contain paired helical filaments and appear early in the course of the disease, granulovacuolar degenerations, diffuse amyloid deposits, and amyloid angiopathy.

Severe neuronal loss in the hippocampal formation and association regions of the neocortex, leaving primary sensory and motor areas relatively spared, is commonly observed in the brain of AD patients, involving the large cortical neurons, and correlated with the presence of NFT in neocortical association areas.[2] Also, synapse loss, together with increased synaptic size, is an early marker of the dementing process because a strong association between loss of neocortical synapses estimated by immunolabeling for the synaptic protein synaptophysin and cognitive impairment has been reported, which appears to be a better correlate of cognitive deficit than NFT densities.[8] Synaptic damage and synapse loss have also been reported in the neocortex of elderly nondemented individuals, suggesting an age-dependent mechanism for the loss or remodeling of synapses in the neocortex.[9]

At the regional level, NFT are more numerous in the temporal cortex, followed in descending order by the frontal cortex, the parietal cortex, and the occipital cortex (Fig. 75.2).[3,4,7] NFT are observed primarily within layers

FIGURE 75.2. Regional distribution of NFT and amyloid deposition in the cerebral cortex in normal aging compared to very mild AD and severe AD.[2–4,7,10–12] NFT appear first in the hippocampal formation and entorhinal cortex. Cases with incipient dementia show low numbers of NFT in the inferior temporal cortex and prefrontal cortex. During subsequent stages in the progression of AD, NFT are found throughout the cerebral cortex, although generally lower densities are present in primary sensory and motor cortices compared with association regions. Senile plaques are present principally in the hippocampal formation and temporal neocortex in normal aging, but it should be noted that the primary visual cortex may contain relatively high levels of amyloid deposition as well. In AD cases, amyloid is present throughout the neocortex. In terms of regional densities it is interesting to note that the hippocampal formation shows somewhat less amyloid deposition than the association neocortex. It should be kept in mind that these patterns are inferred from typical cases and provide a generic overview of the distribution of these lesions from a neuropathologic standpoint, but do not serve as a quantitative measure that can be used as a correlate of the severity of the dementing process, and do reflect the considerable case-to-case variability in numbers of lesions.

NORMAL AGING   **VERY MILD AD**   **SEVERE AD**

Neurofibrillary tangles

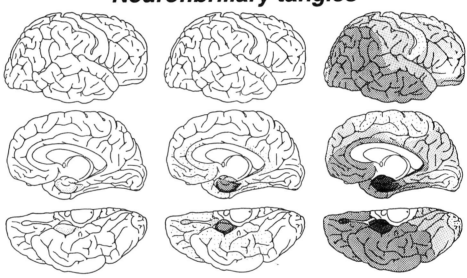

Amyloid deposition

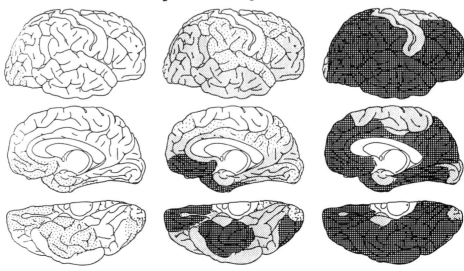

III and V in the neocortex, although their density varies considerably among cortical regions, primary sensory and motor regions having many fewer NFT than association areas.[7,10,11] Similar differences are found in other sensory systems. In addition, considerable differences in laminar NFT distribution exist among neocortical regions. With a few exceptions, SP show a generally comparable distribution among neocortical areas.[11,12] In the medial temporal lobe, layer II of the entorhinal cortex, the subiculum, and the CA1 field of the hippocampus represent particularly vulnerable cortical domains that consistently display very high NFT densities in AD (Fig. 75.2, 75.3).[2,7,13] The distribution of SP in the hippocampal formation is variable, with certain zones displaying high SP densities and amyloid deposition, such as layer III of the entorhinal cortex, the molecular layer of the dentate gyrus, and the superficial layer of the subiculum.[14]

There are strong correlations between the distribution of SP, NFT, and neuron loss among regions and layers of the cerebral cortex and the neurons of origin of certain long corticocortical and hippocampal projections.[10–13,15–17] The neurons of origin of corticocortical projections can be ascribed to three categories, feedforward, feedback, and lateral connections, based on their localization in the cortical layers and the distribution of their axonal terminals in the regions where they project (Fig. 75.4).[18,19] In this scheme, feedforward connections ascend within the hierarchy of a given modality (i.e., from a primary sensory area to an association area), feedback projections descend the same hierarchy, and lateral connections link cortical regions at the same hierarchical level. Feedforward connections originate mostly from neurons located in the superficial layers of the cortex and terminate in the deep portion of layer III and in layer IV of the target cortical region, feedback projection neurons are located principally in layers V and VI and project to layers I and VI, and lateral connections originate from layers V and VI and project to layers III to VI (Fig. 75.4). The distribution of NFT indicates that elements of feedforward, lateral, and feedback projections can all be affected by the degenerating process of AD. Considering that layer V contains generally higher NFT densities than layer III in association areas suggests that feedback as well as lateral projections may be at higher risk in AD than feedforward systems.

Interestingly, most of the projection neurons from the occipital and temporal association cortex to the frontal and from the occipital cortex to the temporal cortex are located in layer III. The regional and laminar distribution of SP suggests that they may be related to NFT formation (see Figs. 75.2, 75.4), in that their distribution appears to reflect the degeneration of the terminations of projections from neurons affected by NFT formation,[10] although multiple neuronal systems are involved in SP formation.[20] The distribution of NFT and SP in the hip-

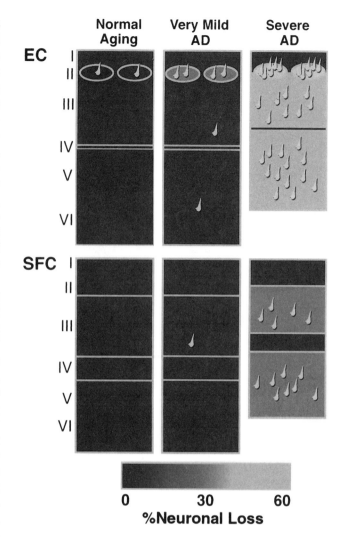

FIGURE 75.3. Regional and laminar NFT formation and neuronal loss in normal aging and AD. The flameshaped structures represent a semiquantitative assessment of NFT densities. An estimate of the percent of neuronal loss is shown by the gray scale (see % equivalent at *bottom*). In normal aging (CDR 0), a few NFT are consistently observed in layer II of the entorhinal cortex (*EC*) and the superior frontal cortex (*SFC*) remains devoid of NFT. There is no neuronal loss in normal aging. In contrast, very early AD (CDR 0.5) is characterized by higher NFT densities in the EC. Very rare NFT are observed in SFC. The neocortical areas show no neuronal loss, but a significant degree of neuronal loss is present in layer II of the EC. In definite AD (CDR 2), NFT are found in very high densities in layer II of the EC, but in moderately high densities in SFC. The degree of neuronal loss parallels NFT densities in these regions. The size of boxes reflects tissue shrinkage, due to neuronal loss, in AD.

pocampal formation also outlines specific projections. The perforant pathway that projects from layers II and III of the entorhinal cortex is affected severely and early during AD, and the presence of NFT in the neurons of origin of this pathway and its termination in the dentate gyrus are correlated with high densities of SP in the molecular layer of the dentate gyrus.[21] High densities of NFT in layer V of the entorhinal cortex are correlated with the degeneration of connections to the amygdala and association cortical areas part of the limbic lobe, and the projections from the hippocampus to the entorhinal cortex, amygdala, and neocortical areas, originating from the CA1 field and the subiculum, are consistently affected, as are amygdala nuclei projecting to the entorhinal cortex and hippocampus.[21]

Molecular Constituents of Neurofibrillary Tangles

The presence of intracellular fibrillar aggregates in certain cerebral regions is a common feature of several neurodegenerative disorders, as well as of aging. Neurofibrillary tangles have been extensively studied as a neuropathologic signature for AD. The molecular dissection has shown that the microtubule-associated proteins (MAP) tau are the main components of these aggregated structures in AD. Tau proteins are derived from a unique human tau gene located on chromosome 17q21–22 (see details in Fig. 75.5). Importantly, exons 2, 3, and 10 are

alternatively spliced, giving rise to six different isoforms in the adult human brain.[22] The expression of these isoforms is developmentally regulated, as only the shortest isoform is present in the fetal brain (called fetal isoform) and all the six tau variants are present in the adult brain. Moreover, the isoforms are differentially distributed among neuronal populations. Also, tau proteins undergo some posttranslational modifications, which is important in the context of pathologic conditions.[22]

Tau proteins belong to the family of the microtubule-associated proteins (MAP), together with MAP1, MAP2, MAP3, and MAP4 in the nervous system. These microtubule-associated proteins are involved in the formation of the cytoskeleton by enhancing the polymerization of tubulin monomers and stabilizing microtubule bundles (Fig. 75.6).[23] The amino-terminal part of tau proteins is referred to as the projection domain, as it forms extensions from the microtubule core. These extensions are able to make connections with cytoskeletal components, such as neurofilaments, and with cytoplasmic elements or the neural plasma membrane. The projection domain is also involved in signal transduction pathways. The carboxy-terminal part of the molecule binds to microtubules through a flexible array of distributed weak sites and is referred to as the microtubule-binding

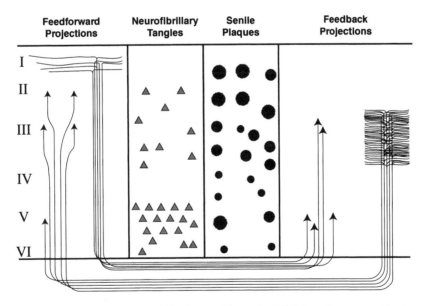

FIGURE 75.4. The laminar distribution of NFT and SP (*black triangles* and *black disks*, respectively, in the *center panels*) matches the distribution of corticocortically projecting neurons along neocortical hierarchies. Feedforward projection ascend the hierarchy, originating from a region involved in primary processing (such as the primary visual cortex), and terminating in an association cortex dealing with more complex types of information (such as a visual region located in the parietal lobe and integrating visual motion). The feedback projections are reciprocal to the feedforward projection and descend the same

hierarchy.[18,19,40] Not shown on this diagram are lateral connections that interconnect cortical regions located at the same functional level in the hierarchy. The NFT are found in the same cortical layers in which the neurons providing feedforward and feedback corticocortical projections are located, and they are slightly more numerous in the deep layers, suggesting a stronger correlation with feedback projections. Senile plaques are observed in higher densities in layer *IV* and the lower portion of layer *III*, which corresponds to the zone of termination of feedforward projection.

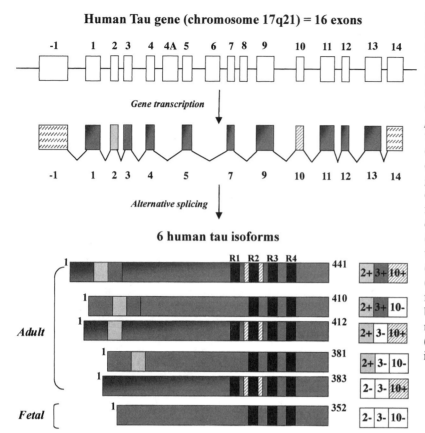

Human Tau gene (chromosome 17q21) = 16 exons

Gene transcription

Alternative splicing

6 human tau isoforms

FIGURE 75.5. Schematic representation of the human Tau gene and the six tau isoforms present in the human brain. The human tau gene is located on the long arm of chromosome 17 at position 17q21. It contains 16 exons, with exon 1 a part of the promoter (*upper panel*). Exons 4A, 6, and 8 are not transcribed in humans (*middle panel*). Exons 1 and 14 are transcribed but not translated. Exons 1, 4, 5, 7, 9, 11, 12, and 13 are essential constitutive elements of the gene, and exons 2, 3, and 10 undergo alternative splicing, giving rise to 6 different mRNAs, translated in 6 different tau isoforms (*lower panel*). These isoforms differ by the absence or presence of one or two 29-amino-acid inserts encoded by exon 2 (*light box*) and 3 (*dotted box*) in the aminoterminal part, in combination with either three (R1, R3, and R4) or four (R1–R4) repeat regions (*black boxes*) in the carboxy-terminal part. The fourth microtubule-binding domain is encoded by exon 10 (*hatched box; lower panel*). The number of amino acid varies between 441 (longest tau isoform) and 352 residues (fetal tau isoform).

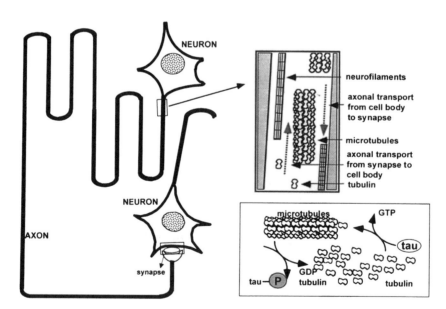

FIGURE 75.6. Neurofilaments and microtubules are the major components of the neuronal cytoskeleton. Microtubules constitute the network responsible for the axonal transport of soluble proteins and vesicles between the neuronal cell body and the synapses (anterograde transport), or between the synapses and the cell body (retrograde transport). In physiologic conditions, a dynamic equilibrium exists such that polymerization of tubulin monomers occurs at one end of the microtubules and depolymerization occurs at the opposite end. Finally, polymers of tubulin are stabilized by specific proteins called microtubule-associated proteins (MAPs). Tau proteins belong to this class. Nonphosphorylated tau proteins promote the polymerization of tubulin monomers into microtubules and also stabilize the bundles of newly formed microtubules. Conversely, phosphorylation of tau proteins abolishes their binding to microtubules and results in depolymerization and eventually NFT formation.

domain. It regulates the rate of microtubule polymerization, stabilizes the forming microtubules, and is also involved in interaction with functional proteins such as protein phosphatase 2A or presenilin 1.[22]

Tau proteins exhibit about 70 potential phosphorylation sites, and at least 30 of them have been described by using different biochemical or immunohistochemical techniques. At any given time, the phosphorylation state of the sites results from the regulated activity of kinases and phosphatases. The binding between tau proteins and microtubules and the subsequent microtubule stabilization depends partially on the phosphorylation state. Hyperphosphorylated tau proteins aggregates have been described in AD, as well as in several other neurodegenerative diseases, the so-called "tauopathies."[22] Extensive studies have shown that a specific distribution of the tau lesions, as well as different electrophoretic patterns of tau proteins, could discriminate among these disorders (Fig. 75.7). In AD, the filamentous tau inclusions are known as paired helical filaments (PHF), based on their ultrastructural appearance. These PHF exhibit specific biochemical properties that distinguish them from the normal tau proteins. PHF form insoluble polymers that are not found in normal samples obtained from biopsy materials. The electrophoretic profile of abnormally phosphorylated tau proteins shows a triplet of bands at 55, 64, and 69 kDa, and a minor band at 72 to 74 kDa. Dephosphorylation of PHF tau proteins before their electrophoretic migration

shows that this triplet results from the aggregation of the six tau isoforms.[22]

In addition to AD, NFT are observed in a variety of neurodegenerative disorders. Remarkably, these disorders can be identified on the basis of their biochemical profile of tau isoforms. Figure 75.7 summarizes the typical tau profiles in postencephalitic parkinsonism (PEP), Guamanian amyotrophic lateral sclerosis/parkinsonism–dementia complex (ALS/PDC), corticobasal degeneration (CBD), progressive supranuclear palsy (PSP), Pick's disease, and frontotemporal dementia with parkinsonism linked to chromosome 17 (FTDP-17). Neurofibrillary tangles are found in variable densities in the brain of patients who survived the influenza pandemic in the years 1916 to 1926 and who later developed PEP. The biochemical analyses have shown that the six isoforms of tau proteins are hyperphosphorylated, aggregate into NFT, and display an AD-like electrophoretic pattern (triplet tau55, tau64, and tau64).[24] Nevertheless, the distribution of these proteins, predominantly in association cortices and subcortical brain regions but also in primary motor cortex and basal ganglia, differs from that in AD, where the triplet of tau proteins is mostly restricted to the hippocampal formation and association neocortex. It should be mentioned that heterogeneity exists among cases. A similar electrophoretic profile of tau proteins has been described in cases with Guamanian ALS/PDC. The regional and laminar distribution of the tau triplet differs

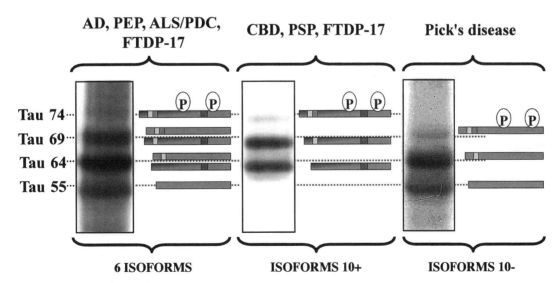

FIGURE 75.7. Schematic representation of the different electrophoretic profiles of pathological tau proteins using a phosphorylation-dependent monoclonal antibody (in *frames*), with their isoforms composition (*right* of each frame). The six tau isoforms are involved in the formation of the tau55, tau64, tau69 AD triplet with the minor tau74 variant. This pattern is also described in postencephalitic parkinsonism (*PEP*), Guamanian amyotrophic lateral sclerosis/parkinsonism–dementia complex (*ALS/PDC*), and some families with *FTDP-17* (*left panel*). The typical progressive supranuclear palsy/corticobasal degeneration (*PSP/CBD*) doublet tau64, 69 is related to the aggregation of hyperphosphorylated tau isoforms with exon 10. The FTDP-17 families with mutations in exon 10 or intron 10 exhibit the same profile (*middle panel*). Hyperphosphorylated tau proteins without exon 10 that aggregate in Pick's disease are detected as a tau55, 64 doublet (*right panel*).

from that in AD cases, as both cortical and subcortical areas are affected, and cortical layers II and III are preferentially involved.[25] In contrast to these two conditions, the electrophoretic pattern of tau proteins in CBD and PSP has been described as two major bands with an apparent molecular weight of 64 and 69 kDa (PSP/CBD tau doublet), although a minor 74-kDa band is also detected.[26–29]

The characteristic lesions described in the brains of patients affected by Pick's disease, the so-called Pick bodies, are also detected with antibodies against phosphorylated sites present within tau proteins. By Western blotting, these antibodies reveal two bands with an apparent molecular weight of 55 and 64 kDa (Pick tau doublet) and a minor band at 69 kDa.[30–32] The importance of tau proteins as the major component of fibrillar lesions has been emphasized by the emergence of a new class of neurologic syndromes called frontotemporal dementia with parkinsonism linked to chromosome 17 (FTDP-17).[33–35] This designation includes different disorders sharing some clinical and pathologic features and for which a genetic linkage with chromosome 17q21–22 has been demonstrated.[36] The neuropathologic features are frontal and temporal atrophy, severe neuronal loss, gliosis affecting both the gray and white matter, and superficial spongiosis. The presence of filamentous inclusions in neuronal cells, or in both neuronal and glial cells, has been described. The presence of these lesions is caused by mutations on the Tau gene that always segregate with the pathology, underlining the direct role of tau proteins in the pathogenic mechanism. At least 17 mutations on the Tau gene have been described in different families. Some mutations result in a tau profile similar to that observed in PSP and CBD (tau64, tau69), whereas others are resolved as a typical AD tau triplet. These disease-specific tau profiles highlight well the fact that various etiopathogenic mechanisms can lead to a comparable neurodegenerative process resulting in the formation of NFT, which can be understood as a general response to neuronal injury.

Neuronal Types Prone to Neurofibrillary Tangle Formation

The number of NFT does not account for the total population of pyramidal neurons, indicating that only certain subpopulations of pyramidal neurons are selectively susceptible to paired helical filament aggregation. The large neocortical pyramidal cells in layers III and V represent the most affected cell class, whereas smaller pyramidal neurons in layers II, VI, and the upper part of layer III are more resistant to NFT formation. Also, the spiny stellate cells and small pyramidal cells in layer IV are not

affected by this process as are the many morphologic types of inhibitory interneurons. The large pyramidal neurons in layers II, III, and V of the entorhinal cortex and those in CA1 field and subiculum are all severely affected. Considering the morphology and connectivity of the vulnerable neurons, it is interesting to note that all are efferent cells that send long projections to other cortical regions or to subcortical structures, and all are large pyramidal neurons.[16,17] However, other cellular characteristics are also linked to vulnerability to the degenerative process because certain large efferent neurons, such as the principal cells in the CA3 field and the large neurons of the dentate hilus, are generally relatively resistant to degeneration in AD, and in subcortical structures, NFT appear in several nuclei that project to the cerebral cortex, such as catecholaminergic cell groups in the brainstem and cholinergic neurons in the nucleus basalis of Meynert.

Certain pyramidal neurons in the human and monkey neocortex have been shown to be enriched in neurofilament protein.[16,17,37] Neurofilament protein immunoreactivity in the primate neocortex is restricted to the perikaryon and dendrites of a subpopulation of large pyramidal neurons. Interestingly, neurofilament proteins, as well as other cytoskeletal proteins, have been implicated in NFT formation,[2,38] and pyramidal cells expressing high levels of nonphosphorylated neurofilament protein appear to be highly susceptible to NFT formation. The distribution of neurofilament protein-containing neurons corresponds to the distribution of corticocortically projecting cells, as demonstrated by studies in the macaque monkey.[39] The correlation between origins of long corticocortical projections and neurofilament protein-containing neurons is particularly visible in the primary visual cortex of monkeys and humans, where layer IVB cells and the Meynert cells are the only large, strongly immunoreactive neurons. These neurons form well-established connections to the parietal lobe and susberve visuomotor functions known to be affected during aging and AD.[40] These observations on visual projections therefore demonstrate the existence of a neurochemically defined neuronal subpopulation that is vulnerable in AD and can be correlated with a functionally characterized projection system.

We have also reported in the macaque monkey that many long association corticocortical projections originate from neurofilament protein-containing neurons, and, in some of them, 90% to 100% of the neurons of origin of the projection contain neurofilament protein,[39] which is particularly the case of projections from the temporal to the prefrontal and parietal neocortex that are known to be involved in networks subserving many aspects of the cognitive functions.[41] In fact, the laminar distribution of neurofilament protein-containing neurons in visual association, prefrontal, and anterior cingulate in

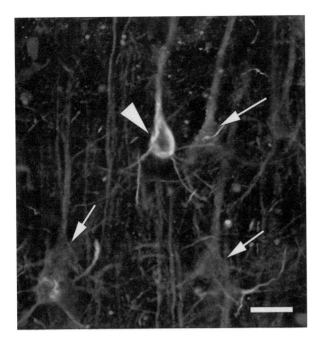

FIGURE 75.8. Involvement of neurofilament protein-immunoreactive pyramidal neurons in layer III of the area 9 in an AD case. In this sample labeled for neurofilament protein and tau protein, a few normal neurons are labeled (*arrows*) and an intracellular NFT is seen developing within a neurofilament protein-immunoreactive neuron (*arrowhead*). *Bar* 30 μm.

human cerebral cortex is very similar to the distribution of NFT in that the layers that have high NFT density in an AD brain no longer contain a high density of neurofilament protein-immunoreactive neurons.[16,17] A comparable situation exists in the hippocampal formation where layers II, III, and V of entorhinal cortex and the pyramidal neurons of the subiculum have a very high density of neurofilament protein-immunoreactive neurons in the normally aging human brain and present with a dramatic loss of these neurons in AD.[2]

These observations demonstrate that neurofilament protein-containing neurons are highly vulnerable in AD, and quantitative analyses have demonstrated a severe loss of neurofilament protein-containing neurons in layers III and V in the inferior temporal and superior frontal cortex (Fig. 75.8). The severity of the loss correlates with the size of these neurons in that the neurofilament protein-containing neurons larger than $6000\,\mu m^3$ of perikaryal volume are the most affected, with up to 60% cell loss, whereas the smaller-size neurons (2000–$6000\,\mu m^3$ of perikaryal volume) are not affected.[16] In addition to regional distribution and relationship to connectivity, NFT identified by antibodies to neurofilament and tau proteins have revealed dynamic cellular alterations in vulnerable neuronal populations during normal aging. Layer II of the entorhinal cortex contains neurofilament protein-immunoreactive neurons and also displays immunoreactivity to tau protein, suggesting the existence of transitional forms of NFT during aging.[2] In AD cases, most NFT in the entorhinal cortex progress to an end stage and are no longer immunoreactive to neurofilament protein, and transitional forms of NFT are observed in the frontal cortex, indicating that a time-dependent process takes place in the formation of NFT in certain neurofilament protein-containing neurons (Fig. 75.9).[2,6,20]

Interestingly, certain neurons, such as the pyramidal neurons of the CA1 field, do not normally express detectable levels of neurofilament protein in young adults but do form NFT in AD. Such neurons show increasing levels of neurofilament protein immunoreactivity during aging before accumulation of tau protein, suggesting that high levels of neurofilament protein are a necessary substrate for the formation of NFT.[42] Thus, one of the neurochemical characteristics of the vulnerable neurons in AD is the presence of high somatic and dendritic concentrations of nonphosphorylated neurofilament proteins, even though this may be only one aspect of the phenotype associated with selective neuronal vulnerability. In addition, when the monkey data are considered together with the distribution of neurofilament protein-containing neurons and NFT in humans, it is likely that the human homologues of the neurofilament protein-containing, corticocortically projecting neurons of the macaque monkey are those that are highly vulnerable in AD.

These neuronal networks use glutamate as their neurotransmitter. Disruption of glutamate metabolism and glutamate receptor-mediated excitotoxicity represents one of the major mechanisms of neuron death in many neurodegenerative disorders. Glutamate receptor-mediated excitotoxicity presumably results from increased calcium flux leading to toxic intracellular concentrations of this ion, and this mechanism is likely associated with all types of ionotropic glutamate receptors that are involved in facilitating or regulating calcium fluxes. Although the *N*-methyl-D-aspartate (NMDA) receptor has been the receptor subtype primarily associated with calcium flux into the neuron, it is now clear that both kainate and α-amino-3-hydroxy-5-methyl-4-isoxazole-propionic acid (AMPA) receptors also modulate calcium influx.[43] Thus, the glutamate receptor profile of cortical neurons and related circuits has emerged as an important parameter when correlating identified neurons and circuits with susceptibility for vulnerability to degeneration through excitotoxicity, because the defining characteristics of a given glutamatergic projection with respect to ion fluxes depends on the subunit composition of the receptors that dominate that system.

Abnormal functioning of glutamatergic receptors and resulting increases in intracellular calcium concentration are also linked to a variety of pathologic molecular events, such as production of free radicals, increased

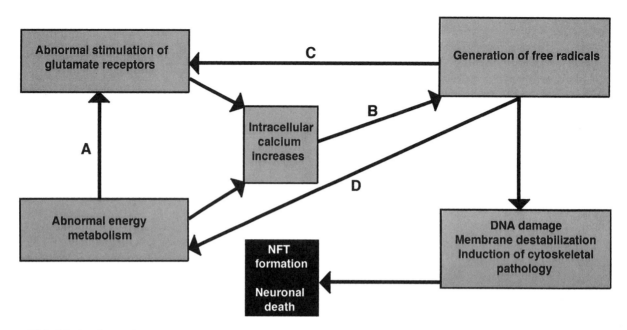

FIGURE 75.9. Mechanisms through which an imbalance in excitatory neurotransmission can induce a molecular cascade resulting in neuronal damage and death. Impaired energy metabolism can result in abnormally elevated stimulation of ionotropic glutamate receptors through depolarization of membranes (A) as well as increasing intracellular calcium. Elevated calcium can trigger the generation of free radicals by activating a number of calcium-dependent enzymatic reactions (B). Free radicals are extremely reactive products that will induce direct damage to cellular structure and result in neuronal death. Free radicals also affect glutamate receptors by further increasing the release of excitatory amino acids (C) as well as energy metabolism by inducing mitochondrial dysfunction (D). It is likely that all these pathways participate in the formation of NFT in the AD brain.

release of excitatory amino acids, destabilization of lipid membranes, and damage to the cytoskeleton, that are all involved in the final processes leading to NFT formation and cell death (see Fig. 75.9). Autoradiographic, immunocytochemical, or in situ hybridization studies have demonstrated severe alterations in the distribution and density of several glutamate receptor subunits in the cerebral cortex in normal aging and AD.[44] In addition, changes in the expression of specific glutamate receptor subunits leading to functional decline without neuronal degeneration are known to occur during normal aging.[45,46] For instance, in aged monkeys, compared to juvenile and young adult monkeys, the NMDA receptor levels decrease specifically and consistently in the outer molecular layer of the dentate gyrus in the hippocampal formation, where the perforant path terminates, but there are no significant differences in expression of AMPA or kainate glutamate receptor subunits and no morphologic reflection of degeneration of the perforant path.[45,46] These data also suggest that the intradendritic parcellation of a particular neurotransmitter receptor is modifiable in an age-related and circuit-specific manner and that such changes may be an underlying condition for age-related memory impairment.[2,45]

It should be noted that several classes of GABAergic interneurons containing the calcium-binding proteins parvalbumin, calbindin, and calretinin, as well as a variety of neuropeptides, are largely resistant to the degenerative process, even in severe cases displaying very high densities of NFT and SP.[3] The cellular distribution of calcium-binding proteins is largely coextensive with that of GABA in cortical interneurons, and these proteins subdivide the GABAergic neurons into nonoverlapping morphologic subtypes that together account for the vast majority of the GABAergic cells.[47] Moreover, parvalbumin-immunoreactive neurons have been shown to be resistant to degeneration in the cerebral cortex of Huntington's disease, Pick's disease, Guamanian ALS/PDC, PEP, PSP, CBD, and frontal lobe dementia, but not in Down syndrome and Creutzfeldt–Jakob disease. Calbindin- and calretinin-containing cells are also resistant in most of these disorders, except in frontal lobe dementia, where calbindin-immunoreactive neurons are vulnerable.[3] The combination of factors such as high cytoplasmic levels of calcium-binding proteins, certain neuropeptides, and GABA with the morphologic features of locally projecting interneurons may confer some resistance to these neurons in many neurodegenerative illnesses and contrasts sharply with the morphologic phenotype of the vulnerable cells.

Molecular Biology of Amyloid and Its Role in Alzheimer's Disease

In addition to the intraneuronal accumulation of PHF, AD is characterized histopathologically by the presence of extracellular deposits of an amyloid peptide (Aβ) in plaques.[48] Plaques are spherical structures 15 to 20μm in diameter, consisting of a peripheral rim of abnormal neuronal processes and glial cells surrounding a core of deposited materials. Brain Aβ has both soluble and insoluble species, with aggregation states from monomer to higher molecular weight oligomers. Soluble brain Aβ is predominantly a random coil and α-helical folded peptide. Insoluble Aβ is β-sheeted and forms either fibrillar or amorphous deposits. These Aβ fibrillar aggregates are thought to act as a nidus for subsequent deposits of other proteins, including α-antichymotrypsin, components of the complement cascade, and apolipoproteins E and J (apoE, apoJ).[49] Aβ production and release are normal physiologic events. Aβ peptides are normally present in the media of amyloid protein precursor-(APP-) expressing cultured cells and in human and rodent cerebrospinal fluid.[50–53] Recently, there have been reports showing evidence there could be two distinct pools of intracellularly generated Aβ: a pool that is eventually secreted and a pool that is destined to remain within the cell.[54,55] The relative importance of intracellular versus extracellular Aβ has not been determined at this point. Level of Aβ, as determined by ELISA, correlates exceptionally well with AD progression.[56]

Aβ is proteolytically derived from a larger integral membrane protein, the amyloid precursor protein (APP). APP is an integral membrane glycoprotein containing the Aβ region, which includes 28 amino acids of the ectodomain and 11 to 14 amino acids of the adjacent transmembrane domain.[48,57] The APP gene is localized on chromosome 21 at 21q21.2.[58,59] APP can be processed by at least three secretases, namely α-, β-, and γ-secretase (Fig. 75.10). In the nonamyloidogenic pathway, α-secretase cleaves the amyloid precursor protein within the Aβ domain, releasing an extracellular portion. The cleavage within the Aβ domain prevents deposition of the intact amyloidogenic peptide. α-Secretase generates a soluble N-terminal fragment of APP known as sAPPα, and its C-terminal counterpart of about 10 to 11kDa remains embedded in the membrane. The 10- to 11-kDa C-terminal product may undergo an additional cleavage by a protease γ-secretase activity. The protease termed "β-secretase" initiates Aβ generation by creating an

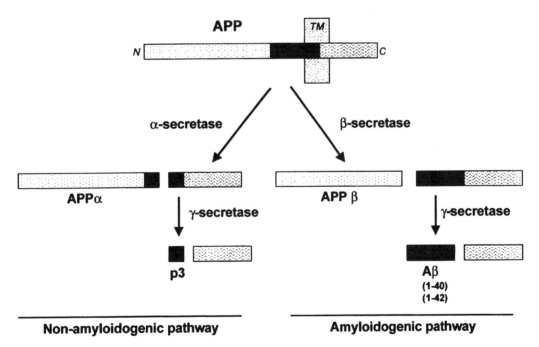

FIGURE 75.10. The amyloid protein precursor (APP) is a single transmembrane domain protein that exists as eight different isoforms transcribed by an alternative splicing mechanisms from a single gene located on chromosome 21. The normal function of APP is still unknown. The differential proteolytic cleavage of APP by α-, β-, or γ-secretase leads to the formation of different proteolytic products, which are involved in two different pathways called the nonamyloidogenic and the amyloidogenic pathway. α-Secretase cleaves APP within the Aβ domain (black box), and the consecutive cleavage by γ-secretase gives rise to the nonamyloidogenic p3 fragment. Conversely, β-secretase cleaves APP before the Aβ domain, and the consecutive cleavage by γ-secretase generates the amyloidogenic Aβ peptides that will aggregate into senile plaques.

approximately 12-kDa C-terminal fragment.[60] This 12-kDa fragment may then undergo "γ-secretase" cleavage within the hydrophobic transmembrane domain to release the 40-, 42-, or 43-residue Aβ peptides.[52] The varying C-terminal of Aβ may be a feature of crucial importance because Aβ peptides display distinct physical properties and, in particular, exhibit aggregation behavior that can vary according to their length.[61] It has been shown recently in fibroblasts with a disrupted TACE (tumor necrosis factor α-converting enzyme) gene that two classes of α-secretase exist, one involved in the basal secretion and the other involved in regulated secretion.[62–64] TACE, a member of the ADAM family (a disintegrin and metalloprotease family) of proteases, has been demonstrated to play a central role in regulated α-secretase cleavage of APP. Four groups have now identified a candidate for β-secretase (BACE), also known as Asp-2.[65–68] Interestingly, presenilin 1 (PS1) appears to facilitate a proteolytic activity that cleaves the integral membrane domain of APP by γ-secretase.[69] It is possible that presenilins are γ-secretase or that they facilitate γ-secretase activity through some other mechanism.

Genes may be related to disease in two ways: through autosomal dominant mutations, by themselves sufficient to cause the disease (i.e., deterministic mutations), or, alternatively, through gene variations (polymorphisms) that may increase disease risk without being sufficient by themselves to cause the disorder. This latter group is referred to as susceptibility genes. Although it is currently thought that most cases of AD occur sporadically, autosomal dominant transmission has been identified in families with early-onset AD, defined as beginning before the age of 65 years. These cases are relatively rare; worldwide, only several hundred families are currently known that carry deterministic mutations.[70] Extensive research carried out during the past two decades has isolated a number of genes that when mutated cause AD, that is, APP on chromosome 21,[71,72] the presenilin 1 (PS1) gene on chromosome 14, and the presenilin 2 (PS2) gene on chromosome 1.[73] Mutations in these genes lead to early-onset AD and only explain a small proportion (5%–10%) of total AD cases. Furthermore, trisomy 21 (Down syndrome) increases the risk of AD, perhaps due to the tripled genetic dosage of APP. In addition, a number of susceptibility genes are also currently being studied, with polymorphisms of the apolipoprotein E gene receiving the most attention. The presence of the apolipoprotein E4 (apoE4-) allele has been identified as a genetic risk factor for sporadic and familial AD with late onset.

Several different pathogenic mutations have been found in exons 16 and 17 of the APP gene to date. These mutations are missense mutations. The early-onset AD mutations are located outside the Aβ amyloid sequence, close to the C-terminal γ-secretase cleavage site,[71] within the transmembrane domain, or at the N-terminal β-

secretase cleavage site within the extracellular part of APP.[74] One mutation is located inside the Aβ amyloid sequence next to the α-secretase cleavage site.[75,76] The localization of mutations led to the hypothesis that they might influence the activity of the respective secretases, resulting in the aberrant processing of APP.[77] Indeed, mutations at codons 716 and 717 lead to a selective increase in the production of Aβ peptides ending at residue 42/43.[78–82] The mutations at codons 670 to 671, on the other hand, appear to augment the production of both Aβ40 and Aβ42(43),[83] whereas the mutation at codon 692 has a more complicated effect on APP processing, causing impaired α-secretase cleavage, increased heterogeneity of secreted Aβ species, and increased hydrophobicity of the Aβ.[80] This mutation also has clinical features in some cases similar to those of cerebral hemorrhage with amyloidosis of the Dutch type and in other cases more similar to AD.

The homologous membrane proteins presenilin 1 (PS1) and presenilin 2 (PS2) were identified in 1995 as the genes responsible for a substantial fraction of early-onset, autosomal dominant AD.[73,84] Mutations in the PS1 gene on chromosome 14 are the most common cause for autosomal dominant familial AD (FAD)[73]; these account for 30% to 50% of all early-onset cases[85] and are the primary cause of AD with onset before the age of 55 years. To date, more than 50 PS1 mutations and 2 PS2 mutations have been reported in FAD. All mutations in the PS are missense mutations, except for the mutation of a splice acceptor site resulting in the deletion of exon 9. Pathogenic mutations in PS modify APP processing, thereby leading to an augmentation of Aβ42(43) secretion. AD patients carrying PS1 or PS2 mutations have significant increase of plasma Aβ42(43) level together with deposition of Aβ42 in the brain.[86–88] In fibroblasts from such patients, the APP metabolism is shifted toward an increase of Aβ42(43) production. Similarly, the presence of mutated PS1 increases Aβ42(43) in transfected cells and in transgenic mice.[89–92] How the mutant PS influences the production of Aβ42(43) peptides remains uncertain. In neurons of PS1-knockout mice, secretion of Aβ is drastically reduced, leading to the accumulation of α- and β-cleaved C-terminus stubs of APP.[69,93] This finding gives evidence that PS1 is obligatory for proteolysis of APP at the γ-secretase cleavage site.

In addition to the deterministic genetic mutations found in APP are the presenilins, genetic factors that modify the risk of getting AD. ApoE alleles on chromosome 19 are considered important risk factors for the development of late-onset AD. ApoE is a 34-kDa component of various lipoproteins, including chylomicrons, very low density lipoproteins (VLDL), and a subset of high-density lipoproteins (HDL).[94] These lipoproteins regulate plasma–lipid transport and clearance by acting as ligand for lipoprotein receptors such as LDLR and low density receptor-related protein (LRP).[95,96] ApoE is polymorphic and is encoded by three alleles (ApoE2, -3, and -4) that differ in two amino acid positions. In general, it seems that E4 allele increases the risk for developing AD by about threefold, and that the E2 allele decreases the risk.[97] The presence of one or two E4 alleles is associated with earlier onset of disease and an enhanced amyloid burden in brain but has little effect on the rate of progression of dementia.[98] Thus, the homozygous E4/E4 subjects have an earlier onset (mean age, >70 years) than heterozygous E4 subjects (mean age of onset for E2/E3, over 90 years).[99]

The most obvious hypothesis is that ApoE E4/E2 polymorphisms might influence the production, distribution, or clearance of Aβ. This hypothesis is supported by observations that first, the subjects with one or more ApoE4 alleles have a higher burden than do subjects with no E4 alleles.[100] Second, there is evidence that both ApoE and Aβ may be cleared through the lipoprotein-related (LRP) receptor and that ApoE4 and Aβ peptide may compete for clearance through the LRP receptor.[95] Third, transgenic mice that overexpress APP develop a significantly lower number of Aβ deposits when bred to an ApoE knockout background.[101] These findings strongly support a role of ApoE in the aggregation or clearance of Aβ in the brain. It should be noted that the ApoE genotype influences the onset of AD in patients with Down syndrome and in those with APP mutations but not in families with presenilin mutations.[101]

In summary, biochemical studies in postmortem tissue support a role for Aβ in AD. In addition, all available genetic evidence support a role for this peptide in AD. For these reasons, therapies targeting Aβ represent important therapeutic avenues for AD.

Conclusions

Clearly, other degenerative processes play an important role in AD, and they may also contribute to the clinical characteristics of the disease. Some cortical networks may be more sensitive to the effects of additional deleterious factors known to be involved in AD, such as inflammation free radicals, and potential amyloid toxicity, which may act in a synergistic manner with their morphologic and molecular phenotype to render them particularly vulnerable.[102] However, the generalized loss of long corticocortical projections emerges functionally as the most devastating component of AD and that most directly related to dementia. Thus, the degeneration of presumed corticocortical circuits within the neocortex appears therefore to be the necessary factor for the clinical expression of the dementia in AD.[2,3]

It should be kept in mind, however, that in sharp contrast to AD patients, many elderly individuals maintain near-normal levels of cognitive performance while sustaining significant compromise of hippocampal circuits and may rely more on neocortical than on hippocampal circuits for memories essential for daily activities.[103] Healthy elders may present with difficulties in learning and retrieving new information, and their major limitation may be the amount of new information they can learn within a given period of time in comparison to younger individuals. Unlike patients with early AD, healthy elders are able to retain the new information after some delay, whereas patients with mild cognitive impairment retain little of it.[103] This impairment in information retention that characterizes the very early stages of AD is correlated to neuronal loss in the entorhinal cortex and to volumetric changes in the temporal lobe. Similarly, the volume of the temporal horn of the lateral ventricle increases in these patients, which may correlate with the selective loss of projections from the entorhinal cortex.[2,3,103–105] In fact, normal brain aging may be defined as intact cognitive abilities in the presence of scarce neurofibrillary pathology in the entorhinal cortex, which may represent a stable age-related asymptomatic AD-like neurofibrillary pathology. This idea points to the differential involvement of hipocampal and neocortical circuits between aging and dementia and indicates that whereas normal brain aging presents as a minimal pathology of discrete medial temporal regions, AD is a disease of the neocortical circuits (see Figs. 75.2, 75.3, 75.4).

This interpretation of the pathologic features of AD suggests that the debilitating effects of dementia result from changes restricted to the association neocortex. Considerable hippocampal alterations may occur in absence of neocortical involvement and with only minor disruptions in activities of daily living of the individual that are not sufficient for a diagnosis of dementia. The cells that provide the most vulnerable projections appear to be highly specialized neurons that share identifiable morphologic and neurochemical features. As the elements of the biochemical and anatomic phenotype that are linked to differential cellular vulnerability in AD are increasingly recognized, functional correlations are likely to emerge between cellular changes, neurochemical characteristics of vulnerability, and affected cortical pathways. It is hoped that this understanding will make it possible to design therapeutic strategies to protect or rescue the neurons at risk in AD. The protection of these neurons appears to be an attractive avenue for intervention in the management of AD and may be more practical than the development of a cure.

References

1. Moss M, Albert M. Alzheimer's disease and other dementing disorders. In: Albert M, Moss M, eds. *Geriatric Neuropsychology*. New York: Guilford Press; 1988:145–177.

2. Morrison JH, Hof PR. Life and death of neurons in the aging brain. *Science.* 1997;278:412–419.

3. Hof PR, Bouras C, Morrison JH. Cortical neuropathology in aging and dementing disorders: neuronal typology, connectivity, and selective vulnerability. In: Peters A, Morrison JH, eds. *Neurodegenerative and Age-Related Changes in Cerebral Cortex, Cerebral Cortex, vol 14.* New York: Kluwer–Plenum; 1999:175–312.

4. Mirra SS, Hart MN, Terry RD. Making the diagnosis of Alzheimer's disease—a primer for practicing neuropathologists. *Arch Pathol Lab Med.* 1993;117:132–144.

5. Brion JP. Molecular pathology of Alzheimer amyloid and neurofibrillary tangles. *Semin Neurosci.* 1990;2:89–100.

6. Vickers JC, Dickson TC, Adlard PA, et al. The cause of neuronal degeneration in Alzheimer's disease. *Prog Neurobiol.* 2000;60:139–165.

7. Arnold SE, Hyman BT, Flory J, et al. The topographical and neuroanatomical distribution of neurofibrillary tangles and neuritic plaques in the cerebral cortex of patients with Alzheimer's disease. *Cereb Cortex.* 1991;1:103–116.

8. Terry RD, Masliah E, Salmon DP, et al. Physical basis of cognitive alterations in Alzheimer's disease: synapse loss is the major correlate of cognitive impairment. *Ann Neurol.* 1991;30:572–580.

9. Masliah E, Mallory M, Hansen L, et al. Quantitative synaptic alterations in the human neocortex during normal aging. *Neurology.* 1993;43:192–197.

10. Pearson RCA, Esiri MM, Hiorns RW, et al. Anatomical correlates of the distribution of the pathological changes in the neocortex in Alzheimer disease. *Proc Natl Acad Sci USA.* 1985;82:4531–4534.

11. Lewis DA, Campbell MJ, Terry RD, et al. Laminar and regional distribution of neurofibrillary tangles and neuritic plaques in Alzheimer's disease: a quantitative study of visual and auditory cortices. *J Neurosci.* 1987;7:1799–1808.

12. Rogers J, Morrison JH. Quantitative morphology and regional and laminar distributions of senile plaques in Alzheimer's disease. *J Neurosci.* 1985;5:2801–2808.

13. Hyman BT, Van Hoesen GW, Kromer LJ, et al. Perforant pathway changes and the memory impairment of Alzheimer's disease. *Ann Neurol.* 1986;20:472–481.

14. Thal DR, Rüb U, Schultz C, et al. Sequence of Aβ-protein deposition in the human medial temporal lobe. *J Neuropathol Exp Neurol.* 2000;59:733–748.

15. Duyckaerts C, Hauw JJ, Bastenaire F, et al. Laminar distribution of neocortical senile plaques in senile dementia of the Alzheimer type. *Acta Neuropathol.* 1986;70:249–256.

16. Hof PR, Cox K, Morrison JH. Quantitative analysis of a vulnerable subset of pyramidal neurons in Alzheimer's disease. I. Superior frontal and inferior temporal cortex. *J Comp Neurol.* 1990;301:45–54.

17. Hof PR, Morrison JH. Quantitative analysis of a vulnerable subset of pyramidal neurons in Alzheimer's disease. II. Primary and secondary visual cortex. *J Comp Neurol.* 1990;301:55–64.

18. Felleman DJ, Van Essen DC. Distributed hierarchical processing in the primate cerebral cortex. *Cereb Cortex.* 1991; 1:1–47.

19. Barbas H. Pattern in the laminar origin of corticocortical connections. *J Comp Neurol.* 1986;252:415–422.

20. Vickers JC. A cellular mechanism for the neuronal changes underlying Alzheimer's disease. *Neuroscience.* 1997;78: 629–639.

21. Hyman BT, Van Hoesen GW, Damasio AR. Memory-related neural systems in Alzheimer's disease: an anatomic study. *Neurology.* 1990;40:1721–1730.

22. Buée L, Bussière T, Buée-Scherrer V, et al. Tau protein isoforms, phosphorylation and role in neurodegenerative disorders. *Brain Res Rev.* 2000;33:95–130.

23. Weingarten MD, Lockwood AH, Hwo SY, et al. A protein factor essential for microtubule assembly. *Proc Natl Acad Sci USA.* 1975;72:1858–1862.

24. Buée-Scherrer V, Buée L, Leveugle B, et al. Pathological tau proteins in postencephalitic parkinsonism: comparison with Alzheimer's disease and other neurodegenerative disorders. *Ann Neurol.* 1997;42:356–359.

25. Buée-Scherrer V, Buée L, Hof PR, et al. Neurofibrillary degeneration in amyotrophic lateral sclerosis/parkinsonism–dementia complex of Guam. Immunochemical characterization of tau proteins. *Am J Pathol.* 1995;146:924–932.

26. Flament S, Delacourte A, Verny M, et al. Abnormal Tau proteins in progressive supranuclear palsy. Similarities and differences with the neurofibrillary degeneration of the Alzheimer type. *Acta Neuropathol.* 1991;81:591–596.

27. Ksiezak-Reding H, Morgan K, Mattiace LA, et al. Ultrastructure and biochemical composition of paired helical filaments in corticobasal degeneration. *Am J Pathol.* 1994; 145:1496–1508.

28. Sergeant N, Wattez A, Delacourte A. Neurofibrillary degeneration in progressive supranuclear palsy and corticobasal degeneration: tau pathologies with exclusively "exon 10" isoforms. *J Neurochem.* 1999;72:1243–1249.

29. Schmidt ML, Huang R, Martin JA, et al. Neurofibrillary tangles in progressive supranuclear palsy contain the same tau epitopes identified in Alzheimer's disease PHF-tau. *J Neuropathol Exp Neurol.* 1996;55:534–539.

30. Delacourte A, Robitaille Y, Sergeant N, et al. Specific pathological Tau protein variants characterize Pick's disease. *J Neuropathol Exp Neurol.* 1996;55:159–168.

31. Probst A, Tolnay M, Langui D, et al. Pick's disease: hyperphosphorylated tau protein segregates to the somatoaxonal compartment. *Acta Neuropathol.* 1996;92:588–596.

32. Sergeant N, David JP, Lefranc D, et al. Different distribution of phosphorylated tau protein isoforms in Alzheimer's and Pick's diseases. *FEBS Lett.* 1997;412:578–582.

33. Foster NL, Wilhelmsen K, Sima AA, et al. Frontotemporal dementia and parkinsonism linked to chromosome 17: a consensus conference. *Ann Neurol.* 1997;41:706–715.

34. Lynch T, Sano M, Marder KS, et al. Clinical characteristics of a family with chromosome 17-linked disinhibition-dementia-parkinsonism-amyotrophy complex. *Neurology.* 1994;44:1878–1884.

35. Wilhelmsen KC, Lynch T, Pavlou E, et al. Localization of disinhibition-dementia-parkinsonism-amyotrophy complex to 17q21-22. *Am J Hum Genet.* 1994;55:1159–1165.

36. Spillantini MG, Bird TD, Ghetti B. Frontotemporal dementia and parkinsonism linked to chromosome 17: a new group of tauopathies. *Brain Pathol.* 1998;8:387–402.

37. Hof PR, Morrison JH. Neurofilament protein defines regional patterns of cortical organization in the macaque monkey visual system: a quantitative immunohistochemical analysis. *J Comp Neurol.* 1995;352:161–186.

38. Trojanowski JQ, Schmidt ML, Shin RW, et al. Altered tau and neurofilament proteins in neurodegenerative diseases: diagnostic implications for Alzheimer's disease and Lewy body dementias. *Brain Pathol.* 1993;3:45–54.

39. Hof PR, Nimchinsky EA, Morrison JH. Neurochemical phenotype of corticocortical connections in the macaque monkey: quantitative analysis of a subset of neurofilament protein-immunoreactive projection neurons in frontal, parietal, temporal, and cingulate cortices. *J Comp Neurol.* 1995;362:109–133.

40. Hof PR, Vogt BA, Bouras C, et al. Atypical form of Alzheimer's disease with prominent posterior cortical atrophy: a review of lesion distribution and circuit disconnection in cortical visual pathways. *Vision Res.* 1997;37:3609–3625.

41. Goldman-Rakic PS. Topography of cognition: parallel distributed networks in primate association cortex. *Annu Rev Neurosci.* 1988;11:137–156.

42. Vickers JC, Riederer BM, Marugg RA, et al. Alterations in neurofilament protein immunoreactivity in human hippocampal neurons related to normal aging and Alzheimer's disease. *Neuroscience.* 1994;62:1–13.

43. Gasic GP, Heinemann S. Determinants of the calcium permeation of ligand-gated cation channels. *Curr Opin Cell Biol.* 1992;4:670–677.

44. Mishizen A, Ikonomovic M, Armstrong DM. Glutamate receptors in aging and Alzheimer's disease. In: Hof PR, Mobbs CV, eds. *Functional Neurobiology of Aging.* San Diego: Academic Press; 2001:283–314.

45. Gazzaley AH, Siegel SJ, Kordower JH, et al. Circuit-specific alterations of N-methyl-D-aspartate subunit 1 in the dentate gyrus of aged monkeys. *Proc Natl Acad Sci USA.* 1996;93:3121–3125.

46. Gazzaley AH, Thakker MM, Hof PR, et al. Preserved number of entorhinal cortex layer II neurons in aged macaque monkeys. *Neurobiol Aging.* 1997;18:549–553.

47. De Felipe J. Types of neurons, synaptic connections and chemical characteristics of cells immunoreactive for calbindin-D28k, parvalbumin and calretinin in the neocortex. *J Chem Neuroanat.* 1997;14:1–19.

48. Glenner GG, Wong CW. Alzheimer's disease: initial report of the purification and characterization of a novel cerebrovascular amyloid protein. *Biochem Biophys Res Commun.* 1984;120:885–890.

49. Snow AD, Mar H, Nochlin D, et al. The presence of heparan sulfate proteoglycans in the neuritic plaques and congophilic angiopathy in Alzheimer's disease. *Am J Pathol.* 1988;133:456–463.

50. Busciglio J, Gabuzda DH, Matsudaira P, et al. Generation of β-amyloid in the secretory pathway in neuronal and nonneuronal cells. *Proc Natl Acad Sci USA.* 1993;90:2092–2096.

51. Haass C, Schlossmacher MG, Hung AY, et al. Amyloid beta-peptide is produced by cultured cells during normal metabolism. *Nature.* 1992;359:322–325.

52. Seubert P, Vigo-Pelfrey C, Esch F, et al. Isolation and quantification of soluble Alzheimer's beta-peptide from biological fluids. *Nature.* 1992;359:325–357.

53. Shoji M, Golde TE, Ghiso J, et al. Production of the Alzheimer amyloid beta protein by normal proteolytic processing. *Science.* 1992;258:126–129.

54. Cook DG, Forman MS, Sung JC, et al. Alzheimer's Aβ(1–42) is generated in the endoplasmic reticulum/intermediate compartment of NT2N cells. *Nat Med.* 1994;3:1021–1023.

55. Skovronsky DM, Doms RW, Lee VMY. Detection of a novel intraneuronal pool of insoluble amyloid beta protein that accumulates with time in culture. *J Cell Biol.* 1998;141:1031–1039.

56. Naslund J, Haroutunian V, Mohs R, et al. Correlation between elevated levels of amyloid beta-peptide in the brain and cognitive decline. *JAMA.* 2000;283:1571–1517.

57. Masters CL, Simms G, Weinman NA, et al. Amyloid plaque core protein in Alzheimer disease and Down syndrome. *Proc Natl Acad Sci USA.* 1985;82:4245–4249.

58. Kang J, Lemaire HG, Unterbeck A, et al. The precursor of Alzheimer's disease amyloid A4 protein resembles a cell-surface receptor. *Nature.* 1987;325:733–736.

59. Tanzi RE, Gusella JF, Watkins PC, et al. Amyloid beta protein gene: cDNA, mRNA distribution, and genetic linkage near the Alzheimer locus. *Science.* 1987;235:880–884.

60. Citron M, Teplow DB, Selkoe DJ. Generation of amyloid beta protein from its precursor is sequence specific. *Neuron.* 1995;14:661–670.

61. Burdick D, Soreghan B, Kwon M, et al. Assembly and aggregation properties of synthetic Alzheimer's A4/beta amyloid peptide analogs. *J Biol Chem.* 1992;267:546–554.

62. Buxbaum JD, Liu KN, Luo Y, et al. Evidence that tumor necrosis factor alpha converting enzyme is involved in regulated alpha-secretase cleavage of the Alzheimer amyloid protein precursor. *J Biol Chem.* 1998;273:27765–27767.

63. Parvathy S, Hussain I, Karran EH, et al. Cleavage of Alzheimer's amyloid precursor protein by alpha-secretase occurs at the surface of neuronal cells. *Biochemistry* 1999;38:9728–9734.

64. Lammich S, Kojro E, Postina R, et al. Constitutive and regulated alpha-secretase cleavage of Alzheimer's amyloid precursor protein by a disintegrin metalloprotease. *Proc Natl Acad Sci USA.* 1999;96:3922–3927.

65. Hussain I, Powell D, Howlett DR, et al. Identification of a novel aspartic protease (Asp 2) as β-secretase. *Mol Cell Neurosci.* 1999;14:419–427.

66. Sinha S, Anderson JP, Barbour R, et al. Purification and cloning of amyloid precursor protein beta-secretase from human brain. *Nature.* 1999;402:537–540.

67. Vassar R, Bennett BD, Babu-Khan S, et al. β-Secretase cleavage of Alzheimer's amyloid precursor protein by the

transmembrane aspartic protease BACE. *Science.* 1999;
286:735–741.

68. Yan R, Bienkowski MJ, Shuck ME, et al. Membrane-anchored aspartyl protease with Alzheimer's disease beta-secretase activity. *Nature.* 1999;402:533–537.

69. De Strooper B, Saftig P, Craessaerts K, et al. Deficiency of presenilin-1 inhibits the normal cleavage of amyloid precursor protein. *Nature.* 1998;391:387–390.

70. St. George-Hyslop S. Role of genetics in test of genotype, status, and disease progression in early-onset Alzheimer's disease. *Neurobiol Aging.* 1998;19:133–137.

71. Goate A, Chartier-Harlin MC, Mullan M, et al. Segregation of a missense mutation in the amyloid precursor protein gene with familial Alzheimer's disease. *Nature.* 1991;349:704–706.

72. Tanzi RE, St George-Hyslop PH, Haines JL, et al. The genetic defect in familial Alzheimer's disease is not tightly linked to the amyloid beta-protein gene. *Nature.* 1987;329: 156–157.

73. Sherrington R, Rogaev EI, Liang Y, et al. Cloning of a gene bearing missense mutations in early-onset familial Alzheimer's disease. *Nature.* 1995;375:754–760.

74. Mullan M, Crawford F, Axelman K, et al. A pathogenic mutation for probable Alzheimer's disease in the APP gene at the N-terminus of beta-amyloid. *Nature Genet.* 1992;1: 345–347.

75. Levy E, Carman MD, Fernandez-Madrid IJ, et al. Mutation of the Alzheimer's disease amyloid gene in hereditary cerebral hemorrhage, Dutch type. *Science.* 1990;248:1124–1126.

76. Van Broeckhoven C, Haan J, Bakker E, et al. Amyloid beta protein precursor gene and hereditary cerebral hemorrhage with amyloidosis (Dutch). *Science.* 1990;248:1120–1122.

77. Hardy J. The Alzheimer family of diseases: many etiologies, one pathogenesis? *Proc Natl Acad Sci USA.* 1997;94: 2095–2097.

78. Cai XD, Golde TE, Younkin SG. Release of excess amyloid beta protein from a mutant amyloid beta protein precursor. *Science.* 1993;259:514–516.

79. Citron M, Oltersdorf T, Haass C, et al. Mutation of the beta-amyloid precursor protein in familial Alzheimer's disease increases beta-protein production. *Nature.* 1992; 360:672–674.

80. Eckman CB, Mehta ND, Crook R, et al. A new pathogenic mutation in the APP gene (I716V) increases the relative proportion of Aβ42(43). *Hum Mol Genet.* 1997;6:2087–2089.

81. Haass C, Hung AY, Selkoe DJ, et al. Mutations associated with a locus for familial Alzheimer's disease result in alternative processing of amyloid beta-protein precursor. *J Biol Chem.* 1994;269:17741–17748.

82. Suzuki N, Cheung TT, Cai XD, et al. An increased percentage of long amyloid beta protein secreted by familial amyloid beta protein precursor (βAPP717) mutants. *Science.* 1994;264:1336–1340.

83. Citron M, Vigo-Pelfrey C, Teplow DB, et al. Excessive production of amyloid beta-protein by peripheral cells of symptomatic and presymptomatic patients carrying the Swedish familial Alzheimer disease mutation. *Proc Natl Acad Sci USA.* 1994;91:11993–11997.

84. Levy-Lahad E, Wijsman EM, Nemens E, et al. A familial Alzheimer's disease locus on chromosome 1. *Science.* 1995; 269:970–973.

85. Cruts M, Hendriks L, Van Broeckhoven C. The presenilin genes: a new gene family involved in Alzheimer disease pathology. *Hum Mol Genet.* 1996;5:1449–1455.

86. Scheuner D, Eckman C, Jensen M, et al. Secreted amyloid beta-protein similar to that in the senile plaques of Alzheimer's disease is increased in vivo by the presenilin 1 and 2 and APP mutations linked to familial Alzheimer's disease. *Nat Med.* 1996;2:864–870.

87. Iwatsubo T. Aβ42, presenilins, and Alzheimer's disease. *Neurobiol Aging.* 1998;19:S11–S13.

88. Lemere CA, Lopera F, Kosik KS, et al. The E280A presenilin 1 Alzheimer mutation produces increased Aβ42 deposition and severe cerebellar pathology. *Nat Med.* 1996;2: 1146–1150.

89. Borchelt DR, Thinakaran G, Eckman CB, et al. Familial Alzheimer's disease-linked presenilin 1 variants elevate Aβ1-42/1-40 ratio *in vitro* and *in vivo*. *Neuron.* 1996;17: 1005–1013.

90. Citron M, Eckman CB, Diehl TS, et al. Additive effects of PS1 and APP mutations on secretion of the 42-residue amyloid beta-protein. *Neurobiol Dis.* 1998;5:107–116.

91. Duff K, Eckman C, Zehr C, et al. Increased amyloid-beta42(43) in brains of mice expressing mutant presenilin 1. *Nature.*1996;383:710–713.

92. Tomita T, Maruyama K, Saido TC, et al. The presenilin 2 mutation (N141I) linked to familial Alzheimer disease (Volga German families) increases the secretion of amyloid beta protein ending at the 42nd (or 43rd) residue. *Proc Natl Acad Sci USA.* 1997;94:2025–2030.

93. Naruse S, Thinakaran G, Luo JJ, et al. Effects of PS1 deficiency on membrane protein trafficking in neurons. *Neuron.* 1998;21:1213–1221.

94. Mahley RW. Apolipoprotein E: cholesterol transport protein with expanding role in cell biology. *Science.* 1988; 240:622–630.

95. Kounnas MZ, Moir RD, Rebeck GW, et al. LDL receptor-related protein, a multifunctional ApoE receptor, binds secreted beta-amyloid precursor protein and mediates its degradation. *Cell.* 1995;82:331–340.

96. Krieger M, Herz J. Structures and functions of multiligand lipoprotein receptors: macrophage scavenger receptors and LDL receptor-related protein (LRP). *Annu Rev Biochem.* 1994;63:601–637.

97. Corder EH, Saunders AM, Strittmatter WJ, et al. Gene dose of apolipoprotein E type 4 allele and the risk of Alzheimer's disease in late onset families. *Science.* 1993; 261:921–923.

98. Gómez-Isla T, West HL, Rebeck GW, et al. Clinical and pathological correlates of apolipoprotein E epsilon 4 in Alzheimer's disease. *Ann Neurol.* 1996;39:62–70.

99. Corder EH, Saunders AM, Risch NJ, et al. Protective effect of apolipoprotein E type 2 allele for late onset Alzheimer disease. *Nat Genet.* 1994;7:180–184.

100. Schmechel DE, Saunders AM, Strittmatter WJ, et al. Increased amyloid beta-peptide deposition in cerebral

cortex as a consequence of apolipoprotein E genotype in late-onset Alzheimer disease. *Proc Natl Acad Sci USA.* 1993;90:9649–9653.

101. Bales KR, Verina T, Cummins DJ, et al. Apolipoprotein E is essential for amyloid deposition in the APP(V717F) transgenic mouse model of Alzheimer's disease. *Proc Natl Acad Sci USA.* 1999;96:15233–15238.

102. Mattson MP. Inflammation, free radicals, glycation, metabolism and apoptosis, and heavy metals. In: Hof PR, Mobbs CV, eds. *Functional Neurobiology of Aging.* San Diego: Academic Press; 2001:349–384.

103. Albert MS. Cognitive and neurobiologic markers of early Alzheimer's disease. *Proc Natl Acad Sci USA.* 1996; 93:13547–13551.

104. Gómez-Isla T, Price JL, McKeel DW Jr, et al. Profound loss of layer II entorhinal cortex neurons occurs in very mild Alzheimer's disease. *J Neurosci.* 1996;16:4491–4500.

105. Bussière T, Hof PR. Morphological changes in human cerebral cortex during normal aging. In: Hof PR, Mobbs CV, eds. *Functional Neurobiology of Aging.* San Diego: Academic Press; 2001:77–84.

76
Delirium

Sharon K. Inouye

Delirium, defined as an acute alteration in attention and cognition, is a common, serious, and potentially preventable source of morbidity and mortality for older persons. Delirium is a clinical diagnosis, based on observation of the patient at the bedside. Although the exact diagnostic criteria continue to evolve, the criteria for delirium appearing in the Diagnostic and Statistical Manual Version IV (DSM-IV) of the American Psychiatric Association are widely used as the current diagnostic standard[1] (Table 76.1). However, these criteria were based on expert opinion, and their diagnostic performance has not been tested. The Confusion Assessment Method (CAM)[2] provides a validated tool, which is currently in widespread use for rapid identification of delirium (see Table 76.1). The CAM algorithm, which is based on the presence of the features of acute onset and fluctuating course, inattention, and either disorganized speech or altered level of consciousness, has a sensitivity of 94% to 100%, specificity of 90% to 95%, positive predictive accuracy of 91% to 94%, and negative predictive accuracy of 90% to 100% for delirium.[2]

Although it can occur in any setting, delirium is most common in settings where the frailty and illness acuity of patients are most severe. The incidence of delirium increases with age, cognitive impairment, frailty, illness severity, comorbidity, and other risk factors for delirium (see following). The emergency room and acute hospital have the highest overall rates of delirium. Acute alteration in mental status represents a leading presenting symptom for acutely ill older persons, accounting for at least 30% of emergency evaluations of older persons. In the hospital setting, the intensive care and postoperative settings have the highest rates of delirium.[3] Although not well studied, delirium occurs with some frequency in nursing home and rehabilitation settings. Although less frequent in the community setting, delirium is an important presenting symptom to community physicians, and can serve as a barometer for underlying health status of elderly persons, often heralding serious underlying disease.

Epidemiology and Risk Factors

Because of its frequency in this setting, most of the epidemiologic studies of delirium have involved hospitalized older patients. Previous studies have measured the prevalence of delirium, that is, cases present at the time of hospital admission, as 14% to 24%, and the incidence of delirium, that is, new cases arising during hospitalization, as 6% to 56%.[4–16] The rates of postoperative delirium range from 10% to 52%.[4–16] Hospital mortality rates in patients with delirium range from 25% to 33%, as high as mortality rates associated with acute myocardial infarction or sepsis.[4,5,10,11,17–24] Delirium has not been well examined in nursing home or community settings. In terms of the costs of delirium, it has been estimated that each year delirium complicates hospital stays for more than 2.3 million older persons, involving more than 17.5 million inpatient days and accounting for more than $4 billion (1994 dollars) of Medicare expenditures related to hospitalization.[25] Moreover, delirium is associated with substantial additional costs after hospital discharge because of the increased need for institutionalization, rehabilitation services, home health care, rehospitalization, and other health care services.

Delirium is usually a multifactorial syndrome,[14] as are many other common geriatric syndromes, such as falls, incontinence, and pressure sores. In some cases, delirium may be caused by a single factor, but more often delirium is the result of the interrelationship between patient vulnerability at the time of admission (i.e., predisposing factors) and the occurrence of noxious insults during hospitalization (i.e., precipitating factors). For example, patients who are highly vulnerable to delirium at baseline (e.g., such as cognitively impaired or severely ill patients), can be pushed into delirium by the presence of only a mild insult, such as a single dose of a sedative medication for sleep. By contrast, patients who are not vulnerable would be relatively resistant, with delirium resulting only after repeated exposure to multiple

TABLE 76.1. Diagnostic criteria for delirium.

Diagnostic and Statistical Manual Version IV (DSM-IV) diagnostic criteria
    A. Disturbance of consciousness (i.e., reduced clarity of awareness of the environment) with reduced ability to focus, sustain, or shift attention.
    B. A change in cognition (such as memory deficit, disorientation, language disturbance) or the development of a perceptual disturbance that is not better accounted for by a preexisting, established, or evolving dementia.
    C. The disturbance develops over a short period of time (usually hours to days) and tends to fluctuate during the course of the day.
    D. There is evidence from the history, physical examination, or laboratory findings that the disturbance is caused by the direct physiologic consequences of a general medical condition.

The Confusion Assessment Method (CAM) Diagnostic Algorithm[a]
    Feature 1. Acute onset and fluctuating course
        This feature is usually obtained from a family member or nurse and is shown by positive responses to the following questions: Is there evidence of an acute change in mental status from the patient's baseline? Did the (abnormal) behavior fluctuate during the day, that is, tend to come and go, or increase and decrease in severity?
    Feature 2. Inattention
        This feature is shown by a positive response to the following question: Did the patient have difficulty focusing attention, for example, being easily distractible, or having difficulty keeping track of what was being said?
    Feature 3. Disorganized thinking
        This feature is shown by a positive response to the following question: Was the patient's thinking disorganized or incoherent, such as rambling or irrelevant conversation, unclear or illogical flow of ideas, or unpredictable switching from subject to subject?
    Feature 4. Altered level of consciousness
        This feature is shown by any answer other than "alert" to the following question: Overall, how would you rate this patient's level of consciousness? (alert [normal], vigilant [hyperalert], lethargic [drowsy, easily aroused], stupor [difficult to arouse], or coma [unarousable]).

[a] The diagnosis of delirium by CAM requires the presence of features 1 and 2 and either 3 or 4.
Source: Adapted with permission from Inouye SK. Delirium and other mental status problems in the older patients. In: Goldman L, Bennett JC. *Cecil Textbook of Medicine, 4th Ed*. Philadelphia: Saunders; 1999:19–22.

noxious insults, such as general anesthesia, major surgery, multiple psychoactive medications, immobilization, and infection. Moreover, the effects of multiple risk factors appear to be cumulative. Clinically, the importance of this multifactorial etiology is that removing or treating one factor alone often is insufficient to resolve the delirium. Attention should be paid to the multifactorial predisposing and precipitating factors that may be contributing to the delirium.

Predisposing or vulnerability factors for delirium include preexisting cognitive impairment or dementia, severe illness, high number of comorbid diseases, functional impairment, advanced age, chronic renal insufficiency, dehydration, malnutrition, depression, and vision or hearing impairment.[8,13,24,26–30] Dementia is a leading risk factor for delirium, consistently identified across studies. Patients with dementia have a two- to five-fold increased risk for delirium. Moreover, one-third to one-half of delirious patients have an underlying dementia. Nearly any chronic medical illness can predispose to delirium, including diseases involving the central nervous system (e.g., Parkinson's disease, cerebrovascular disease, mass lesions, trauma, infection), as well as diseases outside the central nervous system, such as infectious, metabolic, cardiac, pulmonary, endocrine, and neoplastic conditions. The occult presentation of systemic disease—sometimes presenting only with delirium—is an important tenet of geriatric medicine. One validated predictive model,[15] developed to determine delirium risk at the time

of hospital admission, identified the following independent predisposing factors: severe underlying illness, vision impairment, baseline cognitive impairment, and high BUN/creatinine ratio (used as an index of dehydration).

Medications, the most common precipitating factors for delirium, contribute to at least 40% of delirium cases.[14,31,32] Many medications can lead to delirium; the most common are those with recognized psychoactive effects, such as sedative-hypnotics, narcotics, H_2-blockers, and medications with anticholinergic effects. In previous studies, use of any psychoactive medication was associated with a 4-fold increased risk of delirium.[8,14] Sedative-hypnotic drugs have been associated with a 3- to 12-fold increased risk of delirium; narcotics with a 3-fold risk; and anticholinergic drugs with a 5- to 12-fold risk.[24,28–30,33,34] Delirium increases in direct proportion to the number of medications prescribed, an effect that is likely caused by adverse effects of the medications themselves, as well as the increased risk of drug–drug and drug–disease interactions. Recent studies provide strong evidence that inappropriate use and overuse of psychoactive medications are common in older patients, and that many cases of delirium and other related adverse drug events may be preventable.[35–38]

Other precipitating factors for delirium include medical procedures or surgery, intercurrent medical illnesses, infections, immobilization, use of indwelling bladder catheters, use of physical restraints, dehydration, malnutrition, iatrogenic events, electrolyte or metabolic derangement, alcohol or drug intoxication or withdrawal, environmental influences, and psychosocial stress.[10,19,22,26,39–44] Immobilization can lead to delirium and functional decline within just a few days, yet physicians routinely order bedrest or no activity in 57% of patient-days of hospitalization, often without medical justification.[45,46] Moreover, medical devices (e.g., indwelling bladder catheters and physical restraints) can contribute to immobilization, as well as other adverse effects. Iatrogenic events, occurring in 29% to 38%[47–49] of older patients, include complications of diagnostic or therapeutic procedures, transfusion reactions, bleeding due to overanticoagulation, and the like. Insufficiency of any major organ system can precipitate delirium, particularly renal, hepatic, or respiratory failure. Occult respiratory failure is an increasing problem in older patients, who often lack the typical signs and symptoms of dyspnea and tachypnea, and who are easily overlooked by measuring oxygen saturation alone. Acute myocardial infarction or congestive heart failure commonly present as delirium in an elderly patient, without the expected symptoms of chest pain or dyspnea. Occult infection represents another noteworthy cause of delirium, because older patients frequently fail to mount the expected febrile or leukocyte response to severe systemic infections, including pneumonia, urinary tract infection, endocarditis, abdominal abscess, or septic arthritis. Metabolic disorders are important contributors to delirium: these include hyper- or hyponatremia, hypercalcemia, acid–base disorder, hypo- and hyperglycemia, and thyroid or adrenal disorders. A validated predictive model[14] for delirium risk based on exposure to precipitating factors during the course of hospitalization identified the following five independent precipitating factors: physical restraint use, malnutrition, more than three medications added during the previous day (70% of these were psychoactive medications), indwelling bladder catheter, and any iatrogenic event.

Pathogenesis

To date, the fundamental pathophysiologic mechanisms of delirium remain unclear. Delirium has been thought to represent a functional rather than structural lesion, with characteristic electroencephalographic findings demonstrating global functional derangements and generalized slowing of cortical background (alpha) activity.[50,51] Delirium is considered to be the final common pathway of many different pathogenic mechanisms, culminating in the widespread reduction of cerebral oxidative metabolism with failure of cholinergic transmission. Proposed mediators have included adenosine, beta-endorphin, histamine, somatostatin, lymphokines, tryptophan, phenylalanine metabolites, various neuropeptides,

and cortisol.[52–55] A recent study[56] has found that changes in large neutral amino acids, which are precursors of several neurotransmitters, may play a role in delirium. Although delirium has been considered a transient syndrome, several of these basic mechanisms may not be completely reversible, particularly those resulting in hypoxic brain injury. In addition, the dose and duration of the insult, as well as the presence of preexisting cognitive impairment, may greatly influence the reversibility of the delirium.

Clinical Presentation

The key features of delirium are acute onset and inattentiveness. Determining the acuity of onset requires accurate knowledge of the patient's previous level of cognitive functioning. With delirium, the mental status typically changes over hours to days, as distinguished from dementia in which the changes occur more insidiously over weeks to months. Extra effort may be required to ascertain baseline information from a reliable source, such as a family member, caregiver, or nurse. Another key feature is the fluctuating course of delirium, with symptoms tending to come and go or increasing and decreasing in severity over a 24-h period. Lucid intervals are characteristic, and can be misleading even to experienced clinicians. Inattention is recognized as difficulty focusing, maintaining, and shifting attention. Delirious patients appear easily distracted, have difficulty following commands or maintaining a conversation, and often perseverate with an answer to a previous question. On cognitive testing, patients may manifest difficulty with simple repetition tasks, digit spans, or reciting months backward. Other key features include a disorganization of thought and altered level of consciousness. Disorganization of thought is a manifestation of underlying cognitive or perceptual disturbances, and is recognized by disorganized or incoherent speech, rambling or irrelevant conversation, unclear or illogical flow of ideas, or unpredictable switching from subject to subject. Altered level of consciousness is typically manifested by lethargy, with reduced awareness of the environment. Although not cardinal elements, features frequently associated with delirium include disorientation, cognitive deficits (e.g., memory impairment, dysnomia), psychomotor agitation or retardation, perceptual disturbances (e.g., hallucinations, misperceptions, illusions), paranoid delusions, emotional lability, and sleep–wake cycle disruption.

Clinically, delirium can present in either hypoactive or hyperactive forms. The hypoactive form of delirium, which is characterized by lethargy and reduced psychomotor activity, is the most common form in older patients. This form of delirium is often unrecognized and is associated with a poorer overall prognosis.[57–59] The hyperactive form of delirium, in which the patient is agitated, vigilant, and often hallucinating, is rarely missed. Importantly, patients can fluctuate between the hypoactive and hyperactive forms—the mixed type of delirium. Moreover, partial or incomplete forms of delirium have been recognized to be common,[60,61] particularly during the resolution stages of delirium, and have been shown to adversely influence long-term prognosis.

Diagnosis and Differential Diagnosis

Delirium is a clinical diagnosis, relying on astute observation at the bedside, careful cognitive assessment, and history taking from a reliable informant to establish the patient's baseline functioning. Previous studies have documented that clinicians may fail to detect delirium in up to 70% of affected patients.[62–64] Identifying the potentially multifactorial contributors to the delirium is of critical importance, because many of these factors are treatable and, if left unaddressed, may result in substantial morbidity and mortality. Because the potential contributors are innumerable, the search requires keen clinical judgment combined with a thorough medical evaluation. The challenge is enhanced by the frequently nonspecific or atypical presentation of the underlying illness in older persons. In fact, in the elderly population, delirium may be the *only* sign of life-threatening illness such as sepsis, pneumonia, or myocardial infarction.

The first step in evaluation should include formal cognitive assessment and determination of any acute change from the patient's baseline level of cognition. Because cognitive impairment is readily missed during regular conversation, a brief cognitive screening test, such as the Mini-Mental Status Examination,[65] is recommended. Attention should be assessed with simple tests, such as a forward digit span (inattention indicated by inability to repeat five digits forward) or reciting the days of the week or the months backward. A comprehensive history and physical examination remain the cornerstones of the evaluation of delirium. The history should be directed toward establishing the patient's baseline level of cognitive functioning and the course of any mental status changes, as well as obtaining clues about potential precipitating factors or insults, such as recent medication changes, new infections, or medical illnesses. The physical examination should include a detailed neurologic examination for focal deficits and a careful search for signs of falls or head trauma, infection, or other acute medical processes.

Because of the frequent contribution of medications to delirium, review of the medication list, including over-the-counter medications, should be carried out in every patient. The majority of older patients will be on at least several medications during hospitalization, heightening the potential for adverse events as well as drug–drug or drug–disease interactions. In older patients, medications may cause adverse effects even at recommended dosages and at measured serum levels that are within the "therapeutic range." Thus, medications with psychoactive effects should be removed or minimized whenever possible. When these medications cannot be removed, dosage reductions or substitution of less toxic alternatives should be considered. The side effects and interaction profiles of all current drugs should be reviewed. Finally, chronic medication and alcohol use should be assessed specifically to evaluate for any potential withdrawal risk. In older patients, substance use is commonly unrecognized or overlooked, particularly during the early phase of hospitalization.

Evidence-based strategies estimating the predictive value of laboratory tests in delirium assessment are lacking. Thus, the laboratory evaluation must be based on clinical judgment, and should be tailored to the individual situation. An astute history and physical examination, review of medications, targeted laboratory testing (e.g., complete blood count, chemistries, glucose, renal/liver function tests, urinalysis, oxygen saturation), and search for occult infection should assist with identification of the majority of potential contributors to the delirium. The need for further laboratory testing (such as thyroid function tests, B_{12} level, cortisol level, drug levels or toxicology screen, ammonia level) will be determined according to the individual patient's clinical picture. In patients with cardiac or respiratory diseases, or with related symptoms, an electrocardiogram, chest radiograph, and/or arterial blood gas determination may be warranted. The indications for cerebrospinal fluid examination, brain imaging, or electroencephalography remain controversial. Overall, the diagnostic yield for these procedures are low, and they are probably indicated in less than 10% of delirium cases. Cerebrospinal fluid examination is indicated for the febrile delirious patient where meningitis or encephalitis must be excluded. Brain imaging (such as computed tomography or magnetic resonance imaging) should be reserved for cases with new focal neurologic signs, with history or signs of head trauma, or without another identifiable cause of the delirium. Electroencephalography, which has a false-negative rate of 17% and false-positive rate of 22% for distinguishing delirious and nondelirious patients,[51,66] plays a limited role and is most useful to detect occult seizure disorders and to differentiate delirium from nonorganic psychiatric conditions.

The differential diagnoses for delirium include a variety of conditions associated with confusion and altered mental status, most commonly dementia, depression, and nonorganic psychotic disorders. The paramount challenge in differential diagnosis is distinguishing dementia, a chronic confusional state, from delirium alone or delirium superimposed on dementia. The differential diagnosis is crucial, however, because of the prognostic significance of delirium, which often represents a medical emergency. Obtaining the clinical history is critical to making the distinction between delirium and dementia. These two conditions are distinguished by the acuity of symptom onset in delirium (dementia is much more insidious), and the impaired attention and altered level of consciousness associated with delirium. Disorientation and memory impairment, while commonly recognized features, are not useful in differential diagnosis because they may be present with both conditions and may be absent in delirium. Differentiating depression and nonorganic psychotic disorders from delirium can pose other challenges for the clinician. Although paranoia, hallucinations, and affective changes can occur with delirium, the presence of key delirium features of acute onset, inattention, altered level of consciousness, and global cognitive impairment will assist with the diagnosis of delirium. In cases involving an uncooperative patient or where an accurate history is unavailable, establishing the diagnosis with certainty may not be possible. In these cases, because of the potentially life-threatening nature of delirium and its high occurrence rate in the older hospitalized population, the recommendation is to manage the case as a presumptive delirium and search for reversible causes (e.g., intercurrent illness, metabolic derangements, drug toxicity), until further information can be obtained.

Figure 76.1 presents an algorithm for the evaluation of altered mental status in the older patient. The first step in the evaluation is to establish the patient's baseline cognitive functioning and the time-course of any cognitive changes. Chronic impairments, developing or progressing over months to years, are most likely attributable to a dementia, which should be evaluated accordingly (see Chapter 74). Acute alterations occurring over hours to weeks, which may be superimposed on an underlying dementia, should be further evaluated with cognitive assessment to determine whether delirium is present. If delirium features are not present (see Clinical Presentation section above), then further evaluation for major depression, acute psychotic disorder, or other psychiatric disorders (see Chapters 78 and 79) is indicated.

Clinical Course and Prognosis

Delirium has been previously considered to be a transient, reversible condition; however, recent studies[60,61] have documented that delirium may be more persistent than previously believed. A delirium duration of 30 days or more is typical in older patients, and a prolonged transitional phase characterized by cognitive, affective, or behavioral abnormalities is quite common. In fact, as few as 20% of patients had complete resolution of all delirium symptoms at 6-month follow-up in one study.[60] Delirium appears to have greater deleterious effects on long-term cognitive functioning in patients with underlying cognitive impairment or dementia. Long-term detrimental effects are likely related to the duration, severity, and underlying cause(s) of the delirium. Whether delirium itself leads to permanent cognitive impairment or dementia remains controversial; however, previous studies document that at least some patients never recover their baseline level of cognitive functioning.

Delirium had been documented to be an important prognostic determinant.[67] Previous studies[8,10,18,21,28,29,34,60,68–79] have shown that delirium is an independent predictor of prolonged length of hospital stay, increased morbidity and mortality, and higher rates of institutionalization and functional and cognitive decline, even after controlling for age, gender, dementia, illness severity, and baseline functional status.

Prevention and Management

Prevention of Delirium

Primary prevention of delirium, that is, preventing delirium before it occurs, is the most effective strategy to reduce delirium and its attendant complications. Table 76.2 indicates well-documented delirium risk factors and tested preventive interventions for each risk factor. These risk factors were selected because current evidence supports both the clinical relevance and the remediable nature of each risk factor with practical interventions. A controlled clinical trial[80] demonstrated the effectiveness of a delirium prevention strategy targeted toward these risk factors. Implementation of these preventive interventions resulted in a 40% risk reduction for delirium in hospitalized older patients.

Nonpharmacologic Management

Nonpharmacologic approaches should be used for management of every delirious patient. These approaches include strategies for reorientation and behavioral intervention, such as ensuring the presence of family members, orienting influences, use of sitters, and transferring a disruptive patient to a private room or closer to the nurse's station for increased supervision. Personal contact and communication are critical, incorporating reorientation strategies, simple instructions, and frequent eye contact. Patients should be encouraged to participate in decision making about their care as much as possible. Eyeglasses and hearing aids (if needed) should be worn as much as possible to reduce sensory deficits. Mobility, self-care, and independence should be enhanced;

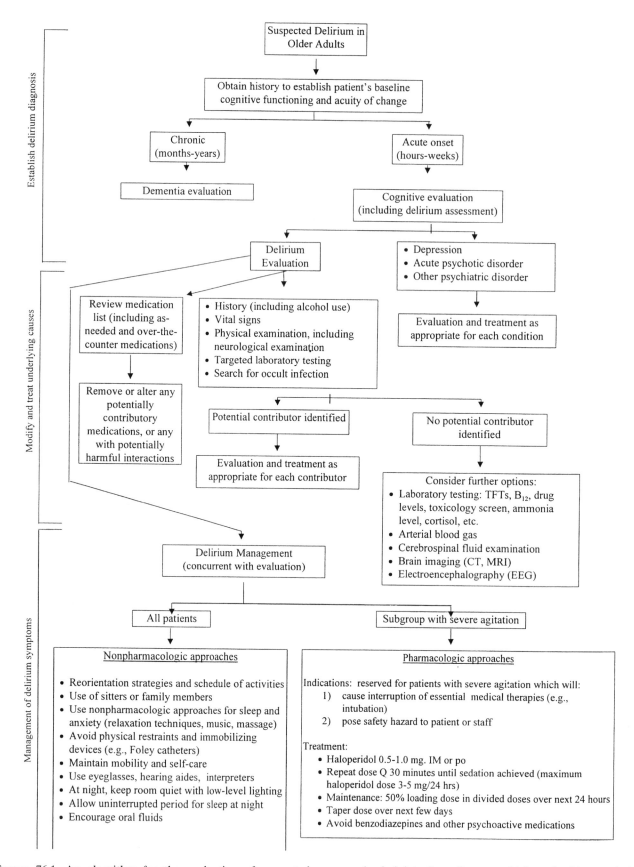

FIGURE 76.1. An algorithm for the evaluation of suspected delirium in the older adult. *TFT*, thyroid function tests; B$_{12}$, vitamin B$_{12}$ assay; *CT*, computed tomography; *MRI*, magnetic resonance imaging; *mg*, milligrams; *IM*, intramuscular injection; *po*, oral administration; *Q*, every. (Adapted with permission from Inouye SK. Delirium and other mental status problems in the older patients. In: Goldman L, Bennett JC. *Cecil Textbook of Medicine, 4th Ed.* Philadelphia: Saunders; 1999:19–22.)

TABLE 76.2. Delirium risk factors and potential interventions.

Risk factor	Interventions
Cognitive impairment	Therapeutic activities program
	Reality orientation program (reorienting techniques, communication)
Sleep deprivation	Noise reduction strategies
	Scheduling of nighttime medications, procedures, and nursing activities to allow uninterrupted period of sleep
Immobilization	Early mobilization (e.g., ambulation or bedside exercises)
	Minimizing immobilizing equipment (e.g., bladder catheters)
Psychoactive medications	Restricted use of prn sleep and psychoactive medications (e.g., sedative-hypnotics, narcotics, anticholinergic medications)
	Nonpharmacologic protocols for management of sleep and anxiety
Vision impairment	Provision of vision aids (e.g., magnifiers, special lighting)
	Provision of adaptive equipment (e.g., illuminated phone dials, large-print books)
Hearing impairment	Provision of amplifying devices
	Repair of hearing aids
Dehydration	Early recognition and volume repletion

Source: Adapted with permission from Inouye SK. Delirium and other mental status problems in the older patients. In: Goldman L, Bennett JC. *Cecil Textbook of Medicine, 4th Ed.* Philadelphia: Saunders; 1999:19–22.

physical restraints should be avoided because of their adverse effects of immobility and increased agitation and their potential to cause injury. Clocks, calendars, and the day's schedule should be provided to assist with orientation. Room and staff changes should be kept to a minimum. A quiet environment with low-level lighting is optimal for the delirious patient. Allowing an uninterrupted period for sleep at night is of key importance in the management of the delirious patient; this requires coordination and scheduling of nursing and medical procedures, such as medications, vital signs, intravenous fluids, and treatments. Hospital-wide changes may be needed to ensure a low level of noise at night, including hallway noise and conversations. Nonpharmacologic approaches for relaxation, including music, relaxation tapes, and massage, can be effective for management of agitation in delirious patients.

Pharmacologic Management

Pharmacologic approaches should be reserved for patients with severe agitation, which may result in the interruption of essential medical therapies (e.g., intubation, intraaortic balloon pumps, dialysis catheters) or which may endanger the safety of the patient, other patients, or staff. However, clinicians must be aware that any drug used for the treatment of delirium will have psychoactive effects and may further cloud mental status and obscure efforts to follow the patient's mental status. Thus, the drug should be given in the lowest possible dose for the shortest duration. Neuroleptics are the preferred agents of treatment, with haloperidol representing the most widely used and tested treatment for delirium.[81] Although newer neuroleptics are available, fewer data are available to support their use. If parenteral adminis-

tration is required, intravenous haloperidol results in rapid onset of action with short duration of effect, whereas intramuscular use will have a more optimal duration of action. The recommended starting dose of haloperidol is 0.5 to 1.0mg orally or parenterally, repeating the dose every 20 to 30min after vital signs have been checked, until sedation has been achieved. The endpoint should be an awake but manageable patient, not a sedated patient. The average elderly patient who has not previously been treated with neuroleptics should require a total loading dose not exceeding 3 to 5mg haloperidol. Subsequently, a maintenance dose of one-half the loading dose should be administered in divided doses over the next 24h, with tapering doses over the next few days. The leading side effects of haloperidol include sedation, hypotension, acute dystonias, extrapyramidal side effects, and anticholinergic effects (e.g., anticholinergic delirium, dry mouth, constipation, urinary retention).

Benzodiazepines are not recommended for treatment of delirium because of their tendency to cause oversedation, respiratory depression, and exacerbation of the confusional state. However, they remain the drugs of choice for treatment of withdrawal syndromes from alcohol and sedative-hypnotic drugs. For geriatric patients, lorazepam (starting dose, 0.5–1.0mg) is the recommended agent of this class, because of its favorable half-life (10–15h), lack of active metabolites, and availability of a parenteral form.

Terminal Phase

Management of delirium at the end of life poses particular challenges for the clinician. Because delirium occurs in more than 80% of patients at the end of life, establishing the goals of care with the patient and family is a crucial step, including discussions about the potential causes of the delirium, intensity of medical evaluations considered appropriate, and—in some cases—the need for titration between alertness and adequate control of pain and agitation. Even in the terminal phase, many causes of delirium are potentially reversible; however, the burdens of evaluation (e.g., invasive testing) or definitive treatment (e.g., surgery for brain metastasis or reduction in narcotic dose) may not be consistent with the goals for care. In all cases, symptom management should begin immediately, while evaluation is under way. Nonpharmacologic approaches should be instituted in all patients, with pharmacologic approaches for selected cases. Haloperidol remains the first-line therapy for delirium in terminally ill patients. In end-of-life care, there is a lower threshold for the use of sedative agents. Sedation may be indicated as an additional therapy for management of severe agitated delirium in the terminally ill patient, which can cause considerable distress for the patient and family. Because sedation poses the risks of decreased meaningful interaction with family, increased confusion, and respiratory depression, this choice should be made in conjunction with the family according to the goals for care. If sedation is indicated, an agent that is short acting and easily titrated to effect is recommended. Lorazepam (starting dose, 0.5–1.0 mg p.o., i.v., s.q.) is the recommended agent of choice; however, midazolam (starting dose, 0.5–1.0 mg i.v. or s.q.) may be useful for short-term sedation where rapid onset and titration are required. Because the risks of respiratory suppression and hypotension with midazolam are great, the patient must be closely monitored.

System-Wide Changes

The optimal management of delirium requires system-wide changes to improve the quality of hospital care for older patients.[82] Interventions needed to reduce delirium rates include education of physicians and nurses to improve recognition and heighten awareness of the clinical implications; encouragement of cognitive assessment of all elderly hospitalized patients; provision of incentives to change practice patterns that lead to delirium (e.g., immobilization, overuse of psychoactive medications, bladder catheters, and physical restraints); and creation of systems that enhance high-quality geriatric care (e.g., geriatric expertise, case management, clinical pathways, and quality monitoring for delirium). With its common occurrence, its frequently iatrogenic nature, and its close linkage to the processes of care, incident delirium serves as a valuable marker for the quality of hospital care and provides an opportunity for overall improvement in care for the older population.

References

1. American Psychiatric Association. *Diagnostic and Statistical Manual of Mental Disorders (DSM-IV), 4th Ed.* Washington, DC: American Psychiatric Association; 1994.
2. Inouye SK, van Dyck CH, Alessi CA, Balkin S, Siegal AP, Horwitz RI. Clarifying confusion: the Confusion Assessment Method, a new method for detection of delirium. *Ann Intern Med.* 1990;113:941–948.
3. Francis J, Kapoor WN. Delirium in hospitalized elderly. *J Gen Intern Med.* 1990;5:65–79.
4. Bergman K, Eastham EJ. Psychogeriatric ascertainment and assessment for treatment in an acute medical ward setting. *Age Ageing.* 1974;3:174–188.
5. Cameron DJ, Thomas TI, Mulvihill M, et al. Delirium: a test of the Diagnostic and Statistical Manual III criteria on medical inpatients. *J Am Geriatr Soc.* 1987;35:1007–1010.
6. Chisholm SE, Deniston OI, Igrisan RM, et al. Prevalence of confusion in elderly hospitalized patients. *J Gerontol Nurs.* 1982;8:87–96.
7. Fields SD, Makenzie CR, Charlson ME, et al. Reversibility of cognitive impairment in medical inpatients. *Arch Intern Med.* 1986;146:1593–1596.
8. Francis J, Martin D, Kapoor WN. A prospective study of delirium in hospitalized elderly. *JAMA.* 1990;263:1097–1101.
9. Henker FO. Acute brain syndromes. *J Clin Psychiatry.* 1979; 40:117–120.
10. Hodkinson HM. Mental impairment in the elderly. *J R Coll Physicians Lond.* 1973;7:305–317.
11. Kay DWK, Norris V, Post F. Prognosis in psychiatric disorders of the elderly: an attempt to define indicators of early death and early recovery. *J Ment Sci.* 1956;120:129–140.
12. Lipowski AJ. *Delirium: Acute Confusion States.* Oxford: Oxford University Press; 1990:141–173.
13. Rockwood K. Acute confusion in elderly medical patients. *J Am Geriatr Soc.* 1989;37:150–154.
14. Inouye SK, Charpentier PA. Precipitating factors for delirium in hospitalized elderly persons: predictive model and interrelationship with baseline vulnerability. *JAMA.* 1996; 275:852–857.
15. Inouye SK, Viscoli CM, Horwitz RI, et al. A predictive model for delirium in hospitalized elderly medical patients based on admission characteristics. *Ann Intern Med.* 1993; 119:474–481.
16. Rosin AJ, Boyd RV. Complications of illness in geriatric patients in hospital. *J Chronic Dis.* 1966;19:307–313.
17. Black DW, Warrack G, Winokur G. The Iowa record-linkage study. II. Excess mortality among patients with organic mental disorders. *Arch Gen Psychiatry.* 1885;42:78–81.
18. Fields SD, Mackenzie DR, Charlson ME, et al. Cognitive impairment: can it predict the course of hospitalized patients? *J Am Geriatr Soc.* 1986;34:579–585.
19. Guze SB, Cantwell DP. The prognosis in "organic brain" syndromes. *Am J Psychiatry.* 1964;120:878–881.
20. Guze SB, Daengsurisri S. Organic brain syndromes: prognostic significance in general medical patients. *Arch Gen Psychiatry.* 1967;17:365–366.
21. Rabins PV, Folstein MF. Delirium and dementia: diagnostic criteria and fatality rates. *Br J Psychiatry.* 1982;140:149–153.

22. Roth M. The natural history of mental disorder in old age. *J Ment Sci.* 1955;101:281–303.

23. Trzepacz PT, Teague GB, Lipowski ZJ. Delirium and other organic mental disorders in a general hospital. *Gen Hosp Psychiatry.* 1985;7:101–106.

24. Williams M, Campbell EB, Raynor WJ, et al. Predictors of acute confusional states in hospitalized elderly patients. *Res Nurs Health.* 1985;8:31–40.

25. U.S. Bureau of the Census. *Statistical Abstract of the United States, 116th Ed.* Washington, DC: U.S. Bureau of the Census; 1996:165.

26. Elie M, Cole MG, Primeau FJ, Bellavance F. Delirium risk factors in elderly hospitalized patients. *J Gen Intern Med.* 1998;13:204–212.

27. Foreman MD. Confusion in the hospitalized elderly: incidence, onset and associated factors. *Res Nurs Health.* 1989;12:21–29.

28. Gustafson Y, Berggen D, Brannstrom B, et al. Acute confusional states in elderly patients treated for femoral fracture. *J Am Geriatr Soc.* 1988;36:525–530.

29. Rogers MP, Liang MH, Daltroy LH, et al. Delirium after elective orthopedic surgery: risk factors and natural history. *Int J Psychiatr Med.* 1989;19:109–121.

30. Schor J, Levkoff SE, Lipsitz LA, et al. Risk factors for delirium in hospitalized elderly. *JAMA.* 1992;267:827–831.

31. Inouye SK. The dilemma of delirium: clinical and research controversies regarding diagnosis and evaluation of delirium in hospitalized elderly medical patients. *Am J Med.* 1994;97:278–288.

32. Koponen H, Partanen J, Paakkonen A, et al. EEG spectral analysis in delirium. *J Neurol Neurosurg Psychiatry.* 1989; 52:980–985.

33. Foy A, O'Connell D, Henry D, et al. Benzodiazepine use as a cause of cognitive impairment in elderly hospital inpatients. *J Gerontol Med Sci.* 1995;50A:M99–M106.

34. Marcantonio ER, Goldman L, Mangione CM, et al. A clinical prediction rule for delirium after elective noncardiac surgery. *JAMA.* 1994;271:134–139.

35. Bates DW, Cullen DJ, Laird N, et al. Incidence of adverse drug events and potential adverse drug events: implications for prevention. *JAMA.* 1995;274:29–34.

36. Lindley CM, Tully MP, Paramsothy V, et al. Inappropriate medication is a major cause of adverse drug reactions in elderly patients. *Age Ageing.* 1992;21:294–300.

37. Brook RH, Kamberg CJ, Mayer-Oakes A, et al. Appropriateness of acute medical care for the elderly: an analysis of the literature. *Health Policy.* 1990;14:225–242.

38. Owens NJ, Sherburne NJ, Silliman RA, et al. The Senior Care Study: the optimal use of medications in acutely ill older patients. *J Am Geriatr Soc.* 1990;38:1082–1087.

39. Millar HR. Psychiatric morbility in elderly surgical patients. *Br J Psychiatry.* 1981;38:17–20.

40. Flint FJ, Richards SM. Organic basis of confusional states in the elderly. *Br Med J.* 1956;2:1537–1539.

41. Sirois F. Delirium: 100 cases. *Can J Psychiatry.* 1988;33:375–378.

42. Seymour DG, Henschke RD, Cape T, et al. Acute confusional states and dementia in the elderly: the role of dehydration/volume depletion, physical illness and age. *Age Ageing.* 1980;8:137–146.

43. Sier HC, Hartnell J, Morley JE, et al. Primary hyperparathyroidism and delirium in the elderly. *J Am Geriatr Soc.* 1988;36:157–170.

44. Blackburn T, Dunn M. Cystocerebral syndrome: acute urinary retention presenting as confusion in elderly patients. *Arch Intern Med.* 1990;150:2577–2578.

45. Creditor MC. Hazards of hospitalization of the elderly. *Ann Intern Med.* 1993;118:219–223.

46. Lazarus BA, Murphy JB, Colletta EM, et al. The provision of physical activity to hospitalized elderly patients. *Arch Intern Med.* 1991;51:2452–2456.

47. Becker PM, McVey LJ, Saltz CC, et al. Hospital-acquired complications in a randomized controlled clinical trial of a geriatric consultation team. *JAMA.* 1982;257:2313–2317.

48. Steel K, Gertman PM, Crescenzi C, et al. Iatrogenic illness on a general medicine service at a university hospital. *N Engl J Med.* 1981;304:638–642.

49. Reichel W. Complications in the care of five hundred elderly hospitalized patients. *J Am Geriatr Soc.* 1965;13:973–981.

50. Romano J, Engel GL. Delirium. I. Electroencephalographic data. *Arch Neurol Psychiatry.* 1944;51:356–377.

51. Pro JD, Wells CE. The use of electroencephalogram in the diagnosis of delirium. *Dis Nerv Syst.* 1977;38:804–808.

52. Trzepacz PT. Is there a final common neural pathway in delirium? Focus on acetylcholine and dopamine. *Semin Clin Neuropsychiatry.* 2000;5:132–148.

53. Van der Mast RC. Pathophysiology of delirium. *J Geriatr Psychiatry Neurol.* 1998;11:138–145.

54. McIntosh TK, Bush HL, Yeston NS, et al. Beta-endorphin, cortisol, and postoperative delirium: a preliminary report. *Psychoneuroendocrinology.* 1985;10:303–313.

55. Blass JP, Gibson GE, Duffy TE, et al. Cholinergic dysfunction: a common denominator in metabolic encephalopathies. In: Pepeu G, Ladinsky H, eds. *Cholinergic Mechanisms.* New York: Plenum Press; 1981;921–928.

56. Flacker JM, Lipsitz LA. Large neutral amino acid changes and delirium in febrile elderly medical patients. *J Gerontol Biol Sci.* 2000;55A:B249–B252.

57. Liptzin B, Levkoff SE. An empirical study of delirium subtypes. *Br J Psychiatry.* 1992;161:843–845.

58. Koponen HJ, Riekkinen PJ. A prospective study of delirium in elderly patients admitted to a psychiatric hospital. *Psychol Med.* 1993;23:103–109.

59. Sandburg O, Gustafson Y, Brannstrom B, Bucht G. Clinical profile of delirium in older patients. *J Am Geriatr Soc.* 1999; 47:1300–1306.

60. Levkoff SE, Evans DA, Liptzin B, et al. Delirium: the occurrence and persistence of symptoms among elderly hospitalized patients. *Arch Intern Med.* 1992;152:334–340.

61. Rockwood K. The occurrence and duration of symptoms in elderly patients with delirium. *J Gerontol Med Sci.* 1993;48: M162–M166.

62. Cameron DJ, Thomas RU, Mulvihill M, Bronhelm H. Delirium: a test of the Diagnostic and Statistical Manual III criteria on medical inpatients. *J Am Geriatr Soc.* 1987;35: 1007–1010.

63. Gustafson Y, Brannstrom B, Norberg A, Bucht G, Winblad B. Underdiagnosis and poor documentation of acute confusional states in elderly hip fracture patients. *J Am Geriatr Soc.* 1991;39:760–765.

64. Rockwood K, Cosway S, Stolee P, et al. Increasing the recognition of delirium in elderly patients. *J Am Geriatr Soc.* 1994;42:252–256.

65. Folstein MR, Folstein SE, McHugh PR. "Mini-Mental State": a practical method for grading the cognitive state of patients for the clinician. *J Psychiatr Res.* 1975;12:189–198.

66. Trzepacz TT, Brenner RP, Coffman G, et al. Delirium in liver transplantation candidates: discriminate analysis of multiple tests variables. *Biol Psychiatry.* 1988;24:3–14.

67. Cole MG, Primeau FJ. Prognosis of delirium in elderly hospital patients. *Can Med Assoc J.* 1993;149:41–46.

68. Inouye SK, Rushing JT, Foreman MD, Palmer RM, Pompei P. Does delirium contribute to poor hospital outcomes? A three-site epidemiologic study. *J Gen Intern Med.* 1998; 13:234–242.

69. O'Keeffe S, Lavan J. The prognostic significance of delirium in older hospital patients. *J Am Geriatr Soc.* 1997;45:174–178.

70. van Hemert AM, van der Mast RC, Hengeveld MW, et al. Excess mortality in general hospital patients with delirium: a 5-year follow-up of 519 patients seen in psychiatric consultation. *J Psychosom Res.* 1994;38(4):339–346.

71. Murray AM, Levkoff SE, Wetle TT, et al. Acute delirium and functional decline in the hospitalized elderly patients. *J Gerontol Med Sci.* 1993;48:M181–M186.

72. Francis J, Kapoor WN. Prognosis after hospital discharge of older medical patients with delirium. *J Am Geriatr Soc.* 1992;40:601–606.

73. Williams-Russo P, Urquhart BL, Sharrock NE, et al. Postoperative delirium: predictors and prognosis in elderly orthopedic patients. *J Am Geriatr Soc.* 1992;40:759–767.

74. Brannstron B, Gustafson Y, Norberg A, et al. ADL performance and dependency on nursing care in patients with hip fractures and acute confusion in a task allocation care system. *Scand J Caring Sci.* 1988;5:3–11.

75. Rockwood K. Delays in the discharge of elderly patients. *J Clin Epidemiol.* 1990;43:971–975.

76. Koponen H, Stenback U, Mattila E, et al. Delirium among elderly persons admitted to a psychiatric hospital: clinical course during the acute stage and one-year follow-up. *Acta Psychiatr Scand.* 1989;79:579–585.

77. Magaziner J, Simonsick EM, Kashner M, et al. Survival experience of aged hip fracture patients. *Am J Public Health.* 1989;79:274–278.

78. Levkoff SE, Safran C, Cleary PD, et al. Identification of factors associated with the diagnosis of delirium in elderly hospitalized patients. *J Am Geriatr Soc.* 1988;36:1099–1104.

79. Thomas RI, Cameron DJ, Fahs MC. A prospective study of delirium and prolonged hospital stay: exploratory study. *Arch Gen Psychiatry.* 1988;45:937–940.

80. Inouye SK, Bogardus ST, Charpentier PA, et al. A multicomponent intervention to prevent delirium in hospitalized older patients. *N Engl J Med.* 1999;340:669–676.

81. Breitbart W, Marotta R, Platt MM, et al. A double-blind trial of haloperidol, chlorpromazine, and lorazepam in the treatment of delirium in hospitalized AIDS patients. *Am J Psychiatry.* 1996;153:231–237.

82. Inouye SK, Schlesinger MF, Lydon TJ. Delirium: a symptom of how hospital care is failing older persons and a window to improve quality of hospital care. *Am J Med.* 1999;106: 565–573.

77
Cerebrovascular Disease and Stroke

Stanley Tuhrim

Stroke is a major public health problem afflicting primarily older adults. It is the third leading cause of death in the United States and is surpassed only by heart disease worldwide.[1,2] In the United States, more than 700,000 new strokes occur annually.[3] Stroke is also the leading cause of disability in the United States, with an estimated 4 million stroke survivors in this country living with stroke-related deficits.[1] Over 70% of stroke survivors remain vocationally impaired, over 30% require help with activities of daily living, and 20% walk only with assistance.[4] Approximately half of stroke survivors return to some form of employment, but this figure declines with age.[5]

The incidence of stroke doubles in each successive decade after age 55 and occurs approximately twice as often in African-Americans as in whites at all ages. It is more common in men under age 75 but is equally common among older men and women.[3,6,7]

Stroke is actually a heterogeneous group of diseases. There are two main categories, hemorrhage and infarction, which result from different pathophysiologic mechanisms: extravasation of blood from a damaged vessel in hemorrhage and ischemia or insufficient blood perfusing brain tissue in infarction. These categories can be further subdivided pathophysiologically. Subarachnoid hemorrhage is leakage of blood at the brain surface into the cerebrospinal fluid, usually the result of rupture of an aneurysm in an artery at the base of the brain (circle of Willis). Less often, the bleeding may be caused by rupture of a vascular malformation or trauma to a surface vessel. Intracerebral hemorrhage (ICH) usually is caused by rupture of a small artery or arteriole with leakage of blood into the brain parenchyma.

Subarachnoid Hemorrhage

Subarachnoid hemorrhage (SAH) accounts for 5% to 10% of all strokes. Incidence rates vary from 6 to 16 per 100,000, with the highest rates reported from Japan and Finland.[8–10] Women are affected more often than men by a ratio of 3:2, and incidence increases with advancing age.[8,11] SAH patients in the Framingham Study averaged 63 years of age.[12] Tobacco use and heavy alcohol consumption have been identified as risk factors for SAH.[13,14] Hypertension does not play as important a role in SAH risk as in other forms of stroke, although use of cocaine and other noradrenergic stimulants has been associated with SAH, possibly by precipitating rupture of an aneurysm during an acute hypertensive espisode.[15]

Arteriovenous malformations (AVMs) can also cause SAH, but frequently produce intraparenchymal hemorrhage as well. They are rarely the cause of SAH in the elderly. Bleeding is less brisk than with ruptured saccular aneurysms, and symptoms may develop more slowly. AVMs usually present in adolescence or early adulthood, causing headache, seizures, or hemorrhage. In the elderly, the cause of SAH is more often undetermined than in younger patients. Amyloid angiopathy or unrecognized head trauma is often thought to be responsible.

Morbidity and mortality are high in SAH. About 12% of SAH patients die before receiving medical attention.[16,17] The 90-day mortality rate among those who do reach medical attention is about 25%, and 40% of survivors suffer residual cognitive, motor, and sensory deficits.[17] Early mortality results from the direct effects of the initial or recurrent bleeding, whereas medical complications or ischemia, secondary to vasospasm induced by subarachnoid blood, are responsible for most deaths beyond the first week.

The Hunt and Hess Scale is widely used to grade the severity of SAH (Table 77.1).[18] Grade 1 and 2 patients have a good prognosis, while grade 4 and 5 patients usually do poorly and are usually not considered candidates for surgical intervention. Grade 3 patients have the most variable outcomes. The Glasgow Outcome Scale (see Table 77.1), originally developed for head trauma, is frequently used to grade outcomes in SAH.[19] The majority of patients with SAH harbor saccular aneurysms as

TABLE 77.1. Global measures in subarachnoid hemorrhage (SAH).

Hunt and Hess Scale

Grade	Neurologic status
1	Asymptomatic
2	Severe headache, stiff neck, no neurologic deficit except cranial nerve palsy
3	Drowsy, minimal neurologic deficit
4	Stuporous, moderate or severe hemiparesis
5	Deep coma, decerebrate

Glasgow Outcome Scale

Category	Outcome
1	Good recovery, independent lifestyle
2	Moderate disability, independent lifestyle
3	Severe disability, conscious but not independent
4	Vegetative
5	Dead

the cause of bleeding. Saccular aneurysms form at the bifurcation of large arteries and are probably caused by a combination of congenital and degenerative changes in arteries. Hemodynamic stresses at arterial bifurcations lead to degenerative changes in the internal elastic lamina, weakening of the arterial wall, and aneurysmal outpouching. The most common sites for aneurysm formation are within the anterior circulation, at the junction or bifurcation of the major cerebral arteries. Posterior circulation aneurysms are less common, the most common sites being the bifurcation of the basilar artery and the vertebral artery–posterior interior cerebellar artery junction.

Diagnosis of SAH

Most aneurysms remain asymptomatic until they bleed, but some larger aneurysms compress adjacent nerves, brain tissue, or meningeal structures, causing headache and neurologic dysfunction. When aneurysms rupture, they leak blood into the cerebrospinal fluid (CSF) under arterial pressure. Patients usually describe a sudden onset of severe headache, often "the worst headache of my life." There is usually some alteration in consciousness, ranging from deep coma with massive bleeding to sleepiness or agitation with lesser amounts of bleeding. Unless bleeding also occurs directly into brain, patients do not have major focal neurologic signs.

When a patient presents with the abrupt onset of severe headache, with or without meningismus or subtle neurologic signs, SAH must be considered. The differential diagnosis may include other causes of headache, such as migraine or infectious meningitis, but if SAH is considered, a computerized tomographic (CT) scan should be obtained; this can show the presence of blood in the subarachnoid space, confirming the diagnosis. The

location of blood may indicate the likely location of the aneurysm and the amount, and the thickness of blood indicates the likelihood of subsequent vasospasm.[20] Because of variability in magnetic resonance scanning techniques and interpretation skills, for the present, CT scan remains more accurate than MR imaging in most centers, with a yield approaching 95% if done within 24 h of stroke onset.[21] If a CT scan cannot be performed or fails to confirm the diagnosis of SAH, a lumbar puncture should be performed to allow examination of the CSF.[22] All patients with SAH have blood in the CSF when tapped within 48 h. Some patients have a small "warning leak" before massive aneurysmal rupture. These small hemorrhages are often missed by CT and will be detected only by lumbar puncture. No patient in whom SAH is suspected should leave the hospital without a lumbar puncture. Findings diagnostic of SAH include the constant red or pink appearance of the CSF on collection. In this instance, the presence of xanthochromia in the supernatant after prompt centrifugation distinguishes pathologic SAH from leakage induced by trauma during the spinal tap. Centrifugation should be performed immediately after collection to avoid hemolysis of red blood cells ex vivo. Red blood cells in the fluid with a cell count that remains constant from the first tube collected to the last, and the presence of white blood cells in greater proportion than that found in the periphery, are also indicative of true SAH. Xanthochromia may not be present if the CSF is collected within 6 h of ictus and may be the only abnormality remaining if lumbar puncture is delayed several days.

Unless the patient's condition precludes treatment, angiography should be performed to determine the cause of bleeding. Conventional (catheter) angiography will detect approximately 95% of aneurysms and all AVMs. If an initial angiogram is negative, a repeat study, usually performed 1 to 2 weeks later, will detect an aneurysm in about 2% of cases.[23] Magnetic resonance angiography (MRA) and CT angiography are useful as complements to conventional angiography and as screening tests in high-risk, asymptomatic individuals, but are not as sensitive in imaging small (<5 mm) aneurysms. Sequential transcranial Doppler (TCD) examinations are useful for detecting vasospasm. It is helpful to obtain a TCD before surgery and as close to the ictus as possible to serve as a basis of comparison for determining if flow velocities begin to rise (preceding the onset of clinical symptoms of ischemia secondary to vasospasm).

Treatment

Obliteration of the aneurysm is the key treatment for aneurysmal SAH. This intervention removes the possibility of recurrent bleeding and allows treatment of vasospasm with hypervolemic, hypertensive therapy. A large international study demonstrated that early operation prevents rebleeding, but overall outcome was no different between those operated within 3 days of initial SAH and those operated from 15 to 32 days afterward. Mortality was higher in patients operated between 4 and 14 days.[17] Recently, endovascular techniques have been developed that allow obliteration of aneurysms via intraluminal embolization with detachable coils, which can usually be accomplished with minimal additional morbidity to the patient. Selection of aneurysms with suitable configurations is crucial. The durability of the procedure requires further evaluation, however.

Delayed cerebral ischemia can develop because of constriction of the major arteries arising at the base of the brain during the first week after SAH. Preventative treatment with nimodipine, a dihydropyridine calcium channel blocker, is begun as soon as ischemic aneurysmal SAH is recognized and continued for 21 to 28 days. In the event that focal or global neurologic deficits develop due to vasospasm, elevation of blood pressure and increasing intravascular volume can be effective therapy.

Intracerebral Hemorrhage

Nontraumatic intracerebral hemorrhage (ICH) is localized bleeding in the brain parenchyma. Approximately 50,000 new cases occur in the United States every year, with a twofold increase expected in coming years due to increasing age and changes in racial composition of the population.[24,25] ICH accounts for 10% to 15% of all strokes and is associated with the highest mortality.[26] ICH can be classified into primary and secondary, depending upon the underlying etiology of bleeding. Primary ICH originates from spontaneous rupture of small vessels pathologically affected by chronic hypertension and accounts for 78% to 88% of all ICH.[27] Secondary ICH occurs in a minority of patients in association with amyloid angiopathy, structural vascular abnormalities, tumors, or impaired blood coagulation.

Epidemiology

The incidence of ICH ranges from 10 to 20 persons per 100,000 overall but increases with age to approximately 100 per 100,000 persons aged greater than 75.[28–30] ICH is more frequent in men, particularly after the age of 55 years,[30,31] and occurs more frequently in African-Americans[28] and Japanese.[32] For example, the incidence of ICH in the African-American cohort was 50 per 100,000, twice that of whites, in the National Health and Nutrition Examination Survey Epidemiologic Follow-up Study.[33]

Hypertension is the most important risk factor for spontaneous ICH.[34,35] Hypertension increases ICH risk most dramatically in persons who are not compliant with antihypertensive medication,[36,37] whereas improved control of hypertension reduces the incidence of ICH.[29] Excessive use of alcohol also increases the risk for ICH, probably by impairing blood coagulation and directly affecting cerebral vessel integrity.[38,39]

Pathophysiology

Intracerebral hemorrhages occur most commonly in the basal ganglia, thalamus, cerebral lobes, and brainstem (predominantly pons).[27] Ventricular extension occurs in 40% of cases, especially in association with deep, large hematomas. Intraparenchymal bleeding usually results from rupture of one of the small penetrating arteries originating from the large superficial arteries. This bleeding was considered a monophasic event that stopped quickly as a result of clotting and tamponade by increased parenchymal pressure in the surrounding regions. As patients have obtained more rapid access to medical care and CT scans have been obtained nearer the time of initial ictus, it has become apparent that hematomas continue to expand over time. For example, Brott et al.[40] observed hematoma expansion in 26% of patients within 1 h and in another 12% by 20 h of initial CT scan. The factors that predispose to hematoma expansion are poorly understood, but it has been attributed to continued bleeding from the primary source and mechanical disruption of surrounding vessels and may be associated with acute hypertension.[41,42] Compression of surrounding structures by the hematoma causes dysfunction and ultimately cell death. This physical damage is compounded by biochemical effects of blood products from the hematoma that initiate pathophysiologic processes in the surrounding parenchyma, producing edema and neuronal damage. Edema formation starts immediately in the perihematoma region and usually persists for up to 5 days. Both vasogenic and cytotoxic edema follow due to disruption of the blood–brain barrier and failure of the Na-K pump with swelling of neuronal and glial cells, causing further damage.[43]

Clinical Features

Decreased level of consciousness is almost always seen with large hematomas,[44] presumably because of raised intracranial pressure and direct compression or distortion of the thalamic and brainstem reticular activating system mediating arousal and attention.[45] In ICH originating in putamen, caudate, and thalamus, contralateral sensorimotor deficits of varying severity usually occur due to involvement of the internal capsule. Higher cortical dysfunction, including aphasia, neglect, gaze deviation, and hemianopia, may occur because of disruption of connection fibers in the subcortical white matter. In infratentorial ICH, signs of brainstem dysfunction include gaze abnormalities, cranial nerve abnormalities, and contra-lateral motor deficits. Ataxia, nystagmus, and dysmetria are prominent when the ICH involves the cerebellum.[46] Common nonspecific symptoms include headache and vomiting due to raised intracranial pressure and meningismus resulting from intraventricular extension of blood.[44,47,48]

Approximately 25% patients who are alert when they reach the hospital deteriorate within the first 24 h after onset. Presence of large hematomas and ventricular blood increases the risk for subsequent deterioration. Hematoma expansion is the most common cause underlying neurologic deterioration within the first 3 h. Worsening cerebral edema is also an important contributor in patients who deteriorate 24 to 48 h after onset.[49,50]

Mortality following spontaneous ICH ranges from 23% to 58%. Clinical severity as measured by the initial Glasgow Coma Scale Score (GCS), hematoma volume, and presence of ventricular blood on initial CT scan have been consistently identified as predictive of high mortality.[51,52] Broderick et al. found that 1-month mortality was best predicted by a combination of initial GCS score and hematoma volume. In this study, patients with GCS less than 9 and hematoma volume greater than 60 mL had a mortality of 90%. Patients with GCS of 9 or greater and hematoma volume less than 30 mL had a mortality of 17%.[51]

The long-term functional outcome in ICH survivors is similar to that observed with cerebral infarction. Approximately 40% of the patients are functionally independent after 1 year.[53] Age, initial GCS, presence of ventricular blood, hematoma volume, and initial disability predict long-term outcome.[53,54] The likelihood of a second ICH is low. Hill et al. reported an annual incidence of 2.4% for recurrent ICH (fourfold higher among lobar hemorrhages) and 3% for ischemic stroke among 307 survivors of primary ICH.[55] The site of ICH is usually different from the first ICH, and the likelihood of recurrence is much greater in those with persistently uncontrolled hypertension.[56]

Diagnostic Investigations

Although clinical features such as headache, smooth rapid onset of focal deficits, and decreased alertness suggest the diagnosis of ICH, distinguishing definitively between cerebral infarction and ICH requires brain imaging.[57] On the initial CT scan, the location and size of the hematoma, presence of ventricular blood, and hydrocephalus should be noted. Selected patients should undergo conventional angiography to look for secondary causes of ICH, such as aneurysms, arteriovenous malformations, and vasculitis. Magnetic resonance imaging with gadolinium and magnetic resonance angiography can also be used for screening secondary causes of ICH,

although their sensitivity is not well established,[58] and may be particularly useful in identifying underlying tumors. American Heart Association (AHA) guidelines recommend angiography for all patients without a clear cause of hemorrhage who are surgical candidates, particularly young, nonhypertensive patients who are clinically stable. Conventional angiography should be considered in patients who have subarachnoid blood associated with parenchymal clot or have recurrent hemorrhages because of the high likelihood of an underlying vascular anomaly.[25]

Management

In the era of thrombolytic treatment, early differentiation between infarction and ICH using CT scan is crucial, so that thrombolysis can be considered for infarct patients. In patients with ICH, emergent neurosurgical consultation should be obtained when there is rapid deterioration, clinical evidence of transtentorial herniation, or hydrocephalus on CT scan. Hyperventilation, intravenous mannitol, and intraventricular catheter placement for cerebrospinal fluid drainage in such circumstances can preserve brain tissue until surgical decompression can be performed, although its benefit has not been proven except in cerebellar hemorrhage (see following).

The risk of neurologic deterioration and cardiovascular instability is highest in the first 24 h after onset. Patients may require intubation for deteriorating level of consciousness. Approximately 30% of patients with supratentorial ICH and almost all patients with brainstem or cerebellar hemorrhage demonstrate decreased consciousness and require intubation.[59] Cardiovascular instability can also occur with increased intracranial pressure and must be treated promptly to avoid the deleterious effects of hypertension or hypotension in the presence of limited autoregulatory capacity.

Mass effect as a result of the volume of clot, perihematoma edema, and obstructive hydrocephalus remain the major secondary causes of mortality in the initial days after ICH. Treatment with osmotic agents and hyperventilation are only transiently effective and should be used only in the presence of impending cerebral herniation. Randomized trials of steroids have failed to demonstrate efficacy in ICH.[60,61]

Management of Blood Pressure

Elevated blood pressure, seen commonly after ICH, is associated with hematoma expansion and poor outcome.[62] Elevated blood pressure may be secondary to uncontrolled chronic hypertension or occurs as a protective response to preserve cerebral perfusion. There is considerable controversy regarding treatment of blood pressure in the acute period after ICH. Most patients with ICH have chronic hypertension with cerebral autoregulation adapted for higher than normal blood pressures.[63] Furthermore, cerebral perfusion pressure and autoregulatory capacity may be compromised due to elevated ICP.[64] AHA guidelines recommend antihypertensive treatment only when mean arterial pressure is 130 mmHg or greater. Intravenous beta-blockers and vasodilators such as hydralazine or angiotensin-converting enzyme (ACE) inhibitors should be used because they have limited effect on cerebral circulation.[25,65]

Ventricular Blood and Hydrocephalus

Presence of ventricular blood is associated with high mortality in patients with ICH.[66,67] This association may be related to the development of obstructive hydrocephalus or direct mass effect of the ventricular blood clot on periventricular structures that is associated with global hypoperfusion of overlying cortex. Ventricular blood also interferes with the normal CSF functions by inducing local lactic acidosis.[67,68] External CSF drainage using ventricular catheters may improve control of ICP, although the beneficial effect on hydrocephalus and neurologic status appears to be marginal. The risk of infection and clotting within the catheter limit prolonged use of external CSF drainage.[69] Pang et al. demonstrated that lysis of ventricular blood using thrombolytic agents administered via intraventricular catheter can rapidly clear blood from the CSF and improve outcome in dogs.[70] The use of intraventricular thrombolysis has been reported in small series of patients with intraventricular extension of ICH. Either tissue plasminogen activator or urokinase has been used. Administration until ventricular blood resolved resulted in improvement in ventricular dilatation and neurologic status in almost all patients.[71–74] A randomized trial testing the safety and efficacy of this procedure is under way.[75]

Surgical Evacuation

The goals of surgical evacuation of hematoma are to reduce mass effect and minimize release of neuropathic products from the clot; however, with the exception of cerebellar hematomas, the benefit of surgical decompression is unclear. Cerebellar hematomas are unique from a surgical perspective because they can be approached without significant damage to higher cortical and primary motor pathways. Morbidity and mortality is related to compression of the brainstem.[46] Patients with large (>3 × 3 cm) hematomas and those with a decreased level of consciousness or clinical evidence of brainstem compression require early craniectomy because greater benefit is observed in patients who undergo surgery before deterioration of consciousness. Studies of surgical evacuation of unselected supratentorial ICH have not demonstrated significant efficacy, although selected patients with large superficial hematomas may be candidates for evacuation.

Recent studies have focused on developing surgical approaches allowing evacuation of clot with minimal damage to overlying normal tissue including stereotactic and endoscopic approaches. Techniques to liquefy the clot by irrigation with fluid at a high pressure or thrombolytics are under investigation. Repeated injection of fibrinolytic agents, usually at 6- or 12-h intervals using a stereotactically placed catheter can result in complete removal of hematoma.[76,77] The observed risk of inducing rebleeding is less than 5%. These efforts have been supplemented by high-pressure ultrasound irrigation systems and special drills to break the clot into easily removable fragments.[78] A recent pilot study of 12 patients whose mean age was 69 years (range, 55–82) demonstrated this approach leads to a 50% clot volume reduction in 3 days with a low rate of additional bleeding or death. This approach may produce successful clot reduction with less morbidity, especially in the elderly or unstable patient, than open craniotomy, but has yet to undergo full evaluation.[79]

Seizures and Epilepsy

Most seizures associated with ICH occur at the onset of intracerebral hemorrhage or within the first 24 h.[80,81] Seizures are most frequently associated with lobar hematomas, with an incidence ranging from 24% to 54%. Recurrent seizures (epilepsy) develop in 13% to 15% of ICH patients. Because there is no clear association between the use of prophylactic anticonvulsants and the subsequent development of epilepsy in these patients, prophylactic anticonvulsants for all patients are not advisable. Anticonvulsants should generally only be administered to patients who have already suffered a seizure or undergo a neurosurgical procedure.[80,81] Anticonvulsants can usually be discontinued after the first month in patients who have had no further seizures, although patients who have a seizure after 2 weeks of onset of ICH are at higher risk for recurrence.[82]

Cerebral Amyloid Angiopathy

Cerebral amyloid angiopathy (CAA) occurs exclusively in older adults (age >60 years), affecting the cerebral vasculature selectively, favoring the superficial lobar regions, and generally sparing deeper structures typically affected in hypertensive ICH. Amyloid deposition can be demonstrated by Congo red or other stains in the small and medium-sized cortical and leptomeningeal vessels. The incidence of CAA rises dramatically with age; in an autopsy series, CAA was present in 5% of those 60 to 69 years of age but rose to 50% in those over age 80.[83] In addition to the lobar location, the other distinctive feature of CAA is the tendency for recurrence, uncommon in hypertensive ICH. As many as eight distinct hemorrhages have been reported in a single individual.[84] CAA occurs with increased frequency in patients with Alzheimer's disease, and at least 40% of patients with CAA-related ICH have histologic changes of Alzheimer's disease at autopsy.[85]

Ischemic Stroke

Infarction accounts for about 80% of strokes. There are three main subcategories of infarction: (1) cardioembolic, (2) large vessel atherothrombotic, and (3) small vessel or lacunar stroke.

Cardioembolic Infarction

Embolism from thrombi that form in the heart or that occur in large veins and pass through the heart via a right-to-left shunt account for approximately 30% of ischemic strokes. A variety of cardiac sources of embolism have been identified including valvular lesions, hemostasis secondary to rhythm disturbances, hypokinesis of the left ventricle, either globally as in a cardiomyopathy or focally secondary to infarction, or rarely tumors. Atrial fibrillation is the most widely recognized cardiac abnormality associated with ischemic stroke. It is a condition of the elderly, occurring in 0.1% of those 50 to 59 years of age and increasing gradually to 4% of those over age 80. The proportion of strokes attributed to atrial fibrillation also increases with age, rising from 7% of strokes in the sixth decade to 36% for those in the ninth decade.[86] The development of transesophageal echocardiography has provided additional insight into the source of cerebral emboli. With this technique it is possible to detect thrombus in the left atrial appendage, which is generally the site that harbors clot in a fibrillating atrium but is not visible on transthoracic echocardiogram. Spontaneous echo contrast ("smoke") is often seen in a fibrillating atrium (and sometimes in other situations) and is thought to represent platelet–fibrin aggregates that are a precursor to thrombus formation. A patent foramen ovale (PFO), the most common conduit for paradoxical emboli, is also readily diagnosed by this procedure.

Transesophageal echocardiography has also led to appreciation of atherosclerotic plaque in the ascending aorta and aortic arch, especially in elderly patients. These plaques can be ulcerated and serve as a nidus for clot formation or protrude into the lumen as a highly mobile peduncle, likely to embolize to more distal arteries. The thickness of this plaque has been correlated with the risk of stroke.[86–88] Because it is a somewhat invasive procedure, transesophageal echo is not done routinely in most centers, but patients who have no obvious source of stroke should undergo transesophageal echocardiography to determine if one of these embolic sources is present.

Lacunar Infarction

Lacunes are small, deep infarcts caused by degenerative changes within small penetrating arteries that bring blood to the internal capsule, basal ganglia, cerebral white matter, thalamus, and pons. Hypertension is the most important cause of lipohyalinosis, the most common mechanism of disease within the media of these microscopic arteries. Sometimes microatheroma originating at the orifice of these penetrating arteries leads to occlusion. Lacunar infarcts are the most common vascular lesions found within the brain at necropsy. In various series and registries, they account for at least 25% of ischemic strokes. The neurologic symptoms depend on the region of ischemia. The most common clinical presentations are (1) pure motor stroke, due to infarction in the pons or internal capsule, characterized by weakness of the face, arm, and leg on one side of the body; (2) pure sensory stroke, due to infarction in the lateral part of the thalamus and/or posterior limb of the internal capsule, characterized by numbness or paresthesia of the face, arm, leg, and trunk on one side of the body without weakness; (3) ataxic hemiparesis, due to infarction in the subcortical white matter or pons, characterized by a combination of incoordination and weakness on one side of the body without other major findings; and (4) clumsy hand-dysarthria due to pontine infarction, characterized by markedly slurred speech and difficulty with fine motor control of one hand.[89]

Patients suffering from these syndromes do not demonstrate prominent visual, cognitive, or behavioral abnormalities. The diagnosis of lacunar infarction is based on the presence of risk factors, the nature of the clinical signs and symptoms, and the results of neuroimaging tests. Most often, patients with lacunar infarction have a history of hypertension or diabetes. The presence of prominent headache, vomiting, or a decreased level of alertness makes lacunar infarction unlikely. The clinical symptoms and signs should be compatible with a small, deep lesion. Aphasia, hemianopia, and signs of anosognosia or inattention are strong evidence against lacunar disease. CT or MRI should show a small, deep infarct or be normal. In some cases, the clinical and neuroimaging tests are equivocal and do not establish a lacunar cause. In these patients, a search for other ischemic causes, such as coagulopathy, an embolism of cardiac origin, and large artery ischemic disease, is warranted.

Large Artery Occlusive Disease

The large vessels that bring blood into the brain are prone to atherosclerotic narrowing most commonly at sites of origin or bifurcation, especially the bifurcation of the common carotid into the internal and external carotid arteries in the neck. Atherosclerotic stenosis leads to infarction by reducing blood flow distal to the point of stenosis and by acting as a nidus for adhesion and aggregation of platelets producing either thrombosis at that location or embolization to and occlusion of more distal, narrower arteries. The neurologic symptoms will depend on the artery affected.

In general terms, symptoms of cerebral ischemia can be divided into those that arise from the anterior circulation, supplying the anterior three-fourths of each hemisphere, and the posterior circulation, supplying the occipital lobes, posterior thalamus, cerebellum, and brainstem.

The anterior circulation consists of the paired internal carotid arteries that give off the ophthalmic arteries and then branch into anterior and middle cerebral arteries. Atherosclerotic lesions are most common at the origin of the internal carotid arteries in the neck and the middle cerebral stem. The posterior circulation consists of the paired vertebral arteries, which give rise to the posterior inferior cerebefiar arteries before joining to form the basilar artery that gives off the paired anterior inferior and superior cerebellar arteries and penetrating branches supplying the brainstem before bifurcating into paired posterior cerebral arteries. Symptoms and signs of posterior circulation ischemia are highly variable and overlap with those of the anterior circulation, but vertigo, diplopia, nausea, and vomiting are common complaints heard in brainstem or cerebellar disease; nystagmus, disconjugate eye movement abnormalities, gait or limb ataxia, crossed (i.e., ipsilateral face and contralateral limb or body) sensory or motor deficits, and hemianopic visual field loss are indicative of posterior circulation ischemia. Confusion and memory loss can be seen, especially in embolic occlusion of the basilar artery, blocking penetrating branches that supply the thalamus.[90]

Diagnosis and Treatment

In June 1996, the FDA approved the use of tissue plasminogen activator (t-PA) in acute ischemic stroke, if given within 3 h of symptom onset. This decision signaled a virtual revolution in the diagnosis and management of acute stroke. For the first time, a proven safe and effective treatment was available, but the time frame for its use required a much more expeditious response than was customary for patients, emergency medical services, doctors, and hospitals. The public needed to be educated to recognize a stroke and react appropriately (only one-third of patients experiencing a stroke recognize it as such), and care providers needed to be educated to respond to stroke as an emergency. When signs or symptoms are recognized, emergency medical services should be contacted and the patient brought to the nearest hospital capable of caring for stroke as an emergency.

Once at the hospital, prompt triage is necessary because of the possibility of life-threatening cardiorespiratory effects. Assessment should begin with evaluation of the patient's airway, breathing, and circulation, followed by a general medical and neurologic history and physical assessment. Determining the time of symptom onset and presence of signs of trauma or medical conditions that would predispose to a particular stroke type or preclude the use of t-PA are crucial. Ancillary tests should include a complete blood count, prothrombin and activated partial thromboplastin times, serum glucose and electrolytes, electrocardiogram, and chest x-ray. A CT scan should be performed as quickly as possible to exclude intracranial hemorrhage or a nonischemic cause of the patient's symptoms. Conditions that may mimic a stroke include encephalitis, hypoglycemia, seizure, brain tumor, subdural hematoma, and migraine. If these conditions are excluded by history, physical, and imaging findings, most patients who arrive within 3 h will be candidates for intravenous thrombolysis. Exclusion criteria are listed in Table 77.2.

The only exclusion criterion that may be altered by treatment is the patient's blood pressure. Consideration for thrombolysis is one of the very few clinical circumstances in which elevated blood pressure should be treated in the setting of acute ischemic stroke. Before

TABLE 77.2. Characteristics of patients with stroke who may be eligible for intravenous tissue plasminogen activator therapy.

Age >18 years
Diagnosis of ischemic stroke causing clinically apparent neurologic deficit
Onset of symptoms <3 h before possible beginning of treatment
No stroke or head trauma during the preceding 3 months
No major surgery during the preceding 144 days
No history of intracranial hemorrhage
Systolic blood pressure <185 mmHg
Diastolic blood pressure <110 mmHg
No rapidly resolving symptoms or only minor symptoms of stroke
No symptoms suggestive of subarachnoid hemorrhage
No gastrointestinal or urinary tract hemorrhage within the preceding 21 days
No arterial puncture at a noncompressible site within the preceding 7 days
No seizure at the onset of stroke
Prothrombin time <15 s or international normalized ratio <1.7, without the use of an anticoagulant drug
Partial thromboplastin time within the normal range, if heparin was given during the preceding 48 h
Platelet count >100,000/mm^3
Blood glucose concentration >50 mg/dL (2.7 mmol/L)

Source: Adapted from TPA Stroke Study Group Protocol Guidelines.

initiation of thrombolysis, the patient's blood pressure should be less than 185/110, which may be accomplished with the intravenous administration of labetolol 10 mg. This dose may be repeated or doubled every 20 to 30 min until the desired blood pressure is attained. Other agents such as enalapril or nitroprusside may also be used.

Intravenous Thrombolytic Therapy

The results of three phase III trials of thrombolysis with intravenous t-PA have been reported. The only one with clear-cut positive results was the NINDS t-PA Stroke Study in which 624 patients were treated with 0.9 mg per kilogram t-PA administrated within 3 h of onset; half were treated within 90 min. Patients treated with t-PA were 30% more likely to have minimal or no disability 3 months later. The major risk of treatment was intra-cerebral hemorrhage, which occurred in 6.4% of patients treated with t-PA but in only 0.6% of those who received placebo. Mortality was similar in both groups (17% t-PA, 20% placebo). Patients with the three major stroke subtypes (lacunar, cardioembolic, large-vessel occlusive) benefited similarly.[91]

In two other large, randomized trials with longer treatment windows, t-PA was not more effective than placebo, although post hoc analyses suggest there may be a benefit beyond three hours if patients are appropriately selected. Subsequent studies have demonstrated that local hospitals can perform thrombolysis with intravenous t-PA given within 3 h with results similar to those in the NINDS trial.[92]

Intra-arterial Thrombolysis

Intra-arterial thrombolysis, in which a microcatheter is advanced to and sometimes through the obstructing clot, is only available at selected centers but has gained increased acceptance because of a recent randomized trial and multiple positive reports of case series. PROACT II demonstrated that patients with arteriographically confirmed occlusion of the middle cerebral artery (MCA) or its two main branches who received intraarterial thrombolysis with prourokinase within 6 h of onset had better outcomes at 3 months poststroke than those who received only low-dose intravenous heparin. No randomized trials of intra-arterial thrombolytic therapy for vertebrobasilar disease have been completed, but several reports of improved outcome relative to the usual poor prognosis in this condition has led many authorities to recommend its use, particularly in patients who cannot be treated with intravenous t-PA within 3 h of onset.[93]

Antithrombotic Therapy

During the past 30 years, anticoagulation with continu-ous infusion of intravenous unfractionated heparin has probably been the most widely used acute stroke treatment, yet no clinical trial to date has adequately tested its efficacy. Recently, several trials of anticoagulation by different methods have reported conflicting results. The International Stroke Trial enrolled nearly 20,000 patients within 48 h of symptom onset in a 3×2 factorial design in which patients received subcutaneous heparin at a dose of 5,000 or 12,500 IU twice daily, or no heparin with or without 300 mg aspirin daily. There were no differences in the primary outcome measures (death at 14 days; death or dependency at 6 months) among any of the treatment groups.[94] There was an increased risk of hemorrhage in the high-dose heparin group. This study has been criticized because of the unconventional (by American standards) method of heparin administration, lack of monitoring of anticoagulant effect, lack of blinding, and failure to obtain neuroimaging before randomization and initiation of treatment.

The Trial of ORG 10172 in Acute Stroke Treatment evaluated the low molecular weight heparinoid (LMWH) danaproid versus placebo in 1281 acute ischemic stroke patients. Patients were treated with continuous intravenous infusion for 7 days beginning within 24 h of symptom onset. There was no significant reduction in stroke progression, 7-day mortality, or risk of stroke recurrence. There was a trend toward a better 3-month outcome in the large-vessel atherosclerotic subgroup (68% versus 55% favorable outcome). Another double-blind placebo-controlled trial randomized 2750 patients to a high or low dose of a different LMWH, nadroparin, or placebo subcutaneously, begun within 48 h of symptom onset. There was a significant dose-dependent effect among the three study groups in favor of the LMWH in the main outcome measure, that is, death or dependency after 6 months.[95]

The Heparin in Acute Embolic Stroke Trial (HAEST) compared the LMWH dalteparin 100 IU/kg twice daily to aspirin 160 mg daily, begun within 30 h of symptom onset in treatment of 449 patients with acute ischemic stroke and atrial fibrillation. There was no difference in the frequency of stroke recurrence in the first 2 weeks following stroke and no difference in functional outcome at 2 weeks or 3 months.[96]

Despite the lack of evidence supporting its use, intravenous unfractionated heparin remains in widespread use in patients not eligible for thrombolysis, especially those with presumed cardioembolic infarction, antiphospholipid-antibody syndrome, extracranial carotid or vertebral artery dissection, cerebral vein thrombosis, and impending large-vessel thrombosis. It is usually given as a continuous intravenous infusion with a goal of maintaining the partial thromboplastin time at 1.5 to 2.0 times normal.

Antiplatelet Therapy

Early treatment with aspirin is commonplace for patients not treated with thrombolysis or anticoagulation. This practice arose because aspirin was of proven benefit in secondary stroke prevention and in the acute management of myocardial ischemia, but recently two trials evaluated its benefit in more than 40,000 patients treated within 48h of stroke onset. In the International Stroke Trial, although there was no difference in the primary outcome measures among treatment groups, secondary analyses demonstrated a small (2.8% versus 3.9%) decrease in the rate of recurrent ischemic stroke in patients treated with aspirin. The Chinese Acute Stroke trial randomized 21,106 patients to aspirin 160mg or placebo for 4 weeks and demonstrated a slightly lower mortality rate (3.3% versus 3.9%) and recurrent stroke rate (1.6% versus 2.1%) in the aspirin group.[97]

Other oral antiplatelet drugs (e.g., clopidogrel, dipyridamole, ticlopidine) effective in secondary prevention have not been studied in acute stroke. A phase II study of abciximab, a GPIIb, IIIa receptor antagonist effective in acute myocardial infarction (MI) and in coronary artery stenting procedures, demonstrated safety and showed a trend toward better outcomes in the treated group. A phase III study is underway.[98]

Neuroprotection

Ischemic neuronal death results from a cascade of events set in motion by insufficient supply of oxygen and nutrients. As the understanding of the process grows, so does interest in drugs that may interfere with one or more steps in the process. However, several approaches that showed promise in laboratory models have foundered in clinical trials. Potentially, neuroprotective agents, such as dihydropyridine calcium channel blockers (nimodipine), N-methyl-D-aspartite-receptor antagonists (aptiganel), antibodies to intercellular adhesion molecules (elinomab), free radical scavengers (lubeluzole), and other agents with multiple putative mechanisms of action (citicholine, clomethiazole) have failed to show efficacy in phase III trials. Various explanations, including adverse effects limiting tolerable doses, inadequate delivery of drug to ischemic tissue, and delay in administration, have been given for the failure to replicate in clinical stroke positive responses shown in laboratory models. Although research continues and enthusiasm is high for the discovery of a potentially effective agent or combination of agents, no effective neuroprotective agent has yet been demonstrated.[99]

Acute Stroke Units

Thrombolysis is currently the most dramatic and effective form of acute stroke therapy, but is applied to only

TABLE 77.3. Effectiveness of different acute stroke interventions.

Intervention	Percent stroke population treatable	Percent absolute risk reduction	NNT
Stroke unit	80	6.6	15
Aspirin	80	1.2	83
Thrombolysis	5	6.5	15

Source: Adapted from Hankey,[100] with permission.

about 2% of all strokes in the United States. Aspirin is more widely applicable, and, while statistically significantly better than placebo in two large trials, its use results in an absolute risk reduction of about 1% in the outcome events measured; this translates into treating 100 patients to prevent one poor outcome. Anticoagulation is still widely used but is of no proven benefit. By far the most widely applicable, effective acute stroke intervention is the use of dedicated acute stroke units. In randomized trials, this approach reduces death or dependency from stroke by as much as thrombolysis but is applicable to all stroke patients.[100] The form that dedicated acute stroke units take varies from site to site and from country to country. Some focus on the initial 48h, whereas others include rehabilitation programs, but numerous studies have demonstrated their effectiveness relative to general medical or neurologic services. Although the characteristics of these units may vary, they share an integrated approach to patient care in which an interdisciplinary team including physician, nurse, and therapist are involved primarily in the care of stroke patients, work together as a team, and provide closer monitoring and more rapid assessment and treatment of the patient. As a result, short-term and long-term mortality rates are lower, hospitalizations are shorter, and patients are more likely to be discharged to home. The overall cost of the illness is also reduced[101] (Table 77.3).

Stroke Prevention

Although effective treatment of acute stroke exists, it is far preferable to prevent its occurrence. Effective prevention encompasses addressing stroke risk factors and treating specific etiopathologic mechanisms identified in a given individual.

Stroke Risk Factors

Hypertension is the most important modifiable stroke risk factor, as was first demonstrated by investigators in the Framingham Heart Study, who found that stroke risk increased proportional to both systolic and diastolic blood pressure throughout the measured range.[102] This effect has been found to be consistent across many

TABLE 77.4. Effectiveness of different secondary stroke prevention strategies.

Intervention	Percent of TIA/ischemic stroke eligible	Absolute risk reduction	Relative risk reduction	NNT
Hypertension control	50	2.2	28	45
Cholesterol lowering	40	1.7	24	60
Anticoagulation	20	8.0	67	12
Antiplatelet therapy[a]	75	1.2	23	83
Carotid endarterctomy	8	3.8	44	26

[a] Aspirin, clopidogrel, or aspirin + dipyridamole.
Source: From Hankey,[100] with permission.

populations.[103] Subsequent studies have demonstrated that reduction of blood pressure lowers stroke risk.[104] Treatment of isolated systolic hypertension is also clearly beneficial, especially in the elderly.[105,106] The choice of specific antihypertensive agent is less important than obtaining satisfactory control and should be determined by individual patient characteristics, although a recent study suggested that an ACE inhibitor may provide stroke protection beyond its antihypertensive effect.[107] Because ACE inhibitors are generally well tolerated in the elderly, this class of agents should be considered as initial antihypertensive treatment in a stroke-prone individual. Recent national guidelines suggest blood pressure of less than 140/85 (135/80 in diabetics) as the appropriate treatment goal.[108]

Hyperlipidemia

Elevated serum cholesterol is an important risk factor for coronary artery disease but its role in stroke is unclear. The Multiple Risk Factor Intervention Trial (MRFIT) screened 351,000 men and demonstrated a curvilinear relationship in which serum cholesterol greater than approximately 240 mg/dL was associated with an increased risk of ischemic stroke mortality, whereas a level less than 140 mg/dL was associated with an increased rate of intracerebral hemorrhage.[109] However, in a meta-analysis of 45 studies, the Prospective Studies Collaboration failed to find a relationship between total cholesterol and stroke among 450,000 individuals.[110] Similarly, neither the Framingham Study[111] nor the Cardiovascular Health Study[112] demonstrated a relationship between cholesterol and stroke. Consistent with these primarily negative findings, early cholesterol reduction studies showed a beneficial effect on heart disease but not stroke.

Surprisingly, the more recent results in trials using hydroxymethylglutaryl coenzyme A (HMG-CoA) reductase inhibitors consistently demonstrated a relative risk reduction of 20% to 30% for stroke, similar to the risk reduction demonstrated for the various cardiovascular

events studied,[113,114] This seemingly paradoxical finding may be explained by the putative beneficial effects of statins on platelets, plaque stabilization, smooth muscle cells, endothelial cell function, or inflammation, in addition to lowering LDL cholesterol.[115] The effect of triglycerides on stroke risk is also unclear, but a recent study of gemfibrozil demonstrated a similar degree of stroke risk reduction with minimal effect on high-density or low-density lipoproteins but significant lowering of triglycerides, suggesting triglycerides may also play a more significant role in stroke than previously recognized.[116] Current guidelines suggest treating individuals with coronary artery disease whose LDL cholesterol is greater than 130 mg/dL with a target less than 100 mg/dL. In view of the results of recent trials, extending these recommendation to patients with cerebrovascular disease seems prudent.

Other Factors

The Framingham Study was also among the first prospective cohort studies to demonstrate an increased stroke risk in cigarette smokers. Smokers had twice the risk of stroke as nonsmokers, but that risk was eliminated within about 2 years of cessation.[117]

Most studies have shown an increased risk of stroke with heavy alcohol consumption, but recently moderate consumption (<2 drinks/day) has been shown to be protective against stroke.[118] While urging heavy drinkers to decrease or eliminate their alcohol consumption is advisable for many reasons, the idea of encouraging nondrinkers to begin is controversial.

Elevated levels of homocysteine in the blood, termed hyperhomocysteinemia, has recently been associated with increased risk of stroke and myocardial infarction.[119] Individuals with levels above 15 μmol/L appear to have five times the risk of stroke of those with levels below 10 μmol/L. The efficacy of reducing stroke risk by lowering blood homocysteine levels with a combination of vitamins B_6, B_{12}, and folic acid is currently being assessed, but recommending the use of a multivitamin containing these elements, especially in the elderly, appears prudent.

Conditions Requiring Treatment

Atrial Fibrillation

As mentioned, atrial fibrillation (AF) is a particularly important risk factor in the elderly. Chronic AF in association with valvular heart disease increases stroke risk 17-fold, while in the absence of valvular disease stroke risk is still increased 5-fold.[120] Recent studies have identified factors that increase stroke risk in nonvalvular AF including older age, hypertension, recent onset of congestive heart failure, diabetes mellitus, a history of systemic embolism, or cerebral ischemia. Poor left ventricular function and increased left atrial size on echocardiogram also increase risk.[121]

Chronic anticoagulation with warfarin has been shown to be very effective in reducing stroke risk in patients in AF with and without a history of stroke. Anticoagulation should be prescribed for all patients who have had cerebral ischemic symptoms in the setting of AF unless there is a specific contraindication, and prophylactically in most patients who have been asymptomatic but have the additional risk factors mentioned, especially those over age 60.[122]

Carotid Stenosis

Narrowing of the lumen of the internal carotid artery is associated with an increased risk of stroke. A residual lumen of less than 20% of normal is highly correlated with the development of total occlusion of the internal artery or the development of symptoms related to that artery.[123] Endarterectomy is the most widely used specific treatment for this condition. In the past decade, several large-scale randomized trials involving symptomatic and asymptomatic individuals have provided data that allow a rational selection of appropriate patients for this procedure. In both the European Carotid Stenosis Trial (ECST)[124] and the North American Symptomatic Carotid Endarterectomy Trial (NASCET),[125] individuals with symptoms referable to a highly stenotic (70%–90%) carotid artery randomized to the nonsurgical arms had an estimated 28% 2-year stroke rate. The ipsilateral stroke rate was 22% in ECST and 26% in NASCET in these patients. Individuals with moderate symptomatic stenosis had stroke rates approximately one-half those of the highly stenotic groups. The benefit of surgery in reducing subsequent stroke risk in the symptomatic highly stenotic groups was clear-cut. This benefit disappeared once the degree of stenosis was less than 50% by NASCET criteria (comparable to approximately 75% by ECST criteria).[126] In the Asymptomatic Carotid Atherosclerosis Study, the benefit of carotid endarterectomy to asymptomatic individuals with at least 60% stenosis was less dramatic, and women with asymptomatic carotid stenosis may not benefit from endarterectomy at all.[127]

The benefit of surgery must be balanced against the risk for each individual. Life expectancy also plays a role in the decision-making process, because early morbidity including stroke and death is associated with the procedure; this should be less than 3% in experienced hands. Given these caveats, endarterectomy can be performed safely even in the very elderly and should be recommended for appropriate individuals of any age whose life expectancy is great enough to anticipate benefit despite the risk of early perioperative morbidity.

Antiplatelet Therapy

Antiplatelet therapy is the most commonly prescribed stroke prevention remedy and is usually appropriate for any symptomatic individual who does not require anticoagulation. Most patients are maintained on enteric-coated aspirin, with 325 mg daily the most commonly prescribed dose in the United States. However, much controversy exists. There is no consensus regarding the optimal dose, with recent recommendations suggesting a range of 50 to 325 mg,[128] although other authorities suggest higher doses are more effective if tolerated.[129] Newer medications such as Aggrenox (a combination of 25 mg aspirin and 200 mg dipyridamole in a sustained-release formulation), ticlopidine, and clopidogrel have been shown to have somewhat greater efficacy than aspirin in randomized trials, but maintenance on these medications currently costs in excess of $1000/year in the United States for an individual purchasing their drugs at a retail pharmacy. Because the differences among various agents are small when compared with the effect of taking no antiplatelet agent and compliance has been shown to be a major problem, attention should be directed at ensuring patients are compliant with whatever regimen is prescribed.

Conclusion

Despite recent advances in stroke treatment, prevention remains the most effective means of reducing the overall burden of stroke. Secondary prevention in patients who have experienced a transient ischemic attack (TIA) or stroke targets those at highest risk, but primary prevention in individuals at high risk because of the presence of the factors discussed here is also of great importance. Even among those with no identified stroke risk factors, on a population basis lower salt intake (accompanied by increased dietary potassium and calcium),[130] a diet high in folic acid and low in saturated fats, and no more than moderate alcohol consumption can forestall the development of vascular disease risk factors and reduce stroke incidence.

References

1. American Heart Association. *1999 Heart and Stroke Statistical Update*. Dallas: American Heart Association; 1998.
2. Murray CJL, Lopez AD. Mortality by cause for eight regions of the world: global burden of disease study. *Lancet*. 1997;349:1269–1276.
3. Broderick J, Brott T, Kothari R, et al. The Greater Cincinnati/Northern Kentucky Stroke Study: preliminary first-ever and total incidence rates of stroke among blacks. *Stroke*. 1998;29:415–421.

4. Gresham GE, Fitzpatrick TE, Wolf PA, et al. Residual disability in survivors of stroke: the Framingham Study. *N Engl J Med.* 1975;293:954–956.

5. Black-Schaffer RM, Osberg JS. Return to work after stroke: development of a predictive model. *Arch Phys Med Rehabil.* 1990;71:285–290.

6. Sacco RL, Boden-Albala B, Gan R, et at. Stroke incidence among white, black, and Hispanic residents of an urban community: the Northern Manhattan Stroke Study. *Am J Epidemiol.* 1998;147:259–268.

7. Sudlow CL, Warlow CP. Comparable studies of the incidence of stroke and its pathological types: results from an international collaboration. International Stroke Incidence Collaboration. *Stroke.* 1997;28:491–499.

8. Ingall TJ, Whisnant JP, Wiebers DO, et al. Has there been a decline in subarachnoid hemorrhage mortality? *Stroke.* 1989;20:718–724.

9. Sarti C, Tuomilehto J, Salomaa V, et al. Epidemiology of subarachnoid hemorrhage in Finland from 1983 to 1985. *Stroke.* 1991;22:848–853.

10. Kiyohara Y, Ueda K, Hasuo Y, et al. Incidence and prognosis of subarachnoid hemorrhage in a Japanese rural community. *Stroke.* 1989;20:1150–1155.

11. Phillips LH, Whisnant JP, O'Fallon WM, et al. The unchanging pattern of subarachnoid hemorrhage in a community. *Neurology.* 1980;30:1034–1040.

12. Sacco RL, Wolf PA, Bharucha NE, et al. Subarachnoid and intracerebral hemorrhage: natural history, prognosis, and precursive factors in the Framingham Study. *Neurology.* 1984;34:847–854.

13. Longstreth WT Jr, Nelson LM, Koepsell TD, et al. Clinical course of spontaneous subarachnoid hemorrhage: a population-based study in King County, Washington. *Neurology.* 1993;43:712–718.

14. Juvela S, Hillbom M, Numminen H, et al. Cigarette smoking and alcohol consumption as risk factors for aneurysmal subarachnoid hemorrhage. *Stroke.* 1993;24:639–646.

15. Oyesiku NM, Colohan AR, Barrow DL, et al. Cocaine-induced aneurysmal rupture: an emergent factor in the natural history of intracranial aneurysms? *Neurosurgery.* 1993;32:518–526.

16. Ingall TJ, Wiebers DO. National history of subarachnoid hemorrhage. In: Whisnant JP, ed. *Stroke: Populations, Cohorts and Clinical Trials.* Oxford: Batterworth-Heimann; 1993:174–186.

17. Kassell NF, Torner JC, Haley EC Jr, et al. The International Cooperative Study on the Timing of Aneurysm Surgery. Part 1: Overall management results. *J Neurosurg.* 1990;73:18–36.

18. Hunt WE, Hess RM. Surgical risk as related to time of intervention in the repair of intracranial aneurysms. *J Neurosurg.* 1968;28:14–20.

19. Jennett B, Bond M. Assessment of outcome after severe brain damage. *Lancet.* 1975;1:480–484.

20. Fisher CM, Kistler JP, Davis JM. Relation of cerebral vasospasm to subarachnoid hemorrhage visualized by computerized tomographic scanning. *Neurosurgery.* 1980;6:1–9.

21. Adams HP Jr, Kassell NF, Torner JC, et al. Predicting cerebral ischemia after aneurysmal subarachnoid hemorrhage: influences of clinical condition, CT results, and antifibrinolytic therapy. A report of the Cooperative Aneurysm Study. *Neurology.* 1987;37:1586–1591.

22. Caplan LR, Flamm ES, Mohr JP, et al. Lumbar puncture and stroke. *Stroke.* 1987;18:540A–544A.

23. Forster DM, Steiner L, Hakanson S, et al. The value of repeat pan-angiography in cases of unexplained subarachnoid hemorrhage. *J Neurosurg.* 1978;48:712–716.

24. Taylor TN, Davis PH, Torner JC. Projected number of strokes by subtypes in the year 2050 in the United States. *Stroke.* 1998;322 [abstract].

25. Broderick JP, Adams HP Jr, Barsan W, et al. Guidelines for the management of spontaneous intracerebral hemorrhage: a statement for healthcare professionals from a special writing group of the Stroke Council, American Heart Association. *Stroke.* 1999;30:905–915.

26. Bamford J, Sandercock P, Dennis M, Burn J, Warlow C. A prospective study of acute cerebrovascular disease in the community: the Oxfordshire Community Stroke Project—1981–1986. 2. Incidence, case fatality rates and overall outcome at one year of cerebral infarction, primary intracerebral and subarachnoid haemorrhage. *J Neurol Neurosurg Psychiatry.* 1990;53:16–22.

27. Foulkes MA, Wolf PA, Price TR, Mohr JP, Hier DB. The Stroke Data Bank: design, methods, and baseline characteristics. *Stroke.* 1988;19:547–554.

28. Broderick JP, Brott T, Tomsick T, Huster G, Miller R. The risk of subarachnoid and intracerebral hemorrhages in blacks as compared to whites. *N Engl J Med.* 1992;326:733–736.

29. Furlan AJ, Whisnant JP, Elveback LR. The decreasing incidence of primary intracerebral hemorrhage: a population study. *Ann Neurol.* 1979;5:367–373.

30. Giroud M, Gras P, Chadan N, et al. Cerebral hemorrhage in a French prospective population study. *J Neurol Neurosurg Psychiatry.* 1991;54:595–598.

31. Sacco RE, Mayer SA. Epidemiology of intracerebral hemorrhage. In: Feldmann E, ed. *Intracerebral Hemorrhage.* New York: Futura; 1994:3–23.

32. Suzuki K, Kutsuzawa T, Takita K, et al. Clinicoepidemiologic study of stroke in Akita, Japan. *Stroke.* 1987;18:402–406.

33. Qureshi Al, Glies WH, Croft JB. Racial differences in the incidence of intracerebral hemorrhage: the effect of blood pressure and education. Results from the First National Health and Nutrition Survey Epidemiologic Follow-up Study. *Neurology.* 1999;52:1617–1621.

34. Brott T, Thalinger K, Hertzberg V. Hypertension as a risk factor for spontaneous intracerebral hemorrhage. *Stroke.* 1986;17:1078–1083.

35. Omae T, Ueda K. Risk factors for cerebral stroke in Japan: prospective epidemiologic study in Hisayama community. In: Katsuki S, Tsubaki T, Toyokura Y, eds. *Proceedings of the 12th World Congress of Neurology.* Amsterdam: Excerpta Medica; 1982:119.

36. Thrift AG, McNeil JJ, Forbes A, Donnan GA. Three important subgroups of hypertensive persons at greater risk of intracerebral hemorrhage. Melbourne Risk Factor Study Group. *Hypertension.* 1998;31:1223–1229.

37. Qureshi AI, Suri MAK, Safdar K, Ottenlips JR, Janssen RS, Frankel MR. Intracerebral hemorrhage in blacks: risk factors, subtypes, and outcome. *Stroke.* 1997;28:961–964.

38. Klatsky AL, Armstrong MA, Friedman GD. Alcohol use and subsequent cerebrovascular disease hospitalizations. *Stroke.* 1989;20:741–746.

39. Gorelick PB. Alcohol and stroke. *Stroke.* 1987;18:268–271.

40. Brott T, Broderick J, Kothari R, et al. Early hemorrhage growth in patients with intracerebral hemorrhage. *Stroke.* 1997;28:1–5.

41. Broderick JP, Brott TG, Tomsick T, Barsan W, Spilker J. Ultra-early evaluation of intracerebral hemorrhage. *J Neurosurg.* 1990;72:195–199.

42. Kazui S, Minematsu K, Yamamoto H, Sawada T, Yamaguchi T. Predisposing factors to enlargement of spontaneous intracerebral hematoma. *Stroke.* 1997;28:2370–2375.

43. Yang GY, Betz AL, Chenevert TL, Brunberg JA, Hoff JT. Experimental intracerebral hemorrhage: relationship between brain edema, blood flow, and blood-brain barrier permeablity in rats. *J Neurosurg.* 1994;81:93–102.

44. Mohr JP, Caplan LR, Melski JW, et al. The Harvard Cooperative Stroke Registry: a prospective registry. *Neurology.* 1978;28:754–762.

45. Andrews BT, Chiles BW III, Olsen WL, Pitts LH. The effect of intracerebral hematoma location on the risk of brain-stem compression and on clinical outcome. *J Neurosurg.* 1998;69:518–522.

46. Ott KH, Kase CS, Ojemann RG, Mohr JP. Cerebellar hemorrhage: diagnosis and treatment. A review of 56 cases. *Arch Neurol.* 1974;31:160–167.

47. Ropper AH, Gress DR. Computerized tomography and clinical features of large cerebral hemorrhages. *Cerebrovasc Dis.* 1991;1:38–42.

48. Melo TP, Pinto AN, Ferro JM. Headache in intracerebral hematomas. *Neurology.* 1996;47:494–500.

49. Qureshi AI, Safdar K, Weil J, et al. Predictors of early deterioration and mortality in black Americans with spontaneous intracerebral hemorrhage. *Stroke.* 1995;26:1764–1767.

50. Mayer SA, Sacco RL, Shi T, Mohr JP. Neurologic deterioration in noncomatose patients with supratentorial intracerebral hemorrhage. *Neurology.* 1994;44:1379–1384.

51. Broderick JP, Brott T, Duldner JE, Tomsick T, Huster G. Volume of intracerebral hemorrhage: a powerful and easy-to-use predictor of 30-day mortality. *Stroke.* 1993;24:987–993.

52. Tuhrim S, Horowitz DR, Sacher M, Godbold JH. Validation and comparison of models predicting survival following intracerebral hemorrhage. *Crit Care Med.* 1995;23:950–954.

53. Juvela S. Risk factors for impaired outcome after spontaneous intracerebral hemorrhage. *Arch Neurol.* 1995;52:1193–1200.

54. Tuhrim S, Dambrosia JM, Price TR, et al. Intracerebral hemorrhage: external validation and extension of a model for prediction of 30-day survival. *Ann Neurol.* 1991;29:658–663.

55. Hill MD, Silver FL, Austin PC, Tu JV. Rate of stroke recurrence in patients with primary intracerebral hemorrhage. *Stroke.* 2000;31:123–127.

56. Arakawa S, Saku Y, Ibayashi S, Nagao T, Fujishima M. Blood pressure control and recurrence of hypertensive brain hemorrhage. *Stroke.* 1998;29:1806–1809.

57. Kim JS, Lee JH, Lee MC. Small primary intracerebral hemorrhage. Clinical presentation of 28 cases. *Stroke.* 1994;25:1500–1506.

58. Huston J, Nichols DA, Luetmer PH, et al. Blinded prospective evaluation of sensitivity of MR angiography to known intracranial aneurysms: importance of aneurysm size. *Am J Neuroradiol.* 1994;15:1607–1614.

59. Gujjar AR, Deibert E, Manno EM, Duff S, Diringer MN. Mechanical ventilation for ischemic stroke and intracerebral hemorrhage: indications, timing, and outcome. *Neurology.* 1998;51:447–451.

60. Poungvarin N, Bhoopat W, Viriyavejakul A, et al. Effects of dexamethasone in primary supra-tentorial intracerebral hemorrhage. *N Engl J Med.* 1987;316:1229–1233.

61. Tellez H, Bauer RB. Dexamethasone as treatment in cerebrovascular disease. 1: A controlled study in intracerebral hemorrhage. *Stroke.* 1973;4:541–546.

62. Carlberg B, Asplund K, Hagg E. The prognostic value of admission blood pressure in patients with acute stroke. *Stroke.* 1993;24:1372–1375.

63. Kuwata N, Kuroda K, Funayama M, Sato N, Kubo N, Ogawa A. Dysautoregulation in patients with hypertensive intracerebral hemorrhage. A SPECT study. *Neurosurg Rev.* 1995;18:237–245.

64. Qureshi AI, Bliwise DL, Bliwise NG, Akbar MS, Uzen G, Frankel MR. Rate of 24-hour blood pressure decline and mortality after spontaneous intracerebral hemorrhage: a retrospective analysis with a random effects regression model. *Crit Care Med.* 1999;27:480–485.

65. Tietjan CS, Hurn PD, Ulatowski JA, Kirsch JR. Treatment modalities for patients with intracranial pathology: options and risks. *Crit Care Med.* 1996;24:311–322.

66. Mutlu N, Berry RG, Alpers BJ. Massive cerebral hemorrhage. Clinical and pathological correlations. *Arch Neurol.* 1963;8:644–661.

67. Tuhrim S, Horowitz DR, Sacher M, Godbold JH. Volume of ventricular blood is an important determinant of outcome in supratentorial intracerebral hemorrhage. *Crit Care Med.* 1999;27:617–621.

68. Mayer SA, Kessler DB, Van Hurtum RL, Thomas CE, Fink ME. Effect of intraventricular blood on global corticol perfusion in acute intracerebral hemorrhage: a single photon emission tomographic study. *Ann Neurol.* 1995;38:228 [abstract].

69. Adams RE, Diringer MN. Response to external ventricular drainage in spontaneous intracerebral hemorrhage with hydrocephalus. *Neurology.* 1998;50:519–523.

70. Pang D, Sclabassi RJ, Horton JA. Lysis of intraventricular blood clot with urokinase in a canine model. Part 3. Effects of intraventricular urokinase on clot lysis and posthemorrhagic hydrocephalus. *Neurosurgery.* 1986;19:553–572.

71. Todo T, Usui M, Takakura K. Treatment of severe intraventricular hemorrhage by intraventricular infusion of urokinase. *J Neurosurg.* 1991;74:81–86.

72. Mayfrank L, Lippitz B, Groth M, Bertalanffy H, Gilsbach JM. Effect of recombinant tissue plasminogen activator on

clot lysis and ventricular dilatation in the treatment of severe intraventricular hemorrhage. *Acta Neurochir.* 1993; 122:32–38.

73. Rohde V, Schaller C, Hassler WE. Intraventricular recombinant tissue plasminogen activator for lysis of intraventricular haemorrhage. *J Neurol Neurosurg Psychiatry.* 1995;58:447–451.

74. Findlay JM, Grace MG, Weir BK. Treatment of intraventricular hemorrhage with tissue plasminogen activator. *Neurosurgery.* 1993;32:941–947.

75. Coplin WM, Vinas FC, Agris JM, et al. A cohort study of the safety and feasibility of intraventricular urokinase for nonaneurysmal spontaneous intraventricular hemorrhage. *Stroke.* 1998;29:1573–1579.

76. Matsumoto K, Hondo H. CT-guided stereotaxic evacuation of hypertensive intracerebral hematomas. *J Neurosurg.* 1984;61:440–448.

77. Niizuma H, Suzuki J. Stereotactic aspiration of putaminal hemorrage using a double track aspiration technique. *Neurosurgery.* 1988;22:432–436.

78. Hondo H, Uno M, Sasaki K, et al. Computed tomography controlled aspiration surgery for hypertensive intracerebral hemorrhage. Experience of more than 400 cases. *Stereotact Funct Neurosurg.* 1990;54–55:432–437.

79. Montes JM, Wong JM, Fayad PB, Arvad IA. Stereotactic computer tomographic-guided aspiration. *Stroke.* 2000;31: 834–840.

80. Faught E, Peters D, Bartolucci A, Moore L, Miller PC. Seizures after primary intracerebral hemorrhage. *Neurology.* 1989;39:1089–1093.

81. Berger AR, Lipton RB, Lesser ML, Lantos G, Portenoy RK. Early seizures following intracerebral hemorrhage: implications for therapy. *Neurology.* 1988;38:1363–1365.

82. Cervoni L, Artico M, Salvati M, Bristot R, Franco C, Delfini R. Epileptic seizures in intracerebral hemorrhage: a clinical and prognostic study of 55 cases. *Neurosurg Rev.* 1994;17:185–188.

83. Gilbert JJ, Vinters HV. Cerebral amyloid angiopathy: incidence and complications in the aging brain. *Stroke.* 1983;4:915–923.

84. Finelli PF, Kaessimian N, Bernstein PW. Cerebral amyloid angiopathy magnifesting as recurrent intracerebral hemorrhage. *Arch Neurol.* 1984;41:330–333.

85. Vinters HV. Cerebral amyloid angiopathy: a critical review. *Stroke.* 1987;18:311–324.

86. Wolf PA, Abbott RD, Kannell AB. Atrial fibrillation as an independent risk factor for stroke: the Framingham Study. *Stroke.* 1991;22:983–988.

87. Alweiss GS, Goldman ME. Transesophaged echocardiography: diagnostic and clinical applications in the evaluation of the stroke patient. *J Stroke Cerebrovasc Dis.* 1997; 6:332–336.

88. Amarenco P, Cohen A, Tzoruirio C, et al. Atherosclerotic disease of the aortic arch and the risk of ischemic stroke. *N Engl J Med.* 1994;331:1474–1479.

89. Fisher CM. Lacunar strokes and infarcts: a review. *Neurology.* 1982;32:871–876.

90. Caplan L. "Top of the basilar" syndrome. *Neurology.* 1980; 30:72–79.

91. Hacke W, Brott T, Caplan L, et al. Thrombolysis in acute ischemic stroke: controlled trials and clinical experience. *Neurology.* 1999;53(suppl 7):S53–S14.

92. Katzan IL, Furlan AJ, Lloyd LE, et al. Use of tissue-type plasminogen activator for acute ischemic stroke: the Cleveland Area Experience. *JAMA.* 2000;283:1151–1158.

93. Furlan A, Higashida R, Wechsler L, et al. Intra-arterial prourokinase for acute ischemic stroke: the PROACT II study. *JAMA.* 1999;282:2003–2011.

94. The International Stroke Trial (IST). A randomized trial of aspirin, subcutaneous heparin, both, or neither among 19,435 patients with acute ischemic stroke. *Lancet.* 1997; 349:1569–1581.

95. The Publications Committee for the Trial of ORG 10172 in Acute Stroke Treatment (TOAST) Investigators. How molecular weight heparinoid, ORG 10172 (danaparoid), and outcome after acute ischemic stroke: a randomized controlled trial. *JAMA.* 1998;279:1265–1272.

96. Berge E, Abdelnoor M, Nahstad PH, Sandset PM, on behalf of the HAEST Study Group. How molecular-weight heparin versus aspirin in patients with acute ischemic stroke and atrial fibrillation: a double-blind randomised study. *Lancet.* 2000;355:1205–1210.

97. CAST (Chinese Acute Stroke Trial) Collaborative Group. CAST: randomised placebo-controlled trial of early aspirin use in 20,000 patients with acute ischaemic stroke. *Lancet.* 1997;349:1641–1649.

98. Adams HP, Bogourslawsky J, Baurathan E, et al. Abciximab in acute ischemic stroke—a randomized, double-blind, placebo-controlled, dose-escalation study. *Stroke.* 2000;31:601–609.

99. Lee J-M, Zipfel GJ, Choi DW. The changing landscape of ischaemic brain injury mechanisms. *Nature.* 1999;399 (suppl):A7–A14.

100. Hankey GJ. Stroke: how large a public health problem and how can the neurologist help? *Arch Neurol.* 1999; 718–754.

101. Stroke Unit Trialists Collaboration. How do stroke units improve patient outcomes? *Stroke.* 1997;28:2139–2144.

102. Kannel WB, Wolf PA, Verter J, McNamara PM. Epidemiologic assessment of the role of blood pressure in stroke. The Framingham Study. *JAMA.* 1970;214:301–310.

103. Collins R, MacMahon S. Blood pressure, antihypertensive drug treatment and the risks of stroke and of coronary heart disease. *Br Med Bull.* 1994;50:272–298.

104. Hypertension Detection and Follow-up Program. III. Reduction in stroke incidence among persons with high blood pressure. *JAMA.* 1982;247:633–638.

105. SHEP Cooperative Research Group. Prevention of stroke by antihypertensive drug treatment in older persons with isolated systolic hypertension. Final results of the Systolic Hypertension in the Elderly Program (SHEP). *JAMA.* 1991;265:3255–3264.

106. Staessen JA, Fagard R, Thijs L, et al. Randomised double-blind comparison of placebo and active treatment for older patients with isolated systolic hypertension. *Lancet.* 1997;350:757–764.

107. The Heart Outcomes Prevention Evaluation Study Investigators. Effects of an angiotension-converting-enzyme inhibitor ramipril on death from cardiovascular causes,

myocardial infarction and stroke in high-risk patients. *N Engl J Med.* 2000;342:145–153.

108. Anonymous. The sixth report of the Joint National Committee on prevention, detection, evaluation and treatment of high blood pressure. *Arch Intern Med.* 1997;157:2413–2446.

109. Iso H, Jacobs DRJ, Wentworth D, et al. Serum cholesterol levels and six year mortality from stroke in 350,977 men screened for the MRFIT. *N Engl J Med.* 1989;320:9804–9810.

110. Prospective Studies Collaboration. Cholesterol diastolic blood pressure and stroke: 13,000 strokes in 450,000 people in 45 prospective cohorts. *Lancet.* 1995;346:1647–1653.

111. Wolf PA, D'Agostino RB, O'Neal MA, et al. Secular trends in stroke incidence and mortality: the Framingham Study. *Stroke.* 1992;23:1551–1555.

112. Fried LP, Borhani NO, Enright P. et al. The Cardiovascular Health Study: design and rationale. *Ann Epidemiol.* 1991;1:263–276.

113. Hebert PR, Gaziano JM, Chan KS, Hennekens CH. Cholesterol lowering with statin drugs, risk of stroke and total mortality: an overview of randomized trials. *JAMA.* 1997;278:313–321.

114. LIPID's Study Group. Prevention of cardiovascular events and death with mavastatin in patients with coronary heart disease and a broad range of initial cholesterol levels. *N Engl J Med.* 1998;339:349–357.

115. Furberg CD. Natural statins and stroke risk. *Circulation.* 1999;99:185–188.

116. Rubins HB, Robins SJ, Collins D, et al. Gemfibrozil for the secondary prevention of coronary heart disease in men with low levels of high density lipoprotein cholesterol. *N Engl J Med.* 1999;341:410–418.

117. Wolf PA, D'Agostino RB, Kanrntel WB, et al. Cigarette smoking as a risk factor for stroke. *JAMA.* 1998;259:1025–1029.

118. Sacco RL, Elkind M, Boden-Albala B, et al. The protective effect of moderate alcohol consumption on ischemic stroke. *JAMA.* 1999;28l:1112–1120.

119. Giles WH, Croft JB, Greenlund KJ, Ford LS, Kittner SJ. Total homocyst(e)ine concentration and the likelihood of nonfatal stroke: results from the Third National Health and Nutrition Examination Survey, 1988–1994. *Stroke.* 1998;29:2473–2477.

120. Wolf PA, Abbott RD, Kannel WB. Atrial fibrillation as an independent risk factor for stroke in the Framingham Study. *Stroke.* 1991;22:983–988.

121. Atrial Fibrillation Investigators. Risk factors for stroke and efficacy of antithrombotic therapy in atrial fibrillation: analysis of pooled data from five randomized trials. *Arch Intern Med.* 1994;154:1449–1457.

122. Ezekowitz MD, Levine JA. Preventing stroke in patients with atrial fibrillation. *JAMA.* 1999;281:1830–1835.

123. Roederer GO, Langlois YE, Jager KA, et al. The natural history of carotid arterial disease in asymptomatic patients with cervical bruits. *Stroke.* 1984;15:605–613.

124. European Carotid Surgery Trialist's Collaborative Group. MRC European Carotid Surgery Trial: interim results for symptomatic patients with severe (70–99%) or with mild (0–19%) carotid stenosis. *Lancet.* 1991;337:1235–1243.

125. North American Symptomatic Carotid Endarterectomy Trial Collaborators. Beneficial effect of carotid endarterectomy in patients with high-grade carotid stenosis. *N Engl J Med.* 1991;325:445–451.

126. Chassin MR. Appropriate use of carotid endarterectomy. *N Engl J Med.* 1998;339:1468–1471.

127. Barnett HJM, Meldrum HE, Eliasziw M. The dilemma of surgical treatment for patients with asymptomatic disease. *Ann Intern Med.* 1995;123:723–725.

128. Albers GW, Easton JD, Sacco RL, Teal P. Antithrombotic and thrombolytic therapy for ischemic stroke. *Chest.* 1998;114:6385–6985.

129. Dyken ML, Barnett HJ, Easton JD, et al. Low-dose aspirin and stroke. "It ain't necessarily so." *Stroke.* 1992;23:1395–1399.

130. Sacks FM, Svetkey LP, Vollmer WM, et al. Effects on blood pressure of reduced dietary sodium and the Dietary Approaches to Stop Hypertension (DASH) diet. *N Engl J Med.* 2001;344:3–10.

78
Abnormalities of Posture and Movement

José C. Masdeu and María Cruz Rodriguez-Oroz

There exists a large group of cases where the gait in old people becomes considerably disordered, although the motor power of the legs is comparatively well preserved. A paradoxical state of affairs is the result: testing of the individual movements of the legs while the patient reclines upon the couch shows little, if any, reduction in the strength . . . But when the patient is instructed to get out of bed and to walk, remarkable defects may be witnessed. The patient, first of all, appears most reluctant to make the attempt. His stance is bowed and uncertain. He props himself against the end of the bed and seeks the aid of the bystanders. Encouraged to take a few steps, he advances warily and hesitatingly. Clutching the arms of two supporters, he takes short, shuffling steps. The legs tend to crumple by giving way suddenly at the knee joints. Progression, as far as it is possible, is slow and tottery.

McDonald Critchley, 1948[1]

Postural abnormalities in older persons lead to falls, which are discussed in Chapter 66. This chapter first reviews the neurologic basis of postural impairment, and its etiology and treatment; it concludes with a review of other movement disorders. Of the topics discussed here, postural impairment has the greatest impact on disability and is by far the most prevalent. Although most older people have preserved distal function of the extremities, so that they can write and brush their teeth, many have poor postural reflexes, a cautious gait, and risk falling. Despite its prevalence, for many physicians, the condition is still as mysterious as it was for Dr. Critchley, whose masterful quote introduces this chapter. For this reason, it is discussed here in some detail.

Postural reflexes become most evident and are most critical when the person stands and walks, but they are also involved in a number of other motor activities. Dr. Critchley noted that his patients fared well while in bed, but had he asked them to move up in bed, he would have witnessed a marked impairment in the ability to perform this simple maneuver. Caregivers to the elderly are instinctively so aware of this fact that they make sure to place the patient in an adequate position in bed. Other-

wise, the patient may remain in an awkward or uncomfortable position, unable to shift in bed as required to correct it. The postural system runs in the background, controlling those movements we do not attend to. This "automatic pilot" of the motor system has its own neural pathways and is affected by specific diseases, the object of this chapter. *Stance, equilibrium,* and *balance* are terms that refer to the ability or act of maintaining the erect posture. Gait or ambulation presupposes the ability to stand, although the neural mechanisms underlying these two motor functions are far from identical. Surprisingly, some patients experience more difficulty standing than walking, for instance, those with orthostatic tremor.[2] The emphasis of this chapter is not so much on the diagnosis of neurologic disorders that secondarily result in ambulation difficulties, such as stroke causing hemiplegia, but on disorders that primarily affect the ability to stand or walk, often without overt weakness, as described in Critchley's quote.[1] Disorders of stance and gait can be the presenting syndrome of many different pathologies along the neuraxis. Clinical localization before the use of ancillary diagnostic testing is essential if ancillary procedures are to be applied in a focused and economical manner that will minimize the likelihood of false-positive findings.[3]

When diagnosing postural disorders, it is useful to think about the neurologic systems underlying the control of gait and balance.[4,5] At the simplest level, gait requires sensory information and a motor output. Sensory information includes proprioception, vision, and vestibular input. On the motor side, the corticospinal, vestibulospinal, and reticulospinal tracts convey to the cord output from higher centers. In their turn, the anterior horn cells through their axons stimulate muscles that turn that output into specific movements.

Sensory systems can be tested by exploring the performance of the patient while one or two varieties of sensory input are removed and the postural reflexes depend on the remaining sensory information. For instance, the Romberg test explores the patient's ability to maintain a steady upright posture with vision removed and the base of support reduced by keeping the feet together. Proprioceptive or vestibular loss will result in difficulty maintaining balance. To test the intactness of the corticospinal tract, spinal cord, peripheral nerves, and muscles, the examiner asks the patient to wiggle her toes, to draw a circle on the floor with each foot, and to extend the big toe against resistance. Proximal muscle strength in the legs can be tested by asking the patient to rise from a low chair without using her arms to prop herself up. Despite the patient's ability to complete quite well all these tasks, they may still have difficulty walking and a propensity to falling. This apparent discrepancy highlights the importance of neural systems critical for posture, which are distinct from the system mediating volitional leg and foot movements.[4] In addition to the vestibular and cerebellar input, the function of the basal ganglia and of several brainstem nuclei, including the pedunculopontine nucleus, plays an important role in the control of postural and locomotor activity. Normally, this activity is unconscious, carried on in the background, for instance, while the person concentrates their attention on fetching something from the refrigerator, rather than on the activity of walking.

Epidemiology

Postural disorders are particularly frequent in the elderly population. The Duke study of normal aging estimated that gait disturbances affect 15% of the elderly, being the most frequent neurologic impairment in this age group.[6] Among the elderly, falls are the leading source of injury-related deaths.[7] In the United States, about 9500 deaths among people age 65 years or older are attributed each year to a falling episode. Falling is also a major cause of morbidity among older people. Eighty-four percent of the approximately 200,000 hip fractures occurring yearly affect people older than 65. Most of these cases are related to a fall. Hip fracture is the most common injury leading to hospitalization in this age group.[8]

Etiology of Postural Disorders in Older Adults

Unlike that in younger adults, postural impairment in older people seldom results from a single etiology. Most often, partial impairment of multiple systems is responsible for the impaired balance and gait witnessed by the clinician. In about one-fourth of the cases, however, one of the factors contributing to postural impairment can be corrected enough to reverse the disability. The task of the clinician is to identify the causes contributing to postural

impairment and to sort out the correctable ones. Still, a large number of elderly patients have idiopathic postural impairment: the identifiable causes do not explain satisfactorily why an individual patient has a tendency to fall.

The multifactorial genesis of postural impairment in the older adult cannot be overemphasized. Studies of falls have illustrated that individuals who fall typically have more than one risk factor for falling.[9] Robbins and coworkers found that the predicted 1-year risk of falling ranged from 12% for persons with none of three risk factors (i.e., hip weakness assessed manually, unstable balance, and taking four or more prescribed medications) to 100% for persons with all three risk factors.[10] It is also likely that older persons with vestibular dysfunction alone will not experience gait difficulties, but the rule is that proprioception and vision are also impaired to some extent. As a result, the vestibular dysfunction becomes symptomatic. To sensory deficits, impairment of central processing is added in many older adults. Corticobasal-ganglionic-thalamocortical mechanisms can be affected by a drop of dopaminergic neurons or neurons belonging to other systems, as in many of the disorders considered later in this chapter, fiber damage by chronic ischemia in the white matter watershed, lateral to the ventricular angles, or other mechanisms still poorly understood.

In some published series, the majority of patients were assigned a primary cause for their gait or postural disorder.[11,12] Other authors failed to find a cause in the majority of patients.[13] This discrepancy may reflect (1) different patient populations; a single diagnosis may be more readily identifiable in a general medical or neurologic practice, whereas in gait disorders clinics the proportion of idiopathic gait disorders is larger, possibly because patients with Parkinson's disease and other readily identifiable disorders are not referred to specialized centers for evaluation; or (2) a different diagnostic approach; sensory deficits, for instance, are very prevalent in the elderly with or without gait disorders; finding a sensory deficit, some clinicians may consider it responsible for the gait disorder, whereas others may think that a different etiology must be at work to explain the clinical picture. Whether a given etiology is the main culprit for the patient's gait difficulties is often not the key question, but rather whether a correctable cause can be found and addressed. Even a modest functional improvement may forestall the dismal consequences of repeated falls.

In a series of 120 older adults referred to a neurologist for an undiagnosed gait disorder, Sudarsky reported the frequency of each etiology.[12] Sensory deficits represented the largest single neurologic cause of postural instability. This etiology, myelopathy, and multiple infarcts accounted for half the cases. In 14% of the cases, the etiology remained undetermined. The rest fell under the categories of parkinsonism, cerebellar degeneration, hydrocephalus, an assortment of other causes (including neoplasms and subdural hematoma), psychogenic gait disorders, and toxic or metabolic causes. In 50 consecutive patients older than 50 years of age admitted to a neurologic service because of walking difficulty, Fuh and coworkers identified the following causes: multiple cerebral infarcts, 24%; myelopathy, 22%; parkinsonism, 12%; cerebellar degeneration, 8%; brain tumor, 6%; Binswanger's, 4%; Alzheimer's, 4%; other diseases, 10%; and unknown etiology, 10%.[14] The miscellaneous category included a patient with chronic inflammatory demyelinating polyneuropathy. Patients with undetermined gait disorder were older than 60 and had "senile gait." Potentially treatable causes of gait impairment were found in nearly one-third of patients.

Following is an anatomic list of the major etiologic categories responsible for postural impairment. They are listed from the more peripheral causes, including muscle weakness, to the etiologies affecting primarily the control centers of the brain.

Muscle Weakness

Many older adults with gait difficulties blame their problem on muscle weakness. With age, muscle mass and strength decrease, even in normal people. Muscle mass is lost at a rate of 0.5% to 1.0% annually in women and men over 60 years, and muscle strength loss ranges from 20% to 40% from the third to the eighth decades and may be even greater in the eighth decade.[15] Weakness is due to loss of muscle mass and contractility (force/cm^2 of muscle cross section). The good news is that vigorous physical activity is associated with maintaining muscle strength, mass, and contractility.[15] Diseases of muscle or the neuromuscular junction are rarely responsible for gait impairment in the older adult. Polymyositis and myasthenia gravis can give rise to limb weakness. In this case, isometric weakness is more pronounced than the gait impairment, alerting the clinician to the possibility of muscle disease. Disorders of muscles and joints are discussed in Chapters 42 through 46.

Sensory Deficits

Sensory deficits ranked first as the responsible etiology in some series of unselected patients referred for postural impairment.[12] While often proprioception, vestibular function, and vision are all affected, there are specific disorders that involve one modality more than the other two.

To clarify testing for sensory function crucial for gait, it is important to review briefly the physiology of sensory postural control. Proprioception, vestibular function, and vision are all required because no single sense can measure directly the position of the center of gravity of the body to place it within the base of support, a condition of stability in bipedal stance and gait.[5] The somatosensory input provides information on the orientation of body parts relative to one another and to the support surface. Vision measures the orientation of the eyes and head in relation to surrounding objects. The vestibular system measures gravitational, linear, and angular accelerations of the head in relation to inertial space. As the person stands or walks, the brain must quickly select the sensory inputs providing accurate information, because often one or more of the three sensory systems may provide information that is misleading for the purposes of balance control. For instance, when a person stands beside a large bus that begins to move slowly, the visual system conveys the false impression that the person is moving in the opposite direction. Nashner has called *sensory organization* the process of selecting and combining sensory information appropriate for balance control.[5] Faulty sensory organization, or one that relies primarily on an impaired sensory system, may lead to unsteadiness when walking. Some simple clinical maneuvers, such as Romberg's, can help sort out gross deficiencies in one sensory modality, and specialized testing with posturography is seldom needed to evidence subtler changes.

Proprioception

Somatosensory input dominates the control of balance when the support surface is steady. Even with vision removed, a patient with bilateral vestibular loss but good proprioception can stand normally.[5] Several disorders that can affect primarily proprioception are reviewed in turn. Many other disorders can affect proprioception in the older adult, including toxic neuropathies induced by cisplatin or nitrous oxide.

Vitamin-Induced Neuropathies

B$_{12}$ Deficiency

Pernicious anemia with deficient production of intrinsic factor is the most common cause of B$_{12}$ deficiency, many cases occurring in older people.[16] B$_{12}$ deficiency is also observed due to chronic intestinal malabsorption and rarely to dietary deficiency. The daily requirement for B$_{12}$ is only 5μg/day. Neuropathy and myelopathy (subacute combined systems degeneration) can occur without hematologic manifestations.

The onset is insidious, beginning with distal paresthesias, weakness, and unsteadiness of gait, particularly difficulty walking in the dark. Proprioceptive loss in the legs and sensory ataxia can grow quite severe. Lhermitte's sign is often present, reflecting damage of the dorsal columns. Tendon reflexes are typically depressed to absent. An extensor plantar response is characteristically observed, and, with time, a spastic-ataxic gait as well.

B$_{12}$ assay is used for screening, and Schilling test for confirmation of true pernicious anemia. The disorder is important to recognize as it is occasionally encountered in the elderly and is a treatable cause of imbalance and gait disorder. With B$_{12}$ therapy, gait improves fully in a majority of patients with duration of neurologic signs under 3 months.[16]

Megadose Pyridoxine Neuropathy

Chronic ingestion of megadoses (2–6 g/day) of *pyridoxine* (vitamin B$_6$) has also been associated with an ataxic peripheral neuropathy.[16] Both proximal and distal parts of the body are simultaneously affected by sensory loss of the large fiber modalities. The other major clinical features are ataxia and pseudoathetosis without severe weakness. Sensory loss may be heralded by Lhermitte's sign, severe paresthesias, or dysesthesias.[17] Pyridoxine intoxication kills dorsal root ganglia cells at high doses and impairs their metabolism at lower toxic doses, so that both their peripherally and centrally directed axons degenerate. Axonal regeneration can occur when excessive pyridoxine is eliminated.[16] Diagnostic testing for this disorder relies on the history and on the improvement subsequent to elimination of excessive pyridoxine intake.

Chronic Immunomediated Disorders

Paraneoplastic Sensory Neuropathy (Anti-Hu)

This disorder affects primarily the dorsal root ganglia cells. Paresthesias or dysesthesias generally move from a distal to proximal direction, but some cases have shown early sensory changes in proximal areas, including the face.[16] Position and vibration sense are most severely affected, with consequent severe sensory ataxia as well as pseudoathetosis in the outstretched limbs.[18] There is early, widespread absence of reflexes. The associated neoplasm is most often a small cell cancer of the lung. The neuropathy may precede the clinical appearance of the carcinoma for longer than 3 years but more often by only a few months. The neuropathy often progresses in a subacute fashion but may then level off. Although treatment of the underlying neoplasm usually has no effect on the neuropathy, there are some rather dramatic single cases associated with reversal after effective treatment of the primary neoplasm. Pathologic observations show a lymphocytic infiltration of dorsal root ganglia with a marked depopulation of dorsal root ganglion cells and Nageotte nodules. The peripheral sensory axons degenerate, but there is also degeneration in the centrally directed axon because the dorsal columns, particularly the gracile sectors, are severely affected.

This type of carcinomatous neuropathy is often associated with cerebrospinal fluid and serum antibodies that react with dorsal root ganglia (IgG anti-Hu antibodies).

These antibodies also react with a brain nuclear protein and an identical antigen that is highly specific for small cell lung cancer.[18] The spinal fluid of these patients often contains a few mononuclear cells (5–50/mm^3) with elevations of protein as high as several grams. Unfortunately, the response to immunosuppression is usually poor.[19]

Sensory Neuropathy of Sjögren's Syndrome

Sjögren's syndrome, characterized by keratoconjunctivitis sicca, xerostomia sicca, and a rheumatoid-like arthritis, is often accompanied by a sensory polyneuropathy or polyganglionopathy.[20,21] More frequent in women, this disorder can present with gait disorder due to deafferentation.[21,22] Minor salivary gland biopsy is frequently positive.[20] Vasculitic neuropathy or nonspecific epineurial inflammation may be found on nerve biopsy. Antibodies to extractable nuclear antigens are the most specific serologic marker of Sjögren's syndrome, but this was present in only 10% of patients with the sicca complex and neuropathy but no arthritis.[20] Treatment with immunosuppression is not satisfactory. There are preliminary data suggesting a better response to low-dose oral alpha-interferon or zidovudine.[23,24]

Chronic Idiopathic Ataxic Neuropathy

Chronic ataxic sensory neuropathy is a slowly progressive illness with distal paresthesias and sensory ataxia, areflexia, normal strength, and a profound loss of proprioceptive and kinesthetic sensation extending up to the most proximal joints.[25] Many of these patients have uncomfortable paresthesias with a severe loss of balance in the dark. The ataxia may be accompanied by pseudoathetosis. Sabin has studied several patients with sensory ganglionopathies who complained bitterly of very uncomfortable "pulling" and "stretching" sensations when they tried to move about and as a result confined themselves to bed and chair existence.[16] Many patients have a serum monoclonal, mostly IgM, or polyclonal gammopathy; and some have elevated cerebrospinal fluid gamma globulin levels in spite of low normal total cerebrospinal fluid protein levels.[25] Response to immunosuppressant strategies has been poor.[25]

GALOP Syndrome

Some of the milder cases of chronic ataxic neuropathy may actually have GALOP (gait disorder; autoantibody; late-age onset; polyneuropathy), a milder syndrome, often responsive to treatment.[26,27] GALOP is characterized by the presence of IgM antibodies reactive with central myelin antigen (CMA). Pestronk and coworkers described nine patients, of an average age of 70 years, with anti-CMA antibodies, eight of whom had disabling difficulty with ambulation, "out of proportion to that expected for age."[27] The gait disorder developed over a period of 2 to 15 years and presented as slow ambulation and frequent falling, particularly backward. Patients walked with small steps and had difficulty turning. Some of them had moderate distal weakness in the legs, but a sensory loss in a stocking distribution was common, although not as pronounced as that seen in ataxic sensory neuropathies. Romberg sign was strikingly positive. Most helpful for diagnostic testing is an ELISA assay detecting very high titers (>1 : 10,000) of serum IgM binding to a central nervous system myelin antigen (CMA) preparation that copurifies with myelin-associated glycoprotein (MAG).[26] Some patients who were treated with intravenous immunoglobulin or cyclophosphamide experienced improvement.[27]

Chronic Inflammatory Demyelinating Polyneuropathy

Although not typically the main presentation, gait impairment can occur in the demyelinating polyneuropathies.[16] Hyperacute Guillain–Barré syndrome (GBS) is misdiagnosed in the emergency room when a healthy-appearing patient is observed to stagger about with a bizarre ataxia and complain of only tingling paresthesias. Examination reveals good strength, which may be sustained only in irregular bursts, damped reflexes, and normal sensation as tested in the usual way. The patient is often released from the emergency room with a diagnosis of hysteria, but hours later may require emergency care for evolving widespread flaccid paralysis. This early ataxic phase of GBS might also be caused by a physiologic effect of large fiber demyelination that is concentrated in the posterior roots. Some patients recovering from GBS go through a phase of ataxia that is out of proportion to loss of strength or position sense. Likewise, chronic inflammatory demyelinating polyneuropathy (CIDP) may present as an ataxic syndrome. The degree of gait impairment corresponds to the degree of motor-sensory loss.[28] Occasionally, CIDP may induce ataxia by causing a vestibular syndrome.[29] CIDP relapses are treated with corticosteroids or intravenous immunoglobulin.[30]

Vestibular Disorders

Older people who complain of unsteadiness when walking often have a normal standard neurologic examination. Fife and Baloh used rotational vestibular testing and quantitative posturography to study 26 such individuals older than 75 years of age and found vestibular impairment in all of them, as compared to age-matched controls.[31] Lesions of the vestibular region may present with unilateral or bilateral findings. Unilateral findings are not uncommon in vascular disorders, such as the

Wallenberg syndrome, which is not rare in older patients. With infarction, patients tend to fall to the side of the infarct. Their gait is broad based and lurching. Removal of vision by environmental darkness or impaired eyesight affects negatively their ability to ambulate and predisposes them to falls. Initially, most of these patients have a prominent headache and are nauseated. In addition to the impairment of balance and ataxia ipsilateral to the lesion, they have a crossed sensory loss (on the ipsilateral face and contralateral body), an ipsilateral Horner's syndrome, and ipsilateral palatal weakness, with hoarseness and dysphagia. Atherosclerotic vascular disease of the vertebral or posteroinferior cerebellar arteries may occlude these vessels and is responsible for this syndrome in about half of the cases.[32] Most the rest are caused by cardiogenic emboli. Spontaneous dissection of the arterial wall is a frequent cause in younger,[33] but not in older, patients, where temporal arteritis should be suspected, particularly in the very old with a high sedimentation rate.[34] In a small autopsy series of patients with temporal or giant cell arteritis, the vertebral arteries were found to be affected in all cases.[35] Polymyalgia rheumatica may be present but is not a universal finding. The superficia temporal arteries are often tender and swollen, with a faint pulse. Temporal arteritis responds well to prednisone therapy.

Bilateral findings are present in Wernicke's encephalopathy of vitamin B_1 deficiency, occasionally seen in elderly with a poor nutritional status.

Vision

Visual loss and, particularly, distorted visual input can have a major effect in the gait of an older person who already has some sensory loss in the other two modalities essential for maintaining balance, namely, proprioception and vestibular function. Before lens implants became commonplace, older adults having cataract surgery often went through a period of time when they found it difficult to walk normally and were afraid of falling. Eventually their brain learned to integrate the new visual information for the purpose of maintaining balance. To a lesser degree, some of the same difficulty can result from a change in prescription glasses in persons who have proprioceptive or vestibular impairment. On the other hand, these patients find it helpful to walk in areas that are well lighted, optimizing the use of visual clues and thus facilitating steadiness. The diagnosis and treatment of visual disorders is discussed in Chapter 60.

Spinal Claudication

The term *spinal claudication* comprises several disorders that cause the patient to experience radicular pain or leg weakness after having walked or stood still for a while. It differs from vascular claudication in the localization and nature of the pain, but more so in that peripheral pulses are not markedly depressed. Spinal claudication generally results from compression of the cauda equina and the lumbosacral roots by a narrow spinal canal, with tight lateral recesses leaving little room for the exiting roots. In some patients, compression of the radicular arteries, and particularly the artery of Adamkiewicz, feeding the conus and epiconus, may cause cord ischemia and leg weakness. Three factors play in this anatomic situation: (1) the patient was born with a narrow canal; (2) degenerative disease of the spine with facet joint and ligament hypertrophy contributes to crowding even further the space available to the cauda equina, roots, and radicular vessels; and (3) exaggeration of the lumbar lordosis in the upright position worsens the compression of these structures.

Although this syndrome is real, it is rare. Unfortunately, some older adults who complain of gait difficulties have a lumbosacral MRI performed "just in case." When this test shows marked degenerative changes in their spine, with a narrow canal, the tendency is to diagnose the disease based on the imaging findings. Particularly in this case, it is extremely important to correlate carefully the imaging findings with the clinical presentation. Severe degenerative changes are the rule in MRI of the lumbosacral spine in persons older than 70 years and may be found in asymptomatic subjects of all ages.[36–38] The clinical history is more important than the imaging findings to make the diagnosis. The history must be scrutinized. Other causes of gait impairment cause "gait claudication" because patients tire from having to attend to their gait and being fearful of a fall. For instance, many patients with parkinsonism have to sit after having stood for a short while because their "legs get heavy." Anxiety over a fall can cause "weak legs." Onset or worsening of characteristic radicular pain, on the other hand, favors spinal claudication. MRI findings are helpful to plan the surgery, but some surgeons prefer to rely on CT, which shows bone changes better than MRI. EMG may show denervation changes in a radicular distribution or, rarely, may be normal in the resting state. By themselves, EMG changes are not diagnostic. The treatment of true spinal claudication is surgical decompression.

Cervical Myelopathy

Although lumbosacral stenosis is seldom the cause of gait difficulties in the older adult, cervical myelopathy from cervical spondylosis was the second most common cause in both Sudarsky's and Fuh's series.[12,14] Because it is potentially treatable, cervical myelopathy should be considered in any older adult presenting with postural impairment in the upright position. Some patients present with the characteristic clinical picture of cervical radicular pain and spastic paraparesis, but most do not have radicular pain. Initially, at the time when surgery is most likely to be successful and prevent further deterioration, the gait impairment may be very subtle, noticeable to the patient but yielding minimal findings on neurologic examination.[39] The paucity of findings may delay the diagnosis. In the Yale series, the investigators believed that the diagnosis had been delayed on average by 6.3 years.[39] The earliest consistent symptom in all their 22 patients was a gait abnormality. These patients may become unsteady when closing their eyes and standing with feet together. They are unable to walk in tandem. The brachioradialis reflex may be depressed and, instead, a brisk finger flexor response is elicited when percussing the brachioradialis tendon (inverted radial reflex). Careful testing of vibratory sense may reveal a sensory level in the cervical region. Sometimes the patient perceives the stimulus better in the thumb than in the small finger. Early diagnosis is important, because the myelopathy of cervical spondylosis is often progressive if untreated.[39]

In terms of diagnostic testing, all the precautions discussed in the previous section on spinal stenosis apply here as well. MRI of the cervical spine is helpful, but, in the absence of the clinical findings, the presence of spondylitic changes by themselves does not make the diagnosis. Rather severe changes can be seen in asymptomatic older adults.[40–43] Plain x-rays are helpful in determining the shape of the cervical spine, the alignment of the vertebrae, the status of the bone, the vertical extent of the disease process, the degree of anterior and posterior osteophytes, and the nature of the disk spaces. Baseline plain x-rays are also quite useful when surgery is being considered for comparison with postoperative x-rays or when the patient cannot undergo MRI, for instance, in the case of someone bearing a pacemaker. Several recent studies agree that MRI is the screening test of choice in most instances.[39,44] Bony osteophytes can be seen as black ridges compressing the canal and, if the compression is severe, causing high-intensity changes in the spinal cord on T_2-weighted images.

In addition to the narrowing of the spinal canal by spondylitic hypertrophy of bones and ligaments, two changes are frequently observed in the cord itself: decreased diameter and a hyperintense signal on T_2-weighted images. How often a hyperintense area is observed depends on the stage of progression, with gliosis and microcavitation of the gray matter, and other poorly understood factors. In some series, as many as 40% of the patients have this finding.[45] Although some have found the presence of this finding and its irreversibility after surgery to predict a poor outcome, others have not.[45,46] MRI may show other changes within the spinal cord itself due to chronic compression such as syrinx formation.

MRI is also of great value in the differential diagnosis of myelopathy, as conditions such as tumor and infection can be easily ruled out. In multiple sclerosis, an abnormal signal may be found in the spinal cord and elsewhere in the brain due to the presence of plaques. MRI is a satisfactory alternative to myelography for most patients with suspected cervical spondylotic myelopathy.[44]

However, MRI scan is not so good as CT in showing osteophytes or ossification of the posterior longitudinal ligament. If surgical treatment is contemplated, thin-slice CT of the cervical spine after intrathecal introduction of a nonionic water-soluble contrast material is of great help. MRI scan, CT scan, and CT myelography are all complementary tests and not mutually exclusive. CT myelography is most valuable when deciding on the surgical approach, either anterior or posterior. CT myelography also allows for accurate measurement of the spinal canal in the axial, sagittal, and coronal planes. A canal diameter less than 12 mm in the anteroposterior plane is considered stenotic. Ossification of the posterior longitudinal ligament (OPLL) is sometimes found in patients with cervical spondylotic myelopathy. OPLL may be segmental or continuous in the cervical spine. CT myelography is particularly useful for diagnosing this entity, which has significant bearing on the type of surgical procedure to be performed.

Somatosensory evoked responses can be normal in half of patients with symptomatic cervical myelopathy.[47] Motor responses from magnetic stimulation and spinal cord evoked potentials are more sensitive.[48–50] Occasionally, these electrophysiologic tests can be useful when the clinical picture is less than conclusive.[51] More often, in mild cases they are inconclusive as well. Postdecompression improvement of somatosensory evoked responses has predicted faster recovery but not the 1-year outcome of surgical patients.[52] Most neurosurgeons do not require these data as part of the presurgical battery.

Cerebellar Disorders

Cerebellar lesions may affect posture by causing disequilibrium and by altering limb and trunk kinematics and interlimb coordination.[53] The cerebellum does not appear to actually generate postural and gait synergies because these automatic responses, albeit very dysmetric, are present in dogs with total cerebellectomies.[54]

Disturbances of gait and balance are primarily caused by lesions of the vestibulocerebellum and spinocerebellum or their connections. Lesions of the cerebellar hemispheres cause irregular timing, force, and cadence of leg movements, leading to inaccurate and variable stepping.[55] Lesions of the *vestibulocerebellum*, or floccular-nodular lobe, can produce balance, and gait disturbances that resemble those caused by vestibular lesions.[53] Tremor of the head and trunk, truncal imbalance, and swaying and falling in all directions are characteristic of vestibulocerebellar lesions. Vestibular nystagmus may be present. The clinical syndrome caused by lesions of the *spinocerebellum* is best characterized by alcoholic cerebellar degeneration, which primarily affects the anterior lobe of the cerebellum but also involves the olivary complex and the vestibular nuclei.[56] Patients with alcoholic cerebellar degeneration have a widened base, instability of the trunk, and a slow and halting gait with irregular steps and superimposed lurching. The gait abnormalities are accentuated at the initiation of gait, on turning, and with changes in gait speed. These patients may have severe gait ataxia without nystagmus, dysarthria, or arm dysmetria. Even the heel-to-shin test may give little inkling of the severity of the gait disturbance. Interestingly, if patients stop drinking and have adequate nutrition, the gait improves such that the steps are no longer irregular and tandem walking or sudden movements are necessary to demonstrate the gait ataxia.[56] Although most often patients with cerebellar lesions tend to fall to the side of the lesion, some patients with lesions in the tonsillar area develop increased tone (and increased reflexes) in the ipsilateral side and fall to the contralateral side.

Ischemic and hemorrhagic strokes are the most frequent causes of cerebellar dysfunction in the older adult.[53] Gait impairment is the most frequent presentation of infarcts in the territory of the superior cerebellar artery.[32] In the older age group, infarction in the territory of the posterior inferior cerebellar artery is caused by atheromatous vascular disease as often as by embolic disease. Presumed cerebral embolism was the predominant stroke mechanism in patients with superior cerebellar artery distribution infarcts.[32]

The clinical presentation of cerebellar hemorrhage may be acute, subacute, or chronic.[57,58] Variations in location, size, and development of the hematoma; brainstem compression; fourth ventricular penetration; and development of hydrocephalus result in variations in the mode of presentation of cerebellar hemorrhage. These hemorrhages most frequently occur in the region of the dentate nucleus. Patients present with occipital or frontal headache, dizziness, vertigo, nausea, repeated vomiting, and inability to stand or walk. They often have truncal or limb ataxia, ipsilateral gaze palsy, and small reactive pupils. Horizontal gaze paresis, paretic nystagmus, and facial weakness are also frequent. Frank hemiparesis is absent. Ocular bobbing and skew deviation may be present. Not all patients present such a dramatic picture; those with small (usually less than 3 cm in diameter) cerebellar hematomas may present only with vomiting and with no headaches, gait instability, or limb ataxia. Anatomic findings that predict deterioration with cerebellar hemorrhage include displacement of the fourth ventricle, brainstem deformity, hydrocephalus, and compression of the basal cisterns.[59,60] In some series, a hematoma larger than 3 cm also worsens prognosis.[60] Clinically, patients fare poorly who have abnormal corneal and oculocephalic responses, a Glasgow coma score less than 8, and motor response less than localization to pain.[60]

Degenerative diseases of the cerebellum include disease restricted to the cerebellum and diseases with extracerebellar involvement, such as olivopontocerebellar ataxia (OPCA) or multisystem atrophies, discussed in greater detail later.[53] Spinocerebellar degenerations typically begin at a younger age.

Paraneoplastic cerebellar syndromes can be seen in bronchial, breast, and ovarian cancer.[53] The symptoms include ataxia of gait and stance, limb ataxia, terminal tremor, gaze-evoked nystagmus, and disturbed smooth pursuit eye movements.

Toxic cerebellar syndromes in older people are frequently caused by slower drug metabolism and reduced tolerance.[53] All centrally acting drugs may lead to cerebellar disturbances of stance and gait. The drugs most frequently responsible for toxic disturbances include alcohol, antiepileptic drugs, lithium, and tranquilizers.

Vascular Disease

Vascular disease of the brain ranks among the top three causes of gait impairment in the older adult.[12,14] Those affected are patients referred for progressive gait impairment, not stroke patients with secondary hemiparesis and gait difficulty. Vascular disease causing this syndrome most often affects the supratentorial compartment in the form of lacunar disease or ischemic disease of the white matter. Less often, it involves the posterior circulation, involving vestibular or cerebellar structures, as already described, and very rarely other brainstem structures important for gait, such as the mesencephalic locomotor center. Lacunar disease is discussed first, followed by white matter disease and finally the syndrome of the mesencephalic locomotor center. CT and MRI are the diagnostic tests most useful for the study of these syndromes.

Lacunar Disease of Gait: Critical Structures

Ischemic brain disease tends to follow one of three patterns, discernible by clinical evaluation and with the help of neuroimaging procedures: (1) cortical infarcts, most often related to embolic disease; (2) subcortical disease, often in the form of widespread lacunes and white matter changes, most often related to arteriolar disease; and (3) a mixture of the two patterns, often related to atheromatous disease of the major vessels.[3] The second and third types of cerebrovascular disease tend to cause gait and

balance impairment early in the course of the disease. Subcortical infarcts strategically located may impair equilibrium and gait with little or no limb weakness on isometric testing. These lesions tend to affect structures with a critical role in gait and balance mechanisms, including the orticobasal-ganglionic-thalamocortical loop. Although acute stroke tends to be associated with overt neurologic findings, gait impairment may be neglected as a neurologic finding and yet be the result of small, "silent" lacunar strokes.[61] In a cohort of clinically asymptomatic patients studied during the Asymptomatic Carotid Artery Stenosis trial, Brott and coworkers documented lacunar strokes with CT in 11% of the patients.[62] These patients were more likely to have gait impairment.

Thalamic Astasia or Disequilibrium

Inability to stand or walk despite minimal weakness has been recorded with thalamic infarction or hemorrhage, particularly when the superior portion of the ventrolateral nucleus or suprathalamic white matter was involved.[63,64] It has also been reported in patients with lesions in the internal capsule or corona radiata who had the syndrome of unilateral ataxia and crural paresis (ataxic hemiparesis).[65] Alert, with normal or near-normal strength on isometric muscle testing and a variable degree of sensory loss, these patients could not stand and some with acute lesions could not sit up unassisted; they fell backward or toward the side contralateral to the lesion. These patients appeared to have a deficit of overlearned motor activity of an axial and postural nature. In the vascular cases, the deficit improved in a few days or weeks. However, these patients had a tendency to sustain falls during the rehabilitation period.

Capsular and Basal Ganglia Lesions

A tendency to fall despite good strength was recorded by Groothuis et al.[66] in a patient with a small medial capsular hemorrhage involving the most lateral portion of the ventrolateral nucleus of the thalamus and by Labadie and coworkers in patients with acute lesions in the basal ganglia.[67] Multiple bilateral lacunae involving the basal ganglia can be attended by gait impairment.

White Matter Disease

In controlled studies of elderly prone to falling, impaired gait and balance correlated with the presence of white matter disease on CT or MRI.[68–72] Periventricular white matter changes were present in cases of "lower body parkinsonism."[73,74]

Because the histology underlying these changes remains elusive in some cases, Hachinski et al. coined the descriptive term leuko-araiosis for the CT findings.[75] Several authors have reported normal histology, but ischemic changes similar to the findings in subcortical arteriosclerotic encephalopathy (SAE) have been present in cases with pronounced changes on T_1-weighted MM or CT.[76] Amyloid angiopathy has been incriminated in the genesis of white matter disease in some elderly individuals.[77,78] In addition to white matter changes, amyloid angiopathy results in subcortical hemorrhages. Some ischemic leukoencephalopathies of middle-aged and older people, such as CADASIL (cerebral autosomal dominant arteriopathy with subcortical infarcts and leukoencephalopathy), are familial.[79]

Pontomesencephalic Gait Failure

The laterodorsal region of the midbrain contains the mesencephalic locomotor region, which plays an important role in locomotion in animals.[80] In humans, loss of neurons in the pedunculopontine nucleus has been found in progressive supranuclear palsy and victims of Parkinson's disease, but not in patients with Alzheimer's disease, implying perhaps a role of this nucleus in ambulatory mechanisms. Discrete vascular damage in this region can give rise to a disorder bearing striking resemblance to the idiopathic gait failure experienced by many elderly individuals, which in most cases does not have a clear anatomic correlate.[81,82]

Toxic or Metabolic Encephalopathies

Because these encephalopathic disorders are often treatable causes of gait impairment, it is important to recognize metabolic or toxic agents, most often in the form of medications. Psychotropic, diuretic, antihypertensive, and antiparkinsonian medications, especially if used in improper doses, may contribute to falls in the elderly by decreasing alertness, depressing psychomotor function, or causing weakness, fatigue, dizziness, or postural hypotension.[83–85] These adverse physiologic effects may be exacerbated by altered drug metabolism in elderly individuals. Although not confirmed by all studies, there is good evidence that hypnotic-anxiolytic drugs, particularly benzodiazepines, increase the risk of falls.[10,86–88] The role of diuretic, antihypertensive, and other medications linked to orthostatic hypotension in increasing the risk of falls is uncertain and needs further investigation.[84] Several studies have found an association of falls with the number of medications being taken; this could reflect synergistic effects among drugs, but could also be related to the poorer health of individuals taking multiple medications.

Patients with metabolic encephalopathy often display an insecure gait and may fall over backward if displaced. This phenomenon is particularly dramatic with uremia and hepatic failure, in which asterixis may impair stance.[12]

Parkinsonian Syndromes

The parkinsonian syndromes share an impairment in posture and gait. Spontaneous movements on the part of the patient are diminished. There is increased resistance to passive range of motion. The concatenation of these clinical findings is known as *parkinsonism*. However, although the most frequent entity responsible for parkinsonism is idiopathic Parkinson's disease, some other disorders can induce a similar disturbance, and a careful differential diagnosis must be considered, as is discussed next.

Parkinson's Disease

Parkinson's disease (PD) is a common disorder among the elderly population. Thus, its incidence increases with age from less than 10 per 100,000 at age 50 to more than 200 per 100,000 at age 80.[89] After the ninth decade, its incidence appears to decline, but these data are likely to be an artifact derived from poor ascertainment and the smaller size of the population of this age. The gender distribution shows a slightly greater incidence in males, and there is no conclusive evidence for race differences. Epidemiologic studies have been conducted trying to identify risk factors for PD. Apart from increasing age, the strongest risk factor associated with PD is the presence of disease in a family member.

Clinical manifestations in PD are caused by the loss of dopaminergic cells in the pars compacta of the substantia nigra (SNpc), and the subsequent loss of nigrostriatal dopaminergic modulation of the neural mechanism for movement control.[90]

Clinical Features

The cardinal manifestations of Parkinson's disease are tremor, rigidity, akinesia, and postural instability with associated gait disorder. Postural and gait disturbances usually appear later in the course of typical Parkinson's disease, whereas they are an early manifestation of the "Parkinson plus" disorders, such as progressive supranuclear palsy, striatonigral degeneration, multisystem atrophy, and corticobasal ganglionic degeneration.[90]

Tremor

The parkinsonian tremor is typically a resting tremor that disappears when a voluntary movement is performed. Electromyographic recording of the muscles involved shows a rhythmic alternating activity at 4 to 6 Hz between agonist and antagonist muscles. Distal joints are preferentially affected (i.e., metacarpophalangeal), and some distracting maneuvers, such as counting, induce an increment in its magnitude. In some patients there is also a postural tremor of higher frequency (7–12 Hz), with additional involvement of more proximal joints.

Rigidity

Parkinsonian rigidity consists of an involuntary increment in muscle tone in flexor and extensor muscle groups. This sign is clinically expressed by stiffness of the muscles at palpation and on passive range of motion, and by the spontaneous flexion of the joints in all extremities. It is caused by a continuous muscle activity that makes relaxation impossible. The most typical feature of rigidity is an augmented resistance to passive joint displacement on examination that can be smooth (lead pipe-like) or rackety (cogwheel-like). Simultaneous movements in other body segments provoke an increment in rigidity (Froment's rigidity sign). It is more evident when the passive movement is slowly executed, a feature that separates it from spasticity, in which the tone increases with a higher velocity of motion. When rigidity is severe, it may even restrict the range of passive displacement of a joint.

Akinesia

Although, strictly speaking, *akinesia* means absence of movements, this term includes both the slowness and clumsiness in the execution of movements and the reduction of spontaneous and induced movements. More specifically, *bradykinesia* refers to the slowness of the movement, which is more evident during complex tasks when several muscle groups are working on a sequence of movements. *Hypokinesia* refers to the poverty of spontaneous movements, a reduction in their amplitude, and their occasional freezing. It is easily recognized in the reduction of the frequency and amplitude of automatic movements such as blinking, arm swing while walking, step length, reaching movements, and writing (micrographia).

The three cardinal features of Parkinson's disease usually appear asymmetrically, affecting first one half of the body and spreading to the contraleral limbs and to the axial muscle in further stages. This pattern is of diagnostic importance, because other parkinsonian syndromes tend to cause rigidity and akinesia of both sides of the body from the inception of the disease.

Postural Instability and Gait Disturbance

These abnormalities begin at a later stage of the disease, usually after other signs have already appeared, and they are responsible to a great extent for the deterioration in the motor condition and quality of life of parkinsonian patients.[91] If posture and gait disturbances start when the cardinal features of Parkinson's disease are already

present, the diagnosis is not difficult. Even when gait is affected early, however, it has characteristics that can help the diagnosis, especially in the early stages.[92] Initially, patients have a mildly flexed posture that slowly worsens, evolving to flexion of the knees, trunk, elbows, wrists, and metacarpophalangeal joints, with the arms adducted to the trunk. Loss of postural reflexes may occur soon after the diagnosis, but it is not disabling until intermediate or advanced stages, when the patient loses the capacity to make rapid postural adjustments and becomes prone to falling forward or backward. On clinical examination, postural reflexes can be tested by standing behind the patient and pulling them backward on the shoulders ("pull test"). Normally, this maneuver only elicits a contraction of the tibialis anterior muscle that will correct the backward tilt. With milder disease, patients may take one or two steps backward until catching themselves, but in more advanced stages they will be unable to maintain their equilibrium, and the examiner must keep them from falling.

As the disease progresses, stride length becomes progressively shortened. At this point shuffling is a common finding, and turning is typically made up of several small steps. In a more advanced stage gait freezing appears. Initially it occurs when starting to walk (start hesitation), turning (turn hesitation), or passing through narrow spaces and in stressful situations. Eventually, this phenomenon may occur at any time, especially with environmental stimuli such as sounds or visual stimuli that attract the patient's attention, causing them to stop.[93] With gait freezing, the patient's feet seem to be stuck to the floor and they become unable to raise their legs. Freezing is caused by the simultaneous contraction of agonist and antagonist muscles in the leg, instead of the alternating sequence necessary for a plantar flexion followed by a dorsal flexion of the foot. The base of support is narrow, and the patient does not accompany the attempt to move the feet with truncal or swing movement. Freezing can be overcome using sensory tricks, mainly visual, for instance, by stepping on a piece of paper on the floor, or with a different motor strategy such as a military march.[94] Once gait has been initiated, the first two or three steps are even shorter than usual. Sometimes the patient may raise her feet a few millimeters, but instead of taking a normal step, she drags her foot forward a few centimeters, developing a shuffling gait. Once gait has been initiated, it is not infrequent that the forward flexor posture, shifting the center of gravity forward, and the failure of postural reflexes make the patient walk faster in a shuffling way trying to restore her center of gravity (festinating gait) and finally falling forward. Forward falls are more frequent than backward falls in Parkinson's disease, whereas in parkinsonian disorders other than idiopathic Parkinson's disease the patient tends to fall backward.

Differential Diagnosis

A parkinsonian gait can be observed in conditions other than idiopathic Parkinson's disease. However, some subtle differences in posture and gait, and the presence of signs not usually present in Parkinson's disease, may help in the diagnosis. Because the disorder of gait and posture in Parkinson's disease is basically induced by a deficit in striatal dopaminergic modulation, any other process disrupting the same mechanism can cause a similar disorder. There are several illnesses in which the degenerative process involves not only the substantia nigra, as in Parkinson's disease, but other structures as well. These entities include multisystem atrophies (i.e., striatonigral degeneration, pontocerebellar atrophy, Shy–Drager), corticobasal ganglionic degeneration, progressive supranuclear palsy (PSP), Alzheimer's disease, diffuse Lewy body disease, Creutzfeldt–Jakob disease, the rigid variant of Huntington's disease, and some even less common disorders. The differential diagnosis is based on the presence of clinical findings that are atypical for Parkinson's disease, such as cerebellar disturbances, severe autonomic failure, limb apraxia, supranuclear ophthalmoplegia, early cognitive impairment, marked postural instability, or absence of response to levodopa treatment. Beside these atypical findings, the characteristics of the parkinsonian syndrome itself often differ from typical Parkinson's disease. For instance, resting tremor is usually absent, and the syndrome conforms to the more rigid akinetic forms of parkinsonism. Some of these disorders affect at onset both halves of the body, including the axial muscles. The facial expression has been compared to a "perplexed face," with a widened palpebral opening and a wrinkled forehead. Postural and gait disturbances occur earlier in the course than in Parkinson's disease, and consist mainly of a marked postural instability, with frequent falls forward and backward, and a shuffling or freezing gait. The base of support is generally wider than in Parkinson's disease. Other differential diagnostic considerations include subcortical vascular disease and normal pressure hydrocephalus.

Beside these primarily neurologic diseases, there are some systemic disorders than can induce a clinical picture similar to that of Parkinson's disease, including gait abnormalities; this is the case with hypothyroidism, hypoparathyroidism, and other endocrine disorders and depression. Drugs easily induce parkinsonism among the geriatric population, so this possibility should be taken into consideration during the differential diagnosis. The most important medications are neuroleptics, antihypertensives (reserpine, alpha-methyldopa, some calcium channel blockers), and other antidopaminergic drugs such as metoclopramide used as antiemetics. Parkinsonism may be also secondary to encephalitis and to toxins such as carbon monoxide, manganese, mercury, methane, cyanide, and MPTP, but these are rarely seen in daily practice.

Treatment

Pharmacologic Therapy

Levodopa, which is transformed into dopamine by the remaining nigral neurons, continues to be the "gold standard" in the treatment of Parkinson's disease. It is administered with a peripheral dopa-decarboxylase inhibitor (benserazide or carbidopa) to prevent its peripheral conversion to dopamine and increase its cerebral bioavailability. Dopamine in the systemic circulation causes a number of side effects, including nausea, vomiting, hypotension, and cardiac arrhythmias. Levodopa treatment, however, is not a panacea. After several years of levodopa treatment, and perhaps due to the natural evolution of the disease, the originally smooth response becomes less than satisfactory. Mobility begins to fluctuate depending on levodopa intake first ("wearing off") and in a random way later ("on-off"), and the patient may experience dyskinesias or involuntary movements during the phase of motor benefit, as well as psychiatric symptoms. The origin of these complications is not completely understood, but the pulsatile administration of levodopa is known to be a risk factor.[95] Recently, therapeutic strategies have been developed to provide a more steady dopaminergic stimulation. Slow-release levodopa formulations and direct dopamine agonists, including bromocriptine, pergolide, lisuride, ropinirole, and pramipexole, maintain more stable striatal dopaminergic stimulation. Direct agonists are being used in the initial stages of the disease, alone or in association with low doses of levodopa, to prevent or delay the development of these complication.[96] The most common side effects of these drugs are nausea, orthostatic hypotension, and psychiatric complications.

Early in the disease, levodopa is generally more effective than direct agonists and, with selegiline (see following), tends to be preferred as the first-line drug. However, a clinical trial using a dopamine agonist as monotherapy in the early stages of the disease has shown a lesser incidence of motor complications than with the use of levodopa alone after 5 years of treatment.[97] Another strategy to maintain steady dopaminergic stimulation involves the use of entacapone, a peripheral inhibitor of catechol-O-methyltransferase (COMT), an enzyme that accelerates the catabolism of levodopa.[98] Its use in association with levodopa prolongs the elimination half-life of levodopa, increasing the time of pharmacologic benefit and providing a more physiologic dopaminergic stimulation. At present, it is used mainly in patients with motor complications.

Gait freezing usually responds to levodopa therapy and dopamine agonists. However, sometimes the benefit is of less magnitude than for the rest of the parkinsonian features. In our experience, the use of amantadine as coadjuvant therapy is useful in these cases. Its mechanism of action is not clear, but it has anticholinergic and antiglutamatergic activity. The main side effects are livedo reticularis and ankle edema, plus the usual anticholinergic side effects. In a few cases freezing can be aggravated by levodopa therapy, and it is then extremely difficult to treat.

Anticholinergic therapy has no clear benefit for parkinsonian gait. These drugs were used mainly to treat sialorrhea and tremor; tremor responds just as well to levodopa therapy. Their adverse effects, more pronounced in an older population (urinary retention, angle-closure glaucoma, constipation, and cognitive and psychiatric deficits), have contributed to making them obsolete.

So far we have considered symptomatic treatments that simply alleviate the motor deficits in Parkinson's disease. However, after the diagnosis of Parkinson's disease is made, the degenerative process of the dopaminergic neurons of the substantia nigra continues and contributes decisively to the patient's worsening. Neuroprotective therapies are being developed, directed at preventing neuronal death and rescuing those neurons in the process of degeneration.[99] No drug has proved its efficacy in clinical trials, but there are several experimental studies showing the neuroprotective activity of selegiline.[100] Because this drug inhibits monoamine oxidase B (MAO B), an enzyme that favors the catabolism of dopamine, it increases the bioavailability of dopamine in the synaptic cleft and symptomatically improves the parkinsonian syndrome. For this potential neuroprotective activity and its demonstrated symptomatic effect, it is generally used as monotherapy in early stages and in later stages as coadjuvant therapy.

Surgical Therapy

Until recently the only surgical indication in Parkinson's disease was disabling drug-resistant tremor, treated with thalamotomy or thalamic stimulation. Other surgical techniques used in the 1950s had been abandoned after dopamine became available because they caused unacceptable side effects, partly because discrete target localization was difficult with the techniques then available. Stereotactic surgery, supported by sophisticated neuroimaging and electrophysiologic techniques, is now used for the treatment of the disease itself. It is known that, in Parkinson's disease, as a consequence of the dopaminergic deficit some structures of the basal ganglia, mainly the subthalamic nucleus and the pars interna of the globus pallidus (GPi), are hyperactive.[101] This hyperactivity induces a decrease of motor cortex activation and explains the typical akinesia of Parkinson's disease. Thus, lesioning or inhibiting the activity of these nuclei affords

a great improvement of many parkinsonian features, including gait and freezing. The first surgical approach of this new era was to lesion the GPi. This procedure, termed pallidotomy, improved the tremor, rigidity, and akinesia in the contralateral limbs and abolished drug-induced dyskinesias, but gait, and particularly freezing, were not uniformly improved.[102] As lesions are not generally undertaken bilaterally, because of the risk of causing cognitive deficits, the therapeutic profile of this technique is limited. Bilateral stimulation of the GPi or subthalamic nucleus is the other neurosurgical approach. This technique allows a bilateral therapy while minimizing the risk of cognitive impairment. When applied to the subthalamic nucleus or GPi, all cardinal features of Parkinson's disease, including slow gait and freezing, are significantly reduced, by 51% for subthalamic nucleus and by 33% for GPi.[103–105] Specifically, the benefit induced in gait and axial symptoms was 50%. Other surgical strategies, such as the grafting of fetal mesencephalic neurons, have shown little usefulness in controlled trials and can cause untoward side effects, such as marked spontaneous dyskinesias.

Physical Therapy

Treatment of the parkinsonian gait at any stage of the disease should not be exclusively pharmacologic or surgical.[92,106] There are specific rehabilitation programs with exercises directed to reduce rigidity and to increase the range of joint motion.[107] More importantly, patients are trained to improve posture and minimize the forward displacement of the center of gravity. Tricks to overcome gait freezing and to lengthen step stride can be very helpful in these patients.

Other Parkinsonian Syndromes

Progressive Supranuclear Palsy

Progressive supranuclear palsy (PSP) is a neurodegenerative illness that involves (1) the nigrostriatopallidal system producing rigidity, bradykinesia, and postural instability; (2) the cerebral cortex, mainly the frontal lobes, inducing cognitive and behavioral changes; and (3) the cholinergic nuclei of the pons and mesencephalon, as well as other areas of the brainstem, inducing supranuclear gaze palsies, axial motor abnormalities, sleep disturbances, dysarthria, and dysphagia.[108,109] Neuropathologically it is characterized by neuronal loss and gliosis of the affected areas. Neurofibrillary tangles, of a type different from the ones found in Alzheimer's disease, appear in some neurons of the affected areas.

The average annual incidence rate (new cases per 100,000 person-years) for ages 50 to 99 years is about 5.3.[110] The age of onset (at the end of the sixth and the beginning of the seventh decades of life) and the initial symptoms are quite similar to those of Parkinson's disease. However, the course is quicker, with survival of around 6 to 9 years. Although this entity shares a number of clinical signs with Parkinson's disease (bradykinesia, rigidity), there are some features that help in the differential diagnosis. Thus, in PSP the most frequent presenting sign (60%) is gait disturbance with instability and frequent falls, in contrast to Parkinson's disease in which this abnormality is prominent only after several years of evolution. Usually the patient does not have the flexed posture of Parkinson's disease and, on the contrary, there is often a dystonic hyperextension of the neck. Although the typical parkinsonian signs may be present to some extent from the beginning, the bilateral presentation with a more prominent involvement of axial musculature is a distinctive feature. Resting tremor is not a common finding, although it may be present in 5% to 10% of cases. Another differential feature is that medication with L-dopa has little effect on the parkinsonian signs of PSP.

Later in the evolution, the diagnosis becomes easier. PSP patients usually have a contracted rather than flaccid face, dysphagia, spastic dysarthria rather than the hypophonia of Parkinson's disease, emotional incontinence, and cognitive decline in frontal and executive functions. Patients with atypical presentation may have a dementia suggestive of Alzheimer's disease. The eye findings are most characteristic. There is a supranuclear paresis of eye movements, with eyelid retraction. Saccades are slow and hypometric, with range limitation in both upward and downward directions. Limitation of upgaze is not uncommon in Parkinson's disease, but in PSP downgaze is often affected earlier and more prominently than upgaze. The restriction of eye movements can be easily overcome by the doll's eye maneuver, indicating damage of the supranuclear mechanisms of eye movement control.

Beside the parkinsonian syndrome, nonspecific changes in personality with irritability, social withdrawal, and emotional lability are frequent in early PSP, and very often they are the presenting features. Thus, an erroneous diagnosis of depression is frequent at this point of evolution and, for the geriatric specialist, it is important to bear this in mind.

The diagnosis is based on the clinical features. There are no specific biologic markers of PSP. In advanced stages, there may be bilateral frontal and midbrain atrophy on MRI. Positron emission tomography (PET) studies demonstrate global cerebral hypometabolism, with more profound involvement of the frontal cortex, and a reduction in the dopaminergic input to the caudate and putamen. The differential diagnosis, beside Parkinson's disease, should include corticobasal ganglionic degeneration (CBGD), multisystem atrophies (MSA), mainly striatonigral degeneration, progressive subcortical gliosis, diffuse Lewy body disease, Creutzfeldt–Jakob disease, Alzheimer's disease, Pick's disease, the rigid form of Huntington's disease, and primary pallidal atrophies. Patients suffering from multiple small-vessel lesions in the brain may also resemble patients with PSP.

Treatments based in the replacement of neurotransmitters or receptor stimulation have been of little benefit. Dopaminergic stimulation with levodopa or, more reliably, with dopaminergic agonists at high doses, such as bromocriptine at more than 10 mg in three or four divided doses, often improves slightly the parkinsonian signs, often at the price of inducing complications such as agitation, confusion, or hallucinations. Anticholinergic, cholinergic, and noradrenergic drugs and antidepressants have been tested with even less benefit. Among them, amantadine seems to be the second most efficient drug following dopaminergic medication. In some trials, it has been reported that gait improves with amitriptyline (100 mg/day in two doses), considered the third choice of drug. Fluoxetine and other blockers of serotonin reuptake have not proved beneficial. In two individual cases, apraxia of eyelid opening improved slightly with desipramine, but the ratio of benefit to adverse events is poor with this drug. Idazoxan, a presynaptic alpha-2-receptor blocker, was given to improve gait, but the side effects make it impractical. Recently, a trial with a better tolerated analogue, efaroxan, has not shown efficacy in motor signs of PSP patients (Rascol). Local infiltration with botulinum toxin is useful in the treatment of dystonic features (retrocollis and blepharospasm).

Physical therapy seems to be of little benefit against instability. It is important, however, to instruct relatives in the physical care these patients require. Surgical treatment is not currently an option for PSP.

Corticobasal Ganglionic Degeneration

Corticobasal ganglionic degeneration (CBD) is a rare neurodegenerative disease affecting, often asymmetrically, the frontoparietal cortex, predominantly involving the perirolandic area where atrophy is maximal.[111,112] The temporal cortex is usually preserved. Other affected regions include the substantia nigra, basal ganglia, thalamus, periaqueductal gray matter, colliculi, oculomotor complex, red nucleus, and dentate nucleus. Neuronal loss and gliosis are prominent in these areas, but the typical neuropathologic feature of CBD is the presence of ballooned or achromatic neurons. Neurofibrillary tangles are also frequently identified.

The incidence of CBD is unknown. It begins after the fifth decade of life, without gender differences. Mean survival is 5 to 10 years, although immobility often occurs 3 to 5 years into the illness. The cause of CBD is unknown. Clinically, it debuts with an asymmetric akinetic rigid syndrome without tremor or with a tremor that is more rapid (6–8 Hz) and jerky than in Parkinson's disease (PD). Rather than resting, it tends to be a postural and action-type tremor. The upper limb is involved first, spreading to the ipsilateral leg in later stages, but it is not rare to begin with gait difficulties because of leg clumsiness, jerking, or stiffness. Less often, the leg and arm are affected simultaneously, or the disease starts with dysarthria or aphasia. Along its course, the contralateral limbs are also affected and the patient develops postural instability, hypomimia, dysarthria, and dysphagia. As with the rest of atypical parkinsonisms, the response to levodopa or dopaminergic agonists is very poor.

Cortical dysfunction gradually emerges between the first and third year of evolution. Apraxia and cortical sensory loss (agraphestesia, astereognosia, impaired two-point discrimination) are the most typical findings, which sometimes may be recognized in the affected limb (usually the hand) from the beginning. Memory loss, personality and behavioral changes, and mild aphasia are less frequent. A purposeless, maintained elevation of the akinetic hand or arm that has been termed "alien hand/limb" is typically, although not exclusively, observed in patients with CBD; it may also be seen in other diseases, such as PSP and AD. As the disease progresses, the arm goes into a dystonic posture, typically with adduction and flexion of the elbow and wrist. Action and reflex myoclonus in the more affected limb develop in later stages in 50% of cases. Eye movement abnormalities are frequent, predominantly in horizontal saccades, but, in contrast to PSP, without limitation of range.

Initially, diagnosis is based on clinical findings. In more advanced stages, PET depicts decreased metabolism and SPECT may show decreased cerebral perfusion in the affected areas, including cortex, basal ganglia, and thalamus of the hemisphere contralateral to the most affected hemibody. As the disease progresses, atrophy in the same areas may become evident on MRI. Electrophysiologic studies may help in elucidating the characteristics of tremor and the presence of myoclonus. When the disease is fully established, it is not difficult to recognize. However, initially it may be misdiagnosed as Parkinson's disease. The presence of signs of cortical dysfunction (apraxia and sensory impairment in the affected limb), and the absence of benefit with levodopa treatment, are suggestive of CBD. The differential diagnosis must be made with progressive supranuclear palsy, Pick's disease, multisystem atrophy, diffuse Lewy body disease, Parkinson's disease with dementia, and the different forms of asymmetric cortical degeneration syndromes (ACDS).

Pharmacologic treatment is not successful. The rigid akinetic symptoms improve little with dopaminergic medication. Baclofen can be tried to help rigidity and tremor. Action tremor may respond in some degree to propranolol in the early stages of the disease, but the benefit vanishes as the disease progresses. The elective drug in the treatment of myoclonus and tremor is clonazepan (0.15 mg/day). Physiotherapy is useful to avoid dystonic painful contractures and to preserve maximum functionality throughout the course of the disease.

Multiple System Atrophy

The term *multiple system atrophy* (MSA) refers to a group of progressive neurodegenerative disorders, clinically characterized by the presence of a rigid akinetic syndrome, poorly responsive to levodopa, and cerebellar and autonomic disturbances combined in different proportions.[113-115] As parkinsonian features are accompanied by these atypical signs, "atypical parkinsonism" or "parkinson-plus" are terms also commonly used for this group of disorders. From a neuropathologic point of view, neuronal loss and gliosis are observed mainly in the substantia nigra, striatum, locus ceruleus, pontine nuclei, cerebellar Purkinje cells, inferior olives, and intermediolateral cell columns of the spinal cord. Glial cytoplasmic inclusions in both astrocytes and oligodendrocytes are always present in MSA, mainly in several areas of the motor cortex, the supraspinal autonomic system, and their areas of projection. These inclusions are not specific for MSA; they can also be seen in other neurodegenerative diseases, including progressive supranuclear palsy and corticobasal ganglionic degeneration.

The average annual incidence rate of MSA for ages 50 to 99 years is about 3.0.[10] The age of onset is usually the end of the fourth and the beginning of the fifth decades of life, with a mean survival of 5 to 6 years. A slight male predominance (1.3 : 1) has been reported in some series. Depending on the relative predominance of the symptoms, three different entities are distinguished in MSA: (1) when the clinical picture is one of levodopa-resistant Parkinson's disease, but without relevant autonomic or cerebellar deficits, the disorder is termed *nigrostriatal degeneration (SND)*; (2) prominent cerebellar dysfunction defines the entity as *olivopontocerebellar atrophy (OPCA)*; and (3) when the autonomic system is preferentially affected, it is called the *Shy–Drager syndrome (SDS)*. Some authors have eliminated the SDS from this classification, grouping all cases with autonomic dysfunction in the other two groups, based on the predominant feature. However, there is a relatively high proportion of patients with an overlapping picture in whom there is no clear preponderance of basal ganglionic, cerebellar, or autonomic findings. Pyramidal signs are also found frequently in the clinical examination of these patients. Depression, personality changes, and an attentional or executive deficit are not rare, but a more pervasive cognitive decline is not a typical finding. A peripheral neuropathy has been documented in about 18% of cases.

The rigid akinetic syndrome is the most common disturbance and the presenting form in the majority of cases. Although the age of presentation is younger than the typical age of onset of Parkinson's disease, it may initially resemble Parkinson's disease. The differential diagnosis is based mainly in the poor response to levodopa therapy, early postural instability, and rapid progression. Besides, and in contrast to Parkinson's disease, the beginning is symmetric (both hemibodies affected), and resting tremor is not a common finding, although it may be present. However, it is important to realize that about one-third of patients suffering from MSA have a moderate improvement in response to levodopa that may be maintained along the course of the disease or may vanish in the following years of progression. Another typical feature of patients with MSA is the early development of levodopa-induced dyskinesias, preferentially in facial and neck musculature, and frequently without relief of the parkinsonian dysfunction.

Early in the disease, the most frequent autonomic disturbances are orthostatic hypotension (defined as a minimun fall of 20 mmHg in the systolic or 10 mmHg in the diastolic blood pressure when the patient stands up from being seated), urinary disorders that simulate outflow obstruction or incontinence in men and incontinence in women, and impotence in men. These symptoms may be the initial complaints in almost 50% of cases. A high proportion of patients (95%) have abnormal electromyography (EMG) of anal and urethral sphincters. During the evolution, 80% to 90% of patients suffer severe autonomic failure. Patients with Parkinson's disease may also have postural hypotension, especially induced by dopaminergic drugs, and urogenital disorders, but usually of a milder intensity. Constipation and decreased sweating are also frequent. The presence of inspiratory stridor, although not as prevalent, is very indicative of MSA.

Ataxia, dysarthria, and kinetic tremor with dysmetria are frequently seen as the expression of the cerebellar involvement. Myoclonus is also a common sign. Abnormalities in ocular movements are typical. Nystagmus, ocular dysmetria, fixation instability, and jerky pursuit are frequently observed, in contrast to the supranuclear ophthalmoplegia that characterizes progressive supranuclear palsy.

The diagnosis is mainly based on the clinical findings and their progression pattern. In SND, T_2-weighted MRI shows hypointense signal in the putamen. Atrophy of the posterior fossa (cerebellum and brainstem) is characteristic of olivopontocerebellar atrophy. Even before structural changes can be seen on MRI, a metabolic reduction in these structures can be detected with PET. This technique, and the less expensive SPECT, can show early in the disease a reduction in putaminal dopaminergic receptors, whereas in Parkinson's disease dopaminergic receptors are upregulated. EMGs are useful to demonstrate a denervation of the anal and urethral sphincters, and the tilt table test may help in the diagnosis of orthostatic hypotension. The differential diagnosis with Parkinson's disease may pose a problem mainly in the initial stages. The most important differences have been described in the previous paragraphs. Progressive supranuclear palsy, corticobasal ganglionic degeneration, and vascular parkinsonism are the other entities to bear in mind whose distinctive features have already been mentioned.

Although the response is not excellent, levodopa and dopamine agonists are the most useful drugs. Parkinsonian features may respond mildly or more strongly in about one-third of patients. To assess the efficacy of these drugs, a dose of 1500 mg/day should be tried, because more than the usual dose for Parkinson's disease patients is sometimes needed to obtain a benefit. When levodopa is not useful, no response is obtained with dopaminergic agonists either. Amantadine, 100 mg twice daily, and anticholinergic drugs also may be tried. It is important to realize that surgery is not indicated in these patients. Orthostatic hypotension may improve with simple measures, such as avoiding large meals or extreme heat, standing up slowly from a seated or recumbent position, increasing salt intake, or wearing pressure stockings. When these preventive strategies are not enough, treatment with fludrocortisone (0.4 mg/day in two doses) or indomethacin (25 mg three times/day) should be tried. Other drugs that may help are ephedrine, midodrine, phenylpropanolamine, caffeine, and ergots. Anticholinergic drugs such as oxybutynin (5–10 mg/day) and more recently tolterodine (2 mg twice a day) may improve urinary incontinence. Desmopressin nasal spray at night may also be helpful. When tremor and myoclonus are prominent, clonazepam or valproate are used, but with scarce benefit.

Late-Life Hydrocephalus

Although not a frequent cause of gait disorders in older people, symptomatic hydrocephalus presents initially with a gait disorder and it should be recognized because it is potentially treatable.[116] Particularly after CT became available, several authors found enlarged ventricles to be frequently present in patients with gait disorders.[117] From this finding they concluded that symptomatic hydrocephalus was common and shunting procedures multiplied. However, even in series with carefully selected patients, some failed to improve after shunting, suggesting that hydrocephalus was not the cause of their gait disorder.[118] For this reason, it is important to apply more sensitive diagnostic criteria in the workup of these patients.[119] The classical syndrome consists of slowly progressive gait impairment, with instability. Urinary incontinence may be present, but is not necessary for the diagnosis. Only very late in the course of the disorder may the patient have cognitive slowness or impaired attention. Onset of cognitive impairment before gait disturbance suggests a different process. The diagnosis is made with CT or MRI, which show enlarged ventricles. The cortical sulci may be compressed or enlarged outside the high parietal convexity.[120,121] In dubious cases, a pattern of decreased perfusion or metabolism in the association cortex of the parietal lobes on SPECT or PET predicts a poor outcome.[119] This pattern is usually seen in Alzheimer's disease and Parkinson's with dementia. CSF manometrics are not predictive of which patients will improve after shunting.[122]

Rare Etiologies: Neoplasms, Subdural Hematoma

Seldom, an older person with a worsening gait disorder may harbor a frontal tumor or a subdural hematoma. Meningiomas carry a better prognosis but are not as common as glioblastomas or metastases in the older age group. By the time the patient becomes symptomatic, these lesions can be easily identified by MRI scanning. CT is less sensitive than MRI, particularly for glioblastoma. Also, poor definition of cortical boundaries may make it difficult to differentiate a glioma from a meningioma on CT on a noncontrast study. On a contrast study, the more homogeneous pattern of a meningioma and the presence of a dural tail help differentiate this lesion from glioblastomas. However, some meningiomas may have cystic areas that enhance poorly. Calcification in a meningioma and changes in the cortical bone are better appreciated on CT, but these characteristics are seldom critical for the diagnosis. Also, in the case of glioblastomas, the extent of the tumor is better visualized by MRI than by CT. Neither technique, however shows accurately the extent of brain infiltrated by malignant glial cells. MRI is also more sensitive than CT for the detection of metastatic brain disease. In patients prone to falls, a subacute deterioration should raise the suspicion of a subdural hematoma, particularly when a worsening in gait is accompanied by changes in mental status. Although MRI depicts these lesions with more accuracy than CT, symptomatic subdural hematomas are well seen with CT and can be adequately managed neurosurgically without the need of MRI.

Psychogenic Postural and Gait Disorders

Psychogenic gait disorders caused are rare and generally do not present a diagnostic dilemma. It is important, however, not to mislabel an organic gait disorder as a psychogenic one, and therefore some of the characteristics of these disorders are reviewed briefly here. On the other hand, psychogenic factors often play a role in aggravating the functional consequences of an organic gait disorder, and sometimes they are amenable to specific treatment.[123]

During panic attacks, patients may feel that their legs are weak and they become unsteady. To protect themselves from a perceived risk of falling, they may adopt a gait pattern described as "walking on ice."[124] They crouch forward, abduct their arms, and shorten their stride. Sometimes these patients cling to walls or furniture and may not venture away from the house.[123] A similar gait pattern, described as cautious gait, is very common in patients with organic gait disorders. A major difference is that the cautious gait in patients with anxiety tends to occur episodically, in the context of a panic attack, whereas organic gait disorders are generally more persistent. Other features that differentiate psychogenic from organic gait disorder include dramatic moment-to-moment fluctuations in performance, excessive hesitation, resembling slow motion or walking through a viscous fluid, and buckling of the knees without falling.[124] A psychogenic Romberg test is characterized by buildup of sway, with a consistent tendency to fall toward the observer. It can often be overcome by distraction, for instance, by examining the pupils while the patient quietly stands.[123]

Of the 60 patients with "hysterical gait disorders" described by Keane,[125] some manifested a hemiparesis or paraparesis, but the largest group had an assortment of ataxic gaits, characterized by dramatically exaggerated sway but avoiding falls. Some patients exhibited "tightrope balancing," walking on a narrow base while keeping their arms abducted. Others were described as "tremblers," not to be confused with patients with orthostatic tremor, an organic disorder.[2] Overall, a neurologic examination can easily pinpoint the nature of the problem in about three-quarters of patients with psychogenic gait disorders.[124]

Excessive Movement Disorders in the Elderly

Excessive movements in the elderly may be rhythmic, in which case they are called *tremor*, or not, in which case they are called *myoclonus* if they are very fast (lightning-like) or hyperkinesias in all other cases. Hyperkinetic movements may have the speed of normal volitional, reaching movements, and then they are called *chorea*, if they are predominantly distal, and ballismus, or *hemiballismus* (it is usually unilateral), when they are predominantly proximal. When the hyperkinesias are very slow and tend to present mainly as abnormal postures, they are called *dystonia* when predominantly proximal and *athetosis* when they involve the hand. However, particularly in adults, the term dystonia is often used to encompass both true dystonia as well as athetosis.

Tremor

Tremor is an involuntary oscillation of a body part produced by alternating or synchronous contractions of reciprocally innervated antagonistic muscles.[126] The clinical presentation of this abnormal movement serves as the basis for its classification and reflects the underlying pathology. *Resting tremor* occurs when the affected body part is resting, inactive, and fully supported against gravity. *Postural tremor* is seen with maintenance of a fixed antigravity posture (i.e., the hand holding a teacup). *Action or kinetic tremor* is a rhythmic discontinuity of a movement present in a limb during goal-directed movements.

Tremor in the elderly is mainly associated with three entities: Parkinson's disease, essential tremor, and metabolic or toxic disorders. From a pathologic point of view, resting tremor is the consequence of damage in the substantia nigra pars compacta (SNpc). Thus, it is typically observed in Parkinson's disease, discussed already. Other neurodegenerative disorders resembling Parkinson's disease (parkinsonism plus) and included in its differential diagnosis may, rarely, present as resting tremor, described earlier. Although vascular lesions, tumors, or infections may involve SNpc and induce resting tremor, they are very uncommon in clinical practice.

Postural tremor in the elderly is a very prevalent disorder with many possible etiologies. It may be associated to metabolic or toxic disorders or may appear without concomitant illness or focal neurologic lesion. In this case, it is termed essential tremor (ET). In *essential tremor*, the most common finding is postural tremor of a limb, usually absent at rest and less evident during movement. Sometimes, it may be accentuated when a goal-directed action is performed provoking an action tremor. It may occur in a wide range of frequencies (4–12 Hz). The hands are the body part most frequently involved, with rhythmic movements consisting of flexion-extension of the wrist and adduction-abduction of the fingers.[127] Frequently, tremor is unilateral at the beginning, spreading later to the contralateral side. Handwriting is tremulous and letters become sharp and angulated, being very different from the typical micrographic letter of Parkinson's disease. The second body segment most frequently involved is the cranial musculature (head, tongue, voice). Although it may appear in isolation, it is more common for tremor in this location to begin in later stages and to be associated with hand tremor.[127]

Involvement of the legs and trunk are rare and late occurrences. During the evolution of the disease, the tremor increases in amplitude and decreases in frequency. The increment in amplitude interferes with the execution of fine movements, inducing more incapacity.[128] Essential tremor may be a familial illness with a younger age of presentation or may occur sporadically, in which case the peak age of onset is later. In both instances it is more frequent with advancing age. Prevalence figures for individuals older than 40 years of age range between 0.4% and 5.6%, affecting at least 5% of people age 65 and older, without gender differences. The etiology of the sporadic cases is unknown. Familiar cases are dominantly inherited, and markers for two genes have been recently identified.[129] One important clinical characteristic is that this type of tremor is ameliorated by alcohol consumption.

Drug treatment of essential tremor may be very effective but not necessarily simple. At present there is no agreement about the drug of choice.[128] Propranolol has been classically considered the first-line drug at daily doses between 80 and 200 mg. It decreases tremor amplitude, but the response is often incomplete. Other β-blockers (metoprolol, nadolol, atenolol, timolol, pindolol) are less effective than propranolol. In elderly people, frequently one can observe concomitant disorders such as atrioventricular block, asthma, or diabetes that are relative contraindications for the use of β-blockers, especially those blocking the β_2-subtype. Patients with bronchospasm may benefit from metoprolol (100–200 mg/day), a selective β_1-antagonist. Primidone (50–250 mg/day in a single dose at bedtime) has been demonstrated to be as effective as propranolol and can be used as the drug of choice, particularly in the case of patients suffering from the aforementioned disorders. However, the sedative effect sometimes constitutes a limiting factor that prevents the achievement of the dose needed for tremor control. Other useful drugs in some cases are phenobarbital (120 mg/day) and the benzodiazepines, such as diazepam or clonazepam (1–3 mg/day).

Recently, it has been suggested that when propranolol and primidone are not efficient, alprazolam could be tried.[128] If treatment with monotherapy does not control tremor, combinations of more than one drug may be considered. Other drugs, such as gabapentin, carbonic anhydrase inhibitors (methazolamide), amantadine, clonidine, clozapine, flunarizine, and nimodipine, have not been proven effective in controlling essential tremor, although they have been reported to be helpful in isolated cases. Patients unsuccessfully controlled with pharmacologic treatments may improve with surgery. Surgery is aimed at blocking the activity of the ventralis intermedium nucleus (Vim) of the thalamus, either by performing a lesion (thalamotomy) or by placing an electrode for high-frequency stimulation that resembles the effect of thalamic ablative surgery. Long-term follow-up studies show that this treatment remains effective for years.[130] However, surgery in elderly patients is not without limitations. The benefit to risk ratio must be weighed carefully, in consultation with centers that specialize in this procedure.

Metabolic or toxic disorders that may be associated with postural tremor must always be taken into consideration.[131] The most frequent are hyperthyroidism, pheochromocytoma, hypoglycemia, uremia, liver failure, alcohol withdrawal, hypothermia, toxicity due to lithium, and tricyclic antidepressants, valproic acid, neuroleptics, steroids, amiodarone, isoproterenol, theophyline, or cyclosporine A.

Postural tremor also may occur in the context of familial and acquired peripheral neuropathies. It has been suggested that tremor in these circumstances represents enhanced physiologic tremor.

From a mechanistic point of view, action tremor originates as the consequence of pathology in the dentatorubrothalamic projection. Vascular lesions or degenerative disease involving the cerebellum are the most frequent causes of action tremor, which is less frequent than resting or postural tremor in the elderly. Available drugs do not ameliorate this type of tremor, and the only effective treatment is the surgical treatment as described for postural tremor.

Chorea

This movement disorder consists of arrhythmic, rapid, often jerky, purposeless movements that may be simple or complex but rarely interfere with voluntary motion. They may affect axial musculature (orofacial, neck, truncal) and the limbs. When the involuntary movement of a limb is proximal, of wider amplitude, and brisker it is termed ballismus. Chorea may be the clinical expression of a degenerative neurologic disease, may appear in the context of a systemic or metabolic illness, be secondary to drugs, or may be induced by a vascular lesion.

Primary Neurologic Diseases

Senile chorea is the most frequent cause of choreic movements in the elderly. Contrary to Huntington's disease, it is an insidiously developing and generalized chorea, primarily involving the limbs, with mental preservation and without a family history. It usually affects people older than 60 years of age. Neuropathology shows caudate and putamen atrophy to a lesser degree than in Huntington's disease, but the genetic study is normal in these individuals.[132]

Huntington's disease is an autosomal dominant inherited disease that tends to become clinically obvious at an earlier age. Only 50% of cases of Huntington's disease develop after age 65 years. In these cases, a milder progression of the disease may be expected. The clinical picture is characterized by the presence of chorea, behavioral and mental decline, and a positive family history.

Among metabolic and systemic illnesses, it is important to note that a number of metabolic disorders may provoke choreic movements.[133] Among them the most relevant are hypocalcemia, hypoglycemia, hyperglycemia, hyponatremia, hypernatremia, hypomagnesemia, hyperthyroidism, hyperparathyroidism, hypoparathyroidism, hepatic encephalopathy, polycythemia vera, and neoplastic metabolic and autoimmune disorders. These entities are relatively frequent in older people and should be recognized and treated. Thus, blood tests carried out to exclude these abnormalities are mandatory when facing chorea in the elderly. Other systemic illnesses such as systemic lupus erythematosus or primary antiphospholipid antibody syndrome may be on occasion associated with chorea, but they are very rare in older people. Chorea may be induced by the chronic consumption of drugs such as neuroleptics (haloperidol, chlorpromazine, thioridazine, etc.), antiparkinsonian drugs, anticonvulsants (phenytoin, carbamazepine), stimulants, steroids, opiates, calcium channel blockers, digoxin, or lithium, to name the most frequent.[133] Although any body segment may be affected, tardive dyskinesias due to chronic treatment with neuroleptics affect mainly the mouth, producing lip-smacking, tongue protrusion, or grimacing.

Cerebrovascular disease (infarction or hemorrhage) involving different parts of the basal ganglia may induce chorea or ballismus, usually affecting the contralateral hemibody (hemiballismus). It has classically been thought that hemiballismus or hemichorea was the consequence of a lesion in the subthalamic nucleus. Nowadays it is known that lesions located in other structures of the basal ganglia (i.e., caudate, putamen, globus pallidum) or in the thalamus may result in hemichorea and that a lesion in the subthalamic nucleus sometimes is not associated with chorea or ballismus.

Mild chorea should not be treated, as the consequences of therapy may be worse than the problem. When necessary, chorea in the older person is treated with very small amounts of antidopaminergic drugs, mainly D_2 antagonists. Haloperidol at 0.5 to 20 mg/day and pimozide at 1 to 10 mg/day at bedtime are the most specific. Keep in mind the risk of inducing parkinsonism and depression.

Dystonia

Dystonia is characterized by involuntary sustained muscle contraction that produces twisting movements and abnormal postures in axial muscles and limbs. Sometimes jerky movements resembling tremor in the affected body segment may be superimposed. Dystonia is classified according to the distribution of body regions affected as *focal*, *segmental*, *multifocal*, and *generalized*.

When a hemibody is affected, it is termed *hemidystonia*. If the cause of the dystonia is known, it is classified as *secondary* or symptomatic. If it is not known, the dystonia is *primary* or idiopathic. Generalized dystonia is rare among the geriatric population. In this age group, most frequent are focal and idiopathic forms.[134] At the beginning, they appear frequently during movement (action dystonia) and disappear at rest. As the process evolves, dystonic contractions may affect muscles not normally activated in a task, causing what is called the "overflow" phenomenon and inducing the patient to adopt bizarre postures. Their onset is usually in the fourth or fifth decades and affect women more often than men. Generally, the initial symptoms are insidious and intermittent, extending in 20% to 30% of cases to neighboring areas. Cranial and cervical structures are most frequently affected (78% of patients with dystonia).

Cranial Dystonia

Blepharospasm is an involuntary, intermittent, or sustained bilateral eye closure produced by spasmodic contractions of the orbicularis oculi muscles, often exacerbated by bright light.[135] A mild contraction of the frontalis is frequently seen when the patients try to open their eyes. Milder forms have only a cosmetic consequence, but in more severe cases blepharospasm interferes with vision and the patients become unable to drive, to read, and, in summary, to lead a normal life. It affects women more often than men, and onset peaks around the sixth decade of life. In *oromandibular dystonia*, spasms occur in the region of the jaw, lower face, and mouth. Typically the dystonia takes the form of jaw closure, opening, protrusion or lateral deviation, lip tightening or pursing, or lingual dystonia. It is frequently triggered by actions that involve the muscles affected, such as biting, chewing, or speaking. Frequently seen in edentulous people with poorly fitting dentures, it may improve when the dentures are fixed.

Craniocervical Dystonia or Meige's Syndrome

This syndrome is the association of blepharospasm and oromandibular dystonia. The most typical, complete clinical picture consists of involuntary eye closure, forced opening of the jaw, and tongue protrusion.[136] However, any sort of oromandibular dystonia as described in the previous paragraph may be observed accompanying blepharospasm. Sometimes cervical dystonia (torticollis, anterocollis, etc.) and even pharyngeal dystonia may be associated. Trunk and limbs are usually preserved. It is almost exclusively an illness of elderly people, with a higher incidence in the sixth and seventh decade, and is more frequent in women. The differential diagnosis is with tardive dyskinesia and the spontaneous buccolingual dyskinesias of the elderly, more frequent in edentulous people. A previous history of neuroleptic consumption and a different phenomenology helps to separate these entities.

Other Focal Dystonias

Cervical dystonia (torticollis, anterocollis, or retrocollis) and limb dystonia (mostly task specific such as writer's cramp) have their onset at younger ages. Leg dystonia is frequently the first sign in children displaying primary dystonia, but is rarely seen in adult patients. When it occurs as an isolated sign in the elderly, a diagnosis of Parkinson's disease must be considered.

Treatment of focal dystonia has shifted in the past few years from the pharmacologic field toward the use of the botulinum toxin, and training guidelines for its use have been established.[137] Botulinum toxin injection in muscles that are tonically contracted induce partial weakness and therefore avoid the sustained abnormal posture that characterizes dystonia. It is especially effective in the treatment of blepharospasm and laterocollis. Oromandibular dystonia is among the most challenging forms of focal dystonia to treat with botulinum toxin. However, in this type of dystonia the pharmacologic treatment is also ineffective.

Pharmacologic therapy includes a number of drugs with variable efficacy.[138] In younger patients, anticholinergic therapy at high doses may be helpful. Although not demonstrably superior, trihexyphenidyl (up to 12 mg/day) is most broadly employed. In older people, the central adverse events associated with this drug, including confusion, hallucinations, drowsiness, and memory loss, are a limiting factor. Benzodiazepines (diazepan, lorazepan, clonazepam) are used as a second-option treatment. Clonazepam is more active in blepharospasm than in other types of dystonia. GABA agonists such as baclofen may be helpful for oromandibular dystonia. Monoamine depleters (tetrabenazine in Europe), lithium, anticonvulsants (carbamazepine, primidone), and a number of other drugs have been used in different combinations with irregular benefit. Dopaminergic antagonists, extensively used in the past, help little in the long run and have a higher risk of inducing parkinsonism, sedation, and tardive dyskinesias in the geriatric population. Surgical treatment has been revitalized in the past few years for the treatment of dystonia. Thalamotomy, pallidotomy, and deep brain stimulation of the thalamus or globus pallidus have been reported to be effective in the treatment of generalized dystonia.[139] However, results are better in cases of hemidystonia or in generalized dystonia. Peripheral denervation surgery was used in the past to treat cervical dystonia. This technique has been essentially abandoned because of the superiority of botulinum toxin in controlling the involuntary muscle contraction.

Myoclonus

Myoclonus is a shocklike involuntary muscle contraction originating in the central nervous system by abnormal neuronal discharges.[140] A physiologic classification of myoclonus can be made by taking into account the location in the neuroaxis of the neurons discharging abnormally and causing the muscle contraction. Thus, myoclonus can be *cortical, reticular, spinal,* or *propiospinal* in origin. From a practical point of view, this movement disorder may be classified on the basis of its clinical presentation as *spontaneous, reflex* when it occurs in response to auditory, visual, or somatosensory stimuli, and *action* when it is driven by a voluntary movement. Depending on the body segment affected by the myoclonic jerks, they may be *focal, segmental, multifocal,* or *generalized.* They may be *physiologic,* such as the typical nocturnal myoclonus; *essential,* usually familial and associated with dystonia; and *secondary* to a high number of metabolic disorders, toxic substances, anoxia, or in the context of a more diffuse neurologic or neurodegenerative disease, in which case they are typically associated with other neurologic abnormalities such as epilepsy, ataxia, or dementia.[141]

In the elderly, the most common form of presentation is spontaneous multifocal or generalized myoclonus, aggravated by action and sometimes aggravated also by sensory stimuli. Severe action myoclonus is very incapacitating. Frequently, the origin is cortical and is secondary to metabolic or toxic encephalopathies, and is a minor proportion to neurodegenerative diseases. Any metabolic abnormality may induce myoclonus, but the most frequent causes are renal failure, hyponatremia, hypokalemia, and liver failure, which may show myoclonus as an initial sign. Vitamin E deficiency secondary to malabsorption may course with action myoclonus and ataxia as prominent signs. In addition to bismuth intoxication, the list of drugs causing myoclonus is long, and in the geriatric population the possibility of drug abuse or an overdose should always be considered. Beside multifocal of generalized myoclonus, reticular reflex myoclonus may be also observed in metabolic and toxic disorders. Treatment always consists of the correction of the metabolic defect or suppression of the toxic agent.

The association of myoclonus and dementia in elderly patients deserves special attention. It is observed in Alzheimer's disease[142] and also in other neurodegenerative diseases such as corticobasal ganglionic degeneration, typically associated to limb apraxia and a parkinsonian syndrome. Huntington's disease, prion-related encephalopathies such as Creutzfeldt–Jakob disease, herpes simplex infections, and subacute sclerosing panencephalitis are less prevalent but may cause myoclonus. Other neurodegenerative diseases (different variants of spinocerebellar degeneration, and olivopontocerebellar atrophy) may feature myoclonus and ataxia, particularly among the geriatric population.

To treat myoclonus, first consider the correction of a metabolic disorder, or the suppression of an offending drug. When that is not an option, a number of medications may help. Clonazepam (2–15 mg/day), piracetam (8–20 mg/day; not available in the United States), sodium valproate (1200–3000 mg/day), and primidone (500–1000 mg/day) are the most useful drugs, particularly in cortical myoclonus.[143] Clonazepam is the most effective, but piracetam is better tolerated. Different combinations of these drugs are frequently needed to control severe myoclonus. Fluoxetine (10–20 mg/day) may be used in combination, especially to treat reticular reflex myoclonus.

References

1. Critchley M. On senile disorders of gait, including the so-called "senile paraplegia." *Geriatrics.* 1948;3:364–370.
2. Britton TC, Thompson PD, van der Kamp W, et al. Primary orthostatic tremor: further observations in six cases. *J Neurol.* 1992;239:209–217.
3. Masdeu J. Disorders of stance and gait. In: Greenberg J, ed. *Neuroimaging: A Companion to Adam's and Victor's Principles of Neurology.* New York: McGraw-Hill; 1995:25–40.
4. Mori S. Neurophysiology of locomotion: recent advances in the study of locomotion. In: Masdeu J, Sudarsky L, Wolfson L, eds. *Gait Disorders of Aging. Falls and Therapeutic Strategies.* Philadelphia: Lippincott & Raven; 1997:55–78.
5. Nashner L. Physiology of balance, with special reference to the healthy elderly. In: Masdeu J, Sudarsky L, Wolfson L, eds. *Gait Disorders of Aging. Falls and Therapeutic Strategies.* Philadelphia: Lippincott & Raven; 1997:37–53.
6. Newman G, Dovenmuehle R, Busse E. Alterations in neurologic status with age. *J Am Geriatr Soc.* 1960;8:915–917.
7. Baker S, Harvey A. Fall injuries in the elderly. In: Radebaugh T, Hadley E, Suzman R, eds. *Falls in the Elderly: Biologic and Behavioral Aspects.* Philadelphia: Saunders; 1985:501–512.
8. Haupt B, Graves E. *Detailed Diagnoses and Surgical Procedures for Patients Discharged from Short-Stay Hospitals.* 1979: United States. DHHS (PHS) 82-1274-1. Washington, DC: Department of Health and Human Services; 1982.
9. Rubenstein L, Josephson K. Interventions to reduce the multifactorial risks for falling. In: Masdeu J, Sudarsky L, Wolfson L, eds. *Gait Disorders of Aging. Falls and Therapeutic Strategies.* Philadelphia: Lippincott & Raven; 1997:309–326.
10. Robbins A, Rubenstein L, Josephson K, et al. Predictors of falls among elderly people. Results of two population-based studies. *Arch Intern Med.* 1989;149:1628–1633.
11. Sudarsky L, Ronthal M. Gait disorders among elderly patients. *Arch Neurol.* 1983;40:740–743.

12. Sudarsky L. Clinical approach to gait disorders of aging: an overview. In: Masdeu J, Sudarsky L, Wolfson L, eds. *Gait Disorders of Aging. Falls and Therapeutic Strategies.* Philadelphia: Lippincott & Raven; 1997:147–157.

13. Achiron A, Ziv I, Goren M, et al. Primary progressive freezing gait. *Movement Disord.* 1993;8:293–297.

14. Fuh JL, Lin KN, Wang SJ, Ju TH, Chang R, Liu HC. Neurologic diseases presenting with gait impairment in the elderly. *J Geriatr Psychiatry Neurol.* 1994;7:89–92.

15. Judge J. Resistance training. In: Masdeu J, Sudarsky L, Wolfson L, eds. *Gait Disorders of Aging. Falls and Therapeutic Strategies.* Philadelphia: Lippincott & Raven; 1997:381–393.

16. Sabin T. Peripheral neuropathy: disorders of proprioception. In: Masdeu J, Sudarsky L, Wolfson L, eds. *Gait Disorders of Aging. Falls and Therapeutic Strategies.* Philadelphia: Lippincott & Raven; 1997:273–282.

17. Albin R, Albers J, Greenberg H, et al. Acute sensory neuropathy-neuronopathy from pyridoxine overdose. *Neurology.* 1987;37:1729–1732.

18. Anderson NE, Rosenblum MK, Graus F, Wiley RG, Posner JB. Autoantibodies in paraneoplastic syndromes associated with small-cell lung cancer. *Neurology.* 1988;38:1391–1398.

19. Dropcho EJ. Paraneoplastic diseases of the nervous system. *Curr Treat Options Neurol.* 1999;1:417–427.

20. Grant IA, Hunder GG, Homburger HA, Dyck PJ. Peripheral neuropathy associated with sicca complex. *Neurology.* 1997;48:855–862.

21. Tajima Y, Mito Y, Owada Y, Tsukishima E, Moriwaka F, Tashiro K. Neurological manifestations of primary Sjogren's syndrome in Japanese patients. *Intern Med.* 1997;36:690–693.

22. Satake M, Yoshimura T, Iwaki T, Yamada T, Kobayashi T. Anti-dorsal root ganglion neuron antibody in a case of dorsal root ganglionitis associated with Sjogren's syndrome. *J Neurol Sci.* 1995;132:122–125.

23. Steinfeld SD, Demols P, Van Vooren JP, Cogan E, Appelboom T. Zidovudine in primary Sjogren's syndrome. *Rheumatology (Oxf).* 1999;38:814–817.

24. Fox RI, Tornwall J, Michelson P. Current issues in the diagnosis and treatment of Sjogren's syndrome. *Curr Opin Rheumatol.* 1999;11:364–371.

25. Dalakas MC. Chronic idiopathic ataxic neuropathy. *Ann Neurol.* 1986;19:545–554.

26. Pestronk A. Chronic immune polyneuropathies and serum autoantibodies. In: Rolak L, Harati Y, eds. *Neuroimmunology for the Clinician.* Boston: Butterworth-Heinemann; 1997:237–251.

27. Pestronk A, Choksi R, Bieser K, et al. Treatable gait disorder and polyneuropathy associated with high titer serum IgM binding to antigens that copurify with myelin-associated glycoprotein. *Muscle Nerve.* 1994;17:1293–1300.

28. Feasby T. Inflammatory-demyelinating polyneuropathies. A review of GBS and CIDP with analysis of clinical, laboratory and pathologic findings in these conditions. *Neurol Clin.* 1992;10:651–670.

29. Frohman EM, Tusa R, Mark AS, Cornblath DR. Vestibular dysfunction in chronic inflammatory demyelinating polyneuropathy. *Ann Neurol.* 1996;39:529–535.

30. Hadden RD, Hughes RA. Treatment of immune-mediated inflammatory neuropathies. *Curr Opin Neurol.* 1999;12:573–579.

31. Fife TD, Baloh RW. Disequilibrium of unknown cause in older people. *Ann Neurol.* 1993;34:694–702.

32. Kase CS, Norrving B, Levine SR, et al. Cerebellar infarction. Clinical and anatomic observations in 66 cases. *Stroke.* 1993;24:76–83.

33. Mokri B, Houser OW, Sandok BA, Piepgras DG. Spontaneous dissections of the vertebral arteries. *Neurology.* 1988;38:880.

34. Reich KA, Giansiracusa DF, Strongwater SL. Neurologic manifestations of giant cell arteritis. *Am J Med.* 1990;89:67–72.

35. Wilkinson I, Russell R. Arteries of the head and neck in giant cell arteritis. *Arch Neurol.* 1972;27:378–391.

36. Savage RA, Whitehouse GH, Roberts N. The relationship between the magnetic resonance imaging appearance of the lumbar spine and low back pain, age and occupation in males. *Eur Spine J.* 1997;6:106–114.

37. Boos N, Rieder R, Schade V, Spratt KF, Semmer N, Aebi M. 1995 Volvo Award in clinical sciences. The diagnostic accuracy of magnetic resonance imaging, work perception, and psychosocial factors in identifying symptomatic disc herniations. *Spine.* 1995;20:2613–2625.

38. Jensen MC, Brant-Zawadzki MN, Obuchowski N, Modic MT, Malkasian D, Ross JS. Magnetic resonance imaging of the lumbar spine in people without back pain. *N Engl J Med.* 1994;331:69–73.

39. Sadasivan KK, Reddy RP, Albright JA. The natural history of cervical spondylotic myelopathy. *Yale J Biol Med.* 1993;66:235–242.

40. Herzog RJ, Wiens JJ, Dillingham MF, Sontag MJ. Normal cervical spine morphometry and cervical spinal stenosis in asymptomatic professional football players. Plain film radiography, multiplanar computed tomography, and magnetic resonance imaging. *Spine.* 1991;16:S178–S186.

41. Healy JF, Healy BB, Wong WH, Olson EM. Cervical and lumbar MRI in asymptomatic older male lifelong athletes: frequency of degenerative findings. *J Comput Assist Tomogr.* 1996;20:107–112.

42. Reul J, Gievers B, Weis J, Thron A. Assessment of the narrow cervical spinal canal: a prospective comparison of MRI, myelography and CT-myelography. *Neuroradiology.* 1995;37:187–191.

43. Weis E Jr. Abnormal magnetic-resonance scans of the cervical spine in asymptomatic subjects. *J Bone Joint Surg [Am].* 1991;73:1113.

44. Statham PF, Hadley DM, Macpherson P, Johnston RA, Bone I, Teasdale GM. MRI in the management of suspected cervical spondylotic myelopathy. *J Neurol Neurosurg Psychiatry.* 1991;54:484–489.

45. Yone K, Sakou T, Yanase M, Ijiri K. Preoperative and postoperative magnetic resonance image evaluations of the spinal cord in cervical myelopathy. *Spine.* 1992;17:S388–S392.

46. Matsuda Y, Miyazaki K, Tada K, et al. Increased MR signal intensity due to cervical myelopathy. Analysis of 29 surgical cases. *J Neurosurg.* 1991;74:887–892.

47. Tang XF, Ren ZY. Magnetic transcranial motor and somatosensory evoked potentials in cervical spondylitic myelopathy. *Chin Med J.* 1991;104:409–415.

48. Baba H, Kawahara N, Tomita K, Imura S. Spinal cord evoked potentials in cervical and thoracic myelopathy. *Int Orthop.* 1993;17:82–86.

49. Baba H, Maezawa Y, Imura S, Kawahara N, Tomita K. Spinal cord evoked potential monitoring for cervical and thoracic compressive myelopathy. *Paraplegia.* 1996;34: 100–106.

50. Maertens de Noordhout A, Remacle JM, Pepin JL, Born JD, Delwaide PJ. Magnetic stimulation of the motor cortex in cervical spondylosis. *Neurology.* 1991;41:75–80.

51. Restuccia D, Valeriani M, Di Lazzaro V, Tonali P, Mauguiere F. Somatosensory evoked potentials after multisegmental upper limb stimulation in diagnosis of cervical spondylotic myelopathy. *J Neurol Neurosurg Psychiatry.* 1994;57:301–308.

52. Bouchard JA, Bohlman HH, Biro C. Intraoperative improvements of somatosensory evoked potentials: correlation to clinical outcome in surgery for cervical spondylitic myelopathy. *Spine.* 1996;21:589–594.

53. Diener H, Nutt J. Vestibular and cerebellar disorders of equilibrium and gait. In: Masdeu J, Sudarsky L, Wolfson L, eds. *Gait Disorders of Aging. Falls and Therapeutic Strategies.* Philadelphia: Lippincott & Raven; 1997:261–272.

54. Rademaker GG. *The Physiology of Standing.* Minneapolis: University of Minnesota Press; 1981.

55. Hallett M, Stanhope S, Thomas S, Massaquoi S. Pathophysiology of posture and gait in cerebellar ataxia. In: Shimamura M, Grillner S, Edgerton V, eds. *Neurobiological Basis of Human Locomotion.* Tokyo: Japan Scientific Societies Press; 1991:275–283.

56. Victor M, Adams R, Mancall E. A restricted form of cerebellar cortical degeneration occurring in alcoholic patients. *Arch Neurol.* 1959;1:577–588.

57. Brennan RW, Bergland RM. Acute cerebellar hemorrhage. Analysis of clinical findings and outcome in 12 cases. *Neurology.* 1977;27:527.

58. Marshall J. Cerebellar vascular syndromes. In: Toole J, ed. *Vascular Diseases. Part III.* New York: Elsevier; 1989:89–94.

59. Koh MG, Phan TG, Atkinson JL, Wijdicks EF. Neuroimaging in deteriorating patients with cerebellar infarcts and mass effect. *Stroke.* 2000;31:2062–2067.

60. St Louis EK, Wijdicks EF, Li H, Atkinson JD. Predictors of poor outcome in patients with a spontaneous cerebellar hematoma. *Can J Neurol Sci.* 2000;27:32–36.

61. Boon A, Lodder J, Heuts-van-Raak L, Kessels F. Silent brain infarcts in 755 consecutive patients with a first-ever supratentorial ischemic stroke. Relationship with index-stroke subtype, vascular risk factors, and mortality. *Stroke.* 1994;25:2384–2390.

62. Brott T, Tomsick T, Feinberg W, et al. Baseline silent cerebral infarction in the Asymptomatic Carotid Atherosclerosis Study. *Stroke.* 1994;25:1122–1129.

63. Masdeu J, Gorelick P. Thalamic astasia: inability to stand after unilateral thalamic lesions. *Ann Neurol.* 1988;23:596–603.

64. Verma A, Maheshwari M. Hypesthetic-ataxic-hemiparesis in thalamic hemorrhage. *Stroke.* 1986;17:49–51.

65. Fisher C, Cole M. Homolateral ataxia and crural paresis; a vascular syndrome. *J Neurol Neurosurg Psychiatry.* 1965; 28:48–55.

66. Groothuis D, Duncan G, Fisher C. The human thalamo-cortical sensory path in the internal capsule: evidence from a small capsular hemorrhage causing a pure sensory stroke. *Ann Neurol.* 1977;2:328–333.

67. Labadie E, Awerbuch G, Hamilton R, Rapcsak S. Falling and postural deficits due to acute unilateral basal ganglia lesions. *Arch Neurol.* 1989;261:492–496.

68. Masdeu JC, Wolfson L, Lantos G, et al. Brain white-matter changes in the elderly prone to falling. *Arch Neurol.* 1989; 46:1292–1296.

69. Baloh RW, Yue Q, Socotch TM, Jacobson KM. White matter lesions and disequilibrium in older people. I. Case-control comparison. *Arch Neurol.* 1995;52:970–974.

70. Camicioli R, Moore MM, Sexton G, Howieson DB, Kaye JA. Age-related brain changes associated with motor function in healthy older people. *J Am Geriatr Soc.* 1999; 47:330–334.

71. Hennerici MG, Oster M, Cohen 5, Schwartz A, Motsch L, Daffertshofer M. Are gait disturbances and white matter degeneration early indicators of vascular dementia? *Dementia.* 1994;5:197–202.

72. Tell GS, Lefkowitz DS, Diehr P, Elster AD. Relationship between balance and abnormalities in cerebral magnetic resonance imaging in older adults. *Arch Neurol.* 1998;55: 73–79.

73. Thompson P, Marsden C. Gait disorder of subcortical arteriosclerotic encephalopathy: Binswanger's disease. *Movement Disord.* 1987;2:1–8.

74. FitzGerald P, Jankovic J. Lower body parkinsonism: evidence for vascular etiology. *Movement Disord.* 1987;4: 249–260.

75. Hachinski V, Potter P, Merskey H. Leuko-araiosis. *Arch Neurol.* 1987;44:21–23.

76. Yamanouchi H. Loss of white matter oligodendrocytes and astrocytes in progressive subcortical vascular encephalopathy of Binswanger type. *Acta Neurol Scand.* 1991;83:301–305.

77. Dubas F, Gray F, Roullet E, Escourolle R. Leucoencéphalopathies artériopathiques (17 cas anatomo-cliniques). *Rev Neurol (Paris).* 1985;141:93–108.

78. Gray F, Dubas F, Roullet E, Escourolle R. Leukoencephalopathy in diffuse hemorrhagic cerebral amyloid angiopathy. *Ann Neurol.* 1985;18:54–59.

79. Sabbadini G, Francia A, Calandriello L, et al. Cerebral autosomal dominant arteriopathy with subcortical infarcts and leucoencephalopathy (CADASIL). Clinical, neuroimaging, pathological and genetic study of a large Italian family. *Brain.* 1995;118:207–215.

80. Garcia-Rill E. The pedunculopontine nucleus. *Prog Neurobiol.* 1991;36:363–389.

81. Masdeu J, Alampur U, Cavaliere R, Tavoulareas G. Astasia and gait failure with damage of the pontomesencephalic locomotor region. *Ann Neurol.* 1994;35:619–621.

82. Nutt J, Marsden C, Thompson P. Human walking and higher-level gait disorders, particularly in the elderly. *Neurology.* 1993;43:268–279.

83. Nevitt M. Falls in the elderly: risk factors and prevention. In: Masdeu J, Sudarsky L, Wolfson L, eds. *Gait Disorders of Aging. Falls and Therapeutic Strategies.* Philadelphia: Lippincott & Raven; 1997:13–36.

84. Ray W, Griffin M. Prescribed medications, falling, and fall-related injuries. In: Weindruch R, Ory M, eds. *Frailty Reconsidered: Reducing Frailty and Fall-Related Injuries in the Elderly.* Springfield: Thomas; 1991:76–89.

85. Ray W, Griffin M, Schaffner W, et al. Psychotropic drug use and the risk of hip fracture. *N Engl J Med.* 1987;316:363–369.

86. Nevitt M, Cummings S, Kidd S, Black D. Risk factors for recurrent nonsyncopal falls: a prospective study. *JAMA.* 1989;261:2663–2668.

87. Lipsitz L, Jonsson P, Kelley M, Koestner J. Causes and correlates of recurrent falls in ambulatory frail elderly. *J Gerontol Med Sci.* 1991;46:M114–M122.

88. Studenski S, Duncan P, Chandler J, et al., Predicting falls: the role of mobility and nonphysical factors. *J Am Geriatr Soc.* 1994;42:297–302.

89. Morens DM, Davis JW, Grandinetti A, Ross GW, Popper JS, White LR. Epidemiologic observations on Parkinson's disease: incidence and mortality in a prospective study of middle-aged men. *Neurology.* 1996;46:1044–1050.

90. Obeso JA, Rodriguez MC, DeLong MR. Basal ganglia pathophysiology. A critical review. *Adv Neurol.* 1997;74:3–18.

91. Klawans HL. Individual manifestations of Parkinson's disease after ten or more years of levodopa. *Movement Disord.* 1986;1:187–192.

92. Pahwa R, Koller W. Gait disorders in parkinsonism and other movement disorders. In: Masdeu J, Sudarsky L, Wolfson L, eds. *Gait Disorders of Aging. Falls and Therapeutic Strategies.* Philadelphia: Lippincott & Raven; 1997:209–220.

93. Mestre D, Blin O, Serratrice G. Contrast sensitivity is increased in a case of nonparkinsonian freezing gait. *Neurology.* 1992;42:189–194.

94. Stern GM, Lander CM, Lees AJ. Akinetic freezing and trick movements in Parkinson's disease. *J Neural Transm Suppl.* 1980:137–141.

95. Obeso JA, Rodriguez-Oroz MC, Chana P, Lera G, Rodriguez M, Olanow CW. The evolution and origin of motor complications in Parkinson's disease. *Neurology* 2000;55:S13–S20; discussion S21–S13.

96. Montastruc JL, Rascol O, Senard JM. Treatment of Parkinson's disease should begin with a dopamine agonist. *Movement Disord.* 1999;14:725–730.

97. Rascol O, Brooks DJ, Korczyn AD, De Deyn PP, Clarke CE, Lang AE. A five-year study of the incidence of dyskinesia in patients with early Parkinson's disease who were treated with ropinirole or levodopa. *N Engl J Med.* 2000;342:1484–1491.

98. Schapira AH, Obeso JA, Olanow CW. The place of COMT inhibitors in the armamentarium of drugs for the treatment of Parkinson's disease. *Neurology.* 2000;55:S65–S68; discussion S69–S71.

99. Rodriguez MC, Obeso JA, Olanow CW. Subthalamic nucleus-mediated excitotoxicity in Parkinson's disease: a target for neuroprotection. *Ann Neurol.* 1998;44:S175–S188.

100. Langston JW, Tanner CM. Selegiline and Parkinson's disease: it's deja vu—again. *Neurology.* 2000;55:1770–1771.

101. Bergman H, Wichmann T, Karmon B, DeLong MR. The primate subthalamic nucleus. II. Neuronal activity in the MPTP model of parkinsonism. *J Neurophysiol.* 1994;72:507–520.

102. Baron MS, Vitek JL, Bakay RA, et al. Treatment of advanced Parkinson's disease by unilateral posterior GPi pallidotomy: 4-year results of a pilot study. *Movement Disord.* 2000;15:230–237.

103. Brown RG, Dowsey PL, Brown P, et al. Impact of deep brain stimulation on upper limb akinesia in Parkinson's disease. *Ann Neurol.* 1999;45:473–488.

104. Jahanshahi M, Ardouin CM, Brown RG, et al. The impact of deep brain stimulation on executive function in Parkinson's disease. *Brain.* 2000;123:1142–1154.

105. Guridi J, Obeso JA. The subthalamic nucleus, hemiballismus and Parkinson's disease: reappraisal of a neurosurgical dogma. *Brain.* 2001;124:5–19.

106. Burleigh-Jacobs A, Horak FB, Nutt JG, Obeso JA. Step initiation in Parkinson's disease: influence of levodopa and external sensory triggers. *Movement Disord.* 1997;12:206–215.

107. Schenkman M, Riegger-Krugh C. Physical intervention for elderly patients with gait disorders. In: Masdeu JC, Sudarsky L, Wolfson L, eds. *Gait Disorders of Aging.* Philadelphia: Lippincott & Raven; 1997:327.

108. Litvan I. Progressive supranuclear palsy revisited. *Acta Neurol Scand.* 1998;98:73–84.

109. Pahwa R. Progressive supranuclear palsy. *Med Clin N Am.* 1999;83:369–379, v–vi.

110. Bower JH, Maraganore DM, McDonnell SK, Rocca WA. Incidence of progressive supranuclear palsy and multiple system atrophy in Olmsted County, Minnesota, 1976 to 1990. *Neurology.* 1997;49:1284–1288.

111. Boeve BF, Maraganore DM, Parisi JE, et al. Pathologic heterogeneity in clinically diagnosed corticobasal degeneration. *Neurology.* 1999;53:795–800.

112. Litvan I, Grimes DA, Lang AE, et al. Clinical features differentiating patients with postmortem confirmed progressive supranuclear palsy and corticobasal degeneration. *J Neurol.* 1999;246:II1–5.

113. Gilman S, Low PA, Quinn N, Albanese A, Ben-Shlomo Y, Fowler CJ, et al. Consensus statement on the diagnosis of multiple system atrophy. *J Neurol Sci.* 1999;163:94–98.

114. Siemers E. Multiple system atrophy. *Med Clin Am.* 1999;83:381–392.

115. Kaufmann H. Multiple system atrophy. *Curr Opin Neurol.* 1998;11:351–355.

116. Weiner HL, Constantini S, Cohen H, Wisoff JH. Current treatment of normal-pressure hydrocephalus: comparison of flow-regulated and differential-pressure shunt valves. *Neurosurgery.* 1995;37:877–884.

117. Fisher C. Hydrocephalus as a cause of disturbances of gait in the elderly. *Neurology.* 1982;32:1358–1363.

118. Graff-Radford N, Godersky J, Jones M. Variables predicting outcome in symptomatic hydrocephalus in the elderly. *Neurology.* 1989;39:1601–1604.

119. Graff-Radford N, Godersky J. A clinical approach to symptomatic hydrocephalus in the elderly. In: Masdeu J, Sudarsky L, Wolfson L, eds. *Gait Disorders of Aging. Falls and Therapeutic Strategies.* Philadelphia: Lippincott & Raven; 1997:245–259.

120. Holodny AI, George AE, de Leon MJ, Golomb J, Kalnin AJ, Cooper PR. Focal dilation and paradoxical collapse of cortical fissures and sulci in patients with normal-pressure hydrocephalus. *J Neurosurg.* 1998;89:742–747.

121. Kitagaki H, Mori E, Ishii K, Yamaji S, Hirono N, Imamura T. CSF spaces in idiopathic normal pressure hydrocephalus: morphology and volumetry. *AJNR Am J Neuroradiol.* 1998;19:1277–1284.

122. Malm J, Kristensen B, Karlsson T, Fagerlund M, Elfverson J, Ekstedt J. The predictive value of cerebrospinal fluid dynamic tests in patients with the idiopathic adult hydrocephalus syndrome. *Arch Neurol.* 1995;52:783–789.

123. Sudarsky L, Tideiksaar R. The cautious gait, fear of falling, and psychogenic gait disorders. In: Masdeu J, Sudarsky L, Wolfson L, eds. *Gait Disorders of Aging. Falls and Therapeutic Strategies.* Philadelphia: Lippincott & Raven; 1997: 283–295.

124. Lempert T, Brandt T, Dieterich M, Huppert D. How to identify psychogenic disorders of stance and gait. *J Neurol.* 1991;238:140–146.

125. Keane J. Hysterical gait disorders. *Neurology.* 1989;39:586–589.

126. Jankovic J, Fahn S. Physiologic and pathologic tremors. Diagnosis, mechanism, and management. *Ann Intern Med.* 1980;93:460–465.

127. Koller WC, Busenbark K, Miner K. The relationship of essential tremor to other movement disorders: report on 678 patients. Essential Tremor Study Group. *Ann Neurol.* 1994;35:717–723.

128. Koller W, Busenbark K. Essential tremor. In: Watts R, Koller W, eds. *Movement Disorders: Neurologic Principles and Practice.* New York: McGraw-Hill; 1997:365–385.

129. Findley LJ. Epidemiology and genetics of essential tremor. *Neurology.* 2000;54:S8–S13.

130. Pahwa R, Lyons K, Koller WC. Surgical treatment of essential tremor. *Neurology.* 2000;54:S39–S44.

131. Manyam B. Uncommon forms of tremor. In: Watts R, Koller W, eds. *Movement Disorders: Neurologic Principles and Practice.* New York: McGraw-Hill; 1997:527–540.

132. Shinotoh H, Calne DB, Snow B, et al. Normal CAG repeat length in the Huntington's disease gene in senile chorea. *Neurology.* 1994;44:2183–2184.

133. Mark M. Other choreatic disorders. In: Watts R, Koller W, eds. *Movement Disorders: Neurologic Principles and Practice.* New York: McGraw-Hill; 1997:527–540.

134. Tolosa E, Martí M. Adult-onset idiopathic torsion dystonia. In: Watts R, Koller W, eds. *Movement Disorders: Neurologic Principles and Practice.* New York: McGraw-Hill; 1997:430–441.

135. Grandas F, Elston J, Quinn N, Marsden CD. Blepharospasm: a review of 264 patients. *J Neurol Neurosurg Psychiatry.* 1988;51:767–772.

136. Tolosa E, Martí M. Blepharospasm-oromandibular dystonia syndrome (Meige's syndrome): Clinical aspects. *Adv Neurol.* 1988;49:73–84.

137. American Academy of Neurology. Training guidelines for the use of botulinum toxin for the treatment of neurologic disorders. Report of the Therapeutics and Technology Assessment Subcommittee of the American Academy of Neurology. *Neurology.* 1994;44:2401–2403.

138. Jankovik J. Treatment of dystonia. In: Watts R, Koller W, eds. *Movement Disorders: Neurologic Principles and Practice.* New York: McGraw-Hill; 1997:443–454.

139. Kumar R, Dagher A, Hutchison WD, Lang AE, Lozano AM. Globus pallidus deep brain stimulation for generalized dystonia: clinical and PET investigation. *Neurology.* 1999;53:871–874.

140. Obeso J. Classification, clinical features, and treatment of myoclonus. In: Watts R, Koller W, eds. *Movement Disorders: Neurologic Principles and Practice.* New York: McGraw-Hill; 1997:541–550.

141. Marsden C, Hallett M, Fahn S. The nosology and pathophysiology of myoclonus. In: *Movement Disorders, vol 1.* London: Butterworth; 1982:196–248.

142. Wilkins DE, Hallett M, Berardelli A, Walshe T, Alvarez N. Physiologic analysis of the myoclonus of Alzheimer's disease. *Neurology.* 1984;34:898–903.

143. Obeso J, Artieda J, Rothwell J. The treatment of severe action myoclonus. *Brain.* 1989;112:765–777.

79
Depression, Anxiety, and Other Mood Disorders

Harold G. Koenig and Dan G. Blazer, II

Depression

Mood disorders are the most common reversible psychiatric conditions in later life, and the vast majority are usually treated by primary care physicians and geriatricians. Depression, the prototype mood disorder, is a painful emotional experience that involves intense suffering which can drain life of meaning, excitement, and pleasure. Early epidemiologic research appeared to show that depression was unusually common among older persons.[1,2] In his description of the psychosocial stages of human development, Erik Erikson identified the struggle between integrity and despair as the primary developmental task in late life.

Although aging is often accompanied by loss and unwanted change, most elders do not suffer from depression. In fact, recent studies indicate that serious depressive disorders are actually less common among older than among younger persons in American society.[3–5] This is surprising, given the many reasons why the elderly should be depressed, such as declining health, loss of function, death of family and loved ones, shrinking financial resources, and biologic changes in the brain that predispose them to emotional disorder. Despite this, however, the current cohort of persons over age 65 experience only about one-quarter the rate of major depression and one-sixteenth the rate of bipolar disorder as do persons under age 45.[6]

Epidemiology of Depression

Major depressive disorder, a clinically significant and persistent depression associated with other symptoms, such as weight loss and insomnia, is less frequently diagnosed in old age than at other stages of the life cycle. The NIMH Epidemiologic Catchment Area (ECA) study surveyed more than 5700 elderly persons at five sites across the United States; major depression was diagnosed in less than 1% (0.4% in men, 1.4% in women).[6] A number of epidemiologic studies among community-dwelling and institutionalized adults have confirmed these findings.[7–12] On the other hand, when depressive *symptoms* are examined (dysphoric feelings that fluctuate from day to day and may or may not interfere with functioning), their prevalence in older adults is relatively high. The proportion of elders scoring above symptom scale cutoffs in studies conducted between 1980 and 1990 has been consistently between 10% and 15%.[4] Persons over 80 years of age have higher rates of depressive symptoms than other age groups, although this is almost completely accounted for by the increased number of chronic illnesses and functional disability.[13] Aging per se, then, does not appear to be associated with depression.

There has been some controversy over the low rates of major depressive disorder diagnosed in older adults by the ECA surveys. These rates have either been rejected and attributed to methodologic problems, or accepted and ascribed to cohort or period effects. Those who argue that rates are falsely low claim that depression is just as common in older as younger persons, but that elders are (1) less likely to report depressive symptoms (because of the stigma of psychiatric illness), (2) less likely to recall symptoms (due to cognitive impairment), (3) less likely to have symptoms that fit nicely into diagnostic categories, and (4) more likely to express emotional symptoms as somatic complaints. In a study of more than 1300 community-dwelling adults age 60 or over, Blazer et al. reported that 27% of participants experienced significant depressive symptomatology, whereas less than 1% fulfilled criteria for a major depression.[5] Blazer concluded that current diagnostic methods for depression are not well suited for assessing older adults.

Even if the foregoing arguments are true, however, they do not fully account for the low rates observed.[14] More likely, age differences in rates are real and can be explained by cohort or period effects. The cohort effect maintains that persons age 65 or over born before 1920 are simply more psychologically healthy (for whatever reason) than either later or earlier cohorts; their low rate of major depression in later life, then, may simply reflect the fact that this cohort never experienced much depression.[15] Alternatively, a period effect argues that most persons now age 65 or older endured hard times during the Great Depression and Second World War; since the war, however, these Americans have experienced a higher quality of life and greater well-being (especially in economic terms) than ever before. On the other hand, the 76 million members of the baby boom generation (born between 1946 and 1968) have been accustomed to high standards of living; as that cohort ages, increased competition over resources, declining economic prosperity, and lower standards of living may have led to increasing rates of depression, alcohol, and drug abuse (as now observed).[16] Finally, lower rates of depression among the elderly may represent an age effect; in other words, older persons may possess a greater capacity to adapt to social stressors as a result of cumulative life experiences.

Although rates of depression among community-dwelling older adults are low, this is not true for those hospitalized with medical illness or living in nursing homes. The rate of major depression in acutely hospitalized elders is about 13% to 20%; moreover, an additional 30% of these patients experience minor depressive disorders.[10,17] Likewise, rates of depression and other mood disorders are high among patients in nursing homes, where rates of major depression commonly exceed 15% and minor depression

ranges from 30% to 35%.[18–21] The prevalence of bipolar disorder, while only about 0.1% in the community, may be as high as 10% in nursing homes.[20] Unfortunately, between 80% and 90% of depressed elders in acute medical settings go undiagnosed, despite the fact that brief self-rated scales exist that readily detect depression within less than 2 min. For example, the Koenig depression scale consists of 11 yes–no items that cover most of the major symptoms of depression and has been validated against depression diagnoses in medical patients (see Appendix).[22] The decision on whether to screen, however, is a complex one that involves many considerations.[23]

Depressive illness complicates the medical management of older patients. An increase in all-cause mortality has been reported in community-dwelling, acutely hospitalized, and chronically institutionalized older adults with depression.[21,24] Mortality has been attributed to decreased social support, poor nutrition from loss of appetite, possible adverse effects of depression on the immune system, increased carelessness, and loss of motivation for self-care. Increased cardiovascular mortality, in particular, has been associated with depression.[25,26]

Etiology

As already indicated, the causes for depression in later life are multiple. Figure 79.1 displays the genetic, biologic,

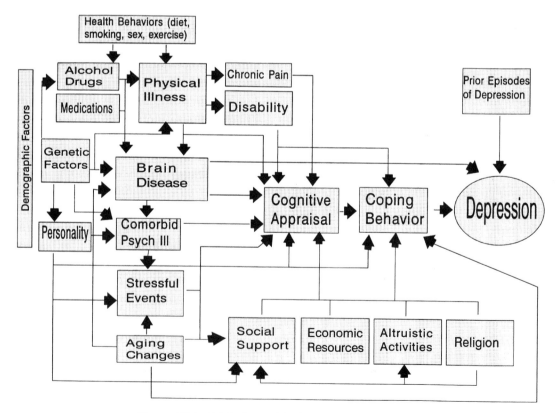

FIGURE 79.1. Etiologic model of depression in later life.

and psychosocial factors that play a role. Genetic factors and brain changes resulting from aging and disease predispose the older adult to depression; stressful life events and health problems can then precipitate a mood disorder if the elder's cognitive appraisal of events is negative and their coping resources inadequate.

Genetic and Biologic Factors

Family studies and molecular genetics suggest that both major depression and bipolar disorders are at least partly inheritable, although the contribution by genetic factors in late-life depression is less than for the early-onset variety. The risk of depression for immediate relatives of index cases with onset after the age of 50 years is only one-half to one-third that of relatives of patients with early-onset disorder (age, <50).[27] The activity and metabolism of neurotransmitters with aging may also affect late-life depression.[28]

Recent interest among clinical investigators has been directed to depression in older adults that is associated with subcortical hyperintensities on magnetic resonance imaging, a syndrome referred to as vascular depression. This depressive syndrome is more common in men, is associated with hypertension, and may have phenomenologic characteristics different from late-life depression not associated with vascular changes.[29] Vascular depression may not be as responsive to long-term intervention as nonvascular depression.

Demographic and Psychosocial Factors

Mood disorders are nearly twice as common among women than men,[6] although this pattern may reverse in later life.[30] Depression is more common in elders with lower incomes and less education,[5,31,32] those who live in rural settings,[32] and those who are divorced or separated.[5,31] Persons with a prior history of psychiatric illness are especially vulnerable when facing the major adjustments required in later life, particularly with health problems.[10] Although many depressions in the elderly are "late onset" (first episode after age 60), a significant minority represent recurrences of mood disorder first diagnosed in young adulthood or middle age.[33]

High social support has been reported to buffer against depression in later life;[5,30] only certain types of support, however, afford such protection. Goldberg and colleagues found that size of the support network was of less importance than its homogeneity (similar age, similar interests), number of confidants, having a husband as a confidant, and level of intimacy.[31] Such support, particularly if perceived by the elder as helpful (high subjective support), may both prevent and facilitate recovery from depression; on the other hand, being married or having a large social network may prolong depression if they exert

a "smothering" effect.[34] A brief social support scale designed specifically for use in chronically ill older adults has now been developed.[35] This scale is included in the Appendix.

Negative life events also commonly precipitate depression in later life.[5] Loss of a spouse is especially difficult for the older person whose marriage has been lifelong and satisfying. Approximately 15% of bereaved adults develop a depressive disorder that requires some form of outside intervention.[36]

Religion, particularly when used regularly to cope with stressful life events, has been associated with greater well-being,[37] lower rates of depression,[38] and faster recovery from depression.[39,40] Many older persons attend church, pray, and read the Bible or other religious scriptures; these behaviors and cognitions are frequently used to cope with the losses associated with aging.[41,42] Studies in both community-dwelling and hospitalized elders have now demonstrated an inverse relationship between religiosity and depressive symptoms.[37,42-46] Active involvement in the religious community and strong religious beliefs appear to reinforce each other and together enhance well-being.[47]

Physical Illness

Physical health has a major impact on the emotional states of older adults. Medical illness often leads to disability, chronic pain, and changes in the brain that both cause distress and limit cognitive flexibility and coping options. Most epidemiologic studies find physical health to be the strongest predictor of well-being and emotional health, regardless of age, sex, or race.[10,31,32] Depressive disorders in physically ill older adults are usually psychologic reactions to progressive disability, chronic pain, side effects from drugs, financial insecurity, or feelings of guilt over being a burden. Less often, depressive disorder results from vascular changes in the brain (vascular depression).[48]

Cognitive Appraisal and Coping

Lazarus[49] emphasized that it is not the particular stress itself (e.g., physical illness, loss of a spouse) that is important in determining the impact of the stressor. Rather, it is the individual's *cognitive appraisal* of the meaning of the event or situation. What is stressful for one older person may not be stressful for another. The cognitive appraisal of the stressor, as well as the perception of adaptive tasks and the selection of coping behaviors, depend heavily on the person's background, health factors, other concurrent stressors, and underlying attitudes toward self, others, current circumstances, and future.

If one feels that one must always be productive to have self-worth, and if illness impairs ability to function and forces dependency, then illness will impose much greater stress than if the person placed less value on productivity and independence. Studies have shown that medical illness can interact with dysfunctional attitudes to precipitate and maintain depression.[50–52] For example, cognitive distortions have been associated with several aspects of disability in patients with chronic low back pain or headache; cognitive variables (in particular, unjustified generalization based on a single incident) account for more disability than would be predicted by severity of pain or number of pain treatments.[53,54] Dysfunctional attitudes, then, may underlie depression in older adults who employ maladaptive rules for interpreting the personal significance of illness-related events.

Clinical and Diagnostic Considerations

The type, number, severity, time course, and combination of symptoms determines whether a depressive disorder is present. Most older persons experience episodes of depressed mood, loss of interest, fatigue, or discouragement that last from hours to days or weeks; yet, these episodes are not severe enough to warrant a diagnosis of major depression or even one of the other affective disorders. These episodes require no more treatment than an encouraging and supportive word from a friend or a good night's rest. Other persons, however, may find themselves locked into a depressive syndrome that will require outside intervention. In a longitudinal study of normal aging, Gianturco and Busse[55] found that 70% of community-dwelling older men experienced some degree of depression at some time during their 17-year study. Differentiating clinically significant depressive disorders from minor mood fluctuations, or from other psychiatric or medical conditions that mimic depression, is not easy.

Major Depressive Disorder

Major depression is defined in the Diagnostic and Statistical Manual of Mental Disorders (DSM-IV) as a depressed mood or a marked loss of interest that is experienced most of the day nearly every day during a 2-week period or longer. In addition, at least four of the following eight symptoms must be present: (1) weight loss (>5% of body weight in a month) or loss of appetite, (2) insomnia or hypersomnia, (3) psychomotor agitation or retardation, (4) fatigue or loss of energy, (5) feelings of worthlessness or guilt, (6) diminished concentration, (7) thoughts of suicide, or (8) loss of interest (including decreased sexual interest). According to DSM-IV, these symptoms must cause clinically significant distress or impairment in social, occupational, or other important areas of functioning.

The symptoms of major depression can be divided into two groups: vegetative (or somatic) and cognitive (or psychologic). Vegetative symptoms include insomnia, anorexia or weight loss, fatigue, concentration difficulties, and psychomotor agitation or retardation. Cognitive symptoms include depressed mood, irritability, hopelessness, guilt, feeling worthless or as a burden, loss of interest, social withdrawal, and suicidal thoughts. Cognitive symptoms can help identify depression in medically ill older patients whose somatic symptoms confuse the diagnostic picture. Somatic symptoms, however, cannot be ignored and may be important for recognizing severe forms of depression. One study found that loss of interest, insomnia, suicidal thoughts, and hypochondriasis best differentiated depressed from nondepressed medically ill older patients; fatigue, weight loss, genital symptoms, and somatic anxiety, on the other hand, were only weakly or not related to depression.[56]

Melancholic and Psychotic Depressions

Melancholic depression is a form of major depression that is associated with weight loss, insomnia, psychomotor retardation, profound loss of interest or pleasure (anhedonia), and a mood that does not fluctuate with external circumstances. Psychotic depression is a major depression that is associated with delusional thinking (bizarre ideas that the person cannot be talked out of), marked paranoia or suspiciousness, and, more rarely, auditory hallucinations. Older persons with depression are more likely to experience delusions than younger persons with depression.[33] Delusions often involve persecution, having an incurable illness, or focus on somatic complaints involving the abdomen. These individuals respond particularly well to electroconvulsive therapy (ECT) as opposed to antidepressants.

Dysthymia

A dysthymia is a chronic depression lasting 2 years or longer that does not fulfill the criteria for major depression. A "double depression" occurs when major depression is superimposed upon chronic dysthymia. Verwoerdt suggested that dysthymic disorder (depressive neurosis) is less frequent in the later part of the life cycle.[57] Community data, however, indicate that dysthymic disorder in the elderly is less frequent, but that the difference in rates between younger and older persons is not so great as for major depression.[6] Although chronic depressions are difficult to treat when they are related to character pathology, studies have shown a good response to adequate doses of tricyclics; psychotherapy may be very helpful to these individuals who may have difficulty relating to others.

Minor Depression

Minor (or subthreshold) depression has received much attention in the literature in recent years. The diagnosis is often one of exclusion, but the condition is defined as a less severe depressive episode than major depression and not as chronic as dysthymia. Criteria for the diagnosis appear in the Appendix (of DSM-IV). The diagnosis involves 2 weeks or more of depressed mood or loss of interest, together with between one and four of the traditional eight symptoms of depression (sleep disturbance, loss of sexual interest, guilt, loss of energy, difficulty concentrating, appetite disturbance, psychomotor agitation or retardation, suicidal thoughts). Beekman and colleagues[58] have estimated the frequency of minor depression in the elderly to be between 8% and 13% in community samples. The clinical significance of minor depression has not been established, nor has the effectiveness of treatment. The syndrome may actually, in most cases, be a prodrome or a residual of major depression (or a less severe manifestation of the same basic psychopathology as major depression). Treatment studies are difficult to perform because the "distance to recovery" in terms of symptom reduction is lower than for major depression. Nevertheless, some large clinical trials have suggested that antidepressant medications may be effective when compared to placebo.

Depression Not Otherwise Specified (NOS)

This depression subtype is often intermittent and unexplained by psychosocial or biologic factors; it is a milder form of mood disorder that does not fulfill either the severity or length criteria for major depression. Two subcategories for depression NOS may be seen by clinicians working with depressed elders. First, the syndrome may fulfill the criteria for dysthymic disorder; however, there are intermittent periods of normal mood lasting more than a few months. Second, some elders may experience a brief episode of depression that does not meet the criteria for major affective disorder and is apparently not reactive to psychosocial stress (so that it cannot be classified as an adjustment disorder). Although not an official diagnostic category, the term "minor depression" is included in the Appendix to DSM-IV. Patients with depression NOS may or may not fulfill DSM-IV criteria for minor depression.

Bereavement

Bereavement, a universal human experience, cannot be classified as a psychiatric disorder. Normal symptoms of grief include sensations of somatic distress such as tightness in the throat, shortness of breath, sighing respirations, lassitude, and loss of appetite. The bereaved may be preoccupied with the image of the deceased. Pathologic grief may occur if the usual symptoms are either delayed, persist beyond the expected period of time, or become unusually severe. Delayed grief can be distinguished from normal grieving by symptoms of overactivity without a sense of loss, frequently accompanied by psy-

chosomatic complaints. When grief is unusually severe it may be associated with marked feelings of worthlessness, hopelessness, or suicidal ideation. Patients who fulfill the symptom criteria for major depression 2 months after bereavement, however, should be treated just like any other patient with major depression.

Adjustment Disorder with Depressed Mood

The DSM-IV category of adjustment disorder with depressed mood is reserved for those individuals who exhibit a maladaptive reaction to an identifiable stressor; here, the relationship of the syndrome to the stressful event is clear. Stressors for older adults may include life events such as retirement, marital problems, difficulty with children, loss of a social role, and an ill-advised change of residence. Depressive symptomatology often develops secondary to physical illness. When an episode of depression accompanies a physical illness and exceeds the level of symptoms expected, then the diagnosis of adjustment disorder is indicated.

Mood Disorder Caused by a General Medical Condition

The essential feature of mood disorder due to a general medical condition (formerly known as organic mood syndrome) is a disturbance in mood that results from direct physiologic effects of a general medical condition. General medical conditions likely to have such physiologic effects include hypothyroidism, hypercalcemia, B_{12} deficiency, and illnesses that directly affect the brain (tumor, some kinds of stroke) (Table 79.1).

Substance-Induced Mood Disorder

Prescription medications such as antihypertensives, antianxiety (benzodiazepines) drugs, chemotherapeutic agents, and other drugs with CNS effects may precipitate a mood disorder (see Table 79.1). Chronic alcohol, cocaine, or other illicit drug use, or withdrawal from these substances, often evoke a depressive-like syndrome and such use must be part of screening.

Differential Diagnosis

Psychiatric conditions with depressive symptoms may be confused with depression; these include hypochondriasis, alcoholism, the organic mental disorders, delusional disorders, and schizophrenia. Hypochondriasis is both a symptom of depression and a separate disorder itself. The essential features are an unrealistic interpretation of physical sensations as abnormal and a preoccupation with the imagined physical illness underlying these sensations. Between 60% and 70% of depressed persons in one study were found to have hypochondriacal symp-

TABLE 79.1. Physical illnesses and medications associated with depression.

Physical illnesses	Medications
End-stage renal disease (especially with uremia)	CNS drugs
	Benzodiazepines
Cardiovascular disease	
Postmyocardial infarction	Alcohol
Postcoronary artery bypass surgery	Levodopa
Cardiomyopathy (congestive or other)	Amantadine
	Major tranquilizers
Endocrine disorders	Stimulants (rebound)
Thyroid (hyper- and hypothyroidism, thyroiditis)	
Parathyroid (hyper- and hypoparathyroidism)	Antihypertensives
Adrenal (Cushing's and Addison's diseases)	Beta-blockers
Disorders of insulin secretion	Clonidine
Hypopituitarism	Reserpine
Metabolic or nutritional disorders	Methyldopa
Hypokalemia or hyperkalemia	Prazosin
Hyponatremia or hypernatremia	Guanethidine
Hypocalcemia or hypercalcemia	
Hypomagnesemia	Chemotherapeutic drugs
Metabolic acidosis or alkalosis	Vincristine
Hypoxemia	L-asparaginase
Vitamin deficiencies (B vitamins, folate)	Interferon
	Tamoxifen
Neurologic diseases	
Parkinson's disease	Steroids
Stroke	Prednisone
Alzheimer's disease	Estrogen preparations
Subdural hematoma	
Amyotrophic lateral sclerosis	Anticonvulsants
Temporal lobe epilepsy	Procarbazine
Multiple sclerosis	Diphenylhydantoin
Normal-pressure hydrocephalus	
	Others
Cancer	Cimetidine
Brain tumors (primary or secondary)	Digitalis
Pancreatic cancer	Nonsteroidal anti-inflammatory drugs
Lung cancer (oat cell)	
Bone metastases with hypercalcemia	
Miscellaneous	
Hepatic failure with encephalopathy	
Anemia	
Infections (particularly viral)	
Chronic pain	

toms.[59] When hypochondriacal complaints appear in later life for the first time, there is a high likelihood that either depression or an undetected physical illness is present.

Hypochondriasis as a disorder is usually distinguishable from depression by (1) the length of the episode (hypochondriasis persisting for years), (2) the degree of suffering by the patient (more among depressed patients), (3) and the waxing and waning course of symptoms in depression, which by nature is cyclic. Differentiating the older adult with hypochondriasis or generalized anxiety disorder from the one who is depressed has therapeutic implications; hypochondriacs often do not tolerate antidepressants because of real or imagined side effects.

Alcoholism, although less frequent in older than in younger persons, still occurs in about 5% to 8% of persons over age 60. A heavy alcohol intake may cause both physical and psychologic symptoms that mimic depression. Conversely, many alcoholics drink to relieve the pain of depression that recurs when they become sober; in this case, depressive disorder has been "masked" by the alcohol problem. The same principles apply to elders who abuse prescription drugs.

The sudden appearance of a psychosis in later life, with paranoid or delusional thinking, may herald the onset of a major depression. Differentiating depression from late-life schizophrenia or delusional disorder may be difficult, but the latter are not usually associated with profound depression. Late-life schizophrenia seldom begins suddenly; instead, it is characterized by gradual withdrawal, bizarre complaints, and paranoia.

Finally, it may be difficult to distinguish an agitated depression from panic disorder with secondary depression. These conditions can often be differentiated by determining which symptoms arose first; patients with a primary panic disorder will report a history of anxiety symptoms that precede the onset of depression, whereas those with primary depression report that their depression came before the onset of panic. The comorbidity between depression and anxiety disorders is discussed further next.

Manic Episodes and Bipolar Disorder

A manic episode is defined as a distinct period of abnormally elevated or expansive mood associated with at least three of the following symptoms: grandiosity, decreased sleep, pressured speech, flight of ideas, distractibility, increased activity, and excessive involvement in pleasurable activities (DSM-IV). A single episode of mania, either by itself or associated with prior episodes of depression, allows for the diagnosis of bipolar disorder (bipolar, type I). Less severe mood swings that have lasted for 2 years or more are termed *cyclothymia*, and other states not meeting any of the criteria for a specific bipolar disorder are labeled *bipolar disorder not otherwise specified*. Bipolar type II is a patient with a history of one or more major depressive episodes and periods of hypomania (but not full-blown mania).

Bipolar disorder is not as common in persons over age 65 as it is in younger persons. The presentation of bipolar disorder in later life may be atypical with a mixture of manic and dysphoric symptoms.[60] Euphoria may be less common and is replaced by irritability or cognitive impairment. The term manic delirium has been used to describe a state of altered consciousness that may be difficult to distinguish from organic brain syndrome, dementia, and even schizophrenia.[61] Older manics may have different symptomatology from younger patients, including less intense levels of overactivity, less intense sexual drive, and less disturbed thought processes.[62] Longer hospitalization, greater residual psychopathology, and a diminished response to pharmacotherapy have also been associated with older age. Increased cerebral vulnerability from stroke, head trauma, or other neurologic disorders is an important etiologic factor in late-onset mania.[63–65]

Diagnostic Evaluation

There is a greater likelihood that mood disorders in later life will be accompanied by physical illness.[66] Diagnostic evaluation, then, should be thorough and comprehensive. A patient's history should focus on the length of the current episode, any history of previous episodes, a history of drug or alcohol abuse, therapies tried in the past, and an assessment of the patient's suffering, particularly with respect to suicidal thoughts. If possible, con-

firmation of the patient's responses should be obtained from a relative or caretaker. In the physical examination, attention should be directed toward such neurologic findings as lateralization, tremor, muscle tone, and slowed reflexes.

Laboratory Workup

Thyroid function studies (T_4, TSH), complete blood cell count, serum electrolytes, vitamin B_{12} level, and drug levels are often helpful in identifying reversible organic causes of depression. Vitamin B_{12} deficiency may present with depressive symptoms, as well as dementia, in the face of a normal serum B_{12} level or hemogram; methylmalonic acid and homocystine levels should be checked in depressed patients with low normal serum B_{12} levels. A head CT scan or MRI scan can rule out brain tumors, although when the history is not suggestive and the neurologic exam is normal, the yield from these tests is very low. Imaging may also identify a vascular depression. Nevertheless, a routine CT or MRI is not indicated in the laboratory workup of late-life depression. An electrocardiogram, as well as renal and liver function tests, can be helpful if psychopharmacologic treatment is contemplated.

Management of Depression

Once a diagnosis has been made and the patient's safety ensured, management includes one or more of the following specific treatments: psychotherapy, pharmacotherapy, or electroconvulsive therapy (ECT). Regardless of which modality is chosen, all depressed elders require psychologic support, which involves listening, empathy, and demonstration of concern, in other words, good clinical care. Many patients with minor depressions or adjustment disorders may improve with this intervention alone. Primary care physicians, nurses, or social workers may provide such support. The clergy may also be a helpful resource, given the important role that religion plays in the lives of many older adults.[67]

Psychotherapy

Psychotherapy avoids the side effects associated with psychoactive drugs.[68] A wide variety of psychotherapies are available to the clinician for use in elderly depressed patients; only a few, however, have proven efficacy in late-life depression. Insight-oriented and psychoanalytic psychotherapy has not been studied systematically with depressed elders. Thus, we focus primarily on cognitive-behavioral and time-limited therapies.

Cognitive therapy (CT) is designed to train patients to identify and correct the negative thinking in depression that contributes to its maintenance.[69] Depressed patients overgeneralize, catastrophize, and think in terms of extremes. It is easy for this negative thinking to convince the patient that he or she is inadequate and ineffective, dissipating hope. Cognitive restructuring helps to break the vicious cycle of depressive thinking. Recall from Figure 79.1 the central role that cognitive appraisal plays in the causal path that leads to depression. Cognitive interventions may enable the older person to view their disabilities and other life stressors in a more positive light, as well as disrupt negative ruminations.

Behavioral therapy (BT), on the other hand, involves positive reinforcement of behaviors that alleviate depression (pleasurable activities) and the negative reinforcement of behaviors that lead to depression (withdrawal, etc.).[70] In BT, the patient is encouraged to keep weekly activity schedules, and mastery and pleasure logs, and to complete other homework assignments. A variant of cognitive-behavioral therapy is interpersonal therapy (IPT).[71] IPT is similar in approach to CT, but the focus of therapy is on the interpersonal interactions of the patient. IPT has been employed in many clinical trials among younger and older subjects, usually in conjunction with medication. Brief dynamic therapy (BDT) stresses the importance of the patient–therapist relationship, emphasizing the realistic collaborative aspects of the therapeutic alliance rather than focusing on the transference as in classical dynamic therapy.[72]

Thompson and colleagues compared the efficacy of CT, BT, and BDT in a study of 91 elders with major depression.[73] After 6 weeks of treatment, 52% of patients were in full remission and 18% showed significant improvement. CT, BT, and BDT were equally effective and significantly superior to the control group. Group psychotherapy, using an educational problem-solving approach, may be a particularly effective, inexpensive, and acceptable form of treatment for older adults, especially those who are socially isolated.[74,75] For elders suffering from unresolved grief reactions following bereavement, mutual self-help groups led by nonclinicians have been shown to be equally effective as participation in formal psychotherapy groups.[76]

Pharmacotherapy

Because of the excellent response of many depressed older adults to drug therapy, antidepressants should always be considered when depressive symptoms threaten the elder's ability to function. The five major classes of medications used to treat mood disorders are (1) selective serotonin reuptake inhibitors (SSRI), (2) other novel antidepressants (venlafaxine, mirtazapine, bupropion, nefazodone), (3) tricyclic antidepressants, (4) monoamine oxidase (MAO) inhibitors, and (5) mood stabilizers (lithium carbonate, carbamazepine, valproic acid). SSRIs and newer non-SSRI antidepressants have taken over as the drugs of choice for depression in late life. These have largely displaced the second-generation tricyclic antidepressants (nortriptyline or desipramine), although the latter continue to have a place in the treatment of late-life depression, particularly severe depression with melancholic symptoms (Table 79.2).

SSRIs such as fluoxetine, sertraline, paroxetine, or citalopram are now the drugs of first choice for geriatric depression. Initial doses must be small (10mg/day or 10mg every other day for fluoxetine; 12.5 or 25mg/day for sertraline; 5–10mg/day for paroxetine) to reduce the likelihood of unpleasant side effects. The newer antidepressants, although generally devoid of the orthostasis, anticholinergic, and cardiac side effects of tricyclic antidepressants, have their own unpleasant effects that affect their use in older patients; these include weight loss, excessive stimulation and agitation, insomnia, gastrointestinal side effects, tremor, and disequilibrium. Because of its long half-life (10–14 days in frail elders), fluoxetine should be used cautiously in older patients, although it may also enable patients to take the drug only three or four times per week, thereby reducing cost. Sertraline, paroxetine, and citalopram with shorter half-lives are more quickly cleared from the body but can create problems when the medication is abruptly discontinued (due to a withdrawal syndrome). Among the oldest-old, inappropriate secretion of antidiuretic hormone (ADH) may occur with the use of these drugs. SSRIs can interfere with the P-450 enzyme system in the liver, and therefore decrease the metabolism of certain drugs such as warfarin. Such potential interactions are present with every SSRI, even the newer ones, although they are purported to be less of a problem with sertraline and citalopram.

Patients who do not respond to traditional SSRIs, or who after being on these drugs for some time lose their responsiveness, may be tried on venlafaxine, which inhibits the reuptake of both serotonin and norepinephrine. Patients may be started on doses of 25mg twice daily, and increased gradually up to 150mg twice daily if necessary. Blood pressure should be monitored because this drug has been associated with worsening of hypertension. Mirtazapine is another novel antidepressant with relatively few side effects that may be tried either initially or after the patient has failed a trial with SSRIs. Mirtazapine has the benefit of being sedating, particularly at low doses. Patients should be started on 15mg at bedtime, and then after a week or two increased to 30mg, the dose at which most older adults respond. A few patients, however, may require as much as 45mg/day given at bedtime. As with venlafaxine, blood pressure should be monitored; also, be aware that agranulocytosis occurs in about 0.1% of patients of all ages.

Until recently, nortriptyline, desipramine, and doxepin were popular drugs for treating older adults with

TABLE 79.2. Recommended doses, reported side effects, and therapeutic blood levels of antidepressants in older persons.

Drug	Dose/day (initial maintenance), mg	Therapeutic serum level, ng/dL	Relative sedation	Relative anticholinergic	Postural hypotension
Heterocyclics					
Doxepin	25–100	>100	++++	++++	++++
Nortriptyline	10–75	50–150	+++	+++	+++
Desipramine	25–125	>125	++	++	+++
Trazodone	50–300	NA	++++	+	+++
Nefazodone	100–600	NA	+++	+	+
SSRIs					
Fluoxetine	5–20	NA	+	+	+
Sertraline	25–100	NA	+	+	+
Paroxetine	10–20	NA	+	++	+
Citalopram	20–40	NA	+	+	+
Others					
Venlafaxine (S/NRI)	25–75	NA	+	+	+
Mirtazapine	15–45	NA	+++	+	+
Bupropion	75–300	NA	+	+	+
MAO inhibitors					
Phenelzine	15–45	>80% inhibition of MAO	+	++	+++
Mood stabilizers					
Lithium carbonate	150–600	0.4–0.7 mmol/L	++	0	0
Valproic acid	250–1250	50–100 ng/mL	++	0	0
Stimulants					
Methylphenidate	5–30	NA	0	0	?

NA, not applicable; four plus signs, strong; three plus signs, moderate; two plus signs, weak; one plus sign, negligible; zero, none; MAO, monoamine oxidase; SSRI, selective serotonin reuptake inhibitor; S/NRI, serotonin/norepinephrine reuptake inhibitor.

endogenous depressions. If used today, lower doses than those for younger adults are preferred, because high blood levels may occur even at reduced dosages.[77] Doses of 10 to 50 mg of nortriptyline or 25 to 75 mg of desipramine at bedtime are often adequate to relieve symptoms, although blood levels should be followed to ensure a therapeutic dose.

For patients with an agitated depression who need sedation, trazodone at doses from 50 to 300 mg/day or nefazodone at doses of 100 to 300 mg/day may be tried. Because they are virtually devoid of anticholinergic side effects, trazodone and nefazodone are attractive drugs for use in elderly patients. Nevertheless, their antidepressant potency is questionable at doses that elders can usually tolerate, and side effects such as excessive drowsiness, orthostasis, and priapism are reasons for caution (although less so for nefazodone than for trazodone).

Bupropion is another antidepressant that may have special advantages in certain patients. Elders who have psychomotor retarding (slowed down in physical movements and mental activity), or are unmotivated, fatigued, frail, and at high risk for falling, may find bupropion helpful. Doses beginning at 75 mg/day and increasing to 225 or 300 mg/day are recommended; any single dose should not exceed 150 mg, usually requiring bid (twice a day) or tid (three times a day) dosing. Toxicity at the higher doses may be manifested by tremor, unpleasant gastrointestinal side effects, or visual hallucinations. Stopping or reducing the dose readily reverses these symptoms. Bupropion has also been associated with an increased risk of seizures, especially in patients with anorexia nervosa or bulimia; thus, a history of seizures should be ruled out before starting this drug.

Combinations of an SSRI and a tricyclic antidepressant, bupropion, or trazadone may help in resistant depressions. For instance, 10 to 20 mg of fluoxetine, 25 to 50 mg of sertraline, or 10 to 20 mg of paroxetine may be used with 10 to 50 mg of nortriptyline or 25 to 50 mg of trazodone at night to achieve the desired antidepressant effect and minimize side effects such as insomnia. Note that all SSRIs interfere with the hepatic metabolism of tricyclics and will increase their blood levels; thus, if an SSRI is added to a regimen that includes a tricyclic antidepressant, the dose of the latter should be reduced by one-half or greater and blood levels carefully monitored. Much attention has been directed toward the cytochrome P-450 group of enzymes and the potential for toxic drug–drug interactions secondary to the effects of the SSRIs upon these enzymes. In general, commonly used medications when used in moderation do not result in side effects. Nevertheless, the clinician should review the specific medications prescribed to the patient, perhaps with a computer-assisted program, to avoid these drug–drug interactions.

St. John's wort is a natural herb that has been used for the treatment of depression, particularly in Europe. The preparations that can be bought over the counter in health food stores in the United States are of uncertain composition and purity. These preparations should not be used for a patient with a clinical diagnosis of depression, because there are known effective treatments that have been tested (antidepressants already described), approved by the FDA, and have careful guidelines and requirements for their preparation. St. John's wort is currently being evaluated in a multisite study funded by the NIH's Office of Alternative Medicine.

Before starting therapy with an antidepressant, the older patient should undergo a thorough history and physical examination to identify contraindications. When using tricyclics, special effort should be employed to elicit a history of closed-angle glaucoma, difficulty with urination, severe dizziness with standing, seizure disorder, severe hypertension, recent myocardial infarction, or unstable angina. The physical examination should include measurement of orthostatic blood pressure changes, as well as examination of the liver and prostate for enlargement. Baseline liver and kidney function test results should also be obtained because most antidepressants are metabolized in the liver and excreted in the urine.

An electrocardiogram should be obtained before starting therapy with antidepressants, especially tricyclics or tetracyclics; even patients on SSRIs may be at increased risk for developing cardiac complications, particularly in the presence of atrial arrhythmias. If a left bundle branch block, bifascicular block, second-degree heart block, or prolongation of the QT interval (>480 ms) are present, antidepressants should not be started until a cardiac consultation has been obtained or the patient is under careful observation in the hospital. Patients with atrial fibrillation may experience an acceleration in heart rate due to anticholinergic side effects that enhance conduction through the atrioventricular (AV) node. Simple first-degree AV block or bundle branch block does not increase the risk of cardiac complications. A follow-up electrocardiogram, after the start of treatment, is essential in all patients with heart disease. The dose should be decreased or the drug should be stopped if there is a marked prolongation of the PR, QT, or QRS durations or if AV block worsens or ventricular arrhythmias increase. Use of tricyclic antidepressants concurrently with quinidine, procainamide hydrochloride (Pronestyl), or other type I antiarrhythmics may produce additive cardiac effects.

To ensure compliance, patients should be informed of possible side effects, such as dizziness with sudden standing, difficulty with urination, dry mouth, and constipation for tricyclic antidepressants, and side effects such as nausea, headache, weight loss, agitation, insomnia, and loss of sexual interest for SSRIs. These effects are often experienced soon after starting the drug therapy, but often gradually improve after a couple weeks of therapy. patients should also be warned that antidepressant effects may not occur before 6 to 8 weeks of treatment. When there is concern over the patient's suicidal potential, no more than 1 g of a tricyclic antidepressant should be dispensed at any one time; fatal overdose with the SSRIs, bupropion, velafaxine, mirtazapine, and nefazodone is much more difficult. Once a response is achieved, antidepressants should be continued for 6 to 9 months and then gradually tapered. Given the high rate of relapse in older adults, some experts are now recommending long-term maintenance therapy at the same dose that achieved a therapeutic response, especially if the elder has experienced a recurrence of a successfully treated episode. Life-long treatment may be indicated for those with a history of one or more relapses.[78] Monoamine oxidase inhibitors are an alternative to the heterocyclic antidepressants and SSRIs, although they are not easy to use in the treatment of depression in older patients.

Lithium carbonate may be useful in preventing the recurrence of unipolar depression, although its efficacy in this regard is not as established as for bipolar disorder. Although lithium alone is a poor antidepressant, it may be used to augment the antidepressant effects of tricyclics. Lithium may sensitize postsynaptic adrenergic receptors, thereby enhancing the effects of tricyclic antidepressants. Anticonvulsants such as carbamazepine or valproic acid are especially useful in treating older patients who rapidly cycle between depressed and manic or agitated moods. In general, the use of lithium or anticonvulsants by nonpsychiatric physicians in the treatment of depression or management of bipolar disorder in older patients is not recommended.

In general, benzodiazepines should not be used to treat geriatric depression as these can induce excessive sedation and may even worsen the depressive state.[79,80] The possible exception is alprazolam, which has been reported to have antidepressant, as well as antianxiety, effects. At doses of 2 to 4 mg/day, the antidepressant effects of this drug have been reported to equal those of imipramine. Nevertheless, elders may easily become dependent on alprazolam, and it is difficult to get them off the drug once started.

Low doses of stimulants such as methylphenidate (5–15 mg two or three times/day) may enhance the appetite and mood of an apathetic older adult. At such doses, side effects are rare (especially if the last dose is given before 2 P.M.), and abuse or addiction is seldom encountered; nevertheless, blood pressure should be monitored and these drugs avoided in patients with unstable angina. Furthermore, tolerance may occur, requiring an escalation of dose to achieve the desired effect. Stimulants have been used to treat depression in medically ill older patients,[10] although it remains unclear whether they actually treat the mood disorder or simply activate retarded patients.

Major depression in patients with dementia should be treated with antidepressant medication. Start with an SSRI, bupropion, or mirtazapine (if sleep is a problem). Avoid tricylics if possible. The starting dose of tricylics, if used, should be low (e.g., 10 mg nortriptyline, increasing slowly to a maximum of 50 mg/day). Anticholinergic effects can worsen dementia and may precipitate an acute delirium.

The treatment of acute mania is best accomplished with lithium carbonate; supplementation with benzodiazepines or phenothiazines may be necessary. The anticonvulsant valproic acid is increasingly being utilized as a first-line agent to control both manic episodes and agitation/aggression in elderly patients. In rare circumstances, a manic episode will respond only to ECT.

Recent studies have demonstrated the effectiveness of combined use of tricyclic antidepressants (specifically nortriptiline) and IPT in both the treatment of a depressive episode and the prevention of relapse once the episode remits.[81] The combination of medications and psychotherapy was especially beneficial in decreasing the likelihood of recurrence once an episode responded to therapy, even in the most severely depressed sample members.

Electroconvulsive Therapy

For severe depressions that are persistent and refractory to psychotherapy and pharmacotherapy, ECT is the most effective treatment.[82] It is particularly effective in major depression with either melancholic or psychotic features. Of the 1400 ECT treatments per year given to psychiatric inpatients at Duke Hospital, 70% are for patients age 60 or over. Despite its remarkable effectiveness and general safety, ECT is still usually performed only after other methods of treatment have failed. In cases where the patient becomes suicidal or attempts to starve to death, ECT is the treatment of choice because of its rapid effect.

For an adequate therapeutic response, treatments are usually given three times per week for a total of 8 to 12 times; this can be done as an inpatient or outpatient. A marked improvement usually is noted after one of the treatments. Following this improvement, two or three further treatments are usually given. The overall success rate for ECT in drug nonresponders is about 80%, a rate similar in both younger and older patients. In the absence of prophylactic drug therapy, the relapse rate 1 year following ECT exceeds 50%. Maintenance ECT (weekly or monthly) or concurrent use of antidepressants decreases the relapse rate to around 20% in the year following ECT.

Confusion following ECT varies from patient to patient, depending on underlying level of cognitive impairment. There is less confusion after unilateral than bilateral electrode placement during ECT and also less confusion after brief pulse stimulation than after sine wave stimulation. It is difficult to evaluate the effects of ECT on memory, because depression itself affects memory. Significant cognitive impairment is not a contraindication to ECT, because if this impairment is caused by depression, it may improve as the depression improves.[83] Most memory impairment induced by ECT disappears by 6 months after treatment.[84]

Prognosis

The natural history of major depression follows a pattern of remission and relapse. Until recently, most follow-up studies indicated that one-third of depressed elders recovered completely from an index episode, one-third experienced a partial recovery or relapsed soon after recovery, and one-third remained continuously ill.[11] The results from follow-up studies, however, depend largely on the sample. British investigators Baldwin and Jolley,[85] however, reported that 60% of depressed elders remained continuously well or had further episodes with complete recovery during a 3- to 8-year follow-up period. Factors associated with better outcome are female sex, current employment, and high level of subjective social support.[3,86] Other positive prognostic factors include an extraverted personality style, absence of severe symptomatology, a family history of depression, a history of recovery from previous episodes, no substance or alcohol abuse, no other comorbid major psychiatric illness, minimal intercurrent life changes, and religious coping style.[38,85,86] On the other hand, poor outcomes have been associated with delusions, significant cognitive impairment, and physical illness.[85,87,88] More recent studies indicate that when antidepressant therapy is combined with psychotherapy or ECT, a remission can be achieved in about 80% of cases (similar to the response rate in younger depressed patients).[89–92]

Little is known concerning the outcome of bipolar disorders in older persons. There is some information to suggest that early-onset bipolar disorder may "burn out" with time. Shulman and Post[93] found that few of their sample of elderly persons with bipolar disorder had the early-onset variety. When mania occurs for the first time in an elder who previously had unipolar depression, the illness may have a poorer prognosis than unipolar depression; the strong association between late-onset mania and progressive neurologic disorders (such as Alzheimer's disease and other dementias) accounts for this.[94]

Suicide and Its Prevention

Cross-sectional epidemiologic studies have shown that suicide rates in later life are higher than at younger ages, and suicide ranks among the top 10 causes of death in persons over age 65.[95] After nearly 40 years of declining suicide rates in the elderly, since 1980 these rates have begun to increase. Risk factors for suicide include sex (male), race (white), marital status (divorced or separated), economic status (low), mental illness, previous suicide attempts, and health. Although men of all ages have a higher suicide rate than women, older men have a higher rate than any other age by sex group;[15] in fact, the higher rate of suicide in the elderly results largely from the higher risk in older white males. Elderly patients with mental illness, particularly depression and schizophrenia, are at high risk for suicide. When depression coexists with other mental disorders, the risk increases further.

The presence of alcohol abuse or dependence is a major risk factor for suicide, especially among elderly white males; this is particularly true for late-onset alcoholics, who often drink in response to psychosocial stressors. Thus, an inquiry about alcohol use is essential when evaluating safety risk in older patients with depression.

Poor health status is another major risk factor for suicide in later life. In 1928, Cavan noted that physical illness led to suicide when a person's capacity to endure severe pain was exceeded.[96] In a review of 391 cases of suicide, she found that 23% had physical illness; in two-thirds of this group, the suicide was directly related to the illness. The close relationship between physical illness and suicide has been repeatedly demonstrated by other investigators, particularly in men and in patients with coexisting depression or organic brain syndrome. MacKenzie and Popkin provide an excellent review of the association between medical illness and suicide.[97]

Involvement of family in helping to monitor an elderly suicidal patient at home is vital in preventing suicide. Inquiry about a "plan" often reveals the means by which the act might be attempted; the family should be instructed to remove from the house weapons such as guns, large knives, and all but necessary medications. If the family cannot assure the physician that at least one family member can be with the patient at all times until the risk of suicide has passed, then hospitalization is the safest course. If hospitalized, the patient should be placed in an environment with windows of shatter-proof glass or safety screens and should not have access to open stairwells or laundry chutes. Potentially harmful devices, such as razors, scissors, knives, forks, ropes, and breakable glass bottles or glasses, should also be removed from the patient's environment. Adequate doses of psychotropic medication should be utilized for the confused or psychotic patient. The quickest and safest form of treatment in the severely depressed and suicidal elder is ECT.

Anxiety Disorders

Anxiety is a common symptom experienced by elderly persons, particularly those with physical health problems.[98] Clinicians evaluating an elderly person with a complaint of anxiety must first decide if the symptom is due to some underlying medical illness. If not, then the clinican must determine whether the anxiety is a result of psychiatric illness or represents a normal response to life events. The signs and symptoms of anxiety are both cognitive and physical, and include difficulty with concentration, dizziness or faintness, tremulousness, insomnia, fears of "going crazy" or dying, tachycardia, diaphoresis, and shortness of breath. Many of these signs and symptoms are also seen in a wide range of medical and other psychiatric disorders from which they must be distinguished.

Epidemiology

Anxiety syndromes typically begin in early life and decrease in frequency after the age of 65. The ECA surveys found that 6% of persons over age 65 fulfilled criteria for an anxiety disorder *within the past month*.[99] Other studies have reported rates of clinically significant anxiety as high as 20% in some elderly populations.[100] Phobia is the most common psychiatric disorder in elderly women, who are also more likely than men to be diagnosed with any of the anxiety disorders.[99] Medical illnesses that increase the vulnerability of older persons to anxiety include Parkinson's disease, chronic obstructive pulmonary disease, and early dementia, where rates of anxiety disorder range from 8% to 38%.[101–103] Elderly persons with anxiety disorder tend to be high utilizers of health services, and therefore commonly come into contact with medical personnel.

Diagnostic Evaluation

Anxiety disorders seldom present for the first time in later life, although generalized anxiety disorder or panic disorder are known to do so.[104] The general rule is that late-onset anxiety is presumed to have a medical cause until proven otherwise. Table 79.3 presents psychiatric and medical causes for anxiety in older patients. Evaluation consists of a comprehensive history, physical examination, and battery of laboratory tests, including electrolytes, thyroid studies, and an electrocardiogram. A history of caffeine intake—tea, colas, or coffee—should be elicited, as well as over-the-counter drug use. Prescription medications that cause anxiety include sympathomimetics, corticosteroids, theophylline, calcium channel blockers, opiates, and amphetamines. Withdrawal from chronic benzodiazepine use may cause a prolonged withdrawal

TABLE 79.3. Medical and psychiatric causes of anxiety in the elderly.

Medical disorders	Psychiatric disorders
Cardiovascular	Anxiety disorders
Myocardial infarction	Panic disorder
Paroxysmal atrial tachycardia	Agoraphobia
Hypothermia	Social phobia
Mitral valve prolapse	Simple phobia
Hyperkalemia	Obsessive-compulsive disorder
	Posttraumatic stress disorder
Dietary	Generalized anxiety disorder
Caffeine	
Vitamin deficiencies	Other psychiatric disorders
	Major depression
Drug-related	Dementia
Anticholinergic toxicity	Psychosis
Akathisia (antipsychotics)	Adjustment disorder to negative life events
Antihypertensive side effects	Sleep disorder
Digitalis toxicity	Somatoform pain disorder
Theophylline	Somatization disorder
Thyroid replacement therapies	Personality disorders
Antidepressants (SSRIs, bupropion)	
	Substance abuse, dependence, withdrawal
Neurologic	Alcohol
Central nervous system infections	Sedative/hypnotics
Central nervous system masses	Prescription drugs
Postconcussion syndrome	Over-the-counter drugs (decongestants, diet aids)
Temporal lobe epilepsy	
Parkinson's disease	
Endocrinologic	
Insulinoma	
Hypoglycemia	
Hypo- or hyperthyroidism	
Hypo- or hypercalcemia	
Pheochromocytoma	
Cushing's disease	
Carcinoid syndrome	
Pulmonary	
Chronic obstructive lung disease with	
hypoxia	
Pneumonia with hypoxia	
Miscellaneous	
Anemia	
Systemic lupus erythematosus	
Toxins	

syndrome in the elderly associated with anxiety. All patients should be asked about alcohol use and when the last drink was taken. When physical and psychiatric symptoms of anxiety overlap in patients with medical problems, a diagnosis of anxiety disorder should be reserved for those who either had anxiety symptoms before the onset of the medical illness or continue to have symptoms after the physical condition has been treated.

Diagnostic assessment is often complicated by a heavy overlap between anxiety disorders and depressive disorders. Although only 2% of older psychiatric inpatients have an isolated anxiety disorder, nearly 40% with major depression fulfill criteria for anxiety disorder.[105]

Clinical Features

The major anxiety disorders noted in DSM-IV include generalized anxiety disorder, panic disorder with and without agoraphobia, posttraumatic stress disorder, obsessive-compulsive disorder, and phobia (social or simple). Because of their prevalence in later life and impact on functioning, we focus here on generalized anxiety disorder (GAD), panic disorder, and obsessive-compulsive disorder (OCD). To meet the DSM-IV criterion for GAD, the person must have experienced excessive or unrealistic anxiety nearly every day for 6 months or longer and have had at least 6 of 18 possible symptoms during that period of time. The 18 symptoms are grouped into symptoms of muscle tension, autonomic hyperactivity, and vigilance or scanning. The 1980–1981 ECA surveys found that the 1-year prevalence of GAD among 5700 persons aged 65 or over was 2.2%, the highest of any anxiety disorder except phobias.[106]

To meet DSM-IV criteria for panic disorder, a person must experience recurrent episodes of severe anxiety or fear, accompanied by at least four of the following symptoms: shortness of breath, palpitations, sweating, dizziness, nausea, choking, depersonalization, numbness or tingling, hot flashes, and chest pain, all usually accompanied by a fear of dying or going crazy; at least four such episodes must have occurred within a 4-week period. These intense periods of anxiety usually occur spontaneously, without warning, and typically last only about 5 to 10 min. Panic disorder may or may not be associated with agoraphobia (the fear of being in public places or situations from which escape may be difficult). The 1-year prevalence of panic disorder in persons over age 65 in the ECA studies was 0.04% in men and 0.41% in women.[107] Although usually a chronic illness that develops in early adulthood, late-onset panic disorder can occur and is characterized by fewer symptoms and less avoidance.[108] Panic disorder in older adults with heart disease is both prevalent and underdiagnosed.[109] Almost one-third of older persons with chest pain and no evidence of coronary artery disease are reported to have late-onset panic disorder.[110]

OCD is characterized by recurrent obsessive thoughts or compulsive behaviors that cause a significant disruption in social or occupational functioning. The person has little control over the obsessive thoughts, which are recurrent and persistent; he or she is often compelled to perform repetitive behaviors or rituals (washing hands, counting, checking locks, etc.) to avoid feeling overwhelmingly anxious. Epidemiologic studies report a 1-year prevalence between 0.9% and 1.5% in the geriatric populations.[111,112] Many older persons with this disorder resist hospitalization for medical problems because it may disrupt their compulsive activities.

Other psychiatric diagnoses, particularly alcoholism, can lead to complaints of anxiety in older patients. Anxiety can be part of an alcohol withdrawal syndrome that occurs when alcohol use is temporarily halted; alternatively, alcohol may be used to self-medicate an underlying anxiety disorder. There is also considerable overlap between the anxiety disorders and dementia, where it may be difficult to distinguish anxiety from agitation.[113]

Management

After treating reversible medical problems and arriving at a specific psychiatric diagnosis, the clinician must choose from a wide range of psychotherapeutic and drug treatment options. If the anxiety symptoms are minor and associated primarily with stressful life circumstances,

treatment largely involves supportive, problem-focused counseling to help the patient choose a healthy coping strategy. If an anxiety disorder is diagnosed, then more specific therapies are indicated.

Behavioral Therapies

Behavioral therapies are commonly used to treat anxiety disorders in both younger and older adults (Table 79.4). Progressive muscle relaxation is commonly used for patients with GAD, panic disorder, or social phobia.[114] This therapy involves the systematic tensing and relaxing of muscle groups, beginning first with the facial muscles and gradually moving down to the neck, upper arms, abdomen, legs, and feet. This technique is often combined with rhythmic breathing and visualization. Studies have shown that progressive muscle relaxation is effective in relieving the anxiety of patients with chronic pulmonary diseases and with cancer.[115,116]

Another behavior technique is called graded exposure; it is used to treat phobias and compulsive behaviors. The person is repeatedly exposed to the feared stimulus until the fear of that stimulus is gradually lost. Systematic desensitization combines progressive muscle relaxation with breathing and visualization; it prevents the stimulus from arousing anxiety by associating it with a deeply relaxed state.[117] Other behavioral techniques include biofeedback, meditation, social skills training, assertiveness training, and participant modeling. Studies have now demonstrated the effectiveness of behavioral therapies for treating anxiety disorders in older adults.[118] Cognitive therapy is commonly used with behavioral techniques to achieve better outcomes.

TABLE 79.4. Management of anxiety disorders in the elderly.

Condition	Treatment
Panic disorder (with or without agoraphobia)	Desipramine, clonazepam, alprazolam, phenelzine, exposure therapy, cognitive-behavioral therapy
Agoraphobia without panic disorder	Cognitive-behavioral therapy, exposure therapy
Social phobia	Cognitive-behavioral therapy, exposure therapy, beta-blockers, phenelzine, serotonin-reuptake inhibitors
Simple phobia	Graded exposure and systematic desensitization
Generalized anxiety disorder	Buspirone, clonazepam, β-blockers, behavioral therapy, psychotherapy
Obsessive-compulsive disorder	Serotonin-reuptake inhibitors, behavioral therapy, psychodynamic therapy
Posttraumatic stress disorder	Psychotherapy, behavior therapy, nortriptyline, clonazepam, phenelzine

Benzodiazepines

The pharmacologic management of anxiety disorders is most successful when used in combination with cognitive and behavioral therapies. Antidepressants and benzodiazepines are the mainstay of pharmacologic treatment for anxiety disorders. Between 17% and 50% of all older adults use benzodiazepines for problems with anxiety or medical problems.[119]

All benzodiazepines work equally well in relieving anxiety; only the side effect profiles of these drugs differ. Elderly persons often respond to low doses of medication. Furthermore, elders are at greater risk for the development of toxicity because of pharmacokinetic changes with aging, such as slowed hepatic metabolism and reduced glomerular filtration rate. Because they bind tightly with plasma albumin (reduced in some elders) and distribute preferentially to fatty tissue (increased in elders), benzodiazepines with a long half-life tend to accumulate and have toxic side effects. The half-lives of diazepam and chlordiazepoxide in older adults is nearly three times that in younger persons.[114] For this reason, short-acting benzodiazepines such as lorazepam and oxazepam arc the drugs of choice. These drugs are conjugated in the liver, eliminated in the urine, and have no active metabolites (as do alprazolam and diazepam). Oxazepam is typically started at a dose of 7.5 mg (1/2 a 15-mg tablet) given three times per day, which can then be gradually increased up to a maximum of 45 mg/day. Lorazepam is usually initiated at a dose of 0.25 mg (1/2 a 0.5-mg tablet) three times per day and tapered upward to a maximum of 3 mg/day.

Alprazolam is a benzodiazepine with an intermediate half-life of 12 to 15 h in the elderly. At a single dose of 0.5 to 2.0 mg, alprazolam is effective for the immediate relief of severe anxiety, particularly during a panic attack. However, it has an active metabolite that can build up in the elderly and cause toxic reactions.[120] As noted earlier, alprazolam can induce dependence, particularly in those with a history of alcohol or benzodiazepine abuse, and is difficult for some elders to discontinue (see following).

It is generally best to use short-acting benzodiazepines in elderly patients; however, there are some indications for using longer-acting agents such as diazepam, chlordiazepoxide, or clonazepam. One indication is where anxiety is constant throughout the day and night and is clearly interfering with ability to function. Many elderly persons have taken these drugs for years and do not abuse them.[121] Of the longer-acting agents, clonazepam is the safest; doses of 0.25 to 1.0 mg twice a day is usually effective, although some patients will do well on a once a day or even once every other day regimen. Clonazepam, however, has been reported to be depressogenic, so it must be used with caution in mixed anxiety-depression states.

When discontinuing benzodiazepines that have been taken regularly for several months or more, the clinician must gradually taper these compounds to avoid inducing seizures or delirium. Alprazolam, in particular, can produce severe dysphoria and psychotic-like symptoms if the drug is tapered too rapidly. The discontinuation of this medication should be accomplished over several months. Alternatively, one might switch to clonazepam (on a mg/mg basis), and then gradually discontinue the clonazepam.

Benzodiazepines can induce a number of side effects about which clinicians must educate their patients. Side effects include oversedation, confusion, memory loss, and disorientation, particularly when used with other CNS suppressants. Benzodiazepines have been shown to cause disequilibrium in older adults and increase the risk of falling and hip fractures; antidepressants and neuroleptics, however, are equally as dangerous in this regard.[122] Benzodiazepines can also impair ventilation during sleep, which may worsen sleep-related breathing disorders such as chronic obstructive pulmonary disease, congestive heart failure, and sleep apnea.[123] Cognitive impairment may also be induced or exacerbated by these drugs.[124] Other problems include disinhibition (particularly in demented elders), impaired driving, and paradoxical agitation.

Antidepressants

Antidepressants are effective and safe treatments for anxiety disorders in older adults. When initiating therapy, we start patients on both antidepressants and benzodiazepines, gradually tapering off the benzodiazepine once the antidepressant has had a chance to take effect. This approach is particularly effective because of the heavy overlap between depressive and anxiety syndromes in later life.[105] We start patients on a low dose of an SSRI and gradually increase the dosage to adults over a period of weeks. All the new SSRIs are effective antianxiety agents if taken at an adequate dose for a sufficient period of time (6–8 weeks). Initially, however, these drugs may exacerbate the patient's symptoms, and therefore should be used concurrently with a benzodiazepine. We typically begin patients on clonazepam at a dose of 0.25 to 1.0 mg twice per day. An alternative to beginning an SSRI is to start 25 mg desipramine per day and increase by 25 mg every 4 days until a therapeutic serum level is achieved (>125 ng/ml). Regardless of antidepressant used, after 6 to 8 weeks, the clonazepam is gradually tapered off over a 4-week period.

Clomipramine, fluoxetine, and fluvoxamine are specifically indicated for obsessive-compulsive disorder. The side effects associated with clomipramine (orthostatic and anticholinergic effects), however, limit its use in the elderly. Fluoxetine, on the other hand, may be associated with gastrointestinal symptoms that make it intolerable unless initiated at a very low dose (10 mg every other day) and gradually increased to 20 or 40 mg per day (if tolerated). Fluvoxamine may be the drug of first choice for older adults with symptoms of OCD. It is typically begun at 25 mg twice daily and increased up to a maximum of 100 mg three times per day as tolerated. Headache can be a problem if the dose is not gradually increased. Unfortunately, fluvoxamine is quite expensive at the doses needed to treat OCD.

Other Drugs

Other treatments for anxiety disorders include buspirone, beta-blockers, and sedating antihistamines. Buspirone is a serotonin agonist that has no cross-tolerance with the benzodiazepines. It has a slow onset of action, and initially may even exacerbate anxiety because of its activating effects. Buspirone is a safe drug to use over the long term given its lack of addictive potential and lack of psychomotor impairment, and it interacts with virtually no other medications. It is specifically indicated for generalized anxiety disorder. At least one study in elderly patients with chronic health problems has demonstrated a significant improvement of anxiety with this drug.[125] A major drawback is cost; the usual dosage of 10 mg three times per day costs about $90 to $180 per month, which may be prohibitive for some elders. Also, buspirone is rarely effective in patients who have taken benzodiazepines previously or have a history of substance abuse.

Beta-blockers are effective in blocking the autonomic symptoms that accompany anxiety (palpitations, sweating, trembling); they do not, however, affect the cognitive aspects of anxiety. Because of this, beta-blockers are not effective in panic disorder, because they do not diminish the psychologic anxiety associated with panic. Propranolol can be very helpful at doses from 10 mg twice a day to 40 mg three times per day in patients with social phobia, performance anxiety, or generalized anxiety disorder. Note, however, that beta-blockers have been associated with depression, and may exacerbate depression if present concurrently with anxiety; furthermore, there are a number of medical contraindications that limit its use in elderly patients.

Antihistamines are frequently used both over-the-counter and by prescription to reduce anxiety. In general, these drugs should not be used to treat anxiety disorders in older adults because of their anticholinergic, drying, and nonspecific sedative effects. Neuroleptics should only be used if anxiety is associated with psychotic symptoms.

Acknowledgment. This work was supported by an NIMH grant R01 MH57662-01 (Dr. Koenig), the Clinical Research Center for the Study of Depression in Late Life (MH40159), and an NIA grant R01 AG12765-03 (Dr. Blazer).

References

1. Srole L, Fischer AK. The Midtown Manhattan Longitudinal Study vs. "The Mental Paradise Lost" doctrine. *Arch Gen Psychiatry.* 37:209–221.
2. Zung WWK. Depression in the normal aged. *Psychosomatics.* 1967;8:287–289.
3. Koenig HG. Depression and dysphoria among the elderly: dispelling a myth. *J Fam Pract.* 1986;23:383–385.
4. Koenig HG, Blazer DG. Epidemiology of geriatric affective disorders. *Clin Geriatr Med.* 8:235–251.
5. Blazer DG, Hughes DC, George LK. The epidemiology of depression in an elderly community population. *Gerontologist.* 1987;27:281–287.
6. Weissman MM, Leaf PJ, Tischler GL, et al. Affective disorders in five United States communities. *Psychol Med.* 1988;18:141–153.
7. Feldman E, Mayo R, Hawton K, et al. Psychiatric disorder in medical impatients. *Q J Med.* 1987;63:405–410.
8. Hagnell O, Lanke J, Rorsman B, et al. Are we entering an age of melancholy? *Psychol Med.* 1982;12(2):279–289.
9. Klerman GL. The current age of youthful melancholia: evidence for increase in depression among adolescents and young adults. *Br J Psychiatry.* 1988;152:4.
10. Koenig HG, Meador KG, Shelp F, et al. Depressive disorders in hospitalized medically ill patients: a comparison of young and elderly men. *J Am Geriatr Soc.* 1991;39:881–890.
11. Weissman MM, Myers JK. Affective disorders in a United States community: the use of research diagnostic criteria in an epidemiological survey. *Arch Gen Psychiatry.* 1978;31(7):1304.
12. Kessler RC, McGonagle KA, Zhao S, et al. Lifetime and 12-month prevalence of DSM-III-R psychiatric disorders in the United States. *Arch Gen Psychiatry.* 1994;51:8–19.
13. Roberts RE, Kaplan GA, Shema SJ, Strawbridge WJ. Does growing old increase the risk for depression? *Am J Psychiatry.* 1997;154:1384–1390.
14. Blazer DG. *Depression in Late Life, 2nd Ed.* St Louis: Mosby; 1993.
15. Blazer DG, Bachar JR, Manton KG. Suicide in late life: review and commentary. *J Am Geriatr Soc.* 1986;34:519–525.
16. Klerman GL, Weissman MM. Increasing rates of depression. *JAMA.* 1989;261:2229–2235.
17. Koenig HG, George LK, Peterson BL, et al. Depression in medically ill hospitalized older adults: prevalence, correlates, and course of symptoms based on six diagnostic schemes. *Am J Psychiatry.* 1997;154:1376–1383.
18. Hyer L, Blazer DG. Depressive symptoms: impact and problems in long term care facilities. *Int J Behav Geriatr.* 1982;1(3):33–35.

19. Parmelee PA, Katz IR, Lawton MP. Depression among institutionalized aged: assessment and prevalence estimation. *J Gerontol.* 1989;44:M22–M29.

20. Weissman MM, Bruce ML, Leaf PJ, et al. Affective disorders. In: Robins LN, Regier DA, eds. *Psychiatric Disorders in America: The Epidemiologic Catchment Area Study.* New York: Free Press; 1991:53.

21. Rovner BW, German P, Brant LJ, et al. Depression and mortality in nursing homes. *JAMA.* 1991;265:993–996.

22. Koenig HG, Cohen HJ, Blazer DG, et al. A brief depression scale for detecting major depression in the medically ill hospitalized patient. *Int J Psychiatry Med.* 1992;22:183–195.

23. Koenig HG, Blazer DG, Ford SM. Should physicians screen for depression in elderly medical inpatients? Results of a decision analysis. *Int J Psychiatry Med.* 1993;23:211–235.

24. Koenig HG, Shelp F, Goli V, et al. Survival and healthcare utilization in elderly medical inpatients with major depression. *J Am Geriatr Soc.* 1989;4:498–505.

25. Musselman DL, Evans DL, Nemeroff CB. The relationship of depression to cardiovascular disease: epidemiology, biology, and treatment. *Arch Gen Psychiatry.* 1998;55:580–592.

26. Glassman AH, Shapiro PA. Depression and the course of coronary artery disease. *Am J Psychiatry.* 1998;155:4–11.

27. Hopkinson G. A genetic study of affective illness in patients over 50. *Br J Psychiatry.* 1964;110:244–254.

28. Robinson DS, Davies JM, Nies A, et al. Relation of sex and aging to monoamine oxidase activity of human plasma and platelets. *Arch Gen Psychiatry.* 1971;24:536–541.

29. Krishnan K, Hays J, Blazer D. MRI-defined vascular depression. *Am J Psychiatry.* 1997;154:497–501.

30. Bebbington PE, Dunn G, Jenkins R, et al. The influence of age and sex on the prevalence of depressive conditions: report from the National Survey of Psychiatric Morbidity. *Psychosom Med.* 1998;28:9–19.

31. Goldberg EL, Van Natta P, Comstock GW. Depressive symptoms, social networks and social support of elderly women. *Am J Epidemiol.* 1985;121:448–456.

32. Murrell SA, Himmelfarb S, Wright K. Prevalence of depression and its correlates in older adults. *Am J Epidemiol.* 1983;117:173–185.

33. Meyers BS, Kalayam B, Mei-Tal V. Late-onset delusional depression: a distinct clinical entity? *J Clin Psychiatry.* 1984;45:347–349.

34. George LK, Blazer DG, Hughes DC, et al. Social support and the outcome of major depression. *Br J Psychiatry.* 1989;154:478–485.

35. Koenig HG, Westlund RE, George LK, et al. Abbreviating the Duke Social Support Index for use in chronically ill older adults. *Psychosomatics.* 1993;34:61–69.

36. Clayton P. Bereavement and depression. *J Clin Psychiatry.* 1990;51(suppl):34.

37. Koenig HG, Kvale IN, Ferrel C. Religion and well-being in later life. *Gerontologist.* 1988;28:18–28.

38. Koenig HG, Cohen HJ, Blazer DG, et al. Religious coping and depression in elderly hospitalized medically ill men. *Am J Psychiatry.* 1992;149:1693–1700.

39. Braam AW, Beckman ATF, Deeg DJH, et al. Religiosity as a protective or prognostic factor of depression in later life;

results from the community survey in the Netherlands. *Acta Psychiatr Scand.* 1997;96:199–205.

40. Koenig HG, George LK, Peterson BL. Religiosity and remission from depression in medically ill older patients. *Am J Psychiatry.* 1998;155:536–542.

41. Koenig HG, George LK, Siegler I. The use of religion and other emotion-regulating coping strategies among older adults. *Gerontologist.* 1988;28:303–310.

42. Koenig HG, Cohen HJ, Blazer DG, et al. Cognitive symptoms of depression and religious coping in elderly medical patients. *Psychosomatics.* 1995;36:369–375.

43. Idler EL, Kasl SV. Religion, disability, depression, and the timing of death. *Am J Sociol.* 1992;97:1052–1079.

44. Idler EL. Religious involvement and the health of the elderly. *Soc Forces.* 1987;66:226–238.

45. Pressman P, Lyons JS, Larson DB, et al. Religious belief, depression, and ambulation status in elderly women with broken hips. *Am J Psychiatry.* 1990;147:758–760.

46. Koenig HG. *Research on Religion and Aging.* Westport, CT: Greenwood Press; 1995.

47. Koenig HG. *The Healing Power of Faith.* New York: Simon & Schuster; 1999.

48. Krishnan KR, Hays JC, George LK, Blazer DG. Six-month outcomes for MRI-related vascular depression. *Depression Anxiety.* 1998;8(4):142–146.

49. Lazarus R. Psychological stress and coping in adaptation & illness. *Int J Psychiatry Med.* 1974;5:321–333.

50. Olinger U, Kuiper N, Shaw B. Dysfunctional attitudes and stressful life events: an interactive model of depression. *Cognit Ther Res.* 1987;11:25–40.

51. Holroyd K, Lazarus R. Stress, coping and somatic adaptation. In: Goldberger L, Breznitz S, eds. *Handbook of Stress.* New York: Free Press; 1982.

52. Bombardier C, D'Amico C, Jordan J. The relationship of appraisal and coping to chronic illness adjustment. *Behav Res Ther.* 1990;28:297–304.

53. Smith T, Follick M, Ahern D, et al. Cognitive distortion and disability in chronic low back pain. *Cognit Ther Res.* 1986;10:201–210.

54. Holroyd K, Andrasik F. Do the effects of cognitive therapy endure? A two-year follow-up of tension headache sufferers treated with cognitive therapy or biofeedback. *Cognit Ther Res.* 1982;6:325–334.

55. Gianturco DT, Busse EW. Psychiatric problems encountered during a long-term study of normal ageing volunteers. In: Issacs AD, Post F, eds. *Studies in Geriatric Psychiatry.* New York: Wiley; 1978:1–16.

56. Koenig HG, Cohen HJ, Blazer DG, et al. Profile of depressive symptoms in younger and older medical inpatients with major depression. *J Am Geriatr Soc.* 1993;41:1699–1176.

57. Verwoerdt A. *Geropsychiatry.* Baltimore: Williams & Wilkins; 1976.

58. Beekman AT, Deeg DJ, Braam AW, Smit JH, Van Tilburg W. Consequences of major and minor depression in later life: a study of disability, well-being and service delivery. *Psychol Med.* 1997;27:1397–1409.

59. De Alarcon R. Hypochondriasis and depression in the aged. *Gerontology.* 1964;6:266–277.

60. Post F. The functional psychoses. In: Isaacs AD, Post F, eds. *Studies in Geriatric Psychiatry.* New York: Wiley 1978:77.

61. Shulman KI. Mania in old age. In: Murphy E, ed. *Affective Disorders in the Elderly*. Edinburgh: Churchill Livingstone; 1986.

62. Post F. Functional disorders. II. Treatment and its relationship to causation. In: Levy R, Post F, eds. *The Psychiatry of Late Life*. London: Blackwell; 1982.

63. Shulman KI. The influence of age and ageing on manic disorder. *Int J Geriatr Psychiatry*. 1989;4:63–65.

64. Young RC, Klerman GL. Mania in late life: focus on age at onset. *Am J Psychiatry*. 1992;149:867–876.

65. Tohen M, Shulman KI, Satlin A. First-episode mania in late life. *Am J Psychiatry*. 1994;151:130–132.

66. Sweer L, Martin DC, Ladd RA, et al. The medical evaluation of elderly patients with major depression. *J Gerontol*. 1988;43:M53–M58.

67. Koenig HG. *Aging and God*. New York: Haworth Press; 1994.

68. Koenig HG, Breitner J. Antidepressant use in the medically ill older person. *Psychosomatics*. 1990;31:22–32.

69. Beck AT, Rush J, Shaw B, et al. *Cognitive Therapy of Depression*. New York: Guilford; 1979.

70. Lewinsohn P. A behavioral approach to depression. In: Friedman R, Katz M, eds. *The Psychology of Depression: Contemporary Theory & Research*. New York: Wiley; 1974:157–176.

71. Klerman GL, Weissman MM, Rounsaville BJ, et al., eds. *Interpersonal Psychotherapy of Depression*. New York: Basic Books; 1984.

72. Horowitz M, Kaltreider N. Brief therapy of the stress response syndrome. *Psychiatr Clin Am*. 1979;2:365–377.

73. Thompson LW, Gallagher D, Breckenridge JS. Comparative effectiveness of psychotherapies for depressed elders. *J Consult Clin Psychol*. 1987;55:385–390.

74. Arean PA, Pen MG, Nezu AM, et al. Comparative effectiveness of social problem-solving therapy and reminiscence therapy as treatments for depression in older adults. *J Consult Clin Psychol*. 1993;61:1003–1010.

75. Myers WA. *New Techniques in the Psychotherapy of Older Patients*. Washington, DC: American Psychiatric Press; 1991.

76. Marmar CR, Horowitz MJ, Weiss DS, et al. A controlled trial of brief psychotherapy and mutual-help group treatment of conjugal bereavement. *Am J Psychiatry*. 1988;145:203–209.

77. Nies A, Robinson DS, Friedman MJ, et al. Relationship between age and tricyclic antidepressant pharmacokinetics and plasma levels. *Am J Psychiatry*. 1977;134:790–793.

78. Greden JF. Antidepressant maintenance medications: when to discontinue and how to stop. *J Clin Psychiatry*. 1993;54(suppl 8):39–45.

79. Tyrer P, Murphy S. The place of benzodiazepines in psychiatric practice. *Br J Psychiatry*. 1987;151:719–723.

80. Greenblatt DJ, Shader RI, Abernathy DR. Current status of benzodiazepines: clinical use of benzodiazepines. *N Engl J Med*. 1983;309:410–405.

81. Reynolds C III, Frank B, Perel I, et al. Nortriptyline and interpersonal psychotherapy as maintenance therapies for recurrent major depression: a randomized controlled trial in patients older than 59 years. *JAMA*. 1999;281:39–45.

82. Abrams R. *Electroconvulsive Therapy, 2nd Ed*. New York: Oxford University Press; 1992.

83. Salzman C. Electroconvulsive therapy in the elderly. *Psychiatr Clin Am*. 1982;5:191–197.

84. Zervas IM, Calev A, Jandorf L. Age-dependent effects of electroconvulsive therapy on memory. *Convulsive Ther*. 1993;9:39–42.

85. Baldwin RC, Jolley DJ. The prognosis of depression in old age. *Br J Psychiatry*. 1986;149:574–583.

86. Post F. The management and nature of depressive illness in late life: a follow-through study. *Br J Psychiatry*. 1972;121:393–404.

87. Murphy E, Smith R, Lindesay J, et al. Increased mortality rates in late-life depression. *Br J Psychiatry*. 1988;152:347–353.

88. Koenig HG, Goli V, Shelp F, et al. Major depression in hospitalized medically ill men: documentation, treatment, and prognosis. *Int J Geriatr Psychiatry*. 1992;7:25–34.

89. Reynolds CF, Frank B, Perel JM, et al. Combined pharmacotherapy and psychotherapy in the acute and continuation treatment of elderly patients with recurrent major depression: a preliminary report. *Am J Psychiatry*. 1992;149:1687–1692.

90. Hinrichsen GA. Recovery and relapse from major depressive disorder in the elderly. *Am J Psychiatry*. 1992;149:1575–1579.

91. Stoudemire A, Hill CD, Morris R, et al. Long-term affective and cognitive outcome in depressed older adults. *Am J Psychiatry*. 1993;150:896–900.

92. Hughes DC, Demallie D, Blazer DG. Does age make a difference in the effects of physical health and social support on the outcome of a major depressive episode? *Am J Psychiatry*. 1993;150:728–733.

93. Shulman K, Post F. Bipolar affective disorder in old age. *Br J Psychiatry*. 1980;136:26–32.

94. Shulman K, Tohen M, Stalin A, et al. Mania compared with unipolar depression in old age. *Am J Psychiatry*. 1992;149:341–345.

95. Conwell Y. Suicide in elderly patients. In: Schneider LS, Reynolds CF, Lebowitz BD, Friedhoff AJ, eds. *Diagnosis and Treatment of Depression in Late Life: Results of the NIH Consensus Development Conference*. Washington, DC: American Psychiatric Press; 1994.

96. Cavan RS. *Suicide*. Chicago: University of Chicago Press; 1928:279–287.

97. MacKenzie TB, Popkin MK. Suicide in the medical patient. *Int J Psychiatry Med*. 1987;17:3–22.

98. Blazer DG. Generalized anxiety disorder and panic disorder in the elderly: a review. *Harvard Rev Psychiatry*. 1997;5:18–27.

99. Regier DA, Boyd JH, Burke JD, et al. One month prevalence of mental disorders in the United States. *Arch Gen Psychiatry*. 1988;45:977–986.

100. Sheikh JI. Anxiety and its disorders in old age. In: Birren J, Sloane R, Cohen G, eds. *Handbook of Mental Health & Aging, 2nd Ed*. San Diego: Academic Press; 1992:409–432.

101. Stein MB, Heuser IJ, Juncos JL, et al. Anxiety disorders in patients with Parkinson's disease. *Am J Psychiatry*. 1990;147:217–220.

102. Karajgi B, Rifkin A, Doddi S, et al. The prevalence of anxiety disorders in patients with chronic obstructive pulmonary disease. *Am J Psychiatry.* 1990;147:200–201.

103. Wands K, Merskey H, Hachinski V, et al. A questionnaire investigation of anxiety and depression in early dementia. *J Am Geriatr Soc.* 1990;38:535–538.

104. Jenike MA. Anxiety disorders of old age. In: Jenike MA, ed. *Geriatric Psychiatry and Psychopharmacology.* Chicago: Year Book; 1989:248–271.

105. Alexopoulas GS. Anxiety and depression in the elderly. In: Salzman C, Uebowitz B, eds. *Anxiety Disorders in the Elderly: Treatment and Research.* New York: Springer; 1991:131–150.

106. Blazer DG, Hughes D, George LK, et al. Generalized anxiety disorder. In: Robins LN, Regier DA, eds. *Psychiatric Disorders in America: The Epidemiologic Catchment Area Study.* New York: Free Press; 1991:180–203.

107. Eaton WW, Dryman A, Weissman MM. Panic and phobia. In: Robins LN, Regier DA, eds. *Psychiatric Disorders in America: The Epidemiologic Catchment Area Study.* New York: Free Press; 1991:155–179.

108. Sheikh J, King R, Taylor CB. Comparative phenomenology of early-onset versus late-onset panic attacks: a pilot survey. *Am J Psychiatry.* 1991;148:1231–1233.

109. Beitman BD, Mukerji V, Alpert M, et al. Panic disorder in cardiology patients. *Psychiatr Med.* 1990;8:67–81.

110. Beitman BD, Kushner M, Grossberg GT. Late onset panic disorder: evidence from a study of patients with chest pain and normal cardiac evaluations. *Int J Psychiatry Med.* 1991; 21:29–35.

111. Blazer DG, George LK, Hughes D. The epidemiology of anxiety disorders: an age comparison. In: Salzman C, Lebowitz B, eds. *Anxiety Disorders in the Elderly: Treatment and Research.* New York: Springer; 1991:17–30.

112. Karno M, Golding JM. Obsessive compulsive disorder. In: Robins LN, Regier DA, eds. *Psychiatric Disorders in America: The Epidemiologic Catchment Area Study.* New York: Free Press; 1991:204–219.

113. Abrams R. Anxiety and personality disorders. In: Sadavoy J, Lazarus U, Jarvik L, eds. *Comprehensive Review of Geriatric Psychiatry.* Washington, DC: American Psychiatric Association; 1991:369–376.

114. Jacobsen E. *Progressive Relaxation, 2nd Ed.* Chicago: Chicago University Press; 1938.

115. Gift AG, Moore T, Soeken K. Relaxation to reduce dyspnea and anxiety in COPD patients. *Nurs Res.* 1992;41:242–246.

116. Holland JC, Morrow GR, Schmale A, et al. A randomized clinical trial of alprazolam versus progressive muscle relaxation in cancer patients with anxiety and depressive symptoms. *J Clin Oncol.* 1991;9:1004–1011.

117. Wolpe J. *The Practice of Behavior Therapy, 2nd Ed.* New York: Pergamon Press; 1973.

118. Hussian RA. *Geriatric Psychology: A Behavioral Perspective.* New York: Van Nostrand Reinhold; 1981.

119. Salzman C, Lebowitz BD. *Anxiety in the Elderly.* New York: Springer; 1991:149–173.

120. Salzman C. Treatment of anxiety. In: Salzman C, ed. *Clinical Geriatric Psychopharmacology, 2nd Ed.* Baltimore: Williams & Wilkins; 1992:189–212.

121. Pinsker H, Suljaga-Petchel K. Use of benzodiazepines in primary care geriatric patients. *J Am Geriatr Soc.* 1984;32: 595–598.

122. Ray WA, Griffin MR, Schaffner W, et al. Psychotropic drug use and the risk of hip fracture. *N Engl J Med.* 1987;316: 363–369.

123. Guilleminault C. Benzodiazepines, breathing, and sleep. *Am I Med.* 1990;88(3A):25S–28S.

124. Salzman C. Anxiety in the elderly: treatment strategies. *J Clin Psychiatry.* 900;51(suppl 10):18–21.

125. Bohm C, Robinson DS, Gammans RE, et al. Buspirone therapy in anxious elderly patients: a controlled clinical trial. *J Clin Psychopharmacol.* 1990;10(suppl 3):47S–51S.

126. Abernathy DR, Greenblatt DJ, Divoll M, et al. Pharmacokinetics of alprazolam. *J Clin Psychiatry.* 1983;44:45–47.

Appendix

11-Item Abbreviated Duke Social Support Index (Self-Administered)

	Number	
1. Other than members of your family, how many persons in this area within one hour's travel (of your home/from here) do you feel you can depend on or feel very close to?

| | None | 00 |

[scoring 0 = 1, 1-2 = 2, >2 = 3]

2. (Other than at work) How many times during the past week did you spend some time with someone who does not live with you, that is, you went to see them or they came to visit you, or you went out together?

	None	00
	Once	01
	Twice	02
	Three times	03
	Four	04
	Five	05
	Six	06
	Seven or more	07

[scoring 0 = 1, 1-2 = 2, >2 = 3]

3. (Other than at work) How many times did you talk to someone—friends, relatives or others—on the telephone in the past week (either they called you, or you called them)?

None	00
Once	01
Twice	02
Three times	03
Four	04
Five	05
Six	06
Seven or more	07

[scoring 0 or 1 = 1, 2-5 = 2, >5 = 3]

4. (Other than at work) About how often did you go to meetings of clubs, religious meetings, or other groups that you belong to in the past week?

None	00
Once	01
Twice	02
Three times	03
Four	04
Five	05
Six	06
Seven or more	07

[scoring 0 or 1 = 1, 2-5 = 2, >5 = 3]

5. Does it seem that your family and friends (i.e., people who are important to you) understand you most of the time, some of the time, or hardly ever?

Hardly ever	1
Some	2
Most	3

6. Do you feel useful to your family and friends (i.e., people important to you) most of the time, some of the time, or hardly ever?

Hardly ever	1
Some	2
Most	3

7. Do you know what is going on with your family and friends most of the time, some of the time, or hardly ever?

Hardly ever	1
Some	2
Most	3

8. When you are talking with your family and friends, do you feel you are being listened to most of the time, some of the time, or hardly ever?

Hardly ever	1
Some	2
Most	3

9. Do you feel you have a definite role (place) in your family and among your friends most of the time, some of the the time, or hardly ever?

Hardly ever	1
Some	2
Most	3

10. Can you talk about your deepest problems with at least some of your family and friends most of the time, some of the the time, or hardly ever?

Hardly ever	1
Some	2
Most	3

11. How satisfied are you with the kinds of relationships you have with your
    family and friends—very dissatisfied, somewhat dissatisfied, or satisfied?

Very dissatisfied	1
Somewhat dissatisfied	2
Satisfied	3

If NO FAMILY OR FRIENDS: Would you say that you are very dissatisfied, somewhat dissatisfied, or satisfied with *not having* any of these relationships?

Brief Koenig Depression Scale

Please answer yes or no to the following statements/questions about how you have been feeling in the past week.

	1	0
1. I often became bored.	Yes	No
2. I often became restless and fidgety.	Yes	No
3. I felt in good spirits.	No	Yes
4. I felt I had more problems with memory than most.	Yes	No
5. I could concentrate easily when reading the papers.	No	Yes
6. I preferred to avoid social gatherings.	Yes	No
7. I felt downhearted and blue.	Yes	No
8. I felt happy most of the time.	No	Yes
9. I often felt helpless.	Yes	No
10. I felt worthless and ashamed about myself.	Yes	No
11. I often wish I were dead.	Yes	No

Scoring: Scores of 3 or higher suggest that further evaluation is necessary for the diagnosis of possible clinical depression. (*Source*: Koenig HG, Blumenthal J, Moore K. New version of brief depression scale. *J Am Geriatr Soc.* 1995;43:1447, with permission.)

80
Late-Life Psychosis

Steven C. Samuels and Deborah B. Marin

Five percent of community elders have paranoid delusions at any given time,[1] and 20% will develop a psychotic episode at some point in their lifetime.[2] Epidemiologic data are limited for late-life psychosis because aged subjects were not included or diagnostic criteria excluded late-onset cases. Females tend to develop psychosis at a later age of onset than males.[3] Psychosis, defined as a delusion or a hallucination, is a symptom rather than a specific disease. A delusion is a fixed false belief, and a hallucination is a sensory perception devoid of any actual stimulus. In the elderly, psychosis is associated with significant morbidity and mortality and negatively affects the quality of life for the patient and caregiver. Patients with psychosis routinely present to health care providers at more advanced stages of disease. The presence of psychosis is associated with increased behavioral disturbance, risk of institutionalization, and health care costs.

The elderly patient with psychosis may have a broad range of diagnoses including delirium, dementia, affective disorders, schizophrenia, delusional disorder, general medical conditions, or substance use. Less common causes of psychosis in the elderly include posttraumatic stress disorder and brief reactive psychosis. Parkinson's disease, chronic obstructive pulmonary disease (COPD), and severe pain are examples of medical conditions that may be complicated by psychosis. Dopaminergic agents, anticholinergic drugs, opiates, and steroids are some of the medications that may cause these symptoms. Psychosis may be related to intoxication or withdrawal from prescription or over-the-counter drugs, herbal preparations, street drugs, and alcohol. Misuse of prescription and over-the-counter drugs is more common in the elderly than illicit drug abuse. Moreover, psychosis attributed to medical conditions or medication is more common in the aged than primary psychiatric causes of psychosis. The astute geriatrician is able to recognize psychosis, determine potential etiologies, initiate a diagnostic workup, and begin treatment. Consultation with a geriatric psychiatrist may be helpful as the interaction between medical illness, brain disease and psychopathology is often complex in the patient with late-life psychosis. Table 80.1 lists the differential diagnosis of psychosis in late life. Common examples of medical conditions that have been associated with psychosis are listed in Table 80.2. Medications and substances associated with psychosis are listed in Table 80.3.

Sites of Care

The patient's treatment setting (inpatient, outpatient, home care, long-term care) may assist the clinician in determining the diagnosis and allocating the available resources when establishing a care plan. For example, in the acute medical, surgical, and intensive care units, psychosis is frequently seen in the context of a delirium. In any setting, a newly diagnosed psychosis should be viewed as a delirium until proven otherwise. The basic principles of delirium management are to determine and treat the underlying cause of the acute confusional state and maintain patient safety. This approach may require symptomatic management with judicious use of antipsychotic agents in combination with environmental modification and reorientation[4] (also see Chapter 77). The reason for an acute admission may give significant clues as to the etiology of the psychosis. For example, a temporal relationship between the onset of the psychosis and initiation or change in a medical condition suggests that the medical condition may be aggravating or causing the psychosis.

The presentation of psychosis in the outpatient setting may falsely lead the clinician to view the psychosis as less serious than in the acute care setting. However, the acute presentation of psychosis in the ambulatory setting still obligates the clinician to consider a general medical condition or substance as potential contributors. The patient's psychoses may fluctuate in relationship to the

TABLE 80.1. Differential diagnosis of psychosis in late life.

Delirium
Schizophrenia
Schizophreniform psychosis
Schizoaffective disorder
Dementia with psychosis
Depression with psychosis
Bipolar disease with psychosis
Posttraumatic stress disorder
Delusional disorder
Brief reactive psychosis
Psychosis secondary to a substance
Psychosis secondary to a medical condition

TABLE 80.2. Examples of medical conditions that are associated with psychosis.

Infections (e.g., urinary tract, meningitis, abscess)
Neoplasms (e.g., primary and metastatic, also paraneoplastic syndromes)
Endocrinopathies (e.g., diabetes, thyroid disease)
Traumatic injury (e.g., subdural; ophthalmologic injury)
Vasculopathies (e.g., CVA, vasculitis)
Degenerative diseases (e.g., Alzheimer's disease, Parkinson's disease)
Nutritional (e.g., vitamin deficiciencies, malnutrition)
Severe pain
Special sense impairment (e.g., decreased acuity, prolonged isolation)
Cardiac disease (e.g., hypoperfusion, postcardiac surgery)
Pulmonary pathology (hypoxia, COPD)
Hepatic failure
Renal disease (e.g., uremia)
Hematologic (e.g., anemia, DIC)
Gastrointestinal (e.g., impaction, obstruction)
Autoimmune diseases

status of the primary psychiatric disorder, medical comorbidity, or medication change. In addition, environmental change, illness, or hospitalization of the caregiver, or nonadherence to medication are psychosocial factors that may contribute to psychosis. Another common scenario in the outpatient setting is the misuse of over-the-counter preparations including herbal remedies. These compounds may have problems with quality control and have significant potential for neuropsychiatric side effects such as psychosis.[5]

The home setting may be the primary site to find psychotic patients, yet it is often difficult for the clinician to make entry into the home. Often, the more severely psychotic patients will not voluntarily visit primary care physicians unless they have somatic delusions. Severely paranoid patients may refuse entry to any "strangers," including home care workers. In the home care setting, psychosis is common and a significant predictor of disability.[6–8] The reported rates of psychosis in the home setting may be artificially low, however, because the more severely psychotic patients may refuse to participate in the surveys that generate these data.

The physical state of a patient's residence provides an exceptional opportunity to infer psychosis in patients who may otherwise go undiagnosed. For example, a severely paranoid patient may have "extra locks" on the door or may have altered the environment in such a way as to imply psychosis. Shades may be drawn, the phone disconnected, or the number changed. The patient who believes "my house is not my home" or "that man is not really my husband" or "someone stole my money" (when it was actually misplaced) are some common scenarios of demented patients with psychosis. In the context of a psychotic patient refusing evaluation, emergency psychiatric evaluation by a mobile crisis team or emergency room team may be necessary. The logistics of getting the patient evaluated are dependent on local ordinances. Most localities allow the patient's individual liberty to be usurped by societal protection with the caveat that the judicial system must review the case. Psychotic patients who remain in the community may benefit from aggressive use of antipsychotic agents, as the presence of psychosis is a consistent predictor of institutionalization in elderly patients with dementia and psychosis.[9]

Long-term care facilities include nursing homes, assisted living facilities, adult homes, and state psychiatric hospitals. The prevalence of psychosis in the nursing home is approximately 10%,[10] including patients with delirium, dementia with psychosis, or affective disorders with psychosis. The relatively high rate of psychopathology in the nursing home aged may result from the transfer of patients from the state psychiatric hospitals to nursing homes and the high percentage of dementia patients who reside in these settings.

Nursing homes are mandated by regulation to follow specific guidelines for assessment and documentation regarding antipsychotic medication use. Proper assessment requires quantifying and objectively identifying the symptoms that are being targeted with the antipsychotic agent. Center for Medicare & Medicaid Services (formerly Health Care Finance Administration) guidelines have been established to defined disruptive behaviors that will justify the use of antipsychotics in the nursing

TABLE 80.3. Examples of substances associated with psychosis.

Steroids
H$_2$ blockers
Quinolones
Analgesics (opiates, NSAIDs)
Alcohol
Benzodiazepines
Anticholinergics
Antihistamines
Dopaminergics
Cardiac (e.g., digoxin)
Heavy metals
Poisons
Other drugs of abuse (cocaine, methamphetamine)

home.[11,12] The guidelines suggest objective documentation of symptoms, quantification of symptoms, persistence of symptoms, a search for a preventable cause, and that symptoms cause a danger to self or others. Other acceptable justifications for antipsychotic use per HCFA guidelines include psychosis that impairs function or causes distress, as continuous yelling, screaming, or pacing that result in functional impairment. Behavioral disturbance and psychosis in nursing home patients is episodic, tend to be mild, and do not worsen over time,[13] suggesting that an empiric attempt at trials of or reduced doses of antipsychotics in these patients makes clinical sense. The HCFA guidelines have resulted in reduction of antipsychotic use in the nursing home.[14]

Adult homes and assisted living facilities are other long-term care facilities that provide less intensive nursing care than nursing homes. Private payment is the most common payment structure for assisted living, whereas nursing or adult homes are increasingly dependent on state-funded entitlements. Prevalence data for psychosis in assisted living facilities and adult homes are sparse, but the prevalence rates of psychosis in the adult home would be expected to be higher than the assisted living facility on the basis of patient mix. Psychosis associated with dementia or depression is expected to be the more common diagnosis in assisted living facilities, whereas severe and persistent mental illness (schizophrenia, schizoaffective disorder) is expected to be the more common diagnosis in the adult homes. One may hypothesize that residents of assisted living facilities have a relatively high functional level before admission compared with the adult home patient, who often has a diagnosis of schizophrenia or schizoaffective disorder. If the patient requires skilled nursing, they may receive care either in the nursing home or in a residence with constant nursing care.

State psychiatric hospital patients have severe functional impairment secondary to psychiatric illness and are unable to survive safely in the community. The "state hospitals" have dramatically decreased in size from a peak in the 1950s due to deinstitutionalization initiatives. The patients who remain are the "sickest of the sick," with prevalence rates of psychosis approaching 75%. Patients in these facilities often receive multiple antipsychotic agents and have relatively high rates of tardive dyskinesia and moderate to severe functional impairment.[15,16] The poor prognosis for schizophrenic and schizoaffective patients who reside in the state hospitals is that they are at advanced risk of developing a progressive dementia after age 65. Risk factors for development of this dementia are low education and high rates of positive (psychosis) and negative symptoms (apathy, amotivation, withdrawal). The cognitive loss correlates with functional impairment and loss of ability to attend to activities of daily living.[17–21]

The following sections review psychosis associated with schizophrenia, dementia, and affective disorders in later life.

Schizophrenia

The community prevalence rates of schizophrenia in individuals over age 65 ranges from 0.1% to 0.5%,[22] and incidence rates in those patients over age 60 years suggest an increase of 11% for each 5-year incremental age increase.[23] One model of differentiating elderly schizophrenic patients is based upon age at disease onset.[24] Late-onset schizophrenia is defined as onset over age 40 and very late onset schizophrenia is defined as onset over age 60. Late-onset schizophrenia is more likely than earlier age onset schizophrenia to present with visual or olfactory hallucinations, persecutory delusions, partition delusions (beliefs that others in a neighboring space are controlling the patient), third-person running commentary, and derogatory auditory hallucinations.[25,26] Compared with earlier-onset schizophrenia, late-onset forms of schizophrenia are less likely to have formal thought disorder, negative symptoms, or soft neurologic signs.[25–28] In contrast, late-onset disease is associated with a higher likelihood of organic causes and sensory impairment.[24] When the geriatrician is considering a diagnosis of schizophrenia in a patient, careful evaluation of cognition and neurologic status including the special senses is warranted.

The practicing geriatrician is likely to treat patients with schizophrenia. The notion that most elderly schizophrenic patients are institutionalized is a myth that probably results from the term dementia praecox used by Kraepelin. This term implied deterioration in cognition for the patients described, and later studies did not confirm this belief.[29] In fact, although most elderly schizophrenic patients have significant symptoms and functional disability, they do not demonstrate significant cognitive impairment or live in an institution.

Dementia

Psychosis may co-occur with several forms of dementia. Psychosis occurs in up to one-third of Alzheimer's disease (AD) patients at any given time[30,31] and has also been associated with vascular dementia, Parkinson's disease, dementia with Lewy bodies, Pick's disease, prion-related dementia, substance-induced persisting dementia, and dementia secondary to medical conditions such as anoxia or head trauma.[32–34]

Psychosis in dementia needs to be differentiated from misidentification or confabulation. An example of misidentification is when a patient with dementia believes that her reflection in the mirror is another person or that individuals in a picture hanging on a wall or on the television are "real." In the first example, the patient may refuse to enter a room with these objects for fear of experiencing these events. Misidentification is best treated with nonpharmacologic interventions rather than antipsychotic medications. Removing the offending structure (mirror, wall hanging, or television) may be effective.

Confabulation is defined as making up an answer or explanation to compensate for deficits in cognition. Distinct from psychosis, confabulation is exemplified by the man who has misplaced his keys and now states "my wife stole them." Misidentification and confabulation may be found in many of the dementia subtypes and appears to be most common in the early to middle stages of AD.

Similar to confabulation, psychosis is more common in the early to middle stages of AD. Although psychosis is a predictor of institutionalization, the intensity of an individual's psychosis may vary. A patient who is neither a danger to themselves or others, nor significantly functionally impaired, may not require the more restrictive setting of an institution.

Psychosis and Alzheimer's Disease

Patients with psychosis and Alzheimer's disease (AD) have a more rapid rate of decline than those AD patients without psychosis.[35] The incidence of psychosis in AD ranges from 5% to 50%, depending on age and the population studied. Although the range of hallucinations and delusions overlaps, the mean rate of hallucinations appears to be less common than delusions.[36] In one large community sample of patients with probable AD, 22% had delusions, 3% had hallucinations, and 9% had both.[37] The patients with hallucinations had less education, increased stage and duration of dementia, and were more likely to be African-American. Hallucinations were associated with falls and anxiolytic use. Delusions were associated with increased age, antihypertensive use, depression, a more impaired health status, and aggression.

Compared to early- or middle-stage patients, the advanced-stage AD patients may be unable to report their psychosis. Behavioral disturbances in the advanced-stage patient may be related to psychosis, although instrumentation to measure psychosis in the advanced-stage AD patient is lacking. Agitation in advanced-stage patients may reflect pain, bladder outlet obstruction, fecal impaction, incontinence, hunger, feeling cold, or overstimulation. Identification of these unmet needs can help delineate the optimal pharmacologic and nonpharmacologic treatment approaches. For example, the advanced-stage AD patient who is in pain may benefit from an empiric trial of analgesic, or the poorly nourished patient who may be hungry should be fed more frequently.

Psychosis in Parkinson's Disease

Psychosis in the context of Parkinson's disease (PD) poses special challenges. Although psychoses occur in 10% to 15% of PD patients, proper attribution of the psychosis to the PD or its treatment may be difficult. The subcortical circuitry that is dysfunctional in PD may also be responsible for the generation of psychotic symptoms in the disease.[38] Anticholinergic and dopaminergic agents, both utilized to treat PD, are notorious for causing psychosis.[39] Because conventional antipsychotic agents may worsen the motor symptoms of PD, atypical antipsychotics have become the choice for treating psychosis associated with PD. Clozaril is the best studied with a clinical trial supporting its use.[40,41] A mean dosage of 25 mg clozaril was significantly better than placebo for drug-induced psychosis in PD. Parkinsonism was not worsened by the medication; in fact, tremor improved in the clozaril-treated group. Clozaril did not significantly change cognitive status during the 4 weeks of the study. Limitations of clozaril include the potential for agranulocytosis and the requirement for blood monitoring. Case reports have described the benefit of risperdal, olanzapine, and quetiapine for psychosis associated with PD, although the motor effects of these medications has not been predictable.[42,43]

Psychosis and Dementia with Lewy Bodies

Much recent press has focused on dementia with Lewy bodies (DLB), with some suggesting that it is the second most common progressive degenerative dementia.[44] Psychosis has been associated with DLB and is one of the proposed core clinical features. Consensus groups have proposed clinical criteria that include parkinsonism, dementia, cognitive fluctuation, and visual hallucinations.[44,45] We recently challenged the validity of these criteria.[46] Visual hallucinations may not be useful in differentiating DLB from other dementia subtypes.[47] In the DLB sample, as in PD, visual hallucinations may be related to medication use. For example, in our review of the DLB literature, 85% of those patients with visual hallucinations were receiving either dopaminergic or anticholinergic medication and 29% of those without visual hallucinations were receiving these medications.[46] Medications and over-the-counter preparations may be related to the psychosis in any elderly patient. The medication list should be carefully reviewed so nonessential medications may be decreased or eliminated.

Psychosis Associated with Vascular Dementia

Hallucinations occur in 1% to 10% of stroke patients and are most commonly associated with right-sided temporoparietal lesions, cerebral atrophy, seizures.[48–50] Other neuroimaging studies suggest that vascular lesions may be important in the pathogenesis of late-life paranoid psychosis.[51] Patients with vascular dementia may be more susceptible to adverse effects (including psychosis) from medications and to subtle changes in chronic medical conditions. Empirical evidence to support one pharmacologic agent over another is lacking for vascular dementia with psychosis. Our practice is the empiric use of atypical antipsychotics such as risperdal, olanzapine, and quetiepine.

Comparison of AD with Psychosis and Late-Life Schizophrenia

Jeste and Finkel recently compared AD with psychosis to late-life schizophrenia.[52] Highlights of the comparison between these conditions revealed that the incidence of AD with psychosis (30%–50%) is much more frequent than the incidence of elderly schizophrenia (less than 1%). Bizarre and well-systematized delusions are rare in psychosis associated with AD whereas they occur frequently in late-life schizophrenia. Hallucinations are more commonly visual in AD and auditory in schizophrenia. Schneiderian first-rank symptoms such as thought insertion, thought broadcasting, or thought withdrawal are more common in schizophrenia than in AD. The misidentification of caregivers is frequent in AD but rare in schizophrenia. A past history of psychosis is very common in schizophrenia, yet rare in AD with psychosis. Psychosis usually remits as AD advances, compared with schizophrenia, where it usually persists. Therefore, the need for years of maintenance antipsychotic use is uncommon in AD with psychosis but common in schizophrenia. Active suicidal ideation is rare in AD with psychosis but present in up to half of schizophrenia patients. Approximately 10% of elderly schizophrenics complete suicide.[53]

Delusional Disorder

Delusional disorder appears to be a distinct diagnostic entity from schizophrenia, schizoaffective disorder, bipolar disease, and dementia with psychosis. This disorder is characterized by nonbizarre delusions of at least 1-month duration. A nonbizarre delusion is a delusion that could happen in real life, such as being followed or loved from a distance. There are no controlled trials of elderly patients with delusional disorder to aid in the management principles for these patients. If delusions are interfering with the patient's social, occupational, or other areas of functioning, we offer a trial of an atypical antipsychotic agent while attempting to build a therapeutic alliance.

Affective Disorders with Psychosis

Affective disorders with psychosis include major depression, bipolar disease, and schizoaffective disorder. Severely depressed patients with psychosis commonly have delusional themes about excessive guilt, being punished, or somatic problems. Manic patients often have grandiose delusions. Elderly patients are at increased risk for completing suicide compared with younger patients,[54] and psychosis is a risk factor for suicide completion.[53] Therefore, psychotic patients should be carefully assessed for suicidal intent and plan.

Patients with major depression and psychosis should be treated with antidepressants and antipsychotics. The specific antidepressant choice is beyond the scope of this chapter. Antidepressants with anticholinergic load or cardiotoxicity should be avoided in elderly patients. After the resolution of psychotic symptoms, the patient may be tapered off the antipsychotic, but should remain on the antidepressant for continuation and maintenance treatment. If the patient's psychosis reappears on removal of the antipsychotic, it may be necessary to continue the patient on an antipsychotic and attempt to reduce or remove this at a later date.

The atypical antipsychotic, olanzapine, has been approved as a stand-alone agent for acute mania but has not been studied in bipolar patients over age 65 for this indication.[55] Electroconvulsive therapy (ECT) is a very effective treatment alternative in elderly patients with affective disorders and psychosis. Although ECT suffers from stigma in the medical and lay communities, it is a safe alternative treatment for affective disorder with psychosis that offers the advantage of a more rapid rate of response than pharmacotherapy. Psychiatric evaluation will assist the patient and the clinician in determining the feasibility of ECT for a particular patient.[56]

Specific Clinical Patterns with Aging

As patients age, the quantity and severity of medical comorbidities and medication use increase and adherence to treatment regimens may decrease. These complexities are compounded by the pharmacokinetic and pharmacodynamic changes that occur with age and the potential for drug–drug interactions.[57,58] Brain changes that occur with aging may contribute to the development or course of the disease associated with psychosis. Additionally, the aging brain may be more susceptible to additional environmental or biologic stressors. The combination of one or several of these factors may contribute to specific clinical patterns of psychosis seen with aging.

Pathogenesis

The pathogenesis of psychosis remains unclear. Theories abound, and there may be several final common pathways leading to psychosis. For example, neurochemical, in vivo imaging, and neuropathologic studies support the relationship between basal ganglia abnormalities and psychosis. Studies attempting to explain the pathophysiology of psychosis are limited by lack of uniformity in patient selection, clinical and neuropathologic diagnoses, psychotic rating methodology, medication and substance use, and medical comorbidity.

Approach to Differential Diagnosis

After the history and examination reveal the presence of hallucinations or delusions, the evaluation should focus on whether medical conditions, their treatments, or other substances (e.g., medications, toxins, over-the-counter preparations, herbal compounds) are contributing factors. The psychosis may also result from substance intoxication or withdrawal. The next step is to determine whether the active phase symptoms of schizophrenia are present, the duration of symptoms, and their relationship to mood symptoms. Figure 80.1 is a decision tree for the differential diagnosis of psychotic disorders based on the DSM-IV.[59]

Treatment Approaches

Treatment for psychosis in late life involves some core principles. The newly diagnosed psychosis in a patient should be viewed as a potential delirium until proven otherwise. General medical conditions and offending substances should be sought as probable contributors. Management should focus on problem behaviors and functional status rather than on the severity or duration of the psychotic symptom per se. Goals of treatment should be realistically defined and reviewed with the patient and caregivers. Adequate time should be given to test whether an intervention is realizing the therapeutic goals set.

In general, the older patient with psychosis requires lower doses of antipsychotic medication compared with the younger patient, with some authors recommending a dosage 15% to 25% of that of a young schizophrenic

patient.[52] Atypical antipsychotics appear to be preferential to conventional antipsychotic agents but are not free from potential adverse effects. Medication treatment in combination with psychological education, environmental manipulation, and behavioral modification appear to be the standard of care in treating elderly patients with psychosis.

Pharmacologic Agents

Traditional Antipsychotics: Do They Still Have a Role?

Haloperidol is the most commonly prescribed antipsychotic agent, and thioridazine is commonly prescribed for agitation because of its sedating effects. These "traditional" agents may no longer be the ideal choices for the management of psychosis in later life.

Cardiac conduction irregularities such as prolongation of QTC and polymorphic ventricular tachycardia (torsades de pointes) have been associated with intravenous haloperidol[60] and oral thioridazine.[61,62] A recent "Dear Doctor" letter issued by the FDA and labeling changes in the product information warn of thioridazine's adverse cardiac conduction profile. These is a black box warning label about the thioridazine's dose-dependent risk of QTC prolongation and the recommendation that EKGs and serum potassium levels be obtained at baseline and periodically monitored.[63]

The traditional antipsychotic agents have variable degrees of dopaminergic, alpha-adrenergic, anticholinergic, and histamine effects. The dopaminergic effects (primarily D_2 blockade) are presumed to result in the therapeutic effects and the extrapyramidal side effects such as tremor, bradykinesia, akathisia, rigidity, and dystonic reactions. The higher potency agents (e.g., haloperidal, fluphenazine) have relatively higher ratios of dopaminergic blockade to adrenergic, anticholinergic, and histaminic effects. The lower-potency agents have higher ratios of anticholinergic, histaminic, and adrenergic effects relative to dopaminergic effects. Adrenergic blockade increases the risk of orthosatic hypotension. The histaminic blockade results in sedation and weight gain. The peripheral and central anticholinergic effects may lead to dry mouth, blurry vision, urinary retention, constipation, and confusion. Aging-related brain changes and disease-related brain changes (e.g., from AD, PD, stroke) place elderly patients at increased risk of side effects from the traditional antipsychotic agents. In one metaanalysis of 16 double-blind controlled studies using conventional antipsychotics for dementia, 20% of patients had a significant side effect (i.e., sedation, orthostatic hypotension, or extrapyramidal effects).[64] The lower-potency agents should be avoided in elderly

FIGURE 80.1. Differential diagnosis of psychotic disorders. (Adapted from DSM IV.)

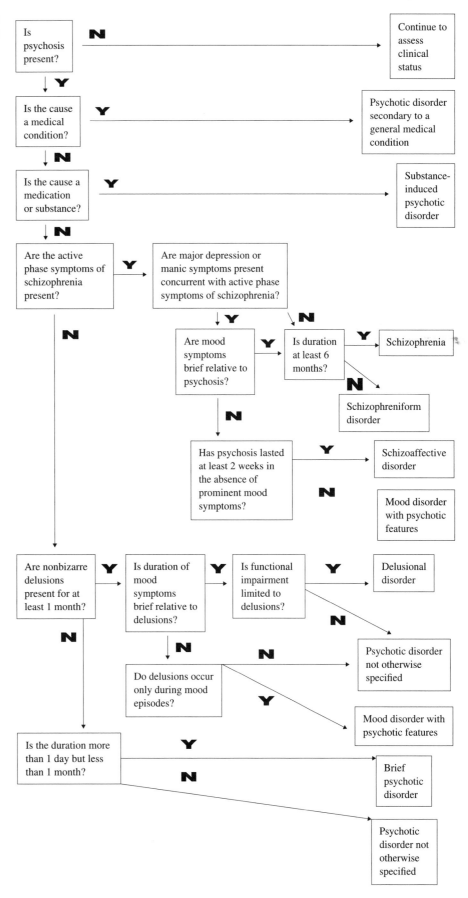

patients who are at increased risk of side effects from these agents.

A meta-analysis of antipsychotic agents used for inpatients with behavioral disturbance associated with dementia or other neurologic conditions demonstrated an effect size of 18%.[65] The placebo group had a 41% response rate and the treatment group had a response rate of 59%. The relatively high placebo response rate may have underrepresented the true differences between groups. Other limitations of the study include heterogeneous groups, generalizability only to inpatients, and dated nature of the study as conventional agents were the only antipsychotics available. Despite their widespread use, there is not a substantial evidence base from which to recommend conventional antipsychotics for behavioral disturbance associated with dementia. One placebo-controlled crossover study compared fixed low-dose haloperidol (0.5–0.75 mg/day) to standard dose haloperidol (2–3 mg/day) for 6 weeks in AD patients with psychosis.[66] Patients receiving standard doses of haloperidol performed superior to low-dose haloperidol or placebo, although there was increased extrapyramidal risk in the standard-dose haloperidol group.

Tardive Dyskinesia

Tardive dyskinesia (TD) is a significant problem in the elderly, leading to functional disability and social stigma. All antipsychotic agents, regardless of potency, carry the risk of tardive dyskinesia. Jeste et al. estimated the 12-month incidence of TD in patients over age 55 years to be 25%, the 2-year incidence to be 34%, and the 3-year cumulative incidence to be 53%.[67] Age, female gender, length of exposure to neuroleptic medication, and the presence of extrapyramidal signs appear to be significant risk factors for TD.[66,68,69]

There was great hope that the introduction of atypical agents would reduce or eliminate the risk of TD from antipsychotic agents. Few studies have compared typical to atypical agents in the risk of TD. Jeste et al. compared haloperidal to risperidone in schizophrenic patients (mean dose, 1 mg/day for both agents) and found that TD was significantly more likely to occur with haloperidol than risperidone.[69] Case reports of TD associated with atypicals are in the literature.[70] Comparing long-term effects of atypical agents to typical ones is not practical because the atypicals have not been available to patients as long. Short-term incidence studies of TD reveal only part of the story. The short-term studies may reveal the development of mild to moderate TD, but moderate to severe TD may develop over the longer term, and the atypical agents have not yet been used long enough. Hence, longer-term studies of the atypical agents are required to determine the rates of side effect development for the atypical agents in the elderly.

Neuroleptic Malignant Syndrome

Neuroleptic malignant syndrome (NMS) is a rare but life-threatening event that has been associated with both typical and atypical antipsychotic agents.[71] Clinical evidence suggestive of the syndrome includes fever, rigidity, mental state changes, autonomic instability, elevated CPK, and previous administration of an antipsychotic agent. The prognosis from NMS is good, with most patients recovering within 2 weeks.[72] Complications arise from prolonged fevers, electrolyte abnormalities, and hypoxia. Treatment for NMS is primarily supportive with conflicting evidence regarding the utility of dopaminergic agonists such as dantroline. The pathophysiology of NMS remains elusive.

Clozapine

Clozapine is primarily indicated for patients with schizophrenia who have not responded to two previous antipsychotic trials. The agent has increased D_2-receptor affinity and specificity for mesolimbic and mesocortical circuits. Agranulocytosis, a rare but fatal side effect from clozapine, is found more commonly in the older than younger patients.[73] The risk of agranulocytosis requires a weekly evaluation of white blood cell and neutrophil counts. The more common side effects from clozapine include sedation, hypersalivation, hypotension, constipation, sweating, nausea/vomiting, urinary incontinence, fever, tachycardia, and weight gain.[74] Discontinuation rate from side effects in elderly patients has approached 25% in some series.[74,75] The emergence of side effects and discontinuation rate from the medication appear related to the rate of dose titration. Starting doses of 6.25 mg clozapine are recommended for elderly patients with slow titration rates (e.g., increase by 6.25 mg q 3–7 days). The doses needed for psychosis associated with dementia appear to be lower than that required for psychotic mood disorders, which are lower than the doses required for primary psychotic disorders.[76] The monitoring requirements for clozapine prevent its use as a first-line agent.

Risperidone

Risperdone is a 5-HTA receptor antagonist in addition to D_2 blocker. It has low histaminic, alpha-1-, and alpha-2-adrenergic effects. This altered mechanism of action may explain its wider therapeutic index compared with conventional antipsychotic agents. Although there are many case reports, open trials, and chart reviews on the effects of risperidone in the elderly,[77] there are only a few controlled double-blind studies with risperidone for agitation and psychosis in the elderly persons with dementia. In one 12-week study of 625 patients with dementia (73% Alzheimer, 15% vascular, and 12% mixed), risperidone at 0.5, 1.0, and 2 mg each day was compared with placebo.[78] The dose of 1 mg per day was optimal for the treatment of psychosis and aggression in patients with dementia and behavioral disturbance. The most common side effects from risperidone included extrapyramidal side effects (EPS), peripheral edema, and somnolence. Hypotension has also been observed in the elderly. Although there was a dose response for therapeutic efficacy with risperidone (2 mg/day > 1 mg/day > 0.5 mg/day), the higher dose (2 mg/day) was associated with elevated dropout rates (42% versus 27% for placebo) from side effects such as EPS and falls.

In a pooled analysis of phase 3 data using risperidone in approximately 1000 demented elderly patients, EPS occurred in 9% of placebo-treated patients, 14% of risperidone-treated patients, and 24% of haloperidol-treated patients.[79] The same group found risperidone to be effective (and superior to haloperidol) in a 13-week trial of 344 patients with behavioral disturbance associated with dementia. The dosage of 1 mg/day was optimal in reducing the severity and frequency of aggression.[80] Taken together, the evidence for using risperidone for behavioral changes associated with dementia suggests an initial dosage of 0.25 to 0.5 mg per day titrated to 1 mg per day. The half-life of 20 h allows for once daily dosing. Risperidone is available in tablets, oral solution, and orally disintegrating tablets, which may facilitate administration to select elderly persons with dementia.

Olanzapine

Olanzapine is an antagonist of dopamine and serotonin and has affinity for histaminic, alpha-1-adrenergic, and M-1 muscarinic receptors.[81] The incidence of parkinsonian side effects is less than 10%. Olanzapine is efficacious in treating both positive symptoms (hallucinations and delusions) and negative symptoms (amotivation, withdrawal, apathy) of schizophrenia. There are limited controlled data in elderly patients with delirium, affective disorder with psychosis, or psychosis associated with Parkinson's disease. The most common side effects associated with olanzapine are somnolence, dizziness, weight gain, and agitation. Other common side effects are constipation, rhinitis, dry mouth, and dyspepsia.

Approximately 10% of patients treated with olanzapine have increases in their ALT and GGT that are dose related and reverse after drug discontinuation. Dysarthria and decreased ADLs have been reported in a case series of four elderly patients who received 5 to 10 mg olanzapine. Their conditions improved after olanzapine was stopped.[82] Dosing adjustments are not required for renal impairment or based solely on age. It appears that the combination of factors that decrease clearance of the drug, such as age, cigarette smoking, and gender, are necessary before a dosing reduction. Weight gain is a significant problem associated with the use of olanzapine. Patients with a low body mass index are more likely to gain weight than those with high pretreatment body mass index.[83] One case series reported a mean gain of 10 kg in 7 months.[84] Increased blood sugar levels and triglyceride levels have also been associated with olanzapine. Olanzapine is 93% protein bound, primarily to alpha-1-glycoprotein and albumin. Time to peak concentration is 6 hours and the elimination half-life is 52 h in those over age 65 years. Careful monitoring is recommended in conjunction with drugs that prolong the QT interval. There have been no cases of agranulocytosis with olanzapine, although long-term use of this agent is limited.

Olanzapine has the potential to interact with other medications. For example, carbamezepine, rifampin, and omeprazole increase the clearance of olanzapine, necessitating dosage adjustments. Ciprofloxacin inhibits the metabolism of olanzapine, increasing the risk of toxicity when the two drugs are coadministered. When olanzapine is added to haloperidol (perhaps in the context of a planned substitution of agents), there appears to be an increased risk of parkinsonism,[85] possibly due to inhibition of cytochrome P-450-2D6 or increased D_2 blockade. Clozapine and olanzapine have not been directly compared in controlled clinical trials in the elderly. One recent study compared olanzapine (5, 10 or 15 mg) to placebo for agitation in AD.[86] Olanzapine was superior in measures of delusions, hallucinations and agitation as measured by the neuropsychiatric inventory (NPI). There was no significant difference in vital signs between the groups.

Quetiapine

Quetiapine, an atypical antipsychotic that is structurally similar to clozapine and olanzapine, has demonstrated efficacy for the positive and negative symptoms of schizophrenia. The agent has high affinity for serotenergic (5HT-2) and moderate affinity for dopaminergic (D_2) receptors, purportedly related to its relatively low potential for parkinsonism. Clinical trials have reported no difference in EPS severity between patients treated with quetiapine or placebo. The agent also has affinity for alpha-1-adrenergic and alpha-2-adrenergic and H_1 histaminic receptors but not muscarinic receptors. The most common side effects observed with quetiapine are dizziness, somnolence, constipation, postural hypotension, dry mouth, dyspepsia, and headache. Additional side effects include agitation, insomnia, tachycardia, and peripheral edema. The elimination half-life of quetiapine is 6 h, necessitating dosing two to three times per day. The peak concentration occurs 1.5 h after administration, and food increases absorption. The drug is 83% protein bound and hepatically metabolized with several active metabolites. Antipsychotic efficacy has been demonstrated in a dose

TABLE 80.4. Comparison of antipsychotic agents used in the elderly.

Drug name (chemical class)	D$_2$ receptor antagonism	5HT2$_a$ receptor antagonism	Anticholinergic effects	Orthostasis	Sedation	Parkinsonism	Effect of food on absorption
Clozapine (dibenzodiazepine)	Low	High	Very high	High	Very high	Rare	None
Risperidone (benzisoxazole)	High	High	Low	Moderate	Low	Low	None
Olanzapine (thienbenzodiazepine)	High	High	Low	Moderate	Moderate	Very low	None
Quetiapine dibenzothiazepine	Moderate	High	Very low	Moderate	Moderate	Rare	Increases
Haloperidol	High	None	Low	Low	Moderate	High	Decreases

range of 150 to 750 mg per day, and clinical trials for schizophrenia have shown effectiveness in dosages of 300 to 400 mg with a maximum dosage of 750 mg per day. Renal impairment does not necessitate dosage adjustment. In contrast, patients with hepatic impairment require a decrease in dosage.

Transient serum transaminasemia may require discontinuation of the agent. The levels normalize after medication discontinuation, and there are no reports of irreversible hepatic damage associated with quetiapine. Patients over age 65 have diminished clearance of quetiapine, and a reduction in dosage may be necessary. Patients who have predisposition to hypotension should have a slower titration schedule to a lower target dose. Leukopenia but not agranulocytosis has been reported with quetiapine. Weight gain of greater than 7% above baseline has occurred in one-quarter of patients.[87] A possible association between quetiapine and cataract formation necessitates ophthalmologic examination at initiation of therapy, shortly theraftereafter, and at 6 months.

Potential drug–drug interactions with erythromycin, fluconazole, phenytoin, and ketoconazole (increased quetiapine levels by P-450 3A4 inhibition) justify a reduction in quetiapine dosing. Close monitoring of international normalized ratio (INR) is required in patients taking warfarin with quetiapine. There are no published clinical trials specific to elderly patients comparing quetiapine to placebo. The response to quetiapine in published clinical trials has been variable; up to one-third of patients have dropped out from studies because of lack of efficacy, and sustained efficacy has been called into question.[88–90] Case reports support the use of quetiapine for psychosis associated with Parkinson's disease without worsening motor symptoms,[43] perhaps suggesting a therapeutic niche.

For agent comparisons, see Table 80.4.

Symptom Treatment in Addition to the Usual Management

Several additional approaches complement pharmacotherapy in the treatment of psychosis in later life. All medical conditions have the potential to aggravate psychosis in a direct or indirect manner. Focus on stabilizing and maintaining patient overall health with preventive screenings, thorough histories, and examinations should have a positive effect on reducing the severity and duration of psychosis in late life.

Treatments for medical problems pose another possible contributing factor. For example, a flare-up of a chronic condition or a new acute medical condition may lead to changes in the medication profile of a patient. The medications list should be frequently reviewed and the clinician should ask, "Are any of these medications nonessential?" An affirmation will lead to a medication adjustment that may substantially reduce the psychosis or even prevent its initiation.

Pragmatic nonpharmacologic approaches for psychosis may include cognitive behavioral approaches to minimize the effect of the psychosis on the patient's interpersonal relationships. For example, a patient may be "coached" to not spontaneously offer the content of a delusional system to others or use the technique of "thought stopping" to temporarily eliminate an internal psychotic

Hepatic metabolism	Protein binding	$T_{\frac{1}{2}}$ (h)	Dosing	Dose/day (mg)	Weight gain	Cost/day	Other
Extensive	97%	8–12	Twice daily	50–900	High	500 mg $22 brand $14 generic	Agranulocytosis; decreased dose in elderly
Extensive P-450	88%	20–30	Once or twice daily	0.25–6	Low	2 mg $3 brand	Decreased dose in elderly; prolactin increase
Weak P-450	93%	31	Once daily	5–20	Significant	10 mg $8.50 brand	Decreased dose in elderly
Extensive P-450	83%	7	Twice daily	100–800	Moderate	600 mg $13 brand	Decreased dose in elderly
Extensive P-450	90%	21	Once or twice daily	0.5–8	Low	3 mg 18 cents (generic)	Decreased dose in elderly; prolactin increase

stimuli. Other general health maintenance measures such as optimal nutrition and exercise regimens may also have benefit, although the evidence base is very limited. Education about late-life psychosis may improve patient adherence to prescribed treatment regimens and offer needed support to overwhelmed caregivers who are at increased risk of excess morbidity and mortality.

References

1. Christenson R, Blazer D. Epidemiology of persecutory ideation in an elderly population in the community. *Am J Psychiatry.* 1984;141:1088–1089.
2. Kendler KS, Gallagher TJ, Abelson JM, Kessler RC. Lifetime prevalence, demographic risk factors, and diagnostic validity of nonaffective psychosis as assessed in a US community sample. The National Comorbidity Survey. *Arch Gen Psychiatry.* 1996;53(11):1022–1031.
3. Howard R, Rabins PV, Seeman MV, Jeste DV. Late-onset schizophrenia and very-late-onset schizophrenia-like psychosis: an international consensus. The International Late-Onset Schizophrenia Group. *Am J Psychiatry.* 2000;157(2): 172–178.
4. Samuels SC, Davis KL. Dementia and delirium. In: Enna SJ, Coyle JT, eds. *Pharmacological Management of Neurological and Psychiatric Disorders.* New York: McGraw-Hill; 267–316.
5. Gardner ER, Hall RC. Psychiatric symptoms produced by over-the-counter drugs. *Psychosomatics.* 1982;23(2):186–190.
6. Bruce ML, McNamara R. Psychiatric status among the homebound elderly: an epidemiologic perspective. *J Am Geriatr Soc.* 1992;40(6):561–566.
7. Currie CT, Moore JT, Friedman SW, Warshaw GA. Assessment of elderly patients at home: a report of fifty cases. *J Am Geriatr Soc.* 1981;29(9):398–401.
8. Levy MT. Psychiatric assessment of elderly patients in the home: a survey of 176 cases. *J Am Geriatr Soc.* 1985;33(1): 9–12.
9. Stern Y, Tang MX, Albert MS, et al. Predicting time to nursing home care and death in individuals with Alzheimer disease. *JAMA.* 1997;277(10):806–812.
10. Junginger J, Phelan E, Cherry K, Levy J. Prevalence of psychopathology in elderly persons in nursing homes and in the community. *Hosp Community Psychiatry.* 1993;44(4): 381–383.
11. Health Care Financing Administration. Medicare and Medicaid: requirements for long-term care facilities final registration. *Fed Reg.* 1991;56:48865–48921.
12. Health Care Financing Administration. Medicare and Medicaid: resident assessment in long-term care facilities. *Fed Red.* 1992;57:61614–61733.
13. Marin DB, Green CR, Schmeidler J, et al. Noncognitive disturbances in Alzheimer's disease: frequency, longitudinal course, and relationship to cognitive symptoms. *J Am Geriatr Soc.* 1997;45(11):1331–1338.
14. Rovner BW, Edelman BA, Cox MP, Shmuely Y. The impact of antipsychotic drug regulations on antipsychotic prescribing practices in nursing homes. *Am J Psychiatry.* 1992;149: 1390–1392.
15. Harvey PD, Jacobsen H, Mancini D, et al. Clinical, cognitive and functional characteristics of long-stay patients with schizophrenia: a comparison of VA and state hospital patients. *Schizophr Res.* 2000;43(1):3–9.
16. Woerner MG, Kane JM, Lieberman JA, et al. The prevalence of tardive dyskinesia. *J Clin Psychopharmacol.* 1991; 11(1):34–42.
17. Harvey PD, Moriarty PJ, Friedman JI, et al. Differential preservation of cognitive functions in geriatric patients

with lifelong chronic schizophrenia: less impairment in reading compared with other skill areas. *Biol Psychiatry.* 2000;47(11):962–968.

18. Purohit DP, Perl DP, Haroutunian V, Powchik P, Davidson M, Davis KL. Alzheimer disease and related neurodegenerative diseases in elderly patients with schizophrenia: a postmortem neuropathologic study of 100 cases. *Arch Gen Psychiatry.* 1998;55(3):205–211.

19. Mathalon DH, Ford JM, Rosenbloom M, Pfefferbaum A. P300 reduction and prolongation with illness duration in schizophrenia. *Biol Psychiatry.* 2000;47(5):413–427.

20. Davidson M, Harvey P, Welsh KA, Powchik P, Putnam KM, Mohs RC. Cognitive functioning in late-life schizophrenia: a comparison of elderly schizophrenic patients and patients with Alzheimer's disease. *Am J Psychiatry.* 1996;153(10): 1274–1279.

21. Friedman JI, Adler DN, Davis KL. The role of norepinephrine in the pathophysiology of cognitive disorders: potential applications to the treatment of cognitive dysfunction in schizophrenia and Alzheimer's disease. *Biol Psychiatry.* 1999;46(9):1243–1252.

22. Copeland JR, Dewey ME, Scott A, et al. Schizophrenia and delusional disorder in older age: community prevalence, incidence, comorbidity, and outcome. *Schizophr Bull.* 1998;24(1):153–161.

23. van Os J, Howard R, Takei N, Murray R. Increasing age is a risk factor for psychosis in the elderly. *Soc Psychiatry Psychiatr Epidemiol.* 1995;30(4):161–164.

24. Howard R, Rabins PV, Seeman MV, Jeste DV. Late-onset schizophrenia and very-late-onset schizophrenia-like psychosis: an international consensus. The International Late-Onset Schizophrenia Group. *Am J Psychiatry.* 2000;157(2): 172–178.

25. Pearlson GD, Kreger L, Rabins PV, et al. A chart review study of late-onset and early-onset schizophrenia. *Am J Psychiatry.* 1989;146(12):1568–1574.

26. Howard R, Castle D, Wessely S, Murray R. A comparative study of 470 cases of early-onset and late-onset schizophrenia. *Br J Psychiatry.* 1993;163:352–357.

27. Almeida OP, Howard RJ, Levy R, David AS. Psychotic states arising in late life (late paraphrenia) psychopathology and nosology. *Br J Psychiatry.* 1995;166(2):205–214.

28. Almeida OP, Howard RJ, Levy R, David AS. Psychotic states arising in late life (late paraphrenia). The role of risk factors. *Br J Psychiatry.* 1995;166(2):215–228.

29. Adityanjee, Aderibigbe YA, Theodoridis D, Vieweg VR. Dementia praecox to schizophrenia: the first 100 years. *Psychiatry Clin Neurosci.* 1999;53(4):437–448.

30. Tariot PN, Podgorski CA, Blazina L, Leibovici A. Mental disorders in the nursing home: another perspective. *Am J Psychiatry.* 1993;150(7):1063–1069.

31. Tariot PN, Mack JL, Patterson MB, et al. The Behavior Rating Scale for Dementia of the Consortium to Establish a Registry for Alzheimer's Disease. The Behavioral Pathology Committee of the Consortium to Establish a Registry for Alzheimer's Disease. *Am J Psychiatry.* 1995; 152(9):1349–1357.

32. Schreiber S, Klag E, Gross Y, Segman RH, Pick CG. Beneficial effect of risperidone on sleep disturbance and

psychosis following traumatic brain injury. *Int Clin Psychopharmacol.* 1998;13(6):273–275.

33. Meyendorf R. Psychopatho-ophthalmology, gnostic disorders, and psychosis in cardiac surgery. Visual disturbances after open heart surgery. *Arch Psychiatr Nervenkr.* 1982; 232(2):119–135.

34. Snow RE, Arnold SE. Psychosis in neurodegenerative disease. *Semin Clin Neuropsychiatry.* 1996;1(4):282–293.

35. Stern Y, Albert M, Brandt J, et al. Utility of extrapyramidal signs and psychosis as predictors of cognitive and functional decline, nursing home admission and death in Alzheimer's disease: prospective analysis from the predictors study. *Neurology.* 1994;44:2300–2307.

36. Wragg RE, Jeste DV. Neuroleptics and alternative treatments. Management of behavioral symptoms and psychosis in Alzheimer's disease and related conditions. *Psychiatr Clin Am.* 1988;11(1):195–213.

37. Bassiony MM, Steinberg MS, Warren A, Rosenblatt A, Baker AS, Lyketsos CG. Delusions and hallucinations in Alzheimer's disease: prevalence and clinical correlates. *Int J Geriatr Psychiatry.* 2000;15(2):99–107.

38. Cummings JL. Vascular subcortical dementias: clinical aspects. *Dementia.* 1994;5(3–4):177–180.

39. Trzepacz PT. Is there a final common neural pathway in delirium? Focus on acetylcholine and dopamine. *Semin Clin Neuropsychiatry.* 2000;5(2):132–148.

40. Parkinson's study group. Low dose clozapine for the treatment of drug-induced psychosis in Parkinson's disease. *N Engl J Med.* 1999;340:757–763.

41. Cummings JL. Managing psychosis in patients with Parkinson's disease. *N Engl J Med.* 1999;340(10):801–803.

42. Friedman JH, Factor SA. Atypical antipsychotics in the treatment of drug-induced psychosis in Parkinson's disease. *Movement Disord.* 2000;15(2):201–211.

43. Parsa MA, Bastani B. Quetiepine (Seroquel) in the treatment of psychosis in the treatment of Parkinson's disease. *J Neuropsychiatry Clin Neurosci.* 1998;10:216–219.

44. McKeith IG, Perry RH, Fairbairn AF, Jabeen S, Perry EK. Operational criteria for senile dementia of Lewy body type (SDLT). *Psychol Med.* 1992;22(4):911–922.

45. McKeith IG, Galasko D, Kosaka K, et al. Consensus guidelines for the clinical and pathologic diagnosis of dementia with Lewy bodies (DLB): report of the consortium on DLB international workshop. *Neurology.* 1996; 47(5):1113–1124.

46. Serby M, Samuels SC. Diagnostic criteria for dementia with Lewy bodies reconsidered. *Am J Geriatr Psychiatry.* 2001;9: 212–216.

47. Serby M, Samuels SC. Visual hallucinations and dementia with Lewy bodies. *Arch Neurol.* 2000;57(12):1792.

48. Brust JC, Behrens MM. "Release hallucinations" as the major symptom of posterior cerebral artery occlusion: a report of 2 cases. *Ann Neurol.* 1977;2(5):432–436.

49. Levine DN, Finklestein S. Delayed psychosis after right temporoparietal stroke or trauma: relation to epilepsy. *Neurology.* 1982;32(3):267–273.

50. Peroutka SJ, Sohmer BH, Kumar AJ, Folstein M, Robinson RG. Hallucinations and delusions following a right temporoparietooccipital infarction. *Johns Hopkins Med J.* 1982; 151(4):181–185.

51. Tonkonogy JM, Geller JL. Late-onset paranoid psychosis as a distinct clinicopathologic entity: magnetic resonance imaging data in elderly patients with paranoid psychosis of late onset and schizophrenia of early onset. *Neuropsychiatry Neuropsychol Behav Neurol.* 1999;12(4):230–235.

52. Jeste DV, Finkel SI. Psychosis of Alzheimer's disease and related dementias. Diagnostic criteria for a distinct syndrome. *Am J Geriatr Psychiatry.* 2000;8(1):29–34.

53. Finkel SI, Rosman M. Six elderly suicides in a 1-year period in a rural midwestern community. *Int Psychogeriatr.* 1995; 7(2):221–230.

54. De Leo D, Conforti D, Carollo G. A century of suicide in Italy: a comparison between the old and the young. *Suicide Life Threat Behav.* 1997;27(3):239–249.

55. Tohen M, Sanger TM, McElroy SL, et al. Olanzapine versus placebo in the treatment of acute mania. Olanzapine HGEH Study Group. *Am J Psychiatry.* 1999;156(5):702–709.

56. Klapheke MM. Electroconvulsive therapy consultation: an update. *Convuls Ther.* 1997;13(4):227–241.

57. Zubenko GS, Sunderland T. Geriatric psychopharmacology: why does age matter? *Harv Rev Psychiatry.* 2000;7(6): 311–333.

58. Catterson ML, Preskorn SH, Martin RL. Pharmocodynamic and pharmacokinetic considerations in geriatric psychopharmacology. *Psychiatr Clin N Am.* 1997;20:205–218.

59. *Diagnostic and Statistical Manual of Mental Disorders, 4th Ed.* Washington, DC: American Psychiatric Association; 1994:694–695.

60. Hunt N, Stern TA. The association between intravenous haloperidol and torsades de pointes. Three cases and a literature review. *Psychosomatics.* 1995;36(6):541–549.

61. Reilly JG. QTc-interval abnormalities and psychotropic drug therapy in psychiatric patients [see comments]. *Lancet.* 2000;355(9209):1048–1052.

62. Hartigan-Go K, Bateman DN, Nyberg G, Martensson E, Thomas SH. Concentration-related pharmacodynamic effects of thioridazine and its metabolites in humans. *Clin Pharmacol Ther.* 1996;60(5):543–553.

63. Thioridazine package insert. Novartis, East Hanover, NJ, June 2000.

64. Lanctot KL, Best TS, Mittmann N, et al. Efficacy and safety of neuroleptics in behavioral disorders associated with dementia. *J Clin Psychiatry.* 1998;59(10):550–561.

65. Schneider LS, Pollock VE, Lyness SA. A meta-analysis of controlled trials of neuroleptic medication in dementia. *J Am Geriatr Soc.* 1990;38:553–563.

66. Devanand DP, Marder K, Michaels KS, et al. A randomized, placebo-controlled dose-comparison trial of haloperidol for psychosis and disruptive behaviors in Alzheimer's disease. *Am J Psychiatry.* 1998;155(11):1512–1520.

67. Jeste DV, Lacro JP, Palmer B, et al. Incidence of tardive dyskinesia in early stages of low-dose treatment with typical neuroleptics in older patients. *Am J Psychiatry.* 1999;156: 309–311.

68. Saltz BL, Woerner MG, Kane JM, et al. Prospective study of tardive dyskinesia incidence in the elderly. *JAMA.* 1991; 266:2402–2406.

69. Jeste DV, Lacro JP, Bailey A, et al. Lower incidence of tardive dyskinesia with risperidone compared to haloperidal in older patients. *J Am Geriatr Soc.* 1999;47:716–719.

70. Ghelmer D, Belmaker RH. Tardive dyskinesia with quetiepine [letter]. *Am J Psychiatry.* 1999;156:796–797.

71. Burkhard PR, Vingerhoets FJG. Olanzapine-induced neuroleptic malignant syndrome. *Arch Gen Psychiatry.* 1999;56:101–102.

72. Pelonero AL, Levenson JL, Pandurangi AK. Neuroleptic malignant syndrome: a review. *Psychiatr Serv.* 1998;49(9): 1163–1172.

73. Lacro JP, Eastham JH, Jeste DV, et al. Newer antipsychotics and antidepressants for elderly people. *Cur Opin Psychiatry.* 1996;9:290–293.

74. Package insert for clozaril.

75. Oberholzer AF, Hendriksen C, Monsch AU, et al. Safety and effectiveness of low dose clozapine in psychogeriatric patients: a preliminary study. *Int Psychogeriatrics.* 1992;4: 187–195.

76. Chengappa KNR, Baker RW, Kreinbrook SB, et al. Clozapine use in female geriatric patients with psychoses. *J Geriatr Psychiatry Neurol.* 1995;8:12–15.

77. Maixner SM, Mellow AM, Tandon R. The efficacy, safety and tolerability of antipsychotics in the elderly. *J Clin Psychiatry.* 1999;60(suppl 8):29–41.

78. De Deyn PP, Katz IR. Control of aggression and agitation in patients with dementia: efficacy and safety of risperidone. *Int J Geriatr Psychiatry.* 2000;15(suppl 1):S14–S22.

79. Katz IR, Jeste DV, Mintzer JE, et al. Comparison of risperidone and placebo for psychosis and behavioral disturbance associated with dementia: a randomized, double-blind trial. *J Clin Psychiatry.* 1999;60:107–115.

80. De Deyn PP, De Smedt G, Brecher M. Efficacy and safety of risperidone in elderly patients with dementia: pooled results from Phase III controlled trials. Presented at the 11th Congress of the European College of Neuropsychopharmacology, Oct 31–Nov 4, 1998, Paris, France.

81. De Deyn PP, Rabheru K, Rasmussen A, et al. A randomized trial of risperidone, placebo, and haloperidol for behavioral symptoms of dementia. *Neurology.* 1999;53:946–955.

82. Beasley CM Jr, Tollefson G, Tran P, et al. Olanzapine versus placebo and haloperizizdol: acute phase results of North American double-blind olanzapine trial. *Neuropsychopharmacology.* 1996;14:111–123.

83. Gaile S, Noviasky JA. Speech disturbance and marked decrease in function seen in several older patients on olanzapine [letter]. *J Am Geriatr Soc.* 1998;46:1330–1331.

84. Tollefson GD, Beasley CM Jr, Tran PV, et al. Olanzapine versus haloperidol in the treatment of schizophrenia and schizoaffective and schizophreniform disorders: results of an international collaborative trial. *Am J Psychiatry.* 1997; 154:457–465.

85. Gupta S, Droney T, Al-Samarrai S, et al. Olanzapine: weight gain and therapeutic efficacy [letter]. *J Clin Psychopharmacol.* 1999;19:273–275.

86. Gomberg RF. Interaction between olanzapine and haloperidol [letter]. *J Clin Psychopharmacol.* 1999;19:272–273.

87. Street JS, Clark WS, Gannon KS, et al. Olanzapine treatment of psychotic and behavioral symptoms in patients with Alzheimer disease in nursing care facilities: a double-blind, randomized, placebo-controlled trial. The HGEU Study Group. *Arch Gen Psychiatry.* 2000;57(10):968–976.

88. Borison RL, Arvanitis LA, Miller BG, et al. ICI 204,636, an atypical antipsychotic: efficacy and safety in a multicenter, placebo controlled trial in patients with schizophrenia. *J Clin Psychopharmacol.* 1996;16:158–169.

89. Fulton B, Goa KL. ICI-204,636: an initial appraisal of its pharmacological properties and clinical potential in the treatment of schizophrenia. *CNS Drugs.* 1995;4:68–78.

90. Wetzel H, Szegedi A, Hain C, et al. Seroquel (ICI 204,636), a putative "atypical" antipsychotic, in schizophrenia with positive symptomotology: results of an open clinical trial and changes of neuroendocrinological and EEG parameters. *Psychopharmacology.* 1995;119:231–238.

Part VII
Ethics and Health Policy Issues for Older Adults

81
Mechanisms of Paying for Health Care*

Bruce C. Vladeck

Although they account for less than 13% of the population of the United States, persons 65 and older incur almost 40% of this nation's total health expenditures, because the burden of illness increases as people age and, on average, older Americans have better access to needed health services than any other age group. The overall levels of health care spending in the United States are so high, and the U.S. population so large, that this also means more money is spent on health care of older people in the United States than is spent on the health care of the entire population of any other nation in the world.[1] Yet the $400 billion we are now spending annually on health services for older Americans still falls far short of providing older people with all the services they need and has clearly not produced a system of care that is entirely satisfactory either to patients or to physicians.

Older Americans are the only class of citizens of this country with an entitlement to universal health insurance, through Medicare. For all its virtues and undeniable successes, however, Medicare has some significant shortcomings, both as a health insurance mechanism and as a major source of financing for the health care delivery system. Thus, any examination of payment for health services for the elderly in America must address what Medicare does and how it does it, what it has accomplished, what it does not do, and the mechanisms that fill in some, but certainly not all, of the gaps. This chapter follows that sequence.

Medicare: Background Considerations

A logical place to begin a discussion of Medicare in a textbook on geriatrics is to acknowledge that an individual's 65th birthday generally tends to be without any particular clinical significance, although it has major implications for health insurance coverage and often for health service arrangements. The significance of age 65 arises, in turn, from Medicare's roots in the Social Security system, from which it arose and to which it remains organically connected. The identification of 65 as "normal" retirement age arose, in turn, from the historical accident of its use in Germany's social insurance scheme implemented in the late nineteenth century, the progenitor of other national social insurance programs. Medicare Hospital Insurance, generally known as Part A, parallels Old Age and Survivors Insurance (what is generally called Social Security) in that it is a compulsory, universal social insurance program, financed by payroll taxes on all wage and salary earners (and a parallel tax on the self-employed), and paying benefits to anyone with a work history or, under differing circumstances depending on the particular program, their dependents or survivors (in the case of Medicare, that includes spouses or widows over age 65 and disabled minor children). Medicare also contains Part B, or Supplemental Medical Insurance, which legally is a purely voluntary insurance program, one-quarter of which is financed by monthly premiums paid by beneficiaries, the balance by general federal revenues. Medicare's connection to Social Security is also reflected in its coverage of roughly 5 million nonelderly disabled persons, who qualify because they receive Social Security Disability Income (SSDI) benefits and have passed the 2-year waiting period between SSDI eligibility and Medicare coverage.

What Medicare Covers—and Does Not Cover

As is widely recognized, Medicare provides health insurance for those services covered in a typical private health insurance package at the time Medicare was enacted in 1965. Due to fiscal constraint, those benefits have not

---

*Prepared with the assistance of Maureen Furletti, MHS

MEDICARE PART A (HOSPITAL INSURANCE) COVERED SERVICES	
COVERED SERVICES...	**IN 2000, THE BENEFICIARY PAYS...**
HOSPITAL STAYS: Semiprivate room, meals, general nursing and other hospital services and supplies.	For each benefit period, the beneficiary pays: • A total of $776 for a hospital stay of 1-60 days. • $194 per day for days 61-90 of a hospital stay. • $388 per day for days 91-150. • All costs each day beyond 150 days.
SKILLED NURSING FACILITY (SNF) CARE: Semiprivate room, meals, skilled nursing and rehabilitative services, and other services and supplies.	For each benefit period, the beneficiary pays: • Nothing for the first 20 days. • Up to $97 per day for days 21-100. • All costs beyond the 100th day in the benefit period.
HOME HEALTH CARE: Intermittent skilled nursing care, physical therapy, speech language pathology services, home health aide services, durable medical equipment and supplies, and other services.	• Nothing for home health care services. • 20% of approved amount for durable medical equipment.
HOSPICE CARE: Pain and management relief, and supportive services for the management of a terminal illness. Home care is provided. Also covers necessary inpatient care and a variety of services otherwise not covered by Medicare.	• Limited costs for outpatient drugs and inpatient respite care.
BLOOD: From a hospital or skilled nursing facility during a covered stay.	• For the first 3 pints.

FIGURE 81.1. Medicare benefits. (*Source*: HCFA. Medicare and You 2000, beneficiary handbook available on www.medicare.gov.)

MEDICARE PART B (MEDICAL INSURANCE) COVERED SERVICES	
COVERED SERVICES...	**IN 2000, THE BENEFICIARY PAYS...**
MEDICAL EXPENSES: Doctors' services, inpatient and outpatient medical and surgical services and supplies, physical, occupational and speech therapy, diagnostic tests, and durable medical equipment (DME).	• $100 deductible (pay once per year). • 20% of approved amount after the deductible, except in the outpatient setting. • 50% for most outpatient mental health. • 20% of first $1,500 for all physical therapy services and 20% of first $1,500 for all occupational therapy services, and all charges thereafter. (Hospital outpatient therapy services do not count towards limit.)
CLINICAL LABORATORY SERVICE: Blood tests, urinalysis, and more.	• Nothing for services.
HOME HEALTH CARE: (for those beneficiaries who do not have Part A) Intermittent skilled care, home health aide services, DME and supplies, and other services.	• No less than 20% of the Medicare payment amount (after the deductible).
BLOOD: As an outpatient, or as part of a Part B covered service.	• For the first 3 pints plus 20% of approved amount for additional pints (after the deductible).
Part B also helps pay for: x-rays, speech language pathology services, artificial limbs, kidney dialysis and kidney transplants, some preventive services, some outpatient drugs, emergency care, limited chiropractic services, breast prostheses following a mastectomy, limited ambulance services, the services of practitioners	

been significantly improved since, although understanding of the medical needs of the elderly, patterns of medical care, the organization of the health system, and private insurance have all changed dramatically in that same period. Thus, although Medicare provides reasonably extensive coverage of acute inpatient hospitalization, for example, it provides essentially no coverage at all for most dental services, correction of refractive error, or hearing aids (Fig. 81.1). The fact that Medicare does not, with a few exceptions, cover outpatient prescription drugs is a problem of such magnitude in itself that it is discussed separately.

Because of these and other limitations on Medicare coverage, because there are such substantial deductibles and copayments, and because—like most private health insurance policies of the 1960s but hardly any today—there is no cap or limit on the total out-of-pocket expenses of beneficiaries, Medicare currently covers, on average, barely half the total medical care costs of its beneficiaries. Thus, essentially every Medicare beneficiary who can seeks some additional or supplemental form of insurance (Fig. 81.2).

Medicare beneficiaries can obtain supplemental coverage in one of four ways. The most fortunate have sup-

FEE-FOR-SERVICE

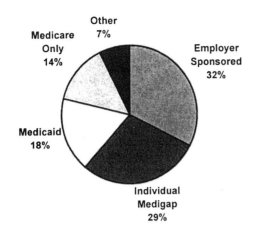

RISK HMO

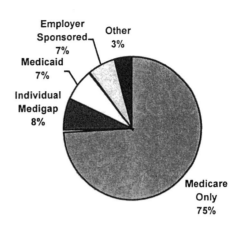

**TOTAL BENEFICIARIES
= 33.3 MILLION**

**TOTAL BENEFICIARIES
= 6.2 MILLION**

FIGURE 81.2. Type of supplemental health insurance held by Medicare beneficiaries, 1998. (*Source*: HCFA. Medicare 2000: 35 Years of Improving Americans' Health and Security, July 2000.)

plemental insurance provided as a retirement benefit by a former employer; in 1997, about a third of beneficiaries had such coverage, but that proportion is dwindling rapidly, as employers seek to cut back on retiree health benefits. Another 27% purchases individual supplemental or "Medigap" policies, the provisions of which are summarized in Figure 81.3. Although the characteristics of the Medigap market differ dramatically from one state to another, premiums for Medigap plans have been rising sharply in most of the nation in the past decade.

About 15% of Medicare beneficiaries have sufficiently low incomes to qualify for either full or partial coverage under Medicaid, the state-administered, federal–state health insurance program for the poor. About the same proportion of beneficiaries is enrolled in Medicare managed care plans, which are permitted considerable freedom in establishing their own premiums, copayments, and deductibles, but which universally have lower out-of-pocket expenses than "traditional" fee-for-service Medicare. Approximately 12% of beneficiaries, or some 4.5 million individuals, are left with Medicare coverage only. Those "Medicare-only" beneficiaries are highly concentrated in the income range just above Medicaid eligibility and tend to have the highest out-of-pocket costs even though their incomes are relatively limited.

In general, the costs of supplemental insurance, in addition to the costs of all those services that are covered neither by Medicare nor by supplemental policies, leaves a significant burden of out-of-pocket expense. The median elderly household spends slightly more than 20% of its income on out-of-pocket health expenses, and even

the most affluent beneficiaries, those in the upper 4% of the income distribution, spend roughly the same proportion of their income on out-of-pocket health costs as the median nonelderly family (Fig. 81.4).

Effects of Medicare

The dramatic improvements in life expectancy, health status, and quality of life among elderly Americans in the past three decades are the result of multiple, interactive factors. Improvements in medical knowledge and technology, in the training and expertise of physicians and other health professionals, and in incomes, education, and nutrition among both the elderly and nonelderly have all played a part. But Medicare has played an independent role as well. Before the enactment of Medicare, persons over the age of 65 actually used fewer hospital and physician services than younger people, despite their greater burden of illness; now, of course, they use substantially more. People 65 and over are now much more likely to have a usual source of medical care—and much less likely to have to rely on clinics or emergency rooms—than other age groups in the population.[2] Also, many medical advances that have helped transform the practice of medical care for the elderly, such as joint replacement, angioplasty, and the use of lasers in ophthalmic surgery, required significant financial investments by hospitals and physicians that were in turn financed, at least in part, by the availability of Medicare reimbursements for the services.

TEN STANDARDIZED MEDIGAP PLANS										
	A	B	C	D	E	F*	G	H	I	J*
BASIC BENEFITS**	2	2	2	2	2	2	2	2	2	2
PART A: INPATIENT HOSPITAL DEDUCTIBLE		2	2	2	2	2	2	2	2	2
PART A: SKILLED NURSING FACILITY COINSURANCE			2	2	2	2	2	2	2	2
PART B: DEDUCTIBLE			2			2				2
FOREIGN TRAVEL EMERGENCY			2	2	2	2	2	2	2	2
AT-HOME RECOVERY				2			2		2	2
PART B: EXCESS CHARGES						100%	80%		100%	100%
PREVENTIVE CARE					2					2
PRESCRIPTION DRUGS								BASIC 2	BASIC 2	EXTENDED 2

FIGURE 81.3. Ten standardized Medigap plans. (*Source*: HCFA. Guide to Health Insurance for People with Medicare, available on www.medicare.gov.) *Plans F and J also have a high deductible option. **Basic benefits include payment of the Part A coinsurance, coverage for 365 additional days during lifetime after Medicare benefits end, payment of Part B coinsurance (generally 20% of Medicare-approved expenses), and coverage of the first three pints of blood.

One of the more interesting attempts to identify the causes of improved health among America's elderly was that of Manton and Vaupel, who noted that the United States had historically done quite poorly on international comparisons of life expectancy, determined from birth or early adulthood, but seemed to catch up as people aged. Using data from five countries with excellent longevity statistics, they then found that, measured from age 80, the United States had the longest life expectancy. They attributed this finding to greater relative and absolute access to medical care for older Americans than their counterparts in other countries, a phenomenon they attributed in part to Medicare policies.[3]

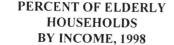

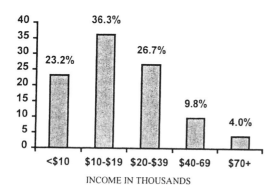

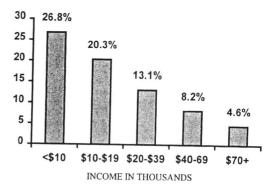

FIGURE 81.4. Elderly health spending as a percentage of income, 1998. (*Source*: HCFA. Medicare 2000: 35 Years of Improving Americans' Health and Security, July 2000.)

Medicare and Providers

Medicare is not only a critical force in the life of its beneficiaries, providing them with their major vehicle of access to medical care, it is also a critical force in the professional life of most providers of medical care in the United States. It is the single largest source of revenue for most American hospitals, home care agencies, clinical laboratories, durable medical equipment suppliers, and practitioners in many medical specialties, including of course, internal medicine and geriatrics, and a significant source of revenue for other physicians, many nursing homes, and other health care organizations as well. Medicare's facility and operational standards, data and reporting requirements, and quality-of-care measures are pervasive not only because of Medicare's importance in itself but because other insurers and public agencies often rely on or defer to them.

Because so much money is involved, and because it is believed that provider behavior and beneficiary access to care are affected not only by the absolute level of payment but also by what is paid for and how it is paid, the mechanisms of Medicare payment receive considerable attention from providers themselves, policy makers, academics, and policy analysts. Medicare's principal payment systems are summarized in Figure 81.5.

The mores of politics essentially require every provider group to insist that its level of payment is woefully inadequate. There is probably no platonically correct level in any event, but where data are available, they permit drawing the following conclusions. Since the Prospective Payment System was adopted in 1993, on average general hospitals have been paid more than their costs for treating Medicare patients, although private insurers frequently paid an even larger premium over costs;[4] before the Balanced Budget Act of 1997, most skilled nursing facilities and home care agencies prospered under Medicare payment arrangements; many have lost money since, although their finances appeared to have stabilized by calendar year 2000;[5] specialty psychiatric and rehabilitation facilities have also done reasonably well; and the provision of clinical laboratory and durable medical equipment services to Medicare has been an extremely profitable business. As for physicians, Medicare has traditionally paid less than private insurers, but the ratio of Medicare payments to average private payments rose rather dramatically during the latter half of the 1990s, more because private payers squeezed their payments than because of Medicare increases. The Physician Fee Schedule was implemented for Medicare in 1992, with the principal objective of shifting a substantial share of Medicare physician payments away from surgery and procedure-intensive specialty care toward more generalist, "cognitive" services. There has been some reallocation of physician spending as a result, but perhaps less than family practitioners, general internists, and geriatricians might have hoped, at least in part because of the inadequacies of the coding/categorization system for Medicare evaluation and management services and the political skills of procedure-oriented specialists.[6] Roughly half of all the physician services for which Medicare pays fall into the fivefold classification of "Evaluation and Management," yet that system fails to adequately capture or describe the full range of noninterventional physician services.[7]

Medicare Managed Care

In the 1990s, when the growth of managed care arrangements dominated the private health insurance sector in the United States, much attention was paid to the relatively smaller role managed care plans continued to occupy in the Medicare program. In fact, health maintenance organizations (HMOs) had been included in Medicare since the program's inception, as traditional prepaid group practices (the term HMO was not even invented until the early 1970s) such as Kaiser-Permanente and Group Health of Puget Sound. These programs were permitted to retain enrollees who had been members before retirement and were paid on a cost-reimbursement method, at a time when cost reimbursement was the dominant mode of payment for all Medicare providers. Beginning in 1985, Medicare began to pay HMOs on a full-risk basis; that is, a flat capitated monthly rate was established by formula for every county in the United States by a formula that, in principle, established the equivalent of 95% of per beneficiary costs in the conventional fee-for-service program. HMOs that were able to provide the basic Medicare benefit package at lower cost were given the option of returning the excess to the government (an option that was never exercised), establishing a stabilization fund, or providing additional benefits—the option that was most widely chosen. Beneficiaries retained the option of enrolling or disenrolling from HMOs at will, thus making it necessary for the plans to offer significant additional benefits to get beneficiaries to forsake free choice of providers and agree to having their access to care "managed."

Medicare enrollments in HMOs grew from roughly 1 million, at the time risk contracting was introduced, to more than 6 million by 1997, although that growth was characterized by peaks and valleys rather than a steady increment. Medicare managed care was highly concentrated in a few areas of the country, notably the West Coast, which has always had higher levels of managed care enrollments since the creation of Kaiser-Permanente during World War II, and south Florida, which has long been characterized by extremely high fee-for-service

PART A

PROVIDER TYPE	SYSTEM	LEGISLATIVE AUTHORITY	YEAR IMPLEMENTED	PAYMENT UNIT	CLASSIFICATION SYSTEM
HOSPITAL INPATIENT[1]	Prospective Payment System (PPS)	Social Security Amendments of 1983	1983	Per discharge	Diagnostic Related Group (DRG)
HOSPITAL CAPITAL	PPS	Omnibus Budget Reconciliation Act of (OBRA) 1987	Phased in 1992-2001	Per discharge	DRG
REHABILITATION HOSPITALS[2]	PPS	Balanced Budget Act (BBA) 1997 and Balanced Budget Refinement Act (BBRA) 1998	Pending implementation April 2001	Per discharge	Functional Related Groups (FRGs)
PSYCHIATRIC HOSPITALS[2]	PPS	BBRA 1998	Pending implementation October 2002	Per diem	Not yet defined
LONG-TERM FACILITIES	PPS	BBA 1997 and BBRA 1998	Pending implementation October 2002	Per discharge	Not yet defined
SKILLED NURSING FACILITIES	PPS	BBA 1997	July 1998	Per diem	Resource Utilization Groups (RUGS III)
HOME HEALTH AGENCIES[3]	PPS	BBA 1997	Pending implementation October 2000	Per 60 day episode	Home Health Resource Groups (HHRGs)
HOSPICE	PPS	Tax Equity and Fiscal Responsibility Act (TEFRA) 1982	November 1983	Per diem based on level of care	Level of Care Day

PART B

PROVIDER TYPE	SYSTEM	LEGISLATIVE AUTHORITY	YEAR IMPLEMENTED	PAYMENT UNIT	CLASSIFICATION SYSTEM
PHYSICIANS	Fee Schedule	OBRA 1992	1993	Per service or procedure	HCFA's Common Procedure Coding System (HCPCS)
HOSPITAL OUTPATIENT[1]	PPS	BBA 1997 and BBRA 1998	August 2000	Per service or procedure	Ambulatory Payment Classification (APC) groups
LABORATORIES	Fee Schedule	Deficit Reduction Act of 1984	1984	Per test	Current Procedural Terminology (CPT) Codes
DURABLE MEDICAL EQUIPMENT	Fee Schedule	OBRA 1987	1989	Per item	HCPCS
AMBULANCES	Fee Schedule	BBA 1997	Pending implementation January 2001	Per ambulance service level	Not yet defined
FREESTANDING AMBULATORY SURGICAL CENTERS (ASCs)	Standard Overhead Amount	OBRA 1980	1981	Per procedure	CPT Codes

FIGURE 81.5. Medicare payment systems. (*Sources*: Medpac June 2000 *Report to Congress*; Ways and Means 1998; *Green Book; Medicare Explained* 1999; and conversations with HCFA staff.) [1] In 1998, Medicare payment to cost ratios for inpatient and outpatient hospital services was 102.6%. Private payers payment to cost ratio was 113.6% for hospital services in 1998. (*Source*: Medpac *Report to Congress*, June 2000.) [2] Until their PPS implementation dates, rehabilitation and psychiatric hospitals are paid on a reasonable cost basis within TEFRA limits. [3] Until implementation of PPS in October 2000, home health agencies receive payment under a cost-based reimbursement system, referred to as the interim payment system.

costs. Extensive study of Medicare managed care plans during this period revealed that they did indeed use fewer days of inpatient hospitalization and more office visits than were typical in fee-for-service arrangements, and that they provided an overall quality of care comparable or in some cases superior to that prevailing in the fee-for-service community in the same areas, but that they probably undersupplied services to the sickest and most chronically ill enrollees.[8] Surveys of beneficiaries showed that the overwhelming proportion of Medicare managed care beneficiaries were highly satisfied with their plans—not a surprising finding when one remembers that dissatisfied beneficiaries were always free to disenroll at will—but the great majority of those not enrolled in HMOs did not want to be—hardly a surprising finding either.[9]

For a growing share of for-profit HMOs, Medicare managed care proved a profitable venture because, although payment was set at 95% of the average costs for fee-for-service enrollees, the HMOs almost invariably enrolled relatively healthier beneficiaries. Some of this risk selection resulted from carefully designed marketing strategies of the HMOs (so-called "cherry-picking"), but most of the phenomenon was attributable to the fact that beneficiaries with the greatest burden of chronic illness were more likely to have established relationships with particular physicians or hospitals who may not have participated in particular HMOs, while restrictions of freedom of provider choice were most acceptable to beneficiaries without established physician relationships, especially those who had recently relocated to retirement areas in Florida, Arizona, or California.[10]

The Balanced Budget Act of 1997 sought to achieve a substantial expansion of Medicare managed care enrollment by creating a new Medicare Part C for capitated plans (renamed "Medicare + Choice"), expanding the types of managed care plans that would be eligible to enroll beneficiaries and receive capitated payments, and establishing an annual open enrollment period with extensive concomitant beneficiary education. At the same time, however, the U.S. Congress fiddled with the payment formula for Medicare + Choice plans to eliminate some of the windfalls from risk selection, to reduce some of the geographic inequities that arose from discrepancies in fee-for-service costs across communities, and to provide incentives for plans to enter more rural communities. The net result was a significant constraint on increases in payment rates in most metropolitan areas that already had considerable Medicare managed care enrollment. Combined with difficult times for the HMO industry in its private business, rapidly rising pharmaceutical costs, and a continuing inability among the plans to effectively manage utilization, this led to a substantial contraction, rather than expansion, of Medicare managed care (Fig. 81.6).

Medicare: Long-Term Financing Issues

During the 1990s, the long-term financing of Medicare became a major political issue. There were several reasons: preoccupation of political leadership with federal budget deficits at a time when Medicare accounted for roughly 10% of the total budget and was the most rapidly growing component; growing recognition of the longer-term implications for Medicare and Social Security financing of the aging of the "baby boom" generation, reinforced by a well-organized and well-financed campaign to convince policy elites and the general public of the existence of a serious impending "entitlements crisis" that required an immediate scaling-back of the national commitment to income support and health insurance programs; and the very rapid rate of increase in Medicare costs in the first 6 years of the 1990s. Most concretely, and most immediately, the Hospital Insurance Trust Fund appeared to be about to run out of money. In the spring of 1997, it was projected that the Fund would be insolvent by 2001 unless major policy changes were undertaken.[11]

The Balanced Budget Act of 1997 reduced future Medicare expenditures by more than $200 billion (although at the time it was enacted it was projected to save only half that much) and created a National Bipartisan Commission on the Future of Medicare to address the long-term financing problems and report back to the Congress. In the period immediately following enactment of the Balanced Budget Act, Medicare expenditures actually fell for the first prolonged period in the program's history. These reductions caused considerable turmoil and financial stress for many nursing homes, teaching hospitals, and especially home health agencies.[12] However, the savings achieved by the Balanced Budget Act and other administrative initiatives, and, more importantly, the enormous economic boom of the late 1990s to which the Balanced Budget Act is believed to have contributed, have combined to dramatically improve the long-term financial prospects of Medicare. By the spring of 2000, the Hospital Insurance Trust Fund was projected to remain solvent for another 25 years, and the financial well-being of the program continued to improve throughout the year.[13]

Thanks in small part to the very rapidity with which Medicare's financial circumstances changed after the Balanced Budget Act was enacted, and in much larger part to serious ideological and philosophical divisions among its members, the National Bipartisan Commission was unable to reach any agreement and issued no report. The recommendations of its cochairmen, however, have subsequently become the basis for further discussions of Medicare "reform" in the early years of the twenty-first century. That "reform," supported by many conservatives who favor a smaller role for government progress, would

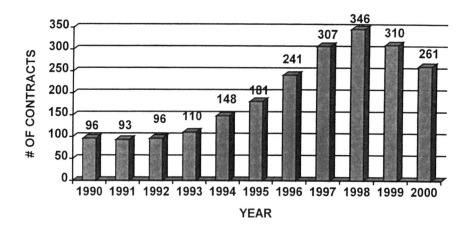

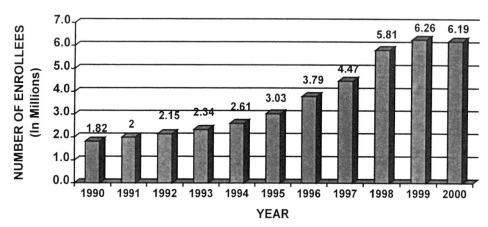

FIGURE 81.6. Medicare risk contracts, 1990–2000. (*Source*: Zarabozo C. "Is the sun setting over Medicare managed care?" presentation at Institute for Medicare Practice, Medicare Seminar, February 2000. *Note*: Number of contracts from December of that year, except in 2000, when June numbers are used. Medicare managed care enrollment, 1990–2000.) (*Source*: Zarabozo C. "Is the sun setting over Medicare managed care?" presentation at Institute for Medicare Practice, Medicare Seminar, February 2000. *Note*: Enrollment numbers are for December of the preceding year, except in 1999, when January 1999 data are used.)

transform Medicare from a defined-benefit, government-operated insurance program to one in which the government annually made a defined contribution toward purchase of a private health plan, with the size of that contribution determined by a bidding process. If private plans offered prices lower than Medicare's current costs, premiums for "traditional" Medicare would increase. Under such a system, the government's contribution to Medicare coverage for any given beneficiary would be determined not by the costs of the services that beneficiary actually consumed, but by some fraction of the average price bid by private insurance plans. Beneficiaries would either have to opt to enroll in low-cost plans, which would likely have very restrictive provider networks or utilization limitations, or pay higher out-of-pocket premiums to maintain their current coverage. There are many practical and conceptual, as well as philosophical, objections to such a scheme, but in the current political environment its adoption remains a possibility.[14]

What Medicare Does Not Cover: Prescription Drugs

When Medicare was enacted in 1965, outpatient prescription drugs played a much smaller role in medical therapeutics than they do today, and they were much less expensive. As a result, most private insurance plans offered limited, if any, coverage for pharmacy, and the failure to include a pharmacy benefit in Medicare was hardly noted. By now, however, the absence of prescription drug coverage in Medicare has become a real crisis. Total spending on prescription drugs for Medicare beneficiaries now averages roughly $1000 per year.[15] Two-thirds of beneficiaries have at least some insurance coverage for prescription drugs through employer-sponsored or individual Medicare supplemental policies, through Medicaid, or through HMO enrollment, but few of those policies cover the full cost of pharmaceuticals,

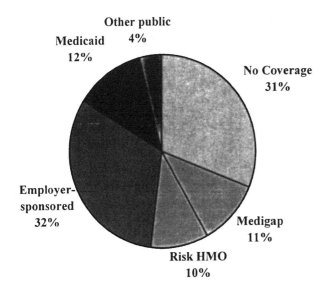

FIGURE 81.7. Distribution of Medicare beneficiaries by drug coverage status and source of coverage, 1996. (*Source*: Davis M, Poisal J, Chulis G, Zarabozo C, Cooper B. Prescription drug coverage, utilization, and spending among Medicare beneficiaries. *Health Affairs*. 1999;18(1)231–243, with permission.)

and thus more than 40% of those expenditures come directly out of pocket. Perhaps more importantly, there is very strong evidence that, although beneficiaries who lack insurance coverage for prescription drugs have poorer health status than those with coverage, they obtain significantly fewer prescriptions—almost 25% fewer. Absence of coverage is thus a significant barrier to access to needed pharmaceuticals, especially among low- and moderate-income beneficiaries (Fig. 81.7).

As of this writing, proposals to provide prescription drug coverage to Medicare beneficiaries are the subject of heated political discussion, but it is not clear what policies will emerge from that process.

What Medicare Does Not Cover: Long-Term Care

As significant as the problem of prescription drug coverage is for many Medicare beneficiaries, the single largest share of out-of-pocket expenditures is attributable not to drugs but to long-term care. Medicare does provide some coverage for skilled nursing facility services, and rather more expansive coverage for home health care, but both were clearly intended to apply only to limited, short-term, postacute episodes, and although a considerable loosening in the definitions of the home health benefit in the 1990s permitted its application to a growing share of real long-term cases, that loosening was largely ended by the Balanced Budget Act (Fig. 81.8).

At any given time, about 4% of all Americans 65 and older reside in nursing homes, but Medicare pays less than 10% of the total costs of nursing home care. Some relatively affluent patients, or those with affluent families, pay for nursing home services entirely from private resources, but for the great majority of nursing home patients, Medicaid is the primary source of financing. Medicaid currently pays for just under half of all national nursing home expenses, but that figure is misleading, for two reasons. First, Medicaid, which by law is always a payor of last resort, pays nursing homes only the *difference* between the approved Medicaid rate for nursing home care and the beneficiary's contribution, generally defined as the person's entire income less $32.50 per month for a "personal needs" allowance. The beneficiary contribution, which generally consists of a monthly Social Security check, is considered "private" expenditure in the National Health Accounts. Second, many long-stay nursing home residents attain Medicaid eligibility only after having exhausted their private resources in the first part of their nursing home stay; nursing homes are thus free to charge particularly high prices to "private" patients, with the perverse effect that that accelerates their spending down to Medicaid eligibility.

Since policy analysts first recognized, some 20 years ago, that Medicaid, which was originally thought of primarily as health insurance for low-income children and their mothers, was spending the lion's share of its money on nursing home care for frail seniors, many of whom had become poor only as a result of their need for long-term care, there has been widespread recognition that *something* should be done to rationalize the financing of long-term care services, especially as the population continues to age and the number of people in their late seventies and

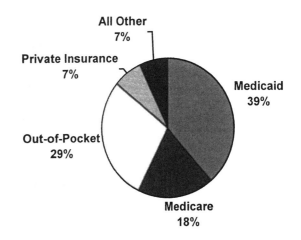

Total = $117 billion

FIGURE 81.8. Long-Term Care Financing, 1998. (*Source*: Graves TN, Kassner E, Mullen F, Coleman B. Long term care fact sheet. Washington, DC: AARP Public Policy Institute; 2000.)

eighties living alone—the population most at risk for needing long-term care services—continued inexorably to increase. But, although there has been a considerable shift in patterns of formal long-term care services away from institutions and toward community-based care, neither the division of responsibility for financing those services nor the intellectual framework within which one could fully reconstitute those financing patterns has changed very much. Solving the problem of financing long-term care thus remains very much a long-term problem.

Medicare's Safety Net

Although Medicaid pays for the greatest share of nursing home costs for the elderly, its role in assisting other Medicare beneficiaries should not be overlooked. Of the 6 million people who are dually eligible for Medicare and Medicaid, perhaps a quarter are receiving formal long-term care services. For the rest, Medicaid is an essential supplemental insurer, covering not only the copayments and deductibles for Medicare, but also those services for which Medicare does not pay at all, including outpatient prescription drugs, dental, vision, and hearing services and medically necessary transportation. Because of the way most states maintain their Medicaid data, it is almost impossible to tell how spending on behalf of dually eligible beneficiaries is allocated between long-term care and acute services, but given the interrelationships among age, poverty, and ill health, it is reasonable to assume that the community-dwelling dual eligibles are relatively high users of acute care services—as are individuals in the long-term care system.

The rules for achieving Medicaid eligibility are bewilderingly complex and vary considerably from one state to another. The relevant point is that, although almost all individuals legally entitled to Medicare have either enrolled or consciously chosen not to, many individuals, including many Medicare beneficiaries, who are legally entitled to Medicaid benefits are not enrolled. Reasons for failure to utilize Medicaid benefits include lack of awareness, the rigors of the enrollment process, and difficulties meeting documentation and other requirements associated with enrollment or because state eligibility officials, themselves confused, fail to enroll individuals who in fact are eligibile. Medicaid is thus a very effective safety net for those it catches, but many still fall through the holes.

Conclusions

America's elderly are the beneficiaries of enormous public expenditures for their health care, which has produced, on average, a level of access to modern, high-technology care unparalleled in the world. At the same time, elderly persons in the United States remain more at risk for crippling out-of-pocket medical expenses or the inability to obtain access to needed care for financial reasons than their counterparts in other industrial nations. The United States spends so much on health care for its elderly because its services are so expensive, not because its public programs are especially generous in design or philosophy.

Within the next 30 years, the number of persons 65 and older in the United States, who are thereby eligible for Medicare, will double. Assuming that health care costs continue to grow more rapidly than general inflation, that means that the real costs of supporting the Medicare program, even as currently defined, may triple. During the same time, the costs of health services that Medicare does not cover, such as outpatient prescription drugs, can be expected to increase even more rapidly than other health care costs. One is reminded of the old joke concerning the review of a bad restaurant: there are only two problems—the food is lousy and the portions are too small. For Medicare, the benefit package is woefully inadequate, but maintaining only those benefits will be increasingly expensive in the years to come.

On the other hand, all those people 65 and over are going to be here 30 years from now, regardless of how Medicare is constituted or whether it exists at all. One can assume, at least for purposes of discussion, that ours will continue to be a society that is generous and socially concerned enough to be unwilling to deny needed health services to elderly people who could benefit from them. Someone, in other words, is going to have to pay. The only real question is who.

Policy debates about the long-term direction and configuration of Medicare touch on many putative subjects. and take many different forms, but the central underlying question is how responsibility for the costs of medical care for the elderly are to be shared. If one believes that the elderly are already bearing an excessive share of their medical costs (especially when compared to younger. more affluent groups in society), then one set of future directions for Medicare is implied. However, that does not appear to be a view that currently controls the commanding heights of the American political debate. Whatever the outcome, the future of Medicare is ultimately and essentially a political question, and the outcome will be politically determined.

References

1. Author's calculations.
2. Medicare Payment Advisory Commission. *Report to the Congress: Medicare Payment Policy.* Washington, DC: U.S. Government Printing Office; 2000:Table 10-2.

3. Manton KG, Vaupel JW. Survival after the age of 80 in the United States, Sweden, France, England and Japan. *N Engl J Med.* 1995;333(18):1232–1235.

4. Medicare Payment Advisory Commission. *Report to the Congress: Selected Medicare Issues.* Washington, DC: U.S. Government Printing Office; 2000: Figure 5-3.

5. Medicare Payment Advisory Commission. *Health Care Spending and the Medicare Program: A Data Book.* Washington, DC: MedPAC; 1998:Charts 4–15, 4–20.

6. Physician Payment Review Commission. *Annual Report to the Congress.* Washington, DC: U.S. Government Printing Office; 2000:Chapter 13.

7. Iezzoni LI. The demand for documentation for Medicare payment. *N Engl J Med.* 1999;341(5):365–367.

8. Luft HS. Medicare and managed care. *Annu Rev Public Health.* 1998;19:459–475.

9. *Medicare 2000: 35 Years of Improving Americans' Health and Security.* Washington, DC: Health Care Financing Administration; 2000: Figure 17.

10. Physician Payment Review Commission. *Annual Report to the Congress.* Washington, DC: U.S. Government Printing Office; 1997: Chapter 3.

11. *1997 Annual Report of The Board of Trustees of the Federal Hospital Insurance Trust Fund.* Washington, DC: U.S. Government Printing Office; 1997.

12. Vladeck BC. The storm before the calm before the storm: Medicare home care in the wake of the Balanced Budget Act. *Care Manag J.* 2000;2(4)232–237.

13. *2000 Annual Report of the Board of Trustees of the Federal Hospital Insurance Trust Fund* (corrected). Washington, DC: U.S. Government Printing Office; 2000.

14. Vladeck BC. Sounding board: plenty of nothing—a report from the Medicare Commission. *N Engl J Med.* 1999;340:1503–1506.

15. Calculated by author from data in: *The Medicare Program: Medicare and Prescription drugs.* Henry J. Kaiser Family Foundation; 2000.

82
Justice and the Allocation of Health Care Resources

Nancy S. Jecker

There is growing concern in the United States, and in many other developed nations, that health care expenditures are too high and are growing too rapidly. Between 1950 and 1990, U.S. health expenditures grew 3% per annum, faster than expenditures for other goods and services. Economists forecast that if health spending in the United States continues to outpace other areas of the economy at this rate, by 2030 health care will consume almost one-third of the gross national product.[1]

One of several factors responsible for increasing health care costs is the changing demographics of populations in most developed countries. Since 1900, the proportion of older people relative to younger people has increased, and demographers predict that this trend will continue well into the twenty-first century. An aging population significantly affects health care costs because elderly individuals, as a group, consume health care at higher levels than other age groups. In the United States, persons 65 and over account for approximately 12% of the population, but they use one-third of the nation's total personal health care expenditures (exclusive of research costs).[2] If present levels of disability remain stable, future spending increases will occur primarily in the areas of chronic, supportive care needed by frail and disabled elderly persons.[3] Although it is sometimes assumed that the high cost of caring for the elderly is due to an "excessive" use of high-technology services at the end of life, recent studies cast doubt on this assumption.[4]

As efforts to reduce health care expenditures are implemented, the impact on patients and physicians is becoming more apparent. Increasingly, physicians must attempt to balance the twin goals of providing the best possible care for patients while simultaneously limiting the use of costly tests and procedures.[5,6] Rationing, often thought to be an inevitable feature of future reforms, is being discussed with growing frequency.

This chapter addresses the general problem of justice in the allocation of scarce health care resources. It looks first at the question of current health care allocation and asks, "According to what criteria are scarce health care resources currently distributed?" Next, it explores proposals for more justly distributing health care resources. The chapter closes by relating decisions about allocating health care to the more general goal of establishing a just society.

De Facto Rationing

Health care rationing refers to the denial of beneficial health care under conditions of fiscal or resource scarcity. Although it is often assumed that rationing is a problem looming in the future, in fact, in the United States, health care is already rationed in many unplanned and informal ways.

Poor and Uninsured Populations

First and foremost, rationing of care occurs for patients who are poor or uninsured. Thus, patients who lack access to mainstream providers often receive health care through an emergency department.[7] There, physicians may be encouraged, for purely economic reasons, either to treat those who have an undesirable reimbursement status as outpatients or to transfer such patients to public hospitals. These policies and other factors place patients without health insurance at greater risk for suffering medical injury due to delayed diagnosis or treatment or otherwise substandard medical care.[8] Such factors may also help to explain why the poor and poorly educated die at higher rates than those with higher incomes or better education.[9,10] Unplanned rationing also takes place when long waits at emergency departments cause persons in need of urgent care to leave without receiving care.[11-14] In a recent survey of 277 public and private hospitals, 38% reported that overcrowding sometimes required holding admitted patients in the emergency department for 24 h or longer until beds in appropriate care units became available. Among responding hospitals, 40% acknowledge diverting ambulances to other hospitals for reasons of overcrowding.[15]

Geographic Variations in Utilization of Health Care Resources

In addition to de facto rationing based on ability to pay for care, unplanned rationing also may occur on the basis of geographic location. Wennberg demonstrates substantial geographic variations in utilization of health care resources, primarily related to differences in the capacity of the local health care system and the practice style of local physicians.[16] For example, capacity influences the intensity of terminal care for Medicare enrollees, with residents of areas with high per capita supplies of acute care beds more likely to die as inpatients in hospitals and more likely to be admitted to intensive care units during their last 6 months of life.[17] Although it is commonly assumed that geographic variations occur as a result of physicians failing to conform their practice to standards of scientific medicine, this assumption is not borne out. Geographic variations are equally present in communities served primarily by academic medical centers. For example, populations living in Boston and New Haven, served by some of the nation's most distinguished teaching hospitals, utilize strikingly different per capita amounts of hospital care, despite remarkable similarities in demographic features and other factors that predict the need for care.[18] For several decades, the per capita amount of care provided to residents of Boston has been about 60% higher than the per capita amount provided to residents of New Haven. These differences are driven by Boston's relatively greater per capita supplies of hospital beds. These findings reinforce the notion that capacity, not medical science, drives the rate of hospitalization.

The phenomenon of geographical variation does not necessarily demonstrate that health care is rationed to patients who reside in geographic areas where medical resources and personnel are less abundant. This disparity occurs because "rationing" does not simply mean reduced access; instead, it implies reduced access to *beneficial* treatments. There is no evidence to suggest, however, that more intensive medical treatments always yield benefits for patients. As Wennberg noted, "There is no scientific evidence that more is always better. There are few studies of the outcomes of hospitalization versus less intensive ways of treating patients with the same disease profiles; and those that have been done show no advantage from more intensive care."[19] For example, outcomes in terms of life expectancy are no different for populations living in Boston and New Haven, despite Boston's greater hospital capacity and despite the fact that Bostonians are more likely to die in the hospital.

What can we conclude about the ethical implications of geographic variability? Certainly, geographic variation makes evident that the distribution of health care occurs in a morally arbitrary and unplanned fashion. The flow of resources often takes place in an unconscious rather than a deliberate and thoughtful manner. Not only do individual patients tend to be unaware of the influence of geographic location, but the influence of supply on utilization occurs without clinicians' explicit knowledge of the relative level of available resources. For example, clinicians serving populations in hospital referral regions where the supply of acute care hospital resources is relatively low do not appear to be aware of constraints on their practice of medicine.[20]

In addition, geographic variation highlights the importance of creating a more explicit, publicly accountable approach to health care allocation because, to the extent that health care allocation occurs in an unplanned fashion, whatever rationing this entails will not be applied consistently. De facto rationing raises serious questions of fairness because it fails to treat patients who are similarly situated in a similar fashion. Therefore, whatever benefits and burdens medical services confer are distributed on the basis of a morally arbitrary fact—where persons happen to live. A more deliberate system can better approximate the ideal of fairness by attempting to specify morally relevant differences between persons and make these the basis for rationing. For example, the quality, length, or likelihood of medical benefit a patient is expected to receive represents more sound criteria for rationing than do morally arbitrary factors, such as whether a patient happens to live in Boston or New Haven. No one would suggest that Bostonians are morally more deserving of medical services by virtue of living in Boston.

Other Examples

Other examples of unplanned rationing include slowing reimbursement and use of health care resources by means of bureaucracies that impede, inconvenience, and confuse providers and patients. The impact of bureaucracy is evident, for example, in statistics revealing that 59.7% of Medicaid or welfare denials result from problems with paperwork or documentation.[21]

Rationing also may be an unplanned outcome of the culture of modern medicine, which trains physicians to cure disease and prolong life while downplaying the significance of care-oriented, low-technology therapies aimed at providing comfort and improving the quality of patients' lives.[22] For example, evidence suggests that adequate palliative care is frequently unavailable for dying patients,[23] infants[24] and children,[25,26] burn patients,[27] cancer patients,[28] postoperative patients, and elderly patients.[29] To the extent that physicians lack the knowledge or skill to offer palliative care services, rationing occurs by default rather than by a deliberate decision for which any individuals are held accountable.[30,31] Within palliative care, more costly, high-technology modalities of pain management are sometimes favored over low-technology modalities, such as oral medication, without differences in patient outcomes.[32,33] Access to palliative care is also restricted for patients who are not terminally ill because needed services have traditionally been reserved for end-of-life care rather than made available to patients and families throughout the illness trajectory.[34]

To the extent that society at large devalues the lives of ethnic minorities, women, the elderly, or other groups, there is every reason to think that this will be reflected, perhaps unconsciously, in health care decisions. Thus, age-based rationing of health care may occur when patient age is discretely factored into decisions to admit patients to the hospital, provide intensive care, terminate therapy, or initiate vigorous treatment.[35]

Discrimination based on group membership can also occur as the result of inattention to the differential effects that policies have for different segments of society. For example, although age-based rationing appears gender neutral, it would, in fact, have a disproportionate effect on women because more women than men fill the ranks of older age groups.[36] Likewise, although the job-based insurance system is not explicitly gender based, it more negatively affects women as a group because women are more likely than men to work on a part-time, part-year, or temporary basis, or in nonunion or low-wage jobs—job categories that offer health care benefits less frequently.[37] Women who work outside the paid labor force, whether caring for children or tending to disabled elderly relatives, are also disadvantaged under a workplace insurance system. Although many women receive workplace health insurance through spouses, this factor can lead to economic dependence and places women at risk of losing coverage through divorce or widowhood.

Likewise, limited awareness of the effects of policies on racial groups may contribute to racial differences in health insurance coverage,[38] infant mortality,[39,40] life expectancy,[41] access and outcome in organ transplantation,[42–44] use of revascularization procedures after coronary angiography,[45] survival following cardiac arrest,[46–48] inadequate emergency department analgesia,[49] and drug therapy for human immunodeficiency virus (HIV) disease.[50]

In summary, although rationing of health care is rarely put forward and defended in a public manner, rationing of health services nonetheless occurs. Unplanned and informal rationing often reflects morally arbitrary criteria, such as geographic location, or medically irrelevant factors, such as the ability to pay.

Proposals for Explicit Health Care Rationing

The problem with the de facto rationing described here is that it does not even aspire to meet ethical standards. Thus, implicit rationing is typically not thought through, not applied consistently, not accountable to the public, not decided democratically, and not insulated from arbitrary and unfair manipulation. In light of these concerns, most would prefer a planned and public system of allocating health care over the present approach. While critics cast doubt on the idea that explicit rationing constitutes proper public policy,[51] most agree about the value of openly debating health care policies and reaching agreement about fundamental principles of justice in health care. In North America, Europe, and other developed countries, public opinion has been solicited regarding rationing of health care and the need to set limits in health coverage. These efforts enable public opinion to become visible and play a role in health policy deliberations.[52,53]

The Oregon Proposal

Various proposals for explicit rationing of health care have been defended as ethically sound. Perhaps the most well known is Oregon's plan to deny Medicaid reimbursement for certain categories of medical services.[54] Oregon's plan was the outgrowth of the 1989 Oregon Basic Health Services Act, a central goal of which was to extend Medicaid to all Oregonians falling below the federal poverty level. The means proposed to pay for this included restricting medical services to current Medicaid eligibles. The Oregon Health Services Commission was responsible for determining the relative priority of medical services. In the Commission's initial plan, a computer generated a list of diseases rated by a formula taking into account the cost of treatment, length of benefit, and quality of well-being after treatment. How far down the list treatments were covered would depend on the availability of funds in each biennium. At some point along the list, a line would be drawn and diseases and injuries that fell below it would not be covered.

After coming under intense criticism, the Commission formed an Alternative Methodology Subcommittee to develop an alternative approach to prioritizing services.[55] The revised approach excluded cost as a significant factor in prioritizing services; instead, it considered the perceived benefit of various treatment categories to individuals and society, as well as their perceived necessity. The revised plan emphasized preventive care and treatable, life-threatening conditions that affect many, rather than conditions that are minor or are fatal and incurable. For example, organ transplants were moved from the bottom to near the middle of the priority list, and familiar ailments, such as pneumonia, were placed near the top.[56]

Oregon's proposal explicitly incorporates rationing, most notably rationing based on the likelihood, quality, or length of medical benefit that a patient will receive from treatment, and rationing based on the imminence of a patient's death. A number of ethical arguments have been adduced in support of each proposal. Rationing based on medical benefit is defended on utilitarian grounds, by arguing that services that generate the greatest amount of benefit merit the highest priority. According to this approach, payoff to patients, and to people generally, is the measure of justice in health care allocation. Medical benefit is also defended on nonutilitarian grounds. For example, it is argued that if people were to devise a just distribution scheme without knowing how such a scheme would affect them, or what their health care needs would be, they would prefer a distribution that assigned people the greatest entitlement to resources when they would have the greatest chance of actually benefiting.[57]

Various ethical reasons can also be advanced in support of rationing based on the imminence of a patient's death. Such an approach arguably has the advantage of saving the greatest number of lives. Alternatively, the justification for applying this criterion may rest on the belief that a patient whose death is imminent is in greater need of health care and that health care should be given first to those with the greatest need.[58]

Critics of both a medical benefit and an imminent death criterion express the concern that these approaches may have adverse effects on elderly persons.[59] As older persons, on average, have a lower life expectancy than younger persons, rationing that takes into account the duration of medical benefit will disproportionately affect older persons. Likewise, to the extent that advanced age correlates with poorer outcomes for medical procedures, rationing based on medical benefit will adversely affect the elderly as a group. Regarding the criterion of imminent death, the elderly are at greater risk of being denied treatment if, as a group, they are found to be at increased risk of mortality for various medical interventions. Thus, although medical benefit and imminent death are age blind, they may be found to have adverse effects on the geriatric population.

Age-Based Rationing

Age is also put forward as an explicit basis for allocating limited health care resources. Perhaps the most prominent proponent of age-based rationing is Daniel Callahan, who argues that "government has a duty, based on our collective social obligation, to help people live out a natural life span, but not actively to help extend life beyond that point."[60] According to this approach, public-

funded life-extending care should not be available to older persons. Instead, government should pay only for medical services intended to improve the quality of life of elderly persons.

Ethical arguments favoring age-based rationing often appeal to society's duty to younger age groups. For example, it is argued that unless age-based limits to health care are set, we will cheat our children and future generations out of adequate health care or other essential goods, such as education.[61,62]

Alternatively, age-based rationing is defended by arguing that although it initially appears to favor one group of people over another, in fact it affects all persons equally over time.[63] This reasoning applies because, over time, each person ages. Therefore, over time, all persons experience both the advantage of greater access when they are young and the disadvantages of reduced access during old age.

Age-based rationing is also justified on utilitarian grounds, by arguing that investing health care dollars in younger persons represents, on average, a better return on investment because the young generally have a greater number of years ahead to live. Another utilitarian defense of age-based rationing points out that a great financial gain could be obtained by limiting health care to the elderly because the elderly use a disproportionate share of health care dollars. According to one estimate, more than 50% of patients hospitalized for myocardial infarction are over age 65.[65] If treatment for this condition were rationed on the basis of age, a major reduction in health care expenditures would be achieved.

Opponents of age-based rationing hold that a just distribution of health care requires meeting the essential needs of all persons, irrespective of age.[65] Thus, if older persons have, on average, a greater need for health care resources, then they are entitled to receive a greater share of such resources. Alternatively, opponents claim that the allocation of health care should depend more on the quality of benefit that medical interventions can produce than on the number of years a patient lives.[66]

In addition, critics of age-based limits maintain that society has special duties to older persons that forbid placing age-based limits on medical care. Such duties may stem from the belief that older persons are more deeply embedded within the fabric of social life. According to this position, "The more personally interwoven a person becomes with others through time, the greater the damage done to the social fabric when that person is torn away by death."[67] Alternatively, special duties may spring from the contributions that older persons as a group have made to the creation of social goods, such as science, technology, medicine, and culture.[68] Proper recognition of these contributions requires ensuring that the elderly themselves reap the benefit that these social goods offer.

Finally, as already noted, age limits on health care adversely affect women because the population of older adults includes more women than men.[69] Among the population aged 65 and over, there are only 68 men per 100 women. The disparity in the numbers of men and women is greatest within the oldest age groups. Thus, for the group aged 85 and over, there are a mere 45 men per 100 women.[70] Denying lifesaving medical care to older women also harms women disproportionately, as women have more future years to live. At age 65, a woman can anticipate living about 18 more years, whereas a man at this age can expect only 14 more years. Women who reach age 75 can look forward to 12 more years of life; by contrast, men at this age will live an average of 9 more years.[71]

National Health Insurance

Age-based rationing focuses on a personal quality of individuals and uses this as a basis for distinguishing between persons, whereas other approaches emphasize similarities rather than differences between persons. For example, those who advocate applying a principle of equality to the distribution of health care insist that, morally speaking, it is not possible to discriminate between individuals and assign people different rights to health care. Instead, whenever anyone enjoys access to a health care service, justice requires making that service equally available to everyone with similar health care needs.[72]

The more precise interpretation of an egalitarian principle depends upon how the concept of "need" is elaborated.[73] Thus, to say that resources must be equally available to everyone who needs them may mean that people should have equal access to every service from which they stand to benefit. Understood in this sense, a principle of equality applies to all areas of health care. Alternatively, if "need" refers only to services that provide especially important benefits, then the principle of equality applies only to "basic" or "essential" services. On the latter interpretation, although nonessential services may be unequally distributed, services that provide very important benefits to people must be equally accessible.

The goal of making basic health care equally available to everyone, irrespective of factors such as a person's income or geographic location, was one of the central aims of the Canadian health care system. The Canadian health care system is a publicly funded system based on the philosophy that health is a right, not a commodity.[74] Thus, in Canada, universal access to provincial health insurance solves the problem of the uninsured by preventing it from occurring. The 1984 Canada Health Act was the first to explicitly state the principles that have become the cornerstone of the Canadian health care

system: accessibility, portability, comprehensiveness, universality, and public administration. Because the Canadian Constitution specifies that health care coverage will be a matter of provincial jurisdiction, to be implemented by individual provinces, these five principles have served as the federal government's criteria for judging the eligibility of provincial health plans to receive federal funding. In Ontario, for example, the criterion of universality is met by provincial regulation establishing that all who "make their home and are ordinarily present in Ontario are eligible for coverage," so long as they reside in the province for 3 months.[75]

Like the United States, Canada's health care system is facing increasing demands that stretch the limits of the public sector. The federal government has reduced its financial contribution, leaving the Canadian provinces that administer health insurance plans in financial crises. These economic limits will challenge the principles of universality and comprehensiveness that form the cornerstone of the Canadian approach to justice in health care. Whether Canada's system of universal coverage can withstand future challenges will depend, in large part, on the strength of its ethical and social foundations. Specifically, the ability to meet future challenges will require restating and reaffirming the reasons for commitment to a principle of equality in health care. It will also call upon Canadians to prioritize competing values, such as universality and comprehensiveness. For example, if limiting benefits and rationing health services is necessary to place the goal of universality on surer footing, are such limits ethically and socially acceptable?

In Canada, support for a principle of equality in health care is generally articulated by emphasizing altruistic and humanitarian concern for others.[76] First, government shoulders the social and ethical responsibility to secure the general social welfare. Thus, Canadian policymakers tend to take for granted that government is responsible to protect the most vulnerable members of the society, even when doing so imposes a cost on other citizens. As expressed by the federal Advisory Committee on Health Insurance, universal access recognizes "the need for the mutual insurance of all members against the more serious dangers, a compulsory insurance so that the more secure cannot stand aside and leave the risks to be loaded on the shoulders of the less secure."[77]

Second, the ethical principle of humanitarianism, or care and concern for fellow citizens, is evident in the historical development of Canada's system of universal health insurance. Reflecting this ethical premise, the Royal Commission on Health Service identifies the factors that support public, as opposed to purely private, interest in health care as including, "A deepening of our humanitarian concern for our fellows," together with, "A recognition of the well-being of members of the population and that the well-being of a proportion of the population at any given time is seriously curtailed because of mental or physical disease."[78]

Generally speaking, support for applying a principle of equality to the distribution of basic health care comes from a variety of sources. First, it can be said that basic health care services provide a very special and important kind of benefit.[79] Unlike other benefits, the preservation of life and health (and the resources necessary to achieve this) is a prerequisite for whatever else a person wants to do in life. Therefore, even if inequalities are ethically tolerable in other areas, they should not be within health care.

Furthermore, although we may consider ourselves as exerting control over many important aspects of our lives, we often lack control over our health and need for health services.[80] For instance, whether one inherits a gene predisposing the person to breast or ovarian cancer, or a gene for Huntington's disease, is the result of the "natural lottery" rather than the result of individual decisions. Likewise, the fact that an individual is born with fetal alcohol syndrome, is injured in a flood, or experiences kidney failure from contaminated meat is not the result of that individual's conscious choices. To the extent that disease is genetically based, or is influenced by choices others make, or occurs as the result of natural disaster, there is no basis for holding people "accountable" for having diseases. In these kinds of cases, allocating health care on the basis of merit lacks ethical underpinning, and a system of treating people equally gains ethical support. Even if merit-based allocation is suitable in other spheres, such as distributing the benefits and burdens associated with offices and positions in a society, it often does not fit the circumstances leading to ill health and the need for health care services.

It is also argued that the value of equal respect requires applying a principle of equality to basic services. Gutmann, for example, maintains that inequality of access to basic health care conveys to people that they are not equally worthy human beings.[81] It is analogous, she argues, to tolerating inequalities in other fundamental areas, such as the right to vote or access to police protection, which are essential to liberty and security. One reason that showing equal respect for persons is important is that it has a profound effect on people's capacity to develop and maintain self-respect. Self-respect, in turn, determines an individual's sense of their own worth; it affects their self-confidence and ability to carry out the important goals they set for themselves.

Summary and Conclusions

In summary, this chapter addressed the problem of how to allocate scarce health care resources between different individuals and groups in society. It demonstrated

that competing conceptions of justice lead to very different distributive approaches. Moreover, the problem of health care rationing is hardly a problem that looms in the future. Instead, rationing occurs as a pervasive feature of present health care systems.

Creating a more just health care system will require societies to engage in open debates about the rationing of health care services. At a deeper level, the choice societies face must be founded on a more fundamental vision of a just society.[82] To what extent does a just society emphasize equality between persons? To what extent must it stress the value of individual freedom? How does a just society balance the value of health with other values, such as the environment or education? These questions lie at the very heart of contemporary health care debates.

References

1. Fuchs V. No pain, no gain: perspectives on cost containment. *JAMA.* 1993;269:631–633.
2. U.S. Senate Special Committee on Aging. *Aging America: Trends and Projections.* Washington, D.C.: Public Health Service, U.S. Department of Health and Human Services; 1985–1986.
3. Schneider EL, Guralnik JM. The aging of America. *JAMA.* 1990;263:2335–2340.
4. Temkin-Greener HA, Meiners MR, Petty EA, Szydlowski JS. The use and cost of health services prior to death: a comparison of the Medicare-only and the Medicare-Medicaid elderly populations. *Milbank Q.* 1992;70:679–701.
5. Angell M. Cost containment and the physician. *JAMA.* 1985;254:1203–1207.
6. Leaf A. The doctor's master. *JAMA.* 1984;311:1573–1575.
7. Stern RS, Weissman JS, Epstein AM. The emergency department as a pathway to admission for poor and high-cost patients. *JAMA.* 1991;266:2238–2243.
8. Burstin HR, Lipsitz SR, Brennan TA. Socioeconomic status and risk for substandard care. *JAMA.* 1992;268:2283–2287.
9. Pappas G, Queen S, Hadden W, Fisher G. The increasing disparity in mortality between socioeconomic groups in the United States, 1960 and 1986. *N Engl J Med.* 1993;329:103–109.
10. Angell M. Privilege and health. *N Engl J Med.* 1993;329:126–127.
11. Baker DW, Stevens CD, Brook RH. Patients who leave a public hospital emergency department without being seen by a physician. *JAMA.* 1991;266:1085-1090.
12. Kellerman AL. Too sick to wait. *JAMA.* 1991;266:1123–1125.
13. Bindman AB, Grumbach K, Keane D, Rauch L, Luce JM. Consequence of queuing for care at a public hospital emergency department. *JAMA.* 1991;266:1091–1096.
14. Olson CM. Hospital admission through the emergency department: an obstructed pathway. *JAMA.* 1991;266:2274.
15. Kellerman AL, Andrulis DP, Hackman BB. Emergency department overcrowding. *Ann Emerg Med.* 1990;19:447.

16. Wennberg JE. *The Dartmouth Atlas of Health Care in the United States: A Report on the Medicare Program.* Dartmouth: Dartmouth Medical School, Center for the Evaluative Clinical Sciences; 1999.

17. Wennberg JE. *The Dartmouth Atlas of Health Care in the United States: A Report on the Medicare Program.* Dartmouth: Dartmouth Medical School, Center for the Evaluative Clinical Sciences; 1999:85.

18. Wennberg JE. *The Dartmouth Atlas of Health Care in the United States: A Report on the Medicare Program.* Dartmouth: Dartmouth Medical School, Center for the Evaluative Clinical Sciences; 1999:88.

19. Wennberg JE. *The Dartmouth Atlas of Health Care in the United States: A Report on the Medicare Program.* Dartmouth: Dartmouth Medical School, Center for the Evaluative Clinical Sciences; 1999:93.

20. Wennberg JE. *The Dartmouth Atlas of Health Care in the United States: A Report on the Medicare Program.* Dartmouth: Dartmouth Medical School, Center for the Evaluative Clinical Sciences; 1999:93.

21. Grumet GW. Health care rationing through inconvenience. *N Engl J Med.* 1989;321:607–611.

22. Jecker NS, Reich WT. Contemporary ethics of care. In: Reich WT, ed. *Encyclopedia of Bioethics.* New York: Simon & Schuster/Macmillan; 1995:336–344.

23. Miettinen TT, Tilvis RS, Karppi P, Arve S. Why is the pain relief of dying patients often unsuccessful? *Palliat Med.* 1998;12(6):429–435.

24. Stevens B, Koren G. Evidence-based pain management for infants. *Curr Opin Pediatr.* 1998;10(2):203–207.

25. Beyer JE. Judging the effectiveness of analgesia for children and adolescents during vaso-occlusive events of sickle cell disease. *J Pain Symptom Manage.* 2000;19(1):63–72.

26. Here's the latest research in pediatric pain control. *ED Manag.* 1999;11(11):128–129.

27. Ulmer JF. Burn pain management: a guideline-based approach. *J Burn Care Rehabil.* 1998;19(2):151–159.

28. Portenoy RK, Lesage P. Management of cancer pain. *Lancet.* 1999;353(9165):1695–1700.

29. Brockopp D, Warden S, Colclough G, Brockopp G. Elderly people's knowledge of and attitudes to pain management. *Br J Nurs.* 1996;5(9):556–558, 560–562.

30. Miner TJ, Tavaf-Motamen H, Shriver CD. Decision making on surgical palliation based on patient outcome data. *Am J Surg.* 1999;177(2):150–154.

31. Higginson IJ. Evidence-based palliative care. There is some evidence—and there needs to be more. *Br Med J.* 1999;319(7208):462–463.

32. Bailes JS. Cost aspects of palliative cancer care. *Semin Oncol.* 1995;22(2 suppl 3):64–66.

33. Warde P, Murphy T. Measuring the cost of palliative radiotherapy. *Can J Oncol.* 1996;6(suppl 1):90–94.

34. Pickett M, Cooley ME, Gordon DB. Palliative care: past, present, and future perspectives. *Semin Oncol Nurs.* 1998 May;14(2):86–94.

35. Barondess JA, Kalb P, Weil WB, Cassel C, Ginzberg E. Clinical decision-making in catastrophic situations: the relevance of age. *J Am Geriatr Soc.* 1988;36:919–937.

36. Jecker NS. Age-based rationing and women. *JAMA.* 1991; 266:3012–3015.

37. Jecker NS. Can an employer based health insurance system be just? *J Health Polit Policy Law.* 1993;18:657–674.

38. Trevino FM, Moyer E, Valdez B, Stroup-Benham CA. Health insurance coverage and utilization of health services by Mexican Americans, Mainland Puerto Ricans, and Cuban Americans. *JAMA.* 1991;265:233–237.

39. Davidson EC, Fukushima T. The racial disparity in infant mortality. *N Engl J Med.* 1992;327:1022–1024.

40. Becerra JE, Hogue CJR, Atrash HK, Perez N. Infant mortality among Hispanics. *JAMA.* 1991;265:217–221.

41. Hilts PJ. Growing gap in life expectancies of blacks and in whites is emerging. *New York Times.* 9 October 1989:Al.

42. Kasiske BL, Neylan JF, Riggio RR, et al. The effect of race on access and outcome in transplantation. *N Engl J Med.* 1991;324:302–307.

43. Kjellstrand CM. Age, sex, and race inequality in renal transplantation. *Arch Intern Med.* 1988;148:1305–1309.

44. Gaston RS, Ayres I, Dooley LG, Dietheim AG. Racial equity in renal transplantation: the disparate impact of HLA-based allocation. *JAMA.* 1993;270:1352–1356.

45. Ayanian JZ, Udvarhelyi S, Gatsonis CA, Pashos CL, Epstein AM. Racial differences in the use of revascularization procedures after coronary angiography. *JAMA.* 1993; 269:2642–2646.

46. Becker LB, Han BH, Meyer PM, et al., and CPR Chicago Project. Racial differences in the incidence of cardiac arrest and subsequent survival. *N Engl J Med.* 1993;329:600–605.

47. Whittle J, Conigliaro J, Good CB, Lofgren RP. Racial differences in the use of invasive cardiovascular procedures in the department of Veterans Affairs medical system. *N Engl J Med.* 1993;329:621–626.

48. Ayanian JZ. Heart disease in black and white. *N Engl J Med.* 1993;329:656–658.

49. Todd KH, Samaroo N, Hoffman JR. Ethnicity as a risk factor for inadequate emergency department analgesia. *JAMA.* 1993;269:1537–1539.

50. Moore RD, Stanton D, Gopalan R, Chaisson RE. Racial differences in the use of drug therapy for HIV disease in an urban community. *N Engl J Med.* 1994;330:763–768.

51. Marmor TR, Boyum D. Medical care and public policy: the benefits and burdens of asking fundamental questions. *Health Policy.* 1999;49(1–2):27–43.

52. Mossialos E, King D. Citizens and rationing: analysis of a European survey. *Health Policy.* 1999;49(1–2):75–135.

53. King D, Maynard A. Public opinion and rationing in the United Kingdom. *Health Policy.* 1999;50(1–2):39–53.

54. Strosberg MA, Wiener JM, Baker R, Fein IA. *Rationing America's Medical Care: The Oregon Plan and Beyond.* Washington, DC: Brookings Institution; 1992.

55. Hadorn D. Setting health care priorities in Oregon. *JAMA.* 1991;265:2218–2225.

56. Egan T. Oregon shakes up pioneering health plan for the poor. *New York Times.* 22 February 1991.

57. Winslow G. *Triage and Justice.* Berkeley: University of California Press; 1982.

58. Kilner J. *Who Lives? Who Dies? Ethical Criteria in Patient Selection.* New Haven: Yale University Press; 1990.

59. Jecker NS, Pearlman RA. An ethical framework for rationing health care. *J Med Philos.* 1992;17:79–96.

60. Callahan D. *Setting Limits*. New York: Simon & Schuster; 1987:137.

61. Lamm RD. Ethical care for the elderly. In: Smeeding TM, ed. *Should Medical Care Be Rationed by Age?* Totowa, NJ: Rowman and Littlefield; 1987:xi–xv.

62. Preston S. Children and the elderly. *Sci Am*. 1984;251:44–49.

63. Daniels N. *Am I My Parents' Keeper?* New York: Oxford University Press; 1988.

64. Wenger NK, O'Rourke RA, Marcus FI. The care of elderly patients with cardiovascular disease. *Ann Intern Med*. 1988; 109:425–428.

65. Jecker NS, Pearman RA. Ethical constraints on rationing medical care by age. *J Am Geriatr Soc*. 1989;37:1067–1075.

66. Jecker NS. Disenfranchising the elderly from life-extending medical care. *Public Aff Q*. 1988;2:51–68.

67. Kilner J. Age as a basis for allocating lifesaving medical resources. *J Health Polit Policy Law*. 1988;13:405.

68. Jonsen A. Resentment and the rights of the elderly. In: Jecker NS, ed. *Aging and Ethics*. Clifton, NJ: Humana Press; 1991:341–352.

69. Jecker NS. Age-based rationing and women. *JAMA*. 1991; 266:3012–3015.

70. Cassel CK, Neugarten BL. A forecast of women's health and longevity. *West J Med*. 1988;149:712–717.

71. Verbrugge LM. An epidemiological profile of older women. In: Haug MR, Amasa B, Ford MS, eds. *The Physical and Mental Health of Aged Women*. New York: Springer; 1985: 41–64.

72. Gutmann A. For and against equal access to health care. In: *President's Commission for the Study of Ethical Problems in Medicine and Biomedical and Behavioral Research. Securing Access to Health Care, vol 2*. Washington, DC: U.S. Government Printing Office; 1983:51–66.

73. Buchanan A. An ethical evaluation of health care in the United States. In: Sass HM, Massey R, eds. *Health Care Systems*. Boston: Kluwer; 1988:39–58.

74. Kluge EH. The Canadian health care system: an analytic perspective. *Health Care Anal*. 1999;7(4):377–391.

75. Health and Welfare Canada. *1984–1985 Canada Health Act: Annual Report*. Ottawa: Minister of Supply and Service; 1986:58–59.

76. Jecker NS, Meslin EM. United States and Canadian approaches to justice in health care: a comparative analysis of health care systems and values. *Theor Med*. 1994;15: 181–200.

77. Advisory Committee on Health Insurance. *Heagarty Report*. Order in Council; p.s., 836, February 5, 1942:143. As cited in Taylor MG. *Health Insurance and Public Policy: The Seven Decisions That Created the Canadian Health Insurance System and Their Outcomes, 2nd Ed*. Montreal: McGill-Queen's University Press; 1988:18.

78. Hall EM, Chair. *Report of the Royal Commission on Health Services*. Ottawa: Queen's Printer, 1964:5.

79. Daniels N. *Just Health Care*. New York: Cambridge University Press; 1985.

80. Outka G. Social justice and equal access to health care. In: Gorovitz S, Macklin R, Jameton AL, O'Connor JM, Sherwin S, eds. *Moral Problems in Medicine, 2nd Ed*. Englewood Cliffs: Prentice-Hall; 1983:544–557.

81. Gutmann A. For and against equal access to health care. In: *President's Commission for the Study of Ethical Problems in Medicine and Biomedical and Behavioral Research. Securing Access to Health Care, vol 2*. Washington, DC: U.S. Government Printing Office; 1983:51–66.

82. Jecker NS, Meslin EM. United States and Canadian approaches to justice in health care. *Theor Med*. 1994;15: 181–200.

83
Medical Treatment and the Physician's Legal Duties

Marshall B. Kapp

Older patients enter into relationships with physicians and other members of the health care team to obtain medical care. These relationships can be characterized as both contractual (i.e., based on a mutual exchange of explicit or implicit promises) and fiduciary (i.e., based on the trust the dependent patient must invest in relying on the more knowledgeable and powerful health care provider). Within either of these frameworks, the resulting relationships implicate a variety of legally enforceable obligations on the part of the physician.

Thus, some familiarity with treatment-related legal requirements and associated potential liabilities is essential to the practicing geriatrician. Additionally, geriatricians often have the opportunity, and sometimes may be required, to contribute medical expertise to the resolution of legal issues, as in cases where a physician's affidavit or testimony is the central piece of evidence regarding mental competence in a contested guardianship or will probate proceeding.

Many legal issues affecting geriatric practice are basically generic. For instance, physicians must be aware of the legal doctrines of informed consent and confidentiality regardless of their patients' age.[1] There is nothing inherently distinctive about older patients from a legal perspective. Many generic legal issues, however, take on unique twists or special urgency when applied to older patients. This difference may be related to a particular older person's physical or mental decline, impaired sensory perception, well-developed life history and set of values, outliving of concerned family members or presence of intermeddling family members, and increased risk of institutionalization. Further, there exists a subset of medically related issues that pertain exclusively to elderly patients, because in some situations legislators have consciously made chronologic age by itself a relevant criterion for some specific purpose. For example, achieving age 65 by itself qualifies one for Social Security retirement benefits,[2] and a person gains protection under the Age Discrimination in Employment Act (ADEA) auto-

matically at age 40.[3] This chapter outlines a few of the most salient legal issues arising within the physician–older patient relationship.

Medical Malpractice

The quality of medical practice is regulated through several means. Important forms of regulation include professional licensure and disciplinary requirements, oversight by Peer Review Organizations (PROs)[4] and other public and private (e.g., Joint Commission on Accreditation of Healthcare Organizations) agencies that audit the quality of care provided to Medicare beneficiaries and others, mandatory reporting of certain adverse actions against physicians to the National Practitioner Data Bank (NPDB),[5] extensive federal and state statutes and regulations governing nursing facilities and home health agencies, and in extreme cases (e.g., when gross neglect is charged), criminal prosecution. Physicians ordinarily are particularly apprehensive about civil medical malpractice tort lawsuits brought by individual patients seeking monetary damages for allegedly negligent care, even though older patients tend to sue their physicians less often than their younger counterparts and with less success.

Much attention has been paid recently to the prevalent phenomenon of medical errors.[6] There have been calls for mandatory reporting of serious errors to a government agency, but fears have been expressed by physicians about the potential ramifications of such reporting in terms of generating an increased rate of malpractice lawsuits.[7]

Another relatively recent development with possible litigation-related implications is the expanding enrollment of Medicare beneficiaries in various forms of managed care organizations (MCOs). This enrollment has been encouraged by the Medicare + Choice (Medicare Part C) program created by the Balanced

Budget Act (BBA) of 1997.[8] Much political discussion has taken place regarding the right of individuals who obtain medical coverage as a fringe benefit of present or prior employment to personally sue their MCO as well as, or instead of, their own physician for alleged negligence;[9] the future of lawsuits brought by Medicare beneficiaries against MCOs for negligence in denying payment for services is, at present, uncertain but bears close watching.

Informed Consent

The fundamental ethical principle of autonomy or self-determination is embodied in the legal doctrine of informed consent. There are three essential elements that must be present for a patient's choices about treatment to be considered legally valid.

First, the patient's participation in the decision-making process and the ultimate decision must be voluntary. The usual definition of voluntariness in the context of consent is that the person giving or withholding consent must be so situated as to be able to exercise free power of choice without the intervention of any element of force, fraud, deceit, duress, overreaching, or other ulterior form of constraint or coercion. It means simply that the person must be free to reject participation in the proposed intervention. The physician must do all possible to minimize any intimidation that might unfavorably affect the quality of the patient–physician relationship, and the patient–institution or patient–agency relationship when applicable, and to make sure that advice and recommendations are conveyed in as nonpressured and empathetic a manner as possible.

The second bedrock requirement for valid consent is that the patient's agreement be sufficiently informed. The informed consent doctrine commands that the health care provider, before undertaking an intervention, must disclose certain information to the person who is the subject of the proposed intervention (or that person's authorized surrogate; see following).

The disclosure standard enforced in a slight majority of American jurisdictions is referred to as the "professional," "reasonable physician," or "community" standard. Under this test, the adequacy of disclosure is judged against the amount and type of information that a reasonable, prudent physician would have disclosed under similar circumstances.

A substantial minority of states have adopted a more expansive standard of information disclosure: the "reasonable patient" or "material risk" standard. This standard dictates that the physician communicate the information that a "reasonable patient" in the same situation would need and want to make a voluntary and knowledgeable decision. Under this approach, the patient must be told about all material risks, that is, those factors that might make a difference to a reasonable, average patient under comparable circumstances.

The patient's age may affect what information is material to that person's decision-making calculations. For instance, a likely side effect that will not manifest itself for another 20 years may not be very important to an older person. However, the probability that a particular intervention will be accompanied by a great amount of physical pain or discomfort may make quite a difference to an old, frail individual. Physicians always should take into account the physical and mental effects of aging, among numerous other factors, when deciding what information regarding an intervention might be material to the specific person and how to communicate that information most usefully.

Within these standards of disclosure, the following informational items have usually been enumerated as essential components of the ideal informed consent process: (1) diagnosis; (2) the general natural and purpose of the proposed intervention; (3) the reasonably foreseeable risks, consequences, and perils of the intervention; (4) the probability of success; (5) reasonable alternatives; (6) the result anticipated if nothing is done; (7) limitations on the professional or health care facility; and (8) advice (i.e., the physician's recommendation).

The third essential element of legally effective consent is that the patient must be mentally able to engage in a rational decision-making process. The topic of evaluating a patient's decisional capacity is discussed in Chapter 84. When the patient lacks sufficient present cognitive and emotional capacity to make medical choices, a proxy or surrogate decision maker must be involved (see following).

The Research Context

The issue of participation by older persons, particularly those residing long term within nursing facilities, in biomedical and behavioral research protocols is a growing ethical (see Chapter 86) and legal concern. Legal questions are especially vexing when the problem being clinically investigated is mental impairment and the proposed human subjects are institutionalized as well as cognitively and emotionally compromised. The policy and practice challenge is to protect impaired elderly persons from exploitation and avoidable harm, while facilitating the conduct of important, high-quality research on problems (such as dementia) that affect older persons disproportionately.

Most biomedical and behavioral research conducted in the United States is regulated under federal law that seeks to protect the rights and well-being of potential human subjects.[10] The Office of Protection from Research

Risks (OPRR) within the Department of Health and Human Services (DHHS) has—and has exercised—the authority to suspend an institution's human subjects research activities for noncompliance with applicable regulations.

At present, there are no particular legal restrictions unique to older research subjects; thus, participation by the elderly in research protocols is governed by the same law that applies to subjects of all ages. For incapacitated persons, consent for research participation may be obtained legally from those individuals who are empowered to make other decisions on the older person's behalf; federal regulations refer to the use of a "legally authorized representative" for consent to research activities.[11]

However, a 1998 report by the National Bioethics Advisory Commission (NBAC) contained a number of recommendations for specially protecting potential human research subjects (of all ages) who have impaired capacity to personally consent to their own research participation.[12,13] Among other items, NBAC recommended:

- Institutional Review Board (IRB) membership should include at least two persons familiar with mental disorders
- A special standing panel of DHHS should be created to handle especially troubling research protocols
- Research using mentally impaired subjects should be disapproved if people without such impairments could be used
- For protocols involving greater than minimal risk, there should be an independent assessment of a potential subject's capacity, and the protocol must detail the assessment process

These recommendations will likely set the agenda for policy discussion in this arena for the foreseeable future.

The endeavor of conducting legally defensible geriatric research, particularly with demented, institutionalized subjects, presents a variety of challenges concerning site and subject selection, capacity evaluations, comprehension and retention of relevant information, choice and authority of proxy decision makers, and minimization of coercive influences. Nonetheless, the geriatric research enterprise is an essential one, and the legal challenges must be met appropriately.

Surrogate Decision Making

As noted, proxy decision making concerning an older person's participation in a research protocol sometimes is necessary when the person lacks sufficient capacity to make their own decisions rationally. Similarly, physicians involved in the diagnosis and treatment of older patients frequently must confront substitute decision makers responsible for intervening on behalf of patients whose cognitive or emotional deficits are so severe that they prevent the patient from personally making and communicating autonomous choices.[14] The topic of surrogate decision making by third parties acting for the incapacitated patient is a complex and legally inexact one.

There are several alternative ways to delegate legally what would ordinarily be the patient's authority to make decisions for the proxy or surrogate to exercise that power on behalf of the incapacitated patient. These delegation mechanisms may be characterized as follows: (1) delegation of authority beforehand by the patient, through methods of advance planning; (2) delegation of authority by operation of statute, regulation, or broad judicial precedent; (3) informal delegation of authority by custom; and (4) delegation of authority by a court order in the specific case.

The two most important current devices for advance health care planning are the living will (in some jurisdictions called a "declaration") and the durable power of attorney for health care.[15] The Patient Self-Determination Act (PSDA) passed by Congress as part of the Omnibus Budget Reconciliation Act (OBRA) of 1990,[16] in the aftermath of the United States Supreme Court's decision in *Cruzan v. Director, Missouri Department of Health*,[17] imposes a number of requirements on hospitals, nursing homes, health maintenance organizations, preferred provider organizations, hospices, and home health agencies that participate in the Medicare and Medicaid programs. Among these are mandates that the provider create and distribute to new patients or their surrogates a written policy on advance directives, consistent with applicable state law; the provider inquire at the time of admission or enrollment whether the patient has previously executed an advance directive; and, if no advance directive has been executed previously and the patient currently retains sufficient decisional capacity, the provider inquire whether the patient wishes to execute such a directive now.[18,19]

In some circumstances, particular facets of decision-making authority may devolve or pass from the patient to someone else by operation of a statute, regulation, or judicial precedent. One well-known example of this form of substitute decision making is the representative payee concept that is utilized to manage regular government benefit payments, including pension and disability checks from the Departments of Veterans Affairs and Defense, Railroad Retirement Board, and Civil Service; Old Age, Survivors, and Disability Insurance benefit payments under Title 2 of the Social Security Act; and Supplemental Security Income benefit payments to the aged, blind, or disabled under Title 16 of the Social Security Act.

As another example of this type of power delegation is found in the federal Medicare-Medicaid requirements for nursing facilities. These regulations provide that, for a facility resident who is (1) adjudicated incompetent in accordance with state law or (2) found by the physician to be medically incapable of understanding his or her rights, the right to make decisions devolves to the resident's guardian, next of kin, sponsoring agencies, or representative payee.

It is in the area of decision making about care of the critically ill patient that statutory, regulatory, and judicial guidance about substitute decision making is clearest. Twenty-seven states and the District of Columbia had enacted legislation generally lumped under the rubric "family consent" or "default" statutes.[20] These statutes set forth legal authority empowering designated relatives, and sometimes others, to make particular kinds of medical decisions on behalf of incapacitated persons who have not executed a living will or durable power of attorney. In addition, courts in many jurisdictions have formally recognized the family's authority to exercise an incapacitated person's rights on his or her behalf and, just as importantly, most of these judicial decisions explicitly establish legal precedent for families to act in future cases without the need for prior court authorization in individual cases.

As a general matter, in the absence of a specific statute, regulation, or court order delegating authority to a substitute decision maker, or a court order finding an individual mentally incompetent and appointing another named person to act as guardian or conservator, neither the family as a whole nor any of its individual members (nor nonrelatives, for that matter) has any automatic legal authority to make decisions on behalf of patients who cannot speak for themselves. Nevertheless, it has long been a widely known and implicitly accepted medical custom or convention to rely on families as decision makers for incompetent persons, even in the absence of express legal power. Even when there is no explicit judicial or legislative authorization in one's own state, the legal risk for a physician or health care institution for a good faith treatment decision made in conjunction with an incompetent patient's family is very slight. In fact, the few courts that have been presented with the question in the context of litigation have virtually unanimously ratified the family's authority.

In some cases, however, informal substitute decision making—that is, the extralegal "muddling through" process that governs a great deal of medical, and especially geriatric, practice—by the physician and family members may not work satisfactorily. The family members may disagree among themselves. They may make decisions that seem to be at odds with the earlier expressed or implied preferences of the patient or that clearly appear not to be in the patient's best interests (e.g., a family's financially or psychologically driven selfish choices). The family may request a course of conduct that seriously contradicts the physician's or facility's own sense of ethical integrity.

When such situations occur, judicial appointment of a guardian or conservator empowered to make decisions on behalf of an incompetent ward may be practically and legally advisable.[21] However, because guardianship usually entails an extensive deprivation of the individual's basic rights, may be imposed in the absence of meaningful procedural safeguards, and involves substantial financial, time, and emotional costs, the "least restrictive alternative" doctrine dictates that it be pursued only as a last resort when less formal mechanisms of substitute decision making have failed or are unavailable.

Additionally, when guardianship is sought, consideration should be paid to the possibility of strictly limiting such guardianship in terms of both duration and extent of transferred powers. Because courts possess the authority to impose such limitations, under either specific state "partial or limited guardianship" statutes or the courts' inherent equity powers, physicians who deal with substitute decision makers who purport to be the patient's legal guardian should request to see a copy of the official court order creating the guardianship, to verify the existence and extent of the guardian's authority.

Institutional Ethics Committees

Standards of the Joint Commission on Accreditation of Healthcare Organizations (JCAHO) require that hospitals have "a mechanism" in place for resolving ethical disputes. One such mechanism is the institutional ethics committee (IEC), variants of which have now been established in many hospitals, as well as nursing homes,[22] hospices, and home health agencies. The IEC is an internal interdisciplinary body that helps an institution or agency and its professional staff to make difficult treatment decisions in an ethically acceptable manner.

Institutional ethics committees differ among institutions and agencies in terms of precise size, composition, structure, procedures, and organizational placement. IEC functions may include policy drafting, staff and public education, and/or case consultation on a concurrent or retrospective basis. Consultation with an IEC probably exerts a legal prophylactic effect, in terms of reducing unnecessary guardianship petitions, deterring possible lawsuits against the institution or agency and its staff, and making it easier to defend against the very rare malpractice cases that might be filed in this context.

"Do Not" Orders

"Do Not" orders from the attending physician to other members of the health care team are predicated on prospectively made decisions to withdraw or withhold certain types of medical interventions from specified patients. Most attention has been devoted, especially in the acute hospital environment, to "do not resuscitate" (DNR) orders (also called "No Codes"), or instructions by the physician to refrain from attempts at cardiopulmonary resuscitation (CPR) in the event of a cardiac arrest. However, other kinds of "do not" orders also are important, particularly in the long-term care environment. Among these are "do not hospitalize" and "do not intubate" orders.

Legally, deciding about implementing "do not" orders should be handled according to the same substantive principles and procedural guidelines that apply to other treatment decisions. In fact, by allowing and encouraging certain decisions to be made prospectively, before a crisis develops, "do not" orders probably reduce any potential legal risk and certainly should curtail legal anxiety.

The legal status of "do not" orders when the patient is mentally competent is unambiguous. It parallels the situation of medical intervention generally, including intervention that would be life prolonging or even lifesaving. In other words, a competent adult patient has the constitutional, common law, and (in many states) statutory right to voluntarily and knowingly refuse basic (e.g., CPR) or advanced cardiac life support or any of its specific components, hospitalization, or any other form of medical intervention and to demand a precisely written "do not" order. Courts have not ordered competent elderly patients to endure medical interventions over their stated objections. The wishes of close family members should be considered by the physician (assuming the competent patient has expressly or by implication authorized family participation in their medical care), but should never be permitted to override the decision of a competent patient.

Under the PSDA, acute and long-term settings should have a written policy statement regarding the institutional or agency philosophy and any relevant technologic and staffing limitations concerning various "do not" situations. A copy of this statement should be presented to every decisionally capable patient or an incapacitated patient's most likely substitute decision maker at or before the time of admission. Extensive, regular staff education should be carried out concerning the provider's policies. Physicians customarily should discuss treatment preferences and objectives openly and honestly with patients who are capable of participating in such decisions. As a matter of course, physicians should document the results of these discussions; such documentation might provide useful evidence later on of the patient's wishes and the good faith quality of the decision-making process.

When a capable patient has made a "do not" decision, he or she must be able to reevaluate and reconsider that decision continually in light of any change in physical or mental condition that materially affects (i.e., that might really make a difference in) the possible benefits and burdens of different treatment alternatives. A "do not" decision can be revoked or modified at any time. It is part of the physician's duty to continually update the patient with new information pertinent to "do not" decisions.

For the mentally incapacitated patient, clarification of respective rights and responsibilities may be available from the patient's previously executed advance directive or from the expressions of a legislatively or judicially designated proxy. Even in the absence of a valid advance directive or explicitly legally authorized proxy, "do not" orders are still permissible for incapacitated patients according to the same general legal principles governing other kinds of decisions about life-sustaining medical treatment, that is, balancing—from the perspective of the patient—the likely benefits and burdens of the particular intervention. The only pertinent distinction between "do not" orders and other decisions to limit the use of life-prolonging medical interventions lies in the prospective nature of the former.

In an effort to clarify this area further, a number of state legislatures have passed specific legislation on this subject. JCAHO standards also address "do not" orders explicitly. Moreover, at least 42 states have in place protocols for writing and implementing Do Not Resuscitate orders pertaining to out-of-hospital situations.[23,24]

The physician's and health care institution's responsibility to adopt, educate about, and communicate concerning a clear policy on "do not" orders applies with full force when presently incapacitated patients are involved. When a patient is not presently capable of participating fully in decision making, the communication and negotiation about potential "do not" management strategies must encompass available, interested family members. The family has the same legal authority to make "do not" decisions for an incapacitated relative as to make other types of medical decisions. Even in the absence of specific legal authorization, in this sphere as elsewhere it is the medical custom or convention to involve families in "do not" decisions. From a practical risk management perspective, extensive interaction with family members concerning such decisions is a prudent, protective practice.

Conversely, whether or not the family possesses the legal authority to veto a physician's proposed "do not" decision has emerged as a controversial issue, as part of the larger "futile treatment" debate.[25,26] Proceeding with entry and implementation of a "do not" order in the face of family opposition entails, from a practical standpoint, a certain risk of legal challenge after the fact. However, the realistic risk of being held liable for this conduct is small when the "do not" order was appropriate in terms of expressed patient wishes, the clinical prognosis, and the imbalance between the likely benefits and burdens of the intervention for the patient.

A communication and negotiation process that is marked by compassion, clarity, and patience should resolve family–physician disagreement peacefully in most situations. When serious disagreement between physician and family or among family members themselves does surface and persist, consultation with an IEC may be advisable; a judicial declaratory judgment and injunction may be sought, but should be considered only as a last resort.[27]

During the communications process, the family should be informed that the continuing propriety of a "do not" order will be reevaluated regularly and that it can be rescinded or modified if prognosis or other factors materially change. As would be true for any clinical action predicated on an inaccurate factual basis, a physician or health care institution might be found legally liable for basing a "do not" order on an incorrect evaluation of the patient's condition and prognosis.

The attending physician should make appropriate use of available professional consultations with relevant clinical specialists, while retaining ultimate medical control and responsibility for the patient. The insight of nurses and other team members who are familiar with the patient also should be sought out and considered.

The wishes of the patient (if ascertainable), the family, and significant others should all be recorded. The judgments of involved health care professionals, as well as the reasoning underlying those judgments, should be documented completely and candidly, as well as any attempts to change the mind of the patient or family. Honesty and accuracy in record keeping is the best defense for the physician and health care facility against any subsequent allegations of negligence or malevolent intent. Failure to put decisions and orders in writing not only exposes the physician to greater legal risk but also engenders possible inappropriate responses by other team members based on the mixed and confused signals that they are given.

Once a "do not" order has been entered into a medical record, it should remain a permanent part of that document. If it is later modified or rescinded, the modification or rescission also should be noted in the record.

Along with documentation, there is the need for communication among appropriate health care team members and institutions once a "do not" order has been written. A decision to refrain from certain interventions needs to be made known to those responsible for carrying out the order because, in the absence of such an order, the health care team normally is obligated to treat the patient with the full medical arsenal available. Communication is chiefly an organizational responsibility, and each hospital, nursing home, and home health agency should have a provision in its written policies detailing its procedures for assuring that all pertinent members of the health care team are informed accurately and promptly

of "do not" orders or other treatment limitations concerning particular patients. Regular interdisciplinary case reviews on various institutional units are one means of communication that should be considered. Special markings on the outside of the medical chart, discreetly but clearly signifying particular treatment restrictions, are also a valuable communicative tool.

Even when a long-term care facility resident needs to be, and with the resident's or surrogate's permission is, transferred to an acute care hospital for treatment of a specific remediable problem (such as acute infection), other treatment limitations may remain appropriate because of the person's other, underlying, nonremediable deficits. In those circumstances, the transferring facility should have a clear, effective, ongoing mechanism in place for communicating "do not" orders directly to hospital personnel. Especially because hospital medical staff (and even more particularly house staff) may have strong preconceptions about resuscitation and other aggressive therapy for older persons who reside in long-term care facilities, it is the facility's duty to transmit to the receiving hospital, at or before the time of the transfer, as much background as feasible concerning preferences, values, and instructions that should guide treatment for that person. The transfer agreement between the long-term care facility and any other health care facility should contain a written provision addressing the communication of this sort of information.

Finally, decisions to limit specific elements of treatment should not signify total disregard or the "writing off" of an older person. Physicians in the past often have been intimidated from providing sufficient pain relief to critically ill patients because they feared criminal prosecution or professional disciplinary action for the overprescription of controlled substances. In the past decade, a number of legal initiatives have been aimed at changing this climate of apprehension to encourage the more appropriate prescribing of pain medications,[28] including the enactment in many states of "Intractable Pain Statutes." Indeed, it is widely recognized today that neglect of continuing palliative care, including effective pain management, could alienate patient and family and expose the physician and health care facility to lawsuits charging abandonment, neglect, or even abuse. Alleviating suffering is a basic goal of medical care and a part of the standard of care legally and ethically owed by health care professionals, even when "cure" of underlying disease is no longer possible. Management goals should consist of the following: remaining in physical and emotional contact with the dying person; relieving terminal symptoms (such as pain, confusion, anxiety, or restlessness); providing nourishment and hydration so long as they are palliative; skin care, bowel and bladder care, and personal grooming; and supporting the family through the period of dying, death, and bereavement. High-dose narcotic agents and sedatives can be used despite the possible risk of suppressed cerebral function and respiratory depression (there is controversy about how real this risk actually is), because the therapeutic intention is to control the symptoms of human suffering, not to precipitate an earlier death.

One disturbing development in 1999 was the introduction in Congress of the Pain Relief Promotion Act (PRPA) (the Hyde–Nickels bill). The bill was designed to override Oregon's physician-assisted suicide law (discussed next), by making it a violation of the federal Controlled Substances Act to administer opioids or other drugs to hasten a patient's death. However, the most likely effect—unintended but foreseeable—of this bill if it were passed and signed into law would be to "chill" responsible pain management by discouraging, for reasons of apprehension about criminal prosecution, all physicians from adequately treating the suffering of their dying patients.[29,30]

Physician-Assisted Suicide

Current U.S. law is unambiguous in its condemnation, particularly through state homicide statutes, of health care providers engaging in active (voluntary, positive) euthanasia (i.e., actively and intentionally doing something such as administering a lethal injection to hasten the death of a patient). In addition, almost all states explicitly legislatively condemn physician-assisted suicide (i.e., actively helping a patient to purposely take his or her own life), through either a specific statute on the subject or judicial interpretations of their general homicide statutes.

In 1997, the U.S. Supreme Court unanimously upheld the validity of state laws making it criminal for physicians or other health care professionals to assist a patient to commit suicide. In these decisions, the Court rejected the notion of any federal constitutional right to physician-assisted sucide.[31,32]

Although the federal Constitution does not require it, the door is open legally for particular states to choose, as a matter of their own respective public policies and politics, to decriminalize physician-assisted suicide or even active euthanasia. Thus far, Oregon is the only state that has accepted this invitation.[33–35]

Adult Protective Services

Every state has assembled an array of programs under the general rubric of adult protective services (APS). The traditional definition of this concept is a system of preventive, supportive, and surrogate services provided to adults living in the community, enabling them to maxi-

mize independence and to avoid abuse and exploitation. APS are characterized by two elements that can be mixed in several different ways: the coordinated delivery of services to adults at risk and the actual or potential authority to provide substitute decision making concerning these services.

The services feature consists of an assortment of health, housing, and social services, such as homemaker, house repair, friendly visits, and meals. Ideally, these services are coordinated by a caseworker who is responsible for assessing an older individual's needs and bringing together the available responses. Many state APS statutes mandate that social service agencies undertake both casework coordination and delivery of services.

The second component of an APS system is authority to intervene on behalf of the client. Ordinarily, the client (if capable of making autonomous decisions), with the encouragement of the physician will consent to a proposed service plan. Alternatively, the decisionally capable client may delegate decision-making authority to someone else through a durable power of attorney instrument. However, if the client refuses offered assistance but some form(s) of intervention appears necessary, the legal system may be invoked to authorize appointment of a surrogate decision maker over the person's objections.

In some states, APS offices rely, in the case of recalcitrant individuals, on the traditional methods of legal intervention in the lives of elderly persons, namely, involuntary commitment and guardianship. Legislation has been enacted in several jurisdictions, however, that creates special procedures to obtain court orders for protective services, for placing the client in an institution, for emergency orders when there is imminent danger to the client's health or safety, or for orders authorizing entry into an uncooperative client's home. These special procedures may be in addition to, or in place of, the existing guardianship apparatus and usually bypass the procedural protections that have been gradually built into extant guardianship laws.

Court orders obtained under an APS statute often are time limited; upon expiration, the APS agency must pursue standard guardianship to continue imposing services over the client's objection. However, during its duration, a court order authorizing APS intervention may be very broad. If the court does not limit it, for example, a protective services order may result in the placement of a person in a hospital, nursing home,[36] assisted living complex, boarding home, hospice, or mental institution. As a matter of standard practice, physicians should ascertain carefully the exact nature and scope of a protective services order before accepting as legally effective the purported informed consent of a public or private social service agency offered on behalf of a patient-client.

Those states that have created new court processes to authorize unconsented-to intervention, on either an emergency or a longer-term basis, also have established standards for identifying candidates for protective services or protective placement. Most of these states follow the same general statutory pattern. First, certain behavioral disabilities are enumerated, such as the inability to care for oneself adequately or to protect oneself from abuse and exploitation by others. Next, a number of causes for this incapacity are listed, most of which involve impairment of mental functioning. "Infirmities of aging," "senility," and "advanced age" were terms often used in earlier statutes to denote impairment in older persons, but such statutory language is rare today. In a very few states, physical impairment alone is considered a sufficient basis for intervention when the condition is likely to lead to self-neglect or victimization by others, even when there is no evidence of mental incompetence; most of these provisions have been invalidated by the courts on constitutional grounds or amended by state legislatures.

In the context of APS, physicians frequently are called on to contribute their expertise and skills in (1) identifying candidates for services; (2) providing evidence if guardianship or commitment litigation takes place; (3) exploring voluntary alternatives; and (4) planning and placement. Physicians often are in a unique, central position to identify initially those individuals who meet the eligibility criteria for, and could significantly benefit from, the intervention of an APS program. Notifying a designated APS agency of the existence and identity of such patients is incumbent on the physician in the more than 40 states with mandatory reporting statutes for suspected adult abuse and neglect (including self-neglect). In states without mandatory reporting laws, physicians making good faith voluntary reports to APS are immune from any liability connected with that reporting.[37]

Just as written reports and live courtroom testimony are sought from physicians in routine guardianship cases, so too is this form of evidence highly valued in special protective services proceedings. The deference paid to physician opinion may be even greater in the latter situation, where less stringent eligibility criteria and procedural formalities often empower the presiding judge with even broader discretion in making findings and fashioning remedies.

As noted, it frequently is best for APS interventions to be accepted voluntarily by older persons who need help to maximize self-control over their lives. The physician has a duty to counsel decisionally capable patients about available long-term care alternatives—both institutional and home- and community based—and their relative advantages and disadvantages, or at least to direct patients to appropriate information sources.

Finally, the physician's potential contribution to service planning and placement activities for the nonindependent elderly patient should not be forgotten. The ultimate goal is not simply to obtain protective services, whether on a voluntary or involuntary basis. Rather, the key is to assure the quality and appropriateness of the services actually provided for the older individual involved. Identification, referral, and evidence presentation should not be the end of physician involvement. Social service agencies are not merely a convenient place to deposit unwanted elders, and it is just as possible for an older person with limited personal resources to be "dumped" harmfully into the community as into a nursing home or public mental institution.

Older individuals are entitled to receive reasonable continuity of care from their physicians. If an older person changes placement (e.g., moves from a private home to an assisted living complex or a nursing facility), the principle of nonabandonment legally obligates the physician to facilitate continuity of medical care either by continuing to treat the patient personally or by making a referral to another competent, willing physician whose services are acceptable to the older person.

Confidentiality

In the course of performing their professional activities, physicians every day learn very personal, intimate information about their older patients. This knowledge of personal patient information imposes certain duties of confidentiality on the physician. Fulfilling these duties can, in specific factual situations, raise substantial legal questions.

As a general legal precept, physicians have the duty to hold in confidence all personal patient information entrusted to them. This obligation has been enforced through civil damage suits based on both statutory (legislative) and common (judge-made) law and embodied in virtually all state professional practice acts and implementing regulations. Some states have enacted statutes that provide monetary damages for physician breach of confidentiality even if the patient is unable to prove any tangible injury. State medical practice acts provide that violation of the duty of confidentiality is a potential ground for revoking, denying, or suspending a physician's license to practice medicine. Detailed federal regulations[38] are being developed to safeguard the privacy of medical records, based on a mandate in the Health Insurance Portability and Accountability Act of 1996.[39] The patient's reasonable expectation of privacy extends to all members of the health care team.

The difficulty in applying this general legal principle to concrete situations involving older patients is that the physician's duty to maintain as confidential the disclosures and medical records of the patient is not an absolute, inflexible obligation. The fact that a duty is not absolute does not mean it is not important. However, when a duty is only *prima facie,* or presumptively applicable, one must consider whether there are relevant factors present that justify or even compel overriding that *prima facie* obligation in a particular case.

The first exception to the usual rule of confidentiality is that a patient may waive, or give up, the right to confidentiality if this is done in a voluntary, competent, and informed manner. This is accomplished daily in the health care area to make information available to third-party payers such as the Health Care Financing Administration that operates Medicare[40] and Medicaid, quality-of-care evaluators and auditors such as JCAHO inspectors or reviewers from the state's Peer Review Organization (PRO), and other public and private entities including long-term care ombudsmen and the patient's legal representatives. The physician has an obligation to cooperate fully in the patient-requested release and transfer of medical information. The patient's waiver of confidentiality and request for release of information should be honored only if it has been documented thoroughly in writing. Further, the identity and legitimate authority of the record seeker should be verified satisfactorily.

Second, when the rights of innocent third parties are jeopardized, the general requirement of confidentiality may yield. For instance, the expressed threat of a dangerous psychiatric patient to kill a specific victim, coupled with the patient's apparent present ability (not hard to imagine even for an elderly person in today's climate of easy handgun availability) and intent to make good on the threat, arguably should be reported to the intended victim and to law enforcement officials.[41]

Questions about confidentiality versus disclosure will arise increasingly in the context of automobile driving by older persons.[42] Once the patient has developed age-related neurodegenerative illness and sensory impairments, the decision to stop driving may develop into an area of tension between patient and physician if informal and noncoercive attempts at persuasion fail to bring about voluntary abstention from the roads.[43] Physicians must be knowledgeable about relevant mandatory reporting requirements regarding unfitness for driving; the law on this point varies among the states.[44] Only a few jurisdictions presently have statutes that expressly mandate physicians to report impaired drivers to public authorities.[45] Even in the absence of a mandatory reporting statute, some physicians have been held civilly liable when they should have foreseen a patient's dangerous driving but did nothing to prevent it and the patient then harmed an innocent third party in a motor vehicle accident.[46] Further, physicians should inform driving-impaired patients of the patients' own legal responsibility to notify the state concerning their impairment.

Third, the patient's expectation of confidentiality must yield when the physician is mandated by state law to report to specified public health authorities the existence of certain enumerated conditions reasonably suspected in a patient. The physician should be familiar with the content of mandatory reporting statutes and regulations in force in their own jurisdiction. Such requirements may be based on the state's inherent police power to protect the health, safety, and welfare of society as a whole. This rationale would support, for example, reporting requirements concerning infectious diseases or vital statistics (e.g., birth and death). Alternatively, reporting of certain conditions may be obligatory under the state's *parens patriae* ("father of the country") power to protect those individuals who are unable to care for their own needs. Mandatory reporting of elder abuse or neglect would be justified on this ground (see Chapter 73).

Finally, the physician may be compelled to reveal otherwise confidential patient information by the force of legal process, that is, by a judge's issuance of a court order requiring such release. This order is a possibility in any type of lawsuit in which the patient's physical or mental condition is in dispute.

The Health Insurance Portability and Accountability Act (HIPAA) of 1996[47] stipulated that if Congress did not enact comprehensive requirements regarding standards with respect to privacy of individually identifiable health information by August 1999, DHHS should issue regulations on this subject. On November 3, 1999, DHHS published proposed comprehensive rules setting federal standards in this sphere[48] after the close of the public comment period on February 17, 2000, DHHS had an opportunity to modify the regulations before they would be issued in final, binding form. Once adopted, the federal rules will supersede state medical records confidentiality laws, unless a state law is more stringent in its protections of patient privacy than the federal requirements.

The right of privacy may be particularly important to today's older individuals who, as part of a cohort predating computers and modern mass communication technologies, often assign an even higher value to personal privacy than do members of subsequent generations. The right of privacy too often is compromised in treating older patients, particularly those with cognitive or emotional deficits.

An older person who has significant mental capacity may, nonetheless, through appearance or demeanor leave the impression that it is appropriate to discuss his or her clinical problems and management with relatives or friends. Every safeguard should be employed to adhere to the ordinary standards of confidentiality unless there is express, or at least unambiguously implied, permission from the patient to do otherwise or the mental condition of the patient is so disabling as to dictate involving relatives or friends within the decision-making circle. Particularly in situations of marginal or questionable patient capacity, the physician should be scrupulous in making sure that the patient has no objection to family or friend involvement. When the family or others with appropriate authority are involved, confidential communications about the patient should be carefully handled to avoid unauthorized disclosure beyond those with a right and a need to have access to the information.

Conclusion

In some respects, as older patients as a group tend to bring disproportionately few malpractice claims against their physicians, legal liability concerns are less of a factor in geriatrics than in many other branches of medicine. In many ways, however, the elderly offer physicians a set of complex and unique legal challenges. This chapter has outlined some of the more salient legal considerations confronting and guiding physicians who care for older patients, in the hope of raising awareness of these issues in a way that will be beneficial both to physicians and to the older individuals who depend on them.

References

1. Liang BA. *Health Law & Policy: A Survival Guide to Medicolegal Issues for Practitioners.* Boston: Butterworth-Heinemann; 2000.
2. 20 Code of Federal Regulations Part 404.
3. 29 United States Code § 621 et seq.
4. 42 United States Code § 1320c.
5. 42 United States Code § 11133–34.
6. Kohn L, Corrigan J, Donaldson M. *To Err Is Human: Building a Safer Health System.* Washington, DC: National Academy Press; 2000.
7. Liang BA. Error in medicine: legal impediments to U.S. reform. *J Health Polit Policy Law.* 1999;24:27–58.
8. Public Law 105–33.
9. Noble AA, Brennan TA. The stages of managed care regulation: developing better rules. *J Health Polit Policy Law.* 1999;24:1275–1305.
10. 45 Code of Federal Regulations Part 46.
11. 45 Code of Federal Regulations § 46.102(d).
12. National Bioethics Advisory Commission. Research Involving Persons with Mental Disorders that May Affect Decisionmaking Capacity. Washington, DC: available at *www.bioethics.gov/capacity.*
13. Kapp MB. Regulating research for the decisionally impaired: implications for mental health professionals. *J Clin Geropsychol.* 2000.
14. Dubler NN, ed. *Symposiun* on the doctor–proxy relationship. *J Law Med Ethics.* 1999;27:5–86.
15. King NMP. *Making Sense of Advance Directives,* rev ed. Washington, DC: Georgetown University Press; 1996.
16. Public Law 101–508, §§ 4206, 4751.
17. 110 S.Ct. 2841 (1990).
18. Bradley EH, Blechner BB, Walker LC, et al. Institutional efforts to promote advance care planning in nursing homes:

challenges and opportunities. *J Law Med Ethics.* 1997;25: 150–159.
19. Molloy DW, Guyatt GH, Russo R, et al. Systematic implementation of an advance directive program in nursing homes: a randomized controlled trial. *JAMA.* 2000;283: 1437–1444.
20. Sabatino CP. The legal and functional status of the medical proxy: suggestions for statutory reform. *J Law Med Ethics.* 1999;27:52–68.
21. Zimny GH, Grossberg GT. *Guardianship of the Elderly: Psychiatric and Judicial Aspects.* New York: Springer; 1998.
22. Hoffmann DE, Boyle P, Levenson SA. *Handbook for Nursing Home Ethics Committees.* Washington, DC: American Association of Homes and Services for the Aging; 1995.
23. Sabatino CP. Survey of state EMS-DNR laws and protocols. *J Law Med Ethics.* 1999;27:297–315.
24. Leon MD, Wilson EM. Development of a statewide protocol for the prehospital identification of DNR patients in Connecticut including new DNR regulations. *Ann Emerg Med* 1999;34:263–274.
25. Council on Ethical and Judicial Affairs, American Medical Association. Medical futility in end-of-life care. *JAMA.* 1999;281:937–941.
26. Leonard CT, Doyle RL, Raffin TA. Do-not-resuscitate orders in the face of patient and family opposition. *Crit Care Med.* 1999;27:1045–1047.
27. Zuckerman C. Looking beyond the law to improve end-of-life care. *Generations.* 1999;13:30–35.
28. Johnson SH, ed. Symposium, on legal and regulatory issues in pain management. *J Law Med Ethics.* 1998;26:265–352.
29. Angell M. Caring for the dying—Congressional mischief. *N Engl J Med.* 1999;341:1923–1925.
30. Orentlicher D, Caplan A. The Pain Relief Promotion Act of 1999: a serious threat to palliative care. *JAMA.* 2000;283: 255–258.
31. Vacco v. Quill, 117 S. Ct. 2293 (1997).
32. Washington v. Glucksberg, 117 S. Ct. 2302 (1997).
33. Or. Rev. Stat. §§ 127.800–.897.
34. Chin AE, Hedberg K, Higginson GK, et al. Legalized physician-assisted suicide in Oregon—the first year's experience. *N Engl-J Med.* 1999;340:577–583.
35. Ganzini L, Nelson HD, Schmidt TA, et al. Physicians' experiences with the Oregon Death With Dignity Act. *N Engl J Med.* 2000;342:557–563.
36. Kapp MB. The "voluntary" nature of nursing facility admissions: legal, practical, and public policy implications. *N Engl J Crim Civil Confine.* 1998;24:1–35.
37. Quinn MJ, Tomita SK. *Elder Abuse and Neglect: Causes, Diagnosis, and Intervention Strategies, 2nd Ed.* New York: Springer; 1997.
38. 64 Federal Register 59,918 (November 3, 1999).
39. 42 United States Code §§ 1320d through 1320d-8.
40. U.S. General Accounting Office. Medicare: Improvements Needed to Enhance Protection of Confidential Health Information. GAO/HEHS-99-140. Washington, DC: USGAO; 1999.
41. Tarasoff v. Regents of the University of California, 17 Cal.3d 425, 551 P.2d 334, 131 Cal.Rptr. 14 (1976).

42. Council on Ethical and Judicial Affairs. *Impaired Drivers and Their Physicians.* Chicago: American Medical Association; 1999.

43. Johnson JE. Urban older adults and the forfeiture of a driver's license. *J Gerontol Nurs.* 1999;25:12–18.

44. Marottoli RA. New laws or better information and communication? *J Am Geriatr Soc.* 2000;48:100–102.

45. Reuben DB, St. George P. Driving and dementia: California's approach to a medical and policy dilemma. *J Am Geriatr Soc.* 1996;164:111–121.

46. Weintraub MI. Driving and Alzheimer disease [letter]. *JAMA.* 1996;275:182.

47. Public Law No. 104–191, 110 Stat. 1936 (1996).

48. 64 Federal Register 59918 (Nov. 3, 1999).

84
Determination of Decision-Making Capacity

Jason H.T. Karlawish and Robert A. Pearlman

An older person's decision-making capacity determines their ability to direct his or her care. They can choose whether to receive a test or a treatment, and even direct others to make choices for them. If the patient lacks decision-making capacity, however, they may not be able to exercise their autonomous choices. Other people may need to decide for them.

Decision-making capacity and the related concept of competency have received extensive conceptual development in bioethics and the law.[1,2] This development has occurred largely because decision-making capacity is one of the essential components of the theory of informed consent. This theory is a robust guide for difficult decisions such as determining whether a person should be hospitalized against their will, have a surrogate assume authority over their own care, or even be enrolled in potentially risky research. Unfortunately, clinical medicine has been slow to adopt this theory into the day-to-day practice of medical decision making.[3]

Two clinical conditions emphasize the need for geriatricians to understand these concepts and to know how to apply them in clinical practice. First, elderly people are more likely than younger adults to experience illnesses that impair their ability to make decisions.[4-6] These illnesses include neurodegenerative dementias, psychiatric illnesses, delirium, and impairments in hearing and vision. In fact, the initial diagnostic clue that a patient has one of these potentially treatable *medical* problems may be the discovery of the *ethically challenging* problem that a patient has difficulty making a decision. Second, an appreciable number of elderly people refuse life-sustaining treatment that their health care providers recommend. Although refusing treatment may be a reasonable clue that a patient has impaired decision-making capacity, disagreement with a physician's recommendation is not the sole grounds for finding a patient incompetent.[7] A physician who is skilled at assessing decision-making capacity will find this clinical circumstance an ideal opportunity to assess the patient's decision-making capacity and to discuss options of care, including palliative care.

Collectively, these points illustrate that the ability to assess decision-making capacity is not simply a matter of reluctantly accommodating the dictates of law into the practice of medicine. It is actually part of the competent and ethical practice of geriatric medicine. A physician who can efficiently practice the skills of assessing how a patient makes a decision has effective skills to foster communication with a patient and to identify clinically significant impairments in a patient's cognition and emotion. In this way, the physician fulfills the roles of the "doctor" as teacher and healer. The purpose of this chapter is to summarize the importance of determining decision-making capacity and to explain the standards for assessing it and judging competency. Following this introductory material, the chapter discusses particularly challenging situations and proposes mechanisms for physicians to improve the quality of their skills.

The Concepts of Competency and Decision-Making Capacity

The terms competency and decision-making capacity are often used interchangably, or they are distinguished on the basis of the person's profession. A common and technically correct distinction is that a judge determines whether a person is competent while a physician determines whether the person has decision-making capacity. Clinical practice, however, illustrates that this distinction collapses. The consequences of a physician's judgment that a patient lacks decision-making capacity are that the patient is not competent to make the decision.[8] Regardless of who is assessing a person's ability to make a choice, however, the terms competency and decision-making capacity do have meaningful differences.

The difference between "decision-making capacity" and "competence" is that the former describes a person's abilities to make a decision. It is assessed according to a number of standards, described next. In contrast, competency describes the judgment that a person's decision-making capacity is adequate to make a particular decision. The former is a condition of a person, whereas the latter is a judgment that integrates information which describes a person's capacities and the context and consequences of the decision.[9]

Competency and decision-making capacity are distinct concepts. It is entirely possible that a physician could determine that a person lacks decision-making capacity but is competent to make a decision, as might happen frequently if physicians took the time to examine, in detail, their patients' choices. For example, a patient who agrees to take hypertension treatment may fail to understand certain facts about that treatment. ("The pills work because they reduce stress.") But, although this misunderstanding represents impaired decision-making capacity, it has harms that are essentially nil. Hence, given the context and consequences, any reasonable practitioner (or judge) would conclude that the person is competent to take the medication. A less common scenario is the patient who has decision-making capacity but is not competent, as would occur in the case of a legal criterion that establishes who is competent. For example, a very bright 12-year-old may fulfill the standards of decision-making capacity but, as a child, as a matter of law, is not competent.

The Importance of Assessing Decision-Making Capacity

The essential attributes that a person needs to make a decision are cognitive skills and a set of values that allow the person to categorize and weigh the importance of information. A number of medical diseases and geriatric syndromes can impair these attributes. These diseases include neurodegenerative dementias such as Alzheimer's disease and frontotemporal dementia, psychiatric diseases such as major depression and anxiety, and medical illnesses that precipitate the common clinical syndrome of delirium.

Data document notable prevalence of incompetency and impairments in decision-making capacity among patients with some of these disorders. Among patients with Alzheimer's disease who have a Mini-Mental Status Examination score between 12 and 30, the inability to understand information needed to make a decision about medical care is extremely common (nearly 90%). Nearly half these patients may retain the ability to appreciate information, however.[10] Moreover, a patient's competency will vary depending upon the decision at hand. In one study, 20% of Alzheimer's disease patients were competent to complete an advance directive.[11] Psychiatric illnesses can also affect decision-making capacity and lead

to incompetency. A study that compared the competency of hospitalized patients with depression and schizophrenia found that the prevalence of incompetency varied from 52% of the patients with schizophrenia to 24% of the patients with depression.[12] Finally, patients without clinically significant impairments in cognition or affect can be incompetent. For example, 12% of hospitalized patients with angina were not competent to make a treatment choice,[12] and among studies of cognitively normal, community-dwelling elderly, 22% were not competent to complete an advance directive[11] and 7% to consent to treatment of a hip fracture.[13]

Three key conclusions can be drawn from these data. First, not all patients with diagnoses that classically affect cognition have impaired decision-making capacity. Second, an affective disorder such as depression can affect decision-making capacity. Finally, some patients with a diagnosis that typically affects cognition may have impaired decision-making capacity. For the clinician, this means that the model of using risk factors to generate pretest probabilities of a diagnosis can be adapted into the practice of assessing decision-making capacity. A patient with an illness such as major depression or mild dementia is more likely to have impaired decision-making capacity than one who does not.

The importance of assessing a patient's decision-making capacity rests in the need to balance two simultaneous ethical commitments to adult patients—to respect an adult person's autonomy and to promote that person's health and well-being. When a person has decision-making capacity, their autonomy is generally honored and decision making occurs in light of medical recommendations and patient values and preferences. In short, a patient gives an informed consent. Patient well-being is assured because a patient who understands a clinical situation and participates in decision making is more likely than the physician to know what is best for their well-being. For example, when a patient refuses a life-sustaining treatment because they give greater weight to quality of life than to the potential quantity of life, this personal choice reflects their assessment of the trade-offs between quality and quantity of life. However, a patient who cannot think through such trade-offs lacks decision-making capacity and may not be competent. If the patient is not competent, respecting that patient's choice as autonomous is both an ethical and medical error. In this situation, the physician's duty is to seek the decision of others, in particular, family or a surrogate, to make the decision.

In summary, it is important to assess decision-making capacity because it serves as a means to balance a physician's simultaneous commitments to respecting a patient's autonomy and promoting their well-being.[14] Having assessed a patient's decision-making capacity, a physician then judges whether the patient is competent to make the decision.

The Standards for Assessing Decision-Making Capacity

At least one of five standards constitutes decision-making capacity.[15] These standards were developed in law and bioethics, and they are intuitively sensible elements of how a rational person ought to make a decision. They provide the foundation for the judgment of a patient's competence. The physician assesses the patient's performance on each standard and then uses the results of these assessments to decide whether a patient's decision-making capacity is inadequate to make the decision.

The five standards of decision-making capacity are listed in Table 84.1. The first is the ability to communicate a choice, which describes a patient's ability to consistently state a choice ("I do not want the surgery."). Unlike the other standards, this standard makes no claim upon the patient's reasons. In a sense, it is the simplest standard. A physician assesses this by asking the patient "What would you like to do?" Much of the day-to-day practice of clinical medicine relies upon this standard or even a weaker version of it, namely, a patient's nonverbal acquiescence to an intervention such as checking their blood pressure. Diseases that can impair a patient's ability to fulfill this standard include communication disorders and extreme states of anxiety that cause a patient to rapidly change choices.

The second standard is the ability to make a reasonable choice. Like the first, this standard is quite simple but unlike the first it introduces content to the choice. The content is the "reasonableness" of the choice in which reasonableness is not necessarily defined by the patient's values but the values a "reasonable person" has; this is obviously a blunt standard to apply. For example, a physician who relies solely upon this standard would likely find that an otherwise healthy patient who refuses a low-risk and likely beneficial intervention such as surgery for a noninvasive breast cancer would have impaired decision-making capacity. Hence, adherence to this standard alone risks a paternalistic practice of medical decision making. Diseases that can impair a patient's ability to fulfill this standard include those that cause delusions and marked deficits in judgment such as dementia and schizophrenia.

Standards three through five are more substantive than the first two because they require the physician to assess the patient's functional cognition. The third standard, appreciation, describes a patient's ability to recognize that, regardless of her choice, the facts of the decision apply to her. These facts include the diagnosis ("I know you said I have cancer and that's what this is.") and the options for treatment ("I can leave it alone or have the surgery."). This standard requires that the patient recognize the relevance of the facts regardless of how the patient values those facts. Diseases that cause delusions or disassociation are likely to impair a patient's ability to fulfill this standard.

The fourth standard of decision-making capacity is reasoning. The ability to reason describes a patient's ability to generate consequences and compare them. ("If I have the surgery, I will have given up on my faith in my ability to heal myself. If I do not have the surgery, I'll take a chance the cancer could spread.") To fulfill this standard a patient has to recognize the different options, generate the consequences of each, and compare them. The ability to achieve this standard is impaired by conditions that reduce executive function, which means the ability to attend to and compare more than one concept. Diseases that impair attention such as delirium and frontal dementia can impair a patient's ability to fulfill this standard.

The fifth standard of decision-making capacity is understanding, the patient's ability to paraphrase back the meaning of the information that the physician disclosed to her. ("A surgery will involve cutting into my skin, removal of my gallbladder, and a 3-week period of recovery.") To fulfill this standard a patient has to "say back" or paraphrase the information the physician disclosed. In doing this, the patient demonstrates that they grasp the meaning of the information. Obviously, the more facts the physician discloses, the more difficult it becomes for the patient to achieve understanding. Indeed, a physician could set the fact content so complex that even a colleague would "fail." Clearly, a judgment is required as to what facts are essential for making the decision. Understanding is most dependent on a patient's memory and language. Hence, diseases that impair memory and language such as Alzheimer's disease and aphasias can significantly impair a patient's ability to fulfill this standard.

In theory, the five standards exist along a continuum from the simplest (communicating a choice) to the hardest (understanding). One study of patients with Alzheimer's disease suggests that this is in fact true.[10] However, patients with depression and schizophrenia have a different pattern of complexity.[12] The significance of this is that the physician cannot simply rely upon the "hardest standard" as a screen for decision-making capacity. Instead, a physician can consider these standards as generally falling into two categories: the first two standards are simpler and the last three are more stringent.

TABLE 84.1. The standards for assessing decision-making capacity.

The ability to make a choice
The ability to make a reasonable choice
The ability to appreciate
The ability to reason
The ability to understand

How to Assess Decision-Making Capacity

The standards of decision-making capacity provide structure to the physician's assessment. The physician uses the results of the assessment to decide what degree of performance on which of the standards is adequate to decide that a patient has decision-making capacity. A physician needs to have set routines to assess the standards and to use the results of the assessment. General rules to assess decision-making capacity are to use open-ended questions that allow the patient to think aloud, to use silent pauses rather than a battery of questions, and to sit face-to-face with a patient rather than at an unequal posture such as standing at the foot of the patient's bed.

To begin an assessment it is sensible to inform the patient of the purpose of the questions that will follow. A useful opening script might be as follows. "I'd like to take some time to go over the options of treating your breast cancer. One of my roles as doctor is as teacher. I'm a doctor of medicine, so my responsibility is to teach you about your health and options for taking care of it." To then focus on the issue of assessing decision-making capacity a physician might say, "I'd like to go over the decision you face. Can we talk about what you see as your medical problems and the options for taking care of them?"

Table 84.2 describes scripted lines to demonstrate how to assess each of the standards. Assessing the abilities to make a choice and a reasonable choice are relatively straightforward. Little skill is needed to assess these standards beyond giving the patient the opportunity to actually make a choice. As simple as this is, in the conduct of a busy office practice, a physician can forget to ask the patient the simple questions listed in Table 84.2.

TABLE 84.2. How to assesses decision-making capacity.

The ability to make a choice:
   "So those are the options. What would you like to do?"

The ability to make a reasonable choice:
   Same as ability to make a choice. Physician judges whether the decision is "reasonable."

The ability to appreciate:
   Appreciate illness: "Can you tell me in your own words what you see as your problem?"
   Appreciate treatments: "Can you tell me in your own words what you see as your options for your problem?"

The ability to reason:
   Comparative reasoning: "Regardless of whether you want to try surgery or medicine, how would taking the medicine be different from having the surgery?"
   Consequential reasoning: "Regardless of whether you want to try surgery or medicine, how would having the surgery affect your daily life? What about the medicine?"

The ability to understand:
   "Can you tell me in your own words what I told you about the reasons for and against having the stress test?"

A key point in the assessment of appreciation is to have the patient separate their choice from their appreciation of its direct relevance to their situation, which is not an immediately obvious task to most patients. Hence (see Table 84.2), a physician asks the patient to separate the choice from appreciation of the options. Open-ended probes can be useful to allow a patient to clarify an answer. A physician assesses reasoning by asking the patient to compare options and generate consequences of options. To assess the ability to understand, the physician should ask the patient to say in their own words the information the physician has disclosed. In the case of complex information, it is sensible to disclose just parts of the information at a time. It is generally not useful to disclose information and then ask a person "Do you understand?" Most people avoid admitting their misunderstanding.

The assessment of decision-making capacity occurs throughout the daily practice of medicine. When a patient participates in the decision, does not evince any cognitive impairment or affective disorders, and agrees to a recommended treatment that has benefits and minimal risk compared with alternative treatments, it is reasonable for the physician to presume that the patient has decision-making capacity. This scenario describes much of outpatient practice. Conversely, when a patient is comatose, delirious, severely demented, or severely psychotic, it is reasonable for the physician to either observe that the patient does not have the capacity to make decisions or decide that further simple questions are needed to assess decision-making capacity.

However, between these two points there is an enormous middle ground. The principal question for a physician is what circumstances or clinical data should suggest an evaluation of a patient's decision-making capacity. Physicians should question a patient's decision-making capacity when the patient's cognition or affect appears out of the ordinary,[16] such as described in Table 84.3.

These conditions fall into several categories: cognitive impairment, behavioral abnormalities, affective disorders, "unreasonable" or unusual choices, and a choice that is antithetical to previously held values and preferences.[2,17,18] These conditions do not signify the lack of decision-making capacity or incompetency, but they do signify clues that there may be impairments in decision-making capacity and even incompetence. For example, a Mini-Mental State score that suggests cognitive impairment does not of itself describe impaired decision-making capacity, and a physician who uses it to do so would produce both false-positive and false-negative assessments of decisional capacity.[7,19] Similarly, problems with behavioral functions may indicate problems that interfere with decisional capacity, yet the link between these two constructs has not been validated.[20] After one of these triggering cues, the physician needs to consider whether to assess the patient's decision-making capacity.

TABLE 84.3. Clues that may warrant an evaluation of decision-making capacity.

Cognition and neurobehavioral functions
  Mini-Mental State examination score suggesting marked cognitive impairment
  Disorientation
  Change in preferences each time patient is approached
  Attention deficits (e.g., somnolence)
  Disability with language
  Impaired short-term memory
  Impaired reasoning
  Impaired recognition

Acute change in functional status
  Diminished independence in activities of daily living
  Functional decline in social activities
  Acute change in behavior

Psychologic modifiers of cognition and reasoning
  Untreated depression
  Distorted patient assessment of self, world, and future
  Anxiety
  Delusions
  Paranoia
  False beliefs

Unreasonable or unusual choices
  Wanting high-burden (e.g., side effects, risks)/low-benefit treatment when available, alternative treatments seem to have better profiles
  Refusing high-benefit/low-burden treatment when available, alternative treatments seem to have worse profiles
  Inability to express a reason for such a choice
  Shift in values or preferences
  Expressing a preference for or against treatment that conflicts with long-standing values or previously expressed preferences
  Family members communicate that the patient is not evincing a choice that makes sense according to the patient's history

How to Make the Judgment of Incompetence

All adult patients are competent until proven otherwise. The burden of proof that the patient is not competent rests upon the physician. The general approach to assessing whether a patient lacks decision-making capacity and is not competent is to use a sliding scale concept of competency assessment.[21] The concept describes the physician's judgment about the adequacy of a patient's decision-making capacity in the context of the consequences of the various alternatives. The physician must categorize the consequences of the various alternatives. Then, given these potential consequences, the physician judges whether the patient has adequate decision-making capacity to make the decision.

With treatments that are relatively safe and likely to provide large benefits, it is reasonable to set a simple standard for assessing the decision-making capacity of a patient who agrees with this treatment. For example, agreement to receive antibiotics for an acute and reversible bacterial infection may be sufficient evidence of capacity to make a competent choice. However, the refusal of this treatment would warrant a close assessment of the patient's appreciation, reasoning, and understanding. Assessing these higher standards is not meant to challenge the patient's decision, but to assure the patient and the physician that the patient's choice respects their values. In general, a high standard should be applied when a patient refuses a high-benefit and low-risk intervention or needs to make a decision about an intervention with high risks.

As in all medical judgments, physicians can make false-positive or false-negative errors. A false-positive error describes judging that a patient is incompetent when, in fact, they are competent. In contrast, a false-negative error describes judging that a patient is competent when, in fact, the person is incompetent. These errors have unique consequences. A false-positive error causes the patient to experience a loss of autonomy, respect, and dignity that can lead to feelings of frustration and loss of control to the degree that a patient feels imprisoned. Second, this type of error threatens trust in the doctor. Third, family members and physicians who are making the decisions for the patient are often inclined to "overtreat" when compared to the preferences of patients.[22,23] This tendency increases the likelihood of iatrogenic complications and unnecessary health care costs. Fourth, it is possible that surrogate decision makers may choose to undertreat the patient. This attitude also may augment the patient's feelings of loss of respect and may result in significant harm, especially if the treatment under consideration is life sustaining and the patient dies as a result. Fifth, this error may result in unnecessary court proceedings and costly delays in treatment.

In contrast, a false-negative error undermines the principle of beneficence. This type of error increases the risk of an incoherent treatment policy. For example, patients with decisional capacity usually make medical choices that conform with personal values about the goals of their health care. When patients who have lost decisional capacity are still making decisions, this coherence is seriously threatened. Finally, false-negative errors undermine the desired societal protections afforded by surrogate decision makers.

To minimize these kinds of errors, physicians should appreciate the value of instruments that measure the patient's ability to perform each of the standards. These instruments can aid the assessment of decision-making capacity and the judgment of competency. In general, these instruments rely upon scoring a patient's answers to questions. There are two possible standards to describe what is a normal score: matching scores to the independent judgment of a clinician who is expert in assessing competency[24–27] or setting a cutoff score based on some degree of deviation from the scores of cognitively normal persons[10,12] or the scores of the subject population.[28] Instruments exist to assist in assessing a patient's ability to execute an advance directive,[11,24,28] enroll in research,[29] refuse emergent medical care,[25] and consent to hospitalization[30] or to treatment of a medical illness.[10,27] Although the value of these instruments has not been demonstrated in day-to-day clinical practice, research suggests that an instrument as simple as operationalized definitions of the standards for assessing decision-making capacity can produce moderate interrater agreement.[31] Clinicians will find these instruments particularly useful in the care of patients who face a common decision such as a geriatrician who cares for nursing home patients who need to execute an advance directive.

The value of instruments is that they can structure an assessment and limit the variability between physicians. In this way, patients are assured a fair assessment, which is particularly important because physicians have poor interrater reliability when they assess a patient's competency.[32] Another potential advantage of instruments is that the range of scores on the instrument can be correlated with scores on a brief and standardized measure of cognition. Knowing this relationship, a patient's score on a measure of cognition allows the physician to estimate the likelihood that the patient is competent. A score that falls below a cutoff signals the need to scrutinize the patient's decision-making capacity.

A final advantage of scales is that they formalize the concept of "marginal competence." The term describes the patient whose performance is impaired but not so much as to be obviously incompetent. In psychometric terms, this is the patient who lies just a few points above the cutoff of incompetence. The clinical significance of this concept is that it identifies a patent who may have limited capacity to make some decisions or who needs particular attention during follow-up care. It also identifies a patient who needs alternative or additional approaches to imparting information and trying to ensure comprehension.

What About When . . . ?

Case 1: Fluctuating Mental Status

History

A physician enters a 76-year-old female patient's room before morning rounds to obtain informed consent for a diagnostic procedure. The physician finds the patient to be somewhat confused. Her Mini-Mental State examination score is 24.

Considerations

The patient's subtle confusion is both a clinical and ethical clue of a potential problem. The patient may have a delirium and may lack decision-making capacity. The

Mini-Mental State score suggests cognitive impairment, but it is an insensitive measure of decisional capacity. An interview is required to assess both the patient's decision-making capacity and the cause of the confusion. If the physician judges that the patient lacks decision-making capacity and is not competent at this time, the nonemergency procedure should be deferred. It would be premature to proceed by obtaining proxy consent.

Case 2: Decisional Capacity for Executing an Advance Directive

History

An older person desires an advance directive. Another physician has communicated that the purpose of a directive is to avoid overtreatment and abuses by the health care "system" near the end of life. The patient states that she wants a directive to avoid any unnecessary treatment.

Considerations

Decisional capacity to choose a treatment is not the same as capacity to complete an advance directive.[33] Choosing a treatment involves a real and immediate decision in the present time. Choosing treatment in a directive is more complicated. Patients need to understand and appreciate that the choices articulated in a directive will be used in the future when they are no longer capable of participating in decision making, that some choices involve medical treatments and designating a proxy, and that their choices may change over time, and if they do, the patient should change their directive. The patient should also be able to reason through the consequences of different treatments and health states.

Case 3: Patient Refusal of Psychiatric Consultation for Evaluation of Competency

History

An older man who resides in a nursing home is refusing oral antibiotics for a lower extremity cellulitis. In preliminary discussions with the physician, he refuses to discuss his problem or the reasons for the treatment. The patient refuses to see a psychiatrist for an evaluation of his competency.

Considerations

Refusal of a minimal risk and beneficial treatment signals a need to examine decision-making capacity. The reasons for the refusal should be explored. The patient may express legitimate concerns that have nothing to do with decision-making capacity. The reasons may extend beyond the nature of the specific decision and pertain to mistrust or loss of autonomy and control in the nursing home. The patient should be informed that the use of a second opinion minimizes the risk of errors in judgment. This communication should not convey a threat; instead, it is information about options. If the patient continues to refuse the assessment, the physician should recalibrate the usual balance between competency and incompetency. Instead of the default case of favoring competency, the physician should set them in equilibrium and seek substantial evidence of decision-making capacity from sources such as caregivers.

Case 4: Depression and Treatment Refusal

History

An 88-year-old female patient involved in a home care program has long-standing depression. Multiple treatment trials have not provided appreciable benefit. She is refusing admission to the hospital for intravenous antibiotics for cellulitis of her lower extremity.

Considerations

The blanket use of a psychiatric diagnosis to determine impaired decision-making capacity is not appropriate. The physician must determine whether the diagnosis is directly affecting the patient's decision making. For example, if the patient does not have any hope, feels worthless, or cannot envision a better future, then this likely would modify their ability to rationally weigh the benefits and burdens of a recommended treatment. It would further suggest that the depression is affecting the patient's decision making and be grounds for the determination of incompetency. On the other hand, if the depression is not severe or due to its chronicity has become an authentic part of the patient's personality, then decision-making capacity might not be compromised.[34,35]

Case 5: Requesting Cardiopulmonary Resuscitation Despite Terminal Illness

History

An older patient with disseminated breast cancer has failed the previous course of chemotherapy. Her physician decides that it would be sensible for the patient to have a "Do Not Resuscitate Order" on the chart. The physician asks the patient whether she would want them to try to restart her heart after it stops. Much to the physician's surprise, the patient states that she wants cardiopulmonary resuscitation (CPR). The physician wonders whether the patient is competent.

Considerations

Many patients consider CPR to be more effective than it is. In the physician–patient interview to assess decision-making capacity, the physician should review the patient's understanding of the likelihood of successful cardiopulmonary resuscitation in their circumstances. If the patient continues to desire CPR despite the likelihood of its failure, the basis for their preference should be explored. Reliance upon hope is not evidence of impaired decision-making capacity.

How Should Physicians Assure Quality Improvement?

The determination of a patient's decision-making capacity is a linchpin to the practice of quality medicine because it promotes patient self-determination and attempts to ensure beneficent outcomes. In general, physician skills and responsibilities have not been subjected to formal quality assurance. However, studies suggest that physicians' knowledge and skills in assessing decision-making capacity and competency may be highly subjective and arbitrary.[36] Thus, physicians need mechanisms to develop their knowledge and skills to determine decision-making capacity and competency.[37]

Physicians and physicians in training have several mechanisms to ensure the quality of their skills to assess decision-making capacity. Education should focus on knowledge of the standards for assessing decision-making capacity and the skills to assess the standards and the patient's cognitive abilities and affect. Physician training of these skills should involve faculty mentoring and role modeling and expert critique from physicians such as psychiatrists. Routine clinical encounters with patients can serve as an opportunity to refresh skills in assessing decision-making capacity. Periodically, a physician should take the time to assess an evidently competent patient's decision using the methods outlined in Table 84.2.

After a physician determines that a patient has impaired decision-making capacity, if the clinical circumstances are nonemergent and the decision can be deferred, opportunities exist to improve a patient's decision-making capacity. Stopping or changing medications, repeating the assessment, or providing decision aids may improve the patient's decision-making capacity.[38] This process of managing decisional incapacity offers opportunities for quality assurance monitoring.

At the level of the hospital or nursing home, quality determinations of decision-making capacity can be ensured by clear policies that define who is responsible for these determinations, how it should be done, where the data should be documented, who should be involved if the determination is ambiguous, and how to resolve conflicting impressions by any of the stakeholders (patient, family, surrogate, physician). Policies should stress the attending physician's responsibility and participation because the determination is grounded, in part, on understanding the patient's situation, prognosis, and psychologic issues. Policies also can support witnessing the information provided in the process of informed consent.

The mistaken judgment that a patient is competent may occur when a physician discloses limited information. Audits can promote quality assurance by reviewing similar cases and situations and identifying and evaluating lack of consistency. Random audits also can ask patients about their understanding of a current or recent treatment. Little attention is given to assessing decisional capacity when a patient or family is not objecting to a recommendation. In other words, there may be unrecognized problems with determination of decisional incapacity in circumstances when all stakeholders in the decision are in agreement.[39] When this type of audit was used in a psychiatric hospital, half the respondents who assented to treatment appeared to have impaired decision-making capacity.[40] Audits that characterize problems determining decision-making capacity can serve as catalysts for educational activities.

Summary

Decision-making capacity is a central determinant of an older person's ability to direct their own care. When a patient has decision-making capacity, patient autonomy and self-determination are generally honored. Decision making occurs in light of medical recommendations, patient preferences, and professional standards. When a patient lacks decision-making capacity, however, the substituted judgment and best interests of the patient are brought to bear.[41] The risks of physical and ethical harms to the patient are substantial if a patient receives treatment without competent consent. In between these situations are patients who have difficulties making a decision but are likely competent. For these patients, assessing decision-making capacity structures the practice of effective communication and will likely reduce encounters with "difficult" or "demanding" patients.

All physicians in clinical practice should be comfortable with assessing decision-making capacity. The physician needs to remember three important considerations: (1) the purpose of assessing decision-making capacity and competency is to resolve the tension between respect for the patient's self-determination and the promotion and protection of their well-being; (2) decision-making capacity and competency both refer to a patient's ability to make a specific decision; and (3) the patient is presumed to be competent unless something triggers a question of impaired decision-making capacity.

When a decision involves choices between interventions that are relatively safe and likely provide large benefits, it is reasonable to accept a low standard of decisional capacity, such as the mere evidence of a choice. However, refusal of these interventions or a decision that involves greater than minimal risks or only marginal benefits should require a higher standard, such as requiring the patient to demonstrate understanding, appreciation, and reasoning. In general, this process will serve the interests of both the patient and physician because it fosters effective communication.

The need for a combination of clinical judgment and common sense in the determination of decision-making capacity raises the possibility of wide variations in clinical practice. Educational programs, role modeling, use of second opinions, provision of advisory feedback from ethics committees, and other quality assurance mechanisms should be implemented to minimize this occurrence.

References

1. Faden RR, Beauchamp TL. Foundations in moral theory. In: *A History and Theory of Informed Consent*. New York: Oxford University Press; 1986:3–22.
2. Appelbaum PS, Grisso T. Assessing patients' capacities to consent to treatment. *N Engl J Med*. 1988;319:1635–1638.
3. Braddock CH, Edwards KA, Hasenberg NM, Laidley TL, Levinson W. Informed decision making in outpatient practice: time to get back to basics. *JAMA*. 1999;282:2313–2320.
4. Brookmeyer R, Gray S, Kawas C. Projections of Alzheimer's disease in the United States and the impact of delaying disease onset. *Am J Public Health*. 1998;88:1337–1342.
5. Berry K, Fleming M, Manwell L, Copeland L, Appel S. Prevalence of and factors associated with current and life depression in older adult primary care patients. *Fam Med*. 1998;30:366–371.
6. Flint AJ. Epidemiology and comorbidity of anxiety disorders in the elderly. *Am J Psychiatry*. 1994;151:640–649.
7. Buchanan AE, Brock DW. *Deciding for Others: The Ethics of Surrogate Decision Making*. Cambridge: Cambridge University Press; 1989:58.
8. Grisso T, Appelbaum PS. Thinking about competence. In: *Assessing Competence to Consent to Treatment. A Guide for Physicians and Other Health Professionals*. New York: Oxford University Press; 1998:17–30.
9. White BC. Current confusion surrounding the concept of competence. In: *Competence to Consent*. Washington, DC: Georgetown University Press; 1994:44–81.
10. Marson DC, Ingram KK, Cody HA, Harrell LE. Assessing the competency of patients with Alzheimer's disease under different legal standards. *Arch Neurol*. 1995;52:949–954.
11. Fazel S, Hope T, Jacoby R. Dementia, intelligence, and the competence to complete advance directives [research letter]. *Lancet*. 1999;354:48.

12. Grisso T, Appelbaum PS. Comparison of standards for assessing patients' capacities to make treatment decisions. *Am J Psychiatry.* 1995;152:1033–1037.

13. Schmand B, Gouwenberg B, Smit JH, Jonker C. Assessment of mental competency in community-dwelling elderly. *Alzheimer Dis Assoc Disord.* 1999;13:80–87.

14. Faden RR, Beauchamp TL. The nature and degrees of competence. In: *A History and Theory of Informed Consent.* New York: Oxford University Press; 1986:288–293.

15. Grisso T, Appelbaum PS. Abilities related to competence. In: *Assessing Competence to Consent to Treatment. A Guide for Physicians and Other Health Professionals.* New York: Oxford University Press; 1998:31–60.

16. Culver C, Gert B. The inadequacy of incompetence. *Milbank Q.* 1990;68:619–643.

17. Sullivan MD, Youngner SJ. Depression, competence, and the right to refuse lifesaving medical treatment. *Am J Psychiatry.* 1994;151:971–978.

18. Searight H. Assessing patient competence for medical decision making. *Am Fam Physician.* 1992;45:751–759.

19. Folstein M, Folstein S, McHugh P. Mini-Mental State: a practical method for grading the cognitive state of patients for the clinician. *J Psychol Res.* 1975;12:189–198.

20. Alexander M. Clinical determination of mental competence: a theory and a retrospective study. *Arch Neurol.* 1988;45:23–26.

21. Beauchamp TL, Childress JF. The sliding-scale strategy. In: *Principles of Biomedical Ethics, 4th Ed.* New York: Oxford University Press; 1994:138–141.

22. Bedell S, Delbanco T. Choices about cardiopulmonary resuscitation in the hospital: when do physicians talk to patients. *N Engl J Med.* 1984;310:1089–1093.

23. Uhlmann R, Pearlman R, Cain K. Ability of physicians and spouses to predict resuscitation preferences of elderly patients. *J Gerontol.* 1988;43:M115–M121.

24. Molloy DW, Silberfeld M, Darzins P, et al. Measuring capacity to complete an advance directive. *J Am Geriatr Soc.* 1996; 44:660–664.

25. Kaufman DM, Zun L. A quantifiable, brief mental status examination for emergency patients. *J Emerg Med.* 1995; 13:449–456.

26. Bean G, Nishisato 5, Rector NA, Glancy G. The psychometric properties of the competency interview schedule. *Can J Psychiatry.* 1994;39:368–376.

27. Etchells E, Darzins P, Silberfeld M, et al. Assessment of patient competency to consent to treatment. *J Gen Intern Med.* 1999;14:27–34.

28. Mezey M, Teresi J, Ramsey G, Mitty E, Bobrowitz T. Decision-making capacity to execute a health care proxy: development and testing of guidelines. *J Am Geriatr Soc.* 2000;48:179–187.

29. Miller CK, O'Donnell DC, Searight R, Barbarash RA. The Deaconess informed consent comprehension test: an assessment tool for clinical research subjects. *Pharmacotherapy.* 1996;16:872–878.

30. Billick SB, Bella PD, et al. Competency to consent to hospitalization in the medical patient. *J Am Acad Psychiatr Law.* 1997;25:191–196.

31. Marson DC, Earnst KS, Jamil F, Bartolucci A, Harrell LE. Consistency of physicians' legal standard and personal judgments of competency in patients with Alzheimer's disease. *J Am Geriatr Soc.* 2000;48:911–918.

32. Marson DC, McInturff B, Hawkins L, Bartolucci A, Harrell LE. Consistency of physician judgments of capacity to consent in mild Alzheimer's disease. *J Am Geriatr Soc.* 1997; 45:453–457.

33. Silberfeld M, Nash C, Singer P. Capacity to complete an advance directive. *J Am Geriatr Soc.* 1993;41:1141–1143.

34. Ganzini L, Lee M, Heintz R. The effect of depression treatment on elderly patients' preferences for life-sustaining medical therapy. *Am J Psychiatry.* 1994;151:1631–1636.

35. Lee M, Ganzini L. The effect of recovery from depression on preferences for life-sustaining therapy in older patients. *J Gerontol.* 1994;49:M15–M21.

36. Markson L, Kern D, Annas G, Glantz L. Physician assessment of patient competence. *J Am Geriatr Soc.* 1994;42: 1074–1080.

37. Kutner J, Ruark J, Raffin T. Defining patient competency for medical decision making. *Chest.* 1991;100:404–409.

38. Krynski MD, Tymchuk AJ, Ouslander JG. How informed can consent be? New light on comprehension among elderly people making decisions about enteral tube feeding. *Gerontologist.* 1994;34:36–43.

39. Kapp M. Liability issues and assessment of decision-making capability in nursing home patients. *Am J Med.* 1990;89:639–642.

40. Appelbaum P, Mirkin 5, Bateman A. Empirical assessment of competency to consent to psychiatric hospitalization. *Am J Psychiatry.* 1981;138:1170–1176.

41. Karlawish JHT, Quill T, Meier DE. A consensus-based approach to practicing palliative care for patients who lack decision-making capacity. *Ann Intern Med.* 1999;130: 835–840.

85
Ethical and Policy Issues in End-of-Life Care

Melissa M. Bottrell, Christine K. Cassel, and Emily R. Felzenberg

Clinical medical ethics combines the disciplines of philosophy, behavioral science, law, and medicine to resolve moral issues and value conflicts in medicine. All physicians face ethical dilemmas, but the practice of geriatric medicine is particularly rich and ethically complex with respect to end-of-life care. Elders often face chronic illnesses for which treatments are costly or risky, have uncertain outcomes, or are unable to offer meaningful disease modification or prolongation of life.[1] The ambiguity regarding beneficial outcomes colors decisions about often difficult trade-offs between treatments that may offer potentially significant reductions in quality of life versus treatments that may not extend life but may increase comfort and thus quality of life. Decisions to change the focus of care from curative interventions to more palliative care can produce anxiety for patients and family members. Additionally, many elders may have conditions that profoundly impair communication and cognition. The result is often uncertainty about who should make health care decisions, what constitutes informed consent, and how to ascertain what decision should be made. Finally, in the broadest sense, care for elders accounts for the largest segment of health care spending, half of which comes from public programs, leading to questions about the relative value of health care compared with other goods available in the market and the value of marginally effective or futile treatments when survival is not likely to be long. Such issues pose ethical questions about intergenerational resource transfers and ultimately moral issues related to rationing of medical resources.

Approaching these difficult ethical issues requires both an awareness of how these concerns intersect the practice of geriatric medicine and a systematic approach to examine the issues. Bioethics offers numerous systematic approaches to ethical analysis of moral dilemmas, for which examples and training can be found in numerous texts.[1–3] Many of these approaches use a set of basic principles that undergird both attitudes of the public as well as personal values of physicians.[4] These principles commonly include beneficence, respect for persons, fidelity, and justice. For purposes of this chapter, discussion of issues in geriatric medicine and end-of-life care is focused through the lenses provided by these principles.

Discussion and implementation of decisions surrounding end-of-life care are critical. Attempts to improve end-of-life care often focus on enhancing the role of patients (and when appropriate, family members) as partners in the decision-making process and resolving conflicts that interfere and may even prevent health care providers from creating a good dying experience for patients and their families.[5] Using the principles of respect for persons, beneficence, fidelity, and justice together with the systematic approach offered by clinical medical ethics, the clinician can better address and resolve issues of ethical importance in end-of-life care, including understanding and appropriately managing ethical conundrums brought forth by issues of patient autonomy, withholding and withdrawing life-sustaining treatment, futility, do not resuscitate (DNR) orders, and physician-assisted suicide.

Transition Decisions: From Life-Sustaining Treatment to Palliative Management

Decisions to forgo life-sustaining treatment occur under a multitude of conditions. They can be provoked when it is decided not to resuscitate a patient with advanced dementia, to maintain a resident in a nursing home rather than transfer them to the hospital for diagnostic or treatment interventions, to replace chemotherapeutic treatments focused on curing cancer with palliative radiation, or not to administer antibiotics to a bedbound elder with severe chronic obstructive pulmonary disorder (COPD). In each case, the decision-making process must use a benefit/burden analysis comparing the benefits of treatment options against potential burdens of the treatment and potential side effects. Such decisions also take place within a larger social context such that benefit/burden analyses may differ for an older patient compared with a younger patient because of personal fears about aging and disability or stereotypes of aging.[6] Some authors claim that advanced age may give persons a different perspective on what remains of life and the so-called closing biography—suggesting greater acceptance of mortality. Yet, providers cannot assume this stance simply because of patient age and must approach each patient individually. Within that analysis, the decision-making team of patient, family, and clinical professionals must consider how to respect the patient's autonomy within their cultural context, support the family, and, to the extent possible, relieve the burden while also recognizing that some treatment courses may be futile.

Respecting Patient Autonomy

Because freedom is so central to our philosophy as a nation, it follows that autonomy is an integral part of medicine in the United States. Mechanisms to respect patient autonomy run throughout the health care endeavor, from patient education materials regarding particular treatments or diseases, to physician training in how to communicate with patients, to forms for informed consent and advance directives. These tools aim to create an environment in which it is possible for the clinician to ascertain the beliefs, perspectives, and concerns of the patient so as to focus health care decisions in a manner that enhances patient autonomy. Autonomy may also conflict with beneficence, as for example, when a patient refuses a proposed treatment despite the physician's best recommendation. Further, in this multicultural nation, not all individuals or families expect to express their autonomy in medical decisions in the manner most typically expected in legal contexts, especially when making the emotionally and technically fraught decisions at the end of life.

Advance Directives

The practical difficulties and ethical dilemmas surrounding patient autonomy can be most obviously seen through examination of advance directives. In the United States, estimates of the percentage of persons who have executed advance directives range from 4% to 20%. Highly educated Caucasians are generally more receptive than other groups to advance directives and tend to forgo life-sustaining treatment at a higher greater rate. Those who are poor and nonwhite, particularly Hispanics and blacks, may feel apprehensive about treatment limitation because they already feel that they have restricted access to care, and thus are hesitant to give the health care system an additional reason to withhold care.[7] Further, elders commonly do not complete an advance directive because they feel they can rely on others, in particular, their families, to make decisions for them, and, in fact, expect family members to help make complex health care decisions. Thus, for many elders, the particularly Western view of autonomy that stems from the individual and is expressed through a legal document does not apply to their expression of autonomy.

For these elders, respect for persons may flow from a broader family perspective that includes considerations of family burdens of care or expectations that a particular family member (i.e., a son or daughter) is the appropriate decision maker.[8] When an elder is cared for by family at home or is a longtime nursing home resident, specialized knowledge of the patient that comes from being surrounded by family members and clinicians who know the patient further helps to ensure that the patient's vision of autonomy is supported. In practice, however, modern medical practice often involves myriad transitions between settings, through which neither the knowledge of the patient nor explicit directives about the patient's end-of-life care preferences through advance directives are transferred.

Inconsistencies in care between settings often result from the patient's inability to communicate, lack of uniformity in advance directives or advance directive policies, fear of liability on the part of the institution, physician, and other health care providers, and absence of an advance directive. Even when advance directives exist and are accessible, they have limitations because the language is often ambiguous or lacks specific directions for the situation at hand. In unclear situations of patient preferences, nursing home staff may transfer residents to hospitals, and emergency medical technicians (EMTs) may administer cardiopulmonary resuscitation (CPR), although this may be contrary to patient wishes. A number of strategies are available to combat the lack of continuity of care and breaches of support for patient autonomy. Physicians should encourage patients to designate a specific health care proxy or surrogate who, depending on state law, can be empowered to speak for the patient when the patient is unable to do so. Further, improved communication between health care professionals and institutions is necessary. For example, hospital physicians and other clinicians should meet staff in nursing homes that regularly admit patients to their service. Doing so could provide contacts to which the clinician could turn when context is missing regarding the preferences or concerns of a particular patient or family and thus provide alternatives means by which to clarify patient's wishes.

As another approach, Oregon developed the Physician Orders for Life-Sustaining Treatment (POLST), a comprehensive, one-page order form to convey preferences for life-sustaining treatments during patient transfer from one care setting to another. The form specifies four categories of care, including (1) do not resuscitate (DNR) orders, (2) comfort care, (3) antibiotic use, and (4) tube feeding.[9] Studies show use of the POLST leads to consistent respect for patient preferences to limit life-sustaining interventions.[9,10] The POLST attempts to overcome problems regarding lack of availability of advance directives, failure to comply with the patient's DNR order because the patient's wishes are not known, and physician fear in signing DNR orders because care may be compromised or cannot be implemented without translation into a physician's order.

A high degree of respect for patient wishes is implied in the POLST. Several features contribute to the form's effectiveness and consistency, including its statewide standardization, the pink color that makes it hard to ignore, easily locatable and clearly stated orders, acceptable and understandable language about the orders, and language specific to comfort care for pain and suffering. Specifically, the POLST, unlike an advance directive, limits specific treatments according to patient wishes and concurrently implements the preferences by putting them into the form of physician orders. The POLST offers a promising way to ensure patient end-of-life treatment preferences are respected.

In addition to the POLST, several state legislatures are considering policies allowing EMTs to accept DNR (do not resuscitate) orders of patients being transferred to hospitals, hospitals are honoring advance registration of DNR orders to ensure compliance of out-of hospital DNR orders (i.e., those written in nursing homes), and advocates are supporting wallet cards, bracelets, or other forms of DNR order identification to increase compliance with patient wishes.

Withholding or Withdrawing Life-Sustaining Treatment

Although patient preferences as expressed in advance directives may provide an outline of how to approach a patient's care, at some point, decisions about treatment plans include hard choices of more than simply adding comfort care but also whether to withhold or withdraw life-sustaining interventions. Patients have a right to refuse treatment even if it is life sustaining.[4] Withholding life support is defined as not providing a patient with medical interventions, such as CPR—the procedure most frequently withheld. Withdrawing life support is defined as removing previously initiated medical interventions, such as mechanical ventilation—the procedure most fre-

quently withdrawn.[11] In the clinical setting, definitional distinctions between withholding and withdrawing are often made. In some cases, it may seem morally and conceptually easier to withhold a particular procedure, such as mechanical ventilation when the outcome of beginning the procedure is less certain, than to withdraw treatment, because although a treatment may not provide meaningful outcomes, treatment withdrawal would result in death. Moreover, the timing of decisions often makes the distinctions between withdrawal and withholding seem relevant. Withholding can occur relatively suddenly if the patient goes into cardiac arrest. Withdrawing is often a gradual process and may involve administering analgesics and sedatives to the patient while removing a treatment. In practice, withdrawing is documented more frequently than withholding.[11,12]

Physicians often become morally, legally, and even psychologically committed to a treatment's completion, once started,[12] especially when the patient has been receiving the intervention for a long time. Thus, intervention withdrawal tends to occur more commonly for treatments that are invasive, expensive, scarce, or lead to a quick death once withdrawn, and tends to occur less often when treatments have been in place for a period of time or for the management of iatrogenic complications.[13] Physicians may be "committed" to the ventilation or dialysis support that they initiated, even though the treatment fails to clearly benefit the patient. Treatment continuation may even cause patients to receive unwanted treatments despite their ethical and legal rights or that of their surrogates to refuse life-prolonging interventions. Health care professionals, including physicians and nurses, often lack training with regard to the clinical aspects of withdrawing intensive life-sustaining treatment, such as palliation of dyspnea. Such skills are necessary to provide effective end-of-life care.

Despite the common use of the terms in practice, the definitional distinction between withholding and withdrawing lacks logical validity and moral relevance. All treatment decisions contain some of the elements of a withhold or withdrawal decision—the morally and legally relevant distinction between treatment decisions is that, irrespective of whether a life-sustaining treatment was withheld or withdrawn, the outcome is the patient's death. The patient's right to remove or not initiate life-sustaining treatments has both a moral and a legal grounding.

Legal Protections for Patient Autonomy

The legal basis for respecting patient decisions at the end of life stems from a variety of sources—most famously from two cases that involved the withdrawal of life support. Karen Ann Quinlan and Nancy Cruzan were young women in persistent vegetative states whose families wished to have their life support removed. In *Quinlan*, the New Jersey Supreme Court recognized the right to withdraw medical interventions from an incompetent patient in accordance with the family's belief that the patient would have wanted treatment withdrawn.[12,14] In *Cruzan*, the U.S. Supreme Court affirmed the right to withdraw artificial life-sustaining treatments once the incompetent patient's wishes are known with relative confidence.[12,14] Many similar cases involve elderly people who lacked capacity because of dementia and in which the family sought to limit life-sustaining interventions. With very few exceptions, the cases all were upheld so long as the decision to limit treatment was consistent with the patient's values. Philosophically, because the state has an interest in protecting and ensuring the continued life of its citizens, these cases validate the state's legal interest and right in interpreting an individual's preference, including those who are incompetent, to forgo life-sustaining treatment.[12]

Artificial Nutrition and Hydration

Within the context of decisions to withdraw or withhold care, decisions regarding forgoing artificial nutrition and hydration often raise special concerns. Legally, intravenous lines or tubes are considered medical procedures and thus are subject to the same benefit to burden analysis as any other technical intervention, such as dialysis or mechanical ventilation; surrogates and patients have the right to refuse them as with any medical treatments.[15] At the same time, providing food and water is felt by some to be a moral duty and an essential form of supportive care.[16] The idea of food and water is also emotionally comforting to a family in their caring for a dying patient.[4] Decisions to forgo nutrition and hydration typically commonly concern patients with moderate to severe loss of cognitive function due to Alzheimer's disease or dementia, strokes resulting in loss of ability to swallow, end-stage diseases (e.g., metastatic cancer), end-stage organ failure, and treatment complications (e.g., infection, aspiration pneumonia).[4] Such situations, in which a family already carries a heavy emotional burden, are only made worse by the emotional feelings often connected to food and water.

However, the eating process is a human contact quite different from intravenous, gastrostomy, or jejunostomy feedings. Continued intervention may result in fluid overload and significant discomfort whereas death after withdrawal may be more comfortable. Therefore, understanding and evaluating the reasons offered to forgo artificial hydration and nutrition and thus withhold or withdraw life-sustaining treatment are essential to pro-

viding effective end-of-life care. Clinicians, patients and family members must consider when artificial nutrition and hydration may prolong dying and patient suffering, acknowledge that these treatments may lead to poor quality of life, and thus make the more humane choice to allow the patient to die.

Do Not Resuscitate Orders

DNR (do not resuscitate) orders are recommended for most terminally ill patients[17] and so require consideration in end-of-life care. People of very advanced age or with multiple advanced chronic illnesses who suffer an unwitnessed, out-of-hospital, cardiac arrest have restorative success approaching zero. Even for witnessed arrests, a return to earlier functioning is unlikely, making the success rate of CPR administered in nursing homes 0% to 5%.[9] A DNR orders clinicians to not pursue efforts to restore cardiac function if the heart stops beating or lungs stop functioning.[17] For patients with primary lung disease, patients may also elect to forgo intubation and mechanical ventilation because it is painful and unlikely to lead to a return to an acceptable quality of life. For these patients, cardiac arrest may be reversed with a quick attempt at resuscitation, such as defibrillation, but the patient may want a DNI (do not intubate) order. For patients with very end stage disease, a DNR/DNI order covers both.

The DNR order does not exclude or prohibit use of other medically suitable interventions. As with other medical decisions to forgo life-sustaining treatment, deciding whether to administer CPR requires evaluation of the ethical considerations such as the potential likelihood of clinical benefit and the patient's preferences. Unlike most medical treatments, however, a presumption in favor of sustaining life exists legally, ethically, and medically, making CPR the correct course of treatment unless a DNR order is in place, or unless the treatment is refused or deemed medically futile. Unlike many treatments, CPR does not require a physician's order but does require a contrary order in the form of a DNR order to withhold it. It is the only medical treatment of this sort, because success depends on immediate response.[1]

Because current policy dictates CPR be attempted for every patient in cardiac arrest who does not have a DNR order, CPR raises unique challenges with regard to decisions to forgo life-sustaining treatments. First, a CPR decision is conditional, depending on whether cardiac arrest actually occurs within a health care setting. Further, the success of CPR depends on factors such as how quickly it is administered after cardiac arrest, the skill of the resuscitation providers, access to a cardiac monitor, the patient's general health and well-being, and the underlying medical conditions. Although CPR may restore life with effective circulation after a cardiac arrest in some patients, CPR is often unsuccessful in patients with advanced disease and contravenes the concept of a gentle or dignified death.

With DNR orders, as for other medical interventions, informed choices are required and must be based on clear information about the benefits, risks, and alternatives available to the patient. In practice, many elders have mistaken perceptions of the effectiveness of CPR as well as mistaken understandings of the procedure based on television or popular media. Some studies have shown that when elders are fully informed about the low probability of restorative success and the actual steps that occur in CPR, such as chest compression and the potential for cracked ribs in frail elders, they opt for DNR status over CPR.[18] Yet, clinicians often fail to comprehensively discuss CPR.[18] Fully informed communication about end-of-life care options must include comprehensive discussion of CPR, other medical interventions, and palliative care options. Recommendations about CPR should be clear and definitive so the patient or surrogate, their families, and other health care providers (such as nursing home nurse aides) understand the decision and have the opportunity to ask questions. To the extent possible, a DNR decision should be made with the support and assistance of the geriatric care team as well as family members to stave off potential conflicts at the last moment. The DNR order must reflect the patient's preferences, values, and beliefs and be careful not to impose the physician's value judgments or the surrogate's wishes. Finally, consulting with social workers, spiritual guidance counselors, or ethics committees can support sound and just decisions and ensures that the patient's wishes are respected.[19]

Futility

Decisions to withhold or withdraw care may be prompted not only by desires to focus on quality of life but also by recognition that some treatments may be futile. Considerations of treatment futility may be more common in geriatrics because older people have limited life expectancies.[20] In terms of justice, ethicists argue that physicians have a responsibility to avoid harm to patients that may result from providing futile treatment, as well as larger social concerns that providing futile treatments limits the availability of scarce resources for use by others for whom treatments would be effective. If futility were a straightforward empirical assessment, many end-of-life decisions could be easier. Many authors have thus examined the concept and proposed decision criteria. Unfortunately, although some futility judgments are justified, applying the concept in practice may not be an appropriate tactic because futility judgments are often fraught

with "confusion, inconsistency and controversy."[1] Nevertheless, the concept is worthy of discussion because the term and the concerns about futile treatments often inform considerations about end-of-life care in the elderly.

Strict and Loose Definitions of Futility

Strict definitions of futility, which could be applied to fairly and uniformly guide decisions to withhold or withdraw life-sustaining treatments, are based on objective criteria and the medical expertise of physicians.[1] Lo proposed three strict criteria, which include the following. (1) *The treatment lacks a pathophysiologic basis*—no ethical or legal justifications can be offered to continue treatment when there is no physiologic benefit for the patient. (2) *Despite maximal treatment, cardiac arrest occurs*—when optimal therapy fails, treatment is medically futile to continue. For example, CPR is ineffective when it would fail to effectively restore circulation to a patient in cardiopulmonary arrest. (3) *When the treatment has already failed for the patient, it is deemed futile and lacks a medical, ethical, or legal reason to continue repeating failed interventions.* For example, the patient does not respond to CPR and remains asystolic even 30 min after CPR was initiated.

Lo also offered four looser definitions for futility that could be applied to end-of-life care for elders. (1) *A small probability of success exists with the treatment.*[1] The difficulty is determining an appropriate cutoff point (i.e., 1% versus 5%) for futility in this probabilistic approach. Even if a quantitative threshold is stated, disagreement between patients and their surrogates may result because no single probability can be applied to define an unacceptable risk in every potential set of circumstances. In addition, although a probability may be small, it still may be considered worthwhile. The concern then becomes how to measure a small probability of survival, especially as data regarding effectiveness of clinical interventions in elders and especially the oldest-old are often unavailable.

(2) Physicians do not believe the treatment will succeed in achieving any desired goals.[1] This determination raises controversial value judgments. Patients or family members may desire treatment to achieve nonmedical, short-term goals, such as allowing family from far distances to see the patient before death. In such circumstances, physicians may have a moral duty to act with compassion and sustain life despite the lack of a legal duty to do so. Experts generally agree that patients should be informed in a comforting matter if even a small chance of success exists because of the need to support fully autonomous decision making on the part of patients or health care proxies. This definition of futility, however, can be used to guide treatment choices for patients when

palliative care becomes the most humane treatment approach.[6]

(3) The patient's quality of life is not acceptable.[1] Treatments may be termed futile when patients, family members, or clinicians judge the patient's quality of life unacceptable, such as when the patient is permanently unconscious and will never regain cognitive functioning. However, use of this definition by physicians exclusively to guide end-of-life decision making runs the risk of paternalistically imposing the physician's values upon patients. Advocates for the disabled and other vulnerable populations, such as the elderly, oppose the quality of life criterion suggestions as being discriminatory and disguised value judgments about the value of the lives of those less able bodied. Moreover, competent elderly patients, having learned to cope with chronic illness and find ways to enjoy life, tend to more highly regard their own quality of life than their family does. Patients with Alzheimer's disease who are incompetent and cannot communicate, but who do not appear to be suffering, create complex quality of life judgments for their family and physician.[1]

(4) The expected efforts and resources required outweigh prospective benefits.[1] The issue is whether the benefits to the patient are worth the costs to society as a whole. This consideration recognizes arguments about rationing in which cost rather than benefit becomes the deciding factor and in which treating patients with poor prognoses of survival may deny treatment to other patients with better prognoses.[21] Use of this criterion may appear to have an objective basis, but moral implications implicit in the definition make it a poor definition to use for final determination of when treatments should or should not be applied for particular patients.

The difficulties inherent in each and every one of the strict and loose definitions and the disagreement among physicians that persist in its application to patient care means that futility, at this time, is only one of many points to consider in making decisions for patients at the end of life. The principle of beneficence speaks to the physician's obligation to do what is best for the patient. Beneficent care requires attention to technical expertise as well as compassionate care, and allows for greater leniency in the physician's response to patient or surrogate requests for interventions decided to be futile, especially when death is imminent. In geriatrics, adequate knowledge of clinical medicine and biomedical science is as important as a caring approach to the patient.

In practice, physicians who are concerned that they are being asked to support futile treatment should focus on ongoing communication, consultation with ethics committees, and second opinions from colleagues to help minimize potential mistakes in futility judgments, keep value judgments in check, and simultaneously protect the professional and moral integrity of physicians and patient

autonomy. Keeping the patient informed and discussing the intervention's futility with the patient or surrogate is an important ethical and legal obligation and the best approach. Such discussions are usually beneficial to patients or surrogates and reinforce the principles of care, including respect for patients. Most patients or surrogates will eventually support the physician's judgment[1] and appreciate unambiguous and compassionate communications and recommendations.

Euthanasia and Physician-Assisted Suicide

In the broadest sense, euthanasia, physician-assisted suicide (PAS) and decisions to withhold or withdraw life-sustaining treatment share common objectives such as relief of pain and suffering and respect for patient autonomy. The importance of these issues in end-of-life care for elders is highlighted by ethical, legal, political, and societal trends that frame the debate, along with religious and philosophical beliefs.[22,23]

Active euthanasia, also called mercy killing, causes death and ends suffering by intentionally administering medication directly to end the patient's life.[17] Euthanasia is generally categorized in three ways: that is, voluntary when a patient requests it, involuntary when a patient expresses opposition, and nonvoluntary when a patient has lost capacity and cannot make decisions or express his or her wishes.[1,23] Involuntary euthanasia, although practiced in the form of lethal injections for death row inmates, is always immoral if considered as part of a health care plan. As respect for patient autonomy is potentially the only acceptable justification for active assistance in dying, nonvoluntary euthanasia is not an acceptable practice.[1]

The fine distinction between euthanasia and physician-assisted suicide involves the physician providing to the patient a lethal dose of medication, on the patient's request, with the intent to allow the patient to end his or her own life.[17] The patient independently must perform the final act. Physician assistance in dying may range from providing the patient with information about committing suicide to prescribing medication. Because the patient must carry out the deed, concerns about compelling a patient against his or her wishes and abusing the powers associated with being a physician and the physician's role are lessened, although still a potential consideration. Still, being relieved of the moral responsibility for the suicidal act does not relieve the physician of further moral responsibility in physician-assisted suicide. Each situation necessitates careful consideration of the intent, motivation, justification, and results of the decision. Again, as with most end-of-life decisions, discussion with the patient and his or her family is critical and allows for more effective and meaningful palliative care practices.[1]

In practice, a physician is not, however, assisting with suicide if the physician is providing treatments to relieve pain and suffering even if the patient's death might be hastened.[17] In such circumstances, the underlying illness, not the treatment provided or withheld, is the cause of the patient's death. The distinction between "killing" in the sense of euthanasia or PAS versus "allowing to die" in the sense of withholding or withdrawing care, or providing high doses of narcotics or sedatives to relieve pain but that also may result in patient death, is useful in practice. However, many philosophers consider the distinction problematic. These authors find the distinction between "killing" and "letting die" to not be a sound basis for moral judgment. Second, the idea that the disease causes the patient's death rather than the withholding/withdrawing of treatment may not be tenable because death may not have occurred in the absence of this factor. Third, assisted suicide and letting die cannot be distinguished by the intent of the patient. A patient who is refusing treatments and who has had adequate informed consent also recognizes death as an outcome and thus the distinction lacks moral weight. Conversely, the U.S. Supreme Court has held that there is a rational distinction between killing and letting die,[24,25] and that those who ask their doctors to commit assisted suicide and those who forgo treatment are not similarly situated.[26]

Concerns about active euthanasia and assisted suicide should not make physicians reluctant to relieve distressful symptoms in terminally ill patients. Indeed, fears that terminal distress will not be adequately relieved impel some people to seek active euthanasia and assisted suicide. Physicians should continue to partner with patients and families to ensure that patients are fully informed of consequences and feel more assured that they will not be abandoned when the plan of care moves from curative to palliative.

Physician-Assisted Suicide and Conflict with the Physician's Role

Physician-assisted suicide and euthanasia cause conflicts for the physician's healing role, because, traditionally, a physician has a duty to preserve life.[1] Arguments against physician-assisted suicide emphasize the sanctity of life,[1] debate the passive (e.g., withholding treatment) versus active (e.g., physician-assisted suicide) killing distinction, discussed earlier, and examine the potentials for abuse, especially with vulnerable populations.[1,25,27] Other authors argue that the physician's professional ethics and integrity may be jeopardized by performing PAS.[25,27] The trust in the physician–patient relationship

could be breached, and patients may forgo seeking a physician's care. Lack of diligence in ensuring that the patient's requests are voluntary and that the appropriate patient receives physician-assisted suicide,[1] as well as inevitable mistakes,[25] are additional concerns. Important, but often inarticulated, are the religious beliefs of ethicists and policymakers on this issue. Respect for religious freedom requires allowing individual choice even if it conflicts with one's own values.

Justifying Physician-Assisted Suicide

Arguments in favor of physician-assisted suicide focus on showing respect for individual autonomy,[1] recognizing the right of competent people to choose the course of their life and death, the importance of comfort and relief of suffering, and a justice argument for treating "like cases alike." If competent, terminally ill patients can refuse treatment and thus hasten death, suicide becomes the only option for patients when treatment refusal will not suffice to hasten death. Physician-assisted suicide then serves as a compassionate alternative to unbearable suffering, because physical and emotional suffering cannot always be relieved.[1] Although society has a strong interest in preserving life, that interest may diminish when a person is terminally ill and has reached his or her "closing biography," has said good-bye to family, and wishes to exit "on his or her own terms," usually described as death with dignity, Personal liberty is limited when there is a complete prohibition on assisted death, warranting the allowance of physician-assisted suicide in certain cases. In circumstances where suicide would happen with or without assistance, PAS allows a more humane and controlled method of end-of-life decision making.[1] Religious tolerance requires respect for personal objections to all killing, but religious tolerance also requires us to respect those whose beliefs support a right to end their own lives, especially in the context of intractable suffering and ultimately terminal illness. The political debates in numerous states and in the U.S. Congress demonstrate the depth of feeling on both sides.

Legal Issues and Physician-Assisted Suicide

Voluntary euthanasia and physician-assisted suicide have been openly condoned in the Netherlands for more than 10 years. Although critics argue that abuses occur, such as euthanasia of disabled infants and elderly persons with dementia, popular support in the Netherlands remains high. In the United States, Oregon has legalized a very limited form of PAS. The U.S. Supreme Court has unanimously ruled that no constitutional right to physician-assisted suicide exists. Statutes prohibiting physicians from providing lethal medication for use by competent, terminally ill patients do not violate the Due Process or Equal Protection Clauses of the Constitution. The Court found no fundamental liberty interest in committing physician-assisted suicide, protected by the Due Process Clause of the 14th Amendment.[24,25,27] The Court also implied a right to adequate palliative care and held state laws constitutionally valid in distinguishing between prohibiting intentional acts to hasten death and permitting acts to relieve pain while unintentionally hastening death. States considering legalization of PAS are required to ensure palliative care is adequate and effectively implemented.[24]

Safeguards and Guidelines for Performance of PAS

Consideration of legalized PAS must include guidelines to balance a humane response to a patient's individual values with providing adequate protection to vulnerable populations. Such guidelines must clarify that a tolerable death and well-controlled pain and suffering should result from comfort care.[28] Thus, physician-assisted suicide is only acceptable for terminally ill patients with incurable conditions whose illnesses are accompanied by severe pain and unrelenting suffering. Adequate palliative care must be provided. The patient's decision must be voluntary and informed, and asking for assistance in dying must be a continuous, clear, and convincing request to end suffering. The patient's ability to make sound decisions must be demonstrated, including identification and treatment of depression. The doctor–patient relationship should have been maintained over a period of time and be meaningful to best understand the patient's desire for physician-assisted suicide. More than one physician should evaluate the patient to confirm that the choice is voluntary, informed, and rationally reached. The concept of such careful guidelines lies behind Oregon's legalizing a narrowly defined form of the practice.[28]

Physician-Assisted Suicide in Oregon

Physician-assisted suicide became an option for terminally ill patients in Oregon with the passage of Oregon's Death with Dignity Act. A terminally ill person can request a prescription to end his or her life if he or she qualifies under the law's requirements.[29] Because care for terminally ill patients is also considered the purview of hospice care, however, conflicts between hospice care philosophy and physician-assisted suicide continue to be the subject of debate.[30] In the first 2 years after the Supreme Court upheld the law, 56 persons received pre-scriptions for a lethal dose. Of those 56, 43 died of the lethal dose, 11 died of the underlying disease, and 2 remained alive as of January 2000.[31] Requesters were, on average, in their early seventies, and cancer was the most common illness. Patients expressed concern over inadequate pain control, losing autonomy due to illness, and losing control over bodily functions. The number of requesters remains small and has not resulted in an overwhelming rise in physician-assisted suicide, as initially anticipated and feared. Moreover, in some local communities, fears that clinicians would be faced with requests for PAS have prompted regional improvements in pain management and other end-of-life care services.[32]

Physician-Assisted Suicide and the Elderly

As life expectancy grows, many older people face years of isolation and decline. Some may want to assert a right to a dignified death on their own terms, making PAS an option. This phenomenon may be responsible for the increase in suicide rates among elderly men in the United States. On the other hand, abuses could occur in this vulnerable population. Pressure could result, including influencing elderly people to choose physician-assisted suicide rather than more expensive palliative care options. Families may choose physician-assisted suicide to relieve caregiving burdens and even encourage physicians to impose value judgments in quality of life on the patient or surrogate.

In one study comparing attitudes of elderly outpatients and their families toward PAS, family members held more favorable attitudes toward PAS than patients in cases of terminal illness (59.3% versus 39.9%), in cases of chronic illness (25.3% versus 18.2%), and in cases of mental incompetence (55.6% versus 34.0%).[33] Moreover, family members poorly predicted patient attitudes toward PAS. Thus, focusing on the patient's interests rather than family preferences or a physician's moral judgments becomes an important direction and goal for end-of-life care decisions.

Conclusion

The particular ethical quandaries posed by geriatric care at the end of life require that physicians, patients, and families candidly discuss and consider end-of-life care. Decisions to withhold and or withdraw life-sustaining treatment are grounded in respect for patient autonomy, beneficence, and considerations of medical futility. Artificial nutrition and hydration and DNR orders pose particular concerns but can be managed by partnering with patients in their care. Physician-assisted suicide may be a final option for some patients in some states but should be approached with awareness of important guidelines for protecting patients against potential abuses. Even without formal ethics training, the practitioner who cares for elders daily manages personal dilemmas brought about by the sensitive issues inherent in end-of-life care. By applying the principles of medical ethics to the thoughtful care of older adults, geriatricians can set an example in the care of patients with difficult ethical problems generally and in end-of-life care specifically.

References

1. Lo B. *Resolving Ethical Dilemmas: A Guide for Clinicians.* Baltimore: Williams & Wilkins; 1995.
2. Purtillo R. *Ethical Dimensions in the Health Professions, 2nd Ed.* Philadelphia: Saunders; 1993.
3. Jonsen AR, Siegler M, Winslade WJ. *Clinical Ethics.* New York: McGraw-Hill; 1998.
4. Ackerman RJ. Withholding and withdrawing life-sustaining treatment. *Am Fam Physician.* 2000;62(7):1555–1560.
5. Basile CM. Advance directives and advocacy in end-of-life decisions. *Nurse Pract.* 1998;23(5):44–60.
6. Cassel CK. Philosophical and ethical issues in geriatrics. In: Kelley WN, ed. *Textbook of Internal Medicine, 4th Ed.* Philadelphia: Lippincott Williams & Wilkins; 2000:3127–3131.
7. Culigari AM, Miller T, Sobol J. Race and health care: an American dilemma? *N Engl J Med.* 1996;155:1893–1898.
8. Wolf SM, ed. *Feminism and Bioethics: Beyond Reproduction.* New York: Oxford University Press; 1996.
9. Tolle S, Tilden VP, Nelson CA, Dunn PM. A prospective study of the efficacy of the physician order form for life-sustaining treatment. *J Am Geriatr Soc.* 1998;46(9):1097–1102.
10. Lee MA, Brummel-Smith K, Meyer J, Drew N, London MR. Physician orders for life-sustaining treatment (POLST): outcomes in a PACE program. *J Am Geriatr Soc.* 2000;48(10):1219–1225.
11. Luce JM. Withholding and withdrawal of life support: ethical, legal, and clinical aspects. *New Horiz.* 1997;5(1):30–37.
12. Ahronheim JC, Moreno J, Zuckerman C. *Ethics in Clinical Practice, 1st Ed.* Boston: Little, Brown, 1994.
13. Brody H, Campbell ML, Faber-Langendon J, Ogle KS. Withdrawing intensive life-sustaining treatment—recommendations for compassionate clinical management. *N Engl J Med.* 1997;336(9):652–657.
14. *In Re.* Quinlan. 70 N.J. 10. 355. A.2d 647: N.J., 1976.
15. Annas GJ, Law SA, Rosenblatt RE, Wing KR. *American Health Law.* Boston: Little, Brown; 1990.
16. Pearlman RA, Back AL. Ethical issues in geriatric care. In: Hazzard WR, Blass JP, eds. *Principles of Geriatric Medicine and Gerontology, vol 40, 4th Ed.* New York: McGraw-Hill; 1999:557–570.
17. Basta LL. *A Graceful Exit: Life and Death on Your Own Terms.* New York: Plenum Press; 1996.
18. Levin JR, Wenger NS, Ouslander JG, et al. Life-sustaining treatment decisions for nursing home residents: who discusses, who decides and what is decided? *J Am Geriatr Soci.* 1999;47(1):82–87.
19. Agich GJ, Arroliga AC. Appropriate use of DNR orders: a practical approach. *Clevel Clin J Med.* 2000;67(6):392–400.
20. van der Steen JT, Muller MT, Ooms ME, van der Wal G, Ribbe MW. Decisions to treat or not to treat pneumonia in demented psychogeriatric nursing home patients: development of a guideline. *J Med Ethics.* 2000;26(2):114–120.
21. Schneiderman LJ, Jecker JS, Jonsen AR. Medical futility: its meaning and ethical implications. *Ann Intern Med.* 1990;112:949–954.
22. Scanlon C. Assisted suicide: the wrong answer. *Home Care Provider.* 1997;2(4):159–161.
23. Young EWD. Physician-assisted suicide: where to draw the line. *Camb Q Healthcare Ethics.* 2000;9:407–410.
24. Burt RA. The Supreme Court Speaks—not assisted suicide but a constitutional right to palliative care. *N Eng J Med.* 1997;337(17):1234–1236.
25. Annas GJ. The bell tolls for a constitutional right to physician-assisted suicide. *N Eng J Med.* 1997;337(15):1098–1103.
26. Sulmasy DP, Ury WA, Ahronheim JC, et al. Publication of papers on assisted suicide and terminal sedation. *Ann Intern Med.* 2000;133(7):564–566.
27. Gostin LO. Deciding life and death in the courtroom. From Quinlan to Cruzan, Gluksberg, and Vacco—a brief history and analysis of consitutional protection of the "right to die." *JAMA.* 1997;278(18):1523–1528.
28. Quill TE, Cassel CK, Meier DE. Care of the hopelessly ill: proposed clinical criteria for physician assisted suicide. *N Engl J Med.* 1992;327:1380–1384.
29. Miller PJ. Life after death with dignity: the Oregon experience. *Soc Work.* 2000;45(3):263–271.
30. Mesler MA, Miller PJ. Hospice and assisted suicide: the structure and process of an inherent dilemma. *Death Studies.* 2000;24(2):135–155.
31. Roscoe LA, Malphurs JE, Dragovic LJ, Cohen D. A comparison of characteristics of Kevorkian euthanasia cases and physician assisted suicide cases in Oregon. *Gerontologist.* 2001;41(4):439–446.
32. Mezey MD, Mezey, Mathy D. Oregon Pain Practice Improvement Cluster Initiative. [e-mail to Melissa M. Bottrell, melissa.bottrell@nyu.edu]. 1 July 2001.
33. Koenig HG, Wildman-Hanlon D, Schmader K. Attitudes of elderly patients and their families toward physician assisted suicide. *Arch Intern Med.* 1996;156(19):2240–2248.

86
Ethical Challenges to Research in Geriatric Medicine

Greg A. Sachs and Harvey Jay Cohen

For many years, one of the main items on the agenda of advocates for improved health care for older people has been the promotion of research on the medical problems that affect the elderly. Until the 1980s, it was quite common for people over age 65 to be excluded from clinical trials, even from studies of disease that disproportionately affect the elderly, such as heart disease and cancer. Many clinical problems of older people received little or no research funding. Clearly, great strides have been made in the past two decades. There is a National Institute of Aging at the National Institutes of Health, geriatric medicine fellowships train investigators in research around the country, journals specializing in geriatric medicine and gerontology are flourishing, general medical journals abound with articles related to the care of the elderly, and clinical trials include older subjects, many even focusing specifically on older adults. Yet, as research involving older human subjects has gone forward, many important ethical challenges to the conduct of this research have either emerged or resurfaced.

In this chapter, we discuss three main aspects of the ethical challenges to research in geriatrics. First, we briefly review the principles of research ethics of the past 50 years as applied to human subjects of all ages. Second, we highlight the ways in which geriatric research presents special challenges. Third, we discuss the most recent developments and controversies in research ethics, many of which challenge the traditional model of research ethics.

Historical Overview

Discussions of the ethics of research involving human subjects for at least the first 40 years following World War II were dominated by concerns about informed consent. This attitude is not surprising, given that, starting with the Nazi experiments on concentration camp prisoners, many of the most egregious abuses of research subjects and most ethically suspect research involved either non-consenting or uninformed subjects. Table 86.1 lists some of the most important of these troubling cases, as well as many of the international and U.S. responses in terms of guidelines and regulations for the ethical conduct of research involving human subjects. It is worth noting that the amount of activity in the last few years, especially with respect to federal oversight and both proposed and actual regulatory action, is greater than at any time since the development of the U.S. research oversight structures in the 1970s. We address many of these regulatory developments in the final sections of this chapter.

In the United States, much of the current institutional review board (IRB) apparatus and attention to informed consent and consent forms flows from federal regulations that were adopted following the reports of the National Commission for the Protection of Human Subjects of Biomedical and Behavioral Research (the National Commission).[1] Although formulating standards relating to informed consent was an important part of the work of the National Commission, it is important to recognize (as the National Commission did) that many other ethical principles need to be addressed when evaluating research.[2] First, informed consent is not a primary level ethics principle, per se. The fundamental principle that gives rise to the attention on informed consent is the principle of respect for persons. This principle, as stated by the philosopher Immanuel Kant, requires treating people as ends rather than as means to an end. To some extent, researchers use their subjects as a means rather than an end, as a means to obtain an answer to their research question. Using people in this fashion becomes ethically permissible only when the individuals are autonomous ("capable of deliberation about personal goals and of acting under the direction of such deliberation") and they give their competent, voluntary, informed, and comprehending consent or permission to be used in this fashion. Another equally important ethical conviction found by

TABLE 86.1. Important events in ethics and regulation of research: 1945–2000.

1945: Uncovering of details of Nazi war crimes, including experimentation on prisoners

1949: Nuremberg Code on medical experimentation

1964: Helsinki Declaration of the World Medical Association on biomedical research involving human subjects

1966: Henry Beecher *New England Journal of Medicine* paper on "unethical or questionably ethical procedures" in the research literature

1972: Story of the Tuskegee Syphilis Study breaks

1974: Federal regulations on research published (45 CFR 46); National Commission for the Protection of Human Subjects of Biomedical and Behavioral Research established

1978: Belmont Report (and other U.S. guidelines and regulations emanating from the work of the National Commission)

1980: President's Commission for the Study of Ethical Problems in Medicine and Biomedical and Behavioral Research formed; worked through 1983

1995: Advisory Committee on Human Radiation Experiments Final Report; National Bioethics Advisory Commission (NBAC) created; Presidential Tuskegee apology

1999: Research suspended at several institutions by FDA or Office of Protection for Research Risks (OPRR); gene therapy trial death; calls for new research ethics regulation, training and certification

the National Commission that flows from the principle of respect for persons is that individuals who have diminished autonomy, whether their capacity for self-determination is diminished by mental illness or by incarceration in a prison, are in need of and should receive special protection. Several of the National Commission's reports specifically address the needs of various vulnerable populations, such as children and prisoners. Importantly, the National Commission and subsequent federal regulations did not specifically address the needs of the two vulnerable populations of most concern in geriatrics research: subjects with dementia and subjects who reside in long-term care facilities.

Two other fundamental ethical principles were identified by the National Commission as central to research: beneficence and justice. Sometimes beneficence is divided into two principles, nonmaleficence and beneficence, the former meaning not inflicting harm on others and the latter referring to the obligation to promote good. Clearly, although investigators do not set out to intentionally harm their subjects, some clinical trials involve invasive testing, drugs, or new surgical procedures that do carry the risk of harm to subjects. Thus, consideration of whether a trial should be done (or for an individual, whether or not they choose to consent to participate), often involves a complex consideration of potential benefits to participants, to others with the condition under study, or to the state of scientific knowledge, weighed against the trial's risks or burdens. Clinicians, of course, are familiar with these concepts in terms of both

the Hippocratic dictum "do no harm" and the general orientation toward doing what will help one's patients. The National Commission discussed an additional obligation for researchers to promote the public good when they accept public support for their research endeavors.

Justice has to do with treating people fairly, giving each individual what is due or owed to him or her. In the research arena, as discussed by the National Commission and others since, the primary concern has been the fair or equitable distribution of both the burdens and benefits of research. There is a general concern about disadvantaged or vulnerable populations being used as research subjects because of convenience or ease of recruitment, resulting in these populations being subjected to a disproportionate amount of the risks of research. Many disadvantaged populations, particularly those without regular access to health care, are simultaneously at risk of not gaining access to the fruits of the research endeavor, such as new and expensive medications or the latest diagnostic testing and surgical procedures. Justice calls for the equitable distribution of research burdens and benefits within the society. An interesting development in this area in the 1990s that was discussed in the third edition of this text was new federal regulations mandating the inclusion of minorities and women in clinical studies to overcome what has been deemed inadequate representation in trials conducted over the past few decades—quite different from the approach that views these groups as vulnerable populations needing special protection from research risks or from exploitation and overuse as subjects.

What Is Different About Research on Older People?

This question is not a trivial one. If one believes that older people are not inherently very different from younger people, why should there be any special concerns, recourse to different ethical principles, or need for special regulations in considering the conduct of research involving older people? In fact, as part of an effort to overcome ageist stereotypes, much has been written about successful aging and the ways in which the vast majority of older people are cognitively intact, functionally independent, and active. Focusing for a moment on this view of aging and older people, one would have to say that there really should be no difference between research on younger subjects and research on older subjects. For research on older subjects, one still needs competent, voluntary, informed, and comprehending consent for a subject to participate. One would still expect investigators to minimize the risk to older subjects and maximize the potential benefits. One would still look for an equitable distribution of the benefits and burdens of the research involving older subjects. Although some potential older subjects may be vulnerable and in need of special protection, most are not. Indeed, one would hope that IRB consideration of studies involving older subjects would focus on expectations of possible harm to subjects based on knowledge of their circumstances and clinical or physiologic condition, not age per se.

Lack of Research on Older People

On the other hand, there are matters relating to the history of clinical investigation, the clinical realities of geriatric medicine and research, and the presence of special populations within the general older population that we argue merit special attention and consideration. The first of these, the history of clinical investigation involving older people, is probably one of the most obvious to clinicians eager to practice what has been called evidence-based medicine, focusing on what the research literature can tell us about the diagnosis, evaluation, and treatment of diseases and clinical syndromes. Quite simply put, there has been little information from clinical trials on older people, especially the oldest-old (those over age 85). It was quite common even in the 1960s and 1970s for large clinical trials on diseases common in older people, such as diabetes mellitus or hypertension, to exclude subjects over the age of 65.[3] It is only in the last several years that many larger clinical trials have enrolled sufficient numbers of older subjects, or, alternatively, that separate trials focusing specifically on older people have been conducted, to be able to answer whether results found in younger populations generalize to older people.

Some of the more gratifying outcomes of many of these trials are findings, as in the Systolic Hypertension in Elderly Program (SHEP) study, demonstrating that older subjects not only often benefit from the same interventions tried in younger patients but that sometimes the marginal benefit is greatest in the oldest.[4] Another recent example is the North American Symptomatic Carotid Endarterectomy Trial (NASCET), a study of carotid endarterectomy that demonstrated the greatest benefits for many severities of carotid stenosis accrued to the oldest subjects, including those over age 85.[5] The relative lack of research information is even more apparent when one considers some conditions that affect predominantly older people or those who reside in nursing homes. It is not clear whether the lack of attention to research on older people was due to practical difficulties in conducting geriatric research (discussed in more detail following), a lack of interest in older people and their problems per se, or other causes. Regardless of the cause, from the perspective of the ethical principle of justice discussed

earlier, older people were not receiving their fair share of either the burdens or the benefits of clinical research. Although this has been changing for the better in recent years, considerable room for improvement remains. A review of the recent experience of the Southwestern Oncology Group, one of the major cancer coperative study groups in the United States still found the typical cancer protocol subject to be much younger than the typical patient with cancer.[6]

Clinical Realities Making Geriatric Research More Difficult

A priori, there may not be major differences in the ethical principles guiding research on older and younger subjects, but it is clear that the clinical realities of geriatric medicine and the older population have a major impact on the actual conduct of research.[7,8] First, because older people are more likely to have comorbid conditions and to be on multiple medications, there is increased tension between selecting subjects who have only the condition of interest (yielding fewer confounding factors) and selecting subjects who will be more representative of typical older adults who have other health problems in addition to the condition under study (yielding results that are more generalizable to the broader population of the elderly). Second, trying to screen, recruit, and formally enroll older subjects may be more complicated because of communication and cognitive problems, such as hearing deficits, strokes, and dementia. Third, several studies, especially population-based studies involving subjects of all ages, suggest that older people have lower participation rates than do younger people. That is, even when eligible and approached for recruitment into a research study, older people may be more likely to refuse. Last, once people are enrolled in a study, there is a greater risk of attrition due to illness or death. Taken together, these clinical realities suggest that conducting research using older human subjects is indeed likely to be more time consuming, more expensive, and more difficult.[7,8]

There is an important caveat to the foregoing formulation. One should not assume that older patients are less willing to participate in research. A recent study of older and younger breast cancer patients found that older women were less likely to be offered the option of participating in clinical trials than younger women. For those who were offered enrollment, however, the older and younger women participated in similar proportions.[9] We must be careful not to let the biases of physicians or researchers drive research participation. The cohort of aging Baby Boomers may have different attitudes toward research from preceding cohorts of older potential subjects.

Special Population No. 1: People with Cognitive Impairment

As discussed earlier, the competent, voluntary, informed, and comprehending consent of an individual is crucial to making that person a research subject. Unfortunately, older people are at considerable risk for conditions in which an altered mental status calls into question the ability to give informed consent. Impaired decision-making capacity and an inability to give informed consent may be a temporary condition, as with a postoperative delirium, or it may be permanent, as with severe Alzheimer's disease. Geriatric medical research is not unique in its need to confront this consent dilemma; researchers in neurosurgery,[10] intensive care medicine,[11] and emergency medicine[12] often want to study potential subjects who are not capable of giving informed consent at the time the study is to be conducted. Researchers in these other fields, however, often do not encounter their potential subjects until they have already lost decision-making capacity. Providers in geriatric medicine and some geriatric researchers, on the other hand, often know patients or potential subjects before the loss of decision-making capacity, raising additional interesting questions about the assessment of decision-making capacity, advance consent for research, and proxy consent. The greatest ethical dilemma arises from cases in which the ultimate choice is between forgoing promising research because informed consent cannot be obtained or making do without the ideal informed consent, perhaps accepting some creative alternatives.

In looking at research on people with cognitive impairment, we restrict our discussion to the consideration of the paradigm presented by research on Alzheimer's disease or other progressive dementias. We choose to limit our discussion to this area because the ethical dilemma is starkest when the condition to be studied is the same as the condition causing the loss of decision-making capacity. While it is true that individual investigators, patients, and families may face challenging decisions, for example, regarding proposed use of an investigational chemotherapy for a cancer that has occurred in a patient with dementia, it is clear that research on cancer could proceed even if it were to be limited to patients who can give informed consent for themselves. Research on Alzheimer's disease, at least studying subjects beyond the earliest stages of the illness, requires using people who cannot give informed consent.

The assessment of individuals' capacity to give informed consent for themselves is an important first step in deciding whether or how to enroll potential subjects in research protocols. It is important to emphasize that declaring someone unable to make decisions or to give consent should not be based on diagnostic labels or categories. That is, giving someone the diagnosis of Alzheimer's disease does not automatically confer the status of incompetence upon that individual. Rather, one should take the approach that the ability to give informed consent for research, like clinical decision-making capacity, is task specific.[13] More complex information and more complicated decisions require greater degrees of cognitive function. For example, a patient with moderate Alzheimer's disease still might be able to give consent for a study involving an interview on symptoms of depression, but it is likely that this patient would not be capable of understanding and giving consent for a protocol involving a reservoir for the intraventricular infusion of a nerve growth factor into the cerebrospinal fluid. Unfortunately, although it is easy to describe the task-specific or "sliding scale" concept of decision-making capacity assessment, at this time there are no standard or widely accepted scales for operationalizing this concept in the conduct of research. The assessment simply must be carried out on a case-by-case basis with each research protocol and each potential subject. Importantly, standard measures of cognition and severity of dementia should not be taken as direct measures of the ability to give consent. Even people with Mini-Mental State Exam scores as low the 10 to 20 range may be able to give valid consent for some projects.

In clinical practice, providers are becoming more familiar with advance directives and the concept of advance care planning for clinical decision making in the event of patient incapacity. Formal advance directives are legal documents that allow patients to indicate specific treatment preferences (living wills, medical directives) or to appoint a proxy to make decisions (durable powers of attorney for health care, health care proxies). It has been suggested that a similar approach be taken with consent for research on dementia.[14–16] Cognitively intact older people or patients with the very earliest stages of Alzheimer's disease, for example, could be encouraged to execute advance directives for research purposes. Similar to clinical advance directives, a research advance directive could indicate the kinds of research projects in which someone would or would not want to participate in the future or could designate a proxy to make research enrollment decisions.

Such an approach appears logical and consistent with clinical decision-making practices, but there are at least three important concerns about research advance directives.[16] First, because it is not clear how helpful clinical advance directives are proving to be and because there has been even less experience with research advance directives, one hesitates to recommend wide adoption of such an unproven policy. Second, the legal status of research advance directives is not clear because most state laws creating advance directives focus on clinical decisions, especially those pertaining to the use of life-sustaining treatments.[15] Third, although information contained in a research advance directive might be useful, there is the concern that promoting their use might create the impression (or even lead to regulations or laws) that they are required to do research on dementia. Because a minority of adults execute clinical advance directives, and one can assume that even fewer would execute research advance directives, one can envision a scenario in which research advance directives actually end up inhibiting rather than promoting dementia research.[16]

What then should be done for cases in which the potential subject is impaired so that informed consent cannot be obtained and research advance directives are either not an option or not present? The current model for obtaining permission to do research on cognitively impaired subjects involves what sometimes is called proxy consent plus subject assent.[17,18] Informed consent is sought from a proxy, usually a close relative, who speaks on behalf of the impaired individual. Ethical support for this part of the process is based on the belief that a family member or other proxy is best suited for giving consent because (1) he or she knows the potential subject best and is most likely to make a decision that would be in keeping with the subject's values and what that subject might have decided for him or herself (making a substituted judgment); (2) the proxy has the best interests of the subject at heart and will make the "best decision"; or (3) as a closely involved family member, the proxy is the person most likely to be affected by the decision, other than the subject, and thus has a stake in making the decision.[19,20] Clearly, in clinical practice, there is a long-established tradition of turning to family members when a patient cannot make decisions.

Concerns about proxy consent center on potential conflicts of interest (proxies volunteering subjects because the proxy hopes to benefit in the future from the research) or data from clinical decision-making studies that demonstrate significant discord between what patients say they would decide for life-sustaining treatment vignettes and what their proxies predict the patients would want.[21,22] In general, it is probably safe to presume that the number of cases in which families will knowingly act contrary to the wishes or interests of a subject are very few in number and one can trust proxy decision making. In addition, because there are other reasons to support proxy decision making besides the ability to construct a substituted judgment, the data on patient–proxy discord need not eliminate proxy consent as a viable option.[20]

The assent of the subject is the other half of the model that is coupled with proxy consent. Assent refers to the willingness of a subject to agree to go along with a research protocol even if the subject cannot provide informed consent. This concept also has been applied to consent for research involving children.[23] This is a

particularly useful construct for approaching dementia research if one thinks of it as an opportunity to try and obtain useful information from a potential subject about their values and preferences that can help guide research participation decisions, rather than just thinking of assent as the lack of objection to research procedures. One empirical study on research decision making for dementia supports the ability of even very impaired subjects with dementia to give strikingly revealing and informative reports on their values and preferences when given information about specific dementia research protocols.[24]

Ethical issues in research on subjects with cognitive impairment received a great deal of attention in the latter part of the 1990s, including position statements by the American Geriatrics Society and the Alzheimer's Association and a report and proposed regulations from the National Bioethics Advisory Commission (NBAC).[25–27] The NBAC report and proposed regulations generated a great deal of controversy. NBAC called for such matters as assessment of potential subjects' decision-making capacity by independent assessors; continued use of a two-tiered approach to risk assessment (minimal risk and greater than minimal risk); significant restrictions on research that does not hold out the potential of direct benefit to subjects; and limited use of advance consent for research.[27] The NBAC proposals were criticized by some as not going far enough in protecting a vulnerable population and by others for potentially inhibiting or prohibiting important research.[28,29] Being assailed from both sides of the debate has contributed to NBAC's proposals not being implemented to date.

Special Population No. 2: Residents of Long-Term Care

The second population that sharply focuses some of the ethical concerns specific to research in geriatric medicine and gerontology is the long-term care population, especially people residing in nursing homes. Because of the high prevalence of dementia in nursing homes, some of the concerns about research in these facilities are identical to the concerns about research on dementia already discussed. There are distinct concerns about research in nursing homes, however, that relate to the nature of life within these institutions.[30]

First, although nursing homes are increasingly used as sites for research, unlike academic hospitals they are not research institutions, nor are they solely medical care delivery sites. Indeed, efforts are made in many nursing homes to emphasize the social nature of the institution, the "nursing home as home," rather than seeing them as stepdown units from hopitals. The bulk of care in nursing homes is provided by nurses' aides and the role of physicians is somewhat limited with respect to day-to-day life. Most of the staff is unlikely to be familiar with standard research procedures and may be uncomfortable with research. Considerable education and encouragement may be needed to gain the trust and cooperation of a nursing home's staff for a research project.

Second, much has been written about the issue of nursing homes as environments in which individual autonomy may be limited.[31,32] Even seemingly simple things such as choosing a roommate or deciding when to get out of bed in the morning or what to eat often are out of the control of a nursing home resident.[33] Life within any "total institution" certainly challenges the ability of even cognitively intact and healthy people to make decisions freely, let alone people who are ill or frail. Thus, it is easy to see why there would be concerns about the ability to obtain voluntary and uncoerced consent in a nursing home, even if it is informed and comprehending consent. Specifically, one wonders if nursing home residents, who are dependent on staff for so much, feel truly free to refuse to participate in research conducted on site. Obviously, these concerns are heightened when nursing home staff or physicians are themselves participating in a research project, especially if they are helping to recruit and enroll subjects. In addition, even if the consent process can be made voluntary and uncoerced, concerns remain about privacy and confidentiality in the research process because nursing homes are places where these two commodities often are in short supply.

A third area of ethical concern in nursing home research relates more to the principles of beneficence and justice than to autonomy and informed consent. Although great progress has been made in the past several years in improving conditions in nursing homes, much remains to be accomplished, and a large gulf exists between the best and worst facilities. An interesting ethical question arises in deciding where to do nursing home research. Should research be limited to only the best facilities, where the residents' needs all are being met, thus avoiding the possibility of exploiting the most vulnerable and needy residents who receive inferior daily care? From the research standpoint, a superb facility probably facilitates efficient conduct of a study, but it may limit the generalizability of one's results to similar top-notch nursing homes. From an ethics standpoint, restricting research to the best facilities may avoid exploiting the most vulnerable, but it also prevents residents in other nursing homes from sharing in the benefits of research participation as well as its burdens. By this we mean not only the benefits derived from the knowledge generated by research studies, but also the benefits provided by research participation that include increased social interaction, increased attention, and the feeling of contributing to something important. Clearly, a balance must be struck between these competing concerns in deciding which nursing facilities to select for research projects.[30]

Evolving Ethical Controversies Within the Research Community

Much of what has been discussed to this point fits within a model of research ethics that was quite stable through most of the 1980s and 1990s: trustworthy researchers interacting with individual subjects, guided by the principles of respect for persons (with a heavy emphasis on autonomy and informed consent), beneficence, and justice. More recently, several problems or concerns have arisen, some of which represent challenges within the foregoing framework and others that challenge the framework itself. We discuss four of these evolving ethical challenges in research at large: (1) trust and the research community; (2) confidentiality in research; (3) research and the private sector; and (4) likely future research ethics challenges. These developments are not unique to research in geriatric medicine, but we believe that they are of such importance that they warrant discussion here.

Trust and the Research Community

In the late 1990s, the Office of Protection for Research Risks (OPRR; subsequently replaced by OHRP, the Office for Human Research Protection) and the Food and Drug Administration (FDA) temporarily suspended the clinical research operations at several universities and medical centers.[34-36] While several of these research suspensions were thought by some in the research community to have been due to technical noncompliance with institutional review board (IRB) and other regulations, and that no research subjects were placed at risk of harm, some cases clearly were more serious. IRB members from one institution, for example, complained of a lack of support and resources for their work, and an audit provided examples of research being conducted without IRB review and of protocols being reviewed by panels that included the researcher.

Following shortly on the heels of several of these research suspensions, a research subject participating in a gene therapy study at the University of Pennsylvania died.[37] This case received significant attention initially because of the death being the first one associated with a gene therapy trial. Subsequent investigations uncovered a host of research protocol irregularities at the University of Pennsylvania and other universities conducting gene therapy trials. These irregularities included deviations from protocols, changes being made in protocols without approval by IRBs or other supervising bodies, and adverse events not being reported to appropriate authorities.

Coupled with the Office of the Inspector General's (OIG) report citing deficiencies in the existing research oversight structure and process,[38] many additional actions and proposals for strengthening research regulation have come from the federal government. These measures have included new requirements for education and certification in research ethics for investigators, research staff, and IRB members; directives to IRBs to take a more active role in monitoring of ongoing research; and NBAC's most recent report proposing a complete overhaul of the federal structure supervising the nation's IRBs.[39]

In response to these developments, many research and professional organizations have made public statements reaffirming their commitment to the ethical conduct of research involving human subjects. Although geriatrics researchers have not played a prominent role in the cases just mentioned, the American Geriatrics Society is one of the organizations that promulgated a position statement on the ethical conduct of research.[40] At the heart of these efforts is the desire to reassure the public that the research community still deserves the trust that it has enjoyed in the past several decades. Some investigators believe that if that basic trust is lost, no amount of regulation or oversight will make up for the harm that will come to the research enterprise.

Confidentiality in Research

Privacy and confidentiality are two things that researchers have always been required to respect in their dealings with their subjects. In the past, this did not place too many demands on most researchers. Most research was conducted at a single institution; investigators controlled the (mostly hard copy) data relating to their own subjects; subjects were promised that their identity would be kept confidential; and separate sheets with subject code numbers and names and locked file cabinets often sufficed. Today, most clinical trials are multicenter studies, sponsored by pharmaceutical or biotechnology firms, with data transmitted to coordinating centers to be reviewed by other investigators and statisticians, a data monitoring and safety board, and eventually the FDA or other regulators. Electronic transmission of research data is becoming commonplace. In addition, medical records in clinical practice are more routinely being kept in electronic formats. The electronic medical record is not only allowing clinicians to more readily communicate important clinical information to all involved in a patient's care, but it is also allowing health services researchers and other clinical investigators to assemble data sets and identify potential subjects in a fraction of the time required previously. By linking data from existing clinical records, research data sets, and administrative data sources such as Medicare claims, researchers are able to ask and answer questions using information on thousands or even hundreds of thousands of subjects.

Clearly, multicenter studies, electronic data transmission, and electronic records all hold great promise for research. Simultaneously, however, they greatly increase the potential for violations of confidentiality for subjects. As of this writing, new federal regulations governing medical records, including stronger requirements for written consent before allowing access to any records, have just been implemented. These controversial regulations, like many other efforts to regulate research, attempt to balance access to the potential benefits of research against the potential harms that might ensue. It remains to be seen if these new restrictions on the flow of medical data result in the proper balance or if research is inhibited excessively.

Research and the Private Sector

One trend in research mentioned in the section immediately above has been the increasing role of for-profit pharmaceutical firms, equipment manufacturers, and biotechnology companies. Not only are these entities financing more of the nation's research than in the past, more research is being conducted, directed, and supervised by commercial research organizations (CROs) outside academic centers. The combination of commercial interests driving research, private control and oversight of research, and increasingly complex relationships between researchers and commercial entities has raised a number of ethical concerns. First, there is concern that the desire of commercial firms to keep information from competitors may inhibit the free exchange of information that is an integral part of how research usually proceeds. Second, there is the concern that commercial firms profit motives will unduly influence the research process. For example, will they be less willing to publish negative studies, an already important challenge in the existing clinical trials literature? Will CROs and private IRBs be less thorough in their scrutiny of protocols because of a conflict of interest? Will this perceived conflict of interest further challenge the public's trust of the research enterprise? Third, many concerns have been raised about the impact of relationships with industry and the potential conflicts of interest created for researchers, clinicians, and academic centers.[41,42] Some concerns exist that greater commercial ties lead to potentially biased presentations of research, such as in review articles or journal supplements. Surveys suggest that most academic centers have not yet formulated adequate policies for dealing with these potential conflicts of interest.[43,44]

Another way in which ethical concerns have been raised by the commercialization of research relates to how many academic researchers and centers have learned to follow many of the practices formerly reserved to the for-profit sector. Researchers have created for-profit biotechnology firms to try and reap the financial gains from results of their work that might lead to successes in the marketplace. Most academic centers have offices or departments devoted to similar ventures and more aggressive patenting practices. International controversy exists around the patenting of genes and gene products. Lawsuits have been filed seeking access to financial gains that may have resulted from research findings. Marcia Angell has argued that these ethical issues surrounding academic centers and the for-profit sector are one of the greatest challenges to the very soul of academic medicine.[41,42]

Likely Future Challenges

Many of the coming ethical dilemmas for research in geriatric medicine are identifiable today. Some of these will certainly be continuations of the issues already discussed, including debates over tighter regulation of human subject research and the evolving relationship between industry and academia. Others may be existing controversies that will take center stage in the public debate. Controversies that we would place in this category would include the use of stem cells in clinical trials (especially relevant for geriatrics as many of the diseases targeted for this kind of work are age-associated diseases such as Alzheimer's disease, Parkinson's disease, and stroke), and debates over both who will pay for research and who will have access to expensive technologies and drugs that result from research successes. Finally, other ethical dilemmas will arise because of advances in technology and the debate over whether we ought to do the things that become possible because of science. Similar to the debate over human cloning, it is likely that the field of aging will face concerns over whether we should pursue research that may extend the life span. We may very well find ourselves in debates over whether it is "right" to pursue antiaging interventions, arguments over the impact on society if such interventions work, and competing claims for access to these therapies versus efforts to protect individuals and society from potential harms.

Conclusion

Research in geriatric medicine is growing in important ways at this time in history. Ethical issues particular to geriatrics research, as well as those challenges facing the broader research community, also loom large at this time. For research on geriatric medicine to continue to make inroads on the health problems of older adults, it is essential that these ethical issues continue to be addressed in a thoughtful and effective manner.

References

1. The National Commission for the Protection of Human Subjects of Biomedical and Behavioral Research. *The Belmont Report: Ethical Principles and Guidelines for the Protection of Human Subjects of Research.* DHEW (OS) 78-0012. Appendix I. DHEW (OS) 78-0013, Appendix II. DHEW (OS) 78-0014. Washington, DC: Department of Health, Education and Welfare; 1978.
2. Levine RJ. *Ethics and Regulation of Clinical Research, 2nd Ed.* New Haven: Yale University Press; 1986.
3. Sachs GA, Cassel CK. Biomedical research involving older human subjects. *Law Med Health Care.* 1990;18:234–243.
4. The Systolic Hypertension in the Elderly Program (SHEP) Cooperative Research Group. Prevention of stroke by anti-hypertensive drug treatment in older patients with isolated systolic hypertension: final results of SHEP. *JAMA.* 1991; 265:3255–3264.
5. Alamowitch S, Eliasziw M, Algra A, Meldrum H, Barnett HJM, for the North American Symptomatic Carotid Endarterectomy Trial (NASCET) Group. Risk, causes, and prevention of ischaemic stroke in elderly patients with symptomatic internal-carotid-artery stenosis. *Lancet.* 2001; 357:1154–1160.
6. Hutchins LF, Unger JM, Crowley JJ, Coltman CA Jr, Albain KS. Underrepresentation of patients 65 years of age or older in cancer-treatment trials. *N Engl J Med.* 1999;341: 2061–2067.
7. Zimmer AW, Calkins E, Hadley E, et al. Conducting clinical research in geriatric populations. *Ann Intern Med.* 1985; 103:276–283.
8. Applegate WB, Curb JD. Designing and executing randomized clinical trials involving elderly persons. *J Am Geriatr Soc.* 1990;38:943–950.
9. Kemeny M, Muss HB, Kornblith AB, Peterson B, Wheeler J, Cohen HJ (CALGB). Barriers to participation of older women with breast cancer in clinical trials. *Proc ASCO.* 2000;19:abstract 2371.
10. Prentice ED, Antonson DL, Leibrock LG, et al. IRB review of a phase II randomized clinical trial involving incompetent patients suffering from severe closed head injury. *IRB Rev Hum Subjects Res.* 1993;15(5):1–7.
11. Fost N, Robertson JA. Deferring consent with incompetent patients in an intensive care unit. *IRB Rev Hum Subjects Res.* 1980;2(7):5–6.
12. Olson CM. The letter or the spirit: consent for research in CPR. *JAMA.* 1994;271:1445–1447.
13. Applebaum PS, Grisso T. Assessing patients' capacities to consent to treatment. *N Engl J Med.* 1988;319:1635–1638.
14. Fletcher JC, Dommel FW Jr, Cowell DD. Consent to research with impaired human subjects. *IRB Rev Hum Subjects Res.* 1985;7:1–6.
15. High DM. Research with Alzheimer's disease subjects: informed consent and proxy decision making. *J Am Geriatr Soc.* 1992;40:950–957.
16. Sachs GA. Advance consent for dementia research. *Alzheimer Dis Assoc Disord.* 1994;8(suppl 4):19–27.
17. American College of Physicians. Cognitively impaired subjects [position paper]. *Ann Intern Med.* 1989;111:843–848.

18. Melnick VL, Dubler NN, Weisbard A, Butler RN. Clinical research in senile dementia of the Alzheimer type: suggested guidelines addressing the ethical and legal issues. *J Am Geriatr Soc.* 1984;32:531–536.

19. Hardwig J. What about the family? *Hastings Cent Rep.* 1990; 20(2):5–10.

20. Nelson HL, Nelson JL. Preferences and other moral sources. *Hastings Cent Rep.* 1994;24(suppl 6):S19–S21.

21. Seckler AB, Meier DE, Mulvihill M, et al. Substituted judgment: how accurate are proxy predictions? *Ann Intern Med.* 1991;115:92–98.

22. Uhlmann RF, Pearlman RA, Cain KA. Physicians' and spouses' predictions of elderly patients' resuscitation preferences. *J Gerontol Med.* 1988;43:M115–M121.

23. National Commission for the Protection of Human Subjects of Biomedical and Behavioral Research. *Research Involving Children: Report and Recommendations.* DHEW (OS) 78-0004, Appendix. DHEW (OS) 78-0005. Washington, DC: DHEW; 1977.

24. Sachs GA, Stocking CB, Stern R, et al. Ethics of dementia research: informed consent and proxy consent. *Clin Res.* 1994;42:403–412.

25. Sachs CA, AGS Ethics Committee, American Geriatrics Society. Informed consent for research on human subjects with dementia. *J Am Geriatr Soc.* 1998;46:1308–1310.

26. Alzheimer's Association. Ethical issues in dementia research (with special emphasis on "informed consent"). Position statement adopted by Alzheimer's Association, May 1997. Available at *www.alz.org/aboutus/overview/statements.htm#ethical.* Accessed 6/24/01.

27. National Bioethics Advisory Commission. *Research Involving Persons with Mental Disorders That May Affect Decisionmaking Capacity, vol I. Report and Recommendations of the National Bioethics Advisory Commission.* Rockville, MD: National Bioethics Advisory Commission; 1998.

28. Michels R. Are research ethics bad for our mental health? *N Engl J Med.* 1999;340:1427–1430.

29. Capron AM. Ethical and human-rights issues in research on mental disorders that may affect decision-making capacity. *N Engl J Med.* 1999;340:1430–1434.

30. Sachs GA, Rhymes J, Cassel CK. The Ethics of Biomedical and Behavioral research in Nursing Homes: Guidelines for Investigators. *J Am Geriatr Soc.* 1993;41:771–777.

31. Hofland B. Autonomy in long term care: background issues and a programmatic response. *Gerontologist.* 1988;28 (suppl):3–9.

32. Collopy BJ. Autonomy in long term care: some crucial distinctions. *Gerontologist.* 1988;28(suppl):10–17.

33. Kane RA, Caplan AL, eds. Everyday ethics: resolving dilemmas in nursing home life. New York: Springer; 1990.

34. Weiss R. U.S. halts research on humans at Duke University. Can't ensure safety, probers find. *Washington Post.* May 12, 1999;A1.

35. Hilts PJ. VA Hospital is told to halt all research. *New York Times.* March 25, 1999.

36. Greenberg DS. Sham oversight. *Washington Post.* May 31, 1999;A23.

37. Stotberg SG. The biotech death of Jesse Gelsinger. *New York Times Sunday Magazine.* November 28, 1999.

38. Department of Health and Human Services, Office of the Inspector General. *Institutional Review Boards: A Time for Reform.* OE1-01-97-00193. Washington, DC: DHHS; 1998.

39. National Bioethics Advisory Commission. Ethical and policy issues in research involving human participants. Final recommendations, May 18, 2001. Available at *http://bioethics.gov/pubs.html#final.* Accessed 6/24/01.

40. American Geriatrics Society. The responsible conduct of geriatrics research [position statement]. In press, *J Am Geriatr Soc.*

41. Angell M. The pharmaceutical industry—to whom is it accountable? *N Engl J Med.* 2000;342:1902–1904.

42. Angell M. Is academic medicine for sale? *N Engl J Med.* 2000;342:1516–1518.

43. Lo B, Wolf LE, Berkeley A. Conflict-of-interest policies for investigators in clinical trials. *N Engl J Med.* 2000;343:1616–1620.

44. Van McCrary S, Anderson CB, Jakovljevic J, et al. A national survey of policies on disclosure of conflicts of interest in biomedical research. *N Engl J Med.* 2000;343:1621–1626.

Index

ISBN 0-387-95514-3

9 780387 955148